FIRST AID & GENERAL EMERGENCY TREATMENT

INGREDIENTS INDEX • THERAPEUTIC INDEX

SUPPORTIVE TREATMENT • TRADEMARK INDEX

GENERAL FORMULATIONS • MANUFACTURERS INDEX

FIRST AID & GENERAL EMERGENCY TREATMENT

INGREDIENTS INDEX • THERAPEUTIC INDEX

TOXICITY RATING CHART

Toxicity Rating or Class	Probable LETHAL Dose (human)	
	mg./kg.	for 70 kg. man (150 lbs.)
6 super toxic	less than 5	a taste (less than 7 drops)
5 extremely toxic	5–50	between 7 drops and 1 teaspoonful
4 very toxic	50–500	between 1 teaspoonful and one ounce
3 moderately toxic	500–5 gm./kg.	between 1 ounce and 1 pint (or 1 lb.)
2 slightly toxic	5–15 gm./kg.	between 1 pint and 1 quart
1 practically non-toxic	above 15 gm./kg.	more than 1 quart

FIRST AID & GENERAL EMERGENCY TREATMENT

INGREDIENTS INDEX • THERAPEUTIC INDEX

SUPPORTIVE TREATMENT • TRADEMARK INDEX

GENERAL FORMULATIONS • MANUFACTURERS INDEX

FIRST AID & GENERAL EMERGENCY TREATMENT

INGREDIENTS INDEX • THERAPEUTIC INDEX

SUPPORTIVE TREATMENT • TRADEMARK INDEX

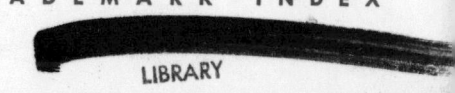

Clinical Toxicology

OF

Commercial Products

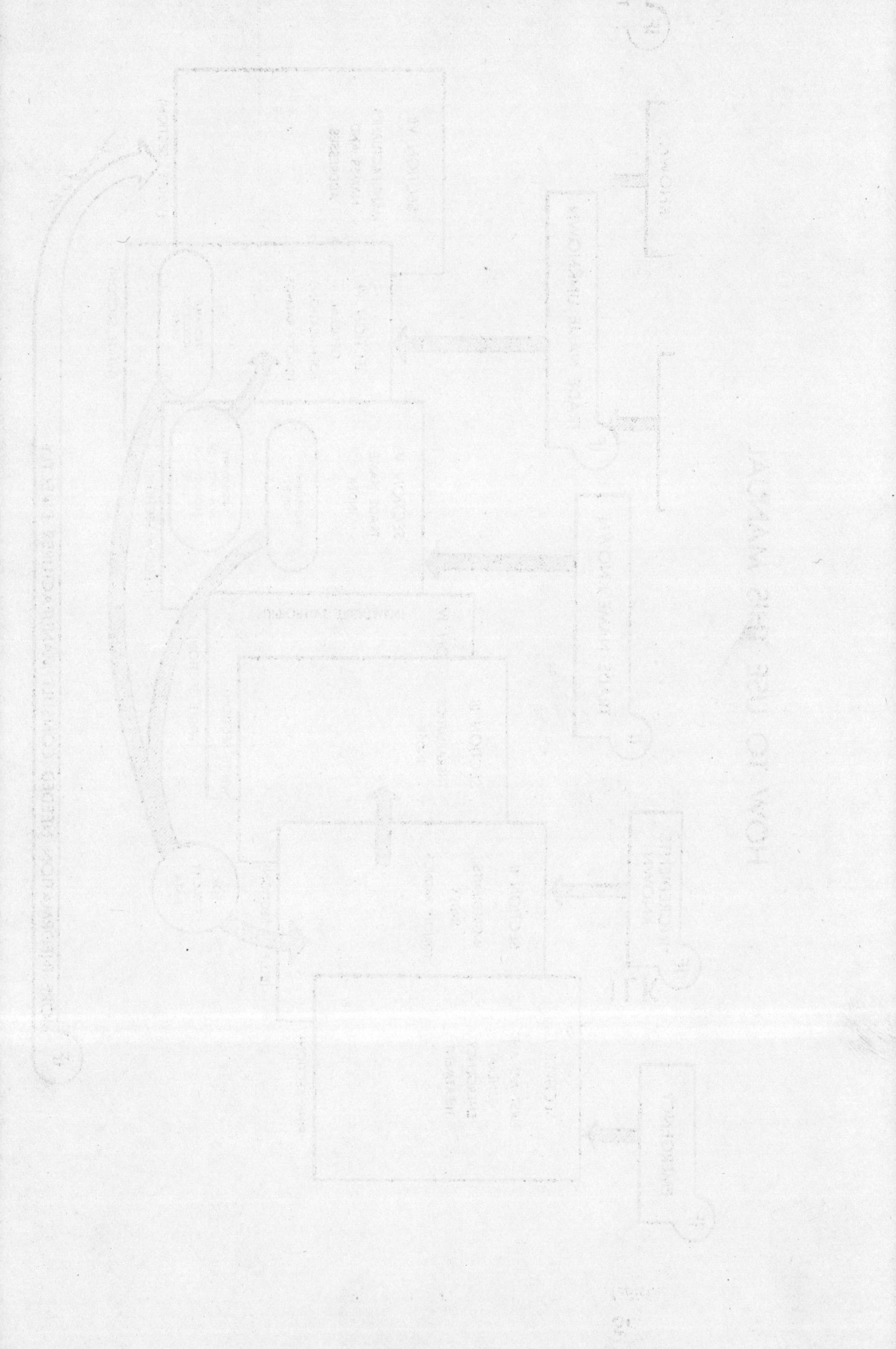

HOW TO USE THIS MANUAL

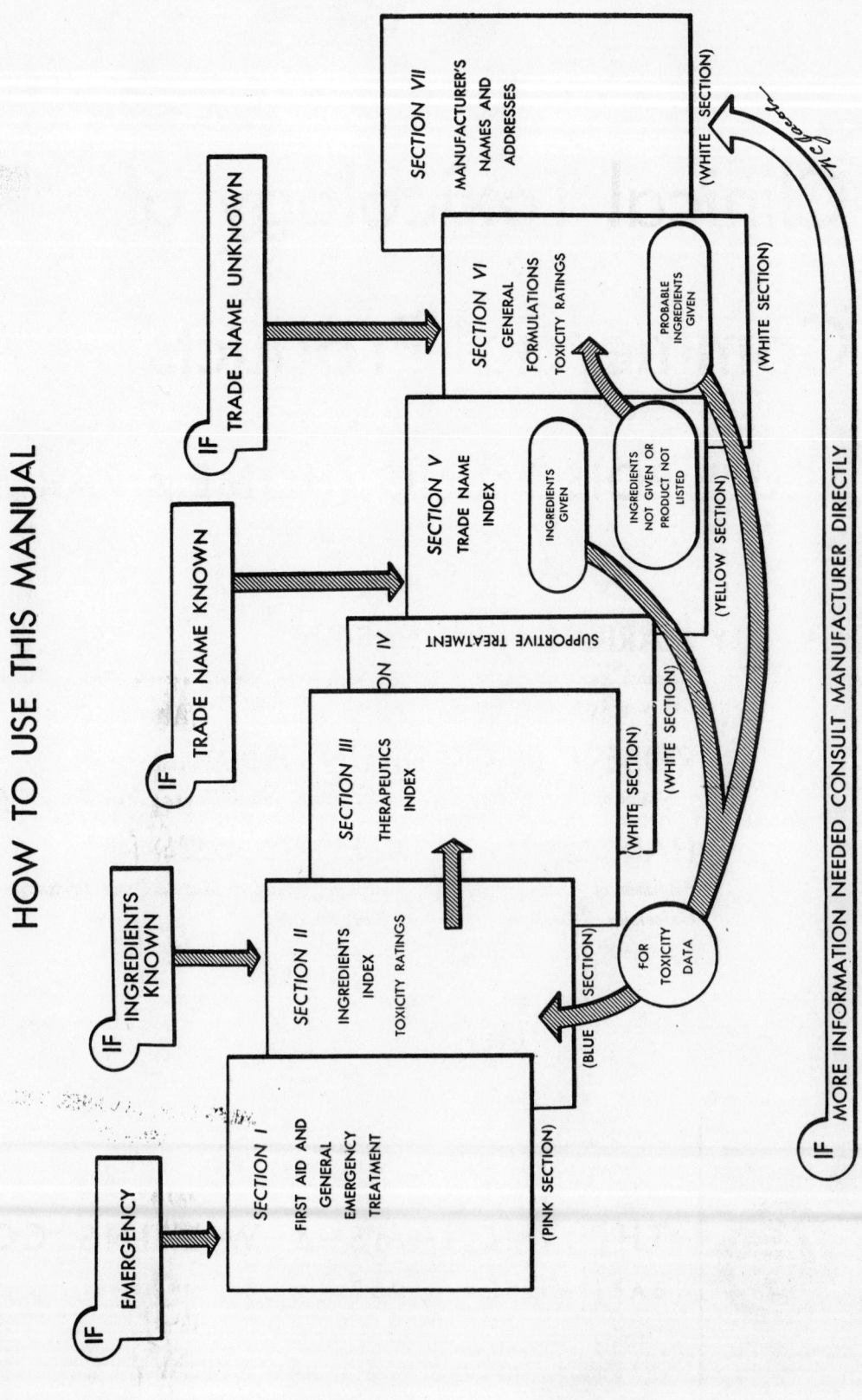

Clinical Toxicology of Commercial Products

ACUTE POISONING (HOME & FARM)

BY **MARION N. GLEASON**

Research Assistant in Pharmacology, School of Medicine and Dentistry, The University of Rochester, Rochester, New York.

ROBERT E. GOSSELIN, M.D., Ph.D.

Professor of Pharmacology, Dartmouth Medical School, Hanover, New Hampshire.

HAROLD C. HODGE, Ph.D., D.Sc.

Professor of Pharmocology and Toxicology, School of Medicine and Dentistry, The University of Rochester, Rochester, New York.

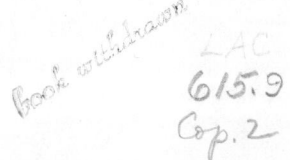
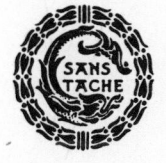

THE WILLIAMS & WILKINS CO.

BALTIMORE · 1957

Foreword

Modern industry is pouring out a steady stream of products designed to make work easier and life more pleasant. Through their use, comforts and leisure once known to few are available to everyone. And advances in medicine offer the possibility of a longer, healthier life in which to enjoy them. The chemical and pharmaceutical industries especially play a major role in the tremendous engineering, medical, and other scientific progress which gives us the many benefits of modern living.

But progress brings with it problems as well as advantages. Witness the problem of accidental poisoning which is growing with the great increase in variety and use of chemical products, especially around the home. The greatest potential accident hazard is among children under five years of age.

The shelves of family shopping centers are conveniently stacked with medicine, cosmetics, pesticides, cleaning agents, and countless other useful products. Weekly if not daily some new brand is added to the list of household agents or home remedies that people are urged to try. Most of them are harmless when used according to instructions but, from aspirin to the newest insecticide, each one can be harmful—even fatal—when misused. Parents need to be cautioned to store *all* such agents safely out of sight and reach of young children.

Although medical, public health, and governmental agencies are working together ceaselessly to develop effective preventive measures, carelessness and misuse still occur. For every day of the year, about eight people in the United States die from accidentally or intentionally swallowing some substance capable of causing death. Evidence is increasing that there are several hundreds of non-fatal cases for every fatality. The great majority of these are children between one and three years of age.

Few practicing physicians have escaped anxiety in treating poisoning cases. They know the worry which accompanies the accidental emergency when the toxic agent cannot be readily identified, or when the ingested material is still so new that effects and treatment have not yet been described in medical literature.

This reference volume, designed to make urgently needed information immediately available, should be most helpful to any physician faced with a patient who has swallowed some possibly toxic trademarked product. Medical libraries, pharmacies, industrial medical departments, public health nursing centers, and any agency frequently called upon for emergency help should also find it helpful as a quick source of information on first aid, treatment procedures, and other questions. Widespread and immediate use of such a reference can help to prevent deaths from chemical poisoning.

The authors have accomplished a colossal task which others, including manufacturers themselves, considered virtually impossible. Yet here it is—practical, concrete evidence that nothing which is needed to save life remains "impossible" to the dedicated men and women in medicine and allied fields.

GEORGE M. WHEATLEY, M.D., M.P.H.
Third Vice-President, Health and Welfare,
Metropolitan Life Insurance Company
and Chairman, Subcommittee on Chemical Poisons,
American Public Health Association

Preface

"In this work, when it shall be found that much is omitted, let it not be forgotten that much likewise is performed."

Dr. Samuel Johnson
(on completion of his *Dictionary*, 1755.)

The purpose of this book is to assist the physician in dealing quickly and effectively with acute chemical poisonings in the home and on the farm, when, through misuse, a patient eats or drinks a harmful amount of a commercial product. The book provides a) a list of trade name products together with their ingredients when these have been available, b) sample formulas of many types of products with an estimate of the toxicity of each formula, c) toxicological information including an estimate of the toxicity of individual ingredients, d) recommendations for treatment, and e) names and addresses of manufacturers.

We suggest that the physician take time to understand the organization of the material in the seven sections of the book before an emergency arises. An illustrative chart, *How to Use This Manual*, serves as a frontispiece. A study of this guide, with hypothetical cases in mind, is recommended. The contents of each section are briefly described below.

Section I. First Aid and General Emergency Treatment

As a synopsis of the physician's role in chemical poisonings from the first phone call to the final disposition, this section outlines in sequence the general emergency procedures and precautions required in all cases of acute poisoning. Included are references to relevant material in other sections.

Section II. Ingredients Index

This section is an alphabetical compilation of chemical substances (ingredients) commonly found in commercial products used by the consumer in and around the home and farm. The acute toxicity of each ingredient has been estimated ("toxicity rating"). Included is a brief description of toxic effects and/or cross references to more detailed information in Sections III and IV.

Section III. Therapeutics Index

Section III summarizes clinical and experimental data on sixty-eight compounds (or classes of compounds) which are named "reference congeners" in Section II because each typifies a group of related substances. This section stresses toxic signs and symptoms and recommended programs of therapy.

Section IV. Supportive Treatment

In this section techniques of supportive treatment are discussed, with particular emphasis on these problems frequently encountered in clinical toxicology.

Section V. Trade Name Index

Here are listed alphabetically over 15,000 trade names of products which might be ingested accidentally or suicidally. For each item the category of use is indicated, e.g., rodenticide, silver polish, hair dye. In most cases the ingredients are stated, with asterisks marking those components expected to be responsible for harmful effects. With each product the manufacturer's name is given. A method of estimating a toxicity rating for each product is described in the introduction to this section.

Section VI. General Formulations

This section presents formulas for the diverse types of products listed in the Trade Name Index. These formulas are believed to be "basic," "typical," or "representative" and give some guidance to physicians when the trade name of an ingested substance is not known, or when information about its ingredients cannot be obtained easily.

The names listed in this index represent a wide sampling of the many thousands of items available on the market to home owners, agriculturists, and operators of small businesses where toxic materials might be accessible to small children. Many of the products are relatively harmless, but an attending physician needs assurance that an ingested substance is innocuous, as well as information concerning the ingredients of a product that is potentially poisonous.

In preparing this material it was recognized that changes in formulas are frequent, that new products are marketed daily and old ones discontinued. To achieve some degree of accuracy in describing the merchandise presented in this index, contributing manufacturers were given the opportunity to edit descriptions of their products, to delete the names of obsolete items, and to add new ones. This was done in December, 1955. The authors plan a similar procedure to keep this index up to date in a subsequent supplement and future editions.

Section VII. Manufacturers' Names and Addresses

The names and addresses of all manufacturers of products appearing in the Trade Name Index are listed for the convenience of physicians who wish to phone or write for further information.

While preparing this material we were often told that the task is an impossible one. If the title were as all-inclusive as it purports to be, *i.e.*, if an attempt had been made to describe all commercial products with toxic potentialities, we would heartily agree with our critics. The coverage is admittedly incomplete. The goal has been to list the hardy perennials and

the current annuals and to omit the obsolescent and evanescent thousands. For example, some 70,000 cosmetic preparations are or have been marketed under individual names; at present it is estimated that 1000 to 2000 new cosmetic products appear each month, but many disappear within a short time. Most products of this type are not listed. How to deal with these rapid-turnover items remains an unsolved problem. On the other hand, where to limit the list of trade names was almost as perplexing as how to collect the data. For instance, our objective, namely to describe products used in homes and on farms, automatically excluded materials marketed for industrial use. However, many of these items can be and are purchased by do-it-yourself workers, hobbyists, and owners of small businesses and so become accessible to small children. Descriptions of such commercial products, when available, are included in this manual.

Beside materials sold exclusively in industrial applications, many other commercial commodities were deliberately excluded. Legend drugs, *i.e.*, those requiring a prescription, have been omitted from the compilation of products and from the general formulations (Sections V and VI), but some of the common therapeutic agents are represented by toxicity data in Sections II and III. Also excluded are all devices, structural materials and objects which are hazardous only because of possible physical injury, *e.g.*, broken glass. Poisonous plants and animal venoms have been omitted. Foods, food products, and dietary supplements are not listed. Chemicals generally have been excluded, except when components of commercial mixtures. No product has been left out solely for its lack of toxicity. The physician and patient often profit by assurance that an ingested substance is harmless.

Much attention and effort were devoted to eliminating errors of both fact and judgment. We apologize for mistakes that have escaped our detection but make no claim of infallability. Another major concern has been the protection of copyrights and trademarks. During the compilation it was discovered that additional security would have been gained by marking with an ® all registered trademarks, but unfortunately this was found to be impractical. We regret that most of the text has not been documented with specific references to exceptionally valuable sources of clinical information. However, *References Useful in Clinical Toxicology* (p. 13) offers some compensation for this deficiency and should be consulted when needed.

With this volume are postal cards addressed to us at the University of Rochester. We hope that these cards will encourage manufacturers to send names of products for inclusion in our supplement. Other cards are designed for physicians and toxicologists who are willing to furnish information about specific poisonings, particularly cases in which an unusual substance or mixture of substances was ingested, whether the resulting illness was mild or severe. We also invite criticisms and suggestions about any and all parts of this work. Finally we urge any physician who is aware of an established or suspected case of poisoning due to an agricultural

chemical (economic poison) to notify *promptly* the nearest of the following laboratories:

U. S. Public Health Service
P. O. Box 769
Savannah, Georgia

U. S. Public Health Service
P. O. Box 73
Wenatchee, Washington

"This direct notification is not to be confused with or intended to be a substitute for the morbidity reports usually sent local and State Health Departments or poisoning control centers."

The preparation of this edition represents a collaboration between a team working at the University of Rochester and 4500 manufacturers. With few exceptions our many letters have been answered with unfailing courtesy and remarkable patience. As a rule the information we solicited was sent us, and valuable suggestions were often volunteered, such as reference sources and useful names and addresses. Deeply appreciated were the words of commendation which appeared in hundreds of letters. Many of these arrived with what seemed to be telepathic insight into the need of a staff for encouragement while harrassed by the many perplexities of this project.

Home and farms should be safe for living and working. It is ironic that the environments in which we expect comfort and protection for ourselves and our children hold so many familiar but cruel hazards. The multiple medical aspects of accident prevention have not been thoroughly explored. This book deals with one restricted phase—acute poisonings in homes and on farms.

Acknowledgments

We wish to express appreciation for the cooperation given us by our consultants: Dr. James H. Sterner, Medical Director of the Eastman Kodak Co., Associate Professor of Medicine, University of Rochester School of Medicine and Dentistry and member of the Council on Industrial Health, American Medical Association; Dr. Donald D. Posson, Assistant Professor of Pediatrics, University of Rochester School of Medicine and Dentistry and member of the Accident Prevention Committee, American Academy of Pediatrics; Dr. Edward Press, Field Director, the American Public Health Association, Chairman, Subcommittee on Poisoning, American Academy of Pediatrics and member of the Committee on Toxicology of the American Medical Association; Dr. Clifford O. Eddy, Manager of the Development Department, Niagara Chemical Division, Food Machinery and Chemical Corp.; Dr. Edward LeB. Gray, Associate in Pharmacology and Toxicology, University of Rochester School of Medicine and Dentistry; and Dr. David W. Fassett, Director, Laboratory of Industrial Medicine, Eastman Kodak Co.

The generous assistance we have received from various groups and organizations and their representatives is gratefully acknowledged. Special thanks are due the following: The Committee on Accident Prevention of the American Academy of Pediatrics; Dr. George M. Wheatley, Third Vice-President, Health and Welfare, Metropolitan Life Insurance Co. and Chairman, Subcommittee on Chemical Poisons of the American Public Health Association; Mr. Bernard E. Conley, Secretary, Committee on Pesticides and Committee on Toxicology, American Medical Association; Mrs. Veronica L. Conley, Secretary, Committee on Cosmetics, American Medical Association; Dr. Franklin M. Foote, Executive Director, National Society for the Prevention of Blindness; Mr. Curt Kornblau, Research and Information Service, Supermarket Institute; Mr. John A. Logan, President, National Association of Food Chains, and its member companies, American Stores Co., Colonial Stores Inc., First National Stores Inc., Grand Union Co., The Great Atlantic and Pacific Tea Co., The Kroger Co., National Tea Co., Red Owl Stores, Inc. and Safeway Stores, Inc.; Mr. Frederick S. Kent, former Chief of Home Safety Activities, Division of Sanitary and Engineering Services, U. S. Department of Health, Education, and Welfare; Dr. Irvin Kerlan, Associate Medical Director and Dr. Karl Brimmer, former Acting Medical Director, Food and Drug Administration; Mr. F. J. Schlink, President, Consumers' Research; Miss Dorothy Fey, Executive Secretary United States Trademark Association; Miss Ruth R. Bien, Chief Chemist, Good Housekeeping Research Bureau; Mr. Charles H. Gertner, Executive Secretary, Automobile Club of Rochester, N. Y.; Safety Councils of Duluth, Minn., Indianapolis, Ind. and Rochester,

N. Y.; and the State Agriculaural Departments of California, Connecticut, Kansas, South Dakota and Winconsin.

The National Agricultural Chemicals Association has given us invaluable assistance by providing data concerning thousands of agricultural products, editing drafts of the material on therapeutics and contributing toxicological information. We cannot express deeply enough our gratitude to the member companies of this organization to its Executive Secretary, Mr. L. S. Hitchner, and to Mr. J. V. Vernon, President of the Niagara Chemical Division of the Food Machinery and Chemical Corporation for his liaison work with our project.

The time-consuming work of many individuals and local organizations throughout the country, such as Parent-Teachers Associations, Boy Scout troops and American Legion groups, deserves our grateful recognition for making pilot surveys and securing lists of products. Especially useful was the cross-country survey of products on the shelves of rural and urban stores made by a group of young members of the Society of Friends under the leadership of Dr. Dirk Spruyt. Our compilation of toxicological information profited greatly from the assistance of Dr. William S. Spector, Managing Editor and Executive Secretary on the Handbook of Biological Data, National Research Council. Dr. Clarence J. Gamble contributed helpful material on contraceptive products. Dr. Chester M. White, Director of Research, and Mr. John F. Bush, President of the Puritan Co., gave us valued data on automotive products. We are particularly indebted to the following companies for much detailed work in our behalf: The Sears Roebuck and Co.; The Procter and Gamble Co. of Cincinnati, Ohio; The G. H. Packwood Co.; and the Shell Chemical Corp. Dr. Alfred Gilman, Professor of Pharmacology at Columbia University, pointed out to us the need for a thorough and balanced exposition of supportive therapy. We thank him for this and other suggestions and for his encouraging interest in our project.

Appreciation is due the work of the technical and secretarial teams associated with this project. Their names include Drs. Peter Gram, Maurice Wertheimer, William A. Little, Robert O. Jensen, Karl M. Johnson, Ruth S. Gosselin, Clarence M. Virtue, Philip S. Chen, Jr., Charles J. Spiegl; Messrs. Clifton Latiolais, Kenneth Lauterbach, John Gabourel, Edward Weigel, Dominic DiVincenzo and Robert Hayes; Ruth Gastel, Elizabeth Cockcroft, Betty Lou Cayley, Sandra Ayers; Mmes. Linda Ellis, Joyce Furchtenicht, Emily Gleason, Clementine Kennedy, Shirley Levene, Sarah Merrill, Bessie Quick, Rosalie Rebhan, Mary June Soffer, Carol Turner, Dorothy Weigel and the Executive Secretary of the project, Elizabeth Nicholl. Other acknowledgements are included in the introductions to the separate sections.

Acknowledgment is gratefully made to the editorial staff of the publisher, especially to Mr. R. Kenneth Bussy and to Mrs. Eleanor Cochrane and the staff who performed the difficult and exacting task of redacting our Trade Name Index and list of manufacturers' names and addresses.

Contents

SECTION II

Ingredients Index

INTRODUCTION AND EXPLANATION

This section with its more than 1,000 entries is an alphabetical compilation of the chemical substances (ingredients) which are commonly found in commercial products used by the consumer in and around the home and farm. For each ingredient a categorical estimate of acute toxicity is recorded (toxicity rating), and when possible each entry is followed by a brief description of toxic symptoms and treatment and/or cross-references to more detailed information in Sections III and IV. A diligent but not exhaustive survey has been made to locate relevant toxicity data for each of the ingredients listed in this compilation.

What Substances are Included

An attempt has been made to list here every compound known to be a prominent ingredient in widely used consumer products (other than medications and foods). In such a naively ambitious project, errors of commission and especially of omission are inevitable. In any case neither the inherent toxicity nor the toxic hazard has dictated the selection of entries for this index. Innocuous materials have been included whenever it appears that medical practicioners may be unfamiliar with the compound and with its lack of significant toxicity.

An effort has been made to list in the basic index (left-hand column) each compound by all of its common names, official names, and chemical synonyms. A few common trade names (notably widely used products with only one active ingredient) are also listed here, but if only the trade name or trademarked name is known, Section V should be consulted first. In many cases drugs and medicinal agents are included (with particular emphasis on non-prescription items used in clinical and veterinary medicine). The drug list is incomplete, however, partly because we believe that adequate sources of information on drug toxicity are readily available to most practicing physicians. Indigenous plants with toxic principles have also been omitted (except for poisonous mushrooms), although the active toxic ingredient may be listed if it is commonly used in commercial formulations (*e.g.*, oil of cedar leaf from arbor vitae). Not included in this compilation are chemicals which are used only by industry in manufacturing processes and which are not found in the final consumer product.

17

How to Consult this Index

To find a specific compound in this alphabetical index (left-hand column), omit from its chemical name all numerals and such abbreviated prefixes as: o-, m-, p-, O-, sec.-, tert.-, n-, N-, α-, β-, etc. (Note that in industry'and commerce these prefixes are commonly omitted and so may be regarded as optional.) On the other hand, in the case of compounds where these prefixes are commonly written out (e.g., ortho, para, iso, beta, bis, di, tetra, etc.), this index should be consulted under the first letter of the prefix. The position of any entry in this alphabetical compilation has been determined strictly by the letter sequence of its name, irrespective of the way in which these letters may be divided or interrupted by word spacings, hyphens, parentheses, numerals, etc. Common abbreviations (e.g., 2,4-D, DDT) have been compiled and included. When an ingredient is designated by numerals without a single letter (e.g., 1080), consult this index under "Compound—." In searching for a particular sodium, ammonium, potassium, or calcium salt, etc., the name of the anion is often best consulted.

Synonyms (Column 1).

For each entry in column 1 a common chemical or commercial synonym (e.g., a common trade name) is recorded. By this device we hope to prevent confusion between two entries with closely related names. If the entry in column 1 is a mixture, the principal active ingredient, rather than a true synonym, is given. When the primary entry is a class name, one or more specific examples may be listed. In practice these distinctions are probably self-evident.

Toxicity Rating (Column 2).

The numerical toxicity rating of column 2 is largely explained in Table II.1. To use the toxicity ratings effectively, their many implications and limitations must be appreciated, as noted below.

1) The rating is based on mortality, not morbidity, i.e., it is really a lethality rating. In general a clinically significant illness may be expected

TABLE II.1*

Toxicity Rating or Class	Probable LETHAL Dose (human)	
	mg./kg.	For 70 kg. man (150 lbs.)
6 Super toxic	Less than 5	A taste (less than 7 drops)
5 Extremely toxic	5–50	Between 7 drops and 1 teaspoonful
4 Very toxic	50–500	Between 1 tsp. and 1 ounce
3 Moderately toxic	500–5 gm./kg.	Between 1 oz. and 1 pint (or 1 lb.)
2 Slightly toxic	5–15 gm./kg.	Between 1 pt. and 1 quart
1 Practically non-toxic	Above 15 gm./kg.	More than 1 quart

* Modified from Hodge and Sterner (Am. Ind. Hyg. Assoc. Quart., **10**: 4, 1949), whose original table was designed for industrial chemicals, not consumer compounds.

after doses of about one-tenth the probable lethal dose (as the latter is reflected in the numerical toxicity rating).

2) Unless otherwise noted, each rating is based on the acute toxicity of a single dose when taken by mouth or gavage. Other dose regimens and other routes of administration are not represented by the rating.

3) The toxicity rating reflects an estimate of the probable or mean lethal dose, not the minimal fatal dose. Perhaps because of personal idiosyncrasy or hypersensitivity or predisposing disease, minimal lethal doses recorded in the clinical literature are usually considerably lower than those implied by the current ratings.

4) With only a few compounds are clinical data adequate to establish a toxicity rating. Most of the values here are based on laboratory determinations of mean lethal doses (LD_{50}) in small laboratory mammals (rat, mouse, guinea pig, rabbit; sometimes cat, dog, and monkey). Implicit in the use of such data is the conventional assumption that the mean lethal dose in man lies in the same class as that of the test animals. Whenever available, however, clinical data and even clinical impressions have been given precedence.

5) Toxicity ratings followed by interrogation points are based on obviously inadequate data; some represent no more than "guesstimates" (in the language of a popular news periodical).

6) For most corrosive agents, such as mineral acids, alkalies, bleaches, *etc.*, no toxicity rating is suggested. In these cases death is usually the result of a severe local tissue injury, with secondary complications such as toxemia, shock, perforation, infection, hemorrhage, and obstruction. The intensity of the local lesion and of its sequelae is often determined by the concentration of the corrosive substance, while the volume and "dose" are secondary considerations. For such agents no single toxicity rating is an appropriate measure of lethality, unless the concentration is also specified. No simple parameter describes this relation in a way which is thought to be clinically useful.

7) In Table II.1 common units of measure are used to describe lethal doses for an adult of average size (body weight of 150 lb. or 70 kg.). For patients who are heavier or lighter, probable lethal doses are proportionately larger or smaller, and they can be readily estimated from values of mg./kg. recorded in the table. While we appreciate that infants and children are not simply small adults, reliable clinical data are so scarce that we are forced to assume that lethal doses are proportional to body weight irrespective of age. Recognized exceptions are noted in Sections II and III.

8) Although all are based on Table II.1, toxicity ratings in this section have a distinctly different meaning from these in Section VI. In Section VI each rating is an estimate of the toxicity of a complete commercial product, as it is marketed and as it is described in Section VI. Here in the Ingredients Index, each rating is a measure of the inherent toxicity of a single ingredient. In establishing the toxicity ratings listed here, each dose has been calculated in terms of a single substance (usually technical grade) and is generally based on experiments in which only an innocuous solvent or

vehicle was used (such as water, corn oil, *etc.),* omitting all solvents, additives, and other ingredients found in the usual commercial formulations. Because many of the ingredients listed here are unavailable to the consumer in pure or undiluted form, the toxicity ratings in Section VI are more realistic in terms of clinical exposure but are inevitably less accurate than those in this section.

Miscellaneous Comments (Column 3).

Although notes about composition, common uses, and related topics are occasionally recorded in column 3, most comments concern toxicity, toxic symptoms, and treatment. Treatment may not be mentioned for one of two reasons: (a) because Section III is thought to provide adequate information (which can be located by consulting the appropriate "reference congener" listed in column 3); or (b) because the only recommended treatment is symptomatic and supportive.

Whenever practical, toxicological distinctions between the entry and its toxic analogue (column 3) are emphasized. Whenever relevant the cutaneous and percutaneous toxicities are indicated because these are not measured by (or necessarily related to) the toxicity ratings of column 2.

"Central nervous depression" often mentioned in column 3 is equivalent to the toxicologists' "narcosis" and must not be confused with the psychiatric syndrome of emotional depression. In its severest form central nervous depression culminates in respiratory arrest from general reflex paralysis. In its milder forms many stages can be distinguished: headache, inattention, vertigo, excitement, confusion, drowsiness, stupor, and coma, often with a terminal convulsion which is probably due to asphyxa. See Section IV for a discussion of supportive treatment in this syndrome.

The Meaning of a Reference Congener (Column 3).

An attempt has been made to group toxicologically related compounds, so that each group can be typified by one of its members, designated here as a "reference congener." Ideally all substances having the same reference congener are chemically related and produce similar toxic effects by mechanisms which are biochemically akin, so that one program of treatment is appropriate to all. This ideal had to be modified in order to restrict the number of reference congeners, which were selected on largely arbitrary grounds. In practice, a compound may differ considerably from its designated congener, both in quantitative and qualitative terms. In spite of its deficiencies, the device of a reference congener is a reasonable attempt to coordinate, correlate, and record succinctly formidable masses of toxicity data.

For information about or relevant to any substance listed in this index, its reference congener should be noted in column 3. This is a reference to Section III, where the toxicology of each congener is discussed in some detail. Within reasonable limits each discussion in Section III is applicable to all substances having the same reference congener; we believe that this is especially true of recommended treatment.

Substance and Synonym or Principal Ingredient	Toxicity Rating (See Inside Cover)	Comments and Reference Congeners
ABALYN Methyl abietate		The toxicity is probably low. See abietic acid below.
ABIETIC ACID Sylvic acid	2(?)	Almost no information. Low intravenous toxicity in mice (presumably low also by other routes). Central nervous paralysis in frogs.
ACETAL Diethylacetal	3	A central nervous depressant, similar to but more toxic than paraldehyde.
ACETALDEHYDE Ethyl aldehyde	3	Less irritating but a stronger central nervous depressant than formaldehyde. Vapor exposures, however, are usually limited by the intense irritation of mucous membranes and conjunctiva. Ingestion produces central nervous depression with symptoms like alcohol intoxication, sometimes with pulmonary edema and albuminuria. Rapidly metabolized. The acute circulatory collapse of the Antabuse-alcohol reaction is thought to be partly due to the metabolic accumulation of acetaldehyde. For treatment of latter, see Disulfuram in Section III.
ACETANILID N-Phenylacetamide	4	Similar to but less toxic than aniline in animals, but clinical experience does not confirm this difference in man. Indeed a toxicity rating of 5 might be a better description of the recorded human fatalities. Perhaps less prominent nervous symptoms than in aniline poisoning. (See also: ANILINE, Reference Congener, in Section III.)
ACETIC ACID		Vinegar and "dilute acetic acid" are about 4 to 6% acetic acid. Essence of vinegar is 14% acetic acid. Glacial acetic acid (100%) is highly corrosive. (See also: ACID, Reference Congener in Section III.)
ACETIN Monoacetin Glyceryl monoacetate (usually contaminated with glycerine)	1	Largely (but not completely) hydrolyzed in bowel to glycerine and acetic acid. May disturb acid-base balance. Given subcutaneously or intramuscularly to lab. animals (including monkeys), it produces vasodilatation, central nervous depression, and death from respiratory failure (mean lethal dose 1 to 5 gm./kg.).
ACETOARSENITE Generally marketed as the copper salt (e.g., Paris Green)	5	A widely used agricultural pesticide. (See also: ARSENIC, Reference Congener in Section III.)
ACETONE Dimethyl ketone Propanone	3	Effects similar to ethyl alcohol for equal blood levels, but the anesthetic potency is greater. Ten to 20 ml. taken by mouth without ill effect. (See also: ETHYL ALCOHOL, Reference Congener in Section III.)
3-(α-ACETONYLBENZYL)-4-HYDROXY-COUMARIN Warfarin	4	Single-dose toxicity is not well defined, but it is probably low relative to the cumulative multiple-dose toxicity. (See also: WARFARIN, Reference Congener in Section III.)
ACETOPHENETIDIN Phenacetin	4	Less toxic than aniline or acetanilid. Cyanosis and methemoglobin are less marked, but severe skin rashes may be more common. (See also: ANILINE, Reference Congener in Section III.)
ACETYLENE TETRACHLORIDE Tetrachloroethane	4	More potent central nervous system effects than chloroform or carbon tetrachloride. On ingestion severe mucosal injury and often liver necrosis, sometimes with late cirrhosis. Can be absorbed through intact skin. (See also: CARBON TETRACHLORIDE, Reference Congener in Section III.)
ACETYLSALICYLIC ACID Aspirin	4	(See also: SALICYLATE, Reference Congener in Section III.)
3-ACETYL-6-METHYL-2,4-PYRANDIONE Dehydroacetic acid and its sodium salt	3	A fungicide used in cosmetics and agriculture. No primary or allergic cutaneous reactions. Humans have ingested 0.01 gm./kg. daily for 150 days without observable ill-effects. At high dosage levels monkeys showed anorexia, vomiting, weakness, stupor, ataxia, and convulsions. The control of convulsions by barbiturates was life-saving in experimental poisoning.
ACIDS Mineral acids		(See also: ACID, Reference Congener in Section III.)
ACONITE The dried powdered root of Monkshood or Wolfsbane	5	Aconitine, an unstable alkaloid, is the chief active ingredient (0.4 to 0.8% of the dried powdered root). Fatal dose is 20 to 40 cc. of a 10% tincture (alcoholic). In mouth and on mucous membranes, solutions produce a peculiar warm and tingling sensation with subsequent numbness. Central nervous stimulation is largely responsible for nausea, vomiting, and diarrhea; also restlessness, ataxia, vertigo, slow and dyspneic breathing, hypothermia, and convulsions. As with digitalis the cardiac effects arise directly and reflexly; they may be severe. (See also: DIGITALIS, Reference Congener in Section III.)

Substance and Synonym or Principal Ingredient	Toxicity Rating (See Inside Cover)	Comments and Reference Congeners
ACRYLONITRILE Vinyl cyanide Carbacryl Propene nitrile	4	Similar to but less toxic than its molecular equivalent in hydrogen cyanide. In sublethal exposures mild jaundice has been reported. Liquid spilled on the skin results in erythema and later painful blisters. Treament measures for cyanide do not protect exposed guinea pigs, suggesting that the release of HCN is too small to account for acrylonitrile poisoning in this species. (See also: CYANIDE, Reference Congener in Section III.)
ACTAMER 2,2'-Bisthio(4,6-dichlorophenol)	2	A germicide of low toxicity. No skin reaction when applied as a 2% ointment (carbowax). (See also: PHENOL, Reference Congener in Section III.)
ACTI-DIONE Cycloheximide	5	An antibiotic fungicide of high toxicity, lying near the borderline between toxicity classes 4 and 5 in monkeys and probably in dogs (rating of 6 in rats). In all 3 species, toxic symptoms include excessive salivation and diarrhea. Blood-stained feces may arise from vascular lesions of the colon (monkey) or stomach and small intestines (dogs). Rat and dog show transient central nervous excitement with tremors and in the dog perhaps meningeal irritation. In all species tested, death is preceded by coma. No antidote is known.
AEROSOLS Trademarked name for a series of commercial surfactants	3	A series of anionic surface-active agents, particularly dialkyl sodium sulfosuccinate. (One exception is Aerosol C-61, which is cationic). Irritating to eyes but not to skin at conc. of 1%.
ALANAP N-1-Naphthyl phthalamic acid (Alanap-1) and its sodium salt (Alanap-3) Alpha naphthyl phthalamic acid	3	A herbicide of low acute toxicity in rats. The free acid is particularly benign when ingested (LD_{50} greater than 8 gm./kg.). No skin irritation described in man or animals.
ALCOHOL, ETHYL Ethanol Grain alcohol Neutral spirits	2	Clinical experience indicates that the lethal dose lies near the borderline between toxicity classes 2 and 3. (See also: ETHYL ALCOHOL, Reference Congener in Section III.)
ALCOHOL, ISOPROPYL 2-Propanol	3	(See also: ISOPROPYL ALCOHOL, Reference Congener in Section III.)
ALCOHOL, METHYL Methanol Wood alcohol	3	(See also: METHYL ALCOHOL, Reference Congener in Section III.)
ALCOHOLS, HIGHER e.g., Butyl, amyl, etc.	3	(See also: ALCOHOLS, HIGHER, Reference Congener in Section III.)
ALCOHOL SULFATE SALTS Usually sodium or triethanolamine salt	3	Often a secondary or branched-chain alcohol (e.g., Tergitols, Teepol). Anionic wetting and emulsifying agents. Skin penetration suspected with some derivatives. No clinical poisonings are known. Also see alkyl sodium sulfates.
ALDRIN Hexachlorohexahydro-endo, exo-dimethano-naphthalene	5	Animal tests place this compound near the border line between toxicity classes 4 and 5. Similar, chemically and toxicologically, to dieldrin. (See also: DIELDRIN, Reference Congener in Section III.)
ALGIN Sodium alginate	1(?)	A polymer of β-d-mannuronic acid with free carboxyl groups (sodium salt), prepared from various seaweeds (kelp), and widely used as an emulsifier and stabilizer in commercial ice cream, pharmaceuticals, etc. Apparently it is not decomposed or absorbed appreciably when ingested, and it does not swell in an acid medium.
ALGINIC ACID	1(?)	A hydrophilic gum prepared from the sodium salt (see "algin"). It is able to absorb and chemically bind sodium and other cations when ingested, but it has proved to be less efficient than synthetic carboxylic-type resins.
ALIPHATIC HYDROCARBONS Straight-chain, saturated hydrocarbons of the methane series, prepared largely from crude petroleum oil	3	Used as fuels, solvents, vehicles, and cleaners. The lower members of this series (e.g., methane, butane) are gases of low anesthetic potency. The liquid fractions are also central nervous depressants when absorbed from the alimentary tract, or severe pulmonary irritants when aspirated. Narcotic potency increases with the chain length at least through octane, but very long molecules like hexadecane and above (as found in liquid petrolatum and solid paraffin) are almost inert. Kerosene is representative of the toxic liquid fractions. (See also: KEROSENE, Reference Congener in Section III.)
ALIPHATIC THIOCYANATES e.g. Lethanes		A series of agricultural insecticides. When tested in animals, various organic thiocyanates differ widely in toxicity. (See also: ALIPHATIC THIOCYANATES, Reference Congener in Section III.)

Substance and Synonym or Principal Ingredient	Toxicity Rating (See Inside Cover)	Comments and Reference Congeners
ALIZARIN 1,2-Dihydroxyanthro- quinone		Occurs in the root of madder plant. It and many derivatives are used as dyes in home and industry. Except for reports of allergic reactions in humans, no toxicity data were located.
ALKALI Corrosive alkalis like lye, sodium and potassium hydroxides, etc.		(See also: ALKALI, Reference Congener in Section III.)
ALKENYL DERIVATIVE		Alkenyl generally designates a long unsaturated hydrocarbon chain (while alkyl refers to a saturated one). See corresponding "alkyl" derivative, which usually has a similar toxicity (at least among the surfactants).
ALKYL ARYL AMMONIUM CHLORIDE (OR BROMIDE)	4	This is a generic name for a large number of quaternary ammonium surfactants, used chiefly as germicides and sanitizers. (See also: QAC, Reference Congener in Section III.)
ALKYL ARYL POLYETHER ALCOHOLS Alternative generic names: Alkyl phenoxy polyethoxy ethanols Alkyl phenol polyglycol ethers Polyethylene glycol alkyl aryl ethers	2 and 3	Non-ionic surfactants used as wetting and emulsifying agents. They are available with a wide variety of physical properties. None is highly toxic in animals and none is appreciably irritating to the skin, even at full-strength. The only symptoms (and lesions) in orally poisoned animals are related to gastrointestinal irritation (e.g., diarrhea, bloating). Little, if any, intestinal absorption or decomposition.
ALKYL ARYL POLYETHER SULFATES AND SULFONATES Marketed as sodium salts, e.g., Triton X-200, X-301, 770	2 and 3	Anionic surfactants prepared by sulfating and sulfonating compounds like those above. Animal tests reveal no consistent difference in acute oral toxicity between the non-ionic product and its anionic derivative, but the latter are always more irritating to eyes and skin, perhaps because solutions of these salts are usually alkaline.
ALKYL ARYL SODIUM SULFONATES Aryl group is usually benzene, naphthalene, toluene, or xylene. e.g., Ultrawets, Santomerse, Nacconals, Aresket, Areskap	3	This is probably the largest and most important class of anionic surfactants, but in general they are unsuitable for household use, because many of them are highly defatting to the skin.
ALKYLATED SODIUM PHOSPHATES e.g., Victawets	3(?)	Toxicity rating is based on the only datum available, namely the intraperitoneal lethal dose of Victawet 12 in rats.
ALKYL DIMETHYL BENZYL AMMONIUM CHLORIDE (OR BROMIDE) Benzalkonium chloride e.g., Triton X-400 or K-60 (where alkyl= stearyl), Roccal, BTC, Zephiran chloride	4	Probably the most widely used cationic surfactant, employed at use concentrations of 0.1% (and less) as a germicide and sanitizer for chemically clean surfaces. Commercially available as concentrated aqueous solutions. Dependent in part upon the length of the alkyl group, the toxicity rating (mice and rats) may be 3 or 4, usually the latter. (See also: QAC, Reference Congener in Section III.)
ALKYL DIMETHYL 3,4-DICHLORO- BENZENE AMMONIUM CHLORIDE Arakonium chloride Dichloran Tetrosan also contains alkenyl groups.	4	A cationic surfactant used at dilutions of 1:1000 to 1:5000 as a germicide and sanitizer for clean surfaces. Based on animal studies this compound lies near the borderline between toxicity classes 3 and 4. (See also: QAC, Reference Congener in Section III.)
ALKYL DIMETHYL ETHYL AMMONIUM CHLORIDE (OR BROMIDE) e.g., Cetylcide Ethyl cetab	4	A cationic surfactant. (See also: QAC, Reference Congener in Section III.)

Substance and Synonym or Principal Ingredient	Toxicity Rating (See Inside Cover)	Comments and Reference Congeners
ALKYL DIMETHYL ETHYL-BENZYL AMMONIUM CHLORIDE (OR BROMIDE) e.g., BTC 471 (BTC 927 is dimethylbenzyl instead or ethylbenzyl)	4	A cationic surfactant. (See also: QAC, Reference Congener in Section III.)
ALKYL HYDROXYETHYL IMIDAZOLINIUM CHLORIDE e.g., Alrosept MB Alrosept MM	4	A cationic surfactant. (See also: QAC, Reference Congener in Section III.)
ALKYL MERCURIC CHLORIDE (OR PHOSPHATE) Alkyl group is usually ethyl or methyl	5	Toxic by all portals. Systemic toxicity almost as high as mercuric chloride. Nervous symptoms are prominent; they include headache, vertigo, ataxia, decrease in visual fields, delirium, and paresis. (See also: MERCURY, Reference Congener in Section III.)
ALKYL NAPHTHYL METHYL PYRIDINIUM CHLORIDE e.g., Emcol 888	4	A cationic surfactant used at concentrations of 0.1% and less as a disinfectant for clean surfaces. (See also: QAC, Reference Congener in Section III.)
ALKYL PHENOL POLYGLYCOL ETHERS e.g., Neutronyx-600	3	The same type of non-ionic surfactant as is described below. For practical purposes these generic names are interchangeable.
ALKYL PHENOXY POLYETHOXY ETHANOLS e.g., Igepals, where alkyl is usually nonyl; Tritons X-45, X-100, X-102, X-114, where alkyl is octyl; Brij products where alkyl is lauryl	2 and 3	Non-ionic surfactants available with a wide variety of physical properties and used as wetting agents and emulsifiers. Even at full-strength, they rarely sensitize or irritate human skin. The only symptoms (and lesions) in orally poisoned animals are related to gastrointestinal irritation (e.g., diarrhea, bloating). Little, if any, intestinal absorption or decomposition.
ALKYL QUATERNARY AMMONIUM CHLORIDE (OR BROMIDE)	4	This is a general name for the largest category of cationic surfactants. Used as germicides and sanitizers. (See also: QAC, Reference Congener in Section III.)
ALKYL SODIUM ISETHIONATE e.g., Igepons AT and AC	2	Anionic surfactants used as wetting agents, detergents, etc. They are fatty acid esters of sodium isethionate $(HO-(CH_2)_2-SO_3-Na)$.
ALKYL SODIUM N-METHYLTAURATE e.g., Igepons T, TK, or TN, or more specifically T-42, T-51, etc.	3	The alkyl group (often oleoyl) is a fatty acid attached to the nitrogen by an amide linkage. Anionic surface-active agents, some of which produce skin irritation at concs. of 5%.
ALKYL SODIUM SULFATES Sodium salts of fatty alcohol sulfates (sometimes a secondary or branched-chain alcohol, as in Tergitols) e.g., Sodium lauryl sulfate (Duponol C), Drene, Dreft, Teel, Gardinols	3	Widely used anionic detergents of low acute and chronic toxicity. A few of the branched-chain products have been shown to have significant percutaneous toxicity. Skin irritation may be encountered with any of these substances. Taken by mouth, sodium lauryl sulfate stimulates gastric mucous production and sometimes inactivates pepsin in test animals. In subacute and chronic feeding tests, even fatally poisoned animals show only diarrhea and intestinal bloating, with no gross lesions outside of the gastrointestinal tract.
ALKYL SODIUM SULFONATES	3	Unlike the -C-O-S- linkage of the alkyl sulfates, the sulfonates have a -C-S- bond. The sulfonates are more stable with respect to hydrolysis than the sulfates but are less soluble in hard water. Although no adequate toxicological comparison has been reported, lethal doses of alkyl sulfonates and sulfates appear to be substantially the same in laboratory animals. See alkyl sodium sulfates above.
ALKYL TOLYL METHYL TRIMETHYL AMMONIUM CHLORIDE e.g., Hyamine 2389	4	A cationic surfactant used in concs. of 1:1000 (or less) to disinfect clean surfaces. Some primary skin irritation from aqueous solutions of 10% or more (See also: QAC, Reference Congener in Section III.)

Substance and Synonym or Principal Ingredient	Toxicity Rating (See Inside Cover)	Comments and Reference Congeners
ALKYL TRIMETHYL AMMONIUM CHLORIDE (OR BROMIDE) e.g., Cetab (where alkyl is cetyl)	4	A cationic surfactant. (See also: QAC, Reference Congener in Section III.)
ALLETHRIN Allyl cinerin	3	Toxic actions similar to pyrethrins. Perhaps 4 is a more accurate estimate of the toxicity rating. (See also: PYRETHRUM, Reference Congener in Section III.)
ALROSEPT MM 1-Tridecyl-2-methyl-2-hydroxyethyl imidazolinium chloride	4	A cationic surfactant used at a conc. of 1:5000 as a germicide for clean surfaces. Other Alrosepts have similar structures and similar toxicities. (See also: QAC, Reference Congener in Section III.)
ALLYL ALCOHOL 1-Propenol-3	4	Vapor and liquid are intensely irritating to skin and mucous membrane. Produces lacrimation and corneal burns. Penetration through intact skin is dangerous. Animal studies place this compound near the borderline between toxicity classes 4 and 5.
ALLYL CINERIN Allethrin	3	Toxic actions similar to pyrethrins. Perhaps 4 is a more accurate estimate of the toxicity rating. (See also: PYRETHRUM, Reference Congener in Section III.)
ALLYL ISOTHIOCYANATE Volatile oil of mustard		Used as a counter-irritant in medicine, a fungicide, an insecticidal fumigant, and a repellent for cats and dogs. A violent irritant unless diluted. Used externally as a rubefacient (0.1-2.0% in 50% ethanol). Aqueous suspensions are more irritating than oil solutions and may produce blisters. Internal toxicity is not described.
ALOIN A mixture of the active principles obtained from aloe	4(?)	An irritant laxative (dose 15 mg.), with bowel actions largely limited to the colon. More irritating than cascara sagrada or senna. May produce renal irritation and discolor an alkaline urine red.
ALPHA-		If not listed below, omit the prefix and try again.
ALPHA NAPHTHOL THIOUREA ANTU	3(?)	(See also: ANTU, Reference Congener in Section III.)
ALUMINUM AMMONIUM (OR POTASSIUM) SULFATE Alum (ammonium or potassium alum)		Low toxicity in experimental animals (toxicity rating of 2), but on two occasions the ingestion of 30 gm. has killed an adult human. Death is probably due to the corrosive action of the sulfuric acid formed by hydrolysis of the salt. Concentrated solutions (e.g., 20%) have produced gingival necrosis and fatal hemorrhagic gastroenteritis. Also incoordination, clonic contractions, and evidence of nephritis. The only recommended treatment is supportive.
ALUMINUM CHLORIDE	3(?)	May cause allergic reactions. Irritating to abraded skin. Corrosive if anhydrous. Ingestion presumably produces the same toxic effects as alum. See above.
ALUMINUM OXIDE AND HYDROXIDE	1	These insoluble salts are essentially harmless by oral administration.
AMANITA e.g., Amanita phalloides	3 or 4	A genus consisting of many toxic species of mushrooms (or toadstools). (See also: AMANITA TOXINS, Reference Congener in Section III.)
2-AMINO-2-HYDROXYMETHYL-1,3-PROPANDIOL Tris (hydroxymethyl) aminomethane	3	A commercial emulsifier. Aqueous solutions are alkaline and consequently irritating. Even after neutralization, large oral doses in laboratory animals cause weakness, collapse, and coma (without convulsions).
2-AMINO-5-NITROTHIAZOLE	4(?)	Used for treatment of blackhead disease (histomoniasis, a protozoan enterohepatitis) in poultry. No toxicity data were located, but a related compound, 2-aminothiazole, has a rating of 4 in several laboratory mammals, and single oral doses produce hyperpnea, dyspnea, weakness, hypotension, mild clonic-tonic and asphyxial convulsions, and death in 6 to 24 hours.
p-AMINOPHENOL 4-Amino-1-hydroxy-benzene Rodinal	4	A photographic developer. Sometimes used in hair dyes. A metabolic product of acetanilid, aniline, and acetophenetidin. Causes methemoglobinemia, but less toxic than aniline in animals. Aqueous solutions on the skin have produced restlessness and convulsions in man, as well as skin irritation. Dilutions used in photography are probably ineffective by skin contact in most cases. (See also: ANILINE, Reference Congener in Section III.)

Substance and Synonym or Principal Ingredient	Toxicity Rating (See Inside Cover)	Comments and Reference Congeners
AMINOPYRINE Amidopyrine Pyramidon	4	Most of the toxicity reported for this drug appears to be due to hypersensitivity, notably an occasional fatal agranulocytosis and angioneurotic edema. No effect on red blood cells or on hemoglobin. Large doses are said to cause convulsions.
3-AMINO-1,2,4-TRIAZOLE Amizol ATA	2(?)	A relatively new herbicide used against poison oak and poison ivy. The toxic hazard to man is not yet established, but rats survive intraperitoneal doses of 1 gm./kg.
AMMATE Ammonium sulfamate	3(?)	Used as a herbicide. Moderately low toxicity in laboratory animals by ingestion and by skin contact. The correct toxicity rating may be 2.
AMMONIA Ammonia water (ammonium hydroxide) or ammonia gas		Dilute ammonia water (U.S.P.) is 9 to 10% (w/v) ammonia (NH_3). Strong ammonia solution (U.S.P.) is 27 to 30% (w/v) NH_3, as are most freshly opened bottles of household ammonia. (See also: AMMONIA, Reference Congener in Section III.)
AMMONIATED MERCURY Mercuric chloride ammoniated Aminomercuric chloride	5	Too vigorous skin application may cause dermatitis and even systemic poisoning. Almost as toxic as the bichloride when ingested. (See also: MERCURY, Reference Congener in Section III.)
AMMONIUM SALTS (OTHER THAN THOSE LISTED HERE)		Consult this index under the name of the anion.
AMMONIUM SULFAMATE Ammate	3(?)	Used as a herbicide. Low toxicity in laboratory animals by ingestion and by skin contact. The correct toxicity rating may be 2.
AMPHETAMINE Beta-phenyl-isopropylamine Benzedrine	5	Acute lethal dose in adults is probably 20 to 25 mg./kg., in children only 5 mg./kg. Overdosage causes restlessness, insomnia, nausea and vomiting, intense mydriasis, confusion, delirium, mania, and collapse. Convulsions and coma are terminal events. Various cardiovascular actions are described: tachycardia, arrhythmias, heart block, hypertension or hypotension, and circulatory collapse. Treatment is symptomatic with emphasis on sedatives (especially barbiturates).
AMYL ACETATE Isoamyl acetate Banana oil Pear oil	3(?)	Like other simple esters, an irritant and central nervous depressant. More narcotic than ethyl acetate and more irritating than butyl. Vapor has produced edema of the glottis. Secondary amyl acetate is thought to be qualitatively (and perhaps quantitatively) similar in toxicity to the commoner isoamyl ester.
AMYL ALCOHOL A mixture of several isomers	3	Can be described as lying near the borderline between toxicity classes 3 and 4. (See also: ALCOHOLS, HIGHER, Reference Congener in Section III.)
AMYL NITRITE		Prompt circulatory collapse from vasodilatation, in addition to methemoglobinemia. (See also: NITRITE, Reference Congener in Section III.)
AMYTAL Amobarbital 5-ethyl-5-isoamyl Barbituric acid	4	A sedative with a moderately long duration of action. Detoxified in vivo. Its actions are very prolonged in the presence of liver damage. (See also: BARBITURATE, Reference Congener in Section III.)
ANABASINE 2-(3'-Pyridyl) piperidine Neonicotine	6	Toxic actions are like nicotine, but toxicity is one-third to one-fifth that of nicotine. Cheaper than the latter as an insecticide. (See also: NICOTINE, Reference Congener in Section III.)
ANILINE Aniline oil Aminobenzene	4	(See also: ANILINE, Reference Congener in Section III.)
ANTABUSE (OR ANTABUS) Disulfiram Bis(diethylthiocarbamyl) disulfide Tetraethylthiuram disulfide	3	Toxicity rating of 3 is based on animal experiments in which no alcohol was given. (See also: DISULFIRAM, Reference Congener in Section III.)
ANTIHISTAMINICS	5	(See also: ANTIHISTAMINICS, Reference Congener in Section III.)

Substance and Synonym or Principal Ingredient	Toxicity Rating (See Inside Cover)	Comments and Reference Congeners
ANTIMONY COMPOUNDS	5	Although it has a slightly better prognosis, antimony poisoning closely parallels arsenic poisoning, except that vomiting from antimony may be more prominent, perhaps because its compounds are less readily absorbed than arsenicals. Trivalent antimony compounds (e.g., tartar emetic) are many times more lethal than pentavalent derivatives. BAL appears to be effective in treating antimony poisoning, at least when it is due to trivalent forms of the metal. Tolerance to antimony is denied. (See also: ARSENIC, Reference Congener in Section III.)
ANTIMONY TRICHLORIDE Butter of antimony	5	A particularly corrosive form of trivalent antimony. See "antimony compounds" above for general comments. (See also: ARSENIC, Reference Congener in Section III.)
ANTIPYONIN "Neutral sodium tetraborate"	3	Borax is sodium bi-, tetra-, or pyroborate. The lethal dose probably lies near the borderline between toxicity classes 3 and 4. (See also: BORATE, Reference Congener in Section III.)
ANTIPYRINE Phenazone	4	Similar to acetanilid poisoning although cyanosis is much rarer. Skin rashes, however, are far more common and may persist for several weeks; they may resemble the erythematous macules seen after phenolphthalein. Probably less toxic than acetanilid but more poisonous than acetophenetidin. (See also: ANILINE, Reference Congener in Section III.)
ANTU Alpha naphthyl thiourea	3(?)	(See also: ANTU, Reference Congener in Section III.)
AR-60 Methylated naphthalenes	3(?)	Presumably less toxic than naphthalene. The only untoward effects reported in man are skin irritation and skin photosensitization. (See also: NAPHTHALENE, Reference Congener in Section III.)
ARAMITE 2-(p-tert.-Butylphenoxy) isopropyl-2-chloroethyl sulfite (Aramite-15W is a 15% wettable powder) Elemite	3	Studies of acute toxicity in laboratory mammals place this pesticide near the borderline between toxicity classes 2 and 3. A large oral dose causes central nervous depression of long duration. (Chronic exposure may present special problems not yet fully evaluated). Undiluted Aramite (an oil) and its concentrated solutions are irritating to the skin and conjunctiva.
ARECOLINE Methyl-1,2,5,6-tetrahydro-1-methylnicotinate, often marketed as the hydrobromide salt, obtained from areca (dried seeds of Areca catechu L.)	5(?)	An alkaloid used in veterinary medicine against tapeworms (taeniacide). Has actions like both pilocarpine (or muscarine) and nicotine. Causes salivation, nausea, vomiting, abdominal cramps, diarrhea, clonic convulsions, and collapse. Treatment includes liberal doses of atropine. (See also: NICOTINE, Reference Congener in Section III.)
AROMATIC(S)		In commerce this name is used to refer to any substance with a fragrant, spicy, or pungent odor. Many are complex mixtures of plant origin (volatile oils). Because they are present in commercial products only in small quantities, they are rarely, if ever, responsible for acute toxic reactions (other than allergies). This class of substances must not be confused with "aromatic hydrocarbons," "aromatic solvents," or "aromatic hydrocarbon solvents," which include benzene and its relatives and which are often present in dangerous amounts.
AROMATIC HYDROCARBON SOLVENT	4	A generic term used to designate any one or any mixture of the following substances: benzene, toluene, xylenes, cumene, ethyl benzene, mesitylene, and related compounds. (See also: XYLENE, Reference Congener in Section III.)
AROMATIC SOLVENT NAPHTHA	4	A mixture of inconstant composition prepared from the distillation of coal (sometimes from petroleum in current practice). Contains xylenes, ethyl benzene, cumene, and perhaps toluene. Traces of benzene and of pyridine derivatives may be present. Inhalation hazard is less than that of benzene or of toluene because of lower volatility. Ingestion toxicity is like that of xylene. (See also: XYLENE, Reference Congener in Section III.)
ARSENATES	5	In animals, arsenates (pentavalent) are less toxic than arsenites (trivalent). (See also: ARSENIC, Reference Congener in Section III.)
ARSENIC	5	Elemental arsenic is less toxic to animals than arsenite or arsenate. (See also: ARSENIC, Reference Congener in Section III.)

Substance and Synonym or Principal Ingredient	Toxicity Rating (See Inside Cover)	Comments and Reference Congeners
ARSENICALS		Organic arsenic compounds vary considerably in toxicity, but the final toxic syndrome is the same in qualitative terms. (See also: ARSENIC, Reference Congener in Section III.)
ARSENIC TRISULFIDE Auripigment Orpiment	5	Gradually decomposes to arsenic oxide. The pure sulfide is said to have a relatively low toxicity. (See also: ARSENIC, Reference Congener in Section III.)
ARSENIC TRIOXIDE White arsenic Arsenious acid anhydride	6	The average fatal oral dose in man probably lies between 0.1 and 0.3 gm. Coarse powders are less toxic than fine ones. (See also: ARSENIC, Reference Congener in Section III.)
ARSENITES	6	Arsenites (trivalent) are more toxic in animals than arsenates (pentavalent). (See also: ARSENIC, Reference Congener in Section III.)
ASP-47 Tetraethyl dithiono- pyrophosphate Sulfotepp	6	Toxicity comparable to parathion in laboratory animals. Relatively resistant to hydrolysis. (See also: PARATHION, Reference Congener in Section III.)
ASPIDIUM	4	Male fern; usually available as an ether extract of dried rhizomes, which yield not less than 6.5% of Oleoresin of Aspidium (U.S.P.). Active ingredients are filicic acid, filicin, and related substances. An anthelmintic. The oleoresin is a gastrointestinal irritant (nausea, vomiting, colic, bloody diarrhea). Produces central nervous excitation (dizziness, vertigo, delirium, tremors, and tonic-clonic convulsions), followed by depression (coma, respiratory or cardiac failure). Visual disturbances may culminate in temporary or permanent blindness. Mild kidney, liver, and cardiac damage may appear. Intestinal absorption and toxicity are enhanced by fats and oils. Supportive treatment includes gastric lavage, saline catharsis, and control of convulsions (see Section IV.)
ASPIRIN Acetylsalicylic acid	4	(See also: SALICYLATE, Reference Congener in Section III.)
ATROPINE dl-Hyoscyamine	6	(See also: ATROPINE, Reference Congener in Section III.)
AZOBENZENE Diphenyl diimide Azobenzide	4	Used as an acaricide in agriculture. The toxicity is not well defined. Chronic ingestion by rats has produced liver damage. (See also: ANILINE, Reference Congener in Section III.)
BAL Dimercaprol 2,3-Dimercapto-1- propanol British Anti-Lewisite	4(?)	(See also: BAL, Reference Congener in Section III.)
BALSAM PERU Peruvian or Indian balsam. It consists chiefly (50 to 60%) of esters of cinnamic and benzoic acids, especially cinnamein (benzyl cinnamate)	3(?)	An oleoresin which is mildly antiseptic and may be mildly irritating to the skin. It has been ingested and even injected intravenously without ill effects. In man cinnamic acid is said to be largely excreted in urine as benzoic and hippuric acids.
BARBITAL Diethylbarbituric acid Veronal	4	Probably lies near the borderline between toxicity classes 4 and 5. The oldest clinically useful barbiturate drug. A hypnotic and central nervous depressant. It has a long duration of action because elimination is dependent on renal excretion and the latter is inherently slow. As discussed in Sec. III, an osmotic diuresis may be a useful therapeutic measure in poisonings. (See also: BARBITURATE, Reference Congener in Section III.)
BARIUM FLUOSILICATE Barium silicofluoride	4	Not as toxic as sodium fluoride because of low solubility in water. Hydrolyzed by alkali to highly toxic fluoride ion. Although not described in test animals (most species being relatively resistant to barium), barium intoxication may here complicate the clinical picture of acute fluoride poisoning, but the fluosilicate is probably one of the less toxic forms of barium. (See also: FLUORIDE, Reference Congener in Section III.)
BARIUM SALTS, INSOLUBLE e.g., Sulfate	1(?)	Sometimes dangerous because of soluble barium impurities. Otherwise inert and insoluble. (See also: BARIUM, Reference Congener in Section III.)

Substance and Synonym or Principal Ingredient	Toxicity Rating (See Inside Cover)	Comments and Reference Congeners
BARIUM SALTS, WATER OR ACID-SOLUBLE e.g., Oxide, chloride, nitrate, carbonate, sulfide, acetate	3,4 or 5	Acute toxicity varies widely with the compound, animal species, and even strain. Toxicity rating of 5 is probably the best description of clinical experience. (See also: BARIUM, Reference Congener in Section III.)
BELLADONNA LEAF OR ROOT Deadly nightshade, from Atropa belladonna L.	4	Toxicity is based on content of atropine and related alkaloids, – usually about 0.5%/w. (See also: ATROPINE, Reference Congener in Section III.)
BEN Benzyl benzoate	3	Converted to hippuric acid in vivo. In laboratory animals ingestion causes progressive incoordination, central nervous excitement, convulsions, and death. Treat symptomatically.
BENADRYL Diphenhydramine hydrochloride	5	According to clinical experience, this antihistaminic drug is probably best described as lying near the borderline between toxicity classes 4 and 5. (See also: ANTIHISTAMINICS, Reference Congener in Section III.)
BENTONITE A hydrated aluminum silicate mineral	1	Biologically inert when ingested. Used as a protective colloid in suspensions. Similar to kaolin but bentonite has smaller particles.
BENZALDEHYDE Benzoic aldehyde Artifical essential oil of almond	3	Subcutaneous lethal dose in rats is about 5 gm./kg., but oral fatal dose in man is estimated to be about 2 oz. Produces central nervous depression with respiratory failure. Epileptiform convulsions observed in rabbits.
BENZALKONIUM CHLORIDE Alkyl benzyl dimethyl ammonium chloride (e.g., Zephiran chloride, BTC, Triton X-400, etc.)	4	Probably the most widely used cationic germicide, usually marketed as aqueous solutions of 2 to 50% but used at concs. of 0.1% or lower. (See also: QAC, Reference Congener in Section III.)
BENZENE Benzol	4	Similar to but more hazardous than xylene. (See also: XYLENE, Reference Congener in Section III.)
BENZENE HEXACHLORIDE Hexachlorocyclohexane (not hexachlorobenzene)	4	(See also: BENZENE HEXACHLORIDE, Reference Congener in Section III.)
BENZETHONIUM CHLORIDE p-Diisobutyl phenoxy-ethoxyethyl dimethyl benzyl ammonium chloride (e.g., Hyamine 1622, Phemerol chloride, etc.)	4	A cationic surfactant used as a germicide, disinfectant, and preservative. (See also: QAC, Reference Congener in Section III.)
BENZIN OR BENZINE Petroleum ether (not the same as benzene)	3	The usual solvent-grade consists largely of C_4 to C_8 petroleum aliphatic hydrocarbons and distills between 40 and 80° C. A high-boiling (80 to 130° C. or 100 to 150° C.) petroleum ether or technical benzin more closely resembles kerosene. (See also: KEROSENE, Reference Congener in Section III.)
BENZOCAINE Ethyl aminobenzoate		Many other aminobenzoates are also used as local anesthetic agents (e.g. butyl, isobutyl, etc.) A local anesthetic of low toxicity. It is poorly absorbed from all sites, probably because it is water insoluble. Systemic effects, if any, presumably include central nervous excitement. Concentrations in most products have no toxic significance.
BENZOIC ACID Benzenecarboxylic acid	3	A 67 kg. man has ingested single doses of 50 gm. without ill effects, although the mean lethal dose in cats and dogs is 2 gm./kg. Large oral doses produce gastric pain, nausea, and vomiting. When injected in rats, tremors, convulsions, and death occur.
BENZYL ALCOHOL Phenylcarbinol Phenylmethanol	3	Pure alcohol is irritating and corrosive but much less toxic than phenol. Aqueous concentrations up to 4% are well tolerated; they produce transient anesthesia of mucous membranes. Ingestion of large volumes is followed by vomiting, diarrhea, and central nervous depression. Converted into benzoic and hippuric acids. A human fatality has been ascribed to the rectal administration of 45 ml.

Substance and Synonym or Principal Ingredient	Toxicity Rating (See Inside Cover)	Comments and Reference Congeners
BENZYL BENZOATE	3	Converted to hippuric acid in vivo. In laboratory animals ingestion causes progressive incoordination, central nervous excitation, convulsions, and death. Treat symptomatically. Has caused skin irritation in humans.
BERBERINE An alkaloid, usually as the sulfate; obtained from the rhizomes and roots of Hydrastis canadensis	5(?)	Used as a bitter stomachic. A mild local anesthetic on mucous membrane. Toxic doses depress the heart (directly and reflexly through the vagus), relax blood vessels, depress respirations, and stimulate smooth muscle in the intestines, bronchi, and possibly uterus. Vigorous supportive treatment may be necessary for circulatory collapse.
BERYLLIUM SALTS		Mixed beryllium metasilicates were used until recently as phosphors in fluorescent lamps. Very low ingestion toxicity, but inhaled dusts may produce an acute pneumonitis or a chronic progressive pulmonary granulomatosis, usually with an insidious and delayed onset. Chronic ulcers occur if soluble beryllium dusts gain entrance into superficial cuts and abrasions. Dermatitis.
BETA-		If not listed below, omit the prefix "beta" and try again.
BETA-BUTOXY-BETA-THIOCYANO-DIETHYL ETHER Lethane 384	4	Toxicity rating is based on the commercial formulation, which is 50%/v light petroleum ether (kerosene). (See also: ALIPHATIC THIOCYANATES, Reference Congener in Section III.)
BETA-DICHLORO-ETHYL ETHER β,β'-Dichloro-ethyl ether Chlorex	4	A strong irritant. Percutaneous absorption can be dangerous. Possibly late effects like carbon tetrachloride (liver and kidney injury). No severe systemic poisonings in man have been reported. (See also: CARBON TETRACHLORIDE, Reference Congener in Section III.)
BETA-NAPHTHOL β-Naphthol β-Hydroxynaphthalene	4	Less toxic than phenol. Absorbed via intact skin or bowel. Toxic doses produce crampy abdominal pain, nausea, vomiting, diarrhea, and sometimes convulsions. May produce a severe nephritis and rarely an acute hemolytic anemia. Lens opacities and retinal changes have been described. Alpha isomer is said to be even more toxic. (See also: PHENOL, Reference Congener in Section III.)
BHC Benzene hexachloride Hexachlorocyclohexane	4	Not hexachlorobenzene (See also: BENZENE HEXACHLORIDE, Reference Congener in Section III.)
BICHLORIDE OF MERCURY Mercuric chloride	5	Act fast! One gram has killed an adult man. (See also: MERCURY, Reference Congener in Section III.)
BIOQUIN Copper quinolinate	2(?)	Said to have a very low toxicity. No skin irritation or corrosive action when ingested. (See also: COPPER, Reference Congener in Section III.)
BIS-		If not located below, substitute Di- for Bis- and try again.
BIS(5-CHLORO-2-HYDROXY-PHENYL) METHANE Dichlorophene G-4	3	Moderately low ingestion toxicity in guinea pigs. A concentration of 1% is not irritating to human skin. (See also: PHENOL, Reference Congener in Section III.)
1,1-BIS(p-CHLORO-PHENYL)ETHANOL Di-(p-chlorophenyl)-methyl carbitol Dimite	3(?)	An acaricide. Effects on humans are not known. Suspect DDT-like actions. Less toxic than DDT in animals. (See also: DDT, Reference Congener in Section III.)
1,1-BIS(p-CHLORO-PHENYL)-2-NITRO-BUTANE (OR-PROPANE) Dilan	3	Symptoms and treatment like DDT poisoning. Can be absorbed through intact skin but probably not in significant amounts. (See also: DDT, Reference Congener in Section III.)
BIS(DIETHYLTHIO-CARBAMYL)DISULFIDE Disulfiram Antabuse	3	Toxicity rating of 3 is based on animal tests in which no alcohol was given. (See also: DISULFIRAM, Reference Congener in Section III.)
BIS(DIMETHYLAMINO) PHOSPHONOUS ANHYDRIDE Schradan Octamethyl pyrophosphoramide OMPA	5	A "systemic" insecticide, i.e., translocated in sap to all parts of plants. Only slightly less toxic than parathion. Not a cholinesterase inhibitor in vitro, but converted to one by liver. Brain cholinesterase, however, is not inhibited in fatally poisoned animals. (See also: PARATHION, Reference Congener in Section III.)

Substance and Synonym or Principal Ingredient	Toxicity Rating (See Inside Cover)	Comments and Reference Congeners
BIS(DIMETHYLTHIO-CARBAMYL) DISULFIDE Thiram, Arasan, Thuad	4	(See also: THIRAM, Reference Congener in Section III.)
BIS(p-ETHYLPHENYL) DICHLOROETHANE Perthane Q-137	2	In animals toxic signs and symptoms are like those in DDT poisoning, but the toxicity is much lower (near the borderline between toxicity classes 2 and 3). There is little, if any, percutaneous absorption, skin irritation, or sensitization. Unlike DDT, feeding tests on rats with radioactive Perthane indicate little tendency for the material to deposit in body fat. (See also: DDT, Reference Congener in Section III.)
BISHYDROXYCOUMARIN Offical U.S.P name for 3,3'-methylene-bis(4-hydroxycoumarin) Dicoumarol or dicumarol		Single therapeutic dose in man is 200 to 300 mg. Single-dose toxicity is not well established but is probably low relative to the cumulative multiple-dose toxicity. (See also: WARFARIN, Reference Congener in Section III.)
BIS(ISOPROPYLAMIDO) FLUOROPHOSPHATE Isopestox	.4	An insecticide and acetylcholinesterase inhibitor, like parathion. After the acute phases of the poisoning, degenerative lesions may become apparent in the central and peripheral nervous systems. (See also: PARATHION, Reference Congener in Section III.)
BIS(ISOPROPYLAMINE) FLUOROPHOSPHINE OXIDE Isopestox	4	See above. (See also: PARATHION, Reference Congener in Section III.)
BISMUTH SALTS Soluble or insoluble	3(?)	Ingestion toxicity is regarded as low. Very poor absorption from bowel. Systemic effects include ulcerative stomatitis, anorexia, headache, skin rashes, kidney tubular damage, and rarely mild jaundice. BAL may be useful if a severe renal lesion is anticipated (see BAL in Section III.)
BISMUTH SUBNITRATE Basic bismuth nitrate Bismuth white	3(?)	Especially in infants, the subnitrate may be reduced by bacteria within the bowel, to yield nitrite, which causes methemoglobinemia after absorption. (See also: NITRITE, Reference Congener in Section III.)
BISMUTH SUBSALICYLATE Basic bismuth salicylate	3(?)	An agricultural fungicide. Used medicinally as an intestinal absorbent (oral dose 1 to 2 gm.) and as an antiluetic drug (i.m. dose 0.2 gm.). Practically insoluble in water but decomposed by alkali, so that salicylate poisoning is conceivable after ingestion. Bismuth poisoning is outlined above.
BIS(PARACHLORO-PHENOXY) METHANE Neotran is a wettable powder with 40% bis(p-chlorophenoxy) methane	2	An agricultural acaricide (e.g., miticide) of very low toxicity. Only slight percutaneous absorption and no skin irritation. It has caused liver pathology in laboratory animals. No human poisonings are known. (See also: DDT, Reference Congener in Section III.)
BIS(PARAMETHOXY-PHENYL)-TRICHLORO-METHANE Methoxychlor	3	Lower toxicity than DDT. Estimated to be one-tenth as toxic in man by ingestion, but this difference may not hold in respiratory exposures to vapor. In animals central nervous depression is more prominent than excitation, and poisonings are slower in onset and longer in duration than in DDT intoxication. (See also: DDT, Reference Congener in Section III.)
2,2'-BISTHIO (4,6-DICHLOROPHENOL) Actamer	2	A germicide of low toxicity. No skin reaction when applied as a 2% ointment (in carbowax). (See also: PHENOL, Reference Congener in Section III.)
BITTER ALMOND, OIL OF 2 to 4% hydrogen cyanide (hydrocyanic acid) and 95% benzaldehyde	4	(See also: CYANIDE, Reference Congener in Section III.)
BLAUD'S PILLS Ferrous carbonate	3	Each pill contains 65 mg. (1 gr.) of ferrous carbonate. (See also: FERROUS SULFATE, Reference Congener in Section III.)
BLUESTONE OR BLUE VITRIOL Cupric sulfate pentahydrate	4	(See also: COPPER, Reference Congener in Section III.)
BORATE SALTS	3	Most of the water-insoluble compounds are complex or mixed salts, many of which are soluble in the dilute acid of gastric juice. Once a tetra-, di-, meta-, ortho-, or pyroborate salt dissolves in a buffered aqueous solution, one borate cannot be distinguished, on chemical or toxicological grounds, from any one of the others. In contrast perborates do not decompose immediately. Hypoborates are reducing reagents and may release hydrogen gas when they decompose. Most of these salts probably lie near the borderline between toxicity classes 3 and 4. (See also: BORATE, Reference Congener in Section III.)

Substance and Synonym or Principal Ingredient	Toxicity Rating (See Inside Cover)	Comments and Reference Congeners
BORAX Sodium tetraborate	3	Like most sodium or potassium borates, solutions of borax are alkaline. Toxicity is essentially the same as that of boric acid, best described as lying near the borderline between toxicity classes 3 and 4. (See also: BORATE, Reference Congener in Section III.)
BORDEAUX MIXTURE Copper sulfate and unslaked lime (sometimes slaked), freshly dissolved and then mixed in various proportions (often equal parts by weight).	4	A gelatinous mass representing a molecular mixture of copper hydroxide and copper sulfate, widely used as a foliage fungicide. Usually components must be freshly dissolved and then mixed, but some pre-mixed formulations are on the market. Less astringent and presumably less toxic than copper sulfate. (See also: COPPER, Reference Congener in Section III.)
BORIC ACID Boracic acid Orthoboric acid	4	(See also: BORATE, Reference Congener in Section III.)
BOROGLYCERIN Glyceryl borate Boroglycerin glycerite (U.S.P.) is about 50% boroglycerin	3	Two parts boric acid and 3 parts glycerin, heated. Its ingestion has caused borate poisoning. (See also: BORATE, Reference Congener in in Section III.)
BORNEOL Bornyl alcohol 2-Camphanol	4	Toxicity is essentially indistinguishable from that of camphor. As with camphor, laboratory animals appear to be much less susceptible than man. (See also: CAMPHOR, Reference Congener in Section III.)
BORNYL CHLORIDE Pinene hydrochloride Chlorocamphane "Turpentine camphor"	4(?)	A synthetic substance resembling camphor, manufactured from turpentine. (See also: CAMPHOR, Reference Congener in Section III.)
BORON TRIOXIDE B_2O_3, the anhydride of boric acid Boron sesquioxide	4	Slowly reacts with water to form boric acid. Like the latter it presumably lies near the borderline between toxicity classes 3 and 4. (See also: BORATE, Reference Congener in Section III.)
BROMATE SALTS e.g., Sodium bromate	5	(See also: BROMATE, Reference Congener in Section III.)
BROMIDE SALTS e.g., Sodium, potassium, ammonium, etc.	3	Acute oral poisoning is rare because single toxic doses are usually promptly rejected by vomiting, but one oz. has been swallowed and absorbed sufficiently to cause death. The systemic effects of bromide ion are chiefly mental: drowsiness, irritability, ataxia, vertigo, confusion, mania, hallucinations, and coma. Other effects include skin rashes, neurological signs, sensory disturbances, and increased spinal fluid pressures. Treatment includes hydration, the maintenance of a mild water diuresis, and sodium or ammonium chloride by any route (10 to 15 gm. daily in divided doses).
2-BROMO-4-PHENYL PHENOL e.g., Dowicide 5	3(?)	(See also: PHENOL, Reference Congener in Section III.)
BROWN MIXTURE Compound mixture of opium and glycyrrhiza (U.S.P.)	2	A cough mixture and sedative. One teaspoonful contains 0.6 ml. paregoric (2.5 mg. opium), 1.2 mg. tartar emetic, and ethyl nitrite. Overdosages produce vomiting due to tartar emetic or systemic antimony poisoning. See antimony compounds in this index.
BRUCINE Usually the sulfate salt	5	A denaturant in alcohols and oils. Probable fatal dose in an adult is estimated at 1 gm. May produce nausea, vomiting, restlessness, excitement, twitching, and rarely convulsions. (See also: STRYCHNINE, Reference Congener in Section III.)
BULAN 1,1-Bis(p-chlorophenyl)-2-nitrobutane	4	Same symptoms and treatment as DDT. Can be absorbed through intact skin. (See also: DDT, Reference Congener in Section III.)
BUROW'S SOLUTION An aqueous solution of aluminum acetate (4.8 to 5.8%)	2(?)	When diluted 10-to 20-fold, it is used as a wet dressing in weeping skin disorders because of its astringent and antiseptic properties. Probably moderately irritating if ingested.
BUTANE A principal ingredient of "bottled gas," e.g., Pyrofax		A mildly anesthetic gas in high concentrations. Principal hazards are those of fire and explosion.

Substance and Synonym or Principal Ingredient	Toxicity Rating (See Inside Cover)	Comments and Reference Congeners
BUTANOL n-Butyl alcohol	3	Acute toxicity is about 3 times that of ethyl alcohol. More irritating than ethyl but less so than amyl alcohol. (See also: ALCOHOLS, HIGHER, Reference Congener in Section III.)
2-BUTANONE Ethyl methyl ketone	3	Similar to but more irritating than acetone. Vapor is irritating to mucous membrane and conjunctiva. Central nerve depression in experimental animals, but irritating odor ordinarily prevents significant clinical exposures. No serious poisonings reported in man, except for dermatitis.
BUTOPYRONOXYL Indalone Butyl mesityl oxide (oxalate)	2	May be mildly irritating to skin on repeated application. Mild focal necrosis in liver and kidneys of rabbits after repeated cutaneous exposures. No human poisonings are known.
BUTOXY POLYPRO- PYLENE GLYCOLS e.g., Crag Fly Repellent	3	A fly repellent especially useful for livestock. No skin irritation. Very low (but significant) percutaneous toxicity. If like the monopropylene glycol ethers, these polyglycols can be expected to produce central nervous depression and kidney injury after ingestion. (See also: ETHYLENE GLYCOL, Reference Congener in Section III.)
β-BUTOXY-β'-THIOCYANO- DIETHYL ETHER Lethane 384	4	Toxicity rating based on the commercial formulation which is approx. 50% kerosene (by volume). (See also: ALIPHATIC THIOCYANATES, Reference Congener in Section III.)
BUTYL ACETATE n-Butyl acetate	3	A mild irritant and central nervous depressant. More irritating than ethyl acetate. It probably lies near the borderline of toxicity classes 2 and 3.
N-BUTYL ALCOHOL Butanol	3	Acute toxicity about 3 times that of ethyl alcohol. More irritating than ethyl but less so than amyl alcohol. (See also: ALCOHOLS, HIGHER, Reference Congener in Section III.)
BUTYL CARBITOL Diethylene glycol monobutyl ether	3	Probably lies near the borderline between toxicity classes 3 and 4. Slightly more toxic than the ethyl derivative (= Carbitol) but otherwise presumably like it. Both resemble ethylene glycol in toxicity and toxic actions. (See also: ETHYLENE GLYCOL, Reference Congener in Section III.)
N-BUTYL "CARBITOL" RHODANATE Lethane 384 β-Butoxy-thiocyano- diethyl ether	4	(See also: ALIPHATIC THIOCYANATES, Reference Congener in Section III.)
(BUTYLCARBITYL)- (6-PROPYL PIPERONYL)ETHER Piperonyl butoxide (technical grade material may contain 20% related compounds)	2	Used as a synergist to increase the insecticidal potency of pyrethrins and rotenone. Very low toxicity in test animals, which show anorexia, vomiting, diarrhea, hemorrhagic enteritis, inanition, and perhaps mild central nervous depression. No skin irritation or significant percutaneous absorption.
BUTYL CELLOSOLVE Ethylene glycol mono-n-butyl ether	4	Probably lies near the borderline between toxicity classes 3 and 4. About twice as toxic as the ethyl derivative (= Cellosolve) but otherwise like it. Consult "Cellosolves" in this index for a brief comparison with ethylene glycol. (See also: ETHYLENE GLYCOL, Reference Congener in Section III.)
N-BUTYL CHLORIDE 1-Chlorobutane	3	Used as an anthelmintic in veterinary medicine. Weaker central nervous depressant actions than ethyl chloride. Dogs tolerate at least 11 ml./kg. without toxic effects. (See also: CARBON TETRACHLORIDE, Reference Congener in Section III.)
BUTYL MESITYL OXIDE Sometimes called butyl mesityl oxide oxalate Butapyronoxyl Indalone	2	May be mildly irritating to skin on repeated application. Mild focal necrosis in liver and kidneys of rabbits after repeated cutaneous exposures. No human poisonings are known.
BUTYLPHENOXY- ISOPROPYL CHLOROETHYL SULFITE Aramite 2-(p-tert.-Butylphenoxy)- isopropyl-2-chloroethyl sulfite (Aramite-15W is a 15% wettable powder)	3	Studies of acute toxicity in laboratory mammals place this pesticide near the borderline between toxicity classes 2 and 3. A large oral dose causes central nervous depression of long duration. (Chronic exposure may present special problems not yet fully evaluated). Undiluted Aramite (an oil) and its concentrated solutions are irritating to the skin and conjunctiva.

Substance and Synonym or Principal Ingredient	Toxicity Rating (See Inside Cover)	Comments and Reference Congeners
CADMIUM SALTS e.g., Chloride, oxide, sulfate, anilinocadmium dilactate	5(?)	Inhaled as a dust or aerosol, cadmium salts (including even the relatively insoluble oxide) probably have a toxicity rating of 6 in man, with death from fatal pulmonary injury. When swallowed, these salts are much less lethal, in part because they induce vomiting and so are not retained. Although as little as 10 mg. of cadmium salts have often produced severe toxic symptoms when ingested, a toxicity rating of 5 is probably a reasonable estimate of cadmium's lethality by the oral route. (See also: CADMIUM, Reference Congener in Section III.)
CAFFEINE 1,3,7-Trimethylxanthine	4	Fatalities are rare. The fatal dose in adults probably exceeds 10 gm. Symptoms include restlessness, excitement, and tinnitis. A rapid pulse and extrasystoles are often evident. Animals react to high doses with convulsions, which have not yet been described in man. Treatment is symptomatic with special emphasis on sedative drugs (e.g., barbiturates).
CALAMINE Zinc oxide with 0.5% ferric oxide	2(?)	No satisfactory data. Large single doses in animals produce gastritis and vomiting, like copper salts. Some calamine formulations contain significant amounts of phenol (1 to 2%); ingestion or repeated application over large areas of skin can and has caused systemic phenol poisoning.
CALCIUM ARSENATE Tricalcium arsenate Cucumber dust	5	The commercial grade is a complex molecular mixture containing 26% arsenic. It is often colored with a small amount of pink dye. (See also: ARSENIC, Reference Congener in Section III.)
CALCIUM ARSENITE	5	In commerce this material has a variable composition. Significantly more toxic in man (perhaps by a factor of 2) than the pentavalent calcium arsenate. Lies near the borderline between toxicity classes 5 and 6. (See also: ARSENIC, Reference Congener in Section III.)
CALCIUM CYANAMIDE "Cyanamide"	3	Reacts with acid to liberate $HN{=}C{=}NH$, a solid with an appreciable vapor pressure. A synthetic agricultural fertilizer. Contains no free cyanide and apparently is not metabolized to cyanide. When absorbed, the cyanamide ion ($CN_2^=$) causes intense cutaneous and mucosal flushing (congestive hyperemia), headache, vertigo, rapid breathing, hypotension, and profound shock. The primary vascular reaction is not correctable by atropine or any known antidote. An attack after a single oral dose is usually transient (1/2 to 2 hours), and the fatal dose in man is estimated at 40 to 50 gm. The vapor is intensely irritating and may produce both pulmonary and systemic signs. After mild exposures, symptoms may be precipitated or intensified by the ingestion of alcohol.
CALCIUM CYANIDE e.g. Cyanogas	6	All inorganic cyanide salts are toxic when ingested. If the free gastric acidity is high, toxic symptoms appear almost immediately. (See also: CYANIDE, Reference Congener in Section III.)
CALCIUM POLYSULFIDES Lime sulfur	4(?)	Irritant and sensitizing agent. May yield hydrogen sulfide by decomposition before or after ingestion. Used in agriculture as an insecticide and fungicide. (See also: HYDROGEN SULFIDE, Reference Congener in Section III.)
CALCIUM SALTS (Other than listed above) e.g. chloride, hydroxide carbonate, sulfate, etc.		Except for gastric irritation caused in part by osmotic disturbances, calcium per se has no significant oral toxicity For specific salts, consult this index under the name of the anion. For the toxicity of the anhydrous sulfate, see plaster of Paris; for the oxide, see lime. Injected subcutaneously or intramuscularly, soluble calcium salts are intensely irritating, and in infants even calcium gluconate may produce sloughing. Injected intravenously, ionized calcium salts may cause slowing of the heart rate, and sinus arrhythmia; in toxic doses heart block, extrasystoles, and ventricular fibrillation are described. Injected calcium may also stimulate in vivo epinephrine release.
CALGON Sodium hexametaphosphate	2(?)	Most preparations are only mildly alkaline. If ingested in large amounts, nausea, vomiting, and diarrhea are probable. Because this salt appears to be hydrolyzed within the bowel to phosphoric acid, a systemic acidosis may result.
CALOMEL Mercurous chloride	5	A cathartic. Rarely causes systemic mercury poisoning. Rarely "calomel sickness" appears after a latency of about one week; it is a benign reaction characterized by fever and rash (scarlatinal or urticarial). In the presence of water (especially if alkaline), calomel slowly decomposes to mercury and to dangerous mercuric chloride. (See also: MERCURY, Reference Congener in Section III.)
CAMBOGIA Gamboge	4	A gum resin. A violent cathartic, leading to severe prostration and death. The ingestion of 4 gm. has proved fatal.

Substance and Synonym or Principal Ingredient	Toxicity Rating (See Inside Cover)	Comments and Reference Congeners
CAMPHOR 2-Camphanone Gum camphor	4	On the basis of clinical experience, man appears to be much more susceptible to camphor poisoning than other species. Toxicity rating in common laboratory animals is 2 or 3, while clinical data places it near the borderline between toxicity classes 4 and 5. (See also: CAMPHOR, Reference Congener in Section III.)
CAMPHOR, TAR Naphthalene	4	Not to be confused with gum camphor. (See also: NAPHTHALENE, Reference Congener in Section III.)
CANTHARIDES The active ingredient is cantharidin (0.6 to 1.0%).	5	Highly irritating to skin and mucous membranes. A vesicant. Produces nausea, vomiting, colic, and bloody diarrhea, when ingested. Systemic actions include a toxic nephritis. Avoid oils because they enhance absorption.
CAPRYLIC ALCOHOL n-Octyl alcohol	3(?)	Thought to have a low ingestion toxicity. Known to be a hemolytic agent in vitro. Does it cause hemolysis when ingested? (See also: ALCOHOLS, HIGHER, Reference Congener in Section III.)
CAPSICUM Oleoresin of capsicum Cayenne pepper Tabasco pepper African chillies	3(?)	Irritating to mucous membranes. Produces severe gastritis and diarrhea. No primary systemic effects are recognized. Treat by lavage and demulcents.
CAPTAN N-Trichloromethyl-mercapto-4-cyclohexene-1,2-dicarboximide Orthocide	2	A fungicide of low toxicity in laboratory and farm animals (near the borderline between toxicity classes 2 and 3). At lethal doses diarrhea and weight loss appear but no histopathological lesions. Low toxicity is thought to derive from lack of appreciable absorption (because of rapid alkaline hydrolysis in bowel?). Chlorine atoms are unusual because readily hydrolyzed to Cl^-. No human poisonings are known.
CARBINOL Methyl alcohol	3	(See also: METHYL ALCOHOL, Reference Congener in Section III.)
CARBITOL Diethylene glycol monoethyl ether	3	About the same acute toxicity by ingestion as ethylene glycol in animals. No adequate data for human comparisons, but the mean lethal dose of ethylene glycol in man is probably 3 to 4 oz. Poisonings produce similar symptoms. Carbitol is essentially non-irritating to human skin; no skin penetration. (See also: ETHYLENE GLYCOL, Reference Congener in Section III.)
CARBITOL ESTERS Diethylene glycol monoethyl ether esters (e.g., acetate, citrate, laurate, phthalate, ricinoleate, stearate)	3	These esters are apparently saponified (e.g., hydrolyzed) in the body to the glycol ether (= Carbitol) and an organic acid. Symptoms which are due to Carbitol are similar to those produced by ethylene glycol. In animals the esters are slightly less toxic than Carbitol by ingestion but more toxic by skin contact. (See also: ETHYLENE GLYCOL, Reference Congener in Section III.)
CARBOLIC ACID Phenol	4	(See also: PHENOL, Reference Congener in Section III.)
CARBOLINEUM A high-boiling coal tar oil, presumably equivalent to "anthracene oils."	3(?)	Used as a wood preservative. Believed to consist chiefly of anthracene, but it is reasonable to infer that phenolic derivatives and naphthalene are also present. See both phenol and naphthalene in Sec. III. (See also: PHENOL, Reference Congener in Section III.)
CARBON DISULFIDE Carbon bisulfide	3	Probably this compound lies near the borderline between toxicity classes 3 and 4. (See also: CARBON DISULFIDE, Reference Congener in Section III.)
CARBON MONOXIDE Exhaust gas Flue gas		(See also: CARBON MONOXIDE, Reference Congener in Section III.)
CARBON TETRACHLORIDE Tetrachloromethane	4	Man appears to be unusually susceptible to poisoning by carbon tetrachloride. In most laboratory animals the toxicity rating is 2. (See also: CARBON TETRACHLORIDE, Reference Congener in Section III.)
CARBOWAX Solid and semi-solid polyethylene glycols	1	A series of waxy substances with mean molecular weights of 1000 and higher (indicated by the numeral following this trademarked name). In animals the toxicity decreases with increasing molecular weight. With massive doses some animals die from kidney injury. No human poisonings are known. (See also: ETHYLENE GLYCOL, Reference Congener in Section III.)
CARBOXYMETHYL-CELLULOSE	1	Usually dispensed as a water-soluble sodium salt, e.g., Carboxymethocel S. A bulk cathartic, not absorbed from the bowel.

Substance and Synonym or Principal Ingredient	Toxicity Rating (See Inside Cover)	Comments and Reference Congeners
CARBROMAL Bromdiethylacetylurea Contains 34% combined bromine	4	A feeble sedative and hypnotic drug. Usual dose 0.3 to 0.6 gm. Recovery after 3.0 gm. Partially decomposed to bromide ion, but the sedative action is presumably due to the intact molecule.
CARVACROL Isopropyl-o-cresol 2-Hydroxy-p-cymene	4	An isomer of thymol. Somewhat more toxic than thymol in rats and rabbits. Same symptoms and treatment as phenol.(See also: PHENOL, Reference Congener in Section III.)
CARYOPHYLLIC ACID Eugenol 4-Allyl-2-methoxy-phenol	3(?)	Obtained from clove oil, which is about 80% eugenol. Possesses properties of local antisepsis and local anesthesia. Used locally in the control of toothache. A rubifacient and irritant. Ingestion presumably results in a gastroenteritis, but systemic toxicity is lower than phenol, probably because of insolubility in water. (See also: PHENOL, Reference Congener in Section III.)
CASCARA SAGRADA Dried bark of Rhamnus Purshiana	3(?)	Active ingredients are hydroxy-methyl anthroquinones. A cathartic which excites peristalsis in the colon. The adult dose is 0.6 to 2.0 gm. or 2 to 4 ml. of the fluidextract. Large doses cause enteritis, but no fatalities are known.
CASTOR OIL Chiefly the glycerides of ricinoleic and iso-ricinoleic acids	2(?)	A purgative, often causing griping. Clinical dose 1/2 to 1 oz. Produces pelvic congestion and may induce abortions. Fatal dose unknown but presumably it is large.
CASTRIX 2-Chloro-4-dimethylamino-6-methylpyrimidine	6	A rodenticide causing fatal convulsions. In laboratory animals symptoms begin 30 to 50 minutes after ingestion. Compound is not chemically related to strychnine, but recommended treatment is the same. (See also: STRYCHNINE, Reference Congener in Section III.)
CATECHOL Pyrocatechol	4	As toxic as phenol. Similar to phenol, but convulsions may be more frequent and blood dyscrasias are described. (See also: PHENOL, Reference Congener in Section III.)
CATIONIC DETERGENT e.g., Benzalkonium chloride		(See also: QAC, Reference Congener in Section III.)
CAUSTIC SODA Sodium hydroxide		(See also: ALKALI, Reference Congener in Section III.)
CAUSTIC POTASH Potassium hydroxide		(See also: ALKALI, Reference Congener in Section III.)
CBP Technical 1-chloro-3-bromopropene-1	4	Intense skin and eye irritation from vapor or liquid, abating rapidly after exposure. Percutaneous absorption is low. (See also: D-D, Reference Congener in Section III.)
CEDILANID Lanatoside C Digilanid C Derived from the leaf of Digitalis lanata	6	Lanatoside C is more often used as a cardiotonic drug than A or B. It has all the therapeutic and toxic actions of digitalis leaf. Its actions are less persistent than those of digitoxin but more prolonged than those of strophanthin. A "digitalizing dose" of lanatoside C is 5 to 10 mg. orally (of which about one tenth is absorbed); the daily maintenance dose is 0.25 to 1.0 mg. The acute lethal dose by mouth is probably 5 to 10 times that of digitoxin; in an average adult this means 15 to 50 mg. of lanatoside C or somewhat less of the usual lanatoside mixture (Digilanid). (See also: DIGITALIS, Reference Congener in Section III.)
CELLOSOLVES Ethylene glycol mono-ethers (e.g., monoethyl ether)	3	Acute toxicities are several times greater than that of ethylene glycol in animals (clinical data are inadequate for valid comparisons). Ether linkage is supposedly stable in vivo. Central nervous depression as with ethylene glycol, but the ether derivatives produce more marked kidney injury and hematuria (apparently without oxalic acid formation or crystalluria). These ethers penetrate intact skin. (See also: ETHYLENE GLYCOL, Reference Congener in Section III.)
CELLOSOLVE ESTERS Ethylene glycol mono-ether esters, e.g., the monoethyl ether acetate	3	In general each monoether ester is somewhat less toxic (in animals) than the corresponding monoether. The esters are apparently saponified in vivo but the ether linkage is stable. Oral toxicity (and toxic actions) is similar to that of ethylene glycol, but percutaneous toxicity is probably higher. (See also: ETHYLENE GLYCOL, Reference Congener in Section III.)
CELLOSOLVE SULFATE Monoethyl ether of ethylene glycol monosulfate		No toxicity data are known, but if the compound hydrolyzes to sulfuric acid (as ethylene glycol sulfate does spontaneously), systemic acidosis may be a serious problem after ingestion. Otherwise toxicology is probably like that of ethylene glycol ethers. (See also: ETHYLENE GLYCOL, Reference Congener in Section III.)
CETYL ALCOHOL 1-Hexadecanol Hexadecyl alcohol Palmityl alcohol	1(?)	Said to be an effective laxative when emulsified. Thought to be a metabolic product which is secreted in small amounts into the intestinal lumen. (See also: ALCOHOLS, HIGHER, Reference Congener in Section III.)

Substance and Synonym or Principal Ingredient	Toxicity Rating (See Inside Cover)	Comments and Reference Congeners
CETYL DERIVATIVES (other than those listed here)		See corresponding "alkyl" derivative in this index.
CETYL PYRIDINIUM CHLORIDE Ceepryn chloride	4	A quaternary ammonium compound used as a germicide on skin and on inanimate surfaces. Available as aqueous or alcohol solutions (e.g., tinctures) in concentrations of 10% or less. (See also: QAC, Reference Congener in Section III.)
CEVADILLA Sabadilla, from the seeds of Schoenocaulon officiale. About 0.3 to 0.5% alkaloids, of which crystalline veratrine (cevadine) and veratridine are the chief members	4	Used as an insecticide (5 to 10% dusts in lime or sulfur carrier). Not to be confused with Veratrum viride or album. Although much less toxic, poisoning resembles that due to aconite: local irritation, emesis, headache, giddiness, weakness, twitching, convulsions, hypothermia, drowsiness but seldom coma. Death due to respiratory or cardiovascular collapse. As with digitalis the cardiac effects arise directly and reflexly and are often severe. (See also: DIGITALIS, Reference Congener in Section III.)
CHENOPODIUM OIL American wormseed; active constituent is an organic peroxide called ascaridol (about 65% of oil). Other ingredients include cymene, camphor, and saponins	4	An anthelmintic with multiple toxic actions. Irritates skin and mucous membrane, inducing vomiting. Depresses bowel, causing constipation. Stimulates briefly and then depresses central nervous systems, producing delirium and coma. Affects special senses, producing diplopia, blindness, tinnitus, deafness (rarely permanent). Causes circulatory collapse due to vasomotor paralysis and sometimes pulmonary edema. Late effects include liver and kidney injuries. Treat symptomatically. Use saline cathartic.
CHLORAL HYDRATE 2,2,2-Trichloro-1,1-ethanediol	4	A central nervous depressant. Mean lethal dose in man is about 10 gm. Large doses or concentrated solutions act as a corrosive agent, producing hemorrhagic gastritis and enteritis. (See also: BARBITURATE, Reference Congener in Section III.)
CHLORAMINE-T Sodium p-toluene-sulfonchloramide Chlorosol Chlorozene	3(?)	Available chlorine is 12.6%. Not usually regarded as toxic but more so than an equivalent amount of chlorine as hypochlorite. An occasional reaction is rapid and violent, suggesting hypersensitivity. Poisoning characterized by pain, vomiting, sudden loss of consciousness, circulatory and respiratory collapse, and death. Treat symptomatically. (See also: HYPOCHLORITE, Reference Congener in Section III.)
CHLORANIL Spergon Tetrachloro-1,4-benzoquinone	3	Low toxicity in laboratory animals. Poorly absorbed. Produces watery diarrhea, central nervous depression, coma, and death. A skin irritant in high concentrations but no percutaneous absorption.
p-CHLORANILINE p-Chloroaniline	5(?)	Said to be more toxic than aniline. Can be absorbed through intact skin. (See also: ANILINE, Reference Congener in Section III.)
CHLORASOL	4	Said to contain 75% ethylene dichloride and 25% carbon tetrachloride. (See also: CARBON TETRACHLORIDE, Reference Congener in Section III.)
CHLORATE SALTS e.g. Sodium chlorate, magnesium chlorate, etc.	4	Susceptibility varies widely among men and animals, but estimated lethal dose for man is about 30 gm., representing about one-tenth the toxicity of bromate. Produces gastritis, methemoglobinemia, and a late toxic nephritis. Less central nervous depression than bromate poisoning but perhaps more methemoglobin. (See also: BROMATE, Reference Congener in Section III.)
CHLORDANE (or chlordan) Octachloro-4,7-methanohydroindane	4	Probably chlordane is best described as lying on the borderline between toxicity classes 3 and 4. (See also: CHLORDANE, Reference Congener in Section III.)
CHLOREX β,β'-Dichloro-ethyl ether	4	A strong irritant. Percutaneous absorption can be dangerous. Possibly late effects on liver and kidneys like carbon tetrachloride. No systemic poisonings have been reported in man. (See also: CARBON TETRACHLORIDE, Reference Congener in Section III.)
CHLORINATED CAMPHENE Toxaphene	4	Believed to lie near the borderline between toxicity classes 4 and 5. (See also: TOXAPHENE, Reference Congener in Section III.)
CHLORINATED DIPHENYL Chlorodiphenyl Chlorinated biphenyl	3	Severe liver fatty infiltration or necrosis has been reported in industrial exposures to vapor. Liver damage in rats exposed to material with 50 to 55% chlorine content; no liver damage in rabbits exposed to material with 42% chlorine content. Toxicity rating is based on an oral dose in rats. Skin effects in man are rare.

Substance and Synonym or Principal Ingredient	Toxicity Rating (See Inside Cover)	Comments and Reference Congeners
CHLORINATED HYDROCARBONS		The chlorinated hydrocarbon solvents are best typified by carbon tetrachloride, while the chlorinated hydrocarbon insecticides are best exemplified by DDT. The typical toxic effects are strikingly different. The chlorinated solvents are liver and kidney poisons and central nervous depressants, whereas DDT and congeners are convulsants. (See also: CARBON TETRACHLORIDE, Reference Congener in Section III.)
CHLORINATED LIME Calcium hypochlorite		The salt has about 35%/w active chlorine. As with other corrosive agents, the toxicity rating of a solution depends upon its concentration. (See also: HYPOCHLORITE, Reference Congener in Section III.)
CHLORINATED NAPHTHALENES Halowax		Acneform rash and liver necrosis from exposure to vapor. Ingestion toxicity is not known, but presumably it increases with the degree of chlorination. The cause of "Virus X" disease in cattle (hyperkeratosis).
CHLORINE WATER		Water dissolves about twice its volume of chlorine gas, forming a mixture of hydrochloric and hypochlorous acids. Corrosive because of acidity and oxidizing potential. Correct acidosis by alkali therapy. If chlorine gas has been inhaled, inhalation of the following spray (or aerosol) has been recommended: an aqueous solution of sodium hyposulfite (2%) and sodium carbonate (0.5%). Also see nitrogen oxides (Sec. III). (See also: HYPOCHLORITE, Reference Congener in Section III.)
CHLOROACETIC ACID (and salts) e.g., Sodium monochloroacetate	4	In addition to corrosive effects of acid, salts are much more toxic than di- or tri-chloroacetates, presumably because the systemic effects are somewhat like monofluoroacetate (although much less toxic than the latter in animal tests). Probably the compound lies near the borderline between toxicity classes 4 and 5. (See also: FLUOROACETATE, Reference Congener in Section III.)
CHLOROANILINE Several isomers	5(?)	Said to be more toxic than aniline. Both meta and para isomers have caused poisonings like aniline. Can be absorbed through intact skin. (See also: ANILINE, Reference Congener in Section III.)
CHLOROBENZENE Monochlorobenzene	3(?)	Sometimes used in dry-cleaning. Ingestion has led, after a latency of several hours, to pallor, cyanosis (with methemoglobinemia), and collapse, strikingly similar to aniline poisoning. (See also: ANILINE, Reference Congener in Section III.)
CHLOROBENZILATE Ethyl di(p-chloro phenyl) glycollate 2-Hydroxy-2,2-bis (4-chlorophenyl) ethyl acetate	3	A relatively new acaricide. Low toxicity in mice and rats. Only a slight tendency to accumulate in the body. Toxic actions are probably like those of DDT. (See also: DDT, Reference Congener in Section III.)
1-CHLORO-3-BROMOPROPENE-1 CBP	4	Intense skin and eye irritation from vapor or liquid, abating rapidly after exposure. Percutaneous absorption is low. (See also: D-D, Reference Congener in Section III.)
CHLOROBUTANOL β,β,β-Trichloro-tert.-butyl alcohol Acetone chloroform Chloretone	4	A central nervous depressant used clinically as a hypnotic drug. Hypnotic oral dose for an adult is 0.3 to 1.0 gm. Resembles chloral hydrate but no gastric irritation. Has a local anesthetic action. (See also: BARBITURATE, Reference Congener in Section III.)
CHLOROCRESOLS Various isomers, e.g., 6-chloro-m-cresol, p-chloro-m-cresol, etc.	4	Used as antiseptics and disinfectants. Not irritating to skin in concentrations of 0.5 to 1.0% in alcohol. Systemic effects are presumably like phenol. (See also: PHENOL, Reference Congener in Section III.)
2-CHLORO-4-DIMETHYLAMINO-6-METHYLPYRIMIDINE Castrix	6	A highly potent rodenticide causing fatal convulsions. In laboratory animals symptoms begin 30 to 50 minutes after ingestion. The compound is not chemically related to strychnine, but recommended treatment is the same. (See also: STRYCHNINE, Reference Congener in Section III.)
2-CHLOROETHANOL Ethylene chlorohydrin	4	Vapor more toxic than ethylene dichloride. Dangerous amounts can be absorbed through intact skin without producing much skin irritation. Various visceral lesions in fatal cases, including severe pulmonary edema, liver and kidney injury. (See also: CARBON TETRACHLORIDE, Reference Congener in Section III.)
CHLOROETHYLENE Vinyl chloride		A refrigerant gas with weak depressant actions on the central nervous system, like ethyl chloride. Effects are usually brief. (See also: CARBON TETRACHLORIDE, Reference Congener in Section III.)
CHLOROFORM Trichloromethane	3	Several times more potent than carbon tetrachloride as a depressant of the central nervous system, but clinical experience suggests that it is less toxic than carbon tetrachloride when swallowed. Even the ingestion of 6 oz. has been survived, while as little as a teaspoonful has produced a serious illness. Mean lethal dose probably lies near 1 fl. oz. (44 gm.). (See also: CARBON TETRACHLORIDE, Reference Congener in Section III.)

Substance and Synonym or Principal Ingredient	Toxicity Rating (See Inside Cover)	Comments and Reference Congeners
CHLORO-IPC Isopropyl-N-(3-chloro-phenyl) carbamate	3	Herbicide of moderately low toxicity in laboratory animals. Human hazard is not well defined.
CHLORONAPHTHALENES		Acneform rash and liver necrosis from exposure to vapors. Ingestion toxicity is not known but it presumably increases with the degree of chlorination. Less toxic than chlorinated diphenyls. The principal cause of hyperkeratosis in cattle.
CHLORONITROBENZENE Several isomers (o-, m-, or p-)	4(?)	Like nitrobenzene, cyanosis, methemoglobinemia, and collapse. Toxic symptoms may be aggravated by ingestion of ethyl alcohol. (See also: ANILINE, Reference Congener in Section III.)
1-CHLORO-1-NITRO-ETHANE (OR -NITROPROPANE)	4	Severe pulmonary edema after inhalation of vapor or ingestion of liquid. No systemic effects from skin application and no significant irritation. 1,1-Dichloro-1-nitroethane also causes pulmonary edema and generalized vascular injury. (See also: NITROGEN OXIDES, Reference Congener in Section III.)
CHLOROPHENOLS Many isomers; chlorine atoms vary in number from 1 to 5.	4	Monochlorophenols are less toxic than phenol but more toxic than chlorobenzene. The ortho isomer is more toxic than the meta or para. Additional chlorination appears to enhance toxicity. Thus pentachlorophenol is as toxic and corrosive as phenol and has the additional property of being a metabolic stimulant like dinitrophenol. (See also: PHENOL, Reference Congener in Section III.)
CHLOROPHENOTHANE The official U.S.P. name for DDT	4	(See also: DDT, Reference Congener in Section III.)
p-CHLOROPHENYL-p CHLOROBENZENE SULFONATE Ovex The active ingredient of Ovotran	3	An acaricide of moderate low oral toxicity in laboratory animals. Liver and kidney damage in chronic exposures. Causes skin irritation in man, but no other symptoms have been reported in man.
p-CHLOROPHENYL PHENYL SULFONE Sulphenone	3	An acaricide of moderately low oral toxicity to laboratory mammals. No skin irritation. No significant tissue storage in chronic feeding tests.
3-(p-CHLOROPHENYL)-1,1-DIMETHYL UREA CMU weed killer	3	No skin irritation. Repeated doses in rats produce anemia. Methemoglobinemia may occur.
2-CHLORO-4-PHENYL-PHENOL e.g. Dowicide 4		(See also: PHENOL, Reference Congener in Section III.)
p-CHLOROPHENYL-p-CHLOROBENZYL SULFIDE	3	A long-lasting acaricide acting primarily against eggs. Its toxicity in laboratory rodents is like that of Ovotran.
CHLOROPICRIN Trichloronitromethane	5	A "war gas" sometimes used as a fumigant and tracer gas. Vapor is intensely irritating to skin, eyes, mucous membrane, and stomach. Called "vomiting gas." Treatment is symptomatic with special attention to the lungs. Ingestion of liquid produces severe gastroenteritis. (See also: NITROGEN OXIDES, Reference Congener in Section III.)
CHLOROTHYMOL 1-Hydroxy-3-methyl-4-chloro-6-isopropyl-benzene	3(?)	A good germicide, but aqueous solutions are irritating to mucous membranes. Systemic effects are presumably like those of thymol and phenol, but it is probably less toxic than either. (See also: PHENOL, Reference Congener in Section III.)
CHLOROTOLOXYACETIC ACID (AND SALTS) 2-Methyl-4-chloro-phenoxyacetic acid, MCP	3	Slightly less toxic than 2,4-D. (See also: 2,4-D, Reference Congener in Section III.)
CHLOROWAX Chlorinated paraffin 70	1	No injury in test animals until doses are reached which produce bowel obstruction.
CHLORO-XYLENOL PCMX, p-Chloro-m-xylenol	3	Penetrates skin but no cutaneous irritation at concentration of 5%. (See also: PHENOL, Reference Congener in Section III.)
CHLORTHION O,O-Dimethyl-O-3-chloro-4-nitrophenyl thio-phosphate	3	Toxic symptoms in animals resemble parathion poisoning. Conflicting reports about experimental lethal doses, but toxicity is low, in spite of high in vitro anti-cholinesterase potency (a distinction ascribed to slow tissue absorption). Little, if any, percutaneous toxicity (in rabbits and guinea pigs). (See also: PARATHION, Reference Congener in Section III.)

Substance and Synonym or Principal Ingredient	Toxicity Rating (See Inside Cover)	Comments and Reference Congeners
CHROMATE SALTS (sol.) e.g., Sodium chromate	4	Corrosive because of its oxidizing potency. Treat local injuries like acid burns; also external lesions may be scrubbed with a dilute sodium hyposulfite solution (2%). If ingested, severe circulatory collapse and toxic nephritis may ensue. A less common source of poisoning than chromic acid or dichromates. See chromic acid in this index. (See also: COPPER, Reference Congener in Section III.)
CHROME GREEN Chromic oxide Cr_2O_3	2(?)	Insoluble in water. Known to have a comparatively low toxicity.
CHROME YELLOW (OR RED) Lead chromate (usually yellow, although some of the basic salts are orange and red)	4	Insoluble in water and dilute acid but appreciably soluble in gastric juice. Said to have a distinctly higher acute ingestion toxicity than most other lead salts, presumably because the acute reaction is largely that of chromate poisoning. Signs of chronic lead poisoning, however, may appear days or weeks after the acute episode. (See also: LEAD, Reference Congener in Section III.)
CHROMIC ACID Chromium trioxide (CrO_3)	4	Mean lethal dose probably lies between 5 and 10 gm. Corrosive because of its oxidizing potency, not its acidity. Treat local injuries (skin and mucous membrane) like acid burns; also external lesions may be scrubbed with a dilute sodium hyposulfite solution (2%). If ingested, violent gastroenteritis, peripheral vascular collapse, vertigo, muscle cramps, coma, and toxic nephritis with glycosuria may ensue. Allergic reactions have been described, and one case of a toxic encephalopathy in a poisoned infant is recorded. On the basis of favorable experimental reports, BAL deserves a therapeutic trial if systemic poisoning develops. (See also: COPPER, Reference Congener in Section III.)
CHROMIUM SULFATE Chromic sulfate	3(?)	Cationic chromium salts (e.g., chrome alum, chromium potassium sulfate etc.) are said to have a low toxicity, in contrast to chromate and dichromate salts. (See also: COPPER, Reference Congener in Section III.)
CINEOL (the d-isomer) Eucalyptol (the dl-isomer). (The major constituent of oil of eucalyptus and oil of cajuput)	4	Poisoning is usually by oil of eucalyptus (70% eucalyptol). As little as 1 gm. has caused coma with recovery. Symptoms include vertigo, ataxia, stupor, respiratory stridor, and miosis. Symptoms may be delayed for 2 hours. (See also: TURPENTINE, Reference Congener in Section III.)
CINNAMALDEHYDE Cinnamic aldehyde 3-Phenylpropenal Phenylacrolein Cinnamal	3(?)	The chief ingredient (up to 90%) of oil of cinnamon. Both the oil and pure aldehyde are irritants; especially if undiluted, they cause inflammation and erosion of gastrointestinal mucosa. Systemic actions are probably few. Presumably oxidized in vivo to cinnamic acid, which is excreted in urine as benzoic and hippuric acids.
CINNAMIC ACID ESTERS e.g., Methyl, ethyl, benzyl, propyl, etc.	3	In laboratory animals the propyl and isopropyl derivatives lie near the borderline between toxicity classes 2 and 3. Dermatitis has been reported. Said to be largely excreted in urine as benzoic and hippuric acids.
CITRONELLA OIL Consists principally (93%) of geraniol and citronellal; also contains methyl heptanone, terpenes, etc.	3(?)	Used in perfumes and insect repellents (the latter property ascribed to methyl heptanone). No toxicity data were located, but toxicity is probably low. By stomach tube in rabbits, citronellol (an alcohol derived from citronellal) produced paralysis, coma, and death in doses of about 1 to 4 ml./kg. (toxicity rating 3).
CLOVE OIL The major constituent is eugenol (about 80%)	3(?)	Possesses properties of local antisepsis and local anesthesia. Used locally in the control of toothaches. A rubifacient and irritant. Ingestion presumably results in a gastroenteritis, but systemic toxicity is lower than phenol, probably because of insolubility in water. (See also: PHENOL, Reference Congener in Section III.)
CMU 3-(p-Chlorophenyl)-1, 1-dimethylurea Karmex W Herbicide	3	A herbicide. No skin irritation. Repeated doses in rats produce anemia. Methemoglobinemia may occur.
COAL TAR		A mixture of condensible volatile products formed during the destructive distillation of bituminous coal. Composition is variable but generally it consists of: 2 to 8% light oils (chiefly benzene, toluene, xylene); 8 to 10% middle oils (chiefly phenols, cresols, and naphthalene); 8 to 10% heavy oils (naphthalene and derivatives); 16 to 20% anthracene oils (mostly anthracene); and about 50% pitch. In this mixture phenol and its congeners have the highest acute toxicity. (See also: PHENOL, Reference Congener in Section III.)

Substance and Synonym or Principal Ingredient	Toxicity Rating (See Inside Cover)	Comments and Reference Congeners
COAL OIL Kerosene Kerosine	3	Prepared by the fractional distillation of petroleum (boiling point range is about 175^0 to 275^0 or 325^0 C.). Consists chiefly of C_{10} to C_{16} hydrocarbons of the methane series, together with a small fraction of aromatic compounds (xylenes etc.) and of saturated rings (naphthenes). See also: KEROSENE, Reference Congener in Section III.)
COBALT SALTS Cobaltic or cobaltous compounds	4(?)	In toxic doses soluble salts act locally on the gastrointestinal tract like copper salts (pain, vomiting, etc.). Systemic effects in man include a peculiar vasodilatation (flushing) of face and ears, mild hypotension, rash, tinnitus, and nerve deafness. Chronic administration of cobaltous chloride has produced a goitre and reduced thyroid activity. Animals also demonstrate an increase in respiration, as well as tremors and convulsions. As with copper, a toxic nephritis may result. BAL should be tried as described in Section III. (See also: COPPER, Reference Congener in Section III.)
COCILLANA Dried bark of Guarea rusbyi (Britt.), containing a small amount of an alkaloid rusbyine	4(?)	Has been used as an expectorant and nauseant. Oral doses over one gram produce vomiting, with prostration and purging. Dull frontal headache, sneezing, and nasal discharge are described. No recognized antidote.
COCS Copper oxychloride sulfate	4	Effects similar to those of other soluble copper salts. (See also: COPPER, Reference Congener in Section III.)
CODEINE Methyl morphine	5	Lethal dose for an adult is about 0.5 to 1.0 gm. (See also: MORPHINE, Reference Congener in Section III.)
COLLODION Pyroxylin (chiefly dinitrocellulose)	3(?)	4% pyroxylin in 70% ether and 24% absolute ethyl alcohol. This solvent mixture is the chief source of toxicity. See "ether" in this index. (See also: ETHYL ALCOHOL, Reference Congener in Section III.)
COMPOUND (CMPD) 42 Warfarin	4	(See also: WARFARIN, Reference Congener in Section III.)
COMPOUND (CMPD) 104 Heptachlor	4	(See also: HEPTACHLOR, Reference Congener in Section III.)
COMPOUND (CMPD) 118 Aldrin	5	Similar, chemically and toxicologically, to dieldrin. Animal tests put this compound near the borderline between toxicity classes 4 and 5. (See also: DIELDRIN, Reference Congener in Section III.)
COMPOUND (CMPD) 497 Dieldrin	5	Believed to lie near the borderline between toxicity classes 4 and 5. (See also: DIELDRIN, Reference Congener in Section III.)
COMPOUND (CMPD) 612 Ethyl hexanediol	3	An insect repellent. Little or no skin absorption. Ingestion causes central nervous depression. Death in rats is accompanied by severe kidney and liver damage. Treat by gastric lavage, artifical respiration, and supportive measures.
COMPOUND (CMPD) 1068 Chlordane	4	Lies near the borderline between toxicity classes 3 and 4. (See also: CHLORDANE, Reference Congener in Section III.)
COMPOUND (CMPD) 1080 Sodium fluoroacetate	6	(See also: FLUOROACETATE, Reference Congener in Section III.)
COMPOUND (CMPD) 3422 Parathion	6	(See also: PARATHION, Reference Congener in Section III.)
COMPOUND (CMPD) 3956 Toxaphene	4	Lies near the borderline between toxicity classes 4 and 5. (See also: TOXAPHENE, Reference Congener in Section III.)
COPPER ACETOARSENITE Paris green Schweinfurth green	5	A substance of complex composition, having an arsenic trioxide equivalent of about 59%. Used as an insecticide, a wood preservative, and a paint pigment. (See also: ARSENIC, Reference Congener in Section III.)
COPPER ARSENATE	5	This is usually a basic copper arsenate, i.e., a mixed salt of cupric hydroxide and cupric arsenate. One preparation used as an agricultural insecticide has an arsenic content of 41% (as arsenic pentoxide). (See also: ARSENIC, Reference Congener in Section III.)
COPPER NAPHTHENATES Copper cyclopentane-carboxylate	3(?)	Usually supplied as a viscous green solution of petroleum oil, containing 8.0% copper (or more). No skin irritation. Little or no corrosive action when ingested. Toxicity is due chiefly to solvent or to impurities. (See also: COPPER, Reference Congener in Section III.)

Substance and Synonym or Principal Ingredient	Toxicity Rating (See Inside Cover)	Comments and Reference Congeners
COPPER OXYCHLORIDE Basic cupric chloride	4	Soluble in dilute acids (e.g., gastric juice). When ingested it is similar in its effects to soluble copper salts (e.g., the sulfate). (See also: COPPER, Reference Congener in Section III.)
COPPER 3-PHENYL-SALICYLATE	3(?)	A fungicide and fungistatic agent. No skin irritation. Little or no corrosive action when ingested. (See also: COPPER, Reference Congener in Section III.)
COPPER QUINOLINOLATE Cupric-8-hydroxy-quinolinate	2(?)	Among copper compounds, a very low toxicity. No irritation on skin and no corrosive action when ingested. (See also: COPPER, Reference Congener in Section III.)
COPPER SALTS (CUPRIC) e.g., Sulfate, acetate, subacetate, chloride, oxychloride	4	Potent emetics. Serious toxicity if retained. (See also: COPPER, Reference Congener in Section III.)
COPPER SALTS (CUPROUS) e.g., Chloride	4	Cuprous chloride is said to be more than twice as toxic as cupric chloride, but there appear to be no major toxicological distinctions between the two valence states of copper, perhaps because many cuprous salts are oxidized quickly by moist air. Other cuprous salts hydrolyze to cuprous oxide on contact with water. See cuprous oxide in this index. (See also: COPPER, Reference Congener in Section III.)
CORROSIVE SUBLIMATE Mercuric chloride	5	Act fast! One gram has killed an adult. (See also: MERCURY, Reference Congener in Section III.)
COUMACHLOR 3-(α-Acetonyl-4-chlorobenzyl)-4-hydroxycoumarin Tomorin		A rodenticide like warfarin, with delayed actions on prothrombin level and blood clotting, resulting in death by hemorrhage. (See also: WARFARIN, Reference Congener in Section III.)
CRAG HERBICIDE 1 Sodium 2,4-dichloro-phenoxyethyl sulfate	3	A herbicide of moderately low toxicity in laboratory mammals. A 5% solution produced necrosis of rabbit skin but a 1% solution was not harmful. Chronic ingestion in rats caused some kidney and liver pathology. (See also: 2,4-D, Reference Congener in Section III.)
CREOLIN Creolin-Pearson	3(?)	Said to contain cresols (about 15%), hydrocarbons (46%), and soap. (See also: PHENOL, Reference Congener in Section III.)
CREOSOL (not cresol) 2-Methoxy-4-methyl phenol	4	One of the active ingredients of wood creosote. Slightly less toxic and less corrosive than phenol. (See also: PHENOL, Reference Congener in Section III.)
CREOSOTE OR CREOSOTE OIL Coal-tar creosote or wood-tar creosote	4	A mixture of phenols, cresols, etc., obtained from coal tar, with essentially the same toxicity as phenol. In contrast wood-tar creosote (especially beechwood) contains no free phenol or cresols; it is composed chiefly of guaiacol, also creosol, etc. with toxicities similar to but less than phenol. (See also: PHENOL, Reference Congener in Section III.)
CREOSOTIC ACID A mixture of isomeric cresotic acids (hydroxytoluic acids)	4	(See also: SALICYLATE, Reference Congener in Section III.)
CRESATIN m-Cresyl acetate	4	Presumably benign until hydrolyzed in the bowel to acetic acid and m-cresol. The latter is less corrosive and less toxic than phenol. (See also: PHENOL, Reference Congener in Section III.)
CRESOLS o-, m-, and p-Hydroxytoluene, usually present as a mixture obtained from coal tar.	4	About the same toxicity and toxic actions as phenol (but ortho and especially para isomers are even more toxic). Perhaps slightly more corrosive than phenol, but systemic effects may be a little milder because of slower absorption. (See also: PHENOL, Reference Congener in Section III.)
CRESYLIC ACID A mixture of 3 isomeric cresols from coal tar, including sometimes various xylenols.	4	See cresols above. (See also: PHENOL, Reference Congener in Section III.)
CROTON OIL Oleum tiglii, the fixed oil from the seed of Croton tiglium	5	The most drastic of all purgatives. Rarely used today. Causes hemorrhagic gastroenteritis. Death has resulted from the ingestion of 20 drops. Even on the skin, vesiculation, necrosis, and sloughing may occur.

Substance and Synonym or Principal Ingredient	Toxicity Rating (See Inside Cover)	Comments and Reference Congeners
CRYOLITE Sodium fluoaluminate Na_3AlF_6	2(?)	Acute toxicity by ingestion is known to be very low (e.g., intraperitoneal lethal dose in rats is 100 times that of sodium fluoride). Much less soluble than sodium fluoride or fluosilicate and more stable than the latter with respect to hydrolysis. (See also: FLUORIDE, Reference Congener in Section III.)
CUBE EXTRACT, EXTRACTIVES, POWDER, ROOT, OR RESIN Cube or cubé refers to several species of plants of the genus Lonchocarpus	2(?)	Toxicity is due principally to the rotenone content (usually 4 to 6% in commercial preparations, although extracts may be much higher). (See also: ROTENONE, Reference Congener in Section III.)
CUCUMBER DUST Tricalcium arsenate	5	The commercial grade is a complex molecular mixture containing 26% arsenic. It is often colored with a small amount of pink dye. (See also: ARSENIC, Reference Congener in Section III.)
CUMENE Isopropylbenzene 2-Phenyl propane Cumol	4(?)	A central nervous depressant like xylene. In mice cumene narcosis develops more slowly and lasts longer than the depression produced by benzene or toluene. No human poisonings are known. (See also: XYLENE, Reference Congener in Section III.)
CUPRIC COMPOUNDS		See Copper compounds in this index.
CUPROUS OXIDE Red copper oxide Very small particles, however, are yellow (e.g. Yellow Cuprocide)	3(?)	A widely used agricultural fungicide. Presumably appreciable amounts dissolve in acidic gastric juice; if insoluble the correct toxicity rating is less than 3. (See also: COPPER, Reference Congener in Section III.)
CYANAMIDE Generated by the action of acid on calcium or sodium cyanamide	3	A synthetic agricultural fertilizer. Contains no free cyanide and apparently is not metabolized to cyanide. When absorbed, the cyanamide ion ($CN_2^=$) causes intense cutaneous and mucosal flushing (congestive hyperemia), headache, vertigo, rapid breathing, hypotension, and profound shock. The primary vascular reaction is not correctable by atropine or any known antidote. An attack after a single oral dose is usually transient (1/2 to 2 hours), and the fatal dose in man is estimated at 40 to 50 gm. The vapor is intensely irritating and may produce both pulmonary and systemic signs. After mild exposures, symptoms may be precipitated or intensified by the ingestion of alcohol.
CYANATES e.g., Potassium cyanate	3	Best described as lying near the borderline between toxicity classes 3 and 4. Toxicity has been ascribed to the slow in vivo conversion of cyanate to cyanide. (See also: CYANIDE, Reference Congener in Section III.)
CYANIDES e.g., Sodium cyanide	6	One of the fastest poisons known. To be effective, treatment must be prompt. (See also: CYANIDE, Reference Congener in Section III.)
CYANO (METHYL-MERCURI) GUANIDINE Methylmercuric dicyandiamide	5	Perhaps slightly less toxic than other organic mercury compounds commonly used in agriculture. Because of its lower vapor pressure, less hazardous than others by inhalation. By the intraperitoneal route in mice, acute toxicity is half that of mercuric chloride. (See also: MERCURY, Reference Congener in Section III.)
CYCLOHEXANE Hexahydrobenzene Hexamethylene	3	Vapor causes weak anesthesia of brief duration but more potent than hexane. High vapor concentrations have produced convulsions in rabbits. Toxic oral doses in rabbits led to severe diarrhea, circulatory collapse, and death, without prominent central nervous depression or anesthesia. Autopsy revealed generalized vascular damage with degenerative lesions in brain and viscera. No effects on blood formation have been described. Mildly irritating to human skin. No systemic poisonings have been reported in man.
CYCLOHEXANOL Hexalin	3	Human toxicity is not well defined. In animals central nervous depression without convulsions. Vomiting may occur. The vapor is irritating. In a suspected clinical poisoning due to the inhalation of vapor, nausea and tremors were prominent.
CYCLOHEXANONE	3(?)	A comparatively harmless solvent. A weak central nervous depressant and a mild or moderate irritant.
CYCLOHEXIMIDE Acti-dione	5	An antibiotic fungicide of high toxicity, lying near the borderline between toxicity classes 4 and 5 in monkeys and probably in dogs (rating of 6 in rats). In all 3 species, toxic symptoms include excessive salivation and diarrhea. Blood-stained feces may arise from vascular lesions of the colon (monkey) or stomach and small intestines (dogs). Rat and dog show transient central nervous excitement with tremors and in the dog perhaps meningeal irritation. In all species tested, death is preceded by coma. No antidote is known.

Substance and Synonym or Principal Ingredient	Toxicity Rating (See Inside Cover)	Comments and Reference Congeners
CYCLOHEXYLAMINE Hexahydroaniline Aminocyclohexane	4	Severe caustic actions on skin and mucous membrane. Systemic effects in man include nausea and vomiting, anxiety, restlessness, and drowsiness. Spinal-type convulsions occur in rabbits. Treat symptomatically.
2-CYCLOHEXYL-4,6-DINITROPHENOL 2,4-Dinitro-6-cyclohexyl phenol	4	Skin contact may lead to local necrosis but rarely if ever to dangerous systemic effects (by this portal). (See also: DINITROPHENOL, Reference Congener in Section III.)
D-3 DDD	3	Less toxic than DDT in animals and poisonings are slower in onset and longer in duration. Lethargy is more prominent and convulsions are less frequent than in DDT poisoning. In chronic feeding experiments, DDD, like DDT, is stored in body fat, but it is mobilized and excreted faster than DDT when a normal diet is resumed. (See also: DDT, Reference Congener in Section III.)
2,4-D 2,4-Dichloro-phenoxyacetic acid	4	A popular herbicide, usually marketed as its salts and esters. (See also: 2,4-D, Reference Congener in Section III.)
2,4-D ESTERS e.g., Isopropyl, butyl, etc.	3	Lies near the borderline between toxicity classes 3 and 4. (See also: 2,4-D, Reference Congener in Section III.)
2,4-D SALTS e.g., Sodium, ammonium, alkylamine, etc.	3	Lies near the borderline between toxicity classes 3 and 4. (See also- 2,4-D, Reference Congener in Section III.)
DACTIN DDH 1,3-Dichloro 5,5-dimethyl hydantoin		An insoluble bleach which slowly releases active chlorine. Less corrosive than inorganic hypochlorites with equal amounts of available chlorine. The only known toxic reactions are those of local corrosion. (See also: HYPOCHLORITE, Reference Congener in Section III.)
DATURINE 1-Hyoscyamine	6	The same toxicity to the central nervous system as atropine (equal parts of d- and l-hyoscyamine), but as a peripheral blocking agent this l-isomer is at least twice as potent as atropine. (See also: ATROPINE, Reference Congener in Section III.)
DBP Dibutyl phthalate	2	An insect repellent used mainly to impregnate clothing. Low toxicity in animals. No clinical data.
DCP Dichlorophenoxy acetic acid 2,4-D	4	The salts and esters are somewhat less toxic and lie near the borderline between toxicity classes 3 and 4. (See also: 2,4-D, Reference Congener in Section III.)
DCPC Di-(p-chlorophenyl) methyl carbitol Dimite	3(?)	No specific toxicity data were located. Less toxic than DDT but toxic actions are probably similar. (See also: DDT, Reference Congener in Section III.)
DCPM Di(chlorophenoxy) methane Neotran	2	A miticide of low toxicity in laboratory mammals. Only slight percutaneous absorption and no skin irritation. (See also: DDT, Reference Congener in Section III.)
D-D Chlorinated propane-propylene mixture	4	(See also: D-D, Reference Congener in Section III.)
DDD Dichloro diphenyl dichloroethane	3	Less toxic than DDT in animals and poisonings are slower in onset and longer in duration. Lethargy is more prominent and convulsions are less frequent than in DDT poisoning. In chronic feeding experiments, DDD, like DDT, is stored in body fat, but it is mobilized and excreted faster than DDT when a normal diet is resumed. (See also: DDT, Reference Congener in Section III.)
DDH 1,3-Dichloro-5,5-dimethyl hydantoin Dactin		Serves as a mild bleach by slowly releasing active chlorine. Presumably less corrosive than hypochlorite solutions with the same concentration of available chlorine. Local tissue injury is the only recognized toxic action. (See also: HYPOCHLORITE, Reference Congener in Section III.)
DDT Dichloro diphenyl trichloroethane (and many other synonyms)	4	(See also: DDT, Reference Congener in Section III.)
DDVP Dimethyl-2,2-dichloro-vinyl phosphate	4	An experimental chlorinated organic phosphate insecticide. One-tenth as toxic as parathion and thus lying near the borderline between toxicity classes 4 and 5. (See also: PARATHION, Reference Congener in Section III.)

Substance and Synonym or Principal Ingredient	Toxicity Rating (See Inside Cover)	Comments and Reference Congeners
DECAHYDRO-NAPHTHALENE Decalin	3(?)	Dermatitis and conjunctival irritation. Systemic toxicity is not well defined but no serious industrial poisonings are known. More toxic than tetrahydronaphthalene in animals. Vapor exposures in guinea pigs cause cataracts and kidney lesions.
DECALIN Decahydronaphthalene	3(?)	See above.
N-DECYL DERIVATIVE		See corresponding "alkyl" derivative in this index.
DEHYDROACETIC ACID 3-Acetyl-6-methyl-2,4-pyrandione (The sodium salt has a similar toxicity)	3	A fungicide used in cosmetics. No primary or allergic skin reactions. Humans ingested 0.01 gm./kg. daily for 150 days without observable ill-effects. At high dosage levels monkeys showed anorexia, vomiting, weakness, stupor, ataxia, and convulsions. The control of convulsions by barbiturates was life-saving in experimental poisonings.
DEMEROL Meperidine Pethidine (usually as the hydrochloride)	5	Believed to lie near the borderline between toxicity classes 4 and 5; this rating is based on poisonings in non-addicts (i.e., no drug tolerance). Causes central nervous excitation: subjective vertigo, apprehension, tremors, ataxia, confusion, hallucinations, and convulsions. These signs and symptoms resemble atropine poisoning, as does mydriasis, tachycardia, and dryness of mouth. Hyperpyrexia, however, is rare. Unlike morphine poisoning, respiratory depression occurs only terminally, but n-allyl-normorphine (nalorphine) is useful in the treatment of severe meperidine poisoning (see morphine). Otherwise symptomatic treatment as in atropine poisoning. (See also: ATROPINE, Reference Congener in Section III.)
DEMETON Systox Ethyl mercaptoethyl diethyl thiophosphate	5	A "systemic" insecticide, i.e., translocated in sap to all parts of plants. Almost as toxic as parathion in animals. Percutaneous toxicity is high. One human fatality has been reported. (See also: PARATHION, Reference Congener in Section III.)
DEOBASE A highly purified kerosene	3	Deodorized but still toxic. Unsaturated and aromatic compounds have been largely removed. (See also: KEROSENE, Reference Congener in Section III.)
DERRIS Tuba-root. Derris is also the name of a botanical genus rich in rotenone, and tuba is the common name of one species.	2(?)	Toxicity is due principally to its rotenone content (usually 5 to 6% in commercial derris). (See also: ROTENONE, Reference Congener in Section III.)
DESLANOSIDE Desacetyl-lanatoside C Cedilanid D	6	A cardiotonic glycoside derived from lanatoside C. More stable than the parent compound in solution. Has the same therapeutic and toxic actions as lanatoside C when given in the same way, but deslanoside is usually injected i.v. (initial dose 1.2 to 1.6 mg.; daily maintenance dose i.v. about 0.4 mg.). Cardiac effects begin in 10 to 30 min., maximal in 1 to 2 hours, finished in 3 to 6 days. The lethal dose by mouth is apparently the same as that of lanatoside C. (See also: DIGITALIS, Reference Congener in Section III.)
DFDT Difluoro diphenyl trichloroethane	3	Similar to but less toxic than DDT. The fluorine atoms within the molecule do not appear to contribute to the symptoms. (See also: DDT, Reference Congener in Section III.)
DFP Diisopropyl fluorophosphate	5	Rarely used today and not at all by the agriculturalist. Occasionally prescribed by physicians (ophthalmologists). Degenerative changes in peripheral and central nervous systems. (See also: PARATHION, Reference Congener in Section III.)
DHA Dehydroacetic acid 3-Acetyl-6-methyl-2,4-pyrandione	3	A fungicide used in cosmetics and agriculture. No skin reactions, either primary or allergic. Men have ingested 0.01 gm./kg. daily for 150 days without observable ill-effects. At high dosage levels, monkeys showed anorexia, vomiting, weakness, stupor, ataxia, and convulsions. The control of convulsions by barbiturates was life-saving in experimental poisonings.
DI-		If not located below, substitute Bis- for Di- and try again.
DIACETONE ALCOHOL 4-Hydroxy-4-methyl-2-pentanone	3(?)	A solvent, hydraulic brake fluid, and a component of some antifreeze mixtures. May cause central nervous depression and possibly renal damage. Liver injury and anemia reported in animals. More toxic than acetone.

Substance and Synonym or Principal Ingredient	Toxicity Rating (See Inside Cover)	Comments and Reference Congeners
DIALKYL DIMETHYL AMMONIUM CHLORIDE (OR BROMIDE) Usually a mixture of alkyl groups, e.g., derived from cocoanut amines	4	Dilute aqueous solutions are used as germicides, deodorizers, and sanitizers on chemically clean surfaces. The dilauryl bromide salt has been used in oil emulsions for moth-proofing. (See also: QAC, Reference Congener in Section III.)
DIALKYL SODIUM SULFOSUCCINATE e.g., Aerosols OT (dioctyl), MA (dihexyl), AY (diamyl), etc.	3	Commercial anionic surfactants which are widely used. Toxicity rating is based on dioctyl derivative tested in rats. Irritating to eyes but human patch tests reveal no skin irritation with 1% aqueous solutions.
2,4-DIAMINOPHENOL HYDROCHLORIDE Amidol	4	A photographic developer, sometimes used in hair dyes. No human poisonings are known. See p-phenylene diamine in this index for effects and treatment.
2,4-DIAMINOTOLUENE	4	No human poisonings are known. See p-phenylene diamine in this index for effects and treatment.
DIAZINON O,O-Diethyl-O-(2-isopropyl-4-methyl pyrimidyl(6)) thiophosphate	4	Relatively new. Less toxic than most organic phosphate insecticides (oral mean lethal dose in rats is 100 to 150 mg./kg.) but a potent cholinesterase inhibitor. (See also: PARATHION, Reference Congener in Section III.)
1,2-DIBROMO-3-CHLORO-PROPANE	4(?)	A soil fumigant (fungicide). No specific toxicity data were located, but presumably this compound is highly irritating to the skin and mucous membranes, like the components of D-D mixture. (See also: D-D, Reference Congener in Section III.)
DIBUTYL PHTHALATE Di-n-butyl phthalate Butyl phthalate	2	An insect repellent used mainly to impregnate clothing. Low toxicity in animals. No clinical data.
DICHLONE 2,3-Dichloro-1,4-naphthoquinone	3	Low toxicity in laboratory animals. Skin irritation is enhanced by fats and oils. Large doses are promptly vomited by dogs.
DICHLORALUREA Bis(1-hydroxy-2,2,2-trichloroethyl) urea	1	A herbicide. Essentially innocuous by mouth in rats. Low skin irritancy.
o-DICHLOROBENZENE Ortho-dichlorobenzene	4(?)	For para isomer, see paradichlorobenzene. Ortho isomer is more toxic: a local irritant, a strong central nervous depressant, and a liver poison. In animals liver destruction is often severe. Lens opacities have been described after known exposures in man and animals. (See also: CARBON TETRACHLORIDE, Reference Congener in Section III.)
DICHLORO-BIS(p-ETHYLPHENYL) ETHANE Perthane Q-137	2	In animals toxic signs and symptoms are like those in DDT poisoning, but the toxicity is much lower (near the borderline between toxicity classes 2 and 3). There is little, if any, percutaneous absorption, skin irritation, or sensitization. Unlike DDT, feeding tests on rats with radioactive Perthane indicate little tendency for the material to deposit in body fat. (See also: DDT, Reference Congener in Section III.)
DICHLORO-BIS (PARACHLOROPHENYL) ETHANE DDD TDE	3	Less toxic than DDT in animals, and poisonings are slower in onset and longer in duration. Lethargy is more prominent and convulsions are less frequent than in DDT poisoning. In chronic feeding experiments DDD, like DDT, is stored in body fat, but it is mobilized and excreted faster than DDT when a normal diet is resumed. (See also: DDT, Reference Congener in Section III.)
DICHLORODIFLUORO-METHANE Freon-12		A propellant in insect aerosol bombs. Not toxic except for lung irritation at very high vapor concentrations. If heated, thermal decomposition products like HCl, Cl_2, HF, F_2, and phosgene are dangerous.
5,5'-DICHLORO-2,2'-DIHYDROXY-DIPHENYL METHANE Dichlorophene	3	Moderately low ingestion toxicity in guinea pigs. No skin irritation in concentrations of 1%. Solutions of the sodium salt are highly alkaline and corrosive. (See also: PHENOL, Reference Congener in Section III.)
1,3-DICHLORO-5,5-DIMETHYL HYDANTOIN DDH Dactin		Serves as a mild bleach by slowly releasing active chlorine. Presumably less corrosive than hypochlorite solutions with the same concentration of available chlorine. Local tissue injury is the only recognized toxic action. (See also: HYPOCHLORITE, Reference Congener in Section III.)

Substance and Synonym or Principal Ingredient	Toxicity Rating (See Inside Cover)	Comments and Reference Congeners
DICHLORO DIPHENYL DICHLOROETHANE DDD	3	Less toxic than DDT in animals and poisonings are slower in onset and longer in duration. Lethargy is more prominent and convulsions are less frequent than in DDT poisoning. In chronic feeding experiments, DDD, like DDT, is stored in body fat, but it is mobilized and excreted faster than DDT when a normal diet is resumed. (See also: DDT, Reference Congener in Section III.)
DICHLORO DIPHENYL TRICHLOROETHANE DDT	4	(See also: DDT, Reference Congener in Section III.)
DICHLOROETHANES e.g., Ethylene dichloride	3	No marked differences in the toxicity of the 1,1- and 1,2-isomers are recognized. See ethylene dichloride in this index. (See also: CARBON TETRACHLORIDE, Reference Congener in Section III.)
1,2-DICHLOROETHYLENE Acetylene dichloride	3	Less toxic than ethylene dichloride. Rapid recovery usually after vapor exposure: central nervous depression or in milder exposures nausea, vomiting, weakness, tremor, and epigastric cramps. Intravenous injection of calcium gluconate has relieved the cramps and vomiting. Reversible corneal clouding is described. (See also: CARBON TETRACHLORIDE, Reference Congener in Section III.)
DICHLOROETHYL ETHER β,β'-Dichloroethyl ether Chlorex	4	Strong irritant and lacrimator. Percutaneous toxicity can be dangerous. Possibly some late effects like carbon tetrachloride (liver and kidney injuries). No severe human poisonings have been reported. (See also: CARBON TETRACHLORIDE, Reference Congener in Section III.)
DICHLOROHYDRIN 1,3-Dichloro-2-propanol	4(?)	Similar to carbon tetrachloride poisoning, but irritant actions (e.g., hemorrhagic gastritis, pharyngitis, etc.) may be even more severe. (See also: CARBON TETRACHLORIDE, Reference Congener in Section III.)
DICHLORO-ISOPROPYL ALCOHOL 1,3-Dichloro-2-propanol	4(?)	Similar to carbon tetrachloride poisoning, but irritant actions (e.g., pharyngitis, hemorrhagic gastritis, etc.) may be even more severe. (See also: CARBON TETRACHLORIDE, Reference Congener in Section III.)
DICHLOROMETHANE Methylene chloride	3	May produce central nervous depression but one of the less toxic chlorinated hydrocarbon solvents. (See also: CARBON TETRACHLORIDE, Reference Congener in Section III.)
DICHLOROMONO-FLUOROMETHANE Freon-21		In high concentrations, it may cause central nervous depression. If heated, thermal decomposition products like HCl, Cl_2, HF, F_2, and phosgene are dangerous.
DICHLORO-NAPHTHOQUINONE Phygon	3	Moderately low toxicity in laboratory animals. Diarrhea and severe central nervous depression in rats. Large doses are promptly vomited by dogs. Skin irritation is enhanced by fats and oils.
1,1-DICHLORO-1-NITROETHANE Ethide	4	A grain fumigant. The vapor usually gives adequate warning (irritation). May produce severe pulmonary edema either by inhalation of vapor or ingestion of liquid. Also skin irritation. (See also: NITROGEN OXIDES, Reference Congener in Section III.)
DICHLOROPHENE Bis(5-chloro-2-hydroxy phenyl) methane. Soluble formulations are marketed as "Cuniphens."	3	Moderately low ingestion toxicity in dogs and guinea pigs. No skin irritation at concentrations of 1% and little at 4%. (See also: PHENOL, Reference Congener in Section III.)
DICHLOROPHENOXY ACETIC ACID 2,4-D	4	The salts and esters are somewhat less toxic and lie near the borderline between toxicity classes 3 and 4. (See also: 2,4-D, Reference Congener in Section III.)
DICHLOROPHENOXY-ETHYL SULFATE, SODIUM SALT Crag Herbicide 1	3	A herbicide of moderately low toxicity in laboratory animals. A 5% solution produced necrosis of rabbit skin, but a 1% solution was harmless. Chronic ingestion in rats caused some kidney and liver pathology. (See also: 2,4-D, Reference Congener in Section III.)
DI-(p-CHLOROPHENOXY) METHANE The active ingredient of Neotran	2	A miticide of very low toxicity in laboratory mammals. Only slight percutaneous absorption and no skin irritation. It has produced liver pathology in laboratory animals. No human poisonings are known. (See also: DDT, Reference Congener in Section III.)
2,4-DICHLOROPHENYL ESTER BENZENE SULFONIC ACID		An agricultural miticide. No toxicity data were located.

Substance and Synonym or Principal Ingredient	Toxicity Rating (See Inside Cover)	Comments and Reference Congeners
DI-(p-CHLOROPHENYL) METHYL CARBINOL (OR ETHANOL) Dimite	3(?)	An acaricide. Said to have a low mammalian toxicity, but no specific data were located. Less toxic than DDT, but toxic actions are probably similar. (See also: DDT, Reference Congener in Section III.)
DICHLOROPROPANE Propylene dichloride	4	One of the most toxic chlorinated hydrocarbons, producing visceral lesions in the liver, heart, and kidneys. Present in D-D mixture. (See also: D-D, Reference Congener in Section III.)
1,3-DICHLORO-2-PROPANOL Dichloro-isopropyl alcohol	4(?)	Similar to carbon tetrachloride poisoning, but irritant actions (e.g., hemorrhagic gastritis, pharyngitis, etc.) may be ever more severe. (See also: CARBON TETRACHLORIDE, Reference Congener in Section III.)
DICHLOROPROPENE 1,3-Dichloro-propene-1	4	Highly irritating to skin, eyes, and all mucous membranes. Present in D-D mixture. (See also: D-D, Reference Congener in Section III.)
2,2-DICHLOROPROPRIONIC ACID αα-Dichloroproprionic acid Dalapon		A new herbicide. No information about mammalian toxicity has been located.
DICHLOROTETRA-FLUOROETHANE Freon-114		Vapor may cause mild and usually transient central nervous depression. Perhaps slightly more toxic than methane analogue. See warning under "Freons".
DICHROMATE SALTS (SOLUBLE) e.g., Sodium or potassium dichromate	4	Mean lethal dose probably about 10 gm. Highly corrosive to skin and mucous membranes (treat like acid burns). In addition external lesions may be scrubbed with a dilute solution of sodium hyposulfite (2%). If ingested, violent gastroenteritis, peripheral vascular collapse, vertigo, muscle cramps, coma, and later toxic nephritis (with glycosuria). Allergic reactions have also been described. (See also: COPPER, Reference Congener in Section III.)
DICUMAROL OR DICOUMAROL Dicumarin Bishydroxycoumarin 3,3'-Methylene-bis (4-hydroxycoumarin)		Single therapeutic human dose is 200 to 300 mg. Single-dose toxicity is not well established, but it is probably low relative to the cumulative multiple-dose toxicity. (See also: WARFARIN, Reference Congener in Section III.)
DICYCLOHEXYLAMINE Dodecahydro-diphenylamine	4	In animals somewhat more toxic than cyclohexylamine, and unlike the latter it can be absorbed in dangerous amounts through skin. Rabbits which ingest it die in convulsions. See cyclohexylamine in this index.
DIELDRIN Hexachloro-epoxy-octahydro-endo, exo-dimethanonaphthalene	5	Believed to lie near the borderline between toxicity classes 4 and 5. (See also: DIELDRIN, Reference Congener in Section III.)
DIETHANOLAMINE AND SALTS e.g., Hydrochloride	2(?)	By analogy with triethanolamine, diethanolamine probably has a low toxicity. In animals given fatal oral doses, the only gross pathology is found within the gastrointestinal tract. It has been suggested (without proof) that these deaths are due to a systemic alkalosis. (This may be true of the free amine but is obviously not true of its salts).
DIETHYLCARBAMAZINE 1-Diethylcarbamyl-4-methylpiperazine hydrochloride or citrate Hetrazan	3(?)	Used against filariasis in man and animals. Especially popular in veterinary medicine. The average adult man tolerates a single dose of 1.5 gm. without ill effects. Untoward reactions include nausea, vomiting, headache, weakness, and (as seen in dogs) muscle tremors and convulsions. Intravenous injection in dogs produces transient rise in blood pressure and heart rate.
DIETHYL 2-CHLORO-VINYL PHOSPHATE Compound 1836	5	A relatively new organic phosphate insecticide, which is almost as toxic in rats as parathion. (See also: PARATHION, Reference Congener in Section III.)
DIETHYL DIPHENYL DICHLOROETHANE Perthane 2,2-Bis(p-ethylphenyl) 1,1-dichloroethane	2	In animals toxic signs and symptoms are like those in DDT poisoning, but the toxicity is much lower (near the borderline between toxicity classes 2 and 3). There is little, if any, percutaneous absorption, skin irritation, or sensitization. Unlike DDT, feeding tests on rats with radioactive Perthane indicate little tendency for the material to deposit in body fat. (See also: DDT, Reference Congener in Section III.)
1,4-DIETHYLENE DIOXIDE (OR OXIDE) Dioxane (a cyclic diether)	3	No human poisonings by ingestion but 5 deaths from vapor exposure are known. Causes central nervous depression and subsequent renal (vascular and parenchymal) necrosis and central liver necrosis. Oxalic acid is not a significant metabolic product (if there is any). Death is due to acute renal failure. Can be absorbed through intact skin of animals. (See also: ETHYLENE GLYCOL, Reference Congener in Section III.)

Substance and Synonym or Principal Ingredient	Toxicity Rating (See Inside Cover)	Comments and Reference Congeners
DIETHYLENE GLYCOL β, β'-Dihydroxy-diethyl-ether	3	In animals slightly less toxic than ethylene glycol, Cellosolve, or Carbitol (toxicity rating in animals = 1 or 2), but probable lethal dose in man is 1 to 2 gm./kg. Causes central nervous depression and hydropic degenerative lesions in liver and kidney (probably without significant oxalate formation). Anuria from tubular degeneration may prove fatal within a few days. (See also: ETHYLENE GLYCOL, Reference Congener in Section III.)
DIETHYLENE GLYCOL MONOETHYL ETHER Carbitol	3	More acutely toxic than diethylene glycol by ingestion (see above), but qualitatively similar to poisonings by ethylene and diethylene glycols. Essentially non-irritating to human skin and no skin penetration (in man). (See also: ETHYLENE GLYCOL, Reference Congener in Section III.)
DIETHYL-O-(2-(ETHYL-MERCAPTO)-ETHYL) THIOPHOSPHATE Systox Demeton	5	A "systemic" insecticide, i.e., translocated in sap to all parts of plants. Almost as toxic as parathion in animals. Percutaneous toxicity is high. One human fatality has been reported. (See also: PARATHION, Reference Congener in Section III.)
O,O-DIETHYL-O-(2-ISOPROPYL-4-METHYL-PYRIMIDYL (6)) THIOPHOSPHATE Diazinon	4	Relatively new. Less toxic than most organic phosphate insecticides (oral mean lethal dose in rats is 100 to 150 mg./kg.), but a potent cholinesterase inhibitor. (See also: PARATHION, Reference Congener in Section III.)
DIETHYL PARANITRO-PHENYL PHOSPHATE Para-oxon	6	One of the most toxic organic phosphate insecticides. Relatively high stability may present residue problems. (See also: PARATHION, Reference Congener in Section III.)
O,O-DIETHYL-O-PARANITROPHENYL THIOPHOSPHATE Parathion	6	(See also: PARATHION, Reference Congener in Section III.)
DIETHYL PHTHALATE Ethyl phthalate	3	Used as a solvent, a fixative for perfume, and a denaturant for alcohol (especially in cosmetics). It serves as a denaturant because of its bitter objectionable taste. Irritating to mucous membranes. Produces central nervous depression when absorbed.
DIETHYL XANTHOGEN DISULFIDE Ethyl xanthogen disulfide	3	A comparatively new herbicide. In several animal species, it lies near the borderline between toxicity classes 3 and 4. A skin irritant and sensitizer. Said to be readily absorbed in toxic amounts through intact skin.
DIFLUORO DIPHENYL TRICHLOROETHANE 1,1,1-Trichloro-2,2-bis(p-fluorophenyl-1) ethane DFDT	3	Similar to but less toxic than DDT. The fluorine atoms within the molecule do not appear to contribute to the symptoms. (See also: DDT, Reference Congener in Section III.)
DIGALEN A soluble amorphous mixture of the cardiotonic glycosides from digitalis leaf (purpurea)	6	Potency is determined by bio-assay. One U.S.P. unit is approximately equivalent, therapeutically and toxicologically, to 0.1 mg. of digitoxin. The initial "digitalizing" dose is usually 10 to 15 U.S.P. units by mouth, 4 U.S.P. units by vein. The single fatal oral dose lies between 20 and 50 U.S.P. units in an average adult. (See also: DIGITALIS, Reference Congener in Section III.)
DIGIFOLIN The natural mixture of cardiac glycosides of digitalis leaf (purpurea), separated from inert material	6	Potency is determined by bio-assay. One U.S.P. unit is approximately equivalent, therapeutically and toxicologically, to 0.1 mg. of digitoxin. The initial "digitalizing" dose is usually 10 to 15 U.S.P. units by mouth, 4 U.S.P. units by vein. The single fatal oral dose lies between 20 and 50 U.S.P. units in an average adult. (See also: DIGITALIS, Reference Congener in Section III.)
DIGILANID Lanatoside The cardiac glycosides from the leaf of Digitalis lanata	6	Digilanid often refers to a mixture of the purified glycosides in their natural proportions (47% A, 17% B, 36% C). In its latency and duration of action, it is faster than digitoxin and slower than ouabain. A single oral "digitalizing" dose (of which only about 20% is absorbed) is 3 to 6 mg., and the average daily maintenance dose is 0.5 mg. An estimated single lethal dose is 15 to 25 mg. (See also: DIGITALIS, Reference Congener in Section III.)
DIGITALIS Foxglove Dried whole leaf of Digitalis purpurea	4	Clinical data place this compound near the borderline between toxicity classes 4 and 5. The powder is available in pills, tablets, capsules, and suppositories. One ml. of the official tincture (70% alcohol) is equivalent in digitalis content to 0.1 gm. of the standard powdered leaf or 1 U.S.P. unit. (See also: DIGITALIS, Reference Congener in Section III.)

Substance and Synonym or Principal Ingredient	Toxicity Rating (See Inside Cover)	Comments and Reference Congeners
DIGITOXIN A crystalline cardiac glycoside derived from the leaves of Digitalis purpurea, often contaminated with gitoxin (a related glycoside)	6	About 1,000 times as potent as standard whole-leaf digitalis. The precursor of digitoxin in the leaf is purpurea glycoside A. Although insoluble in water, digitoxin is rapidly and completely absorbed from the bowel without irritation. A "digitalizing" dose for an average adult is 1 to 1.5 mg. orally or intravenously, and maximal cardiac effects occur in 4 to 12 hours. The action is persistent (2 to 3 weeks) and cumulative, and its maintenance usually requires only 0.1 mg. daily. An estimated single lethal dose is 3 to 10 mg. (See also: DIGITALIS, Reference Congener in Section III.)
DIGOXIN A crystalline glycoside derived from the leaves of Digitalis lanata, specifically from its precursor lanatoside C	6	Has all the therapeutic and most of the toxic actions of whole-leaf digitalis. Absorbed from the bowel with little irritation. After an average oral "digitalizing" dose of 2 to 4 mg. (of which only about half is absorbed), cardiac actions start in 5 to 30 min., are maximal in 1 to 5 hours, and are finished in 2 to 6 days. Because of its comparatively rapid dissipation, the daily maintenance dose is 0.25 to 1 mg. An estimated single lethal dose is 10 to 20 mg. (See also: DIGITALIS, Reference Congener in Section III.)
1,2-DIHYDROPYRIDAZINE-3,6-DIONE Maleic hydrazide, marketed as sodium and diethanolamine salts	3	An inhibitor of plant growth. In animals causes tremors and muscle spasm. No effects on the skin.
DIHYDROROTENONE	4	Said to have 1.5 times the mammalian toxicity of rotenone. (See also: ROTENONE, Reference Congener in Section III.)
DIHYDROXYBENZENE Three isomers (o-, m-, p-)	4	For ortho isomer (o- or 1,2-), see catechol. For meta isomer (m- or 1,3-), see resorcinol. For para isomer (p- or 1,4-), see hydroquinone. In various test-animals, resorcinol has usually proved to have the lowest acute toxicity, but all 3 compounds are similarly hazardous. In animals they are generally somewhat more toxic than phenol.
DIHYDROXY DICHLORO DIPHENYL METHANE Dichlorophene	3	Moderately low ingestion toxicity in dogs and guinea pigs. No skin irritation at concentrations of 1% (human data). (See also: PHENOL, Reference Congener in Section III.)
DI-ISOBUTYL CRESOLYL ETHOXY ETHYL DIMETHYL BENZYL AMMONIUM CHLORIDE MONOHYDRATE Methyl benzethonium chloride e.g., Hyamine 10-X	4	Similar to the compound below in terms of uses and toxicity. In animals it lies near the borderline between toxicity classes 3 and 4. (See also: QAC, Reference Congener in Section III.)
DI-ISOBUTYL PHENOXY ETHOXY ETHYL DIMETHYL BENZYL AMMONIUM CHLORIDE MONOHYDRATE Benzethonium chloride, e.g., Phemerol chloride, Hyamine 1622, etc.	4	A popular cationic surfactant used at concentrations of 0.1 to 0.01% as a germicide, sanitizer, disinfectant, and deodorant for previously cleaned surfaces. Small amounts are found in some parenteral medications. In laboratory animals it lies near the borderline between toxicity classes 3 and 4. (See also: QAC, Reference Congener in Section III.)
DILAN 1,1-Bis(p-chlorophenyl)-2-nitrobutane (2 parts) plus propane analogue (1 part)	3	Same symptoms and treatment as DDT. Can be absorbed through intact skin but probably not in significant amounts. (See also: DDT, Reference Congener in Section III.)
DILAUDID Dihydromorphinone hydrochloride	5	A more potent analgetic drug than morphine and correspondingly more toxic (perhaps 4 times as toxic). In clinical doses dilaudid causes less sedation and more transient analgesia than does morphine. Use n-allyl normorphine (Nalline) to combat respiratory and circulatory depression. (See also: MORPHINE, Reference Congener in Section III.)
DIMERCAPROL Official U.S.P. name for BAL 2,3-Dimercaptopropanol	4(?)	(See also: BAL, Reference Congener in Section III.)
DIMETAN 5,5'-Dimethyl dihydroresorcinol dimethyl carbamate	4	An aphicide. Skin absorption is negligible. Although not described in mice and rats, toxic signs and symptoms presumably resemble those of parathion poisoning, since Dimetan is a reversible inhibitor of the enzyme cholinesterase and is related to physostigmine and neostigmine. No clinical data. (See also: PARATHION, Reference Congener in Section III.)

Substance and Synonym or Principal Ingredient	Toxicity Rating (See Inside Cover)	Comments and Reference Congeners
DIMETHOXY DIPHENYL TRICHLOROETHANE Methoxychlor	3	Lower toxicity than DDT. Estimated to be one-tenth as toxic in man by ingestion, but this difference may not hold in respiratory exposures to vapor. In animals central nervous depression is more prominent than excitation, and poisonings are slower in onset and longer in duration than in DDT intoxication. (See also: DDT, Reference Congener in Section III.)
DIMETHYLAMINE AND SALTS		Aqueous solutions of dimethylamine are highly alkaline, like ammonia water (see Sec. III). Animal toxicity has been ascribed to its caustic actions and to systemic alkalosis. In contrast the amine salts (e.g. hydrochloride) are relatively benign.
DIMETHYL 1-CARBO- METHOXY-1-PROPEN- 2-YL PHOSPHATE	6	A relatively new organic phosphate insecticide. As toxic in rats as parathion. (See also: PARATHION, Reference Congener in Section III.)
O,O-DIMETHYL-O-(3- CHLORO-4-NITRO- PHENYL) THIO- PHOSPHATE Chlorthion	3	Toxic symptoms in animals resemble parathion poisoning. Conflicting reports about experimental lethal doses, but toxicity is low, in spite of high in vitro anti-cholinesterase potency (a distinction ascribed to slow tissue absorption). Little if any percutaneous toxicity (in rabbits and guinea pigs). (See also: PARATHION, Reference Congener in Section III.)
DIMETHYL-2,2- DICHLOROVINYL PHOSPHATE DDVP	5	An experimental chlorinated organic phosphate. One-fifth to one-tenth as toxic as parathion and therefore near the borderline between toxicity classes 4 and 5. (See also: PARATHION, Reference Congener in Section III.)
5,5-DIMETHYL DIHYDRORESORCINOL DIMETHYL CARBAMATE Dimetan	4	An aphicide. Skin absorption is negligible. Although not described in mice and rats, toxic signs and symptoms presumably resemble those of parathion poisoning, since Dimetan is a reversible inhibitor of the enzyme cholinesterase and is related to physostigmine and neostigmine. No clinical data. (See also: PARATHION, Reference Congener in Section III.)
DIMETHYL DITHIO- PHOSPHATE OF DIETHYL MERCAPTOSUCCINATE Malathion Malathon	4	The only organic phosphate insecticide approved for household use (1955). Relatively low mammalian toxicity (on the borderline between toxicity classes 3 and 4) and low anticholinesterase potency, but experimental poisonings resemble parathion. Small but significant percutaneous toxicity in rabbits. (See also: PARATHION, Reference Congener in Section III.)
O,O-DIMETHYL-1- HYDROXY-2,2,2- TRICHLOROETHYL- PHOSPHONATE Dipterex	4	Toxicity relatively low among organic phosphate insecticides, although a potent cholinesterase inhibitor in vitro. Rapid and complete recovery from sublethal doses in laboratory animals. (See also: PARATHION, Reference Congener in Section III.)
O,O-DIMETHYL-O- (p-NITROPHENYL) THIOPHOSPHATE Methyl parathion	5	Slightly less toxic to rats than parathion, but a much less potent cholinesterase inhibitor. Used principally in combination with parathion. (See also: PARATHION, Reference Congener in Section III.)
DIMETHYL PHTHALATE	2	An insect repellent. Not irritating to skin and not absorbed through skin. In eyes or on mucous membranes it is painful but not corrosive. Ingestion may produce central nervous depression. Treat symptomatically.
3,5-DIMETHYLTETRA- HYDRO-1,3,5,2H- THIADIAZINE-2- THIONE Crag Fungicide 974	3	As tested in laboratory animals, it lies near the borderline between toxicity classes 3 and 4. Used as a material protectant against fungi. Slight but significant percutaneous absorption in rabbits. Mild primary skin irritation and some skin sensitization in man. Systemic effects are not known.
DIMITE Di-(p-chlorophenyl)- methyl carbinol (or-ethanol)	3(?)	An acaricide. Said to have a low mammalian toxicity, but no specific data were located. Less toxic than DDT, but toxic actions are probably similar. (See also: DDT, Reference Congener in Section III.)
DINITROBENZENE The ortho, meta, or para isomer	5	Probably slightly more toxic than nitrobenzene (definitely true in animals) and distinctly more toxic than dinitrotoluene. The meta isomer is said to be the most important toxicologically, expecially as methemoglobin former. The principal symptom is cyanosis (like nitrobenzene), not liver necrosis (like dinitrotoluene). In subacute poisoning, symptoms may be precipitated by sunlight or by the ingestion of alcohol. (See also: ANILINE, Reference Congener in Section III.)
DINITRO-BUTYL PHENOL 4,6-Dinitro-2-isobutyl phenol	5	Available as ammonium and amine salts. May produce burns and be absorbed through skin. (See also: DINITROPHENOL, Reference Congener in Section III.)

Substance and Synonym or Principal Ingredient	Toxicity Rating (See Inside Cover)	Comments and Reference Congeners
DINITRO-CAPRYL PHENYL CROTONATE Dinitro-(1-methylheptyl) phenyl crotonate Karathane Arathane	3	An insecticide and acaricide. No detailed data were located, but it is not unreasonable to anticipate toxic actions like dinitrophenol. (See also: DINITROPHENOL, Reference Congener in Section III.)
DINITROCHLORO-BENZENE 1-Chloro-2,4-dinitro-benzene	5(?)	A primary irritant; severe allergic dermatitis in almost everyone after repeated skin contact. Systemic actions include methemoglobinemia. More toxic than nitrochlorobenzene. (See also: ANILINE, Reference Congener in Section III.)
DINITROCRESOL 3,5-Dinitro-o-cresol 4,6-Dinitro-o-cresol	5	More toxic than dinitrophenol. Skin contact may lead to local necrosis and dangerous systemic effects. (See also: DINITROPHENOL, Reference Congener in Section III.)
DINITRO-(1-METHYL HEPTYL) PHENYL CROTONATE Dinitro-capryl phenyl crotonate Karathane Arathane	3	An insecticide and acaricide. No detailed toxicity data were located, but it is not unreasonable to anticipate toxic actions like dinitrophenol. (See also: DINITROPHENOL, Reference Congener in Section III.)
DINITRO ORTHO SEC. AMYL PHENOL	5	Skin contact may lead to local necrosis and dangerous systemic effects. (See also: DINITROPHENOL, Reference Congener in Section III.)
DINITRO ORTHO SEC. BUTYL PHENOL 4,6-Dinitro-2-isobutyl phenol	5	Available as ammonium and amine salts. Skin contact may lead to local necrosis and dangerous systemic effects. (See also: DINITROPHENOL, Reference Congener in Section III.)
DINITRO ORTHO CRESOL 3,5-Dinitro-o-cresol 4,6-Dinitro-o-cresol	5	More toxic than dinitrophenol. Skin contact may lead to local necrosis and dangerous systemic effects. (See also: DINITROPHENOL, Reference Congener in Section III.)
DINITRO ORTHO CYCLOHEXYL PHENOL 2-Cyclohexyl-4,6-dinitrophenol	4	Skin contact may lead to local necrosis but rarely if ever to dangerous systemic effects (by this portal). (See also: DINITROPHENOL, Reference Congener in Section III.)
DINITROPHENOL 2,4-Dinitrophenol Alpha dinitrophenol	5	(See also: DINITROPHENOL, Reference Congener in Section III.)
DINITROTOLUENE	4(?)	Toxicity irregular but said to be much lower than dinitrobenzene. As in TNT poisoning, each (and all) of the following signs has been observed: methemoglobinemia, anemia, leucopenia, and liver necrosis. Liver injury may be more common than cyanosis, especially if diet is deficient in protein. (See also: ANILINE, Reference Congener in Section III.)
DIOCTYL SODIUM SULFOSUCCINATE Bis(2-ethylhexyl) sodium sulfosuccinate, e.g., Aerosol OT	3	A widely used anionic surfactant. One of the most powerful wetting compounds known. Employed as a dispersing and emulsifying agent in various dermatological preparations. Eye irritation when used locally in concentrations above 0.1%. Even in chronic feeding tests, fatally poisoned animals show only diarrhea and intestinal bloating, with no gross lesions outside of the alimentary tract.
DIOXANE 1,4-Diethylene oxide, or dioxide, (a cyclic diether)	3	No human poisonings by ingestion are known but 5 deaths from vapor exposure have been reported. Causes central nervous depression and subsequent renal (vascular and parenchymal) necrosis and central liver necrosis. Oxalic acid is not a significant metabolic product (if there is any). Death is due to acute renal failure. Can be absorbed through the intact skin of animals. (See also: ETHYLENE GLYCOL, Reference Congener in Section III.)
DIPENTENE Limonene Cinene	3(?)	One of the terpene hydrocarbons found in turpentine. A major constituent in oils of orange, lemon, caraway, dill, bergamot, and pine needle. No toxic reactions have been described, other than mild local irritation, but albuminuria and hematuria are probable if ingested in sufficient quantity. (See also: TURPENTINE, Reference Congener in Section III.)
2-DIPHENYLACETYL-1,3-INDANDIONE Dipaxin Diphacinone	4(?)	A new rodenticide with delayed effects on the prothrombin level and consequent disturbances in blood coagulation, resulting in death by hemorrhage. More potent than Warfarin in multiple dose experiments and especially after single-dose exposures. (See also: WARFARIN, Reference Congener in Section III.)

Substance and Synonym or Principal Ingredient	Toxicity Rating (See Inside Cover)	Comments and Reference Congeners
DIPHENYLAMINE N-Phenylamine	3	Used externally in cattle for the treatment of screwworm infestation. When given by mouth (oil solutions) to laboratory animals, it causes persistent anorexia, diarrhea, emaciation, hypothermia, and general debility, presumably from protracted gastroenteritis. Deaths may be delayed 2 to 3 weeks after a single lethal dose. In cats (and probably other species), transient methemoglobinemia is produced but is probably not the cause of death.
DI-n-PROPYL ISOME MALEATE-ISOSAFROLE n-Propyl isome	2	Central nervous depression seen after very high doses in laboratory animals.
DIPTEREX Dimethyl trichloro- hydroxyethyl- phosphonate	4	Toxicity relatively low among organic phosphate insecticides, although a potent cholinesterase inhibitor in vitro. Rapid and complete recovery from sublethal doses in laboratory animals. (See also: PARATHION, Reference Congener in Section III.)
DISODIUM 3,6-ENDOXO- HEXAHYDROPHTHALATE Endothal sodium	5	A herbicide of high oral toxicity in rats, with delayed deaths. No clinical information except for moderate skin irritation and marked irritation of abraded skin, eyes, and mucous membranes, without sensitization. Severe gastrointestinal inflammation with erosion in animals, especially if Endothal is undiluted or unmixed with food. Cold milk or Amphojel (1 oz.) recommended instead of emetics. Systemic actions are obscure; feeding tests in rats produced disorders of gait and convulsions; i.v. administration to dogs produced cardiac failure without neurological signs.
DISODIUM ETHYLENE- BIS-(DITHIOCARBAMATE) Nabam	3	Central nervous depression in animals. Oils increase absorption and toxicity. Mild skin irritation. Alcohol is best avoided after exposures to nabam because some dithiocarbamates are known to induce acetaldehyde poisoning when ethyl alcohol is metabolized (as does Antabuse). For the alcohol-Antabuse reaction, see Disulfiram in Section III.
DISULFIRAM Antabuse Tetraethylthiuram disulfide	3	Toxicity rating based on animal tests in which no alcohol was given. (See also: DISULFIRAM, Reference Congener in Section III.)
DMC Dimite Di-(p-chlorophenyl) ethanol	3(?)	An acaricide. Said to have a low mammalian toxicity, but no specific data were located. Less toxic than DDT, but toxic actions are probably similar. (See also: DDT, Reference Congener in Section III.)
DMDT Methoxychlor	3	Estimated to be one-tenth as toxic as DDT in man. In animals central nervous depression is more prominent than excitation, and poisonings are slower in onset and longer in duration than in DDT intoxication. (See also: DDT, Reference Congener in Section III.)
DMP Dimethyl phthalate	2	An insect repellent. Not irritating and not absorbed through skin. In eyes and on mucous membranes it is painful but not corrosive. Ingestion may produce central nervous depression. Treat symptomatically.
DNOC (ALSO DN) Dinitro ortho cresol	5	More toxic than dinitrophenol. Skin contact may lead to local necrosis and dangerous systemic effects. (See also: DINITROPHENOL, Reference Congener in Section III.)
DNOCHP Dinitro-ortho- cyclohexyl phenol, as the dicyclohexyl- amine salt	4	Skin contact may lead to local necrosis but rarely if ever to dangerous systemic effects. Ingestion (or inhalation) is dangerous however. (See also: DINITROPHENOL, Reference Congener in Section III.)
DNOSAP Dinitro-ortho- sec.-amyl-phenol	5	Skin contact may lead to local necrosis and dangerous systemic effects. (See also: DINITROPHENOL, Reference Congener in Section III.)
DNOSBP Dinitro-ortho-sec.- butyl phenol, usually as the triethanolamine salt	5	Skin contact may lead to local necrosis and dangerous systemic effects. (See also: DINITROPHENOL, Reference Congener in Section III.)
DNP Dinitrophenol	5	(See also: DINITROPHENOL, Reference Congener in Section III.)
DNTP Diethyl-p-nitrophenyl thiophosphate Parathion	6	(See also: PARATHION, Reference Congener in Section III.)

Substance and Synonym or Principal Ingredient	Toxicity Rating (See Inside Cover)	Comments and Reference Congeners
DODECYL DERIVATIVE		See corresponding lauryl or "alkyl" derivative in this index.
DONOVAN'S SOLUTION	3	An aqueous solution, each 100 ml. containing 0.9 to 1.0 gm. arsenious iodide and 1.05 gm. mercuric iodide. Since this solution contains almost equi-toxic amounts of arsenic and mercury, untoward effects can be expected from both. If ingested, the first symptoms are probably due to the mercuric ion, and if vomiting is prompt, arsenic poisoning may never develop. Because of the rapid absorption of mercury, mercurialism is almost inevitable in doses of one or more ounces. (See also: MERCURY, Reference Congener in Section III.)
DOWICIDES e.g., Dowicide 1, A, 4,33, etc.		A series of phenolic substances used as disinfectants, including chlorinated phenols, o-phenylphenol, brominated and chlorinated o-phenyl phenols, and sodium salts of these compounds. As tested in animals the various derivatives lie in toxicity classes 3 and 4. Phenol is a congener common to them all. (See also: PHENOL, Reference Congener in Section III.)
DUBOISINE A mixture of hyoscyamine -hyoscine alkaloids from one of the Solanaceous plants	6	Usually obtained as the acid salts, e.g., sulfates or hydrobromides. (See also: ATROPINE, Reference Congener in Section III.)
DYES AND PIGMENTS		For a tabular summary of dyes and pigments, see Section VI (General Formulations).
E-600 Para-oxon	6	One of the most toxic organic phosphate insecticides. Relatively high stability may present residue problems. (See also: PARATHION, Reference Congener in Section III.)
E-605 Parathion	6	(See also: PARATHION, Reference Congener in Section III.)
E-1059 Systox	5	A "systemic" insecticide, i.e., translocated in sap to all parts of plants. Almost as toxic as parathion in animals. Percutaneous toxicity is high. One human fatality has been reported. (See also: PARATHION, Reference Congener in Section III.)
E-3314 Heptachlor	4	(See also: HEPTACHLOR, Reference Congener in Section III.)
EDATHAMIL CALCIUM-DISODIUM Generic name (N.N.R.) for: Calcium disodium ethyl-enediamine tetraacetate Calcium disodium (ethylenedinitrilo) tetraacetate	2	A drug used intravenously to detoxify and enhance the renal excretion of lead and some other heavy metals. This calcium derivative (chelate) has a low toxicity in experimental animals; in contrast, the sodium salts may cause hypocalcemic tetany and a negative calcium balance. For methods of using this drug in therapy, see discussion of lead poisoning in Section III.
EDC Ethylene dichloride 1,2-Dichloroethane	3	Symptoms like those from chloroform and carbon tetrachloride, i.e., the primary effect is central nervous depression. Death has resulted from the ingestion of 20 to 50 cc. (30 to 70 gm.). Kidney tubular damage and occasionally a mild liver injury have been recognized, but carbon tetra-chloride is more hazardous in both respects. Corneal clouding is described in poisoned dogs, and many species develop hemorrhagic necrosis of the adrenal cortex (Friedericksen-Waterhouse syndrome). Severe injuries to the lungs and skin are uncommon. Nausea in mild exposures. BAL and other sulfhydryl compounds (e.g., methionine) have therapeutic value in poisoned animals. (See also: CARBON TETRA-CHLORIDE, Reference Congener in Section III.)
EDE Ethylene dichloride emulsion	3	Usually 10 to 20% emulsions with mono- and tri- ethanolamine oleates. See above. (See also: CARBON TETRACHLORIDE, Reference Congener in Section III.)
EDTA Ethylenediamine tetraacetic acid		The calcium-disodium salt of this acid is a drug used intravenously to detoxify and enhance the renal excretion of lead and some other heavy metals. This calcium derivative (chelate) has a low toxicity in experimental animals (toxicity rating of 2 in rats), in contrast to the sodium salts which may cause hypocalcemic tetany and a negative calcium balance. For methods of using this drug therapeutically, see lead poisoning in Section III.
EMP Ethyl mercury phosphate	5	Almost as toxic as bichloride of mercury. Nervous symptoms are prominent and severe, though sometimes transitory; they include headache, vertigo, ataxia, decrease in visual fields, delirium, and paresis. (See also: MERCURY, Reference Congener in Section III.)

Substance and Synonym or Principal Ingredient	Toxicity Rating (See Inside Cover)	Comments and Reference Congeners
ENDOTHAL, SODIUM Disodium 3,6-endoxo- hexahydrophthalate and free acid	5	A herbicide of high oral toxicity in rats, with delayed deaths. No clinical information except moderate skin irritation and marked irritation of abraded skin, eyes, and mucous membranes, without sensitization. Severe gastrointestinal inflammation with erosion in animals, especially if Endothal is undiluted or unmixed with food. Cold milk or Amphojel (1 oz.) recommended instead of emetics. Systemic actions are obscure; feeding tests in rats produced disorders of gait and convulsions; i.v. administration to dogs produced cardiac failure without neurological signs.
ENDRIN Hexachlorooctahydro- endo, endo-dimethano- naphthalene	5	A stereoisomer of dieldrin, several times more toxic than the latter but producing similar symptoms. (See also: DIELDRIN, Reference Congener in Section III.)
EPHEDRINE 1-Ephedrine α-Hydroxy-β-methylamine propylbenzene	5	The probable lethal dose in man is 50 mg./kg. Poisoning is characterized by restlessness, anxiety, sweating, tremor, rapid pulse, extrasystoles, confusion, and delirium. Treatment is symptomatic with emphasis on sedatives (e.g., barbiturates).
EPN Ethyl p-nitrophenyl thionobenzene phosphonate	5	An acetylcholinesterase inhibitor which is about one-sixth to one-eighth as toxic as parathion. Skin absorption may be dangerous. (See also: PARATHION, Reference Congener in Section III.)
1,2-EPOXYETHANE Ethylene oxide		A fumigant vapor causing intense irritation of skin, mucous membranes, and lungs, with the production of pulmonary edema. Irritation and pain usually act as adequate warnings but not always. Prompt deaths are thought to be the result of central depression with respiratory arrest; deaths delayed several hours are due to pulmonary edema; those after a few days are due to liver and kidney damage. (See also: NITROGEN OXIDES, Reference Congener in Section III.)
ESSENTIAL OILS e.g., Oils of savin, rue, tansy, nutmeg, pennyroyal, apiol, eucalyptus, juniper, cedarleaf, cajuput	4	Most of these oils are reputed to be ecbolic but abortions cannot be induced by safe doses. Basically symptoms and treatment as after turpentine, but toxicity is greater. In most cases a teaspoonful may cause illness in an adult and less than an ounce may kill (especially if vomiting does not occur promptly). Savin produces more renal damage than turpentine, and pennyroyal more liver degeneration. Also see eucalyptol, oil of sassafras, menthol, pine oil. (See also: TURPENTINE, Reference Congener in Section III.)
ESNN 2-Phenyl cyclohexanol	3	Severe skin irritation in rabbits after repeated application.
ETHAL OR ETHOL Cetyl alcohol 1-Hexadecanol Palmityl alcohol	1(?)	Said to be an effective laxative when emulsified. Thought to be a metabolic product which is secreted in small amounts into the intestinal lumen. (See also: ALCOHOLS, HIGHER, Reference Congener in Section III.)
ETHANOL Ethyl alcohol	2	Best described as lying near the borderline between toxicity classes 2 and 3. (See also: ETHYL ALCOHOL, Reference Congener in Section III.)
ETHER Diethyl ether Ethyl ether	3	One or 2 oz. may be fatal when swallowed. Symptoms are similar to ethyl alcohol intoxication except that onset is more rapid and duration is shorter. Because of its volatility the stomach becomes promptly distended; this may embarrass breathing. Unlike ethanol, ether is not oxidized (or otherwise metabolized) in vivo. (See also: ETHYL ALCOHOL, Reference Congener in Section III.)
ETHIDE 1,1-Dichloro-1- nitroethane	4	A grain fumigant. The vapor usually gives adequate warning (irritation). May produce severe pulmonary edema either by inhalation of vapor or ingestion of liquid. Also skin irritation. (See also: NITROGEN OXIDES, Reference Congener in Section III.)
ETHOHEXADIOL The official U.S.P. name for ethyl hexanediol	3	Insect repellent. Little or no skin absorption. Ingestion causes central nervous depression. Death in rats is accompanied by severe kidney and liver damage. Treat with lavage, artifical respiration, and supportive measures.
ETHYL ACETATE Acetic ether	3	Relatively innocuous (probably near the borderline between toxicity classes 2 and 3). Mild local irritation and central nervous depression.
ETHYL ALCOHOL Ethanol	2	Best described as lying near the borderline between toxicity classes 2 and 3. (See also: ETHYL ALCOHOL, Reference Congener in Section III.)
ETHYL AMINOBENZOATE Benzocaine		A local anesthetic of low toxicity. It is poorly absorbed from all sites, probably because it is water insoluble. Systemic effects, if any, presumably include central nervous excitement. Concentrations in most products have no toxic significance.

Substance and Synonym or Principal Ingredient	Toxicity Rating (See Inside Cover)	Comments and Reference Congeners
ETHYL CHLORIDE Chloroethane		Central nervous depression, usually brief and reversible. Vapor has relatively low potency. (See also: CARBON TETRACHLORIDE, Reference Congener in Section III.)
ETHYL DI-(p-CHLOROPHENYL) GLYCOLLATE Chlorobenzilate	3	A relatively new acaricide. Low toxicity in mice and rats. Toxic actions are probably like those of DDT. Only a slight tendency to accumulate in the body. (See also: DDT, Reference Congener in Section III.)
ETHYLENE CHLOROBROMIDE 1-Bromo-2-chloroethane	4	Toxic actions are like those of ethylene dichloride. Hazardous by all routes, including percutaneous absorption. May produce anesthesia and liver and kidney injuries. No human poisonings recorded. (See also: CARBON TETRACHLORIDE, Reference Congener in Section III.)
ETHYLENE CHLOROHYDRIN 2-Chloroethanol	4	Vapor more toxic than ethylene dichloride. Dangerous amounts can be absorbed through intact skin without irritation to the skin. Various visceral lesions in fatal cases, including severe pulmonary edema, liver and kidney injury. (See also: CARBON TETRACHLORIDE, Reference Congener in Section III.)
ETHYLENE DIBROMIDE Ethylene bromide 1,2-Dibromoethane	4	A severe irritant. Liquid on skin causes blisters if evaporation is delayed. Inhalation causes delayed pulmonary lesions. Drowsiness occurs, but central nervous depression is not as marked as with the dichloride. Death appears to be due to respiratory or circulatory failure, complicated by pulmonary edema. Necrosis of liver and kidneys is not conspicuous, although fatal liver damage has been reported. (See also: CARBON TETRACHLORIDE, Reference Congener in Section III.)
ETHYLENE DICHLORIDE Ethylene chloride 1,2-Dichloroethane	3	Symptoms like those from chloroform and carbon tetrachloride, i.e., the primary effect is central nervous depression. Death has resulted from the ingestion of 20 to 50 cc. (30 to 70 gm.). Kidney tubular damage and occasionally a mild liver injury have been recognized, but probably carbon tetrachloride is more hazardous in both respects. Corneal clouding is described in poisoned dogs, and many species develop hemorrhagic necrosis of the adrenal cortex (Friedericksen-Waterhouse syndrome). Severe injuries to the lungs and skin are uncommon. BAL and other sulfhydryl compounds (e.g. methionine) have therapeutic value in poisoned animals. (See also: CARBON TETRACHLORIDE, Reference Congener in Section III.)
ETHYLENE GLYCOL Ethanediol	3	Toxicity rating of 3 is based on clinical data. In guinea pigs, rats, and mice, the rating is 2. (See also: ETHYLENE GLYCOL, Reference Congener in Section III.)
ETHYLENE GLYCOL ALKYL (AND ARYL) ESTERS e.g., Ethylene glycol diacetate	3	Generally the simple mono- and di-esters have about the same acute toxicity as ethylene glycol. They are readily saponified in the body to glycol and the corresponding organic acid. Special problems arise where the latter is highly toxic (e.g., salicylic acid). (See also: ETHYLENE GLYCOL, Reference Congener in Section III.)
ETHYLENE GLYCOL ALKYL (AND ARYL) ETHERS Cellosolves	3	Acute toxicities are several times greater than that of ethylene glycol in animals (clinical data are inadequate for valid comparisons). Ether linkage is supposedly stable in vivo. Central nervous depression as with ethylene glycol, but the ether derivatives produce more marked kidney injury and hematuria (apparently without oxalic acid formation or crystalluria). These ethers penetrate intact skin. (See also: ETHYLENE GLYCOL, Reference Congener in Section III.)
ETHYLENE OXIDE 1,2-Epoxyethane		A fumigant vapor causing intense irritation of skin (blisters), mucous membranes, and lungs, with the production of pulmonary edema. Irritation and pain usually act as adequate warnings but not always. Prompt deaths are thought to be the result of central depression with respiratory arrest; if delayed several hours, deaths are due to pulmonary edema; those after a few days are due to liver and kidney damage. (See also: NITROGEN OXIDES, Reference Congener in Section III.)
ETHYLENE TETRACHLORIDE Tetrachloroethylene	3	Less toxic than carbon tetrachloride or chloroform. Given therapeutically to adults by mouth (dose 1 to 4 ml.) for hookworm. Widely used in veterinary medicine. (See also: CARBON TETRACHLORIDE, Reference Congener in Section III.)
ETHYL FORMATE	3	Produces irritation and central nervous depression. A much stronger irritant than ethyl acetate, probably because of hydrolysis to formic acid.
ETHYL GASOLINE Leaded gasoline	3	Tetraethyl lead content is not of toxic significance in acute poisonings by ingestion or inhalation, but persons in the gasoline industry who are careless about repeated skin contact have developed lead poisoning (see Sec. III). No non-petroleum additive is believed to be toxic as present in commercial formulations. Also see gasoline in this index. (See also: KEROSENE, Reference Congener in Section III.)

Substance and Synonym or Principal Ingredient	Toxicity Rating (See Inside Cover)	Comments and Reference Congeners
ETHYL HEXANEDIOL 2-Ethyl hexanediol-1,3 Rutger's 612	3	Insect repellent. Little or no skin absorption. Ingestion causes central nervous depression. Death in rats is accompanied by severe kidney and liver damage. Treat with lavage, artificial respiration, and supportive measures.
ETHYL MERCAPTOETHYL DIETHYL THIO-PHOSPHATE Systox Demeton	5	A "systemic" insecticide, i.e., translocated in sap to all parts of plants. Almost as toxic as parathion in animals. Percutaneous toxicity is high. One human fatality has been reported. (See also: PARATHION, Reference Congener in Section III.)
N-(ETHYLMERCURI)-p-TOLUENE SULPHON-ANILIDE e.g., Ceresan M	4	A seed disinfectant which is almost as toxic as mercuric chloride. Less irritating to the skin than ethyl mercury phosphate.(See also: MERCURY, Reference Congener in Section III.)
ETHYL MERCURY CHLORIDE e.g., Ceresan	5	A seed disinfectant which is almost as toxic as bichloride of mercury. Especially dangerous because of its toxic vapors. See ethyl mercury phosphate. (See also: MERCURY, Reference Congener in Section III.)
ETHYL MERCURY PHOSPHATE Ethyl mercuric phosphate	5	A volatile fungicide which is almost as toxic as bichloride of mercury (although solutions are not as corrosive). Nervous symptoms are prominent and severe, though sometimes transitory; they include headache, vertigo, ataxia, decrease in the visual fields, delirium, and paresis. (See also: MERCURY, Reference Congener in Section III.)
ETHYL METHYL KETONE 2-Butanone	3(?)	Similar to but more irritating than acetone. Vapor is irritating to mucous membranes and conjunctiva. Central nervous depression in experimental animals. Irritating odor ordinarily prevents significant clinical exposures. No serious poisonings reported in man, except for dermatitis.
ETHYL NITROPHENYL BENZENE THIO-PHOSPHATE EPN	5	A cholinesterase inhibitor which is about one-sixth to one-eighth as toxic as parathion. Skin absorption may be dangerous. (See also: PARATHION, Reference Congener in Section III.)
ETHYL NITROPHENYL THIONOBENZENE (OR THIOBENZENE) PHOSPHONATE EPN	5	See above. (See also: PARATHION, Reference Congener in Section III.)
O-ETHYL-O-PARANITROPHENYL BENZENETHIO-PHOSPHONATE EPN	5	See above. (See also: PARATHION, Reference Congener in Section III.)
ETHYL PHOSPHATES e.g., Triethyl phosphate	3(?)	A sedative in rats. Some ethyl phosphates (e.g., parathion) are highly toxic cholinesterase inhibitors.
EUCALYPTOL Eucalyptol is the dl form. Cineol is the d-isomer.	4	Eucalyptus oil is about 70% active eucalyptol. As little as 1 ml. has caused a transient coma. Fatalities have followed doses as small as 3.5 ml., and recovery has occurred after a dose of 20 and even 30 ml. Symptoms include epigastric burning with nausea and usually vomiting; vertigo, ataxia, muscle weakness, stupor; pallor and sometimes cyanosis, respiratory stridor (edema), and miosis. Delirium and occasionally convulsions occur. Rarely symptoms may be delayed for 2 hours. (See also: TURPENTINE, Reference Congener in Section III.)
EUDERMOL Nicotine salicylate	6	The salts of nicotine are almost as toxic as the free alkaloidal base, except that the salts do not readily penetrate intact skin. (See also: NICOTINE, Reference Congener in Section III.)
EUGENOL Caryophyllic acid 4-Allyl-2-methoxy-phenol	3(?)	Obtained from clove oil, which is about 80% eugenol. Possesses properties of local antisepsis and local anesthesia. Used locally in the control of toothaches. A rubefacient and irritant. Ingestion presumably results in a gastroenteritis, but systemic toxicity is lower than phenol, probably because of insolubility in water. (See also: PHENOL, Reference Congener in Section III.)
FERBAM Ferric dimethyl dithiocarbamate Fermate	3	In most laboratory animals, this compound lies near the borderline between toxicity classes 2 and 3. Kidney injury is described. May cause irritation to skin and to mucous membranes and rarely skin sensitization in man. Because in animals the sodium salt is known to disturb severely the metabolism of ethyl alcohol (see Disulfiram in Sec. III), alcoholic beverages are best avoided after known exposures to ferbam.

Substance and Synonym or Principal Ingredient	Toxicity Rating (See Inside Cover)	Comments and Reference Congeners
FERMATE Ferric dimethyl dithiocarbamate	3	See Ferbam in this index.
FERRIC DIMETHYL DITHIOCARBAMATE Ferbam Fermate	3	See Ferbam in this index.
FERRIC SALTS e.g., Ferric chloride, subsulfate, ammonium citrate, etc.		Given orally, ferric and ferrous salts induce essentially the same toxic syndrome. (See also: FERROUS SULFATE, Reference Congener in Section III.)
FERROCYANIDE AND FERRICYANIDE SALTS e.g., Sodium, potassium ferric	3(?)	No adequate toxicity data were located, but apparently these salts are comparatively benign. They are not decomposed to cyanide. Rapidly excreted in the urine, apparently without metabolic alteration. Dogs tolerate intravenous injections of 2.5 gm./kg. For ferric ferrocyanide, see ferric salts above.
FERROUS SALTS e.g., Ferrous sulfate, chloride, carbonate, gluconate, etc.		Although iron salts differ considerably in astringency, lethal doses appear to be closely related to the total iron content. (See also: FERROUS SULFATE, Reference Congener in Section III.)
FLUOALUMINATE, SODIUM Cryolite $AlF_3 \cdot 3NaF$ or Na_3AlF_6	2(?)	Acute toxicity by ingestion is said to be very low. Much less soluble than sodium fluoride or fluosilicate and more stable than the latter with respect to hydrolysis. (See also: FLUORIDE, Reference Congener in Section III.)
FLUORIDE SALTS e.g., Sodium, barium, zinc, etc.	4	Clinical data indicate that the sodium salt lies near the borderline between toxicity classes 4 and 5. Although less toxic in animals, barium fluoride may be as toxic in man as the sodium salt (or perhaps slightly more toxic). Calcium fluoride is comparatively benign (toxicity rating 3 ?) because of its low solubility and low ionization. In terms of acute toxicity, most fluorides presumably lie between the sodium and calcium salts. (See also: FLUORIDE, Reference Congener in Section III.)
FLUOROACETATE SALTS e.g., Sodium fluoroacetate	6	A delayed convulsant, with none of the toxic actions of fluorides. (See also: FLUOROACETATE, Reference Congener in Section III.)
FLUOSILICATE SALTS e.g., Sodium, barium. Also known as silicofluorides	4	Generally more soluble than the corresponding fluoride salt (but not true in the case of sodium). Hydrolyzed by alkali to fluoride ion. In experimental animals the fluosilicates appear to be as toxic as the corresponding fluorides. Lavage stomach with lime water (calcium hydroxide). (See also: FLUORIDE, Reference Congener in Section III.)
FORMALDEHYDE SOLUTION Formalin	3	Commercial formaldehyde contains 30 to 37%/w of formaldehyde gas and 0 to 5% methyl alcohol. Because 1 oz. taken by mouth has caused death within 2-1/2 hours, the solution presumably lies near the borderline between toxicity classes 3 and 4. (See also: FORMALDEHYDE, Reference Congener in Section III.)
FORMALIN 30 to 37% aqueous solution of formaldehyde	3	See above. (See also: FORMALDEHYDE, Reference Congener in Section III.)
FORMIC ACID AND FORMATE SALTS		Produces violent burns and local necrosis, like the strong mineral acids. Sodium formate appears to have a low toxicity (10 gm. by mouth without ill-effects in man). Formate ion is extensively oxidized in vivo, but it may have direct actions on brain (cause of convulsions in poisoned animals?). Methemoglobinemia has been reported in poisoned animals. (See also: ACID, Reference Congener in Section III.)
FOWLER'S SOLUTION An aqueous solution of potassium arsenite equivalent to 1% arsenic trioxide	4	The probable lethal dose for an adult lies between 10 and 30 ml. (See also: ARSENIC, Reference Congener in Section III.)
FREONS e.g., Dichlorodifluoro-methane		Trademarked name for a series of fluorinated-chlorinated hydrocarbons, used as refrigerant gases, propellent gases for insecticidal aerosol "bombs," etc. High vapor concentrations (e.g., 20%) may cause confusion, pulmonary irritation, tremors, and rarely coma, but these actions are generally transient and there are no late sequelae. In contact with an open flame or very hot surface, freons may decompose into many highly irritant and toxic gases: chlorine, fluorine, hydrogen fluoride and chloride, and even phosgene.

Substance and Synonym or Principal Ingredient	Toxicity Rating (See Inside Cover)	Comments and Reference Congeners
FUEL OIL OR DIESEL OIL Gas oil "Distillate"	3	Petroleum fraction distilling between 250° and 350° C. or slightly higher than kerosene, which it closely resembles. (See also: KEROSENE, Reference Congener in Section III.)
FURFURALDEHYDE-2 Furfural	3	Said to be about one-third as toxic as formaldehyde. An irritant to mucous membranes. Central nervous depression with brain lesions in animals. Ingested furfural has produced liver cirrhosis in rats. (See also: FORMALDEHYDE, Reference Congener in Section III.)
G-11 Hexachlorophene 2,2'-Methylene bis(3,4,6- trichlorophenol)	3	Used in concentrations of 1 to 2% as a disinfectant in several liquid and solid soap products. Not irritating to the skin, but sensitization has been reported. Systemic effects presumably resemble those of phenol. No poisonings known in man. (See also: PHENOL, Reference Congener in Section III.)
GALLIC ACID 3,4,5-Trihydroxy- benzoic acid	3(?)	Apparently much less toxic than salicylic acid. Fed to men in quantities of 2 to 10 gm. without fatalities and without even severe ill-effects. Readily absorbed from the gastrointestinal tract. In animals it reduces body temperature and causes progressive weakness and perhaps convulsions.
GAMMA BENZENE HEXACHLORIDE GBH Lindane Hexachlorocyclohexane	4	(See also: BENZENE HEXACHLORIDE, Reference Congener in Section III.)
GARDINOL-TYPE DETERGENTS Fatty alcohol sulfates, e.g., Duponals, Drene, Dreft, Teel	3	Widely used anionic detergents of moderately low acute and chronic toxicities. A few of the branched-chain products have been shown to have significant percutaneous toxicity. Skin irritation may be encountered with any of these substances. Taken by mouth, sodium lauryl sulfate stimulates gastric mucus production and sometimes inactivates pepsin in test animals. In subacute and chronic feeding tests, even fatally poisoned animals show only diarrhea and intestinal bloating, with no gross lesions outside of the gastrointestinal tract.
GAMBOGE Cambogia	4	A gum resin and drastic purgative, leading to severe prostration and death. The ingestion of 4 gm. has proved fatal.
GAS (EXHAUST, FLUE, ILLUMINATING OR MANUFACTURED GAS) Carbon monoxide (CO) is the principal toxic ingredient.		Exhaust or flue gases may also contain corrosive oxides of nitrogen and sulfur. Manufactured gas consists chiefly of volatile hydrocarbons of low toxicity (e.g. methane) and of hydrogen; the carbon monoxide (CO) content usually lies between 2 and 15% v. Natural gas contains no CO (unless produced by "cracking" or some related process). (See also: CARBON MONOXIDE, Reference Congener in Section III.)
GASOLINE A mixture chiefly of C_4 to C_{12} aliphatic hydrocarbons obtained as a petroleum distillate, often after "cracking" heavy fractions	3	Boiling point range is approximately 40 to 225° C. Tetraethyl lead content is not of toxic significance in acute exposures by ingestion or inhalation, but persons in the gasoline industry who are careless about repeated skin contact have developed lead poisoning (Sec. III). No non-petroleum additives are believed to be toxic in the commercial formulations. Appreciable amounts of aromatic hydrocarbons (e.g., xylenes) are found in commercial fuels, expecially when the petroleum is from Texas and California (but not from eastern U.S.A. fields). A high content of aromatic hydrocarbons and a consequent high toxicity are also associated with a high "octane rating" (whenever the latter is not due to additives, such as tetraethyl lead or alcohol). See also: KEROSENE, Reference Congener in Section III.)
GBH Gamma benzene hexachloride Lindane	4	(See also: BENZENE HEXACHLORIDE, Reference Congener in Section III.)
GELSEMIUM Yellow jasmine Dried rhizome and roots of Gelsemium sempervirens L.	5(?)	Has been used empirically in the treatment of neuralgias (average dose 30 mg.). Contains at least 3 potent alkaloids: gelsemine, sempervirine, and gelsemicine, each producing features reminiscent of curare, atropine, and strychnine poisonings: weakness, vertigo, tremors, ptosis, jaw drop, diplopia, mydriasis, dyspnea, anxiety, convulsions. No specific treatment has been outlined.
GENTIAN VIOLET Various isomers of methylrosaniline chloride Crystal Violet is relatively pure hexamethyl-pararosaniline chloride.	4(?)	Used medicinally as an intestinal anthelmintic. Ingestion causes nausea, vomiting, diarrhea, and abdominal pain, sometimes even in therapeutic doses (0.06 gm. t.i.d.). Systemic toxicity is not well defined, but kidney and liver disease are traditional contraindications to this drug. No severe poisonings have been reported in man.

Substance and Synonym or Principal Ingredient	Toxicity Rating (See Inside Cover)	Comments and Reference Congeners
GERANIOL One of 3 major alcohols found in rose oil (the others are citronellol and nerol) Also found in geranium oils, citronella, and others	3(?)	Widely used in perfumes, soaps, and cosmetics. No toxicity data were located, but the toxicity is probably low.
GITALIN An amorphous mixture of cardiotonic glycosides obtained from the leaves of Digitalis purpurea The chief constituent, which can be crystallized, is also named gitalin.	6	Has all the therapeutic and toxic actions of whole-leaf digitalis, but said to have a greater margin of safety. In adults the average oral dose for rapid digitalization is about 5.7 mg. (4.5 to 9.0 mg.), while the daily maintenance dose is about 0.5 mg. With respect to duration of action, gitalin is faster than digitoxin and slower than digoxin. The single lethal dose in an adult probably lies between 15 and 50 mg. (See also: DIGITALIS, Reference Congener in Section III.)
GLYCERINE Glycerol	1	An emollient and demulcent on skin. Concentrated solutions are irritating to mucous membrane (e.g., evacuation after rectal suppository). No appreciable oral toxicity, but the injection of large doses may induce convulsions, paralysis, hemolysis, etc.
GLYCERYL MONOSTEARATE Also mono-and di-esters of other fatty acids	1	These partial glycerides are widely used, often in conjunction with a little soap, as surfactants and emulsifiers in cosmetics, medicinals, and food products. Like natural fats they are well digested and assimilated.
GLYCERYL TRIACETATE Triacetin	1	Laboratory animals have tolerated diets consisting of 50% triacetin. If hydrolyzed, systemic acidosis is a possible consequence.
GLYCEROL TRINITRATE Nitroglycerin	6	A fast-acting and much more potent drug than sodium nitrite (100-fold difference in therapeutic doses); this can be explained only partially by rates of absorption, since the fatal intravenous doses in rabbits differ by a factor of at least 2 (expressed as nitrite equivalents). In man it is more potent when absorbed from the mouth (e.g., sublingual) than when swallowed. Can be absorbed through intact skin. (See also: NITRITE, Reference Congener in Section III.)
GLYODIN 2-Heptadecyl glyoxalidine acetate Crag Fruit Fungicide 341	3	A fungicide (or fungostatic) of low toxicity in laboratory animals. Poorly absorbed except in the presence of fat solvents. Concentrated solutions are irritating to the skin.
GLYOXALIDINE Glyodin Crag Fruit Fungicide 341	3	See above.
GOLD SALTS e.g., gold sodium thiosulfate, gold trichloride, gold sodium thiomalate	4(?)	No information on oral toxicity was located. Given intramuscularly at weekly intervals to patients with rheumatoid arthritis, gold salts often induce toxic reactions, (frequently of an allergic nature): dermatitis, nausea, vomiting, diarrhea, nephritis, blood disorders, peripheral neuritis, hepatitis, and encephalitis. Severe reactions respond well to BAL (see BAL in Section III).
GRAPHITE Plumbage Pencil lead Black lead	1	Crystalline carbon, chemically and biologically inert, although allergic symptoms have been described.
GUAIACOL Methylcatechol o-Hydroxyanisole o-Methoxyphenol	4	Slightly less corrosive and less toxic than phenol. In most clinical poisonings, guaiacol was taken as wood-tar creosote. Percutaneous absorption is dangerous. (See also: PHENOL, Reference Congener in Section III.)
GUMS, VEGETABLE e.g., Gum Karaya, acacia (arabic). tragacanth, ghatti, agar, and most other water-soluble gums	1(?)	Aside from an occasional allergic reaction, these drugs can be ingested in large amounts, with little danger or distress except for diarrhea, flatulence, and rarely fecal impaction. They are not absorbed.

Substance and Synonym or Principal Ingredient	Toxicity Rating (See Inside Cover)	Comments and Reference Congeners
HAMAMELIS Dried leaves of Hamamelis virginiana, containing tannin (2 to 9%)	2	The dried leaves (or an extract thereof) are used in ointments and suppositories (dose 2 gm.). The fluidextract (prepared from leaves) has an ethyl alcohol content of 70 to 78% and significant amounts of tannin (dose 2 to 4 ml.). Witch hazel water is a saturated aqueous solution (with 15% ethanol) of volatile products distilled from dried twigs; it presumably contains small but appreciable amounts of terpenes (sequiterpenes). All of these preparations serve as mild astringents and local sedatives. Ethyl alcohol and tannin are the major toxic ingredients.
HALOWAX Chlorinated naphthalenes		Acneform rash and liver necrosis from exposure to vapors. Ingestion toxicity is not known, but it presumably increases with the degree of chlorination. The principal cause of hyperkeratosis in cattle.
HCCH OR HCH Hexachloroacyclohexane Often called benzene hexachloride (although this is technically incorrect)	4	(See also: BENZENE HEXACHLORIDE, Reference Congener in Section III.)
HENBANE Hyoscyamine	3	Dried leaves contain about 0.04% hyoscyamine alkaloids (hyoscine, hyoscyamine). (See also: ATROPINE, Reference Congener in Section III.)
HEPTACHLOR Heptachloro-tetrahydro-4,7-endomethano-indene	4	(See also: HEPTACHLOR, Reference Congener in Section III.)
HEPTACHLORO-CAMPHENE AND -PINENE Strobane	4	Only one-third to one-quarter as acutely toxic as toxaphene in animals, but poisonings are thought to be qualitatively similar in terms of symptoms and treatment. Strobane does not cause skin irritation or sensitization in man. Percutaneous toxicity is very low in rabbits and presumably in man too. (See also: TOXAPHENE, Reference Congener in Section III.)
HEPTACHLORO-DICYCLOPENTADIENE Heptachlor	4	(See also: HEPTACHLOR, Reference Congener in Section III.)
HEPTACHLORO-TETRAHYDRO-4,7-ENDOMETHANO-INDENE Heptachlor	4	(See also: HEPTACHLOR, Reference Congener in Section III.)
HEPTADECYL GLYOXALIDINE (AND ITS ACETATE SALT) Glyodin Crag Fruit Fungicide 341	3	A fungicide of moderately low toxicity in laboratory animals. Poorly absorbed except in the presence of solvents. Concentrated solutions are irritating to the skin.
HEROIN Diacetylmorphine	6	In a non-tolerant adult (i.e., a non-addict), 0.06 gm. is thought to be lethal. Not found in any legitimate product in the U.S.A. (See also: MORPHINE, Reference Congener in Section III.)
HETP Hexaethyl tetraphosphate	6	Slightly more potent than parathion and less so than TEPP. Unstable like TEPP. Not used currently in agriculture. (See also: PARATHION, Reference Congener in Section III.)
HEXACHLOROBENZENE Perchlorobenzene	3(?)	NOT benzene hexachloride (since the latter is always used to designate hexachlorocyclohexane). Occasionally used as a fungicide. The only estimate of lethality is the information that the oral lethal dose in guinea pigs is greater than 3 gm./kg. Very slight exfoliation on prolonged skin contact. Systemic effects are not described. No clinical data.
HEXACHLORO-CYCLOHEXANE Benzene hexachloride	4	(See also: BENZENE HEXACHLORIDE, Reference Congener in Section III.)
HEXACHLOR-EPOXY-OCTAHYDRO-DIMETHANO NAPHTHALENE Dieldrin or its isomer endrin	5	Based on animal tests, endrin lies distinctly within toxicity class 5, while dieldrin lies near the borderline between classes 4 and 5. Toxic signs and symptoms are indistinguishable, however. (See also: DIELDRIN, Reference Congener in Section III.)
HEXACHLOROETHANE Perchloroethane Carbon hexachloride	4	More potent central nervous effects than chloroform or carbon tetrachloride, but slower in action. On ingestion, severe mucosal injury and often liver necrosis. Because of low vapor pressure, no industrial exposures are known. (See also: CARBON TETRACHLORIDE, Reference Congener in Section III.)

Substance and Synonym or Principal Ingredient	Toxicity Rating (See Inside Cover)	Comments and Reference Congeners
HEXACHLORO-HEXAHYDRO-ENDO, EXO-DIMETHANO-NAPHTHALENE Aldrin	5	Based on animal tests, aldrin lies on the borderline between toxicity classes 4 and 5. Its toxic properties are similar to those of dieldrin. (See also: DIELDRIN, Reference Congener in Section III.)
HEXACHLOROPHENE 2,2'-Methylene-bis(3,4,6-trichlorophenol)	3	Used in concentrations of 1 to 2% as a disinfectant in several liquid and solid soap products. Not irritating to the skin, but sensitization has been reported. Systemic effects presumably resemble those of phenol. No poisonings known in man. (See also: PHENOL, Reference Congener in Section III.)
2,4-HEXADIENOIC ACID Sorbic acid	2	Protects materials against fungi. Not a primary irritant or sensitizing agent on the skin.
HEXAETHYL TETRA-PHOSPHATE HETP	6	Slightly more potent than parathion but less so than TEPP. Unstable like TEPP. Not used currently in agriculture. (See also: PARATHION, Reference Congener in Section III.)
HEXAHYDROBENZOIC ACID Cyclohexane carboxylic acid, one of the constituents of commercial naphthenic acids from petroleum		No specific information about toxicity despite long and widespread use. Cyclohexane is a central nervous depressant; this may or may not be true of this acid derivative.
HEXAMETHYLENE-TETRAMINE Methenamine	3(?)	Slowly decomposes into formaldehyde, especially in an acid medium (e.g., stomach, urine). A very large oral dose (usual doses are 1 to 2 gm.) causes gastrointestinal irritation (vomiting and pain), albuminuria, gross hematuria, and dysuria with inflammatory lesions in the renal tubules, renal pelves, and urinary bladder. Repeated use may cause sensitization with urticaria or dermatitis. (See also: FORMALDEHYDE, Reference Congener in Section III.)
n-HEXANE		A mild central nervous depressant. Vapor causes anesthesia of short duration without sequellae.
HEXYLRESORCINOL 4-Hexyl-1,3-dihydroxybenzene	3	Somewhat less toxic than resorcinol or phenol. Effective by all portals including percutaneous absorption. Irritating to skin when in high concentrations. Some cutaneous reactions are due to hypersensitivity. By mouth large doses cause irritation and erosion of gastric and intestinal mucosa. Because of poor absorption, systemic symptoms are unusual but damage to liver and heart has been reported in dogs. (See also: PHENOL, Reference Congener in Section III.)
HOMATROPINE Mandelyltropeine	4(?)	Less effective and less toxic than atropine. One tenth as potent a parasympathomimetic blocking agent as is atropine. Used medicinally only in the eye.
HYAMINES e.g., Hyamine 1622, 10-X, 2389	4	Trademarked name for several cationic surfactants of the quaternary ammonium type, used as disinfectants for clean surfaces. (See also: QAC, Reference Congener in Section III.)
HYDRASTINE An alkaloid, usually as the hydrochloride; obtained from the rhizomes and roots of Hydrastis canadensis	5(?)	Formerly used in the treatment of gastrointestinal inflammation and uterine hemorrhage (dose 10 mg.). Toxic doses cause strychnine-like convulsions due to hyperexcitability of the central nervous system; also relaxation of the gut; and possibly stimulation of the uterus. Treatment as in strychnine poisoning. (See also: STRYCHNINE, Reference Congener in Section III.)
HYDRASTIS Dried rhizomes and roots of Hydrastis canadensis	3(?)	Contains 3 active alkaloids: hydrastine (about 2%), berberine (2 to 4%), and canadine. Hydrastine in toxic doses causes strychnine-like convulsions due to hyperexcitability of the central nervous system; also relaxation of the gut; and possibly stimulation of the uterus. Berberine causes vasodilation, cardiac depression, and broncho-constriction. Canadine has weak morphine-like effects. In toxic doses of the mixture, hydrastine's actions predominate, but the circulatory effects of berberine may also be apparent. The treatment is symptomatic and supportive.

Substance and Synonym or Principal Ingredient	Toxicity Rating (See Inside Cover)	Comments and Reference Congeners
HYDROCHLORIC ACID Hydrogen chloride Muriatic acid		(See also: ACID, Reference Congener in Section III.)
HYDROCYANIC ACID Hydrogen cyanide: prussic acid is a 2% aqueous solution of this acid.	6	Cyanide is one of the fastest poisons known. To be effective, therapeutic measures must be prompt! (See also: CYANIDE, Reference Congener in Section III.)
HYDROFLUORIC ACID Hydrogen fluoride HF		(See also: FLUORIDE, Reference Congener in Section III.)
HYDROGEN PEROXIDE Official aqueous solutions are 3% with respect to H_2O_2.		Said to have a low toxicity. No primary systemic effects when ingested because it is decomposed in the bowel before absorption. Decomposition may release large volumes of oxygen (ten times the volume of solution). Large doses presumably produce gastritis and esophagitis.
HYDROGEN SULFIDE Sulfureted hydrogen Hydrosulfuric acid "Stink damp"		(See also: HYDROGEN SULFIDE, Reference Congener in Section III.)
HYDROQUINONE p-Dihydroxybenzene 1,4-Dihydroxybenzene	4	Irritating but not corrosive. Human poisonings have been reported from a mixture of hydroquinone and metol. Systemic actions like phenol, but in addition tremors and convulsions are prominent, plus an occasional severe hemolytic anemia (subsequent to methemoglobinemia?). Fatal human doses have ranged from 5 to 12 grams, but 300 to 500 mg. have been ingested daily for 3 to 5 months without ill-effects. Lesions of skin (especially depigmentation) and of eyes are described in man, but these effects may have been due to local contact with quinone. (See also: PHENOL and ANILINE, Reference Congeners in Section III.)
HYDROXYBENZENE Phenol	4	(See also: PHENOL, Reference Congener in Section III.)
2-HYDROXY-2,2-BIS (4-CHLOROPHENYL) ETHYL ACETATE Chlorobenzilate	3	A relatively new acaricide. Low toxicity in mice and rats. Feeding tests indicate only a slight tendency to accumulate in body. Toxic actions are probably like those of DDT. (See also: DDT, Reference Congener in Section III.)
7-HYDROXYCOUMARIN Umbelliferone		In sun-screen lotions and creams. No toxicity data located.
2-HYDROXYDIPHENYL o-Phenyl phenol (and its salts)	3	Not absorbed through skin. An oil solution (5%) is well tolerated on human skin, but aqueous solutions of the sodium salt are irritating in concentrations above 0.5%. In rats ingestion causes death from central nervous depression, as does phenol. (See also: PHENOL, Reference Congener in Section III.)
HYDROXYLAMINE and its salts	4	Said to be decomposed in the body to nitrite and ammonia. Systemic poisoning characterized by cyanosis, methemoglobinemia, convulsions, and coma. Locally a severe skin irritant and sensitizer. (See also: NITRITE, Reference Congener in Section III.)
HYDROXYMERCURI-CHLOROPHENOLS 2-Chloro-4-(hydroxymercuri) phenol (chiefly)	5	Semesan contains 20% mercury, equivalent to 30% mixed hydroxy mercuri-chlorophenols, plus diluents which promote water solubility. Less corrosive than mercuric chloride but the systemic toxicity is probably almost as great. Toxic by all portals. Non-volatile and insoluble in water, but soluble in alkali. Oil facilitates absorption from the bowel. Used in agriculture as a fungicide for treating seeds and turf diseases. Strongly irritating to the skin but not a vesicant. (See also: MERCURY, Reference Congener in Section III.)
HYDROXYMERCURI-CRESOL e.g., One of the components in some Semesan products.	5	Similar to and often mixed with hydroxymercurichlorophenol. See latter. (See also: MERCURY, Reference Congener in Section III.)
HYDROXYMERCURI-NITROPHENOL e.g., Semesan Bel is 10% mercury, chiefly in the form of this compound.	5	Similar to and often mixed with hydroxymercurichlorophenol. See latter. Aqueous solutions of the sodium salt have been used in medicine as a disinfectant under the name Mercurophen. Nitromersol (Metaphen) is a closely related medicinal germicide. (See also: MERCURY, Reference Congener in Section III.)

Substance and Synonym or Principal Ingredient	Toxicity Rating (See Inside Cover)	Comments and Reference Congeners
HYDROXYPHENYL- MERCURICHLORIDE Phenol mercuric chloride	5	Contains 61% mercury. Readily soluble in water. Dilute solutions have been used in medicine as a germicide and fungicide. Less corrosive than mercuric chloride but the systemic toxicity is probably almost as great. (See also: MERCURY, Reference Congener in Section III.)
8-HYDROXYQUINOLINE Oxyquinoline Oxine Often used as water soluble salts like the sulfate, citrate, tartrate, or benzoate	3(?)	For the treatment of dysentery, men have received oral doses of 3 gm. in solution, four times daily, without apparent ill-effect. Rabbits tolerate single doses of 3.7 gm./kg. (as the sulfate, mixed with potassium sulfate). Various halogenated derivatives used in treating amebiasis are also comparatively benign (they may cause diarrhea and rarely liver injury). When injected in animals, however, hydroxyquinoline is distinctly toxic and causes marked stimulation of the central nervous system.
HYOSCINE Scopolamine	6	Commonly stated to be more toxic than atropine, but with either drug fatalities are rare. Idiosyncrasies, however, are definitely more common with hyoscine. Clinical doses of hyoscine commonly induce drowsiness or sleep, but large overdosages may produce excitement and psychotic behavior (like atropine). The hyoscine psychosis is followed by more prominent and prolonged central nervous depression. Peripheral actions mimic those of atropine. (See also: ATROPINE, Reference Congener in Section III.)
HYOSCYAMINE 1-Hyoscyamine Daturine	6	The same toxicity to the central nervous system as atropine (equal parts of d-and 1-hyoscyamine), but the 1-isomer is at least twice as potent as a peripheral blocking agent. (See also: ATROPINE, Reference Congener in Section III.)
HYOSCYAMUS Henbane (from leaves and seeds of Hyoscyamine niger)	3	Dried leaves contain about 0.04% hyoscyamine alkaloids (hyoscine, hyoscyamine, etc.) (See also: ATROPINE, Reference Congener in Section III.)
HYPOCHLORITE SALTS e.g., Sodium, calcium magnesium, etc.		(See also: HYPOCHLORITE, Reference Congener in Section III.)
HYPOSULFITE SALTS Thiosulfates e.g., Sodium, potassium	3(?)	Remarkably inert in vivo, except for osmotic disturbances. Poorly absorbed from the alimentary tract and so acts as an osmotic cathartic. In the treatment of cyanide poisoning, 12.5 gm. of highly purified sodium thiosulfate has been injected i.v. without ill-effects.
ICHTHAMMOL Ichthyol Ammonium ichthosulfonate	3(?)	Obtained by sulfonating the distillate of certain bituminous schists and neutralizing with ammonia. Contains about 10% sulfur as alkyl derivatives, notably sulfides and mercaptans (half the sulfur), sulfones, and sulfonates. A feeble skin irritant and antiseptic. Formerly prescribed by mouth (200 mg.) as an expectorant. Large doses cause gastrointestinal irritation and diarrhea. No systemic effects are recognized.
ICHTHYOL Ichthammol Ammonium ichthosulfonate	3(?)	See Ichthammol above.
IGEPAL Igepals-CO are nonyl derivatives Igepals-CA are isooctyl derivatives Igepals-DM are higher alkyl derivatives	2	The trademarked name (some formerly called Antarox) for various condensations of ethylene oxide and nonylphenol (or isooctylphenol), described as polyoxyethylated nonylphenol or nonyl phenoxy polyoxyethylene ethanol. They are non-ionic surfactants used as wetting and emulsifying agents. Even at full-strength, they are not irritants or sensitizing agents on human skin. Animal tests place these compounds near the borderline between toxicity classes 2 and 3. The only gross lesion described in fatally poisoned rats was gastric hyperemia.
IGEPON e.g., Igepon AP, AC, T, TK, TN, CN	2 and 3	Trademarked name for various synthetic surfactants formed by condensing a fatty acid with an organic sulfonate, usually sodium methyl taurine or sodium isethionate. These products are anionic surfactants, used as wetting and dispersing agents in detergents (etc). In solution some are quite alkaline, which may explain why they may produce skin irritation in concentrations of 1 to 10% (in contrast to Igepals above).
IMPERIAL GREEN Copper acetoarsenite	5	A substance of complex composition, having an arsenic trioxide equivalent of about 59%. Used as an insecticide, a wood preservative, and a paint pigment. (See also: ARSENIC, Reference Congener in Section III.)
INDALONE Butopyronoxyl Butyl mesityl oxide (oxalate)	2	May be mildly irritating to the skin on repeated applications. Mild focal necrosis in liver and kidneys of rabbits after repeated cutaneous exposures (90 days). No human poisonings are known.

Substance and Synonym or Principal Ingredient	Toxicity Rating (See Inside Cover)	Comments and Reference Congeners
INERT INGREDIENTS		Ingredients labelled "inert" by the manufacturer are not necessarily inert from the viewpoint of the toxicologist and physician. For example, in many agricultural sprays the chief toxic ingredient is often the "inert" vehicle, which is usually kerosene or one of the petroleum oils. Dusts and powders often consist in large measure of such "inert ingredients" as hydrated lime, calcium carbonate, gypsum, calcium phosphate, magnesium carbonate, bentonite, silica, diatomaceous earth, Fuller's earth, kaolin, walnut shell powder, redwood bark dust, and talc. Some of the liquid fumigants used in agriculture contain carbon tetrachloride as the "inert" solvent.
IODINE	5	Clinical estimates place iodine near the borderline between toxicity classes 4 and 5. (See also: IODINE, Reference Congener in Section III.)
IODIDE SALTS e.g., Sodium, potassium	3(?)	Iodide salts do not share the corrosive actions of free iodine, and no human fatalities are known after single oral doses of the common salts. Ten grams of NaI have been given slowly by the intravenous route without ill-effects. The usual manifestations of "iodism" are salivation, coryza, sneezing, conjunctivitis, headache, laryngitis, bronchitis, stomatitis, parotitis, and various skin rashes. Except for terminating the exposure, treatment is rarely required.
IODOFORM Tri-iodomethane	4	Best described as lying near the borderline between toxicity classes 4 and 5. Poisoning is often due to absorption through wounds when iodoform dressings are used (no more than 2 gm. iodoform should be so used). May cause dermatitis. Systemic effects include vomiting and all degrees of cerebral depression or excitation. A very rapid pulse is characteristic, with or without a slight fever. No useful antidote is recognized.
IPC Isopropyl-N- phenylcarbamate	3	Herbicide of low toxicity in laboratory animals. The human hazard is not well defined.
IRON SALTS Ferrous and ferric	3	In large doses soluble iron salts are corrosive irritants. (See also: FERROUS SULFATE, Reference Congener in Section III.)
ISOAMYL ALCOHOL 3-Methyl-1-butanol Fermentation amyl alcohol	4	Believed to lie near the borderline between toxicity classes 3 and 4. (See also: ALCOHOLS, HIGHER, Reference Congener in Section III.)
ISOAMYL SALICYLATE	4	Used in perfumery and soaps for its pleasant odor. The toxicity rating here is inferred from that of methyl salicylate. See methyl salicylate in this index. (See also: SALICYLATE, Reference Congener in Section III.)
ISOBORNYL THIOCYANOACETATE Thanite	3	Animal studies place this compound near the borderline between toxicity classes 3 and 4. (See also: ALIPHATIC THIOCYANATES, Reference Congener in Section III.)
ISOBUTYL ALCOHOL Fermentation butyl alcohol Isopropyl carbinol	3	Acute toxicity about three times that of ethyl alcohol. More irritating than ethyl but less so than amyl. (See also: ALCOHOLS, HIGHER, Reference Congener in Section III.)
ISODRIN Hexachloro- hexahydro- endo, endo- dimethanonaphthalene	5	Related to aldrin, but at least twice as toxic in laboratory rodents. (See also: DIELDRIN, Reference Congener in Section III.)
ISOLAN		Consult Addendum on p. 104.
ISOOCTYL DERIVATIVES		See corresponding "alkyl" derivative in this index. Probably approximately as toxic as the corresponding octyl derivatives.
ISOPESTOX Bis(isopropylamido)- fluorophosphate	4	An insecticide and acetylcholinesterase inhibitor, like parathion. After the acute phases of the poisoning, degenerative lesions may become apparent in the central and peripheral nervous systems. (See also: PARATHION, Reference Congener in Section III.)
ISOPROPYLACETONE Methyl isobutyl ketone 4-Methyl-2-pentanone	3(?)	Used as a solvent for cellulose lacquer. Similar to methyl ethyl ketone but probably more toxic. Gastroenteritis is expected to be the dominant symptom after ingestion, but central nervous depression may occur.
ISOPROPYL ALCOHOL 2-Propanol Petrohol	3	(See also: ISOPROPYL ALCOHOL, Reference Congener in Section III.)
ISOPROPYL CRESOL Carvacrol 2-Hydroxy-p-cymene	4	An isomer of thymol. Somewhat more toxic than thymol, at least in cats and rabbits. Same symptoms and treatment as phenol. (See also: PHENOL, Reference Congener in Section III.)

Substance and Synonym or Principal Ingredient	Toxicity Rating (See Inside Cover)	Comments and Reference Congeners
ISOPROPYL DERIVATIVES (Other than those listed here)		See corresponding "alkyl" derivative in the index. An exception is: 1-isopropyl-3-methylpyrazolyl-(5)-dimethylcarbamate, which is described in the addendum on p. 104.
ISOPROPYLMETHYL- PYRIMIDYL DIETHYL THIOPHOSPHATE Diazinone	4	Relatively new. Less toxic than most organic phosphate insecticides (oral mean lethal dose in rats is 100 to 150 mg./kg.) but a potent cholinesterase inhibitor. (See also: PARATHION, Reference Congener in Section III.)
ISOPROPYL-N-(3- CHLOROPHENYL) CARBAMATE Chloro-IPC	3	See isopropyl-N-phenylcarbamate below, which it closely resembles.
ISOPROPYL-N- PHENYLCARBAMATE IPC	3	Herbicide of moderately low lethality in laboratory animals. Human hazard is not well defined.
JIMSON WEED Stramonium Thorn apple Jamestown weed Dried leaves and flowering tops of Datura stramonium L.	4	Contains 0.25 to 0.45% alkaloids of the atropine-type (principally hyoscya- mine). Pharmacologically and toxicologically equivalent to belladonna leaf. (See also: ATROPINE, Reference Congener in Section III.)
JAVELLE WATER Solution of chlorinated potash	3(?)	When freshly prepared it contains about 2.5% active chlorine and is therefore about half as concentrated as the official N.F. solution of sodium hypo- chlorite. (See also: HYPOCHLORITE, Reference Congener in Section III.)
KAOLIN Hydrated aluminum silicate	1	Given by mouth in doses of 100 gm. several times a day as an absorbent for intestinal disorders. Inert except for the dangers of obstruction, perfora- tion, and granuloma formation. Cholera patients have been fed 600 gm. of kaolin (plus water) over a 12-hour period without ill-effects. Mice have been successfully fed diets containing 80% kaolin.
KARMEX W HERBICIDE CMU 3-(p-Chlorophenyl)- 1,1-dimethylurea	3	No skin irritation described. Repeated doses in rats produce anemia. Methemoglobinemia may occur.
KEROSENE OR KEROSINE Coal oil	3	Prepared by the fractional distillation of petroleum (boiling point range is about 175 to 275 or 325°C). Consists chiefly of C_{10}-C_{16} hydrocarbons of the methane series, together with a small fraction of aromatic compounds (xylenes etc.) and of saturated rings (naphthenes). (See also: KEROSENE, Reference Congener in Section III.)
LABARRAQUE'S SOLUTION Sodium hypochlorite	3(?)	An aqueous solution: 4 to 6% sodium hypochlorite, 4% sodium chloride, and 0.1 to 1.5% sodium hydroxide or carbonate. The lye contributes to the corrosive action when swallowed. A solution of approximately half the above strength is also described as "Labarraque's solution." (See also: HYPOCHLORITE, Reference Congener in Section III.)
LANATOSIDE(S) Digilanids Glycosides from the leaves of Digitalis lanata, called lanatosides or digilanids A,B, and C	6	Lanatoside C is more often used as a cardiotonic drug than A or B. It has all the therapeutic and toxic actions of digitalis leaf. Its actions are less persistent than those of digitoxin but more prolonged than those of strophanthin. A "digitalizing dose" of lanatoside C is 5 to 10 mg. orally (of which about one-tenth is absorbed); the daily maintenance dose is 0.25 to 1.0 mg. The acute lethal dose by mouth is probably 5 to 10 times that of digitoxin; in an average adult this means 15 to 50 mg. of lanatoside C or somewhat less of the usual lanatoside mixture (Digilanid). (See also: DIGITALIS, Reference Congener in Section III.)
LANOLIN Wool fat, hydrous (25 to 30% water) or anhydrous	1	Contains cholesterol esters of higher fatty acids and other higher alcohols (ceryl). Not absorbed from the alimentary tract.
LARKSPUR ALKALOIDS Delphinium. Crude alkaloids are usually prepared from the seed (or roots)		May be absorbed through skin when in solution, especially if skin is broken. Used since antiquity to treat body lice (ointment or fluidextract). As a poison it resembles aconite. Ingestion produces tingling or burning pain, nausea, vomiting, salivation, bradycardia, hypotension, collapse, incontinence of urine and feces, coma, and death. Treat symptomatically. Atropine may help.
LASSAR'S PASTE A mixture of zinc oxide (1 part), starch (1 part), and petrolatum (2 parts)	2(?)	The ingestion toxicity of zinc oxide is not well established, but probably it is low. If the oxide is appreciably soluble in gastric juice, vomiting and gastritis may be anticipated.

Substance and Synonym or Principal Ingredient	Toxicity Rating (See Inside Cover)	Comments and Reference Congeners
LAUDANUM Tincture of opium	4	A 10% solution of opium in alcohol, equivalent to about 1% morphine. Do not confuse with the much weaker Camporated Tincture of Opium (see Paregoric for the latter). (See also: MORPHINE, in Section III.)
LAURYL ALCOHOL Dodecyl alcohol 1-Dodecanol	2(?)	Thought to have a very low toxicity, but definitive studies were not located. (See also: ALCOHOLS, HIGHERS, Reference Congener in Section III.)
LAURYL OR LAUROYL DERIVATIVES (Other than listed here)		See corresponding "alkyl" derivative in this index.
LAURYL ISOQUINOLINIUM BROMIDE e.g., Isothan Q-15	4	A cationic surfactant which has a slightly greater acute toxicity in rats than benzalkonium chloride. No skin irritation or sensitization at use concentrations of 0.1% and lower. Used as in agricultural fungicide. (See also: QAC, Reference Congener in Section III.)
LAURYL THIOCYANATE Lauryl rhodanate Dodecyl thiocyanate	4(?)	Low toxicity in animals, but a human fatality has resulted from ingestion of a mixture of lauryl thiocyanate (14 gm.) and Lethane 384 (6 gm.). (See also: ALIPHATIC THIOCYANATES, Reference Congener in Section III.)
LEAD ARSENATE Lead acid arsenate or dibasic lead arsenate is approximately $PbHAsO_4$. "Basic lead arsenate" has an indefinite composition.	5	In a single dose, arsenic is a more powerful poison than lead. (See also: ARSENIC, Reference Congener in Section III.)
LEAD ARSENITE	5	More toxic and corrosive than lead arsenate. (See also: ARSENIC, Reference Congener in Section III.)
LEAD CHROMATE Chrome yellow Basic lead chromate is known as chrome red.	4	Insoluble in water and dilute acid but appreciably soluble in gastric juice. Said to have a distinctly higher acute toxicity than most lead salts, presumably because the acute reaction is largely that of chromate poisoning (see chromic acid). Signs of chronic lead poisoning, however, may appear days or weeks after the acute reaction. (See also: LEAD, Reference Congener in Section III.)
LEAD SALTS		Most lead compounds lie in toxicity classes 3 or 4. (See also: LEAD, Reference Congener in Section III.)
LETHANE 60 β-Thiocyanoethyl esters of fatty acids	2	(See also: ALIPHATIC THIOCYANATES, Reference Congener in Section III.)
LETHANE 384 β-Butoxy-β^Lthiocyano diethyl ether	4	Can be absorbed through intact skin. (See also: ALIPHATIC THIOCYANATES, Reference Congener in Section III.)
LIGROIN Refined solvent naphtha	3	A petroleum distillate fraction like petroleum ether but with a higher boiling point range (130 to 155° C). Similiar to but of more uniform composition than high-boiling petroleum ether (or tech. benzin). (See also: KEROSENE, Reference Congener in Section III.)
LIME, SLAKED AND UNSLAKED		Unslaked lime (quicklime) is calcium oxide (CaO); reacts with water with the evolution of heat, to form calcium hydroxide (Ca(OH)2). This reaction on the skin or in the mouth produces both a thermal and caustic burn. Slaked lime (calcium hydroxide) is a simple alkali; because of low solubility its aqueous solutions are not corrosive. (See also: ALKALI, Reference Congener in Section III.)
LIME SULFUR Calcium polysulfides		An irritant and sensitizing agent. It may decompose into hydrogen sulfide before or after ingestion. Used in agriculture as an insecticide and fungicide. (See also: HYDROGEN SULFIDE, Reference Congener in Section III.)
LIMONENE Dipentene	3(?)	One of the terpene hydrocarbons found in turpentine. A major constituent in oils of orange, lemon, caraway, dill, bergamot, and pine needle. No toxic reactions have been described other than mild local irritation and skin sensitization, but albuminuria and hematuria are probable if ingested in sufficient quantity. (See also: TURPENTINE, Reference Congener in Section III.)
LINDANE Gamma isomer of hexachlorocyclohexane ("benzene hexachloride")	4	(See also: BENZENE HEXACHLORIDE, Reference Congener in Section III.)
LINOLEYL DERIVATIVE		See corresponding "alkyl" derivative in this index.

Substance and Synonym or Principal Ingredient	Toxicity Rating (See Inside Cover)	Comments and Reference Congeners

LINSEED OIL
  Flaxseed oil
  Glycerides of linoleic
    oleic, stearic,
    palmitic, and myristic
    acids
	1	A drying oil used in paints, etc. Digestible and nutritious, but it has a disagreeable taste. Large doses (over 1 oz.) are laxative. Boiled linseed oil (e.g., treated with a drier and heated to enhance the oil's ability to react with oxygen and form a hard film) is more dangerous and should never be taken internally, because lead or other toxic elements (e.g., manganese, cobalt) have usually been added.

LITHIUM SALTS	3(?)	Toxic on chronic administration with restricted salt (sodium chloride) diets, but a sodium deficiency was at least partly responsible for the toxic symptoms: drowsiness, weakness, anorexia, nausea, tremors, blurring of vision, coma, and death. A gastroenteritis is described in animals. Acute poisoning in man is reported after 4 doses of 2 gm. each of lithium chloride, causing weakness, prostration, vertigo, tinnitus.

LITHOPONE
  Mixture of zinc sulfide,
    barium sulfate, and
    zinc oxide
	3(?)	If gastric acidity is high, hydrogen sulfide may be formed. (See also: HYDROGEN SULFIDE, Reference Congener in Section III.).

LOBELINE (And its
    salts)
  The chief alkaloidal
    constituent of the
    herb Lobelia inflata
	5(?)	An emetic and expectorant. As with nicotine, central nervous stimulation is followed by severe depression. (See also: NICOTINE, Reference Congener in Section III.)

LYE
  Any strong alkali,
    usually sodium or
    potassium hydroxide
    or carbonate
		A corrosive poison. (See also: ALKALI, Reference Congener in Section III.)

LYSOL
  Lysol Brand
    Disinfectant, a
    registered trade name
    for a popular germicide
	2	According to the manufacturer the current product consists of 7% ethyl alcohol, less than 2% cresylic acid, and unspecified concentrations of o-hydroxydiphenyl and soap. Four ounces of full-strength Lysol have been swallowed by a man without serious ill-effects, and the estimated lethal dose is over a pint. (See also: PHENOL, Reference Congener in Section III.)

MAGNESIUM SALTS
  e.g., Chloride, citrate,
    hydroxide, oxide,
    phosphate, sulfate
	3(?)	Generally magnesium salts are so slowly absorbed that oral administration causes nothing more than purging. If evacuation fails to occur (bowel obstruction or atony), mucosal irritation and absorption occur. Systemically Mg^{++} produces central nervous depression, abolition of reflexes, and death from respiratory paralysis. Intravenous calcium chloride (10 to 20 cc. of 5% solution, diluted if desirable with isotonic saline) counteracts these toxic actions of magnesium. Also physostigmine 0.5 to 1.0 mg. subcutaneously. Use artificial respiration (See Section IV).

MALATHION
  O,O-Dimethyl
    dithiophosphate of
    diethyl mercapto
    succinate
  Malathon
	4	The only organic phosphate insecticide approved (1955) for household use. Relatively low mammalian toxicity (on the borderline between toxicity classes 3 and 4) and low anti-cholinesterase potency, but experimental poisonings resemble parathion. Small but significant percutaneous toxicity in rabbits. (See also: PARATHION, Reference Congener in Section III.)

MALEIC HYDRAZIDE
  1,2-Dihydropyridazine-
    3,6-dione and its
    salts (sodium and
    diethanolamine)
  MH
	3	A growth inhibitor of plants. In animals it causes tremors and muscle spasms. No effect on the skin, except possible sensitization.

MANGANESE SALTS
  (Inorg.)
  Manganous and
    Manganic
  e.g., Manganese sulfate
	3(?)	Because manganese salts are poorly absorbed from the alimentary tract, acute systemic intoxication does not occur after ingestion. (Acute reactions after permanganate are due to local tissue injury from intense oxidation). Systemic poisoning, however, may occur from chronic ingestion or inhalation. As seen after industrial exposures to dusts, nervous symptoms predominate: mask-like facial expression, spastic gait, tremors, slurred speech, fatigability, and insomnia. Treated with scopolamine and amphetamine. Because calcium blood levels are often depressed, large doses of calcium salts are given by mouth.

MANGANESE ETHYLENE
  BIS-DITHIOCARBAMATE
  Maneb
  Manzate
	3	Some irritation to skin, nose, and throat. In animal tests its oral toxicity places it near the borderline between toxicity classes 2 and 3.

MCP or MCPA
  Methyl chlorophenoxy
    acetic acid
	3	Slightly less toxic than 2,4-D. (See also: 2,4-D, Reference Congener in Section III.)

Substance and Synonym or Principal Ingredient	Toxicity Rating (See Inside Cover)	Comments and Reference Congeners
MENTHOL Hexahydrothymol 3-p-Menthanol	4	Obtained principally from oil of peppermint (about 50% menthol). Ingestion causes severe abdominal pain, nausea, vomiting, vertigo, ataxia, drowsiness, and coma. (See also: TURPENTINE, Reference Congener in Section III.)
MERCURIC CHLORIDE Bichloride of mercury	5	Very dangerous by all portals. Act fast! (See also: MERCURY, Reference Congener in Section III.)
MERCUROUS CHLORIDE Calomel	5	Rarely causes systemic mercury poisoning. An irritant cathartic or purgative when ingested. If retained, 30 to 40 mg./kg. may be fatal. Rarely "calomel sickness" appears after a latency of about one week; it is a benign reaction characterized by fever and rash (scarlatinal or urticarial). (See also: MERCURY, Reference Congener in Section III.)
MERCURY COMPOUNDS Organic and inorganic		In general, toxicity depends upon release of the mercuric ion. (See also: MERCURY, Reference Congener in Section III.)
MERCURY OXYCYANIDE The commercial salt is often a mixture of the oxycyanide (1/3) and the cyanide (2/3), to reduce danger of explosion.	5	Symptoms both of mercury and of cyanide poisoning have been described, but at least in dogs the mercury effects have proved more important. It is probable that in man cyanide poisoning appears first, especially if the free gastric acidity is high (stomach empty of food). (See also: MERCURY, Reference Congener in Section III.)
MERPHENYL COMPOUNDS		See corresponding phenylmercuric compound in this index.
MESITYL OXIDE Iso-butenyl ketone Isopropylidenacetone		Inhaled vapor causes progressive, generalized central nervous depression. The vapor is also a moderately strong irritant to conjunctivae and mucous membranes.
METALDEHYDE m-Acetaldehyde Metacetaldehyde "Meta"	4	Probably lies near the borderline between toxicity classes 3 and 4. Used to kill snails and as a dry fuel. After a time lag of 1 to 3 hours, ingestion is followed by severe abdominal pain, nausea, vomiting, diarrhea, a marked rise in body temperature, convulsions, and coma. If death is delayed, renal tubular injury and liver necrosis may appear. Only symptomatic and supportive measures are available.
METAL FUMES		Under intense heat some metals (notably zinc, copper, cadmium, lead, mercury, tin, nickel) may volatilize and burn to finely divided air-borne particles of metal oxide. Inhalation of freshly-formed fumes may produce an influenzal-like illness called "metal fume fever" (also "brass founders' ague," etc.). Signs and symptoms include chills, fever, malaise, generalized aches, dry cough, and sometimes nausea and vomiting. Typically the disease has an acute onset and short duration; permanent damage is rare. Zinc is most commonly responsible and is probably the most benign; fumes of cadmium, lead, and mercury may cause significant systemic poisoning. Treatment is usually symptomatic, although in some cases BAL may be useful (See cadmium, in Section III).
METALLIC SULFIDES Especially alkaline sulfides (sodium, potassium, calcium, etc.)	4	If free gastric acidity is high, the ingestion of these salts may result in their decomposition to hydrogen sulfide in the stomach, with subsequent systemic poisoning. In any case the alkaline sulfides are strong local irritants to mucous membrane (and skin). Treatment: gastric lavage, demulcents, saline cathartic, plus measures outlined under hydrogen sulfide. (See also: HYDROGEN SULFIDE, Reference Congener in Section III.)
METHENAMINE Hexamethylenetetramine	3(?)	Slowly decomposes into formaldehyde, especially in an acid medium (e.g., stomach, urine). A very large oral dose (usual doses are 1 to 2 gm.) causes gastrointestinal irritation (vomiting and pain), albuminuria, gross hematuria, and dysuria, with inflammatory lesions in the renal tubules, renal pelves, and urinary bladder. Repeated use may cause sensitization with urticaria or dermatitis. (See also: FORMALDEHYDE, Reference Congener in Section III.)
METHOXYCHLOR Methoxy-DDT 1,1,1-Trichloro- 2,2-bis(p-methoxy-phenyl) ethane	3	Lower toxicity than DDT. Estimated to be one-tenth as toxic in man by ingestion, but this difference may not hold in respiratory exposures to vapor. In animals central nervous depression is more prominent than excitation, and poisonings are slower in onset and longer in duration than after DDT. (See also: DDT, Reference Congener in Section III.)
METHOXYETHYL-MERCURIACETATE	5	One of several organic mercury compounds used in agriculture as fungicides and seed protectants. (See also: MERCURY, Reference Congener in Section III.)
METHYL ABIETATE Abalyn		Probably low toxicity. See abietic acid in this index.

Substance and Synonym or Principal Ingredient	Toxicity Rating (See Inside Cover)	Comments and Reference Congeners
METHYL ALCOHOL Methanol Wood alcohol	3	(See also: METHYL ALCOHOL, Reference Congener in Section III.)
p-METHYLAMINO-PHENOL SULFATE (OR HYDROCHLORIDE) e.g., Photol Metol	4	Photographic developer, sometimes used in hair dyes. Effects from ingestion by humans are not well established. Deaths from 5 to 15 gm. of mixed metol and hydroquinone, with symptoms like phenol and aniline poisonings. Question of hemolytic anemia is not clear because of possible confusion with phenolic pigments. (See also: PHENOL and ANILINE, Reference Congeners in Section III.)
METHYLATED NAPHTHALENE	3(?)	Presumably less toxic than naphthalene. The only untoward effects reported in man are skin irritation and skin photosensitization. (See also: NAPHTHALENE, Reference Congener in Section III.)
METHYL BROMIDE Monobromomethane	4	(See also: METHYL BROMIDE, Reference Congener in Section III.)
METHYL CELLOSOLVE Ethylene glycol monomethyl ether	3	About the same toxicity as the ethyl analogue (=Cellosolve). Consult "Cellosolves" in this index for a brief comparison with ethylene glycol. (See also: EHTYLENE GLYCOL, Reference Congener in Section III.)
METHYL CELLOSOLVE ACETATE Ethylene glycol mono-methyl ether acetate	3	Slightly less toxic (in animals) than the ether itself. The ester is apparently saponified in vivo, but the ether linkage is stable. About twice as toxic as ethylene glycol but toxic effects are similar. (See also: ETHYLENE GLYCOL, Reference Congener in Section III.)
METHYL CELLULOSE e.g., Methocel	1	Biologically inert aside from mechanical actions. Not absorbed from the bowel. Used as an emulsifying agent, protective colloid, and bulk cathartic.
METHYL CHLORIDE Monochloromethane		A vapor of moderately high toxicity. Rapidly hydrolyzed to hydrochloric acid and methyl alcohol. Signs and symptoms are typical of the latter. Central nervous effects may be irreversible. Persistent post-recovery symptoms include headache, nervousness, insomnia, and intention tremor. (See also: METHYL ALCOHOL, Reference Congener in Section III.)
METHYL CHLORO-PHENOXY ACETIC ACID 2-Methyl-4-chloro-phenoxyacetic acid MCP	3	Slightly less toxic than 2,4-D. (See also: 2,4-D, Reference Congener in Section III.)
METHYLCYCLOHEXANE Hexahydrotoluene Cyclohexylmethane	3(?)	Vapor causes brief central nervous depression like cyclohexane. Oral dose in rabbits causes only mild lethargy, severe diarrhea, and circulatory collapse. Vascular and degenerative lesions are seen in kidney and liver. Perhaps slightly more toxic than cyclohexane by mouth. No systemic poisonings reported in man.
METHYLENE CHLORIDE Dichloromethane	3	One of the least toxic chlorinated hydrocarbons, but it may produce central nervous depression. (See also: CARBON TETRACHLORIDE, Reference Congener in Section III.)
2,2'-METHYLENE-BIS(4-CHLOROPHENOL) Bis(5-chloro-2-hydroxy-phenyl) methane Dichlorophene	3	Moderately low ingestion toxicity in dogs and guinea pigs. A concentration of 1% is not irritating to human skin (occasional irritation at 4%). (See also: PHENOL, Reference Congener in Section III.)

Substance and Synonym or Principal Ingredient	Toxicity Rating (See Inside Cover)	Comments and Reference Congeners
2,2'-METHYLENE BIS (3,4,6-TRICHLORO-PHENOL) Hexachlorophene G-11	3	Used in concentrations of 1 to 2% as a disinfectant in several liquid and solid soap products. Not irritating to the skin, but sensitization has been reported. Systemic effects presumably resemble those of phenol. No poisonings known in man. (See also: PHENOL, Reference Congener in Section III.)
METHYL ETHYL KETONE 2-Butanone	3	Similar to but more irritating than acetone. Vapor is irritating to mucous membranes and conjunctiva. Central nerve depression in experimental animals, but irritating odor ordinarily prevents significant clinical exposures. No serious poisonings reported in man, except for dermatitis.
METHYL FORMATE	3(?)	Vapor produces irritation of mucous membranes and central nervous depression. More toxic than methyl acetate. Symptoms resemble methyl alcohol poisoning. (See also: METHYL ALCOHOL, Reference Congener in Section III.)
METHYL ISOBUTYL KETONE Isopropylacetone	3(?)	Used as a solvent for cellulose lacquer. Similar to methyl ethyl ketone but probably more toxic. Gastroenteritis is expected to be the dominant disorder after ingestion, but central nervous depression may occur.
METHYL p-HYDROXY-BENZOATE Methyl parasept Methylparaben		Not toxic in the small amounts found in most commercial products (0.05 to 0.2%), where it serves as a preservative and antiseptic. Said to be less toxic than salicylic acid and its derivatives.
METHYLMERCURIC DICYANODIAMINE (or -CYANOGUANIDINE) Cyano (methylmercuri) guanidine	5	Perhaps slightly less toxic than other organic mercury compounds commonly used in agriculture. Because of its lower vapor pressure, less hazardous than others by inhalation. By the intraperitoneal route in mice, acute toxicity is half that of mercuric bichloride. (See also: MERCURY, Reference Congener in Section III.)
METHYL PARATHION Dimethyl parathion Dimethyl-O-p-nitrophenyl thiophosphate	5	Slightly less toxic to rats than parathion but a much less potent cholinesterase inhibitor. Used principally in combination with parathion. (See also: PARATHION, Reference Congener in Section III.)
METHYL PHENOL Cresol Hydroxytoluene Three isomers (o-, m-, p-) are usually present as a mixture.	4	About the same toxicity and toxic actions as phenol. Meta isomer is less toxic than phenol but ortho and para derivatives are more so. The mixed isomers may be slightly more corrosive than phenol, but systemic effects are perhaps a little milder because of slower absorption. (See also: PHENOL, Reference Congener in Section III.)
3-METHYL-1-PHENYL-PYRAZOLYL-(5)-DIMETHYLCARBAMATE Pyrolan	5	A relatively new insecticide. In laboratory rodents it lies near the borderline between toxicity classes 4 and 5. Toxic signs and symptoms are not described but presumably resemble those of parathion poisoning, since Pyrolan is a reversible inhibitor of the enzyme cholinesterase and is related to neostigmine. No clinical data. (See also: PARATHION, Reference Congener in Section III.)
METHYLROSANILINE CHLORIDE Gentian violet	4(?)	Used medicinally as an intestinal anthelmintic. Ingestion causes nausea, vomiting, diarrhea, and abdominal pain, sometimes even in therapeutic doses (0.06 gm. t.i.d.). Systemic toxicity is not well defined, but kidney and liver diseases are traditional contraindications to this drug. No severe poisonings have been reported in man.
METHYL SALICYLATE Oil of wintergreen Sweet birch oil Gaultheria oil Betula oil	4	A strong irritant to skin and mucous membranes. Used externally as a counter-irritant. May be absorbed rapidly through intact skin. Bowel absorption is somewhat erratic, and gastric lavage may be beneficial even several hours after ingestion. Absorbed at least in part as the intact ester and small amounts are even excreted as such by the kidneys, but the compound is largely hydrolyzed. Typical systemic effects of salicylate and not of methyl alcohol, but probably more toxic than sodium salicylate. (See also: SALICYLATE, Reference Congener in Section III.)
METOL p-Methylaminophenol sulfate	4	Photographic developer, sometimes used in hair dyes. Effects from ingestion by humans are not well established. Deaths from 5 to 15 gm. of mixed metol and hydroquinone, with symptoms like phenol and like aniline poisonings. Question of hemolytic anemia is not clear because of possible confusion with phenolic pigments. (See also: PHENOL and ANILINE, Reference Congeners in Section III.)
MGK N-Octyl bicycloheptene dicarboximide	3	Insecticide synergist of low toxicity. Not irritating to human skin. In animal tests it has produced hyperexcitability followed by central nervous depression. Treat symptomatically.
MINERAL SPIRITS One of the petroleum naphtha fractions, like Stoddard solvent	3	A petroleum "cut" distilling between approx. 150 and 200° C., consisting chiefly of C_8 to C_{12} aliphatic hydrocarbons. Widely employed as a paint thinner, metal cleaner, etc. (See also: KEROSENE, Reference Congener in Section III.)

Substance and Synonym or Principal Ingredient	Toxicity Rating (See Inside Cover)	Comments and Reference Congeners
MIRBANE, ESSENCE OF OR OIL OF Nitrobenzene	5	Toxic by all routes including skin absorption. Mean lethal dose by mouth probably lies between 1 and 5 gm. Systemic effects may be delayed a few hours. Poisoning closely resembles that due to aniline. Ethyl alcohol aggravates intoxication. Because of bitter almond odor, cyanide poisoning may be suspected, but cyanide acts much faster. (See also: ANILINE, Reference Congener in Section III.)
MONO-		If the compound is not listed here, omit the prefix and try again.
MONOACETIN Acetin Glyceryl monoacetate (usually contaminated with glycerine)	1	Largely (but not completely) hydrolyzed in bowel to glycerine and acetic acid. May produce a systemic acidosis. Subcutaneous and intramuscular injections in laboratory animals (including monkeys) are followed by vasodilatation, central nervous depression, and death from respiratory failure (mean lethal intramuscular dose 1 to 5 gm./kg.).
MONOBUTYL BIPHENYL SODIUM MONOSULFONATE Aresket	3	An anionic surface-active agent used in insecticide sprays. One of the general category of alkyl aryl sodium sulfonates. See latter in this index.
MONOBUTYL PHENYL PHENOL SODIUM MONOSULFONATE Areskap	3	An anionic surface-active agent used in insecticide sprays, embalming fluids, etc. One of the general category of alkyl aryl sodium sulfonates. See latter in this index.
MONOCHLORODIFLUORO-METHANE Freon 22		A gas of low toxicity, but very high concentrations are not entirely inert. Possible lung injury. See also Freons in this index.
MONOCHLOROMETHANE Methyl chloride		A vapor of moderately high toxicity. Rapidly hydrolyzed to hydrochloric acid and methyl alcohol. Signs and symptoms are typical of the latter. Central nervous effects may be irreversible. Persistent post-recovery symptoms include headache, nervousness, insomnia, and intention tremor. (See also: METHYL ALCOHOL, Reference Congener in Section III.)
MONOFLUOROACETATE SALTS e.g., Sodium fluoro-acetate	6	A delayed convulsant. Actions unlike those of fluorides. (See also: FLUOROACETATE, Reference Congener in Section III.)
MONOMETHYL-PARA-AMINOPHENOL SULFATE p-Methylaminophenol sulfate Photol Metol	4	A photographic developer; sometimes used in hair dyes. Effects from ingestion by humans are not well established. Deaths from 5 to 15 gm. of mixed metol and hydroquinone, with symptoms like phenol and aniline poisonings. Question of hemolytic anemia is not clear because of possible confusion with phenolic pigments. (See also: PHENOL and ANILINE, Reference Congeners in Section III.)
MONSEL'S SALT Ferric subsulfate Basic ferric sulfate Approx. formula: $Fe_4(SO_4)_5(OH)_2 \cdot H_2O$	3	Monsel's solution is a nearly saturated aqueous solution of this salt; it is prepared by mixing and boiling ferrous sulfate with sulfuric and nitric acids. This solution, which contains 20 to 22% iron, is used externally as a styptic. (See also: FERROUS SULFATE, Reference Congener in Section III.)
MORPHINE Morphia Morphium	5	(See also: MORPHINE, Reference Congener in Section III.)
MORPHOLINE Tetrahydro-1, 4, 2H-oxazine Diethylenimide oxide	4	A secondary amine used as a corrosion inhibitor, as an antioxidant, and, in the form of salts, as an emulsifying agent. Strongly alkaline. Liquid and vapor are irritating to skin and mucous membranes. In rats pulmonary edema, liver necrosis, and renal tubular degeneration, but only at vapor concs. which are intensely irritating. Moderately high percutaneous toxicity in rabbits. On the skin the liquid may produce necrosis.
MURIATIC ACID Hydrochloric acid An aqueous solution of hydrogen chloride gas, usually marketed in concentrations of about 38, 32, and 10%		(See also: ACID, Reference Congener in Section III.)
MUSCARINE A derivative of choline and the active toxic principle of the poisonous fly mushroom Amanita muscaria		Toxic actions resemble those of pilocarpine, physostigmine, arecoline, and parathion. (See also: AMANITA TOXINS, Reference Congener in Section III.)

Substance and Synonym or Principal Ingredient	Toxicity Rating (See Inside Cover)	Comments and Reference Congeners
MUSHROOMS, POISONOUS	3 or 4	In the U. S. A. most deaths are due to the ingestion of 3 species: Amanita phalloides, A. verna, and A. virosa. (See also: AMANITA TOXINS, Reference Congener in Section III.)
MYRISTYL ALCOHOL Tetradecyl alcohol	2(?)	Thought to have a very low toxicity, but definitive studies have not been located. (See also: ALCOHOLS, HIGHER, Reference Congener in Section III.)
MYRISTYL DERIVATIVE (Other than listed here)		See corresponding "alkyl" derivative in this index.
NABAM Disodium ethylene-bis-dithiocarbamate	3	Central nervous depression in animals. Oils increase absorption and toxicity. Mild skin irritation. Alcohol is best avoided after exposures to nabam because some dithiocarbamates are known to induce acetaldehyde poisoning when ethyl alcohol is metabolized (as does Antabuse). For the alcohol-Antabuse reaction, see Disulfiram in Section III.
NAPHTHA Petroleum naphtha	3	A low-boiling fraction obtained from the distillation of petroleum, consisting chiefly of aliphatic hydrocarbons of the methane series, like kerosene. Note: solvent naphtha or aromatic solvent naphtha is an entirely different product, obtained from coal tar and consisting of xylenes and related compounds (see xylene, Sec. III). (See also: KEROSENE, Reference Congener in Section III.)
NAPHTHALENE Naphthene	4	(See also: NAPHTHALENE, Reference Congener in Section III.)
NAPHTHALENE ACETIC ACID 1-Naphthalene acetic acid Alpha-naphthalene acetic acid (and its esters, e.g., methyl)	3	A synthetic plant hormone. In animals it produces gastroenteritis and central nervous depression. Slight to moderate irritation of rabbit skin after prolonged contact (not so the methyl ester). The dust may cause nasal irritation.
NAPHTHALENES, CHLORINATED e.g., Halowax		Acneform rash and liver necrosis from exposure to vapor. Ingestion toxicity is not known, but presumably it increases with the degree of chlorination. The principal cause of hyperkeratosis in cattle. Less toxic than chlorinated diphenyls.
NAPHTHENES Sometimes used as a synonym of naphthalene but not usually in industry or commerce.		In petroleum industry "naphthenes" mean saturated (or nearly saturated) cyclic hydrocarbons—like methyl-substituted cyclohexanes, etc. Small quantities are found in most of the aliphatic petroleum fractions (like kerosene) but much more is present in aromatic fractions (like crude xylol). Because they are rarely (if ever) prepared free from benzene, etc., the toxicity of petroleum naphthenes is unknown, but cycloparaffins, in general, are central nervous depressants.
β-NAPHTHOL Beta-naphthol β-Hydroxynaphthalene	4	Produces crampy abdominal pain, nausea, vomiting, and sometimes convulsions. Intestinal or percutaneous absorption may lead to a severe nephritis, liver injury, or an acute hemolytic anemia. Lens opacities and retinal changes have been described. Alpha isomer is said to be even more toxic. (See also: PHENOL, Reference Congener in Section III.)
N-1-NAPHTHYL PHTHAMIC ACID AND SODIUM SALT Alanap-1 The sodium salt is available in solution (Alanap-3)	3	A herbicide of low acute toxicity in rats. The free acid (Alanap-1) is particularly benign when ingested (toxicity rating 2). No skin irritation described in man or animals.
N-1-NAPHTHYL PHTHALIMIDE Alanap-2		An experimental herbicide. No toxicity data were located.
NAPHTHENIC ACIDS		In commerce this is the name of acidic petroleum fractions, consisting of cyclic carboxylic acids extractable from kerosene and oil. Cyclopentane carboxylic acid and cyclohexane carboxylic acid are included but most of the molecules are larger (e.g., methyl derivatives and multiple saturated rings). No specific toxicity information is available despite long and widespread use. Crude acids have unpleasant odors but not if purified. Cycloparaffins (like cyclopentanes and cyclohexanes) are central nervous depressants, and the potency is greater the higher the molecular weight. Perhaps the same is true of the naphthenic acids.
1-(1-NAPHTHYL)-2-THIOUREA Antu	3(?)	(See also: ANTU, Reference Congener in Section III.)

Substance and Synonym or Principal Ingredient	Toxicity Rating (See Inside Cover)	Comments and Reference Congeners
NEATSFOOT OIL Prepared by boiling ox feet, yielding the glycerides of oleic and palmitic acids	1	Used as a lubricant and to waterproof and soften leather. Consists of harmless and digestible fats which are found in normal diets.
NEONICOTINE Anabasine 3-(2-Piperidyl) pyridine	6	Toxic actions are like nicotine, but toxicity is about one-third to one-fifth that of nicotine. Cheaper than the latter as an insecticide. (See also: NICOTINE, Reference Congener in Section III.)
NEOTRAN A wettable powder with 40% bis (parachlorophenoxy) methane	2	A miticide of very low toxicity in laboratory mammals. Only slight percutaneous absorption and no skin irritation. It has produced liver pathology in laboratory animals. No human poisonings are known. (See also: DDT, Reference Congener in Section III.)
NICKEL SALTS	4(?)	Partly because of local astringent and irritant actions, nickel salts act as emetics when swallowed (but also by other routes). As with other irritant-emetics, the lethal dose is presumed to vary widely. Absorption from the bowel is poor and systemic poisoning is rare. Systemic effects include capillary damage (especially in brain and adrenals), renal injury, myocardial weakness, and central nervous depression. Pulmonary effects are predominant after a respiratory exposure to gaseous nickel carbonyl. (See also: COPPER, Reference Congener in Section III.)
NICOTINE (And its Salts) 1-Methyl-2-(3-pyridyl) pyrrolidine	6	The probable lethal dose by ingestion is about 0.6 to 0.9 mg./kg. in man. (See also: NICOTINE, Reference Congener in Section III.)
NITRATE SALTS e.g., Sodium nitrate	3	Nitrate salts as such are no more toxic than other neutral salts, but if not promptly absorbed, they may be reduced to nitrites by bacteria in the bowel. (See also: NITRITE, Reference Congener in Section III.)
NITRIC ACID Aqua fortis Commercial nitric acids contain 68% and 56% HNO_3 in water		(See also: ACID, Reference Congener in Section III.)
NITRILE DERIVATIVES Cyano organic compounds		Many organic nitriles (or cyanides) are decomposed in the body to yield highly toxic cyanide (CN^- or HCN). (See also: CYANIDE, Reference Congener in Section III.)
NITRITE SALTS e.g., Sodium nitrite	4	Toxicity rating of 4 describes animal studies, but no adequate clinical data were located. (See also: NITRITE, Reference Congener in Section III.)
NITROANILINE Nitraniline p-Nitroaniline	5(?)	More toxic than aniline and probably more toxic than nitrobenzene. (See also: ANILINE, Reference Congener in Section III.)
NITROBENZENE Essence of or oil of mirbane	5	Toxic by all routes including skin absorption. Mean lethal dose by mouth probably lies between 1 and 5 gm. Systemic effects may be delayed a few hours. Poisoning closely resembles that due to aniline. Ethyl alcohol aggravates intoxication. Because of bitter almond odor, cyanide poisoning may be suspected, but cyanide acts much faster. (See also: ANILINE, Reference Congener in Section III.)
2-NITRO-1,1-BIS(p-CHLOROPHENYL)-BUTANE OR-PROPANE Dilan	3	Probably lies near the borderline between toxicity classes 3 and 4. Same symptoms and treatment as DDT. Can be absorbed through intact skin but probably not in significant amounts. (See also: DDT, Reference Congener in Section III.)
NITROCHLOROBENZENE Usually a mixture of 3 isomeric forms	5(?)	Severe allergic dermatitis frequently after skin contact. Less toxic than dinitrochlorobenzene. Systemic effects are like aniline (methemoglobin) but perhaps cardiac disorders are more severe. Avoid ingestion of ethyl alcohol, which aggravates the intoxication. (See also: ANILINE, Reference Congener in Section III.)
NITROGLYCERINE Nitroglycerol Glyceryl trinitrate	6	A fast-acting and much more potent drug than sodium nitrite (100-fold difference in therapeutic doses); this can be explained only partially by rates of absorption since the fatal intravenous doses in rabbits differ by a factor of at least 2 (expressed as nitrite equivalents). In man more potent when absorbed from the mouth (e.g., sublingual) than when swallowed. Can be absorbed through intact skin. (See also: NITRITE, Reference Congener in Section III.)
NITROMETHANE e.g., Nitrocarbol	3	Mildly irritating to skin and mucous membrane. Less toxic than nitropropane. See nitropropane in this index.

Substance and Synonym or Principal Ingredient	Toxicity Rating (See Inside Cover)	Comments and Reference Congeners
NITROPHENIDE Bis(m-nitrophenyl) disulfide m, m'-Dinitrodiphenyl disulfide		An anticoccidial agent used in veterinary medicine. No human poisonings are known, but dogs which were unintentionally fed nitrophenide in cereal developed a non-fatal illness lasting a week and characterized by ataxia, vertigo, nystagmus, mydriasis, and opisthotonus.
ρ-NITROPHENOL Paranitrophenol	4	A fungicide. Poisonings are assumed to resemble both phenol and aniline. (See also: PHENOL and ANILINE, Reference Congeners in Section III.)
NITROPROPANE 2-Nitropropane	3	Tested in rabbits, it lies near the borderline between toxicity classes 3 and 4. Slightly more toxic than nitromethane or nitroethane. Mildly irritating to mucous membranes but not skin. Reactions described in men exposed to vapor include anorexia, nausea, vomiting, diarrhea, and severe occipital headaches. In several species of animals, high vapor concentrations have produced weakness, ataxia, dyspnea, cyanosis, coma and death (with a few terminal convulsions). In cats and probably other species, these symptoms are partially due to methemoglobinemia caused by the metabolic breakdown of nitropropane into nitrite ions (also true of other nitroparaffins). (See also: NITRITE, Reference Congener in Section III.)
NITROPRUSSIDE SALTS e.g., Sodium nitro-prusside Nitroprussiates Nitroferricyanides	4(?)	Decomposes, especially in alkaline medium, to nitrite ion. Ingestion causes a prompt and sustained fall in blood pressure. Cyanide poisoning from this salt has not been demonstrated and probably never occurs. (See also: NITRITE, Reference Congener in Section III.)
NMRI-448 A mixture of 2 liquids: 2-phenyl cyclohexanol (70%) 2-cyclohexylcyclohexanol 30%	3	An insect repellent for the skin. No clinical data. Symptoms in poisoned animals were not reported, but probably central nervous depression was prominent. Chronic application to rabbit skin (90 days) caused skin necrosis, bone marrow lesions, sometimes adrenal hemorrhage, and perhaps testicular atrophy.
NONYL DERIVATIVE		See corresponding "alkyl" derivative in this index.
NORNICOTINE 2-(3'-Pyridyl) pyrrolidine	6	About one third as toxic as nicotine. (See also: NICOTINE, Reference Congener in Section III.)
NUX VOMICA Dried ripe seeds of Strychnos nux-vomica, containing 1.1 to 1.4% (rarely 2%) strychnine and about an equal amount of brucine	4	The tincture is a 10% solution in 70% alcohol (strychnine conc. 0.12%), and the probable lethal dose is 3 oz. Nux vomica fluidextract (N.F.) is 1.0 to 1.2% strychnine (1.5% in British Pharmacopeia), and the dried powdered extract is 7 to 7.7% strychnine. (See also: STRYCHNINE, Reference Congener in Section III.)
OCTACHLOROCAMPHENE Toxaphene	4	Believed to lie near the borderline between toxicity classes 4 and 5. (See also: TOXAPHENE, Reference Congener in Section III.)
OCTACHLOROCYCLO-HEXENONE Oktane is a 40% solution in petroleum oil.		A herbicide and fungicide. The only known toxicity data (from a preliminary screening test) indicate a mean lethal dose of about 100 mg./kg. in mice, when injected daily for 7 successive days.
OCTACHLORODIHYDRO-DICYCLOPENTADIENE Chlordane	4	Probably chlordane is best described as lying on the borderline between toxicity classes 3 and 4. (See also: CHLORDANE, Reference Congener in Section III.)
OCTACHLORO-4,7-METHANO-TETRA-HYDROINDANE Chlordane	4	See above. (See also: CHLORDANE, Reference Congener in Section III.)
OCTADECYL DERIVA-TIVES		See corresponding "alkyl" derivative in this index.
OCTAMETHYL PYRO-PHOSPHORAMIDE Schradan	5	A "systemic" insecticide, i.e., translocated in sap to all parts of plants. Only slightly less toxic than parathion. Not a cholinesterase inhibitor in vitro, but converted to one by liver. Brain cholinesterase, however, is not inhibited in fatally poisoned animals. (See also: PARATHION, Reference Congener in Section III.)
OCTYL ALCOHOL 2-Ethylhexyl alcohol, unless specified as normal (or primary) octyl or caprylic alcohol.	3(?)	No relevant data on clinical toxicity were located. (See also: ALCOHOLS, HIGHER, Reference Congener in Section III.)

Substance and Synonym or Principal Ingredient	Toxicity Rating (See Inside Cover)	Comments and Reference Congeners
N-OCTYL BICYCLO-HEPTENE DICARBOX-IMIDE Octacide 264 MGK 264	3	A synergist in pyrethrum and rotenone insecticides, slightly more toxic than piperonyl butoxide or n-propyl isome. Not irritating to human skin when applied in full-strength. Systemic effects include central nervous excitation followed by depression. Treat symptomatically.
OCTYL CRESOLS Various isomers (o-, m-, and p-)	3	Low ingestion toxicity in rats (near the borderline between toxicity classes 2 and 3), but necrosis results from cutaneous applications. No clinical data are known. (See also: PHENOL, Reference Congener in Section III.)
OCTYL DERIVATIVE (Other than listed here)		See corresponding "alkyl" derivative in this index.
n-OCTYL SULFOXIDE OF ISOSAFROLE Sulfoxide	3	Used as a synergist to increase insecticidal potency of pyrethrins and possibly rotenone. In laboratory animals it has caused tremors and central nervous depression. Even surviving animals may experience prolonged coma.
OIL, LUBRICATING, FUEL, DIESEL, OR PETROLEUM		See petroleum distillate, petroleum oil (refined), or fuel oil in this index.
OIL OF BITTER ALMONDS Hydrocyanic acid (2 to 4%) and the rest is benzaldehyde	5	Hydrocyanic acid (hydrogen cyanide) is the only significantly toxic ingredient in this solution. (See also: CYANIDE, Reference Congener in Section III.)
OIL OF MIRBANE Nitrobenzene	5	Toxic by all routes including skin absorption. Mean lethal dose by mouth probably lies between 1 and 5 gm. Systemic effects may be delayed a few hours. Poisoning closely resembles that due to aniline. Ethyl alcohol aggravates intoxication. Because of bitter almond odor, cyanide poisoning may be suspected, but cyanide acts much faster. (See also: ANILINE, Reference Congener in Section III.)
OIL OF SASSAFRAS 80% Safrol	5	One of the essential or volatile oils. Thought to lie near the borderline between toxicity classes 4 and 5. Similar to oil of eucalyptus in toxicity (see Eucalyptol), except that vomiting and circulatory collapse are more common and miosis and respiratory symptoms less so. (See also: TURPENTINE, Reference Congener in Section III.)
OIL OF TURPENTINE Turpentine Spirits of turpentine	3	(See also: TURPENTINE, Reference Congener in Section III.)
OIL OF VITRIOL Sulfuric acid		(See also: ACID, Reference Congener in Section III.)
OILS, VOLATILE (OR ESSENTIAL) e.g., Oils of savin, rue, tansy, nutmeg, penny-royal, apiol, eucalyptus, juniper, cedarleaf, cajuput.	4	Most of these oils are reputed to be ecbolic but abortions cannot be induced by safe doses. Basically symptoms and treatment are like turpentine but toxicity is greater. In most cases a teaspoonful may cause illness in an adult and less than an ounce may kill (especially if vomiting does not occur promptly). Savin produces more renal damage than turpentine, and pennyroyal more liver degeneration. Also see eucalyptol, oil of sassafras, menthol, pine oil, wintergreen oil. (See also: TURPENTINE, Reference Congener in Section III.)
OLEIC ACID 9-Octadecenoic acid	1	A common constituent of many animal and vegetable fats and therefore of most normal diets.
OLEYL DERIVATIVE		See corresponding "alkyl" derivative in this index.
OMPA Octamethyl pyrophos-phoramide	5	A "systemic" insecticide, i.e., translocated in sap to all parts of plants. Only slightly less toxic than parathion. Not a cholinesterase inhibitor in vitro but converted to one by the liver. Brain cholinesterase, however, is not inhibited in fatally poisoned animals. (See also: PARATHION, Reference Congener in Section III.)
OPIUM	5	Three grams is considered a fatal dose in the non-addict. (See also: MORPHINE, Reference Congener in Section III.)
ORGANIC PHOSPHORUS INSECTICIDES OPI	6, 5, 4, or 3	Many alkyl phosphates, thiophosphates, and pyrophosphates are used for pest control. Most of them are highly toxic. Toxic effects are referable to the central and autonomic nervous systems and are associated with cholinesterase inhibition. (See also: PARATHION, Reference Congener in Section III.)
ORTHO-BENZYL-PARA-CHLOROPHENOL Santophen	3	Produces diarrhea when ingested by laboratory animals. Skin irritation and absorption at high concentrations. (See also: PHENOL, Reference Congener in Section III.)

Substance and Synonym or Principal Ingredient	Toxicity Rating (See Inside Cover)	Comments and Reference Congeners
ORTHODICHLOROBEN-ZENE 1,2-Dichlorobenzene	4(?)	A local irritant, a strong central nervous depressant, and a liver poison. Para isomer is less toxic. (See also: CARBON TETRACHLORIDE, Reference Congener in Section III.)
ORTHOPHENYLPHENOL 2-Hydroxydiphenyl e.g., Dowicide 1	3	Not absorbed through skin. An oil solution (5%) is well tolerated on human skin, but aqueous solutions of the sodium salt are irritating in concentrations above 0.5%. In rats ingestion causes death from central nervous depression, as does phenol. (See also: PHENOL, Reference Congener in Section III.)
OUABAIN		Consult Addendum on page 104.
OVOTRAN A proprietary name Parachlorophenyl-para-chlorobenzene sulfonate is the active ingredient (50%)	3	An acaricide of moderately low oral toxicity in laboratory animals. Kidney and liver damage in the rat during chronic exposures. Causes skin irritation in man, but no other symptoms have been reported in man.
OXALATE SALTS e.g., Sodium oxalate	4	Soluble salts of oxalic acid have essentially the same toxicity as the acid. (See also: OXALATE, Reference Congener in Section III.)
OXALIC ACID Ethanedioic acid	4	(See also: OXALATE, Reference Congener in Section III.)
OXYQUINOLINE SALT Hydroxyquinoline salt (e.g., sulfate, benzoate, citrate, tartrate, etc.)	3(?)	For the treatment of dysentery, men have received oral doses of 3 gm. in solution, four times daily, without apparent ill-effect. Rabbits tolerate single doses of 3.7 gm/kg. (as the sulfate, mixed with potassium sulfate). Various halogenated derivatives used in treating amebiasis are also comparatively benign (they may cause diarrhea and rarely liver injury). When injected in animals, however, hydroxyquinoline is distinctly toxic and causes marked stimulation of the central nervous system.
P 40 Sodium selenate	6	Used as a systemic insecticide, i.e., accumulates in plants which are thus rendered toxic to many pests and also to mammals. Highly toxic by all routes (probably borderline between toxicity classes 5 and 6), but slightly less toxic than sodium selenite. A general protoplasmic poison attacking sulfhydryl enzymes. Like arsenic it causes degenerative lesions in liver, kidneys, heart, spleen, stomach, bowel, and lungs. Many signs and symptoms are possible. No human fatalities have been reported. Treat like arsenic poisoning, except that BAL appears to be contraindicated. Bromobenzene (oral adult dose 1 gm.) is said to increase the urinary excretion of selenium. (See also: ARSENIC, Reference Congener in Section III.)
PALMITYL DERIVATIVE		See corresponding "alkyl" derivative in this index.
PANTOPON Pantopium Omnopon	6	A mixture of the purified alkaloids of opium in the proportions which occur naturally. On the basis of its morphine content (about 50%), Pantopon probably lies near the borderline between toxicity classes 5 and 6. (See also: MORPHINE, Reference Congener in Section III.)
PARA-		If the compound is not located below, omit the prefix and try again.
PARACHLORO-METACRESOL PCMC	4	Acute toxicity like phenol. No skin irritation at concentrations of 0.1%. (See also: PHENOL, Reference Congener in Section III.)
PARACHLORO-METAXYLENOL PCMX	3	Penetrates skin but no cutaneous irritation in 5% concentrations. (See also: PHENOL, Reference Congener in Section III.)
PARACHLOROPHENYL PARACHLOROBENZENE SULFONATE Ovotran	3	Moderately low oral toxicity in laboratory animals. Liver and kidney damage in chronic exposures. Causes skin irritation in man, but no other symptoms have been reported in man.
PARACHLOROPHENYL PHENYL SULFONE Sulphenone	3	An acaricide of moderately low oral toxicity in laboratory animals. No skin irritation. No significant tissue storage in chronic feeding experiments.
PARADICHLOROBENZENE p-Dichlorobenzene PDB Dichloricide	3	The least toxic active ingredient found in mothballs and related products. Sometimes used as an insecticidal fumigant. The ingestion of 20 gm. has been well tolerated in man. The vapor has caused irritation to skin, eyes, and throat, but no severe clinical poisonings are known after ingestion. Large doses in animals cause liver injury and sometimes tremors (in insects the compound is a nerve stimulant not unlike DDT). Also see o-dichlorobenzene, which appears to be much more toxic.
PARAFFIN, CHLORINATED Chlorcosane	1	No injury in test animals short of doses which produce intestinal obstruction. The same is true of common paraffin.

Substance and Synonym or Principal Ingredient	Toxicity Rating (See Inside Cover)	Comments and Reference Congeners
PARAFORMALDEHYDE Paraform Triformol Trioxymethylene	4	Same internal toxicity as formaldehyde, which it slowly releases at body temperature. (See also: FORMALDEHYDE, Reference Congener in Section III.)
PARAPHENYLENE DIAMINE p-Diaminobenzene Orsin Diolene is the ortho isomer and is less toxic	4	Used for dyeing hair and fur. A potent skin sensitizer. Produces severe local reactions and systemic effects from percutaneous absorption or following ingestion. Local actions include severe dermatitis and urticaria; in the eye chemosis, lacrimation, exophthalmos, ophthalmia, and even permanent blindness. Systemic actions include asthma, gastritis (regardless of portal of entry), rise in blood pressure, transudation into serous cavities, vertigo, tremors, convulsions, and coma. Treatment is symptomatic. Whenever histamine-like effects predominate, a therapeutic trial with an antihistaminic is suggested.
PARA-OXON Diethyl-p-nitrophenyl phosphate	6	One of the most toxic organic phosphate insecticides. Relatively high stability will probably cause residue problems. Toxic effects appear rapidly after exposure. (See also: PARATHION, Reference Congener in Section III.)
PARATHION O,O-Diethyl-O-para-nitrophenyl thiophosphate	6	(See also: PARATHION, Reference Congener in Section III.)
PARATOLUYLENE-DIAMINE p-Toluenediamine	4	Animal tests suggest that it is slightly less toxic but presumably similar to paraphenylenediamine. See latter in this index.
PAREGORIC Camphorated tincture of opium	3	A tincture of 0.4% opium (equivalent to 0.04% morphine). Based on its morphine content, it lies near the borderline between toxicity classes 2 and 3. It has been confused with tincture of opium (laudanum), which is 25 times more potent (toxicity rating 4). (See also: MORPHINE, Reference Congener in Section III.)
PARIS GREEN Copper acetoarsenite Schweinfurth green	5	A substance of complex composition, having an arsenic trioxide equivalent of about 59%. Used as an insecticide, a wood preservative, and a paint pigment. (See also: ARSENIC, Reference Congener in Section III.)
PCH Piperonyl cyclonene	3	In animals it lies on the borderline between toxicity classes 2 and 3. Used as a synergist to increase the insecticidal potency of pyrethrins and rotenone. No known human poisonings. Causes vomiting in animals. Only mild skin irritation, but repeated skin application (5% in dimethyl phthalate) proved fatal to rabbits.
PCMC Parachlorometacresol	4	Acute ingestion toxicity like phenol. No skin irritation at concentration of of 0.1%. (See also: PHENOL, Reference Congener in Section III.)
PCMX Parachlorometaxylenol	3	Penetrates skin but no cutaneous irritation in 5% concentration. (See also: PHENOL, Reference Congener in Section III.)
PCP Pentachlorophenol	4	As dangerous as phenol. Absorption and toxicity increased by oils. A metabolic stimulant like dinitrophenol. Has produced human fatalities due to hyperpyrexia. (See also: DINITROPHENOL, Reference Congener in Section III.)
PDB Paradichlorobenzene	3	The least toxic active ingredient found in mothballs and related products. Sometimes used as an insecticidal fumigant. The ingestion of 20 gm. has been well tolerated in man. The vapor has caused irritation to skin, eyes, and throat, but no severe clinical poisonings are known after ingestion. Large doses in animals cause liver injury and sometimes tremors (in insects the compound is a nerve stimulant not unlike DDT). Also see o-dichlorobenzene, which appears to be much more toxic.
PDU 3-Phenyl-1, 1-dimethyl-urea	2	A herbicide of lower acute toxicity in rats than CMU.
PELLETIERINE TANNATE Punicine tannate. A mixture of alkaloids as tannate salts (equivalent to not less than 20% as hydrochlorides) extracted from pomegranate bark	5(?)	An anthelmintic used chiefly against tapeworm. An ordinary dose (0.3 gm.) often produces mild toxic symptoms. The alkaloids first stimulate and then depress the central nervous system; are selectively toxic to the optic nerve; have veratrine- and curare-like actions on muscle. Overdoses cause nausea, vomiting, diarrhea; twitching, cramps, weakness, and sometimes convulsions; dizziness, headache, mydriasis, partial blindness; paralysis, and death. Treat by lavage, saline catharsis, supportive measures, including artificial respiration.

Substance and Synonym or Principal Ingredient	Toxicity Rating (See Inside Cover)	Comments and Reference Congeners
PENTACHLOROETHANE	4	Very hazardous. More potent central nervous effects than chloroform or even tetrachloroethane. (See also: CARBON TETRACHLORIDE, Reference Congener in Section III.)
PENTACHLOROPHENOL "Penta"	4	As dangerous as phenol. Absorption and toxicity are increased by oils. A metabolic stimulant like dinitrophenol. Has produced human fatalities due to hyperpyrexia. (See also: DINITROPHENOL, Reference Congener in Section III.)
PENTASODIUM TRIPOLYPHOSPHATE Sodium tripolyphosphate	3(?)	Irritating because of alkalinity and hypertonicity. If ingested in large amounts, nausea, vomiting, and diarrhea are probable. Thought to be hydrolyzed to (ortho)phosphate before absorption.
PERACETIC ACID Peroxyacetic acid	4(?)	Commercially available as a 40% solution in acetic acid. Highly corrosive. (See also: ACID, Reference Congener in Section III.)
PERCHLOROETHANE Hexachloroethane	4	More potent central nervous effects than chloroform or carbon tetrachloride but slower in action. On ingestion, severe mucosal injury and often liver necrosis. Because of low vapor pressure, no known industrial exposures. (See also: CARBON TETRACHLORIDE, Reference Congener in Section III.)
PERCHLOROETHYLENE Tetrachloroethylene	3	Less toxic than carbon tetrachloride or chloroform. Given therapeutically (for hookworms) to adults by mouth (dose 1 to 4 ml.). Low solubility in water and poorly absorbed in the absence of fats and oils. Widely used in veterinary medicine. (See also: CARBON TETRACHLORIDE, Reference Congener in Section III.)
PERCHLOROMETHANE Carbon tetrachloride	4	(See also: CARBON TETRACHLORIDE, Reference Congener in Section III.)
PEROXYACETIC ACID Peracetic acid	4(?)	Commercially available as a 40% solution in acetic acid. Highly corrosive. (See also: ACID, Reference Congener in Section III.)
PERTHANE Dichloro-bis(p-ethyl-phenyl) ethane	2	In animals toxic signs and symptoms are like those in DDT poisoning, but the toxicity is much lower (near the borderline between toxicity classes 2 and 3). There is little, if any, percutaneous absorption, skin irritation, or sensitization. Unlike DDT, feeding tests on rats with radioactive Perthane indicate little tendency for the material to deposit in body fat. (See also: DDT, Reference Congener in Section III.)
PETROL		See gasoline in this index.
PETROLEUM BENZIN Petroleum ether	3	Low-boiling petroleum distillate, largely consisting of saturated hydro-carbons C_4H_{10} to C_8H_{18} (principally pentane and hexane), distilling between 35 and 80° C. (See also: KEROSENE, Reference Congener in Section III.)
PETROLEUM DISTILLATE Any one of many fractions varying from petroleum ether to lubricating oils	3	Major fractions in order are: petroleum ether (benzin), gasoline, kerosene, fuel oil, lubricating oils (and mineral oil, etc.), paraffin wax, and asphalt or tar (pitch, coke). All fractions (when impure) tend to produce local skin irritation and skin photosensitization. The latter is revealed by prickling and erythema shortly after exposure to sunlight, often followed by pigmentation. (See also: KEROSENE, Reference Congener in Section III.)
PETROLEUM ETHER Petroleum benzin	3	See petroleum benzin above.
PETROLEUM NAPHTHA Petroleum ether	3	This name is sometimes used to designate a distillate with a slightly higher boiling point range (65 to 120°C.) than petroleum ether. At other times the name refers to any petroleum distillate fraction which is chiefly or ex-clusively composed of aliphatic (straight-chain) hydrocarbons (in contrast to aromatic rings). (See also: KEROSENE, Reference Congener in Section III.)
PETROLEUM OILS (REFINED) Liquid petrolatum, mineral or paraffin oils, white oils, petrole-um jelly, all refined especially to remove unsaturated compounds.	1	Consists largely of saturated aliphatic (C_{14} to C_{18}) and cyclic hydrocarbons. Prepared by refining cruder lubricating oils. Fractions vary in viscosity and other physical properties. When ingested they produce a mild laxative effect. Not absorbed but may inhibit the absorption of nutrient lipids.
PETROLEUM SULFONATE	3(?)	Prepared from any petroleum distillate (especially lubricating oils) which contain unsaturated compounds capable of being sulfonated. See alkyl sodium sulfonates in this index.
PHENACETIN Acetophenetidin	4	Less toxic than aniline or acetanilid. Cyanosis and methemoglobin are less marked, but severe skin rashes may be more frequent. (See also: ANILINE, Reference Congener in Section III.)

Substance and Synonym or Principal Ingredient	Toxicity Rating (See Inside Cover)	Comments and Reference Congeners
PHENETHYL ALCOHOL 2-Phenylethanol β-Phenyl ethyl alcohol	3	A more potent local anesthetic than benzyl alcohol. Found in natural and synthetic oils of rose and distilled rose water. Injected in mice, it causes muscular weakness and incoordination, exophthalmos, coma, and death.
PHENOBARBITAL Phenyl ethyl malonyl urea Luminal	4	Probably lies near the borderline between toxicity classes 4 and 5. The second oldest barbiturate drug. A hypnotic and central nervous depressant. It has a long duration of action because elimination is dependent upon renal excretion and the latter is inherently slow here. As discussed in Sec. III, an osmotic diuresis may be a useful therapeutic measure in phenobarbital poisonings. (See also: BARBITURATE, Reference Congener in Section III.)
PHENOL Carbolic acid	4	(See also: PHENOL, Reference Congener in Section III.)
PHENOL MERCURIC CHLORIDE o-Hydroxyphenyl mercuric chloride Mercarbolide	5	Contains 61% mercury. Readily soluble in water. Dilute solutions have been used in medicine as an external germicide and fungicide. Less corrosive than mercuric chloride but systemic toxicity is probably almost as great. (See also: MERCURY, Reference Congener in Section III.)
PHENOLPHTHALEIN		Consult Addendum on p. 104.
PHENOTHIAZINE Thiodiphenylamine	3	Probably lies near the borderline between toxicity classes 3 and 4. Cumulative therapeutic dose should be kept below 20 gm. Overdosage (and accidental exposures) have caused hemolytic anemia, toxic hepatitis, skin photosensitization, and intense pruritus.
PHENOTHIOXIN Phenoxathrin	4	Used as an insecticide. In rats and guinea pigs it lies near the borderline between toxicity classes 3 and 4. Liver pathology described in chronic feeding tests with rats. Moderate to marked irritation of rabbit skin after prolonged contact. No human data.
PHENOXATHRIN Phenothioxin	4	See above.
2-PHENOXYETHANOL Phenyl cellosolve	4	Probably lies near the borderline between toxicity classes 3 and 4. About twice as toxic as the ethyl derivative (= Cellosolve) but otherwise like it. Consult "Cellosolves" in this index for a brief comparison with ethylene glycol. (See also: ETHYLENE GLYCOL, Reference Congener in Section III.)
N-PHENYLACETAMIDE Acetanilid	4	Similar to but less toxic than aniline in animals, but clinical experience does not confirm this difference in man. Indeed a toxicity rating of 5 might be a better description of the recorded human fatalities. Perhaps there are less prominent nervous symptoms than in aniline poisoning. (See also: ANILINE, Reference Congener in Section III.)
PHENYLAMINE Aniline	4	(See also: ANILINE, Reference Congener in Section III.)
PHENYL CELLOSOLVE Ethylene glycol monophenyl ether	4	Probably lies near the borderline between toxicity classes 3 and 4. About twice as toxic as the ethyl derivative (= Cellosolve) but otherwise like it. Consult "Cellosolves" in this index for a brief comparison with ethylene glycol. (See also: ETHYLENE GLYCOL, Reference Congener in Section III.)
PHENYL CYCLOHEXANOL 2-Phenyl cyclohexanol	3	Severe skin irritation in rabbits after repeated application.
3-PHENYL-1,1-DIMETHYLUREA PDU	2	A herbicide of lower acute toxicity in rats than CMU.
PHENYLENEDIAMINE (o- or p-) e.g., Orsin (para isomer) Diolene (ortho isomer)	4	Used for dyeing hair and fur. A potent skin sensitizer. Produces severe local reactions and systemic effects from percutaneous absorption or following ingestion. Local actions include severe dermatitis and urticaria; in the eye, chemosis, lacrimation, exophthalmos, ophthalmia, and even permanent blindness. Systemic actions include asthma, gastritis (regardless of portal of entry), rise in blood pressure, transudation into serous cavities, vertigo, tremors, convulsions, and coma. Treatment is symptomatic. Whenever histamine-like effects predominate, a therapeutic trial with an antihistaminic is suggested. The ortho isomer is less toxic than the para.
PHENYL ETHYL ALCOHOL 2-Phenethyl alcohol β-Phenyl ethyl alcohol	3	A more potent local anesthetic than benzyl alcohol. Found in natural and synthetic oils of rose and distilled rose water. Injected in mice, it causes muscular weakness and incoordination, exophthalmos, coma, and death.

Substance and Synonym or Principal Ingredient	Toxicity Rating (See Inside Cover)	Comments and Reference Congeners
β-PHENYLISOPROPYL-AMINE Amphetamine	5	Acute lethal dose in adults is probably 20 to 25 mg./ kg., in children only 5 mg./kg. Overdoses cause restlessness, insomnia, nausea and vomiting, intense confusion, delirium, mania, and collapse. Convulsions and coma are terminal events. Various cardiovascular actions are described: tachycardia, arrhythmias, heart block, hypertension or hypotension, and circulatory collapse. Treatment is symptomatic with emphasis on seda-tives (especially barbiturates).
PHENYLMERCURIC ACETATE PMAS Related esters include the salicylate, oleate, benzoate, phthalate, and gluconate. (General formula is $C_6H_5HgOOCR$)	5	An important agricultural and industrial fungicide. Acute lethal dose is per-haps half that of mercuric chloride. Much less corrosive than the latter but prolonged cutaneous contact with the dust leads to vesication. Systemic actions include central nervous disturbances. (See also: MERCURY, Ref-erence Congener in Section III.)
PHENYLMERCURIC SALTS e.g., Borate, nitrate, subnitrate, chloride, and hydroxide (General formula is C_6H_5HgX where X is an anionic group)	5	These salts ionize in solution to yield the phenylmercuric ion, which is less corrosive and less toxic than the mercuric ion. Used in agriculture as fungicides and in medicine as external germicides. (See also: MERCURY, Reference Congener in Section III.)
PHENYLMERCURIC TRIETHANOL AMMONIUM LACTATE Related compounds include phenylmercuri-monoethanolammonium acetate.	5(?)	Used as an agricultural fungicide. Systemic toxicity is probably almost as high as mercuric chloride but less corrosive than the latter. (See also: MERCURY, Reference Congener in Section III.)
1-PHENYL-3-METHYL-PYRAZOLYL-(5)-DIMETHYLCARBAMATE		Consult Addendum on p. 104.
PHENYL PHENOL Orthophenylphenol e.g., Dowicide 1 The sodium salt is available as Dowicide A	3	Not absorbed through skin. An oil solution (5%) is well tolerated on human skin, but aqueous solutions of the sodium salt are irritating in concentra-tions above 0.5%. In rats ingestion causes death from central nervous depression, as does phenol. (See also: PHENOL, Reference Congener in Section III.)
PHENYL SALICYLATE Salol	4	Used for enteric coating of pills, in suntan lotions and creams, and formerly as an intestinal antiseptic. Insoluble in water and gastric juice. Said to be slowly hydrolyzed to phenol (40%) and salicylic acid (60%) by intestinal alkali and enzymes, but recent evidence suggests that much hydrolysis occurs in tissues after absorption. The toxic effects are chiefly those of phenol but without phenol's marked corrosive actions on the gastrointestinal tract. (See also: PHENOL, Reference Congener in Section III.)
PHOSPHORIC ACID Orthophosphoric acid		(See also: ACID, Reference Congener in Section III.)
PHOSPHORUS (YELLOW) White phosphorus	6	(See also: PHOSPHORUS, Reference Congener in Section III.)
PHOSPHORUS PENTASULFIDE Phosphoric sulfide Phosphorus persulfide Thiophosphoric anhydride Formula: P_2S_5 (or P_4S_{10}).		Decomposes on contact with water to phosphoric acid, sulfur dioxide, and hydrogen sulfide. The latter is certainly the most toxic of these decompo-sition products. (See also: HYDROGEN SULFIDE, Reference Congener in Section III.)
PHOSPHORUS PENTOXIDE Phosphoric acid anhydride (P_2O_5)		Reacts with water and aqueous solutions to form phosphoric acid. (See also: ACID, Reference Congener in Section III.)
PHTHALIC ACID ESTERS e.g., Diethyl ("ethyl") phthalate, dibutyl phthalate, dioctyl phthalate, etc.	2 and 3	Used as solvents, fixatives in perfumes, and plasticizers. Because of its objectionable bitter taste, the ethyl (= diethyl) ester is used as a denaturant for alcohol, especially in cosmetics. The dimethyl ester is an insect re-pellent. Each is an irritant on mucous membranes and a central nervous depressant if absorbed.

Substance and Synonym or Principal Ingredient	Toxicity Rating (See Inside Cover)	Comments and Reference Congeners
PHYGON 2,3-Dichloro-1,4-naphthoquinone	3	Moderately low toxicity in laboratory animals. Diarrhea and severe central nervous depression in rats. Large doses are promptly vomited by dogs. Skin irritation is enhanced by fats and oils.
PICRIC ACID 2,4,6-Trinitrophenol	5	Severe poisoning from ingestion of 1 to 2 gm. Severe gastroenteritis, intravascular hemolysis, hemorrhagic nephritis, and sometimes hepatitis. Increased metabolism like dinitrophenol (see Sec. III). Headache, progressive stupor, coma, and death in severe poisonings. (See also: PHENOL, Reference Congener in Section III.)
PIGMENTS AND DYES		For a tabular summary of dyes and pigments, see Section VI (General Formulations).
PINENE α-Pinene	3	The principal ingredient of turpentine, with essentially the same toxicity as turpentine. (See also: TURPENTINE, Reference Congener in Section III.)
PINE OIL Steam-distilled pine oil is a mixture of terpene alcohols, chiefly α-terpineol, plus terpene hydrocarbons (5 to 10%), borneol (5 to 10%), and terpene ethers (5 to 10%)	3	Irritating to eyes and mucous membranes. Produces hemorrhagic gastritis. Systemic effects include weakness and central nervous depression, with hypothermia and respiratory failure. (See also: TURPENTINE, Reference Congener in Section III.)
PIPERAZINE Piperazidine Diethylenediamine	2	Used for the treatment of oxyuriasis in man and animals. Especially popular in veterinary medicine. Lethal doses (in animals) produce convulsions and respiratory depression.
PIPERONYL BUTOXIDE (Butylcarbityl)-(6-propyl piperonyl) ether (technical grade material may contain 20% related compounds)	2	Used as a synergist to increase the insecticidal potency of pyrethrins and rotenone. Very low toxicity in test animals, which show anorexia, vomiting, diarrhea, hemorrhagic enteritis, inanition, and perhaps mild central nervous depression. No skin irritation or significant percutaneous absorption.
PIPERONYL CYCLOHEXENONE (an obsolete name) Piperonyl cyclonene	3	See below.
PIPERONYL CYCLONENE Piperonyl cyclohexenone	3	In animals it lies on the borderline between toxicity classes 2 and 3. Used as a synergist to increase the insecticidal potency of pyrethrins and rotenone. No human poisonings are known. Causes vomiting in test animals. Only mild skin irritation but repeated skin applications (5% in dimethyl phthalate) proved fatal to rabbits.
2-PIVALYL-1,3-INDANDIONE Pival A water-soluble sodium salt of this compound is known as Pivalyn.	4(?)	A new rodenticide with delayed effects on the prothrombin level and consequent disturbances in blood coagulation, producing death by hemorrhage. When tested on rats (single intraperitoneal injections), Pival proved to be more toxic than Warfarin, but it is apparently less potent than Warfarin by multiple daily doses. (See also: WARFARIN, Reference Congener in Section III.)
PLASTER OF PARIS Calcium sulfate anhydrous or with about 5% water (1/2 mol)		Because it hardens quickly after absorbing moisture, its ingestion may result in obstruction, particularly at the pylorus. Mixed with flour (1:2), it has been used as a rodenticide. To delay "setting," drink glycerin or gelatin solutions, or large volumes of water. Surgical relief may be necessary.
PLURONICS Ethylene and propylene oxides chemically reacted with propylene glycol	2	Trademarked name for various non-ionic surfactants with a wide variety of physical forms, used in cosmetics, medicinal ointments, etc. In laboratory animals very low acute toxicity, especially Pluronic F68. No irritation or sensitization of skin or eyes.
PMA Phenyl mercuric acetate PMAS PMAC Related esters include the salicylate, oleate, benzoate, phthalate, and gluconate. General formula is $C_6H_5HgOOCR$).	5	An important agricultural and industrial fungicide. Acute lethal dose is perhaps half that of mercuric chloride. Much less corrosive than the latter but prolonged cutaneous contact with the dust leads to vesication. Systemic actions include central nervous disturbances. (See also: MERCURY, Reference Congener in Section III.)

Substance and Synonym or Principal Ingredient	Toxicity Rating (See Inside Cover)	Comments and Reference Congeners
POLYACRYLONITRILE		A soil conditioner. No reports of toxicity have been found.
POLYALKYL ETHER DERIVATIVES		See corresponding polyethylene glycol derivative in this index.
POLYETHYLENE GLYCOLS	1 and 2	If a numeral is included, it represents the approx. mean molecular weight. Fractions with molecular weights of 600 (and below) are liquid, of 1000 (and above) are solid. The higher molecular weight the lower the toxicity, perhaps partly because the long polymers are so incompletely absorbed from the bowel. Very large doses are required to kill animals and deaths are renal in origin (not due to primary central nervous depression). (See also: ETHYLENE GLYCOL, Reference Congener in Section III.)
POLYETHLENE GLYCOL ALKYL ARYL ETHERS e.g., Triton X-100 Igepals	2 and 3	Non-ionic surfactants available with a wide variety of physical properties and used as wetting agents and emulsifiers. Even at full-strength, they rarely sensitize or irritate human skin. The only symptoms (and lesions) in orally poisoned animals are related to gastrointestinal irritation (e.g., diarrhea, bloating). Little, if any, intestinal absorption or decomposition.
POLYETHYLENE GLYCOL STEARATE (and esters of other fatty acids) e.g., Myrj 52 (etc.) Nonisols Polyoxyl 40 stearate	1	Non-ionic surfactants generally soluble or dispersible in water. Some of these compounds have been proposed as emulsifiers in foods (e.g., bread). These esters are hydrolyzed in the bowel. The fatty acid is absorbed and metabolized; at least the shorter polyoxyethylene residues are also absorbed, but they are excreted unchanged in the urine (no detectable metabolism to oxalic acid in man).
POLYETHYLENE POLYSULFIDE PEPS		Employed as a fungicide and spray adjuvant. A brief trial in mice suggests a low acute toxicity by the oral route of administration.
POLYETHYLENE (20) SORBITAN MONO-STEARATE (and other fatty acid esters) Also called polyoxyethylene etc. e.g., Tween 60 and other Tweens	1	A group of non-ionic surfactants, generally soluble or dispersible in water. Small quantities are used in many foods and beverages, cosmetics, etc. No single oral dose is known to be lethal in animals, and men have been fed 15 gm. daily for several months with impunity. In the bowel the fatty acid is split off and absorbed, and the rest is eliminated in feces. See also Polysorbate 80 below.
POLYGLYCOL DERIVATIVES		See corresponding polyethylene glycol derivative in this index.
POLYOXYETHYLENE AND POLYOXYALKYLENE DERIVATIVES		See corresponding polyethylene glycol derivative in this index. They are usually manufactured by condensing ethylene oxide with many different substances.
POLYPROPYLENE GLYCOLS Name is often followed by a numeral which indicates approx. mean molecular weight.	3	Unaccountably much more toxic than propylene glycol or even ethylene glycol in laboratory animals. Polymers with molecular weights of about 1000 seem to be more toxic than longer or shorter homologues. When ingested or injected in dogs, ventricular extrasystoles result.
POLYSORBATE 80 Polyoxyethylene (20) sorbitan mono-oleate e.g., Tween 80	1	Unintentionally administered to a 4-month infant at a daily dose of 19.2 gm./kg. for two consecutive days. The patient passed 6 loose stools but showed no other evidence of intoxication. Also see polyethylene sorbitan (20) mono-stearate above.
POMEGRANATE BARK Granatum Extracts contain a mixture of active alkaloids called pelletierine.	3(?)	0.5 to 1.0% alkaloids, especially pelletiernine. See latter in this index.
POTASH Potassium hydroxide		(See also: ALKALI, Reference Congener in Section III.)
POTASSIUM CHLORATE	4	An oxidizing agent. More toxic than the sodium salt but less toxic than potassium bromate. Chlorate produces gastritis, methemoglobin, and a toxic nephritis. Less central nervous depression than bromate poisoning but perhaps more methemoglobin. (See also: BROMATE, Reference Congener in Section III.)

Substance and Synonym or Principal Ingredient	Toxicity Rating (See Inside Cover)	Comments and Reference Congeners
POTASSIUM CHROMATE	4	Corrosive because of its oxidizing potency. Treat local injury like acid burns. If ingested, violent gastroenteritis, circulatory collapse, vertigo, coma, and a toxic nephritis. Treat peripheral vascular shock vigorously. Also see chromic acid in this index. (See also: ACID, Reference Congener in Section III.)
POTASSIUM CYANATE	3	Best described as lying near the borderline between toxicity classes 3 and 4. Toxicity has been ascribed to its slow in vivo conversion to cyanide. (See also: CYANIDE, Reference Congener in Section III.)
POTASSIUM CYANIDE	6	Act quickly! (See also: CYANIDE, Reference Congener in Section III.)
POTASSIUM DICHROMATE Potassium bichromate	4	An oxidizing agent. The mean lethal dose is probably about 10 gm. Highly corrosive to skin and mucous membranes (treat like acid burns). If ingested, violent gastroenteritis, peripheral vascular collapse, vertigo, muscle cramps, coma, and later toxic nephritis (with glycosuria). Allergic reactions have also been described. On the basis of favorable experimental reports, BAL deserves a therapeutic trial if systemic poisoning develops (see BAL in Sec. III).(See also: ACID, Reference Congener in Section III.)
POTASSIUM HYDROXIDE Caustic potash		(See also: ALKALI, Reference Congener in Section III.)
POTASSIUM OXALATE The acid potassium salt is sometimes called salt of lemons.	4	(See also: OXALATE, Reference Congener in Section III.)
POTASSIUM PERMANGANATE Condy's crystals		An oxidizing agent. Only mildly irritating in dilute solutions but concentrated solutions and dry crystals are highly corrosive. In at least three oral poisonings, death has resulted from edema of the glottis. Systemic effects are not of primary importance because of poor absorption. Treat by swallowing egg white and by gastric lavage. Preparations should be made for an emergency tracheotomy.
POTASSIUM SALTS e.g., Nitrate (saltpeter), chloride	3	Acute potassium intoxication from oral administration is highly improbable because large doses induce vomiting and because absorbed potassium is rapidly excreted (except in the face of pre-existing kidney damage). Potassium poisoning disturbs the rhythm of the heart (a slow, weak pulse, heightened T wave of ECG, arrhythmias, heart block), and eventually weakens cardiac contractility (fall in blood pressure). Respirations are initially accelerated, but skeletal muscle weakness may advance to the stage of paralysis.
POTASSIUM THIOCYANATE Potassium sulfocyanate Potassium rhodanate	4	Theoretically more toxic than sodium thiocyanate because of possible potassium intoxication, but the major toxic effects after ingestion are probably due to the thiocyanate ion. See thiocyanate salts in this index.
POTASSIUM THIOSULFATE Potassium hyposulfite	3	Cathartic, diuretic, and probably emetic. The thiosulfate ion is remarkably inert in vivo, but potassium is less benign. See potassium salts in this index.
PROLAN 1, 1-Bis(p-chlorophenyl) -2-nitropropane	3	Same symptoms and treatment as DDT. Can be absorbed through intact skin. In rats symptoms may be prolonged for several days (unlike DDT or bulan). (See also: DDT, Reference Congener in Section III.)
1-PROPENOL-3 Allyl alcohol	4	Vapor and liquid are intensely irritating to skin and mucous membrane. Produces lacrimation and corneal burns. Penetration through intact skin is dangerous. Animal studies place this compound near the borderline between toxicity classes 4 and 5.
PROPYL ACETATE n- or iso-Propyl acetate	3	Like other simple esters, mild irritant and central depressant actions. Probably this compound lies near the borderline between toxicity classes 2 and 3.
PROPYL ALCOHOL 1-Propanol	3	Somewhat more toxic than isopropyl alcohol. (See also: ISOPROPYL ALCOHOL, Reference Congener in Section III.)
PROPYLENE DICHLORIDE Dichloropropane	4	One of the most toxic chlorinated hydrocarbons, producing visceral lesions in the liver, heart, and kidneys. Present in D-D mixture. (See also: D-D, Reference Congener in Section III.)
PROPYLENE GLYCOL 1, 2-Propanediol	1	Toxicity is said to be similar to that of glycerine and is therefore practically non-toxic. No untoward reactions described in man, but large oral doses in animals may produce central nervous depression and minimal kidney changes. (See also: ETHYLENE GLYCOL, Reference Congener in Section III.)

Substance and Synonym or Principal Ingredient	Toxicity Rating (See Inside Cover)	Comments and Reference Congeners
PROPYLENE GLYCOL MONOMETHYL ETHER e.g., Dowanol 33B	3(?)	Both alpha and beta isomers have similar toxicities. Central nervous depression and kidney tubular necrosis seen in experimental animals. Less toxic than ethylene glycol monomethyl ether but slightly more toxic than ethylene glycol. (See also: ETHYLENE GLYCOL, Reference Congener in Section III.)
PROPYLENE GLYCOL MONOSTEARATE (and other fatty acid esters) e.g., Atlas G 924	2(?)	Slightly more toxic than propylene glycol in animals. Large doses produce central nervous depression and kidney tubular injury, as does ethylene glycol. (See also: ETHYLENE GLYCOL, Reference Congener in Section III.)
n-PROPYL ISOME Di-n-propyl maleate-isosafrole	2	Central nervous depression seen after very high doses in laboratory animals.
PRUSSIC ACID A 2% aqueous solution of hydrocyanic acid	5	Act fast! The mean lethal dose of this solution is probably 3 cc. (See also: CYANIDE, Reference Congener in Section III.)
PUMICE Complex silicates	1(?)	Insoluble and chemically inert. Intestinal obstructions, perforations, and perhaps local granulomas are conceivable after the ingestion of large quantities.
PYRENONE		Various combinations of pyrethrins and butoxide, used as insecticides. (See also: PYRETHRUM, Reference Congener in Section III.)
PYRETHRIN (I or II)	3	Pyrethrin I is pyrethrolone ester of chrysanthemum monocarboxylic acid. Pyrethrin II is similar. Pyrethrin II is less toxic than Pyrethrin I. (See also: PYRETHRUM, Reference Congener in Section III.)
PYRETHRUM Dried flowers of Chrysanthemum cinerariaefolium	1	Contains about 1% pyrethrins. (See also: PYRETHRUM, Reference Congener in Section III.)
PYRIBENZAMINE HYDROCHLORIDE Tripelennamine hydrochloride	5(?)	Unlike diphenhydramine, convulsions have not been reported, although rigidity, stupor, and circulatory collapse are described in human poisonings. (See also: ANTIHISTAMINICS, Reference Congener in Section III.)
PYRILAMINE MALEATE Neo-antergan maleate	5	A potent antihistaminic drug. It probably lies near the borderline between toxicity classes 4 and 5. (See also: ANTIHISTAMINICS, Reference Congener in Section III.)
PYROCATECHOL o-Dihydroxybenzene Catechol	4	As toxic as phenol. Similar to phenol, but convulsions may be more frequent, and blood dyscrasias are described. (See also: PHENOL, Reference Congener in Section III.)
PYRIDINE	3	Absorbed from the respiratory and gastrointestinal tracts, but probably not significantly from the skin (although a dermatitis may result). In animals central nervous depression; also in man after vapor inhalation. Small oral doses (2 to 3 ml.) in man produce mild anorexia, nausea, fatigue, and mental depression, and after prolonged daily administration hepatorenal damage (in rats prevented by methionine). The ingestion of several ounces has produced severe vomiting, diarrhea, hyperpyrexia, delirium, and death in 43 hours; autopsy revealed pulmonary edema and membranous tracheobronchitis (due to aspiration?).
PYROGALLOL Pyrogallic acid 1,2,3-Trihydroxybenzene	4	Toxicity and toxic actions like phenol, but also methemoglobinemia, hemolysis, and renal injury, as in aniline poisoning. Delayed deaths from uremia have been reported. Percutaneous absorption is dangerous. Mildly caustic to skin and mucous membranes. (See also: ANILINE, Reference Congener in Section III.)
PYROLAN		Consult Addendum on p. 104 under: 1-phenyl-3-methylpyrazolyl-(5)-dimethylcarbamate
PYROLIGNEOUS ACID Wood vinegar; prepared by the destructive distillation of wood		Contains about 6% acetic acid in water and small concentrations of creosote, methyl alcohol, and acetone. (See also: ACID, Reference Congener in Section III.)
Q-137 1,1-Dichloro-2,2-bis(p-ethylphenyl) Perthane	2	In animals toxic signs and symptoms are like those in DDT poisoning, but the toxicity is much lower (near the borderline between toxicity classes 2 and 3). There is little, if any, percutaneous absorption, skin irritation, or sensitization. Unlike DDT, feeding tests on rats with radioactive Perthane indicate little tendency for the material to deposit in body fat. (See also: DDT, Reference Congener in Section III.)

Substance and Synonym or Principal Ingredient	Toxicity Rating (See Inside Cover)	Comments and Reference Congener
QUATERNARY AMMONIUM SALTS Alkyl-substituted ammonium chloride or bromide	4	A wide variety of cationic surfactants used as germicides and sanatizers. (See also: QAC, Reference Congener in Section III.)
QUICKLIME Calcium oxide Burnt lime		Reacts with water with the evolution of heat to form calcium hydroxide. May produce both a thermal and caustic burn. (See also: ALKALI, Reference Congener in Section III.)
QUINCE SEED Cydonium Seed of Cydonia oblonga		Contains amygdalin, emulsin, 15% fatty oil, and 20% gum (cydonin). Emulsin is an enzyme which hydrolyzes amygdalin into benzaldehyde, HCN, and glucose. The amount of available cyanide must be very small because a mucilage prepared from the seeds has long been used in medicine as a demulcent of low toxicity.
QUININE Obtained from the bark of various species of the genus Cinchona	4	The fatal dose is often cited as 8 gm., but a 30 gm. dose has been tolerated. The toxic syndrome, often called cinchonism, closely resembles salicylate poisoning, and recommended supportive treatment is similar. (See also: SALICYLATE, Reference Congener in Section III.)
QUINONE 1, 4-Benzoquinone	4	An oxidizing agent. Has produced ocular and cutaneous lesions in man, but no systemic poisonings are known. In animals single oral doses are said to produce delayed deaths. Toxic effects differ from those of hydroquinone.
RANGE GAS Manufactured gas Stove gas Illuminating gas Coal gas		The principal toxic ingredient is carbon monoxide, which may be present in any concentration between 2 and 15%/v. Natural gas contains none, unless in processing it is produced by "cracking" or is added by mixing with manufactured gas. (See also: CARBON MONOXIDE, Reference Congener in Section III.)
RANGE OIL Kerosene	3	(See also: KEROSENE, Reference Congener in Section III.)
RED OIL A commercial mixture of fatty acids, particularly oleic acid (9-octadecenoic acid)	1	Several grades in commerce vary in color from yellow to red-brown, depending upon the degrees of unsaturation, etc. Used to prepare soft soaps, lubricating and polishing compounds, and Turkey red oil. Unless there are unrecognized impurities, red oil is presumably as benign as any other mixture of dietary fatty acids.
RED SQUILL Consists of the cut and dried inner scales of the sea onion bulb, Scilla (or Urginea) maritima (L.), red variety	4	Unlike the white variety, red squill is an effective rodenticide, but it varies greatly in potency. Symptoms include burning pain in the pharynx, nausea, vomiting, diarrhea, abdominal pain, thirst, restlessness, excitement, paresis, convulsions, and prostration. These symptoms are accompanied by severe disturbances in heart action due to cardiotonic glycosides in the mixture. Rats and mice die of convulsions, perhaps because of the presence of a glycoside called scilliroside, but the dangerous actions in man are presumably those on the the heart. Also consult this index under "squill, red and white" and under "scillaren." (See also: DIGITALIS, Reference Congener in Section III.)
RESORCINOL Resorcin m-Dihydroxybenzene	4	Used on the skin as a bactericidal and fungicidal ointment (usually 5%). About the same toxicity as phenol, but convulsions are more prominent. Perhaps slightly less toxic than catechol or hydroquinone. (See also: PHENOL, Reference Congener in Section III.)
RESORCINOL MONOACETATE	4	Similar to resorcinol but actions are milder and more persistent. Skin ointment vary in concentration from 5 to 20%, lotions from 3 to 5%. (See also: PHENOL, Reference Congener in Section III.)
RHODANATE AND RHODANIDE SALTS (INORG.) Thiocyanates Sulfocyanates e.g. Sodium, potassium, ammonium	4	See thiocyanate salts in this index.
RICIN Ricine A toxic albumin obtained from castor beans (not present in castor oil)	6	Powdered beans have been used as fertilizer. Low-concentration powders (0.3%) are marketed as a mole killer. Five beans have proved fatal in a child, 20 beans in an adult. After administration of ricin by any route there is a latency of many hours (sometimes several days). Ingestion results in a severe gastroenteritis, often hemorrhagic. Later the victim may become drowsy, confused, irrational, and comatose. Convulsions occur. Peripheral vascular collapse (shock) and renal failure may develop. Local inflammatory lesions result from dust in the eyes, nose, and throat. Convalescence is slow. Supportive treatment should be maintained energetically.

Substance and Synonym or Principal Ingredient	Toxicity Rating (See Inside Cover)	Comments and Reference Congeners
RICINOLEIC ACID 12-Hydroxy-9-octa-decenoic acid	2(?)	An unsaturated fatty acid believed to be the active purgative principle in castor oil. Said to produce its cathartic effect by stimulating motor activity through a local action on the small intestinal mucosa. Also absorbed in part within the bowel and apparently metabolized. Used externally as a bland emollient. No reports of fatalities were located.
ROSIN Abietic anhydride Colophony Yellow resin		The residue left after distilling away the volatile oils from pine oleoresins. Gum rosin results from distilling crude turpentine, wood rosin from distilling aged pine stumps (Pinus palustris). Both are water-insoluble. Rosin has been used in medicinal ointments for skin and wounds. Softened with castor oil, it is the usual adhesive on sticky fly-papers. No toxicity data were located, but the toxicity is probably low.
ROSIN OILS Rosinol		A yellow viscous oily liquid obtained by the dry distillation of rosin. Used in lacquers, varnishes, lubricants, inks. No toxicity data were located, but the toxicity is probably low.
ROTENONE Constituent of derris root	4	(See also: ROTENONE, Reference Congener in Section III.)
RUTGER'S 612 2-Ethyl hexanediol-1,3	3	An insect repellent. Little or no skin absorption. Ingestion causes central nervous depression. Death in rats is accompanied by severe kidney and liver damage. Treat by lavage, artificial respiration, and supportive measures.
RYANIA The active insecticidal principle is reported to be an alkaloid ryanodine.	3	After a short latent period in laboratory animals it causes vomiting, weakness, diarrhea, slow deep breathing, tremors, convulsions, and profound central nervous depression, with coma and death. Treatment is strictly symptomatic.
SABADILLA Cevadilla, from the seeds of Schoenocaulon officinale. About 0.3% alkaloids, of which crystalline veratrine (cevadine) and vera-tridine are the chief members.	4	Used as an insecticide (5 to 20% dusts in lime or sulfur carrier). Not to be confused with Veratrum viride or album. Although apparently much less toxic, poisoning resembles that due to aconite: local irritation (e.g., sneezing from dust in nose), emesis, headache, giddiness, weakness, twitching, convulsions, hypothermia, drowsiness but seldom coma. Death is due to respiratory or cardiovascular collapse. As with digitalis the cardiac effects arise directly and reflexly and are often severe. (See also: DIGITALIS, Reference Congener in Section III.)
SACCHARIN 2, 3-Dihydro-3-oxobenz-isosulfonazole Anhydro-o-sulfamine-benzoic acid Often marketed as its sodium salt	2	A sweetening agent or sugar substitute, excreted almost quantitatively without metabolic alternation (75 to 90% in urine). Oral doses of 5 to 25 gm. daily or single doses of 100 gm. may cause anorexia, nausea, vomiting, and diarrhea. Large daily doses may also produce gastric hyperacidity. Rabbits are killed by oral doses of 8 to 10 gm./kg., presumably as a result of gastroenteritis.
SAFFRON Crocus N.F. VII The stigmas of Crocus sativus L., consisting of about 1% picrocrocin (a volatile oil)	2(?)	Used almost exclusively for coloring (yellow) and flavoring of foods, etc. No toxic effects are described. Known to be benign.
SALICYLANILIDE e.g., Ansadol Shirlan (sodium salt) Shirlan Extra	3	A fungicide and anti-mildew substance. Only slight skin irritation and no percutaneous absorption. Systemic effects are not well defined, but when ingested, both aniline poisoning (Sec. III) and salicylism (Sec. III) might be anticipated.
SALICYLATES AND SALICYLIC ACID o-Hydroxybenzoic acid, salts, and esters	4	(See also: SALICYLATE, Reference Congener in Section III.)
SALOL Phenyl salicylate	4	Used for enteric coating of pills, in suntan lotions and creams, and formerly as an intestinal antiseptic. Insoluble in water and gastric juice. Said to be slowly hydrolyzed to phenol (40%) and salicylic acid (60%) by intestinal alkali and enzymes, but recent evidence suggests that much hydrolysis occurs in tissues after absorption. The toxic effects are chiefly those of phenol but without phenol's marked corrosive actions on the alimentary tract. (See also: PHENOL, Reference Congener in Section III.)

Substance and Synonym or Principal Ingredient	Toxicity Rating (See Inside Cover)	Comments and Reference Congeners
SANTONIN The active principle of various species of Artemisia plants (Levant wormseed)	5	A non-irritant and potent anthelmintic. Visual disturbances are common (especially color vision); sometimes disorders of hearing, taste, and smell appear. Large doses stimulate the central nervous system: headache, vomiting, abdominal pain, diarrhea, confusion, muscle twitching, tonic-clonic convulsions. There are subsequent or intermittent periods of depression: coma, fall in body temperature, circulatory or respiratory collapse. Hematuria may be prominent. Treatment is supportive and includes gastric lavage and saline catharsis. See Sec. IV for anti-convulsant therapy.
SAPROL	4	Said to consist of 40% cresols, 40% other coal tar derivatives, and 20% high-boiling hydrocarbons. (See also: PHENOL, Reference Congener in Section III.)
SCHEELE'S GREEN OR SCHEELE'S MINERAL Cupric arsenite	5	Usually 40 to 45% arsenic trioxide equivalent. Used as an insecticide. (See also ARSENIC, Reference Congener in Section III.)
SCHRADAN Octamethyl pyrophosphoramide	5	A "systemic" insecticide, i.e., translocated in sap to all parts of plants. Only slightly less toxic than parathion. Not a cholinesterase inhibitor in vitro, but converted to one by the liver. Brain cholinesterase, however, is not inhibited in fatally poisoned animals. (See also: PARATHION, Reference Congener in Section III.)
SCILLAREN The active cardiotonic glycosides of squill	6	Scillaren-A is a crystalline sterol glycoside, and scillaren-B is an amorphous glycoside fraction. Both have cardiotonic actions and toxic effects like digitalis. Unlike squill and crude extracts, scillarens are well absorbed from the alimentary tract. In terms of "cat units" they are more potent than digitoxin, but they are less toxic because of rapid excretion. A 2:1 mixture of scillarens-A and -B is given orally in a dose of 0.8 mg. one to four times daily to maintain a state of "digitalization." (See also: DIGITALIS, Reference Congener in Section III.)
SCOPOLAMINE Hyoscine	6	Commonly stated to be more toxic than atropine, but with either drug fatalities are rare. Idiosyncrasies, however, are definitely more common with hyoscine. Clinical doses of hyoscine commonly induce drowsiness or sleep, but large overdosages may produce excitement and psychotic behavior, like atropine. The hyoscine psychosis is followed by more prominent and prolonged central nervous depression. Peripheral actions mimic those of atropine. (See also: ATROPINE, Reference Congener in Section III.)
SELENATE, SODIUM	6	Used as a "systemic" insecticide, i.e., accumulates in plants which are thus rendered toxic to many pests, and also to mammals. Highly toxic by all routes (probably borderline between toxicity classes 5 and 6), but slightly less toxic than sodium selenite. A general protoplasmic poison attacking sulfhydryl enzymes. Like arsenic it causes degenerative lesions in liver, kidneys, heart, spleen, stomach, bowel, and lungs. Many signs and symptoms are possible. No human fatalities have been reported. Treat like arsenic poisoning except that BAL appears to be contra-indicated. Bromobenzene (oral adult dose 1 gm.) is said to increase the urinary excretion of selenium. Repeated low doses of sodium arsenate (or arsenite) have been used successfully to control chronic selenium poisoning in farm animals. (See also: ARSENIC, Reference Congener in Section III.)
SELENIUM DERIVATIVES		Closely related to but more toxic than tellurium. A general tissue poison like arsenic, presumably attacking sulfhydryl enzymes. Acute toxicity of soluble selenium compounds is high. In approximate order of decreasing toxicity: soluble selenites, selenates, insoluble inorganic salts (e.g., selenium sulfide), various organic derivatives (some volatile). The oxychloride is a severe vesicant. Metallic selenium is insoluble and not toxic unless finely divided as a fume. Also see "Selenate, sodium" (above). (Also see: ARSENIC, Reference Congener in Section III.)
SELENIUM SULFIDE Selenium monosulfide Selsun sulfide		A water-insoluble compound. Unlike many selenium salts, it is not decomposed by water or dilute acid to selenic or selenious acids. Only traces are absorbed through the skin, but ingestion is hazardous. If swallowed, avoid oils or alcohol which may promote absorption. Lavage and saline catharsis are recommended. For systemic effects, see "selenate, sodium." Local irritation and sensitization are rare.
SESAME OIL Benne, teel or gingilli oil, extracted from the seeds of Sesamum indicum L.	1(?)	A digestible vegetable oil, consisting of glycerides of oleic, stearic, etc., acids, plus about 1% sesamin (a complex cyclic ether). Like other fixed oils it is a laxative in large amounts. Used as a vehicle for intramuscular medication and, because of its sesamin content, as a synergist for pyrethrins.

Substance and Synonym or Principal Ingredient	Toxicity Rating (See Inside Cover)	Comments and Reference Congeners
SHELLAC Lacca Lac		A resinous excretion of certain insects feeding on appropriate host trees, usually in India. As processed for marketing, lacca may be mixed with small amounts of arsenic trisulfide (for color) and of rosin. White shellac is free of arsenic. The usual solvent is methyl alcohol. No toxicity data have been located, but the possible presence of arsenic and of methanol must be considered in suspected poisonings.
SILICA Silicone dioxide	1	Chemically and biologically inert when ingested in any of its many physical forms, such as crystalline quartz, amorphous siliceous earth (diatomaceous earth, diatomite, kieselguhr), or colloidal silica gels. The chronic inhalation of certain samples of crystalline quartz, however, may cause a progressive pneumoconiosis commonly known as silicosis.
SILICOFLUORIDE SALTS Fluosilicates e.g., Sodium, barium	4	Generally more soluble than the corresponding fluoride salt (but not true in the case of sodium). Hydrolyzed by alkali to fluoride ion. In experimental animals the fluosilicates appear to be as toxic as the corresponding fluorides and thus lie near the borderline between toxicity classes 4 and 5. Lavage stomach with lime water (calcium hydroxide). (See also: FLUORIDE, Reference Congener in Section III.)
SILICONE OILS Substituted polysiloxanes		No unequivocal toxic effects are recognized. A large dose of hexamethyl disiloxane by mouth is said to have caused mild inebriation and subsequent transient central nervous depression.
SILVER SALTS e.g., Silver nitrate (lunar caustic)		The insoluble chloride, bromide, iodide, and oxide are generally non-irritating and relatively benign. The ingestion of corrosive silver nitrate (toxicity rating 4) has been responsible for most cases of acute silver poisoning. The symptoms are those of a severe gastroenteritis and shock, with vertigo, coma, convulsions, and death. Treat like acute copper poisoning, except that gastric lavage should be performed with NaCl solutions (table salt). Apparently BAL has not received a therapeutic trial in acute poisoning. Chronic exposure to silver salts (total dose 8 gm.) may cause argyrism, which is solely of cosmetic concern. BAL does not increase the excretion of silver in cases of argyria. (See also: COPPER, Reference Congener in Section III.)
SILVEX 2(2,4,5-Trichloro-phenoxy) proprionic acid	3	Silvex, its amine salt, and its esters, have slightly lower acute toxicities than 2,4-D in laboratory animals. (See also: 2,4-D, Reference Congener in Section III.)
SOAPS Sodium (or potassium) salts of fatty acids, prepared from edible fats	2	Studies of acute oral toxicity in rats place the simple household soaps near the borderline between toxicity classes 1 and 2. They are therefore less lethal than synthetic anionic detergents and even less than most non-ionic detergents. However, soaps with an appreciable content of free alkali (e.g., some laundry soaps) are less benign. By intrauterine injection (as in some criminal abortions), soaps cause hemolysis, emboli, hyperpyrexia, shock, renal damage, and often prompt death.
SODIUM ALGINATE Algin	1(?)	A polymer of β-d-mannuronic acid with free carboxyl groups (sodium salt), prepared from various seaweeds (kelp), and widely used as an emulsifier and stabilizer in commercial ice cream, pharmaceuticals, etc. Apparently it is not decomposed or absorbed appreciably when ingested, and it does not swell in an acid medium.
SODIUM ARSENATE Sodium meta-arsenate	5	Contains at least 50% arsenic. Believed to lie near the borderline between toxicity classes 5 and 6. Dibasic sodium arsenate is almost as toxic; it contains 40% arsenic when anhydrous or 24% arsenic in the case of the usual hydrate. (See also: ARSENIC, Reference Congener in Section III.)
SODIUM ARSENITE Sodium meta-arsenite	6	Highly toxic trivalent arsenic, having an arsenic trioxide equivalent of 76.1%. (See also: ARSENIC, Reference Congener in Section III.)
SODIUM CYANIDE	6	One of the fastest poisons known. To be effective, treatment must be prompt! (See also: CYANIDE, Reference Congener in Section III.)
SODIUM 2,4-DICHLORO-PHENOXY-ETHYL SULFATE Crag Herbicide 1	3	A herbicide of moderately low toxicity in laboratory mammals. A 5% solution produced necrosis of rabbit skin but a 1% solution was not harmful. Chronic ingestion in rats caused some kidney and liver pathology. (See also: 2,4-D, Reference Congener in Section III.)
SODIUM DINITRO-ORTHO-CRESYLATE Sodium salt of 3,5-dinitro-o-cresol	5	Similar to but more toxic than dinitrophenol. (See also: DINITROPHENOL, Reference Congener in Section III.)

Substance and Synonym or Principal Ingredient	Toxicity Rating (See Inside Cover)	Comments and Reference Congeners
SODIUM ETHYL XANTHATE	3	Oral mean lethal dose in mice is 0.73 gm./kg. (about the same in guinea pigs). Concentrated solutions (and presumably dusts) are irritating to rabbit skin and eyes, and percutaneous toxicity is comparatively high (lethal dose less than 1 gm./kg.). Poisoned animals show salivation, loss of righting reflex, pulmonary congestion, pleural effusion, and death. Mild dermatitis is the only lesion observed to date in man.
SODIUM FLUOALUMINATE Cryolite Sodium aluminofluoride $AlF_3 \cdot 3NaF$ or Na_3AlF_6	2(?)	Acute toxicity by ingestion is said to be very low. Much less soluble than sodium fluoride or fluosilicate and more stable than the latter with respect to hydrolysis. (See also: FLUORIDE, Reference Congener in Section III.)
SODIUM FLUOROACETATE Compound 1080	6	A delayed convulsant, not at all like fluorides in toxic actions. (See also: FLUOROACETATE, Reference Congener in Section III.)
SODIUM FLUORIDE	4	Clinical data indicate that this compound lies near the borderline between toxicity classes 4 and 5. (See also: FLUORIDE, Reference Congener in Section III.)
SODIUM FLUOSILICATE Sodium silicofluoride	4	About as toxic as sodium fluoride in experimental animals. If also true in man, this compound lies near the borderline between toxicity classes 4 and and 5. (See also: FLUORIDE, Reference Congener in Section III.)
SODIUM HEXAMETA-PHOSPHATE e.g., Calgon	2(?)	Most preparations are neutral or only mildly alkaline. If ingested in large amounts, nausea, vomiting, and diarrhea are probable. Because this salt appears to be hydrolyzed within the bowel to phosphoric acid, a systemic acidosis may result.
SODIUM HYDROXIDE Caustic soda		(See also: ALKALI, Reference Congener in Section III.)
SODIUM HYPOCHLORITE		The official solution (NF) contains between 4 and 6% sodium hypochlorite (NaOCl), or approx. the same conc. with respect to "available chlorine." Dilute solutions of the Carrel-Dakin type are about 0.5% NaOCl. (See also: HYPOCHLORITE, Reference Congener in Section III.)
SODIUM HYPOSULFITE Sodium thiosulfate "Hypo" Formula: $Na_2S_2O_3$ (anhydrous or with 5 mols of water)	3(?)	Remarkably inert in vivo, except for osmotic disturbances. Poorly absorbed from the bowel. Acts as an osmotic cathartic. In the treatment of cyanide poisoning, 12.5 gm. has been injected intravenously without ill-effects. The thiosulfate ion distributes itself in extracellular fluid. Hyposulfite is not the preferred name because it is occasionally used to refer to the hydrosulfite ion $S_2O_4^{-2}$.
SODIUM ISOPROPYL XANTHATE	3(?)	Toxic properties are assumed to be like those of sodium ethyl xanthate. See latter in this index.
SODIUM N-METHYL DITHIOCARBAMATE DIHYDRATE Vapam	4	Used in solution as a soil fumigant. Irritating to the skin and mucous membranes. Alcohol should be avoided after known exposure to Vapam (see Disulfiram in Section III).
SODIUM MONOFLUOROACETATE Compound 1080	6	A delayed convulsant, not at all like fluorides in toxic actions. (See also: FLUOROACETATE, Reference Congener in Section III.)
SODIUM NITRITE	4	Toxicity rating of 4 describes animal studies, but no adequate clinical data have been located. (See also: NITRITE, Reference Congener in Section III.)
SODIUM OXALATE	4	Soluble salts of oxalic acid have essentially the same toxicity as the free acid. (See also: OXALATE, Reference Congener in Section III.)
SODIUM PENTACHLOROPHENATE Sodium pentachloro-phenolate	4	Lower oral toxicity than the free pentachlorophenol but solutions are highly alkaline and therefore irritating. In two human fatalities both patients developed high fevers and showed profuse sweating, "suffocation," muscular contractions, and death within 24 hours. Animal tests indicate the therapeutic importance of reducing hyperpyrexia. (See also: DINITROPHENOL, Reference Congener in Section III.)
SODIUM PERBORATE Can be represented by either of 2 formulae: $NaBO_3 \cdot 4H_2O$ $NaBO_2 \cdot 3H_2O \cdot H_2O_2$	4	Decomposes to hydrogen peroxide and sodium borate (or metaborate). Strongly alkaline and irritating. Repeated oral use as a mouth wash may cause hypertrophy of filiform papillae of tongue. Systemic effects are like those of boric acid. (See also: BORIC ACID, Reference Congener in Section III.)
SODIUM RHODANIDE Sodium thiocyanate	4	See sodium thiocyanate in this index.

Substance and Synonym or Principal Ingredient	Toxicity Rating (See Inside Cover)	Comments and Reference Congeners
SODIUM SALICYLATE Sodium salt of o-hydroxybenzoic acid	4	(See also: SALICYLATE, Reference Congener in Section III.)
SODIUM SELENATE	6	Used as a "systemic" insecticide, i.e., accumulates in plants which are thus rendered toxic to many pests, and also to mammals. Highly toxic by all routes (probably borderline between toxicity classes 5 and 6), but slightly less toxic than sodium selenite. A general protoplasmic poison attacking sulfhydryl enzymes. Like arsenic it causes degenerative lesions in liver, kidneys, heart, spleen, stomach, bowel, and lungs. Many signs and symptoms are possible. No human fatalities have been reported. Treat like arsenic poisoning except that BAL appears to be contra-indicated. Bromobenzene (oral adult dose 1 gm.) is said to increase the urinary excretion of selenium. (See also: ARSENIC, Reference Congener in Section III.)
SODIUM SILICATE Water glass Generally a mixture of molecular species of variable composition	3(?)	Moderately alkaline. Except for non-specific irritation no toxic actions are recognized. Said to be absorbed and excreted in the urine.
SODIUM SILICOFLUORIDE Sodium fluosilicate	4	About as toxic as sodium fluoride in experimental animals. If also true in man, this compound lies near the borderline between toxicity classes 4 and 5. (See also: FLUORIDE, Reference Congener in Section III.)
SODIUM SULFIDE	4	If free gastric acidity is high, the ingestion of this salt may result in its decomposition to hydrogen sulfide, with subsequent systemic poisoning. In any case the alkaline sulfides are strong local irritants to mucous membrane and skin. Treatment: gastric lavage, demulcents, saline catharsis, plus measures outlined under hydrogen sulfide. (See also: HYDROGEN SULFIDE, Reference Congener in Section III.)
SODIUM SULFITE	3	Used as a preservative in food, a skin lotion for ringworm, and a mouthwash. When ingested, solutions cause gastric irritation by the liberation of sulfurous acid. Because of rapid oxidation to sulfate, sulfites are well tolerated until large doses are reached; then violent colic and diarrhea, circulatory disturbances, central nervous depression, and death are described. Treatment is symptomatic and supportive.
SODIUM SULFOCYANATE Sodium thiocyanate Sodium rhodanate Sodium rhodanide	4	The probable lethal dose in man lies between 15 and 30 gm. (when ingested at one time). Several acute fatalities have been reported, with death in 10 to 48 hours. Large overdoses induce vomiting, extreme cerebral excitement, delirium, convulsions, and spasticity of the extensor muscles (leading to opisthotonus in poisoned animals). The temp., respiration, heart rate, and blood pressure are not directly affected. Anuria or persistent albuminuria in non-fatal cases (dogs and cats). Other toxic effects (which are generally restricted to subacute or chronic poisonings) may mimic iodism or bromide intoxication: coryza, skin rashes, weakness, fatigue, vertigo, nausea, vomiting, diarrhea, confusion, disorientation, aphasias, etc. The thiocyanate ion is slowly excreted in the urine; it is not decomposed to cyanide. The only available treatment is symptomatic and supportive.
SODIUM TETRABORATE, METABORATE, AND (ORTHO) BORATE	3	Once dissolved in any buffered solution, these salts are identical, i.e., there are no chemical or toxicological distinctions between them. They are probably best described as lying on the borderline between toxicity classes 3 and 4. (See also: BORIC ACID, Reference Congener in Section III.)
SODIUM THIOCYANATE Sodium sulfocyanate	4	See sodium sulfocyanate above.
SODIUM THIOGLYCOLLATE Sodium thioglycolate Sodium mercaptoacetate	3(?)	Commonly found in cold-wave hair preparations. Occasionally these products cause a dermatitis of scalp or hands, with erythema, edema, and even subcutaneous hemorrhages. When ingested, the high alkalinity of solutions causes caustic poisoning, but serious systemic effects are not described. Chronic exposure in animals has led to thyroid hyperplasia.
SODIUM THIOSULFATE Sodium hyposulfite "Hypo" Formula: $Na_2S_2O_3$ (anhydrous or with 5 mols of water)	3(?)	Remarkably inert in vivo, except for osmotic disturbances. Poorly absorbed from the bowel. Acts as an osmotic cathartic. In the treatment of cyanide poisoning, 12.5 gm. has been injected intravenously without ill-effects. The thiosulfate ion distributes itself in extracellular fluid.

Substance and Synonym or Principal Ingredient	Toxicity Rating (See Inside Cover	Comments and Reference Congeners
SODIUM TRICHLOROACETATE	3	Di- and trichloroacetate salts have essentially the same acute toxicity in laboratory animals as sodium acetate. Animals quickly become comatous and recover within 36 hours or die in coma. Monochloroacetate is at least 20 times more toxic.
SOLANINE A generic name for a group of glycosidal alkaloids from plants of the genus Solanum, including the common potato	5(?)	The isolated glycosides have been used in the treatment of asthma and epilepsy. Fatal poisoning has been described from the ingestion of sprouting potatoes, but the usual concentration in potatoes (less than 0.01%) has no toxic significance. Alleged toxic signs and symptoms include nausea, vomiting, diarrhea, colic, headache, tachycardia (later a slow pulse), dilated pupils, confusion, coma, and death. No specific treatment is described.
SORBIC ACID 2,4-Hexadienoic acid	2	Used to protect materials against fungi. Not a primary irritant or sensitizing agent on the skin.
SORBITAN MONOSTERATE and other fatty acid esters e.g., Span 60 (Span 80 is the mono-oleate ester) Arlacels	1	Water-insoluble non-ionic surfactants made by esterifying with digestible fatty acids various partial anhydrides of sorbitol. Added in small quantities to many foods, beverages, cosmetics, etc. When digested, both the fatty acid and the polyhydric alcohol sorbitan are absorbed, but the latter is completely excreted in urine. No single oral dose is known to be lethal in laboratory animals, and man has been fed with impunity single doses of 20 gm. or daily doses of 6 gm. for one month.
SPAN Fatty acid monoesters of sorbitan	1	See Sorbitan monostearate above.
SPERGON 2,3,5,6-Tetrachloro-p-benzoquinone	3	Low toxicity in laboratory animals. Poorly absorbed. Produces watery diarrhea, central nervous depression, coma, and death. A skin irritant in high concentrations but no percutaneous absorption.
SPERMACETI Cetaceum. Chief constituent is cetyl palmitate; also free cetyl alcohol and other esters.	1(?)	Used as an emollient and as an ointment base. No ingestion toxicity is described.
SQUILL, RED OR WHITE Sea onion Consists of the cut and dried inner scales of the bulb of Scilla (or Urginea) maritima (L)	3 and 4	The red variety has the higher toxicity rating. Fresh squill contains a crystalline sterol glycoside (scillaren-A) and an amorphous glycoside fraction (scillaren-B). Both have cardiotonic actions like digitalis, but squill is used in medicine today only as a nauseant expectorant. Even official preparations of squill are no longer assayed for their content of cardiac glycosides, but probably scillaren-A and -B constitute less than 0.5% of dried squill. The toxic syndrome mimics that which follows digitalis overdosage. Scillarens appear to be more potent than digitoxin, but the hazard of intoxication is low because the alimentary absorption of squill is uncertain and its urinary excretion is rapid. In addition to scillaren A and B, red squill possesses a glycoside known as scilliroside; it may or may not be responsible for the convulsions seen in rats, by virtue of which red squill serves as a rodenticide. Also see red squill in this index. (See also: DIGITALIS, Reference Congener in Section III.)
STANNIC AND STANNOUS SALTS Tin compounds, e.g., dioxide, dichloride, sulfide, sulfate, etc.		Tin and its salts are relatively non-toxic and poorly absorbed from the gastrointestinal tract. Tin is present in most canned foods to the extent of 20 to 50 ppm (microgm./gm.). When injected in laboratory animals, tin salts produce stimulation and subsequent depression of the central nervous system, as well as vomiting and diarrhea. More than 60 persons in France are said to have died recently from an encephalitis after ingesting a commercial "Vitamin F", consisting of diethyl tin diiodide combined with linoleic acid. Methyl derivatives of tin, lead, and bismuth have also produced encephalopathies. BAL has apparently not been tested as a therapeutic measure in tin poisoning.
STEARIC ACID Octadecanoic acid	1	A basic ingredient in vanishing creams, lotions, etc. Also a constituent of many neutral fats and therefore of most normal diets. No acute systemic ill-effects are recognized after ingestion.
STEARYL ALCOHOL Octadecyl alcohol (and usually related fatty alcohols) e.g. Stenol	1(?)	Thought to have a very low toxicity, but definitive studies were not located. (See also: ALCOHOLS, HIGHER, Reference Congener in Section III.)
STEARYL DERIVATIVE Other than listed here		See corresponding "alkyl" derivative in this index.

Substance and Synonym or Principal Ingredient	Toxicity Rating (See Inside Cover)	Comments and Reference Congeners
STODDARD SOLVENT One of higher-boiling petroleum naphtha fractions, like mineral spirits.	3	A petroleum fraction distilling between approx. 150 and 200ºC, consisting chiefly of C_8 to C_{12} aliphatic hydrocarbons. Used in dry cleaning. (See also: KEROSENE, Reference Congener in Section III.)
STRAMONIUM Thorn apple Jamestown weed Jimson (Jimpson) weed Dried leaves and flowering tops of Datura stramonium L.	4	Contains 0.25 to 0.45% alkaloids of the atropine-type (principally hyoscyamine). Pharmacologically and toxicologically equivalent to belladonna leaf. (See also: ATROPINE, Reference Congener in Section III.)
STROBANE Chlorinated terpenes, especially heptachloro-camphene	4	Only one-third to one-quarter as acutely toxic as toxaphene in animals, but poisonings are thought to be qualitatively similar in terms of symptoms and treatment. Strobane does not cause primary skin irritation or sensitization in man. Percutaneous toxicity is very low in rabbits and presumably in man too. (See also: TOXAPHENE, Reference Congener in Section III.)
STROPHANTHIN A glycoside (K-strophanthin-β) or mixture of glycosides obtained from the seeds of Strophanthus kombé.	6	A cardiac glycoside with a potency officially adjusted so that 1 mg. is equivalent to 0.5 mg. of reference ouabain. Like the latter it is poorly absorbed from the alimentary tract, where much of an oral dose appears to be destroyed. Given intravenously it has potent cardiotonic actions of relatively brief duration (about 24 hours). Except for duration, poisonings resemble those due to digitalis. (See also: DIGITALIS, Reference Congener in Section III.)
STRYCHNINE (AND SALTS) From Nux vomica	6	(See also: STRYCHNINE, Reference Congener in Section III.)
SUCCINCHLORIMIDE N-Chlorosuccinimide	3	Slowly liberates chlorine, producing gastric irritation. (See also: HYPOCHLORITE, Reference Congener in Section III.)
SULFAQUINOXALINE 2-Sulfanilamido-quinoxaline		A sulfonamide drug widely used in veterinary medicine to treat intestinal coccidiosis in fowl. Toxic doses in several animal species produce hypoprothrombinemia with fatal internal hemorrhages. The prothrombin deficit can be successfully treated with vitamin K. No human data are known.
SULFATED FATTY ALCOHOLS Sodium salts of fatty alcohol sulfates (sometimes a secondary or branched-chain alcohol, as in Tergitols) e.g. Sodium lauryl sulfate (Duponol C), Drene, Dreft, Teel, Gardinols	3	Widely used anionic detergents of moderately low acute and chronic toxicity. A few of the branched-chain products have been shown to have significant percutaneous toxicity. Skin irritation may be encountered with any of these substances. Taken by mouth, sodium lauryl sulfate stimulates gastric mucus production and sometimes inactivates pepsin in test animals. In subacute and chronic feeding tests, even fatally poisoned animals show only diarrhea and intestinal bloating, with no gross lesions outside of the gastrointestinal tract.
SULFERROUS Ferrous sulfate	3	(See also: FERROUS SULFATE, Reference Congener in Section III.)
SULFIDE SALTS Alkaline sulfide salts Metal sulfides	4	If free gastric acidity is high, the ingestion of these salts may result in their decomposition to hydrogen sulfide in the stomach, with subsequent systemic poisoning. In any case, the alkaline sulfides are strong local irritants to mucous membrane (and skin). Treatment: gastric lavage, demulcents, saline catharsis, plus measures outlined under hydrogen sulfide. (See also: HYDROGEN SULFIDE, Reference Congener in Section III.)
SULFITE SALTS e.g. Sodium, potassium, ammonium	3	Used as a preservative in food, a skin lotion for ringworm, and a mouthwash. When ingested, solutions cause gastric irritation by the liberation of sulfurous acid. Because of rapid oxidation to sulfate, sulfites are well tolerated until large doses are reached; then violent colic and diarrhea, circulatory disturbances, central nervous depression, and death are described. Treatment is symptomatic and supportive.
SULFOCYANATE SALTS (inorg.) Thiocyanate salts Rhodanates Rhodanides e.g. Sodium, potassium, ammonium	4	See thiocyanate salts in this index.

Substance and Synonym or Principal Ingredient	Toxicity Rating (See Inside Cover)	Comments and Reference Congeners
SULFONATED PETROLEUM OILS Sulfonated petroleum oils, usually marketed as sodium or calcium salts. e.g., "mahogany soaps" Penetrol	3	Anionic surfactants used as diluents and "spreaders" for agricultural sprays. Toxicity rating is based on studies with chemically related alkyl sodium sulfonates. See latter in this index.
SULFONATED CASTOR OIL More properly called sulfated castor oil or the ammonium salt of ricinoleic sulfuric acid ester (since castor oil is 80-85% ricinoleic acid). Turkey red oil	3	One of the earliest commercially important anionic surfactants, still widely used in the textile industry and in agriculture. Has been injected to cause sclerosis of varicose veins. Toxicity rating is inferred from that of simple alkyl sodium sulfates. See latter in this index.
SULFOTEPP Tetraethyl dithiono-pyrophosphate	6	Toxicity comparable to parathion in laboratory animals. Relatively resistant to hydrolysis. (See also: PARATHION, Reference Congener in Section III.)
SULFOXIDE n-Octyl sulfoxide of isosafrole	3	Used as a synergist to increase insecticidal potency of pyrethrins and possibly rotenone. In laboratory animals it has caused tremors and central nervous depression. Even surviving animals may experience prolonged coma.
SULFUR e.g., Precipitated sublimed, or washed	3(?)	Low toxicity but may cause irritation to skin, eye, and respiratory tract. Large doses (15 gm.) by mouth may lead to hydrogen sulfide production in vivo, chiefly due to bacterial action within the colon. Small particles are more toxic than large ones. A man has survived the ingestion of 60 gm. of sulfur over a period of 24 hours. (See also: HYDROGEN SULFIDE, Reference Congener in Section III.)
SULFUR CHLORIDE Sulfur monochloride Sulfur subchloride		A fuming oily liquid used as an agricultural insecticide, wood hardener, etc. Moisture promptly decomposes it to hydrochloric acid and sulfur dioxide. (See also: ACID, Reference Congener in Section III.)
SULFUR DIOXIDE Sulfurous anhydride		A highly irritant gas, often cited as a dangerous atmospheric constituent in smog areas. Inhalation produces all grades of respiratory tract irritation, sometimes with pulmonary edema. The vapor concentration probably determines the mode of death: e.g., suffocation from reflex respiratory arrest (very high conc.), pulmonary edema (moderate conc.), or systemic acidosis (low conc.) (See also: NITROGEN OXIDES, Reference Congener in Section III.)
SULFURIC ACID Oil of vitriol The commercial acid is 93 to 98% H_2SO_4 (the rest is water).		(See also: ACID, Reference Congener in Section III.)
SULFUROUS ACID Sulfur dioxide solution, usually about 6% SO_2 in water		Also see sulfur dioxide in this index. (See also: ACID, Reference Congener in Section III.)
SULPHENONE Parachlorophenyl phenyl sulfone	3	An acaricide of moderately low oral toxicity to laboratory mammals. No skin irritation. No significant tissue storage in chronic feeding tests.
SYLVIC ACID Abietic acid	2(?)	Almost no information. Low intravenous toxicity in mice (presumably also by other routes). Central nervous paralysis in frogs.
SYSTOX Ethyl mercapto-ethyl diethyl thiophosphate Demeton	5	A "systemic" insecticide, i.e. translocated in sap to all parts of plants. Almost as toxic as parathion in animals. Percutaneous toxicity is high. One human fatality has been reported. (See also: PARATHION, Reference Congener in Section III.)
TALC Talcum Finely powdered native hydrous magnesium silicate	1	No acute toxicity is recognized. Mild pneumoconiosis after chronic inhalation.

Substance and Synonym or Principal Ingredient	Toxicity Rating (See Inside Cover)	Comments and Reference Congeners
TANNIC ACID Tannin	3	An astringent of moderately low toxicity. Large doses may produce gastritis (especially if stomach is empty), vomiting, pain, diarrhea, or constipation. Injected tannic acid may produce collapse, convulsions, and death, - or delayed severe focal liver necrosis. The latter is rarely, if ever, seen after ingestion.
TARS, TAR OILS, AND TAR ACIDS The black or dark residue remaining after the destructive distillation of coal, crude petroleum, or wood (usually pine or juniper).	4(?)	Tars, tar oils, and tar acids are closely related. All 3 types of products vary in composition, depending upon the source and method of manufacture. In all cases, however, the principal toxic ingredients are phenol and its congeners, - and other aromatic hydrocarbons (e.g., xylenes, naphthalene, etc.). Toxicity estimates are difficult because even the U.S.P. does not specify the phenol or cresol content of official preparations, - but 1 oz. of most tars, if ingested, would probably jeopardize life. Most medicinal ointments are only 1 to 10% tar. (See also: PHENOL, Reference Congener in Section III.)
TARTAR EMETIC Antimony potassium tartrate	5	The minimum lethal dose in man is 130 mg. (while 15000 mg. have been survived). A strong irritant and emetic, but the emetic dose (e.g., 30 mg. by mouth) is dangerously high if vomiting fails to occur. Also consult this index under "antimony compounds" for general comments. (See also: ARSENIC, Reference Congener in Section III.)
TCA Trichloroacetic acid and its sodium salt		A corrosive organic acid which rapidly penetrates and "fixes" tissues. Systemic effects are presumably secondary to gastrointestinal damage and to acidosis, not due to the trichloroacetate ion which has a low inherent toxicity (i.e., the simple salts are not hazardous). (See also: ACID, Reference Congener in Section III.)
TCE Tetrachloroethane	4	More potent central nervous effects than chloroform or carbon tetrachloride. On ingestion severe mucosal injury and often liver necrosis. Can be absorbed through intact skin. (See also: CARBON TETRACHLORIDE, Reference Congener in Section III.)
TCP Trichlorophenoxyacetic acid 2,4,5-T	3	About the same toxicity as 2,4-D in laboratory animals, -which places this compound near the borderline between toxicity classes 3 and 4. TCP is also an abbreviation for the commercial mixture of tricresyl phosphates; see o-tricresyl phosphate in this index. (See also: 2,4-D, Reference Congener in Section III.)
TDE Dichloro diphenyl dichlorethane Tetrachlorodiphenyl ethane	3	Less toxic than DDT in animals, and poisonings are slower in onset and longer in duration. Lethargy is more prominent and convulsions are less frequent than in DDT poisoning. In chronic feeding experiments, TDE, like DDT, is stored in body fat, but it is mobilized and excreted faster than DDT when a normal diet is resumed. (See also: DDT, Reference Congener in Section III.)
TEP or TEPP Tetraethyl pyrophosphate	6	More potent than parathion, but poisonings may be slightly more transient, because TEPP is detoxified faster and because enzyme inhibition seems to be reversible in large measure. (See also: PARATHION, Reference Congener in Section III.)
TEREBENE Mixture of terpene hydrocarbons, chiefly dipentene, prepared from oil of turpentine.	3(?)	Used as a stimulant expectorant, and formerly for dyspepsia and for chronic urinary tract inflammation. Oral dose 0.12-0.5 ml. (or by inhalation). In excess it may produce albuminuria and hematuria. (See also: TURPENTINE, Reference Congener in Section III.)
TERPENES e.g., Pinene	3	The cyclic hydrocarbons contained in volatile oils are usually designated as terpenes (from turpentine oil). (See also: TURPENTINE, Reference Congener in Section III.)
TERPINEOL Lilacin, a mixture of several isomers	3	The principal constituents of pine oil (about 75% terpineols). Used in perfumery for its lilac odor. As judged by pine oil, terpineols are irritating to eyes and mucous membranes. Produce hemorrhagic gastritis. Systemic effects include weakness and central nervous depression, with hypothermia and respiratory failure. (See also: TURPENTINE, Reference Congener in Section III.)
TERPIN HYDRATE	3	An expectorant said to lessen abundant sputum. Chemically related to the terpenes and terpineols. Said to be more pleasant, less irritant, and less toxic than turpentine (including the rectified oil), but no evidence was located to show that the lethal dose is greater than that of turpentine. (See also: TURPENTINE, Reference Congener in Section III.)
TERPINYL THIOCYANO-ACETATE Isobornyl thiocyanoacetate	3	Animal studies place this compound near the borderline between toxicity classes 3 and 4. (See also: ALIPHATIC THIOCYANATES, Reference Congener in Section III.)

Substance and Synonym or Principal Ingredient	Toxicity Rating (See Inside Cover)	Comments and Reference Congeners
TETRABROMO-o-CRESOL 2-Methyl-3,4,5,6-tetrabromophenol	3	A fungicide of low acute toxicity by mouth in guinea pigs. Concentrated solutions are corrosive to skin. No clinical data. (See also: PHENOL, Reference Congener in Section III.)
TETRACHLORO-BENZOQUINONE Chloranil	3	Moderately low toxicity in laboratory animals. Poorly absorbed. Skin irritation in high concentrations but no percutaneous absorption. After ingestion (animal tests), watery diarrhea, central nervous depression, coma, and death.
TETRACHLORO DIPHENYL ETHANE DDD	3	Less toxic than DDT in animals and poisonings are slower in onset and longer in duration. Lethargy is more prominent and convulsions are less frequent than in DDT poisoning. (See also: DDT, Reference Congener in Section III.)
TETRACHLOROETHANE Acetylene tetrachloride	4	More toxic than carbon tetrachloride and more potent as a central depressant than chloroform. On ingestion severe mucosal injury and often liver necrosis, sometimes with later cirrhosis. Can be absorbed through intact skin. (See also: CARBON TETRACHLORIDE, Reference Congener in Section III.)
TETRACHLOROETHYLENE Ethylene tetrachloride	3	Less toxic than carbon tetrachloride or chloroform. Given therapeutically (for hookworms) to adults by mouth (dose 1-4 ml.). Low solubility in water and poorly absorbed in the absence of fats or oils. Widely used in veterinary medicine. (See also: CARBON TETRACHLORIDE, Reference Congener in Section III.)
TETRACHLORO-QUINONE Chloranil	3	Moderately low toxicity in laboratory animals. Poorly absorbed. Ingestion is followed by watery diarrhea, central nervous depression, coma, and death. A skin irritant in high concentrations.
TETRAETHYL DITHIOPYROPHOS-PHATE Sulfotepp	6	Toxicity is comparable to parathion in laboratory animals. Relatively resistant to hydrolysis. (See also: PARATHION, Reference Congener in Section III.)
TETRAETHYL PYROPHOSPHATE TEPP	6	More potent than parathion, but poisonings may be slightly more transient because TEPP is detoxified faster and because enzyme inhibition seems to be reversible in large measure. (See also: PARATHION, Reference Congener in Section III.)
TETRAETHYLTHIURAM Disulfiram Antabuse	3	Toxicity rating of 3 is based on animal tests in which no alcohol was given. (See also: DISULFIRAM, Reference Congener in Section III.)
TETRAHYDRONAPH-THALENE Tetralin		Vapors are known to produce in man headache, nausea, vomiting, irritation of conjunctiva and of respiratory tract mucosa. Absorbed vapor is excreted by kidneys as tetralol, giving urine a grass-green color. Cataract formation and nephritic lesions are seen in guinea pigs after vapor exposure. No data on ingestion toxicity were located.
TETRALIN Tetrahydronaphthalene		See above.
TETRAMETHYLTHIURAM DISULFIDE Thiram	4	(See also: THIRAM, Reference Congener in Section III.)
TETRANAP Tetrahydronaphthalene		Vapors are known to produce in man headache, nausea, vomiting, irritation of conjunctiva and of respiratory tract mucosa. Absorbed vapor is excreted by kidneys as tetralol, giving urine a grass-green color. Cataract formation and nephritic lesions in guinea pigs after vapor exposure. No data on ingestion toxicity were located.
TETRASODIUM PYROPHOSPHATE Sodium pyrophosphate	3(?)	Alkaline and irritating. Nausea, vomiting, and diarrhea are probable after ingestion. Presumably pyrophosphate is largely hydrolyzed to orthophosphate before absorption. Some animal data suggest that pyrophosphate is considerably (and unaccountably) more toxic than implied by a toxicity rating of 3.
TETRIN TEPP Tetraethyl pyrophosphate	6	More potent than parathion, but poisonings may be slightly more transient because TEPP is detoxified faster and because enzyme inhibition is reversible in large measure. (See also: PARATHION, Reference Congener in Section III.)
THALLIUM SALTS e.g., Sulfate, acetate	5	(See also: THALLIUM, Reference Congener in Section III.)

Substance and Synonym or Principal Ingredient	Toxicity Rating (See Inside Cover)	Comments and Reference Congeners
THANITE Isobornyl thiocyano-acetate	3	Animal studies place this compound near the borderline between toxicity classes 3 and 4. (See also: ALIPHATIC THIOCYANATES, Reference Congener in Section III.)
2,2-THIOBIS (4,6-DICHLORO-PHENOL Actamer	2	A germicide of low toxicity. No skin reaction when applied as 2% ointment (Carbowax). Systemic effects are presumed to be like phenol. (See also: PHENOL, Reference Congener in Section III.)
THIOCARBAMIDE Thiourea		Repeated use may induce agranulocytosis and thrombopenia. Single-dose toxicity is not known but is apparently low. Compound is rapidly excreted, unchanged in urine.
THIOCYANATES, ORGANIC Usually aliphatic derivatives, e.g., lauryl thiocyanate, Lethanes, etc.		Used as agricultural insecticides. When tested in animals, various organic thiocyanates differ widely in toxicity. (See also: ALIPHATIC THIOCYANATES, Reference Congener in Section III.)
THIOCYANATE SALTS (INORG.) e.g., Sodium, potassium ammonium, etc. Sulfocyanates Rhodanates Rhodanides	4	The probable lethal dose in man lies between 15 and 30 gm. (when ingested at one time). Several acute fatalities have been reported, with death in 10 to 48 hours. Large overdoses induce vomiting, extreme cerebral excitement, delirium, convulsions, and spasticity of the extensor muscles (leading to opisthotonus in poisoned animals). The temperature, respirations, heart rate, and blood pressure are not directly affected. Anuria or persistent albuminuria in non-fatal cases (dogs and cats). Other effects (which are generally restricted to subacute or chronic poisonings) may mimic iodism or bromide intoxication: coryza, skin rashes, weakness, fatigue, vertigo, nausea, vomiting, diarrhea, confusion, disorientation, aphasias, etc. The thiocyanate ion is slowly excreted in the urine; it is not decomposed to cyanide. The only available treatment is symptomatic and supportive.
β-THIOCYANOETHYL ESTERS OF FATTY ACIDS e.g., Lethane 60	3	(See also: ALIPHATIC THIOCYANATES, Reference Congener in Section III.)
THIODIPHENYLAMINE Phenothiazine	3	Probably lies near the borderline between toxicity classes 3 and 4. Cumulative therapeutic dose should be kept below 20 gm. Overdosage and accidental exposures have caused hemolytic anemia, toxic hepatitis, skin photosensitization, and intense pruritus.
THIOGLYCOLLATE SALTS Mercaptoacetate salts e.g., Sodium, ammonium potassium thioglycollates or thioglycolates	3(?)	Commonly found in cold-wave hair preparations. Occasionally these produce a dermatitis of scalp or hands, with erythema, edema, and even subcutaneous hemorrhages. When ingested, the high alkalinity of these solutions causes a caustic poisoning, but serious systemic effects are not described. Chronic exposure in animals has led to thyroid hyperplasia.
THIOSULFATE SALTS Hyposulfites e.g., sodium, potassium, etc.	3	Remarkably inert in vivo, except for osmotic disturbances. Poorly absorbed from the alimentary tract and so acts as an osmotic cathartic. In the treatment of cyanide poisoning, 12.5 gm. of highly purified sodium thiosulfate has been injected i.v. without ill-effects.
THIOUREA Thiocarbamide		Repeated use may induce agranulocytosis and thrombopenia. Single-dose toxicity is not known but is apparently low. Compound is rapidly excreted, unchanged in urine.
THIRAM Tetramethylthiuram disulfide	4	(See also: THIRAM, Reference Congener in Section III.)
THYMOL 5-Methyl-2-isopropyl-1-phenol 3-Hydroxy-p-cymene	4	A potent fungicide and anthelmintic, mildly irritating locally. Resembles phenol in its systemic actions but less toxic, partly because it is less soluble. Believed to lie near the borderline between toxicity classes 3 and 4. Produces gastric pain, nausea, vomiting, central hyperactivity (e.g., talkativeness), occasionally convulsions, coma, cardiac and respiratory collapse. Avoid oils and alcohol, which promote absorption. (See also: PHENOL, Reference Congener in Section III.)
TIN COMPOUNDS Simple salts and metal, e.g., tin dioxide, dichloride, sulfide, sulfate, etc.		Tin and its salts are relatively non-toxic and poorly absorbed from the intestinal tract. Tin is present in most canned foods to the extent of 20 to 50 ppm. (or microgm. per gm.). When injected in laboratory animals, tin salts produce stimulation and subsequent depression of the central nervous system, as well as vomiting and diarrhea. More than 60 persons in France are said to have died recently from an encephalitis after ingesting a commercial "Vitamin F", consisting of diethyl tin diiodide combined with linoleic acid. Methyl derivatives of tin, lead, and bismuth have also produced encephalopathies. BAL has apparently not been tested as a therapeutic measure in tin poisoning.

Substance and Synonym or Principal Ingredient	Toxicity Rating (See Inside Cover)	Comments and Reference Congeners
TITANIUM OXIDE Titanium dioxide	1	A pound (16 oz.) has been ingested without apparent harm or distress. It was eliminated in feces in about 24 hours.
TOADSTOOLS, POISONOUS	3 or 4	Most toxic species belong to the genus Amanita. (See also: AMANITA TOXINS, Reference Congener in Section III.)
TOBACCO Dried or partially dessicated leaves of various species of the genus Nicotiana	4	The acute toxicity of tobacco, when eaten or inhaled as smoke, is largely ascribed to its nicotine content. Nicotine, present as salts of organic acids, constitutes 1.0 to 2.5% (by weight) of commercial tobacco as marketed for smoking, - and sometimes as high as 8% of dessicated tobacco. Thus an average cigarette (weight approx. 1 gm.) may contain 25 mg. of nicotine, and 2 or 3 cigarettes contain a fatal dose for an adult. Cigarette smoke, however, contains less than 10 mg., of which only a few milligrams are usually absorbed. Although deaths have been recorded from the ingestion and rectal administration of a few grams of tobacco, even infants have survived after swallowing several cigarettes. Apparently the intestinal absorption of nicotine, as it is present in tobacco, is so slow that spontaneous vomiting eventually removes much unabsorbed alkaloid. Treat like nicotine poisoning. (See also: NICOTINE, Reference Congener in Section III.)
TOLUENE Methyl benzene Toluol	4	Toxicity is very similar to that of xylene. It may produce a mild macrocytic anemia but no leukopenia (as benzene does). (See also: XYLENE, Reference Congener in Section III.)
TOLUENEDIAMINE Partoluylenediamine	4	Animal tests suggest that it is slightly less toxic but presumably similar to paraphenylenediamine. See latter. No human poisonings are known.
TOLUIDINE 4-Methylaniline p-Toluidine	4(?)	Like aniline, but renal injury is more likely. The ortho and meta isomers probably have similar toxicities. (See also: ANILINE, Reference Congener in Section III.)
TOLUOL Toluene Methyl benzene	4	Toxicity is very similar to that of xylene. It may produce a mild macrocytic anemia but, in contrast to benzene, no leucopenia or severe bone marrow lesions. (See also: XYLENE, Reference Congener in Section III.)
N-m-TOLYL PHTHALAMIC ACID e.g., Duraset	3	Acute toxicity measured in rats places this compound near the borderline of toxicity classes 2 and 3. However, chemical data indicate that gastric acid (pH 3) and intestinal alkali (pH 10) may hydrolyze this amide to phthalamic acid (low toxicity) and to m-toluidine (high toxicity in man). See toluidine above. (See also: ANILINE, Reference Congener in Section III.)
TOXAPHENE Chlorinated camphene Octachlorocamphene	4	Believed to lie near the borderline between toxicity classes 4 and 5. (See also: TOXAPHENE, Reference Congener in Section III.)
TRIACETIN Glyceryl triacetate	1	Laboratory rats have tolerated diets consisting of 50% triacetin. If hydrolyzed, systemic acidosis is a possible consequence.
TRIALKYL THIOPHOSPHATE e.g., Parathion	6	Some are among the most toxic materials used for pest control. Rapidly absorbed from all portals. Toxic effects are referable to the central and autonomic nervous systems and are associated with cholinesterase inhibition. (See also: PARATHION, Reference Congener in Section III.)
TRIBASIC COPPER SULFATE A molecular mixture of cupric hydroxide and cupric sulfate, the exact composition of which is uncertain (about 50% copper by weight)	4	The name is apparently applied to several commercially available powders of the pre-mixed Bordeaux-type, used as foliage fungicides. Less astringent and presumably less toxic than copper sulfate, but the copper content may be higher than that of copper sulfate. (See also: COPPER, Reference Congener in Section III.)
TRICHLOROACETIC ACID		A corrosive organic acid which rapidly penetrates and "fixes" tissues. Systemic effects are presumably secondary to gastrointestinal damage and to acidosis, not due to the trichloroacetate ion which has a low inherent toxicity (i.e., the simple salts are not hazardous). (See also: ACID, Reference Congener in Section III.)
TRICHLOROACETONITRILE Formula: CCl_3-CN		A volatile liquid used as a fumigant for treatment of stored grain and households. Lacrimation usually gives adequate warning of vapor exposure. A vesicant on the skin. Causes systemic cyanide poisoning. (See also: CYANIDE, Reference Congener in Section III.)
TRICHLOROBENZENES Usually available as a mixture of three isomers	4(?)	Has been used to combat termites. May irritate the eyes and respiratory tract. Has caused liver injury in man and animals. It is probably less toxic than o-dichlorobenzene.

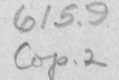

Substance and Synonym or Principal Ingredient	Toxicity Rating (See Inside Cover)	Comments and Reference Congeners
1,1,1-TRICHLORO-2,2-BIS (PARACHLORO-PHENYL) ETHANE DDT	4	(See also: DDT, Reference Congener in Section III.)
1,1,1-TRICHLORO-2,2-BIS(PARAMETHOXY-PHENYL) ETHANE Methoxychlor	3	Lower toxicity than DDT. Estimated to be one tenth as toxic in man by ingestion, but this difference may not hold in respiratory exposures to vapor. In animals central nervous depression is more prominent than excitation, and poisonings are slower in onset and longer in duration than from DDT. (See also: DDT, Reference Congener in Section III.)
TRICHLOROETHYLENE Trichloroethene Ethinyl trichloride e.g. Trilene	4	Acute toxicity like chloroform. Rapid recovery with or without severe sequellae like trigeminal (or other nerve) paralysis or liver necrosis. Can be absorbed through intact skin. (See also: CARBON TETRACHLORIDE, Reference Congener in Section III.)
N-TRICHLOROMETHYL-MERCAPTO-4-CYCLO-HEXENE-1,2-DICARBOX-IMIDE Captan Vancide 89	2	See comments below.
N-TRICHLOROMETHYL-THIO-TETRAHYDRO-PHTHALIMIDE Captan Vancide 89	2	A fungicide of low oral and cutaneous toxicity in laboratory and farm animals (best described as lying near the borderline between toxicity classes 2 and 3). At lethal doses diarrhea and weight loss appear but no histopathological lesions. Low toxicity is thought to derive from lack of appreciable absorption (because of rapid alkaline hydrolysis in bowel?). Chlorine atoms are unusual because readily hydrolyzed to Cl^-.
TRICHLOROMONO-FLUOROMETHANE Freon 11		A gas of low toxicity but not entirely inert. See Freons in this index.
TRICHLORONITRO-METHANE Chloropicrin	5	A "war gas", sometimes used as a fumigant and tracer gas. Vapor is intensely irritating to skin, eyes, mucous membranes, and stomach. Called "vomiting gas". Treatment is symptomatic with special attention to the lungs. Ingestion of liquid produces severe gastroenteritis. (See also: NITROGEN OXIDES, Reference Congener in Section III.)
TRICHLOROPHENOXY-ACETIC ACID 2,4,5-T	3	About the same toxicity as 2,4-D in animals, which place this compound near the borderline between toxicity classes 3 and 4. (See also: 2,4-D, Reference Congener in Section III.)
TRICHLOROPHENOXY PROPRIONIC ACID Silvex	3	This acid, its amine salt, and its esters are slightly less toxic than 2,4-D in most laboratory animals. (See also: 2,4-D, Reference Congener in Section III.)
TRICHLORO-FLUOROETHANE Freon-113		A gas of low toxicity but not entirely inert. See Freons in this index.
TRICHLOROPHENOLS e.g., 2,4,5-Trichloro-phenol (Dowicide 2) 2,4,6-Trichlorophenol (Dowicide 2s)	4	Almost as toxic as phenol. Thought to have an acute toxicity between mono-chlorophenols and pentachlorophenol. (See also: PHENOL, Reference Congener in Section III.)
TRICRESOL Cresol	4	A mixture of 3 isomeric cresols from coal tar. About the same toxicity and toxic actions as phenol. Perhaps slightly more corrosive than phenol, but systemic effects may be a little milder because of slower absorption. (See also: PHENOL, Reference Congener in Section III.)
o-TRICRESYL PHOSPHATE Triorthocresyl phosphate		A unique polyneuritis with flaccid paralysis (but no sensory disturbances), first appearing many days after the exposure ("ginger paralysis"). With large doses, however, the latent period may be very short. Recovery is slow but usually complete. None of the usual toxic effects of cresols or phenols are described in clinical poisonings. Because this substance is also capable of inhibiting the enzyme cholinesterase in vitro and in vivo, treatment as in parathion poisoning may become necessary (see parathion, Sec. III). Meta and para isomers are relatively inactive.
TRIETHANOLAMINE Tri(hydroxyethyl) amine	2	Several ounces can probably be tolerated by man. The principal toxic effect in animals has been ascribed to alkalinization (systemic alkalosis). Gross pathology has been limited to the gastrointestinal tract in fatal oral poisonings in rats and guinea pigs.

Substance and Synonym or Principal Ingredient	Toxicity Rating (See Inside Cover)	Comments and Reference Congeners
TRIETHANOLAMINE OLEATE Also other fatty acid esters of triethanol-amine	2(?)	These esters are synthetic soaps. They form practically neutral aqueous solutions, which are not irritating or injurious to the skin. Widely used as detergents and emulsifiers in medicine and pharmacy. Ingestion toxicity is thought to be low.
TRIETHYLENE GLYCOL	2(?)	This compound has a lower acute toxicity than diethylene glycol but a higher toxicity than propylene glycol. Symptoms are presumably like those due to ethylene glycol, but there is no evidence of decomposition to ethylene glycol in vivo. (See also: ETHYLENE GLYCOL, Reference Congener in Section III.)
TRIFORMOL Paraformaldehyde Paraform Trioxymethylene	4	Same internal toxicity as formaldehyde, which it slowly releases at body temperature. (See also: FORMALDEHYDE, Reference Congener in Section III.)
1,2,3-TRIHYDROXY-BENZENE Pyrogallol	4	Toxicity and toxic actions like phenol, but also methemoglobinemia, hemolysis, and renal injury, - as in aniline poisoning. Delayed deaths from uremia have been reported. Percutaneous absorption is dangerous. Mildly caustic to skin and mucous membranes. (See also: ANILINE, Reference Congener in Section III.)
3,4,5-TRIHYDROXY-BENZOIC ACID Gallic acid	3(?)	Apparently much less toxic than salicylic acid. Fed to men in quantities of 2 to 10 gm. without fatalities and even without severe ill-effects. Readily absorbed from the gastrointestinal tract. In animals it reduces body temperature and causes progressive weakness and perhaps convulsions.
TRIIODOMETHANE Iodoform	4	Best described as lying near the borderline between toxicity classes 4 and 5. Poisoning has been due to absorption through wounds when iodoform dressings were used (no more than 2 gm. iodoform should be so used). May cause dermatitis. Systemic effects include vomiting and all degrees of cerebral depression or excitation. A very rapid pulse is characteristic, with or without a slight fever. No useful antidote is recognized.
TRINITROBENZENE	5(?)	No specific toxicity data were located, but the toxic actions are probably like those of dinitrobenzene. See latter in this index. (See also: ANILINE, Reference Congener in Section III.)
2,4,6-TRINITROPHENOL Picric acid	5	Severe poisoning from ingestion of 1 to 2 gm. Severe gastroenteritis, hemorrhagic nephritis, and sometimes hepatitis. Increased metabolism like dinitrophenol (see Sec. III). Headache, progressive stupor, coma, and death in severe poisoning. (See also: PHENOL, Reference Congener in Section III.)
TRIOXYMETHYLENE Paraformaldehyde	4	Same internal toxicity as formaldehyde, which it slowly releases at body temperature. (See also: FORMALDEHYDE, Reference Congener in Section III.)
TRIPHENYL PHOSPHATE	4(?)	Used as a plasticizer and a fire-proofing agent. A neurotoxic substance like tricresyl phosphate; more potent than the latter in cats but probably not in man. Causes a delayed peripheral neuritis involving motor neurones, resulting in a flaccid paralysis, particularly of the distal muscles. No sensory disturbances. Signs and symptoms of cholinesterase inhibition should also be anticipated and treated as in parathion poisoning (see Section III).
TRIS(HYDROXYMETHYL) AMINOMETHANE 2-Amino-2-hydroxy-methyl-1,3-propanediol	3	A commercial emulsifier. Aqueous solutions are alkaline and consequently irritating. Even after neutralization, large oral doses in laboratory animals cause weakness, collapse, and coma (without convulsions).
TRITONS A trademarked name for a series of commercial surfactants	3	These surface-active agents are non-ionic (alkyl aryl polyether alcohols) or anionic (similar compounds which have been sulfated or sulfonates and marketed as sodium salts), except for cationic Triton K-60 or X-400. None is highly toxic in animals, and none produces significant irritation or sensitization of human skin (except Triton X-400).
TTD Bis(diethylthiocarbamyl) disulfide Disulfiram Antabuse	3	Toxicity rating of 3 is based on animal tests in which no alcohol was given. (See also: DISULFIRAM, Reference Congener in Section III.)

Substance and Synonym or Principal Ingredient	Toxicity Rating (See Inside Cover)	Comments and Reference Congeners
TURKEY RED OIL Principally the ammonium salt of ricinoleic sulfuric acid ester, prepared by sulfating castor oil.	3	One of the earliest commercially important anionic surfactants, still widely used in the textile industry and in agriculture. Has been injected to cause sclerosis of varicose veins. Toxicity rating is inferred from that of simple alkyl sodium sulfates. See latter in this index.
TURPENTINE Oil of turpentine Spirits of turpentine	3	(See also: TURPENTINE, Reference Congener in Section III.)
TWEENS A trademarked name for polyethylene (20) sorbitan mono-laurate and other fatty acid esters	1	A group of non-ionic surfactants, generally soluble or dispersible in water. Small quantities are used in many foods and beverages, cosmetics, etc. No single oral dose is known to be lethal in animals, and men have been fed 15 gm. daily for several months with impunity. In the bowel the fatty acid is split off and absorbed, and the rest is eliminated in feces.
UMBELLIFERONE 7-Hydroxycoumarin		In sun-screen lotions and creams. No toxicity data were located.
UNDECYLENIC ACID 9-Undecylenic acid 10-Undecenoic acid	3	A normal constituent of sweat. Used as a fungicide on skin. Formerly taken by mouth in the treatment of psoriasis. In daily oral doses of 6 to 14 gm., the following transient effects are described in man: gastrointestinal disturbances, headache, fever, dizziness, urticaria, folliculitis, and conjunctivitis. Lethal dose in rats about 2.5 gm./kg.
URGININ Urginin A and B	6	A mixture of two water-insoluble glycosides from squill (Urginea maritima). Has therapeutic and toxic actions like digitalis. The usual daily maintenance dose in an adult is 0.5 to 1.0 mg. by mouth. (See also: DIGITALIS, Reference Congener in Section III.)
UROLOCIDE Dodecyl carbamyl-methyl dimethyl benzyl ammonium chloride	4	A cationic surfactant used as a disinfectant at aqueous concentrations of about 0.1%. A 5% solution is not irritating to human skin. (See also: QAC, Reference Congener in Section III.)
URANIUM NITRATE Uranyl nitrate and other acid-soluble uranyl salts	3(?)	Poorly absorbed by mouth. Given parenterally it is as toxic as mercury or arsenic. Produces severe kidney tubular degeneration and renal failure. See Sec. IV for a discussion of general treatment in this syndrome. BAL is useless. Edathamil calcium-disodium (Ca-EDTA) is recommended intravenously according to the dose schedule for lead poisoning (Sec. III).
UVA URSI Bearberry Dried leaves of Arctostaphylos uva-ursi, containing volatile oil, arbutin, tannin (6-7%), gallic and malic acids, etc.	2(?)	Once used as a diuretic and antiseptic drug. Cleavage of arbutin, a glucoside, liberates hydroquinone, which appears in the urine after large doses. Usual dose 1 gm. three to six times a day, but no ill-effects even after 20 gm.
VANILLIN 3-Methoxy-4-hydroxybenzaldehyde	3	Synthetic or derived from vanilla beans. Used as a flavoring agent in place of vanilla. In laboratory animals ingestion of a single toxic dose causes hyperpnea, muscular weakness, dyspnea, collapse, and death due to circulatory failure. (See also: PHENOL, Reference Congener in Section III.)
VAPAM Sodium N-methyl dithiocarbamate dihydrate		Used in solution as a soil fumigant. Irritating to the skin and mucous membranes. Alcohol should be avoided after known exposures to Vapam (see Disulfiram in Section III).
VERONAL 5,5'-Diethyl barbituric acid Barbital	4	Probably lies near the borderline between toxicity classes 4 and 5. The oldest clinically useful barbiturate drug. A hypnotic and central nervous depressant. It has a long duration of action because elimination is dependent on renal excretion and the latter is inherently slow. As discussed in Sec. III, an osmotic diuresis may be a useful therapeutic measure in poisonings. (See also: BARBITURATES, Reference Congener in Section III.)
VINYL CHLORIDE Chloroethylene		A refrigerant gas with weak depressant actions on central nervous system, like ethyl chloride. Effects are usually brief. (See also: CARBON TETRACHLORIDE, Reference Congener in Section III).

Substance and Synonym or Principal Ingredient	Toxicity Rating (See Inside Cover)	Comments and Reference Congeners
VINYL CYANIDE Acrylonitrite Propene nitrile	4	Similar to but less toxic than its molecular equivalent in hydrogen cyanide. In sublethal exposures mild jaundice has been reported. Liquid spilled on the skin results in erythema and later painful blisters. Treatment measures for cyanide do not protect exposed guinea pigs, suggesting that the release of HCN is too small to account for acrylonitrile poisoning in this species. (See also: CYANIDE, Reference Congener in Section III.)
VITRIOLIC ACID Sulfuric acid		The commercial acid is 93 to 98% H_2SO_4 (the rest is water). (See also: ACID, Reference Congener in Section III.)
VOLATILE OILS Essential oils, e.g., oil of savin, rue tansy, nutmeg, pennyroyal, apiol eucalyptus, juniper, cedarleaf, cajuput	4	Most of these oils are reputed to be ecbolic, but abortions cannot be induced by safe doses. Basically symptoms and treatment as after turpentine but toxicity is greater. In most cases a teaspoonful may cause illness in an adult and less than an ounce may kill (especially if vomiting does not occur promptly). Savin produces more renal damage than turpentine, and pennyroyal more liver degeneration. Also see eucalyptol, oil of sassafras, menthol, pine oil, wintergreen oil. (See also: TURPENTINE, Reference Congener in Section III.)
WARFARIN 3-(a-Acetonylbenzyl) -4-hydroxycoumarin	4	Single-dose toxicity is not well defined, but it is probably low relative to the cumulative multiple-dose toxicity. (See also: WARFARIN, Reference Congener in Section III.)
WATER GLASS Sodium silicate, generally a mixture of molecular species of variable composition	3(?)	Moderately alkaline but no other recognized actions when ingested. Said to be absorbed and excreted in urine.
WHITE ARSENIC Arsenic trioxide	6	The average fatal oral dose in man probably lies between 0.1 and 0.3 gm. Coarse powders are less toxic than fine ones. (See also: ARSENIC, Reference Congener in Section III.)
WINTERGREEN OIL Methyl salicylate	4	A strong irritant on skin and mucous membranes. Used externally as a counter-irritant. May be absorbed rapidly through intact skin. Bowel absorption is somewhat erratic, and gastric lavage may be beneficial even several hours after ingestion. Absorbed at least in part as the intact ester and small amounts are even excreted as such by the kidneys, but the compound is largely hydrolyzed. Typical systemic effects of salicylates, not of methyl alcohol, but probably more toxic than sodium salicylate. (See also: SALICYLATE, Reference Congener in Section III.)
WITCH HAZEL Dried leaves of Hamamelis virginiana, containing tannin (2-9%).	2	The dried leaves (or an extract thereof) are used in ointments and suppositories (dose 2 gm.). The fluidextract (prepared from the leaves) has an ethyl alcohol content of 70-78% and significant amounts of tannin (dose 2-4 ml.). Witch Hazel Water is a saturated aqueous solution (with 15% ethyl alcohol) of volatile products distilled from dried twigs; it presumably contains small but appreciable amounts of terpenes (sesquiterpenes). All of these preparations serve as mild astringents and local sedatives. Ethyl alcohol and tannin are the major toxic ingredients.
WOOD ALCOHOL Methyl alcohol	3	(See also: METHYL ALCOHOL, Reference Congener in Section III.)
XYLENE Xylol	4	(See also: XYLENE, Reference Congener in Section III.)
XYLENOL Dimethylphenol	4(?)	A constituent of cresylic acid. (See also: PHENOL, Reference Congener in Section III.)
XYLOL Xylene; sometimes referred to in industry as "solvent naphtha"	4	(See also: XYLENE, Reference Congener in Section III.)
ZERLATE Zinc dimethyl dithiocarbamate Ziram	4	Toxic in guinea pigs and rabbits, less toxic in rats. Poorly absorbed in the absence of oils. Irritating to skin and mucous membranes, especially in sensitive persons. Alcohol should probably be avoided after known exposures (see disulfiram in Section III).
ZINC ARSENATE AND ARSENITE	5(?)	Presumably zinc has no toxic significance in this combination, poisoning being due to the arsenic content (See also: ARSENIC, Reference Congener in Section III.)
ZINC CYANIDE	6(?)	Presumably zinc has no toxic significance in this combination, poisoning being due to the cyanide content. (See also: CYANIDE, Reference Congener in Section III.)

Substance and Synonym or Principal Ingredient	Toxicity Rating (See Inside Cover)	Comments and Reference Congeners
ZINC DIMETHYL DITHIOCARBAMATE Ziram	4	Toxic in guinea pigs and rabbits, less toxic in rats. Poorly absorbed in the absence of oils. Irritating to skin and mucous membranes, especially in sensitive persons. Alcohol should probably be avoided after known exposures (see disulfiram in Section III).
ZINC ETHYLENE BIS (DITHIOCARBAMATE) Zineb	2	Very low acute toxicity in rats. Some irritation to skin and mucous membranes has been reported in man.
ZINC OXIDE Flowers of zinc Zinc white	3(?)	The usually U.S.P. grade has a high purity, but some technical grades contain a few tenths of 1% lead. No estimates of acute oral toxicity were located, and it is assumed that no human fatalities have resulted from ingestion of the pure oxide. Because it is soluble in dilute mineral acid (presumably including gastric juice), it probably shares to a limited extent the toxic actions of water-soluble "zinc salts" (see latter). For the inhalation toxicity of freshly formed fumes of zinc oxide, see "metal fumes" in this index. (See also: COPPER, Reference Congener in Section III.)
ZINC PHENOL- SULFONATE Zinc sulfocarbolate Zinc sulfophenate	4(?)	Formerly used as an intestinal antiseptic in doses of 60 to 200 mg. Currently found in insecticide formulations. In large doses it has emetic and astringent actions.(See also: COPPER, Reference Congener in Section III.)
ZINC PHOSPHIDE Commercial material is 90 to 95% pure.	4	Employed as a rodenticide. Toxicity is said to be due to phosphine gas (PH_3) released from zinc phosphide by the action of gastric acid. Perhaps this can be minimized by the prompt ingestion of weak alkali. Lavage with 3 to 5% sodium bicarbonate. Phosphine produces dyspnea, nausea and vomiting, bradycardia, and circulatory collapse. See Sec. IV for supportive treatment.
ZINC SALTS, SOLUBLE e.g., Chloride, sulfate acetate	4	Although no longer recommended, the sulfate has been used as an emetic drug (adult dose 0.5-1.0 gm.) Toxicity and toxic actions are like those of copper salts. Produces irritation or corrosion of the alimentary tract with pain, emesis, etc. The chloride appears to be more corrosive and more toxic than the sulfate. A few grams of the chloride has killed an adult, while recovery has been reported after ingestion of 90 gm. Delayed deaths have been ascribed to inanition following severe strictures of the esophagus and pylorus. (See also: COPPER, Reference Congener in Section III.)
ZINC STEARATE Usually a mixture of zinc salts of stearic and palmitic acids, with an excess of zinc oxide	3(?)	This zinc soap is widely used in cosmetic powders because it contributes adhesive properties to the preparation. No information about oral toxicity was located, but aspiration of the powder has produced acute fatal pneumonitis in infants. The lesions resemble those from talc but are generally more severe. In contrast powdered zinc oxide does not produce an appreciable pulmonary reaction, although the freshly formed fume is toxic.
ZINEB Zinc ethylene bis (dithiocarbamate) e.g., Dithane	2	Slightly toxic when ingested by rats. Some irritation to skin and mucous membranes has been reported in man.
ZIRAM Zinc dimethyl dithiocarbamate	4	Toxic in guinea pigs and rabbits, less toxic in rats. Poorly absorbed in the absence of oils. Irritation to skin and mucous membranes, especially in sensitive person. Alcohol should probably be avoided after known exposures (see disulfuram in Section III).

Substance and Synonym or Principal Ingredient	Toxicity Rating (See Inside Cover)	Comments and Reference Congeners
		ADDENDUM
ISOLAN 1-Isopropyl- 3-methylpyrazolyl- (5)-dimethylcarbamate	5	An insecticide particularly effective against aphids. Very toxic to mice and rats. Toxic signs and symptoms are not described but presumably resemble those of parathion poisoning, since Isolan is a reversible inhibitor of the enzyme cholinesterase and is related to neostigmine. No clinical data. (See also: PARATHION, Reference Congener in Section III.)
1-ISOPROPYL-3- METHYLPYRAZOLYL- (5)-DIMETHYL- CARBAMATE Isolan	5	An insectice particularly effective against aphids. Very toxic to mice and rats. Toxic signs and symptoms are not described but presumably resemble those of parathion poisoning, since Isolan is a reversible inhibitor of the enzyme cholinesterase and is related to neostigmine. No clinical data. (See also: PARATHION, Reference Congener in Section III.)
OUABAIN G-strophanthin A crystalline glycoside obtained from the seeds of Strophanthus gratus	6	Given intravenously (occasionally i.m.), it has potent cardiotonic actions of brief duration (12 to 24 hr.). Except for duration, poisonings resemble those of digitalis. It is poorly absorbed from the alimentary tract, where much of an oral dose appears to be destroyed. An average "digitalizing" dose intravenously (0.3 to 0.5 mg.) produces cardiac actions within 5 min., maximal in 0.5 to 2 hr., and complete in about 24 hr. (See also: DIGITALIS, Reference Congener in Section III.)
PHENOLPHTHALEIN		A laxative widely used for the past 50 years. No systemic toxicity from oral doses has been established, - except for rare allergic reactions of the skin. Children have tolerated without distress single oral doses as high as 8 gm. No prophylactic treatment is regarded as necessary, except perhaps the ingestion of activated charcoal. If urine or feces is alkaline, it may acquire a red color; this is not blood.
1-PHENYL-3-METHYL- PYRAZOLYL-(5)- DIMETHYLCARBAMATE Pyrolan	5	A relatively new insecticide. In laboratory rodents it lies near the borderline between toxicity classes 4 and 5. Toxic signs and symptoms are not described but presumably resemble those of parathion poisoning, since Pyrolan is a reversible inhibitor of the enzyme cholinesterase and is related to neostigmine. No clinical data. (See also: PARATHION, Reference Congener in Section III.)

SECTION III

Therapeutics Index

TABLE OF CONTENTS

INTRODUCTION AND EXPLANATION

Section III summarizes clinical and experimental data on 68 compounds (or classes of compounds) which in Section II are named "reference congeners" because each typifies toxicologically a group of related substances. This section stresses toxic signs and symptoms ("Symptomatology") and recommended programs of therapy ("Treatment"). That the identity of the offending toxic agent is established is implicit here.

As elsewhere, the emphasis is on acute poisonings of non-industrial origin; in some instances subacute and chronic intoxications are described. Allergic reactions receive only casual mention, although they constitute a large and important class of clinical cases. With medicinal chemicals no attempt is made here to record the numerous minor "untoward reactions" encountered when drugs are used in the customary doses. Section III concerns only syndromes of frank overdosage, as revealed in accidental, willful, suicidal, and homicidal poisonings. Within these restrictions, parenteral routes of administration are seldom involved. Ingestion, inhalation, and percutaneous absorption are the usual modes of poisoning described here.

Under "Symptomatology," toxic signs and symptoms are grouped into convenient categories and arranged in a sequence. The order is intended to describe approximately the succession of clinical events during progressive intoxication. Since only the severest poisonings reach terminal stages, these lists are useful as scales of reference and as guides for prognosis. In an analogous way, the order of listing under "Treatment" implies a system of priorities which is believed to be appropriate for cases of severe poisoning.

Unless specified otherwise, all doses (both toxic and therapeutic) refer to an adult of average size (70 kg. or 150 lb.). When scaled to the correct body weight, most of these doses are believed to be appropriate to the very young and the very old. Recognized exceptions are specified in the text. Physicians with experience in pediatrics and in geriatrics are probably aware of other exceptions to the body-weight rule and may prefer other empirical methods for translating doses. For details of supportive treatment, Section IV should be consulted (see specific page references in the text).

ACID

Hydrochloric, sulfuric, nitric, acetic, phosphoric, and other corrosive acids are found in many homes in a variety of forms and often in innocent looking containers. For information about oxalic acid; see oxalate (p. 165); for hydrofluoric acid, see fluoride (p. 143); for nitrous fumes, see nitrogen oxides (p. 163); for carbolic acid, see phenol (p. 168); for boric, hydrocyanic, and salicylic acids, see borate, cyanide, and salicylate respectively.

Toxicology: Corrosive burns result from skin contact, from the inhalation of fumes, and from the ingestion of strong acids. For information about respiratory exposures to acid vapors (e.g., HCl, SO_2, NO_2, etc.), see Nitrogen Oxides on p. 163).

Some acids are so corrosive that spasm from the first swallow prevents further ingestion. Indeed because of immediate pain when taken into the mouth, strong mineral acids are probably less often swallowed than are corrosive alkalis. The lethal dose and the interval before death are difficult to predict with any useful degree of accuracy. As with other caustic solutions, concentration is more critical than volume. A few milliliters (less than one dram) of concentrated mineral acid has killed; even a few drops is hazardous if aspirated into the larynx. Hydrochloric (muriatic) acid is less corrosive and therefore less toxic than nitric or sulfuric acids, but because of its volatility, inflammation of the respiratory tract often follows its ingestion. Mineral acids usually produce a more fulminating illness than do the corrosive alkalis; but in both types of poisoning, death results from one or more of the following complications: circulatory shock, asphyxia due to glottic or laryngeal edema, perforation of the stomach or esophagus, intercurrent infections, or inanition from late stricture formation.

Symptomatology (after ingestion or skin contact):

1. Corrosion of mucous membranes of mouth, throat, and esophagus, with immediate pain and dysphagia. The necrotic areas are at first grayish-white but soon acquire a blackish discoloration (yellow in the case of nitric acid) and sometimes a shrunken or wrinkled texture.
2. Epigastric pain, which may be associated with nausea and the vomiting of mucoid and coffee-ground material. Intense thirst.
3. Circulatory collapse with clammy skin, weak and rapid pulse, shallow respirations, and scanty urine. Circulatory shock is often the immediate cause of death.
4. Asphyxial death due to glottic edema.
5. Ulceration of all membranes and tissues with which the acid comes in contact. Ulcerated areas often perforate, leading to mediastinitis or peritonitis.
6. Late esophageal and pyloric strictures may require major surgical repair. Permanent scars may also appear in the cornea, skin, and oropharynx.
7. Uncorrected circulatory collapse of several hours' duration may lead to renal failure and ischemic lesions in the liver and heart.

Treatment:

1. Avoid lavage or emetics.
2. Administer by mouth a neutralizer and diluent such as: magnesium oxide, milk of magnesia, calcium hydroxide (lime water), aluminum hydroxide gel (2 fl. oz.), soap solution. It is best to avoid carbonates and bicarbonates, such as baking soda, chalk, crushed wall plaster, etc., because on contact with strong acids, they release carbon dioxide, which produces gastric distension and sometimes rupture.
3. Drink copious amounts of water if possible.
4. Administer a demulcent: olive oil, milk, egg whites, starch water, mineral oil, melted butter.
5. Opiates for the control of pain (p. 199).
6. Correct circulatory shock with intravenous replacement fluids, such as isotonic saline, serum albumin, and whole blood (p. 193.). Keep the patient warm.
7. Prompt surgical intervention in cases of respiratory obstruction, perforation, and stricture formation.
8. Give nothing by mouth (except perhaps 2-gm. doses of bismuth subcarbonate) after the initial administration of diluents, neutralizers, and demulcents. Parenteral alimentation (p. 222) should be continued until mucosal repair is essentially complete (usually about one week). Then try liquids, soft foods, and finally a regular diet.
9. Broad-spectrum antibiotics as prophylaxis against infections. Cortisone therapy has been recommended in persistent shock.
10. For skin burns, wash with large amounts of water and then apply a paste of sodium bicarbonate. For eye burns hold the lids open and flush immediately with a slow stream of water; continue this procedure for 10 to 15 minutes. For the treatment of severe eye burns, an ophthalomologist should be consulted.

Laboratory:

1. Albuminuria, hematuria, and casts may be observed.
2. Leukocytosis.

ALCOHOLS, HIGHER

The "higher" aliphatic alcohols are defined here to exclude methyl, ethyl, and isopropyl alcohols, which are described elsewhere in this section. Included here are such liquid alcohols as butyl, amyl, isoamyl, ethylhexyl, etc., which are used principally as solvents. Isoamyl alcohol is the chief constituent of "fusel oil" in fermentative distillates. Higher homologues include the solid fatty alcohols, such as lauryl, myristyl, cetyl, and stearyl; they are important as emollients in cosmetics.

Toxicology: The probable order of increasing toxicity by ingestion is as follows: ethyl, isopropyl, propyl, isobutyl, and amyl alcohols. Whereas primary or normal butyl alcohol may belong anomalously early in this list (between ethyl and isopropyl ?), comparative toxicities of the various butyl and amyl isomers have not been adequately defined. Butyl alcohols are generally less irritating than amyl alcohols and less potent as central nervous depressants, but they have about three times the acute toxicity of ethanol. Ingestion of 30 cc. of amyl alcohol has proved fatal in an adult. Toxic symptoms from butyl and amyl alcohols are usually more severe and more prolonged than those in ethanol intoxication.

Whereas the solid aliphatic alcohols (*i.e.*, lauryl and higher homologues) are generally conceded to have very low toxicities by ingestion, no conclusions are available about those homologues lying between amyl and lauryl alcohols, notably the various hexyl and octyl isomers and especially ethylhexyl alcohol. Presumably these solvents are less poisonous than amyl alcohols but share some of the same toxic effects.

Symptomatology:
1. Central nervous system: headache, muscle weakness, giddiness, confusion, delirium, coma.
2. Gastro-intestinal: nausea, vomiting, diarrhea (odor of the alcohol in excreta).
3. Irritation of skin, eyes, throat—from vapor or liquid.
4. Occasional complications:
   a. gastro-intestinal hemorrhage,
   b. renal damage with glycosuria,
   c. liver damage,
   d. cardiac failure,
   e. pulmonary edema,
   f. methemoglobin formation reportedly from amyl alcohols.

Treatment:
1. Lavage with copious amounts of water.
2. Lavage with 100 cc. mineral oil and leave 60 cc. of mineral oil in the stomach.
3. Caffeine sodium benzoate, 0.5 gm., subcutaneously.
4. Oxygen and artificial respiration as needed (p. 185).
5. Electrolyte balance: start 500 cc. M/6 sodium lactate intravenously, but maintain a cautious and conservative attitude toward electrolyte replacement unless shock threatens, because of possible kidney damage (see p. 210).
6. Protect liver with methionine, or cystine and choline (see p. 213). Maintain carbohydrate intake by intravenous infusions of glucose.
7. Vitamin supplements, especially of the B complex.

Laboratory: not generally relevant.

ALIPHATIC THIOCYANATES

Various synthetic aliphatic thiocyanates (rhodanates) are widely used as contact insecticides. Low molecular weight homologues, such as methyl, ethyl, and isopropyl thiocyanates, are volatile liquids sometimes employed as insecticidal fumigants. Long-chain derivatives, such as lauryl thiocyanate and certain ester and ether derivatives, are oily liquids marketed as dusting powders and as kerosene-base sprays, often in combination with pyrethrum and rotenone, for use in fields, gardens, and homes. They have also been used on the skin as delousing preparations and as livestock sprays. The following insecticide products are available commercially: Thanite (isobornyl thiocyanoacetate), Lethane 384 (β-butoxy-β-thiocyano-diethyl ether in an equal volume of petroleum solvent), and Lethane 60 (β-thiocyanoethyl esters of C_{10}-C_{18} fatty acids in an equal volume of petroleum solvent).

Toxicology: As observed in laboratory animals, aliphatic thiocyanates differ widely among themselves in oral and parenteral toxicity. The only human fatality known to us involved an adult who drank a mixture containing no more than 3.5 gm. of Lethane 384 and 10 gm. of lauryl thiocyanate. Of the common thiocyanate insecticides, Lethane 384 has the highest acute toxicity; based on various animal species, the lethal oral dose in an adult person may lie anywhere between 1 teaspoonful and 1 ounce of the concentrated commercial solution (50 per cent active ingredient). Lauryl thiocyanate appears to be considerably less toxic, while Lethane 60 and Thanite possess intermediary toxicities. None of these compounds is as toxic as ethyl or methyl thiocyanate. All derivatives have an appreciable percutaneous toxicity, although this is not regarded as an important hazard with the concentrations usually employed in agriculture.

Primary irritation of skin and eyes due to local contact, however, is not a negligible hazard, and the undiluted liquids may produce very severe cutaneous reactions, particularly lauryl thiocyanate and isobornyl thiocyanoacetate.

Besides these quantitative differences, important qualitative distinctions are recognized among the various organic thiocyanates. For example, methyl, ethyl, and isopropyl thiocyanates are rapidly acting poisons of high potency (the oral mean lethal dose of methyl thiocyanate is less than 20 mg./kg. in rats). They produce central nervous depression, usually with a transient period of respiratory stimulation, progressing promptly to death from respiratory failure. Enzymes in the liver and perhaps in other organs are known to liberate cyanide ion from methyl and ethyl thiocyanates. Because cyanide is probably largely responsible for these poisonings, antidotal measures against cyanide should be instituted promptly (see p. 132). Butyl thiocyanate and higher homologues do not furnish significant amounts of cyanide in vivo.

The mechanism of action of the higher thiocyanates and their ether and ester derivatives is unknown. No toxicological connection between aliphatic and inorganic thiocyanates has been demonstrated. On the basis of SCN content, sodium thiocyanate probably has a lower acute toxicity than any thiocyanate insecticide. In contrast to the hyperexcitability induced by overdoses of the inorganic salts, the principal systemic action of organic thiocyanates is central nervous depression, intense dyspnea, cyanosis, and sometimes convulsions which are probably asphyxial in origin. In some instances, however, tremors, paralysis, spasticity, and even opisthotonos have been described, notably in rabbits given Lethane 384 by various routes. Some toxic effects reported in laboratory studies must be ascribed to the petroleum vehicle (purified kerosene in the case of the Lethanes). Especially with the dilute formulations commonly used in the home (e.g., 4 per cent active ingredient), kerosene is expected to contribute appreciably to any poisonings which may arise from accidental ingestion or other misuse.

Symptomatology (largely inferred from animal tests):

1. The ingestion of concentrated solutions may lead to vomiting because of mucosal irritation.
2. The principal systemic reaction is probably one of central nervous depression, perhaps interrupted by periods of restlessness, hyperpnea, and tonic convulsions. As judged by animal tests, depression may last for many days.
3. The signs and symptoms of kerosene poisoning are often dominant after exposures to dilute solutions of thiocyanate insecticides (see p. 150).
4. Death is usually due to respiratory arrest from paralysis of the medullary centers.
5. Massive skin contamination with organic thiocyanate solutions may produce systemic poisoning as described above and in addition local irritation and dermatitis.
6. In non-fatal cases evidence of injuries to the liver and kidneys may appear.

Treatment:

1. In poisonings due to methyl, ethyl, or isopropyl thiocyanate, proceed immediately as with cyanide poisoning (p. 132). For all other derivatives, proceed as follows.
2. Cautious gastric lavage with copious amounts of water. Observe all precautions to avoid aspiration (p. 6).
3. At the conclusion of lavage, instill 30 to 60 ml. of mineral oil in the stomach, as well as a saline cathartic (e.g., sodium sulfate 15 to 30 gm. in water). Avoid digestible fats, oils, and alcohol, which may promote absorption from the bowel.
4. Symptomatic and supportive measures for central nervous depression (see p. 204). Nikethamide (Coramine) and caffeine sodium benzoate may be useful respiratory stimulants.
5. If severe or persistent, convulsions should be controlled by the intravenous administration of a short-acting barbiturate drug (p. 202).
6. Positive pressure oxygen therapy (p. 192) and the prophylactic administration of antibiotics are advisable if pulmonary edema arises as a toxic response to the petroleum solvent (kerosene).

Laboratory:

1. Function tests should be used to detect and evaluate incipient renal and liver injuries.
2. The concentration of inorganic (ionic) thiocyanate in the blood plasma is said to be elevated in acute poisonings due to thiocyanate insecticides. Thiocyanate analyses in clinical poisonings are highly desirable to confirm this claim.

ALKALI

The strong corrosive alkalis include lye, caustic soda, caustic potash, sodium and potassium hydroxides, carbonates, oxides, and peroxides. They are commonly used as cleansing agents and are present in many washing powders, drain-pipe cleaners, and paint removers. Most of the reported cases of poisoning have resulted from the careless practice of leaving lye solutions in familiar

containers within the reach of a thirsty child. Also see ammonia (p. 112).

Toxicology: The strong alkalis are markedly corrosive and penetrating. This property is due to their solubilizing reaction on proteins, saponifying effect on lipids, and dehydrating action on tissue cells. The corroded areas are soft, gelatinous, and friable, and often exhibit a brownish discoloration.

Usually the first mouthful of lye solution makes further swallowing impossible because of intense pain and spasm. The intensity of the local injury and of the subsequent systemic reaction cannot be dependably predicted from the size of the dose. As with most caustic solutions, concentration is more critical than volume. Systemic reactions are due solely to local tissue injury, and death may result from any one of several complications: circulatory shock, asphyxia due to glottic or laryngeal edema, perforation of the esophagus or stomach, intercurrent infections, or inanition due to the late formation of esophageal strictures. The course of poisoning is usually less rapid than that due to the ingestion of strong mineral acids.

Symptomatology:

1. The ingestion of lye causes swallowing to become painful and difficult almost immediately. A burning pain extends down the esophagus to the stomach. Contaminated areas of the lips, chin, tongue, and pharynx become edematous and covered with exudate. Because of pharyngeal and esophageal edema, it may become impossible after a few hours to swallow even saliva. Mucous membranes are at first white but later brown, edematous, gelatinous, and necrotic.

2. The vomitus is thick and slimy due to mucus; later it may contain blood and shreds of mucous membrane.

3. The pulse is often rapid and feeble; respirations are fast and shallow; the skin is cold and clammy; collapse ensues.

4. Death due to shock, asphyxia from glottic edema, or intercurrent infection (pneumonia) commonly occurs on the second or even the third day.

5. Convalescence may be interrupted during the first week by the sudden onset of pain, abdominal rigidity, and shock, indicating perforation of the stomach or esophagus.

6. If complications do not appear, liquids and soft food can be swallowed with comparative ease within 5 to 7 days. It should be recognized, however, that in most cases this absence of distress merely marks a latent period and that esophageal strictures will develop within weeks or months unless effective treatment is instituted.

Treatment:

1. Dilute ingested alkali by drinking immediately large volumes of water or milk. An attempt should be made to neutralize the caustic with a weak acid (never strong!), such as diluted vinegar, lemon juice, or orange juice. While these solutions are being prepared, wash contaminated skin and accessible areas of mucous membrane extensively with running tap water.

2. Gastric lavage and emetics are contraindicated because of the danger of gastric or esophageal perforation.

3. Olive oil in small quantities (*e.g.*, a teaspoonful) given frequently by mouth and applied to all denuded areas. If swallowing is not impossible, other demulcent drinks may be helpful (*e.g.*, milk, egg white).

4. Analgesics should be given liberally to relieve pain (p. 199).

5. Treat shock by the intravenous administration of electrolyte solutions, plasma, and whole blood (p. 193). Keep the patient warm.

6. Prompt surgical intervention, when indicated, as with severe laryngeal edema or gastric perforation. If asphyxia appears, a tracheotomy may be indicated (p. 185).

7. Liquids and soft foods may be given as tolerated, but in most instances the parenteral administration of fluids and carbohydrates is necessary for the first week.

8. Early careful esophageal dilatations (fourth day or even earlier) may prevent or eventually remedy strictures. Well-lubricated, soft rubber, mercury-filled bougies in graduated sizes (16–30 F for children) are inserted daily into the esophagus; each day a larger size is employed. After 2 weeks the interval between dilatations is gradually lengthened. (For details of technique, see surgical texts.)

9. Cortisone therapy may help to minimize stricture formation.

10. In case of surface burns on skin or eyes, wash with large amounts of cold running water. Probably cortisone should be instilled in the conjunctival sac of an injured eye but, if possible, consult an ophthalmologist.

11. Penicillin and broad-spectrum antibiotics as prophylaxis against secondary infections.

Laboratory: Not generally relevant.

AMANITA TOXINS

Poisoning from toxic mushrooms (toadstools) is called mycetismus. Poisonous species are common in North America and are difficult for the inexperienced to distinguish from edible varieties.

Homespun methods of differentation are fallacious; for example, taste is no adequate criterion since the deadly *Amanita phalloides* is said to have a delicious flavor. In the United States the genus *Amanita* is responsible for most poisonings, but *Helvella* is sometimes imputed. Common species of the *Amanita* are *muscaria*, familiarly called the "fly agaric," and *phalloides*, often called the "destroying angel." In the U. S. A. about 90 per cent of fatal mycetismus (about 50 cases a year) is due to the ingestion of *A. phalloides*.

Toxicology: Two types of poisoning are caused by *Amanita*. A rapid type (mycetismus nervosa) follows the ingestion of *Amanita muscaria*; symptoms occur within a few minutes or a few hours and are due to the toxic effects of muscarine, which mimic intense parasympathetic stimulation. The prognosis is good with prompt and adequate administration of atropine. Delayed poisoning (mycetismus choleriformis) results from the ingestion of *Amanita phalloides* after a latency of 6 to 15 hours. Here at least three toxic polypeptides appear to be responsible for damage to tissue cells, particularly in the liver, kidney, heart, and brain. No satisfactory treatment for poisoning with *A. phalloides* is recognized, and about half the cases end fatally. A toxin antiserum has been described, but its therapeutic value is unproved, and it is reputedly available only at the Pasteur Institute in Paris, France.

More than 70 species of mushrooms are capable of producing toxic reactions in man. Poisonings from most species of *Amanita* resemble the illnesses produced by *muscaria* or by *phalloides*. Another common mushroom, *Helvella esculenta* or the false morel, possesses a hemolytic glycoside, and its ingestion may cause an acute hemolytic anemia. *Amanita phalloides* contains at least 4 toxins: phallin (which is a glycosidal hemolysin, probably destroyed by cooking) and 3 peptides, namely phalloidine, α-amanitine, and β-amanitine. The minimal lethal dose of these peptides in dogs and mice is 0.1 to 0.4 mg./kg., and man is said to be even more susceptible. Since the toxins represent about 0.005 per cent of the fresh mushroom, a few ounces of the latter may contain a fatal dose for an adult person.

Symptomatology:

A. Due to *Amanita phalloides* (onset 6 to 15 hours after ingestion)
  1. Sudden onset of abdominal pain, usually colicky.
  2. Nausea, violent vomiting, and severe bloody or blood-streaked diarrhea.
  3. Rapidly developing weakness.
  4. Dehydration, with extreme thirst.
  5. Cyanosis, cold clammy skin, and other signs of shock. Hypotension and bradycardia may persist for many days.
  6. Restlessness, twitching, delirium, hallucinations, sometimes convulsions, and eventually prostration and coma.
  7. Tender enlargement of the liver, with jaundice apparent within 2 to 3 days, due to hepatic cell degeneration, which may progress to acute yellow atrophy.
  8. Oliguria or anuria, secondary to injury of the kidney parenchyma.
  9. Death in 5 to 8 days may be due to cellular damage in the central nervous system, liver, kidneys, or heart.

B. Due to *Amanita muscaria* (onset a few minutes to a few hours after ingestion).
  1. Salivation, nausea, vomiting, colic, and watery diarrhea.
  2. Dyspnea, wheezing, rales.
  3. Slow, irregular pulse.
  4. Miosis; visual disturbances; lacrimation.
  5. Sweating, cyanosis.
  6. Confusion, excitement, late stupor.
  7. Death may occur in a few hours from cardiac arrest or circulatory collapse.

Treatment:

1. "Universal antidote", 5 to 6 teaspoonsful in water (p. 10).
2. An emetic drug and/or prompt gastric lavage with potassium permanganate solution (1: 5000) or with water. Save the gastric contents.
3. Saline catharsis with sodium sulfate (15 to 30 gm. in water). High colonic enemas may help to stimulate prompt evacuation.
4. Atropine sulfate, 2 mg. subcutaneously, repeated as indicated. Atropine is a specific antagonist for the muscarine in *Amanita muscaria*, but it is ineffective in poisonings due to *A. phalloides*. In every instance of doubt, give atropine because, even if ineffective, it is at least innocuous.
5. Meperidine (Demerol) for the control of pain. Morphine is best avoided because it may delay purging.
6. Correct shock and dehydration by the cautious intravenous administration of replacement fluids (p. 193).
7. Institute supportive treatment for impending renal and hepatic insufficiencies (pp. 210 and 213).
8. Digitalis may be given a trial if hypotension persists after rehydration is complete.
9. With those varieties of poisonous mushrooms which produce an acute hemolytic reaction, blood transfusions may become essential.

Laboratory:

1. Because prognosis and treatment vary drastically with the type of mushroom, a species identification is always desirable. If a large enough piece of the fungus is available, an

expert can recognize it from various botanical characteristics. Recently a rapid and comparatively simple chromatographic isolation of phalloides toxins has been proposed as a practical method of identification (Block *et al.*: Science, *121:* 505, 1955). The procedure

is said to require only 0.1 gm. of fresh *A. phalloides*; it should prove distinctly useful, especially if it can be performed satisfactorily with stomach contents (unproved).

2. Repeated biochemical tests of liver and kidney function are indicated.

AMMONIA

Ammonia in solution (ammonia water) is used in a variety of products such as cleaning agents, liniments, and aromatic spirits.

Toxicology: Ammonium hydroxide differs from other alkalis in its volatility; the vapor (NH_3) is irritating to skin, eyes, and respiratory passages. The ingestion of ammonia solutions produces effects similar to other corrosive alkalis. As with most caustic solutions, concentration is more critical than volume. One teaspoonful (3 to 4 ml.) has been recorded as a fatal oral dose of strong ammonia solution (28 per cent), but as much as 1 fl. oz. has been tolerated in several cases.

Symptomatology:

1. Vapors cause irritation of eyes and respiratory tract. High concentrations may cause conjunctivitis, laryngitis, tracheitis, and rarely pulmonary edema or pneumonitis. A sensation of suffocation may be induced by spasm of the glottis.
2. Contact with skin can cause burns and vesication.
3. Ingestion can lead to all the signs and symptoms, pathological lesions, and complications induced by other corrosive alkalis (see p. 109).

Treatment:

1. Lavage and emetics are contraindicated.
2. If ammonia water is swallowed, the victim should try to drink immediately large quantities of water or weak acids such as: diluted vinegar, lemon juice, orange juice, dilute hydrochloric acid (*e.g.*, 3 to 6 oz. of 0.5 per cent HCl).
3. Administer a demulcent (egg white, olive oil, milk, *etc.*).
4. Control pain with opiates or meperidine (Demerol).
5. Treat shock (p. 193). Keep the patient warm.
6. Contaminated eyes and skin should be washed with copious amounts of tap water. For the definitive treatment of most chemical burns of the eye, an ophthalmologist should be consulted.
7. Tracheotomy may be indicated if signs of asphyxia develop (p. 185).
8. For the management of pulmonary edema, see p. 192.
9. Cortisone therapy has been recommended.
10. Follow-up therapy in cases of perforation, strictures, *etc,* (see Alkali, p. 110).

Laboratory: Not generally relevant.

ANILINE

Aniline is widely used industrially in chemical syntheses. It and its derivatives occur in many products found in the home, such as paints, varnishes, marking inks, stove polishes, and shoe polishes. Many poisonings are reported each year from exposure to aniline and related substances, *e.g.*, to aniline dyes freshly stamped on diapers.

Toxicology: Aniline and related compounds (*e.g.*, nitrobenzenes, aniline dyes, *etc.*) may gain access to the body by skin penetration, by ingestion, or by inhalation. Aniline itself may produce poisoning if ingested in amounts as small as 0.25 gm., particularly if the stomach is empty. As little as 6 gm. has been reported to be a lethal dose, although much larger amounts have been tolerated. The mean lethal dose may lie between 15 and 30 gm. (cc.) of pure aniline. Technical aniline as found in many commercial products may be more dangerous because of toxic impurities (xylidines and toluidines). The outstanding feature of aniline poisoning is

cyanosis, which is due here to methemoglobin and sometimes a small amount of sulfhemoglobin. The result is a functional anemia, since methemoglobin is incapable of binding oxygen for normal gas transport. Oxygen deficits undoubtedly arise in many tissues. In addition, red blood cells with these altered pigments sometimes undergo intravascular hemolysis, which leads to a true anemia, deleterious renal effects, and jaundice. Apparently methemoglobin formation is not due to aniline itself but to metabolic products such as aminophenol and especially phenylhydroxylamine.

The central nervous and cardiac disorders seen in aniline poisoning are unquestionably aggravated by tissue anoxia, but oxygen lack is probably not their primary cause, which remains undefined. Liver disease may follow severe aniline intoxication (especially if aniline is contaminated with xylidines), but it is apparently more frequent in poisonings due to nitrobenzenes and nitrotoluenes.

Except after unusually severe hemolytic episodes, the renal injury is mild and reversible. Even with severe symptoms, final recovery is the rule in aniline poisoning.

Symptomatology:

1. Grayish-blue cyanosis, without signs of cardiac or pulmonary insufficiency.
2. Severe headache, nausea, sometimes vomiting, dryness of throat.
3. Central nervous symptoms: confusion, ataxia, vertigo, tinnitus, weakness, disorientation, lethargy, drowsiness, and finally coma. Convulsions may occur.
4. Cardiac effects: heart blocks, arrhythmias, and shock.
5. Death, while uncommon, is usually due to cardiovascular collapse, and not respiratory paralysis.
6. Urinary signs and symptoms may include painful micturition, hematuria, hemoglobinuria (and methemoglobinuria), oliguria, and renal insufficiency (usually mild).

Treatment:

1. Gastric lavage with water or potassium permanganate solution (1:5000).
2. Leave a solution of magnesium sulfate in the stomach (15 to 30 gm. in water).
3. Administer oxygen (p. 189) and use artificial respiration as indicated (p. 185).
4. Treat shock cautiously because of the uncertain cardiac status (p. 195).
5. Transfusions with whole blood or washed red cells (in saline) may be necessary (p. 194).

6. Stimulants as indicated and sedatives if necessary.
7. For methemoglobinemia, some authors recommend slow intravenous injection of 1 per cent methylene blue (0.2 ml. per kg.). This dye may be made up in a 1.8 per cent sodium sulfate solution. Other authors recommend sodium ascorbate (0.5 gm.) intravenously. Caution: on rare occasions methylene blue may cause hemolysis (it probably often produces Heinz bodies within erythrocytes).
8. If aniline is spilled on clothing, remove immediately and discard. Any contaminated area of skin should be washed for 10 to 15 minutes with soap and running water.

Laboratory:

1. N-acetyl-*p*-aminophenol (the chief metabolite of aniline) may be detected in urine.
2. Spectroscopic methods in clinical laboratories are often too insensitive to show methemoglobin absorption bands, even when cyanosis is clinically evident in aniline poisoning. By the usual clinical test, the hemoglobin level is typically normal, while the blood oxygen-carrying capacity is measurably low, a difference which is a sensitive index of methemoglobinemia. Sometimes freshly drawn blood is grossly chocolate-brown in color.
3. The urinary findings are often compatible with intravascular hemolysis, methemoglobinemia, and kidney injury. The urine is almost always dark.

ANTIHISTAMINICS

The enthusiastic reception of the early antihistaminic drugs (around 1942) promoted a search for new histamine antagonists; many of these efforts were successful. The number of antihistaminics now available through commercial channels is legion. Their hazards are not widely recognized by the layman, and so they are often used indiscriminately.

Toxicology: Although the incidence of side reactions varies from one preparation to another, about 20 per cent of persons receiving current antihistaminic drugs complain of some kind of untoward effects. The most common side effect is sedation in varying degrees, particularly marked with diphenhydramine (Benadryl). While sedation may be an asset in night-time medication, it is often a hazard in the ambulatory patient. Other untoward reactions referable to the central nervous system are dizziness, tinnitus, fatigue, ataxia, and blurred vision. Sometimes clinical doses precipitate central excitation evidenced by euphoria, nervousness, tremors, and insomnia. Anorexia and other gastro-

intestinal symptoms are not uncommon. Miscellaneous complaints include dryness of the mouth, headache, tingling and weakness of the hands, hypotension, palpitations, and dysuria. The paradox of allergic reactions to these anti-allergic drugs is well recognized. Allergic manifestations include dermatitis and rarely leucopenia or agranulocytosis (with the ethylenediamine group of derivatives).

When an antihistaminic drug is ingested in an amount distinctly greater than the customary dose, any one of many toxic syndromes may result. Frequently these reactions represent extensions of the common side effects listed above. Central nervous depression is the dominant response, but an excitement stage often follows. In young children central stimulation and convulsions may precede depression. In fatal cases the terminal phase is one of coma, with death from respiratory arrest. Most severe poisonings have been due to the willful ingestion of these drugs by young children. A considerable margin of safety separates the therapeutic dose from the usual lethal one. Adults have sur-

vived single doses as high as 2500 mg., while as little as 100 mg. has proved fatal. Children may be proportionately more susceptible.

Treatment is strictly symptomatic and supportive, and the proper measures change with each stage of the poisoning. Analeptic drugs are inadvisable in the early phases because of the danger of precipitating convulsions. The depression which follows the excitatory phase is rarely responsive to the analeptics. Fortunately the vital signs are usually well maintained even without support from any arousal drug. Histamine has no place in the treatment of antihistaminic poisoning.

Symptomatology:

1. Central nervous depression is usually the dominant reaction in adults; it is evidenced by drowsiness, lethargy, fatigue, hypnosis, and coma. Related nervous symptoms include vertigo, ataxia, tinnitus, and blurred vision.
2. Central nervous hyperexcitability often follows initial sedation; sometimes excitement is the first evidence of poisoning. The stimulant phase brings tremors, anxiety, insomnia, excitement, delirium, and convulsions.

3. Dangerous hyperpyrexia is reported in poisoned children.
4. Gastrointestinal reactions include a dry mouth, anorexia, nausea, vomiting, abdominal distress, constipation, and/or diarrhea.
5. The terminal phase is one of severe central nervous depression, with death from respiratory arrest or cardiovascular collapse.

Treatment:

1. Gastric lavage (p. 6) with warm tap water.
2. Cautious use of the short-acting barbiturates for the control of central nervous stimulation (p. 202).
3. If used cautiously, caffeine, amphetamine, nikethamide, *etc.*, may occasionally be useful in the supportive treatment of central nervous depression. See p. 204.
4. Ice packs, alcohol sponge baths, *etc.*, (p. 230) for the control of hyperpyrexia. Probably salicylates should be avoided here.
5. Artificial respiration and oxygen therapy as necessary (p. 185).
6. Symptomatic and supportive measures as indicated.

Laboratory: generally irrelevant.

ANTU

ANTU was developed as an outgrowth of the observation that phenylthiourea kills rats but is not toxic to man. Many derivatives were prepared before one was found which had the same high toxicity to rodents without the bitter taste of phenylthiourea. Alpha naphthyl thiourea (ANTU) proved to be the most effective. Some species of rats, however, are not sensitive to it, and others develop resistance rapidly. ANTU is a stable, bluish-gray powder, highly insoluble in water, without perceptible odor, and with only a transient bitter taste. It is used in baits in concentrations of 1 to 3 per cent.

Toxicology: ANTU is probably not toxic to man except in large amounts; the mean lethal dose by mouth is 4 gm./kg. in monkeys and presumably much the same in man. No human fatalities have been reported. Dogs are quite susceptible to ANTU but are usually protected by prompt vomiting. Observations on experimental animals indicate that the only organ affected is the lungs; pulmonary edema and pleural effusion develop due to the action of ANTU on pulmonary capillaries. Both cysteine and thiosorbitol have been given to

ANTU-poisoned rats and found to be promising antidotes under some conditions. ANTU may possess antithyroid activity in chronic sublethal exposures. It is not irritating to the skin.

Symptomatology (as observed in animals):

1. Dyspnea, rales, cyanosis (due to severe pulmonary edema and sometimes pleural effusion).
2. Lowered body temperature (hypothermia).
3. Death from asphyxia.

Treatment:

1. Emetics or prompt gastric lavage with tap water.
2. Saline catharsis with 15 to 30 gm. sodium sulfate in water.
3. Positive-pressure oxygen (see p. 192). Postural drainage. Absolute rest.
4. Avoid fat ingestion, since ANTU may be more readily absorbed in its presence.
5. Use caution in giving oral or intravenous fluids because of the danger of precipitating pulmonary edema.

Laboratory: generally irrelevant.

ARSENIC

Arsenic is a common ingredient of rodenticides, insecticides, herbicides, paints, and other products. Many organic arsenic compounds are employed as

therapeutic agents in clinical and veterinary medicine.

Toxicology: Arsenic was formerly used exten-

sively as a "criminal poison" because it is odorless and nearly tasteless. Accidental poisoning is still common because arsenic compounds are widely used and readily available. The mortality in acute poisoning is high (50 to 75 per cent); death usually occurs within 48 hours. The lethal dose varies with the compound, but 0.2 to 0.3 gm. of the trioxide ("white arsenic") is usually fatal in an adult. Finely subdivided arsenic trioxide is significantly more toxic than coarsely powdered material, since appreciable amounts of the latter may be eliminated in feces without dissolving.

In most cases the presenting symptoms are those of a severe gastritis or gastroenteritis. Because the lesions are due not to local corrosion but to vascular damage from absorbed arsenic, the first symptoms may be delayed several minutes or even a few hours. Eventually a violent hemorrhagic gastroenteritis leads to profound losses of fluid and electrolytes, resulting in collapse, shock, and death. Occasionally the alimentary symptoms are mild or absent, in which case the presenting complaints are usually referable to the central nervous system: headache, vertigo, muscle spasm, stupor, delirium, and sometimes mania.

Subacute and chronic exposures may reveal themselves in these and many other ways. Among the protean manifestations of chronic poisoning are anorexia, mild gastrointestinal disturbances, low-grade fever, pallor, weakness, and a catarrhal inflammation of nose, throat, conjunctivae, and larynx—simulating an infectious coryza. Stomatitis and salivation are common. Skin afflictions are many and varied: erythema, eczema, pigmentation (arsenic melanosis), keratosis (especially of palms and soles), scaling and desquamation, brittle nails, loss of hair and nails, and localized subcutaneous edema (especially of the eyelids). Signs of renal damage develop. Hepatomegaly with jaundice (and sometimes pruritus) may evolve into cirrhosis with ascites. Severe blood dyscrasias result from depression of any and all cellular elements in bone marrow. In advanced poisoning, nervous symptoms are prominent; encephalopathies have been described, but peripheral neuritis is more common. Sensation is involved first (paresthesia, hypesthesia, pain), but eventually paralysis and muscular atrophy appear, usually in the legs.

In all cases it is presumably the ion of arsenious acid, rather than the element itself, which is the toxic principle. The *in vivo* conversion to arsenite explains why all chemical forms of arsenic eventually produce the same toxic syndrome. (One exception is gaseous AsH_3 or arsine, which is a potent hemolytic agent, unlike other arsenic derivatives.) As arsenite the element is an active enzyme inhibitor, presumably because of its attachment to sulfhydryl groups of essential proteins. Absorbed arsenic is excreted largely by the kidneys, but feces,

skin and hair sometimes contain appreciable amounts. After a single dose, excretion is essentially complete within 2 weeks. Urinary excretion is markedly enhanced, without damage to the excretory organs, by the administration of BAL (dimercaprol). If prompt, this treatment suppresses most signs and symptoms of acute poisoning.

Symptomatology (acute poisoning only):

1. Symptoms usually appear one half to one hour after ingestion but may be delayed many hours, especially when arsenic is taken with food.
2. Sweetish metallic taste; garlicky odor of breath and stools.
3. Constriction in the throat and difficulty in swallowing. Burning and colicky pains in esophagus, stomach, and bowel.
4. Vomiting and profuse painful diarrhea. Often the excreta resemble the "rice water" stools of cholera; later the feces become bloody.
5. Dehydration with intense thirst and muscular cramps.
6. Cyanosis, feeble pulse, and cold extremities.
7. Vertigo, frontal headache. In some cases ("cerebral type") vertigo, stupor, delirium, and even mania develop without prominent gastrointestinal signs.
8. Syncope, coma, occasionally convulsions, general paralysis, and death.
9. Various skin eruptions, more often as a late manifestation, or in chronic poisoning (see above).
10. In case of recovery, weakness and diarrhea may persist for weeks, and occasionally a syndrome indistinguishable from chronic poisoning evolves (see above).

Treatment (acute poisoning only):

1. Gastric lavage: 2 to 3 liters of water, followed by 1 glassful of milk or colloidal ferric hydroxide (if freshly prepared) or 1 per cent sodium thiosulfate solution or BAL solution.
2. Saline cathartic: 15 to 30 gm. of sodium sulfate in water.
3. Administer BAL (dimercaprol) intramuscularly as a 10 per cent solution in oil. The dosage schedule recommended below is

	Severe Poisoning	Mild Poisoning
1st day	3.0 mg./kg. q4h (6 inj.)	2.5 mg./kg. q4h (6 inj.)
2nd day	3.0 mg./kg. q4h (6 inj.)	2.5 mg./kg. q6h (4 inj.)
3rd day	3.0 mg./kg. q6h (4 inj.)	2.5 mg./kg. q12h (2 inj.)
Each of the following 10 days or until recovery	3.0 mg./kg. q12h (2 inj.)	2.5 mg./kg. qd (1 inj.)

thought to be adequate for patients of all ages. All doses are expressed as milligrams of BAL (*not* of solution). For the clinical toxicity of BAL, see p. 117.

4. Counteract dehydration by intravenous fluids as needed (p. 215) and correct electrolyte deficiencies.

5. Morphine may be necessary to control abdominal pain.

6. Treat shock vigorously; use blood transfusions and oxygen as necessary (pp. 194, 189).

Laboratory:

1. Save the initial gastric washings and a urine specimen (100 ml.) for arsenic analysis.

2. Urine output is usually diminished. Albuminuria and hematuria may be prominent.

3. Liver function tests may reveal subclinical hepatic injury.

ATROPINE

Atropine (*dl*-hyoscyamine) is an alkaloid widely used in clinical medicine for its ability to block the effects of parasympathetic nerve stimulation. It is prepared by extraction from the powdered roots of *Atropa belladonna, Datura stramonium*, and other solanaceous plants (where it occurs naturally as the *l*-isomer). Active alkaloids related to atropine have been obtained from natural and synthetic sources. Indigenous plants are occasionally responsible for cases of atropine poisoning.

Toxicology: The margin of safety of this drug (and of related alkaloids) is much higher than generally appreciated. Although 10 mg. of atropine usually produces severe distress, many adult persons have recovered from single doses of 100 mg. and more. Indeed, in the absence of predisposing disease, deaths from atropine poisoning are thought to be rare in adults, and the mean lethal dose is not known. Children are more susceptible than adults to this and related alkaloids, but young children are probably more tolerant than implied by the commonly stated lethal estimate of 10 mg.

Neither the fatal dose nor the nature of the toxic syndrome is significantly determined by the route of administration. Although many of the untoward signs and symptoms can be related to paralysis of the glands and smooth muscles innervated by the parasympathetic nervous system, the most dangerous and spectacular manifestations of poisoning arise from intense excitation of the central nervous system. States of idiosyncrasy and hypersensitivity have also been described.

Symptomatology:

1. Dryness of mucous membranes, burning pain in the throat, difficulty in swallowing, and intense thirst.

2. Dilatation of pupils, which become unreactive to light; blurred vision and photophobia.

3. The skin becomes hot, dry, and flushed. A scarlatiniform or maculo-papular rash may appear over the face, neck, and upper trunk, especially in infants and children, and desquamation may follow.

4. Hyperpyrexia.

5. Tachycardia, palpitations, elevated blood pressure.

6. Uncommonly nausea, vomiting, and (in infants) abdominal distension. Urinary urgency and hesitancy.

7. Restlessness, fatigue, excitement, and confusion, progressing to mania and delirium, which may persist for many hours and even several days.

8. In rare instances, coma, depression of medullary centers, circulatory collapse, and death from respiratory failure.

Treatment:

1. Gastric lavage with 4 per cent tannic acid or other alkaloidal antidotes. (Potassium permanganate in safe concentrations is ineffective in destroying atropine.) Emetics may be employed, but lavage is preferable.

2. Pilocarpine may be given orally in doses of 5 mg. and repeated at intervals until the mouth is moist. Pilocarpine may make the patient more comfortable but has no influence on the central nervous effects of atropine. Sips of water may also help to relieve intense thirst.

3. Short-acting barbiturates administered cautiously may control excitement. Avoid large doses. Chloral hydrate or paraldehyde may be substituted for barbiturate drugs.

4. When (and if) depression occurs, central nervous stimulants, such as nikethamide and caffeine may be tried but are not expected to be effective.

5. Artificial respiration and oxygen therapy in cases of respiratory depression (p. 185).

6. Check for urinary retention and catheterize if necessary (p. 210).

7. Antipyretic therapy—alcohol sponges (p. 230). Aspirin and other salicylates are probably best avoided.

8. A miotic drug (*e.g.*, pilocarpine nitrate 0.5 per cent) in the conjunctival sac may be used to counteract mydriasis. Because of photophobia, a darkened room may add to the patient's comfort.

Laboratory: Not generally relevant, but a leukocytosis may be observed.

BAL

BAL (2,3-dimercapto-1-propanol or dimercaprol) has been shown to be of value (often life-saving) in poisoning due to arsenic, mercury, and gold. Further clinical evaluation is necessary to prove its value in poisoning from antimony, bismuth, copper, chromium, cobalt, nickel, and zinc. It appears to be ineffective against tellurium, thallium, and vanadium, and it may enhance the toxicity of uranium, iron, selenium, and cadmium. Although valueless in experimental lead poisoning in animals, there are favorable reports on the treatment of lead encephalopathy in children.

BAL exerts its beneficial effect in heavy metal poisonings by displacing the metal from its combination with sulfhydryl groups of enzyme proteins and by forming a non-toxic metal-BAL complex, which is excreted. A metal ion is more firmly bound by two molecules of BAL (2:1 chelate) than by one molecule (1:1 chelate), but because both types of union are reversible and the complex may dissociate, doses of BAL must be repeated for several days.

BAL is available commercially as a 10 per cent preparation (w/v) in peanut oil, containing 20 per cent benzyl benzoate; it is suitable for intramuscular injection only.

Toxicology: The administration of BAL in therapeutic doses may produce transient side-effects. A dose of 8 mg./kg. will almost always cause untoward symptoms. Doses of 5 mg./kg. repeated every 3 hours for 24 hours usually produce no significant cumulative effects.

The most consistent objective response to BAL in therapeutic doses is a rise in systolic and diastolic blood pressure, accompanied by tachycardia. This rise, which is roughly proportional to the dose, begins promptly and is usually complete within two hours. Children react like adults, except that a persistent fever is frequently observed in children after the second or third injection. Large overdoses in children (e.g., 10, 25, and 40.5 mg./kg.) have caused convulsions and coma, from which recovery was prompt. There is evidence that BAL is less toxic in patients with heavy metal poisoning than in normal subjects.

Symptomatology (in approximate order of frequency):

1. Nausea and sometimes vomiting.
2. Headache.
3. Burning sensation of lips and mouth.
4. Feeling of constriction in throat, chest and hands.
5. Conjunctivitis, tearing, and salivation.
6. Tingling of hands.
7. Burning sensation of penis.
8. Sweating of forehead and hands.
9. Abdominal pain.
10. Tremors.
11. Lower back pain.
12. Positive Chvostek and Trousseau signs occasionally.

Treatment for BAL poisoning: Since reports indicate that the symptoms of BAL poisoning subside in 30 to 90 minutes, no emergency measures are usually required. To relieve unpleasant symptoms, however, some authorities advocate intramuscular use of a 1:1000 solution of epinephrine hydrochloride (0.1 to 0.5 ml.) or an oral dose of ephedrine sulfate (25 to 50 mg.). The latter may also be used prophylactically half an hour before the injection of BAL.

Dosage schedule of BAL in heavy metal poisoning: The following schedules are advocated by the Council on Pharmacy and Chemistry of the American Medical Association, in cases of arsenic and gold intoxication. The Council makes no official recommendations for mercury poisoning. In practice the same doses of BAL are usually used in mercury and arsenic poisoning, although some clinicians prefer a larger initial dose (e.g., 5 mg./kg.) in acute mercurialism (see Mercury, p. 154). The following dose schedules have been used in both adults and children, and they are probably appropriate to infants as well. All doses are expressed as milligrams of BAL (not of solution), and all injections should be intramuscular.

	Severe Metal Poisoning	Mild Metal Poisoning
1st day	3.0 mg./kg. q4h (6 inj.)	2.5 mg./kg. q4h (6 inj.)
2nd day	3.0 mg./kg. q4h (6 inj.)	2.5 mg./kg. q6h (4 inj.)
3rd day	3.0 mg./kg. q6h (4 inj.)	2.5 mg./kg. q12h (2 inj.)
Each of following 10 days (or until recovery)	3.0 mg./kg. q12h (2 inj.)	2.5 mg./kg. qd (1 inj.)

BARBITURATES

Many dialkyl and alkyl-aryl substituted malonylureas are employed in clinical medicine as sedative and hypnotic agents. The oldest of these barbiturates is the diethyl derivative, barbital, first introduced as a drug in 1903. Since then hundreds of derivatives have been synthesized and tested, and several dozen are in current clinical use. Some serve as potent anticonvulsants, others as

intravenous anesthetic agents. Unsubstituted malonylurea (barbituric acid) is widely used by the chemical industry in the manufacture of plastics, *etc.* The annual consumption of barbiturates in the United States is said to approach 300 tons. Acute barbiturate intoxication is common and accounts for about 1500 deaths annually in the U. S. A. No class of drugs is responsible for more acute poisonings. Chronic barbiturate intoxication is an important social and medical problem; together with the treatment of the withdrawal syndrome, however, it is beyond the scope of this manual.

Toxicology: Derivatives of barbituric acid differ from one another in latency of onset, duration of action, and metabolic fate. Differences of potency are comparatively minor (2- to 3-fold). In Table III.1, some of the popular drugs are classified according to the duration of the hypnosis which they induce. Speed of onset (latency) follows the same classes. Differences in metabolic fate can be represented by similar groupings. Specifically, short- and ultrashort-acting barbiturates are almost exclusively detoxified *in vivo* (chiefly in the liver), while long-acting congeners are largely excreted in the urine as pharmacologically active molecules. Recovery from poisoning depends ultimately on the liver in the first instance and on the kidneys in the second. With drugs of intermediate durations of action, both detoxification and excretion are important disposal mechanisms. Thiobarbiturates, like thiopental (Pentothal) and thiamylal (Surital), differ from oxy-derivatives in many respects; besides an ultra-short duration of action, they are

TABLE III.1

Classification of barbiturate drugs

A. Long-acting:
    Barbital (Veronal)
    Phenobarbital (Luminal)
    Mephobarbital (Mebaral)
    Diallylbarbituric acid (Dial)

B. Intermediate duration of action:
    Amobarbital (Amytal)
    Aprobarbital (Alurate)
    Butabarbital (Butisol)
    Butethal (Neonal)
    Hexethal (Ortal)
    Vinbarbital (Delvinal)

C. Short-acting:
    Cyclobarbital (Phanodorn)
    Pentobarbital (Nembutal)
    Secobarbital (Seconal)

D. Ultrashort-acting:
    Hexabarbital sodium (Evipal)
    Thiamylal sodium (Surital)
    Thiopental sodium (Pentothal)

inactive by mouth and can be administered only by the intravenous or rectal routes. Unlike most barbiturates, phenobarbital and mephobarbital (Mebaral) have specific anticonvulsant properties. With the exceptions noted above, the barbiturate drugs closely resemble one another.

Most acute barbiturate poisonings arise from attempted suicide. Sometimes the suicide is unintentional and stems from "automatism," *i.e.*, self-poisoning while in a state of confusion induced by a normal therapeutic dose. Some poisonings arise in the course of normal clinical practice and are due to natural or acquired hypersensitivity. Although the various derivatives differ somewhat in degree of toxicity, an oral dose of 1 gm. of most barbiturates produces serious poisoning in an adult, and death commonly occurs after 2 to 10 gm. Presumably the lethal dose is smaller by parenteral routes of administration. Even mild liver insufficiency enhances markedly the toxicity of all common barbiturates except barbital and phenobarbital. Long-acting barbiturates have been responsible for most fatal poisonings, although in terms of lethal dose they are no more toxic and may be less potent than shorter acting derivatives. While sodium salts of rapidly acting congeners have produced death within an hour after massive oral doses, most barbiturate deaths are delayed for several hours or several days. Fatalities have been reported on the fourth and fifth days, but the prognosis is usually favorable if the patient survives the first 24 or 36 hours. In a limited study, poisoned patients were found to regain consciousness when the drug concentration in blood fell to: 5 to 9 mg./100 ml. with long-acting barbiturates, 2 to 4 mg./100 ml. with drugs of intermediate action, and 1 to 2 mg./100 ml. with short-acting congeners.

An overdose of a barbiturate drug induces the classical picture of progressive central nervous depression. In its severest form this syndrome leads to respiratory arrest as a result of general reflex paralysis; in its milder forms, it may mimic any stage of clinical anesthesia. Except for a rapid (and weak) pulse, vital signs are characteristically reduced. In addition to direct inhibition of vasomotor tone with consequent hypotension, circulatory insufficiency may be aggravated by hypoxia from inadequate pulmonary ventilation. Early deaths are usually due to respiratory arrest, but delayed fatalities may arise from one or any combination of the following complications: hypostatic pneumonia, bronchopneumonia, lung abscess, pulmonary edema, cerebral edema, vasomotor collapse, and irreversible renal shutdown. An occasional patient who survives severe and prolonged hypoxia during the acute phase may suffer residual neurological lesions, but recovery is usually complete. In the U. S. A. the mortality rate

in acute barbiturate poisoning lies between 5 and 10 per cent.

The only recognized treatment is supportive and symptomatic. The alleged antidotal action of sodium succinate and other intermediates in carbohydrate metabolism has not impressed most clinicians. A new barbiturate antagonist, β,β'-methylethyl glutarimide (NP-13), which is a convulsant in normal animals at a dose of 30 mg./kg., has caused prompt arousal after intravenous doses of 50 mg. in men and women under barbiturate anesthesia. The drug has not yet been released for general use, and its effectiveness and specificity in the treatment of barbiturate poisoning have not been demonstrated. The established non-specific analeptic drugs have often been used effectively in barbiturate poisoning, where they serve to increase and maintain the general level of reflex excitability. A beneficial response consists of an increase in the rate or depth of respiration and a return in the blood pressure toward normotensive levels. Large and repeated doses may be necessary, but the analeptic drugs should not be used to restore consciousness because the attempt may precipitate convulsions. Because of the threat of this complication, an ultrashort-acting barbiturate should always be available for immediate intravenous injection. Although each of the common stimulant drugs has its proponents, picrotoxin and pentylenetetrazol (Metrazol) are widely conceded to be the most useful. Because of its more sustained action and perhaps greater effectiveness on the respiratory and vasomotor centers of the medulla, picrotoxin may be preferable to pentylenetetrazol. The popularity of analeptic therapy has recently been challenged by Scandinavian investigators who prefer more conservative measures. Their results emphasize convincingly that analeptic drugs have often been used unnecessarily, but most clinicians are convinced that the judicious use of central nervous stimulants has saved lives in severe barbiturate poisoning. In any case, analeptic therapy should be regarded as only one phase of general supportive treatment and perhaps a minor one.

Among supportive measures used in barbiturate poisoning, the highest priority goes to the correction of anoxia. Any one or combination of the following measures may be necessary: the removal of airway obstruction, oxygen administration, artificial respiration, and analeptic therapy. If anoxia can be minimized, cardiovascular collapse rarely if ever develops. Dehydration must be corrected, but overhydration should be avoided. Hemodialysis with a modern artificial kidney has proved effective in promoting barbiturate excretion and in speeding recovery. Diuretic drugs are seldom if ever useful, but osmotic diuretic agents (such as urea and sodium sulfate) deserve a trial in poisonings due to long-acting drugs such as phenobarbital and barbi-

tal, where recovery is ultimately dependent on drug excretion. At least in the dog, most of the barbital which is filtered in the renal glomerulus is passively resorbed in the proximal tubules, i.e., it moves with the water, which is largely returned to the circulation. Osmotic diuretics enhance barbital excretion in dogs by inhibiting osmotically this resorption of water. Neither water nor mercurial diuretic drugs act in this way, and neither has an appreciable effect on barbiturate excretion in most cases.

Symptomatology:

1. Drowsiness is usually the first symptom. A transient period of confusion, excitement, delirium, and hallucinations is not uncommon.
2. Ataxia, vertigo, slurred speech, headache, paresthesias, and subjective visual disturbances.
3. A stupor progressing through deepening states of coma, with inhibition or absence of superficial and deep reflexes. Responses to painful stimuli gradually cease. The Babinski toe sign may become positive.
4. Respirations may be rapid and shallow or slow and labored, but the minute volume (pulmonary ventilation) is always reduced.
5. Mild but progressive cardiovascular collapse, evidenced by cyanosis, hypotension, a weak rapid pulse, and cold and clammy skin. Circulatory insufficiency is almost always secondary to hypoxia from respiratory depression.
6. The pupils are usually slightly constricted but react to light; they may dilate during terminal asphyxia.
7. Urine formation is slowed or suppressed completely.
8. The body temperature is usually reduced. If a fever develops, it usually signals bronchopneumonia.
9. Respirations become irregular, sometimes Cheyne-Stokes in character, and eventually cease.
10. Although death is usually due to respiratory arrest, hypostatic or aspiration pneumonia late in the course of the illness may prove lethal. Occasionally severe grades of pulmonary edema are encountered (especially early in poisonings from ultrashort-acting barbiturates). Vasomotor collapse and shock often contribute to a lethal outcome, and rarely renal shutdown due to vascular collapse proves to be irreversible.
11. Among survivors, residual damage is rare, but an occasional patient who has suffered prolonged and severe hypoxia during the acute phase may exhibit permanent neurological damage.
12. Sometimes barbiturate poisoning is due to or

complicated by natural or acquired idiosyncrasy. Allergic reactions from acquired hypersensitivity are of the usual types: asthma, urticaria, angioneurotic edema, dermatitis, fever, delirium, liver necrosis. Natural idiosyncrasy commonly expresses itself as an excitement reaction, a prolonged hangover, and as a pain syndrome. The latter consists of paroxysms of localized or diffuse pain of a myalgic, neuralgic, or arthralgic character.

Treatment:

1. Gastric lavage with a potassium permanganate solution (1:5000), if practical within a few hours after ingestion. Precautions against aspiration are essential. See p. 6.

2. Leave in the stomach 15 to 30 gm. of sodium sulfate in water as a saline cathartic.

3. If sensory stimuli (*e.g.*, pinching) arouse the patient even briefly from his coma and if his respirations are full and regular, further treatment is seldom required.

4. Observe and record at 15- to 30-minute intervals the following observations: vital signs (respiration, pulse, blood pressure, and temperature), skin color, cardiac rhythm, pupillary size and light reflex, corneal and gag reflexes, response to pain, and tendon reflexes.

5. Correct airway obstruction. The insertion of an oropharyngeal airway is usually advisable in a comatose patient who has no gag reflex. Suction frequently to remove saliva and mucus. See p. 184.

6. At the slightest suspicion of hypoxia, continuous or intermittent oxygen therapy is warranted.

7. Sometimes the inhalation of oxygen causes an arrest of spontaneous breathing. Artificial respiration is then essential. Do not wait for respiratory arrest; give mechanical assistance whenever the rate or depth of breathing is clearly inadequate. See p. 185.

8. Sometimes inadequate pulmonary ventilation can be improved by the cautious use of such analeptic drugs as caffeine, nikethamide, amphetamine, pentylenetetrazol (Metrazol), and picrotoxin. For doses and techniques of administration, see p. 206. Analeptic therapy should be avoided unless a clear and compelling need exists. One suggested criterion is the patient's response to a small intravenous dose of Metrazol (5 ml. of a 10 per cent solution); any lessening in the depth of coma, however transient, is evidence that analeptic therapy is not needed and that symptomatic care will suffice.

9. The threat of cardiovascular collapse usually disappears when and if hypoxia is corrected. Analeptic drugs may be beneficial in the early stages of shock. A plasma transfusion is sometimes useful.

10. Correct dehydration by the cautious administration of replacement fluids. In the treatment of barbital and phenobarbital poisoning *only*, osmotic diuretic drugs (notably urea and sodium sulfate) may have a legitimate role (see above), but otherwise diuresis is not beneficial. Catheterize the urinary bladder to prevent retention. Measure and record urine output.

11. Good nursing is essential. The body temperature should be maintained if possible. Antibiotic therapy is advisable as prophylaxis against pneumonia. By repeatedly changing the patient's posture, hypostatic pneumonia and decubitus ulcers are avoided. See p. 229.

Laboratory: Qualitative and quantitative analyses for barbiturates are desirable in the management of severe poisonings. The isolation of barbiturate crystals and determination of their melting point (mixed melting point) is the most specific method available but requires large samples. Cobalt color reactions have limited application because of poor specificity. Most current methods of quantitative analysis are based on the influence of pH on the ultra-violet absorption spectrum of drug isolated by solvent extraction.

BARIUM

Barium salts are contained in some rodenticides, depilatories, and fireworks. In any of these forms barium may become available unintentionally to children. Various barium salts have been mistaken for the sulfate and administered by clinical radiologists with fatal results.

Toxicology: The acid-soluble barium salts (carbonate, chloride, hydroxide, nitrate, acetate, sulfide) are highly toxic, while the insoluble barium sulfate is quite benign. The lethal oral dose of barium chloride is said to be about 1.0 gm., but much larger doses have been tolerated. Death occurs within a few hours or a few days. Severe reactions have also been reported from the inhalation of barium carbonate and peroxide dusts.

Barium stimulates smooth, striated, and cardiac muscle; the result is violent peristalsis, arterial hypertension, muscle twitching, and disturbances in cardiac action. The central nervous system may be first stimulated and then depressed. Kidney damage has been described as a late complication, probably a result of circulatory insufficiency.

Symptomatology:

1. Excessive salivation, vomiting, severe abdominal pain, and violent purging with watery and bloody stools.
2. A slow and often irregular pulse and a transient elevation in arterial blood pressure.
3. Tinnitus, giddiness, and vertigo.
4. Muscle twitchings, progressing to convulsions and/or paralysis.
5. Dilated pupils with impaired accommodation.
6. Confusion and increasing somnolence, without coma.
7. Collapse and death from respiratory and cardiac failure.

Treatment:

1. Rapid oral administration of a soluble sulfate in water, such as magnesium or sodium sulfate (2 oz.), alum (4 gm.) or very dilute sulfuric acid (30 ml. of a 10 per cent solution diluted to 1 qt.). These agents precipitate barium as the insoluble sulfate.
2. Gastric lavage or an emetic.
3. Atropine sulfate (0.5 to 1.0 mg.) to alleviate colic. In severe cases morphine (10 to 15 mg.) may be necessary to relieve abdominal pain.
4. Blood pressure may be reduced, if elevated, by sublingual tablets of nitroglycerin ($\frac{1}{100}$ to $\frac{1}{50}$ gr.).
5. Oxygen administration to relieve dyspnea and cyanosis.
6. Isotonic saline (NaCl) intravenously (1000 ml.) to combat dehydration from vomiting and diarrhea.
7. Quinidine sulfate (0.1 to 0.3 gm.) to prevent ventricular fibrillation.
8. Supportive therapy.

Laboratory: not usually relevant.

BENZENE HEXACHLORIDE

Benzene hexachloride or BHC (more properly called hexachlorocyclohexane) in its various forms is a widely used insecticide, especially in the control of cotton insects. Lindane, which is the gamma isomer of benzene hexachloride, is effective against many agricultural pests, not only the leaf-feeding insects but also the soil-infesting types. BHC has been used in some household preparations and is effective against DDT-resistant flies, mosquitoes, and body lice. It is used in the form of powders, emulsions, oil sprays, poison baits, and aerosols. BHC is also used medically as a vermifuge and in an ointment for the treatment of scabies.

Toxicology: Technical BHC (1,2,3,4,5,6-hexachlorocyclohexane) is a mixture with the following approximate isomeric composition: alpha 65 to 70 per cent, beta 6 to 8 per cent, gamma 12 to 15 per cent, delta 2 to 5 per cent, and others 5 to 10 per cent. These isomers differ qualitatively and quantitatively in biological activity. The alpha and gamma isomers are central nervous stimulants; the beta and delta are depressants. In a mixture of these isomers it is possible that one component may antidote another. The mean lethal dose of technical BHC may be about 400 mg./kg. when ingested by man. The gamma isomer (lindane) has the highest acute toxicity; its lethal dose is perhaps 125 mg./kg.

BHC is absorbed through all portals including the intact skin. The rapidity with which symptoms develop after ingestion varies with the isomer: the gamma is fastest (within 1 hour), the alpha slowest (within 24 hours), and the technical or commercial mixture is intermediate (within 2 hours). Death from the pure gamma isomer is prompt (24 hours), while from the others it may be delayed several days. The pathology resembles that caused by DDT; liver damage and hyaline changes in the renal tubules are described most often.

Although symptoms and treatment are similar, lindane is more acutely toxic than DDT, but unlike DDT it is not a chronic or cumulative poison.

Symptomatology (from technical BHC or the gamma isomer):

1. Hyperirritability and central nervous excitation: notably vomiting, restlessness, muscle spasms, ataxia, and clonic and tonic convulsions.
2. Subsequent central nervous depression leading to respiratory failure.
3. Pulmonary edema (with cyanosis and dyspnea) was observed in two fatally poisoned children.
4. From exposure to lindane vapors (and its thermal decomposition products), headache, nausea, vomiting, irritation of eyes, nose, and throat.
5. Dermatitis and urticaria occasionally.

Treatment:

1. Gastric lavage and saline cathartics (not oil laxatives because they promote absorption).
2. Sedatives: pentobarbital or phenobarbital in amounts adequate to control convulsions (p. 201).
3. Calcium gluconate intravenously may be used in conjunction with sedatives in the control of convulsions.
4. Rest and quiet.
5. Do *not* use epinephrine because ventricular fibrillation may result.

Laboratory: generally irrelevant.

BORATE

Borates are widely used as antiseptic agents despite their limited effectiveness. Powders, ointments, and solutions containing boric acid have long been prescribed for dermatologic disorders, eyewashes, gargles, urinary antiseptics, and diaper rinses. Borates have also been used as food preservatives, but they are now largely supplanted by safer agents. Sodium borate (borax) is used in cleaning compounds, wood preservatives, and herbicides. When dissolved in buffered aqueous solution, the various complex salts, such as meta-, di-, tetra-, pyro-, and orthoborate, cannot be differentiated from one another chemically or toxicologically.

Toxicology: The reputation of borates is so firmly entrenched that they are still readily available despite toxic potentialities reported as early as 1881. Acute poisonings have followed ingestion, parenteral injection, enemas, lavage of serous cavities, and application of powders and ointments to burned and abraded skin. Ironically many of these incidents have occurred in hospitals through ignorance or error.

The biochemical mechanism of borate poisoning is unknown. Clinical and pathological findings relate principally to the central nervous system, gastrointestinal tract, kidneys, liver, and skin, and the highest concentrations of boron are found at these sites. Borates are rapidly absorbed from mucous membranes and abraded skin, but toxic symptoms may be delayed for several hours. Borate excretion occurs mainly through the kidneys; about half is excreted in the first 12 hours, and the remainder is eliminated over a period of 5 to 7 days.

Clinical findings commonly consist of gastrointestinal disturbances (hemorrhagic gastroenteritis), erythematous skin eruptions, and signs of central nervous stimulation followed by depression. In an adult the mean lethal dose of boric acid and sodium borate probably exceeds 30 gm. As one phase of treatment for brain tumor, each of ten adults was recently injected intravenously with about 20 gm. of borax ($Na_2B_4O_7 \cdot 10H_2O$); no deaths resulted, but severe untoward reactions included nausea, vomiting, diarrhea, mild peripheral vascular collapse, mental confusion, with subsequent drowsiness, rash, and intermittent retching for several days. Infants and young children are thought to be more susceptible to borate intoxication than are adults. In a study of over 100 cases of accidental poisoning, the over-all fatality rate was 55 per cent, but in infants under one year of age, 70 per cent of the cases ended fatally. Death may occur in a few hours but is usually delayed several days.

Symptomatology:
1. Nausea, vomiting, diarrhea, epigastric pain. Vomiting is often persistent, and the vomitus and feces may contain blood. Hemorrhagic gastroenteritis may develop irrespective of the route of administration.
2. Weakness, lethargy, headache, restlessness, tremors, and intermittent convulsions—with subsequent central nervous depression.
3. Erythematous skin eruptions (giving rise to a boiled lobster appearance) followed by extensive exfoliation. Typical sites of this rash are the palms, soles, buttocks, and scrotum, but no skin surface is immune. The pharynx and tympanic membranes may also be involved.
4. Shock syndrome—cold clammy skin, cyanosis, thready pulse, and low blood pressure.
5. Occasionally kidney injury (oliguria, albuminuria) and rarely liver damage (hepatomegaly, jaundice) have been reported; neither appears to have been the cause of death. Shock may or may not be fully responsible for these lesions.
6. The body temperature is usually normal (or even low), but fevers are described in the absence of recognized intercurrent infection.
7. Death is due to vascular collapse in the early stages or to central nervous depression later in the course of poisoning. Bronchopneumonia, meningitis, and other terminal infections have been described.

Treatment:
1. Gastric lavage with warm tap water (if borate was swallowed).
2. Saline catharsis with 15 to 30 gm. of sodium sulfate in water.
3. Replace water and electrolytes lost through vomiting and diarrhea. Parenteral administration is usually necessary (pp. 215–217).
4. Treat shock with oxygen, intravenous plasma, or blood (p. 193).
5. Control convulsions with a short-acting barbiturate (p. 201).
6. Antibiotics as prophylaxis against infection.
7. Caffeine sodium benzoate and other analeptic drugs as indicated (p. 204).
8. Symptomatic treatment for skin lesions.

Laboratory:
1. Boron is detectable in urine and sometimes in cerebrospinal fluid by the turmeric paper test.
2. Urinalysis may reveal albumin.
3. Biochemical tests of liver function are useful and appropriate.

BROMATE

Bromate poisoning was formerly a clinical rarity, but in recent years potassium (and less often sodium) bromate has been used as a "neutralizer" in home permanent cold wave kits. Several cases of accidental poisoning in children have resulted from the ingestion of bromate solutions. Most manufacturers have now substituted less toxic substances as "neutralizers" (*e.g.*, sodium perborate and sodium hexametaphosphate). Chlorates are less toxic than bromates but produce similar poisonings. Potassium chlorate has been used in throat gargles, some dentifrices, and fireworks.

Toxicology: The mean lethal dose of potassium bromate (KBrO₃) has not been definitely established, but a few ounces of a 2 per cent solution have caused serious and even fatal poisonings (total dose about 5 gm.). Death is apparently due to acute renal failure resulting from the nephrotoxic action of the bromate ion and/or the products of severe intravascular hemolysis. Hemolysis is usually preceded by severe methemoglobinemia, which may not become apparent for several hours after ingestion. Gastrointestinal effects are due to the caustic action of hydrobromic acid and bromine, produced by the action of stomach acid on the bromate ion. The renal lesion, which consists principally of tubular degeneration, is sometimes associated with severe liver necrosis. Convalescence is slow.

Symptomatology:
1. Vomiting, diarrhea, gastric pain.
2. Restlessness and later apathy. Severe central nervous depression is common in poisoned animals, but is not prominent in clinical poisonings until uremia is advanced.
3. Methemoglobin formation and hemolysis, which develop slowly as first. Cyanosis and later icterus, yielding a greenish hue to skin and mucous membranes.

4. Lumbar pain, oliguria, and albuminuria, progressing to anuria and azotemia within a few hours or a few days.
5. Death from renal failure, usually within 1 to 2 weeks.

Treatment:
1. Gastric lavage with tap water or a 1 per cent solution of sodium thiosulfate.
2. Administer a demulcent and an analgesic like meperidine (Demerol). Avoid morphine.
3. Administer oxygen. If methemoglobinemia becomes severe, a replacement transfusion with whole blood may become essential.
4. Do not attempt to correct methemoglobinemia with methylene blue because this dye may enhance the toxicity of bromate (or chlorate).
5. Sodium thiosulfate solution (100 to 500 ml. of 1 per cent) by intravenous drip has been recommended.
6. Correct dehydration by infusing intravenously a glucose solution (5 per cent in water). Avoid electrolytes (except as above) unless acid-base imbalance or shock become severe.
7. Supportive treatment of acute renal failure (see p. 210).

Laboratory:
1. Bromate may be detected in blood and urine. If this test is impractical, an analysis for the presence of bromide may help to establish the diagnosis.
2. Periodic measurements of the oxygen-carrying capacity of blood are desirable.
3. Repeated urinalyses may reveal albumin, hemoglobin, red blood cells, and cellular casts.

CADMIUM

Metallic cadmium is used as a rust-proof plating for iron, as a constituent of various alloys, and in a variety of metallurgic processes. The use of cadmium-lined containers for food and beverage is banned in several states because of the tendency of the metal to dissolve in contact with acid foods and to produce poisonous concentrations of cadmium salts. Cadmium carbonate is found in some silver polishes.

Toxicology: Acute poisoning may result from the inhalation of cadmium dusts and fumes (usually cadmium oxide) and from the ingestion of cadmium salts. Many non-fatal cases of "food poisoning" have followed the ingestion of acid foods kept even for brief periods in coated containers, such as ice

cube trays and metal pitchers. A severe gastroenteritis is the chief response to ingested cadmium, but at least in experimental animals, kidney and liver injuries may occur and the kidney disorder may kill. In contrast the dangerous actions following inhalation of dust or fumes are largely limited to the lungs and respiratory mucosa. Edema and necrosis of the pulmonary epithelium are described, and in the dog three clinical stages have been recognized: 1) acute pulmonary edema developing within 24 hours and reaching its maximum within 3 days; 2) proliferative interstitial pneumonitis lasting from approximately the third to the tenth day; and 3) permanent lung damage consisting of

perivascular and peribronchial fibrosis. A similar sequence is implied by human autopsy material.

Inhaled as dusts or aerosols, cadmium salts (including even the relatively insoluble oxide) are highly toxic. The inhalation of 40 mg. of cadmium, with the pulmonary retention of 4 mg., has been estimated to be fatal in man. When swallowed, cadmium salts are much less lethal, in part because they induce vomiting and so are not retained. Although as little as 10 mg. of soluble cadmium salts has produced severe toxic symptoms when ingested, death probably requires several hundred milligrams by the oral route.

Ionic cadmium inhibits sulfhydryl enzymes, presumably in all accessible tissues. Following inhalation a portion of the retained cadmium is firmly fixed to pulmonary tissue, but relatively large amounts leave the lungs and are distributed to other organs. In rabbits only small quantities are excreted in urine, and fecal excretion over a 5-day period amounts to no more than 10 per cent of a single parenteral dose.

Dimercaprol (BAL) forms a soluble complex with ionic cadmium. In rabbits the administration of BAL markedly increases the fecal excretion of cadmium. Urinary excretion also rises moderately, but the kidney content of fixed cadmium is considerably elevated, apparently because the BAL-cadmium complex bringing metal to the kidney is partially dissociated there. Consequently poisoned rabbits may improve after therapy with BAL, only to die later from renal insufficiency. Because of the threat of kidney damage, BAL is probably inadvisable in clinical cases of cadmium poisoning by ingestion. BAL is recommended, however, for treatment of pulmonary complications which follow an inhalation exposure, because the lungs may be protected by the mobilization of cadmium in amounts which are insufficient to damage the kidneys.

Symptomatology:

A. Inhalation (an asymptomatic period of 4 to 8 hours may precede the clinical illness).
   1. Metallic taste in the mouth, and headache.
   2. Shortness of breath, chest pain, cough with foamy or bloody sputum.
      Pulmonary rales and related physical signs. These signs and symptoms mimic "the flu."
   3. Weakness, leg pains.
   4. An asphyxial death from intense pulmonary edema, or
   5. Gradual resolution of pulmonary edema (over a period of a few days) and development of fever, with persistence of cough, chest pain, and dyspnea for one or more weeks. Physical signs of pneumonic consolidation.

   6. Late liver damage has followed respiratory exposures in industry.
B. Ingestion (an asymptomatic period of ½ to 1 hour may precede the clinical illness).
   1. Severe nausea, vomiting, diarrhea and abdominal cramps, and salivation.
   2. Headache, muscular cramps, vertigo, and perhaps convulsions (rarely).
   3. Exhaustion, collapse, shock, and death, usually within a period of 24 hours.
   4. The gradual evolution of signs and symptoms of liver and kidney damage.
   5. Death in 1 to 2 weeks due to acute renal failure with anuria and uremia.

Treatment:

A. Inhalation
   1. Terminate exposure and remove patient to fresh air.
   2. Codeine sulfate for cough and chest pain.
   3. Treat pulmonary edema by postural drainage, positive-pressure oxygen therapy, and possibly the inhalation of an aerosolized solution of ethyl alcohol or methyl siloxane as a defoaming agent (p. 192).
   4. Dimercaprol (BAL) intramuscularly according to the dosage schedule on p. 117. in order to mobilize cadmium and remove it from the lungs.
   5. Penicillin as prophylaxis against secondary infection and bacterial pneumonia.
   6. Prophylactic and supportive measures for possible liver injury (p. 213).
B. Ingestion
   1. Allay gastrointestinal irritation by swallowing milk or beaten egg whites at frequent intervals.
   2. Gastric lavage with water, milk, or albumin solution, if vomiting is not prompt and intensive.
   3. Administer by mouth sodium or magnesium sulfate in water (15 to 30 gm.).
   4. Avoid dimercaprol (BAL), since its administration might convert a gastroenteritis into a severe toxic nephritis (see above).
   5. Parenteral fluids and electrolytes, given cautiously in order to maintain hydration and acid-base balance.
   6. Prophylactic and supportive measures for possible liver injury (p. 213).
   7. Supportive measures for acute renal failure, as outlined on p. 210.

Laboratory:

1. Function tests may demonstrate subclinical kidney and liver injuries.
2. X-ray findings in the chest after inhalation exposures are consistent with diffuse pulmonary edema; later findings are like those of bronchopneumonia (proliferative interstitial pneumonitis).

CAMPHOR

Camphor (2-camphanone) and camphorated oils are rarely used today as stimulants in clinical medicine. Camphor is widely employed in "camphor ball' moth repellents and flakes. In some lay circles, it is worn as protection against infection (usually in a bag suspended from the neck). Borneol (2-camphanol) is believed to have a similar and perhaps identical toxicity.

Toxicology: Camphor is readily absorbed from all sites of administration. It produces a feeling of coolness on the skin and in the respiratory tract. In contrast a small oral dose causes a sensation of warmth in the stomach; large doses may induce nausea and vomiting. Camphor is a central nervous stimulant; systemic poisoning is characterized by epileptiform convulsions. Post-convulsive depression of the central nervous system follows stimulation. The ingestion of 2 gm. generally produces dangerous effects in an adult, and 0.7 to 1.0 gm. (1 teaspoonful of liniment or camphorated oil) has proved fatal in children.

Symptomatology (within 5 to 90 minutes after ingestion):

1. Nausea and vomiting.
2. Feeling of warmth. Headache.
3. Confusion, vertigo, excitement, restlessness, delirium, and hallucinations.
4. Increased muscular excitability, tremors, and jerky movements.
5. Epileptiform convulsions, followed by depression. Convulsions sometimes occur early in the syndrome and may be severe, but they do not have the grave prognosis of strychnine convulsions.
6. Coma. Depression may at times be the primary symptom.

7. Death results from respiratory failure or from status epilepticus.
8. Slow convalescence (days or weeks), often with persistent gastric distress.

Treatment:

1. Treatment is aimed at preventing convulsions. Intravenous sodium pentabarbital or amytal is effective. The drug should be injected *slowly* until the desired condition is reached, namely a degree of depression sufficient to prevent or stop convulsions and to keep the patient asleep, but not deep enough to depress respirations or blood pressure. (If a barbiturate is not available, ether, chloroform, or avertin may be used temporarily.) For details of anticonvulsant therapy, see pp. 201-204.
2. Gastric lavage (with warm water) may be performed when the patient is asleep or well pre-medicated. In the presymptomatic stage, lavage should take precedence over all measures.
3. The patient should be kept under careful observation for many hours and protected from all possible stimuli. Wakefulness, muscular twitchings, and increased reflex excitability are signs that warn of need for additional barbiturate.
4. Caffeine sodium benzoate 0.5 gm. intramuscularly during the phase of depression.
5. Oxygen therapy, artificial respiration (p. 185).
6. Avoid the ingestion of oils or alcohol, which may promote intestinal absorption of camphor.

Laboratory: Laboratory data are not usually relevant.

CARBON DISULFIDE

Carbon disulfide (or bisulfide) is a clear, colorless, volatile liquid which, in its pure state, smells like ether or chloroform, and in a commercial grade has an offensive odor like decaying cabbage. It is used as a solvent for waxes and resins, as a cleaner for removing grease, and in vapor form, as a disinfectant and insecticide.

Toxicology: Carbon disulfide is hazardous as a liquid or as a vapor. Absorption occurs through all portals, and acute poisoning can be caused by the ingestion of 1 teaspoonful of liquid or the inhalation of vapor concentrations as low as 0.3 per cent. The fatal oral dose is unknown; although more than two ounces has failed to kill when ingested with suicidal intent, 1 to 2 oz. is probably a reasonable estimate of the mean lethal dose in adults.

Like the chlorinated hydrocarbon solvents, acute exposures to carbon disulfide vapor produce central nervous depression after a transient excitement stage; death is usually due to respiratory paralysis, sometimes with terminal convulsions. Unlike the chlorinated hydrocarbon solvents, carbon disulfide has no prominent injurious actions on liver or kidneys, but it is a very dangerous nerve poison. Chronic exposures to low vapor concentrations have resulted in a fantastic variety of signs and symptoms, and even acute exposures may be followed by persistent disability. The outstanding sequelae are neuropsychiatric disorders ranging from irritability to a manic depressive psychosis—with or without evidence of organic nervous disease of peripheral motor nerves, sensory nerves, pyramidal and extrapyramidal tracts, and basal

ganglia. Among the reported clinical manifestations of nerve damage are all grades of emotional and mental disorders, weakness and paralysis, hypesthesias, blindness, and the signs of parkinsonism.

Carbon disulfide vapor is rapidly absorbed when inhaled. About 10 to 15 per cent is excreted through the respiratory tract, and a trace is present in urine. Most absorbed carbon disulfide is metabolized to sulfates and organic sulfur compounds (not hydrogen sulfide), which are eventually excreted by the kidneys.

Symptomatology:

Acute

1. Mild irritation of skin, eyes, and mucous membranes from liquid or concentrated vapors.
2. Headache.
3. Garlicky breath, nausea, vomiting, diarrhea (even after vapor exposures), and occasionally abdominal pain.
4. Weak pulse, palpitations.
5. Fatigue, weakness in the legs, unsteady gait, vertigo.
6. Mania, hallucinations of sight, hearing, taste, and smell.
7. Central nervous depression with respiratory paralysis.
8. Death may occur during coma or after a convulsion.

Chronic

1. Tremors, weakness, paralysis. Multiple peripheral neuritis is often encountered. The absence of a corneal reflex is highly characteristic according to one authority.
2. Emotional instability of all grades, including frank psychoses.
3. Recovery may occur within a few months or a few years, but paralyses may be permanent.

Treatment:

1. Remove patient to fresh air.
2. Artificial respiration (p. 185) and oxygen therapy (p. 189), as necessary.
3. Gastric lavage with warm water (if intoxication is due to ingestion).
4. Strong tea or coffee by mouth or rectum; caffeine sodium benzoate (0.5 gm.) subcutaneously; nikethamide intravenously, and other central nervous stimulants (p. 204), as needed.
5. For severe excitement, a short-acting barbiturate may be given cautiously (see p. 201).

Laboratory:

1. Blood may show a slight increase in lymphocytes, a marked increase in monocytes, and occasionally an eosinophilia.
2. Serum cholinesterase activity is said to be reduced in poisoned patients, but this enzyme inhibition is apparently insufficient to produce characteristic symptoms.

CARBON MONOXIDE

Carbon monoxide (CO) is a combustible, non-irritating, colorless, tasteless, and essentially odorless gas. Having about the same density as air, it readily mixes with air without stratification. It may be found wherever organic material is burned under conditions of incomplete combustion (e.g., dynamite explosions) and is a prominent constituent of flue gas from furnaces and exhaust gas from internal combustion engines (concentrations as high as 30 per cent have been measured in automobile exhaust gas, although 7 per cent is more common). Natural gas associated with petroleum deposits has no carbon monoxide, but in processing natural gas (e.g., cracking), carbon monoxide may be produced. As distributed, manufactured gas commonly has a carbon monoxide content between 2 and 15 per cent (by volume). Carbon monoxide is a hazard in many industrial processes. Among non-industrial workers, firemen, cooks, bakers, chauffeurs, garage mechanics, lineotypists, and furnace repair men bear the greatest risk.

Toxicology: Carbon monoxide is responsible for a larger number of severe chemical poisonings than any other single agent. Under ordinary conditions of poisoning, carbon monoxide is not itself toxic to body cells; it acts only by depriving them of necessary oxygen. Oxygen is effectively excluded from the tissues by the formation of a reversible complex between carbon monoxide and the hemoglobin molecule; this complex, known as carboxyhemoglobin, is incapable of transporting oxygen. Not only is the oxygen-carrying capacity of blood markedly reduced, but also the shape of the dissociation curve of oxyhemoglobin is altered so that a smaller portion of blood oxygen is released in tissue capillaries. The reduction in the oxygen-carrying capacity of blood is proportional to the amount of carboxyhemoglobin formed. The latter depends in turn upon the concentrations of carbon monoxide and of oxygen in inspired air and on the relative affinities of the hemoglobin molecule for these two gases. Because the affinity for carbon monoxide is 200 to 300 times that for oxygen, a small concentration of CO in inspired air can tie up a large proportion of circulating hemoglobin; for example, CO concentrations of 0.01, 0.02, 0.1, and 1.0 per cent eventually saturate 17, 20, 60, and 90 per cent of the hemoglobin, respectively. To reach any of these levels of carboxyhemoglobin requires exposures of appreciable duration; blood-gas equilibrium is attained in 1 to 4 hours in the average adult. All factors which speed respiration

and circulation accelerate this process and so shorten the latent period before toxic signs and symptoms. Thus exercise, fever, and anemia increase the hazard of collapse from carbon monoxide. For much the same reason, young children are more susceptible than adults.

The nature and intensity of toxic signs and symptoms can be correlated, under certain circumstances, with the blood level of carboxyhemoglobin (see Symptomatology below). Any such correlation is clearly impossible when the blood concentration is changing rapidly. In massive exposures, consciousness may be lost with few or no premonitory signs and symptoms. As with other chemical asphyxiants, the critical organs are those which are most sensitive to oxygen lack, notably the brain. Most signs and symptoms are referable to disturbed cerebral metabolism. Myocardial anoxia sometimes becomes sufficient to precipitate untoward reactions. The characteristic cherry-red color of the skin in carbon monoxide poisoning is due to a low concentration of reduced hemoglobin and a high concentration of carboxyhemoglobin in circulating blood.

If the patient is still breathing, biochemical repair begins as soon as he is exposed to fresh air. Carboxyhemoglobin is a completely reversible complex, and essentially all absorbed CO is eventually exhaled; only trace amounts are oxidized to CO_2. The hemoglobin recovered from carboxyhemoglobin is in every way normal, as are the red blood cells which contain it. Carbon monoxide excretion is always fast at first but slows down as the body content of CO decreases. Good therapy is designed to accelerate the dissociation and exhalation of carbon monoxide. If the patient is breathing adequately, the administration of pure oxygen is the most important element in therapy. For a resting adult, half-recovery time (in terms of carboxyhemoglobin) is about 4 hours breathing air and 40 minutes breathing pure oxygen. If respirations have ceased or are inadequate, artificial respiration is essential. Anything which speeds respiration and circulation enhances the rate at which active hemoglobin is regenerated. Analeptic drugs, however, are neither effective nor safe because of the tissue hypoxia which inevitably accompanies carbon monoxide poisoning. Even the addition of CO_2 to oxygen, to serve as a respiratory stimulant, is now regarded as more hazardous than beneficial. The patient should be kept warm and strictly at rest. Sometimes a mild metabolic acidosis deserves attention.

In severe CO poisoning death is usually due to respiratory arrest from severe central nervous depression. This may be associated with cerebral edema and increased intracranial pressure because of excessive transudation through anoxic brain capillaries. Occasionally pulmonary complications are the proximal cause of death; *e.g.,* hypostatic or aspiration pneumonia, pulmonary edema. Myocardial infarction, with or without coronary thrombosis, may be precipitated by carbon monoxide poisoning. Permanent nerve injury may become first evident days or weeks after an acute exposure. Neurological sequelae, however, are very rare and are encountered only after extremely severe intoxications.

Symptomatology (in the following discussion the symbol COHb refers to carboxyhemoglobin and the numeral represents the percentage of circulating hemoglobin which is so modified):

1. No symptoms or shortness of breath during vigorous muscular exercise (0 to 10 per cent COHb).
2. A mild headache ("tightness across the forehead") and breathlessness on moderate exertion (10 to 20 per cent COHb).
3. Throbbing headache, irritability, emotional instability, impaired judgment, defective memory, and rapid fatigue (20 to 30 per cent COHb).
4. Severe headache, weakness, nausea and vomiting, dizziness, dimness of vision, confusion (30 to 40 per cent COHb).
5. Increasing confusion, sometimes hallucinations, severe ataxia, accelerated respirations, and collapse with attempts at exertion (40 to 50 per cent COHb).
6. Syncope or coma, with intermittent convulsions, accelerated respirations, tachycardia with a weak pulse, and a pink or red discoloration of the skin due to the presence (in blood) of carboxyhemoglobin (50 to 60 per cent COHb).
7. Increasing depth of coma, with incontinence of urine and feces (60 to 70 per cent COHb).
8. Profound coma with depressed or absent reflexes, a weak thready pulse, shallow and irregular respiration, and complete quiescence (70 to 80 per cent COHb).
9. Rapid death from respiratory arrest (above 80 per cent COHb).
10. Miscellaneous and atypical reactions include various skin lesions, sweating, hepatomegaly, hyperpyrexia, albuminuria, oliguria, anginal pain, and congestive heart failure.
11. During convalescence a bronchopneumonia may develop because of the aspiration of saliva or vomitus. Even in the absence of frank infection, varying grades of pulmonary edema are reported occasionally.
12. Myocardial infarction, with or without coronary thrombosis, may appear at any time up to a week following an acute poisoning.
13. After an uneventful convalescence, signs of nerve or brain injury may rarely appear at any time within 3 weeks following an acute

exposure. Among the permanent sequelae are neuropathies and various motor and mental defects, some of which mimic multiple sclerosis, Parkinsonism, and schizophrenia. Such permanent injuries, however, are encountered only after severe poisonings; usually there are no sequelae.

Treatment:

1. Terminate exposure immediately.
2. Administer pure oxygen by the best method available. An oronasal mask is usually best (p. 189). Artificial respiration is necessary whenever breathing is inadequate. Apneic patients have often been saved by efficient and persistent artificial respiration (p. 185). As always a patent airway must be carefully maintained (p. 184).
3. Avoid stimulant drugs, including carbon dioxide. Do not inject methylene blue.

4. Protect the patient from cold.
5. Give antibiotics as prophylaxis against pulmonary infection.
6. A whole blood transfusion may be useful if it can be given early in the treatment program.
7. Insure absolute rest in bed for at least 48 hours.
8. Watch for late neurological and/or cardiac complications.

Laboratory:

1. Carbon monoxide analyses of blood and expired air are useful but not usually necessary. Colorimetric, spectroscopic, and gasometric methods are available, but microgasometric techniques (*e.g.*, Scholander-Roughton) are the most sensitive and most practical.
2. Repeated electrocardiograms are desirable.

CARBON TETRACHLORIDE

Because of its excellent solvent properties and non-flammability, carbon tetrachloride (CCl₄) is widely used as a cleaner and a stain remover. In spite of attempts to find a less toxic substitute, this solvent is still found in many commercial products. It is used as a fire extinguisher, degreasing cleaner, non-flammable solvent for polishing waxes, *etc.*, and vehicle for certain agricultural fumigants. In medicine it formerly served as an intestinal anthelmintic. In many respects carbon tetrachloride is representative of a large class of related chlorinated hydrocarbons.

Toxicology: The principal toxic actions of carbon tetrachloride are central nervous depression and cellular necrosis in the kidneys, liver, or both. Death may be due to any one of these lesions, but in non-fatal cases recovery is eventually complete. Occasionally ventricular fibrillation and cardiac arrest are responsible for sudden death in carbon tetrachloride poisoning. Many other visceral lesions have been described as primary responses to carbon tetrachloride, but except for occasional cases of hemorrhagic necrosis of the adrenal cortex, pancreatitis, and optic neuritis, these claims require further substantiation. Much of the edema and hemorrhage described in various tissues is undoubtedly secondary to severe kidney and liver injuries. Although moderately irritating to skin and mucous membrane, carbon tetrachloride rarely if ever produces primary pulmonary edema. As with other chlorinated hydrocarbons, however, intense heat (open flame or very hot metal surface) may cause decomposition into such notorious pulmonary irritants as hydrogen chloride (HCl), chlorine gas (Cl₂) and phosgene (COCl₂).

Carbon tetrachloride is toxic when ingested as a liquid and when inhaled as a vapor. Percutaneous absorption appears to have no practical significance.

Intestinal absorption is aided by fats, oils and alcohol. Some of the absorbed material is eliminated through the lungs, while the unabsorbed portion is excreted in feces. The monkey is known to metabolize much of the absorbed compound to CO_2 and urea. In an adult human the mean lethal dose by mouth appears to lie between 5 and 10 ml., but as little as 2 ml. has killed on several occasions. Susceptibility to carbon tetrachloride poisoning is enhanced by the contemporaneous use of alcohol, by a poor nutritional status, and perhaps by a calcium deficiency. Children, adolescents, and persons with preexisting liver disease are said to be especially sensitive to the hepatotoxic action.

Although there are many exceptions, nervous symptoms are said to predominate in inhalation exposures, while gastrointestinal and hepatorenal injuries are more prominent after ingestion. Whether or not such a generalization is valid, central nervous depression and coma may occur without evidence of visceral injury, and renal failure may develop in cases without nervous involvement. With the exception of nausea and vomiting, symptoms develop more slowly after ingestion (latency 24 to 36 hours) than after inhalation (latency usually a few minutes).

The principal liver lesion is necrosis of the hepatic cells (especially those in the central portion of each lobule), together with fatty infiltration. In the kidneys, fatty degeneration and necrosis of the renal epithelium may be extensive. Although liver injury probably begins first, the kidney lesion is more prominent and more often recognized clinically.

Other chlorinated hydrocarbons share many of the toxic potentialities of carbon tetrachloride. Chloroform, for example, has much more potent depressant actions on the central nervous system

than carbon tetrachloride, although it is less lethal. With volatile compounds like dichloromethane or ethyl chloride, recovery from central depression is very rapid. Tetrachloroethane is a more severe mucosal irritant than carbon tetrachloride and is more toxic in many other respects. Many of the bromine analogues are also severe irritants and in some cases (*e.g.*, methyl bromide, ethylene dibromide), fatal pulmonary edema may terminate vapor exposures. Liver and/or kidney injuries have been ascribed to many halogenated hydrocarbons, and carbon tetrachloride is one of the worst offenders here. Although carbon tetrachloride has a more selective action on the kidneys than on the liver, the opposite appears to be true of tetrachloroethane and chloroform. Even halogenated hydrocarbons like ethyl chloride (which rarely produces visceral lesions) sometimes sensitize the myocardium so that even endogenous epinephrine precipitates fatal ventricular fibrillation.

Symptomatology:

1. Prompt nausea, vomiting, and abdominal pain. Sometimes the pain becomes intense enough to mimic an acute surgical complication. After ingestion, hematemesis and diarrhea.
2. Headache, dizziness, confusion, drowsiness, and occasionally convulsions.
3. Visual disturbances, sometimes consisting of a concentric restriction of the color fields without central scotomata (toxic amblyopia).
4. Rapid progression of central nervous depression with deepening coma and death from respiratory arrest or circulatory collapse.
5. Occasionally sudden death due to ventricular fibrillation.
6. In massive exposures the above symptoms merge with those outlined below, but central nervous depression may subside without

sequelae (especially after a short vapor exposure), or an essentially asymptomatic interval of a few days may precede hepatorenal decompensation.

7. Kidney and/or liver injury, symptomatic or subclinical. Either may occur insidiously after an otherwise unrecognized exposure. The kidney lesion usually produces the more severe disturbance in carbon tetrachloride poisoning.
8. Oliguria, albuminuria, anuria, sudden weight gain, edema. Death may occur within a week in the absence of effective supportive treatment.
9. Anorexia, jaundice, and right upper quadrant pain due to an enlarged and tender liver.

Treatment:

1. Restore patient to fresh air and remove any contaminated clothing.
2. Administer oxygen and artificial respiration as required (p. 185).
3. If swallowed, remove by gastric lavage with water or saline solution and instill a saline cathartic such as sodium or magnesium sulfate in water (15 to 30 gm.).
4. Do not administer fats, oils, alcohol, epinephrine, or ephedrine.
5. Respiratory stimulants such as caffeine and nikethamide should be given a trial if central nervous depression is severe (p. 204).
6. Fluids and electrolytes should be administered only cautiously, if at all.
7. Adopt prophylactic measures for possible liver injury, as outlined on p. 213.
8. For the management of acute renal failure, see pp. 210–212.

Laboratory: Repeated function tests are desirable to detect and evaluate kidney and liver injuries.

CHLORDANE

Chlordane, a mixture of various isomers of octachloro-4,7-methanohydroindane and related compounds, is an amber viscous liquid that is soluble in practically all petroleum solvents. It may be formulated as emulsifiable concentrates, wettable powders, dusts, and granules. Chlordane has been found useful as an insecticide in agriculture and in the control of such household pests as flies, mosquitos, and roaches.

Toxicology: Chlordane is toxic to humans by ingestion, skin absorption, and perhaps by the inhalation of large quantities of mist. It has been estimated that the fatal oral dose for an adult lies somewhere between 6 and 60 gm., with onset of symptoms within 45 minutes after ingestion. A single skin application of 110 gm. is estimated to be dangerous to an adult because of percutaneous absorption; skin irritation and sensitization are rare.

Chlordane is a stimulant to the central nervous system but its exact mode of action is unknown. In general chlordane produces symptoms similar to but of longer duration than those of DDT. Chronic poisoning in animals produces inanition and degenerative lesions in the liver and renal tubules.

Symptomatology:

1. Earliest signs of poisoning are increased sensitivity and hyperexcitability due to irritation of the central nervous system. Convulsions and tremors are followed by depression. Cycles of excitement and depression may be repeated several times.
2. Liver damage as a possible late manifestation.
3. Anorexia and weight loss.

4. Severe gastroenteritis has been described in one of the fatal human poisonings.

Treatment:

1. Gastric lavage with warm tap water.

2. Sodium sulfate catharsis (half an ounce in 6 to 8 oz. of water). Avoid oil laxatives.

3. A rapidly acting barbiturate or ether may aid in controlling convulsions, but care must be taken not to augment any respiratory depression. See p. 202.

4. Oxygen therapy and artificial respiration may be necessary (p. 185).

5. Avoid epinephrine.

6. Since no specific antidotes are known, symptomatic therapy must be accompanied by complete rest.

7. Use soap and water in adequate quantities to wash off any compound spilled on the skin. If spilled in eyes, wash repeatedly with water.

Laboratory: Function tests to detect and evaluate possible liver and kidney disturbances.

COPPER

Soluble and insoluble copper salts are used extensively in agriculture as fungicides and insecticides. Copper arsenates and arsenites (*e.g.*, copper acetoarsenite or paris green) are principally dangerous for their arsenic content; consult arsenic poisoning (p. 114). Copper sulfate (cupric sulfate) is occasionally used in clinical medicine as an emetic drug; the adult dose is 0.25 to 0.5 gm. in water repeated no more than once (after an interval of 15 minutes, if necessary). This use cannot be recommended since toxic effects appear if vomiting does not.

Toxicology: Acute poisoning from the ingestion of copper salts is rarely severe, if the metal is removed promptly by emesis. Vomiting is provoked chiefly by the local irritant and astringent action of ionic copper on stomach and bowel. Emesis usually begins within 5 to 10 minutes, but if the stomach is full of food, it may be delayed for half an hour or more. If vomiting fails to occur, gradual absorption from the bowel may cause systemic copper poisoning. Copper resembles many other heavy metals in its systemic toxic effects: widespread capillary damage, kidney injury, and central nervous excitation followed by depression. Copper appears to be less deleterious than most heavy metals when ingested continuously in small amounts, but chronic feeding to animals results in a pigmentary cirrhosis of the liver. Jaundice and pain over the liver have been described even in an acute human poisoning.

In general the soluble ionized salts of copper are much more toxic than the insoluble or slightly dissociated compounds. Probably the most poisonous salts are the chloride and the subacetate. Cuprous chloride is said to be twice as toxic as the more common cupric salt, but no *major* toxicological distinctions are recognized between the two valence states of copper. As with other irritant emetics, the lethal dose of any copper salt varies widely (from less than 1 gm. to several oz. in adults); the *mean* lethal dose of the sulfate probably lies near 15 gm. Treatment is largely symptomatic. Further clinical trials are required to evaluate BAL as a therapeutic measure in copper poisoning; the same is true of intoxications due to zinc, nickel, chromium, and bismuth. Presumably a trial with BAL should be reserved for cases of systemic poisoning, *e.g.*, when the effects are not the result solely of severe gastroenteritis.

Symptomatology:

1. Prompt emesis (usually within 5 to 10 min.).

2. Pain in mouth, esophagus, and stomach.

3. Diarrhea with colicky abdominal pain.

4. Metallic taste in mouth.

5. Severe headache, cold sweat, weak pulse, and other signs of shock.

6. Death may be preceded by convulsions, paralysis, or coma.

Treatment:

1. Empty stomach by lavage with milk or preferably a 1 per cent solution of potassium ferrocyanide (the resulting copper ferrocyanide is insoluble).

2. Administer egg white and other demulcents.

3. Maintain electrolyte and fluid balances (see p. 215).

4. Morphine or meperidine (Demerol) may be necessary for the control of pain.

5. If symptoms persist or intensify (especially circulatory collapse or cerebral disturbances), try BAL intramuscularly according to the following dosage schedule:

	Severe Poisoning	Mild Poisoning
1st day...........	3.0 mg./kg. q4h (6 inj.)	2.5 mg./kg. q4h (6 inj.)
2nd day.........	3.0 mg./kg. q4h (6 inj.)	2.5 mg./kg. q6h (4 inj.)
3rd day...........	3.0 mg./kg. q6h (4 inj.)	2.5 mg./kg. q12h (2 inj.)
Each of the following 10 days or until recovery	3.0 mg./kg. q12h (2 inj.)	2.5 mg./kg. qd (1 inj.)

Laboratory: Liver function tests may be indicated.

CYANIDE

Hydrocyanic acid (prussic acid) and alkali salts like sodium and potassium cyanide are found in vermicidal fumigants, insecticides, rodenticides, metal polishes (especially silver polish), electroplating solutions, and in various metallurgical and photographic processes. As a fumigant, particularly for such structures as greenhouses, ships, mills, and warehouses, hydrogen cyanide (HCN) is applied directly as a solution (hydrocyanic acid), or the gas is generated from one of the cyanide salts by the action of dilute mineral acid. These fumigations should be performed only by expert exterminators. Organically bound cyanides (*e.g.*, acrylonitrile) are sometimes used as fumigant gases, especially for grains. Naturally occurring nitriles are found in many plants, particularly in certain fruits and beans. Amygdalin, for example, is a chemical combination of glucose, benzaldehyde, and hydrogen cyanide, found in the bark, leaves, fruit, and flowers of the cherry laurel and in the seeds of cherry, plum, peach, apricot, apple, and pear. On rare occasions plants have been sources of cyanide poisoning, but most recognized poisonings have been traced to the accidental, suicidal, or homicidal ingestion of hydrocyanic acid or one of its alkali salts. Cyanide poisoning appears to be less prevalent now than in the past; about 50 years ago it was a major cause of chemical intoxication, particularly in Europe. Chronic cyanide poisoning is unknown.

Toxicology: Poisoning may arise from any substance which releases the cyanide ion. Cyanide is a potent and rapidly acting chemical asphyxiant; it deprives tissues of necessary oxygen by inhibiting reversibly such oxidative enzymes as cytochrome oxidase. Because oxygen cannot be utilized, venous blood retains the bright red color of oxyhemoglobin. Cyanide does not react to an appreciable extent with the hemoglobin molecule. As with other chemical asphyxiants, the critical organs are those which are most sensitive to oxygen lack, notably the brain. A transient stage of central nervous stimulation is followed by central nervous depression and finally hypoxic convulsions and death due to respiratory arrest. Cardiac irregularities are commonly observed, but the heart beat invariably outlasts breathing movements.

Few poisons are more rapidly lethal than cyanide. The inhalation of hydrogen cyanide and the ingestion of cyanide salts commonly produce reactions within a few minutes and death within an hour. The prognosis is fairly good if the patient is still alive 1 hour after swallowing a dose of cyanide, but fatal relapses have been described after periods as long as 4 hours. If the stomach is empty and the free gastric acidity is high, poisoning is especially fast. After large doses some victims have had time only for a warning cry before sudden loss of consciousness. Hydrogen cyanide in aqueous solution (hydrocyanic acid) is readily absorbed from the skin and from all mucous membranes (such as the rectum and vagina), but the alkali salts are usually toxic only when ingested. The average lethal dose of HCN taken by mouth is believed to lie between 60 and 90 mg. (1 to 1½ grains); this corresponds to about 1 teaspoonful of a 2 per cent solution of hydrocyanic acid and to about 200 mg. of potassium cyanide (KCN). Prompt treatment, however, has saved a person who swallowed 6000 mg. of KCN. The lethality of most derivatives is regarded as proportional to the content of readily available cyanide. The mortality rate is high, but in nonfatal cases recovery is generally complete. Rarely neuropsychiatric sequelae are observed, as in carbon monoxide poisoning (p. 126).

Absorbed cyanide is in small measure excreted unchanged by the lungs; most is converted to the comparatively harmless thiocyanate ion by an enzymatic reaction which is accelerated by thiosulfate and by some sources of available sulfur. To protect tissue cells until the cyanide ion is detoxified, the therapist tries to convert a portion of the circulating hemoglobin into methemoglobin, because the latter can compete effectively with cytochrome oxidase for cyanide. The cyanmethemoglobin so formed is gradually changed to normal hemoglobin as the cyanide ion is converted to relatively nontoxic thiocyanate. Amyl nitrite is perhaps the fastest way to produce appreciable concentrations of circulating methemoglobin. The inhalation of amyl nitrite is followed by the intravenous injection of sodium nitrite. Methylene blue has been used but is less satisfactory than the nitrite ion for producing methemoglobinemia. Para-aminopropriophenone (PAPP) is too slow to be an effective antidote. When combined with artificial respiration and general supportive treatment, the above antidotes have saved the lives of cyanide victims even after the onset of apnea.

Symptomatology:

1. Massive doses may produce, without warning, sudden loss of consciousness and prompt death from respiratory arrest. With smaller but still lethal doses, the illness may be prolonged for 1 or more hours.

2. Upon ingestion, a bitter, acrid, burning taste is sometimes noted, followed by a feeling of constriction or numbness in the throat. Salivation and nausea are not unusual, but vomiting rarely occurs except after concentrated solutions of sodium and potassium cyanide, which are corrosive because of their

high alkalinity. Other symptoms follow in rapid progression.

3. Anxiety, confusion, vertigo, giddiness, and often a sensation of stiffness in the lower jaw.

4. Hyperpnea and dyspnea. Respirations become very rapid and then slow and irregular. Inspiration is characteristically short while expiration is greatly prolonged.

5. The odor of bitter almonds may be noted on the breath or vomitus. This characteristic odor is sometimes a diagnostic help.

6. In the early phases of poisoning, an increase in vasoconstrictor tone causes a rise in blood pressure and reflex slowing of the heart rate. Thereafter the pulse becomes rapid, weak, and sometimes irregular. The victim notes palpitations and a sensation of constriction in the chest.

7. Unconsciousness, followed promptly by violent convulsions, epileptiform or tonic, sometimes localized but usually generalized. Opisthotonos and trismus may develop. Involuntary micturition and defecation occur.

8. Paralysis follows the convulsive stage. The skin is covered with sweat. The eyeballs protrude, and the pupils are dilated and unreactive. The mouth is covered with foam, which is sometimes blood-stained. The skin color may be brick-red. Cyanosis is not prominent in spite of weak and irregular gasping.

9. Death from respiratory arrest. As long as the heart beat continues, prompt and vigorous treatment offers some promise of survival.

Treatment (must be prompt):

1. If the patient is apneic, start artificial respiration immediately. Keep the airway clear.

2. Administer by inhalation amyl nitrite (amyl nitrite perles) for 15 to 30 seconds of every minute, while a sodium nitrite solution is being prepared.

3. Discontinue amyl nitrite and immediately inject intravenously 10 ml. of a 3 per cent solution of sodium nitrite over a period of 2 to 4 minutes. If necessary, inject a non-sterile solution. Do not remove the needle.

4. Through the same needle infuse intravenously 50 ml. of a 25 per cent aqueous solution of sodium thiosulfate. The injection should take about 10 minutes. Other concentrations (5 to 50 per cent) are permissible if the total dose is held at approximately 12 gm.

5. If symptoms recur, the injections of nitrite and thiosulfate may be repeated at half the above doses.

6. Because of the speed of absorption and the rapidity with which symptoms appear, gastric lavage is seldom a practical procedure and should be postponed at least until after procedures 1–4. Probably the best lavage fluid is a dilute solution of potassium permanganate (1:5000).

7. Oxygen therapy and a whole blood transfusion may become necessary if nitrite-induced methemoglobinemia becomes too severe.

Laboratory: In cyanide poisoning laboratory tests are seldom useful in prognosis or treatment, but specimens (e.g., gastric contents) should be saved in case of legal need for a chemical analysis.

2 , 4-D (2 , 4-DICHLOROPHENOXYACETIC ACID)

2,4-D and its derivatives are among the most widely used substances in weed control. They are particularly effective in weeding grain crops because of their selective action on broad-leafed plants. Millions of pounds are used each year (1952—28 million pounds). At present the acid itself is not used as a herbicide but is the basic material from which soluble esters and salts are produced (e.g., sodium 2,4-dichlorophenoxyacetate).

Toxicology: The mammalian pharmacology is not well known, and no unequivocal poisonings have been described in man. Both acute and chronic toxicity in laboratory mammals is low. Oral administration of the water-soluble sodium salt has established the following acute mean lethal doses (LD$_{50}$): 380 mg./kg. in mice, 670 to 800 mg./kg. in rats, 800 mg./kg. in rabbits, and 550 to 1000 mg./kg. in guinea pigs. Monkeys appear to be comparable to these laboratory rodents in terms of susceptibility to 2,4-D, and presumably man is too. All species which have been tested react similarly, and there seems to be no significant differences in potency between crude and purified preparations, or between sodium and ammonium salts, or between water-soluble salts and oil-soluble esters. The free acid, however, is somewhat more toxic (e.g., LD$_{50}$ 380 mg./kg. in rats, 100 mg./kg. in dogs, as administered in olive oil or undiluted). Death after large doses of all preparations is believed to be due to ventricular fibrillation, and if death is delayed, myotonia (muscle stiffness or spasticity) occurs, especially in the hind limbs, as well as ataxia, paralysis, and coma. Mild pathological lesions have been described in kidney and liver.

Symptomatology (no poisonings, acute or chronic, observed in man):

1. Weakness and perhaps lethargy.

2. Anorexia, diarrhea, weight loss.

3. Myotonia-like condition which responds to quinidine. Spasticity may involve the muscles of mastication and swallowing.

4. Possibly sudden death due to ventricular fibrillation and subsequent cardiac arrest.

Treatment:

1. Removal of agent by gastric lavage.
2. Supportive treatment.
3. Quinidine sulfate or quinine (0.2 gm. orally

every 2 hours for the first 10 to 12 hours), to relieve myotonia, if present, and to suppress ventricular cardiac rhythms.

Laboratory: Repeated electrocardiograms might prove helpful.

D-D (CHLORINATED PROPANE-PROPYLENE MIXTURE)

D-D consists exclusively of chlorinated C_3 hydrocarbons, including 1,3-dichloropropene-1, 1,2-dichloropropane, and related compounds. The mixture has a dark brown color and a pungent garlic-like odor. It is soluble in most organic solvents but only slightly in water. D-D is a soil fumigant and is used at full strength by injection into the soil.

Toxicology: D-D is highly toxic to mammals by ingestion and inhalation, and moderately toxic by skin absorption. Its odor and intense irritation of eyes, skin, and respiratory mucosa warn of danger and reduce the exposure hazard. The mean lethal dose in rats is about 140 mg./kg. by ingestion. In continued exposures inhalation is the chief hazard. The symptoms abate promptly after exposure ceases. In animals visceral lesions of liver, heart, and kidneys have been described:

Symptomatology:

1. Inhalation, acute: gasping, refusal to breathe, coughing, substernal pain, and extreme respiratory distress at vapor concentrations over 1,500 p.p.m. Irritation of eyes and upper respiratory mucosa appears promptly after exposure to concentrated vapors. Lacrimation is prominent.

Inhalation, chronic: central nervous depression and moderate irritation of respiratory system.
2. Dermal: severe skin irritation with marked inflammatory response of epidermis and underlying tissues.
3. Oral: acute gastrointestinal distress with pulmonary congestion and edema.

Treatment:

1. Remove ingested material by gastric aspiration and lavage. Use water as a lavage fluid.
2. Demulcents like alumina gels, but no fats or oils.
3. Opiates and atropine for the control of pain and intestinal spasm.
4. Aminophyllin (theophyllin-ethylenediamine) 0.25 gm. i.v. slowly to correct bronchospasm.
5. Oxygen, especially under positive pressure, for the relief of cyanosis. See page 192 for the treatment of pulmonary edema.
6. Wash extensively any contaminated areas of skin with soap and water. Discard contaminated clothing.

Laboratory: Repeated function tests are desirable to detect and evaluate possible liver and kidney injuries.

DDT

DDT is probably the most widely used insecticide at the present time. It has an important role in many phases of agriculture, in the control of insects of public health significance, and in the eradication of household pests. Chlorophenothane is the official U.S.P. name for the pharmaceutical grade of DDT, but for most uses a technical grade is available. Technical DDT, which has 48 to 51 per cent organic chlorine by weight, contains various isomers, of which two-thirds to three-quarters (by weight) is 1,1,1-trichloro-2,2-bis(p-chlorophenyl) ethane. It is formulated as wettable powders, solutions, emulsions, aerosols, and dusts, in concentrations varying from 1 to 75 per cent. Most common household insecticidal sprays consist of a 5 per cent solution of DDT in purified kerosene (e.g., Deobase).

Toxicology: DDT has a wide margin of safety when judiciously used, and few if any adequately documented cases of DDT poisoning in man have ended fatally. The dry powder and aqueous suspensions are poorly absorbed from the gastrointestinal and respiratory tracts, and they do not penetrate the skin appreciably. Oils, fats, and lipid

solvents from any source, however, enhance the absorption of DDT from all sites, including intact skin.

The single oral dose of DDT necessary to produce untoward symptoms in man is about 10 mg./kg. After a dose of 16 mg./kg. or more, there are sometimes convulsions in the absence of effective treatment. Amounts at least as high as 285 mg./kg. have been ingested without fatalities, but since these doses lead promptly to vomiting, the amount actually retained is not known. The value generally accepted as an acute mean lethal dose (LD_{50}) in rats is 250 mg./kg.; it is perhaps a reasonable estimate for man. Fats and oils enhance toxicity by promoting absorption. In many instances of alleged poisoning the principal symptoms have been due to the commercial vehicle (usually kerosene), not to DDT.

DDT acts primarily on the central nervous system of man; the cerebellum and higher motor cortex appear to be the chief sites of action. Clinical manifestations include paresthesias, tremors, and convulsions. The mechanism of action is not yet understood. Most pathologists deny the existence

of histopathological lesions in the brain of DDT-poisoned animals, with the exception of small petechnal hemorrhages resulting from convulsions. Only in animals given large and/or repeated doses of DDT is it possible to find consistent pathological lesions, namely non-specific liver cell necrosis and mild degeneration of kidney tubular epithelium. Liver and kidney dysfunction have not been described in human poisonings (with perhaps one exception). Primary skin irritation is rarely if ever due to DDT, and allergic dermatitis has been reported only occasionally.

In acute exposures, recovery is usually complete or well advanced in 24 hours. No clinical syndrome of chronic intoxication is recognized in man. After a single dose or small repeated doses, however, DDT and some of its metabolic degradation products (e.g., DDE) accumulate in body fat, where they remain in a largely inactive form for long periods of time. Biopsy specimens of human subcutaneous fat and other adipose tissues can be analyzed for DDT. DDT and derivatives are excreted in urine and milk.

Symptomatology (onset is usually 2 to 3 hours after ingestion):

1. Very large doses are followed promptly by vomiting, due to local gastric irritation. Delayed emesis and/or diarrhea may occur (the mechanism is not understood).
2. Paresthesias, usually first of lips, tongue, and face.
3. Malaise, headache, sore throat, fatigue.
4. Coarse tremors (usually first of the neck and head and particularly of the eyelids), apprehension, ataxia, and confusion.
5. Convulsions, both clonic and tonic. Convulsions may alternate with periods of coma and paresis.
6. Vital signs are essentially normal, but in severe poisoning the pulse may be irregular and abnormally slow. Because DDT sensitizes the heart to endogenous epinephrine, ventricular fibrillation and sudden death may occur at any time during the acute phase.
7. If pulmonary edema supervenes, it is probably an expression of solvent intoxication (see kerosene poisoning).
8. Death is usually due to respiratory failure from medullary paralysis.

Treatment:

1. Gastric lavage with tap water (if convulsions are not imminent).
2. Saline cathartic, e.g., sodium sulfate (15 to 30 gm.) left in the stomach.
3. Phenobarbital 0.1 gm. prophylactically in the absence of central nervous signs and symptoms. Parenteral barbiturate therapy if tremors or convulsions develop (e.g., pentobarbital, pentothal). See page 201.
4. Calcium gluconate (10 cc. of 10 per cent solution given slowly by intravenous injection) is useful (in addition to sedation) to control DDT convulsions in experimental animals.
5. Avoid fats, oils, and fat solvents, epinephrine, sudden strong external stimuli.
6. Rest and observation for at least 24 hours. Give parenteral fluids as needed.

Laboratory:

1. When the diagnosis is uncertain, the urine can be examined for the presence of DDA [bis(p-chlorophenyl) acetic acid].
2. Biochemical tests to detect liver and kidney dysfunction should be performed repeatedly.

DIELDRIN

Technical dieldrin (hexachloro epoxy octahydro-endo,exo-dimethano naphthalene) has a minimal purity of 90 to 95 per cent (including related active products) as labelled. Alone or in combination with other insecticides, it is used in insect control, where it has an advantage in terms of unusually long persistence. Dieldrin is applicable to the control of a wide variety of economic pests, but it is not recommended for use on edible leaf crops, or where residues will appear in foods for man or animals. It is prepared commercially as powders for dusting, wettable powders for use as emulsion sprays, oil solutions, aerosols, and granules for use as bait.

Toxicology: Dieldrin, particularly in oil solution, is absorbed very readily through the skin, the respiratory mucosa, and the gastrointestinal tract. Untoward symptoms are known to occur in man after oral doses as small as 10 mg./kg. The mean lethal dose by the oral route is approximately 65 mg./kg. in white rats, and this value is thought to be a reasonable estimate of lethality in man. In animals the percutaneous toxicity of dieldrin is almost as high as its oral toxicity (much higher according to one laboratory). Dermal exposures result in systemic poisoning without skin irritation or local sensitization (except secondary to the solvent or vehicle, which is usually kerosene or xylene).

The actions of dieldrin and of a related substance, aldrin, are similar both qualitatively and quantitatively in animals and apparently also in man. In both cases the principal site of action is the central nervous system, and the principal symptom is a series of convulsions. The convulsions are self-remitting but recur with increasing severity; they characteristically alternate with periods of severe depression. In contrast, after repeated exposures several spray-men developed a syndrome

indistinguishable from idiopathic epilepsy, except that it ceased when the exposure was terminated. In the usual acute intoxication, recovery is complete or well advanced within 24 hours, but animal experiments suggest the possibility of seizures for many days after a single dose or repeated doses. Mild and transient kidney and liver injuries have been described.

Symptomatology (onset of symptoms between 20 minutes and 12 hours after ingestion):

1. Malaise, headache, nausea, vomiting, dizziness, and tremors.
2. Clonic and tonic convulsions, sometimes without premonitory symptoms.
3. Convulsive episodes may alternate with periods of severe central nervous depression. Death from respiratory arrest may occur during coma.
4. During the acute phases a leukocytosis and rise in blood pressure have been described.

Treatment:

1. Decontaminate any suspicious areas of skin promptly by washing extensively with soap and running water. If skin and clothing are obviously contaminated, the therapist should protect himself by wearing gloves of Neoprene or artificial rubber.
2. After ingestion evacuate and lavage stomach with warm water (unless convulsions are imminent).
3. Administer a saline cathartic. Avoid oils or oil laxatives.
4. Barbiturates are the treatment of choice in the prevention and control of tremors and convulsions (p. 201). Large doses are surprisingly well tolerated. Phenobarbital is preferable as a prophylactic measure, but a short-acting drug (e.g., pentothal, pentobarbital, Seconal) is preferable after convulsions have begun. As soon as the intensity of the post-convulsive depression can be judged, the patient should be continued on adequate maintenance doses of a barbiturate drug. Anti-convulsive therapy may have to be continued for a week.
5. Avoid sudden physical stimuli which may precipitate convulsions during periods of central hyperirritability.
6. Oxygen therapy and artificial respiration if needed during periods of depression (p. 185).
7. Any patient who experiences a convulsion should be observed carefully for at least one week.

Laboratory: In severe intoxications laboratory tests may reveal kidney and liver injuries, which according to present evidence remit spontaneously during recovery.

Repeated electroencephalograms (EEG) are useful to detect prolonged cortical dysfunction.

DIGITALIS

Digitalis and other so-called cardiac glycosides are a group of pharmacologically and chemically related substances derived from various plants; each consists of a characteristic steroid (known as the aglycone or genin) coupled with one or more types of sugar molecules. Single crystalline glycosides and mixtures are available from many botanical sources and in many physical forms. They are widely used in clinical medicine because of their inotropic and chronotropic actions on the diseased heart. Extracardiac actions are sometimes sought, such as the use of squill as a nauseant expectorant. A non-medicinal variety of squill, known as red squill, is used in the form of the powdered dry bulb as a potent rodenticide. The accidental and suicidal ingestion of red squill and of other digitalis preparations has caused fatal poisonings in man, but most poisonings are due to overdosage in therapy.

Toxicology: The therapeutic and toxic actions of the various cardiac glycosides are basically similar; the differences relate principally to potency, latency, and persistency. These distinctions imply that the various drugs differ from one another in stability, absorbability, penetrability, tissue fixation, metabolic degradation, and excretion. Because the chief actions of the cardiac glycosides are common to them all, the toxicity of these compounds is additive. This discussion concerns principally whole-leaf digitalis (powdered leaves of *Digitalis purpurea*) or digitoxin (a pure glycoside which can be derived from it). Qualitative distinctions between digitoxin and several other cardiac glycosides are outlined in Section II (Ingredients Index).

In toxic doses digitalis produces nervous and mental disturbances, including persistent nausea and vomiting of reflex origin, but the most definitive and most dangerous actions concern the rate and rhythm of the heart and the mechanism of the heart beat. These disorders, which are simply extensions of therapeutic actions, are best detected and analyzed with the aid of an electrocardiogram. Digitalis and its glycosides have been responsible for the production of every known type of cardiac arrhythmia and all grades of impaired conduction at the auriculo-ventricular junction. The more common disturbances revealed by the ECG are listed in Fig. III.1; arrows indicate some of the recognized sequences of events during progressive digitalis poisoning. Although the expert cardiologist can detect and correctly diagnose by physical signs many of these disturbances, serial electro-

Fig. III. 1. Progressive effects of digitalis on ECG

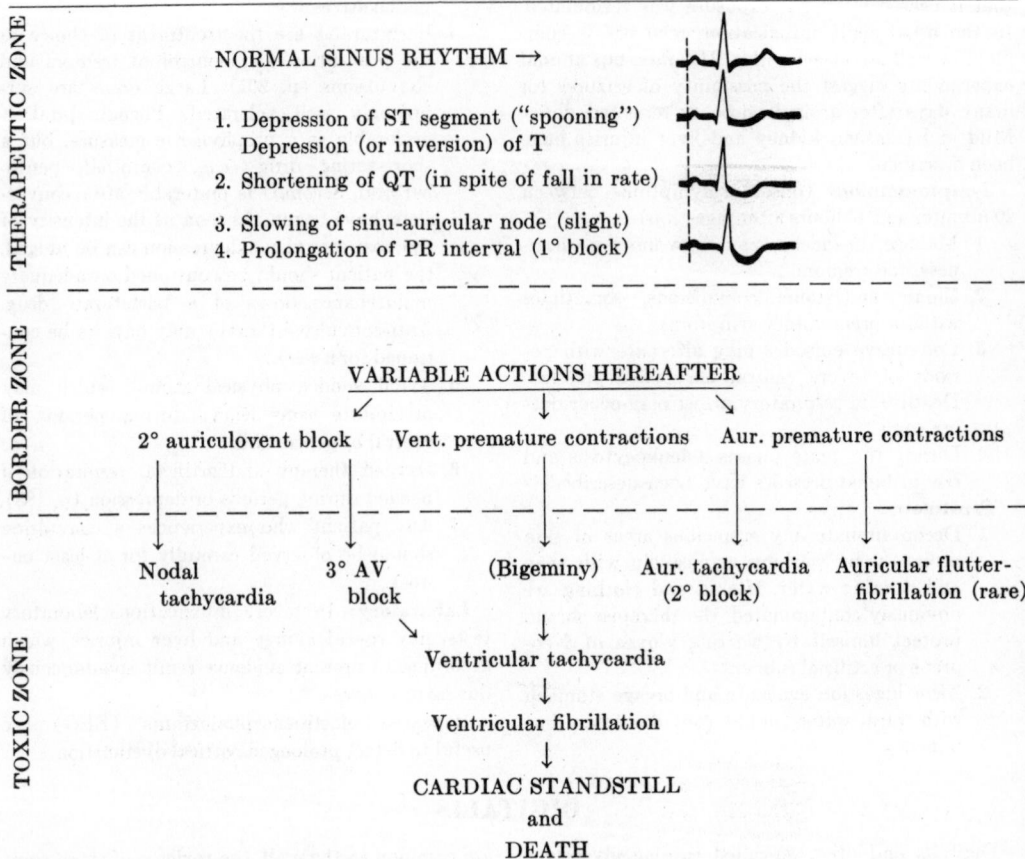

THERAPEUTIC ZONE

NORMAL SINUS RHYTHM →

1. Depression of ST segment ("spooning")
   Depression (or inversion) of T

2. Shortening of QT (in spite of fall in rate)

3. Slowing of sinu-auricular node (slight)
4. Prolongation of PR interval (1° block)

BORDER ZONE

VARIABLE ACTIONS HEREAFTER

2° auriculovent block   Vent. premature contractions   Aur. premature contractions

TOXIC ZONE

Nodal   3° AV   (Bigeminy)   Aur. tachycardia   Auricular flutter-
tachycardia   block   (2° block)   fibrillation (rare)

Ventricular tachycardia

Ventricular fibrillation

CARDIAC STANDSTILL
and
DEATH

cardiograms are usually necessary for the intelligent management of digitalis poisoning.

Whenever a cardiac glycoside is responsible for any of the disturbances listed at the bottom of Fig. III.1 ("toxic zone"), the drug should be immediately discontinued; at least a reduction in dosage is warranted whenever the "border zone" is reached. When these same derangements in mechanism of beat are due to causes other than digitalis, cardiac glycosides are not necessarily contraindicated. For example, digitalis may be administered in the presence of a complete heart block from causes other than drug; in contrast ventricular bigeminy and ventricular tachycardia are probably valid contraindications to digitalis irrespective of their origin. In all cases the ECG should be regarded only as a diagnostic and prognostic aid. It is the patient and not the electrocardiogram which needs treatment, but the ECG is emphasized because it may reveal signs of severe intoxication in patients who are almost asymptomatic (in borderline poisonings the converse may be true, i.e., symptoms may precede electrocardiographic signs).

The toxic dose is subject to a wide range of variation, but toxicity is often encountered when the therapeutic dose is even slightly exceeded. In spite of frequent claims that one or another of the cardiac glycosides has a greater margin of safety, only small differences in this respect exist among the common drugs. Most deaths have followed multiple doses, and the single oral lethal dose is not well established, but it probably lies between 20 and 50 times the usual daily maintenance dose. Other things being equal, a drug of long persistency is a greater toxic hazard than a drug with a rapid rate of dissipation; digitoxin and whole-leaf digitalis are among the worst offenders in this respect. Probably persons differ in the efficiency with which they absorb oral doses of digitalis, and certainly the various cardiac glycosides differ from one another in this respect. Because experimental and clinical data suggest that the glycosides and calcium may have additive or synergistic actions on the heart, the intravenous use of calcium salts is regarded as unwise in a digitalized patient. Perhaps ephedrine also enhances the toxicity of digitalis. Diuretic therapy sometimes precipitates digitalis poisoning,

perhaps by depleting tissues of potassium and so inducing hypokalemia. Elderly patients are comparatively intolerant of cardiac glycosides and are prone to manifest toxic reactions (especially arrhythmias) with supposedly safe doses. The factors outlined above (and probably many others) are responsible for the wide range of lethal doses which are observed in clinical practice; drug allergy or hypersensitivity is rarely implicated.

The ingestion of large doses of whole-leaf digitalis often produces prompt vomiting due to local irritation, but with digitoxin and other purified glycosides, emesis is delayed because it arises only from actions on the central nervous system. Irrespective of the route of administration, a cardiac glycoside must be fixed to the myocardium before its cardiac effects begin. With digitoxin and digitalis leaf, the latency varies between ½ and 2 hours; the cardiac actions are maximal in 4 to 12 hours and disappear only after 2 to 3 weeks. In most poisonings the danger period lasts for several days. About 20 per cent of the glycosides in an oral dose of whole-leaf digitalis is absorbed (whether given as the powder or tincture), in contrast to the essentially complete absorption of digitoxin. The biological fate of cardiac glycosides is not well understood. With digitoxin only about 10 per cent of a dose is excreted unchanged, but an appreciable fraction (perhaps 30 per cent) is found in the urine as biologically active metabolites. Much of the excretion occurs within the first 48 hours, but small amounts can be detected in the urine for several weeks.

The treatment of digitalis poisoning is generally unsatisfactory. Aside from discontinuing the drug and all related cardiac glycosides, none of the therapeutic procedures suggested below is accepted by all authorities, and none produces uniformly good results. In specific situations, atropine, quinidine, procaineamide, potassium salts, and perhaps magnesium salts may produce beneficial effects, but none of these drugs is consistently effective and none is entirely safe.

Symptomatology:

1. An asymptomatic period of several minutes to several hours follows a single oral toxic dose.
2. Anorexia is often the first complaint. Nausea, salivation, and vomiting follow. Sometimes abdominal pain or discomfort accompanies these symptoms. Diarrhea is occasionally observed.
3. Nausea and vomiting occur irrespective of the route of administration; they are often persistent.
4. Early electrocardiographic changes are illustrated in Fig. III.1 (1 through 4); taken together they are diagnostic of a "digitalis action" on the heart. In severe intoxications, however, these subtle ECG changes can seldom be recognized because of gross disturbances in the rhythmicity and location of the pacemaker and in the conduction pathway. The disorders listed in the diagram (Fig. III.1) are not mutually exclusive and do not exhaust all the known possibilities. Associated with these disturbances in the rate and rhythm of the pulse, the patient may experience palpitations.
5. Headache, malaise, fatigue, weakness, and drowsiness without coma. Neuritic pain, especially that resembling trigeminal neuralgia, is described. Paresthesias are not uncommon.
6. Mental and emotional disorders include confusion, disorientation, aphasia, delirium, hallucinations, and rarely convulsions.
7. Visual disturbances include all grades of transient amblyopia, diplopia, blurring, and disturbances in color vision.
8. Skin rashes of various types are noted rarely; they are usually accompanied by eosinophilia.
9. Death is often due to ventricular fibrillation (during which the heart pumps no blood).

Treatment:

1. If overdosage is recognized promptly, the use of an emetic drug and/or gastric lavage is advisable. In most cases these measures are pointless once toxic signs and symptoms appear.
2. Nausea and vomiting are difficult, if not impossible, to suppress in digitalis poisoning, but sedation is sometimes useful in this regard.
3. Restlessness and excitement should be corrected by the cautious administration of sedative drugs, repeated as necessary.
4. Disturbances in the rate and rhythm of the heart may be modified at least transiently by one or more of the following drugs: atropine, potassium salts, magnesium salts, procaineamide, and quinidine, as noted below. These measures represent largely empirical attempts to control the mechanism of heart beat until the body can eliminate the offending cardiac glycoside.
   a. Moderately large doses of atropine sulfate (e.g., 2 mg. in an adult) serve to block the influence of exaggerated vagal tone. The result may be some acceleration of a digitalis-induced sinus bradycardia and a reduction in the intensity of an auriculoventricular block. There is no evidence, however, that atropine has a beneficial effect on the dangerous complications of digitalis poisoning, and its use is not often warranted.
   b. The oral administration of potassium salts

(usually the chloride, nitrate, or acetate) has been recommended in an amount of 2 to 10 gm.; it is usually taken in divided doses as a 25 per cent aqueous solution diluted with milk. In some clinics potassium is given intravenously, but this is a dangerous procedure and should be reserved for those with special training. After the acute phase, the oral dose may be reduced to 1 gram three times daily until the effects of digitalis have been entirely dissipated. The rationale for this treatment is an alleged deficit of intracellular potassium in the over-digitalized heart. When seen, the beneficial effects appear within 40 minutes and last up to 8 hours; they consist principally of a suppression of ectopic rhythms, including ventricular tachycardia and extrasystoles of all kinds. Auricular flutter and fibrillation are rarely modified, and most conduction disturbances are intensified by this treatment. Potassium therapy may be effective without producing a measurable rise in the level of plasma potassium.

c. Rarely magnesium sulfate is given intravenously in doses of 10 to 20 ml. of a 20 per cent aqueous solution. In digitalis poisoning, ionic magnesium shares some of the same actions as potassium, i.e., a suppression of premature beats and of paroxysmal tachycardias and an accentuation of conduction defects. In many cases, however, the beneficial effects have proved to be highly transient, and the original disorder has recurred within a few minutes.

d. Procaineamide hydrochloride and quinidine sulfate or lactate have been recommended. These drugs are similar in their actions on the heart, and there is little basis for choosing between them. A large number of untoward reactions can be precipitated by both drugs, especially when they are used parenterally. For example, both compounds have successfully stopped primary ventricular rhythms in digitalis poisoning, only to result in fatal cardiac stand-still because of an unrecognized but co-existent conduction block between the normal auricular pacemaker and the ventricle. This same complication is theoretically possible in the therapeutic use of potassium salts. Perhaps procaineamide and quinidine should be reserved for those cases of digitalis poisoning in which impaired renal function makes potassium therapy unwise.

5. Although not described in man, lesions suggestive of myocardial ischemia are described in fatally poisoned animals. If anginal pain develops in a patient who is poisoned with digitalis, a therapeutic trial with recognized coronary vasodilators is recommended (e.g., sublingual nitroglycerin, intravenous or oral aminophyllin or papaverine, etc.).

6. Dehydration and ionic imbalances (due to vomiting and diarrhea) should be cautiously corrected by the parenteral administration of water, glucose, and the appropriate mixture of electrolytes.

Laboratory:

1. Serial electrocardiograms are essential for proper diagnosis, prognosis, and treatment evaluation.

2. An occasional eosinophilia is the only abnormality described in routine laboratory tests.

3. The serum level of potassium should be checked in order that hypokalemia may be corrected by replacement therapy.

DINITROPHENOL

Alpha dinitrophenol (2,4-dinitrophenol) is used as a spray against aphids and mites, as a fungicide for certain molds and mildews, and occasionally as a weedkiller. Various substituted derivatives (e.g., 4,6-dinitro-o-cresol) have similar uses and similar toxicities. These compounds are available as oil solutions, wettable powders and as salts of aliphatic amines and sodium. At one time dinitrophenol was used as a weight-reducing drug, especially in nostrums of secret composition, but this use has been abandoned because of its toxicity.

Toxicology: Dinitrophenol is rapidly absorbed from all portals (gastro-intestinal tract, respiratory tract, and intact skin). The fatal dose in adults is about 1 to 3 gm. by mouth, and 3 gm. has proved fatal even in divided doses over a period of 5 days. Unlike rats and rabbits, man does not detoxify or eliminate dinitrophenol rapidly.

The metabolism of all body cells is stimulated by contact with dinitrophenol, which appears to act by blocking oxidative phosphorylation. In a poisoned person, the result is an almost immediate increase in oxygen consumption, body temperature, breathing rate, and heart rate. Because circulation and respiration do not accelerate in proportion to the metabolic demand, anoxia and acidosis develop. Body fat is the major, if not the exclusive fuel for this extra metabolism. In addition to this metabolic action, dinitrophenol shares many of phenol's toxic properties: it is corrosive to skin and mucous membrane (milder than phenol); it exerts direct actions on the cerebrum and lower brain centers (consisting

of stimulation followed by depression); it often produces a necrotizing tubular injury of the kidneys. If the acute phase of poisoning is survived, the patient usually tolerates successfully the later complications, which may include renal insufficiency and a toxic hepatitis.

The fulminating type of poisoning is characterized by sudden onset, severe symptoms, and prompt death (within 24 hours). Death is due to respiratory or circulatory collapse, especially the former. Many factors undoubtedly contribute to this collapse, notably hyperpyrexia, anoxia, acidosis, dehydration, muscle rigor (due to heat and/or lactic acid), and occasionally pulmonary edema.

In subacute poisoning due to repeated daily exposures, some individuals complain of lassitude, headache, and malaise, while others experience a disarming sense of well-being, energy, and drive. To terminate the exposure and administer small doses of phenobarbital usually constitute adequate therapy in these cases. All patients should be warned against overheating, since the metabolic actions and consequent toxicity of dinitrophenol are exaggerated by heat. Indeed at low ambient air temperatures (below 16°C), hypermetabolism cannot be produced in animals by this compound. Most clinical poisonings have occurred on hot days.

Symptomatology:

1. Marked fatigue, tremendous thirst, profuse sweating, flushing of face.
2. Nausea, vomiting, abdominal pain, and occasionally diarrhea.
3. Restlessness, anxiety, excitement, occasionally leading to convulsions.
4. A rise in body temperature which is roughly proportional to the toxic dose, often leading to severe hyperpyrexia (e.g., 110°F.).
5. Tachycardia, hyperpnea, dyspnea, cyanosis, and sometimes muscle cramps.
6. Loss of consciousness, cessation of breathing, and death.
7. Late complications:

a. Decreased urine output with albuminuria, casts, pigment, sometimes blood cells, due to toxic nephritis.
b. Jaundice and tenderness in liver region due to toxic hepatitis.
8. Occasional hypersensitivity reactions after repeated exposures (or in chronic poisoning) include agranulocytic angina, skin rashes, peripheral neuritis, and late cataract formation.

Treatment:

1. Gastric lavage with large quantities of 5 per cent sodium bicarbonate solution, leaving 1 to 2 pints in the stomach.
2. Saline cathartics, e.g., 15 to 30 gm. sodium or magnesium sulfate in water.
3. Ice packs and alcohol sponges to reduce body temperature. Antipyretic drugs are ineffective here. Cold water enemas have been used. Intensive efforts to correct a dinitrophenol fever are justified. If it can be accomplished, mild hypothermia (rectal temperature between 92 and 97°F.) is probably desirable because dinitrophenol appears to lose much of its metabolic toxicity at these reduced temperatures.
4. Fluids, orally or intravenously (e.g., 5 per cent glucose in saline, 1000 ml.), to correct dehydration and acidosis (p. 215).
5. Stimulants: caffeine sodium benzoate 0.5 gm. subcutaneously.
6. Oxygen therapy. Artificial respiration as needed (see p. 185).
7. Prophylactic measures in anticipation of kidney and liver insufficiencies (see pp. 210 and 213 respectively).

Laboratory:

1. The urine may contain albumin, casts, bile pigment, sometimes blood. It darkens rapidly on contact with the air. Dinitrophenol and 2-amino-4-nitrophenol may be present in urine.
2. Repeated tests are desirable to detect and evaluate possible disturbances of kidney and liver function.

DISULFIRAM

Disulfiram (tetraethylthiuram disulfide or Antabuse) is used in clinical medicine to establish and reinforce a conditioned reflex by which many chronic alcoholics are able to refuse alcoholic beverages. The drug acts by interfering with alcohol metabolism, so that the ingestion of alcohol is followed by distressing and occasionally dangerous symptoms.

To some extent this property is shared by many related compounds which are used for various purposes in industry and agriculture. For example, the methyl analogue of disulfiram (tetramethylthiuram disulfide or thiram) has been used as a rubber accelerator (Thuads) and as an important agricul-

tural fungicide. Also, thiram and similar compounds have served as successful insecticides and are marketed as repellents against the Japanese beetle. The monosulfide derivatives of these disulfides also possess fungicidal and insecticidal properties, and the monosulfide analogue of Antabuse has been incorporated in a medicinal soap for the treatment of human scabies. Closely related to these monosulfides are the substituted dithiocarbamates, which are marketed as sodium, iron, zinc, and manganese salts and are widely used as agricultural fungicides.

Toxicology: None of these compounds appears to have a high inherent toxicity in either acute or

chronic exposures; most of them are moderately or very slightly toxic. The major hazard of disulfiram (Antabuse), and probably of most related substances, is the reaction which comparatively small doses induce in persons who ingest even modest amounts of ethyl alcohol. Below is summarized the symptom complex precipitated by ethyl alcohol in those who have taken otherwise insignificant amounts of disulfiram.

Only the alcohol reaction is described here. The primary toxicity of disulfiram in the absence of alcohol is a different problem in all respects, including dose, symptoms, and treatment. *For the inherent toxicity of disulfiram, see discussion of thiram on page 179.*

The disulfiram-alcohol reaction is apparently due to a drug-induced disturbance in alcohol metabolism and is not a simple intensification of alcoholic intoxication. The acute reaction coincides with the appearance of excessive concentrations of acetaldehyde in the blood. Acetaldehyde accumulates presumably because disulfiram inhibits enzymes which normally oxidize this intermediary product of alcohol metabolism. Other factors must be involved too, because injected acetaldehyde does not completely mimic the disulfiram-alcohol reaction. About 1 gram of disulfiram daily for a few days sensitizes an adult of average size to as little as half an ounce of whiskey. With less safety, a large single dose of disulfiram can establish this reactive state, which may persist for more than a week. The greater the doses of drug and of alcohol the more violent is the reaction. In mild cases the effects last only an hour, in severe cases several hours. In persons receiving disulfiram a few deaths have occurred following the ingestion of alcoholic beverages.

In animal tests with rabbits, several compounds related to disulfiram have been found to share this property of promoting acetaldehyde accumulation during ethanol metabolism. Thiram was even more potent than disulfiram in this reaction, but the propyl and butyl analogues were inactive. The monosulfides (*e.g.*, tetraethylthiuram monosulfide)

showed marked and prolonged effects. Soluble diethyl and dimethyl dithiocarbamates (*e.g.*, sodium and potassium salts) had a potent but transient capacity to sensitize to alcohol, while the insoluble salts (*e.g.*, ferric, zinc, *etc.*) were not tested in this way. Presumably an accidental exposure to any one of these substances might escape detection or even suspicion until the ingestion of alcohol.

Symptomatology (the alcohol-induced reaction only):

1. Sensation of heat, flushing, vasodilatation.
2. Fall in blood pressure, tachycardia, palpitations.
3. Severe pulsating headache, nausea and vomiting.
4. Dyspnea, sensation of constriction in the neck, chest pain.
5. Hypotension, sweating, thirst, weakness, vertigo, and confusion.
6. Circulatory collapse, coma, and death.
7. Severe atypical reactions include myocardial infarction, acute congestive heart failure, cardiac arrhythmias, marked respiratory depression, and convulsions.

Treatment:

1. Gastric lavage but only if it can be done promptly.
2. Oxygen inhalation may relieve many of the distressing symptoms.
3. Rapid intravenous infusion of 5 per cent glucose in water (about 500 ml.).
4. Ascorbic acid (sodium ascorbate) 1 gm. intravenously (slowly).
5. Ephedrine sulfate 30 mg. intramuscularly.
6. Diphenhydramine hydrochloride (Benadryl) 100 mg. intravenously.
7. In severe cases the slow and cautious intravenous injection of saccharated iron has been recommended (100 mg. in 5 ml.).
8. The rigorous prohibition of any ethyl alcohol for at least 10 days after the last dose of disulfiram.

Laboratory: Blood analyses for acetaldehyde may aid in diagnosis.

ETHYL ALCOHOL

Ethyl alcohol (ethanol, grain alcohol, neutral spirits) in concentrations up to 50 per cent (100 proof) is often available in the home in drug formulations (*e.g.*, tinctures), cosmetic preparations, rubbing alcohol, and intoxicating beverages. All except the latter are commonly "denatured" by the addition of substances intended to induce prompt vomiting (*e.g.*, brucine) or to discourage consumption by a bitter and objectionable taste (*e.g.*, diethyl phthalate).

Toxicology: If ingested within a short period (*e.g.*, a few minutes), the fatal dose in an average

adult is considered to be 1½ to 2 pints of whiskey or gin (40 to 55 per cent alcohol).

Intoxication with alcohol may be simulated by many pathologic conditions, including diabetic acidosis, the post-convulsive depression of epilepsy, uremia, head injuries, and poisonings by any other central nervous depressant and some stimulants (*e.g.*, atropine). A diagnosis of acute alcoholism should not be made casually; a chemical test of blood, urine, or expired air is always desirable. Although a general relationship between symptoms and blood alcohol concentration cannot be stated

with precision, even a drinker with tolerance is unequivocally intoxicated when his blood alcohol level reaches 0.15 per cent (a common legal limit). A blood concentration between 0.3 and 0.4 per cent is commonly associated with stupor or coma, and 0.5 per cent is often fatal. Every patient in an alcoholic coma should be considered critically ill. The prognosis is especially poor if coma persists for more than 12 hours.

Ethyl alcohol is absorbed through gastric and intestinal mucosae, and its absorption is complete within 30 to 90 minutes. On rare occasions inebriation has been ascribed to the inhalation of vapor, but ingestion is the widely preferred route. Percutaneous absorption is said to be negligible. Ethanol is distributed throughout the body water, and over 90 per cent of a dose is metabolized by oxidation to acetaldehyde, to acetate, and to carbon dioxide and water, in that order. The rate of metabolic degradation is unexpectedly constant, and within wide limits it is independent of the amount consumed; an average adult is said to be able to oxidize each hour the equivalent of 2/3 oz. of 100-proof whiskey. Most authorities no longer hold that this rate can be materially increased by the administration of insulin, glucose, or vitamins, even if a hypoglycemic reaction is intentionally precipitated. Less than 10 per cent of the absorbed alcohol is excreted, chiefly in urine, measurably in expired air, and detectably in sweat. Excretion cannot be accelerated to a beneficial degree by diuretic drugs, by hyperventilation, or by the induction of sweating.

Only acute ethanol intoxication is considered here. For the symptoms and treatment induced by alcohol in a person premedicated with Antabuse (disulfiram), see discussion of disulfiram (p. 139). Denatured alcohol seldom presents special problems in therapy unless the denaturant is methyl alcohol, which is rarely used now for this purpose. If denaturation or contamination with even small amounts of methanol is suspected, see discussion of methyl alcohol (p. 155). Chronic alcoholism presents many special and perplexing problems to the therapist, who should consult standard textbooks in medicine and psychiatry.

Symptomatology (acute intoxication):

1. Early emotional lability: exhilaration, boastfulness, talkativeness, remorse, and belligerency.

2. Impaired motor coordination: slowed reaction time, slurred speech, ataxia.
3. Sensory disturbances: diplopia, vertigo.
4. Flushing of face, rapid pulse, sweating.
5. Nausea and vomiting, progressing to incontinence of urine and feces.
6. Drowsiness, stupor, and finally coma, with impaired or absent tendon reflexes.
7. Pupils dilated or normal.
8. Peripheral vascular collapse (shock): hypotension, tachycardia, cold pale skin, hypothermia.
9. Slow stertorous respirations.
10. Death from respiratory or circulatory failure.
11. During convalescence: postalcoholic headache and gastritis; infections (e.g., pneumonia, septicemia); alcoholic psychoses (e.g., delirium tremens).

Treatment:

1. Gastric lavage with warm water or sodium bicarbonate solution (3 to 5 per cent), —unless more than 2 hours have elapsed since alcohol was ingested. Do not use apomorphine.
2. Stimulants such as subcutaneous caffeine sodium benzoate or strong coffee by mouth or rectum. Oxygen and artificial respiration as needed (p. 189, 185).
3. Treat circulatory collapse, dehydration, and acidosis by intravenous infusions of isotonic sodium chloride or sodium lactate (M/6).
4. Optional: 5 to 10 per cent glucose in water (500 to 1000 ml.) plus 10 to 20 units of insulin and thiamin chloride 20 mg., given by slow intravenous infusion.
5. Multivitamin preparations, especially B complex, are widely used parenterally in the treatment of acute alcoholism; the practice is harmless but not unequivocally beneficial or relevant.
6. Keep patient warm. Avoid the aspiration of vomitus. Good nursing care (p. 229) minimizes the incidence of pneumonia.

Laboratory: Quantitative analyses for ethyl alcohol on samples of blood and/or urine. Various modifications of the Bogen test are usually employed. Positive reactions may be elicited by methanol, isopropyl alcohol, formaldehyde, acetaldehyde, and acetone or ether in large amounts, but *not* by paraldehyde, chloral hydrate, carbon tetrachloride, chloroform, or diabetic acidemia.

ETHYLENE GLYCOL

Ethylene glycol is a colorless, almost odorless liquid. In industry it finds many uses as a solvent and as a starting material in chemical syntheses. Around the home it is found in a few cosmetic

preparations, but "permanent type" automobile anti-freeze is the principal source of poisonings.

Toxicology: More than 40 human fatalities from the ingestion of ethylene glycol have been

reported, and the mean lethal dose appears to lie between 3 and 4 oz. in an adult. Inhalation is not generally hazardous because the glycol has a low vapor pressure. Only minor skin irritation and skin penetration are described, but the Food and Drug Administration have ruled that preparations intended for repeated topical application should contain no more than 5 per cent of this glycol.

In man ethylene glycol is a central nervous depressant and a kidney poison. It is largely oxidized *in vivo*, and like ethyl alcohol it apparently passes through an acetaldehyde stage. Less than 5 per cent of an ingested dose is metabolized to and excreted as urinary oxalate, but this is no longer regarded as sufficient to explain the hydropic degeneration of renal tubular epithelium seen in acutely poisoned animals and man. In contrast, when animals are fed small quantities of ethylene glycol over a period of several months, kidney tubular atrophy is undoubtedly aggravated by and perhaps caused by oxalate production and retention as calcium oxalate stones in renal tubules, kidney pelvis, and urinary bladder. In clinical poisonings by ethylene glycol, deaths from central nervous depression and respiratory arrest are more common than those from renal failure.

Toxicology of Ethylene Glycol Derivatives: In acute (but not chronic) studies, the various ether derivatives of ethylene glycol are several times more toxic than the parent compound. One relevant difference is the more prominent kidney injury, which is manifest one or more days after the ingestion of ethylene glycol ethers. In contrast most mono- and di-esters of ethylene glycol have about the same acute toxicity as the parent compound, to which they are hydrolyzed in the body. Mixed monoether-ester derivatives are similar in toxicity and toxic actions to the corresponding monoethers.

With one exception the generalizations above also apply to diethylene glycol and its derivatives, all of which are slightly less toxic than their ethylene glycol analogues. The exception is the high toxicity, relative to diethylene glycol, of its simple esters. Data are inadequate to demonstrate similar parallelisms among the derivatives of triethylene glycol and among those of higher polymers.

When ethylene glycol is compared with its simple polymers (*e.g.*, di-, tri-, and poly-ethylene glycols), the acute toxicity in animals appears to be less the higher the degree of polymerization (*i.e.*, the higher the molecular weight). Thus triethylene glycol is less toxic than diethylene glycol, and among the polyethylene glycols the solid preparations (molecular weights of 1000 and higher) are less toxic than the liquid samples (molecular weights of 600 and less). In animals very large doses are required to kill and deaths appear to be renal in origin (not due to primary central nervous depression). Probably most of these generalizations are valid for man, but clinical data suggest that diethylene glycol is almost as toxic as ethylene glycol or perhaps slightly more so; both compounds elicit similar signs and symptoms.

Symptomatology:
1. Transient exhilaration.
2. Nausea, vomiting (sometimes progressing to hematemesis), and abdominal cramps. Diarrhea has been reported in diethylene glycol poisoning.
3. Extreme weakness and perhaps muscle cramps.
4. Ataxia, vertigo, progressing to stupor and finally coma, with or without an intermediary stage of convulsions.
5. Death by respiratory paralysis, or recovery from coma.
6. Lumbar pain, albuminuria, hematuria, oliguria, progressing to anuria.
7. Acute renal failure with uremia, peripheral edema, ascites, pulmonary edema, drowsiness, cyanosis, coma, and death within a week or 10 days.

Treatment:
1. Gastric lavage with 1:5000 potassium permanganate solution.
2. Caffeine sodium benzoate subcutaneously for central nervous depression. Oxygen and artificial respiration as needed (p. 185).
3. Short-acting barbiturate intravenously if convulsions supervene (see p. 201).
4. Avoid the administration of electrolytes by any route, unless shock or severe acidosis threatens.
5. Supportive measures (prophylactic and therapeutic) for acute renal failure (see pp. 210–212).

Laboratory: Repeated urinalyses, blood analyses, and kidney function tests are desirable for evaluation of the renal lesion.

FERROUS SULFATE

Ferrous salts are widely used in the treatment of iron-deficiency anemias. Ferrous carbonate, chloride, gluconate, lactate, and glutamate have been prescribed, but the sulfate is the most popular iron preparation in the United States. It is available as the official hydrate (0.3 gm. $FeSO_4 \cdot 7H_2O$ or 0.2 gm. of the exsiccated salt), as a syrup, and as elixirs. Occasionally metallic iron powder (Reduced Iron N.F.) and ferric salts (*e.g.*, the ammonium citrate and hydroxide) are used in the clinical treatment of anemia.

Toxicology: Although the oral administration

of iron does not cause chronic systemic poisoning, acute intoxications are not infrequent. Apparently *all* forms of iron are potentially toxic, but most of the reported deaths have occurred in infants and young children who ingested ferrous sulfate tablets because of the sweet coating. Adults are not immune to acute iron poisoning; death has been reported in an adult who ingested at one time one quarter of a pound of the sulfate. Infants and young children have been killed by 7 to 25 common tablets of ferrous sulfate (0.3 gm. each), while doses of 4.5 to 15 gm. have been survived, perhaps because substantial but unknown portions were promptly removed by vomiting.

Iron preparations have an intensely corrosive action on the gastric mucosa, particularly at the pyloric end. Vomiting begins within 10 to 60 minutes, followed by shock, coma, and death within a few hours. Postmortem examination usually reveals liver damage consisting of periportal hemorrhagic necrosis. Among some survivors delicate fibrosis of the liver (mild cirrhosis) and pyloric stenosis have been described. The mechanism of acute iron poisoning is unknown. No methemoglobin is formed.

Rats receiving massive amounts of ferrous sulfate by stomach tube tolerate two lethal doses if given promptly a soluble phosphate. This is the basis for the phosphate treatment recommended below; its effectiveness has not been tested in patients. BAL increases the mortality of experimental animals given near-lethal doses of iron. Edathamil calcium-disodium (EDTA) does not appear to alter the lethality of iron in rats, but it probably deserves a trial in poisoned children.

Symptomatology:

1. Severe gastritis or gastroenteritis with abdominal pain, retching, and prolonged vomiting, beginning 10 to 60 minutes after ingestion. Vomitus may become bloody. Diarrhea is sometimes violent; the feces are watery and later tarry. Dehydration becomes intense.

2. Shock, pallor, cyanosis, and coldness. Rapid, weak or imperceptible pulse, low blood pressure, rapid and shallow respirations.

3. Drowsiness, hyporeflexia, dilated pupils, coma.

4. Liver injury, consisting of hemorrhagic necrosis which is usually reversible.

5. Death from shock, usually in 4 to 5 hours. Sometimes following apparent recovery, pneumonia with fever may cause fatal collapse 1 to 3 days later.

6. Among survivors pyloric stenosis and mild hepatic cirrhosis may be encountered as persistent sequelae, but recovery is usually complete.

Treatment:

1. Give milk immediately and then induce vomiting by stroking the pharynx with a blunt object (*e.g.*, spoon handle).

2. Gastric lavage with one pint of a 5 per cent aqueous solution of mono- or di-sodium phosphate. After lavage, leave 2 to 3 oz. of phosphate solution in the stomach (this quantity is proper for a 1- or 2-year-old child; use proportionately more in an adult).

3. Bismuth subcarbonate 0.2 gm. every 4 hours in young children.

4. Intravenous 5 per cent glucose in saline to correct dehydration.

5. Transfusion with plasma or whole blood if shock becomes severe (p. 193).

6. Oxygen therapy as indicated.

7. In severe poisonings, try edathamil calcium-disodium intravenously according to the dosage schedule on p. 153. Do not use BAL.

8. For supportive treatment of liver injury, see p. 213.

9. Antibiotics as prophylaxis against pneumonia and other intercurrent infections.

10. Observe the patient carefully for 48 hours.

Laboratory: Laboratory data are not generally relevant. No methemoglobinemia occurs.

FLUORIDE

Sodium fluoride (NaF) and sodium fluosilicate (Na$_2$SiF$_6$) are used commonly as insecticides (ant, roach, and beetle powders) and rarely as rodenticides. Sodium fluoride has been used internally as an anthelmintic in swine (*never* in man) and externally as a delousing powder on poultry and cattle. Cryolite, an insoluble sodium fluoaluminate, is sometimes dusted on vegetable and fruit crops as an insecticide. Although infrequently found outside of laboratories and various industries, HF as a gas (hydrogen fluoride) and as an aqueous solution (hydrofluoric acid) warrants consideration because it is a very hazardous form of fluoride.

Toxicology: In spite of several fatalities, the lethal dose of sodium fluoride in man is not accurately known. Less than 1 gm. by mouth has caused dangerous poisoning, but the mean lethal dose is probably close to 5 gm., and 8 to 10 gm. are almost certainly lethal in untreated cases. The toxicity of sodium fluosilicate is about the same. Hydrofluoric acid is probably more toxic than sodium fluoride, while cryolite is certainly much less toxic.

Fluoride is a "general protoplasmic poison." When present as a soluble salt, it is readily absorbed from the alimentary tract. A 2 per cent solution of sodium fluoride kills mucosal cells, and its ingestion leads to a severe hemorrhagic gastroenteritis; in part this corrosiveness is due to a toxic

action on mucosal capillaries and is seen even after parenteral administration. Hydrofluoric acid is corrosive even on intact skin, where it causes painful penetrating ulcers which heal slowly.

The systemic actions of fluoride are presumably related to the inhibition of one or more enzymes controlling cellular glycolysis (and perhaps respiration) and to the binding or precipitation of calcium as CaF_2. If death is not prompt, systemic symptoms are many and varied. Severe shock is due not alone to gastrointestinal damage but also to central vasomotor depression and to cardiac disturbances. At least in dogs, fluoride interferes with both the contractile power of the heart and the mechanism of beat, in a way that cannot be ascribed to hypocalcemia. The central nervous system is also poisoned, and perhaps this is responsible for the occasional epileptiform convulsions and eventual respiratory failure. Death is usually due to respiratory arrest or to cardiovascular collapse. The role of calcium binding in these phenomena is not clearly established. Many victims die without overt manifestations of hypocalcemia (e.g., tetany). Nevertheless the repeated administration of soluble calcium salts is appropriate therapy, not only to prevent or correct hypocalcemia but also to attempt the inactivation of the toxic fluoride ion by binding or precipitating it.

Symptomatology:

A. Ingestion of neutral fluorides (e.g., NaF)
  1. Salty or soapy taste, salivation, nausea, burning or crampy abdominal pain, vomiting, diarrhea (may be bloody). Dehydration and thirst.
  2. Muscle weakness, tremors, and rarely transient epileptiform convulsions, followed by central nervous depression.
  3. Shock characterized by pallor, weak and thready pulse (sometimes irregular), shallow unlabored respiration, weak heart tones, wet cold skin, cyanosis, dilated pupils, followed almost invariably by death in 2 to 4 hours.
  4. When death is delayed, paralysis of the muscles of deglutition, carpopedal spasm, and spasm of the extremities.
  5. Occasionally local or generalized urticaria.
B. Local actions of HF vapor or aqueous solutions.
  1. Superficial or deep burns of the skin and mucous membranes of the digestive and/or respiratory tracts. Necrotic ulcers are painful and heal slowly.
  2. For symptoms (and treatment) after the inhalation of HF or F_2, see Nitrogen Oxides on p. 163.

Treatment:

A. Ingestion of neutral fluorides (e.g., NaF)
  1. Start intravenous infusion of glucose in isotonic saline.
  2. Inject intravenously 10 ml. of 10 per cent calcium gluconate solution. Repeat in about 1 hour and/or whenever tetany appears.
  3. Gentle gastric lavage with lime water or a 1 per cent solution of calcium chloride (saline is a poor substitute but better than nothing). Then give orally several oz. of lime water at frequent intervals; if necessary large quantities of milk may be substituted. Aluminum hydroxide gels should be exceptionally effective for binding fluoride.
  4. Inject intramuscularly 10 ml. of 10 per cent calcium gluconate at 4 to 6 hour intervals until recovery is complete (p. 220).
  5. Treat shock vigorously by the administration of saline, plasma, or whole blood (p. 193). Norepinephrine is probably useful. Give oxygen as needed. Keep the patient warm.
  6. Correct dehydration and attempt to maintain a mild diuresis, but discontinue fluids and electrolytes (except calcium) if anuria develops (p. 210).
B. Treatment of HF burns of skin
  1. Houston Baker of the Corning Glass Co. recommends the immediate local application of the following solution: boric acid, 1 part; borax, 1 part; water, 30 parts.
  2. Dr. E. E. Evans of the DuPont Co. gives the following directions for treating HF burns:
  a. Wash thoroughly with clean cold water and apply magnesium oxide paste.
  b. Soak the affected area for at least an hour in 70 per cent alcohol and ice. Apply magnesium oxide paste and bandage. Pain developing late may be relieved by infiltrating with 10 per cent calcium gluconate into and around such areas.
  c. In extensive burns with blisters, debride completely, cutting away all white raised tissue. Apply magnesium oxide paste for 24 to 48 hours and, if there is no further extension of the burned area, apply a mild ointment. Pressure dressings are satisfactory.

Laboratory:

1. Signs of renal injury may arise as a direct toxic action or as a consequence of shock.
2. Electrocardiograms are desirable.

FLUOROACETATE

Sodium fluoroacetate or Compound 1080 is a synthetic, water soluble, non-volatile salt, with a faint odor like vinegar; it is usually mixed with a black dye. As an experimental rodenticide, it has no equal in terms of potency, stability, and acceptability in rodent baits and drinking water. However, because of its very high toxicity for mammals, including man and domestic animals, this substance should be used only by professional exterminators and other experts. Certain derivatives of 2-fluoro-ethanol are potent insecticides and are toxic to mammals presumably because of metabolic oxidation to fluoroacetate.

Toxicology: Chronic intoxication with sodium fluoroacetate is improbable, but the very high acute toxicity constitutes a real hazard, and at least 14 human fatalities have been reported. As little as 0.1 mg./kg. has proved lethal for dogs and cats. Estimates of the mean lethal dose in man range from 1 to 5 mg./kg.; 2 mg./kg. is probably the best single value. In experimental studies the lethal dose is essentially the same by all routes of administration. Ingestion is certainly the most likely mode of poisoning, but there is one report of a non-fatal intoxication due to the inhalation of sodium fluoroacetate powder. The compound appears to be absorbed promptly from the alimentary tract, but initial symptoms are commonly delayed for one or several hours.

Fluoroacetate is a "delayed convulsant." The fluoroacetate ion is not poisonous itself but is converted to fluorocitric acid, which blocks the tricarboxylic acid cycle, an essential mechanism of energy production in mammalian cells. Toxic effects do not appear immediately; time is required for the "lethal synthesis" of fluorocitrate. This metabolic lesion manifests itself principally in disturbed activities of the central nervous system and of the heart. Dogs die of convulsions or of subsequent respiratory paralysis, but in man, monkeys and rabbits the central nervous excitation is usually incidental, and the dangerous and fatal complication is ventricular fibrillation. In experimental poisonings in monkeys, parenteral monoacetin (glyceryl monoacetate) has proved to be an effective antidote. It appears to serve as an acetate donor to antagonize the fluoroacetate ion in a competitive manner. This antidote has had no clinical trial, as far as we know.

Symptomatology:
1. Vomiting.
2. Apprehension, auditory hallucinations, nystagmus, tingling sensation of nose, facial twitching, numbness of face.
3. Central nervous excitation, progressing to epileptiform convulsions.
4. Severe central nervous depression between and subsequent to the convulsive episodes, but death is not often due to respiratory failure in humans poisoned with fluoroacetate.
5. Disturbances in the mechanism of the heart beat usually appear only after the convulsive phase.
6. Pulsus alternans, long sequences of ectopic beats (often multifocal), and ventricular tachycardia may disintegrate into ventricular fibrillation and death.

Treatment:
1. Induce vomiting immediately if possible.
2. Gastric lavage with tap water unless convulsions make this impractical.
3. Instill into the stomach sodium or magnesium sulfate in water (15 to 30 gm.).
4. Administer parenterally monoacetin (glyceryl monoacetate) if available. The recommended dose is 0.5 ml./kg. of undiluted fluid intramuscularly every half hour for several hours and then at a reduced level for at least 12 hours. In the same dose monoacetin may also be given intravenously after dilution with 5 parts of sterile isotonic saline. No preparation of monoacetin is known to be available on the pharmaceutical market. The usual commercial fluid has large amounts of free glycerine (due to hydrolysis favored by heat and exposure to sunlight), and the assay is seldom better than 70 per cent. The exigency of an overt poisoning, however, probably warrants the use of even non-sterile commercial material. Irrespective of impurities, injections may be expected to produce some sedation and vasodilatation. The site of intramuscular injection must be varied because of local pain and edema.
5. A short acting barbiturate drug may be tried in the control of convulsions (p. 201).
6. Oxygen therapy and artificial respiration, as required (p. 185).
7. It is doubtful that digitalis is ever warranted. Parenteral procaine amide, quinidine, or papaverine may be given a therapeutic trial (p. 197), but in experimental poisonings these drugs have proved much less successful than monoacetin in controlling cardiac arrhythmias.

Laboratory:
1. The cardiac status should be repeatedly monitored by an electrocardiogram. Any pattern of alteration in the mechanical or electrical heart beat indicates a need for more monoacetin.
2. Hyperglycemia and glycosuria have been noted in some experimental studies.

FORMALDEHYDE

Formaldehyde gas (HCHO) in solution may be present around the home as a constituent of antiseptics, deodorizing preparations, and fumigants. It has a pungent odor with a suffocating effect. Formalin is an aqueous solution containing not less than 37 per cent (by weight) of formaldehyde and small amounts of methanol, ethanol, or both (0 to 5 per cent, to prevent polymerization).

Toxicology: Formaldehyde is quickly absorbed from the alimentary tract and lungs. It is oxidized to formic acid in various tissues, especially the liver. Some formic acid may appear in the urine, but much of it is completely destroyed. According to one hypothesis, some of the absorbed formaldehyde undergoes metabolic reduction to methyl alcohol. A part of the formaldehyde is probably transformed into methenamine (hexamethylenetetramine).

Inhaled vapors are very irritating to the eyes, nose, and upper respiratory tract; high concentrations may produce edema or spasm of the larynx. Tracheobronchitis may result from inhalation, but pulmonary edema is uncommon. The susceptibility of mucous membranes to the irritative actions of formaldehyde is diminished by repeated exposure. Contact with vapor or solutions causes the skin to become white, rough, hard, and anesthetic, due to superficial coagulation necrosis; with long exposure dermatitis and hypersensitivity frequently result.

The ingestion of formalin (37 per cent formaldehyde solution) leads promptly to inflammation and ulceration of the gastrointestinal mucosa, to circulatory collapse, and to kidney damage. Absorbed formaldehyde appears to have its principal effect on the central nervous system, as is evidenced by convulsions and stupor. The mechanism of these reactions is unknown, but acidosis and circulatory collapse are probably contributory.

The largest dose of formalin from which recovery has been reported is 4 oz., while the ingestion of 1 oz. has caused death within 3 hours. Probably the mean lethal dose in an adult is about 2 oz. If the patient survives the first 48 hours, the prognosis is good, and a very rapid recovery is the rule.

Symptomatology:

A. Inhalation

1. Irritation of mucous membranes, especially of eyes, nose, and upper respiratory tract.
2. With higher concentration, cough, dysphagia, bronchitis, pneumonia, edema or spasm of the larynx. Pulmonary edema is uncommon.

B. Ingestion

3. Immediate intense pain in mouth, pharynx, and stomach.
4. Nausea, vomiting, hematemesis, abdominal pain, and occasionally diarrhea (which may be bloody).
5. Pale, clammy skin, and other signs of shock.
6. Difficult micturition, hematuria, anuria.
7. Vertigo, convulsions, stupor, and coma.
8. Death due to respiratory failure.

C. Skin contact

9. Irritation and hardening of skin. Strong solutions produce coagulation necrosis.
10. Dermatitis and hypersensitivity from prolonged exposure.

Treatment:

1. Administer by mouth one or more of the following: water, milk, 0.2 per cent ammonia water (1 teaspoonful of strong ammonia water diluted with one pint of water), ammonium acetate (3 teaspoonsful in water), egg whites, universal antidote. Ammonium salts are probably best because they transform formaldehyde into methenamine. Then try to induce vomiting.
2. Gastric lavage with a very dilute ammonia solution (0.2 per cent, see above), if pain and spasm do not prevent gentle passage of a gastric tube.
3. Demulcents: milk, eggs, aluminum hydroxide gels.
4. Spirits of ammonia, 8 ml. diluted with water, by mouth.
5. Morphine for the control of pain.
6. Combat shock by the intravenous administration of isotonic saline, plasma, or whole blood (p. 193).
7. To correct acidosis, give sodium bicarbonate orally, or M/6 sodium lactate solution intravenously (p. 217).
8. Artificial respiration, if indicated (p. $$$).
9. Penicillin to prevent pneumonia and other secondary infections.
10. Wash affected skin with large quantities of soap and water.

Laboratory: Urinalysis may reveal red blood cells (sometimes gross hematuria) and casts.

HEPTACHLOR

Heptachlor or heptachloro-tetrahydro-4,7-endo-methanoindane (the usual technical product also contains related compounds) is a white crystalline solid readily soluble in petroleum distillates, alcohols, and ketones. It may be formulated commercially as emulsifiable concentrates, wettable powders, dusts, or granular preparations. Heptachlor is used as an insecticide for combatting grass-

hoppers, cotton weevils, soil insects, and many others.

Toxicology: No human fatalities have been reported, but in animals heptachlor is more toxic than chlordane, to which it is related. When ingested by rats or rabbits, the acute mean lethal dose has been established at 80 to 90 mg./kg. (toxicity rating 4). Heptachlor is dangerous by ingestion, skin absorption, or spray inhalation. Liver necrosis is the only pathological lesion found in acutely poisoned animals. Chronic exposures produce inanition in animals. Like DDT, heptachlor accumulates in body fat.

Symptomatology:

1. The earliest signs of poisoning arise from irritation of the central nervous system. Hyperexcitability is evidenced by tremors and eventually by convulsions. Depression and paralysis may follow.

2. Liver damage as a possible late manifestation.

3. Moderate local irritation is probable after dermal exposures.

Treatment:

1. Remove materials spilled on the skin by a thorough washing with soap and water. If spilled in eyes, wash repeatedly with water.

2. If ingested, lavage stomach with warm tap water (unless convulsions are imminent).

3. Saline catharsis, e.g., 15 to 30 gm. sodium sulfate with 6 to 8 oz. of water.

4. Avoid epinephrine and oil laxatives.

5. A rapidly acting barbiturate may aid in controlling convulsions, but care must be taken not to augment respiratory depression. See p. 201.

6. Oxygen therapy and artificial respiration may be necessary (p. 185).

7. Since no specific antidotes are known, symptomatic therapy must be accompanied by complete rest.

Laboratory: Periodic examination for incipient liver injury (e.g., liver function tests).

HYDROGEN SULFIDE

Hydrogen sulfide (H_2S) is a colorless gas, heavier than air, possessing the odor of rotten eggs. It is a rapid and powerful systemic poison. It is found in several industries, but its importance for this compilation arises from its presence in sewers and cesspools and among the products of putrefaction everywhere. Moreover, it may be formed in significant amounts within the gastrointestinal tract after the ingestion of inorganic sulfide salts or elemental sulfur (due to the actions of gastric acid and of colonic bacteria, respectively).

Toxicology: Vapor concentrations as low as 0.005 per cent (50 ppm) in air may cause toxic symptoms, and 0.1 to 0.2 per cent is usually fatal within a few minutes. Odor is not a dependable way to detect this gas because the sense of smell is very quickly dulled. Susceptibility to hydrogen sulfide varies with the individual and may be increased by previous exposure, but no truly cumulative effects are recognized.

With low concentrations of hydrogen sulfide, the toxic symptoms are due largely to tissue irritation, especially of the respiratory tract mucosa. High concentrations also cause systemic reactions, which involve mainly the central nervous system. A transient excitement stage may occur, but the dominant reaction is one of central nervous depression with death from respiratory arrest. Other organ systems may also be involved. Indeed hydrogen sulfide is believed to be a general tissue enzyme poison that produces histotoxic anoxia by mechanisms that are perhaps analogous to those caused by cyanide. Even the hemoglobin molecule is attacked, with a consequent reduction in the oxygen-carrying capacity of blood, but no sulfhemoglobin is formed. The only recognized treatment is supportive and symptomatic. If tissue oxygenation can be maintained, tissue cells soon oxidize toxic sulfide to innocuous sulfate.

Symptomatology:

A. Subacute poisoning:

1. *Irritant actions*

   Eyes: painful conjunctivitis, photophobia, lacrimation, and corneal opacity.

   Respiratory tract: rhinitis with anosmia, tracheobronchitis with pain and cough, pulmonary edema with dyspnea, sometimes late bronchopneumonia.

   Skin: direct contact (as a solution) may produce erythema and pain.

2. *Gastrointestinal effects:* profuse salivation, nausea, vomiting, diarrhea.

3. *Central nervous effects:* giddiness, headache, vertigo, somnolence, amnesia, confusion, and unconsciousness.

4. *Miscellaneous:* tachypnea, palpitation, tachycardia, arrhythmia, sweating, weakness, and muscle cramps.

B. Acute poisoning:

1. Sudden collapse and unconsciousness, with or without a warning cry.

2. Death from prompt respiratory paralysis, perhaps with a terminal asphyxial convulsion.

3. After sublethal exposures recovery is usually slow; the patient may have a residual

cough, cardiac dilatation, slow pulse, peripheral neuritis, albuminuria, and some degree of amnesia or of psychic disturbance. Recovery is eventually complete in most non-fatal cases.

Treatment:

1. Remove immediately to fresh air. Keep at rest and comfortably warm.

2. If respirations are depressed, artificial respiration without interruption until normal breathing is restored or until rigor ensues. See p. 185.

3. Administer oxygen (p. 189) and maintain it even after spontaneous breathing is established. If pulmonary edema ensues, see p. 192.

4. For central nervous depression, nikethamide (1 to 2 ml. of a 25 per cent solution) or Metrazol (1 to 4 ml. of a 10 per cent solution) intravenously; caffeine sodium benzoate (0.5 gm.) intramuscularly. See p. 204.

5. Atropine sulfate (0.0006 gm. intramuscularly) may contribute some symptomatic relief.

6. Conjunctivitis may be relieved by the instillation of one drop of olive oil in each eye and sometimes by 3 to 4 drops of epinephrine solution (1:1000) at frequent intervals (e.g., 5 minutes). Occasionally local anesthetics and hot or cold compresses are necessary to control the pain.

7. Antibiotics as prophylaxis against lung infections.

Laboratory: Urine may contain albumin, casts, and a few red blood cells. No simple chemical test is diagnostic of poisoning by hydrogen sulfide, but the odor is sometimes recognizable in the victim's breath. The presence of H_2S in air can be detected by lead-acetate test paper.

HYPOCHLORITE

Hypochlorite salts (e.g., sodium, potassium, calcium, magnesium) serve as disinfectants, bleaches, and deodorizers. Specifically they are used to disinfect contaminated utensils, large masses of organic matter (excreta), and occasionally water for drinking. Under a host of trade names, dilute hypochlorites are found in almost every home in the form of laundry bleach. Dilute aqueous solutions (5 to 10 per cent) are sometimes used medicinally as foot baths. Hypochlorites are unstable, especially when in solution; slowly decomposing, they become less toxic with age. The concentration of a hypochlorite solution is often stated in terms of "available chlorine" or "active chlorine." This is the percentage of gaseous chlorine (gm. Cl_2 per 100 ml. solution or per 100 gm. solid) which can be released by the hypochlorite if it oxidizes chloride ions that are present in excess in these preparations (often as added sodium chloride). While in chlorinated soda the stated concentrations of sodium hypochlorite and of available chlorine are essentially equal, only about one-third of chlorinated lime is available chlorine. These values vary with the method of preparation, the age, the technique of storage, etc.

Toxicology: The toxicity of hypochlorites arises from their corrosive actions on skin and mucous membranes. Most of this corrosiveness stems from the oxidizing potency of the hypochlorite itself, a capacity which is measured in terms of "available chlorine." The acidity of some hypochlorite preparations and the alkalinity of others may contribute to the tissue injury and mucosal erosion. According to some authorities, acid preparations are more dangerous than alkaline ones because of the presence of hypochlorous acid (HOCl). Due to its low ionization and consequent lack of charge, this acid is probably able to penetrate mucous membrane more deeply than does the hypochlorite ion. Both the acid and salt appear to be rapidly inactivated (reduced) by protein and other tissue constituents, and probably little, if any, reaches the systemic circulation. All systemic symptoms, therefore, are thought to be secondary to local tissue injury and shock.

As with other strictly corrosive agents, lethality is more intimately related to concentration than to dose (i.e., conc. × vol.). The ingestion of hypochlorite solutions with "available chlorine" concentrations as low as 0.5 per cent is rarely a threat to life. Although no exact clinical data are available, solutions with 4 to 6 per cent available chlorine are probably lethal to adults only in oral doses of many ounces, but as little as one ounce may be dangerous if the concentration is 15 per cent or more. With bleaches, as well as other caustic agents, death is usually due to complications of severe local injury, such as toxemia, shock, perforation, hemorrhage, infection, and obstruction.

Only symptomatic and supportive measures are available in the treatment of hypochlorite poisoning. A solution of sodium thiosulfate (hyposulfite) will reduce any unreacted material with which it comes in contact. Since even neutral or alkaline hypochlorite salts may be converted to hypochlorous acid by the acidity of gastric juice, mild alkali therapy by mouth may be beneficial, if given promptly. When indicated, surgical measures such as tracheotomy or gastrectomy may be life-saving.

Symptomatology:

1. Pain and inflammation of the mouth, pharynx, esophagus, and stomach. Erosion of mucous membrane.

2. Vomiting. The vomitus may resemble coffee grounds (hemorrhage).

3. Circulatory collapse, with cold and clammy skin, cyanosis, and shallow respirations.

4. Confusion, delirium, coma.

5. Edema of pharynx and larynx, with stridor and obstruction.

6. Perforation of the esophagus or stomach, with mediastinitis or peritonitis.

7. The inhalation of hypochlorous acid fumes causes severe respiratory tract irritation and pulmonary edema.

8. Skin contact may cause vesicular eruptions and eczematoid dermatitis.

Treatment:

1. Swallow immediately milk, egg white, starch paste, milk of magnesia, aluminum hydroxide gel, or magnesium trisilicate gel. Avoid sodium bicarbonate because of the release of carbon dioxide. Do not use acidic antidotes.

2. Cautious gastric lavage with tap water or a solution of sodium thiosulfate (2 per cent).

3. Milk of magnesia (1 oz.) left in the stomach is useful as a mild antacid, adsorbent, demulcent, and cathartic.

4. Demulcents, such as starch, egg white, milk, gruel.

5. Opiates for the control of pain (p. 199).

6. Treat shock vigorously with intravenous fluids (p. 193).

7. Prompt surgical intervention when indicated, e.g., tracheotomy, gastrectomy.

8. If spilled on skin, wash with liberal quantities of water and apply a paste of baking soda.

Laboratory: Generally irrelevant.

IODINE

Iodine, one of the oldest antiseptics in modern medicine, still maintains its popularity because it is economical and effective as a skin antiseptic, bactericide, fungicide, amebicide, and counterirritant. It is used most frequently as the official U.S.P. tincture (2 per cent iodine and 2 per cent NaI in 50 per cent alcohol), but it is also available as strong iodine tincture (7 per cent iodine and 5 per cent KI in 83 per cent alcohol), Lugol's solution (5 per cent iodine and 10 per cent KI in aqueous solution), and iodine ointment (4 per cent iodine).

Toxicology:

Accidental and suicidal poisonings from iodine are not uncommon, but fatalities are rare. Reported lethal doses in adults range from a few tenths of a gram to more than 20 gm. Probably the mean lethal dose lies between 2 and 4 gm. of free iodine or 1 to 2 oz. of the strong tincture.

Poisoning is largely due to the highly corrosive action of iodine on the gastrointestinal tract, an action which is due at least partly to the oxidizing potential of this element. Food present in the digestive tract rapidly inactivates iodine by converting it to comparatively harmless iodide. If death intervenes, it usually occurs within 48 hours (except in a rare case of delayed death due to esophageal stenosis). Other routes of administration are occasionally a source of poisoning. Inhalation of iodine vapor is very irritating to mucous membranes. Application of iodine to the skin may rarely give rise to a hypersensitivity reaction in the form of fever and a generalized skin eruption. Local inflammatory reactions (burns) are not uncommon after cutaneous application of the strong tincture.

The nervous, circulatory, and renal disturbances which follow the ingestion of iodine are ascribed to corrosive gastroenteritis and attending shock. Although free iodine may remain in the alimentary tract for several hours after ingestion, most if not all is converted to inorganic iodide or organically-bound iodine before or during intestinal absorption. The blood plasma reveals principally iodide and a small amount of protein-bound iodine. The evidence is insufficient, however, to rule out the possibility that small amounts of free iodine reach the circulation and exert direct systemic effects on parenchymal organs. Traces of free iodine have been reported in saliva, sweat, and urine.

The iodide ion probably plays no significant role in the acute toxicity of iodine. Simple iodide salts are non-corrosive and relatively benign. They are principally active as expectorants and diuretics. A mild toxic syndrome called "iodism" results from chronic iodide overdoses and from the repeated administration of small amounts of iodine. Iodism is characterized by salivation, coryza, sneezing, conjunctivitis, headache, laryngitis, bronchitis, stomatitis, parotitis, and skin rashes. Except for discontinuing the medication, treatment is rarely required.

Symptomatology:

1. Burning pain of the oral mucosa and esophagus. The lips and mucous membranes are stained brown.

2. Severe corrosive gastroenteritis evidenced by vomiting, abdominal pain, and diarrhea. The vomitus is blue if starch is present in the stomach. Occasionally the stools become bloody.

3. Hypotension, tachycardia, cyanosis, and other signs of shock.

4. Headache, dizziness, delirium, collapse, and stupor.

5. Death may be due to circulatory collapse, asphyxiation from edema of the glottis, aspiration pneumonia, or pulmonary edema.

6. Occasionally hemorrhagic nephritis (with

oliguria or anuria) becomes apparent within one to three days.

7. Late esophageal stenosis has been reported at least once.

Treatment:

1. Swallow *promptly* milk, starch, flour, or eggs. Starch paste is excellent.
2. Gastric lavage with a solution of starch (1 to 10 per cent), of sodium thiosulfate (5 per cent), or of protein (egg white, milk).
3. Fluid and electrolyte replacement for the correction of dehydration, shock, and acid-base imbalances (p. 215—219).
4. Supportive measures for the treatment of circulatory collapse (p. 193).
5. Opiates for the control of pain (p. 199).
6. Preparations for an emergency tracheotomy in case signs of laryngeal obstruction appear (p. 185).
7. Prophylactic antibiotic therapy.

Laboratory: The urine may reveal albumin, casts, and red blood cells.

ISOPROPYL ALCOHOL

Isopropyl alcohol (2-propanol) is a solvent and a disinfectant, but in the home it is found principally in rubbing alcohol and in hand lotions.

Toxicology: By clinical criteria isopropyl alcohol is less toxic than methyl alcohol; it is metabolized largely to acetone and excreted quickly. Its acute potency as a central nervous depressant is about twice that of ethyl alcohol. The probable lethal oral dose for an adult is about 8 ounces. The symptoms are similar to those of ethanol intoxication, but gastric irritation with nausea and vomiting is said to be more prominent. Indeed vomiting with aspiration is a serious threat and a dangerous complication in isopropyl alcohol poisoning.

Symptomatology:

1. Dizziness, incoordination, headache, confusion, stupor, and coma.
2. Gastroenteritis with vomiting, hematemesis, and diarrhea.
3. Bradycardia, hypotension, and sometimes severe circulatory collapse.
4. Death by respiratory paralysis.
5. Late manifestations: aspiration pneumonia; kidney and liver dysfunctions, which are usually mild and transient.

Treatment:

1. Gastric lavage with water.
2. Caffeine sodium benzoate 0.5 gm. subcutaneously, to counteract central nervous depression. Oxygen and artificial respiration as needed (see p. 185).
3. Intravenous glucose and saline to correct dehydration, electrolyte deficiencies, acidosis, and shock (pp. 215—219).
4. Prophylactic measures in anticipation of disturbances in liver (p. 213) and kidney (p. 210) function.

Laboratory: Severe acetonuria (isopropyl alcohol is oxidized to acetone *in vivo*). Function tests to detect and evaluate possible liver and kidney disturbances.

KEROSENE

Kerosene (kerosine) is one of several petroleum distillates prepared by the fractionation of crude petroleum oil. In order of decreasing volatility the major fractions are: petroleum ether or benzine, gasoline, mineral spirits, kerosene, fuel oil, lubricating oils, paraffin wax, and asphalt or tar. These fractions consist chiefly of aliphatic or straight-chain hydrocarbons of the methane series. Petroleum ether or benzine is composed largely of pentane and hexane, while kerosene is predominantly hydrocarbons lying between nonane and hexadecane. All fractions and particularly kerosene contain appreciable amounts of aromatic or unsaturated ring hydrocarbons (*e.g.*, toluene and xylene) and saturated rings or cycloparaffins (sometimes called naphthenes). Petroleum products obtained by "cracking" processes also contain unsaturated straight-chain molecules (olefins and diolefins). Kerosene and related compounds are used as illuminating fuels, heating fuels, motor fuels, vehicles for many insecticides and fungicides, cleaning agents, and paint thinners. Kerosene and gasoline can often be found around homes, garages and farms in containers originally designed for milk and other beverages. The ingestion of these hydrocarbon mixtures has caused numerous fatalities, particularly in children and infants.

Toxicology: The chief systemic reaction to kerosene and related petroleum hydrocarbons is central nervous depression. Because of its low volatility, kerosene is seldom hazardous as a vapor, but gasoline is poisonous at a concentration of 0.2 per cent in air. There appears to be a narrow margin between the anesthetic and lethal doses, but in non-fatal poisonings serious after-effects are almost never encountered.

Less kerosene is required to produce anesthesia when it is inhaled as a vapor than when it is ingested as a liquid, apparently because absorption from the bowel is slow and incomplete. Oral ad-

ministration, however, entails an additional hazard in that vomiting and eructation predispose to the aspiration of liquid kerosene into the respiratory tract. Because these hydrocarbons are irritants, aspiration almost invariably results in severe and often fatal pulmonary edema. Although probably less important than aspiration, a similar pulmonary lesion may arise from petroleum hydrocarbons which have been absorbed from the alimentary tract and carried to the lungs by the circulation. Besides central nervous depression and local irritation, mild and presumably reversible lesions of a degenerative and sometimes hemorrhagic nature are occasionally reported in visceral organs such as the lungs, liver, kidneys, bone marrow, and spleen. Sometimes the myocardium is so sensitized that small amounts of endogenous epinephrine precipitate ventricular fibrillation and sudden death, but aromatic solvents like benzene are probably more hazardous in this respect.

The mean lethal dose cannot be stated with certainty. By the oral route, 3 to 4 oz. is probably a reasonable estimate for an average adult, although at least twice this amount has been tolerated and as little as half an ounce has caused death. Small quantities are often lethal in those cases with pulmonary lesions secondary to aspiration, a complication to which infants and children are particularly susceptible. In fatal poisoning death usually occurs within 2 to 24 hours after ingestion.

The relation between toxic signs and symptoms and the chemical composition of petroleum distillates has not been adequately established. Although pure samples of aliphatic hydrocarbons like hexane have been used experimentally to induce typical toxic reactions, unsaturated hydrocarbons, aromatic rings, and naphthenes undoubtedly contribute to the usual clinical intoxication. For example, the aromatic constituents are particularly irritating to skin and mucous membranes. Hydrocarbons of all types induce central nervous depression, but the aliphatic hydrocarbons (which predominate in petroleum distillates) are said to produce profound coma with an inhibition of deep tendon reflexes, while the coma from aromatic hydrocarbons is characterized by motor restlessness, tremors, and hyperactive reflexes. In the aliphatic series, narcotic potency increases with the chain length at least through octane, but very large molecules (hexadecane and above) are essentially innocuous, apparently because they are not absorbed from the alimentary tract. Consequently petroleum fractions above kerosene (*e.g.*, lubricating oils and paraffin oils) are much less toxic than kerosene itself, and are essentially benign if refined by the removal of unsaturated derivatives. In experimental animals, cyclo-paraffins (naphthenes) have a greater narcotic potency and lethality than do aliphatic hydro-

carbons with the same boiling point. Gasoline (plain or leaded) is said to be more toxic than kerosene in children. If this distinction is valid, it may be due to differences in aliphatic chain length or to differences in non-aliphatic constituents. In any case, gasoline additives such as tetraethyl lead do not contribute appreciably to the acute toxicity. In view of the variation in molecular composition among different petroleum fractions and among different samples of the same fraction, it is surprising that the clinical syndrome of acute intoxication is as uniform as described.

The only recommended treatment is symptomatic and supportive. Because of the danger of aspiration, emetics should never be prescribed. For the same reason, some clinicians believe that gastric lavage is inadvisable. With proper caution and correct technique, however, the risk of aspiration is minimized, and if done promptly, lavage is probably always advisable after a large quantity of kerosene has been swallowed.

Symptomatology (also see discussion of aromatic solvents on p. 181).

A. Inhalation
1. Transient euphoria ("naphtha jag"), resembling alcoholic intoxication.
2. Burning sensation in the chest.
3. Headache, tinnitus, nausea.
4. Weakness, restlessness, and incoordination.
5. Confusion and disorientation, leading to drowsiness and eventually coma, sometimes with convulsions.
6. Vasomotor disturbances causing, for example, cyanosis of the extremities.
7. Rarely sudden death, presumably due to ventricular fibrillation.
8. Death usually due to respiratory arrest.

B. Ingestion.
1. Local irritation with burning sensation in mouth, esophagus, and stomach.
2. Vomiting, eructation, and diarrhea with blood-tinged stools.
3. Drowsiness and any of the other signs and symptoms described above may be observed after ingestion, but the usual clinical course is quite benign unless liquid hydrocarbon is aspirated into the respiratory tract.
4. The sudden development of rapid breathing, cyanosis, tachycardia, and low-grade fever are the usual signs of pulmonary involvement, generally secondary to unrecognized aspiration. Basilar rales rapidly progress to massive pulmonary edema or to pneumonic hemorrhage, infiltration, and secondary infection. Death may result from asphyxia.
5. Severe or untreated cases may develop confluent pneumonia, cardiac dilatation, he-

patosplenomegaly, urinary changes consisting of albumin, cells and casts, and auricular fibrillation-flutter associated with cardiac failure.

Treatment:

1. Emetics are definitely contraindicated.
2. Cautious gastric lavage with copious amount of water or a weak sodium bicarbonate solution (3 per cent). Observe all precautions prescribed on p. 6. At the conclusion of lavage, instill 30 to 60 ml. of mineral oil in the stomach, as well as a saline cathartic in water (e.g., sodium sulfate).
3. If central nervous depression is prominent, nikethamide (Coramine) or caffeine sodium benzoate may be employed parenterally.
4. Parenteral antibiotic therapy as prophylaxis against bacterial invasion of the lungs.
5. Supportive treatment of pulmonary edema

by the use of positive pressure oxygen therapy (p. 192).

6. Avoid epinephrine because of its possible adverse effects on the sensitized myocardium. Avoid digestible fats, oils, and alcohol, which may promote absorption from the bowel.

Laboratory:

1. Repeated electrocardiograms are desirable to detect myocardial damage and conduction defects.
2. An unexpected and unexplained hemoglobinemia has been reported occasionally in man and experimental animals. When possible, an attempt should be made to detect it.
3. Blood disorders are rarely seen in acute poisonings; in chronic exposures they are presumably due to the small content of benzene which is present in all except highly purified samples.

LEAD

Lead and its salts are used in a wide variety of processes in and out of industry. For example the metal is used in printer's type, storage battery plates, solder, electric cable covering, bearing alloys, pipes, and gun shot. The carbonate, chromate, and various oxides are found in paints and pottery glaze ("white lead" is the carbonate). Salts like the arsenate are used in agriculture as insecticidal sprays. Occasionally solutions of the subacetate serve in medicine as external astringents. Cases of lead poisoning have been traced to tetraethyl lead in gasolene.

Toxicology: Lead is poisonous in all forms. It is one of the most hazardous of the toxic metals because the poison is cumulative and the toxic effects are many and severe. Acute intoxications from a single dose are unusual, but they have resulted from the accidental ingestion of solutions of soluble lead salts. After the immediate reaction subsides, a threat remains that severe and even fatal attacks may reappear within days or weeks. These delayed and persistent reactions are usually indistinguishable from the signs and symptoms of typical chronic plumbism, where intoxication arises from the cumulative retention of lead from repeated small exposures. Like the latter, the delayed reaction may develop insidiously or with dramatic suddenness. Thus the acute and chronic syndromes may merge, and both are discussed below.

Following ingestion of a large amount of any soluble lead salt (especially the acetate, carbonate, or chromate), the signs and symptoms are due largely to local irritation of the alimentary tract. If absorption is sufficient, pain, leg cramps, muscle weakness, paresthesias, depression, coma, and death may follow within one or two days. An acute hemolytic crisis and/or severe renal damage may compli-

cate the illness. Fatal poisonings of this type have been described after the ingestion of lead acetate and carbonate in doses which usually exceed 30 gm.

Another type of acute lead poisoning has followed industrial exposures to tetraethyl lead vapor. As with volatile mercury compounds, the chief derangement here occurs within the central nervous system and manifests itself as insomnia, headache, restlessness, irritability, ataxia, delusions, mania and sometimes convulsions. This type of intoxication appears to have a better prognosis than the closely related encephalopathy of chronic plumbism (see below).

If sufficient lead is retained after a single exposure, a syndrome identical with chronic intoxication may develop within weeks or months. Many acute poisonings, however, subside without sequelae, since the absorption of lead from the bowel is inherently slow and incomplete. Presumably this outcome is also favored by vigorous treatment. As long as the body, however, contains excessive amounts of lead fixed in the tissues (notably bone), symptomatic recurrences are an everpresent threat. Whether insidious or sudden in onset, a recurrence may occur without an exciting incident, or may be precipitated by any stressful situation. In all cases these episodes are regularly associated with a definite and characteristic rise in the lead concentration of the body fluids and excreta.

In spite of the multiplicity of symptoms, acute crises in chronic plumbism are treated in essentially the same way as acute lead poisoning, according to the outline below. These measures are designed to reduce the concentration of free lead in blood and body fluids in any of three ways: a) by preventing the absorption or resorption of lead from the alimentary tract; b) by promoting the urinary and

biliary excretion of lead without damage to the excretory organs, and c) by accelerating the deposition of lead in bone. The asymptomatic patient with a high body content of lead is a special problem beyond the scope of this discussion, especially since the desirability and practicability of de-leading procedures in such a patient are subjects of controversy. In symptomatic episodes the most effective single therapeutic agent appears to be the calcium disodium salt of ethylenediamine tetraacetic acid (EDTA) or edathamil calcium-disodium. This compound forms a stable, soluble, non-toxic, virtually non-ionic complex with lead ions. The result of administration is usually a considerable rise in the urinary excretion of lead and at least a transient suppression of toxic signs and symptoms, including even the manifestations of lead encephalopathy. Dimercaprol (BAL) also forms a complex with lead, but for reasons that are not fully understood, BAL has seldom proved useful in the treatment of clinical lead poisoning.

The diagnosis of chronic plumbism is beyond the scope of this discussion, but in brief, three clinical syndromes are recognized. The alimentary type is characterized by anorexia, a metallic taste, constipation, and severe abdominal cramps (lead colic) due to intestinal spasm and sometimes associated with rigidity of the abdominal wall, leading to misdiagnoses and even surgical intervention. The neuromuscular type consists of peripheral neuritis which is usually painless and limited to the extensor muscles. A wrist drop is the most characteristic lesion of lead palsy. Weakness or paralysis may occasionally be accompanied by arthralgia and myalgia, but sensation is otherwise unaffected. The cerebral type of lead poisoning has been called lead encephalopathy and is the most common type in children; it is described below. In any one of these types of chronic plumbism, the patient may show facial pallor, a gingival lead line, mild jaundice, anemia, basophilic stippling of the red blood cells, albuminuria, cylindruria, porphyrinuria, and excessive urinary concentrations of lead.

Symptomatology:
A. Acute poisoning by ingestion only
  1. An astringent and metallic taste in the mouth, dry throat, thirst.
  2. Burning abdominal pain, nausea, and vomiting. The vomitus may appear milky due to the presence of lead chloride. The abdominal pain may become colicky and severe.
  3. Sometimes diarrhea, less often constipation. The stools may be bloody, or black due to the presence of lead sulfide.
  4. Peripheral circulatory collapse (shock).
  5. Neuromuscular symptoms include muscular weakness, pain, and cramps, especially in the legs.

6. Central nervous system manifestations include headache, insomnia, paresthesias, depression, coma, and death.
7. Though usually of secondary concern, kidney damage may result in oliguria, albuminuria, and cylindruria. The renal lesion may be due to the mildly nephrotoxic action of lead, to disturbances in kidney circulation, or to the products of intravascular hemolysis.
8. An acute hemolytic crisis sometimes develops and results in anemia and hemoglobinuria.
9. Death may occur within one or two days, but recovery is the rule. Convalescence is slow and may be interrupted by episodes like those seen in typical chronic poisoning (see above).

B. Lead encephalopathy in chronic lead poisoning (as described in children)
  1. Headache and insomnia.
  2. Persistent vomiting, which is sometimes projectile. A typical lead colic may or may not be present.
  3. Visual disturbances, choked optic disks.
  4. Irritability, restlessness, delirium, hallucinations.
  5. Convulsions and coma.
  6. The intracranial pressure is characteristically high. The cerebrospinal fluid is generally unremarkable except for an elevation of total protein.
  7. Death from exhaustion and respiratory failure. The mortality rate is high; recovery is slow and frequently incomplete.

Treatment:
A. Acute poisoning by ingestion
  1. Gastric lavage with a 1 per cent solution of sodium or magnesium sulfate. Leave 15 to 30 gm. of magnesium sulfate in 6 to 8 ounces of water in the stomach, both as an antidote and as a cathartic.
  2. Egg white, milk, and tannin are useful demulcents.
  3. For abdominal pain atropine sulfate and other antispasmodics should be given a trial, but morphine may become necessary.
  4. Intravenous calcium chloride (5 ml. of a 10 per cent solution) or calcium gluconate (10 ml. of a 20 per cent solution) may cause a temporary suppression of lead colic and other untoward symptoms.
  5. Dehydration, shock, and electrolyte disturbances should be treated by the parenteral administration of isotonic saline (p. 215).
  6. Give edathamil calcium-disodium (Ca-Na$_2$-EDTA) by slow intravenous drip in concentrations of 3 per cent or less. A satisfactory solution can be prepared by dilut-

ing a 5-ml. ampul (containing 1 gm.) to a volume of about 50 ml. with isotonic saline or 5 per cent dextrose solution. Two infusions may be given a day, at an injection rate not in excess of 0.17 gm./hr. (or 0.33 gm./day) for each 10 lb. (4.5 kg.) of body weight. This program may be continued for a maximum of 5 to 7 days (maximum total dose 2.5 gm./10 lb.). If necessary this course of therapy may be repeated once, after a rest period of 7 days. With these precautions untoward reactions from edathamil are virtually unknown, but because the drug is still relatively new, caution is advisable.

B. Treatment of lead encephalopathy: The treat-ment measures outlined above are generally appropriate. In addition, large doses of barbiturate drugs may be necessary to control extreme degrees of central nervous excitation. Occasionally intracranial decompression by the cautious removal of cerebrospinal fluid may become advisable.

Laboratory: The many laboratory aids for the diagnosis of chronic lead poisoning (*e.g.*, stippling of red blood cells) are beyond the scope of this discussion. In general a 24-hour specimen of urine is always desirable for a chemical determination of lead and of porphyrins. A blood analysis for lead is helpful if the blood sample is taken and stored in specially cleaned glassware.

MERCURY

A host of mercury compounds have served in clinical medicine as antiseptics, antisyphilitics, cathartics, and diuretics. Modern agriculture also employs many organic and inorganic derivatives of mercury in the form of dusts, wettable powders, solutions, and fumigant vapors; these preparations serve as fungicides and as seed and cereal protectants.

Toxicology: All forms of mercury are poisonous if absorbed. When ingested the bichloride is probably the most dangerous; fatalities have resulted from as little as 0.5 gm., although the mean lethal dose in adults probably lies between 1 and 4 gm. Every known class of mercury compound is potentially hazardous, and each has given rise to typical mercury intoxication under appropriate circumstances; this includes the free metal, calomel, modern mercurial antiseptic dyes, and mercurial diuretic drugs. Most of the poisonous actions are associated with the mercuric ion, which these inorganic and organic materials furnish rapidly or slowly. Acute poisoning is the major threat in the home and on the farm, but because mercury is a cumulative poison, subacute and chronic intoxications are recognized, particularly in industry.

The alimentary absorption of many mercury compounds (notably mercuric chloride) is so rapid that the course and prognosis are determined largely by events within the first 10 to 15 minutes, particularly by the intervention of vomiting or a therapeutic lavage. Many mercury compounds (including mercuric chloride in concentrations of 1 to 5 per cent) are irritating to the skin and may produce dermatitis with or without vesication. Absorption from intact skin is sometimes sufficient to produce systemic poisoning. Contact with the eyes causes ulceration of the conjunctiva and cornea. The respiratory tract is the usual portal in accidental exposures to volatile mercury compounds, including the metal (quicksilver). Acute mercurialism may end fatally within a few minutes, but death (in uremia) is usually delayed 5 to 12 days.

When corrosive preparations are ingested (*e.g.*, ionizable mercuric salts), necrosis begins immediately in the mouth, throat, esophagus, and stomach. Within a few minutes violent pain, profuse vomiting, and severe purging are experienced, and the patient may die within a few hours from peripheral vascular collapse secondary to fluid and electrolyte losses. If the patient survives this phase, the primary gastroenteritis subsides spontaneously within a few days. A second phase, developing within 1 to 3 days after the exposure, is characterized by stomatitis, membranous colitis, and tubular nephritis (nephrosis). This second phase, which is seen even with noncorrosive preparations of mercury and is independent of the portal of entry, is associated with a slow and prolonged excretion of mercury by the salivary glands, the gastrointestinal mucosa, and the kidneys. Death in this phase is usually the result of complete renal failure.

Mental and nervous symptoms are not common in acute mercurialism (in contrast to chronic mercury and acute arsenic poisonings). One important exception should be noted. Many organic mercury compounds used in agriculture (*e.g.*, alkyl mercuric salts, phenylmercuric derivatives) produce prompt and marked nervous symptoms, which include ataxia, restriction of the visual fields, paresis, and delirium. These effects are associated with the deposition of mercury in the brain and spinal cord. While alarming, these signs and symptoms may be surprisingly transient.

Symptomatology:

A. First phase

1. Burning pain, sense of constriction, and ashen discoloration of the mucous membrane in mouth and pharynx, occurring immediately after the ingestion of corrosive mercury salts.

2. Within a few minutes intense epigastric pain, followed by diffuse abdominal pain and associated with almost continuous vomiting of mucoid material, which frequently contains blood and shreds of mucous membrane.

3. Severe purging, with liquid, bloody stools and considerable tenesmus.

4. Metallic taste, with excessive salivation and thirst.

5. A rapid, weak pulse; shallow breathing; pallor; prostration, collapse, and death.

6. Most organic mercurial fumigants, when inhaled, are capable of inducing prompt nervous symptoms: ataxia, restriction of visual field, paresis, and delirium.

7. Signs and symptoms listed above (except for no. 6) are not encountered with mercury compounds of low irritancy or with portals of entry other than the mouth. In these cases the first clinical evidence of poisoning may be phase 2 (see B).

B. Second phase. If death does not intervene, phase 2 begins in 1 to 3 days (unless vomiting so effectively removed the poison that absorption was negligible).

8. The gastroenteritis described above tends to subside in about 36 hours under the influence of local treatment.

9. Mercurial stomatitis may appear within 24 to 36 hours. It is characterized by a glossitis and ulcerative gingivitis. Salivation is marked (ptyalism). Severe infections, loosening of teeth, and necrosis of the jaw are major complications.

10. Necrosis of the renal tubules is evident within 2 to 3 days. In sequence the results are transient polyuria, albuminuria, cylindruria, anuria, and eventual death associated with azotemia and renal acidosis, or recovery within 10 to 14 days.

11. A membranous colitis first appears many days after the original exposure. It is evidenced by dysentery, tenesmus, ulceration of the colonic mucosa, and hemorrhage. Liver necrosis sometimes develops. In neglected cases collapse and death may occur weeks after the start of the illness.

Treatment (Emergency):

1. Give egg whites, milk, or "universal antidote" (see p. 10) to help precipitate mercury in the stomach. Then induce vomiting (see p. 2).

2. Gastric lavage with egg white solution, 5 per cent solution of sodium formaldehyde sulfoxalate, or 2 to 5 per cent solution of sodium bicarbonate.

3. Administer one-half to one ounce of sodium or magnesium sulfate in 6 to 8 oz. of water (unless spontaneous purging has already begun).

4. Administer BAL (dimercaprol) intramuscularly as a 10 per cent solution in oil. If given within 3 hours after ingestion, severe renal damage may be prevented. Dosage schedules are suggested below. In severe poisoning many clinicians prefer an initial dose of 5.0 mg. BAL/kg. and maintenance doses of 2.5 mg./kg. every 3 hours during the first 24 hours (see p. 117 for the clinical toxicity of BAL).

	Severe Metal Poisoning	Mild Metal Poisoning
1st day	3.0 mg./kg. q4h (6 inj.)	2.5 mg./kg. q4h (6 inj.)
2nd day	3.0 mg./kg. q4h (6 inj.)	2.5 mg./kg. q6h (4 inj.)
3rd day	3.0 mg./kg. q6h (4 inj.)	2.5 mg./kg. q12h (2 inj.)
Each of the following 10 days (or until recovery)	3.0 mg./kg. q12h (2 inj.)	2.5 mg./kg. qd (1 inj.)

5. Demulcents (e.g., milk of magnesia, starch, bismuth subcarbonate) and analgetic drugs may be useful and necessary.

6. Treat shock (peripheral vascular collapse) by correcting dehydration and electrolyte imbalances (see p. 215).

7. If renal insufficiency develops, see p. $$$ for the management of acute renal failure.

8. The maintenance of an adequate nutritional status (see p. 222) may be troublesome if colitis becomes severe or persistent.

Laboratory: Mercury analyses of blood and urine are available in special laboratories, but there is no simple reliable method of analysis.

METHYL ALCOHOL

Methyl alcohol (methanol, wood alcohol) is a widely used solvent in paints, varnishes and paint removers. It is used alone as an antifreeze fluid and with ethanol and soap as a solid canned fuel.

Toxicology: Methyl alcohol is readily absorbed from the gastrointestinal and respiratory tracts. As little as 2 teaspoonsful is considered toxic if ingested. The fatal dose in man lies between 2 and 8 ounces; this range implies a high variation in individual susceptibility. Death may be prompt, but it

is usually delayed for several days, and the mortality rate is high. The prognosis improves if treatment is instituted before visual disturbances appear.

When methanol consumption is uncomplicated by the intake of ethyl alcohol, inebriation and subsequent drowsiness are said to be mild and transient. This phase may be followed by an entirely asymptomatic interval. The characteristic signs and symptoms develop in rapid succession after a latency of 6 to 30 hours (usually 12 to 18) following the initial intake. Because these late effects are produced by pure samples, impurities are thought to play no important role in the toxicity of methyl alcohol.

The symptoms of methyl alcohol poisoning result from a combination of factors, of which a characteristic metabolic acidosis appears to be the trigger. Central nervous depression is due partly to this acidosis and partly to cerebral edema. Acidosis is the result of methanol oxidation to formic acid, which accumulates and reduces severely the body's alkali reserve. For unknown reasons other organic acids also tend to accumulate. The severity of essentially all symptoms in methanol poisoning is said to be proportional to the intensity of this delayed acidosis. In contrast to human exposures, a long latent period, relatively high toxicity, acidosis, and ocular injury are *not* features of methyl alcohol intoxication in laboratory animals.

Visual disturbances, which are the most distinctive aspect of methanol poisoning in man, may become evident soon after the severe phase begins. Dilated, unreactive pupils and dimness of vision are characteristic. The ocular lesion, which involves chiefly the ganglion cells of the retina, is a destructive inflammation followed by atrophy. In the acute phase the retina is congested and edematous, and the edges of the optic disk may be blurred. The result is bilateral blindness, which is usually permanent unless treatment is prompt and energetic. Even if complete blindness is avoided, residual scotomata are common.

Ethyl alcohol, when consumed at the same time as methyl alcohol, prolongs the latent period before toxic symptoms appear. It has also been observed that even severe symptoms of methanol poisoning are alleviated by the ingestion of ethanol, and for this reason, the recommended treatment includes ethanol in small quantities (*e.g.*, whiskey, 1 oz. every 3 to 4 hours by mouth or stomach tube). The mechanism of this protection may lie in the ability of ethyl alcohol to inhibit the metabolic oxidation of methanol, even though this rate is inherently slow. This hypothesis has been proved in rats by using radioactively labelled alcohols.

Symptomatology (after a latency usually of 12 to 18 hours):

1. Headache, anorexia, weakness, leg cramps, vertigo, progressing either to apathy and coma or less frequently to excitement, mania, and convulsions.
2. Nausea and vomiting. Violent abdominal pain, back pain, leg pain.
3. Dimness of vision with dilated pupils, reacting poorly, if at all, to light, followed often by bilateral blindness (transient or permanent). Eyes are often sensitive to pressure, and eye movements are painful.
4. Breathing: rapid and shallow, or deep and labored (Kussmaul type).
5. Weak, rapid pulse; hypotension, cyanosis. The cyanosis may be due to abnormal blood pigments.
6. Death is due to respiratory failure or rarely to circulatory collapse.
7. Protracted convalescence with asthenia, blindness, and impaired renal function.

Treatment:

1. Gastric lavage with 3 to 5 per cent sodium bicarbonate, leaving some solution in the stomach after the lavage.
2. Whiskey (or 50 per cent ethanol in water) 1 oz. every 3 to 4 hours by mouth or by stomach tube, until acidosis is corrected by alkali and perhaps for 24 hours thereafter.
3. The treatment of acidosis may be life-saving and sight-saving. Give 4 gm. sodium bicarbonate by mouth (or by stomach tube if necessary) every 15 minutes until the urine becomes alkaline or the plasma CO_2 combining power is normal. Repeat the course of alkali treatment as indicated. Even when fully corrected, the acidosis may recur at any time during the first several days. Avoid sodium lactate as an alkalinizing agent since lactate metabolism may be impaired in these patients. Check plasma CO_2 combining power, preferably every hour. Also see p. 217–219.
4. Nikethamide, caffeine, oxygen, and artificial respiration (p. 185), if respirations become weak and insufficient.
5. Protect patient's eyes from light.
6. Morphine for abdominal pain (unless respiration is depressed).
7. Dextrose and saline may be administered intravenously.

Laboratory: Check blood alcohol level and plasma CO_2 combining power (or urine acidity) at repeated intervals (preferably every hour, since relapses are common).

METHYL BROMIDE

Methyl bromide is a gas at ordinary temperatures (boiling point of 40.1°F or 4.6°C at atmospheric pressure); it is usually sold as a liquid under pressure. It is widely used in fire extinguishers, as a re-

frigerant gas, and as an insecticidal fumigant. At low vapor concentrations (which may produce poisonings over a long period of time), methyl bromide is not detectable by taste or odor.

Toxicology: Even at high vapor concentrations the symptoms are characteristically delayed. The usual latency after inhalation is between 4 and 12 hours. Any one of the following acute toxic reactions may be the immediate cause of death: coma, convulsions, and pulmonary edema. Renal failure due to tubular necrosis, bronchopneumonia, and paralysis have all been reported as late sequelae. When spilled on the skin, liquid methyl bromide produces blisters if evaporation is delayed in any way, for example by gloves or other clothing.

Unlike methyl chloride, no biochemical evidence exists that the toxicity of methyl bromide is due to its hydrolysis to methyl alcohol. Many of the toxic symptoms, however, are similar to those from methanol, notably the characteristic latent period, abdominal pain, nausea, vomiting, mental confusion, occasional visual disturbance, and metabolic acidosis. However the characteristically severe acidosis of methanol intoxication has not been described in poisonings due to methyl bromide; vomiting is probably adequate to explain the comparatively mild acidosis in methyl bromide poisoning. Similarly visual disturbances appear to be much milder and more transient than those due to methyl alcohol or methyl chloride. Another property not shared by the chloride or alcohol is the bromide's ability to methylate various protein molecules. *In vitro* this reaction has been studied particularly with sulfhydryl enzymes. Indeed, dimercaprol (BAL) has been shown to have prophylactic activity in mice experimentally poisoned with methyl bromide, and probably BAL should have a clinical trial if it can be administered in the latent period preceding toxic symptoms. From these considerations it appears unlikely that the toxicity of methyl bromide is due to its hydrolysis to methyl alcohol.

Symptomatology (4 to 12 hours after inhalation of vapor):

1. Dizziness and headache.
2. Anorexia, nausea, vomiting, and abdominal pain.
3. Lassitude, profound weakness, slurring of speech, and staggering gait.
4. Transient blurring of vision, diplopia, sometimes strabismus, and even temporary blindness.
5. Mental confusion, mania, tremors, and epileptiform convulsions.
6. Rapid respirations, associated with signs of severe pulmonary edema, cyanosis, pallor, and collapse. The pulmonary edema, convulsions, and mental confusion may occur independently of one another.
7. Coma, areflexia, and death from respiratory or circulatory collapse.
8. Late sequelae include bronchopneumonia after severe pulmonary lesions, renal failure with anuria due to tubular degeneration, and severe weakness with or without evidence of paralysis. These difficulties, however, tend to subside within one or two weeks, and complete recovery is the rule.

Treatment:

1. Remove promptly from a contaminated atmosphere.
2. If the patient is first seen in the asymptomatic (latent) period, a therapeutic trial with dimercaprol (BAL) should be considered. Use the dosage schedule on p. 117.
3. Quickly remove any contaminated clothing. Methyl bromide can penetrate ordinary rubber gloves. (All contaminated clothing should be carefully aerated before being reworn.) Wash contaminated skin carefully with water. Blistered areas are best covered with a sterile vaseline dressing, which should be changed as indicated.
4. Restrain the confused or maniacal patient (p. 201). Treat convulsions by the parenteral administration of anticonvulsive drugs. See p. 202 for the technique of administering barbiturates.
5. Any marked metabolic acidosis must be corrected by the cautious administration of alkali. The problem is complicated by the threat of pulmonary edema and of renal shutdown; except for these complications, acidosis should be treated vigorously. See p. 217.
6. Administer positive pressure oxygen for impending pulmonary edema. See p. 192 for supportive treatment in this syndrome.
7. Because of central nervous depression with coma and respiratory paralysis, artificial respiration may become necessary (p. 185).
8. Even if asymptomatic, the patient should be kept under observation for at least 48 hours.
9. Treat renal failure (with anuria) according to the principals on p. 210.

Laboratory:

1. Frequent chemical determinations of the blood electrolytes, particularly the plasma CO_2 and chloride levels, to detect and measure a metabolic acidosis. The urine, if any, may contain albumin, cells, and casts.
2. No simple chemical tests are available for the diagnosis of methyl bromide poisoning.

MORPHINE

Morphine and other natural alkaloids of opium serve many uses in clinical medicine. These materials are commonly prescribed as powdered opium, tincture of opium (laudanum), camphorated tinc-

ture of opium (paregoric), pantopon, and various acid salts and solutions of morphine. Codeine, dihydromorphinone (dilaudid), and methyldihydromorphinone (metopon) are common derivatives of morphine currently used in therapy. Heroine, an illegal derivative of morphine, is important because it is the favorite opiate of narcotic addicts in eastern United States, but the management of chronic addiction and of the withdrawal syndrome are beyond the scope of this manual.

Toxicology: Acute morphine poisoning may arise from a suicidal act, from an error in an addict's estimation of his own tolerance, or from accidental overdosage in therapy. Homicidal poisoning is rare. Iatrogenic intoxication has been reported often in victims of traumatic shock, who may appear to require large or repeated doses only because the drug is poorly absorbed from parenteral sites until an adequate circulation is re-established. In a normal adult who is not in pain, 60 mg. of morphine is generally a toxic dose; 100 mg. is always dangerous, and the probable lethal dose lies between 120 and 250 mg. (2 to 4 grains). Infants and young children are thought to be more susceptible on a body weight basis, but this time-honored impression has recently been denied by at least one competent investigator. Elderly persons and patients with myxedema are comparatively intolerant of morphine and other opiates, while patients with hyperthyroidism and those in severe pain have a high tolerance. The highest levels of tolerance, however, are encountered in narcotic addicts, some of whom take more than 1000 mg. of morphine daily, with few objective signs other than miosis and constipation.

Morphine is absorbed through all mucous membranes, including the buccal, nasal, and respiratory mucosae, but ingestion is the commonest mode of administration. The nature of the toxic syndrome is not determined by the portal of entry. Signs and symptoms begin within 20 to 40 minutes after ingestion. Once established, morphine poisoning presents most of the classical features of central nervous depression. Although not diagnostic, the triad of coma, pinpoint pupils, and profoundly depressed respiration strongly suggests morphine poisoning. In acute morphinism death occurs typically within 6 to 12 hours. The patient who survives the first 24 hours has a favorable prognosis. Death is nearly always due to respiratory failure. If not the cause of death, circulatory insufficiency is at least often contributory. When present, cardiovascular collapse is usually a consequence of severe anoxia from inadequate lung ventilation. Sometimes pulmonary complications such as edema or pneumonia are responsible for death in morphine poisoning.

Opium, laudanum, paregoric, and pantopon owe their toxicity to their contents of morphine. Alkaloids related to morphine have qualitatively similar actions, but many of them are weaker depressants and stronger stimulants. For example, thebain is a weak narcotic and a potent convulsant, and toxic doses of codeine produce restlessness and excitement rather than coma.

A vigorous program of symptomatic and supportive treatment has saved many victims of morphine poisoning. The single most important element in therapy is the correction of anoxia by all available means: the maintenance of a patent airway, the administration of oxygen, the use of artificial respiration, and the injection of analeptic drugs which stimulate respiratory activity. Because morphine is a potential convulsant, recognized convulsants like strychnine and picrotoxin are avoided in the treatment of morphinism, but caffeine, amphetamine, ephedrine, and metrazol are sometimes used. In most clinics, however, the conventional analeptic drugs have been displaced by N-allylnormorphine (nalorphine or Nalline). Given parenterally, this morphine analogue promptly antagonizes the respiratory depression, coma, and hypotension of morphine poisoning. Under appropriate conditions most of the other recognized actions of morphine have been reduced or abolished. The beneficial effects of nalorphine in the treatment of morphinism have been ascribed to a competition between the two substances for hypothetical receptor sites in critical tissues. Although this hypothesis has many satisfactory features, it is not entirely adequate.

The following miscellaneous observations on nalorphine are of particular interest to the therapist. In the absence of morphine, nalorphine has many of the actions of morphine, though to a lesser degree. Among the central nervous effects described in normal man are nausea, giddiness, sweating, lightheadedness, euphoria, itching, drowsiness, crying, anxiety, postural hypotension, a depression in the respiratory minute volume (without a consistent change in the respiratory rate), and an inhibition of the normal respiratory response to carbon dioxide. In a compensated morphine or opium addict, a small dose of nalorphine (3 mg. subcutaneously) is usually sufficient to precipitate an unequivocal withdrawal syndrome. Morphine antagonism in not always demonstrable with nalorphine, especially in patients who receive only small doses of morphine. A therapeutic failure with this antidote, therefore, does not rule out a diagnosis of morphinism. Conversely, a positive response cannot be regarded as diagnostic of morphine or opium poisoning. For example, nalorphine has been shown to antagonize in man many of the depressant actions of heroine, dilaudid, methadone, metapon, and meperidine (Demerol); its action against codeine is not described. With the possible exception of the thiobarbiturates, nal-

orphine is ineffective against such central nervous depressants as the barbiturates, paraldehyde, nitrous oxide, *etc.*

Symptomatology:

1. Supralethal doses of morphine produce prompt coma, but sublethal doses usually lead to a transient period of euphoria and exhilaration, characterized by a sensation of warmth and comfort, appearing within half an hour after ingestion.
2. Gradual drowsiness, dizziness, heaviness of the head, weariness, diminution of sensibility, loss of pain and other modalities of sensation.
3. Nausea and vomiting.
4. A transient excitement stage, characterized by extreme restlessness, delirium, and rarely epileptiform convulsions, is sometimes seen in children and rarely in adult women.
5. Bilateral miosis, progressing to pinpoint pupils, which do not react to light or accommodation. The pupils may dilate during terminal asphyxia.
6. Itching of the skin and nose, sometimes with skin rashes and urticaria.
7. Coma, with muscular relaxation and depressed or absent superficial and deep reflexes. A Babinski toe sign may appear.
8. Marked slowing of the respiratory rate with inadequate pulmonary ventilation and consequent cyanosis. Breathing becomes stertorous and irregular (Cheyne-Stokes or Biot).
9. The pulse is slow and the blood pressure gradually falls to shock levels. Urine formation ceases or is reduced to a very low rate.
10. The skin is cold and pale and shows a mottled cyanosis. The body temperature falls.
11. Death within 6 to 12 hours is usually due to respiratory arrest and consequent asphyxia. Sometimes shock, pulmonary edema, hypostatic or aspiration pneumonia contribute significantly to the fatal outcome.
12. During the recovery phase, itching, headache, nausea, vomiting, confusion, and obstipation may require attention. A symptomatic relapse may signal developing bronchopneumonia.

Treatment:

1. Even several hours after the ingestion of morphine, gastric lavage may be beneficial, because the drug often induces pylorospasm. A potassium permanganate solution (1:5000) or 1 ml. of tincture of iodine in a liter (quart) of water makes a satisfactory lavage fluid. Precautions against aspiration are essential. Emetics are rarely successful and are potentially dangerous. Save gastric contents for analysis.
2. Leave in the stomach 15 to 30 gm. of sodium sulfate in water as a saline cathartic.
3. In morphine overdosage due to subcutaneous or intramuscular injection, a tourniquet or ice bag may be used to delay absorption.
4. Try to keep the patient awake by mild continuous stimulation that arouses but does not exhaust him. Moderately intense stimuli constitute an effective antidote against an impending morphine coma.
5. Correct airway obstruction. The insertion of an oropharyngeal airway is usually advisable in a comatous patient who has no gag reflex. See p. 184.
6. Continuous or intermittent oxygen therapy is usually indicated, but there is rarely, if ever, justification for the use of O_2-CO_2 mixtures. See p. 189.
7. Sometimes the inhalation of oxygen causes an arrest of spontaneous breathing. Artificial respiration is then essential. Do not wait for respiratory arrest, but give mechanical assistance whenever the rate or depth of breathing is clearly inadequate.
8. Respirations can sometimes be maintained by the cautious use of such analeptic drugs as caffeine, nikethamide, pentylenetetrazol, ephedrine, and amphetamine (p. 204). Strychnine and picrotoxin should never be used. Probably the most effective drug, however, is nalorphine (see below).
9. The usual adult dose of nalorphine is 5 to 10 mg. intravenously, but single doses as high as 30 and 40 mg. have been employed. If the rise in pulmonary ventilation is judged inadequate, the dose may be repeated within 10 to 15 minutes, but the cumulative dose probably should not exceed 40 mg. in any four-hour period. In most cases of morphinism, additional injections of nalorphine are necessary within 2 to 3 hours. The therapeutic goal of nalorphine is the correction of respiratory depression and of hypotension associated with morphine intoxication. Superficial and deep reflexes usually improve and sometimes consciousness returns, but no attempt should be made to restore the level of consciousness with this or any other analeptic drugs. See p. 158 for a description of the clinical toxicity of nalorphine.
10. Maintain hydration and electrolyte balance by the modest administration of fluid and salts, but avoid overhydration. Diuretic drugs are without beneficial effects.
11. Hypotension is treated indirectly by the administration of oxygen and the use of such analeptic drugs as ephedrine and ampheta-

mine. Sometimes a plasma transfusion is useful.

12. Good nursing is essential. The body temperature should be maintained if possible. Antibiotic therapy is advisable as prophylaxis against pneumonia. By repeatedly changing the patient's posture, hypostatic pneumonia and decubitus ulcers are avoided. See p. 229.

Laboratory: None of the routine laboratory tests have diagnostic or prognostic significance in acute morphinism. A variety of chemical tests and at least one bioassay procedure are practical ways of detecting morphine and related alkaloids in biological fluids and excreta. Tests are described in most texts on forensic medicine.

NAPHTHALENE

Naphthalene (naphthalin or tar camphor) is a white crystalline solid of very low solubility in water. It is an ingredient of some moth repellents and was formerly used as an intestinal vermifuge.

Toxicology: With the exception of dermatitis due to hypersensitivity, reports of naphthalene poisoning in industry are rare. This record and naphthalene's insolubility and poor absorbability have led many to underestimate its toxicity. Recent accidental poisonings in children reemphasize that small quantities of naphthalene may cause severe gastrointestinal and neurological symptoms, together with acute intravascular hemolysis. Routine questioning rarely reveals the cause of symptoms, but the diagnosis can usually be established by a detailed clinical history and/or toxicological examination of the urine (see below).

Naphthalene is toxic by ingestion, by vapor inhalation, and by skin contact. Cutaneous exposure, however, rarely if ever produces systemic effects, although dermatitis and ocular irritation may be severe. The ingestion of 2 gm. has proved fatal in a child, and the probable lethal dose in an adult lies between 5 and 15 gm. There appear to be marked variations both in individual susceptibility and in the character of the toxic response. Some of the reactions imply states of hypersensitivity, and this impression can often be confirmed by patch testing. A hemolytic crisis constitutes the most spectacular reaction in naphthalene poisoning; it may be followed by renal tubular blockade and acute renal failure. In at least one case liver necrosis and severe jaundice have been reported, without evidence of hemolysis. Various states of central nervous excitation and depression are described, and one of the few long term sequelae is a rare instance of optic neuritis.

In contrast to naphthalene, the only reported effects of methylated naphthalene in man are skin irritation and skin photosensitization. Chlorinated derivatives of naphthalene frequently produce an acneform eruption of the skin and various degrees of liver necrosis.

There is no specific treatment for poisoning by naphthalene or by its derivatives. Absorbed naphthalene is apparently oxidized to α-naphthol, which is found in the urine as naphthol glucuronate and ethereal sulfate.

Symptomatology:

A. Surface contact

1. Ocular irritation but no serious eye injuries are described. Naphthalene cataracts produced experimentally in rabbits have not been described in man.

2. Skin irritation and, in the case of a sensitized person, severe dermatitis. Lesions clear spontaneously as soon as the exposure is terminated.

3. Percutaneous absorption is apparently inadequate to produce acute systemic reactions.

B. Inhalation of vapor

1. Headache, confusion, and excitement.

2. Nausea and sometimes vomiting, and extensive sweating.

3. Occasionally dysuria, hematuria, *etc.*, but an acute hemolytic reaction has not been described after inhalation exposures.

4. Rarely optic neuritis is encountered.

C. Ingestion

1. Abdominal cramps with nausea, vomiting, and diarrhea.

2. Headache, profuse perspiration, listlessness, confusion.

3. In severe poisoning, coma with or without convulsions.

4. Irritation of the urinary bladder, presumably due to excretory products of naphthalene metabolism. Signs and symptoms include urgency, dysuria, and the passage of a brown or black urine with or without albumin and casts; usually these effects disappear within a few days, and they should be distinguished from a hemolytic reaction.

5. Acute intravascular hemolysis may or may not appear. It often begins on the third day and is accompanied by anemia, leucocytosis, fever, hemoglobinuria, jaundice, renal insufficiency, and sometimes disturbances in liver function.

6. In the absence of adequate supportive treatment, death may result from acute renal failure.

Treatment:

1. Induce emesis and perform gastric lavage

with large amounts of warm water, whenever poisoning by mouth is suspected.

2. Instill a saline cathartic such as magnesium or sodium sulfate in water (15 to 30 gm.).

3. Demulcents such as milk, egg white, gelatin, or other protein solutions may be useful, but oils should be avoided because they may promote absorption.

4. Contaminated eyes or skin should be flushed with warm water, followed by the application of a bland ointment.

5. Stimulants such as caffeine sodium benzoate, intramuscularly, as required.

6. A severe anemia due to hemolysis may require small repeated blood transfusions. Cortisone therapy (p. 235) appears to have been beneficial in at least two cases of naphthalene hemolysis.

7. In the event of hemoglobinuria, alkalinize the urine by giving small amounts of sodium bicarbonate (the efficacy of this measure in preventing blockage of renal tubules is doubted by many investigators).

8. Supportive measures in the case of acute renal failure (see p. 210). For the management of a patient with liver necrosis, see p. 213.

Laboratory:

1. Laboratory findings are often compatible with a severe hemolytic anemia.

2. Alpha naphthol is present in the urine, and its detection may be necessary for a definitive diagnosis.

NICOTINE

Nicotine (1-methyl-2-(3-pyridyl) pyrrolidine) is a colorless, volatile, and strongly alkaline liquid, which on exposure to air acquires a brown color and a tobacco-like odor. It is readily soluble in water and forms salts with acids. The alkaloid is obtained from the dried leaves and stems of *Nicotiana tobacum* and *rustica*, where it occurs in concentrations of 2 to 8 per cent with citric and malic acids. Nicotine is encountered most frequently in tobacco products and insecticide preparations. For use as an insecticide it is usually marketed as a 40 per cent solution of the sulfate, but free nicotine is available and is sometimes used. Tobacco is employed not only for smoking and chewing, but it has been used in snuff, enemas, and poultices. Cigarette tobacco varies in its nicotine content, but common blends contain 15 to 20 mg. per cigarette. Cigarette smoke, however, contains less than 10 mg. per cigarette, of which only a few milligrams are usually absorbed. Reactions from chronic exposure to tobacco and nicotine are not considered in this manual.

Toxicology: Nicotine is one of the most toxic of all poisons and acts with great rapidity. It is absorbed from the alimentary canal, respiratory tract, and intact skin. Percutaneous absorption is many times faster with the free alkaloid than with its acid salts. The major effects of nicotine, aside from local caustic actions, are a transient stimulation and subsequent depression or paralysis of the central nervous system, all peripheral autonomic ganglia, and nerve endings in skeletal muscles. In addition smooth muscle cells are perhaps directly excited by the alkaloid, an action which may be partly responsible for the observed vasoconstriction and intestinal movements. These phasic neural and neuromuscular actions of nicotine lead to complex and variegated clinical syndromes.

Taken by mouth the mean lethal dose of nicotine is about 60 mg. in an adult (1 mg./kg.), but marked tolerance to the alkaloid is developed by confirmed smokers. Tobacco is much less toxic than expected from its nicotine content; apparently intestinal absorption is so slow that spontaneous vomiting removes much unabsorbed alkaloid as it is present in tobacco. In fatal cases of nicotine poisoning, death is usually rapid; it occurs nearly always within an hour and occasionally within 5 minutes. Generally death is due to paralysis of the respiratory muscles; paralysis of medullary centers controlling respiration requires a larger dose. If the patient survives 4 hours, the prognosis is good. The elimination of nicotine is complete within sixteen hours; about 80 to 90 per cent is detoxified and the remainder is excreted unchanged in the urine.

Symptomatology:

1. Burning sensation in mouth and throat, salivation, nausea, abdominal pain, vomiting, and diarrhea. (Gastrointestinal reactions are less severe but do occur after cutaneous and respiratory exposures.)

2. Systemic effects include headache, sweating, dizziness, auditory and visual disturbances, confusion, weakness, and incoordination.

3. At first respirations are deep and rapid, the blood pressure is high, and the pulse is slow. Intense vagal stimulation may cause transient cardiac standstill. The pupils are generally constricted. Central nervous excitation is also evidenced by tremors and sometimes by clonic-tonic convulsions.

4. As depression develops, the pupils dilate, the blood pressure falls, and the pulse becomes rapid and often irregular. Faintness, prostration, and dyspnea progress to collapse with terminal convulsions and loss of reflexes.

5. Death from paralysis of respiratory muscles.

Treatment (speed is *imperative*):

1. For ingested poison, administer 6 to 8 heaping teaspoonfuls of "universal antidote" (p. 10) as a slurry in water.
2. Gastric lavage with 0.5 per cent solution of tannic acid or a 1:5000 solution of potassium permanganate.
3. If nicotine is spilled on the skin, wash thoroughly and *immediately* with cold water.
4. Artificial respiration (p. 185) and oxygen therapy (p. 189) until spontaneous breathing is adequate or until the heart ceases to beat. Central respiratory stimulants are rarely if ever indicated. Keep the airway clear (p. 184).
5. If severe or persistent, convulsions may be controlled with small intravenous doses of barbiturates (p. 201).
6. Most of the visceral manifestations can be controlled by various combinations of autonomic blocking drugs, such as atropine and dibenamine. Caramiphen (parpanit) hydrochloride and diethazine (diparcol) hydrochloride, two drugs with complex actions on the central and autonomic nervous systems, have been extolled in the control of experimental nicotine poisoning. Given intravenously in large doses, the latter compound has protected dogs against 100 to 200 lethal doses of nicotine. Although this degree of effectiveness cannot be anticipated in man for many reasons, caramiphen and diethazine deserve clinical trials in acute nicotine poisoning. Only oral preparations are currently available.

Laboratory: Secretion of the adrenal medulla may cause an elevation of blood sugar, but laboratory data are rarely of diagnostic or prognostic help in acute nicotine poisoning.

NITRITE

Nitrites and toxic nitrates are available in many homes as medicinal agents, such as amyl nitrite, nitroglycerin, sodium nitrite, spirit of niter, and bismuth subnitrate. In some rural areas sufficient nitrite and nitrate may be present in contaminated well water to poison infants given this water. Poisonings have also resulted when sodium nitrite was mistaken for sodium chloride in the preparation of food.

Toxicology: The two basic actions of nitrites *in vivo* are the relaxation of smooth muscle, especially in small blood vessels, and in toxic doses the conversion of hemoglobin to methemoglobin. Both organic and inorganc nitrites exhibit this "nitrite" syndrome, but among the nitrates only organic derivatives produce the typical reaction. One exception is bismuth subnitrate, an antidiarrheal agent which may be converted to nitrite by the action of coliform bacteria in the intestines. In contrast, most inorganic nitrates (*e.g.*, sodium, potassium, *etc.*) are rapidly absorbed and excreted unchanged, causing few reactions other than diuresis and perhaps catharsis. Presumably any inorganic nitrate salt which is not promptly absorbed in the upper alimentary tract may be reduced to a toxic nitrite in the colon.

The nitrites are effective by various portals of entry. Amyl nitrite vapor is readily absorbed from the lungs, but the liquid is inactive when ingested. Nitroglycerin is absorbed when placed on the skin or when swallowed, but a prompt and potent action is best obtained by absorption through the oral or buccal mucosa. Sodium nitrite must be swallowed (or injected) to produce poisoning. Absorbed nitrite disappears rapidly from the blood stream, but this rate cannot be correlated with the duration of vasodilatation. Absorbed nitrites are largely oxidized to inactive nitrates.

Deaths from nitrite poisoning are unusual. Recorded lethal doses span a wide range because of real variations in individual susceptibility. In part these variations arise from acquired tolerance, but many other phenomena are probably involved too. For example, the relatively marked susceptibility of infants to bismuth subnitrate poisoning is said to arise from the prevalence of nitrate-reducing bacteria high in the infants' intestines.

Nitrite syncope or shock is due initially to the pooling of blood in dilated post-arteriolar vessels, notably capillaries, venules, and even large veins. This vasodilatation is not blocked by atropine or by any known drug. Epinephrine, whose principal vascular action is the constriction of dilated arterioles, is ineffective here. Probably epinephrine and related compounds should be strictly prohibited, since spontaneous reflexes usually generate and maintain arteriolar constriction in a nitrite-poisoned patient. Reflex bradycardia may also arise, but this can be blocked by atropine. Eventually this shock-like state is complicated by oxygen lack, whch arises from circulatory inadequacy (stagnant anoxia) and from a reduction in the oxygen-carrying capacity of blood. The latter is due to the action of nitrite in converting hemoglobin to methemoglobin. The therapist attempts to reverse this hemoglobin reaction (*e.g.*, by methylene blue) or to compensate for it (*e.g.*, by blood transfusion).

Symptomatology:

1. A prompt fall in blood pressure.
2. A headache which is persistent and throbbing, with associated vertigo, palpitations, and visual disturbances.

3. The skin is flushed and perspiring, later cold and cyanotic.

4. Nausea and vomiting. The ingestion of nitrites may also cause colic and even bloody diarrhea.

5. Syncope, especially when attempting to stand upright.

6. Methemoglobinemia, with attendant cyanosis and anoxia.

7. Hyperpnea; later dyspnea and slow breathing.

8. The pulse may be slow, dicrotic, and intermittent.

9. Increased intraocular tension.

10. Paralysis, followed by clonic convulsions.

11. Death due to respiratory arrest.

Treatment:

1. Keep patient recumbent in a shock position and comfortably warm.

2. Gastric lavage with a 1:5000 solution of potassium permanganate (if the nitrite was taken orally).

3. Administer oxygen (p. 189) and artificial respiration if necessary (p. 185).

4. Methylene blue (1 per cent solution) 1 to 2 mg./kg. intravenously, or 50 mg./kg. orally in less severe cases of methemoglobinemia.

5. Ascorbic acid (0.5 to 1.0 gm.) by slow intravenous injection has been recommended in place of methylene blue but is probably much less effective.

6. Transfusion with whole blood or plasma expanders (p. 194).

7. Caffeine sodium benzoate (0.5 gm.) intravenously or subcutaneously.

Laboratory: Spectroscopic methods in clinical laboratories are often too insensitive to show methemoglobin absorption bands, even when cyanosis is clinically evident. By the customary clinical test (formation of acid hematin), the blood hemoglobin level is typically normal, while the blood oxygen-carrying capacity is measurably low, a difference which is a sensitive and practical index of methemoglobinemia in nitrite poisoning.

NITROGEN OXIDES

Gaseous mixtures of the oxides of nitrogen, commonly called nitrous fumes, contain varying proportions of the following five oxides: nitrous oxide (N_2O), nitric oxide (NO), nitrogen trioxide (N_2O_3), nitrogen dioxide (NO_2, with its dimer N_2O_4), and nitrogen pentoxide (N_2O_5). Of these constituents, NO and NO_2 are the principal hazards. Nitric oxide is a colorless gas, rapidly oxidized by O_2 in air to nitrogen dioxide. The latter is the chief constituent of nitrous fumes; it is a reddish-brown gas, which exists at low temperatures as the colorless tetroxide. The conversion of NO_2 to N_2O_4 is a rapid and reversible reaction, and the equilibrium depends only upon the temperature; at 35°C the mixture consists of about 70 per cent N_2O_4 and 30 per cent NO_2.

Numerous industrial and non-industrial sources of nitrous fumes are recognized. The oxides are released in the reaction between nitric acid and any organic material, in the exhaust from metal cleaning processes, in the gases from electric arc welding, in electroplating, engraving, and photogravure operations, in dynamite blasting, in diesel engine exhaust, and in the burning of nitrocellulose (*e.g.*, non-safety photographic and x-ray film). Although nitrous fumes from these and other sources are sometimes encountered in the home, barn, garage, and workshop, nitrogen oxides are emphasized in this compilation chiefly because they typify a large number of irritant gases which produce acute pulmonary reactions when inhaled: *viz.*, chlorine (Cl_2), fluorine (F_2), bromine (Br_2), sulfur dioxide (SO_2), hydrogen chloride (HCl), hydrogen fluoride (HF), hydrogen sulfide (H_2S), phosgene ($COCl_2$), chloropicrin ($CCl_3\text{-}NO_2$), 1-chloro-1-nitroethane and -ni-

tropropane, dichloro-nitroethane (Ethide), perfluoro-isobutylene, and ethylene oxide. These and many other gaseous irritants have been studied as potential chemical warfare agents. Several of them are currently used as agricultural fumigants. In the discussion below, reference is made to various gases besides nitrogen oxides, since all produce similar poisonings. Also see hydrogen sulfide on p. 147.

Toxicology: Of the five principal oxides of nitrogen, nitrous oxide (N_2O) is a mild anesthetic used in medicine and dentistry and is comparatively harmless. Nitric oxide (NO) is absorbed in the lungs and reacts with blood hemoglobin to form methemoglobin, with a consequent reduction in the oxygen-carrying capacity of circulating blood. With nitrous fumes, this is a minor effect because NO is a minor constituent (except in gases from electric arc welding). Little is known about the toxicology of nitrogen trioxide and of nitrogen pentoxide. Nitrogen dioxide, with its dimer N_2O_4, is the largest component of most fumes and causes most of the damage.

Only very high vapor concentrations induce prompt or immediate distress. Usually there are no symptoms at the time of exposure, except perhaps for a slight and transient cough, mild fatigue, and brief nausea. The acute danger period arises 5 to 72 hours later, when a slowly evolving but progressive inflammation of the lungs causes profuse exudation into the alveolar spaces. Fluid loss from the blood produces massive pulmonary edema and severe hemoconcentration. Because of impaired gas exchange in the lungs, breathing becomes rapid and cyanosis becomes intense. Death is usually due

to asphyxia within a few hours after respiratory symptoms begin. The relation between vapor concentration and duration of lethal exposure has been defined in laboratory animals, but these data are seldom useful to the physician who has no convenient way of estimating the intensity of exposure except in terms of the clinical response. In non-fatal cases, infectious pneumonia and bronchitis may severely complicate convalescence.

The typical reaction to nitrous fumes is delayed and insidious because nitrogen oxides are absorbed by and react with pulmonary alveolar structures only. The upper respiratory tract is largely spared, perhaps because these gases have a low solubility in aqueous media. This is not true of many irritant gases. For example, ammonia, hydrochloric, sulfuric, and hydrofluoric acids, and formaldehyde are said to act mainly on the upper portions of the respiratory tract; chlorine, fluorine, bromine, chloropicrin, dichloro-nitroethane, hydrogen sulfide, sulfur dioxide, acrolein, and ethylene oxide act on all portions; nitrous fumes, phosgene, ozone, phosphorus trioxide, and phosphorus chlorides act chiefly on the alveolar walls.

Unlike nitrogen oxides, those irritant vapors that attack the mucosa of the upper respiratory tract (see above) usually give prompt and adequate warning. Irritation of mucous membranes results in conjunctivitis, rhinitis, pharyngitis, and bronchitis. High vapor concentrations cause immediate pain and choking, temporary reflex arrest of breathing (in expiration), spasmodic closure of the glottis, bronchoconstriction, reflex slowing of the heart, and prompt asphyxial syncope. Excessive spasm or edema of the glottis may be directly fatal. Asthmatic breathing and violent coughing may lead to disruptive emphysema, with the appearance of subcutaneous blebs of air in the neck. Although some of these agents produce a metabolic acidosis, as well as CO_2 retention, the alkali reserve of blood and tissues is not seriously depleted. In non-fatal cases convalescence is usually slow and often complicated by general asthenia, various respiratory infections, weak and irregular cardiac action, cardiac dilatation, recurrent asthmatic attacks, chronic bronchitis, and rarely diffuse pulmonary fibrosis and emphysema.

The treatment of pulmonary edema outlined below is appropriate after an exposure to any fume or vapor which is a primary irritant.

Symptomatology:

1. Usually no symptoms occur at the time of exposure, with the exception of a slight cough and perhaps fatigue and nausea.
2. Only very concentrated nitrous fumes produce prompt coughing, choking, headache, nausea, abdominal pain, and dyspnea (tightness and burning pain in the chest).
3. A symptom-free period follows and lasts for 5 to 72 hours.
4. Fatigue, uneasiness, restlessness, cough, hyperpnea, and dyspnea appear insidiously, as pulmonary edema gradually develops.
5. Increasingly rapid and shallow respirations, cyanosis, mild or violent coughing with frothy expectoration, and physical signs of pulmonary edema (e.g., rales and rhonchi). The vital capacity is rapidly reduced. A serous exudate may develop in the pleural cavity, but its volume is usually small.
6. Anxiety, mental confusion, lethargy, and finally loss of consciousness.
7. A weak, rapid pulse, dilated heart, venous congestion, intense cyanosis, and severe hemoconcentration. Circulatory collapse is secondary to anoxia and hemoconcentration.
8. An asphyxial death due to blockade of gas exchange in the lungs. Death commonly occurs within a few hours after the first evidence of pulmonary edema.
9. In non-fatal cases, convalescence may be complicated by infectious bronchitis, pneumonia, and general asthenia.

Treatment:

1. Terminate the exposure immediately.
2. Enforce *complete* rest (bed or chair) for 24 to 48 hours, whether toxic signs and symptoms are recognized or not. Keep the victim comfortably warm.
3. As soon as he begins to cough, has difficulty breathing, or feels slightly fatigued, start oxygen therapy. Pure oxygen should be administered by any method which insures high inspiratory concentrations. An oronasal mask is usually best. A slightly positive gas pressure in the mask is desirable (p. 189).
4. A small dose of morphine (e.g., 10 mg.) is safe and desirable to diminish anxiety and dyspnea. The deeper and slower respirations which are induced by morphine frequently create better gas exchange in the lungs.
5. The removal of frothy exudate from the respiratory tract is a major therapeutic problem. Suctioning, postural drainage, and antifoaming agents are discussed on p. 192.
6. Most drugs are ineffective and possibly harmful; in this category are atropine, epinephrine, expectorants, emetics, sedative drugs (except for small doses of morphine), and usually cardiac glycosides. In a few instances rapid digitalization with a drug like ouabain may be advisable. The intravenous administration of hypertonic solutions (e.g., 50 per cent glucose or sucrose solution) has only a transient effect, if beneficial at all.
7. Cardiovascular collapse is strictly secondary

to anoxia and to hemoconcentration. Venesection and replacement of blood by isotonic saline are regarded as useful measures in some clinics and as dangerous procedures in others. Venesection should certainly be avoided once circulatory collapse has become established. The use of rotating tourniquets (as described on p. 192) may be beneficial during the stage of intense venous congestion.

8. An emergency tracheotomy under local anesthesia (p. 185) may make it possible to remove foam more efficiently by a suctioning catheter, but it usually complicates the administration of oxygen.

9. Artificial respiration may become necessary, but unless airway obstruction can be corrected, it is seldom effective.

10. Give penicillin and/or other antibiotics as prophylaxis against respiratory infections.

Laboratory:

1. Methemoglobinemia may be detected by comparing the oxygen-carrying capacity of blood with the concentration of hemoglobin measured by the color of acid hematin. A mild grade of methemoglobinemia sometimes results from inhalation of nitrogen oxides, particularly nitric oxide, but it is rarely sufficient to contribute appreciably to tissue anoxia.

2. In addition to CO_2 retention, a mild metabolic acidosis may be detectable. It seldom warrants specific treatment.

3. Various methods have been devised for sampling and analyzing air samples for nitrogen oxides, but these are seldom available to the non-industrial physician.

OXALATE

Oxalic acid and its salts are commonly used as bleaches, rust and ink eradicators, and metal cleaners. Their presence around the home has led to frequent accidental poisoning, particularly because of the resemblance between oxalic acid and Epsom salts, and between potassium hydrogen oxalate and cream of tartar. On a few occasions death has been ascribed to eating boiled oxalate-rich rhubarb leaves as a spinach substitute.

Toxicology: When ingested in large doses, oxalic acid and its soluble salts act as severe corrosive agents on the gastrointestinal mucosa. Although this corrosive action may be slightly more marked with the free acid than with its soluble salts, acidity itself is not responsible, and the administration of dilute alkali is unwarranted and unwise. Symptoms appear almost immediately and death may occur within a few minutes, apparently as a result of severe gastroenteritis and secondary shock.

If the patient does not die quickly from the local injury, absorption and consequent systemic intoxication may become manifest. With dilute oxalate solutions, the local gastrointestinal symptoms may be entirely absent; symptoms are then delayed, and the first evidence of poisoning may be muscle twitching, cramps, or central nervous depression. The systemic effects can be explained largely by the calcium-complexing action of oxalate which depresses the level of ionized calcium in body fluids. This hypocalcemia produces severe disturbances in the actions of the heart and of the nervous system; death may result from either of these disorders. Renal injury is usually demonstrable in acute oxalate poisoning, but it is rarely the cause of death. Kidney damage may have a dual origin: the oxalate ion chemically damages the renal tubule, and a mechanical injury may result from crystals of calcium and magnesium oxalate which precipitate within the kidneys and urinary tract.

The mean lethal dose for an adult probably lies between 15 and 30 gm., and death usually occurs within a few hours. Convalescence is characteristically slow, especially if there is much damage to the gastrointestinal tract. Esophageal strictures are apparently an uncommon complication.

Symptomatology:

1. Burning pain in throat, esophagus, and stomach. Exposed areas of mucous membrane turn almost immediately an opaque white, but unlike the mineral acids there are no corrosive actions on the lips and face.

2. Vomiting (often bloody or with a coffee-ground appearance), intense burning pain, severe purging.

3. The pulse becomes weak, irregular, and sometimes imperceptible. Hypotension and the usual signs of cardiovascular collapse appear.

4. If death is delayed for a few hours, nervous or neuromuscular symptoms develop: headache, muscle cramps (particularly of the jaw and extremities), tetany, sometimes convulsions, stupor, coma, and death.

5. Renal damage, as evidenced by oliguria, albuminuria, and hematuria.

Treatment (must be prompt):

1. Give immediately by mouth a dilute solution of any soluble calcium salt: milk of magnesia, calcium lactate, lime water, finely pulverized chalk or plaster (suspended in a large volume of water), or even milk.

2. Perform gastric lavage carefully, or not at all if severe mucosal injury is already evident. Dilute lime water (calcium hydroxide) makes a good lavage fluid.

3. Administer by slow intravenous injection 10 to 20 ml. of calcium gluconate (10 per cent solution) or of calcium chloride (5 per cent solution). This injection may have to be repeated frequently to prevent hypocalcemic tetany. Calcium gluconate (10 ml.) may also be given intramuscularly every four hours. Calcium compounds are never given subcutaneously; even the intramuscular route is hazardous in infants because of the incidence of sloughing. See also p. 221.
4. In severe cases parathyroid extract (100 U.S.P. units) given intramuscularly.

5. Morphine may be necessary for the control of pain.
6. Treat shock by the cautious intravenous injection of isotonic saline solution.
7. Watch for edema of the glottis and the late formation of esophageal strictures.
8. Useful demulcents by mouth include milk of magnesia, bismuth subcarbonate, and mineral oil.

Laboratory: Hematuria and albuminuria may be prominent. Oxalate crystals are probably always present in the urine of a poisoned patient, but they cannot be considered diagnostic.

PARATHION

Parathion (*O, O*-diethyl-*O*-*p*-nitrophenyl thiophosphate) is one of several related organic phosphate insecticides which possess great potency and a wide range of usefulness in modern agriculture. Parathion is a yellow to dark brown liquid of low vapor pressure, insoluble in water and kerosene, stable in the presence of moisture but hydrolyzed rapidly by alkali. Technical parathion is available commercially as the active ingredient of various dusts, wettable powders, emulsifiable concentrates, and aerosols, all of which act on the insect as contact and stomach poisons. The chemical is retained on the surface of plants and fruit, which may remain toxic for days. Because of its high toxicity parathion is not used in the home or barn.

Toxicology: Organic phosphate insecticides are among the most toxic materials commonly used for pest control. In terms of toxic actions to man, they are related to one another and also to a group of chemical warfare agents known as the nerve gases. Among these compounds parathion has an intermediary toxicity. Absorption to a dangerous degree can occur through any portal including the intact skin. Although several human fatalities have been traced unequivocally to parathion, the probable lethal dose in man is best inferred from animal experimentation. On this basis 10 to 20 mg. is an estimate of the *minimal* oral dose which is acutely lethal to an adult, while the *mean* lethal dose is probably 300 mg. (4 mg./kg.). Based again on animal tests, the acute lethal dose by the dermal route may be three times the latter value. As little as one drop of concentrated material represents a very real danger if splashed in the eye. Obviously great caution is necessary in handling parathion and related compounds, and the therapist should certainly protect himself, at least by wearing rubber gloves, if the patient's skin or clothing appear to be contaminated with active material.

Parathion and its relatives are known to inhibit the enzyme cholinesterase in all parts of the body. Toxic signs and symptoms are regarded as an indirect consequence of this enzyme inactivation.

According to this interpretation a poisoned tissue is unable to prevent local accumulations of acetylcholine, which acts as an excitatory substance in low concentration and a paralytic substance in high concentration. Although this explanation is a useful one, it is well to recognize that it is little more than a working hypothesis. During both poisoning and convalescence, experimental animals exhibit poor correlations between the severity of toxic signs and symptoms on the one hand and tissue levels of enzyme activity or of acetylcholine on the other hand, even in such target organs as the brain. For example, cholinesterase inhibition appears before and lasts much longer than clinically detectable evidences of poisoning. Although the inhibition of cholinesterase appears to be partially reversible for several hours after an acute exposure, there is a progressive and irreversible inactivation of enzyme following repeated exposures. It is probable that this cumulative biochemical lesion is repaired chiefly through the regeneration of new enzyme. Under these circumstances a clinical intoxication is possible from small repeated subclinical exposures. The situation is particularly hazardous because of the narrow margin between the dose which is just sufficient to produce symptoms and that which is adequate to kill.

Based on the above hypothesis toxic signs and symptoms can be classified with respect to the tissue site of enzyme inhibition; thus the pharmacologist refers to the muscarinic, nicotinic, and central nervous effects of organic phosphate insecticides. Such a classification is not particularly useful to the clinical toxicologist, whose principal concern is the sequence and intensity of signs and symptoms. Both sequence and latency depend to some extent on the portal of entry. For example, respiratory tract symptoms appear first during an inhalation exposure to parathion, while gastrointestinal effects are more prominent when the poison is swallowed. A skin exposure may reveal itself before systemic manifestations by the appearance of local sweating and local twitching or

fasciculations (but no erythema or skin irritation). An ocular exposure with liquid parathion is always manifested by prompt miosis and other ocular disturbances. The onset of symptoms is probably quickest after inhalation (a few minutes) and slowest after a primary cutaneous exposure (insidious onset after a latency of one or more hours). In contrast, poisonings by TEPP, para-oxon, and nerve gases always develop at a rapid rate. In part this difference may arise from the fact that pure parathion and several related insecticides are not true cholinesterase poisons until they are converted *in vivo* to active products.

Whatever the portal of entry, severe respiratory distress eventually appears in major intoxications. While mucus secretion, bronchospasm, and pulmonary edema may contribute, fatalities in man are usually due to respiratory failure on the basis of central nervous paralysis. Even coma, arreflexia, and apnea do not preclude a favorable outcome if immediate and energetic treatment is instituted. Two major principles of therapy are artificial respiration when needed and the administration of atropine in large doses to control the visceral actions of the poison, including the cardiovascular effects and probably some of the central nervous actions (but not skeletal muscle paralysis). Common errors in therapy include insufficient doses of atropine, failure to establish a patent airway, ineffective artificial respiration, and neglect of the patient after signs and symptoms have been temporarily controlled. Any severely poisoned patient is in danger for at least 24 hours.

Symptomatology:

1. Nausea is often the first symptom, followed by vomiting, abdominal cramps, diarrhea, and excessive salivation (sialorrhea).
2. Headache, giddiness, vertigo, and weakness.
3. Rhinorrhea and a sensation of tightness in the chest are common in inhalation exposures.
4. Blurring or dimness of vision, miosis (with fixed pinpoint pupils), tearing, ciliary muscle spasm, loss of accommodation, and ocular pain. None of these eye effects is diagnostically dependable except in primary ocular exposures.
5. Loss of muscle coordination, slurring of speech, fasciculations and twitching of muscles (particularly of the tongue and eyelids), and generalized profound weakness.
6. Mental confusion, disorientation, and drowsiness.
7. Difficulty in breathing, excessive secretion of saliva and of respiratory tract mucus, oronasal frothing, cyanosis, pulmonary rales and rhonchi, and hypertension (presumably due to asphyxia).
8. Random jerky movements, incontinence, convulsions, and coma.

9. Death primarily due to respiratory failure.

Treatment:

1. Atropinize the patient immediately. In an adult the usual dose is 1 to 4 mg. of the sulfate (or other salt) given intramuscularly or intravenously. The maintenance of full atropinization may require 2 mg. doses at intervals of 15 to 60 minutes for many hours. Because of their high tolerance, poisoned patients commonly receive too little atropine, rarely too much. The need for more atropine can be recognized by the continuation or recurrence of those toxic symptoms described above; excessive salivation is a particularly useful criterion (but not eye signs).
2. Relieve upper airway obstruction (see p. 184). Mucus and other respiratory tract secretions may have to be aspirated continuously. Endotracheal intubation or tracheotomy may become necessary (see p. 184).
3. Give oxygen and artificial respiration as needed (see p. 185).
4. Gastric lavage with 5 per cent sodium bicarbonate solution may be warranted after the ingestion of parathion, if vomiting is not prompt and profuse.
5. Wash any contaminated areas of skin with soap and water. Irrigate the eyes with water or saline solution.
6. Administer cautiously by the intravenous route isotonic saline to correct dehydration and electrolyte imbalances.
7. Never give morphine, theophyllin, or theophylline-ethylenediamine (aminophyllin). Rarely, if ever, are even short-acting barbiturates justified in the management of the convulsive phase, since the latter can generally be prevented or treated by adequate atropinization and the correction of asphyxia.
8. Keep the patient under constant observation for a period from 24 to 36 hours.

Laboratory:

1. Repeated blood analyses for cholinesterase activity are invaluable in establishing the diagnosis and formulating a long-range prognosis. The test can now be done in the laboratories of most general hospitals. Collect and heparinize about 10 ml. of venous blood (sodium citrate if heparin is unavailable). Centrifuge, separate, and save plasma. The cell layer should be resuspended in 3 times its volume of isotonic saline and recentrifuged. In this way the cells should be washed several times. After 20 minutes of centrifugation at 2000 r.p.m., the volume of packed cells is noted and an equal volume of isotonic saline (0.9 per cent) is added. This red blood cell suspension and the sample of plasma are refrigerated until their cholinesterase activi-

ties can be measured by one of several published procedures. Atropine does not interfere with this test.

2. ECG records are useful, although cardiac blocks rarely occur in clinical poisonings in the absence of asphyxia.

PHENOL

Phenol (carbolic acid) and cresols are marketed in many forms and sold widely for their antiseptic activity. They are often used in homes and on farms as disinfectants, barn deodorants, sanitizers, *etc.* Dilute phenol solutions (1 to 2 per cent) are used medicinally in antipruritic preparations for the skin; repeated use over large skin areas should be avoided *unless* the product also contains camphor (which interacts with phenol to reduce the percutaneous toxicity).

Toxicology: Phenol gains ready access to the body from all routes of administration, including the intact skin. It is a general protoplasmic poison and toxic to all cells. Concentrated solutions (*e.g.*, 10 per cent) are highly corrosive, and even solutions as dilute as 2 per cent occasionally cause skin necrosis. Systemically phenol first stimulates and then depresses the central nervous system. Central depression reveals itself in many ways, notably by coma, hypothermia, loss of vasoconstrictor tone, and respiratory arrest. The heart and circulation are also depressed by phenol.

The lethal dose for adults is estimated at 8 to 15 gm. by mouth and even less by uterine douche or by absorption from wounds and body cavities. Absorption from the bowel begins promptly (although appreciable amounts may remain in the stomach for some hours). Sudden collapse and death from respiratory failure may occur within 15 minutes or may be delayed several days, but the dangerous phase of the poisoning is usually complete within 24 hours. The only available treatment is symptomatic and supportive.

Symptomatology:

1. White corrosive burns of mucous membranes in mouth, esophagus, stomach; abdominal pain, vomiting (less common than with other corrosives), and bloody diarrhea.
2. Pallor, sweating, weakness, headache, dizziness, tinnitus.
3. Shock: weak irregular pulse, hypotension, shallow respirations, cyanosis, and a profound fall in body temperature.
4. Possibly fleeting excitement (delirium), followed by unconsciousness. Convulsions are rarely seen except in children (and most animals).

5. Scanty, dark-colored or "smoky" urine. If death does not occur promptly, moderately severe renal insufficiency may appear.
6. Death from respiratory failure.
7. If spilled on skin, pain is followed promptly by numbness. The skin becomes blanched, and a dry opaque eschar forms over the burn. When the eschar sloughs off, a brown stain remains.

Treatment:

1. Careful gastric lavage with olive oil or similar vegetable oils (salad oils). Castor oil and cottonseed oil have been used. Probably inferior as lavage fluids are 10 per cent glycerin in water, potassium permanganate solution, and lime water. Avoid mineral oil (a poor solvent for phenol) and alcohol (which facilitates the gastric absorption of phenol).
2. Remove contaminated clothing instantly. Wash external burns promptly with copious amounts of running water or with olive oil or castor oil. Alcohol-water mixtures may serve only to spread the area of contamination.
3. Demulcents: egg white, milk, gruel.
4. External heat in moderation.
5. Morphine or meperidine for pain.
6. Respiratory stimulants such as nikethamide or caffeine sodium benzoate (p. 204).
7. Oxygen therapy and artificial respiration as needed (p. 185).
8. Treat shock conservatively because of uncertain cardiac and renal status. Only severe circulatory collapse demands infusions. Digitalis is seldom effective. See p. 195.
9. Supportive measures for impending renal insufficiency (p. 210).
10. Watch for esophageal stricture, even though it occurs only rarely after phenol poisoning.

Laboratory:

1. Phenol can be detected in urine, where it is excreted unchanged or as a glucuronide or ethereal sulfate. A small fraction is oxidized to hydroquinone, pyrocatechol, and unknown substances.
2. Frequent urinalyses to reveal albumin, red blood cells, and casts.

PHOSPHORUS

Acute phosphorus poisoning was common early in this century when yellow (also called white)

phosphorus was used in the manufacture of match tips and fireworks and in the preparation of various

drug products. There is no scientific basis for its medicinal use, and legislation has largely eliminated it from household products. Matches and fireworks imported from China and Japan are still a potential hazard. At present most poisonings result from ingestion of rat poisons or roach powders which contain 1 to 4 per cent yellow phosphorus. Chronic intoxication by inhalation of phosphorus fumes occasionally occurs in industry.

Toxicology: Elemental phosphorus occurs in two common forms. "Red" phosphorus is nonvolatile, insoluble, unabsorbable, and thus nontoxic when ingested, unless it contains traces of yellow phosphorus (sometimes 0.6 per cent). Yellow (or white) phosphorus is a translucent solid, which has a distinct odor resembling garlic. It is practically insoluble in water but readily soluble in most oils. On exposure to air, phosphorus fumes and may flame spontaneously as it oxidizes to the sesquioxide (P_2O_3). Although stable under water, the element is converted by boiling alkali to the hypophosphorous ion ($H_2PO_2^+$) and phosphine (PH_3). In the alimentary tract and other tissues, phosphorus is relatively stable for long periods of time. Some phosphorus is thought to be oxidized slowly to relatively harmless acids which are gradually excreted by the kidneys. The free element itself is presumably the toxic form in tissues.

Phosphorus is a general protoplasmic poison which is slowly absorbed through the gastrointestinal and respiratory mucosae. Toxicity is enhanced when the element is in solution or is finely divided in the form of an emulsion. The classical picture of acute phosphorus poisoning develops in three stages. Gastrointestinal symptoms occurring shortly after ingestion arise from severe mucosal irritation. A relatively symptom-free period of several days (stage 2) is followed by a third stage of systemic intoxication. Gastrointestinal symptoms are severe, and the liver undergoes acute degeneration and fatty infiltration with accompanying metabolic disturbances. Cellular damage is also demonstrable in the kidneys, heart, and brain. Chronic poisoning, seen mostly in factory workers exposed repeatedly to phosphorus vapors, is manifest by cachexia, anemia, bronchitis, and necrosis of the mandible ("phossy jaw"). The inhalation of phosphorus fumes can also cause an acute poisoning like that following ingestion.

The acute fatal dose of phosphorus for an adult is between 50 and 100 mg. or about 1 mg./kg. Recovery, however, has occurred after the ingestion of 825 mg., whereas only 3 mg. has proved lethal to a 2-year-old child. The prognosis is generally poor and the fatality rate is over 50 per cent. Deaths in the first two days are due to peripheral vascular collapse; later in the course of poisoning, death is due to hepatic, renal, or cardiac failure or rarely to post-convulsive central nervous depression.

Symptomatology:

A. Acute poisoning—typically in 3 stages
1. First stage—symptoms due to local irritation, occurring within a few minutes or few hours after exposure and lasting from 8 hours to 3 days.
   a. Skin contact produces painful penetrating 2° and 3° burns, which heal slowly. These lesions represent both chemical and thermal damage.
   b. Ingestion produces burning in the throat and abdomen, with intense thirst.
   c. Nausea, vomiting, diarrhea, severe abdominal pain. A garlic odor from breath and excreta is highly suggestive of phosphorus poisoning (garlic, Lewisite, and arsenic must be ruled out). Luminescent vomitus and feces are essentially diagnostic of phosphorus.
   d. Shock may be severe enough to cause death in 24 to 48 hours.
2. Second stage—symptom-free period of several days (8 hours to several weeks), during which the patient seems to be recovering.
3. Third stage—symptoms of systemic toxicity from absorbed poison.
   a. Nausea, protracted vomiting, diarrhea; massive hematemesis may occur.
   b. Liver tenderness and enlargement, jaundice, pruritus.
   c. Hemorrhages into skin, mucous membranes, and viscera, due to injury of blood vessels and inhibition of blood clotting (low plasma levels of prothrombin and fibrogen).
   d. Renal damage is evidenced by oliguria, hematuria, casts, albuminuria, and sometimes anuria.
   e. Cardiovascular collapse, due to a direct, toxic action of phosphorus on heart muscle and blood vessels.
   f. Central nervous involvement resulting in convulsions, delirium, and coma. If the patient survives, cerebral symptoms may persist for a long time.
   g. Death occurs usually in 4 to 8 days, but it may be delayed 3 weeks. Irreversible shock, hepatic failure, central nervous system damage, massive hematemesis, or renal insufficiency may be the proximal cause of death.

B. Chronic poisoning (from ingestion or inhalation). Cachexia, anemia, bronchitis, general debility, necrosis of mandible—all associated with lowered resistance to infection and defective tissue repair.

Treatment:
1. Care should be taken to protect both patient and attendant from vomitus, gastric wash-

ings, and feces, since the phosphorus in them can cause burns of skin and eyes.

2. Gastric lavage, using copious quantities of one of the following solutions:

   a. Cupric sulfate solution (0.2 per cent) acts as an emetic and as an antidote by coating the phosphorus particles with insoluble copper phosphide.

   b. Potassium permanganate (1:5000) or hydrogen peroxide (2 per cent) may convert phosphorus to various oxides (acids), which are comparatively harmless.

3. Liquid petrolatum (100 to 200 ml.) should be introduced into stomach following lavage and left there. Avoid digestible fats and oils.

4. Isotonic solutions of sodium chloride and of sodium lactate parenterally to combat shock, dehydration, and acidosis (pp. 193, 215).

5. Morphine and other opiates to control pain.

6. Vitamin K_1 in large doses (e.g., 65 mg. slowly by intravenous drip) may in part combat hypoprothrombinemia, but transfusions with *fresh* whole blood may be necessary to correct the coagulation defect and anemia.

7. Supportive treatment for delirium and convulsions (p. 201).

8. General supportive measures for hepatic insufficiency (p. 213) and renal failure (p. 210).

9. Cortisone therapy has been recommended for severe shock.

10. Treat skin burns by washing with warm water or with 1 per cent cupric sulfate solution, and then apply bland ointments. As long as unoxidized phosphorus remains embedded in the skin, the contaminated area should be kept submerged in water or copper sulfate solution. Visible pieces of phosphorus should be removed surgically.

Laboratory:

1. Phosphorus can be demonstrated chemically in vomitus and feces.

2. Urine may contain albumin, bile pigments, casts, blood, and amino acids. Measure and record the output of urine.

3. Blood chemistry: low blood sugar, high nonprotein nitrogen, high icterus index, low fibrinogen, low prothrombin. Both hypo- and hyperphosphatemia have been described.

4. Hematological data are variable: leukopenia or leukocytosis, anemia or polycythemia, monocytosis.

PYRETHRUM

Pyrethrum has been known and used as an insecticide for many years. Even with the advent of many new agents, pyrethrum is still considered so effective that about 2000 brands of pyrethrum-base household sprays are available in this country. The source of this material is the flowers of the pyrethrum plant, *Chrysanthemum cinerariaefolium*. The insecticide can be prepared by drying and grinding the flowers to a powder, which contains about 1 per cent active material. A more efficient method is the extraction of active ingredients with a solvent such as alcohol, kerosene, or naphtha. The activity and toxicity of pyrethrum resides in at least four esters of complex alcohols and acids, called Pyrethrin I and II and Cinerin I and II, known collectively as pyrethrins. When isolated these esters are viscous liquids, insoluble in water, and quickly decomposed by mild acid and alkali.

Pyrethrum is sometimes used as a dust, and the term "insect powder" on a label is legally proper only if the product contains pyrethrum powder. A more common formulation is the extract in a suitable solvent or vehicle for use as a household, garden, or livestock spray. Pyrethrum preparations frequently contain a synergist which is added to increase their stability and insecticidal effectiveness; these include sesamin, piperonyl butoxide, piperonyl cyclonene, n-octyl sulfoxide of isosafrole, n-propyl isome, and N-isobutylundecyleneamide.

Toxicology: Pyrethrins are only moderately toxic to warm-blooded animals by oral administration but highly toxic by parenteral routes. The material is rapidly detoxified, presumably by hydrolysis; thus rats can ingest over a 24-hour period a dose which is lethal if taken at one time, and can maintain this intake every day of their lives without apparent injury. The fatal oral dose in man, as inferred from data on rats and guinea pigs, is 1 to 2 gm./kg., expressed as pyrethrin. Since the pyrethrin concentration of pyrethrum powder is about 1 per cent and of insecticide sprays is usually 0.1 per cent, serious poisonings are highly improbable. Kerosene and naphtha, the common solvents in pyrethrum sprays, are generally more hazardous than the "active ingredients."

The synergists commonly found in pyrethrum formulations (as listed above) possess even lower acute toxicities in laboratory mammals than do pyrethrins. Although these additives enhance insecticidal potency, there is no evidence that they increase the mammalian toxicity of fresh pyrethrum.

In spite of the low primary toxicity of pyrethrins, skin contact and inhalation may cause allergic attacks in sensitive people; severe dermatitis and anaphylactoid reactions have been reported. Persons sensitive to ragweed pollen are particularly prone to react to pyrethrins.

Symptomatology (largely inferred from animal studies):

1. Numbness of lips and tongue, sneezing, nausea, vomiting, and diarrhea.
2. Headache, restlessness, tinnitus, incoordination, clonic convulsions, stupor, and prostration.
3. Death due to respiratory paralysis.
4. Skin contact may cause dermatitis, sometimes with an associated eosinophilia.
5. Hydrocarbon solvents such as kerosene may produce pulmonary edema (p. 150).

Treatment:

1. "Universal antidote" (p. 10) followed by gastric lavage with tap water.
2. Symptomatic and supportive treatment with oxygen (p. 189), artificial respiration (p. 185), barbiturates (p. 200), and parenteral fluids.
3. Wash skin promptly with generous quantities of water.
4. See treatment of kerosene and naphtha poisoning (p. 150), if symptoms are due to the vehicle.

Laboratory: No common laboratory tests have diagnostic or prognostic value.

QAC (QUATERNARY AMMONIUM COMPOUNDS)

Many modern germicides are synthetic derivatives of ammonium chloride, in which the four hydrogens of the ammonium cation have been replaced by organic groups, at least one of which is a long-chain aliphatic residue. One popular compound of this type is lauryl benzyl dimethyl ammonium chloride (U.S.P. name benzalkonium chloride). In a related group of substances, the nitrogen atom is included in a heterocyclic ring (*e.g.*, cetyl pyridinium chloride). While most of these substances are marketed as chloride salts, some are available as bromides, iodides, nitrates, *etc.* These salts are often called cationic surfactants or cationic detergents because their aqueous solutions have low surface tensions.

Over a dozen quaternary ammonium germicides are available commercially as powders, ointments, jellies, aqueous solutions, and tinctures. At concentrations between 0.01 and 1.0 per cent, they are used as antiseptics, bactericides, fungicides, sanitizers, and deodorants. In restaurants, dairies, food plants, laundries, and operating rooms, they are popular disinfectants for utensils, containers, instruments, *etc.* Because they react with soap and most proteins, their maximal germicidal effectiveness is attained only on chemically clean surfaces. Dilute solutions have been employed in medicine to sterilize the skin, conjunctivae, and mucous membranes, and rarely to irrigate the urinary bladder and other body cavities. They have been used to keep bodies of water free of slime mold, algae, fish pathogens, and certain mollusks. Some derivatives have served as moth-proofing agents, oil preservatives, soil pathogen eradicators, and foliage sprays.

Toxicology: The mammalian toxicity of quaternary ammonium germicides is not well established, although at least two human fatalities have been ascribed to them (one due to ingestion and the other to vaginal instillation). Probably all common derivatives produce similar toxic reactions, but as tested in laboratory mammals, the oral mean lethal dose varies with the compound between the approximate limits of 100 and 700 mg./kg. Perhaps humans are more susceptible than small laboratory animals; at least an adult woman died within 30 minutes after drinking one ounce of a 10 per cent solution (3 gm.) of Hyamine 2389. Some of these substances are several hundred times more toxic by the intravenous than by the oral route, while the oral and parenteral toxicities of other congeners differ only slightly. Although concentrated aqueous solutions are primary skin irritants, percutaneous absorption is probably insignificant.

When on the alkaline side of their isoelectric points, all proteins can be precipitated by quaternary ammonium detergents. Strong aqueous solutions commonly produce superficial necrosis of visceral organs with which they come in contact. Concentrated solutions (10 per cent and sometimes less) are primary skin irritants, and concentrations as low as 0.1 per cent are often irritating to conjunctivae and mucous membranes, although benzalkonium chloride is said to be well tolerated at this concentration. According to the available evidence, which is admittedly scanty, fatal poisoning may arise from the ingestion of concentrations which create no recognized pathological lesions except visceral congestion, cloudy swelling, mild pulmonary edema, and varying degrees of gastrointestinal irritation. Even in chronic exposures of several weeks' duration, the only lesion found in fatally ill rats was focal hemorrhagic necrosis of the gastric mucosa, and these animals apparently died of inanition associated with chronic diarrhea. It is doubtful, however, that acute fatalities can be ascribed to corrosive actions on the alimentary tract; in the one recorded human fatality from the ingestion of a cationic detergent, no mucosal ulceration was detected at postmortem examination.

Although a definitive biochemical and pharmacologic effect is probably responsible for systemic poisoning by quaternary ammonium germicides, the nature of this specific disorder is not established. On highly circumstantial evidence, the suggestion has been made that the ingestion of methyl dodecyl benzyl trimethyl ammonium chloride (Hyamine 2389) may cause a fatal inhibition of the enzyme

cholinesterase. Inhibition of this enzyme has been produced *in vitro* by several quaternary ammonium surfactants, but presumably many other protein precipitants would serve as well. In isolated observations in this laboratory, no inhibition of plasma cholinesterase was found in rats sacrificed *in extremis* after an intraperitoneal injection of benzalkonium chloride or cetyl pyridinium chloride. A 50 per cent inhibition of the red cell cholinesterase was noted, but such a depression is not expected to produce untoward reactions. It is improbable that toxic signs and symptoms arising from quaternary ammonium compounds can be ascribed to cholinesterase inhibition.

A curare-like paralysis of skeletal muscles has been ascribed to quaternary ammonium salts, specifically to cetyl pyridinium chloride and benzalkonium chloride. Parenteral injections in rats, rabbits, and dogs have resulted in prompt but transient limb paralysis and sometimes fatal paresis of the respiratory muscles. This effect appears to be highly transient, and to our knowledge it has not been demonstrated after oral administration. These observations, however, are not inconsistent with the signs and symptoms reported in two fatally poisoned women, of whom one drank Hyamine 2389 and the other received benzalkonium chloride by vaginal instillation (in the course of an abortion). Besides a curare-like paralysis of the motor-end plates in skeletal muscle, severe central nervous depression, sometimes preceded by excitement and convulsions, has been reported in poisoned animals. These multiple actions are reminiscent of nicotine poisoning (p. 161). The impressions and inferences outlined above receive support from the structural analogy between quaternary ammonium germicides and decamethonium (a recognized neuromuscular blocking agent) and hexamethonium (an acknowledged gangionic blocking agent).

Symptomatology (largely inferred from animal studies):

1. The ingestion of a concentrated solution leads to immediate burning pain in the mouth and throat.
2. Rapidly developing apprehension, restlessness, confusion, and weakness.
3. Specific muscle weakness, perhaps associated with a transient period of muscle fasciculation.
4. Central nervous depression may or may not be preceded by weak convulsive movements.
5. Labored breathing and cyanosis due to weakness of the respiratory muscles.
6. An asphyxial death, with or without a terminal convulsion, due to paralysis of the muscles of respiration. In fatal cases, death is expected to occur promptly, *i.e.*, within an hour or two after ingestion.

Treatment:

1. Swallow promptly a large quantity of milk, egg whites, or perhaps a mild soap solution. Avoid alcohol, which has been shown to increase the oral toxicity of at least one quaternary ammonium germicide (cetyl pyridinium chloride), presumably by promoting absorption.
2. Gastric lavage if it can be done promptly. Milk, gelatin solution, and a mild soap solution make good lavage fluids.
3. Skeletal muscle weakness or paralysis can be detected by a loss in grip strength, inability to stand, perhaps ptosis, and diminution or absence of tendon reflexes. Curare antagonists such as neostigmine and edrophonium (Tensilon) are probably of no value and may enhance the paralysis (as in decamethonium poisoning). Presumably central nervous stimulants are also ineffective.
4. If respirations become labored, administer oxygen (p. 189) and support breathing mechanically by manual or other methods of artificial respiration (p. 185). In the absence of a gag reflex, an oronasal airway should be interested (p. 184).
5. If persistent, convulsions may be controlled by the cautious intravenous injection of a short-acting barbiturate drug (p. 201).
6. If a quaternary ammonium drug is spilled on the skin, wash promptly with soap and water.

Laboratory: Probably irrelevant.

ROTENONE

Rotenone is a widely used insecticide, combining the qualities of effectiveness against insects and low toxicity for plants and mammals. It is used in dusts and sprays, alone and in combination with DDT, pyrethrins, and fungicides. It has also been employed clinically for the external treatment of chiggers (2 per cent lotion) and scabies (10 per cent emulsion).

Many plant sources of rotenone are known, particularly *Derris* grown in Malaya and the East Indies, and *Lonchocarpus* (familiarly known as cubé) grown in Central and South America. These plants have been known for many centuries and used for poisoning arrow heads, for poisoning fish, and even for suicide. (Apparently the fresh derris root has a much higher toxicity than the dried powdered root from which rotenone is extracted.) Only in recent years, however, have the active principles been iso-

lated and widely utilized. The roots are dried, ground, and extracted with solvents such as chloroform and benzene.

The so-called fish poison plants contain other active ingredients besides rotenone, namely deguelin, toxicarol, tephrosin, and sumatrol—all chemically related to rotenone but less effective as insecticidal agents. Besides these natural rotenoids, several derivatives of rotenone have been chemically prepared—dihydrorotenone isorotenone, dehydrorotenone, etc., each of which is more active against certain insects than is the parent compound, but none of which is in common use at the present time. Most, if not all, of these substances are less toxic to mammals than is rotenone.

Toxicology: Rotenone is relatively free of hazards in normal use, because of 1) the low percentage (0.75 to 1.0 per cent) commonly used in formulations; 2) the unstable nature of rotenone (it decomposes rapidly in light and air); and 3) its irritant actions when ingested, causing prompt vomiting. No human fatalities have been reported.

Rotenone, however, is more toxic to mammals than pyrethrins and approaches the toxicity of DDT. Although the mean lethal dose by mouth varies widely among common species of laboratory mammals, a reasonable estimate (guesstimate) for man is 0.3 to 0.5 gm./kg. Since in animals rotenone is hundreds of times more toxic intravenously than orally, gastrointestinal absorption is presumably slow and incomplete. Because of poor absorption, coarse particles of solid rotenone are much less toxic than fine powders. Fats and oils promote absorption and so enhance toxicity.

Symptomatology (largely inferred from animal studies):

1. Numbness of oral mucous membranes, nausea, vomiting, and gastric pain.
2. Muscle tremors, incoordination, clonic convulsions, and stupor. At least in rabbits and dogs, some of these effects are due to severe hypoglycemia.
3. Respiratory stimulation, followed by depression. The immediate cause of death is asphyxia from respiratory arrest.
4. Skin irritation from local application.
5. Severe pulmonary irritation from inhalation of dust.

Treatment:

1. Swallow "universal antidote" (p. 10) and/or induce vomiting.
2. Gastric lavage with tap water.
3. Administer a saline cathartic, e.g., 15 to 30 gm. sodium sulfate in water). Avoid all oils and fats, which promote intestinal absorption of rotenone.
4. Symptomatic and supportive treatment with oxygen (p. 189), artificial respiration (p. 185), barbiturates (p. 200), and parenteral fluids.
5. Administer glucose intravenously to correct hypoglycemia.
6. Wash skin with liberal quantities of water.
7. Treat pulmonary complications in the same way as those arising from the aspiration of kerosene (p. 150) or the inhalation of nitrogen oxides (p. 163).

Laboratory: Because severe hypoglycemia has been reported in some animals, a blood sugar test is desirable.

SALICYLATE

Salicylic acid (ortho hydroxy benzoic acid) and its derivatives (e.g., aspirin) are an important class of compounds widely used in clinical medicine as analgetics, antipyretics, fungistatics, keratolytics, rubefacients, and antirheumatics. The annual consumption exceeds that of any other group of drugs. Salicylate poisoning is encountered frequently; in children it is usually due to willful ingestion and in adults to suicidal or therapeutic administration.

Toxicology: The common derivatives of salicylic acid produce substantially the same toxic syndrome ("salicylism"). Phenyl salicylate (salol) poisoning is unique in that the chief effects are due to phenol, which is liberated by hydrolysis in the intestinal tract and probably in other tissues too. In toxic doses, salicylamide (which is not metabolized to salicylic acid) produces more central nervous depression than is seen in typical salicylism. Except for severe local irritation, methyl salicylate (oil of wintergreen) is not notably different in its toxic actions, but metabolic acidosis may be a more prominent complication with the methyl ester than with other common derivatives.

Toxic effects usually appear whenever 10 gm. or more of any salicylate are ingested in single or divided doses over a period of 12 to 24 hours, or whenever the blood plasma salicylate level exceeds 30 mg. per 100 ml. The mean lethal dose of sodium salicylate and of acetylsalicylate (aspirin) probably lies between 20 and 30 gm. in an adult, although less than 1 gm. (aspirin) has killed and 130 gm. has been tolerated. Methyl salicylate may be slightly more toxic than the sodium salt (twice as lethal in mice), and salicylamide is probably less toxic. The impression persists that children (especially under the age of 3 years) are proportionately more susceptible than adults to the toxic actions of all salicylates. Although many rheumatic

patients have been poisoned by the intravenous administration of salicylates, most cases of salicylism are due to ingestion. While methyl and phenyl salicylates sometimes produce systemic poisoning by penetrating intact skin, the percutaneous absorption of salicylic acid and its other derivatives reaches toxic levels only when large skin areas are covered with the drug in a suitable base (e.g., lanolin).

The major toxic signs and symptoms arise from stimulation and terminal depression of the central nervous system. Central excitation reveals itself in many ways: emesis, hyperpnea, headache, tinnitus, confusion, mania, and generalized convulsions. The patient usually dies from respiratory failure or from cardiovascular collapse while in a state of coma. Less common features include fever, sweating, skin eruptions, hemorrhages and renal disturbances. In addition to these dose-dependent reactions, signs of idiosyncrasy or drug hypersensitivity are sometimes encountered. In spite of severe sensory disturbances during the acute phase, such as tinnitus, deafness, and dimness of vision, permanent neurological lesions are rarely encountered; indeed no persistent sequelae are generally recognized.

Many of the toxic effects outlined above are due to or aggravated by a severe disturbance in acid-base balance. Many factors contribute to this imbalance, but the chief cause is prolonged hyperventilation from central stimulation, resulting in varying degrees of respiratory alkalosis. This disorder may be aggravated by a metabolic alkalosis which results from vomiting. In the poisoned adult, alkalosis commonly persists until the stage of terminal respiratory failure, but in children a profound ketosis usually converts the initial alkalosis into an uncompensated acidosis. Salicylate also causes a significant rise in oxygen consumption. In the dog this increase (which may be two-fold) is apparently associated with a metabolic stimulation of skeletal muscle; it is not due to epinephrine release and is not dependent on the central or peripheral nervous system. Because of this metabolic stimulation, a small decrease in tissue oxygen tension develops, in spite of hyperpnea and accelerated blood flow (increased cardiac output).

With salicylate overdosage, young children react differently from adults in one important respect, namely the prompt development of ketosis. As a result metabolic acidosis is usually well established in the salicylate-poisoned child before he is seen by the physician, while the adult patient is commonly in a state of respiratory alkalosis under the same circumstances. Another distinction may be the higher incidence of fever and convulsions in the poisoned infant and child.

Therapy for salicylism is symptomatic and supportive, with major emphasis on correction of the acid-base imbalance. In the final analysis recovery depends upon urinary excretion, since 70 to 80 per cent of a given dose can eventually be retrieved in the urine in the form of salicylate and its metabolites. In order to improve renal function, prompt attempts should be made to correct dehydration and shock. Excretion, however, is inherently slow; about 50 per cent of a given dose is eliminated in 24 hours. Elimination is distinctly faster if the urine is alkaline (pH above 7.0) than if it is acid. The administration of sufficient sodium bicarbonate to alkalinize the urine is always a useful procedure if the urine is acid, but the poisoned adult almost invariably has an alkaline urine because of his respiratory alkalosis. Under these circumstances the therapeutic administration of alkali is unwarranted and dangerous.

Symptomatology:

1. A large oral dose of salicylate, particularly of the acid or the methyl ester, causes mild burning pain in the throat and stomach and usually prompt vomiting. An asymptomatic interval of several hours may follow these initial symptoms.
2. Deep and rapid breathing (hyperpnea), anorexia, apathy, and lassitude are important early signs of systemic poisoning.
3. Nausea, vomiting, thirst, and occasionally diarrhea, probably all of central nervous origin.
4. Headache, fullness in the head, dizziness, tinnitus, difficulty in hearing, and dimness of vision.
5. Irritability, restlessness, confusion, disorientation.
6. Delirium, mania, hallucinations, generalized convulsions.
7. Deep coma and death due to respiratory failure and/or cardiovascular collapse.
8. Miscellaneous reactions which are occasionally encountered:
   a. High fever, especially in children, with associated thirst and profuse perspiration.
   b. Hemorrhagic phenomena, usually associated with hypoprothrombinemia, commonly evidenced by petechiae in the skin and mucous membranes, hematemesis, or melena.
   c. A variety of skin eruptions are described, usually only after chronic medication. Some of these lesions may represent drug allergies.
9. Instead of typical salicylism as described above, an occasional patient exhibits a true idiosyncrasy or acquired hypersensitivity. The following allergic responses to salicylate have been described: angioneurotic edema, hives, laryngeal edema and consequent asphyxia, and especially asthma.

Treatment:

1. Pending gastric lavage, use emetics or delay gastric emptying and absorption by swallowing milk or a slurry of "universal antidote" (see p. 10).

2. Gastric lavage with water or perhaps soduim bicarbonate solution (3 to 5 per cent). Mild alkali delays salicylate absorption from the stomach and perhaps slightly from the duodenum, but if alkali promotes gastric emptying, the net effect may be an increased rate of absorption.

3. Saline catharsis with sodium or magnesium sulfate (15 to 30 gm. in water).

4. Take an immediate blood sample for an appraisal of the patient's acid-base status. A pH determination on an anaerobic sample of arterial blood is best. For alternative laboratory procedures, see below. An analysis of the plasma salicylate concentration should be made at the same time. Laboratory controls are almost essential for the proper management of severe salicylism.

5. In the presence of an established acidosis, alkali therapy is essential, but at least in the adult, alkali should be withheld until its need is demonstrated chemically. The intensity of treatment depends upon the intensity of the acidosis (see p. 219). In the presence of vomiting, intravenous sodium lactate (M/6) is the most satisfactory form of alkali therapy.

6. Correct dehydration and hypoglycemia (if present) by the intravenous administration of glucose in water or in isotonic saline. The administration of glucose or lactate may also serve to remedy the ketosis which is often seen in poisoned children.

7. Renal function should be supported by correcting dehydration and incipient shock. Overhydration and diuretic therapy are not justified. An alkaline urine should be maintained by the administration of alkali if necessary, with care to prevent a systemic alkalosis.

8. Small doses of barbiturates, chloral hydrate, paraldehyde, or other sedative drugs (but probably not morphine) may be required to suppress extreme restlessness and convulsions (see p. 201).

9. For hyperpyrexia, use sponge baths (see p. 230).

10. The presence of petechiae or other signs of a hemorrhagic tendency calls for large doses of vitamin K and perhaps ascorbic acid. See p. 181 for a discussion of the treatment of hypoprothrombinemia. Small transfusions may be necessary, since bleeding in salicylism is not always due to a prothrombin deficit.

11. Hemodialysis by means of an artificial kidney has proved useful in salicylate poisoning.

12. In the late stages of central nervous depression, stimulants such as caffeine and nikethamide may be beneficial.

Laboratory:

1. In toxic patients the blood plasma salicylate concentration usually exceeds 30 mg./100 ml.

2. The patient's acid-base status must be appraised by the best methods available, and determinations should be repeated at frequent intervals. An analysis of the CO_2 content of venous blood is rarely adequate and may be distinctly misleading. The best method for measuring an uncompensated acidosis or alkalosis is a pH determination on an anaerobic sample of arterial blood. Instead of a direct measurement, this value can be estimated with reasonable accuracy from any two of the following three laboratory determinations: the alveolar CO_2 tension (measured on an end-tidal sample of expired air), the CO_2 content of arterial blood, and the CO_2-combining power of a blood sample (venous or arterial). If blood analyses cannot be accomplished, a poor but useful substitute is litmus paper to determine the reaction of freshly voided urine; catheterize if necessary and repeat the determination with frequent urine samples. The general significance of these tests is outlined on pp. 217–219.

3. Blood analyses may also reveal any or all of the following:
   a. Ketosis,
   b. Hypoglycemia,
   c. Hypoprothrombinemia,
   d. Prolonged blood coagulation time (rare).

4. Urinalysis may reveal albumin, casts, red blood cells and white blood cells; acetone and diacetic acid; a positive Ebhart's test.

STRYCHNINE

Strychnine is prepared from dried ripe seeds of *Strychnos Nux-vomica*, which contain 1.1 to 1.4 per cent (rarely 2 per cent) strychnine and about an equal amount of brucine (a closely related alkaloid). In clinical medicine strychnine is used traditionally as a stomachic and unjustifiably as a stimulant and tonic, in the form of alkaloidal salts (nitrate, sulfate, phosphate), various elixirs and syrups, nux vomica tincture (0.12 per cent strychnine), nux vomica fluidextract (1.0 to 1.2 per cent strychnine), and the dried powdered extract of *Strychnos Nux-vomica* (7 to 7.7 per cent strychnine). Cathartic and tonic tablets, containing irrational mixtures of cathartics, belladonna, and

strychnine, are still obtainable; attracted by their sugar coating many children have poisoned themselves with these tablets. Strychnine is a long established vermicide, commonly used at bait concentrations of about 0.5 per cent. Although such bait is usually refused by rats, the material is useful in the control of mice, gophers, squirrels, prairie dogs, porcupines, rabbits, moles, and other predatory animals, and birds. The ingestion of strychnine bait has caused human poisoning. Strychnine was formerly an important source of suicidal and homicidal poisonings, but recognized cases are now comparatively infrequent.

Toxicology: Strychnine is a potent convulsant. When taken by mouth, the mean lethal dose in man probably lies between 100 and 120 mg. (1½ to 2 grains). A dose as small as 16 mg. has killed an adult, and 30 mg. is usually a threat to life; in contrast recovery has followed the ingestion of more than 2000 mg. When administererd by the subcutaneous route, the lethal dose is less by one-half to two-thirds. On a body weight basis, children may be slightly more refractory to strychnine than are adults. The lethality of nux vomica is believed to parallel its content of strychnine. Brucine is not a major toxicological problem; although it may act as a local anesthetic agent and perhaps as a paralytic substance, it produces convulsions only in relatively large doses (40 times the effective dose of strychnine, according to one report).

After the ingestion of strychnine or nux vomica, untoward symptoms commonly begin within 10 to 30 minutes (occasionally after a delay of 1 hour). Often without warning of any kind, the patient falls in a violent convulsion, but usually there are prodromal signs and symptoms. Soon any mild sensory stimulus triggers a violent generalized convulsion. A transient clonic phase is quickly followed by spasm of all skeletal muscles; the stronger muscles dominate and produce a posture characteristic of spinal convulsions (see Symptomatology). Tetanic contractions of the diaphragm, thoracic and abdominal muscles stop respiration, so that anoxia and cyanosis develop quickly. After the convulsion, the victim is relaxed, depressed, and exhausted. Because sensation is unaffected, the convulsions are painful and engender overwhelming fear. As many as ten convulsions, separated by intervals of 10 to 15 minutes, may be experienced, but death commonly occurs between the second and fifth paroxysm. The exact mechanism of strychnine's action on the cerebrospinal axis is not clearly established, but the drug apparently acts similarly on all portions of the central and peripheral nervous systems to increase excitability. Effects on other organ systems appear to be entirely secondary to these nerve actions.

Included in the differential diagnosis of strychnine convulsions are the following clinical entities:

tetanus, hydrophobia, spinal meningitis, epilepsy, and hysteria. Infectious tetanus and hydrophobia (rabies) produce prodromal malaise and a less fulminating course than strychnine poisoning. Pharyngeal and glottic spasm are more marked in hydrophobia than in strychnine intoxication. The high fever of spinal meningitis is distinctive. In convulsive attacks of epilepsy, consciousness is always lost. Some cases of hysteria are very difficult to distinguish from strychnine poisoning.

Death is commonly due to asphyxia from respiratory arrest during or between convulsions. Respiratory failure may arise from anoxic damage cumulating during each convulsive episode or from exhaustion of medullary nerve centers because of overstimulation. Both types of injury can be prevented if convulsions are aborted early in the course of poisoning. For this purpose rapidly acting intravenous barbiturate drugs are probably the most satisfactory central nervous depressants. Strychnine is largely detoxified in the liver, but approximately 20 per cent of a sublethal dose escapes in the urine unchanged. Since both detoxification and excretion are comparatively fast, the prognosis in strychnine poisoning is good if the patient can be kept alive for the first 5 to 6 hours.

Symptomatology (beginning 15 to 30 minutes after ingestion):

1. Without warning the patient may fall into a violent convulsion, but often prodromal symptoms are described, such as restlessness, apprehension, heightened acuity of perception (hearing, vision, feeling, *etc.*), abrupt movements, hyperreflexia, and especially muscular stiffness of the face and legs. Rarely vomiting occurs.

2. A minor sensory stimulus may suddenly trigger a violent generalized convulsion which lasts from 0.5 to 2 minutes. At first the movements are intermittent (clonic), but a spinal tetanic phase quickly intervenes. The body typically arches in hyperextension (opisthotonos), so that in a supine position the body is supported by the heels and head. The legs are adducted and extended, the arms are flexed over the chest or rigidly extended, and the fists are tightly clenched. The jaw is rigidly clamped (trismus), the face is fixed in a grin (risus sardonicus), and the eyes protrude in a fixed stare. Because the muscles of respiration are involved in a sustained spasm, breathing ceases and deep cyanosis appears. Consciousness is retained during the convulsion, which is painful, and the patient remains apprehensive and fearful throughout the illness.

3. Between convulsions, muscular relaxation is typically complete. Breathing resumes and the cyanosis lessens. Cold perspiration covers the

skin. Dilated pupils may contract. The patient sometimes falls asleep from exhaustion. Reflex irritability usually remains low for a period of 10 to 15 minutes, when hyperexcitability quickly returns, and sudden stimuli such as a noise or even a draft of air may precipitate another paroxysm.

4. One to ten such attacks occur before recovery or death from respiratory arrest. In the absence of effective treatment, most victims do not tolerate more than 5 convulsions, and death commonly occurs within 1 to 3 hours after the ingestion of a fatal dose. As the poisoning progresses, the convulsions may become more violent and the intermissions shorter.

5. If the patient survives the first 5 to 6 hours, the prognosis is good. There are no serious sequelae among survivors.

Treatment:

1. Treatment is designed primarily to prevent convulsions and thus to protect medullary centers from excessive stimulation and from anoxia.

2. If it can be done before the development of reflex hyperexcitability, the induction of emesis is desirable, but a safer procedure is the ingestion of a slurry of 6 to 8 heaping teaspoonsful of "universal antidote" (p. 10) in a few ounces of water. Gastric lavage is postponed until the patient is fully premedicated.

3. Protect patient from harming himself during convulsions and reduce all sensory stimulation to a minimum by keeping him in a comfortably warm, quiet, and darkened room. Avoid all unessential procedures, and exclude all visitors. Each succeeding convulsion reduces the patient's chances of survival.

4. Inject intravenously sufficient amounts of a barbiturate drug to prevent further convulsive paroxysms. A short acting drug such as amobarbital sodium (Amytal) or pentobarbital sodium (Nembutal) is best. An adequate dose

usually produces loss of consciousness, and more than 0.5 gm. by slow intravenous injection may be necessary (p. 202).

5. If a satisfactory barbiturate is not immediately available, convulsions can often be temporarily controlled by the inhalation of chloroform or ether or by the rectal administration of Avertin (tribromoethanol). See p. 203.

6. Neuromuscular blocking agents (*e.g.*, curare) may have adjunctive value in the management of strychnine convulsions, but limited experience with curariform drugs has not been encouraging. Similarly muscle relaxants with central sites of action (*e.g.*, mephensin) have proved disappointing in the control of strychnine-like convulsions. However, the therapist who has experience with these drugs may find them useful adjuvants (see p. 204).

7. If post-convulsive depression or an overdose of an anticonvulsant drug causes apnea, artificial respiration becomes essential. Keep the airway clear and administer oxygen (p. 184 and 189).

8. The patient must be kept under constant observation for many hours. Wakefulness, hyperreflexia, and muscular twitching signal a need for additional doses of barbiturate.

9. After convulsions and reflex irritability have been suppressed, gastric lavage can be safely performed. A dilute potassium permanganate solution (1:5000) is probably best. The iodide in tincture of iodine (1 teaspoonful in a glass of water) forms an insoluble strychnine salt, which may temporarily delay absorption.

Laboratory: Laboratory data are seldom useful in the diagnosis or prognosis of strychnine poisoning. A leukocytosis is commonly observed; it is presumably associated with the release of epinephrine from the adrenal medulla. Methods are available for the isolation and identification of strychnine in stomach contents and other organs.

THALLIUM

Salts of thallium serve as active ingredients in some rodenticides and ant poisons (usually as thallous sulfate). In spite of high toxicity, thallium acetate has been and occasionally is still used internally as a temporary depilatory in cases of ringworm of the scalp and externally as a cream depilatory in cases of hypertrichosis.

Toxicology: As evidenced by its trivalent compounds, the element thallium belongs in the aluminum family, but monovalent thallium salts are more closely related, chemically and toxicologically, to divalent lead, although the acute toxicity of thallium compounds is much higher. The ingestion of

any thallous salt is followed, after a latent period of 12 to 24 hours, by a severe hemorrhagic gastroenteritis. Probably this phenomenon is due to vascular actions of absorbed thallium. Delirium, convulsions, and coma may appear rapidly, but more often the acute reaction subsides, only to be replaced by the gradual development of the following (in any combination): mild gastrointestinal disorders, polyneuritis, encephalopathy, skin eruptions, and hepatorenal injury. The most characteristic sign, however, is alopecia, but this appears only in cases where death is delayed for at least 20 days. These delayed effects are usually persistent and may

prove fatal. Convalescence is slow. As with lead, this subacute syndrome may develop without a recognized acute illness, especially if small quantities of thallium salts are ingested daily. Subacute and chronic intòxications are associated with the cumulative tissue retention of thallium, presumably in the form of sparingly soluble thallous chloride. Over a period of one month about 70 per cent of an administered dose is excreted, largely in urine and partly in bile.

The mean lethal dose in an adult is probably about 1 gm. Single doses of 8 to 10 mg. of thallium acetate per kg. of body weight have killed a few children. The difference between a depilating and a toxic dose is small and allows no margin for idiosyncrasy. Thallium preparations are unnecessary and dangerous, and their use in clinical medicine should be entirely discontinued. There is no satisfactory treatment for thallium poisoning. Dimercaprol (BAL) may have some beneficial actions, but the effects are not dramatic and are probably not worthwhile.

Symptomatology:

1. Symptoms usually appear within 12 to 24 hours after a single toxic dose or after several weeks of small daily doses.
2. In acute poisonings gastrointestinal effects are dominant: severe paroxysmal abdominal pain (colic), vomiting, and diarrhea. The vomitus and stools are often bloody. In severe cases tremors, delirium, convulsions, paralysis, coma, and death often within 1 to 2 days.
3. In subacute poisonings, signs and symptoms referable to the alimentary tract include intermittent intestinal colic, nausea, vomiting, diarrhea, achlorhydria, stomatitis, excessive salivation, and gingival discoloration (comparable to the lead line).
4. Neuromuscular symptoms include tremors, leg pains, paresthesias of the hands and feet, and a frank peripheral polyneuritis, principally in the legs.
5. Ocular and facial palsies and retrobulbar neuritis lead to severe and sometimes permanent disability.
6. A toxic psychosis, delirium, convulsions, and other signs of encephalopathy.
7. Skin eruptions, including keratinization, petechiae, and ecchymoses.
8. Central necrosis of the liver and damage to the renal tubular epithelium. The hepatorenal lesions per se are rarely fatal.
9. The loss of hair (alopecia) is usually reversible unless repeated exposures are allowed. The lesion is apparently due to a metabolic disturbance in the hair follicle, perhaps of circulatory or neurotropic origin.

Treatment:

1. Immediate measures include administration of an emetic, or gastric lavage with a 1 per cent solution of sodium or potassium iodide (in order to form insoluble thallium iodide).
2. Unless diarrhea is already established, produce catharsis with sodium or magnesium sulfate (15 to 30 gm.) in water or with castor oil (1 oz.).
3. Administer orally demulcents such as milk, starch paste, aluminum oxide gels, bismuth subcarbonate, etc.
4. Intramuscular dimercaprol (BAL) may be of some benefit if it can be started promptly, but this treatment is not widely accepted. For dosage schedule see p. 117.
5. Peripheral vascular collapse (shock) should be treated with parenteral fluids and electrolytes (p. 193).
6. The daily intravenous administration of 0.3 to 1.0 gm. of sodium iodide has been recommended. It presumably promotes the formation and precipitation of insoluble thallous iodide in tissues.
7. The daily intravenous injection of 10 to 20 ml. of a 3 per cent aqueous solution of sodium thiosulfate has been recommended to bring about the gradual excretion of fixed tissue thallium. This treatment is stopped after 3 days if the urine is found to contain no thallium or only a trace. If acute symptoms are reactivated by this procedure, thiosulfate treatment is stopped and iodide substituted. Neither the rationale nor efficacy of treatment programs using iodide, thiosulfate, or both is well established.
8. Symptomatic and supportive treatment for the various signs and symptoms of central nervous origin.
9. Cystine, methionine, and brewer's yeast have been found beneficial in acute and chronic thallium poisoning in rats. For a therapeutic trial in man, an adult should receive 10 to 20 gm. of brewer's yeast daily.
10. Because of possible disturbances in calcium metabolism, the daily ingestion of several grams of calcium gluconate, lactate, or chloride is recommended. Ample quantities of milk may be substituted.
11. If achlorhydria develops, nutrition may be improved by the administration of diluted hydrochloric acid (4 ml.) before each meal.

Laboratory:

1. Urinalysis may reveal albuminuria and an increase in cells and casts.
2. A definitive diagnosis may require chemical or spectrographic analysis of body fluids or excreta for thallium.

THIRAM

Thiram (tetramethylthiuram disulfide) is the methyl analogue of disulfiram or Antabuse; it is a white powder which is almost insoluble in water. Thiram is an important agricultural fungicide and is used in industry as a rubber accelerator. Together with related compounds, it has served successfully as an insecticide and as a repellent against the Japanese beetle.

Toxicology: No systemic poisonings in man have been reported to our knowledge. Animal tests suggest two toxic syndromes: that due to the inherent toxicity of thiram and that induced by ethyl alcohol in those who have ingested otherwise insignificant amounts of thiram. The latter, which is equivalent to the disulfiram(Antabuse)-alcohol reaction, is not described here; for its symptomatology and treatment, *see the discussion of disulfiram on page 139.*

Thiram is a moderately severe irritant of mucous membranes and a mild irritant of intact skin. On the basis of single oral doses (aqueous suspensions) in laboratory animals, the mean lethal dose lies near 0.5 gm./kg. (higher in rats, lower in rabbits). The toxicity is known to be greater in the presence of fats, oils, and fat solvents, which promote absorption. The ethyl analogue (tetraethylthiuram disulfide or disulfiram) is several times less toxic than thiram and is a much weaker irritant. Both compounds, however, produce similar toxic effects, and many of the following observations are abstracted from reports about disulfiram, which has been more extensively studied. Animals killed by single oral doses of disulfiram or thiram show hyperemia and focal ulceration of the gastrointestinal tract, focal necrosis of liver and renal tubules, and patchy demyelinization seen first in the cerebellum and medulla. The mechanism of poisoning is unknown; no carbon disulfide can be detected in the blood of animals fed disulfiram and the same is presumably true after thiram.

Single oral doses of 6 gm. disulfiram (Antabuse) have been well tolerated in man, but the usual clinical doses have occasionally produced severe dermatitis, mild gastrointestinal disorders, and minor psychic disturbances.

Symptomatology (the primary toxic reaction, *not* that induced by alcohol):

1. Nausea, vomiting, diarrhea, anorexia, weight loss. Nausea and emesis may be persistent and the diarrhea copious.
2. Ataxia, hyperexcitability.
3. Hypothermia.
4. Hypotonia and, within a few hours or a few days, flaccid paralysis. In animals this disorder appears first in the hind limbs and is a type of ascending paralysis (Landry's syndrome). The muscles retain responsiveness to mechanical and electrical stimulation. If death does not occur, recovery tends to be complete within one or two weeks.
5. Respiratory paralysis and death.

Treatment:

1. Lavage stomach with tap water.
2. Avoid fats, oils, and lipid solvents, which enhance absorption.
3. Rigorously prohibit ethyl alcohol in all forms for at least 10 days.
4. Symptomatic and supportive treatment for various gastrointestinal symptoms and neurological complications.

Laboratory: Repeated tests are desirable to detect and evaluate possible disturbances of liver and kidney function.

TOXAPHENE

Toxaphene is a chlorinated derivative of camphene, principally octachlorocamphene. The technical or insecticidal grade is an amber-colored waxy solid with a mild pine odor. It is prepared commercially as dusts, sprays, and wettable powders. It is a relatively slow-acting residual insecticide, which has been used extensively against cotton insects and grasshoppers. It has also been used for the control of insects resistant to DDT, but it is not considered safe for household application.

Toxicology: The compound is absorbed through the intact skin, respiratory tract, and the gastrointestinal tract. Intestinal absorption is increased by the presence of digestible oils, and liquid preparations (oil solvents) penetrate the skin far more readily than do dusts or powders. Several human fatalities have occurred. Although not definitely ascertained, the lethal oral dose for an adult is estimated to be 2 to 7 gm., representing a toxicity about 4 times that of DDT. Toxic symptoms in acute poisoning usually appear within one hour, and death occurs within four to eight hours. Lesions arise in the liver and renal tubules of chronically exposed animals. Toxaphene is less readily stored in body fat than is DDT. Measures which are used to combat camphor poisoning may be useful in toxaphene poisoning too, but therapy has not been fully evaluated in human intoxications.

Symptomatology:

1. Reflex hyperexcitability, evidenced by tremor, salivation, and vomiting. When present, emesis is apparently always secondary to reflex

excitation and not to local gastrointestinal irritation.

2. Generalized epileptiform convulsions of variable duration. Symptoms are precipitated or aggravated by external stimuli.

3. Death due to exhaustion and respiratory failure.

4. Mild irritation of skin after dermal exposures, but little if any sensitization.

Treatment:

1. Lavage with tap water and/or use emetics.

2. Saline cathartics, *e.g.*, sodium or magnesium sulfate (15 to 30 gm.) in water.

3. Demulcents, but avoid oils.

4. Barbiturates to control convulsions (pentothal, phenobarbital, or pentobarbital). Convulsions are best managed if treatment is begun before their appearance; if convulsions have already developed, use a short-acting drug like sodium pentothal, and give a full anesthetic dose. See p. 202.

5. Wash off any poison which may have contacted the skin. Use liberal amounts of soap and running water.

6. Avoid epinephrine, as a precaution against possible ventricular fibrillation.

7. Protect patient from strong external stimuli, which may precipitate convulsions.

Laboratory: Repeated tests are desirable to detect and evaluate possible disturbances in liver and kidney function.

TURPENTINE

Turpentine, gum turpentine, oil of turpentine, and spirits of turpentine are essentially synonomous names. Turpentine is a common solvent found in many homes, workshops, and barns, often in a container which was originally intended for a beverage. Samples vary in composition but all consist principally of terpenes, the chief one being a-pinene. Turpentine is used in mixing paints and in removing paint stains. Medicinally it has been used externally as a "stupe," internally for "worms," and in various forms as an expectorant and abortifacient. It is a solvent for waxes and is found in various kinds of polish.

Toxicology: Turpentine is readily absorbed from the gastrointestinal tract, skin, and respiratory tract. Many accidental poisonings through ingestion have been reported and include several fatalities. As little as 15 ml. (½ oz.) has proved fatal to a child, but the mean lethal dose in adults probably lies between 4 and 6 oz. Prolonged respiratory exposure to turpentine fumes or chronic skin contact with the liquid may lead to a toxic nephritis, as is suggested by the urinary findings in acute poisonings. The acute toxicity of turpentine is less than that of most volatile oils (*e.g.*, eucalyptus, sassafras, camphor, wintergreen).

Symptomatology:

1. Abdominal pain, colic, nausea, vomiting and diarrhea.

2. Transient excitement, delirium, ataxia, and finally stupor, which is the commonest severe symptom. Convulsions occur occasionally, usually not until several hours after ingestion, when they may interrupt a deep coma.

3. Painful urination, albuminuria, hematuria. Urine may have an odor resembling that of violets (also in eucalyptol poisoning).

4. Odor of turpentine on breath and in vomitus.

5. Fever and tachycardia are common.

6. Mild respiratory tract symptoms are occasionally seen (*e.g.*, stertor).

7. Death is usually one of respiratory failure.

Treatment:

1. Gastric lavage with tap water or weak sodium bicarbonate solution. It is always worthwhile to perform lavage because appreciable amounts of turpentine can be recovered many hours after ingestion. It may be useful to give a few ounces of mineral oil just before the lavage.

2. Saline catharsis with sodium or magnesium sulfate (15 to 30 gm.) in water.

3. Demulcents such as milk or beaten egg white.

4. Force fluids.

5. Codeine for pain. Avoid morphine because of possible respiratory depression.

6. Stimulants (*e.g.*, caffeine sodium benzoate) may be necessary to counteract severe depression (see p. 205).

Laboratory: Glycosuria, hematuria, and albuminuria may be demonstrated.

WARFARIN

Warfarin is an effective rodenticide available commercially as a powdered concentrate with 0.5 per cent active material. It was developed at the University of Wisconsin as an outgrowth of studies on hydroxycoumarin derivatives in relation to hemorrhagic disease in cattle. Recently warfarin has been used in clinical medicine as a therapeutic anticoagulant.

Toxicology: Warfarin is absorbed from the alimentary tract but not through the skin. It acts upon the liver specifically to inhibit prothrombin formation. In toxic doses it is also injurious to blood ves-

sels, as evidenced by widespread dilatation and engorgement and by an increase in capillary fragility. Both hypoprothrombinemia and vascular injury predispose to fatal internal hemorrhage, which is the basis of its effectiveness as a rodenticide and of its potential toxicity to man.

The inhibition of prothrombin formation does not become apparent until the body's prothrombin reserves are consumed. Multiple doses are usually required to maintain the inhibition of synthesis until these reservoirs are depleted, but if sufficiently large, a single dose may prove effective after a latency of several days. For example, in common laboratory animals the single mean lethal dose ranges between 200 and 400 mg./kg., except for the female rat which is sometimes killed at a level of 50 mg./kg. For an intake of 50 mg./kg., the average adult man would have to eat 1.5 lbs. of a warfarin concentrate (0.5 per cent) or about 30 lbs. of a strong rat bait (0.025 per cent). In contrast the daily ingestion for six days of as little as 1 to 2 mg./kg. (corresponding to about 1 lb. of 0.025 per cent bait per day) has produced a near fatal illness in an adult person. A Korean family of 14 persons lived for a period of 15 days on a diet of warfarinized cornmeal with an estimated individual intake of warfarin which varied between 1 and 2 mg./kg./day; all of these persons became severely ill with hemorrhages and two died.

In its effect on the blood coagulation mechanism, warfarin is the most potent hydroxycoumarin derivative tested. According to some, vascular lesions are also more prominent with warfarin than with its congeners. A single large dose produces no untoward signs or symptoms until clinical evidence of hemorrhage, which is usually apparent on the second, third, or fourth day, but a significant change in the blood prothrombin level can be detected within 24 hours. After a single intravenous injection of the sodium salt (about 1 mg./kg.); the maximum response in man is usually reached in 48 hours, and recovery is essentially complete by the fifth day. Except for potency, warfarin does not differ markedly from other inhibitors of prothrombin formation, such as bishydroxycoumarin (dicumarol). Vitamin K specifically antagonizes this hypoprothrombinemia; it also has a beneficial effect on the vascular lesions. Large and repeated doses of vitamin K are necessary for effective treatment.

Symptomatology (onset after a few days or few weeks of repeated ingestion):

1. Epistaxis and bleeding gums.
2. Pallor and sometimes petechial rash.
3. Massive ecchymoses and/or hematomata, es-

pecially of the elbows, knees, and buttocks.
4. Blood in urine and feces.
5. Occasionally paralysis due to cerebral hemorrhage.
6. Hemorrhagic shock and death.

Treatment:

1. Gastric lavage with tap water, if it is within a few hours after ingestion (single dose).
2. Vitamin K is a specific antidote. Vitamin K_1 emulsion is the preferred form. On the first day of treatment a poisoned adult should receive a dose of 65 mg., given by slow intravenous drip at a rate no faster than 10 mg./min. If necessary on subsequent days, vitamin K_1 should be continued at a reduced level until the prothrombin time returns to normal. Vitamin K_1 is preferable to K_1 oxide (dose 0.5 to 2.5 mg.) and certainly preferable to menadione or menadione sodium bisulfite.
3. Small transfusions of carefully matched whole blood may be necessary as a temporary source of prothrombin and of red blood cells. Fresh blood is preferable to stored blood to supply accessory coagulation factors.
4. Vitamin C is no substitute for Vitamin K, but ascorbic acid may be a useful adjunct to K therapy, as judged by animal studies. At least a dose of 100 mg. of ascorbic acid several time a day can do no harm.
5. After the control of hemorrhage and repair of the coagulation defect, replacement iron therapy is desirable to correct any secondary anemia. Ferrous sulfate at a dose of 0.3 gm. t.i.d. is recommended.
6. In some cases accessible hematomata should be aspirated after the clotting power of the the blood is restored to normal.

Laboratory:

1. The principal diagnostic test is a demonstration of markedly reduced prothrombin activity in blood plasma, as measured by the method of Quick or one of its modifications. The test should be repeated at least twice daily until a normal prothrombin time is established.
2. The blood clotting time and the bleeding time may be prolonged, but these values are not necessarily abnormal.
3. Blood is often demonstrable in urine and feces.
4. Secondary anemia (hypochromic, microcytic) may be marked.

XYLENE

Xylene (including its 3 isomers) is taken here as representative of aromatic hydrocarbon solvents such as benzene, toluene, cumene, and mesitylene. In commerce these substances are often found as

contaminants of one another; associated with them may be trace amounts of carbon bisulfide, pyridine, thiophene, *etc.* These mixtures and the purified hydrocarbons are widely used in industry; around the home they may be found in paint removers, degreasing cleaners, lacquers, insecticides, and pesticides. For many years the principal commercial source of aromatic hydrocarbons has been the destructive distillation of bituminous coal, but petroleum is now an important source.

Toxicology: These volatile solvents are toxic by all portals of entry, but percutaneous absorption is generally too slow to produce acute systemic poisoning. Essentially the same train of symptoms follows the ingestion of liquid and the inhalation of vapor, but in respiratory exposures bronchial and laryngeal irritation are usually more prominent. All of these aromatic hydrocarbons produce basically similar toxic reactions, namely local irritation, central nervous excitation and depression, and bone marrow inhibition.

The lethal dose of xylene is not known, and no fatal cases are recorded. Xylene and toluene, however, are thought to resemble benzene in acute toxicity, and in adults the mean lethal dose of benzene is probably about 15 ml. by mouth. Opinions still differ about the relative toxicities of pure benzene, crude benzene, toluene, and xylene. Whatever the differences in inherent toxicity, clinical experience demonstrates unequivocally that benzene is more hazardous than its alkyl derivatives. The principal distinction between these compounds, however, is seen only in chronic poisoning, where benzene commonly produces severe and fatal bone marrow damage, evidenced first by a leucopenia and later by thrombocytopenia and anemia. These blood dyscrasias, however, are rarely, if ever, seen in poisonings due to pure xylene or toluene or after single exposures to benzene—where death is prompt or recovery is complete.

In acute poisonings death results from one of two phenomena. Occasionally sudden death has been reported in vapor exposures under circumstances which impute the heart as the critical organ. Animal experiments show that benzene vapor sensitizes the myocardium to epinephrine, so that even the endogenous hormone may precipitate sudden and fatal ventricular fibrillation. Usually, however, death is due to respiratory arrest and consequent asphyxia. Unlike the aliphatic petroleum hydrocarbons, where deep coma is associated with depressed reflexes, aromatic hydrocarbons induce states of unconsciousness which are accompanied by tremors, motor restlessness, hypertonus, jactitations, and generally hyperactive reflexes. In animals loss of consciousness and areflexia do not occur until almost fatal doses are reached. Benzene is a more prominent neuroirritant than xylene or toluene, but it is probably less irritating to the eyes and mucous

membranes of the nose and respiratory tract. Xylenes and toluene do not appear to differ from one another in any important respects. When tested in animals at equal vapor concentrations, xylene (as aromatic solvent naphtha) produced a more delayed and a more prolonged central nervous depression than did toluene.

After absorption the volatile aromatic solvents are largely eliminated through the lungs. In part, benzene undergoes oxidative degradation with the formation of phenol, pyrocatechol, hydroquinone, and mucic acid, but alkyl derivatives of benzene are oxidized only to benzoic acid, toluic acid, *etc.* In all cases the only recommended treatment is symptomatic and supportive.

Symptomatology:

1. Ingestion causes a burning sensation in the mouth and stomach, also nausea, vomiting, and salivation.
2. Substernal pain, cough, and hoarseness are described.
3. In vapor exposures a transient euphoria is sometimes observed.
4. Headache, giddiness, vertigo, ataxia, and tinnitus.
5. Confusion, stupefaction, and coma.
6. Associated with this coma are often tremors, motor restlessness, hypertonus, and hyperactive reflexes, but frank convulsions rarely occur except in association with terminal asphyxia.
7. Death from respiratory failure or from sudden ventricular fibrillation.
8. Contact with liquid may cause erythema and blisters of the skin and hemorrhagic inflammatory lesions of mucous membrane.

Treatment:

1. Cautious gastric lavage with warm water. Observe all precautions described on p. 6. One or two ounces of mineral oil may be instilled and left in the stomach at the completion of lavage.
2. Sodium or magnesium sulfate (15 to 30 gm. dissolved in water) as a saline cathartic.
3. Ascorbic acid (50 to 100 mg. intravenously) has been reported as beneficial in the treatment of benzene poisoning.
4. General supportive measures, including oxygen administration (p. 189), artificial respiration (p. 185), and parenteral fluids, as indicated.
5. Avoid epinephrine because of its possible adverse effect on the sensitized myocardium. Avoid all digestible fats, oils, and alcohol, which might promote intestinal absorption.
6. If eyes or skin are affected, wash thoroughly and apply a bland analgetic ointment.

Laboratory: Complete hematological and bone marrow studies are always appropriate.

Section IV

Supportive Treatment in Acute Chemical Poisoning

TABLE OF CONTENTS

INTRODUCTION

In clinical toxicology, good patient management involves much more than terminating the toxic exposure and administering a chemical antidote or pharmacological antagonist. The alert physician is attentive to every symptom that arises during the course of an entire illness, symptoms that contribute to the patient's suffering whether they have serious prognostic import or not. In the course of offering symptomatic relief, the therapist inevitably gives support to those organ systems that are working to preserve physical and chemical homeostasis. The maintenance of homeostasis, which operates spontaneously and automatically in health, often becomes so inadequate in a poison victim that the physician must attempt to regulate many physiological parameters at the same time. It is this attempt that is called supportive treatment. In most poisonings good supportive therapy is more important than the "correct" antidote.

This section describes those measures of suppor-

tive treatment which are believed to be most appropriate in cases of acute chemical poisoning. The material is presented as a series of topics under the relevant organ system (see Table of Contents). Although functional pathology is briefly outlined, the emphasis in this section is on therapy and the techniques of therapy. Specific poisons are mentioned only to illustrate special clinical problems. Unless indicated to the contrary, all recommended doses are designed for an adult person of average size. In children, doses are usually reduced in proportion to the body weight or body surface area. The details of treatment must be conditioned always by the facilities, the training and experience of the therapist, and those many features which are unique to each patient's intoxication. Every clinical situation is influenced by so many indeterminant and intangible factors that there is no place for dogma-

tism in therapeutics. In this spirit the following remarks are offered as suggestions, not as rigorous prescriptions and prohibitions.

The following physicians on the staff of the University of Rochester School of Medicine and Dentistry read portions of this manuscript and/or offered important suggestions and criticisms: W. Andrew Dale, Frank W. Heggeness, Elihu S. Howland, John R. Jaenike, S. Marsh Tenney, and D. Vern Thomas. Dr. Nicholas M. Greene of the Yale University School of Medicine and Capt. James O. Elam, MC., AUS., furnished advice about various phases of resuscitation. Dr. Ruth S. Gosselin assembled much of the material in this section, and Miss June Boss compiled the data on nutrition. For the help of these experts the authors are grateful.

RESPIRATION

Respiratory Obstruction·

It is always imperative to assure a free and patent airway. As long as spontaneous breathing continues, signs of airway obstruction include respiratory retraction at the neck or intercostal spaces, dissociation of diaphragmatic from intercostal movements ("rocking boat respiration"), audible wheezes or rhonchi, and large quantities of secretions in the oropharynx. A variety of signs and symptoms arise from the attending anoxia; they include cyanosis, restlessness, depression, confusion, and lethargy. Restlessness is a particularly common early symptom; cyanosis is an unreliable sign until late in the course of asphyxia.

The following measures in sequence are employed to relieve obstruction in various parts of the respiratory tract:

1. position the patient in a lateral Trendelenburg
2. establish an oropharyngeal or nasopharyngeal airway
3. suction the pharynx, larynx, and trachea, as necessary, through the mouth or nose
4. pass an endotracheal tube if the above measures are insufficient
5. perform a tracheotomy if endotracheal intubation is impossible or the need is expected to continue for more than two or three days
6. remove mucus under direct observation with a bronchoscope
7. relieve patchy atelectasis by pounding the chest, rolling the patient periodically, using a cough machine, *etc.*

These procedures are discussed in detail below.

Obstruction of the oropharynx is often due to a relaxed tongue and other soft tissues. This complication can usually be avoided by keeping the victim on his side with his head low. This lateral

head-down position is also valuable in minimizing the aspiration of vomitus. If the tongue has already slipped into the pharynx, it must be pulled forward. Often this can be done by grasping the chin or by reaching behind the angle of the mandible on both sides (fig. IV.2) and pulling the mandible forward while the neck is extended slightly. If this maneuver does not succeed, the physician can often reach inside the victim's mouth, firmly grasp the tongue with a clamp or fingers, and pull it forward. In the absence of a vomiting reflex, the tongue is best held in place by the insertion of a hard-rubber or plastic oropharyngeal airway; this device is merely slid along the roof of the mouth until its ventral curvature hooks the root of the tongue and carries it forward. A No. 5 airway is suitable for adults, a No. 3 for children, and a No. 1 for infants. If trismus prevents instrumentation through the mouth, a nasopharyngeal airway is used instead. A soft rubber urethral catheter (14 to 30 F) makes a satisfactory airway if 2 or 3 holes are cut in it at half-inch intervals.

Suctioning the airway is necessary to remove mucus and other secretions from the hypopharynx and tracheobronchial tree. A small flexible catheter attached to a suction machine is best, but a large syringe (50 or 100 ml.) can be used, if necessary, to produce a negative pressure. Sometimes the oropharynx can be wiped out with a finger covered with a gauze pad. If the patient is deeply narcotized, the larynx and trachea can usually be entered blindly with a suctioning catheter. If the coma is not intense, this maneuver may induce reflex laryngeal spasm, which is usually transient, but if it persists and completely occludes the airway, the physician must proceed to endotracheal intubation.

Endotracheal intubation. If the conservative

measures outlined above fail to establish a good airway, endotracheal intubation or tracheotomy becomes advisable. The former is usually tried first unless the airway obstruction is expected to be a threat for more than 2 or 3 days. Unlike a pharyngeal airway, an indwelling tube in the trachea prevents respiratory obstruction due to spasm or edema of the vocal cords; it also allows the trachea and even the major bronchi to be suctioned with considerable efficiency by a small catheter passed periodically through the endotracheal tube.

A semi-rigid catheter, No. 34 F and about 10 inches long, makes a satisfactory endotracheal tube for most adults. After removing an oro- or naso-pharyngeal airway, the tube may be passed into the mouth and through the glottis under direct observation with the aid of a laryngoscope. Because of the dangers of trauma, this procedure is best reserved for the physician with special training, but this injunction may have to be ignored in critical emergencies. If masseter spasm prevents instrumentation through the mouth, passage of the endotracheal tube may be attempted blindly through the nose. In any case the bevelled tip of the tube should lie just beyond the larynx (i.e., below the vocal cords); if passed too far it may become impacted in the right main bronchus. A properly positioned endotracheal tube offers no certain guarantee against respiratory obstruction. The tube may kink, or it may become occluded by mucous plugs either complication may arise insidiously or with alarming rapidity. It may be necessary to pass a suction catheter down the tube every few minutes or only infrequently, but a trained person should be in constant attendance as long as intubation is continued. In all cases the endotracheal tube should be removed every 12 to 24 hours, cleaned and re-inserted, or replaced with a new tube. Intubation is usually continued as long as the patient tolerates it. The tube is removed when the victim begins to cough or "buck on the airway." By this time his cough reflex is usually sufficient to insure the expulsion of secretions. In any case it is undesirable to leave an endotracheal tube in place any longer than necessary, because the irritation it produces leads to contraction of the laryngeal muscles around the tube and eventually to laryngeal edema. When a tube is finally removed, a patient should be kept under careful observation for several hours because laryngeal spasm or edema may appear.

Tracheotomy. Surgical relief of upper airway obstruction is necessary if more conservative measures are unsuccessful. Tracheotomy is used instead of endotracheal intubation when the latter cannot be accomplished or when the threat of obstruction is expected to last more than two to three days. Tracheotomy is sometimes preferred to endotracheal intubation because the former considerably reduces respiratory deadspace. Provided that the incision is made promptly enough, tracheotomy can be and should be an orderly surgical procedure, involving sterile technique and local anesthesia. However, in near-terminal asphyxia due to or complicated by upper airway obstruction, the physician must not hesitate about performing an emergency tracheotomy without anesthesia and without sterile equipment. An incision is made through the skin and subcutaneous tissues from the laryngeal prominence (Adam's apple) to the suprasternal notch. The fingers of the left hand locate the trachea by following downward from the larynx. The tissues overlying the trachea are pushed downward. The thyroid isthmus may be torn or cut out if it cannot be avoided. With the left index finger palpating the trachea and acting as a guide, the scalpel is slid down along it and two or three tracheal rings are opened anteriorly by a vertical incision. If available a tracheotomy tube is inserted; otherwise the incision is held open by a hemostat or any other convenient object (e.g., flat key, broken tongue depressor). Only then is bleeding attended to and a dressing applied.

Bronchoscopy. Even in a tracheotomized patient, bronchoscopy with suctioning under direct observation sometimes proves to be the only satisfactory way of cleaning the major bronchi of obstructive plugs. In spite of bronchoscopy, secretions, edema, and foreign bodies may remain in the smaller air passages to produce scattered regions of obstruction and consequent atelectasis. These regions may be identified by the absence of breath sounds over corresponding areas of the chest wall. Pounding these areas energetically with the fist helps to dislodge mucous plugs. Forceful hyperventilation by rebreathing or inspiring 5 per cent CO_2 in oxygen may help. Drainage of the lower air passages is also promoted by rolling the patient from one side to the other periodically and by elevating the foot of the bed. Pneumonia is an almost inevitable complication unless prevented by vigorous antibiotic therapy (see p. 231).

Artificial Respiration

If breathing movements are inadequate or absent, artificial respiration is imperative; it becomes possible only after all major airway obstruction has been corrected. Because they are always available, manual methods of artificial respiration are generally employed first in an emergency. If the introduction of artificial respiration does not cause cyanosis to disappear or subside markedly within a few minutes, an explanation should be sought promptly. If the circulation remains adequate by clinical criteria, persistent cyanosis suggests unrecognized respiratory obstruction. Sometimes the fault is the technique of the therapist. If unexplained difficulties continue, other approved meth-

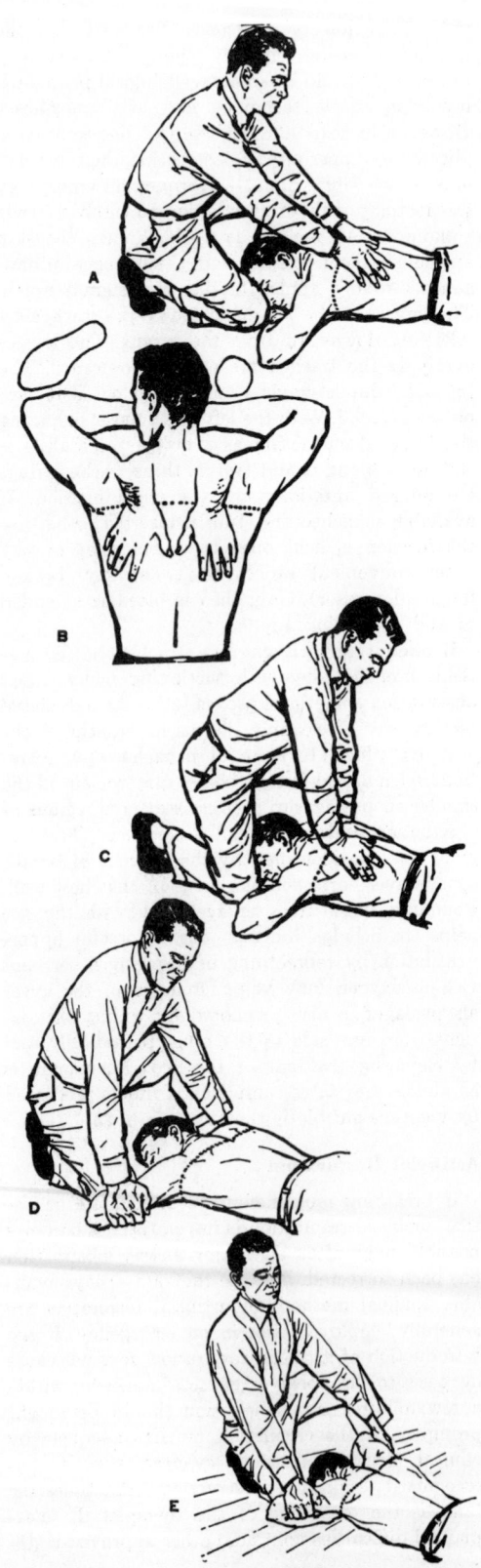

ods of artificial respiration should be given brief trials. Once the physician has assured himself that his procedure of artificial respiration is the best available, it must be continued until cardiac action has ceased beyond any reasonable doubt. Below are summarized clinically useful methods of artificial respiration.

The back-pressure arm-lift method is probably the most satisfactory manual technique of artificial respiration. At a conference in 1951 it was adopted as the official method by the American Red Cross, the U. S. Public Health Service, the National Research Council, and others. The method is preferred because it is easy to learn, is relatively non-fatiguing, requires only one operator, and gives active assistance to both inspiration and expiration. The technique is described below as a series of instructions, which are illustrated in Fig. IV.1.

Position of the subject. (Fig. IV.1A) Place the subject in the face-down prone position with his elbows bent and with the hands placed one upon the other. Turn his face slightly to one side and rest his cheek upon his hands.

Position of the operator. (Fig. IV.1A & B) Kneel on either the right or left knee or, if more comfortable, on both, at the head of the subject facing him. Place your knee or knees at the side of the subject's head close to his forearm. Place your hands upon the flat of the victim's back in such a way that the heels of the hands lie just below a line running between the axillae. With the tips of the thumbs just touching, spread the fingers downward and outward.

Compression phase. (Fig. IV.1C) Keeping your elbows straight, rock forward until your arms are approximately vertical and allow the weight of the upper half of your body to exert slow, steady, even pressure downward upon the hands. This forces air out of the victim's lungs.

Expansion phase. (Fig. IV.1D & E) Release the pressure, avoiding a final thrust, and commence to rock backward slowly. Then place your hands upon the subject's arms, just above his elbows, and draw his arms upward and toward you. Apply just enough lift to feel resistance and tension at the subject's shoulders. Do not bend your elbows, and as you rock backwards the subject's arms will be drawn toward you. This act constitutes active inspiration on the part of the subject. Then lower the arms gently to the ground. This completes the cycle. The arm lift expands the chest by pulling on the chest muscles, arching the back, and relieving the weight on the chest.

Additional directions. The cycle should be repeated twelve times per minute at a steady, uniform rate. The compression and expansion phases

Fig. IV.1. Artificial respiration by the back-pressure arm-lift method (drawings reproduced with permission of the American Red Cross).

should occupy about equal time, the release periods being of minimal duration. If the victim begins to breath on his own, adjust your timing to assist him. Do not fight the victim's attempt to breathe. With children of 4 years old or more, the procedure is the same except that pressure is applied to the shoulder blades with the tips of the fingers only. When a child is under 4 years of age, then his arms are placed alongside of his body, and his head is placed face down on a support consisting of a roll of cloth under his forehead. Pressure is applied to the back of the thorax with the thumbs only and inspiration is effected when the trunk is slightly elevated by lifting at the shoulders. The rate is 15 times per minute.

Mouth-to-mouth or mouth-to-nose insufflation (sometimes called direct inflation methods) are ancient techniques of artificial respiration, which have never become popular because of obvious hygienic and esthetic objections. These procedures are probably more effective, however, than most of the manual methods of resuscitation. Recent evidence indicates that in the presence of resistance to pulmonary ventilation, mouth-to-mouth insufflation is more effective than the back-pressure arm-lift method. In any case, these procedures are always available, and except for the obstetrician, the physician has largely ignored them. In the absence of special equipment, probably the mouth-to-nose method is more easily accomplished by an adult operator with an adult victim than is mouth-to-mouth resuscitation. By pinching the lips of a flaccid, unconscious subject, it is possible to seal his mouth against a reasonably high intra-oral pressure. Once this has been done, the operator leans over and places his mouth over the victim's nose. At this point the operator exhales a normal, or somewhat greater than normal, tidal volume. The operator's expired air is thus used to inflate the patient's chest. The latter expires as soon as his mouth or nose are left free; this passive expiration can be aided by manual compression of the chest. The entire procedure is repeated approximately 12 times per minute. The operator must hyperventilate moderately in order to perform this method properly, but dizziness and other signs of hypocapnea have not been observed in operators even after long periods of resuscitation.

Figures IV.2–IV.5 illustrate how mouth-to-mouth insufflation can be facilitated by comparatively simple equipment. An oronasal mask like that used for clinical anesthesia is employed. With its inflated rubber cuff to act as an air seal, the mask is applied to the face as illustrated in Fig. IV.2. To prevent collapse of the pharynx and hypopharynx with consequent obstruction, note how the mandible is held forward and how the soft tissues of the floor of the mouth are supported. According to the simplest procedure, the resuscitator takes a breath of about twice normal volume and then ex-

hales directly into the mask (Fig. IV.3). In a related procedure the operator both exhales and inhales through a flexible rubber tubing connected directly to the face mask. Here the mask must be modified by drilling in it an air vent which can be alternately opened and blocked by the operator's thumb, as illustrated in Fig. IV.4. In this technique the operator necessarily rebreathes to some extent and so hypocapnea and respiratory alkalosis are avoided. If the therapist also has a gas mask and canister, the procedure can be so modified as to be practical while both victim and operator are in a toxic atmosphere (Fig. IV.5).

Mechanical devices for resuscitation. Artificial respiration by mechanical devices is easier and generally more efficient than that by manual methods. In all instances a patent airway must first be established. A great many mechanical appliances are available commercially. One of the simplest and most effective is a hand-operated Kreiselman bellows respirator or any one of similar design. Another type of simple resuscitative apparatus can be found in the emergency room of most hospitals; it consists of an anesthesia face mask connected by means of a right-angle elbow with a nipple for the oxygen supply to a reservoir bag. With the mask on the face and oxygen running to fill the bag, active inflation of the lungs can be obtained by manual compression of the bag. The degree of inflation can be readily ascertained by watching the chest wall.

In addition to these manually operated devices, many automatic or semi-automatic portable resuscitators can be obtained through commercial channels. In general, each of these is accompanied by relatively simple instructions designed to be read and understood under conditions of duress. Almost all machines involve a positive-pressure inspiratory phase and a passive expiratory one, but with some designs expiration can be active or passive at the discretion of the operator. Most of the appliances operate on the principle that pressure from a cylinder of oxygen, properly reduced, forcefully inflates the lungs. Inflation is controlled by a release valve which is actuated at a predetermined pressure and interrupts the flow of oxygen. With most commercial models the inflationary positive pressure does not exceed 20 mm. of mercury, and there are not fewer than 10 cycles per minute at a flow of 500 ml. per minute. If the mechanical respirator provides as well for active deflation by suction, the negative phase should not exceed 9 mm. of mercury. The chest wall should be watched to check on inflation. If resistance to the flow of oxygen is encountered, the pressure releases too early to effect lung ventilation, and the device starts to recycle at a high frequency, in some cases with a chattering sound. Portable resuscitators of this general design are carried in the vehicles of most municipal fire departments. Finally there are

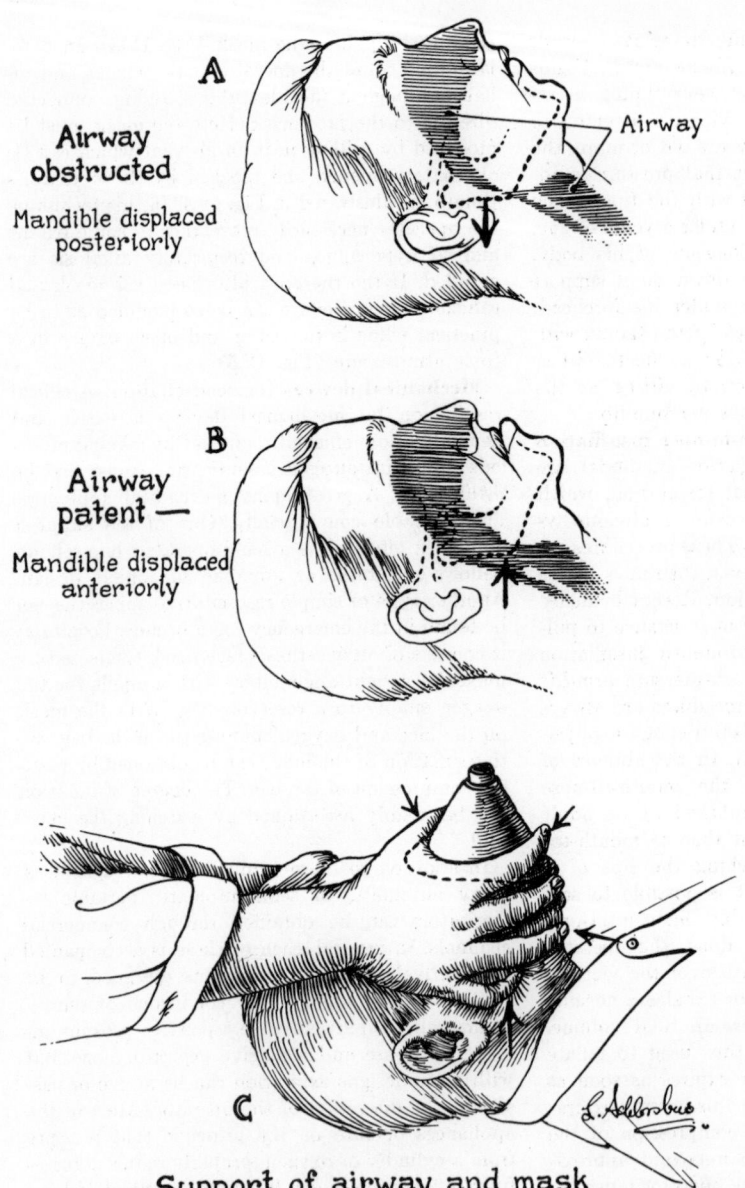

A

Airway obstructed

Mandible displaced posteriorly

Airway

B

Airway patent —

Mandible displaced anteriorly

C

Support of airway and mask

Fig. IV.2 (Courtesy of Directorate of Medical Research, Chemical Warfare Laboratories, Army Chemical Center.) See p. 187.

Drinker or tank-type respirators, which are useful because they require little supervision after they have been properly adjusted. When available, electrophrenic stimulators may be effective in the management of apnea of central nervous origin, but success with this method apparently requires much practice. For an excellent summary of available resuscitation equipment, with operating characteristics, instructions for use and for maintenance, etc., see *Handbook of Poisons*, by R. H. Dreisbach, Lange Medical Publications, Los Alto, California, 1955.

Except for the electrophrenic respirator, all of the resuscitation devices listed above employ positive-pressure inspiration, *i.e.*, pressure within the mask or mouth exceeds that outside the chest. One consequence is the possibility that air or oxygen is forced down the esophagus into the stomach, *particularly if* ventilatory resistance is encountered at or below the larynx. The physician must check for this complication by examining the epigastrium periodically; when distended, it must be decompressed immediately. Occasionally this can be accomplished by passing a Levine tube, but a stiffer gastric tube is preferable. Sometimes a long nasotracheal tube is introduced intentionally into the esophagus, and a Levine tube is then easily threaded through it. With modern methods of resuscitation,

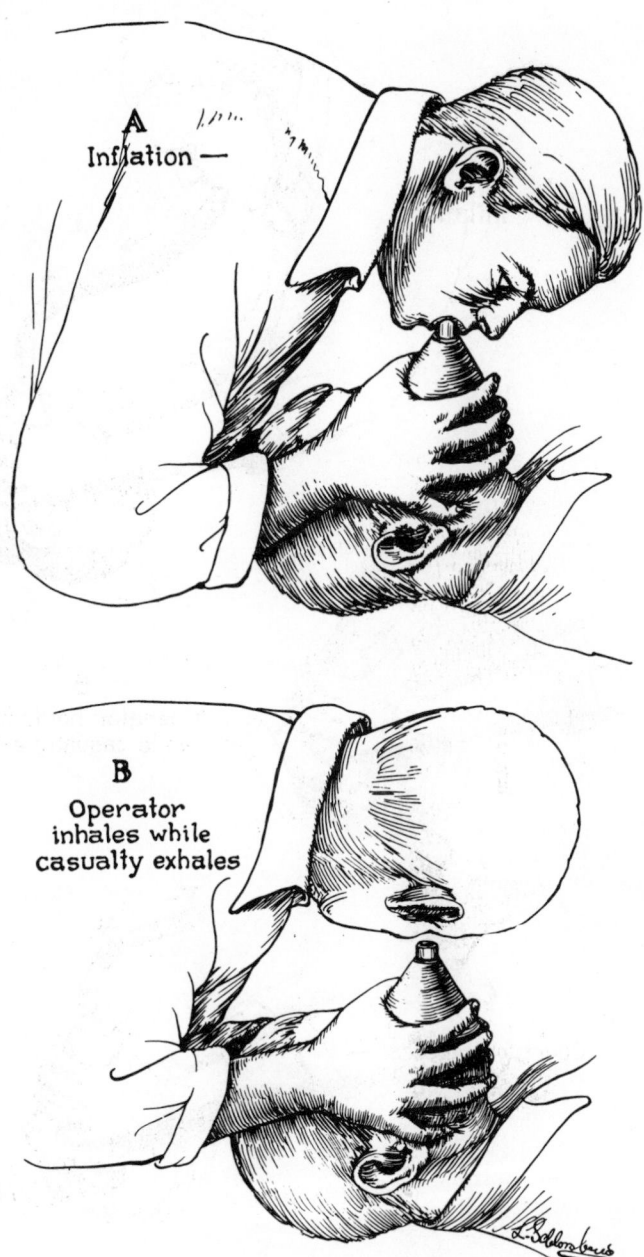

A
Inflation —

B
Operator
inhales while
casualty exhales

Fig. IV.3 (Courtesy of Directorate of Medical Research, Chemical Warfare Laboratories, Army Chemical Center.) See p. 187.

gastric dilatation is regarded as a major problem since any procedure effective in ventilating the lungs in the presence of abnormal airway resistance is necessarily capable of inflating the stomach.

Oxygen Therapy

Most patients who require artificial respiration can profit by the simultaneous administration of oxygen, preferably at a concentration of 40 per cent or above in the inspired air. The lower value is most expeditiously achieved by feeding pure oxygen at a rate of 6 to 8 liters per minute through a nasal catheter which terminates just behind the soft palate. An ordinary soft rubber urethral catheter (10 to 14 F) is satisfactory as a temporary measure, if several holes are cut into it at half-inch intervals. The catheter should be lubricated with water or a water-soluble gel. With the O_2 flowing, the catheter is introduced into that nostril with the wider lumen, and it is inserted for a distance 1½ inches less than that measured between the external auditory meatus and the nostril. The posi-

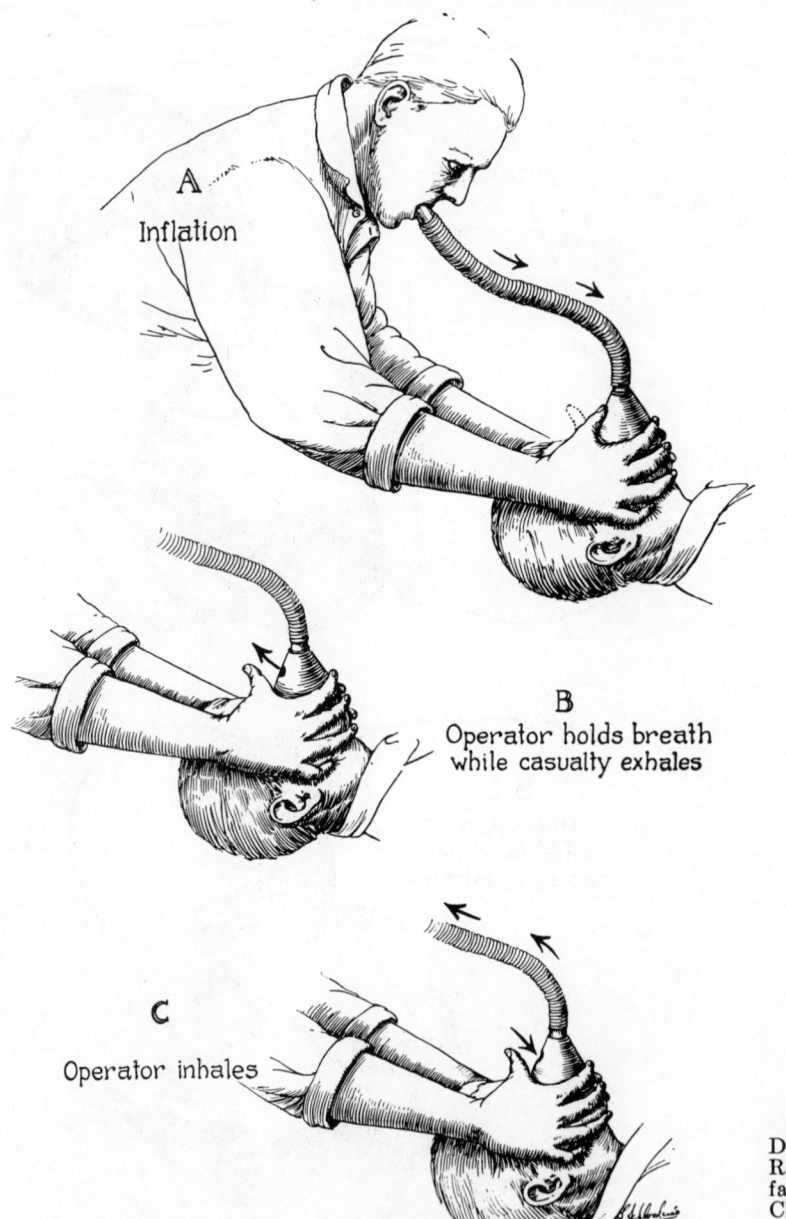

A
Inflation

B
Operator holds breath
while casualty exhales

C
Operator inhales

Fig. IV.4. (Courtesy of
Directorate of Medical
Research, Chemical War-
fare Laboratories, Army
Chemical Center.) See p.
187.

tion of the tube can be checked by looking into the mouth, where the tip of the catheter should be just visible behind the soft palate; if the tube is too low, the risk of inflating the esophagus and stomach is considerable. When properly positioned, the tube is held in place by adhesive tape across the face or forehead. With nasal administration the oxygen should be humidified by bubbling it through water before it enters the catheter.

Many commercial resuscitative devices make provision for oxygen administration through face masks. Only with full-face or oronasal masks can oxygen concentrations as high as 100 per cent be attained regularly in inspired air. Masks of many designs are available. In general, pure oxygen is fed to them at a rate fast enough to prevent deflation of the reservoir bag even during inspiration. Some designs allow positive pressures to be created intentionally within the mask during expiration (see *Pulmonary Edema*, p. 192, for discussion of positive pressure oxygen therapy). Most delirious patients tolerate hoods and tents better

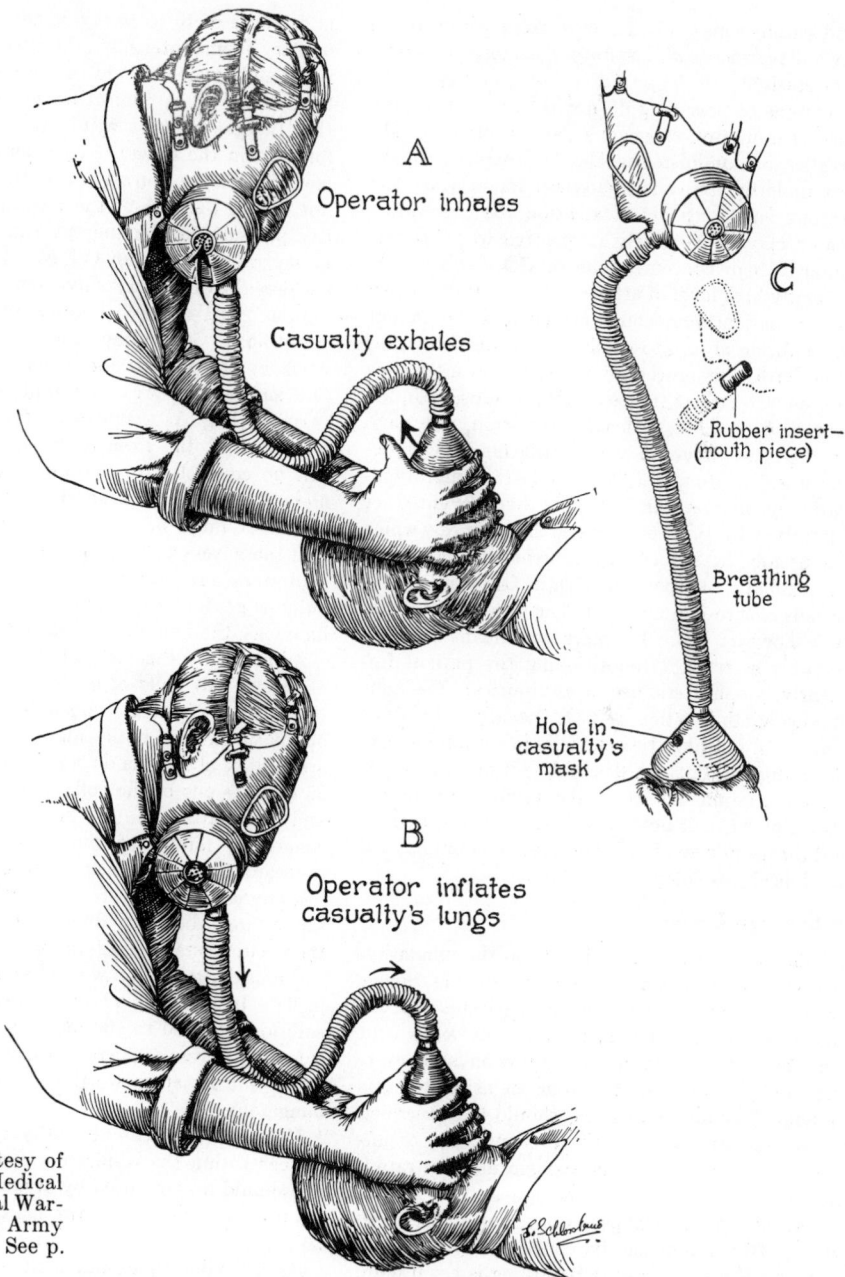

A

Operator inhales

Casualty exhales

C

Rubber insert—
(mouth piece)

Breathing
tube

Hole in
casualty's
mask

B

Operator inflates
casualty's lungs

Fig. IV.5. (Courtesy of Directorate of Medical Research, Chemical Warfare Laboratories, Army Chemical Center.) See p. 187.

than face masks; the former are particularly satisfactory for children and infants. When properly used, hoods and tents allow inspiratory oxygen concentrations of about 60 per cent.

In almost all patients the administration of pure oxygen is safe for at least several hours. Without good indications, inspiratory O_2 concentrations should not be held at 100 per cent for more than 12 hours, because inflammation may develop within

the respiratory tract (cough, sputum, substernal pain). If oxygen therapy is expected to be prolonged, a concentration of 60 per cent is generally preferable to 100 per cent, or the two levels can be used alternately. The lower concentration is entirely satisfactory in many cases, but sometimes pure oxygen is essential (e.g., pulmonary edema, CO poisoning). Even during short periods some patients with chronic pulmonary disease (fibrosis

and emphysema) tolerate pure oxygen poorly for several reasons (*e.g.*, respiratory acidosis, marginal atelectasis).

Victims of poisoning do not require the respiratory stimulus of exogenous carbon dioxide. The practice of administering CO_2-O_2 mixtures to correct underbreathing is ill-advised for at least two reasons; in states of intoxication the respiratory center may be relatively insensitive to even dangerously high concentrations of CO_2, and an abnormally high level of arterial CO_2 inevitably exists in any patient who underventilates. Even though the addition of CO_2 to inspired air leads to marked hyperpnea, the procedure produces or intensifies, but never corrects, a respiratory acidosis. Underbreathing requires artificial respiration, not CO_2. On the other hand, uneven ventilation may represent a legitimate use of CO_2. Atelectasis and hypostatic pneumonia can probably be prevented or minimized by brief episodes of hyperpnea (which can usually be induced by rebreathing or by gas mixtures of 5 to 7 per cent CO_2 in O_2 presented for periods of 2 to 5 minutes). Other preventive measures, however, may be more important and are certainly safer (*e.g.*, repositioning the patient frequently, prophylactic use of antibiotics). The continuous administration of CO_2 (usually 2 to 5 per cent in O_2) is said to be beneficial in carbon monoxide poisoning, but the desirable action here is on the dissociation curves of the various circulating hemoglobins; it is not a respiratory action. In general the usefulness of CO_2 has been overemphasized in clinical toxicology.

Pulmonary Edema

Pulmonary edema may arise from the inhalation of a variety of poisonous gases and vapors. Sometimes a latency of many hours separates the exposure from the first appearance of signs and symptoms. After a known exposure physical exercise must be avoided. Even in an asymptomatic individual, complete bed rest should be prescribed for at least 24 hours. At the first evidence of impending pulmonary edema, oxygen administration should be commenced by the quickest and most expeditious means. Oxygen concentrations between 80 and 100 per cent can be conveniently delivered by oronasal mask. Pressure breathing is not usually necessary in mild situations. Atropine sulfate (0.5 to 1.0 mg. *s.c.*) may prove helpful in suppressing reflex bronchospasm, but this is often accomplished better by intravenous aminophyllin (0.25 to 0.5 gm. *slowly*) or by the brief inhalation of an aerosolized epinephrine solution (1:100). Mild sedation is usually advisable; for this purpose the barbiturate drugs are usually satisfactory; paraldehyde should be avoided under these circumstances. Unless the pulmonary disturbance is of cardiac origin, morphine is used only with great caution.

and a dose of 10 to 15 mg. is not exceeded. If pulmonary edema intensifies, the patient should sit upright, and oxygen should be delivered under "positive pressure." In clinical usage this phrase means that the gas pressure within the mask (and therefore within the lungs) is considerably above barometric pressure during expiration but generally not during the rest of the respiratory cycle. Positive pressure oxygen therapy can be accomplished in several ways. In an O.E.M. mask a metal disc encloses the expiratory valve and is perforated with various sized orifices; because of this partial obstruction to expiration, the pressure within the mask lies between 0 and 4 cm. of water at a gas flow sufficient to prevent complete deflation of the reservoir bag. As a substitute for these or equivalent devices, the exhalation port of some masks can be connected to a rubber tube which is immersed in water to a depth of 4 cm. In all cases the mask must be closely applied to the face so that there is no leakage. Oxygen is started at a peak expiratory pressure of 4 cm. of water, and this value is gradually lowered over a period of several hours as the pulmonary edema clears.

Additional measures include either phlebotomy of one or two pints of blood or blood trapping by the use of rotating venous tourniquets, starting on one arm and both thighs. The cuff pressures are held at about the diastolic arterial level. Every 20 minutes one of the cuffs in sequence is removed and re-inflated on the unoccupied limb. Acute congestive failure of the heart may arise from myocardial decompensation secondary to altered hemodynamics within the pulmonary circuit; heart failure may be very difficult to recognize under these circumstances. In cases of doubt, rapid but cautious digitalization would seem appropriate (see p. 196). Intravenous administration of a hypertonic solution (*e.g.*, 50 to 100 ml. of a 50 per cent solution of glucose or sucrose) may have a transient effect but is rarely worthwhile and is sometimes dangerous.

If large quantities of frothy or foamy exudate appear within the respiratory tract, gravity drainage should be promoted by laying the patient with his body sloping head down on an incline of 15 to 20°. The upper tract can often be kept clear by using a flexible suctioning catheter. Opinions differ on the adjuvant use of antifoam agents. Ethyl alcohol has been promoted in this role, and 30 to 40 per cent aqueous solutions are sometimes put into the humidifier of the oxygen line. Favorable results, however, can be explained largely by the systemic effect of absorbed alcohol on the central nervous system, an action more efficiently and more safely accomplished with conventional hypnotic drugs. In a recent promising demonstration, dimethylpolysiloxane emulsions were found to reduce the volume of respiratory tract foam and the death

rate of rabbits and rats in experimental pulmonary edema (Nickerson and Curry: J. Pharmacol. & Exper. Therap., *114:* 138, 1955). A commercial emulsion (XEC 151, Dow Corning Corp., Midland, Mich.) was diluted 1:10 with water and aerosolized ("nebulized") to produce a fine mist which was inhaled continuously by test animals. Clinical trials are in progress and are reputedly promising, but no adequate clinical evaluation of this group of antifoaming agents has been reported.

CIRCULATION

Two major categories of circulatory disorders follow exposures to toxic chemicals: those due to faulty vasomotor tone or abnormal capillary permeability, and those due to inadequacy of the heart as a pump.

Blood Vessels

Various poisons cause angiitis, thrombosis, internal bleeding, excessive capillary transudation, and all degrees of vasodilatation or vasoconstriction. The most common complication is profound and persistent hypotension, leading to the familiar syndrome of peripheral vascular collapse or shock. Two major types must be distinguished, to be designated in this report as vasogenic shock and oligemic shock. In both instances there is believed to be a disparity between the circulating blood volume and the volume capacity of the vascular circuit. In vasogenic shock the vascular volume is too large, and in oligemic shock the blood volume is too small. In both cases the return of venous blood is insufficient to enable the heart to maintain an adequate cardiac output.

Vasogenic shock is usually the result of depressed activity in the vasomotor centers of the brain stem and medulla oblongata, resulting in widespread vasodilatation without primary loss of circulating fluid. In chemical poisonings this vasomotor paralysis is characteristically associated with generalized central nervous depression (*e.g.*, barbiturate coma). Paralytic hypotension cannot be distinguished from oligemic shock by physical signs, although the former is not invariably accompanied by thirst or profound hemoconcentration and the skin is not always cold and clammy.

Two types of pharmacological agents are available in the control of this disorder: sympathomimetic vasoconstrictor drugs and analeptic drugs. The latter are employed to raise the level of spontaneous or reflex activity in vasomotor centers of the central nervous system. In subconvulsive doses they are effective only when the central nervous system is depressed or inhibited. The actions of analeptic drugs are complex and variable; their effects on the blood pressure are usually transient and frequently undependable. Repeated doses may lead to central nervous depression rather than stimulation. Drugs in this category include nikethamide (Coramine), pentylenetetrazol (Metrazol), picrotoxin, and caffeine. In an adult of average size, recommended doses are as follows: nikethamide, 1 to 3 ml. of a 25 per cent solution *i.v.* or *s.c.*; Metrazol, 0.1 to 0.2 gm. *i.v.* or *s.c.*; picrotoxin, 3 to 10 mg. *i.v.* or *i.m.*; and caffeine sodium benzoate, 0.5 gm. *s.c.* In deep coma these doses may be doubled or even tripled and repeated at intervals of 5 to 20 minutes, if reflexes and vital signs are checked continuously. For more detailed information about the use of these drugs, see Table IV.2 (p. 206).

More precise and perhaps safer control of paralytic hypotension can be secured by the administration of peripheral vasoconstrictor drugs. For example, phenylephrine (Neosynephrine) in doses of 2 to 10 mg. or methoxamine in doses of 15 mg. can be injected intramuscularly; Neosynephrine has also been given by slow intravenous infusion. Probably the drug of choice, however, is l-nor-epinephrine. It lacks the cardio-accelerator and probably some of the vasodilator properties of epinephrine. Given intravenously its effects are immediate but transient. Excellent control of the arterial blood pressure can be obtained by the slow infusion of nor-epinephrine (*e.g.*, Levophed, 4 ml. or 4 mg. in 1 liter of saline or glucose solution, given *i.v.* at an approximate rate of 1 ml. per minute). It is apparent that this procedure demands frequent observations of the blood pressure, preferably at 5- to 10-minute intervals. Cardiac arrhythmias are seldom encountered but are a potential source of danger. Severe local lesions occur if the solution is allowed to extravasate. Because no cumulative effects are recognized at the recommended rate of administration, these infusions can be continued almost indefinitely. The procedure, however, cannot be recommended without reservations because neither cardiac nor renal responses have been thoroughly explored.

Oligemic shock is related, at least in its therapeutic requirements, to surgical shock, hemorrhagic shock, and traumatic shock. In chemical intoxications abnormal permeability of blood vessels may cause the leakage of prodigious amounts of plasma, with or without red blood cells, into tissues, serous cavities, and particularly the lumen of the gastrointestinal tract. The extent of concealed hemorrhage and of plasma depletion by leakage is frequently underestimated. The usual progression of signs and symptoms includes restlessness, thirst, hemoconcentration, hypotension, oliguria, grayish pallor, and a cold moist skin. The mental state may vary from excitement to stupor. Peripheral pulses are usually weak and rapid. These classical signs

and symptoms, however, may not appear until the venous return and cardiac output become severely reduced. One of the earliest manifestations of shock is a decline in blood pressure when the subject changes from the recumbent to the sitting position (this sign is more significant in a young patient than an elderly one). In contrast the arterial pressure is generally well maintained while the patient stays recumbent, until the blood loss exceeds 20 per cent of the normal volume.

Therapy is principally an endeavor to repair and to maintain an adequate circulation by restoring the circulating volume, whether the deficit is due to loss of blood or to exudation of plasma. Vasoconstrictor drugs are rarely effective because compensatory reflexes generate and usually maintain maximal vasoconstriction in this syndrome. Late in the course of oligemic shock, however, vasodilatation may occur. Peripheral vasoconstrictor drugs should be tried only if hypotension persists after liberal intravenous replacement therapy.

The ideal replacement fluid in the treatment of oligemic shock is blood plasma or whole blood. Until the specific need of each patient can be determined, transfusions with whole blood are preferable. If a rise in the venous hematocrit is subsequently demonstrable, plasma or a plasma expander should be substituted for blood. Isotonic saline (0.85 or 0.9 per cent NaCl) is less valuable than plasma; although it may correct hemoconcentration and restore the circulating volume, these actions are usually transient. Isotonic saline, however, has an invaluable role in the emergency control of shock while preparations are made for transfusions with blood, plasma, or plasma substitute. In fully established oligemic shock, the average patient probably requires about 20 ml. of whole blood or plasma expander per kilogram of body weight; in some cases 10 ml. per kg. are sufficient.

Because the virus of serum hepatitis is found in many dried (lyophilized) samples of pooled human plasma, where it cannot be successfully eradicated by present methods, pooled plasma should be given only if substitutes are unavailable. This injunction may not apply to liquid plasma, since the hepatitis virus dies out when human plasma is stored in the liquid state at room temperature from 6 to 12 months. During this aging some of the globulin molecules appear to be hydrolyzed to smaller units, but this decomposition does not impair the product as a useful replacement fluid in the treatment of shock. One excellent, though expensive, substitute for plasma is human serum albumin; commercial samples are freed of hepatitis virus by gentle heat sterilization. Except for the expense of serum albumin and the danger of hepatitis with blood plasma, these proteins are thought to be preferable to all synthetic plasma expanders. Among the latter, the current favorites are polyvinylpyrrolidone,

gelatin, and dextran. Globin, the protein derived from hemoglobin, has proved inferior to the other colloids, and many lots are nephrotoxic. Polyvinylpyrrolidone (PVP) is an inert plastic polymer and the cheapest of all plasma expanders. It is said to have been used extensively by German troops in World War II and is an effective and apparently safe therapeutic agent in the control of shock. Although no tissue injury has yet been ascribed to PVP, a potential hazard must be acknowledged because this polymer is not metabolized and yet is excreted only slowly by the kidneys. Consequently large amounts are stored chiefly in the reticuloendothelial system for periods of many years, and chronic disease arising from this tissue retention has not been thoroughly excluded. By acid hydrolysis, bone gelatin can be hydrolyzed to molecular sizes which are appropriate for intravenous use. When so processed, gelatin is a safe, stable, and cheap plasma expander, which is well retained in the circulation but is eventually metabolized completely to amino acids of nutritional value. Because of gelation at room temperature, the infusion equipment must be kept warm during the administration of this material. Dextran, a mixture of large polymers of glucose, is a cheap, stable and apparently safe plasma expander. It is well retained in the circulation for at least 12 hours; eventually part of it is excreted in the urine and part is metabolized to glucose. There appears to be no long-term storage in tissues. Dextrans are being stockpiled for national defense. Only further clinical experience, however, can clarify the proper roles of PVP, gelatin, and dextran in the management of shock.

Any available peripheral vein is adequate for the administration of replacement fluid in shock. Intra-arterial transfusions have no compelling advantages over intravenous ones. Subcutaneous routes of fluid administration are distinctly undependable in peripheral vascular collapse. When transfusions are administered intermittently through a needle, a superficial vein at one of the following sites is usually chosen: back of hands, forearms, antecubital fossa, or ankle. Only a large needle should be used (15 to 18 gauge), and it should be taped to the skin. It is usually advisable to restrain the limb as well. If a satisfactory superficial vein cannot be seen or palpated, even after use of a tourniquet, a surgical cut-down is necessary. After surgical exposure, the vein should be cannulated, preferably with a polyethylene tube rather than a metal needle because the latter is likely to produce local phlebitis and thrombosis if kept in situ for long periods. A polyethylene catheter is useful, therefore, in two situations: when one is unable to insert and maintain within a vein a needle of proper size, and when one anticipates a need for frequent or continuous intravenous therapy over a period of one or more days. Superficial veins at many

sites have been catheterized successfully, particularly veins in the forearm, the cephalic vein at the shoulder, the external jugular vein, and in infants various scalp veins. The preferred vessel, however, is probably the saphenous vein, which is often palpable on the antero-medial aspect of the lower leg or on the dorsum of the foot, and which in the adult can be located specifically one centimeter anterior to and one centimeter superior to the medial malleolus. At this site the saphenous vein is found superficial to the fascia by dissecting through the skin and subcutaneous tissues. The vein is tied, and a small incision is made in the vessel wall proximal to this tie. A polyethylene tube is chosen with a diameter as large as can be accommodated easily by the exposed vein. To insure sterility, catheters are best stored in a 0.1 per cent aqueous solution of benzalkonium chloride (*e.g.*, Zephiran). The appropriate catheter is inserted into the vein through the incision and threaded for a distance of several inches toward the heart. The tube should be held in place by a tight ligature encircling the cannulated portion of the vein. A second tie anchors the catheter to the body surface where it passes through the skin incision. Between infusions, the cannula is left *in situ* filled with a dilute heparin solution and sealed with a short stylus in the free end.

The rate of administration of intravenous replacement fluid depends upon the severity of the deficit. In routine blood transfusions, a slow rate is always employed, especially for the first 50 ml., which are best injected no faster than 2 ml. per minute. In oligemic shock, however, fast rates of administration are frequently required. Provided that whole blood has been properly cross-matched, it may be given to the patient in severe shock as rapidly as the cardiac action allows. The gravity method may prove too slow, even when a large needle is used and when the container of blood is elevated as high as possible. The rate of flow can be hastened by stripping the tube from above downward with a lubricated thumb and forefinger. Sometimes a three-way metal stopcock and syringe can be used to pump blood into a peripheral vein. In most cases, however, the conventional gravity method of transfusion is satisfactory because an injection rate of 1 liter per hour usually serves to maintain an adequate circulation. The transfusion is stopped when signs of shock disappear and when urine flow is resumed at a rate of at least 40 ml. per hour. The transfusion should also be terminated if rapid or labored breathing, flushed facies, venous distention, a gallop rhythm, or pulmonary rales develop.

Another procedure commonly employed in the treatment of shock is to elevate the foot of the bed or the patient's feet so that his head is several inches lower than his legs. This measure promotes the return of blood from the large venous reservoirs of the legs and abdomen. The patient is covered with one or more blankets, but all attempts to restore a normal skin temperature by the local application of heat should be strictly prohibited. Oxygen inhalation (p. 189) is frequently employed; not all authorities agree that it is a useful measure, but with proper technique it certainly can do no harm. Drugs should be used only cautiously and sparingly in these patients, and the only dependable route of administration in the presence of severe circulatory collapse is the intravenous channel.

Heart

Heart failure. Chemical agents may impair the circulation by the production of many types of cardiac lesions. The mechanisms that initiate and control the beat may become deranged (see discussion of cardiac arrhythmias), or the heart muscle itself may lose some of its contractile strength. A myocardial injury may be direct or indirect, diffuse or focal, reversible or irreversible. Regardless of the nature of the cardiac disorder, heart failure appears whenever the pumping action does not keep pace with the circulatory requirements of the body. Cardiac failure manifests itself in many ways. Any one of at least three clinical syndromes may result from a cardiac injury of toxic origin. The three syndromes are a hypotensive shock-like state, congestive heart failure, and acute pulmonary edema. Although the distinctions are somewhat artificial, this classification serves to emphasize that three different programs of therapy are available. The clinical management of each syndrome is outlined below.

Hypotension of cardiac origin must be distinguished from vasomotor paralysis and from oligemic shock, because treatments differ even though these conditions present many clinical features in common. In the shock-like state of diffuse myocarditis or focal myocardial infarction, various signs and symptoms usually direct attention to the heart. For example, pain, anxiety, and a sensation of oppression in the chest are common. The arterial blood pressure is low, and the peripheral veins are often collapsed. The arterial pulse is soft, small, and readily compressible. The heart rate is usually fast and often irregular. Electrocardiograms may reveal conduction defects, disturbances in the origin of beat, and injury currents. The heart sounds have a poor quality, and a gallop rhythm may be present. Perhaps the most specific finding, however, is cardiac dilatation; it may be evidenced by a diffuse and feeble apex thrust which is displaced to the left or is lost entirely. Dilatation of the left ventricle sometimes causes relative insufficiency of the mitral valve and a consequent systolic murmur. The signs and symptoms of congestive heart failure may

appear gradually. Any shock-like syndrome accompanied by venous hypertension is clearly of cardiac origin. With the exception of venous congestion, the cardiac disorders outlined above may be either causes or consequences of peripheral vascular collapse, but whenever they appear early in the course of circulatory insufficiency the primary defect is presumably within the heart.

The first and principal aim of treatment is a reduction of all circulatory stresses so as to insure maximal rest for the heart. Oxygen consumption and tissue metabolism are minimized by the maintenance of complete bed rest. If recumbency causes labored breathing or other distress, rest in a chair is prescribed. A patient's evaluation of his own comfort is probably the best index to the proper resting posture. Even the mildest exercise (*e.g.*, self-feeding) is usually prohibited. Among other attempts to decrease the circulatory load, the therapist prevents or corrects any abnormal elevations in the circulating blood volume. In contrast to hypotension of peripheral vascular collapse, vasoconstrictor drugs and intravenous fluids are strictly prohibited in the usual conservative regimen, although vasoconstrictors are sometimes employed when the diastolic pressure becomes so low that coronary blood flow is prejudiced. Sodium chloride in any form is withheld, and even the intake of water is sometimes restricted. Elevations of body temperature are corrected by antipyretic drugs and by other appropriate measures, because a fever raises the circulatory requirements of all tissues. For the same reason infections are suppressed by intensive antibiotic therapy. Whenever possible, all types of mental excitement are avoided and anxieties are minimized. Mental and physical repose and adequate sleep can usually be insured by the regular administration of simple sedatives such as the bromides. Pain is vigorously inhibited with analgetic drugs. Occasionally pain of cardiac origin justifies a trial with such coronary vasodilators as intravenous aminophyllin (0.2 to 0.5 gm.) or sometimes intravenous papaverine (0.1 gm.), but epinephrine and its congeners are too dangerous. Cyanosis calls for prompt oxygen therapy (p. 189), which may also correct pain and dyspnea. Severe arrhythmias and tachycardias require one of the antifibrillatory drugs (see p. 198). Any systemic metabolic disorder that might contribute to myocardial weakness must be corrected, including such disturbances as hypoglycemia, hypocalcemia, and severe acidosis. Digitalis and other cardiac glycosides are generally ineffective or even dangerous in cases of diffuse myocarditis or myocardial infarction. Only when and if congestive heart failure develops is digitalis prescribed.

Congestive heart failure is a familiar syndrome arising from subacute or chronic inadequacy of the heart as a pump, due to valvular disease, to weakness of the myocardium, or sometimes to an excessive frequency of cardiac contraction. Associated with a low cardiac output and insufficient tissue blood flow, the renal excretion of water and electrolytes becomes defective. Over a period of several days or several weeks, salt and water accumulate in the body in excessive amounts. These events lead to edema, congestion, cough, dyspnea, orthopnea, anorexia, nausea, venous distension, anxiety, and profound weakness, among many other signs and symptoms.

Whatever the original cause of congestive failure, the chief corrective measure, aside from removing this cause whenever feasible, is the administration of digitalis or a related glycoside. When properly used, these drugs are safe and usually effective; in the presence of congestive heart failure, the only contraindication to their use is digitalis poisoning itself. Standardized preparations of whole-leaf digitalis (from *Digitalis purpura*) are often given orally and can be employed rectally, but the isolated and purified glycosides are often preferred in current practice and are essential for parenteral administration. With digitalis and its congeners, the proper dose must be individualized. For optimal effect this dose must often approach the toxic range, but no rational excuse exists for maintaining a patient in digitalis poisoning (for its recognition and treatment, see p. 135). For each of the common purified cardiac glycosides and popular mixtures thereof, an average "digitalizing dose" and a maintenance dose have been suggested in Section II. In most cases the initial digitalizing dose should be divided and given as aliquots over a period of a few hours or a few days. With standardized (U.S.P. XV) whole-leaf digitalis by mouth, a common dosage schedule in adults is 0.2 gm. three times daily for 2 days, then twice daily for 2 days, and finally 0.1 to 0.2 gm. each day. In more urgent cases, a prompter action can be secured by giving 1.5 gm. in divided doses over a period of 18 to 24 hours, followed by 0.1 to 0.2 gm. daily. In very urgent cases, intravenous ouabain (G-strophanthin) should be substituted. An average "digitalizing dose" of ouabain (0.3 to 0.5 mg. in adults) produces cardiac actions which begin within 5 minutes, are maximal in 0.5 to 2 hours, and are over in about 24 hours. No single dose schedule is adequate for all patients, but because these drugs are often life-saving, they should never be withheld from a patient in congestive heart failure.

Ancillary treatment includes all of the measures specified under "hypotension of cardiac origin" (p. 195). Specifically, rest, oxygen therapy, sedation, and restrictions on the intake of salt (and rarely of water) are proper and useful procedures. In addition diuretic drugs are usually appropriate, even though the improved renal blood flow which results from digitalis may itself stimulate the ex-

cretion of extra salt and water. Oral doses of urea, theophyllin, theobromine, acidifying salts such as ammonium chloride, and acetazoleamide (Diamox) are all capable of promoting a clinically useful diuresis, but the most sustained and most dependable diuresis is that following administration of one of the modern organic mercurial drugs. Although derivatives being developed currently are safe and effective by the oral route, an intramuscular injection is the preferred mode of administration in emergency situations. Intravenous injection is seldom used now because this avenue offers several dangers but no convincing advantages. Meralluride sodium injection U.S.P. (solution mercuhydrin sodium) and mercaptomerin sodium U.S.P. (thiomerin sodium) are commonly administered in single doses of 1 to 2 ml. of 13 to 14 per cent aqueous solutions. Allergic reactions to these and other mercurial drugs are sometimes encountered, and a state of refractoriness to their diuretic action may develop whenever the chloride concentration of plasma is abnormally low (hypochloremia). The daily administration of ammonium chloride (8 to 12 gm. in divided doses by mouth) or Diamox (0.25 to 0.5 gm.) usually corrects this situation. Even with a good diuretic response, a massive pleural effusion and ascites generally warrant thoracentesis and abdominal paracentesis respectively.

Acute pulmonary edema of cardiac origin may develop as one aspect of congestive heart failure, but it often occurs in persons who show no signs of systemic visceral congestion or peripheral edema. The etiology of this condition is not simple and much remains to be explained, but according to one acceptable hypothesis, pulmonary congestion and eventual edema develop because the injured or diseased left ventricle pumps less blood than the right. If this explanation is adequate, the condition is properly called acute left ventricular failure. Probably pulmonary edema of cardiac origin is always preceded by a period of hypertension and vascular congestion in the pulmonary circuit. Sometimes pathological reflexes arising from congested lungs cause bronchoconstriction and wheezing ("cardiac asthma"). With or without recognized prodromata, pulmonary edema may appear with dramatic suddenness and alarming intensity. Good supportive treatment involves all of the measures outlined for pulmonary edema due to irritant gases (p. 192): specifically, rest, oxygen under pressure, morphine or other sedation, phlebotomy or venous trapping with tourniquets, removal of respiratory tract secretions by suctioning, and perhaps use of antifoaming substances. Of these procedures, oxygen, morphine (with atropine), and phlebotomy are probably of greatest value in the control of pulmonary edema of cardiac origin. In addition rapid "digitalization", preferably with intravenous ouabain (p. 196), is usually desirable but probably not

essential. The intravenous administration of mercurial diuretic drugs (*e.g.*, 1 to 2 ml. of a 13 per cent solution of mercuhydrin sodium) has been extolled in Europe in the treatment of acute pulmonary edema, but with these compounds the alleged advantages of the intravenous route over the intramuscular one probably do not compensate for the extra hazard.

Cardiac arrhythmias. Many abnormalities of rate and rhythm are encountered in victims of poison. These disturbances may be due to diffuse or focal myocarditis, with or without necrosis, but often there is no intrinsic cardiac lesion. In these instances the primary derangement lies within those portions of the autonomic nervous system that control the cardiac mechanism. An electrocardiogram is required for a definitive diagnosis of most abnormal rhythms, but a competent bedside examination is often adequate to rule out the more dangerous abnormalities. In any case an ECG tells nothing about the etiology of the disorder; it does not distinguish between those of toxic and those of non-toxic origin.

An abnormal mechanism of beat is comparatively benign if the ventricles are driven at a tolerable rate by an auricular pacemaker (or by the auriculoventricular node). In this category are most cases of auricular (atrial) tachycardia, auricular premature beats, auricular fibrillation, and all types of sinus rhythm. Most patients with these disorders require no treatment directed specifically toward the heart. The offending chemical agent, if any, should be removed, and rest and sedation are generally indicated. Sometimes digitalization with one of the cardiac glycosides is advisable to protect the ventricles from an excessive rate of stimulation by overactive atria.

In two types of situations, specific treatment is necessary for disordered mechanisms of beat. The first category includes any patient with an extremely fast or slow ventricular rate, whether regular or not. In these situations the circulation may become severely impaired. Thus extremes of bradycardia induce syncope, and extremes of tachycardia lead to congestive heart failure. Treatment of the latter is outlined above. Syncope due to transient cardiac standstill (Adams-Stokes syndrome) may be prevented by drugs which enhance the rate. For example, the sinus bradycardia of anticholinesterase poisoning (*e.g.*, parathion) responds to large doses of atropine (about 2 mg. for each subcutaneous or intravenous dose). In cases of complete heart block, a slow ectopic pacemaker in the ventricle can often be accelerated by the cautious administration of epinephrine (0.1 to 0.4 ml. of 1:1000 epinephrine *i.m.*) or other sympathomimetic drug (*e.g.*, ephedrine 30 mg. *p.o.*). In states of intoxication, however, epinephrine and its derivatives are best avoided because many toxic agents (*e.g.*, halogenated hydro-

carbons) sensitize the heart to even conventional doses of epinephrine, with the occasional disastrous production of ventricuar fibrillation.

The second category of cases requiring specific treatment is composed of those rhythms which tend to deteriorate into ventricular fibrillation and consequent death, even without the mediation of exogenous epinephrine. Frequent premature beats of ventricular origin and ventricular tachycardia are recognized to be dangerous in this respect, and generally these conditions should be treated promptly with one of the so-called antifibrillatory drugs. Quinidine hydrochloride is the usual choice when oral medication can be tolerated. One satisfactory dosage schedule in the adult consists of a test dose of 0.2 gm. for the detection of hypersensitivity; in the absence of an untoward reaction it is followed by a large single dose (0.8 gm.) and then small maintenance doses (0.2 gm. every 2 hours), until the cumulative dose has reached 2 to 4 gm. This regimen is interrupted if the disordered rhythm reverts to normal or if severe toxicity develops. For intramuscular use, special preparations of quinidine (e.g., the lactate) are available commercially or procainamide hydrochloride (Pronestyl) may be given a trial by the oral, intramuscular, or rarely the intravenous route. The oral or intramuscular dose of procainamide for an average adult is 1 gm., followed by a maintenance dose of 0.5 to 1.0 gm. every 2 to 4 hours. Intravenous procainamide is too toxic for all except severe emergencies. Procainamide and quinidine are similar in their actions on the heart, and there is little basis for choosing between them. In addition to hypersensitivity or drug allergy, both compounds may precipitate severe functional disturbances in cardiac action, especially when they are administered parenterally. For example, these drugs have successfully arrested primary ventricular rhythms only to result in fatal cardiac standstill because of an unrecognized but coexistent conduction block between the normal auricular pacemaker and the ventricles. The same complication is theoretically possible in the therapeutic use of any antifibrillatory drug.

Cardiac arrhythmias caused by digitalis overdosage (see pp. 135–138) are the same as those mentioned above and require generally the same treatment. Potassium salts by mouth, however, are frequently effective in this condition and are probably more rational than quinidine or procainamide, for which potassium therapy is a proper substitute. For the doses and techniques of administering potassium, see p. 220.

Cardiac arrest. Severe myocardial anoxia and profound vagal inhibition are the two factors most often responsible for the sudden cessation of effective contractions in a structurally sound heart. These factors often arise in chemical poisonings, and occasionally produce cardiac arrest. Given prompt and vigorous resuscitation, many of these victims can probably be saved. A presumptive diagnosis of cardiac arrest is proper when peripheral pulses suddenly disappear, the blood pressure becomes undetectable, and auscultation fails to reveal audible heart sounds. Any one of three cardiac states may exist: feeble but regular beating, ventricular fibrillation, or total standstill. The true situation becomes evident when an electrocardiogram is recorded or when the heart is exposed to view. Differentiation is important for choosing the proper definitive treatment but is unnecessary for initiating emergency resuscitation. Since cardiac arrest must be resolved within two to three minutes, if the patient is to recover without residual brain damage, a predetermined plan of action and a fully equipped kit must be available almost immediately. The following program of resuscitation is based chiefly on suggestions of Dr. S. E. Leeds (J. A. M. A., *152:* 1408, 1953).

If heart sounds are audible over the precordium after detectable arterial pulsations have ceased, a 1:1000 aqueous solution of epinephrine (adrenaline) should be diluted ten-fold with isotonic saline, and 0.5 to 2.0 ml. of the diluted solution should be injected intravenously. The closer to the heart the more effective is this injection. The right jugular vein is usually a satisfactory site, but if the chest is open, the needle is inserted directly into the right atrium. Since this injection occasionally precipitates ventricular fibrillation, the therapist must be prepared to deal with this complication. Epinephrine is ineffective against fibrillation and contraindicated in its presence.

With a silent precordium and absent arterial pulsations, the first maneuver is to prick the heart, preferably in the wall of the right atrium, by plunging through the chest wall a needle mounted on an empty syringe. Occasionally, in cases of true cardiac standstill, this mechanical stimulus causes the heart to resume beating, but it is ineffective if the ventricles are fibrillating. No more than 15 seconds should be spent on this stratagem.

If a pinprick is not promptly effective, the heart is exposed in order to institute cardiac massage. Even without sterile precautions, an incision is made in the fourth or fifth left intercostal space reaching from the left sternal border to the axilla. Because of the very low arterial blood pressure, there is essentially no bleeding. The ribs are spread and held apart by an assistant or by a self-retaining rib retractor. The therapist inserts his hand into the chest and firmly squeezes the ventricles to express as much blood as possible with each contraction of his hand. The rate and frequency of manual compression should be as fast as possible. Sometimes two hands are used at the same time. In some cases the procedure is more efficient if the peri-

cardial sac is opened first. Because effective cardiac massage quickly tires the operator, a qualified assistant should be available to relieve him.

In the meantime, an anesthetist or other qualified person begins artificial respiration. Pure oxygen under positive pressure should be delivered through an anesthesia mask or preferably an endotracheal tube. A modern anesthesia machine is the most efficient way of maintaining pulmonary ventilation. In its absence mouth-to-mouth resuscitation (p. 187) is preferred to other methods because it allows free access to the chest. With both cardiac massage and artificial respiration in operation, fluids (e.g., 5 per cent dextrose in water) are infused to promote venous return. As the patient begins to revive under these intensive supportive measures, a large dose of morphine is usually indicated, unless the original chemical intoxication renders it unnecessary or inadvisable.

As soon as respirations and blood flow are reestablished and artificially maintained, attempts at definitive treatment become practical. Through the thoracotomy incision, it is usually possible to recognize whether the myocardium is quiescent or in a state of fibrillation, even without opening the pericardium. Simple asystole sometimes responds to epinephrine injected into the right atrium, as described above. The injection may be repeated at intervals of a few minutes. Occasionally calcium chloride (e.g., 2 to 4 ml. of a 10 per cent solution infused into the left ventricular cavity) revives a heart which does not respond to epinephrine. Intravenous or intracardiac atropine sulfate in comparatively large doses (e.g., 2 mg.) is sometimes effective when asystole is due to a vagovagal reflex. Procainamide and quinidine, however, are contraindicated in cardiac standstill because they depress all pacemaker activity. Similarly analeptic and sympathomimetic drugs such as caffeine, nikethamide, pentylenetetrazol, amphetamine, and phenylephrine are ineffective or contraindicated. Digitalis and strophanthin are also avoided. Because active attempts to stimulate the quiescent heart often precipitate ventricular fibrillation, the safest procedure is to continue cardiac massage and artificial respiration until myocardial excitability returns spontaneously.

With ventricular fibrillation, active efforts at defibrillation are often necessary, although rarely a normal rhythm returns with massage alone. The best and often the only effective measure is the application of single or multiple electric shocks. Preferred for this purpose is a defibrillator which can deliver a pulse of 110 or 130 volts with a duration of about 0.1 seconds. Electrodes, which are made from large metal plates covered with gauze and saturated with a NaCl solution, are pressed firmly against the ventricles, preferably inside the pericardial sac. To deliver the shock, each of two operators wearing rubber gloves holds a single electrode by its insulated handle and stands on a dry floor, avoiding contact with the metal bed or treatment table. If a single shock or a series of 5 to 10 impulses at 1-second intervals are unsuccessful at terminating the fibrillation and at restoring a normal rhythm, 200 mg. of procainamide (Pronestyl) hydrochloride is administered intravenously or directly into the atrium. After such premedication, a defibrillating shock is usually effective. When a normal rhythm is restored, the chest is closed with absorbable surgical sutures. Oxygen and a broad-spectrum antibiotic are administered for several days.

It is apparent that these heroic measures are not recommended as a routine procedure. Probably attempts at cardiac resuscitation are not worthwhile in an elderly person whose heart is known to have serious structural damage. Before opening the chest, the physician should have at hand all requisite equipment. Useful apparatus and drugs have been listed by S. E. Leeds (op. cit.). A simple defibrillator has been described by R. S. Mackay (J. A. M. A., 154: 1421, 1954). All equipment for cardiac resuscitation, preferably in the form of a kit, should be available for immediate use in every emergency treatment station and surgical operating room.

CENTRAL NERVOUS SYSTEM

Pain

The suppression of pain is one of the first and most essential elements in supportive treatment. Universal humanitarian standards are adequate justification for its high priority. Pain, especially persistent pain, often generates fear, anxiety, irritability, exhaustion, and emotional depression. Besides preventing psychic disturbances, the control of pain may forestall the disorganization of many somatic functions, since through reflex and hormonal control intense pain exerts noxious influences on many organ systems. Sometimes these undesirable reactions to pain serve to perpetuate the offending stimulus, creating so-called "vicious cycles." A simple if somewhat mundane example is the pain of muscle spasm which generates more spasm and so more pain. Certain types of visceral pain (e.g., from myocardial ischemia) may potentiate and perhaps cause severe vasomotor collapse. Of course pain is not always detrimental, and a physician should hesitate to suppress it completely, until its diagnostic and prognostic values have been fully exploited.

The systemic administration of analgesic drugs

is not always necessary to control pain. Thus many types of visceral pain are effectively erased by spasmolytic drugs. For example, atropine sulfate eradicates the pain of colic by inhibiting the intestinal spasm which generates it. Similarly nitrites and other antispasmodics are often effective against biliary and renal colic. Isolated neuritic pain can usually be controlled by infiltration with a local anesthetic solution, such as 1 per cent procaine hydrochloride. Topical anesthetic drugs in the form of ointments and solutions may effectively inhibit pain arising from localized cutaneous and mucosal lesions. Pain from integumentary structures often responds to the local application of heat, especially moist heat. Sometimes cold applications are preferable, notably when an inflamed or itching skin is the source of distress.

In most cases, however, pain requires the administration of a true analgesic drug, i.e., one which exerts its principal or sole actions on the central nervous system. Among the safest and most effective compounds of this type are the salicylates, notably acetylsalicylic acid or aspirin. Oral doses of 0.3 to 0.6 gm. every 2 to 4 hours are often adequate to control superficial pain and particularly pain of a neuralgic, myalgic, or arthralgic character. Often acetophenetidin is given in conjunction with salicylates. When pain is not effectively controlled by these mixtures, they are often supplemented by small amounts of codeine phosphate (e.g., 8 to 30 mg.). Unfortunately, the oral route is the only appropriate channel for administering aspirin and its congeners. Absorption from the rectum is slow and undependable, and while the intravenous route is available for solutions of sodium salicylate, these infusions are somewhat hazardous and distinctly inconvenient. In many chemical poisonings, gastrointestinal damage precludes oral medication. Since salicylates are often irritating to even the normal gastric mucosa, salicylate therapy is of limited value in clinical toxicology.

The narcotic alkaloids furnish dependable and intense analgesia by various routes of administration. Their use should be restricted to patients in whom the non-narcotic analgesic drugs are inadequate. Morphine therapy, for example, may be complicated by such problems as addiction, physical dependence, tolerance, medullary depression (especially of the respiratory tract), spasm of smooth muscle, reflex vomiting, constipation, urinary retention, idiosyncrasies, pruritus, and urticaria. With respect to physical dependence, addiction, and tolerance, all of the narcotic alkaloids share the liabilities of morphine. Codeine is probably the drug of choice in most cases where the non-narcotic analgesics are insufficient. At first small oral doses (8 to 32 mg.) of codeine sulfate or phosphate are tried in conjunction with salicylates. If this is inadequate, codeine salts are given in parenteral doses as high as 65 mg. (i.m. or s.c.) and repeated every 3 to 4 hours as required. If a more powerful analgesic is necessary, one of the following is tried: meperidine (Demerol) hydrochloride, 50 to 100 mg., p.o. or i.m., every 2 to 4 hours as necessary; methadone hydrochloride 5 to 10 mg., p.o., i.m., or s.c., at intervals of 4 to 8 hours as required; dihydromorphinone (Dilaudid) hydrochloride, 1 to 2 mg., p.o., or s.c., every 3 or 4 hours as necessary; methyldihydromorphinone (Metopon) hydrochloride, 3 to 9 mg., p.o., every few hours as necessary. Because of its slightly greater tendency to produce stupefaction, euphoria, and addiction, morphine is best reserved for cases where a euphoric tranquillity is desired, as well as relief from pain. The average adult dose of morphine sulfate is 5 to 15 mg. s.c. or 8 to 20 mg. p.o., but in the presence of severe pain larger amounts may be necessary.

All of the narcotic analgesics are detoxified principally in the liver. They should be prescribed sparingly if at all in cases of liver disease, myxedema, adrenal insufficiency, and other states of reduced metabolism. If poisoning results from overdosages of morphine or its congeners, institute treatment according to the scheme on p. 159. Narcotics should never be administered according to a fixed schedule but should be given only at times of actual need. As soon as the severe phase of a painful illness ceases, all narcotics should be withdrawn. In some patients an iatrogenic addiction can arise after a few days of repeated medication, and so the physician should be alert for withdrawal symptoms as soon as any narcotic drug is discontinued.

Some people who are anxious and fearful complain repeatedly of bizarre and transient pain. Others use the word "pain" to denote any unpleasant sensation, including states of nervous tension. Whether their problems are psychosomatic or semantic, these individuals often respond to simple sedation without the use of an analgesic drug. Thus small repeated doses of one of the barbiturates or of chloral hydrate may serve to allay fear and associated pain. In "true" (!) pain, however, sedative drugs alone are inappropriate because, unless combined with a pain killer, sedatives may produce restlessness and even delirium.

Central Nervous Hyperexcitability

Central nervous hyperexcitability may reveal itself in many ways. Two of the commonest syndromes are delirium and convulsions, representing different types of central stimulation; sometimes they coexist. Delirium is principally a disturbance in cerebral activity, while convulsions usually represent dysfunction of the brain stem or spinal cord. Both syndromes occur frequently in acute chemical poisonings, and both present difficult problems

of therapy. In its most general form, this is the problem of sedation.

Delirium. The following comments about the care of the delirious patient are reprinted from *Principles of Internal Medicine*, editor Harrison, copyright 1954, by permission of Blakiston Div., McGraw-Hill Book Company, Inc., New York City.

"The first objectives are to quiet the patient and to protect him against injury. A private nurse, an attendant or a member of the family should be with the patient at all times, if this can be arranged. Depending on how active and confused the patient is, various types of restraints must be employed. If extremely active and vigorous, a locked room, screened windows that cannot be opened by the patient, and a low bed or mattress on the floor should be arranged. It is often better to let the patient walk about the room than to tie him into bed; this may excite or frighten him so that he struggles to the point of complete exhaustion and collapse. If less active, the patient can usually be kept in bed by leather wrist restraints, a restraining sheet, or a net thrown over the bed. Unless contraindicated by the primary disease, the patient should be permitted to sit up or walk about the room for part of the day.

"All drugs that could possibly be responsible for delirium—particularly opiates, barbiturates, bromides, atropine, hyoscine, cortisone, adrenocorticotropic hormone (ACTH), and salicylates in large doses—should be discontinued. Paraldehyde and chloral hydrate are the only sedatives that can be trusted under these circumstances. Paraldehyde, which is preferred, may be given orally or rectally in doses of 10 to 20 ml. For oral administration mixing it with fruit juices makes it more palatable, though alcoholic patients will take it in any form and seem to enjoy it. One must be cautious in attempting to suppress the agitation completely. To accomplish this may require the use of very large doses of drugs, and vital functions may be dangerously impaired. The purpose of sedation is to secure rest and sleep so that the patient does not exhaust himself. Continuous warm baths or warm packs are also effective in quieting the delirious patient, but very few general hospitals have proper facilities for this valuable method of treatment.

"A fluid intake and output chart should be kept and any fluid and electrolyte deficiency should be corrected. ... The pulse and blood pressure should be recorded at intervals of two hours in anticipation of circulatory collapse, which is sometimes the cause of death, particularly in delirium tremens. In the event of circulatory collapse, transfusions of whole blood and vasopressor drugs may be lifesaving.

"Finally, the physician should be aware of many small therapeutic measures which may allay fear and suspicion and reduce the tendency to hallucinations. The room should be kept well lighted, and if possible, the patient should not be moved from one room to another."

Convulsions. The present discussion is restricted to the acute convulsive episodes seen in chemical poisonings. Omitted are the many problems of managing chronic convulsive disorders such as idiopathic or traumatic epilepsy. One must acknowledge, however, that a poison victim may also suffer from epilepsy and that any convulsion may represent the chemical activation of latent epilepsy. Many metabolic disturbances, for example, can be induced by chemical agents, and such disorders as hypocapnea from hyperventilation, cerebral anoxia, cortisone overdosage, water intoxication, and hypoglycemia are more apt to precipitate convulsions in an epileptic than in a non-epileptic. Even in persons with no stigma of epilepsy, the following compounds regularly induce convulsions if ingested in sufficient amounts: strychnine, picrotoxin, pentylenetetrazol (Metrazol), amphetamine, camphor, DDT and many other chlorinated insecticides, and parathion and its congeners. Often toxic doses of cocaine, tetracaine, various antihistaminic drugs, salicylates, and fluoroacetate salts cause generalized convulsions. Occasionally a general anesthetic is responsible. If one includes atypical cases, almost all drugs and common chemicals have been reported as the cause of seizures, but in many fatal poisonings terminal convulsions are simply anoxic or asphyxial in origin.

Although there are many different ways in which chemicals induce hyperexcitability and consequent convulsions, a single program of supportive treatment is applicable to all cases, if supplemented by appropriate specific therapy. In every case the first consideration is to prevent the patient from injuring himself during those periods when a seizure renders him helpless. For example, he should be laid on the floor or at least prevented from rolling off the bed. His collar is loosened, and artificial dentures and detachable dental bridges are removed between convulsive paroxysms. If the patient has no gag reflex, an oropharyngeal airway is best used to hold the tongue forward; this prevents it from occluding the oropharynx and also from being chewed; the removal of saliva and other secretions is made easier by the use of this device. For the correct technique of insertion, see p. 184. To minimize the aspiration of vomitus the patient is kept on his side, if possible with his head facing downward. All diagnostic and therapeutic procedures are held to a minimum; for example, gastric lavage is postponed until adequate premedication suppresses all convulsive activity. Since paroxysms are precipitated in some victims by very mild stimuli, sensory stimulation should be reduced to a minimum by keeping the patient in a comfortably warm, quiet, and darkened room. Even visits by professional

assistants are held to a minimum. Anoxia and an oxygen debt can be corrected more rapidly by administering oxygen between convulsions if this can be accomplished without triggering another paroxysm. If natural breathing is not resumed as soon as the skeletal muscles relax at the end of a seizure, artificial respiration (p. 185) must be initiated immediately. If convulsions recur at frequent intervals over a long period, the parenteral administration of water, salt, and glucose becomes advisable, usually by hypodermoclysis (p. 215–217).

In most cases these supportive measures must be accompanied by appropriate specific treatment. Examples of definitive treatment include atropine in poisoning by parathion and other anticholinesterase substances, glucose in hypoglycemic attacks, oxygen in anoxic convulsions, the cautious drainage of cerebrospinal fluid in cases of cerebral edema, and vigorous measures to reduce the body temperature in fever convulsions. Many patients, however, also require anticonvulsant drugs, i.e., agents which depress the central nervous system generally or the motor apparatus specifically, without regard to the cause of central nervous hyperexcitability. If continuous or intermittent seizures are allowed to persist, an asphyxial death from respiratory arrest becomes inevitable, because convulsions cause progressive damage to the respiratory center in two ways: from exhaustion which attends violent overstimulation and from anoxia which develops each time tetanic contractions of the respiratory muscles stop breathing movements. By preventing or aborting convulsions early in the course of poisoning, both types of injury are prevented, and time is gained during which specific treatment can be instituted or natural mechanisms of detoxification can be mobilized.

Drugs useful in preventing or reducing the frequency of seizures in chronic epilepsy are seldom effective in treating an actual convulsion or aborting an imminent one, whatever its cause. For example, even when injected intravenously, phenobarbital and mephobarbital act too slowly to be of major benefit to a convulsing patient. Although trimethadione (Tridione) protects animals against experimental seizures of many types and has been recommended in the clinical management of tetanus and status epilepticus, it is seldom used in the treatment of convulsant poisoning. Mesantoin and phenacemide (Phenurone) are known to prevent or modify drug-induced convulsions in experimental animals, but their value as treatment agents does not appear to match their effectiveness as prophylactic drugs. Diphenylhydantoin (Dilantin) sodium is inactive not only in treating but also in preventing convulsions induced by analeptic drugs and by electroshock, although a parenteral preparation (100 to 250 mg. i.v. or i.m.) has recently been recommended in the management of status epilepticus

and postoperative convulsions in neurosurgical patients.

In the presence of an actual or an impending convulsion, the best treatment in most cases is the immediate parenteral administration of any barbiturate drug with a short latency and short duration of action. The intramuscular route is often satisfactory and always safer than the intravenous channel. Because solutions of the sodium salts are locally irritating due to their alkalinity, no more than 5 ml. should be injected at any one intramuscular site. A violent and persistent convulsion usually warrants intravenous therapy. Solutions of the sodium salts of thiopental, pentobarbital, and amobarbital are usually employed; phenobarbital sodium is hazardous by the intravenous route chiefly because the delay in its onset of action often misleads the therapist into giving too much. The effective duration of action is the principal distinction between these drugs (see p. 118); in the dose ranges recommended in Table IV.1, amobarbital is most persistent (except for phenobarbital) and thiopental is most transient. If thiopental sodium is used to counteract a convulsant poison for more than 15 to 30 minutes, more drug is usually required than is recommended in Table IV.1. The larger the cumulative dose of thiopental the slower is the recovery from its effects; if enough is given to saturate body storage depots (chiefly adipose tissue), thiopental's actions are as persistent as those of pentobarbital.

Appropriate doses and proper techniques for injecting barbiturates into convulsing patients are outlined in Table IV.1. Smaller amounts are sometimes adequate, and for this reason all doses are administered fractionally. No more than a just adequate dose is ever used, because the barbiturate effect should not be allowed to extend into the phase of central nervous depression which most convulsant poisons eventually induce. Except for phenobarbital, the doses in Table IV.1 are usually sufficient to anesthetize normal adults—but not all victims of stimulant poisons. On the other hand, anesthesia is often unnecessary to control convulsions. For treating infants and children, the proper adult dose is reduced in proportion to the body weight or to the body surface area. Elderly persons and those with parenchymal liver disease require much less than recommended in Table IV.1. Overdosages with barbiturates require treatment as outlined on p. 120. After convulsions have been controlled, wakefulness, twitching, and hyperreflexia signal a need for more anticonvulsant drug.

Because of its ultra-short duration of action, thiopental (pentothal sodium) is often preferred when the convulsive phase is expected to be transient (i.e., up to 30 minutes). This barbiturate, however, produces more untoward reactions than its congeners; among the occasional alarming ef-

TABLE IV. 1

Parenteral barbiturate therapy for the control of convulsions

Drug	Form	Route	Dose (Adult)	Technique
Thiopental sodium (*e.g.*, Pentothal sodium)	2.5% soln. (sterile). Only freshly prepared aqueous solutions are suitable	*i.v. only* (avoid extravasation)	0.1–0.2 gm. (4–8 ml.)	In an average adult, 2–4 ml. can be injected *i.v.* without delay. Then wait 0.5–1 minute and repeat injection *if necessary*. Supplemental doses of 2–4 ml. are given as required (*e.g.*, every 5 min.), but the total cumulative dose should be kept below 1.0 or 1.5 gm.
Pentobarbital sodium (*e.g.*, Nembutal sodium)	5% soln. (sterile) containing water, propylene glycol, and alcohol, or a freshly prepared aqueous solution	*i.v.* or *i.m.*	0.2–0.5 gm. (4–10 ml.) or 3–7 mg./kg.	In an adult the first 2 to 3 ml. can be injected *i.v.* without delay. Then wait 1 to 5 min. and repeat once or twice *if necessary*
Amobarbital sodium (*e.g.*, Amytal sodium)	5% soln. (sterile). Only freshly prepared aqueous solutions are suitable	*i.m.* or *i.v.*	0.3–0.6 gm. (5–12 ml.)	For *i.v.* injection, use approximately the same volumes and timing as for pentobarbital. For *i.m.* injections 10% solutions are preferable (but not required)
Phenobarbital sodium	5 to 10% soln. (sterile). Aqueous solutions must be freshly prepared, but propylene glycol-water solutions are stable	*i.m.*	0.1–0.2 gm.	Start with 0.1 gm. or less and repeat once in 30 minutes *if necessary*

fects observed during intravenous administration are a profound fall in arterial blood pressure, severe respiratory depression with cyanosis, varying degrees of laryngospasm, bronchospasm, hiccuping, sneezing, and coughing. The anesthesiologist who administers this drug in preparation for surgery minimizes the incidence of these reactions by premedication with intramuscular atropine and a conventional barbiturate like pentobarbital, but premedication is obviously impractical in the emergency treatment of convulsions. Clearly one should hesitate to use thiopental unless equipment is available for the administration of oxygen and artificial respiration. Shock and a history of asthma are also important contraindications. Thiopental-induced laryngospasm and bronchospasm are usually self-limiting, but whenever these reactions are encountered, thiopental injections are best replaced by the inhalation of ether. Sometimes endotracheal in-

tubation is practical in the presence of laryngospasm, but in general the procedure should be reserved for a trained anesthetist. If its longer duration of action is not expected to be critical, pentobarbital sodium is probably preferable to thiopental sodium in the hands of everyone except the expert. If these barbiturates fail to control convulsions without producing excessive depression, trimethadione solution (20 per cent with urethane) should be given a trial by the intravenous, intramuscular, or deep subcutaneous routes, in a dose of 1 or 2 gm., repeated as necessary.

Safer and sometimes as satisfactory as an intravenous barbiturate is ether (diethyl ether) administered by inhalation. For most physicians the open-drop method is easiest, and a satisfactory anesthesia cone can usually be fashioned from make-shift materials. Induction is not simple in the presence of convulsions, but with reasonably

good technique the procedure is safe, even though unpleasant. In a good induction the patient is carried rapidly through the excitement stage of anesthesia. Surgical anesthesia is then maintained while an intramuscular dose of one of the barbiturate drugs (Table IV.1) is given time to become effective. Within a few minutes the level of ether anesthesia is allowed to lessen gradually as the barbiturate effect intensifies. By the open-drop method the depth of ether anesthesia can be changed quickly in either direction. In a young child a less stormy induction and a more prolonged duration of action can be secured by the rectal administration of ether as a mixture of equal parts of ether and olive oil. Sometimes paraldehyde is used instead, in which case two parts of olive oil (or mineral oil) are used. Both of these solutions are given as a retention enema in a dose of 0.5 to 1 ml. of the mixture per kilogram of body weight. Because the level of anesthesia cannot be effectively controlled when the rectum is used as the route of administration, supplemental doses of barbiturates are best avoided.

Substances which relax skeletal muscle are recommended occasionally as adjuvants to the anticonvulsive drugs. Two categories of muscle relaxants are recognized: those which act on central nervous synapses, such as mephenesin, and those which act peripherally to produce a neuromuscular blockade, such as curare (d-tubocurarine), gallamine (Flaxedil), decamethonium (C-10, Syncurine), and succinylcholine (Arectine). Each of these drugs has received clinical trials in cases of electroshock therapy, tetanus, or status epilepticus. With the possible exception of mephenesin, these compounds have no effect on fundamental neurological disturbances. They act only to modify convulsions by weakening or paralyzing skeletal muscles and so prevent the fractures, luxations, and pain of violent seizures. Because the intensity of the drug response cannot be accurately predicted or controlled, a complete flaccid paralysis sometimes results. This is not necessarily a tragic complication, since artificial respiration is practicable when apnea is due to flaccid paralysis and not when due to convulsive spasm. However, all equipment necessary for rapid resuscitation, such as endotracheal intubation, controlled artificial respiration, oxygen administration, and suction, should be available immediately. The therapist without special apparatus and special training is ill-advised to use any of these skeletal muscle relaxants in the control of convulsions.

Central Nervous Depression

As used here, the phrase "central nervous depression" is equivalent to the toxicologists' "narcosis" and is not related to the syndrome of psychic depression or melancholia. Central nervous depression follows overdoses of many drugs and toxic chemicals, all of which presumably interfere with brain metabolism. In its severest form, this syndrome culminates in respiratory arrest as a result of general reflex paralysis. In its milder forms it may mimic any stage of clinical anesthesia: headache, inattention, vertigo, excitement, convulsions, drowsiness, stupor, and coma—often with a terminal convulsion which is probably due to anoxia or asphyxia. The vital signs are characteristically reduced, and reflexes are depressed or absent. Various regulatory centers in the medullary oblongata are commonly inhibited, notably the vasomotor center with consequent vasodilatation and hypotension, and the respiratory center with consequent underbreathing and cyanosis. Circulatory insufficiency may be aggravated by the hypoxia which stems from inadequate pulmonary ventilation. Early deaths are usually due to respiratory arrest or to cardiovascular collapse, but delayed fatalities may arise from any one or any aggregate of the following complications: cerebral edema, pulmonary edema, hypostatic pneumonia, lung abscess, and irreversible renal failure. An occasional patient who survives severe and prolonged hypoxia during the acute phase of poisoning may suffer residual neurological lesions.

Every patient in severe central nervous depression requires prompt, intensive, sustained, and multidimensional treatment. Almost the whole armamentarium of the therapist may be needed. The highest priority goes usually to the correction of anoxia. Any one or group of the following measures may be necessary: the removal of airway obstruction (p. 184), oxygen administration (p. 189), artificial respiration (p. 185), and analeptic therapy (see below). If anoxia can be minimized, cardiovascular collapse is often avoided. Mild degrees of hypotension are properly ignored, but severe circulatory failure deserves treatment as outlined under vasogenic shock (p. 193). Dehydration and electrolyte disturbances must be corrected (pp. 215, 217), and if coma persists, a program of parenteral alimentation is instituted (p. 222). The periodic intake of even small amounts of glucose or other carbohydrate is usually sufficient to prevent ketosis and acidosis. The parenteral administration of a wide-spectrum antibiotic (p. 231) is generally an advisable prophylactic measure. The patient must be examined repeatedly for signs of urinary retention, and if the bladder is distended, it should be emptied by catheterization (p. 210). To prevent hardening of the colonic contents and fecal impactions, an occasional oil retention enema is desirable. Defects in temperature regulation must be compensated artificially (p. 230); hypothermia due to abnormally rapid heat loss and minimal production is the usual problem requiring attention. Repositioning the patient in his bed at frequent intervals minimizes the occurrence of such com-

plications as hypostatic pneumonia, decubitus ulcers, and venous thrombosis (p. 229).

The proper role of stimulant or analeptic drugs is a topic of controversy. With the exception of N-allylnormorphine in the treatment of morphinism, the analeptics are regarded by some therapists as unnecessary and perhaps hazardous because they distract attention from the essential elements of supportive treatment. The recent success of Dr. E. Nilsson in treating barbiturate poisoning without stimulants emphasizes by indirection that analeptics are often used unnecessarily. The comatose patient who moves in response to a painful stimulus, whose respirations and blood pressure are not depressed severely, and whose swallowing and cough reflexes are intact, has no need of an arousal drug and none should be given. Most clinicians, however, are convinced that the judicious use of analeptics has saved lives in severe grades of central nervous depression. To distinguish between patients who do and those who do not require stimulant therapy, one suggested criterion is the response to a small intravenous dose of pentylenetetrazol (Metrazol, 5 ml. of a 10 per cent solution); any lessening in the depth of coma, however transient, is regarded as evidence that analeptics are unnecessary and that symptomatic care will suffice. Although designed for barbiturate poisoning, this test is presumably applicable to other states of central nervous depression. Even with a clear and compelling need, analeptic therapy is never a substitute for the supportive measures described above; it is properly regarded as only one and perhaps a minor phase of general supportive treatment.

The central nervous stimulants of therapeutic value are caffeine and related xanthines, pentylenetetrazol, picrotoxin, nikethamide, ephedrine, amphetamine, strychnine, and camphor. Because it is not a general excitatory drug, N-allylnormorphine (nalorphine, Nalline) is not included in this list; however, in poisonings by morphine and many of its congeners (e.g., heroine, Dilaudid, methadone, metopon, meperidine), nalorphine is a potent analeptic, and its use is discussed under morphine poisoning (p. 158). Camphor and strychnine are no longer popular therapeutic agents in this country. Table IV.2 lists doses and methods of administering pentylenetetrazol, picrotoxin, nikethamide, caffeine, ephedrine, and amphetamine—in cases of severe central nervous depression. Regardless of the cause of depression, these drugs are given with the intent of raising and maintaining the general level of reflex excitability, until sufficient time passes to allow detoxification and excretion of the original poison. A beneficial response consists of an increase in the rate or depth of breathing and a rise in the blood pressure toward normotensive levels. Thus the major therapeutic value of these medicinals is their analeptic actions on the medullary centers of respiration and vasomotion. To be effective, large and repeated doses may be required, but these drugs should not be used to restore consciousness because the attempt may precipitate convulsions. Any convulsive seizure induced by an analeptic drug is followed by a phase of depression which may dangerously aggravate the primary intoxication. Because of the threat of this complication, an ultra-short acting barbiturate such as thiopental sodium (p. 202) should always be available for immediate intravenous injection.

None of the analeptic drugs (Table IV.2) has a mechanism of action which is properly understood. Presumably each serves to compensate for and not to correct whatever metabolic disturbances may be responsible for narcosis. Because the stimulant drugs probably differ from one another in their modes of action on the central nervous system (with the possible exception of ephedrine and amphetamine), more than one preparation is commonly prescribed. The use of several drugs in combination or in alternation serves also to reduce the danger of cumulative toxicity. In terms of therapeutic effectiveness, differences among these drugs are not so great that any one is generally recognized as outstanding. In some clinics picrotoxin or pentylenetetrazol (but not both) is used as the primary analeptic, while nikethamide, ephedrine, caffeine, and amphetamine are regarded as adjuvants, but evidence to support this attitude is not impressive. Perhaps pentylenetetrazol is less effective than picrotoxin (except in its actions on the cerebrum), but it is generally safer because of its faster detoxification. Overdoses of pentylenetetrazol and of picrotoxin cause coordinated, clonic convulsions, typically associated with stimulation of higher motor centers, but like morphine, large doses of picrotoxin also cause dangerous hyperactivity of the spinal cord. As commonly used, nikethamide may be less prone to produce convulsions, but it is probably less effective than picrotoxin or pentylenetetrazol against barbiturate poisoning, although it may have special merit in tribromoethanol (Avertin) intoxication. Caffeine is often used effectively in alternation with ephedrine or amphetamine. Dextroamphetamine (Dexedrine) sulfate and methamphetamine hydrochloride are somewhat more potent than amphetamine and may be used as substitutes for it.

Ephedrine and in large doses amphetamine produce rises in blood pressure by direct actions on the myocardium and on peripheral blood vessels, as well as by analeptic actions on the medullary vasomotor center. Caffeine too may stimulate the heart directly, but its direct vascular actions are less important in states of central depression than its reflex actions. The only significant circulatory effects of nikethamide, pentylenetetrazol, and picro-

TABLE IV. 2

Analeptic therapy in central nervous depression

Drug	Form	Route	Adult Dose*	Comment
Pentylenetetrazol (Metrazol)	Sterile soln.: 10%	*i.v.*, *i.m.* (*p.o.*)	a) Test dose: 5 ml. *i.v.* b) Intensive treatment: 10–20 ml., *i.v.*, and *i.m.* simultaneously; repeat as necessary, using progressively smaller doses by both routes	Use intensive treatment when and only when *no* response to the test dose. Analeptic effects are usually transient, but overdoses may produce convulsions
Picrotoxin	Sterile soln: 3 mg./ml.	*i.v.*, *i.m.* (*p.o.*)	a) 1 mg./min. (1 ml. in 3 min.) by *i.v.* infusion until corneal reflex active or until 6–12 mg. given; then maintenance by 3–6 mg. *i.m.* every 20 to 30 min.–or b) 3–12 mg. (1–4 ml.) *i.v.* slowly and repeat every 10 to 20 min. as necessary	Overdoses may produce dangerous and prolonged convulsions, but several grams have been given safely over a period of a few days to patients in deep coma
Nikethamide (Coramine)	Sterile soln.: 25%	*i.v.*, *i.m.*, *s.c.* (*p.o.*)	1–5 ml. by any route	Probably safer but less effective than the above in most situations
Caffeine	Mixed salt with sodium benzoate. Sterile soln: 0.25 or 0.50 gm./2 ml.	*i.v.*, *i.m.* (*p.o.*) (rectal)	0.5 to 1.0 gm. every 1 to 3 hours as necessary, usually by the intramuscular route.	Generally safe, but a single dose may remain effective for several hours. When doses are repeated too often, cumulative toxicity may become manifest if the primary poison is detoxified first
Ephedrine	Hydrochloride or sulfate salt as a sterile solution	*i.v.*, *i.m.*, *s.c.* (*p.o.*)	30 to 50 mg., usually *i.m.*, every 30 min. to 2 hours as required	Can be effectively alternated with caffeine
Amphetamine (Benzedrine)	Sulfate or phosphate. Powder or sterile solution, usually 10%	*i.v.*, *i.m.*, *s.c.* (*p.o.*)	10 to 30 mg., usually *s.c.*, repeated in 30 min. to 2 hours as necessary	Dextro-amphetamine (Dexedrine) is more potent but is usually used in the same dose. These drugs are less prone to induce convulsions than the other analeptics

* These doses are regarded as appropriate in severe grades of depression; they should be adjusted for the depth of coma and the response to treatment.

toxin are those mediated through the central nervous system.

Although convulsions rarely result from overdoses of amphetamine and its congeners, any of the clinically useful analeptics may produce a convulsive seizure if given in immoderate amounts. In case of a drug-induced convulsion or convulsive prodromata (such as violent twitching), an ultrafast barbiturate drug (p. 118, 202) should be available for immediate intravenous injection. Parenteral trimethadione (20 per cent, with urethane) may have specific value in the control of pentylenetetrazol convulsions.

In a few cases of coma due to poison (*e.g.*, carbon monoxide poisoning, methyl alcohol intoxication), cerebral edema and a high cerebrospinal fluid pressure contribute to the central nervous depression. Under these circumstances cautious cranial decompression sometimes raises the level of reflex excitability and improves the vital signs. The intravenous administration of such hypertonic solutions as 50 per cent glucose or sucrose may be of transient benefit, but a more dependable procedure is the slow removal of cerebrospinal fluid through a needle inserted between lumbar vertebrae into the subarachnoid space. In this way the cerebrospinal fluid pressure is gradually reduced to normal over a period of about one hour. This decompression may have to be repeated several times during the acute phase of the intoxication.

Psychic Disturbances and Suicide

As judged by admissions to municipal hospitals, a large proportion of acute chemical poisonings in adults arises from acts of suicidal intent. As soon as treatment removes any immediate threat to the patient's life, the attending physician must appraise the risk of a second suicide trial. This judgment requires at least an elementary understanding of the personality types with suicidal tendencies and a recognition of the clinical signs of latent self-destructive impulses. Even the physician without special psychiatric training can learn to make a reasonably reliable prediction in this regard. For a specific psychiatric diagnosis, an understanding of the mechanics of the personality disorder, and details of definitive treatment, the advice and help of a trained psychiatrist are imperative.

In western culture, acts of suicide (in contrast to thoughts of suicide) arise from severe emotional disturbances, which are of many types and reveal themselves in many ways. According to Dr. Maurice Levine (Psychotherapy in Medical Practice, the MacMillan Company, New York, 1942), practicing physicians too regularly associate suicide with a diagnosis of manic-depressive psychosis or other states of depression. The following comments reflect in large measure the analysis of Dr. Levine.

In practice suicidal behavior is often encountered in persons with hysterical psychopathic personalities. Probably more than any other group of individuals, the hysterical psychopaths engage in unsuccessful and sometimes blatantly incompetent acts of self-destruction by chemical poisoning. The hysterical psychopath may or may not have overt physical manifestations of hysteria, but in all cases there exists a deep-seated and immature need to be melodramatic and to gain sympathy in what appears to be a spiteful and revengeful attempt to control environment and coerce associates. Thus the suicide gesture becomes a device to frighten others into submission and at the same time to satisfy more obscure neurotic goals. In patients of this type, self-poisoning is usually impulsive and sometimes quickly regretted. Once the chemical intoxication is controlled and convalescence begins, there is rarely any *immediate* threat of a second suicidal act. Whatever danger exists is mitigated by the physician who manages during his ministrations to control or avoid anxieties of his own and who is careful not to be provoked by the patient into anger or criticism. Although these patients need follow-up psychiatric care, hospitalization is not always necessary.

Delirious patients are far less predictable suicidal risks, whether delirium is due to traumatic brain injury, fever, infectious disease, or chemical intoxication. The delirious person is confused, disoriented, and often fearful. He misinterprets things which he hears and sees and sometimes experiences frank hallucinations. His fears and confusion may cause him to jump out of his hospital window or to engage in other unintentional acts of self-destruction. The clinical management of the delirious patient is described on p. 201.

If a suicidal impulse arises in a psychotic person, it is apt to be much more profound and more durable than in the psychopath. For example, some schizophrenics have auditory hallucinations and believe that they are ordered by an outside agency to perform specific acts which sometimes include self-mutilation and suicide. A paranoid individual may commit suicide in an attempt to escape the painful persecution which he mistakenly ascribes to a real or fictitious individual or group. Panic, whatever its psychomechanics, may cause its victim to become so overwhelmed by fear of a genuine or fanciful situation that he injures or kills himself unintentionally. Finally, states of emotional depression may be so severe that suicide is a genuine possibility.

Whatever the etiology of melancholia, its victim experiences exaggerated worry over real or imaginary situations, focused or diffuse anxiety, a sense of unworthiness, of guilt, and of incompetence—all leading to severe frustration and sometimes to suicide. Typically the patient is withdrawn, inactive, uncommunicative, and undemonstrative, but

these are not essential elements in the clinical picture. States of emotional depression may occur at specific stages of various organic diseases. For example, the prolonged convalescence from acute or chronic arsenic poisoning is sometimes associated with severe melancholia; luetic paresis and pernicious anemia are said to be other examples. Another type of person who presents at least a mild risk of suicide is one who suffers a so-called reactive depression. This patient's distress is a response to a real external situation, not an imaginary one; although the circumstances may be truly unfortunate, the emotional reaction is exaggerated out of proportion to the precipitating stimulus.

The most severe and the most persistent of the suicidal urges occur in psychotically depressed patients, notably those with manic-depressive psychoses. A person of this type is always a threat to himself, even during the convalescent period following an unsuccessful suicide. The perseverance of these patients is extraordinary. Any one of them may engage suddenly in such violent acts of self-destruction as throwing himself from a window ledge, hanging himself with bed clothing, mutilating himself with a knife, or raiding a hospital pharmacy for poisons. It is the duty of the medical practitioner to restrain this type of patient and in every other way to curtail his opportunities for violence. The intensity of this suicidal motive is said to stem from profound although largely subconscious sensations of guilt over imaginary wrongs and crimes. In this type of distorted personality, therefore, suicide represents the only adequate retribution, a dramatic and needful attempt to expiate the sin. The manic-depressive psychotic needs psychiatric care, almost always in an institution, long after he has recovered from a chemical poisoning or other suicidal injury. Although it is not always easy, every medical practitioner must attempt to distinguish between psychotically depressed patients and those in other depressive states.

Dr. Levine (*op. cit.*) lists several clinically recognizable signals of an impending suicide in depressed persons of all types. One obvious warning that should keep every attending physician alert is a past history of repeated suicide trials. Such repeated attempts are apt to increase in severity until the individual finally succeeds in killing himself. Another danger signal concerns the intensity of the patient's depression as expressed in his mood. In this evaluation the physician must depend largely upon his own clinical experience. Perhaps the most reliable indices to gauge the depth of melancholia and the associated risk of suicide are a group of somatic or vegetative manifestations which include persistent loss of appetite, serious weight loss, intractable insomnia, enduring constipation, absence of sexual desire or potency, and cessation or diminution of menstruation. The persistence and especially the intensification of any of these signs should prove adequate warning to the alert physician. Another danger signal is the patient's concealment of thoughts about suicide. A great deal of talk about suicide, particularly if the talk is dramatic, does not often lead to a serious attempt. Like other generalizations, this rule cannot be relied upon in any particular case. The risk of suicide by a depressed patient is also enhanced if he develops definite delusions of a depressive nature, such as morbid guilt or impoverishment. Sometimes an impending suicide is signaled by an increasing tendency of the patient to brood, to withdraw within himself, and to cease to display friendly feelings toward others. The same is true of any rise in the patient's tension or anxiety as evidenced by his expressions, his behavior, his pulse rate, *etc.*, and particularly if the increased anxiety is associated with feelings of unreality or frank delusions. On the other hand, a manic patient, whose euphoric defense against depression is shaky at best, may at any time be overcome by guilt all the more enhanced by his period of uninhibited behavior, and so attempt suicide with little or no warning. In very severe emotional depressions, suicides are said to be more frequent during the early stage of seeming recovery than during the phase of deepest melancholy. Clearly vigilance cannot be relaxed during an apparent convalescence. In a depressed patient the fewer the manifestations of a hysterical psychopathic personality the more serious is the prognosis from the viewpoint of suicide. For example, the patient who talks dramatically and strives to gain attention to his problems, who seems inclined to arouse sympathy, and who acts in a spiteful and threatening way, is less likely to make a serious suicidal move than a patient who betrays only quiet desperation.

These remarks are intended to serve as a guide for the medical practitioner, not as a substitute for expert professional opinion. If practical, a psychiatrist should be consulted whenever *any* patient has engaged in an unsuccessful act of suicide.

GASTROINTESTINAL TRACT

Mouth Care

After emergency decontamination (Section I), the local treatment of acid and alkali burns in the mouth involves scrupulous oral hygiene. The practice of oral hygiene is also beneficial to many other types of patients, notably those who are comatose or in whom intubation is being maintained. Dryness of the mouth is best avoided by insuring systemic hydration (p. 215). Dried secretions within the mouth are removed by swabbing with cotton

pledgets moistened with a mild alkaline mouth wash. Cracking of the lips is prevented by the use of cold cream. Stomatitis can sometimes be controlled locally by mouth washes of 0.02 per cent potassium permanganate, but infectious stomatitis also deserves systemic antibiotic therapy (p. 231). The latter is an important prophylactic measure in patients with chemical burns of the mouth and throat.

Nausea and Vomiting

The treatment of severe gastritis, which frequently accompanies chemical poisonings, depends upon the nature of the toxic agent (see Section II). Associated with gastritis, there is often severe nausea and vomiting. If the patient is semiconscious or unconscious, the aspiration of vomitus into the trachea is a major hazard; it can be minimized by keeping the victim on his side with his head slightly lower than his trunk. However distressing to a conscious patient, no attempt (except perhaps gastric lavage—techniques and precautions of which are described in Section I) should be made to stop repeated emesis until it is reasonably certain that the vomitus no longer contains appreciable amounts of the ingested poison. The decision usually depends upon the duration of emesis and the volume of vomitus. In any case, the control of nausea and vomiting may be very difficult or even impossible in these cases. Mild nausea associated with gastric irritation sometimes responds to sips of warm water, mild tea, or bland antacid preparations like alumina gels or milk of magnesia. Atropine sulfate, given subcutaneously in doses of 0.3 to 1.2 mg., is often helpful. In some cases relief follows parenteral sedation (e.g., i.m. sodium phenobarbital or sodium Seconal), but morphine and other opium derivatives should be withheld. Many of the antihistaminic drugs have a mildly anti-emetic action. Recent experience indicates the efficacy of chlorpromazine (Thorazine) in the control of nausea and vomiting from a variety of causes; this drug may be given intramuscularly in a dose of about 25 mg. three of four times a day, but it is best avoided after exposure to hepatic toxins. In the presence of abdominal distension, nausea and vomiting may prove intractable to all measures except abdominal decompression.

Losses of essential electrolytes through intensive vomiting can and *must* be corrected promptly by replacement therapy. Among the individual deficits which may arise are dehydration (p. 215), salt depletion (p. 216), hypochloremic alkalosis (p. 219), rarely metabolic acidosis (p. 219), and hypopotassemia (p. 220). Especially in young children, these deficiencies may reach alarming proportions within a short time. After water and electrolyte balances are restored, the administration of simple

nutrients is usually desirable. As long as gastritis and vomiting persist, parenteral alimentation must be maintained (p. 222).

In general, sips of warm water or tea may be offered within 12 to 24 hours after the nausea of acute gastritis subsides. Milk or strained gruel is sometimes preferred. At first the intake should be limited to one or two teaspoonsful every half hour. If tolerated, a few salted crackers or dry toast may be added. Eventually small servings of a bland diet are given a trial. Although vomiting may be precipitated if oral feedings are inaugurated too soon or too zealously, eating should be resumed as soon as tolerated because parenteral alimentation is generally inadequate, expensive, and annoying to the patient. For more detailed suggestions about the resumption of oral feedings, see p. 223.

Abdominal Distension

In acute chemical poisoning abdominal distension is usually paralytic in origin, and may indicate rupture of the stomach or bowel with generalized peritonitis. In any case prompt recognition is imperative. If the problem is one of simple paralytic ileus, gastric decompression is a useful prophylactic and therapeutic measure. If begun promptly no other treatment is required. Continuous gastric decompression is accomplished by nasogastric intubation. A no. 18 F Levine tube is appropriate for adults; plastic tubes are better tolerated than those made of rubber. A constant negative pressure is maintained by Wangensteen bottles or by a suction machine. The single-bore wide-lumen Levine tube is usually preferable to the double-lumen Miller-Abbott tube in the treatment of paralytic ileus because the inflated balloon of the Miller-Abbott tube is not carried into the small intestine when there is no effective peristalsis. With a nasogastric tube, abdominal decompression is usually effected within 12 to 18 hours, if at all, but suction may have to be continued prophylactically for several days. As long as it is maintained, the physician must correct repeatedly an inevitable hypochloremic alkalosis by administering parenterally isotonic saline or balanced salt solution (p. 217). In addition to gastric intubation, deflation of the colon may be promoted by rectal tubes, usually a no. 38 F catheter. The procedures described above are usually more effective and safer than the administration of cholinergic drugs (see management of urinary retention, p. 210).

Diarrhea

As in the case of emesis, the physician must hesitate to suppress diarrhea which may be useful in removing ingested toxic material. It is difficult to evaluate the importance of this excretory route in toxicology, but reasonably prompt evacuation would seem to be desirable in most cases of in-

gested poison. Fecal excretion may even account for some of the toxic substance originally absorbed from the gastrointestinal tract. Thus appreciable quantities of many alkaloids, and perhaps of most, can be found in bile irrespective of the route of administration. To some extent this biliary excretion is nullified by the intestinal resorption of active poison. To minimize this phenomenon, a brisk passage of intestinal contents is thought to be desirable. Saline cathartics can be used to accomplish this purpose (e.g., sodium or magnesium sulfate in doses of 15 to 30 gm. in water). High colonic irrigation is seldom warranted.

On the other hand, violent purging undoubtedly does more harm than good. At least mild attempts should be made to suppress any diarrhea which becomes persistent and copious. If it is reflex in origin, subcutaneous atropine sulfate (dose 0.3 to 1.2 mg.) is helpful. Good relief of pain and intestinal spasm is often provided by intramuscular meperidine (Demerol) hydrochloride in doses of 50 to 100 mg. every 3 hours. Hot or cold compresses on the abdomen may be of some value. If oral medication is not contraindicated, a mild anti-diarrheal action can be obtained from kaolin (10 gm. with one ounce of water), activated charcoal (one or more teaspoonsful), bismuth subcarbonate (1.0 gm.), or aluminum oxide gels. These agents also serve as adsorbents and may delay passage of toxic chemicals across the intestinal mucosa. Paregoric (camphorated tincture of opium) and other morphine preparations should be withheld or used only sparingly to control the pain of severe cramps. The paramount consideration, however, is the correction of dehydration and electrolyte imbalances which often result from persistent diarrhea (p. 215–220).

URINARY SYSTEM

Urinary Retention

Toxic agents may cause acute urinary retention by producing either bladder atony or vesicle neck spasm. In either instance a full bladder demands prompt drainage. This can be accomplished almost always by urethral catheterization; only rarely is suprapubic cystotomy necessary. If possible a Foley catheter with a 5-ml. bag should be used, and the catheter should remain indwelling. A continuous urine sample is invaluable to the physician treating a victim of poison, because it provides material for toxicological examination and a means of appraising the patient's renal function, state of hydration, acid-base balance, etc. (p. 215). If the bladder is suspected to contain more than 500 ml. of urine, decompression should be accomplished slowly over a period of a few hours. Inability to catheterize the patient usually means errors in technique or a poor choice of catheter. The male urethra has the form of an S curve. If the penis is held under slight tension at right angles to the legs and abdomen, one curve of the S is thereby eliminated. Lubricate the catheter well. Avoid catheters which are too large for the urethral lumen and also those which are so small that they buckle within the urethra. No. 18, 20, and 22 F appear to be most easily introduced in most adult patients by most physicians. The use of a stylet in the hands of the inexperienced operator is inadvisable, as it frequently results in urethral tears or perforations. If continuous drainage is maintained through an indwelling catheter, a broad-spectrum antibacterial agent should be used as prophylaxis against urinary infection. Sulfisoxazole (Gantrisin) is satisfactory in a dose of 0.5 gm. given four times a day. Other useful drugs are chlortetracycline (Aureomycin), oxytetracycline (Terramycin), and tetracycline (Polycycline), as available in doses of 200 to 250 mg. four times a day. The bladder should be irrigated two or three times a day with sterile saline solution, and the catheter should be changed every five to seven days.

Although urethral catheterization is usually preferable, urinary retention from bladder atony or vesicle neck spasm can sometimes be controlled by drugs. The three most widely used are bethanechol chloride (Urecholine), furtrethonium iodide (Furmethide), and neostigmine methylsulfate. Urecholine and Furmethide are employed in doses of 10 to 30 mg. orally or 2.5 to 5 mg. subcutaneously; neostigmine is given subcutaneously in doses of 0.5 to 1.0 mg. While these drugs may be given several times daily, their actions are uncertain and frequently include unpleasant parasympathomimetic side-effects such as sweating, lacrimation, salivation, and intestinal cramps. In some patients these unwanted actions may be controlled by the simultaneous administration of atropine (0.3 to 0.6 mg.) without materially reducing the drug's effectiveness. In any case parasympathomimetic agents should never be tried in patients who are known or suspected to have asthma, heart disease, or any mechanical obstruction within the bowel or urinary tract.

Acute Renal Failure

Inflammation of the kidney, particularly of the renal tubule, occurs often in chemical poisonings. Attempts have been made to distinguish between two types of tubular lesions. Specific tubular necrosis has long been recognized as a local effect of certain nephrotoxic agents; typically its appearance is

delayed 3 to 4 days after exposure. Once established, the disorder is generally present in all the nephrons of both kidneys, but the process tends to be self-limited and completely reversible within one or two weeks. In contrast to this specific reversible effect, there may be an unpredictable and partially irreversible tubular injury, which has been called a tubulorhexic lesion. It is characterized by disruption of the renal tubules and dissolution of the basement membrane with the eventual formation of patchy scars. This disorder is thought to have a vascular origin, since it usually arises after an acute insufficiency of several hours' duration in the renal circulation. Renal ischemia in turn is generally secondary to severe dehydration and peripheral vascular collapse. Insofar as shock is preventable or promptly correctable, this type of tubular injury can be avoided. As seen in clinical practice both varieties of renal lesions frequently coexist in the poisoned patient.

The first and principal consideration in therapy is the correction of shock as quickly as possible. The shorter the duration of circulatory collapse, the less is the eventual renal damage. The management of shock is outlined on p. 193. Once an adequate blood pressure and circulation are restored, the therapist is well advised to adopt a conservative attitude in his efforts to support the patient. When indicated and when available, specific therapy (e.g., BAL) should of course be instituted, but some physicians are too zealous in their attempts at non-specific support of these patients. Overtreatment is a distinct danger to the person with an acute renal lesion. Even if urine flow returns with the restoration of an adequate circulation, tubular necrosis may develop later and lead to oliguria or anuria. In the pre-oliguric stage some patients experience polyuria. Good clinical management requires that this and any other fluid losses are replaced, but no attempt should be made to induce diuresis by the administration of large amounts of water or any other diuretic agent. There is no convincing evidence that a water diuresis speeds the excretion of any toxic substance. While some theoretical advantages are apparent in maintaining a dilute tubular fluid during the excretion of a primary nephrotoxic chemical, this hypothetical benefit may be outweighed by the very real danger of overhydration and eventual congestive heart failure. Unlike the production of a diuresis, cautious alkalinization of the urine may have some protective action on the kidney in the pre-oliguric phase (e.g., sulfonamide poisoning, uranium poisoning). In general, however, the intake of fluid and electrolyte is limited to simple replacement (pp. 215–219).

The same principle dominates clinical management during the oliguric or anuric phase. In the adult, the daily intake of water is limited to tangible losses through the gastrointestinal and urinary tracts, plus 800 to 1000 ml. of water to cover insensible losses (vaporization from skin and respiratory mucosa). At room temperatures of 80°F. and above, active sweating contributes considerably to the water loss, and under these circumstances a daily observation of the patient's body weight offers the best basis for estimating the replacement fluid volume. Underreplacement of the body weight to the extent of 100 to 200 grams of water a day is recommended, because oxidative metabolism of tissue stores manufactures body water at about this rate. The intake of most electrolytes and particularly potassum is kept as low as possible. Dietary sodium chloride is restricted to the simple replacement of losses from the gastrointestinal tract; urinary excretion of salt in the oliguric patient is generally so small that is can be ignored.

Protein is completely excluded from the diet, but a daily caloric intake of 1500 to 2000 calories is maintained, if possible, by the ingestion of carbohydrate and fat. It is important that these foodstuffs are essentially electrolyte-free. If gastrointestinal pathology or vomiting prevents oral feeding, parenteral routes of administration must be utilized (p. 222). Under these circumstances, restrictions on the water allowance limit the daily carbohydrate intake to about 100 gm. This limitation arises because glucose and other sugars can seldom be infused in concentrations above 10 per cent without danger of thrombophlebitis. No fat emulsion suitable for parenteral injection is yet available commercially. For these reasons the oral route is distinctly preferable, even if the control of nausea requires the judicious use of drugs (p. 209). A full normal complement of vitamins (p. 225) should be met by daily supplementation.

On this regimen, patients invariably develop some degree of metabolic acidosis before the restoration of renal tubular function. This acidosis is usually not severe, and no attempt is made to correct it unless it becomes marked and leads to distressing symptoms. Even in a patient who is markedly hyperpneic, with a plasma bicarbonate concentration below 12 mEq. per L., only partial correction of this acidosis should be attempted. One practice is to administer small repeated doses of sodium citrate by mouth or sodium lactate by vein until the severer symptoms subside. In addition to metabolic acidosis, hyponatremia and to à lesser degree hypochloremia develop frequently during the oliguric state, even on a regimen where daily salt losses are replaced. This hyponatremia, like the acidosis, is usually well tolerated, whereas all attempts to correct it by increasing the salt intake are apt to precipitate cardiac failure.

Cardiac disturbances represent the most serious complication in acute renal failure and the principal cause of death. The commonest form is intractable pulmonary edema with or without pe-

ripheral edema or hypertension. The emergency treatment of acute pulmonary edema has been outlined on pp. 192 and 197. Rapid digitalization should always be tried when pulmonary edema appears in a patient with acute renal failure, even though the cardiac glycosides are frequently ineffective in this cardiovascular crisis. The other type of cardiac disorder often encountered in renal failure is caused by potassium intoxication. During the oliguric state, the plasma potassium level always rises, but hyperkalemia becomes a major complication in considerably less than half of these patients. When the potassium concentration reaches 2 to 4 times normal (on the average about 8 mEq. per L.), muscle weakness, hyporeflexia, paresthesias, anxiety, restlessness, and disturbances of cardiac rhythm commonly develop. Because these signs are not invariable, and because they rarely occur soon enough for the initiation of effective therapy, the early detection and proper management of potassium intoxication demand frequent chemical analyses for K^+ in plasma or serum. If an adequate laboratory is unavailable, repeated electrocardiograms may help to detect hyperkalemia but furnish no information from which the extracellular K^+ concentration can be estimated quantitatively. The earliest electrocardiographic sign of potassium intoxication is an increase in the amplitude of the T wave; eventually various cardiac arrhythmias, including episodes of asystole, presage complete cardiac arrest.

The quickest and easiest way of depressing the plasma K^+ concentration is the administration of glucose (1 liter of 10 per cent glucose in water), preferably with the addition to the infusion fluid of crystalline insulin (25 units per 100 gm. of glucose). This measure is not invariably successful, and at best its effectiveness is only transient. The oral and rectal administration of cation exchange resins (in the ammonium or hydrogen form) has been used in an attempt to rob extracellular fluid of potassium. This procedure is seldom effective and may contribute appreciably to the patient's acidosis. The administration of diaphoretic agents and purgatives is dangerous or useless. Intestinal perfusion, colonic irrigation, and peritoneal lavage have all been employed with some success, but none of these procedures is popular today. (The technique of peritoneal lavage has been reviewed by Odel, Ferris and Power, M. Clin. North America, *32:* 939, 1948). These procedures are largely outmoded by hemodialysis through "artificial kidneys," which are commercially available devices that are now found in many general hospitals. Hemodialysis can be used in acute renal failure to reduce azotemia, but its principal role is the control of hyperkalemia and the removal of an excess sodium or

water load. Whereas the artificial kidney can be a lifesaving device, most patients with acute renal failure do not require this type of support.

The therapeutic regimen outlined above clearly requires good clinical and laboratory controls. Whenever possible, all excretions and secretions should be collected, measured, and analyzed for electrolytes. If the patient is incontinent, an indwelling catheter in the urinary bladder is essential. As a desirable minimum for good clinical management, the chemistry laboratory must furnish a daily analysis of blood plasma or serum for potassium, bicarbonate, chloride, and probably sodium. The degree of azotemia, as measured by the blood urea nitrogen or non-protein nitrogen, is also a valuable general guide to the course of the disease.

Oliguria may persist for a period ranging from a few hours to 3 weeks (average 10 to 12 days), but as the renal tubules begin to regenerate, oliguria is gradually replaced by a phase of diuresis. The polyuric phase is also associated with a high mortality and demands careful clinical attention. Because this polyuria does not produce clinical dehydration, a true excess of body water and electrolyte is presumed to exist at the end of the oliguric phase even when no edema is clinically demonstrable. Even after the conservative therapeutic regimen outlined above, weight loss due to fluid excretion is often considerable during the first week or two after the resumption of urine flow. It is apparent that complete fluid and electrolyte replacement therapy during this polyuria is unwarranted and serves only to perpetuate the diuresis.

Miscellaneous clinical problems during acute renal failure include the following gastrointestinal disturbances: anorexia, nausea, vomiting, diarrhea, and abdominal distension. The diarrhea, which usually occurs late in the oliguric state, may be profuse and persistent. These intestinal losses of electrolyte and water must be replaced in like measure through parenteral routes (pp. 215–219). The symptomatic control of these disorders is outlined on pp. 209–210. The commonest mental symptom in acute renal failure is somnolence; to attempt its correction by drugs is generally unwise. A rapidly developing anemia, which is usually normochromic and normocytic, is a constant feature of renal insufficiency. Apparently it is self-limiting and usually well tolerated, in contrast to the blood transfusions which are sometimes used to correct or ameliorate it. Transfusions are hazardous because of the ease with which congestive heart failure can be precipitated in these patients. At no stage of the disease are the following measures employed today: diuretic drugs to "force" renal excretion, surgical denervation of the kidney, or renal decapsulation.

LIVER

Many chemicals have a direct injurious action on the liver, producing all grades of hepatic inflammation and necrosis. The pathological picture may be indistinguishable from that of infectious hepatitis, but the chemical lesion typically consists of a coagulation type of necrosis, in contrast to the autolytic debridement of infectious hepatitis; moreover the pattern of destruction in a toxic injury is more often diffuse than zonal. A mild exposure may produce an asymptomatic lesion, but in another patient the same exposure may lead to acute yellow atrophy and death. In general these variations in individual susceptibility can be neither predicted nor explained.

The injury from a hepatotoxic chemical is characteristically detectable only after a period of latency. For many substances (*e.g.*, chlorinated hydrocarbons, phosphorus, mushroom toxins), this latency persists for 1 to 7 days. With other substances (*e.g.*, certain nitrobenzene derivatives, cinchophen, organic arsenicals), the latent period sometimes lasts several months, and the clinical illness then arises insidiously. Every person in whom exposure to a liver poison is suspected should have repeated and multiple tests of liver function.

Mild Liver Injury

The period between a hepatotoxic exposure and liver decompensation offers the physician an opportunity to establish a prophylactic regimen. Unfortunately no uniformly successful or even reasonably satisfactory system of management has been formulated yet. Although far from perfected, a program of diet and dietary supplements, as outlined below, is regarded as practical and beneficial in the following situations:

a. prophylaxis after a known acute exposure to a hepatotoxic agent,

b. treatment in mild or subacute hepatic necrosis,

c. treatment during the convalescent or reparative phase of all types of liver parenchymal injury.

After a recognized acute exposure, the most important principle of clinical management is believed to be complete bed rest. Even with an asymptomatic patient, strict bed rest is enforced immediately. The second consideration is proper nutrition, which may limit the extent of liver injury as well as favor rapid recovery. If gastrointestinal symptoms do not preclude eating, oral feedings are by far the most satisfactory mode of intake.

Diets of widely varying composition have been employed successfully, but most therapists prefer a high caloric diet, with a large amount of carbohydrate and protein and a moderate or small quantity of fat. A detailed diet and representative menu are suggested on pp. 225–226. In liver cell injury one of the major problems is the acceptability of any high caloric diet. Intake is often erratic and limited by severe anorexia. If nausea and vomiting are not prominent, the nutrition of an uncooperative or anorexic patient can often be maintained by tube feeding; a high protein formula for tube feeding is described in Table IV.7 (p. 227). The quantity and regularity of intake are claimed to be the most important dietary considerations. If a meal is rejected or a feeding is vomited, the loss should be compensated for promptly by an intravenous infusion of glucose (100 gm. in 1 liter of water). The purpose here is to maintain liver glycogen, since the resistance of liver to a chemical injury is conceded to vary directly as its glycogen content. Glucose by any route promotes glycogenesis, and fructose and invert sugar are said to be even more efficient precursors of liver glycogen. An attempt is made to maintain the daily carbohydrate intake between 350 and 500 gm. Even if this quantity can be tolerated by mouth, some therapists prefer to cover part of the allowance by a daily infusion of glucose. In patients with liver disease, insulin is not usually used as an adjuvant to intense carbohydrate therapy. Except in the stage of severe hepatic failure, patients tolerate most dietary proteins and fats, especially fats that are well emulsified (*e.g.*, ice cream, butter). Widely divergent opinions are held on the usefulness of protein hydrolysates and other amino acid mixtures. Their administration by mouth and vein has been restricted generally to patients with severe anorexia. Because amino acids occasionally induce nausea and other untoward reactions and because they do not stimulate protein synthesis except when the caloric needs are well satisfied by carbohydrates and fats, amino acid therapy is not widely used (p. 223).

A large variety of dietary supplements has been employed in the control of liver disease. A high caloric diet demands a correspondingly generous intake of vitamin C and B complex. Dr. S. Lichtman recommends the following daily supplements: thiamine 100 mg., niacinamide 100 mg., vitamin B complex as crude liver or yeast (*e.g.*, 2 to 3 heaping teaspoonsful of Brewers' yeast), ascorbic acid 100 mg., and menadione 2 mg. (The latter is intended as prophylaxis against hypoprothrombinemia.) Except for the thiamine value, these recommendations are almost the same as the standard therapeutic formula of the National Research Council (Table IV.6, p. 226). Many substances have been extolled for their ability to prevent the deposition or to accelerate the removal of fat from the liver; these

lipotropic agents include choline, methionine, cystine, inositol, lipocaic, liver extract, and vitamin B_{12}. In spite of impressive demonstrations in the laboratory, clinicians have seldom found anything favorable to say about these substances. Nevertheless two of these agents, choline and methionine, retain some popularity in the management of hepatic disease, perhaps only because they are safe and relatively cheap. Choline is best taken by mouth as the dihydrogen citrate salt in the form of tablets, capsules or a 25% syrup; a typical dose is 1 gm. (or 1 teaspoonful) 3 times a day. Methionine is given in daily doses of 3 to 6 gm.

Patients in all stages of hepatic cell insufficiency have a reduced tolerance for water and salt. Whereas edema, effusions, and ascites are frequently major complications in subacute or chronic liver disease, especially in the presence of fibrosis, they are not common in acute hepatitis. In the clinical management of the acute injury, however, good judgment dictates against an unrestrictedly liberal intake of fluid and electrolytes. The safest procedure is the simple replacement of losses, so that intake and output are balanced, but control here does not need to be as strict as in acute renal insufficiency. In acute hepatitis water restriction is undoubtedly less important than a generous carbohydrate intake.

Hepatic Coma

The regimen outlined above is distinctly impractical and even undesirable in the management of severe grades of acute liver insufficiency. The latter are evidenced by a rapid biochemical deterioration, usually with mounting icterus, intense anorexia (with or without nausea), and deepening somnolence, culminating in the syndrome of hepatic coma. During this sequence a high caloric diet is more and more emphatically refused.

With the development of severe liver failure the protein content of the diet should be reduced immediately, since a high protein intake may precipitate or intensify hepatic coma. A daily dietary allowance of 50 gm. of protein or amino acid has been recommended. Tube feeding (p. 227) usually becomes necessary or at least desirable; it is generally practical because uncontrollable vomiting is uncommon at this stage of the disease. The main dietary constituent is still carbohydrate. Vitamin supplements are continued. If the oral route is available, lipotropic agents may be introduced or continued in the diet. If oral feeding, with or without the aid of intubation, becomes impractical for any reason, the nutritive intake is limited essentially to glucose by the intravenous route. It is an almost universal practice to give these patients daily infusions of 1 to 3 liters of 5 or 10 per cent glucose in water, often as a continuous drip. Protein hydrolysates and synthetic amino mixtures

have only a limited role under these circumstances, as is discussed under Nutrition (p. 223). Transfusions with whole blood and plasma have been used to control anemia and hypoproteinemia. Fresh whole blood is of value in the management of hypoprothrombinemia when and if the latter becomes refractory to vitamin K therapy. Transfusion reactions, however, are said to be common and especially dangerous in patients with severe liver disease. Human serum albumin, especially a salt-poor preparation, is usually well tolerated by slow intravenous infusion.

In near-terminal liver disease, hyponatremia and hypochloremia are often encountered, and hypokalemia has been recognized recently in some cases of liver disease, even those without severe vomiting or diarrhea. These low serum levels are ignored, if mild, or are corrected cautiously and incompletely by administering the appropriate electrolyte (p. 215). The same conservatism applies to the mild acidosis which sometimes appears. The occasional development of renal insufficiency at a late stage of acute liver disease requires even more rigorous restrictions on the intake of fluid, electrolytes, and nitrogen (see discussion of acute renal failure, p. 210).

In addition to the general supportive measures described above, many procedures have been employed in attempts to terminate hepatic coma and to initiate liver regeneration. Empirical programs occasionally described as successful include intravenous injections of the following substances usually in large doses: liver extract, methionine, serum albumin, Aureomycin, and nicotinic acid. In isolated cases massive doses of cortisone and ACTH, with or without wide-spectrum antibiotics, are also said to have been effective. None of these measures is dependable, none is entirely safe, and none is widely accepted.

Drug metabolism and detoxification are severely impaired in most patients with extensive liver parenchymal disease. Consequent drug intolerances are often encountered, particularly with sedative drugs. Morphine should be strictly withheld from patients with liver disease. Codeine is said to be better tolerated, but some risk is involved here too. Barbiturates are generally contraindicated since a profound and persistent coma may result from even small doses, including those derivatives which normally have actions of short duration (e.g., Pentothal, Seconal, Amytal). Paraldehyde and even chloral hydrate are probably less dangerous, but the dose should be limited to one-half to one-third the customary one. Fortunately most of the distressing symptoms in uncomplicated hepatitis can be controlled by bed rest and diet; there is usually no pressing need for hypnotic, sedative, or analgesic drugs. (Even pruritus is uncommon in toxic hepatitis.) The magnitude of drug intolerance in

liver disease has not been adequately delineated, but there is no reason to believe that it is restricted to analgesics and sedatives. Caution is therefore imperative in the administration of any drug; doses should be kept small and prescriptions should be limited to strict necessity.

ELECTROLYTES AND WATER BALANCE

In a variety of clinical situations, the intake of water and minerals becomes insufficient to meet normal or exaggerated metabolic needs or to correct excessive losses. Imbalances of water and salt create such states as dehydration, edema, acidosis, alkalosis, shock, muscle cramps, oliguria, and fever. Each of these conditions is frequently encountered in acute chemical poisonings. Many of these disorders are interdependent. The several processes which work to maintain constancy in the chemical composition of tissues and body fluids are so closely allied that no one component can be disturbed without inducing shifts in others. Thus a metabolic acidosis almost invariably leads to dehydration, and severe dehydration is not infrequently responsible for a state of acidosis. For simplicity in presentation, however, disorders in the metabolism of water and specific electrolytes are discussed separately. Only deficiency states are described. In the following discussion, the emphasis is placed on diagnosis and treatment, but at least a rudimentary appreciation of mechanism is essential for the rational management of patients with disturbances in salt and water metabolism.

Dehydration

Even when no fluid is admitted, the body continues to excrete water. This elimination occurs at the expense of stored water and water of oxidation. For excretory needs, stored water is extracted from the blood, interstitial liquid, and intracellular fluid. Water produced metabolically by the oxidation of food or tissue fuels amounts to about 300 ml. daily in an average adult. The daily obligatory water expenditure of a healthy person includes 500 to 700 ml. for urinary excretion, 500 to 600 ml. as insensible evaporation from the skin, 400 to 500 ml. as vapor exhaled in expired air, and perhaps 100 ml. in feces. These values represent minimal estimates for an inactive, afebrile, adult patient resting in bed in a temperate environment. Physical activity, elevation of air temperature, or exposure to a source of radiant energy such as the sun, immediately raises the basal water loss through the skin. An air temperature of 80°F. induces active sweating even in a resting person. Water losses in sweat have been known to exceed 14 liters a day under conditions of extreme work and heat.

Many pathological states create unavoidable losses of fluid. Two to 5 liters of water may be eliminated daily in any one of the following ways: vomiting, diarrhea, febrile sweating, and draining of an intestinal fistula or of a suctioning catheter in the stomach or bowel. Tubular lesions may so impair the concentrating power of the kidney that the irreducible volume of urine exceeds 2 liters daily. Draining fistulas in the abdominal and thoracic cavities are sometimes major sources of fluid loss, and the weeping of exudate into dressings over burned or otherwise injured areas of skin may contribute substantially to the total output of water.

In infants and children both physiological and pathological losses of fluid are greater in proportion to the body weight than in adults. This differential is due to the higher metabolic rate of the child, to his proportionately larger surface area through which water vaporizes, to his extra metabolic demands for growth, and in the very young to the reduced capacity of the immature kidney to produce a concentrated urine. If water expenditure is compared with body metabolism instead of body weight, minimal losses are about the same in infants and adults and amount to 80 to 170 ml. (depending upon the urine specific gravity) per 100 calories of metabolic heat. This means that the average, healthy, 10-kg. baby eliminates per kg. of body weight 3 to 4 times as much fluid as the adult of average size.

Pure water depletion is uncommon. It arises in an otherwise healthy person only when he is physically deprived of potable water, as when lost in the desert or at sea. In contrast the sick or poisoned patient may suffer a simple water deficit because of lesions which prevent him from ingesting fluid. Disorders such as pharyngitis, esophagitis, cardiospasm, stricture, and generalized weakness may make it impossible to drink, while apathy, drowsiness, stupor, and coma may erase any desire for needed water. In contrast to combined salt and water deficits described later, simple water depletion is due almost always to inadequate intake, not to excessive loss.

The signs and symptoms of dehydration depend upon any associated deficits of electrolyte. Simple water depletion generates thirst and often little else. Salivary secretions become thick and scanty, and the mucous membranes of the mouth and throat become dry. Subcutaneous tissues lose much of their turgor and elasticity. Progressive weakness arises, and in severe grades of dehydration mental confusion and hallucinations may occur. Until dehydration is advanced, the blood volume is well maintained at the expense of intracellular fluid, and hemoconcentration is not marked. A water deficit which equals 2 per cent of the body weight constitutes a clinically mild dehydration, 4 per cent a

moderate dehydration, and 6 per cent a severe dehydration. A water starvation which reaches about 15 per cent of the body weight, or 20 to 22 per cent of the body water, is believed to be fatal in most cases.

The treatment of dehydration is simply the administration of water in amounts sufficient to correct the deficit. The oral route is preferred, but all channels of administration are appropriate. For parenteral use, water must be rendered isotonic or at least isosmotic; when there is no deficit of body salt, this is usually accomplished by the addition of 5 per cent glucose. The route of administration is a less important decision than the quantity of fluid. Unfortunately the extent of a water deficit can seldom be established with accuracy at the bedside or even in the laboratory. The patient's body weight is the most useful single index, but it cannot be interpreted unless his normal or hydrated weight is known. In most cases this information becomes available only after a cure. With healthy kidneys a daily urine volume in excess of 1 liter or a rate of urine flow above 0.6 ml. per hr. per kg. (2 ml. per hr. per kg. in infants) is inconsistent with a significant depletion of body water. In the absence of cardiac or renal disease, water intake is properly continued to the stage of mild diuresis.

Dehydration should be prevented as well as corrected. In most severe poisonings, it is desirable to delineate fluid requirements carefully by maintaining a chart of daily expenditures through all channels. Continuous losses of water from the skin, respiratory tract, and urine cannot be prevented or even depressed beyond a certain level. For the average afebrile adult resting in bed on a low caloric diet, this irreducible minimum lies between 1500 and 2000 ml. each day. Even in such a patient, the intake should exceed this minimal loss to provide a margin of safety. Any difference between intake and obligatory loss is excreted harmlessly as extra urine.

Salt Depletion

Body deficits of sodium chloride arise almost invariably from extraordinary losses of salt, not from primary restrictions of intake. Salt is never eliminated without water, but unlike water the obligatory losses of sodium chloride are very small in a healthy person. For example, if salt is removed from the diet, normal kidneys conserve this electrolyte by excreting a salt-free urine. The normal salt content of feces is small, and water lost by vaporization in a temperate environment is essentially salt-free. The secretion of sweat, however, normally robs the body of sodium chloride, which is present in concentrations of 0.1 to 0.4 per cent. Under conditions of extreme heat, more than 20 gm. of salt can be lost in a day by this avenue. Furthermore substantial amounts of sodium chloride are present in most pathological excretions, including vomitus, diarrheal stools, the drainage from various fistulas, the chyme from an ileostomy opening, the transudate from burned and eroded areas of skin, the returns from a suctioning catheter in the stomach or bowel, and the urine from any kidney which cannot conserve salt. Daily losses of NaCl in these fluids may total more than 30 gm.

Since water is always removed when an electrolyte is excreted, a simple salt deficit is a rarity. One example is the patient who washes salt out of his body by drinking water while his stomach is being emptied constantly by a suctioning catheter. A more common example is the person who compensates for severe water loss by drinking but does nothing about contemporaneous losses of sodium chloride. Thus men working in the heat may suffer primary salt depletion if they replace the water lost in sweat but not the salt. In contrast, if neither deficit is corrected, a syndrome like that of primary water depletion gradually evolves, since sweat is a hypotonic solution, e.g., it is less salty than blood plasma. Losses of hypertonic gastric and intestinal secretions, however, usually cause severer disturbances in electrolyte metabolism than in water balance. In most cases coexisting deficits of water and of salt are both significant and are often accompanied by profound disorders of acid-base balance.

In contrast to primary water depletion, which represents in large measure cellular dehydration, a salt deficit leads to a reduction in the volume and tonicity of extracellular fluids. Thirst is mild or absent, and the mucous membranes are not characteristically desiccated. Anorexia and nausea are common, and vomiting often prevents the repletion of body salt by ingestion. Headache, giddiness, tendency to orthostatic fainting, and a profound sense of exhaustion are often described. A reduction in the blood pressure and in the volume of the pulse may progress to a typical state of oligemic shock. Factors which incline to circulatory collapse include not only the reduction in blood volume but also the marked rise in blood viscosity because of hemoconcentration. The most distinctive clinical features of primary salt depletion, however, are muscle weakness and painful muscle spasms. These so-called heat cramps often occur in the calf muscles, abdominal muscles, and intrinsic muscles of the hand, particularly during periods of physical activity.

In principle, sodium chloride is all that is necessary to correct a simple salt deficit. Since large doses of salt are poorly tolerated by mouth, especially in the presence of nausea, saline solutions by parenteral channels are preferred. Although hypertonic solutions (e.g., 3 per cent NaCl) have been used successfully, overdoses produce such adverse effects on the circulation that these solutions are not recommended. In any case, normal physiological saline

(0.85 to 0.9 per cent NaCl) is adequate since the body retains the salt that it needs and quickly excretes the excess fluid as urine. To avoid overloading the heart, the intravenous infusion of isotonic saline should probably be restricted to a rate of about 500 ml. per hour in an average adult except in cases of frank shock. Physiological saline is a poor replacement fluid in primary *water* deprivation and it may even aggravate the symptoms; in these cases, only water and electrolyte-free solutions are appropriate reparations.

Deficits of water and salt commonly coexist. The proper replacement fluid depends on the nature of the shortage. When losses arise from vomiting, physiological saline is usually sufficient; when due to extensive sweating, hypotonic saline is required. It can be obtained by mixing isotonic saline and 5 per cent glucose in water in an appropriate ratio, or the two solutions can be administered alternately. Within broad limits, the proper proportions are not critical.

As outlined above, the clinical history and physical examination aid in evaluating the nature and intensity of mixed deficits. Laboratory determinations are also helpful. A small urine volume of high specific gravity is characteristic of patients whose principal defect is a lack of body water. Except in Addison's disease and some types of renal disease, a salt deficiency is denoted by the absence or near absence of NaCl in urine. Plasma levels of sodium and chloride may be moderately low, but a salt deficit is accommodated chiefly by reductions in the volume of blood and extracellular fluid and not by reductions in electrolyte concentration. Hemoconcentration, as evidenced by high plasma levels of protein and of non-protein nitrogen, is usually more striking in states of salt depletion than in water deficits of comparable intensity. Methods for determining the plasma and extracellular fluid volumes are too complicated for extensive or routine application. No test and no series of tests defines precisely the extent of any deficit. The response of the patient to treatment and the clinical judgment of the therapist are the best guides. The patient who excretes 1500 ml. of urine daily with a chloride content in excess of 5 gm. per liter has presumably recovered from any shortages of either water or salt.

Acidosis and Alkalosis

States of acidosis and of alkalosis are frequently superimposed upon deficits or excesses of both water and salt. Although acid-base imbalances are associated with alterations in the concentration of many ions, only variations in the hydrogen ion concentration (pH) are important in generating untoward signs and symptoms. Much of the confusion in the medical literature about the mechanics of acid-base disorders arises from the circuity of the chemical methods commonly used for the detection and evaluation of these disturbances. Misunderstanding would diminish if present methods were largely replaced with reliable determinations of pH on anaerobic samples of arterial blood. Venous blood is unsatisfactory because specimens from different sites vary in hydrogen ion concentration and so reflect only local tissue conditions. In contrast, arterial blood has the same composition in all parts of the body. If properly measured in arterial blood or plasma, a hydrogen ion concentration below 3.5×10^{-8} M (pH above 7.45) is diagnostic of alkalosis, while a hydrogen ion concentration above 4.5×10^{-8} M (pH below 7.35) is pathognomonic of acidosis. As stated here the limits are arbitrary, but the generalization is valid irrespective of the etiology of the disorder. Although the physician cannot distinguish by this test between a respiratory and a metabolic acidosis, at least he cannot confuse acidosis with alkalosis.

Because of practical difficulties in the technique of measuring arterial pH, plasma concentrations of other ions are analyzed instead, with the implicit intent of using these data to infer the existence of deviations in hydrogen ion concentration. In this respect the ions of major interest are sodium (Na^+), chloride (Cl^-), and bicarbonate (HCO_3^-). Together with a clinical history and physical examination, these chemical determinations are adequate guides in most clinical situations. In cases of respiratory acidosis or alkalosis, however, these data may be misleading if not dangerously deceptive, and have been responsible for the mistreatment of many patients with salicylate poisoning. In contrast to the uncertain inferences based upon plasma levels of Na^+, Cl^- and HCO_3^-, the arterial plasma pH can always be estimated with reasonable accuracy from any two of the following three laboratory determinations: the alveolar CO_2 tension (measured on an end-tidal sample of expired air), the CO_2 content of *arterial* blood, and the CO_2-combining power of a blood specimen (venous or arterial). If no facilities are available for the chemical analysis of blood, a poor but useful substitute is litmus paper to determine the reaction of freshly voided urine. If necessary the urinary bladder is catheterized, and repeated specimens are tested. Except in urinary tract infections (where urea may be converted to ammonia), an alkaline urine (litmus paper blue) demonstrates systemic alkalosis (metabolic or respiratory). An acid reaction is at least consistent with systemic acidosis and excludes alkalosis, except in terminal stages of the latter when sodium depletion may become so severe that an acid urine is secreted.

Table IV.3 is a conventional classification of acid-base disorders. Examples of each type can be found in the realm of clinical toxicology. From this table it is apparent, for example, that a meta-

TABLE IV.3

Classification of acid-base disturbances *

ACIDOSIS

1. Respiratory acidosis: increased plasma carbonic acid
    a) Conditions in which there is interference with the excretion of CO_2
        Pulmonary and cardiac disease
        Anesthesia
        Asphyxial states
    b) Breathing in an atmosphere containing excessive quantities of CO_2
2. Metabolic acidosis: depletion of plasma sodium bicarbonate
    a) Accumulation of non-volatile acids
        Medication with HCl, NH_4Cl, ammonium mandelate, *etc.*
        Ingestion or inhalation of acids or acid anhydrides
        Increased production of metabolic acids
            Diabetes mellitus
            Starvation
            Cyclic vomiting of children
            Methyl alcohol poisoning
        Decreased excretion of metabolic acids
            Toxic nephritis
            Renal insufficiency from any cause
    b) Excessive loss of sodium bicarbonate
        Diarrhea
        Losses through intestinal fistulas or catheters

ALKALOSIS

1. Respiratory alkalosis: depletion of plasma carbonic acid
        Overbreathing
        Hysteria
        Encephalitis (sometimes)
        Anoxic anoxemia
        Poisoning with salicylate, quinine, phenol, *etc.*
2. Metabolic alkalosis: increased plasma sodium bicarbonate
        Immoderate intake of alkalies
        Excessive loss of hydrochloric acid
        Vomiting
        Continuous gastric lavage

* Reproduced with slight modifications from James A. Dauphinee, Chap. 12, p. 354, *Clinical Nutrition*, edited by N. Jolliffe, F. F. Tisdall and P. R. Cannon, 1950, with permission of the publisher, Paul B. Hoeber, Inc. New York City.

bolic acidosis may arise in three ways: a) the retention of non-volatile acids or acid-forming salts as a result of immoderate intake or defective excretion; b) the excessive metabolic production of physiological acids, such as carbonic acid, or of abnormal metabolites such as formic acid; c) the depletion of sodium bicarbonate stores by the elimination of alkaline body fluids, as in certain cases of profuse diarrhea. Similarly, a metabolic alkalosis might arise in three ways but only two are recognized: a) excessive intakes of alkali or alkalinizing salts; b) the elimination of chloride ion as hydrochloric acid and the consequent retention of sodium as $NaHCO_3$, as during the extensive vomiting of gastric acid. Respiratory acidosis and alkalosis are due to underbreathing and overbreathing respectively and are associated with changes in the plasma con-

centration of carbonic acid. These changes, however, are not reflected in any predictable way by alterations in the plasma levels of Na^+, Cl^-, or HCO_3^-; any ionic shifts that are observed are usually efforts at renal compensation for the primary disorder. Respiratory alkalosis is a response to toxic doses of many central nervous stimulants, notably salicylates, phenol, quinine and sometimes antihistaminics. Respiratory acidosis probably occurs as a terminal event in every fatal poisoning when breathing ceases or becomes grossly inadequate. Anoxia, however, is much more important than the acidosis which accompanies it.

If the laboratory diagnosis of acid-base disorders is difficult, recognition by physical diagnosis is thoroughly impractical. On the other hand, once the nature of the disturbance has been established

by combining the evidence from the laboratory, from the bedside, and from the history, then changing signs and symptoms are often helpful in evaluating the progress of therapy. Except in respiratory acidosis, where symptoms of anoxia are usually dominant, the acidotic patient commonly complains of generalized malaise, weakness, dull headache, abdominal pain, nausea, and vomiting. Signs of dehydration, circulatory insufficiency, and various grades of stupor or coma are often present. Hyperpnea is a common sign; respirations are usually rapid but sometimes slow and deep (Kussmaul). An established alkalosis is characterized clinically by abnormal irritability, restlessness, and neuromuscular hyperexcitability which is indistinguishable from that of hypocalcemic tetany (see p. 221). Forceful vomiting is common, and a considerable degree of dehydration may accompany the disturbance. Respirations are either enhanced, as in respiratory alkalosis, or moderately depressed as in many cases of metabolic alkalosis. Note that a patient who is hyperventilating may be suffering from respiratory alkalosis or from severe metabolic acidosis. It is apparent that water and salt depletions may coexist with and contribute to the symptomatology of acid-base disorders.

Prompt and effective treatment is often lifesaving in cases where the acidity or alkalinity of the body is severely deranged. When respiratory acidosis arises from acute respiratory depression, asphyxia, or pulmonary edema, acidosis is generally incidental to hypoxia, and treatment is directed chiefly at the relief of this associated oxygen lack (p. 189). Tetany due to hyperventilation (respiratory alkalosis) is usually best controlled by rebreathing into a paper bag. Parenteral calcium therapy (p. 221) may become necessary. Hyperpnea can often be suppressed by sedation and in the case of hysteria by reassurance or more sophisticated forms of psychotherapy. In metabolic alkalosis, as seen after persistent vomiting, physiological saline with or without glucose is always an excellent replacement fluid because in this situation bicarbonate excess is accompanied by hypochloremia and usually by a sodium deficiency. When salt is administered, the chloride deficit is corrected by the retention of Cl^-, and the bicarbonate surplus is eliminated as urinary $NaHCO_3$. Acidifying agents such as ammonium chloride or hydrochloric acid are much less useful because they fail to rectify the salt deficit which almost invariably accompanies a metabolic alkalosis. The details of treatment are essentially the same as for salt and water depletion (see p. 215). Only dangerous levels of alkalosis require the ingestion of diluted hydrochloric acid.

Metabolic acidosis too is associated with dehydration and a salt deficit and frequently responds to the same therapeutic measures (p. 215). In severe acidosis, alkali therapy is usually necessary.

In addition, the syndrome of potassium deficiency (p. 220) often complicates acidosis and requires special attention. When the production of ketone bodies (organic acids and ketones derived from fat metabolism) becomes excessive because of depletion of tissue glycogen reservoirs, the administration of glucose is also beneficial. The diabetic also requires large doses of insulin. The two common alkalinizing salts are sodium bicarbonate and sodium lactate, the latter being metabolized to sodium bicarbonate in the body. If there is no vomiting, the salts are given best by mouth. For parenteral use, sodium lactate is preferred to $NaHCO_3$ because it is more easily sterilized and the lactate ion is useful in replenishing tissue glycogen stores. If lactate metabolism is impaired, as perhaps is true in methyl alcohol poisoning, sodium bicarbonate is obviously preferable. For intravenous infusions, sodium r-lactate is marketed as a 1/6 molar solution (M/6 or 1.75 per cent). Sterile solutions of sodium bicarbonate (available in ampules) are commonly injected in concentrations up to 5 per cent (usually 1.2 per cent or M/7), either alone or mixed with isotonic saline. The intravenous route is usually chosen in preference to the subcutaneous path.

In whatever way one classifies the severity of acidosis, the more extreme the disorder the more alkali therapy is required. No criteria, however, are available for predicting with a useful degree of accuracy the alkali needs of acidotic patients. The intensity and duration of therapy must be controlled by the progression of signs and symptoms, by repeated analyses of plasma sodium, chloride, and bicarbonate (as CO_2-combining power), and/or by measurements of the alkalinity of the urine. As a general rule, whenever the CO_2-combining power is below 20 mEq. per liter (45 vol. per cent), a reasonable initial dose of M/6 sodium lactate or M/6 $NaHCO_3$ is 25 ml. per kg. of body weight (or 6.0 ml. per kg. with 5 per cent $NaHCO_3$). Given by slow intravenous drip, this dose may have to be repeated several times, but as the CO_2-combining power of plasma approaches 20 mEq. per liter, parenteral and probably even oral alkali therapy should be discontinued to avoid over-alkalinization. Infusions of physiological saline, however, are properly continued until deficits of salt are entirely erased (p. 216).

Disorders of Potassium Balance

Both hypo- and hyperkalemia are encountered in victims of poison. Dangerously high levels of potassium are rarely found except in patients with defective renal function. Because of rapid excretion simple potassium salts have a low oral toxicity in a normal person. In severe grades of renal injury and particularly in states of anuria, dietary potassium accumulates in the body. Even when no potassium

is ingested, catabolism gradually releases intracellular potassium and causes a progressive rise in the extracellular concentration. When the level in blood plasma reaches 2 to 4 times normal or about 8 mEq. per liter, the patient commonly exhibits muscle weakness, hyporeflexia, paresthesias, anxiety, restlessness, and disturbances of cardiac rhythm. Because these signs are variable and often occur too late for effective therapy, the early detection and proper management of potassium intoxication demands frequent chemical analyses of plasma or serum. If reliable laboratory measurements are unavailable, repeated electrocardiograms may help to detect hyperkalemia, but they furnish no information from which a quantitative value of the extracellular K^+ concentration can be estimated. The first electrocardiographic sign of potassium intoxication is usually an increase in the amplitude of the T-wave; eventually various cardiac arrhythmias, including episodes of asystole, presage complete cardiac arrest. The clinical management of this syndrome is described on p. 212.

Hypokalemia is evidenced by plasma or serum potassium concentrations below the normal range of 3.5 to 5.5 mEq. per liter (or 14 to 22 mg. per cent). Probably a profound intracellular deficit of potassium always accompanies hypokalemia. Because this cation is plentiful in all ordinary foods, deficiency states arise only when losses are excessive. Partial depletion of cellular potassium and its incomplete replacement by the cellular penetration of extracellular sodium has been described in many pathological states, including diarrhea, hemorrhage, shock, trauma, diabetic coma, metabolic acidosis, hypochloremic alkalosis, and severe dehydration. In the patient with diabetic acidosis, hypokalemia is sometimes induced by intensive treatment (insulin, fluids, sodium chloride, etc.). Particularly in infants and children, the alkalosis and dehydration of profuse vomiting and the acidosis and dehydration of severe diarrhea are both accompanied by substantial losses of potassium.

The clinical manifestations of potassium depletion include weakness, lethargy, and abdominal distention. The most distinctive sign, however, is muscle atony progressing to flaccid paralysis. Cardiac disturbances include tachycardia, arrhythmias, and ventricular dilatation. Subacute and chronic potassium deficiencies lead to a recently recognized but well established nephropathy. These effects are not sufficiently definitive to suggest the correct diagnosis unless the physician is alert to the possibility of this complication. In any conditions that promote excessive losses of potassium, the blood plasma level should be analyzed repeatedly. If no adequate laboratory facilities are available, a suspicion of hypokalemia is strongly supported by electrocardiographic findings of flattening of the T-wave, prolongation of the apparent QT interval, and depression of the ST segment.

The correction of a potassium deficit requires considerable caution, particularly if the renal status is uncertain. The oral route is the safest way to administer potassium salts but is clearly impractical in the presence of vomiting or severe diarrhea. By intravenous or other parenteral channels, potassium must be infused very slowly to avoid even transient periods of hyperkalemia which might produce heart block and cardiac arrest. A hypodermoclysis is safer than an infusion. Even a potassium deficient adult should be given KCl no faster than 1.0 gm. per hr., and the total dose rarely needs to exceed 5 gm. (67 mEq.). Potassium is administered usually as the chloride, either alone or in a balanced salt solution such as Ringer, the Lactate Ringer Solution of Hartmann, or Darrow's Solution. The latter, which contains NaCl, sodium lactate, and KCl (2.7 gm. per liter), has proved particularly effective in infants by hypodermoclysis; the recommended maximal dose is 80 ml. per kg., and it should be spaced over a period of 4 to 8 hours.

Disorders of Blood Calcium

Calcium retention and depletion are dependent on many complex factors, including the dietary levels of calcium and vitamin D, endogenous vitamin D, parathyroid activity, acid-base balance, bone growth and mineralization, bone resorption and disease, renal function, lactation, and many other circumstances. Within broad limits the dietary calcium level is comparatively unimportant, but mild deficiency states during active growth, pregnancy, and lactation have been ascribed to inadequate calcium intake. Indeed calcium and iron are the only minerals in which American diets are sometimes regarded as defective. Probably milk is the best dietary source of calcium; one quart contains about 1.3 gm., which equals the daily requirement of the average child. Milk-free diets, unless carefully designed, tend to be deficient in absorbable calcium. For example, due to the oxalic acid of spinach and the phytic acid of cereals, most calcium in these foods cannot be assimilated.

Probably vitamin D is more often a critical dietary component than is calcium. Inadequate intake of vitamin D is responsible for infantile and juvenile rickets. Persistent overdoses of vitamin D, when accompanied by high calcium diets, lead to hypercalcemia and metastatic calcification of soft tissues. In states of calcium deficiency, however, vitamin D sometimes produces hypocalcemia by promoting the mineralization of bone (e.g., in the ricketic child given vitamin D but not extra calcium). In addition to diet, parathyroid disease and many metabolic disorders of bone lead to profound alterations of calcium balance.

Chronic defects in calcium metabolism are less often of concern to the toxicologist than are acute disturbances. The latter are not often recognized

unless accompanied by abnormally high or low levels of ionic calcium in blood and extracellular fluid. Of the total calcium in blood plasma (10 mg. per cent or 2.50 mM.), only about half is present as the simple ion Ca^{++}. According to recent estimates (W. F. Neuman, personal communication), the calcium in normal blood plasma is partitioned as follows: ionic 53 per cent, protein-bound 34 per cent (7 per cent attached to globulins and 27 per cent to albumin), 7 per cent as a bicarbonate complex, 3 per cent as a citrate complex, and 3 per cent as a soluble phosphate complex. Since only the protein-bound element is non-diffusible, 66 per cent of the total calcium can be found in ultrafiltrates. Variations in this normal pattern over long periods of time may have many metabolic consequences, but only the level of ionic calcium is important for short-term effects.

The chief effects of transient hypercalcemia are those on the heart. If the plasma concentration of ionic calcium rises to twice its normal value (concentrations of total and ionic calcium tend to parallel each other in this range), vagal bradycardia occurs. Eventually, as the calcium reaches levels 2 to 5 times normal, sinus arrhythmia, shifting pacemaker, varying degrees of heart block, ventricular premature beats, ventricular tachycardia, and finally ventricular fibrillation may develop. Actions on somatic nerve and skeletal muscle are minimal. This syndrome can be produced by the parenteral administration of soluble, ionizable calcium salts, but in practice dangerous hypercalcemia cannot be induced by ingestion, even when massive doses are swallowed.

Any considerable reduction in the ionic calcium activity produces tetany. When the total blood calcium is low, as well as the level of Ca^{++}, the condition is called hypocalcemic tetany. When the concentration of chemically bound calcium rises in proportion to the fall in the ionic fraction, the condition is called normocalcemic tetany. The distinction is important only because clinical chemistry laboratories report values of total calcium only, since no simple method is available for the measurement of the ion Ca^{++}.

An impending or latent tetany may be detected with the aid of several diagnostic procedures. The Chvostek sign, Trousseau phenomenon, and peroneal sign are useful ways of exposing neuromuscular hyperexcitability. Electrical stimulation of a motor nerve (the Erb test) is used occasionally. Both the rheobase and chronaxie of peripheral nerve are increased when the extracellular level of ionic calcium is low. Frank or manifest tetany reveals itself as carpal and pedal spasm, laryngospasm, tremors and twitching, pain (probably due to muscle spasm), convulsive seizures of all types, gastrointestinal disorders such as cardiospasm and vomiting, and occasionally many other signs and symptoms. In the neonatal period, cyanosis and irritability are sometimes the only manifestations. Tetany may have a sudden onset and alarming intensity, or the disturbance may be mild and persistent.

Hypocalcemic tetany is due to dietary inadequacies of calcium and vitamin D as in rickets and some forms of osteomalacia, to certain types of gastrointestinal tract disease such as the coeliac syndrome, to excessive utilization as in pregnancy, to excessive loss as in lactation, to hypoparathyroidism, and to idiopathic states such as neonatal tetany. Normocalcemic tetany occurs in metabolic and respiratory alkalosis (see p. 219), because a rise in pH allows the plasma proteins to bind more calcium and so reduce the Ca^{++} concentration. Toxic doses of soluble fluorides and oxalates may also cause normocalcemic tetany (p. 143 and 165). Under some poorly defined circumstances, infusions of sodium phosphate and of sodium citrate produce tetany.

The prompt and vigorous administration of ionic calcium is sufficient to control both hypocalcemic and normocalcemic tetany. Other measures are also useful. For example, rebreathing, as into a paper bag, may suppress the alkalotic tetany of hyperventilation. A single injection of parathyroid extract (Injection, U.S.P.) is sometimes sufficient, after a latency of a few hours, to control mild hypocalcemia for a period of several days. Given by mouth, calcium salts act too slowly to employ in manifest tetany, but the oral route is preferred in states of latent tetany. Calcium chloride, gluconate, and lactate are the common medicinal salts. The recommended oral dose in an adult is 1 to 2 gm. of $CaCl_2 \cdot 2H_2O$, 2 to 4 gm. of calcium lactate, and 4 to 8 gm. of calcium gluconate, repeated every few hours as necessary. Of these preparations, probably the chloride produces irritation most often; to avoid vomiting, it should be given only in a highly diluted formula. Calcium salts should never be injected subcutaneously, and the intramuscular route is sometimes dangerous, particularly in infants. For example even calcium gluconate, which is the least irritating preparation, occasionally produces sloughing when injected intramuscularly as a 10 per cent solution. For this reason the only acceptable route for parenteral administration is the intravenous channel. The usual adult dose of calcium gluconate is 10 to 30 ml. of a 10 per cent sterile solution, injected slowly to avoid severe tachycardia and flushing. Calcium chloride is sometimes infused in concentrations of 5 to 10 per cent; for example, 5 to 20 ml. of a 5 per cent solution can be administered if the rate is kept below 2 ml. per minute. Unlike the lactate or gluconate which are metabolized, repeated doses of calcium chloride may produce a systemic acidosis. In an acidotic patient, e.g., with renal insufficiency, the gluconate is always preferred to the chloride.

NUTRITION

The subject of nutrition has multifold significance for the clinical toxicologist. Good nutrition is protective against many poisons, notably hepatotoxic substances. Whatever the causative agent, acute injury is accompanied by large losses of nutrients, while at the same time tissue damage creates extraordinary metabolic demands for many dietary factors. Damage to the gastrointestinal mucosa sometimes impairs digestion and absorption severely. Liver damage leads to poor utilization of those nutrients which are absorbed. Protein and vitamin deficiences lead to anorexia, which intensely complicates the efforts of the therapist. Finally poor nutrition is almost always instrumental in prolonging convalescence well beyond that of the well-nourished patient.

Physiological and psychological stresses alter body metabolism. One type of reaction is a nonspecific response described by H. Selye and called the "general adaptation syndrome." The pituitary-adrenal system is known to be involved in all reactions to stress and specifically in the acquisition and maintenance of the general adaptation syndrome. While the nutritional status of experimental animals affects the course of the adaptation syndrome, the converse is also true. In chemical poisonings, however, the major metabolic alterations are not stereotyped, but arise from specific physiological effects of the particular toxin causing the stress. In the laboratory, diets protective against one type of poison are found to enhance the harmful effects of another. For example, diets rich in fat increase the toxicity of 2,4,6-trinitrotoluene (TNT) but diminish the toxicity of cyanide. The acute toxicity of rotenone is augmented by a fatty diet, but the chronic toxicity is decreased. In selenium and arsphenamine poisonings liver glycogen appears to be spared better by dietary protein than by carbohydrate, while in carbon tetrachloride poisoning a high carbohydrate diet with a moderate amount of protein is judged to be best. Although it would be inexcusably naïve to translate these laboratory demonstrations directly into clinical practice, eventually special diets may become available to the physician for protection against and supportive treatment for specific chemical insults. Perhaps a diet which is optimally effective against all forms of poisoning may be evolved, but none is yet recognized.

Parenteral Feeding

In many severe poisonings, mucosal lesions of the alimentary tract prevent the patient from retaining, digesting, or assimilating ingested food or fluid. Only parenteral channels are then available for the administration of nutrient substances. Oral feedings, however, should be resumed as soon as possible because parenteral alimentation in current practice is expensive, inconvenient, annoying to the patient, and nutritionally inadequate.

In the adult the intravenous route is the only parenteral channel suitable for the efficient administration of nourishment. Particularly with hypertonic solutions, hypodermoclyses are uncomfortable and unsatisfactory because both water and solute are absorbed slowly from subcutaneous depots. In infants and young children, however, this route is often preferred; especially when the area is infiltrated with hyaluronidase, the mobilization of fluid and solute is comparatively fast. The water and electrolyte requirements of adult and pediatric patients are outlined on pp. 215–220. Besides water and salts, intravenous feedings are limited largely to the administration of glucose or other monosaccharides, vitamins, amino acid mixtures, sodium lactate, alcohol, and serum proteins. To meet high caloric requirements fat emulsions have been administered successfully, but no dependably stable, non-hemolytic preparation for intravenous use has been devised.

Unlike the young child or infant, the well-nourished adult person is well endowed to tolerate short periods of fasting. Of the 1600 to 2000 calories needed daily by the average adult resting in bed, glucose from tissue glycogen is the major metabolic fuel during the initial hours of fasting. After glycogen is depleted, tissue stores of fat and protein are consumed. The result is at least a mild ketosis, a negative nitrogen balance, and a gradual wasting of all tissues. Although the daily administration of 100 gm. of glucose furnishes only a quarter to a fifth of the caloric requirement, this amount of carbohydrate is sufficient to prevent ketosis and to reduce the catabolism of tissue proteins to a minimal level. For 100 gm. of glucose (d-glucose or dextrose), 1 liter of a 10 per cent aqueous solution can be administered intravenously. To prevent sugar from spilling into the urine, about 2 hours is required for this infusion in an average sized person, because the maximal rate of glucose utilization lies between 0.5 and 0.7 gm. per kg. per hour. Invert sugar and levulose are said to be utilized faster than d-glucose and may be substituted for it. In addition to carbohydrate, a parenteral preparation of the water-soluble vitamins (B-complex and ascorbic acid) is desirable in amounts which match the standard maintenance recommendations of the National Research Council (p. 226). Of course daily losses of water and electrolytes must be replaced, but in other respects a modest amount of glucose with vitamin supplements is an acceptable parenteral feeding for an illness of short duration.

No practical solution is yet available for the problem of maintaining a patient's nutrition over

a period of many days solely by parenteral alimentation. Raising the carbohydrate intake to match the caloric needs is a difficult task and one of limited value (except in the patient with parenchymal liver disease). The repeated injection of glucose in concentrations above 10 per cent often induces phlebitis, although under special circumstances concentrations up to 50 per cent have been administered without complications through a small plastic cannula threaded into one of the larger veins (e.g., jugular, inferior vena cava). In assimilating carbohydrate, intracellular stores of potassium are replenished at the expense of the extracellular fluid; to prevent hypokalemia during high carbohydrate feedings, potassium in the form of a balanced salt solution (e.g., Ringer) is serviceable. For its food value ethyl alcohol has been given intravenously in concentrations of 5 to 6 per cent, but its intoxicating potential is a hazard, and it is never safe in an unconscious patient. Sodium lactate furnishes calories, but its alkalinizing action precludes its use except in states of acidosis. Aside from human plasma proteins, mixtures of amino acids and small polypeptides are the only effective sources of nitrogen when only parenteral routes of administration are available. Acid and enzymatic hydrolysates of casein and of other proteins (e.g., bovine blood, yeast, beef) have been employed intravenously and subcutaneously, usually in concentrations of 5 per cent in water. In general these commercial mixtures furnish all 10 amino acids which are essential for man (tryptophane is destroyed by acid hydrolyses and so must be added). If injected too rapidly, these sterile mixtures sometimes induce untoward reactions such as nausea, vomiting, abdominal pain, flushing, chills, and fever. Two to 3 hours should be allowed for the intravenous injection of 1 liter of a 5 per cent amino acid solution. The parenteral use of protein hydrolysates, however, is of limited value because the amino acids are largely deaminated and oxidized whenever the caloric intake in the form of carbohydrate and fat is insufficient. Because an adequate number of calories can rarely be given by parenteral channels only, a negative nitrogen balance usually appears even when liberal quantities of amino acids are infused intravenously. When a commercial fat emulsion satisfactory for intravenous administration is developed, interest in amino acid therapy will revive.

Resumption of Oral Feeding—Bland Diet

Because of the generally unsatisfactory status of parenteral alimentation, oral feedings should be reinstituted as soon as possible. The best treatment for acute gastritis, however, is absolute rest for the stomach for several days. The only reliable criterion for determining when to start feeding is the patient's response to a test meal. To prepare the stomach for food, lavage with warm water containing a small amount of sodium bicarbonate is sometimes advantageous. Unless severe mucosal lesions of the alimentary tract are suspected, a trial feeding is usually safe after a period of 12 to 24 hours without nausea or pain. The initial feeding is limited to a few sips (about a teaspoonful) of warm water, dilute tea, or milk. If well tolerated, a teaspoonful of milk or strained gruel is offered every half hour. The size and frequency of feedings are gradually increased as the patient's tolerance to food rises. A few salted crackers or dry toast are added to the diet. Eventually small servings of cooked cereal, soft boiled eggs, mashed potatoes, and other bland foods are offered. As described later (p. 225), vitamin requirements are best met by daily supplementation. Any food which might stimulate gastric acid unduly is avoided, including acid foods, coarse foods, alcoholic beverages, condiments and spices, meat extracts, and meat soups. All fried and greasy foods are withheld, as are items which tend to produce flatulence. The patient's own appetite is one excellent guide in determining how fast to restore a normal menu, but a bland diet with little or no residue is usually required for 1 to 2 weeks.

To maintain the nutrition of a severely poisoned patient, treatment must be individualized. The physician should check frequently the patient's reactions to feeding and should determine whether the food prescribed is actually served and eaten. Too early or too zealous resumption of oral feeding after a long abstinence may precipitate nausea, vomiting, pain, intestinal distention, and diarrhea. For the management of nausea and vomiting, see p. 209. For diarrhea induced by diet, canned applesauce or commercial pectin, fed alone or with meals, is generally effective, but a diarrhea caused by indiscreet feeding must be distinguished from that due to poison (p. 210), to undernutrition, and to infection. Even when no complications are encountered, it is advisable at the resumption of oral feedings for someone to sit beside the patient at meals to help and encourage him. Because food acquires profound emotional significance during periods of stress, feeding problems, which so often complicate convalescence, can often be prevented by the physician who spends a few minutes with the patient at meal times.

General Diets

A mild intoxication of short duration only rarely disturbs the nutrition of an otherwise healthy person to an extent that is clinically significant. The Committee on Therapeutic Nutrition of the Food and Nutrition Board, National Research Council, considers that any illness or injury is minor when the patient is ambulatory, consumes food by mouth, and is hospitalized less than 10 days. In these cases a diet which meets normal requirements is suffi-

cient. If any nutritional inadequacy is suspected, a high protein supplement and one or two maintenance multivitamin tablets (p. 225) may be added to the regular diet each day. General hospital diets are designed to meet the Recommended Daily Allowances of the National Research Council; these recommendations are judged to be appropriate for the average normal adult person. A general hospital diet contains approximately 2200 calories, 75 gm. of protein, 100 gm. of fat, and 250 gm. of carbohydrate. Vitamins and minerals are present in the recommended amounts (p. 226).

No diet is adequate if it is not consumed. Although everyone agrees that hospital patients rarely eat all foods served, data on actual intake is scanty. Duncan (J. Amer. Diet. Assoc. 25: 330, April 1949) analyzed 6 successive meals of 78 patients on a medical ward. The average daily consumption was 1870 calories out of the 2430 calories which were served. Of the 105 gm. of protein which were presented daily, only 81 gm. were ingested. Of 49 patients who received supplementary feedings, only 14 ingested 100 gm. or more of protein. Of the 29 patients not receiving supplementary feedings, only 1 patient consumed more than 100 gm. of protein. Studies of patients on surgical and obstetrical wards showed still lower intakes of food and protein. Duncan believes that food consumption was best in those patients whose illness directed attention to the diet.

Probably the food intake of any patient can be improved by heeding his individual needs. The management of anorexia is discussed below under the topic of high caloric diets. These general considerations are not usually applicable to the infant. Although nutrition is often a crucial factor in the survival of a poisoned baby, the topic of infant feeding during periods of illness cannot be reduced to simple generalizations—except for the rule that sudden and frequent changes of formula and alternate periods of fasting and gorging must be avoided. If a baby or young child has persistent diarrhea, tolerates food poorly, or does not gain weight, a pediatric specialist should be consulted.

Perhaps the most important consideration in the nutrition of an accidentally poisoned child is the prevention of undesirable attitudes toward food. Many cases of chronic anorexia stem from an illness during which the child was forced to eat so that he could be "built up." Coaxing and cajoling are not likely to have beneficial effects. Some parents need to be reassured that a child's lack of appetite is temporary and that given a choice of good foods the child will eat enough to maintain good nutrition. They should be told too that no one food need be forced upon a reluctant child. The mother should try to serve vegetables which the child likes and to find substitutes for those which he resists. If fruits are consumed in quantity, a temporary diet with

no vegetables is probably more desirable than a life-long aversion to these dietary staples. Milk is practically essential for an adequate supply of calcium. By the use of dry skim milk, some of the daily milk requirement can be incorporated into solid food such as custards, mashed potatoes, and cereals. Milk shakes served with straws are often accepted when plain milk is not. Every child should be encouraged and given an opportunity to feed himself at meals. Interest in eating is often stimulated by letting him plan his own menu on special occasions. For the small child large portions of food and large glasses of milk are overwhelming to the psyche if not to the stomach. Modest servings at frequent intervals are preferable.

High Caloric Diets

A daily intake of 1600 to 2000 calories is sufficient for the average afebrile inactive adult patient with a minor injury or illness, but 2500 to 4000 calories may be required after severe trauma or disease. A large number of calories is necessary not only to meet energy demands but also to insure efficient utilization of dietary protein. Of the dozens of established therapeutic diets, none is more useful to the clinical toxicologist than a high caloric, high protein diet. In one form or another this dietary regimen is used widely for the nutritional rehabilitation of patients convalescing from serious disease, surgery, trauma, and similar stressful conditions that cause the destruction of body protein and the depletion of vitamin stores. Probably a high protein intake should be started even during the catabolic stage of injury since the end of the catabolic stage and the beginning of the anabolic phase cannot be determined accurately by clinical criteria. Although assimilation is poor in the early stages of convalescence, the over-all benefit to the patient easily justifies the effort and expense of establishing a protein-rich diet.

The Recommended Dietary Allowance for a normal 65-kg. man is 65 gm. of protein daily (1 gm. per kg.). For tissue synthesis in injury and disease, however, 2 to 4 gm. per kg. is recommended, or as much as 130 to 260 gm. for a 65-kg. man. The poisoned child needs protein for growth as well as repair. The N.R.C. allowance for the normal child is 2.5 to 3 gm. per kg. per day in early childhood to 1.5 to 2 gm. per kg. in late childhood and adolescence. Little reliable information is available about the long-range effects of acute injury upon growth. In practice an injured child may be given as much protein food as he can tolerate. Four cups of milk, 2 ounces of meat, 1 egg, 2 slices of bread, and 2 servings of vegetables contains approximately 60 gm. of protein, which meets the N.R.C. allowance for the 8-year-old child weighing 27 kg. (59 lb.). It can be seen that high intakes of protein require careful

TABLE IV.4

High-protein, high-carbohydrate, moderate-fat diet—daily allowance for adults

	Servings	Grams	Calories	Approximate Composition		
				Protein	Carbohydrate	Fat
				gm.	gm.	gm.
Milk..............	6 cups	1440	990	51	72	54
Meat or fish........	2 (large)	180	575	46	—	43
Eggs..............	2	100	160	13	—	12
Fruit..............	2	200	140	1	30	—
Vegetables..........	2	200	50	3	10	—
Potato............	1	150	125	3	30	—
Bread, cereal.......	5	—	400	13	75	—
Butter.............	1 tbs.	15	105	—	—	11
Jam, jelly,......... sugar, honey	5 tbs.	—	275	—	70	—
Dessert............	—	—	175	3	30	5
Total............			3000	133	317	125

Figures from "Food Composition Table for Short Method of Dietary Analysis," by J. M. Leichaenring and E. D. Wilson: J. Am. Dietetic A. *27*: 386, 1951.

planning and that considerable ingenuity may become necessary to stimulate appetite.

Table IV.4 outlines an adult diet which is rich in protein and carbohydrate and moderately plentiful in fat. A representative menu is found in Table IV.5. This diet supplies 3000 calories daily, of which approximately a third is derived from fat. Higher levels of fat are undesirable because they delay absorption, depress appetite, and sometimes cause gastrointestinal disturbances, particularly in patients with liver disease. In liver disease, therefore, dietary fat should be restricted when practical to about 80 gm. without reducing the level of protein. To keep down the fat content, skim milk can be substituted for some or all of the whole milk. Gravies and salad dressings are usually eliminated in these high-caloric diets; vinegar or lemon juice and sugar may be used on salads. The amount and proportion of carbohydrate can be raised easily by the addition of more jelly, sugar, or hard candy. In liver disease carbohydrate levels between 350 and 500 gm. daily are sought. It can be seen in Table IV.5 that a protein intake over 130 gm. daily is difficult to achieve. If the patient fails to eat the prescribed amount of meat or other bulky protein foods, or if a still higher protein intake is desired, the incorporation of dry skim milk is an acceptable and comparatively inexpensive way of fortifying liquid milk, fruit drinks, cereal, and desserts. Despite the enthusiasm of some physicians for oral mixtures of amino acids, they are generally unpalatable and expensive, and offer no nutritional advantages over food protein except in patients who lack proteolytic enzymes. Even in these patients amino acids are properly considered short-range therapy and are best presented as medicine, not as food.

A high caloric intake requires correspondingly large amounts of dietary supplements, notably the water-soluble vitamins. In severe injury the same catabolic reaction which raises the caloric and protein requirements, also depletes tissue vitamin stores. Table IV.6 lists the recommended vitamin allowances in health (usually contained in a general hospital diet) and in conditions of stress. Clearly the allowances for a severely ill patient are about 5 times the recommendations for normal maintenance. In any abnormal state with an intense catabolic reaction, one or two *therapeutic* tablets or capsules is administered daily for the first two or three days; then one tablet a day is given until convalescence is well established, when one or two of the standard *maintenance* tablets becomes adequate and is continued until the patient is released from medical supervision. Brewers' yeast is an inexpensive source of B vitamins and is also rich in protein. It is best dispensed as a medicine; 1 or 2 ounces mixed with water can be consumed with a chaser of fruit or vegetable juice. If oral feeding is impractical in the acute phase of an illness, these vitamin allowances can usually be satisfied by parenteral preparations. Very little is known about the specific vitamin requirements of a poisoned person. In acute intoxications of short duration, supplementary vitamin A is probably unnecessary, except in hepatic disease where storage or availability may be subnormal. Even in liver disease a daily supplement of more than 5000 units of vitamin A is unnecessary, and very large doses are toxic. As

TABLE IV.5

High-protein, high-carbohydrate, moderate-fat diet for adults

Suggested Meal Pattern	Sample Menu
Breakfast	*Breakfast*
Citrus fruit	Orange juice
Cereal	Oatmeal, brown sugar
Two eggs	Soft-cooked eggs
Toast, butter, jelly	Toast, butter, jelly
Milk	Milk
Beverage, if desired	Coffee, sugar
10 A.M. Glass of milk	Milk
Lunch	*Lunch*
Meat	Pot roast
Potato	Mashed potato
Vegetable	Green beans
Bread, butter, jelly	Bread, butter, jelly
Dessert	Rice pudding
Milk	Milk
Beverage, if desired	
3 P.M. Glass of milk	Vanilla malted milk
Dinner	*Dinner*
Soup	Beef broth with rice
Meat or meat substi- tute	Baked hash
Vegetable	Carrot and celery sticks
Bread, butter, jelly	Bread, butter, jelly
Fruit	Applesauce
Milk	Milk
Beverage, if desired	Tea
Bedtime	
Milk	*Bedtime*
Sandwich	Milk
	Liverwurst sandwich

TABLE IV.6

Formula for a standard maintenance vitamin tablet or capsule

(Suggested by Committee on Therapeutic Nutrition, Food and Nutrition Board, 1952)

Thiamine hydrochloride	2	mg.
Riboflavin	2	mg.
Niacinamide	20	mg.
Calcium pantothenate	5	mg.
Pyridoxine hydrochloride	0.5	mg.
Folic acid	0.25	mg.
Ascorbic acid	50	mg.
Vitamin B_{12}	2	µg.
Vitamin A	5000	units
Vitamin D	400	units
Vitamin K*	2	mg.

* Separate tablet or capsule.

Formula for a standard therapeutic vitamin tablet or capsule

(Suggested by Committee on Therapeutic Nutrition, Food and Nutrition Board, 1952)

Thiamine hydrochloride	10	mg.
Riboflavin	10	mg.
Niacinamide	100	mg.
Calcium pantothenate	20	mg.
Pyridoxine hydrochloride	2	mg.
Folic acid	1.5	mg.
Ascorbic acid	300	mg.
Vitamin B_{12}	4	µg.
Vitamin K*	—	

* Separate tablet or capsule.

described on p. 181, vitamin K is essential in correcting hypoprothrombinemia induced by certain therapeutic and toxic substances (*e.g.*, dicumarol, warfarin). Ascorbic acid (cevitamic acid), however, is the vitamin which has attracted the most attention in clinical toxicology. Subclinical deficiency states of vitamin C have been blamed for poor resistance to infection, refective immunological responses, and impaired detoxification reactions. Although these claims are not well substantiated, a chemically demonstrable depletion of plasma and tissue vitamin C is adequate justification for daily supplementation. Single doses as high as 1 gm. have been recommended. In general, however, massive doses of vitamins are unnecessary, and this practice diverts attention from the importance of an adequate diet and the need of educating the patient in good eating habits.

In prescribing a high caloric diet the chief problem is usually the difficulty which the patient has in consuming it. Occasionally an insulin-induced hypoglycemia can be used to produce sensations of hunger in a patient whose appetite flags; when successful, 10 units of regular insulin, given subcutaneously 15 to 30 minutes before meals, is sufficient. Although high caloric supplementary feedings are generally recommended (and necessary) in a high-protein, high-carbohydrate diet, they are clearly undesirable if they depress the appetite severely. Whenever appetite becomes a serious limitation, concentrated sugar and fruits should not be served between meals. A small meal at bedtime is probably best; milk with a sandwich or cereal adds appreciably to the daily intake, especially if the milk is fortified by the addition of dried skim milk or an emulsified fat preparation. Sometimes a patient with anorexia responds to a regimen of two meals a day. If practical, these meals should be served at

8:00 A.M. and 4:30 P.M. to coincide with possible periods of maximal hunger contractions. No between-meal feedings are then served. At meal time the patient is told to eat all the food offered. When he does so, the quantity served is gradually increased. When the patient shows that he is willing and able to eat another meal, it can then be introduced at noon. Later, as a normal appetite is regained, meal times can be altered to fit the hospital or family routine.

Tube Feeding

Tube feeding (gavage) is the only satisfactory way of providing adequate nourishment for some patients, notably those with obstacles to eating, such as severe anorexia, corrosive lesions of the mouth and perhaps of the esophagus, paralysis of the swallowing muscles, and varying grades of stupor or coma. For the clinical toxicologist the most frequent indication for tube feeding is probably intractable anorexia, such as that sometimes encountered during the prolonged convalescence from various debilitating poisons like arsenic. To counteract severe anorexia, conservative methods, which include specially prepared appetizing dishes, good nursing care, persuasion, and fortified liquid drinks, are often inadequate. Under these circumstances, tube feeding is a practical and effective way of insuring an appropriate diet whenever the alimentary tract is able to digest and assimilate food.

The usual technique involves intubation of the stomach with a nasogastric tube. Gavage is generally impractical, however, in the presence of severe gastric lesions, and as a substitute in some clinics duodenal feeding has been accomplished by the use of an Einhorn tube threaded into the duodenum. Nutrient enemas are rarely worthwhile and never satisfy metabolic needs. Water and salt are undoubtedly absorbed from the large intestine, and probably also alcohol and glucose in very small amounts, but no other nutritional factors are believed to pass through the colonic mucosa.

The success of tube feedings depends greatly on the attitude and cooperation of the patient. If possible the procedure is explained carefully to the patient, and his consent is obtained. Several sources of difficulty may be encountered. A major danger is the regurgitation and aspiration of a feeding into the trachea; with proper technique this should never occur, except rarely in patients with no swallowing reflex (when tube feeding is inevitably hazardous). During continuous tube feeding, care is taken to prevent the accumulation of food in the stomach, with consequent gastric dilatation and upper abdominal fullness. When the liquid formula is administered intermittently, any gastric residue can be aspirated before a fresh feeding is added. The diarrhea frequently induced by high caloric formulas can usually be controlled by reducing the quantity fed, by adding applesauce or commercial pectin. Liquid diets grossly contaminated with putrefactive bacteria sometimes cause violent untoward gastrointestinal reactions. Although formerly a source of difficulty, gastric tubes seldom become

TABLE IV.7

Tube feeding—high-protein, moderate-carbohydrate, low-fat formula*—daily allowance for adults

	Quantity		Calories	Approximate Composition		
				Protein	Carbohydrate	Fat
				gm.	*gm.*	*gm.*
Skim milk.............	2 qt.	2000 gm.	720	70	102	2
Skim milk powder (dried).............	6 oz.	180 gm.	652	64	94	2
Brewers' yeast powder..	1 oz.	30 gm.	82	11	11	1
Whites of 2 eggs........	—	—	30	7	—	—
Corn syrup (*e.g.*, Karo)..	4 oz.	120 gm.	343	—	89	—
Ascorbic acid (ground tablet).............	—	100 mg.				
Fish liver oil concentrate Vitamin A.............		5000 I.U.				
Vitamin D...........		1000 I.U.				
Total...............			1827	152	296	5

Directions: Beat up whites of eggs and add corn syrup. Make a paste by adding a small amount of skim milk to dried skim milk powder and brewers' yeast powder. The beaten egg whites and paste can then be stirred into the remaining amount of skim milk.

* F. J. Ingelfinger and C. L. Holt: M. Clin. North America, *30*, 1024, 1946. Reproduced (with modifications) by permission of the publishers, W. B. Saunders Co., Philadelphia.

clogged with modern liquid formulas. In spite of the best professional care, some patients cannot or will not tolerate continual intubation. In these exceptional patients the anxiety, hostility, or restlessness induced by a gastric tube probably does not warrant its use.

A small (2 to 3 mm. external diameter) nasogastric tube is preferred. Plastic tubes cause less irritation than soft rubber tubes. A polyvinyl catheter which is softer and more flexible than one of polyethylene is said to be preferable; to insert this tube its rigidity must be increased temporarily by chilling it. In most patients the tube can be left in place almost indefinitely, or it may be passed for each feeding and then withdrawn. Continuous or intermittent feeding is permissible. For example, liquid formulas may be administered at a rate of 100 ml. per hour, for a total of 2400 ml. in 24 hours, providing that the epigastrium is observed frequently for signs of gastric distension. For interval feeding the total daily quantity is divided into 4 to 8 equal aliquots, each of which is injected into the tube by use of a 50 ml. syringe through a no. 15 gauge needle which is fitted tightly into the lumen of the tube. If limited to 300 ml., an individual feeding need take only a few minutes in an adult. All formulas should be warmed to body temperature before administration. Concentrated mixtures should not be fed abruptly or in great quantity to patients who have been fasting. For the first few days of feeding, a diluted formula is used, and only one-third to one-half of the total daily allowance is administered. Tube feeding is discontinued as soon as a patient recovers an adequate appetite.

Many satisfactory liquid formulas have been described for administration by gastric tube. One representative example is outlined in Table IV.7. Although more costly, a powdered concentrate which can be suspended in water is more convenient, and mixtures of this type are available on the commercial market. One product (Sustagen, by Mead, Johnson and Co.) contains in a recommended daily ration (900 gm. suspended in 1.5 to 2.5 liters of water) 210 gm. of protein, 600 gm. of carbohydrate, and 30 gm. of fat, along with adequate minerals and vitamins. With such high protein intakes, it is essential to give the patient ample opportunity to satisfy his thirst by supplementary drinking. Unless the water intake is adequate, a high protein intake leads occasionally to severe azotemia and hypernatremia. These complications are not uncommon in comatose patients who fail to receive extra fluids.

MISCELLANEOUS

Nursing Care

In a severely poisoned patient, no adequate program of supportive treatment can be managed without the active cooperation of a well-trained nurse. In current practice, the busy physician makes many crucial decisions but often leaves their implementation to others. This is proper and appropriate whenever trained nurses are available. On the other hand, every medical practitioner should be reasonably familiar with nursing procedures, if only because he is often required to instruct members of the patient's family in the techniques of patient care in the home. It is not possible or appropriate to describe here the art and science of nursing, but it is proper to outline some of the nursing services that have proved to be so beneficial both to severely ill and convalescing patients. The most effective way for the physician to review this topic is to spend a few days as a patient in a hospital bed.

A capable and diligent nurse exerts many beneficial influences on her patient and on the course of his illness. First she (or he) performs all services specified by the physician with respect to medications, activity, diet, fluids, etc. She observes and records periodically the patient's vital signs and any other relevant clinical data. These general and specific observations supplement and often complement the physician's own examinations. In such areas as the patient's response to food, consumption of fluids, urine output, number of bowel movements, duration of sleep, vital signs during sleep, etc., the nurses' report is often the only source of reliable information. Particularly for the seriously ill person, a nurse performs many services. She protects his skin by keeping him clean and dry. She makes him comfortable and relaxed by massaging his back and limbs, by repositioning him frequently in bed, by rearranging his pillow, and by passive exercises when appropriate. She furnishes blankets and hot packs when he is chilled, and alcohol sponging, ice packs and fanning when he is hot. She spares his strength by giving physical support whenever he must be moved, and she furnishes encouragement and if necessary assistance when he eats, drinks, voids, etc. She keeps indwelling catheters clean and patent, and insures the proper functioning of venoclysis sets and other equipment. She is not only the ally of the physician but often the chief confidante of the patient. In her role as a sympathetic helper, she often becomes one of the principal supports of the patient's morale. A good nurse almost invariably acts as an intermediary between patient, family, physician, and hospital. Finally, the trained nurse is qualified to perform in an emergency most of the life-saving procedures of resuscitation available to physicians.

Problems of Stasis

The word "stasis" is used here to include all physiological disturbances arising from immobilization in bed. Among the more common problems of prolonged and complete bed rest are hypostatic pneumonia, venous thrombosis, decubitus ulcers, constipation, cystitis, muscle atrophy and contractures, and demineralization of bone with associated nephrolithiasis. Directly or indirectly, most of these complications are due to the stagnation of blood.

The major emphasis is prevention. Bed rest should not be enforced when unnecessary or any longer than essential—particularly in elderly patients, since they are more susceptible to disorders of stasis than are the young. Even in the acute phase of an intoxication or illness, most patients can be properly allowed to sit upright for bowel movements and perhaps to get out of bed briefly. In most cases a patient with adequate strength can and should be encouraged to spend several hours each day sitting in a chair and to take mild and graded exercise. In cases of paralysis and of coma, the hazards of stasis can be minimized by repositioning the victim in bed at frequent intervals (perhaps every hour) and by passive exercise of the limbs, together with vigorous massage.

In some situations specific prophylactic measures are available. The systemic administration of antibiotics is useful in preventing hypostatic pneumonia in those who are comatose, whose cough reflex is depressed, or who have been exposed to an irritant vapor. Brief periods of hyperventilation, artificially induced by rebreathing into a paper bag, are useful in promoting the circulation and lymphatic drainage of the lungs and in expelling mucous plugs which create regions of atelectasis. Both rebreathing and the administration of 5 per cent carbon dioxide in oxygen, however, are hazardous in acidotic patients. To forestall venous thrombosis, which occurs most often in the vessels of the limbs and pelvis, one avoids tight dressings and constrictive clothing (e.g., garters), and prevents gaseous distension of the bowel, fecal impaction, urinary retention, dehydration, shock, bruising and other forms of blunt trauma, and septicemia. Any person on prolonged bed rest should move his legs often; if this is impossible, passive exercise and massage become essential. To prevent rashes and bed sores, cleanliness is insured by washing frequently with a hard soap of good quality. To avoid maceration, the skin is kept dry, if necessary by applying rubbing alcohol and then talcum powder or a bland ointment, especially in intertriginous areas and regions subject to pressure. Bed sheets are kept clean, dry, and free of wrinkles and crumbs. By changing the patient's position repeatedly and by

giving him support on inflated rings, one protects areas over bony prominences which are particularly vulnerable to pressure necrosis, such as the buttocks, back, elbows, and knees.

In spite of customary care, disorders of stasis cannot always be prevented. The appropriate treatment varies with the specific complication, but all relevant curative measures should be pursued vigorously. Bronchopneumonia arising in an area of hypostatic congestion requires intensive antibiotic therapy (p. 231). With any evidence of phlebothrombosis (e.g., pain or tenderness in an extremity, unexplained fever, tachycardia), an immediate surgical consultation is desirable. To be effective, high ligation of the superficial femoral veins must be accomplished promptly. Even with no signs of infection, a trial with one of the broad-spectrum antibiotics or sulfonamides is advisable. Anticoagulant therapy is usually instituted with heparin, which acts immediately, and dicumarol or a related drug, which becomes effective 24 to 48 hours after administration. Neither anticoagulant therapy nor ligation is usually necessary in thrombophlebitis, and neither is done except in the rare event of a pulmonary embolus. With bland thrombosis (phlebothrombosis), however, the risk is so great that one cannot afford to wait for embolic complications. In phlebitis the affected limb is usually kept slightly elevated, and even passive motion is minimized until all signs of inflammation have subsided. For uninfected bed sores, a bland ointment (e.g., equal parts of olive oil and balsam of Peru) will often stimulate healing if the area is kept free of pressure. In the event of infection, systemic and perhaps local antibiotic therapy is indicated. All necrotic tissue is carefully removed. If regeneration continues to be abnormally slow, the diet should be investigated and if necessary nutritional supplements prescribed. In a few cases where the ulcer is clean, skin grafts are used to accelerate epithelialization and healing.

Disturbances of Body Temperature

The control of hyperpyrexia and of hypothermia has occasionally been life-saving. In each case, proper therapy depends upon the mechanism of the derangement in body temperature. Fevers may arise from many causes, including infections, parenterally introduced foreign proteins (e.g., milk, peptone), bacterial pyrogens, intravascular hemolysis and other types of rapid tissue breakdown, some central nervous lesions (e.g., basilar hemorrhages), severe dehydration, and the application of intense heat (e.g., sun, hot air, diathermy). Febrile states are also induced by toxic doses of many drugs, including the convulsants, cocaine, atropine, dinitrophenol and derivatives, thyroid hormone, epinephrine and ephedrine, and some samples of methylene blue. Whenever the air is cooler than the body, a fall in deep body temperature to hypothermic levels may result from severe chilling (e.g., cold air, ice water), destruction of vasoconstrictor tone (e.g., spinal cord section), drugs which depress heat production (e.g., anesthetics and central depressants), and peripherally acting vasodilator drugs (e.g., nitrites, magnesium salts, anesthetic agents). In contrast, specific antipyretic drugs such as salicylates, quinine, antipyrine, etc., do not produce hypothermia because they lower an elevated body temperature only to normothermic levels.

Aside from its diagnostic and prognostic value, fever has little clinical significance. Only rarely does it threaten a patient's life or even contribute appreciably to his malaise. In general, only when a fever exceeds 105° or 106°F. are direct and energetic attempts to reduce the temperature justified. Valid exceptions to this conservative rule are recognized, notably in poisonings due to such metabolic stimulants as dinitrophenol and its many derivatives used in modern agriculture. Hot weather and a mild elevation of body temperature appear to enhance the toxicity of these agents, and vigorous efforts to hold the temperature at a normal or even subnormal level are warranted. Like the problem of fever, the hypothermic patient does not usually require treatment designed specifically to raise his body temperature. For example, the person who has spent a winter night outdoors in an alcoholic coma is often seriously ill, but in most cases reduction in body temperature is not a crucial factor in his survival. Provided that the circulation is maintained, bed rest in a conventionally warm room is sufficient to produce gradual restoration of a normal body temperature. In profound hypothermia (rectal temperature below 80°F.), however, specific attempts at artificial rewarming are probably advisable. The safest and most efficacious procedure for heating the hypothermic person has not yet been defined.

Until recent times many ritualistic forms of hydrotherapy were performed on patients with abnormally high and low body temperatures. Today the procedures are simpler, and the therapeutic claims for them are more modest. For example, in extreme fever (hyperpyrexia), various cooling applications are used; these include sponging the skin with tepid water or with alcohol, the application of cold compresses on the forehead and neck, sprinkling water on the skin while it is being fanned, and immersion in baths of cool water. Water temperatures below 78°F. are rarely used, not only because they are sometimes painful but also because they generate reflex vasoconstriction which impairs their effectiveness. To reduce the deep body temperature, a brisk cutaneous circulation must be promoted and maintained, usually by vigorous massage. Ice packs, ice water baths, and ice water enemas are unnecessarily violent and dangerous. In many cases of ex-

treme hyperpyrexia (*e.g.*, cerebral hemorrhage), antipyretic drugs are ineffective and in some cases are potentially dangerous (*e.g.*, atropine poisoning), but if other measures fail, they should be tried. When oral medication is not retained or cannot be tolerated, sodium salicylate can be administered rectally as a 2 per cent solution (usually containing a little starch or acacia as an emollient), but absorption is not dependable by this route.

Infections

In probably no area of supportive treatment does the physician have at his disposal so many effective and safe drugs as in the control of bacterial infections. The modern revolution in the chemotherapy of infectious disease has brought spectacular opportunities and responsibilities. As evidenced by the continuing high consumption of antibiotics and other antibacterial agents, there is no lack of awareness of these drugs or of their therapeutic potential. It is appropriate here only to emphasize that the control of infection is an important aspect of clinical toxicology and to mention some of the problems that arise in the therapeutic use of current antibacterial drugs. Victims of poison are abnormally susceptible to intercurrent infections for many reasons; *e.g.*, damage to mucous membranes and other physical barriers to infection, inadequate drainage of the tracheobronchial tree and other duct systems (*e.g.*, urinary bladder), impaired circulation to critical tissues, defective nutrition, leukopenia or agranulocytosis, *etc.* Infection enhances appreciably the morbidity and even the mortality rate in chemical intoxications.

An unnecessarily large number of sulfonamide drugs is currently marketed. For most systemic infections due to susceptible bacteria, oral doses of sulfadiazine, sulfamerazine, or sulfisoxazole (Gantrisin) are used. Sulfacetamide and sulfadimetine (Elkosin) are also effective, but are commonly reserved for urinary tract infections. For enteric infections poorly absorbed drugs are sometimes preferred to insure high local concentrations within the intestinal tract; the common enteric "sulfas" today are succinylsulfathiazole (Sulfasuxidine), phthalylsulfathiazole, and phthalylsulfacetimide (Thalamyd). The dose varies with the preparation and with the nature and location of the infectious process, but a typical adult dose of a systemically active sulfonamide drug is 3 to 6 gm. initially, followed by 1 gm. every 4 to 6 hours. Children are sometimes given relatively larger doses, namely 0.06 to 0.12 gm. per pound of body weight for the first 24 hours, half as an initial dose and half as six equal maintenance doses. If oral medication cannot be tolerated, sodium salts of most systemically effective sulfonamides (the diethanolamine salt in the case of sulfisoxazole) are available as sterile solutions for intravenous administration. All clinically useful sulfonamides are remarkably innocuous to common laboratory animals, but untoward reactions of the hypersensitivity type are not uncommon in clinical patients. Such reactions as headache, dizziness, mild confusion, and nausea do not necessarily warrant withdrawal of the drug. On the other hand the offending compound should be discontinued and perhaps another sulfonamide derivative substituted cautiously if any of the following disturbances appear: vomiting, diarrhea, fever, dermatitis, leukopenia, and microscopic hematuria. Immediate, complete, and unqualified cessation of all sulfonamide therapy is imperative if any of the following severe reactions are encountered: gross hematuria, renal colic, anuria, hepatitis, peripheral neuritis, agranulocytosis, hemolytic anemia, and aplastic anemia.

Bacterial species and even strains vary widely in sensitivity to various antibiotics. One compound is not clearly superior to another in the treatment of many common infections. Penicillin is still the most extensively used antibiotic. Although its comparatively narrow antibacterial spectrum is a defect, the combination of high effectiveness and low toxicity explains its popularity. Preparations of penicillin are available for essentially every route of administration. In common current practice, repository forms are often used, such as 300,000 to 600,000 units of procaine penicillin G intramuscularly each day. Pain at the site of intramuscular injection is rarely encountered with procaine penicillin. Phlebitis at the site of infusions can be avoided by using highly diluted solutions of crystalline penicillin. All other reactions are rare and belong in the category of idiosyncrasy or hypersensitivity (p. 232); they include pruritus, urticaria (sometimes associated with mild exfoliative dermatitis), other dermal and mucosal lesions, serum sickness pattern, and very rarely anaphylactoid shock and other miscellaneous disorders. Streptomycin is another widely used "narrow spectrum" antibiotic. In short-term therapy (*e.g.*, up to 2 months), dihydrostreptomycin is preferred to streptomycin because it is less intensely neurotoxic to the vestibular apparatus. The dihydro derivative, however, may be more toxic to the auditory portion of the eighth cranial nerve, but this injury becomes significant only after long-continued therapy with high doses. Damage to both portions of the eighth nerve is the only truly toxic effect definitely ascribed to streptomycin and its dihydro derivative. Other untoward reactions resemble the allergic manifestations induced by penicillin. If renal function is adequate, most adults can tolerate 1 gm. of dihydrostreptomycin sulfate injected intramuscularly twice daily for 10 to 14 days without appreciable hazard.

Penicillin and streptomycin are sometimes given in conjunction with one of several broad-spectrum

antibiotics, notably chlorotetracycline (Aureomycin), oxytetracycline (Terramycin), and tetracycline (Achromycin). Because of rare but severe blood dyscrasias, chloramphenicol (Chloromycetin) is usually reserved in current practice for cases of typhoid fever, where it is probably the drug of choice. Erythromycin, a relatively new antibiotic which is stable and effective by mouth, is most useful in treating infections due to Gram-positive organisms that are resistant to penicillin; the average adult dose is 0.3 gm. (3 tablets) every six hours, and as much as 0.5 gm. can usually be tolerated without gastrointestinal distress. The tetracyclines are usually given by mouth as capsules containing 0.25 gm.; a typical adult dose is 1.5 to 3.0 gm. administered over a period of 24 hours as six aliquots. These drugs are too irritating for intramuscular injection, but at least Aureomycin has been successfully infused intravenously in a very dilute solution (0.5 gm. twice daily). All three tetracycline antibiotics display essentially the same toxicity. Especially after Aureomycin, gastrointestinal irritation (leading to nausea and vomiting) can generally be suppressed by drinking promptly (or, better, simultaneously) a glass of cold milk or some other antacid, but aluminum hydroxide gels are contraindicated because they impair absorption of the drug. Diarrhea is not uncommon, particularly after continued medication with any tetracycline, and is sometimes prostrating. This diarrhea, like the occasional proctitis, pruritus ani, and vulval irritation, is thought to be due to an unphysiological change in the intestinal flora. Dermal and other hypersensitivity reactions are comparatively rare.

Idiosyncrasies

The terms drug or chemical allergy, hypersensitivity, and idiosyncrasy are often used interchangeably. In general all of these names refer to untoward reactions which are *not* exclusively dose-dependent, i.e., which cannot be produced regularly in anyone who is given an adequate amount. Only rarely is the term drug hypersensitivity used in reference to an abnormally low threshold for an otherwise predictable response (e.g., tinnitus from quinine). Whenever subtle distinctions are made, the term drug idiosyncrasy is reserved for qualitatively abnormal reactions. For reasons noted below, the overwhelming majority of lesions of hypersensitivity and idiosyncrasy are probably mediated by allergic mechanisms. Although the phrase "drug reaction" is often used in the following discussion, all generalizations are equally applicable to nonmedicinal compounds.

Nature and scope. The emphasis in Sections II and III of this manual rests on syndromes of frank overdosage, consisting of those psychic and somatic reactions which are strictly dose-dependent and so

are largely predictable. In the case of drugs, many of these toxic syndromes reflect undesirable extensions or exaggerations of effects which in proper intensity are therapeutically useful. Omitted from the summaries in Sections II and III are most untoward reactions after customary doses; these infrequent and erratic effects generally belong in the category of idiosyncrasy or hypersensitivity. With many substances, and particularly nonmedicinal chemicals, the distinction between idiosyncratic and toxic responses is obscure. Because the techniques of clinical and laboratory diagnosis furnish no *certain* clues, differentiation is ultimately dependent upon statistical analyses of actual poisonings both in laboratory animals and clinical patients.

If only to determine the appropriate supportive treatment, it is important to try to distinguish between those reactions which are inherent in the toxicity of the offending chemical and those responses which are equally inherent in and peculiar to the poisoned individual. With only an isolated case of poisoning, a proper evaluation is often impossible. Many kinds of obstacles block an unequivocal conclusion. First, both types of reactions may coexist after a massive exposure. The intensity of the clinical response is not a relevant criterion since many of the most dangerous reactions described in the clinical literature bear the stigma of allergy (e.g., the hemolytic crisis of naphthalene poisoning). On the other hand, a negative skin test has no diagnostic significance, since most idiosyncratic reactions to drugs occur in patients whose skin exhibits no prompt response to an intradermal injection of the offending chemical. Passive transfer tests are also diagnostically undependable. Eosinophilia is rarely encountered.

At the statistical level the most useful data to the clinical toxicologist are the true incidence and nature of the untoward reactions to each dosage level of each drug or chemical. Although the available informaion about any single compound is inadequate, the following general impressions are commonly accepted. High doses of any substance regularly produce a toxic syndrome which is similar, at least in a qualitative sense, from one person to the next. Lower doses, in the so-called pharmacological range, also produce a group of effects that develop uniformly in almost everyone. In addition, these and even smaller doses of each substance are associated with a *low* incidence of reactions that often bear the imprint of allergy. This group of phenomena are more stereotyped in their clinical manifestations than are the pharmacological and toxicological responses. The character of the lesion is usually a more distinctive property of the patient than a specific attribute of the agent, in the sense that one patient often reacts in the same way to

various unrelated chemicals while a single agent may induce radically different syndromes in different individuals. At least for some compounds, however, both the frequency of these hypersensitivity reactions and to a lesser degree the patterns of response are predictable in a statistical sense.

An opinion is commonly held that any type of lesion in any target organ of any person may have an allergic origin. Although such an all-encompassing assertion may never be disproved, it is a misleadingly pessimistic evaluation of the difficulties of diagnosis in current clinical practice. At the other end of a spectrum of opinions, H. L. Alexander (Reactions with Drug Therapy, W. B. Saunders Co., Philadelphia, 1955) insists, for example, that only a few hundred drugs are recorded in the medical literature as causes of hypersensitivity and that most of these have been imputed only infrequently or are now obsolete. As noted below, the implication that the true or even the relative incidence of drug hypersensitivity can be gauged from the clinical literature may be naive. In spite of other areas of disagreement, most authorities apparently agree that chemicals differ significantly in their capacities to induce sensitization and that these differences are revealed by the frequency of untoward reactions and to a limited extent also by the nature of the lesions and the target organs of damage. While genuine differences surely exist, it is not definitely established that certain current drugs deserve a good reputation any more than some others warrant a bad reputation with respect to untoward reactions. E. A. Brown (Annals of Allergy 14: 206, 1956) is concerned about the erroneous impressions that arise because of current methods of reporting drug toxicity. When reported in the literature, a single case of a rare but severe illness such as aplastic anemia arising during and allegedly due to the administration of a drug has been known to prejudice many physicians against the drug, especially if it is a new one. This prejudice often stimulates publication of other isolated case reports and also promotes the indiscriminate damning of the drug for a host of poorly documented reactions. Collecting such case histories into review articles tends to compound the suspicions of the uncritical reader. Thus the original case report may act as the trigger for a chain reaction that reflects discredit on a drug and implies at the same time that alternative drugs are relatively free of risk. In most instances, however, the original case, like isolated cases generally, is almost impossible to evaluate without statistical data that are rarely available. For example, to interpret intelligently the allegedly causal role of a drug in the production of aplastic anemia, one must usually know the incidence of this dyscrasia in both the presence and absence of the drug, as encountered in the general population, in patients with diseases commonly treated by the drug, and in patients with and without histories of other allergies. Even if the drug's guilt can be established by statistically valid correlations, the magnitude of the risk must be measured against the hazard and effectiveness of alternative drugs or of no drugs at all. The complaint has been raised that therapeutic nihilists are counterattacking under the banner of drug allergy.

The following criteria are listed by H. L. Alexander (op. cit.) as useful in the diagnosis of drug hypersensitivity: (a) recognition of a reaction which conforms to the pattern of drug hypersensitivity, (b) history of exposure to a drug, particularly a drug which has been identified as a frequent offender, (c) prompt disappearance of the reaction (usually) when exposure to a drug is discontinued, and its reproduction when the drug is readministered (sometimes a dangerous diagnostic test), and (d) history of allergy or other evidence of allergic disease. The latter evidence includes the similarity between reactions to drugs and reactions to conventional allergens, the occasional demonstration of a positive skin test, the marked sensitivity and specificity of the patient's acquired capacity to react to a drug, and finally the success of anti-allergy therapy and sometimes of desensitization procedures. On the basis of these and related criteria, C. A. Dragstedt (J. A. M. A. 135: 133, 1947) concludes that drug reactions consisting of urticaria, angioneurotic edema, certain types of dermatitis, and asthma are usually allergic in origin; jaundice, acute yellow atrophy, and optic neuritis are probably non-allergic; and granulocytopenia, thrombocytopenia, anemia, and polyneuritis may belong in one or the other category. In all cases the reaction is most likely allergic when a priming or sensitizing dose has preceded the toxic episode and is more likely non-allergic when long-continued administration or the use of large doses appears to have played an essential role.

The reaction pattern is sufficiently stereotyped in most cases of drug hypersensitivity to be an aid in diagnosis. Skin eruptions are the commonest clinical manifestation, particularly contact-type dermatitis, urticaria, and various exanthemal rashes. Less frequent skin expressions of drug hypersensitivity are exfoliative dermatitis, erythema multiforme-like rashes, acneform eruptions, bullous lesions, purpura simplex, photosensitizations, simple pruritus, and fixed eruptions. Systemic syndromes are comparatively rare; they are usually represented by one or more of the following reactions: bronchial asthma, fever, serum-sickness type of illness, shock of the anaphylactic variety, hepatitis, all kinds of blood dyscrasias, polyneuritis, and periarteritis nodosum. With each of these lesions, any one of a constellation of medicinal agents is com-

monly associated. The particular drugs which are held to be frequently responsible for each type of reaction are listed by Alexander (*op. cit.*), by Brown (Progress in Allergy *3:* 500–530, 1952) and by others. Such lists are never exhaustive and, for reasons noted before, some examples probably represent erroneous associations, but these compilations are useful guides in alerting the physician to the areas of greatest risk. For example, Alexander reports that the drugs responsible for the greatest variety of hypersensitivity reactions, as judged by published reports, are sulfonamides, mercurials, penicillin, iodides, arsenicals, gold salts, streptomycin, barbiturates, and quinine.

Anti-allergic therapy. Having arrived at a presumptive diagnosis of chemical or drug hypersensitivity and having recognized that its mechanism is probably allergic, the physician is ready to institute anti-allergic supportive treatment. In all severe and most mild reactions, the first practical measure is the rigorous exclusion of the presumptive allergen or allergens. Insofar as practical, no drug with a high allergenic liability is used in treating these reactions. This precaution helps avoid the superimposition of one allergy on another, with the confusion that inevitably attends this complication. In addition, skin and mucous membranes in the process of reacting actively to one allergen appear to be more susceptible to sensitization by others, perhaps only because normal physical barriers are temporarily impaired during many allergic crises.

In most cases discomfort subsides and repair begins soon after the exclusion of the offending drug or chemical. In these cases no other treatment is warranted. The universal temptation to treat skin lesions with topical applications of various medicaments should particularly be suppressed. Only if considerable distress persists after removal of the allergen does the potential benefit from local treatment justify the risk. Only drugs whose external allergenicities are known to be low should be considered—such as glycerin, mineral oil, lanolin, zinc oxide, some cold creams, ichthyol, talc, and perhaps boric acid, potassium permanganate, and phenol.

Some hypersensitivity crises warrant systemic drug therapy. Allergic bronchial asthma, urticaria, giant hives, and anaphylactoid shock often respond most quickly to an intramuscular injection of epinephrine. Unnecessarily large doses of this drug are frequently used. Except for the occasional person who is slightly refractory because of repeated use, any amount in excess of 0.5 ml. of 1:1000 aqueous epinephrine contributes little or nothing except unpleasant side-effects; often 0.2 ml. is a therapeutically effective single dose in the adult. Sometimes a slow intravenous injection of aminophyllin is beneficial, particularly in the severely distressed or epinephrine-resistant asthmatic. For longer durations of action, intramuscular injections of epinephrine in oil (usual adult dose 1 ml. of 1:1000 solution) are occasionally useful. Antihistaminic drugs also have relatively persistent effects. Except for bronchial asthma, the same types of allergic reactions responsive to epinephrine can be controlled occasionally by antihistaminic drugs; the latter are also useful in the serum-sickness syndrome and particularly in allergic rhinitis and conjunctivitis. Many hypersensitivity disorders that do not respond appreciably to antihistamine therapy can be successfully prevented by administering the drug before exposure to the allergen. Antihistaminics, however, are not innocuous, and many cases of skin sensitization have been ascribed to both their local and systemic administration. Probably because it is more extensively used, Pyribenzamine has been blamed for more untoward reactions than have its competitors, but none is free of risk. Many clinicians and particularly dermatologists believe that the adverse effects of antihistaminic drugs outweigh the beneficial results.

Among anti-allergic drugs the greatest popularity currently rests on ACTH and the various adrenal corticoids. Essentially every type of allergic lesion has been reported to respond to these agents with dramatic improvement. Not every case benefits, however, and both ACTH which is a protein and corticoids which are steroids have produced in some patients sensitization phenomena, notably urticaria and even severe systemic reactions on rare occasions. The mechanisms by which these hormones accomplish their beneficial actions are not understood, but presumably they suppress tissue reactivity only, without disturbing the underlying allergic state. This suppression persists only as long as hormone treatment is continued, unless the allergic mechanism subsides spontaneously in the interim. The need of some patients for prolonged and intensive therapy enhances the risk of metabolic side-effects. While receiving large doses of corticotropin (ACTH) and cortisone, most patients are best maintained on a low-sodium diet with daily supplements of potassium chloride (*e.g.*, about 4 gm. in divided doses). Special corticoids under current investigation may possess anti-allergic potency without unwanted actions on electrolyte metabolism. ACTH and cortisone are often used interchangeably. Cortisone has the longer duration of action and is more convenient because it is effective when taken orally. On the other hand ACTH (given intravenously in an aqueous solution or intramuscularly in a gel) is sometimes effective when cortisone fails; the converse is seldom true. For the first day or two, either of these drugs is usually prescribed in relatively large doses. The proper maintenance dose is then established by

trial; it is usually the lowest level adequate to control manifestations of the allergic state. In most adult patients, 50 to 100 mg. of cortisone, given in divided doses each day, is sufficient, but some individuals require 400 mg. and more for effective relief. In some types of cutaneous, conjunctival, and mucosal sensitization, the topical application of adrenocorticoids in the form of ointments and solutions is sufficient. For example, hydrocortisone is marketed in concentrations of 1 and 2.5 per cent in a bland ointment. Because of high effectiveness, broad spectrum of action, and relative freedom from severe toxicity, this group of drugs represents a major advance in the pharmacological control of allergic disease.

Blood dyscrasias. Essentially every known variety of blood dyscrasia has been reported as an expression of drug idiosyncrasy. Unlike most lesions due to hypersensitivity, presumptive evidence of an allergic origin is lacking in most of these cases, and anti-allergic therapy is usually completely ineffective. Although the incidence is low, many of these hematological disturbances are a severe threat to life. Several unique problems of supportive treatment arise in the clinical management of these patients.

Recognized idiosyncratic responses to drugs and chemicals include the following blood dyscrasias: granulocytopenia, agranulocytosis, thrombocytopenic purpura, hemolytic anemia, and aplastic anemia. Various mechanisms operating singly or jointly appear to be responsible for these disturbances in the cellular composition of blood. The pathological events include maturation arrest, peripheral mechanisms of autoagglutination, sequestration, hemolysis, hemophagocytosis, and secondary hypersplenism. It is difficult if not impossible to evaluate each of these mechanisms in an isolated case; in current practice the attempt is impractical and unnecessary. To identify and then remove the chemical substance which triggered these events, however, is always a worthwhile and even essential procedure, although even with this precaution spontaneous recovery may be delayed for a discouragingly long period. When a case of hemocytopenia is suspected to be induced by a drug, the only conclusive proof is the administration of a small test dose after the patient has fully recovered. The procedure is distinctly risky and is obviously unavailable when information is most needed. Ordinary skin tests are essentially worthless.

The principles of supportive treatment in cases of blood dyscrasia are the exclusion of the causative agent, replacement therapy, protection against infection, stimulation of hematopoiesis, and suppression of the metabolic processes responsible for the abnormality. Replacement therapy usually entails transfusions with whole blood. In thrombocytopenic purpura and perhaps some other hemorrhagic diatheses, bank blood should be rejected in favor of blood freshly obtained from a donor. With special equipment and notably special containers, platelets from fresh donor blood can be concentrated and transfused as platelet-rich plasma. Although the beneficial effects are of short duration, repeated platelet transfusions have controlled severe hemorrhagic crises in thrombocytopenic patients. To protect the leukopenic person against infection is always a major concern because even simple infections tend to explode into alarming septicemias when the blood possesses few or no granulocytes. The practice of keeping these patients under a heavy blanket of antibiotics, however, is no longer universally accepted. The long continued administration of broad-spectrum antibacterial drugs or mixtures of various narrow-spectrum agents leads inevitably to profound changes in the microbial flora of the skin and mucous membranes. Drug-resistant organisms and particularly fungi emerge as the dominant forms. An uncontrollable systemic infection from the invasion of these pathogens then becomes probable. The alternative procedure is to withhold prophylactic chemotherapy. Even the agranulocytic patient often keeps free of clinically significant infection for long periods if he practices simple measures of personal hygiene and if he is kept in a protective environment. Of course intensive antibiotic therapy is prescribed at the earliest sign of infection, preferably with massive doses of several drugs at the same time. All attempts to stimulate activity in a depressed bone marrow or to accelerate directly the output of an active marrow have probably failed. At least no convincing demonstrations are available.

Attempts to combat or suppress the morbid physiology which presumably underlies every blood disorder have revealed two measures which are occasionally effective singly or together, namely corticoid therapy and splenectomy. The former has proved beneficial only infrequently in thrombocytopenic purpura and acquired hemolytic anemia and almost never in the other disorders. Presumably processes of allergy are operating in the cases responsive to corticoids and corticotropin. Since there is no other way to differentiate these cases, a therapeutic trial with cortisone or a related hormone is advisable whenever a severe hemolytic or thrombocytopenic reaction is precipitated by a drug or chemical. Even in susceptible cases, large doses of cortisone are usually necessary (e.g., 400 mg. daily in divided doses), and the beneficial effects do not outlast treatment unless a spontaneous remission intervenes. Although sometimes sufficient to carry a patient through a hemolytic or hemorrhagic

crisis, cortisone is perhaps most useful in preparing the subject for splenectomy. On the other hand, this operation has a limited scope. For example, acquired hemolytic anemia is less responsive than is the congenital type. In acute thrombocytopenic purpura, splenectomy is often effective but as often unnecessary, since the process is usually self-limiting within a short time. In any case surgical re-moval of the spleen is hazardous unless hemolytic and hemorrhagic processes are first controlled with cortisone. Rarely, under poorly defined circumstances, neutropenia and pancytopenia are benefited by splenectomy, but most cases of aplastic anemia are refractory to all current efforts to reverse the process.

SECTION V

Trade Name Index

Here can be found over 15,000 trade names of products which might be ingested accidentally or suicidally. For each product the category of use, *e.g.*, rodenticide, silver polish, hair dye, is indicated, and the manufacturer's name is given. The ingredients of a large number of the products are supplied, with asterisks placed after those components which are expected to be responsible for toxic effects. Many proprietary medications are listed, but only a few drugs that require prescriptions are included. As a rule veterinary items can be purchased without a prescription.

The description of the products given here were, for the most part, contributed by the manufacturers. Every effort has been made to record all information that could be useful in treating acute chemical poisonings essentially as it was presented on labels or described in personal communications from manufacturers.

Many items appear without a description of ingredients. An alphabetical search in Section VI, *General Formulation*, for the type of commodity ingested will, in most cases, provide the physician with information as to what ingredients are most commonly used in commercial formulations of the category under consideration, with the exception of pharmaceutical preparations. When trade names of drugs appear here without their constituents the physician is directed to Section VII where the names and addresses of the manufacturers can be found, when a wire or phone call for information is necessary.

In this section the names of products are arranged in alphabetical order. Spacings, periods, hyphens, parentheses, symbols, percentages, etc. have been disregarded. Names which are numerals are listed as though spelled out, e.g., "6-12" under "S." All other numerals are placed at the end of a name, *e.g.*, "Farm Bureau General Dust No. 12." The abbreviation of the title "Dr." is ignored, *e.g.*, "Dr. Salsbury's Louse Powder" is filed under "S." Where "Doctor" appears, it is filed under "D," *e.g.*, "Doctor Roper's Formula." When first and last names are given, the first name is used for alphabetizing in this section, *e.g.*, "Elizabeth Arden Face Powder." It should be noted that in Section VII companies are listed by their surnames, *e.g.*, "Arden, Elizabeth."

How to Use the Asterisks in this Index

For every commercial product listed, an asterisk has been assigned to that ingredient (or class of ingredients) which in our opinion might be responsible for toxic signs and symptoms if the product were ingested rapidly in harmful amounts. In all cases this situation implies unequivocal

237

misuse of the product; no attempt has been made to evaluate the toxic hazard, if any, arising from proper or recommended methods of use. However innocuous a commercial mixture, there exists almost invariably an amount sufficient to provide a toxic dose of each ingredient. The asterisk, however, marks only that single ingredient whose lethal dose is contained in the least quantity of any mixture. Obviously uncertainties arose in assigning some asterisks, and in many mixtures several constituents were starred because the concentration of each was believed to be significant relative to its intrinsic toxicity. On the other hand all components of some products were judged to be so benign that no attempt was made to assign an asterisk to any of them. Obviously no absolute toxicity is implied by any asterisk since no fixed limits were established for issuing them.

For specific toxicity information, Section II should be consulted under the name of each ingredient that possesses an asterisk in Section V. Most of them are listed in Section II (sometimes only by a class name), but for any that are missing, and this includes many medicinal compounds, other toxicity references should be consulted (*e.g.*, p. 13). For each toxic ingredient and by inference for every product in which this ingredient is starred, Section II outlines a possible and, as closely as we can predict, the probable toxic syndrome and, by suitable reference to Section III, directs attention to an appropriate program of treatment. Section II also provides a categorical estimate of the lethality of each separate ingredient in terms of a numerical "toxicity rating" (see Introduction to Section II). Given the percentage composition of a commercial formula (Section V) and the intrinsic toxicities of its starred ingredients (Section II,) the physician has adequate information to reach provisional answers to such questions as: how much of this product can be ingested without endangering life?—or, how much probably will kill? Unfortunately these questions can seldom if ever be answered with the desired degree of precision or reliability, but even approximate and tentative answers are useful in formulating a realistic prognosis whenever the physician knows how much of a potential intoxicant has been ingested.

To reach any useful estimates of the toxicity of a product (in the absence of direct clinical data), the chemical composition of any commodity (Section V) must be evaluated in terms of the known toxicities of its ingredients individually (Section II), notably those ingredients which are starred (Section V). One of the best ways to organize one's efforts is to try to assign a toxicity rating to each product (in contradistinction to the ratings of Section II, which describe only isolated ingredients). To do this, basic assumptions are required. The following subsection (How to Assign Toxicity Ratings to Products) outlines various rules and conventions that we have evolved in selecting toxicity ratings for the sample formulas of Section VI. In our contacts with medical practitioners, we have become convinced that these ratings are a practical way of answering the physicians' question: how toxic is it? That the assignment of toxicity ratings is a feasible procedure is attested by the examples in Section VI (General Formulations).

Each trade name item listed in Section V was also assigned a toxicity

rating, but all of these were deleted in proof. This late revision arose from a realization that many of our ratings could not be justified as exact because of uncertainties both in the information and in the principles upon which they were prédicated. The nature and source of these uncertainties are outlined subsequently. Several manufacturers pointed out the legal responsibility that we would assume in publishing ratings when a few of them would almost inevitably be proved inaccurate. Unfortunately no practical way has been evolved for furnishing physicans with meaningful appraisals of toxicity—without the risk of libeling an occasional product. Under current study are possible solutions to this problem of reconciling the legitimate interests of manufacturers with the demands of physicians for uncomplicated, readily available, and clinically realistic answers to the question: how toxic is it? For the degree that the omission of toxicity ratings has reduced the usefulness of this compilation, we are sincerely sorry. At least asterisks have been retained here to aid the physician who chooses to make his own ratings. We are aware from recent experience of the concern and attention which manufacturers are giving the toxicities of their products. We are encouraged by and pay tribute to the current trend to market consumer goods that are as nearly harmless as possible, even when grossly misused.

How to Assign Toxicity Ratings to Products

The following remarks are designed for the physician or toxicologist who proposes to ascertain an appropriate toxicity rating for any commercial product. As described in detail in the introduction to Section II, toxicity ratings are actually estimates of lethality and reflect the approximate amount of any "poison" that must be ingested for each kilogram of body weight to kill a typical victim. The exact but arbitrary limits that define each numerical toxicity class are specified in Table V.1. The techniques outlined below were used to select the ratings in Section VI, as well as all unpublished ratings in our file.

Two ways are available for assessing the toxicity of commercial mixtures (when the most meaningful data—the effects of known doses in the human—are unknown). First the product itself can be tested in a series of laboratory animals to obtain estimates of the mean lethal dose, the nature of the toxic syndrome, and the target organ of damage, if any. Many alert manufacturers have secured these data about their own merchandise, and

TABLE V.1

Toxicity Rating or Class	Probable Lethal Dose (human)	
	mg. per kg.	for 70-kg. man (150 lbs.)
6 "super" toxic	less than 5	a taste (less than 7 drops)
5 extremely toxic	5–50	between 7 drops and 1 teaspoonful
4 highly toxic	50–500	between 1 tsp. and 1 ounce
3 moderately toxic	500–5 gm./kg.	between 1 oz. and 1 pint (or 1 lb.)
2 slightly toxic	5–15 gm./kg.	between 1 pt. and 1 quart
1 practically non-toxic	above 15 gm./kg.	more than 1 quart

several have furnished this information to us. Most toxicity ratings in our files, however, are based on a second method of estimation, which requires a toxicological appraisal of each ingredient in the commercial mixture. Ideally the identity of every constitutent and the complete composition should be known; in practice, full information is seldom available and seldom essential. Whenever Section II contains information about the lethality of single ingredients when tested separately, the probable lethal dose of a commercial product can be inferred if one is willing to assume that all constituents act independently and have neither additive nor antagonistic effects. Except when two or more ingredients are chemically related, this simplifying assumption is believed to be permissible in most cases, because the final estimates are not intended to be precise. Another way of stating our working hypothesis is this: the presumptive lethal dose of a commercial mixture may be gauged as the smallest quantity which contains a fatal amount of any one of its constituents. By this operational definition, the toxicity of a mixture is determined solely by one of its ingredients (or one group of chemically related ingredients), all others being regarded as diluents. This critical ingredient is designated in Sections V and VI by an asterisk.

To illustrate these remarks, hypothetical examples are useful. Because of inadequate data, the acute toxicity of xylene cannot be specified precisely, but the mean lethal dose is generally believed to lie somewhere within toxicity class 4. Any product containing xylene as the only significantly toxic ingredient would be assigned a) a toxicity rating of 4 if the concentration of xylene were 20 per cent or more, b) a rating of 3 if the concentration lay between 2 and 20 per cent, or c) a rating of 2 if the concentration lay between 0.2 and 2 per cent. Obviously these limits are arbitrary, but a convention of this kind is an operational necessity in most cases. Of course these boundary values are unnecessary and so are ignored whenever the mean lethal dose of the only starred ingredient is comparatively well established (e.g., 0.3 to 0.4 gm./kg. for aspirin). As another example, a product composed half of benzene and half of carbon tetrachloride would be assigned a rating of 4, and both components would receive an asterisk. A product made of half benzene and half *kerosene* would also be rated 4, but only the *benzene* would be starred, since the rating of pure kerosene is 3, *i.e.*, it is approximately one-tenth as toxic as benzene.

For products whose percentage composition has not been revealed by the manufacturer, the assignment of a toxicity rating becomes an elaborate guess. If the most toxic ingredient is thought to be present in substantial amounts (perhaps 20 per cent or over), the product is rated as though that ingredient were present in pure form. Whenever it is obvious that the critical substance is a minor constituent, the rating is lowered as seems best to fit the circumstances. Doubt is always resolved in favor of the higher rating. Many so-called "inert ingredients" are potentially toxic and often constitute the bulk of a commercial mixture. Insecticidal sprays are a good example. In many cases the active ingredients are negligibly toxic, but whenever the "inert" vehicle is suspected to be petroleum ether or a naphtha-like solvent, a toxicity rating of 3 is assigned. When a product not listed

in Section V is encountered or a product for which the manufacturer has not revealed the ingredients, any rating is clearly a guess. We have decided to base these guesses solely upon information about other products that are presumed to be similar because they are marketed for the same purposes. In other words, the rating matches that of the appropriate "representative" formula in Section VI (General Formulations).

We believe that toxicity ratings are useful devices for designating the lethality of bulk products, such as powders, solutions, emulsions, ointments, *etc.*, where the composition is commonly stated as percentages. Where a product is marketed in the form of single units, such as tablets, pills, capsules, suppositories, troches, *etc.*, the percentage composition is seldom revealed. For example, the composition of a tablet is commonly designated by the number of milligrams of active ingredient per tablet, without regard to the nature or amount of inactive binder, filler, *etc.* Both the physician and the layman are conditioned to specify the dose by the number of tablets, and this is true of toxic as well as therapeutic doses. From the number of tablets consumed and the quantity of drug in each, the total dose is revealed; this can be compared with the lethal dose published in Section II for several of the commoner drugs. In this scheme a toxicity rating is unnecessary and awkward, but for the purposes of product research it was thought worthwhile to assign toxicity ratings to these unit-dose medicaments. To do this it was necessary first to estimate the total weight of each pill, tablet, capsule, *etc.*, so that the concentrations of active ingredients could be calculated. Mr. C. J. Latiolais, then pharmacist at the Strong Memorial Hospital, reported the unit sizes that are usually encountered in standard pharmaceuticals, and selected an average or typical unit weight for each item. These values are presented in Table V.2. By pretending, for example, that all capsules weigh the same (0.25 gm. according to the average in Table V.2), toxicity ratings were assigned to all drug products in this compilation.

To summarize: the toxicity rating of a product is intended to describe its degree of acute lethality when ingested. Any rating assigned by the methods described here is necessarily provisional and should never be treated as a constant or a known value. At least three kinds of uncertainty are commonly encountered, *viz.*, unknown are 1) the exact and complete composition of the product, 2) the precise toxicity of each separate ingre-

TABLE V.2

	Weight range	Average
	gm.	*gm.*
Capsules	0.1 –1.4	0.25
Tablets (compressed)	0.04–2.4	0.35
Tablets (enteric-coated)	0.1 –1.7	0.80
Tablets (sugar coated)	0.1 –1.0	0.40
Pills	0.15–0.4	0.32
Troches	1.0 –2.5	1.5
Suppositories		2.0
Granules, effervescent contain 80% inert ingredients		

dient, and 3) the possibility of chemical or biological interactions between the various constituents. As with all judgment values, honest differences of opinion are inevitable, and most borderline products could readily be up or down-graded by one toxicity class. Obviously one must avoid the error of pretending that all products with the same rating are equally toxic. Toxicity ratings are only guideposts, intended to supplement but never to substitute for special knowledge, common sense, or sound clinical judgment.

Name & Use Manufacturer	Ingredients		Name & Use Manufacturer	Ingredients	
ABAC For Children Analgesic (Massengill)	Each tablet: Potassium bromide Sodium bromide Aspirin (acetylsalicylic acid)* Caffeine Aromatics	3.2 mg. 3.2 mg. 65 mg. 6.5 mg. q.s.	ACCLAIM ESSENCE GLACÉE Cosmetic (Parfums Ciro)		
A.A.A. PASTE NO. 1 Antiseptic, external (Jenkins)	Ammoniated mercury* Acid salicylic Acid boric Zinc oxide	2% 1.25% 1% 15%	ACCLAIM EXTRACT Cosmetic (Parfums Ciro)		
A.A.A. PASTE NO.2 Antiseptic, external (Jenkins)	Ammoniated mercury* Salicylic acid Boric acid Zinc oxide	5% 1.25% 1% 15%	ACCO SAPONIFIED CRESYLIC SOLUTION Disinfectant (Amalg. Chem.)	Cresylic acid*	
ABC ALUMINUM WELDING FLUX NO. 8 (Anti-Borax)	Potassium chloride Sodium chloride Lithium fluoride		ACE EAR DROPS (Bailin)		
A.B.C. WAX (Griffin)			ACE-72 M.Q. TUBES Prepared developer (Ace)		
ABDAC DISINFECTANT (Sanis)	Alkyl-dimethyl-benzyl ammonium chloride		ACETAFEINE, NO. 4 Analgesic, tablets (Cappenin)	Acetophenetidin* Aspirin* Caffeine alkaloid	2 gr. 2-3/4 gr. 1/4 gr.
ABESTO CHEMICAL TERMITE CONTROL Wood preservative, soil poisoner (Abesto)	Pentachlorophenol* Orthodichlorobenzene*	5% 5%	ACETIDINE Capsules or Tablets Analgesic (Sharp & Dohe)	Aspirin (acetylsalicylic acid)* 0.1770 gm. Acetophenetidin (phenacetin)* 0.1176 gm. Caffeine 0.0294 gm.	
ABESTO CLEARTOX Wood preservative (Abesto)	Pentachlorophenol*	5%	ACIDINE Antacid (Consolid.Royal)	Magnesium trisilicate Dried aluminum hydroxide gel Calcium carbonate Sodium bicarbonate Oil peppermint Small amounts of: Malt diatase, bismuth subcarbonate and papain	
ABESTO STAINTOX Wood preservative (Abesto)	Pentachlorophenol*	5%	ACID-KLENZ FORMULA LC-10 Detergent (Klenzade)	Organic acids*	
A-BOMB LIQUID FIRE EXTINGUISHER (Pure Drug)			ACID MANTLE CREME Anti-alkali protective skin ointment (Dome)	Aluminum acetate in hydrophilic base (pH 4.2)	
AB-SCENT DEODORANT CREAM Cream or liquid (Jordeau)			ACID MANTLE LOTION Skin acidifier (Dome)	Aluminum acetate	
ABSORBENE Wallpaper cleaner (Glidden Co.)			ACIDOLATE Skin cleanser (White Labs.)	Sulfated vegetable oils Liquid petrolatum Water	
ABSORBINE JR. Rubefacient, counter-irritant solution (Young)	Wormwood Thymol* Menthol* Acetone* Essential oils and tinctures		ACIDOX Intestinal germicidal (veterinary) (Lee, G.)	3-Nitro-4-hydroxy phenylarsonic acid* (arsenic derivative); each fluid ounce contains 2.0 gr. arsenic trioxide 1.07% Acetic acid 3.5% Picolines 1.02% Salt 12% Cert. color 0.01% Water 82.4%	
ACCLAIM EAU de TOILETTE Toilet water (Parfums Ciro)					

*Consult Sec. II., Ingredients Index. This ingredient may be responsible for major toxic effects if poisonous amounts of this product are ingested.

Name & Use Manufacturer	Ingredients	
ACID SEAL PAINT (Goodrich, B.F.)	Toluol* (small amt.)	
ACIDUSOL Acid douche solution (Texas Pharm.)	Oxyquinoline sulfate* Lactic acid Zinc sulfocarbolate* Citric acid Dextrose Buffer solution	3.5% 6.0% 6.8% 7.5% 25.0% q.s.
ACITAMIN, BROWN TOPS Hydrochloric acid replacement (Massengill)	Each capsule: Glutamic acid hydrochloride 0.3 gm. Thiamine hydrochloride 1 mg. Riboflavin 1 mg. Niacinamide 5 mg.	
ACK-ACK INSECT SPRAY W/DDT 5% (Howell Co.)	DDT*	5%
ACME ALL ROUND BOMB Insecticide (Acme Q.P.)	Pyrethrins 0.025% Rotenone & other cube extractives 0.364% Piperonyl cyclonene 0.256% Solvents & propellants*	
ACME ALL ROUND DUST Insecticide, fungicide (Acme Q.P.)	Rotenone and other cube extractives 2.25% Methoxychlor 5% Ferbam 4% Ziram 4%	
ACME ALL ROUND SPRAY Insecticide, fungicide (Acme Q.P.)	Rotenone & other cube extractives 2.25% DDT* 5% Ziram 15% Sulfur 20% Talc & wetting agent	
ACME ARSENATE OF LEAD Insecticide (Acme Q.P.)	Arsenate of lead* (30% is arsenic pentoxide and 58% is metallic lead) 98%	
ACME 3% BHC - 5% DDT Insecticide (Acme Fertilizer)	Gamma isomer of BHC 3.00% DDT* 5.00%	
ACME BORDEAUX MIXTURE Fungicide (Acme Q.P.)	Copper sulfate* (12.75% metallic copper) 50% Lime 50%	
ACME 6% CHLORDANE DUST Insecticide (Acme Q.P.)	Tech. chlordane* 6% Inert ingredients	
ACME CHLORINATED LIME (Babbitt)	Chlorine* 24%	
ACME DIELDRIN "18" Insecticide (Acme Q.P.)	Dieldrin* Tech. 18.62%	
ACME DIMITE Insecticide (Acme Q.P.)	Di-(p-chlorophenyl)-methyl-carbinol (D.M.C.)* 25%	
ACME DURADUST NO. 50 Insecticide (Acme Q.P.)	DDT* 50% Diluent and wetting agent	
ACME EMO-NIK Insecticide (Acme Q.P.)	Hydrocarbon oil 80%/w Nicotine alkaloid* 1.50%	
ACME FERTILIZER 3% BHC - 5% DDT Insecticide (Acme Fertilizer)	Gamma isomer of BHC* 3.00% DDT* 5.00%	
ACME FERTILIZER 10% DITHANE Insecticide (Acme Fertilizer)	Zinc ethylene bisdithiocarbamate 6.50	
ACME FERTILIZER 1.00% ROTENONE Insecticide (Acme Fertilizer)	Rotenone 1.00	
ACME FERTILIZER 10% TDE Insecticide (Acme Fertilizer)	DDD* 10.00%	
ACME FERTILIZER 20% TOXAPHENE DUST Insecticide (Acme Fertilizer)	Toxaphene* 20.00%	
ACME FLY BAIT Insecticide (Acme Q.P.)	Tech. malathion attractants 2% Attractants	
ACME GARDEN FUNGICIDE (Acme Q.P.)	Captan 30% Karathane 3%	
ACME GARDEN GUARD Insecticide (Acme Q.P.)	Rotenone 1% Other extractives of cube 2% Talc carrier and wetting agent	
ACME GARDEN SPRAY Insecticide (Acme White Lead)	Arsenate of lead*	
ACME LIME SULFUR Fungicide (powdered form) (Acme Q.P.)	Calcium polysulfides* 65% Calcium thiosulfate 5% Sulfur 5%	
ACME 5% LINDANE SPRAY Insecticide (Acme Q.P.)	Gamma isomer of benzene hexachloride (from lindane)* 5%	

Name & Use Manufacturer	Ingredients	
ACME 50% MALATHION SPRAY Insecticide (Acme Q.P.)	Tech. malathion Xylene*	50% 38%
ACME PARIS GREEN (Acme Q.P.)	Arsenic trioxide* Copper	50% 24%
ACME RED RIVER POTATO MIX Insecticide, fungicide (Acme Q.P.)	DDT Metallic copper Metallic arsenic* Carrier and wetting agents	9.5% 25.7% 15.1%
ACME ROSE DUST Insecticide, fungicide (Acme Q.P)	Captan Karathane Malathion DDT*	7% 0.75% 4% 5%
ACME 10% TDE Insecticide (Acme Fertilizer)	DDD*	10.00%
ACME TOMATO DUST Insecticide, fungicide (Acme Q.P.)	Metallic copper* Metallic arsenic*	15.0% 4.8%
ACME WEED KILLER Herbicide (Acme Q.P.)	Sodium arsenite*	40%
ACME WETTABLE DUSTING SULFUR Fungicide (Acme Q.P.)	Sulfur* Wetting agent	95%
ACNE CREAM S.F. MFR. NO. 701 Antiseptic skin cream (Specialists)	Colloidal sulfur*	
ACNOID Keratolytic (Sargeant)	Salicylic acid* Camphor* Calamine Balsam of fir Boric acid* Menthol* Chlorthymol* Salol*	
ACNOLAC Antiseptic ointment for acne (Almar)	Zinc sulfide* Polysulfides*	
ACNOMEL CAKE For acne (Smith, Kline & French)	Resoucinol Sulfur Hexachlorophene (w/w)	1% 4% 0.25%
ACNOMEL CREAM Antiseptic cream for acne (Smith, Kline & French)	Resorcinol* Sulfur Hexachlorophene Alcohol	2% 8% 0.25% 11%(w/w)
ACNOPHILL For acne (Torch)	Sulfur Potassa sulfurata Zinc oxide Monobase	5% 5% 10%
ACNYL Antiseptic cream for acne (Pharmex)	Resorcinol* Sulfur Hexachlorophene	2% 8% 0.25%
ACOBEL Antipyretic (veterinary) (Daniels, Dr. A.C.)	Each tablet: Acetophenetidin* Quinine sulfate	
ACP AMID-THIN Insecticide (Am.Chemical)	Naphthylacetamide (76 gm. per gal.)	2.14%
ACP CRAB GRASS KILLER WITH MCP (Am.Chemical)	Potassium cyanate* 2-Methyl -4- chlorophenoxyacetic acid sodium salt	53.8% 11.1%
ACP FRUIT TREE SPRAY (Am.Chemical)	DDT* Dimethoxy diphenyl trichlorethane Sulfur* Ferbam	5% 10% 30% 3.80%
ACP GARDEN DOCTOR Insecticide, fungicide (Am.Chemical)	Methoxychlor Malathion Captan	15.00% 5.00% 10.00%
ACP GRASS KILLER (TCA 90%) (Am.Chemical)	Sodium trichloracetate*	90%
ACP 20-20-20 GRO-STUFF Soluble plant food (Am.Chemical)	Organic nitrogen Phosphoric acid Potash Avail. nitrogen from urea Avail. phosphoric acid from mono potassium and sodium tripoly phosphate Avail. soluble potash from potassium chloride and mono potassium phosphate	20% 20% 20% 20% 20% 20%
ACP POISON IVY KILLER (Am.Chemical)	Amizol (3-amino-1,2,4-triazole)	12.5%
ACP POISON OAK KILLER (Am.Chemical)	Amizol (3-amino-1,2,4-triazole)	12.5%
ACP ROSE AND FLORAL DUST (Am.Chemical)	Ferbam Sulfur* DDT* Lindane Ovotran	7.6% 20.0% 5.0% 0.5% 2.5%
ACP SOIL CONDITIONER (Am.Chemical)	PAC (modified polyacrylonitrile) VAMA (vinyl acetate maleic polymer) Trace elements Plant hormones	
ACRISAN Antiseptic throat spray (Recsei)	Amino-acridine*ascorbate Benzyl alcohol*	0.2% 0.5%
AC-SO TABLETS Cathartic (Mac Donald's)	Aloin* Ext. of cascara sagrada* Podophyllin*	
ACTEEN (Modern Supply)	Coconut oil soap Mapon Sequestering agent	40%

*Consult Sec. II., Ingredients Index. This ingredient may be responsible for major toxic effects if poisonous amounts of this product are ingested.

Name & Use Manufacturer	Ingredients		Name & Use Manufacturer	Ingredients	
ACTIVATOR Photographic supply (Super-Tomic)			**ACTRITE INSECTOKOTE WITH DDT** (Pioneer)	Petroleum distillates* DDT* Methylated aromatic petroleum deriv.	82% 5% 12%
ACT-ON RUB Counter- irritant liquid (Berjon)	Methyl salicylate* Camphor Menthol syn. Oil eucalyptus Oil mustard syn.	10% 1-1/2% 1-1/2% 1-1/2% 0.47%	**ACTRITE INSECTOKOTE WITH 5% DDT** (Pioneer)	DDT*	5%
ACT-ON TABLETS Analgesic (Berjon)	Sodium salicylate* Potassium iodide Sodium bicarbonate Salicylamide		**ACTRITE LIQUID TOILET SOAP** (Pioneer)	Cochin cocoanut oil	
ACTRITE BOWL POWDER For toilet bowls (Pioneer)			**ACTRITE METAL POLISH** (Pioneer)		
ACTRITE COAL TAR DISIN- FECTANT (Pioneer)			**ACTRITE NOXSTAIN LIQUID** For toilet bowls (Pioneer)		
ACTRITE DE-MOTH Insecticide (Pioneer)	Petroleum distillates* 96.877% Methylated petroleum derris 0.185% Pyrethrins 0.048%		**ACTRITE PERFUMED CRYSTALS** Deodorant (Pioneer)		
ACTRITE DE-MOTH WITH 5% DDT Insecticide (Pioneer)	DDT	5%	**ACTRITE PINE CLEANER** (Pioneer)		
ACTRITE DEODORANT DISCS (Pioneer)			**ACTRITE PINE OIL DISIN- FECTANT** (Pioneer)	Steam distilled pine oil*	
ACTRITE DE-ODOR BLOX Deodorant (Pioneer)			**ACTRITE PIPE OPENER** (Pioneer)		
ACTRITE DIFFUSING LIQUID Insecticide (Pioneer)	7-1 Pyrethrum* concentrated liquid		**ACTRITE ROACH AND ANT POWDER** (Pioneer)	Pyrethrins* Sodium fluoride*	
ACTRITE FLOR-DRESS Floor treat- ment (Pioneer)			**ACTRITE ROACH POWDER** (Pioneer)	Pyrethrum*	
ACTRITE FOAM-O- KLEEN Upholstery cleaner (Pioneer)			**ACRITE SASSA CLEANER** (Pioneer)		
ACTRITE ICE-THAW (Pioneer)			**ACTRITE SEAL** Floor seal (Pioneer)		
			ACTRITE SPOT REMOVER (Pioneer)		
ACTRITE INSECT KILLER (Pioneer)	DDT Pyrethrins Petroleum distillates* Sesame oil extractives Methylated aromatic petroleum deriv.	1% 0.034% 95% 1.25% 3.7%	**ACTRITE TILE & PORCELAIN CLEANER** (Pioneer)		
			A-C TROCHES (Abbott)	Anesthesin Calcidin Ext. of licorice Oil of anise Sugar	1/4 gr.
ACTRITE INSECT KILLER WITH 1% DDT (Pioneer)			**ACTRON** Analgesic tablet (Haack)	Acid acetylsalicylic* (aspirin) 5 gr. Calcium carbonate prec. 1-1/2 gr. Aluminum hydroxide gel dried 1 gr. Acid citric anhyd. 1/2 gr.	

*Consult Sec. II., Ingredients Index. This ingredient may be responsible for major toxic effects if poisonous amounts of this product are ingested.

Name & Use Manufacturer	Ingredients	
ACZOL Wood preservative (Zinsser)	Zinc formate	5%
	Copper cresylate *	12%
ADAMSON'S BALSAM Antitussive (Myers)	Lobelia Bloodroot Tartar emetic Rio-ipecac Gum camphor Capsicum Resin cuaiac Gum resin myrrh Balsam tolu Glycerin syrup Molasses	
ADBAC DISINFECTANT (Sanis)	Alkyl-dimethyl-benzyl ammonium chloride*	
ADCO DETERGENT-DRYCLEANER (Adco)		
ADCO ETHERIZED LIQUID SHAMPOO For rugs and upholstery (Adco)		
ADCO-FUME Insecticide (Adco)		
ADCO GENERAL FORMULA Drycleaning (Adco)		
ADCO SHOWER PRUF Water repellent (Adco)		
ADCO SIZE Drycleaning size (Adco)		
ADCO ZEST Powdered detergent for wet cleaning (Adco)		
A.D.D.'S LINIMENT Udder decongestant (veterinary) (Driscoll)	Linseed oil Turpentine Sulfuric acid Sodium nitrate Camphor Lead acetate*	
AD-EL-ITE #24 Paint remover (Glidden Co.)	Benzol*	25%
ADELITE Hygienic kalsomine (Glidden Co.)		
AD-EL-ITE Non-inflammable paint and varnish remover (Glidden Co.)		

Name & Use Manufacturer	Ingredients
AD-EL-ITE Paint & varnish remover (Glidden Co.)	Benzol* Acetone*
AD-EL-ITE Paste wax (Glidden Co.)	
ADGESIC Rubifaciant, counter-irritant (Am. Druggists)	Camphor* Synthetic menthol liquid (not U.S.P.) Oil of peppermint Synthetic oil of wintergreen Oleoresin Capsicum Acetone*
ADGUENTUM Ointment (Chester Baker)	
ADHESIVEASE For removal of adhesive tape from body (Durst, S.F.)	Oxyquinoline Diethylene glycol ethyl ether acetate In petroleum distillate*
ADHES-OFF Solvent for removal of adhesive tape from body (Harvey Labs.)	Trichlorethylene* In petroleum base*
ADIOS Nail polish remover (Gena)	
ADLA TABLETS Antacid (Chester-Kent)	Bismuth subcarbonate Magnesium carbonate Calcium carbonate Sodium bicarbonate Oil of peppermint
ADLERIKA Cathartic (Chester-Kent)	Magnesium sulfate (epsom salts, U.S.P.) Cascara Anise seed Licorice Fennel Sassafras Ginger Carbonate of magnesia Oil of cinnamon Methyl salicylate* Glycerin
ADMALT Tonic (Hance)	Calcium Sodium Potassium Maganese Iron Malt extract Wild cherry bark Aromatics
ADMIRACION FOAMY SHAMPOO (Turner Hall)	Detergents
ADMIRACION OIL SHAMPOO TREATMENT (Turner Hall)	Emulsified mixture of oils* and sulfonated oils*
ADMIRALTY LIQUID WEED KILLER 1-300 Conc. (Admiralty)	Pentachlorophenol* mixture

*Consult Sec. II., Ingredients Index. This ingredient may be responsible for major toxic effects if poisonous amounts of this product are ingested.

Name & Use Manufacturer	Ingredients		Name & Use Manufacturer	Ingredients	
ADMIRALTY PENTAWOOD 1-10 Wood preservative conc. (Admiralty)	Pentachlorophenol* Other chlorophenols Aromatic petroleum solvents*	36.08% 4.92% 34.00%	**ADS-KOL** Analgesic (Am.Druggists)	Each capsule: Acentalilid Powdered extract belladonna leaves* (1.25% total alkaloids) Aspirin* Phenolphthalein Oleo-resin capsicum	1 gr. 1/50 gr.
ADMIRALTY PENTAWOOD 77 Wood preservative (Admiralty)	Pentachlorophenol* Other chlorophenols Petroleum solvents	4.25% 0.75% 89.26%	**ADSPEP RUB** Astringent (Am.Druggists)	Isopropyl alcohol*	91%
ADMIRALTY PERMAWOOD 20 Wood preservative (Admiralty)	Pentachlorophenol* Other chlorophenols Petroleum solvents*	4.40% 0.60% 89.26%	**A.D.S. POISON IVY & POISON OAK LOTION** (Am.Druggists)	Gelsemium Witch hazel Phenol* Lead acetate*	1.5%
ADMIROLA CREAMS (Glenn Prod.)			**A.D.S. SYRUP COCILCOMP** Antitussive (Am.Druggists)	Alcohol Each fluid ounce: Tinct. euphorbia pilulifera Syrup wild lettuce Tincture cocillana Syrup squill compound Cascarin Tartar emetic Menthol	6% 120 m. 120 m. 40 m. 24 m.
A.D.S. AMMONIATED MERCURY OINTMENT Antiseptic (Am.Druggists)	Ammoniated mercury* Ointment base	5% 95%			
A.D.S. ANALGESIC BALM Rubefacient counter-irritant (Am.Druggists)	Methyl salicylate* Camphor* Menthol Oil of cajeput Oil of mustard		**A.D.S. WHITE LINIMENT** Rubifacient, counter-irritant (Am.Druggists)	Spirits of turpentine* Oil of origanum Oil of camphor* Castile soap Ammonium carbonate Ammonia	
A.D.S. BURN OINTMENT Antiseptic, external (Am.Druggists)	Carbolic acid* Zinc oxide Aluminum hydroxide Calendula Balsam Peru Ichthammol Methyl ester parahydroxy benzoic acid Benzoic acid Ethyl amino benzoate Aromatic oils		**ADU LOTION** (Wirth)		
			AERIZON "SILBE" IN-HALANT Nasal deconges-tant (Radin)	Chlorbutanol* Ephedrine* hydrochloride Epinephrine Glycerine	12-1/2 gr./ fl. oz.
A.D.S. CORN TREATMENT Keratolytic (Am.Druggists)	Alcohol Ether* Salicylic acid*	23% 55%	**AERO BRAND CCS' DUST** (Heidt)	Cryolite Copper*	
ADSCREOSE Antitussive (Am.Druggists)	Creosote Syrup of white pine compound Cascara Wild cherry Ipecac Ammonium chloride Sodium benzoate Honey Menthol Tar Aromatics		**AERO BRAND HI-CHLOR** Insecticide (Heidt)	Chlordane*	
			AERO BRAND HI-COP 7 (Melon Dust) (Heidt)	Copper*	7%
A.D.S. EYE BATH Antiseptic (Am.Druggists)	Boric acid* Borax* Berberine sulfate Methyl parahydroxybenzoate		**AERO BRAND HI-COP 10** (Melon Dust) (Heidt)	Copper*	10%
A.D.S. EYE DROPS Antiseptic (Am.Druggists)	Boric acid* Borax* Berberine sulfate Methyl para-hydroxy-benzoate		**AERO BRAND HI-D** Insecticide (Heidt)	DDT*	
ADSIVE CREAM Antiseptic and anesthetic, external (Am.Druggists)	Calcium hydroxide Zinc oxide* Liquid carbolic acid* (carbolic acid 1.8%) Glycerin Camphor F.E.Grindelia soluble Menthol		**AERO BRAND HI-D-S** Insecticide (Heidt)	DDT* Sulfur*	
			AERO BRAND HI-HEX 3-5 (Cotton Dust) (Heidt)	BHC* DDT*	

*Consult Sec. II., Ingredients Index. This ingredient may be responsible for major toxic effects if poisonous amounts of this product are ingested.

Name & Use Manufacturer	Ingredients	
AERO BRAND HI-HEX 3-5-40 Insecticide (Heidt)	BHC* DDT* Sulfur*	
AERO BRAND HI-RONE Insecticide (Heidt)	Rotenone* Sulfur*	
AERO BRAND HI-THANE 8 Insecticide (Heidt)	Zineb	8%
AERO BRAND HI-THOX 5 Insecticide (Heidt)	Methoxychlor*	
AERO BRAND HI-THOX S-5 Insecticide (Heidt)	Methoxychlor* Sulfur*	
AERO BRAND HI-THOX 10 Insecticide (Heidt)	Methoxychlor*	
AERO BRAND HI-TOX 20 Cotton Dust (Heidt)	Toxaphene*	
AERO BRAND HI-TOX 30-40 Cotton Dust (Heidt)	Toxaphene* Sulfur*	
AERO CYANAMID, GRANULAR Herbicide (Am.Cyan.)	Calcium cyanamide* Nitrogen	46% 20.6%
AERO CYANAMID, SPECIAL GRADE Herbicide (Am. Cyan.)	Calcium cyanamide* Nitrogen	57% 21%
AERO DEFOLIANT (Am.Cyan.)	Calcium cyanamide*	
AERO DX SPRAY Insecticide (Pratt, B.)	Pyrethrins Rotenone Other cube extracts Tech. piperonyl cyclonene	0.025% 0.128% 0.236% 0.256%
AERO HCN DISCOIDS Insecticide, fungicide (Am.Cyan.)	Hydrocyanic acid*	96-98%
AERO-KING HIGH PRESS- URE INSECTI- CIDE (Am. Aerosol)	Pyrethrins DDT Tech. piperonyl butoxide Methylated naphthalenes* Petroleum distillate	0.20% 3% 0.80% 8% 8%
AERO LIQUID HCN Fungicide (Am.Cyan.)	Hydrocyanic acid*	96-98%

Name & Use Manufacturer	Ingredients	
AERO-MASTER FOGGING INSECTICIDE- Mill Fogging Formula (Aero-San.)	Petroleum oils* Tech. piperonyl butoxide Pyrethrins*	
AERO METAL CEMENT (Boyle-Midway)	Nitrocellulose lacquer Resins Organic solvents* Aluminum dust	
AEROMIST Glass Cleaner (Boyle-Midway)	Water Alcohol* Diacetone* Wetting agent Anti-oxidant Color (trace)	
AERO NO RUBBING WHITE FURNITURE CREAM (Boyle-Midway)	Petroleum oil* Wax Emulsifiers	
AEROSECT Insecticide (Pennsylv. Eng.)	Pyrethrins Tech. piperonyl butoxide Mineral oil Sesame oil Freon (11 and 12)	0.25% 2.00% 1.00% 11.75% 85%
AEROSECT ANT PREVENTIVE (Pennsylv.Eng.)	Pyrethrins Petroleum distillate Sesame oil	2% 8% 90%
AEROSECT GOLDEN MOTH CRYSTALS (Pennsylv.Eng.)	Paradichlorobenzene* Pyrethrins	99.99% 0.01%
AEROSECT GOLDEN MOTH NUGGETS (Pennsylv.Eng.)	Paradichlorobenzene* Pyrethrins	99.99% 0.01%
AEROSECT GOLDEN SOLID MOTH CAKES (Pennsylv.Eng.)	Paradichlorobenzene* Pyrethrins	99.99% 0.01%
AEROSECT WONDER INSECTICIDE (Pennsylv.Eng)	Pyrethrins Sesame oil Mineral oil	0.4% 8.0% 1.6%
AERO SHAVE (Boyle-Midway)	Soap Humectics Perfume Freon propellents	
AERO SNOW FLAKES Spray for Xmas trees (Boyle-Midway)	Fatty acid Resin Freon gas propellents	
AEROSOL DOMESTIC INSECT KILLER (Domestic)	Pyrethrins*	
AEROSOL HESS BOMB Insecticide (Hess, Dr.)	Petroleum distillates* Terpene polychlorinates Piperonyl butoxide Pyrethrins	11.975% 2% 0.80% 0.20%
AEROSOL INSEKIL Insecticide (Holcomb)	Strobane* Pyrethrins* Piperonyl butoxide	

*Consult Sec. II., Ingredients Index. This ingredient may be responsible for major toxic effects if poisonous amounts of this product are ingested.

Name & Use Manufacturer	Ingredients		Name & Use Manufacturer	Ingredients	
AEROSOL LARVACIDE Fungicide (Larvacide)	Chloropicrin*	50%	A-GENE DI-RETIC TABLETS Diuretic (A-Gene)		
AERO TRANSPARENT CEMENT (Boyle-Midway)	Nitrocellulose lacquer Resins Organic* solvents		A-GENE HYGIENIC POWDER (A-Gene)		
AERO WASH & CLEANER #7480 (Fuller,W.P.)			A-GENE PILE OINTMENT (A-Gene)		
AEROWAX (Boyle-Midway)	Solids: Vegetable and/or mineral waxes Emulsifiers of the fatty acid amine type Borax* Resins	10-15%	AGICIDE ANT POWDER (Agicide)	Gamma isomer of benzene hexachloride (from lindane)	1%
A-FIL CREAM (Hypo-Aller-genic) Prevents sunburn (Texas Pharm.)	Menthyl anthranilate* Titanium dioxide	5% 5%	AGICIDE CATTLE GRUB & LOUSE POW-DER (Agicide)	Rotenone Other cube resins	1.50% 4%
A-FIL SUN STICK Lipstick for protection against sun-burn (Texas Pharm.)	Digalloyl trioleate	2.50%	AGICIDE COPPER DUST Fungicide (Agicide)	Cuprous oxide*	4.60%
AFRICANO Insecticide and rodenticides (Africano)			AGICIDE CRABGRASS KILLER (Agicide)	Potassium cyanate*	46%
AFRICAN VIOLET & HOUSE PLANT INSECT SPRAY (Bostwick)	Pyrethrins Rotenone Other cube extractives Tech. piperonyl cyclonene Methoxychlor	0.025% 0.128% 0.236% 0.256% 3%	AGICIDE 50% DDT WET-TABLE POW-DER Insecticide (Agicide)	DDT* (dichloro diphenyl tri-chloroethane)	50%
AGA-REX WITH PHENOLPHTH-ALEIN Cathartic (Rexall)	Mineral oil Phenolphthalein*		AGICIDE DOG & CAT FLEA POWDER (Agicide)	Rotenone Other cube resins	1.25% 3.30%
AG-A-TON Anthelmintic (veterinary) (Gland-O-Lac)	Nicotine (as alkaloid) Inactive ingredients: Areca nut Nux vomica (containing strychnine) Copper sulfate* Iron sulfate Quassia Wild mustard Gentian Anise oil Tobacco	1.10% 7.5% 0.09%	AGICIDE EVERGREEN DUST OR SPRAY Insecticide, fungicide (Agicide)	Rotenone Other cube resins Pyrethrins Sulfur*	0.75% 2% 0.05% 32%
			AGICIDE FLOWER GARDEN DUSTING POW-DER Insecticide, fungicide (Agicide)	Rotenone Other cube resins Beta butoxy beta' thiocyano diethyl ether Pyrethrins Zineb	0.75% 2% 0.50% 0.10% 3.90%
AGAVA BOILER AND RADIATOR CONDITIONERS (Agava)			AGICIDE FRUIT TREE SPRAY Insecticide, fungicide (Agicide)	DDT (dichloro diphenyl tri-chloroethane)* Rotenone DDD (dichloro diphenyl dichloroethane) Zineb Sulfur*	5% 1% 2.50% 10% 25%
AGAVA BOILER WATER TREAT-MENT (Agava)			AGICIDE GOLD DOT GARDEN DUST Insecticide (Agicide)	DDT (dichloro diphenyl trichloro-ethane)	3%
A-GENE ALKALINE TABLETS (A-Gene)			AGICIDE GOLD DOT POTATO DUST Insecticide (Agicide)	DDT (dichloro diphenyl tri-chloroethane)* Cuprous oxide	5% 4.60%

*Consult Sec. II., Ingredients Index. This ingredient may be responsible for major toxic effects if poisonous amounts of this product are ingested.

Name & Use Manufacturer	Ingredients	
AGICIDE HOG LOUSE, SHEEP TICK DUST POWDER Insecticide, fumigant (Agicide)	Gamma insomer of benzene hexachloride* Other isomers of benzene hexachloride*	1% 6.15%
AGICIDE 1% LINDANE GARDEN DUST Insecticide (Agicide)	Gamma isomer of benzene hexachloride(from lindane)	1%
AGICIDE MAGGOT KILLER (Agicide)	Hexachloro hexahydro dimethano naphthalene* Related compounds	0.95% 0.68%
AGICIDE ORGANIC FUNGICIDE (Agicide)	Zineb	3.9%
AGICIDE PICKLE DUST Insecticide, fungicide (Agicide)	Rotenone Other cube resins Beta-butoxy-beta'-thiocyano diethyl ether Pyrethrins Zineb	0.75% 2% 0.50% 0.10% 3.90%
AGICIDE ROACH AND ANT POW- DER (Agicide)	Gamma isomer of benzene hexachloride(from lindane)0.5%	
AGICIDE ROSE DUST Insecticide, fungicide (Agricide)	Rotenone Other cube resins Beta-butoxy-beta'-thiocyano diethyl ether Pyrethrins Zineb	0.75% 2% 0.50% 0.10% 3.90%
AGICIDE SABADUST Insecticide (Agicide)	Sabadilla seed*	10%
AGICIDE TOMATO DUST Insecticide, fungicide (Agicide)	Zineb DDD (dichloro diphenyl dichloroethane)	3.9% 5%
AGICIDE 20% TOXAPHENE GARDEN IN- SECTICIDE (Agicide)	Toxaphene*	20%
AGICIDE WARFARIN BASE Rodenticide (Agicide)	Warfarin	0.25%
AGICIDE WARFARIN RAT & MOUSE BAIT (Agicide)	Warfarin	0.025%
AGICIDE WEED WILT (Agicide)	2,4-Dichlorophenoxyacetic acid* 5%	
AGNES MAC GREGOR AFTER SHAVE LOTION (MacGregor)		

Name & Use Manufacturer	Ingredients	
AGNES MAC GREGOR COLOGNE (MacGregor)		
AGORAL Cathartic (Warner-Chil- cott)	Mineral oil Phenolphthalein	
AGRICO COUNTRY CLUB FERTILIZER 6-10-4 For fairways (Am. Agric. Chem.)	Nitrogen Phosphorus Potash	6% 10% 4%
AGRICO COUNTRY CLUB FERTILIZER 8-6-4 25% organic for greens (Am. Agric. Chem.)	Nitrogen Phosphorus Potash	8% 6% 4%
AGRICO FOR GARDENS Fertilizer (Am. Agric. Chem.)	Nitrogen Phosphorus Potash	5% 10% 5%
AGRICO FOR LAWNS, TREES & SHRUBS Fertilizer (Am. Agric. Chem.)	Nitrogen Phosphorus Potash	6% 10% 4%
AGRICO FOR TURF 6-8-2 Fertilizer (Am. Agric. Chem.)	Nitrogen Phosphorus Potash Organic nitrogen	6% 8% 2% 50%
AGRICO ROSE FOOD 5-9-6 Fertilizer (Am. Agric. Chem.)	Nitrogen Phosphorus Potash Organic nitrogen	5% 9% 6% 50%
AGRIKLOR Insecticide (Dianol)	Chlordane*	
AGRI-MYCIN 100 Fungicide (Chipman Chem.)	Streptomycin* Oxytetracyline	15% 1.5%
AGRINITE Fertilizer (Am. Agric. Chem.)	Nitrogen	8-1/4%
AGROX Seed disinfec- tant (Chipman Chem.)	Phenyl mercury urea*	6.70%
AGROX C Seed disinfec- tant (Chipman Ltd.)	Phenyl mercury acetate* Ethyl mercury chloride* Total mercury equiv.	7.06% 1.06% 5%
AGROXONE DUST (5%) Herbicide (Plant Prod.)	Sodium 2-methyl-4-chlorophene oxyacetate (Methoxone)* 5%	
AIK AID CAPSULES (Concialdi)		

*Consult Sec. II., Ingredients Index. This ingredient may be responsible for major toxic effects if poisonous amounts of this product are ingested.

Name & Use Manufacturer	Ingredients	Name & Use Manufacturer	Ingredients
AIRCRAFT - MARINE FORMULA "21" (Aircraft)	Methylene chloride* Ethyl alcohol Kerosene* Paraffin Ammonia Plastic thickener Non-toxic rust retardant	AIROSOL MOTH PROOFER (Airosol Co.)	Methylated naphthalenes* 10% Petroleum distillate* 21% DDT (dichloro diphenyl trichloroethane)* 5% Methoxychlor tech. 3% Dibutyl phthalate 1%
AIRCRAFT - MARINE FORMULA "22" (Aircraft)	Methylene chloride* Ethyl alcohol Kerosene* Paraffin Ammonia Butyl acetate Methyl ethyl ketone Plastic thickener Non-toxic rust retardant	AIROSOL SCREW WORM BOMB (Airosol Co.)	Gamma isomer of benzene hexachloride (from lindane)* 3% Pine oil* 15%
		AIR-PURE Germicide Antiseptic deodorant (Chaplin)	Alcohol* (by vol.) 92% Oil of pine Cajeput Thyme Eucalyptus Rosemary Spike lavender Menthol
AIR-DRYETTE Chemical air dryer (Solvay)			
AIRE FRESH Deodorant (Chandler)		AIR-SCENT SPRAY Room deodorant (General Prod.)	Isopropyl alcohol* Triethylene glycol* Propylene glycol Para di-isobutyl phenoxy ethoxy ethyl dimethyl benzyl ammonium chloride*
AIREX Household deodorizer (Gen.Chem.)	Pyrethrins* DDT*		
AIR FRESH Deodorizer (Fuld)		AIRTONA (Thayer)	Ethyl alcohol* Isopropyl alcohol* Essential oils Wetting agents Quaternary ammonium compound
AIR FRESHENER Deodorizer (Stanley home)	Deobase* Perfume Freon (Freon 11 and 12, 50-50 mixture)		
		AIR-TOX Insecticide (Bonide)	Pyrethrins* 25% Tech. piperonyl butoxide 2% Petroleum distillate* 12.75%
AIR FRESH WITH THE MAGIC WICK Deodorizer (Veltex)		AIR-TREAD For corns (Corn Off)	
AIR-GENE Air deodorant and sanitizer (Bostwick)	Isopropanol* Triethylene glycol* Propylene glycol Essential oils Methyldodecylbenzyl trimethyl ammonium chloride*	AIR WICK Deodorizer (Seeman)	No formaldehyde
		AJAX Abrasive cleaner (Colgate-Palmolive)	
AIRKEM Deodorizer (Airkem)	No formaldehyde	AJAX BUG SPRAY (Aerosol Prod.)	
AIRO-KILL Insecticide (Airosol Co.)	Allethrin (allyl homolog of cinerin 1) 0.100% n-Octyl bicycloheptene dicarboximide .166% Dichloro diphenyl trichloroethane* 1% Methoxychlor tech. 1% Beta-butoxy-beta-thiocyano diethyl ether 1% Methylated aromatic petroleum derivative* 6% Petroleum distillate* 10.7%	AKWAPINE Disinfectant (Selig)	Steam distilled pine oil* Sodium soaps
		ALA For malaria (Wood Chem.)	Quinine sulfate* solution of iron chloride Magnesium sulfate Citric acid
		ALBAGAR WITH PHENOL PHTHALEIN Laxative (McKesson)	Each tsp.: Phenolphthalein 3/4 gr. Mineral oil
AIROSOL Automatic insecticide atomizer (Airosol Co.)	Pyrethrum extract purified (20% pyrethrins) 6% DDT* (Aerosol grade) 2% Solvent 8%	ALABASTINE KALSOMINE (Alabastine)	
AIROSOL Insect repellent bomb (Airosol Co.)	2-Ethylhexanediol-1,3* 20%	ALABASTINE WALL COATINGS (Alabastine)	

*Consult Sec. II., Ingredients Index. This ingredient may be responsible for major toxic effects if poisonous amounts of this product are ingested.

Name & Use Manufacturer	Ingredients	Name & Use Manufacturer	Ingredients
ALABASTINE WALL SIZE (Alabastine)		**ALBATUM** Counter-irritant, analgesic (McKesson)	1-Methyl-3-dimethyl-cyclohexanol-5* Camphor* Eucalyptus* oil Thyme oil* Nutmeg oil Rectified oil of turpentine* Oil of cedar leaf
ALABASTRINE Cuticle cream (Beecham)			
ALABIN Antiseptic, rubefacient (Aseptico)	Menthol Thymol* Eucalyptol* Menthyl-salicylate* Parachlorometaxylenol* Sodium bicarbonate Sodium borate* Sodium chloride	**ALBECA PILLS** Cathartic (Bartz)	Each pill: Ext. belladonna leaves, average 1/16 gr. Total alkaloids 1/1280 gr. Powdered strychnine* 1/120 gr. Aloin Extract cascara sagrada*
ALABIN OINTMENT Rubefacient, counter-irritant (Aseptico)	Menthol Eucalyptol* Synthetic oil of wintergreen* Thymol* Petrolatum Sunbleached white beeswax	**ALBEN PILLS** Laxative (Success)	Each pill: Phenolphthalein 1/2 gr. Aloin* 1/4 gr. Extract of belladonna* (contains 1/2000 gr. total alkaloids) 1/24 gr. American ipecac (Indian physic root) 1/15 gr.
ALADDIN TABLETS For throat irritation (Royal Mfg.)	Benzocaine Menthol* Oil of anise* Cream of tartar	**ALBERTO BRY-TAL** For use with peroxide as aid to better hair bleaching (Alberto-C.)	
ALANAP-1 Herbicide (Naugatuck)	N-1-naphthyl phthalamic acid* 90%	**ALBERTO VO5** Hair and scalp conditioner (Alberto-C)	Lanolin Cholestrol Vital oils
ALANAP-3 Herbicide (Naugatuck)	N-1-naphthyl phthalamic acid 22%	**ALBO** Large white shoe cleaner (Whittemore)	
ALANAP TECHNICAL Insecticide (Naugatuck)	N-1-naphthyl phthalamic acid* 95%	**ALBORUM** Deodorant astringent (Whitehouse)	Boric acid* Potash* alum Carbolic acid* Oil of peppermint
ALARINE (Ca Phenin)	Sodium bicarbonate 5 gr. Table salt 5 gr. Sodium salicylate* 7/24 gr. Menthol Methyl salicylate Sodium borate* 5 gr. Sodium benzoate 7/24 gr. Thymol* Eucalyptol*	**ALBORUM POWDER** For douche, gargle, chafing (Whitehouse)	Boric acid* Potash alum* Carbolic acid* Oil of peppermint
ALASKA DEODORIZED FISH FERTILIZER (Alaska)	Organic nitrogen 4% Ammoniacal nitrogen 1% Total nitrogen 5% Available phosphoric acid 2% Water-soluble potash 2%	**ALBRIGHT NOSE DROPS** (Alma)	
ALBA CREAM Local skin antiseptic (C & M)	Sulfurated potash* 5% Sulfur 5% Zinc oxide 10% Solumol washable base	**AL-CAROID ANTACID POWDER** Gastric antacid (Am.Ferment)	Sodium bicarbonate Calcium carbonate Bismuth subcarbonate Magnesium carbonate Magnesium oxide Papain Aromatics
ALBASULPHIDI Local skin antiseptic (Hartz,J.F.)	Alcohol 1/8 of 1% Each fl. oz.: Zinc sulfide* 8 gr. Zinc sulfate 1 gr. Sulfur precip.* 20 gr. Aromatic oils q.s.	**AL-CAROID ANTACID TABLETS** Gastric antacid (Am.Ferment)	Calcium carbonate Bismuth subcarbonate Magnesium carbonate Magnesium oxide Sodium bicarbonate Papain
ALBATAN For intestinal irritation (Supreme Pharm.)	Each fl. oz.: Tannin albuminate 13.5 gr. Kaolin 90.0 gr. Pectin 2.0 gr.	**ALCHESEAL** Primer sealer & latex under-coater (Bisonite)	

*Consult Sec. II., Ingredients Index. This ingredient may be responsible for major toxic effects if poisonous amounts of this product are ingested.

- 253 -

Name & Use Manufacturer	Ingredients		Name & Use Manufacturer	Ingredients	
ALCOA CRYOLITE Insecticide (Aluminum Co.)	Sodium fluoaluminate* (fluorine equivalent 49%)	90%	ALEPHED (CAPSULES, YELLOW Bronchial antispasmodic, decongestant (Massengill)	Each capsule: Allylphenyl-barbituric acid* Ephedrine sulfate*	3/8 gr. 3/8 gr.
ALCOA SODIUM FLUORIDE Insecticide (Aluminum Co.)	Sodium fluoride*		ALERT FIRE EXTINGUISHER (Am.-La France)		
ALCON-EFRIN Nasal decongestant (Alcon)	Phenylephrine* Benzalkonium chloride*		ALERTON MEDICAL SKIN CREAM (Armand)		
ALCON ISOPTO ALKALINE Ophthalmic emollient (Alcon)	Methyl cellulose	1%	ALERT TABLETS (Duncan)		
ALCON ISOPTO-FRIN Ophthalmic emollient (Alcon)	Methyl cellulose Phenylephrine HC1*	0.5% 1/8%	ALFO CRAB GRASS KILLER (Am. Liquid)	Arsenic pentoxide* Arsenic, all in water soluble form, expressed as metallic Ammonium sulfate	41.4% 27.0% 2.0%
ALCO-REX Rubefacient (Rexall)	Absolute alcohol*	70%	ALFCO FARM AND GARDEN SPRAY Insecticide (Am. Liquid)	DDT (dichloro diphenyl trichloro-ethane) Methyl naphthalenes* Alkyl aromatic amine sulfate Vegetable oil Alkyl phenoxy polyethoxy ethanol Isopropanol Phthalic glycerol alkyd resin Organic solvent	13% 40.3% 19% 18.2% 1.44% 0.36% 6.16% 1.54%
ALCORUB With derma-sep Astringent (Purepac)	Di-isobutyl cresoxy ethoxy ethyl dimethyl benzyl ammonium chloride* Ethyl alcohol* by volume	70%			
ALCOTONE Casein paint (Alcatraz)			ALFCO FERTILIZER (Am. Liquid)		
ALCOVAR Paint (Louisville Varnish)			ALFCO SPIDER SPRAY Insecticide (Am. Liquid)	Methyl naphthalenes Tetraethyl pyrophosphate* Other ethyl phosphates Phthalic glycerol alkyd resin Alkyl phenoxy polyethoxy ethanol Isopropanol	56.5% 12% 18% 6.16% 1.44% 0.36%
ALCYION CARBON BLACK PAINT (Garland)					
ALDIBAC Antiseptic (Greever's)	Alkyl (C_8H_{17} to $C_{18}H_{37}$) dimethyl benzyl ammonium chloride*	10%	ALFOAM FIRE EXTINGUISHER (Am.-La France)		
ALDINE Analgesic, rubefacient (Thomas, W.G.)	Chloroform* Oil of wintergreen* Tincture belladonna Camphor* Menthol Aspirin Alcohol*		ALFRESCO PAINTS (Reardon Co.)		
			ALGETOX Fungicide (Speekman)	Sodium salt of pentachlorophenol*	15%
ALEMITE Lubricating grease (Stewart-Warner)			ALGEX CONCENTRATE Rubefacient (Approved)	Menthol Oil of eucalyptus* Methyl salicylate* Camphor*	
			ALGITABS Cathartic (Barnes-Hind)	Each tablet: Sodium and calcium alginates	0.5 gm.

*Consult Sec. II., Ingredients Index. This ingredient may be responsible for major toxic effects if poisonous amounts of this product are ingested.

Name & Use Manufacturer	Ingredients		Name & Use Manufacturer	Ingredients	
ALGRAN 2 1/2 Insecticide (Chipman Chem.)	Hexachloro hexahydro-endo, exo-dimethano naphthalene*	2.38%	ALKA LITHIA Granular effervescent (Alkalithia)	Effervescent salt of lithium citrate	
ALGRAN 20 Insecticide (Chipman Chem.)	Hexachloro hexahydro-endo exo-dimethano naphthalene*	19%	ALKALOL Oral antiseptic (Alkalol)	Alcohol Thymol* Eucalyptol*	5/100 of 1%
ALIDOL Skin emollient, antiseptic (Bredenbeck)	Calamine Phenol Aluminum hydroxide Menthol* Aromatics* Zinc oxide* Petrolatum Lanolin	0.3%		Menthol Camphor* Benzoin Potassium alum. Potassium chlorate* Sodium bicarbonate Sodium chloride Oils	
ALIPCO PULVOID (S.C. Orange) Cathartic (Drug Prod., N.Y.)	Strychnine sulfate Ext. belladonna leaves Total belladonna alkaloids Phenolphthalein Aloin Podophyllin Ipecac Oleoresin capsicum	0.5 mg. 5.4 mg. 0.06 mg. 32 mg. 13 mg. 4 mg. 4 mg. 2.6 mg	ALKALON ALKALI PROOF PAINT (Heil)		
			ALKAMINTS Digestant, antacid (Jenkins)	Each tablet: Papain Magnesium carbonate Sodium bicarbonate Pancreatin Calcium carbonate Corrective carminatives	
ALIVIOL Analgesic (San Pedro)	Aspirin* Caffeine Phenacetin*				
ALKA-DEX Antacid (Ames Drug)	Bismuth subcarbonate Magnesium carbonate Calcium carbonate Sodium bicarbonate Aromatics		ALKANOS (Hudnut, A.)	Sodium benzoate Eucalyptol Menthol Sodium chloride Sodium carbonate	
ALKAIDS Antacid (Alkaid)	Powdered dextrose Calcium carbonate Magnesium carbonate Magnesium trisilicate		ALKANTIS Antacid (La Fayette)	Cerium oxalate Bismuth subcarbonate Oil of peppermint Calcium carbonate Magnesium carbonate	
ALKA-JETS Antacid (Chilton)	Chlorophyll Calcium carbonate Magnesium carbonate Magnesium trisilicate Essential oils Sugar		ALKARINSE Antiseptic rinse (Massengill)	Each tablet: Sodium bicarbonate Sodium borate* Sodium chloride Sodium benzoate Sodium salicylate Oil eucalyptus Methyl salicylate Thymol Menthol	0.32 gm. 0.32 gm. 0.32 gm. 18.8 mg. 18.8 mg. 0.009 cc. 0.0450 cc. 3.9 mg. 1.4 mg.
ALKALI, LAUNDRY MIL- A-11705 Detergent (Wyandotte)	Concentrated alkali*				
			ALKASTRIP Paint stripper (Whitfield)		
ALKALINE DIGESTANTS Antacid, digestant (Jenkins)	Papain Magnesium carbonate with corrective Carminatives Pancreatin Sodium bicarbonate Calcium carbonate		ALKATONE Analgesic, antacid, cholere- tic, cathartic (Jenkins)	Sodium salicylate* Sodium benzoate Fluid extract cascara aromatic	32 gr. 8 gr. 80 min.
ALKALINE EFFERVES- CENT NO. 16 Digestant, antacid (CaPhenin)	Sodium bicarbonate Papain Pancreatin Jamaica ginger Oil peppermint Tartaric acid	10 gr. 1/2 gr. 1/2 gr.			

*Consult Sec. II., Ingredients Index. This ingredient may be responsible for major toxic effects if poisonous amounts of this product are ingested.

Name & Use Manufacturer	Ingredients	Name & Use Manufacturer	Ingredients
ALKA-VITA TABLETS Antacid (Alka-Vita)	Alum hydroxide Magnesium trisilicate Magnesium oxide Bismuth subcarbonate Dried yeast Dried irradiated yeast Oil of wintergreen flavor Vitamin B$_1$ 3 mg. Vitamin D 435 U.S.P. units	ALLEN'S LUBRICATING OIL (Allen, L.B.)	
		ALLEN'S ULLERINE SALVE For skin irritation (Myers Lab.)	Linseed oil Ethyl abietate Turpentine* Petrolatum Paraffin Oil of tar* Balsam Peru Aluminum stearate Oxyquinoline benzoate
ALKA-ZANE Antacid (Warner-Chilcott)	1 heaping tsp.: Sodium citrate 2.7 gm. Sodium bicarbonate 1.6 gm. Potassium citrate 0.50 gm. Calcium phosphate 0.25 gm. Magnesium phosphate 0.25 gm. Calcium glycerophosphate 0.11 gm.		
		ALLERCREME BODY LOTION Hypo-allergenic (Texas Pharm.)	Cholesterol derivatives of lanolin Mineral oil Sorbitol Triethanolamine stearate Butyl para-hydroxybenzoate Cetyl alcohol
AL-KED ENAMEL (Nat. Paint)			

AL-KOL Astringent (Am. Druggists)	Di-isobutyl cresoxy ethoxy
	  ethyl dimethyl benzyl
	  ammonium chloride*
	Ethyl alcohol* 70%
		ALLERCREME CAKE ROUGE Hypo-allergenic (Texas Pharm.)	Talc
			Precipitated calcium carbonate
			Colloidal kaolin
			Certified colors

		ALLERCREME CLEANSING CREAM Hypo-allergenic (Texas Pharm.)	White beeswax (depollenized) Microcrystalline paraffin Light mineral oil Borax*
ALKRON-4E Insecticide (Eston)	Parathion*(4 lb./gal) 47% Aromatic petroleum solvent 48%		
ALKRON-50E Insecticides (Eston)	Parathion* (4 lb./gal) 41.5%	ALLERCREME CREME ROUGE Hypo-allergenic (Texas Pharm.)	Mineral oil Petrolatum Ozokerite Certified colors
ALKRON-100 Insecticide (Eston)	Parathion*	ALLERCREME DEODORANT CREAM Hypo-allergenic (Texas Pharm.)	Glyceryl monostearate (acid emulsifying) Spermaceti Sorbitol Aluminum chlorhydroxide complex* Butyl para-hydroxybenzoate
ALLANTOIN, 2% Antiseptic ointment (Massengill)	Allantoin 2%		
		ALLERCREME DUSTING POWDER Hypo-allergenic (Texas Pharm.)	Titanium dioxide Light calcium carbonate Colloidal kaolin Purified talc
ALLEN'S ANTACID POW-DER (Tampa)			
ALLEN'S BROWN RAT KILLER (Allen)	Alpha-naphthyl-thiourea* 23%	ALLERCREME FLUFF-CREME SHAMPOO Hypo-allergenic (Texas Pharm.)	Sodium lauryl sulfate Cholesterol derivative of lanolin Butyl para-hydroxybenzoate Sodium stearate Cetyl alcohol
ALLEN'S CEMENT FOR CHINA, CROCK-ERY, GLASS & TILE (Allen, L.B.)		ALLERCREME LIPSTICK Hypo-allergenic (Texas Pharm.)	Castor oil Glyceryl monostearate Candelilla wax Bromo acid Certified colors
ALLEN'S FOOT EASE For skin irrit-ation (United Sales)	Aluminum potassium* sulfate Orthoboric acid* Hydrous magnesium silicate	ALLERCREME LIQUID CLEAN-SER Hypo-allergenic (Texas Pharm.)	Sorbitan monolaurate derivative Acetone Alcohol

*Consult Sec. II., Ingredients Index. This ingredient may be responsible for major toxic effects if poisonous amounts of this product are ingested.

Name & Use Manufacturer	Ingredients	Name & Use Manufacturer	Ingredients
ALLERCREME LIQUID DEODORANT Hypo-allergenic (Texas Pharm.)	Aluminum chlorhydroxide complex* Propylene glycol Alcohol* Non-aniline color (a trace)	ALLERCREME SPECIAL FORMULA LUBRICATING CREAM WITHOUT LANOLIN Hypo-allergenic (Texas Pharm.)	Sorbitol Light mineral oil Petrolatum Cetyl alcohol Sorbitan sesquioleate Triethanolamine stearate Butyl para-hydroxybenzoate Propyl para-hydroxybenzoate
ALLERCREME LUBRICATING CREME WITH LANOLIN Hypo- allergenic (Texas Pharm.)	Sorbitol Light mineral oil Anhydrous lanolin Cetyl alcohol Cholesterol derivatives of lanolin Triethanolamine stearate Butyl para-hydroxybenzoate Propyl para-hydroxybenzoate	ALLERG-ADE EYE DROPS Antihistamine (Binday)	Thenylpyramine* HCl
		ALLERG-ADE NOSE DROPS Antihistamine, decongestant (Binday)	Thenylpyramine* HCl 1/2 fl. oz. Ephedrine* HCl
ALLERCREME MILD ASTRINGENT Hypo-allergenic (Texas Pharm.)	Aluminum chlorhydroxide* complex Propylene glycol Alcohol Certified color (a trace)	ALLERG-ADE TABLETS Antihistamine (Binday)	Pyranisamine maleate*
ALLERCREME NURSERY LOTION Hypo-allergenic (Texas Pharm.)	Triethanolamine stearate Mineral oil Oxycholesterin (lanolin derivatives) Sorbitol Cetyl alcohol	ALLERHIST TABLETS Antihistamine (Pharmex)	Pyrilamine maleate* 25 mg.
ALLERCREME NURSERY POWDER Hypo-allergenic (Texas Pharm.)	Titanium dioxide Corn starch Colloidal kaolin Calcium carbonate Purified talc	ALLEXCEL 20 Insecticide (Penick)	Petroleum distillate* Butoxy ethanol* Di-n-propyl maleate-isosafrole condensate Allethrin (allyl homolog of cinerin 1)
ALLERCREME PETAL LOTION Hypo-allergenic (Texas Pharm.)	Triethanolamine stearate Cetyl alcohol Cholesterol derivatives of lanolin Isopropyl palmitate-myristate Glycerin Butyl para-hydroxybenzoate Propyl para-hydroxybenzoate Certified color (a trace)	ALLIED BRAND ANTISPETIC POWDER Antiseptic (Allied Drug)	Boracic acid* Alum Zinc oxide* Yellow dock
		ALLIED BRAND 20% ANTU BROWN RAT POISON (Allied Drug)	ANTU (alpha naphthyl thiourea)* 20%
ALLERCREME SATIN FINISH MAKE-UP Hypo- allergenic (Texas Pharm.)	Magnesium carbonate Titanium dioxide Candelilla wax Absorption base: Isopropyl palmitate-myristate Butyl stearate Certified colors	ALLIED BRAND AROMATIC SPIRIT OF AMMONIA (Allied drug)	Alcohol* 63% Ammonia*
ALLERCREME SKIN LOTION Hypo-allergenic (Texas Pharm.)	Stearic acid Triethanolamine stearate Cetyl alcohol Cholesterol derivatives of lanolin Mineral oil Glycerin Butyl para-hydroxybenzoate Propyl para-hydroxybenzoate	ALLIED BRAND DAIRY SPRAY Insecticide (Allied Drug)	Pyrethrins 0.032%/w Octyl sulfoxide of isosafrole 0.256%/w Butoxyethanol 0.512%/w B-butoxy-B' thiocyanodiethyl ether 2.200%/w Odorless petroleum distillate* 97%/w
ALLERCREME SOAP (Texas Pharm.)	Olive oil Coconut oil Refined tallow	ALLIED BRAND 50% DDT DUST Insecticide (Allied Drug)	DDT* 50%

*Consult Sec. II., Ingredients Index. This ingredient may be responsible for major toxic effects if poisonous amounts of this product are ingested.

Name & Use Manufacturer	Ingredients		Name & Use Manufacturer	Ingredients	
ALLIED BRAND HOUSEHOLD SPRAY (Allied Drug)	Pyrethrins Octyl sulfoxide of isosafrole Butoxyethanol B-butoxy-B' thiocyanodiethyl ether Odorless petroleum distillate*	0.032%/w 0.256%/w 0.512%/w 2.200%/w 97%/w	ALLIED DRUG DDT RESIDUAL SPRAY Insecticide (Allied Drug)	DDT*	5%
ALLIED BRAND INSECT POW-DER (Allied Drug)	Pyrethrins	0.7%	ALLIED DRUG DDT WETTABLE POWDER Insecticide (Allied Drug)	DDT*	50%
ALLIED BRAND LICE KILLER (Allied Drug)	Sodium fluoride Sulfur Nicotine*	5% 10% 0.7%	ALLIED DRUG MOUTH WASH & DEODOR-ANT GA91 Also for skin irritation (Allied Drug)	Boric acid Menthol Oil of thyme Eucalyptol Methyl salicylate Benzoic acid Alcohol	25%/v
ALLIED BRAND PINE OIL DISINFECTANT Disinfectant, deodorant, cleaner (Allied Drug)	Steam distilled pine oil* Anhydrous soap	80% 10%	ALLIED DRUG ROACH POW-DER (Allied Drug)	Sodium fluoride*	95%
ALLIED BRAND ROACH POW-DER (Allied Drug)	Sodium fluoride*	95%	ALLIED DRUG ROACH POW-DER WITH DDT DUST (Allied Drug)	DDT* Pyrethrins Sesame oil extractives	10% 0.08% 0.30%
ALLIED BRAND SCREW-WORM KILLER SMEAR 62 (Allied Drug)	Benzol* Diphenylamine Turkey red oil	35% 35% 6.8%	ALLIED DURALOX Resurfacing composition for concrete (Allied Comp.)		
ALLIED BRAND XTRA-KILL Residual sur-face spray (Allied Drug)	DDT* B-butoxy B'-thiocyanodiethyl ether B-thiocyanoethyl esters of aliphatic acids containing 10 to 18 carbon atoms Petroleum distillate*	5%/w 0.3%/w 0.9%/w 93.8%/w	ALLIED EYE WATER Ophthalmic local anes-thetic (Allied Drug)	Chlorobutanol (chloroform deriv-ative) each fl. oz. 0.333 gr. Boracic acid* Sodium chloride Sodium borate Methyl para hydroxybenzoate	
ALLIED BRAND XTRA-KILL Emulsion concentrate (Allied Drug)	DDT*	25%/w	ALLIED HOME PRODUCTS MOTH PROOF-ING SPRAY (Allied Home)	Methoxychlor tech.* Petroleum distillates *	5% 26%
ALLIED DRUG CALAMINE LOTION For skin irritations (Allied Drug)	Calamine Zinc oxide Polyethylene glycol P.G. monostearate	36.5 gr. 36.5 gr. 38.5 m. 9.12 gr.	ALLIED MILK OF MAGNESIA Laxative, antacid (Allied Drug)		
ALLIED DRUG DDT CONCEN-TRATE Insecticide (Allied Drug)	DDT*	25%	ALLIED PHARMACAL MOSQUITO LOTION (Allied Pharm.)	Oil of citronella* Lavender* Camphor*	
ALLIED DRUG DDT DUST Insecticide (Allied Drug)	DDT*	50%	ALLIED PRODUCTS DIP AND DISINFECTANT (Allied Drug)		
			ALLIED PRODUCTS EYE WATER (Allied Drug)		

*Consult Sec. II., Ingredients Index. This ingredient may be responsible for major toxic effects if poisonous amounts of this product are ingested.

Name & Use Manufacturer	Ingredients		Name & Use Manufacturer	Ingredients	
ALLIED PRODUCTS INSECTICIDES (Allied Drug)			**ALL-PURPOSE FLOWER & GARDEN DUST** Insecticide, fungicide (Chipman)	Captan Methoxychlor Malathion	5% 3% 4%
ALLIED PRODUCTS LIGHTER FLUID (Allied Drug)			**ALL PURPOSE FRUIT & GARDEN SPRAY** Insecticide, fungicide (Chipman)	Captan Methoxychlor Malathion*	10% 5% 10%
ALLIED PRODUCTS PINE OIL Disinfectant (Allied Drug)			**ALL-SHINE** Shoe Polish (Manhattan Kreole)		
ALLIED SEAL-CRAX CV-7 (Allied Comp.)			**ALL STAR PAINTS** (Chicago Paints)		
ALLIED VAPORTEX Cement Paint (Allied Comp.)			**ALLSTATE MOTOR OIL** (Sears)		
ALLIED VAPORTITE Damp-proof coating for basement walls (Allied Comp.)			**ALLTOX 5 BAIT** Insecticide (Calif.Spray)	Toxaphene*	5%
ALL-OVA Insecticide (Jones Prod.)	DDT*		**ALLTOX CUTWORM BAIT** (Calif.Spray)	Toxaphene*	5%
ALL-O-VAR Paint product (Briggs-Maroney)			**ALLTOX-DDT 8-4 DUST** Insecticide (Calif.Spray)	Toxaphene* DDT*	8% 4%
ALL OVER FLEA POWDER (Dill)	Thiocyanates*		**ALLTOX-DDT 10-10 DUST** Insecticide (Calif.Spray)	Toxaphene* DDT*	10% 10%
ALLOX Antiseptic (Standard Medical)	Boric acid* Alum Sodium chloride Menthol* Sodium borate* Aromatics Oxyquinoline sulfate 1/10 of 1%		**ALLTOX-DDT 15-5 DUST** Insecticide (Calif.Spray)	Toxaphene* DDT	15% 5%
ALL-PLAN Insecticide (Planetary Chem.)	Hexachloro hexahydro dimethano naphthalene* 23.10% Related compounds 17.37% Petroleum hydrocarbons 52.03%		**ALLTOX-DDT-S 8-4-50 DUST** Insecticide (Calif.Spray)	Toxaphene* DDT* Sulfur*	8% 4% 50%
ALL PURPOSE CREAM Cosmetic (Stanley Home)	Water Mineral oil Beeswax (cosmetic grade) Ceresin (cosmetic grade) Stearic acid Triethanolamine Cetyl alcohol Deltyl extra Perfume Tegosept		**ALLTOX-DDT-S 15-5-40 DUST** Insecticide, fungicide (Calif.Spray)	Toxaphene* DDT Sulfur	15% 5% 40%
			ALLTOX-DDT 2-1 SPRAY Insecticide (Calif. Spray)	Toxaphene* DDT* Aromatic petroleum derivative solvent *	39.6% 19.8% 33%

*Consult Sec. II., Ingredients Index. This ingredient may be responsible for major toxic effects if poisonous amounts of this product are ingested.

- 259 -

Name & Use Manufacturer	Ingredients		Name & Use Manufacturer	Ingredients	
ALLTOX DDT 4-2 SPRAY Insecticide (Calif.Spray)	Toxaphene* DDT* Aromatic petroleum derivative* solvent	39.6% 19.8% 36%	ALLTOX-S 20-40 DUST Insecticide (Calif. Spray)	Toxaphene* Sulfur	20% 40%
ALLTOX 7.5 DUST Insecticide (Calif.Spray)	Toxaphene*	7.5%	ALLTOX 4.8 SPRAY Insecticide (Calif.Spray)	Toxaphene* Petroleum distillate	50% 39%
ALLTOX 10 DUST Insecticide (Calif.Spray)	Toxaphene*	10%	ALLTOX 6 SPRAY Insecticide (Calif.Spray)	Toxaphene*	58.5%
ALTOX 15 DUST Insecticide (Calif.Spray)	Toxaphene*	15%	ALLTOX 8 SPRAY Insecticide (Calif.Spray)	Toxaphene*	71%
ALLTOX 20 DUST Insecticide (Calif.Spray)	Toxaphene*	20%	ALLTOX 40 WETTABLE Insecticide (Calif.Spray)	Toxaphene*	40%
ALLTOX 40 MICRO CONCENTRATE Insecticide (Calif.Spray)	Toxaphene*	40%	ALL-WAY COLD CAPS For colds (Pharmex)	Salicylamide* Acetophenetidine* Camphor mono.* Caffeine Phenolphthalein Atropine sulf. Quinine sulf.	1 gr. 1 1/4 gr. 1/2 gr. 1/4 gr. 1/5 gr. 1/1000 gr. 1/4 gr.
ALLTOX-MITE DDT 8-3-4 DUST Insecticide (Calif. Spray)	Toxaphene* Aramite DDT*	8% 3% 4%	ALL-WEATHER PAINT (Continental Prod.)		
ALLTOX-MITE 7.5-3 DUST Insecticide (Calif.Spray)	Toxaphene* Aramite	7.5% 3%	ALLWITE Shoe cleaner, whitener (Griffin)		
ALLTOX-MITE 10-3 DUST Insecticide (Calif. Spray)	Toxaphene* Aramite	10% 3%	ALL-WINTER Anti-freeze compound (All-Winter)		
ALLTOX-MITE 15-3 DUST (Calif.Spray)	Toxaphene* Aramite	15% 3%	ALLYN'S HAIR STRAIGHT CREAM For hair (Allyn)		
ALLTOX-S 7.5-50 DUST Insecticide (Calif. Spray)	Toxaphene* (tech. chlorinated camphene, chlorine content 67%-69%)* Sulfur*	7.5% 50%	ALMAG PULVOID Antacid, adsorbent (Drug Prod., N.Y.)	Aluminum hydroxide Magnesium trisilicate Aromatics	0.5 gm. 0.5 gm.
ALLTOX-S 10-50 DUST Insecticide (Calif.Spray)	Toxaphene* Sulfur	10% 50%	ALMAROL Cathartic (Almar)	Castor oil emulsion	
ALLTOX-S 10-70 DUST Insecticide (Calif.Spray)	Toxaphene* Sulfur	10% 70%	ALMA-TAR OINTMENT Dermatologic therapeutic (Almay)	Juniper tar* Potassium stearate cream Stearin monoglycerol ester Cetyl alcohol Propylene glycol	4%
ALLTOX-S 15-50 DUST Insecticide (Calif. Spray)	Toxaphene* Sulfur	15% 50%			

*Consult Sec. II., Ingredients Index. This ingredient may be responsible for major toxic effects if poisonous amounts of this product are ingested.

Name & Use Manufacturer	Ingredients	Name & Use Manufacturer	Ingredients
ALMA-TAR SHAMPOO (Almay)	Coconut oil 4% Oil of cade* Alkyl aryl polyoxyethylene glycol Triethanolamine* Ethylene diamine tetraacetic acid*	ALMAY HAND CREAM Hypo-allergenic (Almay)	Potassium soap of stearic acid Cetyl alcohol Fatty acid esters Propylene glycol
ALMAY ALMATONE Emollient night cream hypo-allergenic (Almay)	Oxycholesterin Lanolin Spermaceti Petrolatum	ALMAY L.C.D. COMPOUND OINTMENT For contact dermatitis (Almay)	Coal tar solution N.F. (1.2% crude coal tar) 5.83% Menthol 0.1% Lanolin
ALMAY AQUA-LO Hypo-allergenic lotion cleanser (Almay)	Ammonium lauryl sulfate* Magnesium lauryl sulfate* Oleyl alcohol (grain alcohol)* Methyl parasept Propyl parasept	ALMAY L.C.D. SOLUTION Dermatologic therapeutic (Almay)	Crude coal tar* approx. 20%/w Alcohol 85%/v Quillaja
ALMAY CLEANSING OINTMENT Dermatologic therapeutic (Almay)	Potassium hydroxide Stearic acid Stearin monoglycerol ester Cetyl alcohol Propylene glycol	ALMAY LIQUID CLEANSER Hypo-allergenic (Almay)	Sulfated fatty alcohols Oleyl alcohol Methyl parahydroxybenzoate Propyl parahydroxybenzoate
ALMAY COLD CREAM Hypo-allergenic (Almay)	Liquid petrolatum Spermaceti Borax* Depollenized beeswax	ALMAY MAKE READY Cream found-ation Hypo-allergenic (Almay)	Talc Titanium dioxide Petrolatum Stearic acid Cetyl alcohol Polyhydric alcohol Fatty acid ester Sorbitol Triethanolamine Methyl and propyl para-hydroxybenzoate Inorganic pigments
ALMAY DEODORANT Hypo-allergenic (Almay)	Calamine Polyglycol esters Ethyl alcohol Hexachlorophene Oil of lavender		
ALMAY DUSTING POWDER Hypo-allergenic (Almay)	Talc Kaolin Magnesium stearate Titanium dioxide	ALMAY MASCARA Hypo-allergenic (Almay)	Lamp black or brown pigment (iron oxide) Hydrated chromium oxide* Clay Silicates Propylene glycol
ALMAY EYE SHADOW Hypo-allergenic (Almay)	Iron oxides Hydrated chromium oxide* Carmine		
ALMAY FACE POWDER Hypo-allergenic (Almay)	Talc Kaolin Magnesium stearate Titanium dioxide Non-sensitizing inorganic pigments*	ALMAY NAIL POLISH Hypo-allergenic (Almay)	Butyl alcohol* Butyl acetate Ethyl acetate Cellulose nitrate Xylol* Camphor Plasticizer Resin
ALMAY FACE POWDER WITH SULFUR (Almay)	Precipitated sulfur 5% Talc Kaolin Magnesium stearate Titanium dioxide Inorganic pigments*	ALMAY NAIL POLISH REMOVER Hypo-allergenic (Almay)	Oleyl alcohol Isopropyl alcohol* Ethyl acetate Acetone*
ALMAY FOUNDATION LOTION Hypo-allergenic (Almay)	Talc Zinc oxide Neutracolor (brand of Bentonite and oxide of iron powder, Almay) Polyglycol esters Glycerin ethyl alcohol Oil of lavender	ALMAY POWDER BASE Hypo-allergenic (Almay)	Spermaceti Almay face powder (white) Polyhydric alcohol* Fatty acid esters Sorbitol Methyl parahydroxybenzoate Propyl parahydroxybenzoate
ALMAY GREASELESS CREAM Hypo-allergenic skin cleanser (Almay)	Potassium soaps of stearic and oleic acids Propylene glycol		

*Consult Sec. II., Ingredients Index. This ingredient may be responsible for major toxic effects if poisonous amounts of this product are ingested.

Name & Use Manufacturer	Ingredients
ALMAY SHAMPOO Hypo-aller- genic (Almay)	Ammonium lauryl sulfate* Magnesium lauryl sulfate* Oleyl alcohol* Alcohol SD40* Methyl parasept Propyl parasept
ALMAY SKIN FRESHENER Hypo-aller- genic astrin- gent (Almay)	Polyglycol esters Ethyl alcohol* Oil of lavender
ALMAY SKIN LOTION Hypo-aller- genic (Almay)	Stearic acid Polyhydric alcohol Fatty acid esters Triethanolamine Cholesterols Cetyl alcohol Glycerin Ethyl alcohol Methyl parahydroxybenzoate Propyl parahydroxybenzoate
ALMAY SUNBURN PREVENTIVE (Almay)	Tannic acid Salol* Propylene glycol* Ethyl alcohol* Oil of lavender
ALMAY TALCUM POWDER WITH SULFUR (Almay)	Precipitated sulfur 5% Talc Magnesium stearate Titanium dioxide Bentonite Iron oxide pigments
ALMAY WAVE SET Hypo-aller- genic (Almay)	Algin Glycerin Propylene glycol* Methyl parahydroxybenzoate
ALMAY ZIRCAL CREAM Dermatologic therapeutic (Almay)	Hydrous zirconium oxide 4% Merbak (2-acetoxy mercuri-4-di- isobutylphenol) 0.1% Ethyl aminobenzoate 1.0% Calamine Bentonite Menthol 0.2% Propylene glycol
ALMEDERM ANTISEPTIC (Meyer)	Hexachlorophene 1%
ALMEGESIC Analgesic, antihistamine (Meyer & Co.)	Each tablet: Pyrilamine maleate 25 mg. Hyoscyamine hydrobromide 0.04 mg. Hyoscine hydrobromide 0.008 mg. Aspirin* 3.5 gr. Phenacetin* 2.5 gr. Caffeine 0.5 gr.
ALMELOSE Laxative (Meyer & Co.)	Each tablet: Sodium carboxymethyl cellulose 0.5 gm.
ALMINATE Antacid (Bristol Lab.)	Dihydroxy aluminum aminoacetate
ALMKLOV'S ITCH SPECIFIC (Almklov)	
ALMOLINE BALM (Almoline)	

Name & Use Manufacturer	Ingredients
ALMYCIL SOLUTION 1% Local fungicide (Meyer)	2, 4, 5-Trichlorophenol (special grade) 1% Alcohol* 56% Propylene glycol*
ALOE OINTMENT For skin burns (Better Way)	Aloe vera* 55-60% Petrolatum-lanolin
ALOE SKIN THERAPY Emollient, rubefacient (Better Way)	Aloe vera* 60% Petrolatum-lanolin
ALOHA COLOGNES AND PER- FUMES (Tattoo)	
ALOMAN PILLS Cathartic (Evert's)	Aloin* Belladonna extract* Powdered ipecac Podophyllin Phenolphthalein Strychnine sulfate* 1/20 gr./pill
ALOMIN Antacid, adsorbent (Lilly)	Kaolin 24 gm. Aluminum hydroxide 24 gm. Calcium carbonate 16 gm. Bismuth subcarbonate 16 gm. Sodium chloride 3 gm. Arcacia 6 gm. Aromatics q.s. Dextrose q.s. to make 100 gm.
ALOPHEN PILLS Cathartic (Parke, Davis)	Aloin 1/4 gr. Extract belladonna* (1/1920 gr. total alkaloids) 1/24 gr. Powdered ipecac 1/15 gr. Phenolphthalein* 1/2 gr.
ALOX 707 Rust preventive (Alox)	Lead* Mixed organic acids
ALPACO PAINT THINNER (Allied Paint)	Petroleum hydro carbon* Pine oil* Turpene* derivatives
ALPHA CHALKBOARD CHALK (Weber Costello)	Calcium carbonate 95% Vegetable binder 5%
ALPHACOLOR BRILLIANTS Art material (Weber Costello)	Earth oxides or non-toxic organic pigments
ALPHACOLOR CHALK PASTELS (Weber Costello)	Earth oxides or non-toxic organic pigments
ALPHACOLOR DRY TEMPERA Art material (Weber Costello)	Earth oxides or non-toxic organic pigments

*Consult Sec. II., Ingredients Index. This ingredient may be responsible for major toxic effects if poisonous amounts of this product are ingested.

- 262 -

Name & Use Manufacturer	Ingredients
ALPHASITE CHALKBOARD CHALK (Weber Costello)	Calcium carbonate 95% Vegetable binder 5%
ALPROCOLS (Rectal suppository) For hemorrhoids (Drug Prod., N.Y.)	Aluminum acetate Acid benzoic Ichthammol Ergotin Nutgall Ext. belladonna (total 4 mg. belladonna alkaloids 1/1250 gr.) Ext. stramonium leaves 16 mg. (total stramonium alkaloids* 1.380 gr.) Procaine hydrochloride 16 mg. Mentholated cocoa butter Aromatic oils
ALSCO METAL POLISH (Antiseptal)	
ALSIZBRONZ PAINT PIGMENT (Franklin Mineral)	
ALTERNATIVE PILLS Dog prep. (Clayton)	
ALTERNATIVE TABLETS Cat prep. (Clayton)	
ALTON'S FORMULA FOR HAIR & SCALP (Alton)	
ALUCAINE Skin ointment (Jenkins)	Benzocaine 5% Carbolic acid* 1.39% Ichthammol 1.39% Balsam Peru 0.46% Exsiccated alum 3.7% Oil cade Oil eucalyptus
ALUCAINE SUPPOSITORIES (Rectal) (Jenkins)	Benzocaine Ephedrine* Carbolic acid Powdered nutgall Desiccated alum
ALUDROX Antacid tablets (Wyeth Lab.)	Each tablet: Aluminum hydroxide gel 1 tsp. Milk of magnesia 1/4 tsp.
AL-U-JEL Antacid (Horton & Converse)	Each tablet: Dried aluminum hydroxide gel U.S.P. 10 gr.
ALUMIKOTE PAINT (Vita-Var)	
ALUMINALL PAINT (Kepec)	
ALUMIN-NU LIQUID (NuSteel)	Refined petroleum oil Vegetable oil soap Pine oil* Tripoli powder

Name & Use Manufacturer	Ingredients
ALUMINUM FINISH WOOD PRESERVATIVE (Smith-Alsop)	Copper naphthanate 18.50% Aluminum powder 3.10%
ALUMINUM HYDROXIDE GEL Antacid, adsorbent (Lilly)	Aluminum hydroxide
ALUMINUM PAINT 91033 (General Paint Okla.)	
ALUMINUM PAINTS (Pittsburgh Plate Glass Paint Div.)	
ALUMIN-NU PASTE (NuSteel)	Refined petroleum oil Stearic acid Ammonia Tripoli powder
ALURT TABLETS (Baker, W.A.)	
ALVARLAC Shellac sub. (Stille-Young)	
AL-VI-CO Decongestant, antispasmodic (Richard Drug)	Ephedrine sulfate 1% Potassium iodide*
ALVCO AMERLITH Varnish (Am. Lithog.)	
AL-X PAINT (Studebaker)	
AMACENE Seed protectant (Pearson & Co.)	Mercury pentanedione* not less than 5.0%
AMACO ARTISTS' PASTELS (Am. Art Clay)	
AMACO CASTING COMPOUND (Am. Art Clay)	
AMACO CHALK For blackboards (Am. Art Clay)	
AMACO CLAY Artists' material (Am. Art Clay)	
AMACO CLAY FLOUR (Am. Art Clay)	
AMACO COLORFAST FABRIC PAINT (Am. Art Clay)	

*Consult Sec. II., Ingredients Index. This ingredient may be responsible for major toxic effects if poisonous amounts of this product are ingested.

Name & Use Manufacturer	Ingredients	Name & Use Manufacturer	Ingredients
AMACO CRAYONS (Am. Art Clay)		AMBASSADOR PAINT BRUSH CLEANER (Ambassador)	
AMACO FINGER PAINT (Am. Art Clay)		AMBASSADOR PAINT & VARNISH CLEANER (Ambassador)	
AMACO GLAZE SURFACER (Am. Art Clay)		AMBERLAC HAIR LACQUER (Lustray)	
AMACO MODELING & DECORATING KIT (Am. Art Clay)		AMBER LION Dandruff remover (Amber Lion)	Boric acid* Potassium carbonate Tincture of benzoin Glycerin Brucine sulfate* Alcohol 42%
AMACO POWDERED TEMPERA (Am. Art Clay)		AMBER LIQUID Fungicide, keratolytic (Kinreco)	Metaphen (mercurial derivative) 0.0038% Ethyl alcohol* 65%/v Salicylic acid*
AMACO SCHOOL PASTELS (Am. Art Clay)		AMBERLYTE PAINT (Martin Varnish)	
AMACO SEMI-MOIST WATER COLORS (Am. Art Clay)		AMBER SUN TAN CREAM (Van-S)	Stearic acid triple pressed U.S.P. Glyceryl monostearate Propylene glycol U.S.P. Methyl para-hydroxy benzoate Mineral oil U.S.P. Lanolin U.S.P. Homo menthyl salicylate* Isobutyl para-amino benzoate
AMACO SHOWCARD COLORS (Am. Art Clay)			
AMAGLAZE COMPOUNDS (Am. Asbestos)		AMBEST General purpose cleaner (Apex Chem.)	Tri-sodium phosphate Sodium carbonate Sodium bicarbonate Complex sodium phosphates Pine oil Butyl cellosolve Wetting agents of alkyl aryl sulfonate type
AMALGAMATED PAINTS (Amalg. Paint)			
AMANIZE PAINT For galvanized metal (Am. Asbestos)			
AMATONE PAINTS (Am. Asbestos)		AMBRITE CHALK CRAYON (Am. Crayon)	
AMAZA PAINT (Lancaster Paint)		AMBROID CEMENT Nitrocellulose- based adhesive (Ambroid)	Camphor* Aniline dye* Alcohols* Ketones* Aromatic hydrocarbons*
AMAZOL ANTISEPTIC (Amazol)		AMBROSIA CLEANER (Hinze)	
AMAZOL OINTMENT (Amazol)		AMBROSIA COLOGNE (Hinze)	
AMBASSADOR DRAIN PIPE & TRAP CLEANER (Ambassador)		AMBROSIA TIGHTENER Astringent (Hinze)	
AMBASSADOR KALSOMINE (Ambassador)		A-MEAN WEED KILLER (Planetary Chem.)	Dimethylamine salt of 2, 4- dichlorophenoxyacetic acid* 49.4%

*Consult Sec. II., Ingredients Index. This ingredient may be responsible for major toxic effects if poisonous amounts of this product are ingested.

- 264 -

Name & Use Manufacturer	Ingredients
AMEND DUAL PURPOSE FACE CREAM (Amend)	White wax Solid alboline White mineral oil Borax*
AMEND SKIN LOTION (Amend)	Stearic acid Mineral oil Lanolin anhydrous Cetyl alcohol Quince seed solution Triethanolamine
AMEND SUN TAN LOTION (Amend)	Stearic acid Menthyl salicylate* Mineral oil Triethanolamine Lanolin hydrous
AMERICAINE OINTMENT Antiseptic, local anesthetic (Arnar-Stone)	Benzocaine Oxyquinoline benzoate Glycols
AMERICAN AGRICULTURAL POTATO POWDER NO. 1 Fungicide (Am. Agric. Chem.)	Arsenate* Copper* Lime
AMERICANA INTERIOR FLAT WALL PAINT (du Pont)	
AMERICANA SPICE BERRY SHAVE LOTION (Lustray)	
AMERICAN BEAUTY ENAMELS (Armstrong Paint)	
AMERICAN BEAUTY HAIR TONIC (Odell)	
AMERICAN CHEMICAL WEED KILLER 566 (Am. Chemical)	Sodium salt of 2, 4-Dichloro-phenoxyacetic acid, butyl ester* 39.2%
AMERICAN CHEMICAL WEED KILLER 650 (Am. Chemical)	2, 4-Dichlorophenoxyacetic acid, isopropyl ester* 45%
AMERICAN CYANAMID MALATHON 4% DUST Insecticide (Am. Cyan.)	Malathon* (malathion) 4%

Name & Use Manufacturer	Ingredients
AMERICAN CYANAMID MALATHON EMULSIFIABLE LIQUID Insecticide (Am. Cyan.)	Malathon* (malathion) 57% Xylene* 32%
AMERICAN CYANAMID MALATHON TECHNICAL Insecticide (Am. Cyan.)	Malathon (malathion)* 95%
AMERICAN CYANAMID MALATHON 25% WETTABLE POWDER Insecticide (Am. Cyan.)	Malathion (malathion)*, 0, 0-dimethyl dithiophosphate of diethyl mercaptosuccinate 25%
AMERICAN EMBALMING FLUID (Am. Fluid)	
AMERICAN FERMENT CAROID & BILE SALTS (Am. Ferment)	Ext. nux vomica* (strychnine 1/217 gr.) Phenolphthalien* Bile salts comp. Ext. cascara sagrada Capsicum Caroid (digestive ferment of carcia papaya)
AMERICAN FERMENT CAROID & CHARCOAL Antacid, carminative (Am. Ferment)	Sodium bicarbonate Activated charcoal Caroid Aromatics
AMERICAN FERMENT CAROID & DIASTASE Digestant (Am. Ferment)	Sodium bicarbonate Diastase Caroid Aromatics
AMERICAN FERMENT CAROID PLAIN TABLETS Digestant (Am. Ferment)	Caroid 1-1/2 gr. Aromatics q.s.
AMERICAN FERMENT CAROID POWDER Digestant (Am. Ferment)	Digestive enzyme from carica papaya
AMERICAN FERMENT CAROID & SODA BICARB. Antacid (Am. Ferment)	Sodium bicarbonate Caroid Aromatics
AMERICAN FUMIGATING AGRI-SPRAY Insecticide (Am. Ferment)	Rotenone*

*Consult Sec. II., Ingredients Index. This ingredient may be responsible for major toxic effects if poisonous amounts of this product are ingested.

Name & Use Manufacturer	Ingredients	Name & Use Manufacturer	Ingredients
AMERICAN GREASE STICK DOOR-EASE Lubricant (Am. Grease Stick)	Microcrystalline waxes Carnauba wax Motor oil	AMES S-L-P TABLETS Sedative (Ames Drug)	Each tablet: Ext. valerian Ext. sumbul Ext. Jamaica dogwood Sodium bromide 7 gr.
AMERICAN LUSTRE PAINT FINISH (Am. Floor)		AMEXO ROOF COATING (Am. Marietta)	
AMERICAN LYE (Penn. Salt.)	Sodium hydroxide*	AMFEX INHALER Nasal astringent (Approved)	Amphetamine* racemic (dl-alpha-methyl phenyl- ethylamine 250 mg. Menthol 12.5 mg.
AMERICAN PENTRA-SEAL FINISH (Am. Floor)		A/M FLY SPRAY (Aero-San.)	Petroleum oil* Piperonyl butoxide tech. Pyrethrins
AMERICAN SERUM DEHORNING PASTE (Am. Serum)		AMFRECIN Douche powder (Amfre)	Sodium lauryl sulfate Lactose Papain Citric acid Methyl salicylate* Menthol*
AMERICAN SERUM LOUSE & TICK POWDER (Am. Serum)		AMICIDE Disinfectant (Watters)	Alkyl dimethyl-benzyl ammonium chloride*
AMERICAN SERUM POULTRY WORM TABLETS (Am. Serum)		AMIDAL Veterinary (Inorganic)	Iodine * 5%
AMERICAN SERUM SODIUM FLUORIDE (Am. Serum)	Sodium fluoride*	AMIDOL Photographic supply (General Photo.)	
		AMILINK INK (General Printing)	
AMERICAN SERUM WORM OIL (Am. Serum)		AMINECTIN POWDER Antacid, adsorbent (Veltex)	Gastric mustic 10 gr. Aminoacetic acid 4.5 gr. Magnesium trisilicate 30 gr. Pectin 2 gr. Aluminum hydroxide gel dried, U.S.P. 31.25 gr. Kaolin colloidal, N.F. 194.50 gr.
AMEROID CARBURETOR & PARTS CLEANER (Drew, E.F.)	Coal tar distillates* Petroleum solvents* Corrosion inhibitors Detergents Chlorinated hydrocarbons*	AMINE WEED KILLER NO. 40 (Pittsburgh Coke)	Dimethylamine salt of 2, 4- dichlorophenoxy acetic acid* 49.4%
AMERSE Germicide (Vestal)	Quaternary ammonium salt 5-gm. tablet: Di-isobutyl cresoxy ethoxy ethyl dimethyl benzyl ammonium chloride monohydrate* 30%	AMINE WEED KILLER NO. 60 (Pittsburgh Coke)	Dimethylamine salt of 2, 4- dichlorophenoxy acetic acid* 69.8%
AMERTAN Antiseptic ointment for burns (Lilly)	Tannic acid 5% Merthiolate* 1-5000	AMINO-FERRO Hematic tonic (Pedrick)	Each oz.: Aminoacetic acid (glycocoll) 2 gm. Ferrous sulfate 775 mg. Sodium glycerophosphate 337 mg. Thiamine hydrochloride 12 mg. Niacin 50 mg. Riboflavine 2 mg.
AMES G-P TABLETS Analgesic (Ames Drug)	Acetophenetidin* 2-1/2 gr. Aspirin* Caffeine		
AMES I-Z-E For eye irritation (Ames Drug) irritation (Ames Drug)	Antipyrine Ephedrine* Sodium borate* Boric acid* Camphor* Sodium chloride Benzalkonium chloride*	AMINO-MOR SOLUBLE For prevention and control of blackhead in turkeys. Use in drinking water (Hilltop)	2-Amino-5-nitrothiazole* 45%

*Consult Sec. II., Ingredients Index. This ingredient may be responsible for major toxic effects if poisonous amounts of this product are ingested.

Name & Use Manufacturer	Ingredients	
AMITONE Antacid (Norex)	Calcium carbonate Glycerine	
AMLEX Laxative (Amlex)	Karaya gum Senna leaves	
AMMENS MEDICATED POWDER For minor skin irritations (Bristol-Myers)	Zinc oxide Boric acid* Starch Talc 8-hydroxyquinolin Aromatic oils	
AMM-I-DENT Chlorophyll Toothpaste (Amm-I-Dent)	Glycerine	10%
	Carboxymethylcellulose	1%
	Soluble saccharin	0.23%
	Aminoacetic acid	0.34%
	Urea	13%
	Sorbitol syrup	10%
	Calcium phosphate and carbonate	45%
	Alkyl sarcosinate	1.7%
	Sodium copper chlorophyllin solution	0.15%
	Methyl and propyl parahydroxybenzoate	0.1%
AMMATE WEED & BRUSH KILLER (du Pont)	Ammonium sulfamate*	
A/M MILL SPRAY Insecticide (Aero-San.)	Petroleum distillate* N-Octylbicycloheptene dicarboximide (264) Allethrin (allyl homolog of cinerin 1)	
AMMO Cleaner (Sapolio)		
AMMONIATED TOOTHPASTE (Comfort)	Glycerine C.P. Gum Detergent Saccharin Urea Dibasic ammonium phosphate Dicalcium phosphate Tricalcium phosphate	
AMNIZOL SOLUBLE For intestinal and liver irritation (veterinary) (Gland-O-Lac)	2-Amino-5-nitrothiazole*	45%
AMOCAL NO. 1 Antitussive (Jenkins)	Each tablet: Glycyrrhiza compound (no opium)	30 m.
	Powdered ipecac	1/16 gr.
	Ammonium chloride	1 gr.
	Iodized calcium	1/2 gr.
	Extract licorice and cane sugar base	
AMOCAL NO. 2 Antitussive (Jenkins)	Each tablet: Glycyrrhiza compound (no opium)	30 m.
	Powdered ipecac	1/16 gr.
	Ammonium chloride	1 gr.
	Iodized calcium	1/2 gr.
	Benzocaine	1/4 gr.
	Extract licorice and cane sugar base	

Name & Use Manufacturer	Ingredients	
AMOCAL JR. Antitussive (Jenkins)	Each tablet: Glycyrrhiza compound (no opium)	30 m.
	Powdered ipecac	1/16 gr.
	Ammonium chloride	1/4 gr.
	Iodized calcium	1/16 gr.
	Ext. licorice and cane sugar base	
AMOCO DRY CLEANER COMPOUND (Am. Oil)		
AMOCO LIGHTER FLUID (Am. Oil)		
AMOUR SAUVAGE PERFUMES (Ybry)		
AMPHOJEL Suspension and tablets Antacid (Wyeth Labs.)	2 types of alumina gels, equivalent to 4% aluminum oxide	
AMPOLEX Adhesive (Aircraft)	Inert filler material Thermo-plastic resin	
AMPOLLINA AEROSOL INSECT BOMB Insecticide (Baribeau)	Pyrethrins	0.15%
	Piperonyl butoxide	1.2%
	DDT	2.0%
AMPOLLINA EMULSION (Baribeau)	DDT*	25%
	Emulsifier	7-1/2%
	Solvent*	67-1/2%
AMPOLLINA OIL SPRAY Insecticide (Baribeau)	DDT*	5%
	Solvent E-407	10%
	Thanite	2%
	Varsol* 3139	83%
AMPOLLINA WETTABLE POWDER Insecticide (Baribeau)	DDT*	10%
	Decallite white filler	60%
	Silica 200 meshes	30%
AM-REN For skin irritation (Carma)	Zinc oxide* Camphor* Phenol* Menthol* Alum Lanolin and petrolatum base	
A.M.R. LIGHTER FLUID (A-M-R)		
A.M.R. MOTHPROOFING (A-M-R)		
A/M ROACH SPRAY (Aero-San.)	Petroleum oil* Piperonyl butoxide tech. Pyrethrins*	

*Consult Sec. II., Ingredients Index. This ingredient may be responsible for major toxic effects if poisonous amounts of this product are ingested.

Name & Use Manufacturer	Ingredients
A.M.R. WONDER DRY CLEANING COMPOUND (A-M-R)	
AMSCO ANTI-FREEZE COMPOUND (Amsco)	
AMSCO STA Anti-freeze (Amsco)	Methanol*
A M SOLUTION Fungicide (medical, external) (Kenton)	Alcohol 64.6% Acid salicylic* Acid benzoic Hydroxy methyl-butyl-benzene Tea tree oil Menthol
AMTABS Cathartic (Cowley Pharm.)	Natural leaf senna 5 gr. Senna ext. 1 gr. Cassia fistula (the ripe fruit) Tamarinds Figs Prunes Dates Apples St. Johns bread
AMYTHOL Poultry inhalant (Whitmoyer)	Steam distilled pine oil* Oil of eucalyptus Creosote U.S.P. (containing guaiacol) Camphor* Menthol
A-M-T TABLETS Gastric antacid (Wyeth Labs.)	Each tablet: Aluminum hydroxide gel 0.15 gm. Magnesium trisilicate 0.25 gm.
AMVETLA Veterinary drug (Am. Vet.)	
ANA-AMID SOLUTION (Thompson Chem.)	Naphthylacetamide
ANACAINE OINTMENT Topical anesthetic (Gordon Labs.)	Benzocaine 10%
ANACIN ANALGESIC TABLETS (Whitehall)	Acetophenetidin* 3 gr./tablet Aspirin* Caffeine*
ANADEX SULFA-KAPS For intestinal irritation (veterinary) (Holt)	Each: Sulfathiazole 1 gm. Vitamin A (from fish liver oil) 12,500 U.S.P. units
ANAGAINE Analgesic, antipyretic (Massengill)	Each capsule: Acetophenetidin* 0.22 gm. Atropine sulfate* 0.2 mg. Aspirin* (acetylsalicylic acid) 0.3 gm. Caffeine 30 mg.
ANAGILL (Liquid) Analgesic (Massengill)	Each 5 cc.: Aspirin* 6-2/3 gr. Caffeine 1/3 gr. Tinct. gelsemium 1-1/3 m. Aromatics q.s.
ANAHIST TABLETS Antihistamine (Anahist)	Thonzylamine HC1* 25 mg.
ANALGEMUL Rubefacient, counter-irritant (Tilden)	Methyl salicylate* (synthetic) Camphor* Menthol*
ANALGESIC EMBROCA-TION Rubefacient, counter-irritant (Clapp, Otis)	Menthol* Methyl salicylate* Oleo resin of capsicum
AN-AL-JEE Rubefacient (Erie)	Methyl salicylate* Menthol* Lanolin
ANAPAC TABLETS Antihistamine analgesic (Rexall)	Pyrilamine maleate* 25 mg. Aspirin* 3-1/2 gr. Phenacetin* 2-1/2 gr. Caffeine 1/2 gr.
ANATOLE ROBBINS AMARANTH OIL (Robbins, A.)	
ANATOLE ROBBINS AUTUMN LEAVES PERFUME (Robbins, A.)	
ANATOLE ROBBINS BATH OIL (Robbins, A.)	
ANATOLE ROBBINS BODY POWDERS (Robbins, A.)	
ANATOLE ROBBINS CLEANSING CREAMS (Robbins, A.)	
ANATOLE ROBBINS COLOGNES AND PERFUMES (Robbins, A.)	
ANATOLE ROBBINS COSMETIC LOTIONS (Robbins, A.)	
ANAYODIN Antiseptic for amebiasis (Ames Co.)	Chiniofon 0.25 gm. Iodine* 26.5-29.0%

*Consult Sec. II., Ingredients Index. This ingredient may be responsible for major toxic effects if poisonous amounts of this product are ingested.

Name & Use Manufacturer	Ingredients	
ANBESOL Antiseptic, anesthetic (Anbesol)	Alcohol* Benzocaine Phenol Iodine	70% 280 gr./gal. 90 gr./gal.
ANCHOR CALF SCOUR COMPOUND For intestinal irritation (veterinary) (Anchor Serum)	Per fl. oz.: Sulfaguanidine U.S.P. Sulfathiazole U.S.P. Kaolin Bismuth subcarbonate U.S.P. Pectin	10 gr. 10 gr. 80 gr. 5.2 gr. 4 gr.
ANCHOR GREEN Skin antiseptic (Anchor Serum)	Camphor Cresol Tannic acid Isopropyl alcohol* Acetone Malachite green and water	1.0% w/v 0.85% w/v 1.0% w/v 60.0% v/v 4.0% w/v q.s.
ANCHOR GROUND GLUE (Cudahy)	Animal protein Sodium pentachlorophenate* Zinc sulfate*	
ANCHOR GWY-KREE For intestinal irritation (veterinary) (Anchor Serum)	Guaiacol* Cresol* Camphor Oils of eucalyptus and pine	10% w/v 10% w/v 1% w/v
ANCHOR SERUM BLOOD STOPPER Anti-hemorrhagic (veterinary) (Anchor Serum)	Ferrous sulfate* Potassium alum Diphenylamine Talc	84.0% 6.0% 1.0% 9.0%
ANCHOR SERUM CATTLE PURGE POWDER (Anchor Serum)	Each 6 oz.: Nux vomica* Barium chloride* Tartar emetic* Gamboge Salt	25 gr. 150 gr. 25 gr. 20 gr. q.s.
ANCHOR SERUM E.Q. 335 Veterinary (Anchor Serum)	Gamma isomer of benzene hexachloride (from lindane)* Pine oil*	3% 35%
ANCHOR SERUM HOG WORMER (Anchor Serum)	Sodium fluoride*	227 gm.
ANCHOR SERUM PHENOTHIAZINE DRENCH Veterinary (Anchor Serum)	Phenothiazine N.F.*	38.70%/w
ANCHOR SERUM PINKEYE POWDER Veterinary (Anchor Serum)	Tyrothricin Proflavine hydrochloride Phenacaine hydrochloride Sulfathiazole* Sulfanilamide*	0.05% 0.1% 1.0% 20.0% 78.85%
ANCHOR SERUM UDDER OINTMENT (Anchor Serum)	Oil eucalyptus* Phenol Methyl salicylate* Camphor Lanolin-petrolatum	
ANCHOR SERUM WOUND DRESSING POWDER Veterinary (Anchor Serum)	Phenol Sulfathiazole Sulfanilamide Starch Urea	1.0% 1.0% 5.0% 5.0% 88.0%
ANCHOR SMEAR 62 Antiseptic (veterinary) (Anchor Serum)	Diphenylamine* Benzol* Lamp black Turkey red oil	35% w/v 35% w/v 20% w/v 10% w/v
ANCHOR WALL SIZE (Cudahy)		
ANCHOR WOUND DRESSING LOTION Antiseptic (Anchor Serum)	Phenol* U.S.P. Tannic acid Methyl violet Isopropyl alcohol*	2.0% w/v 4.0% w/v 0.4% w/v 37.5% v/v
ANCLICIDE, NO. 1 Anthelmintic (veterinary) (Massengill)	Each perle: Parabis* (2,2' methylene-bis (p-chlorophenol)) Methylbenzene*	1 gm. 1.2 gm.
ANCLICIDE, NO. 2 Anthelmintic (veterinary) (Massengill)	Each perle: Parabis* (2,2' methylene-bis (p-chlorophenol)) Methylbenzene*	0.25 gm. 0.30 gm.
ANDALUSIA EAU DE PARFUME (Harris, B.)		
ANDERSEN'S BRUSH TREET Paint brush cleaner (Andersen)	Stoddard's solvent*	
ANDERSEN'S LIQUID WALLPAPER REMOVER (Andersen)	Detergent	
ANDERSEN'S RE-FINIS-HR Floor cleaner (Andersen)	Bleach	
ANDERSEN'S WOOD REPLACER (Andersen)		
ANDERSEN'S ZIP-OFF Paint remover (Andersen)	Methylene chloride* (paint-remover grade) Methanol*	
ANDICAL CREAM LOTION (Andical)		
AN-DU-SEPTIC COLORED CHALK (Binney & Smith)	Levigated whiting Pigments	

---

*Consult Sec. II., Ingredients Index. This ingredient may be responsible for major toxic effects if poisonous amounts of this product are ingested.

Name & Use Manufacturer	Toxicity	Ingredients	Name & Use Manufacturer	Toxicity	Ingredients
AN-DU-SEPTIC DUSTLESS SIGHT SAVER CRAYON (Binney & Smith)			ANESTOL LINIMENT Analgesic, counter-irritant (Norwich)		Methyl salicylate* synthetic Menthol* Alcohol* 64%
AN-DU-SEPTIC WHITE CHALK (Binney & Smith)		Levigated whiting	ANGEL SKIN HAND CREAM (Pond's Extr.)		
ANDY LOTSHAW ALL-PURPOSE BODY RUB Liniment (Lotshaw)		Triethanolamine Mineral oil Stearic acid Carbitol* Menthol* Oxyquinoline sulfate*	ANILINK KLEENSOLVE Solvent (General Printing)		
ANDICAL SCALP LOTION (Andical)			ANIMAL KOPERTOX Fungicide, external (veterinary) (Kopertox)		Copper naphthenate*
ANDREWS AFTER-SHAVE LOTION (Lady Andres)			ANIMAL REGULATOR Veterinary (Pratt Food, Phila.)		Manganese sulfate Potassium iodide Iron sulfate Copper sulfate Oxide of iron Salt Cobalt carbonate 200 mesh limestone flour (calcium and magnesium carbonate) Irradiated yeast Zinc sulfate
ANDREWS FACE AND HAND LOTION (Lady Andres)					
ANDREWS LILAC HAIR LOTION (Lady Andres)			ANNAPOLIS HAIR TONIC (Assoc. Brands)		
ANDREWS MEDICATED CREAM (Lady Andres)			ANN HAVILAND PERFUMES AND TOILET WATERS (Haviland, A.)		
ANDREWS SAGE AND SULPHUR HAIR CREAM (Lady Andres)			ANOCOMP Analgesic (Cowley Pharm.)		Aspirin* 2 gr. Phenacetin* 1 gr. Tr. Gelsemium 1 m. Caffeine citrate 1/10 gr. Phenobarbital 1/40 gr. Soluble saccaharin 1/10 gr.
AND ROL Liquid detergent (Kent Chem.)		Alkyl aryl sulfonate Lanolin	ANODYNE JR. Analgesic (Jenkins)		Each tablet: Acetophenetidin 1/2 gr. Caffeine alkaloid 1/10 gr. Sodium bicarbonate 1/5 gr. Ammonium carbonate 1/32 gr. Ext. licorice 1 gr. Oil anise "star" q.s.
ANESTOL CREAM Analgesic, counter-irritant (Norwich)		Methyl salicylate* synthetic Menthol*	ANOGESIC Rubefacient, counter-irritant (Carroll Chem.)		Alcohol* 70% Methyl salicylate* Menthol* Camphor* Thymol* Eucalyptol Capsicum
			ANOLINE OINTMENT (Carbozine)		

Name & Use Manufacturer	Ingredients	
ANSAC (coated brown) Cardiac preparation and diuretic (Massengill)	Digitalin*, German process	1/50 gr.
	Ext. oxydendron arboreum (sourwood)	1/2 gr.
	Ext. sambucus canadensis (elder flower)	1/2 gr.
	Squillin (conc.)	1/4 gr.
	Sparteine sulfate	1/4 gr.
ANSAC (coated brown) Cardiac stimulant (Massengill	Each tablet: Digitalin*	1/50 gr.
	Ext. oxydendron arboreum (sourwood)	1/2 gr.
	Ext. sambucus canadensis (elder flower)	1/2 gr.
	Squillin (conc.)	1/4 gr.
	Sparteine sulfate	1/4 gr.
ANSCO ARDOL Photographic supply (Ansco)		
ANSCO COLOR PRINTING Photographic supply (Ansco)		
ANSCO PERMADOL Photographic supply (Ansco)		
ANSCO VIVIDOL Photographic supply (Ansco)		
ANSEMCO, NO. 1, Pink Analgesic (Massengill)	Each capsule: Acetophenetidin*	0.15 gm.
	Aspirin (acetylsalicylic acid)*	0.23 gm.
	Caffeine	30 mg.
ANSEMCO, NO. 1, Green, gray or white Analgesic (Massengill)	Each tablet: Acetophenetidin*	0.165 gm.
	Acetylsalicylic acid*	0.23 gm.
	Caffeine	32 mg.
ANSEMCO, NO. 4 (for children) Pink Analgesic (Massengill)	Each tablet: Acetophenetidin*	65 mg.
	Acetylsalicylic acid*	0.13 gm.
	Caffeine	8 mg.
ANSEMCO, NO. 7, Yellow Analgesic, cathartic (Massengill)	Each tablet: Acetophenetidin*	0.165 gm.
	Aspirin (acetylsalicylic acid)*	0.23 gm.
	Caffeine	32 mg.
	Phenolphthalein	16 mg.
ANSUL FIRE EXTINGUISHER (Ansul)	Sodium bicarbonate	
ANTACID NO. 4 (Massengill)	Each tablet: Calcium carbonate, precipitated	0.23 gm.
	Magnesium carbonate	0.13 gm.
	Bismuth subnitrate	32 mg.
	Oil peppermint	q.s.
ANTAWAY ANT POWDER (Suretox)	Rotenone	3/4%

Name & Use Manufacturer	Ingredients	
ANT-B-GON (Calif. Spray)	Sodium arsenite*	0.2%
	Inert ingredients*	
ANT BUTTONS (Harris' original) (Harris Prods.)	Sodium arsenate* (total arsenic as metallic in all water-soluble form 0.62%)	1.71%
ANT CHEK (Chek)		
ANTCHEK (Rotenone)	Thallium sulfate*	1.25%
ANT DOOM (Murray, E.)	Sodium fluoride*	90%
ANT DOPE (Ni-Late)	Sodium arsenate*	not over 2%
ANTE-FIRMIN (adult) Antacid, digestant (Ante-Fermen)	Alcohol	6%
	Rhubarb	
	Bismuth subnitrate	
	Calcium carbonate	
	Zinc phenol sulfonate	
	Tinc. capsicum	
	Cinnamon	
	Oil of peppermint	
ANTE-FIRMIN (children) Antacid, digestant (Ante-Fermen)	Alcohol	4%
	Rhubarb	
	Bismuth subnitrate	
	Calcium carbonate	
	Zinc phenol sulfonate	
	Cinnamon	
	Oil of peppermint	
ANT-ENE ANT KILLER (McPhail)		
ANT & GRUB KILLER (Chipman, Ltd.)	Aldrin*	5.0%
ANTH-OLA CARBOLINEUM Insecticide (Rockland)	Anthracene* oil	
	Coal tar distillate*	
ANTH-OLA WOOD PRESERVATIVE (Rockland)		
ANTHOL CAPSULES Analgesic (Agol)	Acetophenetidin*	3-1/2 gr.
	Caffeine	
	Starch	
	Phloxine B to color	
ANTI-BACCO LOZENGES To combat tobacco habit (Pharmex)	Lobeline sulfate	1/64 gr.
ANTI-BORAX BRAZING FLUX #2 (Anti-Borax)	Borax*	
	Boracic acid*	
ANTI-BORAX SILVER SOLDER PASTE FLUX #16 (Anti-Borax)	Potassium carbonate	
	Potassium fluoborate*	
	Boracic acid*	

*Consult Sec. II., Ingredients Index. This ingredient may be responsible for major toxic effects if poisonous amounts of this product are ingested.

Name & Use Manufacturer	Ingredients		Name & Use Manufacturer	Ingredients	
ANTI-CALCIUM Photographic supply (Eastman)			ANTIPHLOG-ISTINE RUB A-535 Rubefacient, counter-irritant (Denver Chem.)	Methyl salicylate* Camphor* Menthol* Oil of eucalyptus*	
ANTI-COAGULANT & WATER SOFTENER For embalming (Eckels)			ANTI-PYREXOL For skin burns (Kip, Inc.)	Oil of spearmint Oil of bay wintergreen (syn.) Salicyclic acid* Lanolin Zinc oxide Carbolic acid (phenol) Ortho-hydroxyphenyl mercuric chloride Petrolatum Paraffine	0.44% 0.056%
ANTI-FOAM Photographic supply (Eastman)					
ANTI-FOG Photographic supply (Eastman)			ANTI-ROLL Semi-pressed crayon (Binney & Smith)		
ANTI-FOULING PAINTS (Baltimore Copper Paint)	Cuprous oxide* Mercuric oxide* Arsenic compounds* Coal tar Phenols and cresols* Polyvinyl chloride acetate binder Ketone solvents*		ANTIROT 10X Wood preservative (Woolfolk)	Pentachlorophenol*	42%
			ANTISEPTOL CREME (La-Mo)		
ANTIHEMM CONCEN-TRATE Anti-hemor-rhagic for drinking water (veterinary, avian) (Vineland)	Stabilized menadione sodium bisulfite solution*		ANTISTINE PRIVINE Nasal de-congestant (Ciba)	Antistine Privine Phenyl mercuric acetate (as a preservative)	0.5% 0.025% 1-50,000
ANTIHISTAMINE WITH A.P.C. (capsules) Antihistaminic, analgesic (West-Ward)	Each capsule: Pyranisamine maleate Aspirin* Phenacetin* Caffeine	10 mg. 3-1/2 gr. 2-1/2 gr. 1/2 gr.	ANT KILLER (Kelley)	Chlordane	5%
			ANT-KIL POWDER (Durham's)	Tech. chlordane*	10%
ANTIHISTAMINE WITH A.P.C. (tablets) Antihistaminic, analgesic (West-Ward)	Each tablet: Pyranisamine maleate Aspirin* Phenacetin* Caffeine	25 mg. 3-1/2 gr. 2-1/2 gr. 1/2 gr.	ANTNOX KILLS ANTS (Wisconsin Pharm.)	DDT* Pyrethrins Sesame oil extractives Petroleum hydrocarbons	10.00% 0.08% 0.30% 3.00%
			ANT-O (City Fum.)	Thallium sulfate*	
ANTI-HISTAMINE WITH HESPERIDIN (Capsules) Antihistamine, analgesic (West-Ward)	Pyrilamine maleate Hesperidin purified Ascorbic acid Salicylamide* Phenacetin* Caffeine	25 gr. 50 mg. 50 mg. 3-1/2 gr. 2-1/2 gr. 1/2 gr.	ANTOMINE Antihistamine, analgesic (Grove)	Acetophenetidin* Caffeine Quinine hydrobromide Pyrilamine maleate*	1-7/8 gr. 3/8 gr.
			ANT-ROACH FIX (Thompson Chem.)	Tech. chlordane Tech. piperonyl butoxide Pyrethrins Petroleum distillate* Propellent gas	2.00% 0.115% 0.046% 72.839% 25.00%
ANTINA FOOT REMEDY (Altone)		
ANTI-PAC-HIST (Capsules) Antihistamine, analgesic (Preston Lab.)	Thenylpyramine HCL Acetophenetidin* Aspirin* Caffeine alkaloid	25 mg. 2-1/2 gr. 3-1/2 gr. 1/2 gr.	ANT & ROACH KILLER (Bostwick)	Tech. chlordane Pyrethrins Tech. piperonyl butoxide Petroleum distillates*	2.0% 0.046% 0.115% 72.839%
			ANT ROACH POWDER (Ant-Roach)		
ANTIPHLOG-ISTINE Medicated poultice dressing (Denver Chem.)	Syrup of glycerine Iodine Boric acid Salicylic acid Methyl salicylate Oil of eucalyptus Kaolin Oil of peppermint	45.000 0.01 0.1 0.02 0.002 0.002 54.864 0.002	ANTROL ANT KILLERS (Boyle-Midway)	Sodium arsenite*	0.61%

*Consult Sec. II., Ingredients Index. This ingredient may be responsible for major toxic effects if poisonous amounts of this product are ingested.

Name & Use Manufacturer	Ingredients	
ANTROL ANT POWDER (Boyle- Midway)	Tech. chlordane Tech. piperonyl cyclonene Pyrethrins	1.50% 0.35% 0.06%
ANTROL ANT SPRAY (Boyle- Midway)	Chlordane	2-1/2%
ANTROL ANT SYRUP (Boyle- Midway)	Sodium arsenite*	0.61%
ANTROL ANT TRAP (Boyle- Midway)	Thallium sulfate*	1.17%
ANTROL SOWBUG CUTWORM CONTROL (Boyle- Midway)	Copper aceto-arsenite*	8.55%
ANT SLAYER (Pfeiffer)	Sodium arsenite*	0.16%
ANT STICK (Walbuck)	Tech. chlordane	2%
ANTURAT Rodenticide (Hess, Dr.)	Alpha-naphthyl thiourea*	20%
ANTU RAT POISON (Glenn County)	ANTU (alpha-naphthyl- thiourea)*	
ANT WITCH (Interstate Med.)	DDT* Pyrethrum* Talcum	
ANT-X ANT TRAP (Nott)	Thallium sulfate*	1.25%
ANT-X JELLY BAIT (Nott)	Thallium sulfate*	1%
ANT-X POWDER (Nott)	Chlordane	5%
ANTZIX ANT KILLER (Bonide)	Thallium sulfate*	1%
ANVITA Antiseptic vaginal sup- positories (Schmidt)	Boric acid* Alum Thymol* Berberine hydrochloride Monochlorthymol Aromatics Cocoa butter	
A-1 SALVE Antiseptic, external (Wizard)	Petrolatum Lanolin Zinc oxide* Sulfur* Salicylic acid*	
A-1 SALVE NO. 2 Astringent, external (Wizard)	Ichthammol Tannic acid (U.S.P.)	
APACHE Detergent (Wyandotte)	Concentrated alkali*	

Name & Use Manufacturer	Ingredients	
APADEX Antacid, adsorbent (Commerce)	Pectin Kaolin Bismuth subsalicylate* Zinc sulfocarbolate* Salol* Methyl salicylate*	
A.P.C. Analgesic (Superior Pharm.)	Each tablet: Acetophenetidin* Aspirin* Caffeine alkaloid	2-1/2 gr. 3-1/2 gr. 1/2 gr.
APCO 125 Deodorized solvent (Anderson- Prichard)	Paraffins Naphthenes* Aromatics*	69.3% 27.7% 3.0%
APCO 467 Solvent (Anderson- Prichard)	Paraffins plus naphthenes* Aromatics Olefins	90.8% 8.2% 1.0%
APCO 467 Deodorized solvent (Anderson- Prichard)	Paraffins plus naphthenes* 100.0%	
APCO NO. 10 MINERAL SPIRITS Solvent to thin paints, etc. (Anderson- Prichard)	Paraffins Naphthenes* Aromatics*	56.8% 30.6% 12.6%
APCO PILLS Cathartic (Hance)	Each pill: Ext. belladonna leaves* (total alkaloids bella- donna leaves, 0.001 gr.) Phenolphthalein* Aloin* Powd. ipecac	1/12 gr. 1/2 gr. 1/2 gr. 1/4 gr.
AP-CO TABLETS Analgesic (Drobinski)	Each tablet: Acetophenetidin* Acetyl salicylic acid* Caffeine	2-1/2 gr.
APCO THINNER For paints, etc. (Anderson- Prichard)	Paraffins Naphthenes* Aromatics*	56.0% 30.1% 13.9%
APCO WET-EGE SPIRITS Paint thinner (Anderson- Prichard)	Paraffins Naphthenes* Aromatics*	57.4% 30.2% 12.4%
A-PENN FURNITURE POLISH CREAM WAX (A-Penn)	Grease solvent* & wood preservative General detergent Emulsifier	46.0% 46.0% 8.0%
APEX CHEMICAL DITHANE 10%-Z 78 (Apex Chem.)	Zinc ethylene bisdithio- carbamate	6.50
APEX INSECTICIDE (Clean Home)	DDT* Isobornyl thiocyanoacetate*	
APEX MOTH CRYSTALS AND NUGGETS (Clean Home)	Paradichlorobenzene*	

*Consult Sec. II., Ingredients Index. This ingredient may be responsible for major toxic effects if poisonous amounts of this product are ingested.

Name & Use Manufacturer	Ingredients		Name & Use Manufacturer	Ingredients	
APEX MOTH CAKES (Clean Home)	Paradichlorobenzene*		API 25% DDT SPRAY CON-CENTRATE Insecticide (Agric. Proc.)	DDT (dichloro diphenyl trichloroethane)* Aromatic petroleum derivatives*	25% 70%
APEX MOTH TABLETS (Clean Home)	Paradichlorobenzene*		API 50% DDT WETTABLE POWDER Insecticide (Agric. Proc.)	DDT (dichloro diphenyl trichloroethane)*	50.0%
APEX PAINT (Monroe Co.)					
APEX TAILORS CRAYONS (Hershkowitz)			API DIELDRIN 15 (A) Insecticide (Agric. Proc.)	Hexachloro-epoxy-octahydro-dimethano-naphthalene* Related compounds Aromatic petroleum derivative*	15.83% 2.79% 73.38%
APEX TDE TOBACCO DUST Insecticide (Apex Chem.)	DDD*	10.00	API ESTER "6" Herbicide (Agric. Proc.)	Butyl ester of 2, 4-dichlorophenoxy acetic acid*	80%
APEX WALL SIZE (Cleveland C. & P.)			API ESTER OIL "4" 2,4-D CONCEN-TRATE Herbicide (Agric. Proc.)	Butyl 2, 4-dichlorophenoxy acetate*	54.4%
APHAMITE Insecticide, supplement to DDT in fruit spraying (Green Cross)	Wettable parathion* powder	15%	API ESTER-OIL "6" 2,4-D CONCEN-TRATE Herbicide (Agric. Proc.)	Butyl 2, 4-dichlorophenoxy acetate* Petroleum hydrocarbons	80.1% 18.0%
APHEDA Analgesic, antispasmodic for dysmenor-rhea (Western Pharm.)	Acid acetylsal.* Acetophenetidin* Ephedrin sulf.*	2 gr. 2 gr. 1/8 gr.	API GRUB BAR (Agric. Proc.)	Rotenone* Other cube resins*	5.0% 5.8%
			API HEPTACHLOR "2" Insecticide (Agric. Proc.)	Heptachlor* Related compounds Petroleum distillate*	22.4% 8.7% 62.9%
APHINE DISINFECTANT (Aphine)			API 44% ISOPROPYL ESTER 2,4-D EMULSION Herbicide (Agric. Proc.)	Isopropyl ester of 2, 4-dichlorophenoxyacetic acid*	44.0%
APHINE FERTILIZER (Aphine)					
APHINE INSECTICIDE (Aphine)	Nicotine (absolute)* Cedar oil Pine oil Dry soap	0.90% 0.95% 0.95% 4.00%	API LINDANE 25 Insecticide (Agric. Proc.)	Gamma isomer of benzene hexachloride (lindane)*	25%
APHIS DUST (Bonide)	Gamma isomer of benzene hexachloride (from lindane)	1%	API LINDANE 75 Insecticide (Agric. Proc.)	Gamma isomer of benzene hexachloride (lindane)*	75%
API AIR-ESTER "8" 2, 4-D CONCENTRATE TRATE Herbicide (Agric. Proc.)	Butyl 2, 4-dichlorophenoxy acetate*	99.0%	API LIVESTOCK SPRAY Insecticide (Agric. Proc.)	Chlordane* DDT (dichloro-diphenyl-trichloroethane)* Petroleum hydrocarbons*	45% 2% 43%
API ALDRIN EMULSIFI-ABLE CON-CENTRATE Insecticide (Agric. Proc.)	Hexachloro-hexahydro-dimethanonaphthalene* Related compounds Petroleum hydrocarbons*	23.10% 17.37% 52.03%	API LV BRUSH KILLER 20-20 (Agric. Proc.)	Butoxy ethoxy propanol ester of 2, 4-dichlorophenoxy-acetic acid* Butoxy ethoxy propanol ester of 2, 4, 5-tri-chlorophenoxyacetic acid*	37.00% 35.00%
API BEN-HEX Insecticide (Agric. Proc.)	Gamma isomer of benzene hexachloride* Other isomers of benzene hexachloride	12.0% 87.6%			
API BUTYL ESTER "4" EMULSIFI-ABLE 2, 4-D CONCENTRATE Herbicide (Agric. Proc.)	Butyl 2, 4-dichlorophenoxy acetate*	54.4%	API LV-4 ESTER WEED KILLER (Agric. Proc.)	Butoxy ethoxy propanol ester of 2, 4-dichlorophenoxy-acetic acid*	74.00%

*Consult Sec. II., Ingredients Index. This ingredient may be responsible for major toxic effects if poisonous amounts of this product are ingested.

Name & Use Manufacturer	Ingredients	
API 55% MALATHION EMULSIFI- ABLE CON- CENTRATE Insecticide (Agric. Proc.)	Malathion* Xylene*	55.4% 24.0%
API 25% PARATHION Insecticide (Agric. Proc.)	Parathion* Xylene	25% 65%
API PYRENONE DAIRY SPRAY CONCEN- TRATE Insecticide (Agric. Proc.)	Piperonyl butoxide tech. Pyrethrins Polyoxyethylene sorbitol mixed with ether ester Petroleum oil*	10.0% 1.0% 7.0% 82.0%
API PYRENONE MILL & BIN SPRAY Insecticide (Agric. Proc.)	Piperonyl butoxide tech. Pyrethrins Petroleum oil*	10.0% 1.0% 82.0%
API ROTOXIDE 240 LIVE- STOCK SPRAY Insecticide (Agric. Proc.)	Rotenone Other cube resins Piperonyl butoxide tech. Mono-di-isopropyl cresols* Dipentene Pine oil, steam distilled Aromatic petroleum distillate*	2.40% 4.80% 2.00% 10.32% 11.76% 15.00% 43.72%
API TOXAPHENE 6 Insecticide (Agric. Proc.)	Toxaphene* Petroleum distillate	60.00% 30.00%
API TOXAPHENE 40% WET- TABLE POWDER Insecticide (Agric. Proc.)	Tech. chlorinated camphene*	40.0%
API 2, 4-D AMINE CON- CENTRATE Herbicide (Agric. Proc.)	Dimethylamine salt of 2, 4-dichlorophenoxyacetic acid*	49.4%
API 2, 4-D 40% BUTYL ESTER CON- CENTRATE Herbicide (Agric. Proc.)	Butyl 2, 4-dichlorophenoxy- acetate*	40%
API WETTABLE CHLORDANE DUST CON- CENTRATE Insecticide (Agric. Proc.)	Tech. chlordane* Atta clay Santomerse D	40.0% 59.5% 0.5%
APPLE BLOSSOM COLOGNE, DEODORANT, PERFUME, TOILET WATER (Rubinstein)		
APPLETONE DETERGENT COMPOUND (Appleton)		

Name & Use Manufacturer	Ingredients	
APPLETON HAIR AND SCALP OINTMENT (Appleton)		
APPLETON PRESSING OIL COM- POUND (Appleton)		
APPLETON SKIN CREAM OINTMENT (Appleton)		
APPLETON SPECIAL TONIC (Appleton)		
APPLETON VEGETABLE OIL SHAMPOO (Appleton)		
APPLEX Insecticide (Destruxol)	Sodium fluosilicate*	6.00%
APP-L-SET For preharvest drop of apples (Dow)	Sodium 1-naphthaleneacetate*	
APPROVED PHARMA- CEUTICAL EQ-53 MOTH PROOFING COMPOUND (Approved)	DDT (dichloro-diphenyl- trichloroethane)*	25%
APRIL SHOWERS BATH SOFTENER (Cheramy)		
APRIL SHOWERS BRILLIAN- TINE (Liquid, solid) (Cheramy)		
APRIL SHOWERS COLOGNE, DEODORANT, PERFUME, TOILET WATER (Cheramy)		
APRO- HEMOR- RHOIDAL COMBINATION TREATMENT Ointment (Approved)	Tannic acid Benzocaine Phenol crystals* Quinine and urea hydrochloride Powdered nutgalls	
APRO- HEMOR- RHOIDAL SUPPOSI- TORIES (Approved)	Bismuth subgallate Bismuth oxyiodide Resorcin* Peru balsam Zinc oxide Boric acid*	

*Consult Sec. II., Ingredients Index. This ingredient may be responsible for major toxic effects if poisonous amounts of this product are ingested.

Name & Use Manufacturer	Ingredients		Name & Use Manufacturer	Ingredients	
APROPOS PERFUME, COLOGNE (Parfums Anjou)			AQUANON Insecticide (Speekman)	Chlorinated benzenes*	100.00%
A & P SAIL Detergent (Great Atlantic)			AQUAPROOF PAINTS (Preservative)		
APTIKONS Antiseptic vaginal suppositories (Jewell Pharm.)	Chinosol Boric acid*		AQUA-PRUF Water repellent (Anderson-Campbell)	Wax Carbon tetrachloride*	
A-200 PYRINATE LIQUID Ectoparasiticide, external (McKesson & Robbins)	Pyrethrins Dinitroanisole Oleoresin parsley fruit Sesamin Oleic acid Benzyl alcohol	1.0% 1.0% 0.5% 0.037% 3.5% 8.0%	AQUA-SAN Herbicide (Collins Feed)	Olefins Diolefins Toluene* Paraffins Naphthenes Trichlorobenzene* Benzene* Higher boiling aromatic emulsifiers	
AQUA-CLEAR RUST PREVENTATIVE COMPOUND (Sudbury)			AQUA-SEPT Oral antiseptic (Horton & Converse)	Thymol* Menthol* Methyl salicylate* Boric acid* Chlorothymol Eucalyptol Thyme oil	
AQUA-DETH WATER SOLUBLE Rodenticide (Hopkins Agric.)	Sodium salt of warfarin	0.54%	AQUASPAR VARNISH (DeVoe)		
AQUADOW Liquid fertilizer (Dow)			AQUASPRAY Insecticide (Florida Chem.)	DDT* Petroleum oil* Non-ionic emulsifier	25% 70% 5%
AQUA DRIN Nasal decongestant (McKesson & Robbins)	Alcohol Ephedrine (as the lactate) Sodium ethyl mercuric thiosalicylate	0.1% 1% 0.004%	AQUATONE SWIMMING POOL TREATMENT Algaecide (Creative Chem.)		
AQUAFLO Herbicide (Speekman)	Chlorinated benzenes*	83%	AQUA VELVA SHAVING LOTION (Williams, J.B.)	Alcohol* denatured with colocynth	
AQUA FLOR Astringent lotion (San Pedro)	Alcohol*	70%	AQUA-WHITE Whiting (Reliance Whiting)		
AQUALENE SOLUBLE OIL (Crescent Oil)	Mineral oil Petroleum sulfonate		AQUEOUS CALENDULA Antiseptic for wounds (Boericke & Runyon)	Alcohol*	20%
AQUAMARINE HAND CREAM (Revlon)	Lecithin Stearic acid Glycol Glycol ethers and esters Inorganic alkali Preservative Perfume		AQUET Detergent (Greiner)	Alkyl aryl polyethylene glycol	
AQUAMARINE LOTION DEODORANT (Revlon)	Polyoxyethylene ethers and esters Cetyl alcohol Cholesterol absorption bases Fatty acid amide derivative Aluminum chlorhydrate		ARABESQUE COLORS (Ruxton)		
AQUAMARINE MIST Scent (Revlon)	Oils Alcohol		ARABIAN NIGHTS PERFUME, TOILET WATER (Scherk)		

*Consult Sec. II., Ingredients Index. This ingredient may be responsible for major toxic effects if poisonous amounts of this product are ingested.

Name & Use Manufacturer	Ingredients		Name & Use Manufacturer	Ingredients	
ARAB LIQUID RAT AND MOUSE KILLER (Federal Chem.)	Arsenic trioxide*		ARBOR FOOT SALVE (Washington Hom.)	Thuya occidentalis* H.P.U.S.	
ARAB MOTH KILLER (Federal Chem.)	Isobornyl thiocyanoacetate*	2.05%	ARCADIAN WATER COLORS (Binney & Smith)		
	Related terpenes	0.45%			
	Petroleum hydrocarbons*	97.50%	ARCOGON PAINT (Arco)		
ARAB NO ODOR MOTH PROOF (Federal Chem.)	Sodium arsenite* (total arsenic expressed as metallic all in water soluble form 0.4%)	0.65%	ARCOL Tonic, intestinal germicide (veterinary) (Gland-O-Lac)	Each fl. oz: Ammonium arsanilate* (arsenic derivative) (arsenic as metallic 9.6 gr.)	
ARABOL MUCILAGE (Arabol)	Tapioca dextrine base				30 gr.
ARAB RAT-DETH READY MIXED (Federal Chem.)	Warfarin (3-(a-acetonylbenzyl)-4-hydroxycoumarin)	0.025%	ARCOTONE PAINT (Arco)		
			ARCO VARNISH (Arco)		
ARAB RESIDUAL SPRAY Insecticide (Federal Chem.)	DDT* Petroleum hydrocarbons*	5% 95%	ARCO VEL-LURE Paint (Arco)		
ARAB ROACH KILLER (Federal Chem.)	Tech. chlordane Gamma isomer of benzene hexachloride (from lindane) Xylene	2.00% 0.10% 0.50%	ARCTIC ANTI FREEZE (Am. LaFrance)		
			ARCTIC GARGLE Antitussive (Standard Medicines)	Beechwood creosote* Ammonium Alum Antiseptic solution N.F.	
ARAB U-DO-IT CONCEN-TRATE TERMITE CONTROL (Federal Chem.)	Tech. chlordane* Gamma isomer of benzene hexachloride (from lindane) Xylene* Petroleum hydrocarbons*	45.00% 1.00% 5.00% 43.00%	ARCTIC SNOW FLAKES Spray for Christmas trees, etc. (Bliz)	Lucite Hydrofol base Methylene chloride* Perfume Freon*	
ARACAIN RECTAL SUPPOSI-TORIES Emollient, local anes-thetic (Commerce)	Benzocaine Bismuth subgallate Zinc oxide Boric acid*		ARDENA SUN-PRUF CREAM, NO. 2 (Arden)		
			AREN MASSAGE LOTION (Athea)	Triethanolamine stearate Lanolin Petrolatum Hexadecanol Olive oil	
ARASAN SFX THIRAM SEED DISINFECT-ANT (du Pont)	Thiram (tetramethyl thiuramdisulfide)*		AR-EX R-M-S LOTION (Ar-Ex)	Resorcinol monoacetate Precipitated sulfur	3% 5%
ARATONE Nasal de-congestant (Technical Prod.)	Alcohol Ephedrine Chlorobutanol derivative of chloral Potassium bicarbonate Sodium borate Thymol Eucalyptol Methyl salicylate Cudbear glycerine	2% 1% 1/2%	AR-EX SCALP LOTION (Ar-Ex)	Resorcinol monoacetate N.F. Salicylic acid U.S.P. Glycerine C.P. Alcohol Oil of bay	1.5 gm. 1.5 gm. 1.0 gm. 50%
ARBE DUAL PURPOSE POLISH RE-MOVER AND CUTICLE SOFTENER (R-B)			AR-EX SCALP LOTION WITH OIL (Ar-Ex)	Resorcinol monoacetate N.F. Salicylic acid U.S.P. Castor oil U.S.P. Alcohol* Oil of bay	1.5 gm. 1.5 gm. 1.5 gm. 85%

*Consult Sec. II., Ingredients Index. This ingredient may be responsible for major toxic effects if poisonous amounts of this product are ingested.

Name & Use Manufacturer	Ingredients	Name & Use Manufacturer	Ingredients
AR-EX SHAMPOO Soapless, hypo-allergenic (Ar-Ex)		AR-KI-TOCK PAINTS (Rockford)	
AR-EX SKIN DETERGENT (Ar-Ex)	Esterified protein derivative (pH 6.8)	ARLAC Detergent (Wyandotte)	Concentrated alkali*
AR-EX SORSIS ALPHA Rubefacient, antiseptic, local (Ar-Ex)	Ammoniated mercury* Salicylic acid* Phenol* Tar	ARMAND BRILLIAN-TINE (Armand)	
		ARMAND CREAMS For hands and face (Armand)	
AR-EX SORSIS BETA Rubefacient, antiseptic (Ar-Ex)	Ammoniated mercury* Ichthammol Tar* Boric acid*	ARMAND HAIR OIL (Armand)	
AR-EX TAR BATH (Ar-Ex)	Juniper tar* (oil of cade, U.S.P. XIII) 35% Sulfonated castor oil	ARMAND HAND LOTION (Armand)	
AR-EX TAR SHAMPOO (Ar-Ex)	Juniper tar (oil of cade, U.S.P. XIII) 2% Conc. saponified coconut oil	ARMAND POWDER (Armand)	
ARGOSHEEN HAND CLEANER (Argo)		ARMATOL WOOD PRES-ERVATIVE (Huttig)	
ARGYNATE Antiseptic (Horton & Converse)	Silver protein U.S.P. containing metallic silver* 20%	ARMORBAND PAINTS (Sipe)	
ARIDCLEAR Coating for masonry walls (Anti-Hydro)	Resins in coal tar solvents*	ARMORED ROOF & BARN PAINT (United Gilson.)	Fish oil Tall oil Red iron oxide Mineral spirits*
ARISOD Herbicide (General Chem.)	Sodium arsenite* 35.5%	ARMORIZE ALUMINUM METAL & MASONRY PAINT (Carter Paint)	Volatile* 44.9% Non-volatile: 55.1% Oils Resins Aluminum Drier
ARISTOCRAT BRAND PAINTS (Donahue)		ARMORIZE-BLACK Paint (Carter Paint)	Pigment: Carbon black 100% Vehicle: Non-volatile 53.0% Volatile* 47.0%
ARISTOCRAT EMBALMING FLUID (Huncke)			
ARISTOCRAT FIRE EX-TINGUISHER (Snyder)		ARMORIZE-BLUE NO. 1209 Paint (Carter Paint)	Pigment: Iron blue 55.9% Magnesium silicate 8.8% Titanated calcium carbonate 35.3% Vehicle: Non-volatile 43.0% Volatile* 57.0%
ARISTOCRAT VARNISH (Monroe Co.)			
ARISTOLITE PAINTS (Dunn)		ARMORIZE-BROWN Paint (Carter Paint)	Pigment: Burnt umber 38.9% Burnt sienna 44.4% Iron oxide 8.3% Chrome orange* 8.4% Vehicle: Non-volatile 42.3% Volatile* 57.7%
ARISTO MOTOR OIL (Union Oil)			
AR-JAY HAIR RINSE (Ar-Jay)			

*Consult Sec. II., Ingredients Index. This ingredient may be responsible for major toxic effects if poisonous amounts of this product are ingested.

Name & Use Manufacturer	Ingredients	
ARMORIZE- FIRE PLUG RED Paint (Carter Paint)	Vehicle: Non-volatile Volatile* Pigment: Para red Lithol red Titanated calcium carbonate	41.5% 58.5% 58.6% 15.5% 25.9%
ARMORIZE- GRAY Paint (Carter Paint)	Pigment: Zinc odixe Barium sulfate Titanium dioxide Titanium calcium Carbon black Vehicle: Non-volatile Votatile*	24.5% 22.3% 3.4% 46.2% 0.3% 43.0% 57.0%
ARMORIZE- GREEN Paint (Carter Paint)	Vehicle: Non-volatile Volatile* Pigment: Chrome green* Magnesium silicate	48.18% 51.82% 78.85% 21.15%
ARMORIZE- NATIONAL GREEN Paint (Carter Paint)	Pigment: Chrome green* Magnesium silicate Vehicle: Non-volatile Volatile*	78.9% 21.1% 48.2% 51.8%
ARMORIZE- RED Paint (Carter Paint)	Pigment: Toluidine red Chrome orange* Vehicle: Non-volatile Volatile*	72.4% 27.6% 52.0% 48.0%
ARMORIZE- WHITE Paint (Carter Paint)	Pigment: Titanium dioxide Calcium carbonate Vehicle: Non-volatile Volatile*	93.8% 6.2% 51.5% 48.5%
ARMORIZE- YELLOW Paint (Carter Paint)	Vehicle: Non-volatile Volatile* Pigment: Chrome yellow* Magnesium silicate Titanium dioxide Zinc sulfide Barium sulfate*	42.3% 57.7% 76.9% 15.4% 1.2% 1.8% 4.7%
ARMORIZE- ZINC CHRO- MATE-METAL PRIMER Paint (Carter Paint)	Vehicle: Phenolic resins Driers Vegetable oils Pigment: Zinc-lead chromate* Titanated calcium carbonate Diatomaceous silica	29.2% 0.7% 70.1% 42.8% 43.1% 14.1%
ARMORTEC RESIN EMULSION PAINT (Armor)		
ARMOUR VELVET GREEN (Armour Fert.)		

Name & Use Manufacturer	Ingredients	
ARM-R DUX-TOX Prepared wood pre- servative (General Finishes)	Pentachlorophenol* Other chlorophenols	4.41% 0.64%
ARM-R PENTA POST TREAT- MENT Wood pre- servative (General Finishes)	Pentachlorophenol* Other chlorophenols	4.43% 0.65%
ARM-R REDWOOD DUX-TOX Prepared wood pre- servative (General Finishes)	Pentachlorophenol* Other chlorophenols	4.41% 0.64%
ARM-R SEAL-TOX Prepared wood pre- servative (General Finishes)	Pentachlorophenol* Other chlorophenols	4.42% 0.64%
ARMSTRONG CAULKING COMPOUND (Armstrong)		
ARMSTRONG F-1402 ADHESIVE (Armstrong Cork)	Drying oils Naphtha* Alcohol*	
ARMSTRONG ROOFING CEMENT (Armstrong Co.)		
ARMSTRONG S-214 CEMENT (Armstrong Cork)	Denatured alcohol* Phenolic resin	
ARMSTRONG WATERGLASS (Armstrong Co.)		
ARNESTO PAINT (Arnesto)		
ARNOLD ARSEN-O- SPRAY Insecticide (Garden Hose)	Lead arsenate* (acid type) not less than 80%	
ARNOLD 40% CHLORDANE- SPRAY Insecticide (Garden Hose)	Tech. chlordane*	40%
ARNOLD CRYOLITE- SPRAY Insecticide (Garden Hose)	Sodium fluoaluminate* Fluorine	80% 44.5%

*Consult Sec. II., Ingredients Index. This ingredient may be responsible for major toxic effects if poisonous amounts of this product are ingested.

Name & Use Manufacturer	Ingredients		Name & Use Manufacturer	Ingredients	
ARNOLD 33% DDT CART-RIDGE Insecticide (Garden Hose)	DDT*	33.3%	AROMATIC FOOT POWDER For skin irritation (Gordon Labs.)	Menthol* Thymol* Camphor* Boric acid* Oil of eucalyptus Salicylic acid* Alum Magnesium Trisilicate Talc	
ARNOLD FUNGUSPRAY (Garden Hose)	Tri basic copper sulfate*	85%			
ARNOLD 18% LINDANE-SPRAY CART-RIDGE Insecticide (Garden Hose)	Gamma isomer of benzene hexachloride (from lindane)*	18.2%	AROMAZONE Disinfectant (Florozone)		
			ARRESTINE TABLETS To combat tobacco habit (Arrestine)	Lobeline sulfate*	1/64 gr.
ARNOLD NIC-O-SPRAY Insecticide (Garden Hose)	Nicotine* added as alkaloid Fish oil soap (anhydrous)	35% 28%			
ARNOLD PYR-O-SPRAY Insecticide (Garden Hose)	Pyrethrins Soap	1.08% 65%	ARRID Deodorant (Carter Prod.)	Aluminum sulfate Emulsifiers Organic buffer	
			ARROW FIRE EXTINGUISHER (Snyder)		
ARNOLD SULPH-O-SPRAY Fungicide (Garden Hose)	Sulfur*	65%	ARROWHEAD CEMENT For china, crockery, glass, fabric (Webb)		
ARNOLD WEED-O-SPRAY (Garden Hose)	Sodium-2, 4-dichloro-phenoxyacetate* mono-hydrate	55%			
			ARROWHEAD CEMENT WATERPROOF FILLER (Webb)		
AROBON Cathartic (Nestle Co.)	Carob flour				
ARO DIANA LINIMENT (Sachs Mfg.)			ARROWHEAD PAINT (Am. Paint Corp.)		
AROMA BLACK MOTH DESTROYER (Victory Chem.)			ARRYL Antiseptic oral wash (Rogers Park)	Carbamide (synthetic urea) Sodium alkyl aryl sulfonate	
AROMA BLACK MOTH KRYSTALS & DEODORIZER (Victory Chem.)			ARSEN-O-SPRAY CART-RIDGE Insecticide (Garden Hose)	Lead arsenate* (metallic arsenic 16.1%, metallic lead 50%)	80%
AROMANT Inhalant (Otis Clapp)	Alcohol* Camphor* Menthol* Eugenol*	23%	ARTCO ARLIN Insecticide (Artco)	Gamma isomer of benzene hexachloride (from lindane)* Aromatic petroleum derivative solvent*	12.9% 80.3%
AROMATIC FOOTBATH CRYSTALS For skin irritation (Gordon Labs.)	Sod. borate* Sod. bicarbonate Sod. chloride Thymol* Menthol* Oil of eucalyptus		ARTCO ARTOX Insecticide (Artco)	Gamma isomer of benzene hexachloride (from lindane)*	11.7
			ARTCO 2-1/2% CHLORDANE Insecticide (Artco)	Tech. chlordane	2.50%
			ARTCO 45% CHLORDANE Insecticide (Artco)	Tech. chlordane* Petroleum hydrocarbon*	45% 46%

*Consult Sec. II., Ingredients Index. This ingredient may be responsible for major toxic effects if poisonous amounts of this product are ingested.

Name & Use Manufacturer	Ingredients		Name & Use Manufacturer	Ingredients	
ARTCO 72% CHLORDANE Insecticide (Artco)	Tech. chlordane*	72%	ARTHONUL Analgesic (Ray Drug)	Each tablet: Sodium salicylate Salicylamide* Thiamin chloride Ascorbic acid Para-aminobenzoic acid Niacin	3.0 gr. 3.5 gr. 1 mg. 50 mg. 10 mg. 1 mg.
ARTCO EMULSIFIABLE CHLORDANE Insecticide (Artco)	Tech. chlordane*	50%			
			ARTHRISAL-C Analgesic, antirheumatic (Ethical)	Each tablet: Sodium salicylate* 0.3 gm. Para-aminobenzoic acid 0.3 gm. (as sodium para-aminobenzoate) Ascorbic acid (vitamin C) 50.0 mg.	
ARTCO EMULSIFIABLE DIELDRIN Insecticide (Artco)	Hexachloro-epoxy-octahydro-dimethano naphthalene* 15.83% Related compounds 2.79% Petroleum hydrocarbons* 71.38%				
ARTCO FLY KILLER (Artco)	Malathion* Dieldrin* Aromatic petroleum derivative solvent*	15% 5% 70%	ARTISOL TABLETS Analgesic, antirheumatic (Wile)	Sodium salicylate* 5 gr. Aspirin* (acetylsalicylic acid) 5 gr. Vitamin B$_1$ (thiamin hydrochloride) 5 mg. Vitamin C (ascorbic acid) 20 mg.	
ARTCO KALO DUST Wood preservative (Artco)	Tricalcium arsenate*	35%	ARTISTA POWDER PAINT (Binney & Smith)		
ARTCO KALA-FUMIGANT (Artco)	Orthodichlorobenzene* Carbon tetrachloride* Pentachlorophenol* Petroleum hydrocarbon oil	41% 59%	ARTISTA TEMPERA SHOW CARD COLORS (Binney & Smith)		
ARTCO MILL SPRAY Insecticide (Artco)	Piperonyl butoxide Pyrethrins	6.35% 0.635%	ARTISTA WATER COLORS (Binney & Smith)		
ARTCO PENTA 40 Wood preservative (Artco)	Pentachlorophenol* Other chlorophenols Petroleum hydrocarbons	36.5% 5.3% 58.2%	ARTOX Herbicide (Nott)	Disodium monomethyl arsenate* 31.5% Arsenic as metallic 12.75%	
ARTCO SOIL FUMIGANT (Artco)	Hydrocarbon oil* Orthodichlorobenzene Pentachlorophenol* Other pentachlorophenols Carbon tetrachloride* Diacetone alcohol	3%	ARTRUSAL Analgesic (Veltex)	Each tablet: Salicylamide* Sodium salicylate* Manganese salicylate* Caffeine* Niacin	
ARTCO TERMITREAT EMULSIFIABLE COMPOUND Insecticide (Artco)	Copper naphthenate* Petroleum hydrocarbon oil*	50% 46%	ARZENE COMPOUND Internal germicide (veterinary) (Lee)	Arsenosobenzene* (arsenic derivative; each oz. contains 14.6 gr. arsenic trioxide) 5%	
ARTCO TERMITROL Wood preservative (Artco)	Copper naphthenate* Petroleum hydrocarbon oil*	12% 88%	ARZEN NASAL OIL (Arzen-Ardent)		
ARTCO TERMITREAT SOIL TREATMENT Insecticide (Artco)	Sodium pentachlorophenate*	12%			
ARTCO 20 Insecticide (Artco)	Gamma isomer of benzene hexachloride (from lindane)*	20%			

*Consult Sec. II., Ingredients Index. This ingredient may be responsible for major toxic effects if poisonous amounts of this product are ingested.

Name & Use Manufacturer	Ingredients		Name & Use Manufacturer	Ingredients	
A.S.A. COMPOUND Antipyretic, analgesic, antirheumatic (Lilly)	Each pulvule: Acetophenetidin* Acetylsalicylic acid* Caffeine	0.16 gm. 0.227 gm. 0.0325 gm.	ASEPTICO Antiseptic (Aseptico)	Menthol Thymol* Eucalyptol* Menthyl-salicylate* Parachlormetaxylenol* Sodium bicarbonate Sodium borate* Sodium chloride	
ASALCO NO. 1 Analgesic (Jenkins)	Each tablet: Acetyisalicylic acid* Acetophenetidin* Caffeine	3-1/2 gr. 2-1/2 gr. 1/2 gr.			
ASBESTOS FIBRE PLASTIC CEMENT (Pioneer)			ASEPTINOL For skin irritation (Aspetinol)	Zinc oxide* Lanolin anhydrous Oil cade* Calamine Resorcin* Petroleum base	
ASCACEK Anthelmintic (veterinary) (McClellan)	Phenothiazine Nicotine* (expressed as alkaloid) Gentian, iron sulfate and bentonite	30% 5% 65%	ASEPTO SOAP (Embalmers')	Hexachlorophene	2%
ASCADIN PULVOID (WHITE OR GREEN TABLET) Analgesic Antipyretic (Drug Prod.)	Aspirin* Acetophenetidin* Caffeine alkaloid	0.23 gm. 0.16 gm. 32 mg.	ASEPTUM HYGENE POWDER Antiseptic powder (Am. Druggists)	Sodium chloride Menthol* Eucalyptol* Thymol* Borax* Methyl ester of parahydroxy benzoic acid	
ASCARICIDE WATER WORMER Anthelmintic (veterinary) (Anchor Serum)	Piperazine citrate	32% w/v	ASGELIN Analgesic (Cowley Pharm.)	Aspirin* Phenacetin* Caffeine Equiv. tr. gelsemium (green)	3-3/4 gr. 1-1/2 gr. 1/2 gr. 1/2 m.
			ASHTONE Hair bleach powder (Kroy)	Ammonium phosphate Ammonium chloride Ammonium carbonate Calcium carbonate	

*Consult Sec. II., Ingredients Index. This ingredient may be responsible for major toxic effects if poisonous amounts of this product are ingested.

Name & Use Manufacturer	Ingredients		Name & Use Manufacturer	Ingredients	
ASL BANAFLY PYRENONE EMULSION CONCENTRATE Insecticide (Am.Scient.)	Tech. piperonyl butoxide Pyrethrins Refined petroleum oil*	10% 1% 78%	ASL R-SEN-O For intestinal irritation (veterinary) (Am.Scient.)	Arsanilic acid*	10%
ASL BANAGERM Disinfectant, deodorant (Am.Scient.)	Para di-isobutyl phenoxy ethoxy ethyl dimethyl benzyl ammonium chloride monohydrate*	10%	ASL SULFA-R DRESSING POWDER Fungicide, antiseptic (veterinary) (Am.Scient.)	Sulfanilamide* Sulfathiazole Urea Calcium carbonate Sodium bicarbonate Boric acid	10% 2% 50% 5% 30% 3%
ASL BANAGRUB ROTENONE DUST Insecticide (Am.Scient.)	Rotenone Other extractives of cube root	1.5% 3.0%	ASL SWIVERMA Anthelmintic (veterinary) (Am.Scient.)	Piperazine base	19.2 gm.
ASL BANAPEST LINDANE EMULSION CONCENTRATE Insecticide (Am.Scient.)	Gamma isomer of benzene hexachloride (from lindane)* Xylene*	10% 84%	ASLUM OINTMENT For skin irritations (Drug Prod., N.Y.)	Carbolic acid* Aluminum acetate Ichthammol Zinc oxide Aromatic oils* Petrolatum-stearin base	1%
ASL BANARAT WARFARIN BITS (Am.Scient.)	Warfarin (3-(a-acetonylbenzyl)-4-hydroxycoumarin)	0.025%	ASL 5/50 WORMER Anthelmintic (veterinary) (Am.Scient.)	Nicotine* (as alkaloid) Phenothiazine Nux vomica (containing 1.15% strychnine) Colloidal clay	5% 50% 10% 35%
ASL BANARAT WARFARIN PREMIX Rodenticide (Am.Scient.)	Warfarin (3-(a-acetonylbenzyl)-4-hydroxycoumarin)	0.5%	AS-MA Antispasmodic for asthma (Wood Chem.)	Ephedrine hyd.* Iodide potash Tinct. lobelia* Elix. lactated pepsin F.E. cascara arom.	3/4 gr./tsp.
ASL GALLIVERMA Anthelmintic (veterinary) (Am.Scient.)	Each 100 cc.: Piperazine base	22 gm.	AS-MA AID (Sacramento)		
ASL HEPTROL FEEDMIX Poultry remedy (Am.Scient.)	2-Amino-5-nitrothiazole*	20%	A-SOL-A S.F. NO. 920 Wet dressing (Specialists)	Ascorbic acid Benzoic acid* Tartaric acid	
ASL HEPTROL SOLUBLE CONCENTRATE Poultry remedy (Am.Scient.)	2-Amino-5-nitrothiazole*	100%	ASPAPOPS Analgesic (G.I.)	Each lollypop: Aspirin* Benzocaine	2 gr. 1/8 gr.
ASL LAXEPTIC Poultry remedy (Am.Scient.)	Di-isobutyl phenoxy ethoxy ethyl dimethyl benzyl ammonium chloride, monohydrate* Sodium sulfate Magnesium sulfate*	4% 45% 40%	ASPECAF COMPOUND Analgesic (Halperin)	Each tablet: Acetylsalicylic acid* Acetophenetidin* Caffeine	3-1/2 gr. 2-1/2 gr. 1/2 gr.
			ASPERGUM Analgesic (White Lab.)	Aspirin*	3-1/2 gr.
ASL LOUSE POWDER Poultry remedy (Am.Scient.)	Orthophenylphenol Sulfur Soap	7% 10% 1%	ASPIRIN COMPOUND Analgesic (Tutag)	Acetylsalicylic acid* Acetophenetidin* Caffeine	3-1/2 gr. 2-1/2 gr. 1/2 gr.
ASL NICO-5 WORMER Anthelmintic (veterinary) (Am.Scient.)	Nicotine* (as alkaloid)	5%	ASPIROIDS For colds, analgesic (Rexall)	Aspirin* Calcium carbonate Phenolphthalein* Capsicum Ipecac Caffeine	

*Consult Sec. II., Ingredients Index. This ingredient may be responsible for major toxic effects if poisonous amounts of this product are ingested.

Name & Use Manufacturer	Ingredients	Name & Use Manufacturer	Ingredients
ASPIROIDS WITH ANTIHISTA-MINE For colds (Rexall)	Pyrilamine maleate* Salicylamide* Calcium carbonate Caffeine Ipecac Capsicum	ASTARTE BACK & SHOULDER TEXTURE LOTION (Allied Dist.)	Menthol* Acetone* Alcohol* 50%
ASSOCIATED BRANDS HAIR LACQUER (Assoc.Brands)		ASTARTE B.P. & S. OINT-MENT (Allied Dist.)	Balsam Peru* Sulfur*
ASSOCIATED BRANDS HAIR TRAINER (Assoc.Brands)		ASTARTE #42 CA YELLOW CONCENTRATE Foot bath (Allied Dist.)	Calcium lactate
ASSOCIATED BRANDS LIQUID CREME RINSE For hair (Assoc.Brands)		ASTARTE COOLING LOTION (Allied Dist.)	Menthol* Salicylic acid* Benzoic acid* Ethyl alcohol* 50%/v
ASSOCIATED BRANDS LIQUID CREME SHAMPOO (Assoc.Brands)		ASTARTE #27 CU GREEN CONCENTRATE Foot bath (Allied Dist.)	Copper sulfate*
ASSOCIATED BRANDS SHAMPOO & HAIR TRAINER (Assoc.Brands)		ASTARTE DEODORANT COMPOUND Hypoallergenic (Allied Dist.)	Magnesium carbonate Magnesium oxide Sodium biborate* Sodium bicarbonate
ASSOCIATED BRANDS SPECIAL SCALP SALVE (Assoc.Brands)		ASTARTE DEODORANT COMP. POW-DER SET (Allied Dist.)	
ASSOCIATED BRANDS SPECIAL SKIN ASTRINGENT (Assoc.Brands)		ASTARTE DESICCANT (Allied Dist.)	
ASSOCIATED BRANDS WAVE SETTING LOTION (Assoc.Brands)		ASTARTE FACE LOTION (Allied Dist.)	
		ASTARTE FOOT CREAM (Allied Dist.)	
ASSOCIATED PRODUCTS LARKSPUR LOTION For head and crab lice (Assoc.Prod.)	Larkspur alkaloids* Propylene glycol Glacial acetic acid Isopropyl alcohol	ASTARTE HYDROPHYLIC PASTE (Allied Dist.)	
		ASTARTE #35 KA RED CONCENTRATE Foot bath (Allied Dist.)	Potassium sulfate*
ASTARTE ACNE CREAM (Allied Dist.)		ASTARTE LIQUID COOL CREAM (Allied Dist.)	Menthol*
ASTARTE ASTRINGENT (Allied Dist.)			

*Consult Sec. II., Ingredients Index. This ingredient may be responsible for major toxic effects if poisonous amounts of this product are ingested.

Name & Use Manufacturer	Ingredients		Name & Use Manufacturer	Ingredients	
ASTARTE LIQUID FOOT CREAM For skin irritation (Allied Dist.)	Menthol* Tr. benzoin compound		ASTERMA Protective Skin Cream (Astra)	Anhydrous lanolin Olive oil Petrolatum Propylene glycol Persic oil Mineral oil Beeswax Sodium chloride Ferric phosphate Calcium phosphate Ceresine	
ASTARTE LIQUID SCALP CREAM (Allied Dist.)	Sodium thiosulfate Menthol*				
ASTARTE LOTION (Allied Dist.)			ASTEROL DIHYDROCHLOR- IDE ROCHE DUSTING POW- DER Fungicide (medical) (Hoffmann-La- Roche)	Diamthazole (the dihydrochloride of 2-dimethylamino-6-(beta- diethylamino-ethoxy)-benzo- thiazole)* 5%	
ASTARTE #32 Mg blue concentrate Foot bath (Allied Dist.)	Magnesium sulfate				
ASTARTE MILD ASTRING- ENT (Allied Dist.)	Alcohol 10%/v		ASTHENE Nasal decon- gestant (Univ.Med.)	Ephedrine sulfate* 1/8 gr. Ortho-iodo-benzoic acid Calcium lactate	
ASTARTE MILD PASTE For skin (Allied Dist.)	Zinc oxide Amylum Calcium lactate Sodium phosphate Petrolatum Adeps lanae Liquor carbonis detergens		ASTOL MATADOE Insecticide (Nova)		
ASTARTE #1 Na brown concentrate Hand baths (Allied Dist.)	Sodium chloride		ASTOR-X ANT BRUSH (Astor)	Thallium sulfate* .001%	
ASTARTE RINSE (Allied Dist.)			ASTOR-X ANT POWDER (Astor)	Tech. chlordane* 5%	
ASTARTE SCALE EMOLLIENT (Allied Dist.)			ASTOR-X ANTU BROWN RAT KILLER (Astor)	ANTU 5.52%	
ASTARTE SCALP CREAM (Allied Dist.)			ASTOR-X DDT EMULSION CONCENTRATE (Astor)	DDT* 25% Aromatic petroleum derivative solvent* 70%	
ASTARTE SCALP LOTION (Allied Dist.)	Menthol* Alcohol* 50%				
ASTARTE SUNBURN LOTION (Allied Dist.)			ASTOR-X 50% DDT WET- TABLE POW- DER (Astor)	DDT* 50%	

---

*Consult Sec. II., Ingredients Index. This ingredient may be responsible for major toxic effects if poisonous amounts of this product are ingested.

Name & Use Manufacturer	Ingredients		Name & Use Manufacturer	Ingredients	
ASTOR-X DU-AWAY PEST SPRAY (Astor)	Tech. chlordane	2%	ASTOR-X ROACH KILLA (Astor)	Sodium fluoride* Pyrethrins	47.50% 0.18%
ASTOR-X INSECT KILLA PLUS 10% DDT (Astor)	DDT* Pyrethrins	10% 0.27%	ASTOR-X SAF-SPRAY BRAND (Astor)	Tech. piperonyl butoxide Pyrethrins Petroleum distillates*	1.5% 0.15% 98.35%
ASTOR-X INSECT SPRAY PLUS 5% DDT (Astor)	DDT* Beta thiocyano-ethyl esters of aliphatic acids containing 10-18 carbon atoms Beta-butoxy-beta-thiocyano diethyl ether Petroleum distillate*	5% 1.125% 0.375% 93.5%	ASTOR -X SAF-BRAND VAPORIZING CONC. (Astor)	Tech. piperonyl butoxide Pyrethrins Petroleum distillate*	3.00% 0.30% 96.70%
ASTOR-X MALATHION FLY SPRAY CONCENTRATE (Astor)	Malathion* Xylol*	50% 42.4%	ASTOR-X SUPER-SPRAY (O.B.) (Astor)	Gamma isomer of benzene hexachloride (from lindane) Petroleum distillate*	0.5% 99.5%
ASTOR-X MOTH CRYSTALS (Astor)	Paradichlorobenzene*	100%	ASTOR-X TERMICIDE Wood preserver, insecticide (Astor)	Tech. chlordane* Pentachlorophenol* 2-Chlororthophenylphenol* Tetrachlorophenol* Orthodichlorobenzene* Petroleum solvents*	3% 2% 2% 1% 5% 87%
ASTOR-X MOTH SPRAY & PROOFER (Astor)	Petroleum distillate* Methylated naphthalene* DDT* n-octyl bicycloheptene dicarboximide Pyrethrins	89.868% 5.00% 5.00% 0.120% 0.012%	ASTOR-X WARFARIN MOUSE KILLA (Astor)	Warfarin (3(a-acetonylbenzyl)- 4-hydroxycoumarin)	0.025%
ASTOR-X MOUSE KILLA (Astor)	Strychnine*	0.76%	ASTOR-X WARFARIN RAT-MOUSE KILLA CONCENTRATE (Astor)	Warfarin	0.5%
ASTOR-X MOUSE TRACKING POWDER (Astor)	Micronized dichloro diphenyl trichloroethane*	50%	ASTRINGENT POWDER & DEODORANT (Wade)	Zinc sulfate* Blue vitriol* Alum potassium	
ASTOR-X PASTOXINE (Astor)	Red squill powder (fortified)*	30%	ASTRINGENT (Veterinary) (Massengill)	Each tablet: Powdered rhatany Iron sulfate, dried Copper sulfate* Calcium carbonate	0.97 gm. 0.97 gm. 0.97 gm. 0.97 gm.
ASTOR-X RAT KILLA (Astor)	Warfarin	0.025%	ASTRING-O-SOL Astringent (Am. Ferment)	Hydroalcoholic solution of zinc chloride Fluid ext. myrrh Synthetic oil wintergreen* Alcohol*	70%
ASTOR-X RED SQUILL POW-DER CONCEN-TRATE (Astor)	Red squill*	100%	A SUMA EXTRACT Cosmetic (Coty)		
ASTOR-X ROACH AND PEST SPRAY (Astor)	Tech. chlordane Petroleum distillate*	2% 98%	ASURE RAT KILLER (Warren Chem.)	ANTU (alpha naphthyl thiourea)*	20%

*Consult Sec. II., Ingredients Index. This ingredient may be responsible for major toxic effects if poisonous amounts of this product are ingested.

Name & Use Manufacturer	Ingredients		Name & Use Manufacturer	Ingredients	
AT-ASEPTO POWDER Antiseptic surgical dressing (Steinmann)	Thymol iodide Boric acid* Salicylic acid* Bismuth subnitrate Talc		ATHETE LIQUID Skin fungicide (medical) (Thomas, W. G.)	Alcohol* Benzoic acid Menthol* Thymol* Salicylic acid* Balsam Peru	66%
ATAXO (Embalmers')			ATHETE OINTMENT Skin fungicide (medical) (Thomas, W. G.)	Salicylic acid* Benzoic acid Menthol* Zinc oxide Thymol* Ammoniated mercury*	2-1/2%
ATHA-LETO Skin fungicide (medical) (Inman)	Salicylic acid* Resorcin* Oil tar*				
ATHA LU CREME SHAMPOO ("42" Prod.)			ATHLECAINE Fungicide (medical, external (Haynes, P.)	Ethyl alcohol Isopropyl alcohol* Salicylic acid* Thymol* Ethyl aminobenzoate Phenolic and sandarac resin	13% wt. 57%
ATHA-TONE LINIMENT Rubefacient, counterirritant (Gardner Co.)	Methyl salicylate* Menthol-camphor* Oleoresin capsicum				
ATHEA BABY LOTION (Athea)	Triethanolamine stearate Lanolin Petrolatum Hexadecanol Olive oil		ATHLEXOL Fungicide (medical, external) (Allied Drug)	Carbolic acid Oxyquinolin benzoate Salicylic acid* Benzoic acid* Chrysarobin Chlorobutanol Isopropanol*	1%
ATHEA FOOT LOTION (Athea)	Triethanolamine stearate Lanolin Petrolatum Hexadecanol Olive oil		ATHLFOOT Fungicide (medical, external) (McIllwain)	Ether Rubbing alcohol* Salicylic acid* Iodine* Benzoic acid	
ATHEA HAND LOTION (Athea)	Lanolin Petrolatum Vegetable oil Stearic acid Hexadecanol Magnesium stearate Propylene glycol Cetyl alcohol		ATH-LOID OINTMENT Fungicide (medical, external) (Ath-Loid)	Undecylenic acid Zinc undecylenate Triethanolamine	
			ATH-LOID POWDER Fungicide (medical, external) (Athloid)	Undecylenic acid Zinc undecylenate Purified talc U.S.P.	
ATHEA LOTION CREAM SHAMPOO (Athea)	Sodium lauryl sulfate		ATHOSAL Fungicide (medical, external) (Bethesda)	Alcohol Benzoic acid Thymol* Acetone Dimethyldiphenylene disulfide Salicylic acid* Chlorobutanol (5.) chloroform derivate	50%
ATHEA SOAP SHAMPOO (Athea)	Potassium oleate Potassium laurate				
ATHEA SUN RAY Sun tan lotion (Athea)	Triethanolamine stearate Lanolin Petrolatum Hexadecanol Olive oil		ASCATCO Antispasmodic for asthma (Ascatco)	Stramonium alkaloids* Chlorobutanol* Alcohol*	0.017 gr. 0.281 gr. 82%
ATHEA SYNTHETIC SHAMPOO (Athea)	Sodium lauryl sulfate		ATLACIDE Herbicide (Chipman Chem.)	Sodium chlorate*	58.00%
ATHELINE Rubefacient, counterirritant (Caragol)	Menthol .046% Camphor 1.5% Oil of wintergreen syn * 5.0% Extract capsicum .035% Tween 60 0.3% Butyl stearate 0.3% Polyglycol 0.3% Propylene glycol 0.3% Water and vegetable oils 92.0%		ATLACIDE LIQUID Herbicide (Chipman Chem.)	Calcium chlorate* Sodium chloride	25.00% 14.00%

*Consult Sec. II., Ingredients Index. This ingredient may be responsible for major toxic effects if poisonous amounts of this product are ingested.

Name & Use Manufacturer	Ingredients		Name & Use Manufacturer	Ingredients	
ATLACIDE WITH 2, 4-D Herbicide (Chipman Chem.)	Sodium chlorate* 2, 4-D acid	58.00% 0.60%	ATOX DERRIS INSECTICIDE DUST (Chipman Ltd.)	Rotenone	0.75%
ATLANTIC TEXTILE MILL CRAYON (Binney & Smith)			A TO Z LOZENGES Antitussive (Estes)	Benzocaine Eucalyptol* Menthol* Oil anise	
ATLANTIC WHITE BLACK- BOARD CHALK (Binney & Smith)			A.T.R. Fungicide (medical, external) (Wood Chem.)	Phenol Camphor gum Ether Alcohol*	1.5% 61%/v
ATLAS A Herbicide (Chipman Chem.)	Sodium arsenite*	40.00%		Chloral hydrate* Acid salicylic* Glycerine U.S.P.	
ATLAS A DEBARKING COMPOUND (Chipman Chem.)	Sodium arsenite*	40.00%	ATROCAL PULVOID (Yellow) Antispasmodic antacid (Drug Prod., N.Y.)	Atropine sulfate Calcium carbonate precipitated	0.1 mg. 0.65 gm.
ATLAS A6 Herbicide (Chipman Chem.)	Arsenic trioxide*	42.52%			
ATLAS CATTLE DIP IMPROVED Insecticide (Chipman Chem.)	Soap Sodium cresylate Sodium arsenite*	10.00% 11.00% 51.00%	ATROHIST Antihistamine, analgesic (Ethical)	Each tablet: Pyrilamine maleate Atropine sulfate Salicylamide* Acetophenetidin* Caffeine hydrous	25 mg. 1/500 gr. 1-1/2 gr. 2 gr. 1/4 gr.
ATLAS COMPOUND Cathartic (Mac Donald's)	Sodium bicarbonate Powdered ginger Gentian* Aloin Powdered ipecac	4 gr. 3/4 gr. 3/4 gr. 3/16 gr. 1/50 gr.	ATROPAN Analgesic, antispasmodic (Strasenburgh)	Acetanilid* Aspirin* Tar emetic Atropine sulfate	30 mg. 60 mg. 0.3 mg. 0.065 mg.
ATLAS D Herbicide (Chipman Chem.)	Sodium arsenite* Cresylic animal repellent	40.0%	ATRO-SALCO Analgesic (Pitman-Moore)	Each pulvo-cap: Dover's powder (opium 1/40 gr.)	1/4 gr.
ATLAS D DEBARKING COMPOUND (Chipman Chem.)	Sodium arsenite* Cresylic animal repellent	40.0%		Atropine sulfate* Acetophenetidin* Acetylsalicylic acid* (aspirin)	1/1000 gr. 2-1/2 gr. 3-1/2 gr.
ATLAS 60 Herbicide (Chipman Chem.)	Sodium arsenite*	60.0%		Tr. gelsemium (ext. equiv.) 2 m. Camphor monobromated 1/4 gr.	
ATLAS WOOD PRESERVATIVE & CLEANER (Chipman Chem.).			ATTAR OF PETALS COLOGNE DEODORANT, TOILET WATER, PERFUME (Vivaudou)		
ATHLETA Fungicide (medical, external) (Douglas Prod.)	Prec. sulfur Acid salicylic* Oil of cade*		AUBRY SISTERS ROUGE (Aubry)		
ATHO LINIMENT (Dunwody)			AUBRY SISTERS SKIN BEAUTI- FIER (Aubry)		
ATOLAK Cleaning compound (Atomix)			AUDACIOUS COLOGNE & PERFUME (Miahati)		
			AUNT LOU MEDICINE (Aunt Lou)		

*Consult Sec. II., Ingredients Index. This ingredient may be responsible for major toxic effects if poisonous amounts of this product are ingested.

Name & Use Manufacturer	Ingredients		Name & Use Manufacturer	Ingredients	
AUNTY BURNS For skin burns (Priceless)	Oil pine Oil lemon Oil cloves Menthol* Stearic acid Glycerine Oil wintergreen* Oil thyme Ethyl salicylate* Camphor* Boric acid* Potassium hydroxide		**AUTOSAN AUTO SOAP** (Huntington)		
			AUTO TOP PRESERVER (Protection)	Petroleum solvents*	
			AUXILODERM C OINTMENT Fungicide (veterinary) (Paraderm)	Iodine* Salicylic acid* Thymol* Methyl salicylate* Zinc phenolsulfonate Formaldehyde solution Cresol* Menthol Chloroform	3%
AURAGREEN Fungicide (Mallinckrodt)	Malachite green Auramine Crystal violet* (gentian violet)				
AURAL ANALGESIC (Tampa)	Glycerite antipyrine Chlorobutanol* compound		**AUXILODERM H OINTMENT** For skin irritations (veterinary) (Paraderm)	Iodine* Cresol* Menthol* Chloroform Formaldehyde solution Thymol Methyl salicylate* Zinc phenolsulfonate	3%
AURILAVE Antiseptic powder (Partola)	Each oz.: Chlorobutanol* Phenol* Sodium bicarbonate Methyl salicylate* Sodium borate* Boric acid* Menthol* Eucalyptol*	11 gr.			
			AUXILODERM OINTMENT For skin irritations (Paraderm)	Iodine Cresol Methyl salicylate* Formaldehyde solution Zinc phenolsulfonate Menthol Thymol	0.7% 0.3% 9% 0.3% 0.7% 2% 1%
AURO EAR DROPS (Wright, M.)	Benzocaine Propylene glycol Camphor* Thymol*				
AUSTIN'S SYRUP HYDROLE COMP. Antitussive (Austin)	Chloroform Alcohol Hyoscyamus chloroform alcohol Peppermint Ginger Syr. tar Dilute hydrocyanic acid* Dilute hydrochloric acid	4 m. 7%	**AVALANCHE HEAVY ANIMAL SALVE** (Chemurgic)	Di-isobutyl-phenoxy-ethoxy- ethyl-dimethyl-benzyl ammonium chloride monohydrate*	
			AVAMIST Inhalant (avian, veterinary) (Gland-O-Lac)	Formaldehyde solution* U.S.P. Normal butyl alcohol * Isopropyl alcohol* Extract of capsicum	10%/v 14%/v
AUTO RITE Polish (Boyle-Midway)	Silicone oil Petroleum naphtha* Emulsifiers Silicous abrasives		**AVENARIUS CARBOLINEUM** Wood preserva- tive (Carbolineum)	Chlorinated coal tar oils*	
AUTOMATIC SOAP FLAKES (Fitzpatrick)	Vegetable and animal oils				
AUTO MIST Sanitizer, deodorizer (Allied Home)	Triethylene glycol Isopropyl alcohol Di-isobutyl-phenoxy-ethoxy- ethyl-dimethyl-benzyl ammonium chloride Perfume oil	5.6% 0.9% 0.1% 0.3%	**AVENGER MOTHICIDE LIQUID** (Warren Chem.)	DDT*	25.0%
			AVEX Avian expector- ant (veterinary) (Wilke)	Potassium guaiacol sulfonate* Ammonium chloride Iodine* Beechwood creosote* Potassium dichromate Glycerine Acacia	
AUTO POLISH (Stanley Home)	Hydrocarbon solvent* Snow floss Silicone Red oil Carnauba wax Morpholine* Bentonite Butoben		**AVICOL FOR POULTRY** (Tablets) Bacteriacide for drinking water (Burrell-Dugger)	Ortho-phenylphenol* Sulfocarbolates of sodium, calcium, zinc Glauber's salts	

*Consult Sec. II., Ingredients Index. This ingredient may be responsible for major toxic effects if poisonous amounts of this product are ingested.

Name & Use Manufacturer	Ingredients	
AVI-TAB Tonic (veterinary, avian) (Salsbury's)	Copper sulfate* (copper metallic 5.3%) Ext. nux vomica (strychnine 1.2 gr./oz.) Areca nut Kamala Mustard Oleoresin capsicum Anise oil Potassium iodide Sulfates of cobalt, iron, manganese, zinc Starch Glucose	21% 4% 10% 1.4% 4% 14%
AVI-TON Anthelmintic (veterinary) (Salsbury's)	Nicotine* Phenothiazine Nux vomica Strychnine Gentian Calumba Mustard Anise Copper sulfate Copper metallic Ferrous sulfate	0.6% 3.0% 5% 0.057% 3% 0.75%
AVON ANNALOS 7 WEEDKILLER (Parrot Chem.)	Petroleum oil*	
AVON COSMETICS (Avon Prod.)		
AVON CREAMS AND LOTIONS (Avon Prod.)		
AVON FACE AND BODY POWDERS (Avon Prod.)		
AVON SOAPS (Avon Prod.)		
AVON TALCUM POWDER (Avon Prod.)		
AVON TOILET SOAP (Avon Prod.)		
AXAR TABLETS Analgesic (McKesson & Robbins)	Acetophenetidin* (acetanilid derivative) Aspirin* Caffeine	3 gr. 2-1/2 gr. 1/8 gr.
AXILLA CREAM DEODORANT (Keeber)		
AXTELL POWDERED HAND SOAP Mechanic's (La Rue-Axtell)	Pumice Dry oils	

Name & Use Manufacturer	Ingredients	
AYER'S PECTORAL For coughs, bronchial irritations (Sterling Prod.)	Alcohol Chloroform Terpin hydrate Benzaldehyde Wild cherry White pine Ipecac	16-1/2% 2 m./ oz.
A-ZEE-O OINTMENT & POWDER (A-Zee-O)		
AZMA MIST Bronchial decongestant (Nephron)		
AZORB DEOD. POWDER (Airline)		
A-Z SANITIZER Bathroom deodorant (Reliable Chem.)	Naphthalene	
AZURENE SHAKE LOTION S.F. MFR. NO. 825 For skin irritation (Specialists)	Azulene Sesquiterpenes* Sesquiterpene alcohols Sodium benzoate Glycerine Paraffin hydrocarbons Menthol Umbellifore methylether Furfurol* Zinc oxide* Fatty acid	
BAALMANN'S GAS TABLETS (Baalmann)		
BABBITT'S CLEANSER (Babbitt)		
BABBITT'S COLD WATER DRAIN PIPE SOLVENT (Babbitt)	Sodium hydroxide*	
BABE-EEZ (Babe-Eez)	Calamine Starch Castor oil Zinc oxide	
BAB-O CLEANSER (Babbitt)		
BABY BRECK LAVO For washing babies (Breck, J.H.)	Low-alkalinity soap (pH 8)	

Name & Use Manufacturer	Ingredients		Name & Use Manufacturer	Ingredients	
BABY COUGH SYRUP Antitussive (Royal Mfg.)	Alcohol Ext. of white pine Wild cherry Aralia Poplar buds Blood root Sassafras Menthol	6%/v	BACORN'S VAPORIZING FORKOLA JELL Decongestant, external (Bacorn)	Camphor* Thymol Menthol Cocoa butter Oils of eucalyptus* Methyl salicylate* Peppermint Turpentine* Nutmeg Cedar leaf Pinus sylvestris Thyme Petrolatum foundation	
BABYLON PERFUME, COLOGNE, TOILET- WATER (Duvelle)	Alcohol* denatured with di- ethyl phthalate				
			BACOTOL To combat tobacco habit (Ray Drug)	Lobeline sulfate* P.E. gentian P.E. taraxacum P.E. glycyrrhiza	
BABY OINTMENT (Massengill)	Aluminum hydrate Zinc odixe* Boric acid* Tinct. benzoin comp. Carbolic acid	0.2%	BAC-STOP LOZENGES To combat tobacco habit (Davin)		
BABY SYRUP Cough syrup (Hance)	Alcohol Fl. ext. ipecac Fl. ext. squill Cherry bark	1-1/2%/v	BACTA-LIFE Septic tank activator (Blue Seal)	Yeast (nutmeg) Dehydrated enzymes	98% 2%
BACON'S C-K-TEA Cathartic (Wells, S.C.)	Senna leaves Mandrake root Aromatic herbs				

BACO ANTISEPTIC POWDER (Baer Drugs)			BACTINE ANTISEPTIC Germicide, fungicide, de- odorizer (Miles)	Alcohol
				Di-isobutyl cresoxy ethoxy ethyl
				  dimethyl benzyl ammonium
				  chloride*
				Polyethylene glycol mono-iso-octyl
				  phenyl ether
				Chlorothymol
				Propylene glycol
				Essential oils
					4%

BACO DIURETIC SPECIAL (Baer Drugs)					
BACO EYE LOTION (Baer Drugs)			BACTOX PINE ODOR DISIN- FECTANT (Lester)	Soap Pine oil* Sodium orthobenzyl-para-chloro- phenate* Isopropanol*	
BACO FOOT SALTS (Baer Drugs)			BADGER 10% DDT INSECT POWDER (Wisconsin Pharm.)	DDT*	10%
BACON'S C-K-TEA Cathartic (Wells, S.C.)	Senna leaves Mandrake root Aromatic herbs				
BACO NUVITA SCALP OINTMENT (Baer Drugs			BAE-BEE Baby skin Cream (Astra)	Anhydrous lanolin U.S.P. Petrolatum U.S.P. Cetal U.S.P. Olive and mineral oil U.S.P. Beeswax U.S.P. Ferric phosphate U.S.P. Potassium chloride U.S.P.	
BACO OINTMENTS NOS. 2 & 3 (Baer Drugs)			BAER'S LACQUERS (Baer Bros. (Paint))	Isopropyl alcohol* Ethyl alcohol Butyl alcohol Butyl acetate* Methyl isobutyl ketone Petroleum naphtha* Toluol* Ethylene glycol monobutyl ether* Ethyl acetate Nitrocellulose Various resins Castor oil Dibutyl phthalate Soya bean oil	
BACO PILE SUPPOSITORIES (Baer Drugs)					
BACO POLISH (Baer Drugs)					

*Consult Sec. II., Ingredients Index. This ingredient may be responsible for major toxic effects if poisonous amounts of this product are ingested.

Name & Use Manufacturer	Ingredients
BAER'S LACQUER THINNERS (Baer Bros. (Paint))	Isopropyl alcohol* Ethyl alcohol Butyl alcohol* Butyl acetate Methyl isobutyl ketone* Petroleum naphtha* Toluol* Ethylene glycol monobutyl ether* Ethyl acetate*
BAER'S PAINTS AND PAINT PRODUCTS (Baer Bros. (Paint))	
BAG BALM Ointment, veterinary (Dairy Assoc.)	Petrolatum U.S.P. Lanolin U.S.P. Ethylated mercury sterols containing 0.005% mercury and sanitas oil (distilled pine oil)
BAHIM OIL For skin irritation (Jamol)	Cajuput oil Pine oil* Eucalyptus oil* Vegetable oil
BAILES AFTER SHAVE LOTION (Bailes)	
BAILES 3-WAY HAIR TONIC (Bailes)	
BAINICIDE Insect Spray (Lester)	Petroleum distillates* Piperonyl butoxide Pyrethrins* Essential oils*
BAIT-M Insecticide (Acme Q.P.)	Calcium arsenate* 5% Metaldehyde 1.75%
BAKER CALOMEL, RHUBARB & COLOCYNTH COMPOUND Cathartic (Nelson Baker)	Calomel* 2 gr. Rhubarb Aloe* Myrrh Extract of colocynth Resin scammony Essential oils
BAKER'S AUTO BODY CLEANER & POLISH (Baker,C.P.)	Infusorial earth Glycerine Refined petroleum oil Solvent*
BAKER'S CLEANER & SHAMPOO (Baker,C.P.)	Alcohol* Alcohol sulfate*
BAKER'S FURNITURE POLISH (Baker,C.P.)	Sulfonated vegetable oil Neutral petroleum oil*
BAKER'S INSTANTANE- OUS SILVER POLISH (Baker,C.P.)	Infusorial earth Soap Glycerine
BAKER'S METAL POL- ISH (Baker,C.P.)	Oleic acid Alcohol Ammonia* Silica

Name & Use Manufacturer	Ingredients
BALANCEL Mineral supplement (Meyer)	Each tablet: Calcium phosphate, tribasic 343.43 mg. Cobalt chloride 0.048 mg. Copper sulfate 1.0 mg. Ferrous sulfate 18.87 mg. Magnesium sulfate 20.05 mg. Manganese sulfate 9.35 mg. Potassium phosphate, monobasic 272.2 mg. Sodium molybdate 0.012 mg. Potassium iodide 0.109 mg. Zinc chloride 0.545 mg.
BALDWIN'S NO. 10 FLY KILLER (Baldwin)	Malathion (o,o-dimthyl dithiophosphate of diethyl mercaptosuccinate) 1.00%
BALL PEN SCRIPTO INK (Scripto)	Methanol (maximum content less than 2%)
BALL'S HAIR COLOR PREPARATION (Dolle)	
BALM BARR CREME SHAMPOO (Balm Barr)	Lanolin U.S.P. Duponol WA paste Perfume Stearic acid Ninol 737
BALM BARR LOTION (Balm Barr)	Triethanolamine Glycerine U.S.P. Mineral oil U.S.P. Stearic acid Quince mucilage Perfume Lanolin U.S.P. Methyl parasept
BALMIAL Antitussive (Clapp,Otis)	Alcohol 15% Chloroform 3.3 m/fl.oz. Balm of Gilead buds Wild cherry bark White pine bark Sanguinaria (blood root) Ipecac Ammonium chloride Sassafras bark
BALMZANE Rubefacient, counter-irritant (Bryan Labs.)	Methyl salicylate* Camphor* Menthol* with E-4 (Bis-(5-chloro-2-hydroxyphenyl) methane)
BALTIMORE BROWN COPPER PAINT (Balt.Copper)	
BALTIMORE EYE DROPS (Caswell- Massey)	
BALTIMORE GREEN COPPER PAINT (Balt.Copper)	

---

*Consult Sec. II., Ingredients Index. This ingredient may be responsible for major toxic effects if poisonous amounts of this product are ingested.

Name & Use Manufacturer	Ingredients	
BALTIMORE RED COPPER PAINT (Balt.Copper)		
BALTIMORE X253 RED COPPER PLASTIC PAINT (Balt.Copper)		
BAMBOLITE VARNISH NO. 383 (Enterprise Paint)		
BAMTONA For hemorrhoids and skin irritation (Flores)	Camphor* Pyroligneous acid Witch hazel ext. Oil rosemary	
BAMTONA RECTAL SUPPOSITORIES For hemmorhoids (Flores)	Ephedrine sulfate Benzocaine Zinc oxide Bismuth subgallate Balsam Peru Oxyquinoline sulfate	1/16 gr. 2 gr.
BAN Liquid deodorant (Bristol-Myers)		
BAN-A-BUG Residual spray (Wipp)	Tech. chlordane	2%
BANALG LINIMENT Rubefacient, counter-irritant (Cole)	Menthol* Camphor* Methyl salicylate* Oil eucalyptus	
BANARAT BITS Rodenticide (Am.Serum)		
BANAY TABLETS For uterine tension (Banay)	Each tablet: Magnesium glutamate	7 1/2 gr.
BANDINI 5% CHLORDANE DUST Insecticide (Bandini)	Tech. chlordane* Beta butoxy beta' thiocyanodiethyl ether	5.0% 1.0%
BANDINI CHLORDANE SPRAY Insecticide (Bandini)	Tech. chlordane * Petroleum oil* Pine oil Tech. piperonyl butoxide Pyrethrins	25.00% 53.35% 5.00% 1.50% 0.15%
BANDINI DUAL SPRAY Insecticide, fungicide (Bandini)	Copper oleate* Rotenone Other ether extractives of cube	24.00% 1.50% 3.00%
BANDINI FUNGICIDE SPRAY (Bandini)	Sodium polysulfide* Sodium thiosulfate	15.00% 3.75%

Name & Use Manufacturer	Ingredients	
BANDINI 50% MALATHION SPRAY Insecticide (Bandini)	Malathion*	
BANDINI SCALE SPRAY (Bandini)	Petroleum oil*	85.0%
BANDINI SOIL & WATER ACIDIFIER (Bandini)	Ferrous sulfate Magnesium sulfate Ammoniacal nitrogen Phosphoric acid Nitric acid Sulfuric acid	5.0% 5.0% 0.50% 2.00% 0.50% 2.00%
BANDOLINE Hair grooming preparation (Colgate-Palmolive)		
BANISHEE DEODORANT (Haines)		
BANTRON Combat tobacco habit (Carlay)	Lobeline sulfate* Tricalcium phosphate Magnesium carbonate	
BARBARA GOULD COSMETICS (Gould)		
BARBARA GOULD CREAMS (Gould)		
BARBARA GOULD DEODORANTS (Gould)		
BARBARA GOULD LOTIONS (Gould)		
BARBARA GOULD POWDERS (Gould)		
BARBARA GOULD SHAMPOOS (Gould)		
BARBARA KAREN ASTRINGENT (French-Bell)		
BARBARA KAREN BEAUTY FOAM SHAMPOO (French-Bell)		

*Consult Sec. II., Ingredients Index. This ingredient may be responsible for major toxic effects if poisonous amounts of this product are ingested.

Name & Use Manufacturer	Ingredients	Name & Use Manufacturer	Ingredients
BARBARA GOULD EYEBROW PENCIL (Gould)		BARBARA GOULD REVITAL (Gould)	
BARBARA GOULD EYE SHADOW (Gould)		BARBARA GOULD ROSE GERANIUM LIQUID DEODORANT (Gould)	
BARBARA GOULD HAND CREAM (Gould)		BARBARA GOULD ROUGE (Gould)	
BARBARA GOULD HAND LOTION (Gould)		BARBARA GOULD SHAMPOO (Gould)	
BARBARA GOULD LIQUID CONDITIONER SHAMPOO (Gould)		BARBARA GOULD SKIN FRESHENER (Gould)	
BARBARA GOULD MASCARA (Gould)		BARBARA GOULD SPECIAL CLEANSING CREAM (Gould)	
BARBARA GOULD MILD ASTRINGENT CREAM & LIQUID (Gould)		BARBARA GOULD SPECIAL DRY SKIN CREAM (Gould)	
BARBARA GOULD MOISONE CREAM & OIL (Gould)		BARBARA GOULD STARS IN YOUR EYES (Gould)	
BARBARA GOULD NAIL POLISH FOUNDATION (Gould)		BARBARA GOULD THROAT CREAM (Gould)	
BARBARA GOULD NIGHT CREAM (Gould)		BARBARA GOULD VELVET OF PEACHES CREAM & LIQUID FOUNDATION (Gould)	
BARBARA GOULD PERSONAL TOUCH ANTI-PERSPIRANT CREAM (Gould)		BARBARA GOULD VELVET OF ROSES DRY SKIN CREAM (Gould)	
BARBARA GOULD PINE OIL BATH (Gould)		BARBARA KAREN ASTRINGENT (French-Bell)	
BARBARA GOULD PLASTIC CREAM MASQUE (Gould)		BARBARA KAREN BEAUTY FOAM SHAMPOO (French-Bell)	
BARBARA GOULD POMPOM CREAM (Gould)			

*Consult Sec. II., Ingredients Index. This ingredient may be responsible for major toxic effects if poisonous amounts of this product are ingested.

- 294 -

Name & Use Manufacturer	Ingredients	Name & Use Manufacturer	Ingredients
BARBARA KAREN COMPLEXION CLEANSER CREAM (French-Bell)		BARC GREASELESS CREAM For lice, nits, crablice (Wright, M.)	Isobornyl thiocyanoacetate* 4.1% Other related terpenes 0.9% Dioctyl sodium sulfosuccinate 0.6%
BARBARA KAREN DUAL CREAM (French-Bell)		BARCO AM-40 2,4-D WEED KILLER (40% Amine Concentrate) Herbicide (Barco Chemical Inc.)	Triethylamine salt of 2,4-dichloro-phenoxyacetic acid* 61%
BARBARA KAREN ESTROGENIC HORMONE CREAM, OIL (French-Bell)		BARDEX LINIMENT (Bardex)	
BARBARA KAREN GLOW POWDER BASE (French-Bell)		BAR-F LEATHER CREAM (Bar-F)	Beeswax Carnauba wax Neatsfoot oil Lanolin Stearic acid Triethanolamine
BARBARA KAREN HAND CREAM & LOTION (French-Bell)		BARFRED HYPNOCAINE LOTION For burns (Barfred)	Hypnocaine (n-propanol para-amino benzyl carboxylate) Benzyl alcohol* Menthol* Camphor*
BARBARA KAREN MASQUE (French-Bell)		BARFRED HYPNOCAINE OINTMENT For burns and sunburn (Barfred)	Hypnocaine (n-propanol para-amino benzyl) carboxylate 3% Benzyl alcohol 1%
BARBARA KAREN ODOREX Deodorant (French-Bell)		BAR GLOSS Polish (Gisler)	
BARBARA KAREN POWDER (French-Bell)		BARKEEPER'S FRIEND METAL POLISH (Gisler)	
BARBARA KAREN RETIRING CREAM (French-Bell)		BARKER'S INSECTICIDE Veterinary (Barker, M.&M.)	
BARBARA KAREN SPECIAL FORMULA CREAM (French-Bell)		BARKER'S LINIMENT FOR MAN OR BEAST (Barker, M.&M.)	
BARBARA KAREN SUNTAN LOTION (French-Bell)		BARKER'S LIVESTOCK PRODUCTS Veterinary medicines (Barker, M.&M.)	
BARBASOL Shaving cream (Barbasol	Hydrogenated vegetable oil Liquid petrolatum Boric acid* Lanolin	BARNES-HIND A.P.C. TABLETS Analagesic (Barnes-Hind)	Each tablet: Aspirin* 0.227 gm. Acetophenetidin* 0.162 gm. Caffeine citrate 0.0324 gm.
BARBO COMPOUND Coloring for gray hair (Barbo)		BARNES-HIND GERMICIDAL WETTING SOLUTION For use with plastic contact lenses (Barnes-Hind)	Alkyl dimethylbenzyl ammonium chloride 1-50,000
BARBO (Instant) Coloring for gray hair (Barbo)	Alcohol 20%		

*Consult Sec. II., Ingredients Index. This ingredient may be responsible for major toxic effects if poisonous amounts of this product are ingested.

- 295 -

Name & Use Manufacturer	Ingredients		Name & Use Manufacturer	Ingredients	
BAR-O-DANE Insecticide (Bartlett, F.A.)	Tech. chlordane	2%	BARRINGTON HAND CREAM (North American)	Stearic acid Cocoa butter Lanolin Tegosepts	
BARON Herbicide (Dow)	2 (2,4,5-Trichlorophenoxy) ethyl-2,2-dichloropropionate*		BARRINGTON SUPRA SOFNING LOTION (North American)	Stearic acid Cocoa butter Lanolin Tegosepts	
BARRELED SUNLIGHT CHINALINE ENAMELS (Barreled Sunlight)			BAR RUST RUST PREV. & REMOVER COMPOUND (Sharp, J.C.)		
BARRELL'S SPEC. FORMULA LINIMENT (H.G.O.)			BARRY'S AFTER SHAVE LOTION (Lanman)		
BARRETT CARBOSOTA Wood preservative (Barrett Div.)	Coal-tar creosote*	98 1/2%	BARRY'S ANTISEPTIC TOILET CREAM For skin irritation (Suwannee)	Boric acid* Glycerinum Gum tragacanth Alcohol	8%/v
BARRETT PAINT THINNER (Barrett Div.)	Naphtha*		BARRY'S SULFO-SEAL (Veterinary) Screw-worm killer (Suwanee)	Benzol* Coal tar* Neutral oils Tar camphor Chloroform Sulfur	65% 9.7% 7% 3% 2% 6.6%
BARRETT'S ADHESIVE #1 (Barrett V.)	Casein Borax* Oleic acid Glue Ammonia*				
BARRETT'S ADHESIVE #2 (Barrett V.)	Casein Borax* Oleic acid Glue Ammonia*		BARTELDES 2,4-D WEED KILLER (Barteldes)	Sodium salt of 2,4-D*	70%
BARRETT'S ANTSAULT Insecticide (Barrett Chem.)	Chlordane*	5%	BARTLETT'S BORAX-CELITE DUST FOR TURNIPS (Bartlett, N.M.)	Borax*	50%
BARRETT'S CEMENT PATCHING (Wittekind)			BARTLETT'S DUSTING SULFUR (80-10-10) (Microscopic) Insecticide (Bartlett, N.M.)	Sulfur Lead arsenate*	
BARRETT'S MOUSESAULT Rodenticide (Barrett Chem.)	Strychnine sulfate	0.5%	BARTLETT'S DUSTING SULFUR (95-5) (Microscopic) Fungicide (Bartlett, N.M.)	Sulfur*	
BARRETT'S RATSAULT Rodenticide (Barrett Chem.)	ANTU	20%			
BARRETT'S ROACHSAULT Insecticide (Barrett Chem.)	DDT* Chlordane*	10% 5%	BARTLETT'S DUSTING SULFUR WITH 5% DDT Insecticide (Bartlett, N.M.)	Sulfur* DDT*	5%
BARRETT'S RODENT KILLER (Barrett Chem.)					
BARRINGTON COLD CREAM CLEANSING (North American)	Stearic acid Cocoa butter Lanolin Tegosepts		BARTLETT'S 7% FIXED COPPER DUST Fungicide (Bartlett, N.M.)	Copper*	7%

*Consult Sec. II., Ingredients Index. This ingredient may be responsible for major toxic effects if poisonous amounts of this product are ingested.

Name & Use Manufacturer	Ingredients		Name & Use Manufacturer	Ingredients	
BARTLETT'S 7% FIXED COPPER DUST WITH 3% DDT Insecticide (Bartlett,N.M.)	Copper* DDT	7% 3%	BAUGH'S NO. 37 DUAL PURPOSE DUST Insecticide (Baugh)	DDT* Copper*	
BARTLETT'S GYPSUM DUST WITH ARSENATE OF LIME Insecticide (Bartlett,N.M.)	Arsenate of lime *	10%	BAUGH'S NO. 75 DUST Insecticide (Baugh)	Rotenone* Other cube resins	
BARTLETT'S NICOTINE DUST Insecticide (Bartlett,N.M.)	Nicotine sulfate*		BAUMODYNE Rubefacient, counter- irritant (Chicago Pharm.)	Methyl salicylate* Oil of eucalyptus Menthol*	
BARTON'S SAFETY LEATHER DYE (Barton Mfg.)	Alcohol* Dyes (coal tar derivatives related to D&C) Dye solvent (diethylene glycol or o-Dichlorobenzene*—in black leather dye only		BAYCINE Antacid (Battle Creek)	Basic aluminum glycinate Glycine	5 gr. 1 gr.
			BAYER ASPIRIN HEADACHE TABLETS (Bayer)	Acetyl salicylic acid*	
BASSORAN LAXATIVE (Merrell)	Sterculia gum Magnesium trisilicate		BAYER MULSIFIED COCOANUT OIL SHAMPOO (Bayer)	Potassium soap of cocoanut oil Alcohol 3%	
BATH-ADOL For toilet and bath (Great Lakes Labs.)	Alcohol*	92%			
			BAY ROMA HAIR COLORING (Assoc. Brands)		
BATH BUBBLES (Clark,R.)	Sodium sulfate Sodium alkyl aryl sulfonate Sodium alkyl lauryl sulfonate Perfume D&C color		BAY RUM Astringent (Am. Druggists)	Alcohol*	50%/v
BATH-O- FOAM BUBBLE BATH (Clark,R.)	Sodium sulfate Sodium alkyl aryl sulfonate Sodium alkyl lauryl sulfonate Perfume D&C color		BAY RUM (Imported) Astringent (Peoples)	Alcohol*	50%/v
BATH-O-VEL Bath oil, water softener (Torch)			B-B-S (formerly Betacide) Emollient and antiseptic ointment (CaPhenin)	Betanaphthol* Sulfur* Balsam Peru Petrolatum	
BATH PEARLS Bath oil capsules (Delagar)	Mineral oil Perfume	3%	BC Analgesic (B.C.)	Acetophenetidin* Aspirin* Caffeine	2-1/2 gr.
BATHSHEBA COLOGNE & PERFUME (Wolff)			BCC STOCK SPRAY Insecticide (Bonide)	Petroleum distillates* Beta-thiocyano-B'-butoxy diethyl ether	
BATTLE CREEK ACIDONE TABLETS For hypochlor- hydria (Battle Creek)	Each tablet: Hydrochloric acid (10%) 1/10 cc.		B-D ACE ADHERENT (Becton)	Non-oxidizing rosin Alcohol* approx 60%/w Acid tannic approx 1%/w Gum camphor approx 1%/w Oil turpentine approx 1%/w	
			BEACON AMMONIA (Hood)	Ammonia*	5-10%
BAUGH'S AGRICULTURAL 3% DDT DUST (Baugh)	DDT	3%			
BAUGH'S AGRICULTUR- AL 5% DDT DUST (Baugh)	DDT*	5%	BEACON DISINFECTANT BLEACH (Hood)	Sodium hypochlorite* 5 1/4%/w Sodium chloride 5 1/4%/w Sodium hydroxide and/or sodium carbonate 0.2 to 0.3%	

*Consult Sec. II., Ingredients Index. This ingredient may be responsible for major toxic effects if poisonous amounts of this product are ingested.

Name & Use Manufacturer	Ingredients	Name & Use Manufacturer	Ingredients
BEACON LAUNDRY STARCH (Hood)	Pure starch Preservative less than 0.1%	BEATSOL BLACK-EYE BLEACH (G.&W.)	Ammonium chloride Pot. nitrate* Glacial acetic acid Butyl ester of parahydroxy benzoic acid
BEACON PASTE WAX (Beacon)	Natural waxes Terpenic, paraffinic solvents*	BEATSOL B-NO-VERMIN Ectoparasiti-cide (G.&W.)	Larkspur* Sabadilla seed* Alcohol * 90%
BEACON QUIK GLOSS WAX (Beacon)	Natural waxes	BEATSOL COLD SORE LOTION Rubefacient, antiseptic (G.&W.)	Benzoin Storax Tolu Camphor* Alcohol*
BEACON WAX (Beacon)			
BEACON WAX & DIRT REMOVER (Beacon)	Raw material non-toxic, alkaline	BEATSOL CONCEN-TRATED MEDICINAL POWDER Douche pow-der (G.&W.)	Sodium borate* Sodium chloride Thymol* Menthol* Eucalyptol*
BEADS O'BLEACH (Purex Corp.	Organic chlorine compound* Organic surfactant*		
BEAMAX SELF POLISHING WAX (Davies-Young)		BEATSOL CORN RE-MOVER Keratolytic (G.&W.)	Salicylic acid* Flexible collodion
BEAR LAMP BLACK (Monsanto)	Soot	BEATSOL GLYCERINE SUPPOSITOR-IES Emollient, cathartic (G.&W.)	Glycerine U.S.P. 95%
BEAR'S JACK FROST Rubefacient (Bear)	Menthol* Camphor* Oil of peppermint		
BEAUTY LOTION (Stanley Home)	Deltyl extra Triethanolamine Cetyl alcohol N.F. flakes Perfume Tegosept M Certified dye Stearic acid Propylene glycol Lanolin Hexachlorophene Tegosept P Versene	BEATSOL GLYCERINE SUPPOSITOR-IES (For in-fants & child-ren) (G.&W.)	Glycerine U.S.P. 95%
		BEATSOL MEDICATED SALVE Antiseptic (G.&W.)	Oil linseed Petrolatum Zinc oxide Starch Phenol* Acid boric *
BEATSALL D INSECT SPRAY (Meyer)	DDT (dichloro diphenyl trichloroethane)* 5%	BEATSOL HEMORRHOI-DAL SUPPOSI-TORIES (G.&W.)	Istrian nutgalls Zinc oxide Ethyl aminobenzoate Cocoa butter
BEATSALL INSECT SPRAY (Meyer)	B-butoxy-B'-thiocyanodiethyl ether 0.5% B-thiocyano ethyl ethers of aliphatic acid containing 10-18 carbon atoms 1.5% Petroleum distillate* 97.9% Gamma isomer of benzene hexachloride 0.1%	BEATSOL SALVE Emollient, Antiseptic for skin (G.&W.)	Rosin Ichthammol Petrolatum Whitewax
BEATSOL ACTION LINIMENT Rubefacient, counter-irritant (G.&W.)	Gum camphor Alcohol* Methyl salicylate* Rectified spirit of turpentine* Oil of sassafras	BEATSOL SODIUM PERBORATE Oral antiseptic (G.&W.)	Sodium perborate*
BEATSOL ANTISEPTIC VAGINAL CONES (G.&W.)	Oxyquinoline base Benzoic acid Boric acid* Cocoa butter	BEATSOL TEETHING LOTION Local anesthe-tic (G.&W.)	Benzocaine Iodine* Alcohol*

*Consult Sec. II., Ingredients Index. This ingredient may be responsible for major toxic effects if poisonous amounts of this product are ingested.

Name & Use Manufacturer	Ingredients		Name & Use Manufacturer	Ingredients
BEATSOL TOOTHACHE OUTFIT LIQUID Local antiseptic (G.&W.)	Oil of cloves Benzocaine Iodine Isopropyl alcohol* 95%		BEAUTY COUNSELOR EYE SHADOW (Beauty Couns.)	
BEATSOL WART LIQUID Keratolytic (G.&W.)	Ricinic acid Oil castor Isopropyl alcohol*		BEAUTY COUNSELOR FACE LOTION (Beauty Couns.)	
BEATSOL WITCH HAZEL OINTMENT Antiseptic, rubefacient (G.&W.)	Powdered extract witch hazel leaves 2.5% Phenol 1.8% Gum camphor* 3.0% Ointment base 92.7%		BEAUTY COUNSELOR FACE POWDER (Beauty Couns.)	
BEAU KREML HAIR DRESSING (Williams,J.B.)	Brucine sulfate denaturant Polyalkalene glycols*		BEAUTY COUNSELOR HAND CREAM (Beauty Couns.)	
BEAUTIFLOR Floor finisher (Johnson, S.C.)	Petroleum naphtha* Animal, vegetable and petroleum waxes		BEAUTY COUNSELOR HAND LOTION (Beauty Couns.)	
BEAUTY BATH FOR DOGS Insecticide (Huston)	Gamma isomer of benzene hexachloride (from lindane) 0.99% Bis (5-chloro-2-hydroxyphenyl)-methane 0.25% N-(Lauroyl calomino formylmethyl) pyridinium chloride 3.00%		BEAUTY COUNSELOR LEG MAKE-UP (Beauty Couns.)	
BEAUTY BRAND FLOOR WAX (Welmaid)	Wax Resin		BEAUTY COUNSELOR LIPSTICK (Beauty Couns.)	
BEAUTY BRAND PASTE POLISH (Welmaid)	Waxes Petroleum solvent* Oil-soluble dye		BEAUTY COUNSELOR MAKE-UP BASE (Beauty Couns.)	
BEAUTY BRAND SADDLE SOAP (Welmaid)	Soap Wax Neatsfoot oil Shirlan extra* (duPont) Perfume Dye		BEAUTY COUNSELOR MASCARA (Beauty Couns.)	
BEAUTY BRAND SHOE DYE (Welmaid)	Isopropyl alcohol* Orthodichlorobenzene* Dye		BEAUTY COUNSELOR MOUTHWASH (Beauty Couns.)	
BEAUTY COUNSELOR COSMETICS (Beauty Couns.)			BEAUTY COUNSELOR NAIL POLISH (Beauty Couns.)	
BEAUTY COUNSELOR CUTICLE OIL (Beauty Couns.)			BEAUTY COUNSELOR NAIL WHITE (Beauty Couns.)	
BEAUTY COUNSELOR ESTRA-CREAM HORMONE, LUBRICATING FORMULA, NIGHT CREAM, & OILY SKIN FORMULA (Beauty Couns.)			BEAUTY COUNSELOR PERFUME, COLOGNE & TOILET WATER (Beauty Couns.)	
			BEAUTY COUNSELOR ROUGE (Beauty Couns.)	
			BEAUTY COUNSELOR SHAMPOO (Liquid) (Beauty Couns.)	

*Consult Sec. II., Ingredients Index. This ingredient may be responsible for major toxic effects if poisonous amounts of this product are ingested.

Name & Use Manufacturer	Ingredients		Name & Use Manufacturer	Ingredients	
BEAUTY COUNSELOR SKIN FRESHENER (Beauty Couns.)			BEECHEM CHLORDANE Insecticide (Beechem)	Chlordane*	
BEAUTY COUNSELOR TALCUM POWDER (Beauty Couns.)			BEECHEM CHLOROPICRIN Insecticide (Beechem)	Chloropicrin*	
BEAUTY COUNSELOR TOILET SOAP (Beauty Couns.)			BEECHEM DDT, EMULSIFIABLE Insecticide (Beechem)	DDT*	
BEAUTY COUNSELOR TOOTH PASTE (Beauty Couns.)			BEECHEM METHYL BROMIDE Insecticide (Beechem)	Methyl bromide*	
DR. BECKER'S EYE WASH Antiseptic (Olliffe)	Zinc sulfate Camphor water Hamamelis water Sat. sol. boric acid*	12 gr. 3 oz. 2 oz. 11 oz.	BEECHEM PENTACHLOROPHENOL Wood preservative (Beechem)	Pentachlorophenol*	
BECOMING PERFUME, COLOGNE (Parfums de Renel)			BEECHEM WARFARIN PREPARED Rodenticide (Beechem)	Warfarin ((3-(α-acetonylbenzyl)- 4-hydroxycoumarin)) 0.025%	
BEEBE POULTRY LOUSE POWDER Ectoparasiticide (veterinary) (Beebe Labs.)	Sodium orthophenylphenate* 7.0% Sulfur 5.0%		BEEDACOL-KAPS Analgesic (Rafea)	Acetyl salicylic acid* 3 1/2 gr. Acetophenetidin* (acetanilid derivative) 2 1/2 gr. Caffeine alkaloid 1/2 gr. Pyranisamine maleate 25 mg.	
BEE BRAND ANT KILLER (Mc Cormick)	Rotenone* Other cube resins	5% 10%	BEE DEE FOR POULTRY & STOCK Cathartic (veterinary) (Bee Dee)	Senna Sulfur 5% Gentian Ferrous sulfate	
BEE BRAND FLEA KILLER (Mc Cormick)	Rotenone Other cube resins	1% 2%			
BEE BRAND FLEA & TICK KILLER (Mc Cormick)	DDT*	10%	BEEMAN'S B-G-O OINTMENT Emollient, antiseptic for skin (Beeman's)	Carbolic acid* 5.54 m./oz. Iodoform* Zinc oxide Calomine sulfur Salicylic acid* Menthol* Petroleum jelly Lanolin	
BEE BRAND INSECTICIDAL SHAMPOO (Mc Cormick)	Vegetable oil soap 30.00% Camphor oil 1.75% Rotenone 0.10% Other cube resins 0.20% Pyrethrins 0.10% Tech. piperonyl cyclonene 0.50%				
BEE BRAND INSECT POWDER (McCormick)	Pyrethrins 0.75%		BEEMAN'S COUGH SYRUP Antitussive (Beeman's)	Chloroform 5 m./fl. oz. Tartar emetic* Menthol* Potassium quaiacolsulfonate Ammonium chloride Citric acid Imitation wild cherry flavor	
BEE BRAND ROACH KILLER (Mc Cormick)	Pyrethrins 0.33% Piperonyl cyclonene, tech 2.00% Boric acid* 15.00%		BEER BOB HAIR SET (G.W.)		
BEE BRAND ROSE AND FLOWER DUST Fungicide, insecticide (Mc Cormick)	Rotenone 1.00% Cube resins 2.00% Ferbam 8.75% Sulfur* 59.00% Gamma isomer of benzene hexachloride (from lindane) 1.00%		BEETSOL CLEANER & SANITIZER (Sugar Beet)	Quaternary disinfectant*	
			BEETSOL HEAVY DUTY ALL SOLUBLE BORAX HAND SOAP (Sugar Beet)	Soda soaps Borax*	

*Consult Sec. II., Ingredients Index. This ingredient may be responsible for major toxic effects if poisonous amounts of this product are ingested.

Name & Use Manufacturer	Ingredients		Name & Use Manufacturer	Ingredients	
BEETSOL WATERLESS HAND CLEANER (Sugar Beet)	Paraffin hydrocarbon Fatty acid-alkylol soap Polyglycol Lanolin Cellulose gum Titanox Perfume		BELL'S EAR WAX DROPS (Bell Chem. Co. (Chic.))		
			BELL'S EYE DROPS (Bell Chem. Co. (Chic.))		
BE-GONE DETERGENT SHAMPOO (Gordon Thomas)			BELL'S MEDICINE Bronchial, antispasmodic (Bell, H.O.)	Iodide of potassium* Tincture of lobelia* Tincture of rosin weed Alcohol	14%
BE-GONE HAIR COLORING POMADE (Gordon Thomas)			BELL'S SYRUP Antitussive (Hollings-Smith)	Codeine* (opium derivative) 1 gr./oz. Ammonium chloride Ipecac Glycerine Senna Sugar	
BE-GONE MARKHIDE SKIN-TONE (Gordon Thomas)			BELMONT ENGLISH HAIR TONIC (Castilla)	Denatured alcohol* 84% Castor oil Citrus oils	
BE-GONE OIL SHAMPOO TINT (Gordon Thomas)			BELOPHEN PILLS Cathartic (Veltex)	Each pill: Fxtract of belladonna* 1/8 gr. Extract cascara sagrada 1/8 gr. Powd. ipecac 1/16 gr. Phenolphthalein* 1/4 gr. Aloin* 1/4 gr.	
BE-GONE SKIN TREATMENT OINTMENT (Gordon Thomas)			BELURIN (Dayton Pharm.)	Eupatorium Pareira brava Lappa Uva ursi Zea mais Senna Acidum tannicum* Sodii boras* Taraxacum Juglans Inula Spiroea Chimaphila Eriodictyon Potassi nitras	
BELINE LOZENGES To combat tobacco habit (New Eng. Pharm.)	Lobeline sulfate * 1/64 gr.				
BELL-ANS Antacid, digestant (Bell & Co.)	Sodium bicarbonate U.S.P. Willow charcoal Ginger Capsicum* Wintergreen* Saccharin				
BELLODGIA EXTRACT & LOTION (Caron)			BELVA PIN CURL COLD WAVE CREAM (Belva)		
BELL-O-SAL Antirheumatic (Bell-O-Sal Mfg. Co.)	Alcohol 15% Potassium iodide Methenamine Poke root Sodium salicylate* Mercury biniodide* Nux vomica* Belladonna leaves Cascara sagrada Lactated pepsin		BEMALT PALATABLE TONIC (Hance)	Alcohol 12% Vitamin B1 (thiamin chloride) Malt Calcium Sodium Potassium Manganese Iron Wild cherry bark Aromatics	
BELL'S CLEANING FLUID (Bell Chem. Co.(Chic.))			BEN-BAR SCALP APPLICATION (Bennetts-B.)		
BELL'S CORN RE-MOVER (Bell Chem. Co. (Chic.))			BENCHLOPHEN SOLUTION Disinfectant (Hockwald)	Phenols	

*Consult Sec. II., Ingredients Index. This ingredient may be responsible for major toxic effects if poisonous amounts of this product are ingested.

Name & Use Manufacturer	Ingredients
BENDIX METALCLENE (Bendix)	Cresylic acid* Petroleum hydrocarbon* Ethylene dichloride* Potassium soap Small amts: isopropyl alcohol, perchloroethylene, sodium dichromate
BENEAT HAIR DRESSING (Assoc.Brands.)	
BENECIN Analgesic, antirheumatic (Supreme Pharm.)	Calcium succinate Aspirin*
BENEDICT'S QUALITATIVE REAGENT For testing sugar in urine (Peoples)	Copper sulfate* Sodium citrate Sodium carbonate
BENEKOL WITH BENZENE HEXACHLOR-IDE Ectoparasiti-cide (veterinary) (Lloyd)	Benzyl benzoate 27% Cyclohexane hexachloride* (benzene hexachloride), gamma isomer 1% Ethyl aminobenzoate (benzocaine) 0.97% Extract of echinacea
BENESAN Insecticide, seed treatment (Chipman,Ltd.)	Gamma isomer of benzene hexachloride* (from lindane) 50%
BENETRYCIN Antihistamine, analgesic (Supreme Pharm.)	Pyrilamine maleate 12.5 mg. Acetophenetidin* 1.25 gr. Salicylamide* 1.0 gr. Caffeine 0.25 gr.
BENEXANE 5 Insecticide (Chipman,Ltd.)	Gamma isomer of BHC (from lindane) 0.5%
BENEXANE 50 Insecticide (Chipman,Ltd.)	Benzene hexachloride* 50.0% Gamma isomer of BHC* 6.0%
BENGAL'S CEMENT FOR CHINA, CROCKERY & GLASS (Bengal)	
BENGAL'S RUG & UPHOLSTERY CLEANER (Bengal)	
BEN-GAY Rubefacient, counter-irritant (Bengue)	Menthol* Lanolin Methyl salicylate*
BENNY-HEX CONCENTRATE Insecticide (Anzio)	
BENNY-HEX INSECT POWDER (Anzio)	

Name & Use Manufacturer	Ingredients
BENNY-HEX INSECT SPRAY (Anzio)	
BEN-O-LAC TABLETS (Advance Research)	
BEN-SILIC COMPOUND Fungicide (medical, external) (Lockhart)	Benzoic acid* Salicylic acid* Thymol* Alcohol* 70%
BEN-THOL VAPORIZING COMPOUND Antitussive (Ben-Thol)	Camphor* 3 Menthol* 3 Spts. chloroform* 47 Tr. benzoin comp. 0.50
BENTICAL SHAKE LOTION (Lamond)	Zinc oxide Zinc carbonate Titanium oxide
BENZAHEX D-12 Insecticide (Chipman Chem.)	Gamma isomer of benzene hexachloride* 12.00% Other isomers of benzene hexachloride and related compounds* 18.00%
BENZAHEX-DDT 9-15 LIQUID Insecticide (Chipman Chem.)	Gamma isomer of benzene hexachloride* 9.6% Other isomers of benzene hexachloride and related compounds* 14.4% DDT 16.0% Aromatic petroleum derivative* 52.00%
BENZAHEX 1% DUST Insecticide (Chipman Chem.)	Gamma isomer of benzene hexachloride 1.00% other isomers of benzene hexachloride and related compounds 1.75%
BENZAHEX 2% DUST Insecticide (Chipman Chem.)	Gamma isomer of benzene hexachloride* 2.00% Other isomers of benzene hexachloride and related compounds 3.50%
BENZAHEX 3-10 DUST Insecticide (Chipman Chem.)	DDT* 10.00% Gamma isomer of benzene hexachloride* 3.00% Other isomers of benzene hexachloride and related compounds 5.25%
BENZAHEX 3-10-40 DUST Insecticide (Chipman Chem.)	Gamma isomer of benzene hexachloride* 3.00% Other isomers of benzene hexachloride and related compounds 5.25% DDT* 10.00% Sulfur* 40.00%
BENZAHEX 2L Insecticide (Chipman Chem.)	Gamma isomer of benzene hexachloride* 23.20% Other isomers of benzene hexachloride and related compounds 2.20% Aromatic petroleum derivative* 28.00%

*Consult Sec. II., Ingredients Index. This ingredient may be responsible for major toxic effects if poisonous amounts of this product are ingested.

Name & Use Manufacturer	Ingredients
BENZAHEX LIQUID Insecticide (Chipman. Chem.)	Gamma isomer of benzene hexachloride* 11.3% Other isomers of benzene hexachloride* and related compounds 13.7% Aromatic petroleum derivatives* 60.0%
BENZAHEX W-12 Insecticide (Chipman Chem.)	Gamma isomer of benzene hexachloride* 12.00% Other isomers of benzene hexachloride and related compounds* 18.0%
BENZAPHRINE JR. Nasal decongestant (Approved)	Phenylephrine HCl U.S.P. 1/4% Benzalkonium chloride 1-5000
BENZEDREX INHALER Decongestant (Smith, Kline & French)	Propylhexedrine* SKF 250 mg. Menthol* 12.5 mg.
BENZEX Insecticide (Woolfolk)	Gamma BHC* Other isomers
BENZOCAINE-ACID CARBOLIC OINTMENT Antiseptic, local anesthetic (CaPhenin)	Benzocaine 10% Phenol, liq. 1%
BENZOCAINE OINTMENT Surface anesthetic (Massengill)	Benzocaine 2%
BENZODERM Local anesthetic, antiseptic (Jenkins)	Benzocaine 1% Carbolic acid 1% Zinc oxide 5%
BENZO FUME PRESSURE FUMIGATOR Insecticide (Diamond Black)	Azobenzene* 17.5%
BENZO-GUAIATONE Antitussive (Horton & Converse)	Sodium monobenzyl succinate 8 gr. Potassium guaiacol sulfonate 8 gr. Ammonium chloride 8 gr. Antimony and potassium tartrate 1/12 gr. Chloroform 2 m. Menthol 1/10 gr.
BENZOJEN Fungicide (medical, external) (Jenkins)	Acid benzoic* 40 gr./oz. Acid salicylic* 20 gr. Thymol 4 gr. Lanolin and petrolatum aa q.s.
BENZOTHOL Intestinal antiseptic (Jenkins)	Each tablet: Bismuth subgallate 2 gr. Zinc phenolsulfonate 1/2 gr. Betanaphthol benzoate* 1/2 gr. Papain 1 gr.
BERA SKIN LOTION (Assoc. Brands)	
BERGAMOT AFTER SHAVE LOTION (Vivaudou)	
BERGAMOT COLOGNE (Vivaudou)	
BERGAMOT DEODORANT CREAM OR LIQUID (Vivaudou)	
BERGAMOT HAIR DRESSING (Vivaudou)	
BERGAMOT SCALP & HAIR OINTMENT (Vivaudou)	
BERGER'S PURE PARIS GREEN Insecticide (Green Cross)	Arsenic* 39.0% Copper 24.0%
BERLOU MOTHSPRAY (Berlou)	Zinc silicofluoride* 1% Thiocarbamide 0.5%
BERRY BROTHERS LACQUERS (Berry Bros.)	Nitrocellulose Dibutyl phthalate Tricresyl, phosphate* Alkyd, phenolic or other resin Castor oil Alcohols* Ketones* Acetates Petroleum Aliphatic hydrocarbons* Aromatic hydrocarbons*
BERRY BROTHERS VARNISHES (Berry Bros.)	Fossil, alkyd, phenolic, maleic urea, and melamine resins Vinyls Linseed, Chinawood, oiticica, dehydrated castor and tall oils Aliphatic* and aromatic hydrocarbons*
BERRY'S BLACK RUBBER DRESSING (Berry, C.H.)	Rubber paint and solvent*
DR. BERRY'S FRECKLE OINTMENT (Plough)	
BESCO PRESSED CRAYON (Binney & Smith)	

Name & Use Manufacturer	Ingredients
BES-GLO DEODORANT SPRAY (Newcomb)	
BES-GLO PINE DISINFECTANT (Newcomb)	
BES-GLO SKIN TONE (Newcomb)	
BES-GLO WAX POLISH (Newcomb)	
BE SQUARE MONAMOTOR Lubricating grease (Barnsdall)	
"BESTINE" SOLVENT AND THINNER (Union Rubber)	Hexane*
BESTOSEAL CAULKING COMPOUND (Bestoseal)	
BESTOSEAL CHINA, CROCKERY, GLASS CEMENT (Bestoseal)	
BESTOSEAL ROOFING CEMENT (Bestoseal)	
"BEST-TEST" WHITE RUBBER PAPER CEMENT (Union Rubber)	Hexane*
BETA CIBUS DOUCHE POWDER (Beta)	
BETA CREAM COLD WAVES Waving lotion (Vienna)	Ammonium thioglycolate 7 1/2%
BETA CREAM COLD WAVES (Neutralizer) (Vienna)	Potassium bromate 12 gm.
BETALAC PAINTS (Briggs-Maroney)	
BETALAX Laxative (Jewell Pharm.)	Magnesium hydroxide Betanaphthol benzoate* Salol* Papain Malt diastase Magnesium carbonate Lactose Oil of peppermint Oil of anise
BETA-QUINOL FOR SCALP & HAIR (Eptol)	Betanaphthol* Quinine sulfate Fl. ext. jaborandi Fl. ext. capsicum Tinct. cantharides Caramel color Alcohol*

Name & Use Manufacturer	Ingredients
BETA-TROL FOR BACTERIAL CONTROL Disinfectant (Varley)	Beta terpineol* Vegetable oil soap Isopropyl alcohol*
BETHIAPHOS (Elixir) Tonic (Massengill)	Each 5 cc.: Strychnine glycerophosphate* 0.6 mg. Sodium glycerophosphate 80 mg. Calcium glycerophosphate 80 mg. Thiamine hydrochloride (B$_1$) 1.6 mg. Phosphoric acid 0.06 cc.
BETTY ELIZABETH SHAMPOO (Davi)	
BET-U-LOL Rubefacient (Huxley)	Chloral hydrate* 8 gr./fl.oz. Methyl salicylate* Menthol* U.S.P.
BEUCKMAN'S SPOT CLEANER (Ring)	
BEX CURTAIN MAJ-IK (Beck Prod.)	Tech. gelatin
BEXOIN Emollient, antiseptic for skin (Bullock-Walker)	Calomel* 13.13 gr./oz. Salicylic acid 13.13 gr./oz. Bismuth subnitrate Zinc oxide Camphor Starch q.s.
BF-1 Laxative (Vegetrates)	Senna Parsley Irish moss Alfalfa Asparagus Okra Yeast Dulse
B-F-35 Bactericide, fungicide (Greever's)	Dihydroxydichlorodiphenyl methane 2.75% Isopropyl alcohol*(91%) 97.25%
B-G-O OINTMENT Emollient, antiseptic for skin (Beeman's)	Carbolic acid* 5.54 m./oz Iodoform* Zinc oxide Calomine sulfur Salicylic acid* Menthol* Petroleum jelly Lanolin

*Consult Sec. II., Ingredients Index. This ingredient may be responsible for major toxic effects if poisonous amounts of this product are ingested.

Name & Use Manufacturer	Ingredients	Name & Use Manufacturer	Ingredients
B. H. TURKEY TABS Fungicide (veterinary) (Lee, G.)	Sodium arsanilate* and sodium para benzarsonate* (1.32 gr. arsenic* per tablet expressed as arsenic trioxide) Ammonium phenolsulfonate Boric acid	**BICKMORINE TWO-PURPOSE POWDER** Antiseptic (veterinary) (Bickmore)	
BIALIN Laxative (Veltex)	Each tablet: Desiccated ox bile 1/2 gr. Phenolphthalein, yellow 1/2 gr. Extract cascara sagrada 1/2 gr. Aloin 1/8 gr. Podophyllin 1/20 gr.	**BICKUM'S KIT-CAT** (Bickum)	Alcohol 4%
BI CA MINT AND MINT POWDER Antacid (Gratny)	Bismuth subcarbonate Calcium carbonate Colloidal kaolin Magnesium carbonate Sodium bicarbonate Bismuth subgallate Wood charcoal Diastase Oil peppermint	**BICOLAGILL, NO. 8** (Sugar-coated purple) Laxative, choleretic (Massengill)	Each tablet: Ext. nux vomica* (represents strychnine 0.0046 gr.) 4 mg. Sodium taurocholate 65 mg. Ext. ox bile 65 mg. Sodium salicylate* 0.1 gm. Oleoresin capsicum 1.6 mg.
BICAREX Laxative choleretic (Massengill)	Each tablet: Papain 2 gr. Ext. ox bile 1 gr. Ext. cascara sagrada 1/2 gr. Phenolphthalein* 1/2 gr. Ext. nux vomica* 1/16 gr. Oleoresin capsicum 1/40 gr.	**BICOLAGILL, NO. 10** Laxative, choleretic (Massengill)	Each tablet: Sodium glycocholate 16 mg. Sodium taurocholate 16 mg. Phenolphthalein 8 mg. Ext. cascara sagrada 16 mg. Aloin 2.8 mg. Pancreatin 65 mg. Pepsin (1-3000) 32 mg. Oil peppermint q.s.
BICEBIN Gastric sedative (Massengill)	Each tablet: Bismuth subnitrate 0.13 gm. Cerium oxalate 0.13 gm. Benzocaine 16 mg.	**BIDEFIN** Cathartic (Cowley Pharm.)	Ext. ox bile U.S.P. 1 gr. Phenolphthalein* 1/2 gr. Diastase 2 gr. Ext. cascara sagrada 1/2 gr. Oleoresin of capsicum 1/40 gr.
BICHOLAX Cathartic (Massengill)	Each tablet: Sodium glycocholate 16 mg. Sodium taurocholate 16 mg. Phenolphthalein* 32 mg. Ext. cascara sagrada 32 mg. Aloin* 8 mg.	**BIDETAL** Antiseptic for feminine hygiene (Bidetal)	Alcohol 2% Lactic acid Zinc sulfate Ammonium alum
BICKMORE CREAM INSECT REPELLENT (Bickmore)	Dimethyl phthalate Alpha, alpha-dimethyl alpha'-carbobutoxydihydro gamma-pyrone 2-Ethylhexanediol-1, 3* Bicyclo-(2, 2, 1)-5-heptene-2, 3-dicarboxylic acid, dimethyl ester Ethyl cellulose Candelilla wax	**BIF AEROSOL INSECT BOMB** (Wilco)	Pyrethrins Piperonyl butoxide Methoxychlor* Petroleum distillate* Methylene chloride* Mixed Freons
BICKMORE GALL SALVE Antiseptic (veterinary) (Bickmore)	Alum Borax* Oxyquinoline sulfate Sulfur*	**BIF ANT & ROACH SPRAY** (Wilco)	Chlordane*
BICKMORE LIQUID INSECT RE-PELLENT (Bickmore)	Dimethyl phthalate Alpha, alpha-dimethyl alpha'-carbobutoxydihydro gamma-pyrone 2-Ethylhexanediol-1, 3* Bicyclo-(2, 2, 1)-5-heptene-2, 3-dicarboxylic acid, dimethyl ester	**BIFF DEPILATORY POWDER** (Burnham Labs.)	
		BIFF OINTMENT FOR ATH-LETE'S FOOT Fungicide, medical (Hill Labs. Tex.)	Benzoic acid* Salicylic acid* Thymol
BICKMORE X Y Z OINTMENT (Bickmore)	White petrolatum Lanolin Paraffin Camphor* Boric acid* Wettable sulfur* Alum Oxyquinoline sulfate* Oil of spike lavender	**BIF GARDEN SPRAY** (Wilco)	Pyrethrins* Piperonyl cyclonene Rotenone*
		BIF INSECT SPRAY (Wilco)	Pyrethrins* Piperonyl butoxide Petroleum of kerosene* boiling range
		BIF INSECTICIDE POWDER (Wilco)	Pyrethrins Chlordane* DDT*

*Consult Sec. II., Ingredients Index. This ingredient may be responsible for major toxic effects if poisonous amounts of this product are ingested.

Name & Use Manufacturer	Ingredients		Name & Use Manufacturer	Ingredients	
BIF RED BAIT PELLETS Snail and slug exterminator (Wilco)	Metaldehyde*		BILAPHEN TABLETS Cathartic, choleretic (Victoria)	Bile salts Phenolphthalein* Cascara ext. Aloin* Ginger Belladonna* Ext. nux vomica*	
BIF SPRA-COTE INSECT KILLER (Wilco)	DDT* Organic thiocyanates Methylated naphthalenes* Petroleum fraction of kerosene* boiling range		BI-LETS Cathartic (Bi-Lets)	Powdered extract colocynth* Aloes Resin impomoea Powdered extract oxgall Jalap Calomel* Gamboge	60 mg.
BIG CHIEF FLY PAPER (Tongue, R.E.)			BILLEY'S HAIR DRESSING (Exelento)		
BIG D Deodorant (LeFevre Chem.)					
BIG DRIP CHEMICAL AIR DRYER (Big Drip)			BILLOWING BATH (Clark, R.)	Sodium sulfate Sodium alkyl aryl sulfonate Sodium alkyl lauryl sulfonate Perfume D & C color	
BIG-HED LINIMENT (Humco)	Chlorthymol* Gum camphor* Oils origanum artificial Camphor sassafrassy Sassafras artificial Pine oil Spirits turpentine* Mineral spirits*		BILOBLETS TABLETS Laxative (Chase Chem.)	Each tablet: Papain Ox bile extract Ext. cascara sagrada Phenolphthalein* Ext. nux vomica* Oleoresin capsicum	1 gr. 1 gr. 1/2 gr. 1/2 gr. 1/16 gr. 1/40 gr.
BIG JACK LAUNDRY SOAP (Fitzpatrick)	Vegetable and animal oil soaps		BILOS (Enteric-coated blue) Laxative, choleretic (Massengill)	Each tablet: Ext. ox bile	0.324 gm.
BIG JIM Cathartic (Tampa)	Burdock (aretium lappa) Queen's delight (stillingia sylvatica) Cascara sagrada Iodide potash* Alcohol	10%	BIMACAL Antacid (Veltex)	Magnesium trisilicate Calcium carbonate Bismuth subnitrate	
BIG K WALLPAPER CLEANER (Cincy)	Wheat flour Refined kerosene oil* Vegetable dye Salt Preservatives		BIMACAL POWDER Antacid (Veltex)	Magnesium trisilicate Magnesium carbonate Calcium carbonate Sodium bicarbonate Bismuth subnitrate Oil of peppermint	
BIG STINKY FLY TRAP (Dioptron)	Parachlorophenyl parachloro- benzene sulfonate DDT Isopropanol	1.50% 1.50% 35%	BIMA FOR THE STOMACH Antacid (Douglas Pharmacal)	Magma of bismuth Magnesia hydroxide Sodium bicarbonate Fl. ext. rhubarb Fl. ext. ipecac Oil peppermint	
B & I IRON TONIC TABLETS (Cel-Ton-Sa)	Iron (ferrous sulfate)* Gentian root		BINDAY'S BURNADE For skin burns (Binday)	Calcium oleate Bentonite Phenyl salicylate* Phenol	1/2%
BIKINI FLOOR WAX (Uncle Sam)	Resins Waxes Ammonia* Oleic acid Morpholene* Plasticizer		BINDAY'S SCALPADE HAIR TONIC (Binday)	Alcohol Salicylic acid* Resorcinol* monoacetate Oleum ricini	60%
BILAGOG IMPROVED Choleretic (Tailby)	Dehydrocholic acid Bile salts	1 gr. 5 gr.	BINDAY'S SCALPADE SHAMPOO (Binday)	Alcohol* Oil of cade Tr. green soap	about 30%

*Consult Sec. II., Ingredients Index. This ingredient may be responsible for major toxic effects if poisonous amounts of this product are ingested.

Name & Use Manufacturer	Ingredients		Name & Use Manufacturer	Ingredients	
BINDAY'S TAN-ADE For suntan (Binday)	Salol,* in a hydro-alcoholic mixture		BIS-MASTER Antacid (Nat'l. Package)	Calcium carbonate Sodium bicarbonate Bismuth subcarbonate Aromatics Magnesium carbonate Magnesium trisilicate Chlorophyllin	
BIRD ROOF COATINGS AND CEMENT (Bird)	Asphalt Petroleum solvents* (substantially aliphatic) Fillers such as rock dust, talc, soapstone, asbestos		BISMOGILL Astringent, antiemetic, gastroin- testinal sedative (Massengill)	Each tablet: Bismuth subgallate Bismuth subsalicylate* Bismuth betanaphthol* Bismuth sulfocarbolate* Resorcinol* Cerium oxalate	49 mg. 49 mg. 32 mg. 32 mg. 32 mg. 65 mg.
BIRD TONIC Veterinary (Clayton)					
BI-SALO Intestinal antiseptic (Jenkins)	Glycerite of bismuth 78 m. Pepsin U.S.P. 4 gr. Zinc phenolsulfonate 1 gr. Sodium benzoate* 4 gr.		BISMOPAP Intestinal antiseptic (Premo Pharm. Labs.)	Bismuth subsalicylate* Salol* Zinc phenolsulfonate	
BISALPHEN TABLETS Laxative, cholagogue (Boyle & Co.)	Bile salts comp. (ext. ox bile U.S.P.) Ext. cascara sagrada Phenolphthalein Capsicum Papain Ext. nux vomica 1/16 gr.		BISMU-KINO Intestinal antiseptic (Wampole)	Alcohol 1% Bismuth oxycarbonate Zinc phenolsulfonate Camphor* Menthol Carminative oils (clove and nutmeg Chloroform 2 m./fl. oz.	
BISCALOX NO. 4 Antacid (Jeffrey-Fell)	Each tablet: Cerium oxalate 1 gr. Bismuth subnitrate 2 gr. Magnesium carbonate levis 4 gr. Anesthesin 1/4 gr.		BISOCAL POWDER Antacid powder (Horton & Converse)	Each oz.: Bismuth subnitrate 43 gr. Magnesium carbonate 162 gr. Calcium carbonate 104 gr. Sodium bicarbonate 126 gr. Aromatics q.s.	
BIS-KIT K-R-O Ready-mixed form Rodenticide (K-R-O)	Extractives of red squill* 10%		BIS-O-CARB ANTACID TABLETS (Assoc. Prod.)	Calcium carbonate Magnesium carbonate Magnesium trisilicate Oil of peppermint	
BISLAC Antacid, adsorbent (Myers Lab.)	Magnesium carbonate Bismuth subcarbonate Colloidal kaolin Activated charcoal Sodium bicarbonate Lactose Pepsin		BISODOL MINTS Antacid (Whitehall)	Magnesium trisilicate Calcium carbonate Magnesium hydroxide Peppermint	
BIS-MA-CAL Antacid powder (Claflin)	Bismuth subcarbonate Calcium carbonate Magnesium carbonate Sodium bicarbonate Diastase Oil peppermint		BISODOL POWDER Antacid (Whitehall)	Sodium bicarbonate Magnesium carbonate Bismuth subnitrate Oil of peppermint	
BISMA-REX GEL Antacid, adsorbent (Rexall)	Aluminum hydroxide Magnesium trisilicate Bismuth subcarbonate Magnesium carbonate Oil of peppermint		BITE-AID Anti-nail biting and thumb sucking (Binday)	Oleoresin capsicum Sucrose octa-acetate Volatile solvent*	
BISMA-REX MATES Antacid (Rexall)	Precipitated calcium carbonate Magnesium carbonate Magnesium trisilicate Oil of peppermint		BITEX acid & alkali resisting paint coatings (Knight)		
BISMA-REX TABLETS Antacid (Rexall)	Calcium carbonate Magnesium carbonate Magnesium trisilicate Peppermint oil		BITURINE coal tar pipe line enamel #7004 (General Paint Okla.)		
			BIXBY'S SHOE POLISH (Best)		

*Consult Sec. II., Ingredients Index. This ingredient may be responsible for major toxic effects if poisonous amounts of this product are ingested.

- 307 -

Name & Use Manufacturer	Ingredients
BK-BK Cleaner (Pennsylv. Salt)	Sodium hydroxide*
B-K—C.C.A. Abrasive cleaner (Pennsylv. Salt)	Soda ash Alkali silicate Alkali phosphate
B-K CHLORINE-BEARING POWDER Bactericide, disinfectant, deodorant (Pennsylv. Salt)	Calcium hypochlorite* 50%
B.K.F. FLOOR WAX (Gisler)	
B-KLEER Abrasive cleaner (Pennsylv. Salt)	Sodium hydroxide* Alkaline phosphate
B-K LIQUID Bactericide (Pennsylv. Salt)	Sodium hypochlorite* 5.40%
BLACK AIR DRYING VARNISH (George, P.D.)	
BLACK BEAUTY SHOE DRESSING (Welmaid)	Garnet shellac Borax* Dye
BLACKBERRY MIXTURE For intestinal irritation (Hance)	Tannic acid Benzoic acid* Blackberry conc. Blackberry root Cinnamon Nutmeg Cloves Caramel color
BLACKBERRY ROOT GINGER Carminative, digestant (Pfeiffer, S.)	Cinnamon Clove Anise compound
BLACK-CAPS (Safety Rem.)	
BLACK CAT Fungicide, keratolytic (Black Cat)	Salicylic acid* Sol. chloride of iron Ether 12% Alcohol* 50%
BLACK CAT PERFUME (Boyd)	
BLACK-DRAUGHT Laxative (Chattanooga)	Senna Other vegetable products
BLACK EAGLE BRAND COMPOUND Laxative (Cel-Ton-Sa)	Aloe Senna Cascara sagrada Buckthorn

Name & Use Manufacturer	Tox-icity	Ingredients
BLACK FLAG BUG KILLER (Boyle-Midway)		Gamma isomer of benzene hexachloride (from lindane) 0.50% Tech. piperonyl butoxide 0.10% Pyrethrins 0.04% Petroleum distillates* 99.36%
BLACK FLAG EMULSION CONC. WITH 25% DDT Insecticide (Boyle-Midway)		DDT* 25% Petroleum solvent*
BLACK FLAG FLEA, TICK & LOUSE POWDER (Boyle-Midway)		Piperonyl cyclonene tech. 1.00% Pyrethrins 0.10% Rotenone 0.50% Other cube extractives 1.00%
BLACK FLAG FLOWER BOMB (Boyle-Midway)		Gamma isomer of benzene hexachloride (from lindane) 1.000% Rotenone 0.400% Other cube resins 0.600% Pyrethrins 0.025% Tech. piperonyl butoxide 0.250% Petroleum distillate 0.104% Freon propellants
BLACK FLAG INSECTICIDE POWDER (Boyle-Midway)		Tech. chlordane 1.50% Piperonyl cyclonene tech. 0.35% Pyrethrins 0.06%
BLACK FLAG INSECT SPRAY (Boyle-Midway)		DDT* 5% Methylated naphthalenes* 8.5% Beta-butoxy-beta-thiocyanodiethyl ether 1% Essential oils 0.5% Petroleum distillates* 85%
BLACK FLAG MOTH DED (Boyle-Midway)		Terpene polychlorinates (66% chlorine)* 5.0% Paradichlorobenzene* 5.0% Petroleum distillates* 50.0%
BLACK FLAG PINE SCENT DISINFECT-ANT (Boyle-Midway)		Potassium chlorophenyl phenate 5.4% Pine oil* 8.9% Soap 5.1%
BLACK FLAG PUSH-BUTTON INSECT BOMB (Boyle-Midway)		DDT 1.00% Methoxychlor tech. 1.00% Allethrin 0.22% Tech. piperonyl butoxide 0.25% Petroleum distillates* 12.53%
BLACK FLAG PUSH BUTTON ROACH & ANT KILLER (Boyle-Midway)		Gamma isomer of benzene hexachloride (from lindane) 0.30% Pyrethrins 0.05% Piperonyl butoxide tech. 0.40% Petroleum distillates* 34.25%
BLACK FLAG ROACH SPRAY (Boyle-Midway)		Chlordane tech. 2% Petroleum distillates* 98%

---

*Consult Sec. II., Ingredients Index. This ingredient may be responsible for major toxic effects if poisonous amounts of this product are ingested.

Name & Use Manufacturer	Ingredients		Name & Use Manufacturer	Ingredients	
BLACK FLAG SUPER IN-SECT SPRAY (Boyle-Midway)	DDT*	5%	BLACK LEAF ARAMITE EMULSIFI-ABLE CONC. Insecticide (Diamond Black)	2-(p-tert.-butylphenoxy) isopropyl 2-chloroethyl sulfite	25.5%
	Chlordane	0.5%			
	Beta-butoxy-beta-thiocyano-diethyl ether (lethane)	0.65%		Xylene*	66.0%
	Pyrethrins	0.04%			
	Piperonyl butoxide	0.35%			
	Methylated naphthalenes	10%			
	Essential oils	0.4%	BLACK LEAF 15% ARAMITE WETTABLE POWDER Insecticide (Diamond Black)	2-(p-tert.-butylphenoxy) isopropyl 2-chloroethyl sulfite	15%
	Petroleum distillates*	83.06%			
BLACK GLOSS ENAMEL (United Gilson.)	Asphalt				
	Gilsonite				
	Varnish				
	Mineral spirits*		BLACK LEAF ARSENICAL WEED KIL-LER (Diamond Black)	Arsenic trioxide*	40%
BLACK IRON STOVE POLISH (Prescott)					
BLACK JACK ENAMEL (du Pont)			BLACK LEAF BASIC COP-PER SUL-PHATE Fungicide (Diamond Black)	Copper* expressed as metallic	53%
BLACK JACK ROOF COAT-ING (Gibson)					
BLACK JACK ROOFING CEMENT (Gibson)			BLACK LEAF BHC-DDT EMUL. CONC. Insecticide (Diamond Black)	Gamma isomer of benzene hexachloride* (BHC)	9.9%
				Other isomers of benzene hexachloride (BHC)	14.2%
BLACK LEAF 40 Insecticide (Diamond Black)	Nicotine*, expressed as alkaloid	40%		DDT*	16.5%
				Xylene*	53.0%
BLACK LEAF 253 Insecticide (Diamond Black)	DDT* (dichloro diphenyl trichloroethane)	25%	BLACK LEAF 11.4% BHC EMULSIFI-ABLE CON-CENTRATE Insecticide (Diamond Black)	Gamma isomer of benzene hexachloride* (BHC)	11.4%
	Parathion*	3%		Other isomers of benzene hexachloride (BHC)	19.4%
				Xylene*	25.2%
				Aromatic petroleum derivative solvent*	40.0%
BLACK LEAF 258 Insecticide (Diamond Black)	DDT* (dichloro diphenyl trichloroethane)	25%	BLACK LEAF CALCIUM ARSENATE Insecticide (Diamond Black)	Tricalcium arsenate*	70.00%
	Malathion*	8%		Arsenate expressed as metallic	26.00%
				Arsenic in water soluble forms expressed as metallic	0.50%
BLACK LEAF 5% ALDRIN DUST Insecticide (Diamond Black)	Hexachloro-hexahydro-dimethano-naphthalene*	4.75%	BLACK LEAF CALCIUM ARSENATE WITH NICOTINE Insecticide (Diamond Black)	Tricalcium arsenate*	59.08%
	Related compounds	0.80%		Nicotine* expressed as alkaloid	1.70%
				Arsenic expressed as metallic	21.94%
BLACK LEAF ALDRIN EMULSIFI-ABLE CON-CENTRATE Insecticide (Diamond Black)	Hexachloro-hexahydro-dimethano-naphthalene*	22.42%		Arsenic in water soluble forms expressed as metallic	0.50%
	Related compounds	16.91%			
	Xylene	9.50%	BLACK LEAF 5% CHLOR-DANE DUST Insecticide (Diamond Black)	Tech. chlordane	5%
	Petroleum distillate	39.50%			
BLACK LEAF 5% ALDRIN EQUIVALENT GRANULAR INSECTICIDE (Diamond Black)	Hexachloro-hexahydro-dimethano-naphthalene*	4.75%	BLACK LEAF 10% CHLOR-DANE DUST Insecticide (Diamond Black)	Tech. chlordane*	10%
	Related compounds	3.58%			
BLACK LEAF 2% ALDRIN GRANULAR INSECTICIDE (Diamond Black)	Hexachloro-hexahydro-dimethano-naphthalene*	1.90%	BLACK LEAF 45% CHLOR-DANE EMULSI-FIABLE CONC. Insecticide (Diamond Black)	Tech. chlordane*	45.0%
	Related compounds	1.43%		Petroleum distillate*	49.0%

*Consult Sec. II., Ingredients Index. This ingredient may be responsible for major toxic effects if poisonous amounts of this product are ingested.

Name & Use Manufacturer	Ingredients		Name & Use Manufacturer	Ingredients	
BLACK LEAF 72% CHLOR-DANE EMUL-SIFIABLE CONC. Insecticide (Diamond Black)	Tech. chlordane* Petroleum distillate	72.0% 16.5%	BLACK LEAF 0-10-40 COTTON DUST Insecticide (Diamond Black)	DDT* (dichloro diphenyl trichloroethane) Sulfur*	10% 40%
BLACK LEAF 5% CHLOR-DANE GRANULAR INSECTICIDE (Diamond Black)	Tech. chlordane	5%	BLACK LEAF 1-1/2 to 5 to 1 COTTON DUST Insecticide (Diamond Black)	Hexachloro-epoxy-octahydro-dimethanonaphthalene Related compounds DDT Parathion*	1.275% 0.225% 5.000% 1.000%
BLACK LEAF 45% CHLOR-DANE SPRAY Insecticide (Diamond Black)	Tech. chlordane* Petroleum distillate*	45.0% 43.5%	BLACK LEAF 2-1/2H to 5 to 0 COTTON DUST Insecticide (Diamond Black)	Heptachlor Related compounds DDT*	2.50% 0.97% 5.00%
BLACK LEAF 40% CHLOR-DANE WETTABLE POWDER Insecticide (Diamond Black)	Tech. chlordane*	40%	BLACK LEAF 2-1/2H to 10 to 40 COTTON DUST Insecticide (Diamond Black)	Heptachlor Related compounds DDT* Sulfur*	2.50% 0.97% 10.00% 40.00%
BLACK LEAF CHLORO IPC WEED KILLER (Diamond Black)	Isopropyl n-(3-chlorophenyl) carbamate*	47.5%	BLACK LEAF 2-1/2H to 5 to 40 COTTON DUST Insecticide (Diamond Black)	Heptachlor Related compounds DDT* Sulfur*	2.50% 0.97% 5.00% 40.00%
BLACK LEAF 6.5% COPPER-3% DDT DUST Fungicide, insecticide (Diamond Black)	DDT (dichloro diphenyl trichloroethane) Copper*	3.0% 6.5%	BLACK LEAF 3-5-0 COTTON DUST Insecticide (Diamond Black)	Gamma isomer of BHC* Other isomers of BHC DDT*	3.00% 18.00% 5.00%
BLACK LEAF 6.5% COPPER DUST Fungicide, insecticide (Diamond Black)	Copper* (in basic copper sulfate) expressed as metallic	6.5%	BLACK LEAF 3-5-1 COTTON DUST Insecticide (Diamond Black)	Gamma isomer of benzene hexachloride Other isomers of benzene hexachloride DDT (dichloro diphenyl trichloroethane) Parathion*	3% 18% 5% 1%
BLACK LEAF 7% COPPER DUST Fungicide, insecticide (Diamond Black)	Copper*	7%	BLACK LEAF 3-5-40 COTTON DUST Insecticide (Diamond Black)	Gamma isomer of BHC* Other isomers of BHC DDT* Sulfur*	3.00% 18.00% 5.00% 40.00%
BLACK LEAF 9% COPPER DUST Fungicide, (Diamond Black)	Copper*	9%	BLACK LEAF 3-10-0 COTTON DUST Insecticide (Diamond Black)	Gamma isomer of benzene hexachloride* Other isomers of benzene hexachloride DDT* (dichloro diphenyl trichloroethane)	3% 18% 10%
			BLACK LEAF CPR INSECT KILLER Insecticide (Diamond Black)	Pyrethrins Rotenone Other cube extractives Tech. piperonyl cyclonene Petroleum distillate	0.025% 0.128% 0.236% 0.256% 0.102%
BLACK LEAF 0-5-40 COTTON DUST Insecticide (Diamond Black)	DDT* (dichloro diphenyl trichloroethane) Sulfur*	5% 40%	BLACK LEAF 3% DDT-3% CHLORDANE DUST Insecticide (Diamond Black)	DDT (dichloro diphenyl trichloroethane) Tech. chlordane	3% 3%

*Consult Sec. II., Ingredients Index. This ingredient may be responsible for major toxic effects if poisonous amounts of this product are ingested.

Name & Use Manufacturer	Ingredients	
BLACK LEAF 3% DDT-7% COPPER DUST Fungicide, insecticide (Diamond Black)	DDT (dichloro diphenyl trichloroethane) Copper* expressed as metallic	3% 7%
BLACK LEAF 5% DDT DUST Insecticide (Diamond Black)	DDT*	5%
BLACK LEAF 5% DDT-6.5% COPPER DUST Fungicide, insecticide (Diamond Black)	DDT (dichloro diphenyl trichloroethane) Copper*	5.0% 6.5%
BLACK LEAF 5% DDT-9% COPPER DUST Fungicide, insecticide (Diamond Black)	DDT (dichloro diphenyl trichloroethane) Copper* (in basic copper sulfate) expressed as metallic	5% 9%
BLACK LEAF 3% DDT-10% DITHANE DUST Fungicide, insecticide (Diamond Black)	DDT (dichloro diphenyl trichloroethane) Zineb	3.0% 6.5%
BLACK LEAF 3% DDT DUST Insecticide (Diamond Black)	DDT (dichloro diphenyl trichloroethane)	3%
BLACK LEAF 10% DDT DUST Insecticide (Diamond Black)	DDT* (dichloro diphenyl trichloroethane)	10%
BLACK LEAF 25% DDT EMULSIFI- ABLE CONC. Insecticide (Diamond Black)	DDT* Xylene*	25% 69%
BLACK LEAF 10% DDT GRANULAR INSECTICIDE (Diamond Black)	DDT* (dichloro diphenyl trichloroethane)	10%
BLACK LEAF 3% DDT-60% SULPHUR DUST Fungicide, insecticide (Diamond Black)	DDT* (dichloro diphenyl trichloroethane) Sulfur*	3% 60%
BLACK LEAF 50% DDT WETTABLE POWDER Insecticide (Diamond Black)	DDT (dichloro diphenyl trichloroethane)*	50%

Name & Use Manufacturer	Ingredients	
BLACK LEAF DIELDRIN EMUL. CONC. Insecticide (Diamond Black)	Hexachloro-epoxy-octahydro- dimethano-naphthalene* Related compounds Xylene*	15.81% 2.79% 74.00%
BLACK LEAF 5% DIELDRIN GRANULAR INSECTICIDE (Diamond Black)	Hexachloro-epoxy-octahydro- dimethano-naphthalene* Related compounds	4.25% 0.75%
BLACK LEAF 50% DIELDRIN WETTABLE POWDER Insecticide (Diamond Black)	Hexachloro-epoxy-octahydro- endo, exo-dimethano- naphthalene* Related compounds	42.5% 7.5%
BLACK LEAF 5% DITHANE- 3% DDT DUST Fungicide, insecticide (Diamond Black)	DDT (dichloro diphenyl trichloroethane)* Zineb	3.00% 3.25%
BLACK LEAF 5% DITHANE- 5% DDT DUST Fungicide, insecticide (Diamond Black)	DDT* (dichloro diphenyl trichloroethane) Zineb	5.00% 3.25%
BLACK LEAF 5% DITHANE DUST Fungicide, insecticide (Diamond Black)	Zineb	3.25%
BLACK LEAF 6% DITHANE DUST Fungicide, insecticide (Diamond Black)	Zineb	3.9%
BLACK LEAF 10% DITHANE DUST Fungicide insecticide (Diamond Black)	Zineb	6.5%
BLACK LEAF 5% DITHANE- 60% SULPHUR DUST Fungicide, insecticide (Diamond Black)	Zineb Sulfur*	3.25% 60.00%
BLACK LEAF 1-1/2 to 0 to 0 DUST Insecticide (Diamond Black)	Hexachloro-epoxy-octahydro- dimethano-naphthalene* Related compounds	1.275% 0.225%

*Consult Sec. II., Ingredients Index. This ingredient may be responsible for major toxic effects if poisonous amounts of this product are ingested.

Name & Use Manufacturer	Ingredients		Name & Use Manufacturer	Ingredients	
BLACK LEAF 1-1/2 to 5 to 0 DUST Insecticide (Diamond Black)	Hexachloro-epoxy-octahydro-dimethano-naphthalene* Related compounds DDT*	1.275% 0.225% 5.000%	BLACK LEAF 2-1/2D to 5 to 40 DUST Insecticide (Diamond Black)	Hexachloro-epoxy-octahydro-dimethano-naphthalene* Related compounds DDT* Sulfur*	2.125% 0.375% 5.000% 40.000%
BLACK LEAF 1-1/2 to 5 to 40 DUST Insecticide (Diamond Black)	Hexachloro-epoxy-octahydro-dimethano-naphthalene* Related compounds DDT* Sulfur*	1.275% 0.225% 5.000% 40.000%	BLACK LEAF DUSTING SULPHUR WITH 1% DDT Insecticide, fungicide (Diamond Black)	Sulfur* DDT	82.0% 1.0%
BLACK LEAF 1-1/2 to 10 to 0 DUST Insecticide (Diamond Black)	Hexachloro-epoxy-octahydro-dimethano-naphthalene* Related compounds DDT*	1.275% 0.225% 10.000%	BLACK LEAF 1% ENDRIN DUST Insecticide (Diamond Black)	Hexachloro-epoxy-octahydro-endo, endo-dimethano-naphthalene*	1%
BLACK LEAF 1-1/2 to 10 to 40 DUST Insecticide (Diamond Black)	Hexachloro-epoxy-octahydro-dimethano-naphthalene* Related compounds DDT* Sulfur*	1.275% 0.225% 10.000% 40.000%	BLACK LEAF 1-1/2% ENDRIN DUST Insecticide (Diamond Black)	Hexachloro-epoxy-octahydro-endo, endo-dimethano-naphthalene*	1.5%
BLACK LEAF 2-1/2 to 0 to 0 DUST Insecticide (Diamond Black)	Hexachloro-hexahydro-dimethano-naphthalene* Related compounds	2.375% 1.791%	BLACK LEAF 2% ENDRIN DUST Insecticide (Diamond Black)	Hexachloro-epoxy-octahydro-endo, endo-dimethano-naphthalene*	2%
BLACK LEAF 2-1/2 to 5 to 0 DUST Insecticide (Diamond Black)	Hexachloro-hexahydro-dimethano-naphthalene Related compounds DDT* (dichloro diphenyl trichloroethane)	2.4% 0.4% 5.0%	BLACK LEAF ENDRIN EMUL. CONC. Insecticide (Diamond Black)	Hexachloro-epoxy-octahydro-endo, endo-dimethano-naphthalene* Petroleum hydrocarbons	19.8% 73.7%
BLACK LEAF 2-1/2 to 5 to 40 DUST Insecticide (Diamond Black)	Hexachloro-hexahydro-dimethano-naphthalene Related compounds DDT* (dichloro diphenyl trichloroethane) Sulfur*	2.4% 0.4% 5.0% 40.00%	BLACK LEAF FERBAM Fungicide (Diamond Black)	Ferbam	76%
BLACK LEAF 2-1/2 to 10 to 0 DUST Insecticide (Diamond Black)	Hexachloro-hexahydro-dimethano-naphthalene* Related compounds DDT* (dichloro diphenyl trichloroethane)	2.375% 1.791% 10.000%	BLACK LEAF FERBAM DUST Fungicide (Diamond Black)	Ferric dimethyl dithiocarbamate	11.4%
BLACK LEAF 5-10-40 DUST Insecticide (Diamond Black)	Hexachloro-hexahydro-dimethano-naphthalene* Related compounds DDT* Sulfur*	4.750% 3.582% 10.000% 40.000%	BLACK LEAF FLY SPRAY Insecticide (Diamond Black)	Tech. methoxychlor Pyrethrins Tech. piperonyl butoxide Isobornyl thiocyanoacetate Other related terpenes Refined petroleum distillate*	0.500% 0.012% 0.100% 1.152% 0.253% 97.983%
BLACK LEAF 2-1/2D to 0 to 0 DUST Insecticide (Diamond Black)	Hexachloro-epoxy-octahydro-dimethano-naphthalene* Related compounds	2.125% 0.375%	BLACK LEAF 1% GAMMA BHC DUST Insecticide (Diamond Black)	Gamma isomer of benzene hexachloride* Other isomers of benzene hexachloride	1% 6%
BLACK LEAF 2-1/2D to 0 to 40 DUST Insecticide (Diamond Black)	Hexachloro-epoxy-octahydro-dimethano-naphthalene* Related compounds Sulfur* (93% through 325 mesh)	2.125% 0.375% 40.000%	BLACK LEAF 1-1/2% GAMMA BHC DUST Insecticide (Diamond Black)	Gamma isomer of benzene hexachloride* Other isomers of benzene hexachloride	1.5% 10.0%
BLACK LEAF 2-1/2D to 5 to 0 DUST Insecticide (Diamond Black)	Hexachloro-epoxy-octahydro-dimethano-naphthalene* Related compounds DDT* (dichloro diphenyl trichloroethane)	2.125% 0.375% 5.000%			

*Consult Sec. II., Ingredients Index. This ingredient may be responsible for major toxic effects if poisonous amounts of this product are ingested.

Name & Use Manufacturer	Ingredients		Name & Use Manufacturer	Ingredients	
BLACK LEAF 3% GAMMA BHC DUST Insecticide (Diamond Black)	Gamma isomer of benzene hexachloride* Other isomers of benzene hexachloride	3% 18%	BLACK LEAF 1.5% LINDANE- 5% COPPER DUST Fungicide, insecticide (Diamond Black)	Gamma isomer of benzene hexachloride Copper*	1.5% 5.0%
BLACK LEAF 1% GAMMA BHC-60% SULPHUR DUST Fungicide, insecticide (Diamond Black)	Gamma isomer of benzene hexachloride* Other isomers of benzene hexachloride Sulfur*	1% 6% 60%	BLACK LEAF 1% LINDANE- 5% DITHANE DUST Fungicide, insecticide (Diamond Black)	Zineb Gamma isomer of benzene hexachloride (from lindane)	3.25% 1.00%
BLACK LEAF 10% GAMMA BHC WET- TABLE Insecticide (Diamond Black)	Gamma isomer of benzene hexachloride* Other isomers of benzene hexachloride	10.0% 61.4%	BLACK LEAF 20% LINDANE EMULSIFI- ABLE CONC. Insecticide (Diamond Black)	Gamma isomer of benzene hexachloride (from lindane)* Xylene*	20% 49%
BLACK LEAF GRANULATED 15% RHO- THANE DUST Insecticide (Diamond Black)	TDE* (dichloro diphenyl dichloroethane)	15%	BLACK LEAF 10% LINDANE SPRAY Insecticide (Diamond Black)	Gamma isomer of benzene hexachloride (from lindane) Xylene* Methyl isobutyl ketone	10% 48% 32%
BLACK LEAF 2-1/2% HEPTACHLOR DUST Insecticide (Diamond Black)	Heptachlor* Related compounds	2.50% 0.97%	BLACK LEAF 1% LINDANE- 60% SULPHUR DUST Insecticide (Diamond Black)	Gamma isomer of benzene hexachloride Sulfur*	1% 60%
BLACK LEAF HEPTACHLOR EMULSIFI- ABLE CONC. Insecticide (Diamond Black)	Heptachlor* Related compounds Aromatic petroleum derivative solvent*	22.30% 8.67% 63.00%	BLACK LEAF 5% MALA- THION DUST Insecticide (Diamond Black)	Malathion	5%
BLACK LEAF 11-36 INSECT KILLER (Diamond Black)	DDT Tech. piperonyl butoxide Beta-butoxy-beta-thiocyano- diethyl ether Allethrin Methylated aromatic petroleum derivatives Petroleum distillate*	2.00% 0.25% 1.00% 0.10% 4.50% 12.15%	BLACK LEAF 50% MALA- THION EMUL. CONC. Insecticide (Diamond Black)	Malathion* Xylene*	50% 39%
BLACK LEAF LIME SUL- PHUR SPRAY Fungicide, insecticide (Diamond Black)	Calcium polysulfides*	26%	BLACK LEAF 50% MALA- THION SPRAY Insecticide (Diamond Black)	Malathion* Xylene*	50% 39%
BLACK LEAF 1% LINDANE DUST Insecticide (Diamond Black)	Gamma isomer of benzene hexachloride	1%	BLACK LEAF 25% MALA- THION WET- TABLE POWDER (Diamond Black)	Malathion*	25%
BLACK LEAF 1.5% LINDANE DUST Insecticide (Diamond Black)	Gamma isomer of benzene hexachloride (from lindane)	1.5%	BLACK LEAF MASH NIC NICOTIZED PELLETS Vermifuge (Diamond Black)	Nicotine* expressed as alkaloid	5%

*Consult Sec. II., Ingredients Index. This ingredient may be responsible for major toxic effects if poisonous amounts of this product are ingested.

- 313 -

Name & Use Manufacturer	Ingredients		Name & Use Manufacturer	Ingredients	
BLACK LEAF MCP Herbicide (Diamond Black)	Alkanolamine salts (of the ethanol and isopropanol series) of 2-methyl-4-chlorophenoxy-acetic acid*	69.1%	BLACK LEAF 1% PARA-THION-10% DITHANE DUST Insecticide (Diamond Black)	Parathion* Zineb	1.0% 6.5%
BLACK LEAF MOUSE KIL-LER BAIT (Diamond Black)	2-Pivalyl-1, 3-indandione 0.025%		BLACK LEAF 1% PARA-THION DUST Insecticide (Diamond Black)	Parathion*	1%
BLACK LEAF MULTI-PURPOSE GARDEN DUST Fungicide, insecticide (Diamond Black)	Nicotine* expressed as alkaloid Rotenone Other cube extractives Pyrethrins Ferbam (ferric dimethyl dithiocarbamate)	1.00% 1.00% 2.00% 0.10% 7.60%	BLACK LEAF 2% PARA-THION-5% DDT DUST Insecticide (Diamond Black)	Parathion* DDT	2% 5%
BLACK LEAF 25% NICOTINE WETTABLE POWDER Insecticide (Diamond Black)	Nicotine*, expressed as alkaloid	25%	BLACK LEAF 2% PARA-THION DUST Insecticide (Diamond Black)	Parathion*	2%
BLACK LEAF OVOTRAN WETTABLE POWDER Insecticide (Diamond Black)	p-Chlorophenyl p-chlorobenzene sulfonate*	50%	BLACK LEAF 25% PARA-THION EMUL. CONC. Insecticide (Diamond Black)	Parathion (O, O-diethyl-o-p-nitrophenyl thiophosphate)* Xylene	25% 68%
BLACK LEAF 1% PARA-THION-7% COPPER DUST Fungicide, insecticide (Diamond Black)	Parathion* Copper, expressed as metallic	1% 7%	BLACK LEAF 1% PARA-THION-60% SULPHUR DUST Insecticide (Diamond Black)	Parathion* Sulfur	1% 60%
BLACK LEAF 1% PARA-THION-3% DDT DUST Insecticide (Diamond Black)	Parathion* DDT (dichloro diphenyl trichloroethane)	1% 3%	BLACK LEAF 1% PARA-THION-5% TDE DUST Insecticide (Diamond Black)	Parathion* TDE (dichloro diphenyl dichloroethane)	1% 5%
BLACK LEAF 1% PARA-THION-5% DDT DUST Insecticide (Diamond Black)	Parathion* DDT (dichloro diphenyl trichloroethane)	1% 5%	BLACK LEAF 1% PARA-THION-10% TDE DUST Insecticide (Diamond Black)	Parathion* TDE (dichloro diphenyl dichloroethane)	1% 10%
BLACK LEAF 1% PARA-THION-5% DDT-10% TOXAPHENE DUST Insecticide (Diamond Black)	Parathion* DDT Toxaphene*	1% 5% 10%	BLACK LEAF 15% PARA-THION WETTABLE POWDER Insecticide (Diamond Black)	Parathion*	15%
BLACK LEAF 1% PARA-THION-10% DDT DUST Insecticide (Diamond Black)	Parathion* DDT (dichloro diphenyl trichloroethane)	1% 10%	BLACK LEAF 25% PARA-THION WETTABLE POWDER Insecticide (Diamond Black)	Parathion*	25%

*Consult Sec. II., Ingredients Index. This ingredient may be responsible for major toxic effects if poisonous amounts of this product are ingested.

Name & Use Manufacturer	Ingredients	
BLACK LEAF PEANUT DUST NO. 1 (90-10-5) Insecticide (Diamond Black)	Sulfur* Copper* expressed as metallic DDT (dichloro diphenyl trichloroethane)*	75.0% 3.4% 5.0%
BLACK LEAF 25% LINDANE WETTABLE POWDER Insecticide (Diamond Black)	Gamma isomer of benzene hexachloride (from lindane)*	25%
BLACK LEAF PEANUT DUST NO. 2 (90 to 10 to 2-1/2) Fungicide, Insecticide (Diamond Black)	Sulfur* Copper* DDT (dichloro diphenyl trichloreothane)*	82.0% 3.4% 2.5%
BLACK LEAF PEANUT DUST NO. 3 (90-10-0) Fungicide (Diamond Black)	Sulfur* Copper*	82.0% 3.4%
BLACK LEAF PEANUT DUST NO. 4 (90-0-10) Fungicide, insecticide (Diamond Black)	Sulfur* DDT* (dichloro diphenyl trichloroethane)	74.0% 10.0%
BLACK LEAF PEANUT DUST NO. 5 (90-0-5) Fungicide, insecticide (Diamond Black)	Sulfur* DDT* (dichloro diphenyl trichloroethane)	82.0% 5.0%
BLACK LEAF PEANUT DUST NO. 6 (90-0-2-1/2) Fungicide, insecticide (Diamond Black)	Sulfur* DDT (dichloro diphenyl trichloroethane)	82.0% 2.5%
BLACK LEAF PEANUT DUST NO. 7 Fungicide, insecticide (Diamond Black)	Sulfur* Copper*	82.0% 4.0%
BLACK LEAF 25% PHYGON FUNGICIDE (Diamond Black)	2, 3-Dichloro-1, 4-naphthoquinone*	25%
BLACK LEAF 50% PHYGON WETTABLE POWDER Fungicide (Diamond Black)	2, 3-Dichloro-1, 4-naphthoquinone*	50%
BLACK LEAF POTASSIUM CYANATE CRABGRASS KILLER (Diamond Black)	Potassium cyanate*	77.35%
BLACK LEAF PYRENONE INSECT KILLER (Diamond Black)	Pyrethrins Tech. piperonyl butoxide Refined petroleum distillate*	0.450% 1.125% 13.425%
BLACK LEAF READY-MIXED WARFARIN RAT BAIT (Diamond Black)	Warfarin (3-(a-acetonyl-benzyl)-4-hydroxycoumarin)	0.025%
BLACK LEAF 1% ROTE-NONE-3% DDT DUST Insecticide (Diamond Black)	Rotenone Other cube extractives DDT*	1% 2% 5%
BLACK LEAF 0.75% ROTE-NONE DUST Insecticide (Diamond Black)	Rotenone Other cube extractives	0.75% 1.50%
BLACK LEAF 1% ROTE-NONE DUST Insecticide (Diamond Black)	Rotenone Other cube extractives	1.00% 2.00%
BLACK LEAF 1% ROTE-NONE-0.1% PYRETHRUM DUST Insecticide (Diamond Black)	Rotenone Other cube extractives Pyrethrins	1.00% 2.00% 0.10%
BLACK LEAF 1% ROTE-NONE-40% SULPHUR DUST Insecticide (Diamond Black)	Rotenone Other cube extractives Sulfur*	1.00% 2.00% 40.00%
BLACK LEAF 5% ROTE-NONE WETTABLE POWDER Insecticide (Diamond Black)	Rotenone* Other cube resins	5% 10%
BLACK LEAF SLUG & SNAIL PELLETS Molluscacide (Diamond Black)	Calcium arsenate* Metaldehyde	5% 2%

*Consult Sec. II., Ingredients Index. This ingredient may be responsible for major toxic effects if poisonous amounts of this product are ingested.

Name & Use Manufacturer	Ingredients	
BLACK LEAF 90% SODIUM T C A GRASS KILLER Insecticide (Diamond Black)	Sodium trichloroacetate*	90%
BLACK LEAF STANDARD ARSENATE OF LEAD (COLORED) Insecticide (Diamond Black)	Standard lead arsenate*	96%
BLACK LEAF 5% TDE DUST Insecticide (Diamond Black)	TDE* (dichloro diphenyl dichloroethane)	5%
BLACK LEAF 10% TDE DUST Insecticide (Diamond Black)	TDE (dichloro diphenyl dichloroethane)	10%
BLACK LEAF 25% TDE EMULSIFIABLE CONCENTRATE Insecticide (Diamond Black)	TDE (dichloro diphenyl dichloroethane) Xylene*	25% 70%
BLACK LEAF 10% TDE GRANULAR INSECTICIDE (Diamond Black)	TDE (dichloro diphenyl dichloroethane)	10%
BLACK LEAF 50% TDE WETTABLE POWDER Insecticide (Diamond Black)	TDE* (dichloro diphenyl dichloroethane)	50%
BLACK LEAF 1% TEPP DUST Insecticide (Diamond Black)	Tetraethyl pyrophosphate* Other ethyl phosphates	1.0% 1.5%
BLACK LEAF "TOBACCO FORMULA" 5% DDT-25% DITHANE DUST Fungicide, insecticide (Diamond Black)	DDT* (dichloro diphenyl trichloroethane) Zineb	5.00% 16.25%
BLACK LEAF "TOBACCO FORMULA" 10% DDT-10% DITHANE DUST Fungicide, insecticide (Southern Chem.)	DDT* (dichloro diphenyl trichloroethane) Zineb	10.0% 6.5%
BLACK LEAF "TOBACCO FORMULA" 5% DDT DUST Insecticide (Diamond Black)	DDT* (dichloro diphenyl trichloroethane)	5%
BLACK LEAF "TOBACCO FORMULA" 10% DDT DUST Insecticide (Southern Chem.)	DDT* (dichloro diphenyl trichloroethane)	10%
BLACK LEAF "TOBACCO FORMULA" 10% DITHANE DUST Insecticide (Southern Chem.)	Zineb	6.5%
BLACK LEAF "TOBACCO FORMULA" 15% DITHANE DUST Fungicide (Diamond Black)	Zineb	9.75%
BLACK LEAF "TOBACCO FORMULA" 25% DITHANE DUST Fungicide (Diamond Black)	Zineb	16.25%
BLACK LEAF "TOBACCO FORMULA" 1% PARATHION-5% DDT-15% DITHANE DUST Fungicide, insecticide (Diamond Black)	Parathion* DDT (dichloro diphenyl trichloroethane) Zineb	1.00% 5.00% 9.75%
BLACK LEAF "TOBACCO FORMULA" 5% TDE DUST Insecticide (Diamond Black)	TDE (dichloro diphenyl dichloroethane)	5%
BLACK LEAF "TOBACCO FORMULA" 1% PARATHION-5% DDT-20% DITHANE DUST Insecticide, fungicide (Diamond Black)	Parathion* DDT Zineb	1% 5% 13%

*Consult Sec. II., Ingredients Index. This ingredient may be responsible for major toxic effects if poisonous amounts of this product are ingested.

Name & Use Manufacturer	Ingredients		Name & Use Manufacturer	Ingredients	
BLACK LEAF "TOBACCO FORMULA" 1% PARA-THION-5% DDT-25% DITHANE DUST Fungicide, insecticide (Diamond Black)	Parathion* DDT (dichloro diphenyl trichloroethane) Zineb	1.00% 5.00% 16.25%	BLACK LEAF "TOBACCO FORMULA" 2% PARA-THION DUST Insecticide (Diamond Black)	Parathion*	2%
BLACK LEAF "TOBACCO FORMULA" 1% PARA-THION-3% DDT DUST Insecticide (Diamond Black)	Parathion* DDT (dichloro diphenyl trichloroethane)	1% 3%	BLACK LEAF "TOBACCO FORMULA" 1% PARA-THION-10% TDE-10% DITHANE DUST Fungicide, insecticide (Southern Chem.)	Parathion* TDE (dichloro diphenyl dichloroethane) Zineb	1% 10% 6.5%
BLACK LEAF "TOBACCO FORMULA" 1% PARA-THION-5% DDT DUST Insecticide (Diamond Black)	Parathion* DDT (dichloro diphenyl trichloroethane)	1% Min. 5% Min.	BLACK LEAF "TOBACCO FORMULA" 1% PARA-THION-5% TDE DUST Insecticide (Diamond Black)	Parathion* TDE (dichloro diphenyl dichloroethane)	1% 5%
BLACK LEAF "TOBACCO FORMULA" 1% PARA-THION-10% DDT DUST Insecticide (Diamond Black)	Parathion* DDT	1% 10%	BLACK LEAF "TOBACCO FORMULA" 1% PARA-THION-10% TDE DUST Insecticide (Southern Chem.)	Parathion* TDE (dichloro diphenyl dichloroethane)	1% 10%
BLACK LEAF "TOBACCO FORMULA" 1% PARA-THION-10% DDT-10% DITHANE DUST Fungicide, insecticide (Southern Chem.)	Parathion* DDT (dichloro diphenyl trichloroethane) Zineb	1.0% 10.0% 6.5%	BLACK LEAF "TOBACCO FORMULA" 10% TDE-10% DITHANE DUST Fungicide, insecticide (Diamond Black)	TDE (dichloro diphenyl dichloroethane) Zineb	10.0% 6.5%
BLACK LEAF "TOBACCO FORMULA" 1% PARA-THION-10% DITHANE DUST Fungicide, insecticide (Diamond Black)	Parathion* Zineb	1.0% 6.5%	BLACK LEAF "TOBACCO FORMULA" 10% TDE DUST Insecticide (Diamond Black)	TDE (dichloro diphenyl dichloroethane)	10%
			BLACK LEAF "TOBACCO FORMULA" 20% TDE DUST Insecticide (Diamond Black)	TDE (dichloro diphenyl dichloroethane)*	20%
BLACK LEAF "TOBACCO FORMULA" 1% PARA-THION DUST Insecticide (Diamond Black)	Parathion*	1%	BLACK LEAF TOMATO DUST Fungicide, insecticide (Diamond Black)	Copper* (in basic copper sulfate) expressed as metallic	7%
			BLACK LEAF TOXAPHENE-DDT DUST 20-5 Insecticide (Diamond Black)	Toxaphene* DDT (dichloro diphenyl trichloroethane)	20% 5%

*Consult Sec. II., Ingredients Index. This ingredient may be responsible for major toxic effects if poisonous amounts of this product are ingested.

Name & Use Manufacturer	Ingredients	
BLACK LEAF 20% TOX- APHENE DUST Insecticide (Diamond Black)	Toxaphene*	20%
BLACK LEAF TOXAPHENE EMULSIFI- ABLE CON- CENTRATE Insecticide (Diamond Black)	Toxaphene* Petroleum distillate	45.0% 43.5%
BLACK LEAF TOXAPHENE EMULSIFI- ABLE CON- CENTRATE Insecticide (Diamond Black)	Toxaphene* Petroleum distillate	72.0% 16.5%
BLACK LEAF 60% TOX- APHENE EMUL. CONC. Insecticide (Diamond Black)	Toxaphene* Petroleum distillate	60% 35%
BLACK LEAF 20% TOX- APHENE WETTABLE POWDER Insecticide (Diamond Black)	Toxaphene*	20%
BLACK LEAF 40% TOX- APHENE WETTABLE POWDER Insecticide (Diamond Black)	Toxaphene*	40%
BLACK LEAF 2, 4-D AMINE WEED KILLER (Diamond Black)	Mixed isopropyl and di- isopropanolamine salts of 2, 4-dichlorophenoxyacetic acid*	56%
BLACK LEAF 2,4-D ESTER WEED KILLER (Diamond Black)	2, 4-Dichlorophenoxyacetic acid, isopropyl ester* 44%	
BLACK LEAF 2,4-D LOW VOL. ESTER WEED KILLER (Diamond Black)	2-Ethylhexyl (iso-octyl) ester of 2,4-dichlorophenoxyacetic acid*	69.2%
BLACK LEAF 2, 4-D/2, 4, 5-T BRUSH KILLER Herbicide (Diamond Black)	2-Ethylhexyl (iso-octyl) ester of 2, 4-dichlorophenoxyacetic acid* 34.3% 2-Ethylhexyl (iso-octyl) ester of 2, 4, 5-trichlorophenoxy- acetic acid* 32.7%	

Name & Use Manufacturer	Tox- icity	Ingredients
BLACK LEAF 2, 4, 5-T BRUSH KILLER Herbicide (Diamond Black)		2-Ethylhexyl (iso-octyl) ester of 2, 4, 5-trichlorophenoxy- acetic acid* 64.9%
BLACK LEAF WARFARIN CONCEN- TRATE Rodenticide (Diamond Black)		Warfarin (3-(a-acetonylbenzyl)- 4-hydroxycoumarin) 00.5%
BLACK LEAF WARFARIN RAT BAIT (Diamond Black)		Warfarin (3-(a-acetonylbenzyl)- 4-hydroxycoumarin) 0.025%
BLACK LEAF WHITE OIL SPRAY Insecticide (Diamond Black)		Petroleum oils* 90%
BLACK LEAF ZIRAM Fungicide (Diamond Black)		Ziram (zinc dimethyldithio- carbamate) 76%
BLACK MAGIC Adhesive (Miracle)		Resinous materials Pigments* Aliphatic petroleum hydrocarbon*
BLACK MAGIC BLOSSOM BOOSTER Plant nutrient (Parks-Barnes)		Nitrogen, organic 4% Phosphoric acid, available 10% Potash 10%
BLACK MAGIC LIQUID FERTILIZER (Parks-Barnes)		Nitrogen, organic 10% Phosphoric acid, available 5% Potash 5%
BLACK MAGIC PLANTER MIX (Parks-Barnes)		Organic matter (derived from charcoal, processed leaf molds and peats) 65% Perlite (aluminum silicate) 35%
BLACK MAGIC PLANT FOOD (Parks-Barnes)		Nitrogen, organic 2% Total nitrogen 2% Phosphoric acid, available 3% Potash, water soluble 2%
BLACKMAN'S LICE POWDER Insecticide (Blackman Stock)		Sodium fluoride 10.00% Sulfur 10.00% DDT 5.00% Nicotine* 0.30%

*Consult Sec. II., Ingredients Index. This ingredient may be responsible for major toxic effects if poisonous amounts of this product are ingested.

Name & Use Manufacturer	Ingredients		Name & Use Manufacturer	Ingredients	
BLACKMAN'S PILLS Diuretic (H. Blackman)	Uva ursi Potassium nitrate Oleoresin capsicum Stone root Purified aloe Buchu Oil juniper berry Methylene blue		BLACK PANTHER RAT & MOUSE KILLER (Black Panther)	Warfarin (3-(a-acetonylbenzyl) 4-hydroxy comarin) 0.025%	
BLACKMANS VETERINARY PRODUCTS (Blackman Stock)			BLACK PANTHER SUPER DUST OR SPRAY Insecticide (Black Panther)	Rotenone 1.00% Other cube extractives 1.50% Sulfur 10.00% Sodium isopropyl naphthalene sulfonate 0.50%	
BLACKO DIURETIC TABLETS (Blacko)	Each tablet: Ext. triticum (couch grass) Methenamine Ext. corn silk Ext. uva ursi (bearberry) Boric acid* Methylene blue Potassium nitrate		BLACK PERFECTION SALVE Astringent, rubefacient (veterinary) (Energy)	Tannic acid Sulfur* Charcoal Spirits camphor* Lead solution* Lard	
BLACKO TABLETS Laxative (Blacko)	Each tablet: Ext. belladonna lvs. 1/32 gr. Total alkaloid 1/2560 gr. Aloin Oleoresin Ginger Ipecac Phenolphthalein Ext. cascara sagrada		DR. BLACK'S EYE WATER Ophthalmic antiseptic (Dunmire)	Boracic acid* Berberine sulfate* Camphor*	
BLACK-OUT INSECT KILLER (Miami)	DDT* Petroleum distillates* Beta thiocyano ethyl esters of aliphatic acids Beta-butoxy-beta-thiocyano- diethyl ether*		BLACK STRAND & BROWN STRAND HAIR COLOR- ING (Strand)	Capsules: Para-phenylenediamine Resorcinol* Duponal C Bottle: hydrogen peroxide, 10-volume strength*	
BLACK PANTHER BUG KILLER Insecticide (Black Panther)	Petroleum distillates* 97.839% Tech. chlordane 2.000% Tech. piperonyl butoxide 0.115% Pyrethrins 0.046%		BLACK SWAN Glazing compound (Glidden Co.)		
BLACK PANTHER 25% DDT Insecticide (Black Panther)	DDT* 25.00%		BLACK & WHITE BLEACHING CREAM (Black & White Chem.)	Ammoniated mercury* 4% Zinc oxide Bismuth subnitrate	
BLACK PANTHER 10% DITHANE Insecticide (Black Panther)	Zinc ethylene bis-dithio- carbamate 6.50%		BLACK & WHITE PLUKO AMBER OR WHITE Hair dressing (Black & White Chem.)		
BLACK PANTHER DUST Insecticide (Black Panther)	Rotenone 0.75% Other cube extractives 1.50% Sulfur 10.00% Beta-beta-dithiocyano- diethyl ether 0.20% Sodium isopropyl naphthalene sulfonate 0.50%		BLACK & WHITE VANISHING CREAM (Black & White Chem.)		
			BLAISDELL CRAYONS (Blaisdell)	Waxes Dry colors Cellulose nitrate lacquer	
BLACK PANTHER INSECT SPRAY (Black Panther)	DDT* 6.00% Beta-butoxy-beta-thiocyano- diethyl ether 1.00%		BLAISDELL GREASE MARKERS (Blaisdell)	Waxes Dry colors Cellulose nitrate lacquer	
			BLAKE'S MASSAGING COMPOUND Rubefacient, counter- irritant (Louisiana)	Isopropyl alcohol* Boric acid* Chloroform* Methyl salicylate*	

*Consult Sec. II., Ingredients Index. This ingredient may be responsible for major toxic effects if poisonous amounts of this product are ingested.

Name & Use Manufacturer	Ingredients	Name & Use Manufacturer	Ingredients
BLAK-RAY FLUORES-CENT PAINTS (Ultra-Violet)	Zinc oxide Zinc sulfide* Cadmium sulfide* Mineral spirits type solvent* Alkyd type resin	BLEACHRITE Bleach con-centrate (Elk)	Sodium hypochlorite solution*
BLANCHARD BATH OIL (Blanchard)		BLEECKER'S EASY CLEAN-ING FLUID (Bleecker)	Carbon tetrachloride* Ether* Chloroform* Naphtha*
BLANCHARD BUBBLE BATH (Blanchard)		BLEM For furniture blemishes (Johnson, S.C.)	Abrasives Petroleum Vegetable oils Metallic soaps Phenolic preservative (no free phenol)
BLANCHARD CREAMS FOR HANDS AND FACE (Blanchard)		BLEMO Ointment For skin irritation (Blemo)	Red mercuric oxide* 2%
BLANCHARD EAU DE TOILETTE (Blanchard)		BLENSOL COLOR SHAMPOO (Rapidol)	
BLANCHARD'S LOTION For skin irritation (Blanchard, J.)	Alcohol 19% Camphor* Methyl salicylate* Corrosive sublimate (mercuric chloride corrosive) 0.15% Boric acid Quince mucilage	BLENSOL STEEL BLUE RINSE For hair (Rapidol)	
BLAND BABY OIL (Horton & Converse)	Lanolin Mineral oil	BLENZ Color toner for hair (Kroy)	Triethanolamine Rhotex Wetting agent D & C color
BLANDITE Liquid hand soap (Lester)		BLIGHT BUSTER Herbicide (Parrot Chem.)	Copper* 6%
BLANDOXADE OINTMENT Antiseptic, emollient (Haslam)	Zinc oxide Coal tar solution Ichthammol Menthol* Phenol*	BLIGHTROL A Wettable fungicidal powder (Destruxol)	Copper zinc chromate* complex (copper 27.7%, zinc 19.1%, chromium 9.1%) 89%
BLAND'S AEROSOL BOMB Insecticide (Bland)	Pyrethrum DDT*	BLIND-X PAINT & VARNISH CLEANER (Blind-X)	
BLAST-OFF CLEANER (Park Chem.)	Kerosene* Soap Pine oil* Abrasives	BLIND-X VENETIAN BLIND CLEANER (Blind-X)	
BLAUCOP (Sugar-coated red) Tonic, cathartic (Massengill)	Each tablet: Blaud's pill mass 0.26 gm. Copper sulfate 3 mg. Ext. gentian 16 mg. Ext. cascara sagrada 8 mg. Phenolphthalein 4 mg.	BLIND-X WINDOW CLEANER (Blind-X)	
BLAZE FURNITURE CEMENT (Gibson-Homans)		BLISS NATIVE HERB TABLETS Laxative (Bliss)	Aloes Licorice Mandrake Gentian Galangal N.F.V. Burdock Cayenne pepper Uva ursi Buchu
BLAZON Insecticide, liquid (Warren Chem.)	DDT* 10% Chlordane 2%	BLISS RUBBING LINIMENT (Bliss)	

*Consult Sec. II., Ingredients Index. This ingredient may be responsible for major toxic effects if poisonous amounts of this product are ingested.

- 320 -

Name & Use Manufacturer	Ingredients		Name & Use Manufacturer	Ingredients
BLISTEX For cold sores, chapped lips, fever blisters (Blistex)	Menthol* Ammonia*		BLOSSER'S CIGARETTES Anti-spasmodic for asthma (Blosser)	Each cigarette: Stramonium* (total stramonium alkaloids 0.012 grains) Cubeb Yerba santa Eucalyptus Thyme Saw palmetto
BLISTOL, JR. Tate's liniment (Tate-Lax)	Ether 2 fl. dr./fl. oz. Oleoresin capsicum Turpentine* Castor oil			
BLITEX DI-6, T-7, T-10 Fungicides (Agsco)	Copper sulfate tribasic*		BLOSSOM BATH Bubble bath (Clark, R.)	Sodium sulfate Sodium alkyl aryl sulfonate Sodium alkyl lauryl sulfonate Perfume D & C color
BLITZ ANT & ROACH KILLER (Blitz)	DDT 4.0% Tech. chlordane 1.0% Aromatic petroleum derivatives* 16.0% Petroleum distillate 10.0%		BLOT-X Wallpaper grease spot remover (Blotex)	Kaolin SR solvent (100 octane naphtha*) Carbon tetrachloride*
BLITZ BUG KILLER (Blitz)	Tech. methoxychlor 1.0% DDT 1.0% Isobornyl thiocyanoacetate 0.82% Other related terpenes 0.18% n-Octyl bicycloheptene dicarboximide 0.166% Allethrin (allyl homolog of cinerin 1) 0.1% Aromatic petroleum derivatives* 6.0% Petroleum distillate* 10.734%		BLOX-ODOR CRYSTALS For deodorizing rooms (Hillyard Chem.)	Paradichlorobenzene*
			BLUE AND WHITE TABS Diuretic (Oliver's S-O)	Methenamine (white tablet) Sodium acid phosphate (blue tablet) Methylene blue Copaiba Santal oil
BLITZ 48 CHLORDANE INSECTICIDE (Am. Liquid)	Tech. chlordane* 48% Petroleum distillate* 44%		BLUE BALL ANT LIQUID (Blue Ball)	
BLITZ 10 PMA Herbicide (Am. Liquid)	Phenyl mercuric acetate* 10%		BLUE BALL RAT POISON (Blue Ball)	
BLOAT DOSE Carminative, astringent (veterinary) (Roberts, Dr.)	Raw linseed oil Turpentine* Nux vomica (strychnine 0.083 gr.)* Aromatic spirits of ammonium Peppermint oil Paraffine oil		BLUE BALL ROACH POWDER (Blue Ball)	
			BLUE BIRD HAIR PREPARATIONS (Assoc. Brands)	
BLOAT-I-DOTE Carminative (veterinary) (Anchor Serum)	Methyl silicone 2.5 gm. Oil of turpentine* 1 oz.		BLUE BIRD NAIL POLISH REMOVER (Assoc. Brands)	
BLONDEX Hair preparations (Swedish)			BLUE BOND CEMENT (So-Lo)	Rubber Petroleum naphtha*
BLONDEX HOME PERMANENT WAVE KIT (Swedish)			BLUE BONNET RUNFLY Fly smear, healing repellent (James, L.)	Pine tar Pine tar oil* Monsel powder
BLONDIT Hair lightener (Am. Brands)	Concentrated hydrogen peroxide* (20 volume)			

*Consult Sec. II., Ingredients Index. This ingredient may be responsible for major toxic effects if poisonous amounts of this product are ingested.

- 321 -

Name & Use Manufacturer	Ingredients		Name & Use Manufacturer	Ingredients	
BLUE BONNET SIXTY-TWO SCREW-WORM KILLER & FLY SMEAR (James, L.)	Diphenylamine* Benzol* Turkey red oil Lamp black	35% 35% 10% 20%	BLUE CROSS SYRUP OF THENYLATE Antihistaminic, antitussive (Blue Cross)	Ephedrine hydrochloride Thenylpyramine fumarate* Ammonium chloride Chloroform Menthol Alcohol	1/2 gr. 1-1/3 gr. 10 gr. 2 m. 5%/v
BLUE CHEVRON PAINT (General Paint Corp., Okla.)			BLUE CROSS TEETHING LOTION (Blue Cross)	Alcohol Benzocaine Menthol* Camphor* Oil of anise* Propylene glycol*	23%/v
BLUE CROSS ALL PURPOSE BOQUET Astringent (Halsey)	Alcohol (denatured with brucine*)	92%	BLUE CROSS TINCTURE BENSOL (Halsey)	Alcohol Gum benzoin* Tolu balsam Styrax Aloes*	34-38%
BLUE CROSS AMBER SOLUTION Antiseptic mouth wash (Blue Cross)	Alcohol Menthol thyme Thymol Eucalyptol* Methyl salicylate* Boric acid*	28%	BLUE DAWN COLOGNE, PERFUME (Gloria-Fay)		
BLUE CROSS ANALGESIC LOTION Rubefacient, counter-irritant (Blue Cross)	Eucalyptol camphor* Menthol* Methyl salicylate*		BLUE DAWN COSMETIC STICK (Gloria-Fay)		
			BLUE DAWN HAND CREAM (Gloria-Fay)		
BLUE CROSS ANTACID POWDER Antacid, adsorbent (Blue Cross)	Sodium bicarbonate Calcium and magnesium carbonates Bismuth subgallate Subcarbonate papain Kaolin (colloidal)		BLUE DAWN LIPSTICK (Gloria-Fay)		
BLUE CROSS ANTI-CAL For skin irritations (Halsey)	Calamine lotion U.S.P. Menthol* Pyrilamine maleate* Isopropyl alcohol	 1% 1%/v	BLUE DEATH RAT POISON PASTE (Bonide)	Phosphorus*	2%
BLUE CROSS BABY COUGH SYRUP Antitussive (Blue Cross)	Each fl. oz.: Alcohol Cacillana Euphorbia pilulifera Wild lettuce Squill compound Menthol Cascarin	6%	BLUE DEVIL LINIMENT (Blue Devil)		
			BLUE FOAM (Park Chem.)	Cocoanut oil soap Dye	
			BLUE FOX COLOGNE & PERFUME (Miahati)		
BLUE CROSS COLD SORE LOTION (Halsey)	Isopropyl alcohol* Gum benzoin* Camphor* Menthol*	73%/v	BLUE GEM CREAM (House of Lowell)	Petrolatum Mineral oil Beeswax Ceresin wax Oxycholesterin Lanolin Borax	
BLUE CROSS HYGIENIC POWDER (Blue Cross)					
BLUE CROSS MOUTH WASH (Blue Cross)	Zinc chloride Menthol* Oil caryoph Formalin Saccharin Oil cinnamon Alcohol	 5%	BLUE GRASS DEODORANT SPRAY (Arden)		
			BLUE GRAY #439-51-388 PAINT (George, P.D.)		
BLUE CROSS RUBBING ALCOHOL COMPOUND Rubefacient (Blue Cross)	Alcohol*	70%/v	BLUE-JAY FOOT BALM (Blue-Jay)		

*Consult Sec. II., Ingredients Index. This ingredient may be responsible for major toxic effects if poisonous amounts of this product are ingested.

Name & Use Manufacturer	Ingredients	
BLUE JAY FOOT POWDER Adsorbent, astringent (Blue-Jay)	Aluminum sulfate Barium chloride* Salicylic acid*	
BLUE JAY LIQUID CORN REMOVER (Blue-Jay)	Ether* Ethyl alcohol Isopropanol Acetone Phenoxyacetic acid*	
BLUE LOTION Antiseptic (Globe)	Crystal violet* Tannic acid Carbolic acid* Isopropyl alcohol*	 21%/v
BLUE LUSTRE Rug and upholstery cleaner (Grissmer)		
BLUE MAGIC CLEANER (Triple-X)		
BLUE MAGIC DRAIN PIPE SOLVENT FORMULA 6692 (Triple-X)		
BLUE RIBBON CREAM METAL POLISH (Internat. Metal)	Naphtha liquid solvent* Silica abrasives	
BLUE RIBBON NEATSFOOT COMPOUND (Internat. Metal)	Petroleum oil* Neatsfoot animal oil	
BLUE RIBBON PAINTS (Hemmerdinger)		
BLUE RIBBON SADDLE SOAP (Internat. Metal)	Neutral soap Animal oils	
BLUE RIBBON SAFETY INK (Davids, T.)		
BLUE RIBBON SOOT DESTROYER (Internat. Metal)		
BLUE RIBBON STOVE POLISH (Internat. Metal)	Naphtha* Graphite Carbon black	
BLUE SEAL BACTA-LIFE Septic tank activator (Blue Seal)	Yeast (nutmeg) Dehydrated enzymes	98% 2%
BLUE SEAL BOILER CLEANER (Blue Seal)	Tri-sodium phosphate* Sodium sulfate anhydrous Sodium dichromate	66-1/2% 33% 1/2%

Name & Use Manufacturer	Tox-icity	Ingredients	
BLUE SEAL BOILER STOP-LEAK COMPOUND (Blue Seal)		Rust inhibitors	
BLUE SEAL CESSPOOL CLEANER (Blue Seal)		Sodium hydroxide*	100%
BLUE SEAL CLOSET BOWL CLEANER (Blue Seal)		Sodium bi-sulfate*	100%
BLUE SEAL CUTTING OIL (Blue Seal)		Mineral oils Sulfur* Chlorine*	
BLUE SEAL DRAIN PIPE SOLVENT (Blue Seal)		Sodium hydroxide Sodium nitrate Aluminum dross	85% 7-1/2% 7%
BLUE SEAL ENAMEL CLEANER (Blue Seal)		Abrasive Sodium tri-poly phosphate (fines) Alkyl aryl sulfonate Tri-sodium phosphate (fines)	88% 5% 5% 2%
BLUE SEAL PIPE JOINT CEMENT (Blue Seal)		Silicates Carbonates Oxides and sulfates of calcium, magnesium and barium Mineral and vegetable oils	
BLUE SEAL ROOT RAIDER (Blue Seal)		Sodium hydroxide* Aluminum dross	96-1/2% 3-1/2%
BLUE STAR OINTMENT For skin irritations (Bourland)		Salicylic acid* Benzoic acid* Synthetic oil of wintergreen* Anhydrous wool fat Yellow petrolatum Camphor*	
BLUESTONE INSTANT POWDERED FUNGICIDE (Tenn. Corp.)		Copper sulfate* Copper	 25.2%
BLUE STREAK SCREW-WORM KILLER (Globe)		Chloroform* Amyl acetate Benzol* Light coal tar oil	23.00% 0.9% 68.77% 5.01%
BLUE SUDS Soap powder (Blue Suds)		Blue aniline dye	1/4 of 1%
BLUE TOPS For colds (Reese Chem.)		Each capsule: Salicylamide* Caffeine Camphor monobromated* Aloin* Powdered ext. of cascara sagrada	
BLUE WOUND DRESSING Antiseptic (veterinary) (Fidelity Labs.)		Each ounce: Aniline methyl violet Tannic acid Phenol* Oil of cloves Isopropyl alcohol*	 2.0% 2.0% 3.0% 50.0%

*Consult Sec. II., Ingredients Index. This ingredient may be responsible for major toxic effects if poisonous amounts of this product are ingested.

Name & Use Manufacturer	Ingredients		Name & Use Manufacturer	Ingredients	
BLUSTERY WEATHER LOTION Hand and body lotion (Gray, D.)			BOJER KAPS Analgesic (Horowitz)	Acetophenetidin* Caffeine Acetylsalicylic acid*	2-1/2 gr. 1/4 gr. 3-1/2 gr.
BLU-TABS Nasal de- congestant (Reese Chem.)	Each tablet: Ephedrine sulfate Vitamin C Ortho-iodo-benzoic acid* Calcium lactate	1/8 gr. 50 mg.	BOLT BUG KILLER PUSH BUT- TON SPRAY (U.S. Packag- ing)	Allethrin n-Octyl bicycloheptene- dicarboximide Isobornyl thiocyanoacetate Related terpenes DDT* Petroleum distillate* Methylated naphthalene*	0.10% 0.50% 0.82% 0.18% 2.00% 46.733% 4.667%
BLU-WHITE FLAKES Laundry soap (Manhattan Soap)	Sodium tallow-cocoanut oil soap Dyes and optical bleaches	less than 0.5%	BOLWHITE Toilet bowl bleach (Central Chem.)		
B & M LINIMENT (Rollins)	Turpentine* Oil of mustard* Methyl salicylate* Coal tar disinfectant* Balm of Gilead extract Eggs Formaldehyde* Ammonia		BON-AMI CLEANSER, CAKE (Bon Ami)	Fatty soda soap Feldspar Caustic soda or soda ash	
BOATWRIGHT PAINT (Boatwright)			BONASEPTIC FOOT LOTION Fungicide, medical (Bonaseptic)	Alcohol* Acid salicylic* Resorcin* Balsam Peru	78%
BOBBI Home permanent (Bobbi)			BONCHOTOME Antitussive (Goode-Cage)	Beechwood creosote* Sodium iodide* Sodium glycerophosphate Glycerin Alcohol	9-1/2%
BOBBY BRITE ALUMINUM PAINT (Claronex)			BONCLOR 5% CHLORDANE Insecticide (Bonide)	Chlordane	5%
BOB WHITE SHOE DRESSING (Weilmaid)	Pigment Hide glue Glycerine Dowicide*		BONCLOR DUST Insecticide (Bonide)	Tech. chlordane	5%
BO-CAR-AL HYGIENIC POWDER Douche powder (Sharp & Dohme)	Boric acid* Potassium alum Phenol* Oil of eucalyptus* Methyl salicylate* Thymol Menthol*		BONCOP Insecticide (Bonide)	Copper* Methyl naphthalenes* Cube resins	5% 1%
BOCHNER'S COMPOUND Laxative (Bochner)	Aloes Po. gentian Po. hydrastics Bicarb. soda Ess. peppermint		BONDANE Insecticide (Bonide)	Gamma isomer of benzene hexachloride* (from lindane) 	5%
BODY SMOOTH Hand and body lotion (Rubinstein)			BONDEX CEMENT PAINT (Glidden Co.)		
BOEHMER'S PAINT (Boehmer)			BONDITE PAINT (Stonhard)		
BOHMAN'S POISON SEEDS Rodenticide (Bohman)	Strychnine*		BONDKOTE PAINT (Nat'l. Mfg.)		
			BONDWOOD GLUE (Franklin Glue)		
BOILER NEVERLEAK (Liquid)			BONEWITZ 372 GENERAL CLEANER (Bonewitz)	Trisodium phosphate Sodium metasilicate Sodium carbonate Complex phosphates	
			BONEWITZ SAIL Laundry compound (Bonewitz)	Soap Tetrasodium pyrophosphate* Trisodium phosphate* Sodium metasilicate	

*Consult Sec. II., Ingredients Index. This ingredient may be responsible for major toxic effects if poisonous amounts of this product are ingested.

Name & Use Manufacturer	Ingredients	
BONIDE ANT-DUST (Bonide)	Tech. chlordane	6%
BONIDE CUTWORM DUST (Bonide)	Tech. chlordane*	10%
BONIDE DD-IDE SPRAY CONCENTRATE Insecticide (Bonide)	DDT Methyl naphthalenes* Isopropanol Dialkyl-phenoxy-polyethoxy ethanol	20% 74% 1.20% 4.80%
BONIDE 3% DDT Insecticide (Bonide)	DDT	3%
BONIDE 2% DDT DUSTING INSECTICIDE (Bonide)	DDT	2%
BONIDE DIOWEED Herbicide (Bonide)	2, 4-D triethanolamine salt* 2, 4-D acid*	 16.7% 10%
BONIDE DIOWEED DUST Herbicide (Bonide)	Triethanolamine salt of 2,4-dichlorophenoxyacetic acid*	 8.35%
BONIDE DIOWEED LIQUID Herbicide (Bonide)	2, 4-D triethanolamine salt* 2, 4-D acid*	 33.4% 20%
BONIDE DIOWEED 40% LIQUID Herbicide (Bonide)	2, 4-D triethanolamine salt* 2, 4-D acid*	 66.8% 40%
BONIDE Q-B DUST NO. 1 Insecticide (Bonide)	Rotenone Other cube resins	1.0% 2.0%
BONIDE ROACH PAINT (Bonide)	Petroleum distillate* Tech. chlordane*	97.5% 2.5%
BONIDE ROTENONE INSECT DUST 75 (Bonide)	Rotenone Other cube resins	0.75% 1.5%
BONIDE TOMATO DUST Fungicide (Bonide)	Copper oxychloride* (copper cont. 7%)	 12%
BONIDE 2, 4-DIOWEED POWDER Herbicide (Bonide)	2, 4-D acid*	70%

Name & Use Manufacturer	Ingredients	
BONIDE 2, 4-DIOWEED WEED KILLER (Bonide)	Triethanolamine 2, 4-dichloro-phenoxyacetate*	 33.4%
BONIDE WOOD PRESERVER Termite killer (Bonide)	Anthracene oil carbolineum*	
BONKIL INSECTICIDE POWDER (Bonide)	DDT (dichloro diphenyl trichloroethane)*	 10%
BONNEAU DYES (Bonneau)	Aniline dyes* Sodium chloride Sodium sulfate	
BONN'S MANGE CREAM FOR DOGS For skin irritation (veterinary) (Bonaseptic)	Resorcin* Sulfur* Benzalkonium chloride*	
BON-OPTO Astringent, eye-wash (Valmas)	Each tablet: Chlorobutanol* Zinc sulfate Sodium chloride Boric acid* Essence of peppermint Menthol*	 3/50 gr.
BONROTE BEAN DUST Insecticide, fungicide (Bonide)	Cube resins, including rotenone Methyl naphthalenes Sulfur* (325 mesh)	1.00% 1.30% 23.25%
BONSUL SPRAY-DUST Fungicide (Bonide)	Sulfur* (4-5 microns)	95%
BON TON STAIN BOOT POLISH (Whittemore)		
BON TON WHITE SHOE SOAP (Whittemore)		
BONTOX Insecticide, fungicide (Bonide)	Dichloro diphenyl trichloroethane Copper oxychloride* (total copper content 7%) Rotenone Other cube resins Methyl naphthalenes	3.00% 12.00% 0.22% 0.53% 0.85%
BONZER Fungicide (Bonide)	Ferbam	10%
BOO CORN REMOVER Keratolytic (McCambridge)	Salicylic acid* Oil of turpentine Glacial acetic acid Collodion* (ether) Benzocaine	

*Consult Sec. II., Ingredients Index. This ingredient may be responsible for major toxic effects if poisonous amounts of this product are ingested.

Name & Use Manufacturer	Ingredients		Name & Use Manufacturer	Ingredients	
BORALINE Mouth Wash (Penslar)	Zinc chloride* Solution of formaldehyde* Oil of cassia Menthol* Oil of cloves Methyl salicylate* Santophen Alcohol	25%	**BOROCAINE WITH A & D** For skin burns and irritations (Halperin)	Ethyl aminobenzoate U.S.P. Boric acid* U.S.P. Cod liver oil U.S.P.	2%
BORAPAX REGULAR Skin cleanser (Packwood)	Soap Borax*		**BOROCREME** Emollient, ointment (Horton & Converse)	Boric acid*	10%
BORAPAX SUPREME Skin cleanser (Packwood)	Soap Borax* Lanolin		**BOROCYL FOOT-BATH** Antiseptic, astringent (Borocyl)	Salicylic acid* Zinc carbonate Boric acid*	
BORASCU Herbicide (Pacific Coast)	Sodium oxide Boron trioxide Water of crystallization Equivalent borax*	15.2% 34.2% 43.7% 93.6%	**BOROCYL OIL** Emollient, skin (Borocyl)	Live shale oil Sulfonated hydrocarbons*	
BORASCU-44 Herbicide (Pacific Coast)	Sodium oxide Boron trioxide Equiv. borax pentahydrate*	20.0% 44.8% 93.7%	**BOROCYL OINTMENT** (Borocyl)	Benzocaine Balsam Peru Salicylic acid* Zinc carbonate Zinc oxide Boric acid* Glycerine Castor oil Oil of cade Adeps benz. petrolatum	
BORAXO Powdered Hand Soap (Pacific Coast)	Soap Borax*				
BORDOW Fungicide (Dow)	Copper*	12.75%	**BOROCYL SOLUTION** Antiseptic, astringent (Borocyl)	Salicylic acid* Boric acid* Zinc carbonate	
BOR-DOX COPPER FUNGICIDE (Lebanon)	Copper*	12.75%	**BOROFAX OINTMENT** Emollient (Burroughs-Wellcome)	Boric acid* Lanolin	5%
BORER-SOL Insecticide (Destruxol)	Ethylene dichloride*	50%	**BORO-KOLLESOL** Antiseptic powder (Kansas City)	8-Hydroxyquinoline sulfate Boracic acid* C.P.	
BORE-TOX Insecticide (Miller Chem. & Fert.)	Paradichlorobenzene*		**BOROLEUM** For nasal congestion, skin irritation (Sinclair Pharm.)	Menthol U.S.P. Camphor U.S.P. Eucalyptol* U.S.P. Methyl salicylate* U.S.P. Boracic acid* U.S.P. Petroleum U.S.P.	
BORITHOL OINTMENT Antiseptic (Yates Drug)	Each avoir. oz.: Phenol Boric acid Paraffin Lead plaster Petrolatum Resorcin Ammonium ichthyol sulfonate Lavender oil	4-2/3 m. 4-2/3 gr. 4-2/3 gr. 1-1/2 gr.	**BOROLID** Antiseptic Solution (Whorton)	Benzoic acid Acetanilid Thymol Oil cassia Methyl salicylate* Oil peppermint Oil eucalyptus* Boric acid* Zinc chloride	
BOR-LAC COMPOUND S.F. MFR. NO. 610 For skin irritation (Specialists)	Boric acid* Lactic acid		**BORO PHENIQUE** Antiseptic, local anesthetic for mouth and throat (Boro Phenique)	Carbolic acid* Borax* Sodium bicarbonate Menthol*	4.5%
BORNATE LOTION Ectoparasiticide (Wyeth)	Isobornyl thiocyanoacetate* and other related terpenes 5% Dioctylsodium sulfosuccinate 0.6%				

*Consult Sec. II., Ingredients Index. This ingredient may be responsible for major toxic effects if poisonous amounts of this product are ingested.

- 326 -

Name & Use Manufacturer	Ingredients	
BOROPTIC Eye drops (Borotar)	Berberine sulf.* Boric acid* Camphor* Sodium borate Sodium chloride Chlorobutanol	0.25%
BORO- QUINOLINE CALAMINE COMPOUND LOTION Local as- tringent, antiseptic (Humphreys)	Alcohol Boric acid* Oxyquinoline sulfate Prepared calamine Thymol eucalyptol* Menthol* Methyl salicylate* Oil of thyme	12%/v
BOROSORB Emollient (Torch)	Boric acid*	10%
BOSS GROUND GLUE (Cudahy)	Animal protein Sodium pentachlorophenate* Zinc sulfate* Formaldehyde*	
BOSS PAINTER Paint (Armstrong Paint)		
BOSTONIAN SHOE CLEAN- ERS AND SPOT RE- MOVER (Whittemore)		
BOSTWICK DYNOL MOTH- PROOFING (Bostwick)		
BOSTWICK METAL & WOOD COATING (Bostwick)		
BOSTWICK PLASTIC COATING (Bostwick)		
BOSTWICK PLASTIC SPRAY Rust pre- ventive (Bostwick)	Acrylic base Freon Inert ingredients	
BOSTWICK ROSE AND FLOWER GARDEN IN- SECT SPRAY (Bostwick)	Pyrethrins Rotenone Other cube extractives Tech. piperonyl cyclonene Dichlone Petroleum distillates	0.025% 0.128% 0.236% 0.256% 0.120% 0.102%
BOSTWICK SPRAY- KLEEN SPOT REMOVER (Bostwick)	Trichlorethylene* VMP naphtha* Tetrahydrofurfural* Perchlorethylene*	
BOTANO DE LUXE GARDEN DUST Insecticide (Calif. Spray)	Rotenone Pyrethrins Sulfur* Basic copper-zinc sulfates Copper* as metallic Zinc as metallic	0.50 0.10 20.00 16.60 3.50 3.50

Name & Use Manufacturer	Ingredients	
BOTANO LIQUID SPRAY Insecticide (Calif. Spray)	Rotenone* Other cube resins Pyrethrins* Petroleum oils*	
BOTANO-PY 0.2 DUST Insecticide (Calif. Spray)	Pyrethrins	0.2%
BOTANO-R 75 DUST Insecticide (Calif. Spray)	Rotenone* Other resins from cube Beta thiocyano ethyl esters of aliphatic fatty acids averaging 10-18 carbon atoms	
BOTANO-R 1 DUST Insecticide (Calif. Spray)	Rotenone* Other resins from cube	
BOTANO-R 2.5 DUST Insecticide (Calif. Spray)	Inert ingredients Rotenone Other resins from cube	 2.5% 2.5%
BOTANO-R 5 SPRAY Insecticide (Calif. Spray)	Rotenone from cube* Other cube resins Inert ingredients*	5% 5% 90%
"BOTANY" BRAND FACE POWDER (with Lanolin) (Botany)		
BO-TOX ROACH FOOD (Southland)	Boric acid*	40%
BOTTLE CLEAR Cleaner (Armstrong Chem.)		
BOTTLER'S X SPECIAL Cleaner (Wyandotte)	Conc. alkali*	
BOTTLE WASH NO. 3 (Wyandotte)	Conc. alkali*	
BOTTS STENCIL INK (Botts)		
BOVAC BOWEL EVACUANT Cathartic (Bovac)	Psyllium ovata Linum contusum Figs, prunes, raisins, apples Kelp Lactose	
BOVIMIDE For intestinal irritation (veterinary) (Sharp & Dohme)	Each 100 cc.: Sulfathalidine (phthalylsulfa- thiazole) Sulfamerazine Sulfamethazine Kaolin Alcohol Benzoic acid	 6.8 gm. 0.6 gm. 0.6 gm. 10.0 gm. 5% 0.3%

---

*Consult Sec. II., Ingredients Index. This ingredient may be responsible for major toxic effects if poisonous amounts of this product are ingested.

Name & Use Manufacturer	Ingredients		Name & Use Manufacturer	Ingredients	
BOVINATE For ketosis (veterinary) (Holt)	Sodium propionate		BOWE'S TABLETS For relief of sour stomach, etc. (Service Drug)	Magnesium oxide (heavy) Calcium carbonate Bismuth subcarbonate Colloidal kaolin Peppermint oil	

BOVINE
PURGATIVE
NO. 1
Cathartic
(veterinary)
(Massengill)
	Each 5 oz. package:
	Powd. gamboge
	Barium chloride*
	Starch
	Powd. capsicum
	Sodium chloride, magnesium
	  carbonate and white mineral
	  oil
		14.2 gm.
		9.7 gm.
		14.2 gm.
		1.3 gm.
		
		q.s.
			BOWKER'S
			LEAD
			ARSENATE
			Insecticide
			(Am. Agric.
			Chem.)
				Lead arsenate*
				Arsenic as metallic
				Water soluble arsenic
				Lead as metallic
					98.00
					19.50
					0.50
					58.00

BOVIN LIVESTOCK SPRAY Insecticide (Solarine)			BOWLCLEAN (U.S. Sanitary)		
BOVOC PINK-EYE POWDER For keratitis (veterinary) (Sharp & Dohme)	Tyrothricin Sulfanilamide* Sulfathiazole* Phenacaine hydrochloride	0.05% 78.95% 20.0% 1.0%	BOWL CLEAN (New im- proved super) (Hillyard Chem.)	Hydrochloric acid*	
			BOWL CLEAN, POWDERED (Hillyard Chem.)	Sodium bisulfite*	
BOWEL-TONE (Sacramento)					
BOWEN'S CORN REM- EDY OINT- MENT (Bowen)			BOWLENE Toilet bowl cleaner (Climalene)	Sodium bisulfate*	90%
BOWES AUTO POLISH (Bowes)	Carbolic acid	1%	BOWL-GLO Toilet bowl cleaner (Wambaugh)	Bisulfate of soda*	
BOWES AUTO WAX (Bowes)	Vegetable wax Petroleum solvent*		BOWLING ALLEY DUL-GLO FURNITURE POLISH (Nash, C. A.)		
BOWES LIQUID WHITE SIDEWALL CLEANER (Bowes)	Caustic* (pH approx. 11)		BOWLING CHALK (Hershkowitz)		
BOWES RUST PREVENTA- TIVE (Bowes)	Water soluble oil		BOWLITE Cleaner (Gisler)		
BOWES STOP-LEAK Automobile radiator sealer (Bowes)	Sulfonate base Alcohol				

*Consult Sec. II., Ingredients Index. This ingredient may be responsible for major toxic effects if poisonous amounts of this product are ingested.

Name & Use Manufacturer	Ingredients	
BOWL-KLEEN (No-Dust)		
BOW-WOW FLEA KILLER (Sweeney, W.R.)	Pyrethrins	0.5%
BOYD CREAM DEODORANT (Boyd)		
BOYD WHITE LINIMENT (Boyd)		
BOYER 3B CLOSET BOWL CLEANER (Boyer Chem.)		
BOYER 3B PAINT BRUSH CLEANER (Boyer Chem.)		
BOYER 3B TRAP & DRAIN PIPE CLEANER (Boyer Chem.)		
BOYER SOLDERING SALTS #32 (Boyer Chem.)	Zinc chlorate*	
BOYLE A-H TABLETS Antihistamine (Boyle & Co.)	Pyrilamine maleate*	25 mg.
BOYLE ANALGESIC BALM Analgesic, counter- irritant (Boyle & Co.)	Menthol* Methyl salicylate* Lanolin	
BOYLE BENZOIN COMPOUND Antitussive (Boyle & Co.)	Benzoin compound tincture U.S.P. Alcohol* 78%	
BOYLE BRITE EYE LOTION Antiseptic eye wash (Boyle & Co.)	Boric acid* Ephedrine sulfate 1-5000 Sodium ethylmercurithiosal- icylate 1-100,000 Sodium borate Sodium chloride Berberine hydrochloride Camphor*	
BOYLE BUQUETS Stimulant diuretic (Boyle & Co.)	Theobromine sodio salicylate* Oleoresin capsicum Extract buchu Extract uva ursi Extract juniper berries	

Name & Use Manufacturer	Ingredients	
BOYLE CALATEX LOTION Poison oak, skin irritation (Boyle & Co.)	Calamine lotion Menthol* Phenol*	
BOYLE CALSA Analgesic (Boyle & Co.)	Each tablet: Salicylamide* 2 gr. Sodium salicylate* 3 gr. Aluminum hydroxide 2 gr. Calcium carbonate 1 gr. Calcium ascorbate 30 mg. Para-aminobenzoic acid 10 mg.	
BOYLE C-CAPS COLD CAPSULES (Boyle & Co.)	Each capsule: Acetanilid* 1 gr. Podophyllin creosote* Capsicum Camphor*	
BOYLE CERODINE Expectorant (Boyle & Co.)	Each fl. oz.: Codeine phosphate* 1 gr. Chloroform* 2 m. Potassium guaiacolsulfonate 8 gr. Ammonium chloride 8 gr. Antimony potassium tartrate* 1/12 gr. White pine and wild cherry bark	
BOYLE CREMOSUL Antitussive (Boyle & Co.)	White pine* Beechwood creosote* Ipecac Antimony potassium tartrate* Alcohol 2% Tar Cascara Menthol*	
BOYLE DRAWING SALVE For skin irritations (Boyle & Co.)	Ammonium ichthosulfonate Methyl salicylate* Pine tar* Chloral hydrate* 4.3 gr./oz.	
BOYLE DUOCAINE OINTMENT Antiseptic, local (Boyle & Co.)	Benzocaine Menthol* Oxyquinoline benzoate Petrolatum Chlorobutanol 0.5% Zinc oxide Boric acid*	
BOYLE HEATABS For excessive perspiration (Boyle & Co.)	Each tablet: Sodium chloride 7 gr. Sucrose 3 gr. Thiamine mononitrate 0.05 mg. Ascorbic acid 1.5 mg.	
BOYLE HEMASTHESIA OINTMENT For hemorr- hoids (Boyle & Co.)	Benzocaine Phenol* Boric acid* Zinc oxide Bismuth subnitrate Resorcin* Balsam Peru	
BOYLE HEMASTHESIA SUPPOSITORIES (Rectal) (Boyle & Co.)	Bismuth subgallate Boric acid* Tannic acid Balsam Peru Zinc oxide Resorcin* Benzocaine	

*Consult Sec. II., Ingredients Index. This ingredient may be responsible for major toxic effects if poisonous amounts of this product are ingested.

Name & Use Manufacturer	Ingredients	
BOYLE HINKLE'S TABLETS Laxative (Boyle & Co.)	Ext. casc. sag. Aloin Podophylium Ext. belladonna leaf* Glycyrrhiza Oleoresin ginger	16 mg. 16 mg. 10 mg. 8 mg. 10 mg. 4 mg.
BOYLE KAO-GEL Adsorbent (Boyle & Co.)	Each fluid oz.: Kaolin N.F. Pectin N.F. Bismuth subcarbonate	90 gr. 4-1/2 gr. 5 gr.
BOYLE K-KIL Ectoparasiticide (Boyle & Co.)	Carbolic acid Camphor* Light liquid petrolatum	1.4%
BOYLE-MIDWAY PLASTIC WOOD (Boyle-Midway)	Nitrocellulose lacquer Organic solvents* Wood flour filler Plasticizer Resins	
BOYLE-MIDWAY SANI-FLUSH Detergent (Boyle-Midway)		
BOYLE-MIDWAY SCRATCH COVER POLISH (Boyle-Midway)	Petroleum oils*	
BOYLE-MIDWAY RUG & UPHOLSTERY CLEANER (Boyle-Midway)		
BOYLE NATONE NOSE DROPS Nasal deconges-tant (Boyle & Co.)	Ephedrine sulfate* Chlorobutanol Aqueous-isotonic mentholated solution	1% 0.5%
BOYLENE Anesthetic brown salve (Commerce)	Benzocaine Resin cerate Ichthammol Carbolic acid* Thymol* Camphor* Juniper tar Hexachlorophene	
BOYLE PHAROAH HENNA For tinting hair (Boyle & Co.)		
BOYLE 77 SOLUTION Antiseptic mouth wash (Boyle & Co.)	Alcohol Menthol* Boric acid* Eucalyptol* Oil thyme Thymol* Benzoic acid Sodium borate Methyl salicylate* Oil peppermint	25%
BOYLE SYCOCIL COUGH MIXTURE Antitussive (Boyle & Co.)	Cocillana Euphorbia White squill* Wild lettuce Cascarin bitterless Tartar emetic* Senega Menthol*	

Name & Use Manufacturer	Ingredients	
BOYLE SYCOCIL WITH CODEINE COUGH SYRUP Expectorant (Boyle & Co.)	Each fluid oz.: Codeine phosphate* Cocillana* Euphorbia White squill Wild lettuce Cascarin bitterless Tartar emetic* Senega Menthol	9/10 gr.
BOYLE THERAHIST Antihistaminic, analgesic (Boyle & Co.)	Each capsule: Salicylamide* Phenacetin* Caffeine alkaloid Atropine sulfate Pyrilamine maleate* Quinine sulfate	3 gr. 2 gr. 1/2 gr. 1/600 gr. 25 mg. 1/2 gr.
BOYLE WHITFIELD'S OINTMENT Fungicide (Boyle & Co.)	Benzoic acid Salicylic acid*	12% 6%
BOYLE W-P-T COUGH SYRUP Antitussive (Boyle & Co.)	Alcohol White pine Wild cherry Sanguinaria Sassafras Ammonium chloride Chloroform Tar Aralia Poplar bud Menthol* Beechwood creosote	1% 1-1/2 m.
BOZEMAN'S PREPARA-TIONS FOR ATHLETE'S FOOT (Bozeman)		
B. P. & S. OINTMENT S.F. MFR. NO. 725 For skin irritation (Specialists)	Balsam Peru Sulfur*	
B. Q. R. For colds (Beeman's)	Alcohol Chloroform Fluid extract cascara sagrada aromatic Sodium salicylate* Syrup of ipecac Menthol* Balsam Peru Elixir lactated pepsin	8-1/2% 1/8 m./tsp.
BRACELET EAU DE PARFUM (Harris, B.)		
BRACINE JUNIOR Bracing Liniment (James, L.)	Alcohol* Oil wormwood* Acetone	85%
BRACINE SENIOR Bracing liniment (veterinary) (James, L.)	Alcohol* Oil wormwood* Acetone	84%

*Consult Sec. II., Ingredients Index. This ingredient may be responsible for major toxic effects if poisonous amounts of this product are ingested.

Name & Use Manufacturer	Ingredients		Name & Use Manufacturer	Ingredients	
BRADLEY BLOCK PRINTING INK (Bradley, M.)			BRATER'S ASNARETTES Antispasmodic for asthma (Brater, John K.)	Stramonium (containing in each "cigarette" 0.043 gr. of alkaloids) Lobelia Saltpetre	
BRADLEY TRAFFIC CRAYONS (Bradley, M.)			BRATER'S POWDER Antispasmodic for asthma (Brater, John K.)	Stramonium* Lobelia* Saltpetre	
BRADLYNE CRAYONS (Bradley, M.)					
BRAMBLCIDE B.E.P. BRUSH KILLER (Thompson Chem.)	Butoxy ethoxy propyl 2,4,5-trichlorophenoxy acetate*	69.01%	BRAUN ARSENIC, WHITE Herbicide (Braun Corp.)	Arsenic trioxide*	
			BRAUN POTASSIUM CHLORATE POWDER Herbicide (Braun Corp.)	Potassium chlorate*	
BRAMBLCIDE ISO-OCTYL BRUSH KILLER (Thompson Chem.)	Iso-octyl 2,4,5-trichlorophenoxy acetate*	63%	BRAYTON EMULSIFI- ABLE PYRENONE CONC. T-143 OR 10-1 Insecticide (Brayton)	Tech. piperonyl butoxide 11.84% Pyrethrins 1.18% Polyoxyethylene sorbitol mixed ether ester 14.81% Petroleum oil* 72.17%	
BRAMBLE WEEDICIDE ISO-OCTYL BRUSH KILLER (Thomspon's Chem.)	Iso-octyl 2,4,5-trichlorophenoxy acetate* 32% Iso-octyl 2,4-dichlorophenoxy acetate* 33%				
			BRAYTONE SCALP LOTION (Bray)		
BRANDENFELS' 5 WEEKS SCALP & HAIR TREAT- MENT (Brandenfels)			BRAYTON INDUSTRIAL K.D.K. SPRAY Insecticide (Brayton)	Tech. piperonyl butoxide 1.02% Pyrethrins 0.20% Deodorized base oil* 98.78%	
BRANDRETH'S PILLS Laxative (Allcock)	Aloes 0.0547 gr. White castile soap 0.0044 gr. Gum guiac 0.0212 gr. Gum arabic 0.0071 gr. Capsicum 0.0026 gr. Colocynth 0.0132 gr. Cascarin 0.0212 gr. Ext. sarsaparilla 0.0052 gr.		BRAYTON INDUSTRIAL PYRENONE SPRAY Insecticide (Brayton)	Tech. piperonyl butoxide 1.53% Pyrethrins 0.30% Deodorized base oil* 98.17%	
BRANDT'S EAU DENNA HAIR COLORER (Hair Specialty)			BRAYTON MILL-BIN- WAREHOUSE SPRAY Insecticide (Brayton)	n-Octyl bicycloheptene dicarboxi- mide 0.666% Tech. piperonyl butoxide 0.400% Pyrethrins 0.200% Deodorized base oil* 98.734%	
BRANDT'S HAIR WHITENER (Hair Specialty)			BRAYTON P-B INSECT SPRAY (Brayton)	Pyrethrins 0.25% Tech. piperonyl butoxide 0.20% Deodorized base oil* 99.55%	
BRANNIGAN'S CORN SALVE (Lester Drug)	Benzoic acid Salicylic acid⁊ Thymol* Petrolatum		BRAYTON P-M DAIRY FARM SPRAY Insecticide (Brayton)	Petroleum hydrocarbons* 58.40% Aromatic petroleum deriv. solv.* 20.88% Polyoxyethylene sorbitol mixed ether ester 10.00% Methoxychlor tech. 5.22% Piperonyl butoxide tech. 5.00% Pyrethrins 0.50%	
BRASSO METAL POLISH (French, R.T.)	Petroleum solvent* Fatty acids Ammonia* Polishing earth Nitrobenzene 0.3%				
BRATE IMITATION VANILLA (Brate, W.C.)	Vanillin Ethyl vanillin Coumarin* Glycerin Caramel		BRAYTON PYRENONE SPACE SPRAY Insecticide (Brayton)	Petroleum solvents* 99.541% Tech. piperonyl butoxide 0.383% Pyrethrins 0.076%	

*Consult Sec. II., Ingredients Index. This ingredient may be responsible for major toxic effects if poisonous amounts of this product are ingested.

- 331 -

Name & Use Manufacturer	Ingredients	Name & Use Manufacturer	Ingredients
B & R BRAND OF RECTAL SUPPOSITORIES (Humphreys)	Aesculus with hamamelis and collinsonia 1-1/2 gr. Cocoa butter	BREEZY WICK DEODORIZER (Uncle Sam)	Perfume Emulsifier Formaldehyde* Dye
B & R C.C.C. TONIC Stomachic (Humphreys)	Each fl. oz: Alcohol 8%/v Quinine sulfate 1/5 gr. Cinchonidine sulfate 1/4 gr. Berberine sulfate 1/16 gr. Potassium hypophosphite 2 gr. Calcium hypophosphite 3 gr. Sodium hypophosphite 5 gr. Thiamine hydrochloride 500 I.U.	BREINIG SEALER WOOD PRESERVATIVE (Breinig)	Linseed oil Pentachlorophenol* Mineral spirits
		BRENNAN'S LOTION For sunburn, windburn (Brennan)	Isopropyl alcohol* Boracic acid* Chondrus Cydonium Glycerol
		BRENNAN'S OINTMENT For skin irritation (Brennan)	Phenol 1-1/2% Zinc oxide Petrolatum Tannin* Benzocaine
BRE-A-COL Antitussive (Sterling Prod.)	Chloroform 0.02 cc./5 cc. Ammonium chloride White pine Lobelium* Bloodroot F.E. horehound Menthol* Oil of eucalyptus* Honey Pine tar*	BRENNAN'S RECTAL OINTMENT (Brennan)	Phenol 1-1/2% Zinc oxide Petrolatum Tannin* Benzocaine
BREAKSTONE FIRE EXTINGUISHERS (Stempel)		BRENNESSEL HAARWASSER Hair preparation (Germadol)	
BREATHLESS PERFUMES, COLOGNES, DEODORANTS (Parfums Charbert)		BRET-O-LIN OINTMENT (Bretocol)	
		BRET-O-NERVINE (Bretocol)	
BREATH OF THE FOREST AROMATIC For use in hot-vapor-type inhalator (Pinolator)	Oil of fir siperian Menthol* Camphor* Benzoic acid Thymol* Alcohol* 69%	B & R EXPECTORANT (Boericke & Runyon)	Alcohol 9%/v Tincture of belladonna* (total belladonna alk., 0.0006 gr.) 2 m. Tincture of hyoscyamus (total hyoscy. alk., 0.00008 gr.) 2 m. Tartar emetic* 1/8 gr. Ipecac, sanguinaria, senega, bryonia, cimicifuga, and cubeb
BREATH-O-PINE Disinfectant, deodorant (Brondow)	Pine oil* Soap		
BREATH-O-PINE DISINFECTANT Deodorant, cleanser (Carpenter)	Pine oil* 70% Soap 10%	B & R EYE LOTION Antiseptic for eye (Boericke & Runyon)	Sodium chloride Hydrastine hydrochloride Camphor Boric acid
BRECK SHAMPOO (Breck, J.H.)	Low-alkalinity soaps (pH 8)	B & R HOMEOPATHIC POISON OAK PELLETS NO. 1 (Boericke & Runyon)	Rhus toxicodendron 30
BREEZE Detergent (Lever)	Sodium alkaryl sulfonate* Sodium polyphosphates* Fatty amide Sodium sulfate Silicate Perfume Optical dye	B & R HOMEOPATHIC POISON OAK PELLETS NO. 2 (Boericke & Runyon)	Croton tiglium 6x

---

*Consult Sec. II., Ingredients Index. This ingredient may be responsible for major toxic effects if poisonous amounts of this product are ingested.

Name & Use Manufacturer	Ingredients		Name & Use Manufacturer	Ingredients	
B & R HOMEOPATHIC TABLETS NO. 1 For catarrhal irritations (Boericke & Runyon)	Hydrastis canadensis Kali bichromicum* Calcarea carbonica	3x 3x	B & R HOMEOPATHIC TABLETS NO. 45A For colds (Boericke & Runyon)	Arsenicum iodatum 3x-1/3000 gr. Gelsemium sempervirens* -ө- Eupatorium perfoliatum -ө-	
B & R HOMEOPATHIC TABLETS NO. 9 Carminative (Boericke & Runyon)	Nux moschata Asafoetida Ignatia amara (strychnine content 0.000004 gr.)	1x 3x 3x	B & R HOMEOPATHIC TABLETS NO. 72 For hay fever (Boericke & Runyon)	Arsenicum iodatum 2x-1/400 gr. Quillaia saponaria -ө- Sabadilla 2x Chininum arsenicum 2x-1/400 gr.	
B & R HOMEOPATHIC TABLETS NO. 10 For climacteric disturbances (Boericke & Runyon)	Sanguinaria canadensis Lachesis Amyl nitrite	3x 8x 3x	B & R HOMEOPATHIC TABLETS NO. 75 Analgesic (Boericke & Runyon)	Macrotin Sabina Rhus toxicodendron Euonymin	2x 2x 3x 2x
B & R HOMEOPATHIC TABLETS NO. 11 For biliousness (Boericke & Runyon)	Myrica cerifera Chelidonium majus Natrum sulfuricum	-ө- -ө- 3x	B & R HOMEOPATHIC TABLETS NO. 83 For skin conditions (Boericke & Runyon)	Echinacea angustifolia Graphites Sulfur Silicea	3x 3x 3x
B & R HOMEOPATHIC TABLETS NO. 14 For hoarseness (Boericke & Runyon)	Bryonia alba Causticum	3x 3x	B & R HOMEOPATHIC TABLETS NO. 90 For colds (Boericke & Runyon)	Aconitum napellus* Belladonna* Bryonia alba Gelsemium sempervirens*	2x 2x 2x 2x
B & R HOMEOPATHIC TABLETS NO. 18 Antipyretic (Boericke & Runyon)	Aconitum napellus* Bryonia alba Sanguinaria canadensis	2x 2x 3x	B & R HOMEOPATHIC TABLETS NO. 94 (Boericke & Runyon)	Barosma crenata Salix nigra Thlaspi bursa pastoris Triticum repens	1x -ө- -ө- -ө-
B & R HOMEOPATHIC TABLETS NO. 20 Analgesic (Boericke & Runyon)	Spigelia Magnesia phosphorica Belladonna (total belladonna alkaloids 0.000001 gr.)	3x 6x 3x	B & R HOMEOPATHIC TABLETS NO. 99 Anti-rheumatic (Boericke & Runyon)	Acidum benzoicum Rhus toxicodendron* Sulfur	3x 3x 3x
B & R HOMEOPATHIC TABLETS NO. 28A For sore throat (Boericke & Runyon)	Mercurius iodatus ruber 3x-1/3000 gr. Ferrum phosphoricum Belladonna*	3x 3x	B & R HOMEOPATHIC TABLETS NO. 100 (Boericke & Runyon)	Berberis vulgaris Lycopodium clavatum Terebinthinae oleum	-ө- 3x 2x
B & R HOMEOPATHIC TABLETS NO. 33 Digestant (Boericke & Runyon)	Garbo vegetabilis Nux vomica (strychnine content 0.00004 grain) Pepsinum	2x 2x 1/8 gr.	B & R HOMEOPATHIC TABLETS NO. 154 For eye irritation (Boericke & Runyon)	Gelsemium sempervieons 3x Natrum muriaticum 12x Physostigma venenosum 3x Senega -ө-	
B & R HOMEOPATHIC TABLETS NO. 41 Sedative (Boericke & Runyon)	Ignatia amara (strychnine content 0.00004 gr.) Hyoscyamus niger (total hyoscyamus alkaloids 0.00001 gr.) Chamamilla	2x 1x	B & R HOMEOPATHIC TABLETS NO. 180 (Boericke & Runyon)	Sabal serrulata Oleum santoli Triticum repens Stigmata maydis	

*Consult Sec. II., Ingredients Index. This ingredient may be responsible for major toxic effects if poisonous amounts of this product are ingested.

Name & Use Manufacturer	Ingredients		Name & Use Manufacturer	Ingredients
B & R HOMEOPATHIC TABLETS NO. 183 (Boericke & Runyon)	Calcarea phosphorica 3x Ferrum phosphoricum 3x Kali phosphoricum 3x Magnesia phosphorica 3x Natrum phosphoricum 3x		BRIGHT BEAUTY FLOOR POLISH (Candy)	
B & R HOMEOPATHIC TABLETS NO. 195A For throat irritation (Boericke & Runyon)	Mercurius iodatus ruber 2x-1/300 gr. Phytolacca decandra -ө- Belladonna 1/100 gr.		BRIGHTGLO CLEANERS (Merson)	
			BRIGHTLAC FINISH (Phelan-Faust)	
B & R HOMEOPATHIC TABLETS NO. 213-A For catarrhal disturbances (Boericke & Runyon)	Allium cepa -ө- Euphrasia officinalis 1x Camphora* 1x Aconitum napellus 2x Arsenicum iodatum 2x-1/500 gr.		BRIGHT LEAF 10% DITHANE DUST Insecticide (Black Panther)	Zinc ethylene bisdithiocarbamate 6.00
B & R HOMEOPATHIC TABLETS NO. 227 Sedative in laryngitis and bronchitis (Boericke & Runyon)	Rumex crispus -ө- Sanguinaria canadensis -ө- Eriodictyon glutinosum Tartarus emeticus* 2x		BRIGHTO POLISH AND CLEANERS (Brighto)	
			BRIGHTO ROACH SPRAY & POWDER (Brighto)	
B & R HOMEOPATHIC TABLETS NO. 232A For colds (Boericke & Runyon)	Bryonia alba -ө-/m. Eupatorium perfoliatum -ө-/m. Gelsemium sempervirens* -ө-/m. Arsenicum Iodatum 1/1000 gr.		BRIGHTOP Aluminum roof paint (Acorn Ref.)	
			BRIGHT SAIL AIR PURIFIER (Great Atlantic)	Isopropyl alcohol less than 10% Perfume oils* Formaldehyde* Phenol*
B & R HOMEOPATHIC TABLETS NO. 243 For neuritis, rheumatism (Boericke & Runyon)	Rhus toxicodendron* 4x Hypericum perforatum 3x Kali phosphoricum 3x Arsenicum album (arsenic content, trace) 6x		BRIGHT SAIL AMMONIA (Great Atlantic)	Ammonium hydroxide*
B & R HOMEOPATHIC TABLETS NO. 263 For catarrhal disturbances (Boericke & Runyon)	Gelsemium* -ө- Aconite* -ө- Camphor* -ө-		BRIGHT SAIL INSECT KILLER (Great Atlantic)	DDT* n-Octyl bicycloheptene dicarboximide Beta-butoxy-beta-thiocyanodi-diethyl ether Allethrin (allyl homolog of cinerin-1) Methylated aromatic petroleum derivatives* Petroleum distillate
BRIDGEPORT AER-A-SOL INSECTICIDE (Bridgeport)	Pyrethrum 10% Piperonyl butoxide 80% DDT 2.00% Beta-butoxy-beta-thiocyanodi-ethyl ether 1.06% Petrol. deriv. solv. & petr.* 11.04		BRIGHT SAIL LAUNDRY BLEACH (Great Atlantic)	Sodium hypochlorite* Sodium chloride Sodium hydroxide
BRIDGEPORT BUG BOMBS Insecticide (Bridgeport)	Beta-butoxy-beta thiocyanodi-ethyl ether 1.06% Allethrin* n-Octyl bicycloheptene dicarboximide* Dichlorodiphenyltri-chlorethane*		BRIGHT SAIL LIQUID BLUE Bluing (Great Atlantic)	Prussian Blue* Oxalic acid* Acetic acid
BRIGGS OIL COLORS, MARVNEY PAINTS (Briggs Marvney)			BRIGHT SAIL LIQUID LAUNDRY STARCH (Great Atlantic)	Starches Sodium chloride Terpineol Perfume oils o-Phenylphenol

*Consult Sec. II., Ingredients Index. This ingredient may be responsible for major toxic effects if poisonous amounts of this product are ingested.

Name & Use Manufacturer	Ingredients
BRIGHT SAIL PASTE WAX (Great Atlantic)	Waxes Petroleum solvents* Turpentine*
BRIGHT SAIL PORCELAIN CLEANER & METAL POLISH (Great Atlantic)	Silica abrasive Soda soap Pine oil Ammonia Oxalates
BRIGHT SAIL SELF-POLISH-ING FLOOR WAX (Great Atlantic)	Shellac* Wax Synthetic resin Amines* Borax Ammonia
BRIGHT SAIL SOAP FLAKES (Great Atlantic)	
BRIGHT SAIL WINDOW CLEANER (BLUE) (Great Atlantic)	Detergent Wetting agent Isopropyl alcohol less than 10%
BRIGHT SAIL WINDOW WAX (Great Atlantic)	Silica abrasive Amine soaps* Waxes Petroleum solvents* Ammonia
BRIGHT SPOT Household ammonia (McDonald)	Ammonium hydroxide*
BRILLIANT-SHINE Metal polish (Bennett, E.W.)	Thinner* Silica Stearic acid Ammonia Elaine oil
BRILLITE ONE COAT ENAMEL (Red Spot Paint)	
BRILUMINUM Aluminum Coating (Breinig)	
BRI-MAR PAINTS (Briggs Maroney)	
BRIOSCHI Antacid (Ceribelli)	Tartaric acid Sodium bicarbonate
BRISK Detergent (U.S.Sanitary)	
BRISK CLEANING FLUID (Feiner)	

Name & Use Manufacturer	Ingredients
BRISK MEN'S AFTER SHAVE COLOGNE (Armand)	
BRISK MEN'S HAIR DRESS (Armand)	
BRISKSOLVE CLEANERS (Feiner)	
BRISK TABLETS Stimulant (Pharmex)	Each tablet: Caffeine . 1.5 gm. Dextrose 5 gm.
BRISTALIN (Bristol Labs.)	Each fl. oz.: Bristamin dihydrogen citrate 0.075 gm. Fluid ext. of ipecac, U.S.P. 0.06 cc. Ammonium chloride U.S.P. 0.347 gm. Sodium citrate U.S.P. 0.322 gm. Menthol U.S.P. 0.0033 gm. Sodium benzoate 0.1%
BRISTAMIN* APC TABLETS For colds (Bristol Labs.)	Each tablet: Bristamin dihydrogen citrate Acetylsalicylic acid* 210 mg. Phenacetin* 150 mg. Caffeine 30 mg.
BRISTAMIN LOTION For skin irritations (Bristol Labs.)	Bristamin dihydrogen citrate 1%
BRISTAMIN TABLETS Antihistamine (Bristol Labs.)	Each tablet: Bristamin* dihydrogen citrate
BRITE MAGIC Adhesive (Miracle)	Resinous materials Pigments Aliphatic petroleum hydrocarbon*
BRITE METAL POLISH (Worrell)	
BRITE-N-KLEAN Washing com-pound (Puritan Chem.)	
BRITE-N-SWEET Scented Cleaning Powder (Varn-O)	
BRITE SILVER POLISH (Copper Brite)	
BRITE-WOOD Furniture polish (Feiner)	

*Consult Sec. II., Ingredients Index. This ingredient may be responsible for major toxic effects if poisonous amounts of this product are ingested.

- 335 -

Name & Use Manufacturer	Ingredients		Name & Use Manufacturer	Ingredients	
BRIT-TEX For brittle nails (Thomas Prod.)	Lanolin White wax Cocoa butter Spermaceti		BROMIDROSIS FOOT POW- DER Astringent (Gordon Labs.)	Potassium alum Boric acid* Magnesium trisilicate Talc	
BRITISH HAIR LOTION (Page Barker)			BROMO CAFFEINE Analgesic (Alkalithia)	Each heaping tsp.: Sodium bromide Caffeine Sodium bicarbonate Citric acid	6 gr.
BRITTON'S FAMILY OINTMENT (Britton)			BROMOFUME- 40 Fumigant (Eston)	Ethylene dibromide*	38.0%
BRITTON'S FAMOUS CORN REMOVER (Britton)			BROMO QUININE For colds (Grove)	Acetophenetidin* Ext. belladonna Ext. hyoscyamus (0.155% total alkaloids) Quinine hydrobromide Caffeine Yellow phenolphthalein Oleoresin capsicum	1-3/4 gr. 1/50 gr. 1/16 gr. 3/8 gr.
BRITTON'S FAMOUS LINIMENT (Britton)					
BROADY'S FOOT POWDER Fungicide (Broady)	Oxyquinoline sulfate Boric acid* Kaolin Sodium perborate*		BROMO-SAL Analgesic (Mediphar)	Each 6 gm.: Acetanilid Sodium bromide Caffeine Saccharin Sodium bicarbonate Citric & tartaric acids	0.15 gm. 0.3 gm.
BROADY'S OINTMENT Fungicide, medical (Broady)	Benzoic and salicylic acids* Other gums and resins				
BRODIE'S CORDIAL For intestinal irritation (Lyons, I.L.)	Tincture catechu Tannic acid Oil cinnamon Oil peppermint Alcohol 10%		BROMO- SELTZER Analgesic, antacid (Emerson)	Each heaping tsp.: Acetanilid* Sodium bromide* Caffeine Sodium bicarbonate Citric acid	2-1/2 gr. 5 gr.
BROEMMEL POISON OAK EXTRACT (Liquid) (Broemmel)	Alcoholic ext. of poison oak (1.8% extractive standard) Alcohol 22%		BROMOTOX Fumigant (Eston)	Ethylene dibromide* Methyl bromide*	30.0% 69.5%

BROEMMEL
POISON OAK
EXTRACT
(Tablets)
(Broemmel)
	Each tablet:
	Poison oak extract 1 gr.
			BRONAHIST
			Antitussive
			(Veltex)
				Each fl. oz.:
				Pyranisamine maleate* 25 mg.
				Chloroform 2 m.
				Potassium guaiacol sulfonate
				  8 gr.
				Ammonium chloride 8 gr.
				Tartar emetic 1/12 gr.
				Wild cherry and white pine
				  compound	

BROLITE LACQUERS AND ENAMELS (Brown, A.)	Pure alkyd resin*				
BROLITE Z-SPAR (Brown, A.)	Long oil resin base Inactive ingredients*		BRONCHIAL LOZENGES Antitussive (Royal Pharm.)	Powdered extract licorice Powdered cubeb Capsicum Menthol	
BROMA CHROME FINISH ALUMINUM PAINT (Master Bronze)			BRONCHIBALM (Leslie Pharm.)		
			BRONCHI- LYPTUS Antitussive (Bronchi- Lyptus)	Oil of eucalyptus Pure glycerine Syrup	
			BRONCHO AFTER SHAVE LOTION (French-Bell)		
BROMEX Soil Fumigant (Larvacide)	Methyl bromide* 26%		BRONCHO COMPLEXION MEDIC (French-Bell)		
BROMIDROSIS CRYSTALS Astringent (Gordon Labs.)	Zinc sulfate* Sod. chloride		BRONCHO HAND LOTION (French-Bell)		

*Consult Sec. II., Ingredients Index. This ingredient may be responsible for major toxic effects if poisonous amounts of this product are ingested.

Name & Use Manufacturer	Ingredients
BRONCHOLA COUGH SYRUP Antitussive (Sutliff)	Each fl. oz.: Sanguinaria — 6 m. Lobelia — 3-3/4 m. Ipecac — 54/64 m. Squill — 58/64 m. Senega — 58/64 m. Menthol — 1/10 gr. Alcohol — 6%/v
BRONCHO ODOREX (French-Bell)	
BRONCHO SHAMPOO (French-Bell)	
BRONCHO SHAVING CREAM (French-Bell)	
BRON-CHU-LINE EMULSION Antitussive (Internat. Labs.)	Benzylic alcohol — less than 1/2 of 1% Guaiacol Creosote* Calcium hypophosphite* Sodium hypophosphite Acacia Synthetic wintergreen*
BRON-COLE LOZENGES Antitussive (Hance)	Coltsfoot Cubeb Licorice Balsam tolu Capsicum Oil of peppermint Oil of anise Sugar
BRONIACIN Sedative (Massengill)	Each tablet: Ammonium bromide* — 0.25 gm. Potassium bromide* — 0.25 gm. Niacinamide hydrobromide — 10 mg.
BRONZITE Paint (Colonial Works)	
BRONZTAN Sunscreen preparation (Shulton)	Silicone
BROOKS' LINIMENT Anti-rheumatic (Brooks Med.)	Isopropyl alcohol* — 80% Oleoresin capsicum Oil wintergreen* (syn.) Spirits turpentine* Camphor*
BROOKS PYRENONE SPRAY INSECTICIDE FORMULA NO. 920 (Brooks Chem.)	Piperonyl butoxide tech. — 1.90% Pyrethrins — 0.19% Petroleum base oil* — 97.91%
BROOKS PYRENONE SPRAY INSECTICIDE FORMULA NO. 923 (Brooks Chem.)	Piperonyl butoxide tech. — 0.635% Pyrethrins — 0.065% Petroleum base oil* — 99.300%
BROOMATIC MIXTURE Anti-rheumatic (Brooks Med.)	Sodium salicylate* Potassium iodide Sodium acetate

Name & Use Manufacturer	Tox-icity	Ingredients
BROVAL TABLETS Sedative (Morton Pharm.)		Each tablet: Potassium bromide* — 3 gr. Ammonium bromide — 3 gr. Sodium bromide — 1-1/2 gr. Powdered ext. valerian — 1 gr.
BROWNATONE Blonde to Medium Brown hair dye (Kenton)		Copper chloride* Pyrogallic acid* Caustic soda* Alcohol (190 proof) Oil lavender Oil bergamot
BROWNATONE Dark Brown to Black hair dye (Kenton)		Pyrogallic acid* Copper chloride* Ferric chloride Caustic soda* Alcohol (190 proof) Oil lavender Oil bergamot
BROWNATONE HENNAPAC Hair dye (Kenton)		Clay Ferrous sulfate Copper chloride* Calcium carbonate* Henna Pyrogallic acid*
BROWNELL'S PERMA BLUE (Casey Chem.)		Selenium* Nitric acid* Methanol*
BROWN LOZENGES (Compound) Antitussive (Purepac)		Extract of licorice Tartar emetic* Ammonium chloride
BROWN LOZENGES (Plain) Antitussive (Purepac)		Extract of licorice Tartar emetic*
BROWN RAT KILLER (Allen)		Alpha-naphthyl-thiourea* — 23% Flour Talc
BROWN'S DOPE THINNER (Brown, A.)		Ethyl alcohol — 5% Butanol* — 10% Butyl acetate* — 20% Ethyl acetate — 20% Toluene — 25% Aliphatic petroleum hydrocarbons — 20%
BROWN'S MEDICATED BABY OIL (Cort-Livingston)		
BROWN TOPS For colds (Reese Chem.)		Each capsule: Aspirin U.S.P.* Camphor monobromated* Ephedrine sulfate 1/8 gr. Acetophenetidin* — 2 gr.
B & R SCHUSSLER'S TRITURATED TISSUE SALTS (Boericke & Runyon)		Kali phosphoricum — 3x Calcarea phosphorica — 3x Magnesia phosphorica — 3x
B & R TABLETS NO. 156 Digestant (Boericke & Runyon)		Abies nigra Carbo vegetabilis — 2x Hydrastis canadensis Kali carbonicum — 3x Nux vomica (strychnine content 0.000003 gr.) — 3x

*Consult Sec. II., Ingredients Index. This ingredient may be responsible for major toxic effects if poisonous amounts of this product are ingested.

Name & Use Manufacturer	Ingredients		Name & Use Manufacturer	Ingredients	
B & R TABLETS NO. 171A Analgesic (Boericke & Runyon)	Henatyne Acetylsalicylic acid* Macrotin Bryonin	1-3/10 gr. 1 gr. 1/200 gr. 1/200 gr.	B & R TABLETS NO. 279 Analgesic (Boericke & Runyon)	Acetophenetidin* Acetylsalicylic acid* Caffeine	2-1/2 gr. 2-1/2 gr. 1/2 gr.
B & R TABLETS NO. 184 Laxative (Boericke & Runyon)	Extract of cascara sagrada Nux vomica (strychnine content 0.000115 gr.)	2 gr. 1/100 gr.	BRUCE ASPHALT TILE CLEAN- ER (Bruce)	Alkyl aryl polyether alcohol Alkyl aryl sodium sulfonate* Carboxy methyl cellulose	
B & R TABLETS NO. 200 Analgesic (Boericke & Runyon)	Acetanilid* Sodium bicarbonate Iris versicolor Aromatics Caffeine Calomel Nux vomica (strychnine content 0.00015 gr.)	2 gr. 1/2 gr. 1/75 gr. 1/2 gr. 1/10 gr. 1/75 gr.	BRUCE ASPHALT TILE WAX (Bruce)	Vegetable waxes Synthetic waxes Shellac Synthetic resins Oleic acid Emulsifying agents such as morpholine*	
B & R TABLETS NO. 205-A Digestant (Boericke & Runyon)	Papain Sodium salicylate* Rhubarb Nux vomica (strychine content 0.0005 gr.) Bismuth subgallate Pepsin Phenolphthalein Ginger	3/4 gr. 3/4 gr. 1/2 gr. 1/20 gr. 3/4 gr. 1/4 gr. 1/4 gr. 1/2 gr.	BRUCE CLEANING WAX (Bruce)	Petroleum solvent* (mineral spirits) Vegetable waxes Paraffin waxes Microcrystalline waxes Polyethylene	
B & R TABLETS NO. 217A Cathartic (Boericke & Runyon)	Cascarin Aloin Est. of belladonna* (total belladonna alkaloids 0.0015 gr.) Irisin Podophyllin*	1/4 gr. 1/5 gr. 1/8 gr. 1/10 gr. 1/10 gr.	BRUCE FLOOR CLEANER (Bruce)	Petroleum solvent* (mineral spirits) Vegetable waxes Paraffin wax Microcrystalline wax Polyethylene Zinc stearate	
B & R TABLETS NO. 240A For colds (Boericke & Runyon)	Belladonna tincture Bryonia tincture Gelsemium tincture Camphor Oil anise	1/2 drop 1/2 drop 1/2 drop 1/10 gr. q.s.	BRUCE PASTE WAX (Bruce)	Petroleum solvent* (mineral spirits) Paraffin waxes Microcrystalline waxes Polyethylene	
B & R TABLETS NO. 241 Antitussive (Boericke & Runyon)	Terpin hydrate Ipecac Antimony and potassium tartrate Tincture of bryonia Tincture of drosera Tincture of belladonna (total belladonna alkaloids 0.00015 gr.)	1 gr. 1/20 gr. 1/100 gr. 1 m. 3/4 m. 1/2 m.	BRUCE SELF POLISHING WAX (Bruce)	Vegetable waxes Synthetic waxes Shellac Synthetic resins Oleic acid Emulsifying agents such as morpholine*	
B & R TABLETS NO. 249 Gastric antacid (Boericke & Runyon)	Calcium carbonate Magnesium carbonate Bismuth subnitrate Aromatics	3-1/2 gr. 2-1/2 gr. 1/2 gr.	BRUCE TUF-LUSTRE WAX (Bruce)	Petroleum solvents* (mineral spirits and naphtha) Paraffin waxes Microcrystalline waxes Polyethylene	
B & R TABLETS NO. 257 Cathartic (Boericke & Runyon)	Phenolphthalein* Podophyllin Cascarin Aloin* Extract of belladonna* (total belladonna alkaloids 0.0015 gr.)	1/2 gr. 1/4 gr. 1/4 gr. 1/4 gr. 1/8 gr.	BRUIN PAINT (Baer Bros. Paint)		
			BRULAX For colds (Burrough)	Each tablet: Acetanilid* Extract belladonna (alkaloids 0.00062 gr.) Caffeine Aloin Podophyllin Aspirin*	1 gr. 1/20 gr.
B & R TABLETS NO. 259 Sedative (Boericke & Runyon)	Hyoscyamus tincture (total hyoscyamus alkaloids 0.00008 gr.) Nux vomica tincture (total strychnine content 0.00114 gr.) Passiflora tincture Chamomilla tincture Lupulin Moschus	2 m. 1 m. 1 m. 1 m. 1/10 gr. 1/1000 gr.	BRUSH-CAP SPOT RE- MOVER (Norton)	Stoddard solvent* Carbon tetrachloride*	
			BRUSH-DAY- LITE Paint (Glidden Co.)		
			BRUSH FIX Herbicide (Thompson Chem.)	Tetrahydrofurfuryl ester of 2,4-D* Tetrahydrofurfuryl ester of 2,4,5-T*	

*Consult Sec. II., Ingredients Index. This ingredient may be responsible for major toxic effects if poisonous amounts of this product are ingested.

Name & Use Manufacturer	Ingredients
BRUSHKIL 64 Herbicide (Green Cross)	2,4-D acid* equiv. 32 oz./gal. 2,4,5-T acid* equiv. 32 oz./gal.
BRUSH-NU PAINT BRUSH CLEANER (Brush-Nu)	
BRUSHON PAINTS (Liebich)	
BRUSH-RE- NU-ER Paint brush cleaner (Andersen)	
BRUSH RITE GLUE (Standard Paste)	
BRUSH TREET Paint brush cleaner (Andersen)	Stoddard's solvent*
BRUSH-WASH CLEANER (Ames Labs.)	
BRU-WEED Herbicide (Planetary Chem.)	Butyl ester of 2,4-dichloropheno- xyacetic acid* 27.5% Amyl ester of 2,4,5-trichloro- phenoxyacetic acid* 28.0% Aromatic petroleum naphtha 39.0%
BRYKO (Pennsylv. Salt)	Non-ionic detergent*
B & S BRAND CHALK CRAYON (Binney & Smith)	
B-75 GOLDEN (ALL SOLUBLE BORAX BASE INDUSTRIAL) SKIN CLEAN- SER (Sugar Beet)	Soap 25% Borax formulation* 75%
B-SHUR TABLETS (Danmar)	
BSP LIQUID Astringent (Glidden,O.)	Isopropyl alcohol 4% Ringers solution Calamine U.S.P. Methylcellulose
BTC 50% U.S.P. Insecticide (Onyx)	Alkyl dimethyl benzyl ammonium chloride* U.S.P.
BUBBLE BATH (Stanley Home)	Synthetic detergent Perfume Versene Certified dye
BUBBLE BATH PACKAGE (Glenway)	Sodium sulfate anhydrous Alkyl aryl sulfonate* D&C colors Perfume

Name & Use Manufacturer	Tox- icity	Ingredients
BUBBLING ZOO BUBBLE BATH (Glenway)		Sodium sulfate anhydrous Alkyl lauryl sulfonate* Certified color Perfume pH approx. 7
BUCHAN'S OINTMENT Antiseptic (veterinary) (Myers Labs.)		Coal tar phenols* 15% Coal tar neutral oils 20% Resin 15% Soap 20% Tallow 15%
BUCHU, JUNIPER AND POTASSIUM ACETATE N.F. (Lilly)		Alcohol 36% Buchu 15 gm./100 cc. Juniper* 7.5 gm./100cc. Potassium acetate 5 gm./100 cc.
BUCKEYE ANTUBE Insecticide (Buckeye Chem.)		Sodium arsenate* 8.2%
BUCKEYE BOL-CLEAN Toilet bowl cleaner (Davies-Young)		Hydrochloric acid*
BUCKEYE CORN SALVE Keratolytic agent (Balm Barr)		Salicylic acid*
BUCKEYE PAINTS (Buckeye P.&V.)		
BUCKEYE PINE OIL DISIN- FECTANT Coefficients 3 and 4, FDA (Davies-Young)		Distilled pine oil* 70.00% Soap 13.36% Isopropyl alcohol 6.64%
BUCKEYE PINE OIL DISIN- FECTANT Coefficient 5, FDA (Davies-Young)		Distilled pine oil* 80.00% Soap 7.03% Isopropyl alcohol 3.48%
BUCKEYE SELF POLISHING BEAMAX WAX (Davies-Young)		
BUCKLEY'S ASTRINGENT Oral (Crosby Lab.)		Iodine* Zinc phenosulfonate Potassium iodide* Menthol Thymol Glycerine
BUCKLEY'S BENZOCAINE PASTE Topical anesthetic, antiseptic (Buckley)		Benzocaine 15% Thymol iodide* 20% Urea 5%
BUCKLEY'S DENTAL GLYCERITE Astringent, stimulant, antiseptic (Crosby Labs.)		Iodine* Zinc sulfocarbolate Potassium iodide* Menthol Thymol Glycerine

---

*Consult Sec. II., Ingredients Index. This ingredient may be responsible for major toxic effects if poisonous amounts of this product are ingested.

Name & Use Manufacturer	Ingredients	
BUCKLEY'S EUCALYPTOL Antiseptic, stimulant, solvent for gutta percha (Crosby Labs.)	Eucalyptol* Menthol Thymol	93% 3% 4%
BUCKLEY'S LINIMENT Local sedative (Crosby Labs.)	Menthol Iodine* Chloroform* Tincture aconite*	
BUCKLEY'S PHENOL Analgesic, antiseptic (Crosby Labs.)	Liquid phenol* Menthol* Camphor*	
BUCKLEY'S Z. O. LIQUID (Crosby Labs.)	Isopropyl alcohol* Oil of cloves	
BUCKSKIN TOILET WATERS (Parfum L'Orle)		
BUCOPIN Urinary sedative (Jenkins)	Each tablet: Ext. buchu Ext. cornsilk Ext. triticum Potassium bitartrate Atropine sulfate Acid tartaric Sodium bicarbonate	1-1/2 gr. 1/2 gr. 1/4 gr. 2-1/2 gr. 1/500 gr. 1/8 gr. 1/2 gr.
BUDDA COSMETICS (Assoc. Brands)		
BUDDA TOILET WATER (Assoc. Brands)		
BUDERMA OINTMENT (Buckman)		
BU-DU POULTRY WORMER Anthelmintic (veterinary) (Burrell-Dugger)	Phenothiazine Nicotine alkaloid*	21% 2%
BUFETS Analgesic (Pharmex)	Each tablet: Salicylamide* Mag. glycinate Cal. carbonate	5 gr.
BUFFALO BETTER-BUILT CARBON DIOXIDE EXTINGUISHER (Buffalo Fire)	Carbon dioxide gas*	
BUFFALO BETTER-BUILT CB LIQUID FOR FIRE EXTINGUISHERS (Buffalo Fire)	Chlorobromomethane*	

Name & Use Manufacturer	Ingredients
BUFFALO BETTER-BUILT DRY CHEMICAL RECHARGE For fire extinguishers (Buffalo Fire)	Sodium bicarbonate Magnesium stearate Tricalcium phosphate
BUFFALO BETTER-BUILT FOAM RECHARGE For fire extinguishers (Buffalo Fire)	Aluminum sulfate Sodium bicarbonate Beta-naphthol Licorice Potassium Phosphate monobasic
BUFFALO BETTER-BUILT NON-CORROSIVE ANTI-FREEZE RECHARGE For fire extinguishers (Buffalo Fire)	Calcium chloride
BUFFALO BETTER-BUILT RECHARGE FOR SODA-ACID FIRE EXTINGUISHER (Buffalo Fire)	Sodium bicarbonate Conc. sulfuric acid*
BUFFALO BETTER-BUILT VAPORIZING LIQUID For fire extinguishers (Buffalo Fire)	Carbon tetrachloride* Trichloroethylene*
BUFFALO BRAND AMMONIA (Clear) (Robinson Bros.)	Ammonia*
BUFFALO BRAND AQUA AMMONIA 26° (Technical) (Robinson Bros.)	Aqua ammonia* tech. 26°
BUFFALO BRAND CARBON TETRACHLOR-IDE (Robinson Bros.)	Carbon tetrachloride*
BUFFALO BRAND CAR WASH (Robinson Bros.)	
BUFFALO BRAND MURIATIC ACID (Robinson Bros.)	Muriatic acid*

*Consult Sec. II., Ingredients Index. This ingredient may be responsible for major toxic effects if poisonous amounts of this product are ingested.

Name & Use Manufacturer	Ingredients		Name & Use Manufacturer	Ingredients	
BUFFALO BRAND OXALIC ACID (Robinson Bros.)	Oxalic acid*		BUG BOMB (Bridgeport)	Beta-butoxy-beta'-thiocyano diethyl ether	1.06%
				Allethrin (allyl homolog of cinerin #1)	0.10%
BUFFALO BRAND SOLDERING FLUX (Robinson Bros.)	Zinc* ammonium chloride			Petroleum distillate	5.09%
				Aromatic petroleum derivative solvent*	6.00%
				n-Octyl bicycloheptene dicarboximide	0.75%
BUFFALO FURNITURE POLISH (Buffalo Scient.)				Dichlorodiphenyltrichloroethane	2.00%
			BUG CHEK Insecticide (Chek)		
BUFFERIN Antacid, Analgesic (Bristol-Myers)	Each tablet: Aspirin*	5 gr.	BUGDEATH (Wettable Powder) (Hanson, H.)	DDT*	
	Aluminum glycinate				
	Magnesium carbonate		BUG DEVIL Fumigant (Lester)	Ethylene dichloride*	
BUFF PRESERVO Wood preservative (Robeson)	Copper naphthenate	8%		Carbon tetrachloride*	
	Mercury didodecenyl succinate*		BUG DUST Insecticide (Greever's)	Rotenone	0.75%
				Other cube resins	1.50%
BUFF'S BOWL CLEANSE (Buff)				Dusting sulfur*	
			BUG-GETA PELLETS Insecticide (Calif. Spray)	Calcium arsenate*	5.00%
BUG A BOMB HIGH PRESSURE BUG KILLER (Am.Aerosol)	DDT	3.0%		Arsenic as metallic	1.88%
	Tech. methoxychlor	1.0%		Water soluble arsenic	1.88%
	Isobornyl thiocyanoacetate	0.82%		Metaldehyde	2.00%
	Other related terpenes	0.18%	BUG-FIX Insecticide (Thompson Chem.)	Piperonyl butoxide tech.	0.25%
	n-Octyl bicycloheptene dicarboximide	0.166%		Allethrin	0.10%
	Allethrin (allyl homolog of cinerin 1)	0.10%		Dichloro diphenyl trichloro-ethane	2.00%
	Petroleum distillate	2.734%		Beta-butoxy-beta'-thiocyano diethyl ether	1.00%
	Aromatic petroleum derivatives*	12.00%		Xylene*	5.00%
				Petroleum distillate	11.63%
				Perfume	0.02%
BUG-A-BOO MOTH CRYSTALS (Bug-A-Boo)	Paradichlorobenzene *	100%	BUGINE BOMB Insecticide spray (Royal Pharm.)	DDT	2.00%
				Allethrin	0.10%
BUGACIDE Insecticide (Southwest Distrib.)	Chlordane*			n-Octyl bicycloheptene dicarboximide	0.50%
				Petroleum hydrocarbon*	16.40%
				Beta-butoxy-beta-thiocyano diethyl ether	1.00%
BUG-ANT DOOM POWDER (Murray,E.)	Pyrethrins	0.97%	BUGINE INSECT REPELLENT (Royal Pharm.)	2-Ethyl hexanediol-1,3*	20.00%
	Boric acid*	25.5%			
BUG-A-WAY Insecticide (Southland)	Butoxy polypropylene glycol	10.00%	BUG-O-BLITZ (Blitz)	Tech. methoxychlor	1.0%
	Piperonyl butoxide	0.60%		DDT	1.0%
	Pyrethrins	0.12%		Isobornyl thiocyanoacetate	0.82%
	Petroleum distillates*	88.28%		Other related terpenes	0.18%
BUG BLITZ (Am. Aerosol	DDT	3.0%		n-Octyl bicycloheptene dicarboximide	0.166%
	Tech. methoxychlor	1.0%		Allethrin (allyl homolog of cinerin 1)	0.1%
	Isobornyl thiocyanoacetate	0.82%		Aromatic petroleum derivatives*	6.0%
	Other related terpenes	0.18%		Petroleum distillate*	10.734%
	n-Octyl bicycloheptene dicarboximide	0.166%	BUGONE Insecticide (Central Chem.)	Petroleum oil*	
	Allethrin (allyl homolog of cinerin 1)	0.10%		Isobornyl thiocyanoacetate*	
	Petroleum distillate	2.734%		Other related terpenes	
	Aromatic petroleum derivatives*	12.00%	BUG-GONE LIQUID & POWDER Insecticide (Peres)		

*Consult Sec. II., Ingredients Index. This ingredient may be responsible for major toxic effects if poisonous amounts of this product are ingested.

Name & Use Manufacturer	Ingredients		Name & Use Manufacturer	Ingredients
BUG SLAYER (Slayer)	Chlordane tech. 2% Pyrethrins 1% Inert ingredients* 97%		BULL DOG VENETIAN BLIND CLEANER (Gillespie)	
BUG-STOP (Southland)	DDT* 5.00% Butoxy polypropylene glycol 5.00% Tech. piperonyl butoxide 0.40% Pyrethrins 0.08% Petroleum distillates* 89.52%		BULLDOG WART REMOVER Keratolytic (Commerce)	Flexible collodion Salicylic acid*
BUGZOOKA (For Flowers) Insecticide, Fungicide (Ampion)	DDT* 5.00% Lindane 1.00% Tech. chlordane 2.00% Ferbam 7.50% Sulfur* 25.00%		BULL FROG BRAND CLEANSERS (Berman)	
BUG-ZOOKA Insecticide (Haines)			DR. JOHN BULL'S COMPOUND (Bull)	Alcohol 13.37% Sarsaparilla root Yellow dock root Wild cherry bark Poke root Licorice root Sodium carbonate Sugar Oil sassafras
BUHACH INSECT POWDER (Internat. Labs.)	Pyrethrins 0.9%			
BUILDERS BRAND SEMI-PASTE PAINT (Longman)			BULLS EYE SHELLAC (Zinsser)	
			BUNT NO MORE SEED DISINFECTANT Insecticide (Green Cross)	Hexachlorobenzene* 40%
BUKETS Diuretic (Keller)				
BULK-TABS (Clarke, H.)	Methyl cellulose		BU-PA-CO PAINTS (Buckeye P.& V.)	
BULLARD'S FOB (FIRST ON BURNS) (Bullard)	Oxyquinoline sulfate Liquid petrolatum U.S.P. Rosemary oil U.S.P.* Oil of linseed Oil of geranium*		BUR-CO PIVAL READY TO USE RAT & MOUSE KILLER (Burr)	Pival(2-pivalyl-1,3-indandione) 0.025%
BULLARD'S FORMULA For poison oak, poison ivy) (Bullard)	Hectorite Zinc oxide Iron calamine Glycerine		BUR-CO READY TO USE RODENTICIDE CONTAINING WARFARIN (Burr)	Warfarin (3-(a-acetonylbenzyl)-4 hydroxycoumarin) 0.025%
BULL DOG BRAND SEMI-PASTE PAINT (Longman)			BURFEIND'S BLACK CAPSULES For tapeworm (dogs and cats) (Chem. Prod.) (Minn.)	Areca nut* American wormseed* Charcoal Kamala Tobacco* Sucrose
BULL DOG LIQUID LAUNDRY BLUE (Prescott)				
BULL DOG PAINT & VARNISH CLEANER (Gillespie)			BURGEE MARINE FINISHES (Republic)	
BULL DOG REMOVER Paint remover (Gillespie)				

---

*Consult Sec. II., Ingredients Index. This ingredient may be responsible for major toxic effects if poisonous amounts of this product are ingested.

Name & Use Manufacturer	Ingredients		Name & Use Manufacturer	Ingredients	
BURMA-SHAVE (Burma-Vita)	Stearates, sodium, potassium, ammonium less than 5% Free stearic acid, glyceryl monostearate, lanolin less than 20% Petrolatum Zinc stearate Boric acid less than 1% Propyl-P-hydroxy benzoate 0.15%		BURROUGH SAN HYGIENIC POWDER Douche powder (Burrough)	Phenol* Boric acid* Alum Menthol	4.6%
BURNADE For skin burns (Binday)	Calcium oleate Bentonite Phenyl salicylate* Phenol 1/2%		BURROUGHS EMPIRIN COMPOUND (Tabloid) Analgesic (Burroughs-Wellcome)	Acetophenetidin* Acetylsalicylic acid* Caffeine*	2.5 gr. 3.5 gr. 0.5 gr.
BURN-AIDE (Morgan, H. Labs.)	Camphor* Phenol* Tannin Preservative Gums		BURSAR PASTE (Gordon Labs.)	Burow's solution Lassar's paste Aquaphor base	10%
BURN-A-LAY For burns (Bauer & Black)	Benzocaine Chlorobutanol* Thymol* Oxyquinoline benzoate Zinc oxide*		BURSOLINE Water Purifying Tablets (Burnham Sol.)		
BURN EASE For minor burns, sunburn (Nelson Baker)	Carbolic acid 1% Zinc oxide Benzocaine Ichthammol Boric acid*		BURTON MIRACLE FOAM Cleaner for rugs and upholstery (Burton)		
BURNISHINE Silver polishing cream (Paul, J.C.)	Soap Silica Soda ash Camphor* Sassafras		BUSY BEE FL. WAX PASTE (United Chem.)		
BUR-NO For burns, sunburn (Carolina)	Boric acid* Carbolic acid 0.93% Glycerine Menthol* Zinc oxide Isopropyl alcohol 7%		BUTCHER'S BOSTON POLISH Wax (Butcher)	Waxes Solvent (Socony-Vacuum Sovasol #5)* Gum turpentine* Oil soluble dye	
BURNODYNE For burns, sunburn, abrasions (Hance)	Cycloform 3% Benzalkonium chloride 0.1% Isopropyl alcohol 10%		BUTCHER'S CAR WAX (Butcher)	Waxes Petroleum solvent Diatomacious earth	
BURNTANIK For burns (Horton & Converse)	Tannic acid 5% Pentaseptic 1-5,000 Benzyl alcohol 4% Ethyl alcohol 5% Sodium chloride Calcium chloride Potassium chloride		BUTCHER'S COMMERCE BRAND SELF-POLISHING WAX (Butcher)	Waxes Oleic acid Morpholine Borax* Caustic soda Bleached shellac emulsified with ammonia	
BURNTONE For burns (McKesson)	Chlorobutanol (chloroform deriv.) 1% Oxyquinoline tannate and tannic acid Gum-gel base		BUTCHER'S FLOOR CLEANER (Butcher)	Waxes Solvent*(Socony-Vacuum Sovasol #5) Oil soluble dye	
BURNTONE IMPROVED For sunburn, minor burns (McKesson)	Benzocaine 3% Pyrilamine maleate 1.5% Di-isobutyl cresoxy ethoxy ethyl dimethyl benzyl ammonium chloride 0.2% Menthol Polyvinylpyrolidone		BUTCHER'S FLOORBATH Detergent (Butcher)	Oleic acid Carbide and carbon tergitol NPX Monoethanolamine Boric acid* Tri-sodium phosphate	
			BUTCHER'S GREEN STRIPE SELF-POLISHING WAX (Butcher)	Waxes Oleic acid Morpholine* Borax* Caustic soda Bleached shellac emulsified with ammonia	
BUROW'S SOLUTION Astringent (Royal Pharm.)	Aluminum acetate N.F.		BUTCHER'S KITCHEN CREAM Wax polish (Butcher)	Waxes Oleic acid Monoethanolamine* Sovasol #5* General Electric silicone fluid	

*Consult Sec. II., Ingredients Index. This ingredient may be responsible for major toxic effects if poisonous amounts of this product are ingested.

- 343 -

Name & Use Manufacturer	Ingredients		Name & Use Manufacturer	Ingredients	
BUTCHER'S LIQUID WAX (Butcher)	Waxes Solvent*(Socony-Vacuum Sovasol #5) Oil soluble dye		CABELL CRYOLITE- TALC DUST Insecticide (Cabell)	Sodium fluoaluminate*	30%
BUTCHER'S #3 REVIVER Paint product (Butcher)	Linseed oil Japan drier Petroleum solvent*		CABELL DUSTOX Insecticide (Cabell)	Rotenone Other cube extractives	3/4% 1.5%
BUTCHER'S RUBLESS ANTI-SLIP SELF- POLISHING WAX (Butcher)	Waxes Oleic acid Morpholine* Borax* Caustic soda* Industrial resin Ammonia		CABELL ROSE DUST Insecticide, fungicide (Cabell)	Ferric dimethyldithiocarbamate Benzene hexachloride, gamma isomer Sulfur*	11.4% 1.0% 15.0%
BUTCHER'S WHITE DIAMOND Wax (Butcher)	Waxes Solvent*(Socony-Vacuum Sovasol #5) Gum turpentine*		CABELL ROSE DUST & SPRAY Insecticide, fungicide (Cabell)	Zineb Sulfur* Lindane* Inert ingredients*	9.0% 15.0% 1.5% 74.5%
BUTCHER'S WOOD & FLOOR SEAL (Butcher)	Synthetic and natural resins Varnish oils Petroleum solvent*		CABELL TOMATO DUST Insecticide (Cabell)	Calcium arsenate* Copper	4.1% 7%
BU-TEE-WAVE HOME PERMANENT (Halgar)			CABINET-SAN DEODORANT Toiletry (Huntington)		
BU-VAR-CO VARNISH (Buckeye P.&V.)			CABODEX FLOOR FINISH (Devoe)		
BUG-X Insecticide (Davis, O. D.)	Petroleum distillate* Gamma isomer of benzene hexachloride Xylene	98% 0.5% 1.16%	CABOT'S BRUSH CLEANER (Cabot)	Caustic soda Creosote oil Cresylic acid* Rosin Tall oil	10%
BUZZ 1% DDT INSECT SPRAY (Triangle)	Petroleum distillate* DDT* Beta butoxy beta thiocyano-diethyl ether* Beta thiocyano ethyl esters of aliphatic acids containing 10-18 carbon atoms		CABOT'S SYLPHO NATHOL (originally Sulpho-Napthol) Disinfectant (Sulpho-Napthol)	Coal tar neutral oil cresylic acids* Soaps Water and phenol*	90% 10%
BVH VINYL CEMENT (Barrett)	Toluol* Methyl ethyl ketone C. P. acetone* Vinyl resin		CACTALIS NO. 2 Cardiac stimulant (Jenkins)	Each tablet: Digitalis leaves* F.F. and P.T. Caffeine Tinc. Cactus grandiflorous Tinc. Strophanthus	1 gr. 1/2 gr. 5 m. 1 m.
B W C AND B W X Specialized cleaning products (Wyandotte)	Conc. alkali*		CACTUS BUFFING WAX (Thornton, L. M.)	Carnauba wax Petroleum wax Naphtha*	
BYE-BYE-FLY CATTLE SPRAY Insecticide (Warren Chem.)	Lindane Pyrenone*	1/4-1/2% 8%	CACTUS CORN CALLOUS COMPOUND Corn remedy (Cactus)		
BYE NOW DEW OILS DANDRUFF RINSE (Esamar)	Isoquinolinium bromide Polyethylene glycol* 400 monolaurate Preservative		CACTUS CREME POLISH (Thornton, L.M.)	Tech. petroleum* Artificial lemon oil	
BYONAL TABLETS Antispasmodic (Byon)	Phenobarbital* Hyoscyamine sulf Atropine sulf. Hyoscine hydrobromide	16.2 mg. 0.1036 mg. 0.0193 0.0065	CACTUS FLOOR CLEANER (Thornton, L.M.)	Soap Sodium trisulfide*	

*Consult Sec. II., Ingredients Index. This ingredient may be responsible for major toxic effects if poisonous amounts of this product are ingested.

Name & Use Manufacturer	Ingredients	
CACTUS GLASS CLEANER (Thornton, L.M.)	Alcohol* Carbitol*	
CACTUS LIQUID SCRATCH REMOVER (Thornton, L.M.)	Stains Petroleum spirits* Carbon tetrachloride*	
CACTUS PASTE WAX (Thornton, L.M.)	Carnauba wax Petroleum wax Naphtha*	
CACTUS POLISH & CLEANER (Thornton, L.M.)	Tech. petroleum* Camphor oil artifice*	
CACTUS RUG & UPHOLST- ERY SHAMPOO (Thornton, L.M.)		
CACTUS SCRATCH REMOVER POLISH (Thornton, L.M.)	Stains Petroleum spirits*	
CACTUS SELF- POLISHING WAX (Thornton, L.M)	Carnauba wax Oleic acid	
CACTUS SILICONE SHEEN Polish (Thornton, L.M.)	Naphtha Toluol* Silicone	
CACTUS UPHOLSTERY CLEANER (Thornton, L.M.)	Naphtha Carbon tetrachloride*	
CADET OIL WAX SHOE POLISH (Whittemore)		
CAD-I-CIDE Anthelmintic (Parsons Chem.)	Cadmiun oxide*	1.5%
CADMINATE Turf fungicide (Mallinckrodt)	Cadmium succinate*	60%
CADMIUM HOG WORMER (Hess, Dr.)	Cadmium anthranilate*	4.4%
CADO INKS (Cushman)	Coal tar naphtha* Coumarone-indene resin Aniline dyes* Phenol camphor* Picric acid* Amino acids Asphalt in black ink	
CADOPHILL Skin ointment (Torch)	Oil of cade Sulfur Salicylic acid*	5% 5% 3%
CAFAGEN TABLETS Analgesic (Halperin)	Acetophenetidin* Aspirin * Caffeine Salicylamide	1 gr. 3 gr. 1/2 gr. 1-1/2 gr.

Name & Use Manufacturer	Ingredients	
CAFEDIN Analgesic (Veltex)	Each tablet: Acetylsalicylic acid* Acetophenetidin Caffeine alkaloid	1-1/2 gr. 1/2 gr. 1/20 gr.
CAFETAN Analgesic (Strasenburgh)	Acetanilid* Caffeine Tartaric acid Capsicum Sodium bicarbonate	150 mg. 30 mg. 30 mg. 8 mg. 120 mg.
CAFO INSECTICIDES (Flash)		
CAKE A LITE Mechanical dishwash (Armstrong)		
CALABAR GRAINS Cathartic (Richards Bros.)	Calabar bean Gamboge * Podophyllin* Ipecac Capsicum Hydrargyri bichloridum* 1/270 gr. Strychnia* 1/270 gr. Jalap Juglandin Aloes Betanaphthol* Castor oil	
CALACOMP CREAM Skin antipruritic (Jeffrey-Fell)	Calamine Zinc oxide Phenol Camphor	19% 15% 0.5% 0.5%
CALA CREAM Antipruritic (McKesson)	Benzocaine Phenol Prepared calamine Zinc oxide Bentonite Solution of coal tar and lime water	2-1/2% 2%
CALAFOR Skin ointment (Mako)	Prepared calamine Aluminum hydroxide Methyl salicylate* Glycerin Zinc oxide Carbolic acid 1/10 of 1% Synthetic menthol In a base of oleostearates, lanolin and petroleum.	
CAL-A-GRIN LOTION Skin astringent (Rogers Park)	Prepared neo-calamine Magma of bentonite Carbolic acid* liquified Grindelia robusta fl. ext. Sulfur precipitated	
CALAJEN Skin astrigent (Jenkins)	Calamine Zinc oxide Carbolic acid Camphor	5% 5% 0.5% 0.5%
CALAMATUM OINTMENT Antipruritic (Tailby)	Calamine Zinc oxide Camphophenol*	
CALAMATUM OINTMENT WITH ANTIHISTA- MINE Antipruritic (Tailby)	Calamine Zinc oxide Camphophenol* Antihistamine*	

*Consult Sec. II., Ingredients Index. This ingredient may be responsible for major toxic effects if poisonous amounts of this product are ingested.

Name & Use Manufacturer	Ingredients		Name & Use Manufacturer	Ingredients	
CALAMATUM OINTMENT WITH BENZOCAINE Antipruritic (Tailby)	Calamine Zinc oxide Camphophenol* Benzocaine		CALDWELL'S DR. W. B. SENNA LAXATIVE (Centaur- Caldwell)	Alcohol* Senna Peppermint oil Syrup pepsin	4-1/2%
CALAMOIN Skin ointment (Upjohn)	Calamine Zinc oxide Camphor-phenol	5% 5% 1%	CALENDO- PINUS CERATE (SOFT) Nasal emollient (Boericke & Runyon)	Oil of dwarf pine* needles	
CAL-A-SAL Soldering fluid (Callahan)	Pure ammonium chloride* over 99%				
CALBAR AQUARIUM CEMENT (Calbar)			CALENDULA SALVOL Emollient (Clapp, Otis)	Calendula oil*	
CALBAR CAULK-O- SEAL, CALBAR COLD-BAR, CALBAR MASTER CAULK Caulking compounds (Calbar)	Heat-treated oil, such as soya bean oil, linseed oil, etc. Asbestos fiber Calcium carbonate Titanium (when tinted)		CALFALFA, GRANULAR SOIL SULFUR Insecticide, fungicide (Calif. Spray)	Sulfur*	99.5%
			CALFALFA SOIL SULFUR (Calif. Spray)	Sulfur*	99.5%
CAL-BIS-MA Antacid (Warner- Chilcott)	Sodium bicarbonate 585.0 mg. Calcium carbonate 325.0 mg. Magnesium carbonate 195 mg. Magnesium trisilicate 146.2 mg. Bismuth subcarbonate 16.2 mg.		CALF-EZ NO. 2 Intestinal irritation (veterinary) (Wilke)	Sulfaguanidine* 8.82% Bismuth subnitrate 3.12% Thymosol (pine oil 32.3%, soap anhydrous 23.0%, isopropyl alcohol 16.0%) 3.12% Desiccated blood flour 84.94%	
CALCIMO, DUTCH, MURALO KALSOMINE Paint (Muralo)			CALGON, CALGON BOUQUET Detergent (Calgon)	Vitreous sodium phosphate* (sodium hexametaphosphate)	
CALCIMO, DUTCH, MURALO WALL COATING (Muralo)			CALGONITE Detergent, water softener (Calgon)	Alkaline sodium silicate Alkaline sodium polyphosphates*	
			CALGREEN Insecticide (Chipman Chem.)	Cuprous arsenite* 7% Calcium arsenate* 64.43%	
CALCIMUL Calcium therapy (Prescription Spec.)	Each oz.: Calcium phosphate dibasic 120 gr. Sodium benzoate 1-10% Alcohol 5.5%		CALICARB Antacid (Jenkins)	Each tablet: Calcium carbonate 4 gr. Magnesium carbonate 2-1/2 gr. Bismuth subnitrate 1 gr. Powdered ipecac 1/250 gr. Aromatics q.s.	
CALCINATE WITH DEXTROSE Food supple- ment (veter- inary) (Wilke)	Each 100 cc.: Calcium borogluconate*(23% w/v calcium, 4.5% w/v Boric acid) 21.80 gm. Dextrose 9.8 gm.		CAL-ICE Skin cream (Wright, M.)	Benzocaine Digidex (2,2'-di hydroxy 3,5,6, 3',5',6',-hexachlorid phenyl- methane)* Calamine Menthol* Camphor*	
CALCIPIL Nutritive supplement (Stevens Chem.)	Each tablet: Dicalcium phosphate 7.5 gr. Viosterol 333 U.S.P. units		CALICO TABS Rodenticide (Rat Lunches)	Warfarin (3-(a-acetonylbenzyl)- 4-hydroxycoumarin) 0.025%	
CALCITINE CALCIMINE Paint (Fox)			CALI FIG Laxative (Sterling Prod. Div.)	Elixir of senna Syrup of figs Alcohol* 6% Peppermint	
CALCY DROPS FOR DOGS & CATS Diuretic (veterinary) (Daniels, Dr. A.C.)	Methenamine Saw palmetto berries Sandalwood Corn silk Dog grass		CALIFORNIA SINOX-W Herbicide) (Calif. Spray)	Ammonium dinitro ortho secondary butyl phenol* 13%	

*Consult Sec. II., Ingredients Index. This ingredient may be responsible for major toxic effects if poisonous amounts of this product are ingested.

Name & Use Manufacturer	Ingredients
CALIFORNIA SYSTOX 2 SPRAY Insecticide (Calif.Spray)	o,o-diethyl-o-2-(ethylmercapto)-ethyl thiophosphate* 21.8% Related organic phosphates 1.8%
CALIGESIC OINTMENT Antipruritic (Sharp & Dohme)	Each 100 gm.: Calamine, prepared 8.00 gm. Benzocaine 3.00 gm. Hexylated metacresol 0.05 gm.
CALLAHAN'S SOLDERING FLUID (Callahan)	Zincammonium chloride*
CALMACARB Gastric antacid (Vernon)	Calcium carbonate 3-1/2 gr. Magnesium carbonate 2 gr. Bismuth subnitrate 1/2 gr. Aromatics q.s.
CALMAR Analgesic (Am. Apoth.)	Each tablet: Phenacetin* 0.15 gm. Caffeine 0.03 gm. Aspirin* 0.37 gm.
CALMATONE BABY COUGH SYRUP (Commerce)	Alcohol 2.0% Spruce Wild cherry Sanguinaria Ammonium chloride Honey Menthol
CALMIRIN Analgesic (Kremers)	Each tablet: Aspirin* 0.25 gm. Calcium glutamate 0.12 gm.
CALMITOL LIQUID Skin astringent, analgesic (Leeming)	Each fl. oz.: Hyoscyamine oleate 0.55 mg (0.28 mg. hyoscyamine alkaloid) Alcohol 14.3 cc. Camphor* 1.64 gm. Ether 5.1 cc. Chloroform 1.9 cc. Chloral hydrate 1.3 gm. Menthol 1.7 gm.
CALMITOL OINTMENT Skin analagesic, astringent (Leeming)	Each oz.: Calmitol liquid 10% Hyoscyamine olseate 0.055 mg. (0.028 mg. hyocyanus alkaloid) Alcohol 1.4 cc. Camphor 0.16 gm. Ether 0.5 cc. Chloroform 0.19 cc. Chloral hydrate 0.13 gm. Menthol 0.17 gm.
CALMIX C-D-M-P Food supplement (veterinary) (Wilke)	Each 100 cc.: Calcium borogluconate (23% w/v calcium and boric acid 4.2%) 21.80 gm. Dextrose 9.8 gm. Magnesium chloride 3.04 gm. Phosphorus 1.0 gm. Calcium hypophosphite
CALNATES Tonic (Hance)	Each 2 fl. dr.: Strychnine glycerophosphate* 1/64 gr. Sodium glycerophosphate 2 gr. Calcium glycerophosphate 2 gr. Phosphoric acid 1.5 m.

Name & Use Manufacturer	Ingredients
CALOCAINE CREME Skin ointment (Wisconsin Pharm.)	Calamine Zinc oxide Benzocaine Menthol
CALOCIDE Skin astringent (Consolid. Royal)	Ammonium alum Zinc sulfate Tannic acid*
CALO-CURE Turf fungicide (Mallinckrodt)	Mercurous chloride 30% Mercuric chloride* 15%
CALOCYLATE Analgesic (Kremers)	Aspirin* 0.3 gm. Ascorbic acid 15 mg. Calcium glutamate 0.12 gm.
CAL-O-DYNE Analgesic (C. A. L.)	Aspirin* 3.25 gr. Caffein 0.32 gr. Phenolphthalein U.S.P. 0.12 gr. Acetophenetidin* 2.65 gr.
CALOGREEN Turf fungicide (Mallinckrodt)	Mercurous chloride* 90%
CAL-O-MINE Skin astringent (Penslar)	Carbolic acid 1% Prepared calamine Zinc oxide
CAL-O-SECT FLY SPRAY (Calif.Chem.)	Thiocyanate* Inert ingredients*
CALOTABS Cathartic (Calotabs)	Calomel* 2 gr. Aloes* Orizaba jalap Extr. bitter apple Oils of cloves and peppermint Rhubarb Myrrh
CALOTEX Skin astringent (Texas Pharm.)	Calamine Zinc oxide Corn starch Glycerin
CALOX Tooth powder (McKesson)	Amyl phenol* Heptyl phenol* Octyl phenol* Benzoic acid Sodium chloride
CAL-SAL Analgesic (Commerce)	Salicylamide Sodium salicylate* Caffeine alkaloid Phenacetin* 3/4 gr. Manganese salicylate Thiamine chloride
CAL-SAL COMPOUND (Pulvoid) Gastric antacid, laxative (Drug Prod., N.Y.)	Calcium carbonate precipitated 0.16 gm. Calcium salicylate* 80 mg. Powdered rhubarb 65 mg. Lithium carbonate 65 mg. Powdered ipecac 6.5 mg.
CALSAMATE Analgesic (Trout)	Acetylsalicylic acid* 0.3 gm. Calcium glutamate 0.13 gm. Ascorbic acid 15 mg.
CALSOLITE CALSOMINE Paint (Sterling Paint)	

*Consult Sec. II., Ingredients Index. This ingredient may be responsible for major toxic effects if poisonous amounts of this product are ingested.

Name & Use Manufacturer	Ingredients	Name & Use Manufacturer	Ingredients
CALSO WATER Antacid (Calso)	Sodium phosphate Sodium chloride Bicarbonates of calcium, magnesium, and sodium	CAMEO Copper cleaner (Cameo Corp.)	
CALSECOF Antitussive, sedative (Massengill)	Each 5 cc.: Chloroform 20 mg. Ethylmorphine hydrochloride 2.5 mg. Lobelia 75 mg. Tartar emetic 1.3 mg. Aromatics q.s.	CAMEO ALUMINUM, POTTERY CLEANER (Cameo Corp.)	
		CAMEO ENAMELS Paint (Denny)	
CALSOM & MURESCO KALSOMINE (Moore, B.)		CAMEO STARCHING POWDER (Staley)	Borax*
CALSUL EMULSION Fungicide (Dextruxol)	Mineral oil 67.0% Pine oil 0.9% Ammonia 0.9% Soap 2.1% Calcium polysulfide 1.0%	CAMICIDE CATTLE SPRAY (Oil type) Insecticide (Campbell Labs.)	Refined petroleum oil Tech. piperonyl butoxide Pyrethrins
CALSUS LOTION Skin astringent (Wisconsin Pharm.)	Each fl. oz.: Calamine 40 gr. Zinc oxide 20 gr. Glycerin 20 m. Carbolic acid 4 m.	CAMICIDE DAIRY CATTLE SPRAY CONCENTRATE Insecticide (Campbell Chem.)	Refined petroleum oil Polyoxyethylene sorbitol mixed ether ester Tech. piperonyl butoxide Pyrethrins
CAL TAN LOTION Cosmetic (Schram)			
CAL-TRI-HIST CREAM Antipruritic (Pharmex)	Calamine Tyrothricin Antihistamine* Benzocaine Benzalkonium chloride	CAMICIDE GARDEN SPRAY (Aerosol) (Campbell Chem.)	Pyrethrins Rotenone Cube extractives Tech. piperonyl cyclonene Petroleum distillate* Freon 11 and 12
CALUMET BROWN COPPER OXIDE FUNGICIDE (Calumet Div.)	Copper material* 75%	CAMICIDE INSECT SPRAY (Campbell Chem.)	Refined petroleum oil Tech. piperonyl butoxide Pyrethrins n-Octyl bicycloheptene dicarboxiamide*
CALUMET COPPER OXIDE Fertilizer (Calumet Div.)	Copper*(50% available only in Florida) 80%	CAMICIDE NO. 15 PYRENONE MILL SPRAY CONCENTRATE Insecticide (Campbell Chem.)	Refined petroleum oil Polyoxyethylene sorbitol mixed ether ester Tech. piperonyl butoxide Pyrethrins
CALVES CORDIAL Intestinal astringent (veterinary) (Our Husbands)	Alum Charcoal Ginger Calcium carbonate	CAMICIDE PYRENONE LIVESTOCK SPRAY CONCENTRATE Insecticide (Campbell Chem.)	Tech. piperonyl butoxide 11.90% Pyrethrins 0.59% Polyoxyethylene sorbitol mixed ether ester 14.87% Petroleum oil 72.64%
CALZINOCAINE Skin protective, analgesic (Pitman-Moore)	Zinc oxide 6.80% Calamine 7.70% Phenol 0.85% Benzocaine 1.00%		
CAMAY BAR Soap (Procter & Gamble)	Soaps of animal and vegetable fats Cold cream	CAMICIDE REPELLENT (Campbell Chem.)	Dimethyl phthalate Ethylhexanediol* Butyl dimethyl dihydro gamma pyrone carboxylate Freon 11 and 12* Isopropanol*
CAMDEN FLOTATION SULPHUR PASTE Insecticide (Camden)	Sulfur*	CAMICIDE ROACH SPRAY (Campbell Chem.)	Petroleum oil Tech. piperonyl butoxide Pyrethrins
CAMELLIA COLOGNES (Assoc. Brands)			

Name & Use Manufacturer	Ingredients		Name & Use Manufacturer	Ingredients	
CAMPANA ITALIAN BALM Cosmetic (Campana)	Essential oils Alcohol* Phenol* Benzoic acid Gum tragacanth Glycerin Sorbitol		CAMTHOL Skin emmollient, counter-irritant (Shuptrine)	Oil of eucalyptus* Oil of peppermint Menthol Camphor* Thymol* Lanolin Petrolatum	
CAMPBELL'S NO. 782 WASH THINNER (Campbell, M.L.)	Isopropyl acetate* Toluol* VM and P naphtha*	27.2% 27.2% 45.6%	CAMTOX EC-71 Insecticide (Arizona)	Toxaphene* Tech. chlorinated camphene*	71.0%
CAMP DRAIN PIPE & TRAP CLEANER (Camp)			CAMZINOL BALM CREAM Analgesic (Continental Labs.)	Camphor* Zinc oxide Vegetable oils and volatile oils* Carbolic acid* analgesic compounds Menthol* Balsam Peru	
CAMPHEMEN-THOL LOZEN-GES (Hancock's) Antitussive (Hancock, J.)	Camphor* Menthol* Thymol Phenol* Slippery elm Licorice Oil of eucalyptus* Methyl salicylate*		CANARADYNE For wheezing (veterinary, avian) (Spratts)	Capsici B.P. Cubeba Glycerin Benzoin Sp. aeth. nit.	
CAMPHE THYMEN Skin ointment (Arlo)	Carbolic acid* with 3% camphor-phenol Thymol Menthol* Aromatic oils	2%	CANARY PULVEX Insecticide (Cooper)	Rotenone Other cube resins	0.5% 1.5%
CAMPHOLIN Counter-irritant (Jenkins)	Oleoresin capsicum Camphor* Oil of turpentine* Croton oil* Oil of sassafras Oil of origanum		CANCEL DEODORANT CREAM Hypo-allergenic (Peau Seche)	Aluminum salt	
CAMPHO-PHENIQUE Antiseptic (Sterling Prod. Div.)			CANDLE SURPRISE Toilet water (Pessel)		
CAMPHO-PHENIQUE LIQUID Skin astringent (Centaur-Caldwell)	Carbolic acid Camphor*	4.75% 10.86%	CANDO METAL POLISH (Cando)	Infusorial earth Silica Oleic acid (Red Oil) Oxalic acid* Ammonia Pine oil*	
CAMPHO-PHENIQUE POWDER Skin astringent (Centaur-Caldwell)	Carbolic acid* Camphor* Boric acid*	2.0% 4.375%	CANDO SILVER POLISH (Cando)	Water Infusorial earth Pure soap Carbonate of soda Antiseptic oil	
CAMPHOR CREAM Astringent skin cream (C & M)	Camphor* Menthol Phenol Aluminum acetate Solumol	1.5% 0.5% 0.5% 0.5%	CANISEAR For ear cankers (veterinary) (Erwin)	Phenol* Sulfanilamide* Carbonyldiamide in glycol base Malachite green Methylcatechol* Ethylaminobenzoic acid Metacresyl acetate*	1%
CAMPHOR-DISKOIDS (Homeopathic) (Clapp, Otis)	Pure cane sugar Tincture of camphor		CANIS-EYE Eye, nose irritation (veterinary) (Erwin)	Procaine Hydrochloride 0.15% Ethylaminobenzoic acid Metacresyl acetate Methylcatechol* Phenol Sulfanilamide* Carbonyldiamide Malachite green	1%
CAMPHORETTE BLOCKS Insecticide (Reliable (Chem.)	Refined naphthalene* Perfume oils	99-1/2% 1/2%	CANISKIN External fungicide (veterinary) (Erwin)	Ethylaminobenzoicacid Metacresyl acetate* 2-β-mercaptobenzothiazole* acidified in formalinized glycol base	

*Consult Sec. II., Ingredients Index. This ingredient may be responsible for major toxic effects if poisonous amounts of this product are ingested.

Name & Use Manufacturer	Ingredients		Name & Use Manufacturer	Ingredients	
CANISOL LOTION Antipruritic (veterinary) (Canisol)			CAPITOL ROACH SPRAY (Capitol Chem.)	Tech. chlordane Petroleum distillate*	2% 98%
CANKERINE for cankers (veterinary) (McCleillan	Mineral oil Phenol* Oil of eucalyptus* Thymol F. D. & C. coloring Pine oil Oil of camphor* Menthol		CAPROKOL JELLY Vaginal antiseptic (Sharp & Dohme)	Hexylresorcinol Tragacanth Quince seed Glycerin	1-1000 5%
CANNED PLUMBER Drain pipe cleaner (Puritan Chem.)			CAPRONEX FUNGICIDAL OINTMENT (Medical) (Horton & Converse)	Copper caprylate Sodium caprylate Caprylic acid	0.5% 10% 3%
CANNIBAL DRAIN PIPE CLEANER (Sunshine)	Sodium hydroxide*		CAPRONEX POWDER Skin fungicide (Medical) (Horton & Converse)	Calcium caprylate Zinc caprylate Copper caprylate	10% 8% 0.5%
CANOE GLUE NO. 180 (Ferdinand)			CAPROVINE DRENCH Veterinary (Anchor Serum)	Phenothiazine* N.F. Lead arsenate*	37.92% 0.72%
CAN-PHO-SAL BOMB Inhalant, nasal decongestant (poultry) (Salsbury's)	Ortho-hydroxydiphenyl Creosote* Guaiacol Oils of pine*, camphor*, and eucalyptus Dichlorodifluoromethane* and trichloromonofluoromethane* 70%		CAPSAN Ectoparasiti- cide (Vogel)	Phenyl cellosolve Isopropyl alcohol* Aerosol OT Methyl salicylate*	5% 50%
			CAPSICOLA Counter- irritant, rube- facient (Wisconsin Pharm.)	Capsicum Camphor* Eucalyptol*	
CANVASEAL WATER- PROOFING (Everseal)			CAPSOLIN Counter- irritant (Parke, Davis)	Oleoresin capsicum Camphor* Oil of turpentine* Cajuput oil Croton oil*	
CAPHENIN CALAMINE- ZINC-CARBOL- IC CAMPHOR Skin ointment (CaPhenin)	Calamine and zinc oxide 10% Camphor* and carbolic acid 1%		CAPSONAMINE (formerly Capsicum Compound) Counter- irritant (CaPhenin)	Oleoresin capsicum Croton oil* Camphor* Oil of turpentine* Aromatic oils	
CAPHENIN MENTHOL & METHYL SALICYLATE Skin ointment (CaPhenin)	Menthol 10% Methyl salicylate* 20%		CAPSTAN MARINE PAINTS (Reeder)		
CAPHENIN MERCURY AMMONIATED Skin ointment (CaPhenin)	Ammoniated mercury* U.S.P. 10%		CAPUDINE LIQUID Analgesic (Capudine)	Each tsp.: Antipyrine* Sodium salicylate* Caffeine	1-1/2 gr.
CAPILOR HAIR OIL (Germadol)			CARAGOL Counter- irritant (Caragol)	Menthol* Camphor* Oil of wintergreen*	
CAPITOL CEMENT Household adhesive (Capitol Cem.)			CARA NOME BATH SALTS, CLEANSING CREAM, COLD CREAM (Cara Nome)		
CAPITOL DEVELOPER Photographic supply (General Photo.)					

*Consult Sec. II., Ingredients Index. This ingredient may be responsible for major toxic effects if poisonous amounts of this product are ingested.

Name & Use Manufacturer	Ingredients		Name & Use Manufacturer	Ingredients	
CARA NOME COMPRESSED DEODORANT BATH POWDER (Cara Nome)			CARBOLA DISINFECTING WHITE PAINT Insecticide (Carbola)	Phenol Coal tar oils Lindane Malathion	1.60% 1.40% 0.22% 0.66%
CARA NOME CREAM DEODORANT (Cara Nome)	Aluminum chlorhydrate Benzoic acid		CARBOLA DRY FLY BAIT Insecticide (Carbola)	Malathion	2.00%
CARA NOME CREAM MASQUE (Cara Nome)			CARBOLASTIC ROOF PAINT (Thompson & Co.)		
CARA NOME ESTROGENIC HORMONE CREAM (Cara Nome)	Natural estrogenic hormones (principally Estrone and estradiol) 10,000 I.U./oz.		CARBOLATED LYCOZINE (HUMMEL'S) Skin astringent (Park Pharm.)	Zinc oxide Lycopodium Magnesium carbonate Carbolic acid*	
CARA NOME EYE CREAM, FOUNDATION CREAM, HAND CREAM, SKIN CREAM (Cara Nome)			CAR-BO-LAX Cathartic (Carbozine)		
CARA NOME VANISHING CREAM (Cara Nome)			CARBOLEUM DISINFEC- TANT (Pacific Chem.)		
CAR-A-SOL SOLVENT CLEANER (Whitfield)			CARBOLIC ACID OINT- MENT Antiseptic, emollient (Allied Drug)	Carbolic acid* Glycerin White ointment	2%
CARBENSUL Antiseptic (veterinary) (Lloyd)	Each fl. oz.: Sulfanilamide* 40 gr. Urea 40 gr. Benzyl alcohol* 15 gr. Propylene glycol-acetone base		CARBOLINE Disinfectant (Germo)		
CARBEX BELL TABLETS Gastric, antacid (Hollings- Smith)	Sodium bicarbonate Ginger Aromatics		CARBOLINEUM Insecticide (Carbolineum)	Coal tar oils* Carbon	97% 1-1/2%
CARB MASTER Carburetor conditioner (Rust Master)			CARBOMIDE Sedative (Welin-Sater)	Potassium bromide* 5 gr./tablet Charcoal Pepsin	
CARBO-COL Insecticide (Globe)	Coal tar creosote* 98.5%		CARBONA CLEANING FLUID (Carbona)		
CARBO CREAM Skin antiseptic (Jeffrey-Fell)	Liquid carbonis detergent 5.0% Phenol 0.5% Menthol 0.01% Lanum 5.0%		CARBONA INSTANT LATHER (Carbona)		
CARBO DUSTLESS CRAYON (Andrews,A.H.)			CARBONA SHOE POLISH & SHOE WHITENER (Carbona)		
			CARBONA SOAPLESS LATHER (Carbona)		
CARBOFORM Antacid, carminative (Massengill)	Chloroform 20 mg. Bismuth subcarbonate 0.22 gm. Magnesium carbonate 0.22 gm. Prepared chalk 0.11 gm.		CARBONA WALL-WIPE (Carbona)		
			CARBON BISULFIDE Rodenticide (Santa Clara)	Carbon bisulfide*	100%

*Consult Sec. II., Ingredients Index. This ingredient may be responsible for major toxic effects if poisonous amounts of this product are ingested.

Name & Use Manufacturer	Ingredients	Name & Use Manufacturer	Ingredients
CARBON EATER WINDOW CLEANING COMPOUND (Zapo)		CAR CARE CAR FINISHER (Cannon)	

CARBONOEL
LIQUID
Toiletry
(Gordon
Thomas)
		CARCO
		CATTLE
		SPRAY
		(Carpenter)
			Light petroleum oil
			Beta butoxy beta thiocyano
			  diethyl ether*
			Aromatic petroleum derivative
			  solvent*
			Methoxychlor-bis-(methoxy-
			  trichlorethane

CARBONOEL PINE NEEDLE TAR SHAMPOO CREAM (Gordon Thomas)		CARCO ROACH SPRAY (Carpenter)	Chlordane tech. 2% Petroleum distillate* 98%
		CARDINELL Ink eradicator (Cardinell)	
CARBONOEL PRESSING COMPOUND Hair conditioner (Gordon Thomas)		CARDOSIPTEC Douche tablets (Chattanooga)	Acetylsalicylic acid* Sodium acid pyrophosphate Boric acid* Methyl salicylate* Thymol* Chlorothymol Menthol*
CARBONOEL SCALP OINTMENT, SKIN OINTMENT (Gordon Thomas)		CARDUI Tonic, antispasmodic (Chattanooga)	Blessed thistle Black haw Alcohol 19%/v Golden seal

CARBO-
RESIN
(CARBACRYLA-
MINE RESINS)
Diuretic
(Lilly)
	Alkylene polyamine resin
	    12%
	Potassium carbacrylic resin
	    29%
	Carbacrylic resin 59%
		CARESS CREME
		Skin emollient
		(Airem)
			Phenol less than 1%
			Bismuth subnitrate
			Boric acid
			Zinc oxide
			Glycerin

		CARFOAM AUTO CLEANER (Magnus)	
CARBO- SEPTIC Antiseptic gargle (Carbo-Septic)	Glyceric-tannic* acid Phenol* 3.3%	CARFUSIN RORER Fungicide (external) medical (Rorer)	Alcohol 10% Boric acid 1% Carbolic acid 4.5% Resorcinol* 10% Fuchsin 0.3% Acetone 5%
CARBOSOL NO. 2 Herbicide (Indust.Mat.)	Sodium arsenite* 26% Soap 11% Potassium cresylate 10%	CAR GLO AUTO POLISH (Jones Prod.)	
CARBOSOTA CREOSOTE OIL Wood preserva- tive (Barrett Div.)	Creosote*	CARMESAL Analgesic (Carmel)	Carmel salicylamide* 5 gr.

		CARMETHOSE
		Gastric antacid
		(Ciba)
			Each 15 ml.:
			Sodium carboxymethylcellulose
			    750 mg.
			Methyl parahydroxybenzoate
			    0.16%

CARBOSOTA WOOD PRESERVATIVE (Barrett Div.)	Coal-tar creosote* oil		

CARBOWAX
COMPOUND
1500
Emollient
(Barnes-Hind)
	Polyethylene glycol 300 50%
	Carbowax compound 1540
	    50%
		CARMETHOSE
		WITH
		MAGNESIUM
		OXIDE
		Gastric antacid
		(Ciba)
			Each tablet:
			Sodium carboxymethyl cellulose
			    225 mg.
			Magnesium oxide 75 mg.

CARBOXIDE FUMIGANT (Carbide)	Carbon dioxide 90% Ethylene oxide* 10%	CARMEX Cold sores chapped lips (Carma)	Menthol* Camphor* Phenol* Salicylic acid* Lanolin and petrolatum base
CARBURET PAINT PRODUCTS (Jewell P.&V.)		CARMOLIN SKIN OIL FOR DRY SKIN (Carmel)	Liquid lanolin

*Consult Sec. II., Ingredients Index. This ingredient may be responsible for major toxic effects if poisonous amounts of this product are ingested.

Name & Use Manufacturer	Ingredients	Name & Use Manufacturer	Ingredients
CAR-NA-LAC Floor wax (Continental Car-Na-Var)		CARPINE FACE LOTION, FACE POWDER, HAIR TONIC, SHAMPOO JELLY (Hudson & Co.)	
CARN-NA-ORETE Rubber enamel (Continental Car-Na-Var)		CAR PLATE Cleaner (Johnson, S.C.)	
CAR-NA-SEAL Floor sealer (Continental Car-Na-Var)		CARROLL PAINT BRUSH CLEANER (Carrol S.&V.)	
CARNICA SALVE Emollient (Burrough)	Carbolic acid* Witch hazel Arnica* Zinc oxide	CARROLL'S BABY COUGH SYRUP (Carroll Chem.)	Extr. cocillana Euphorbia Wild lettuce Cascara* Squill* Sodium citrate Ammonium chloride Honey and sugar
CARNU Polish (Johnson, S. C.)			
CAR-O-DENE Skin astringent (Carolina)	Boric acid* Tannic acid* Carbolic acid* Zinc sulfate Glycerin	CARROLL'S DIURETIC COMPOUND (Carroll Chem.)	Buchu Couch grass Uva ursi Saw palmetto berries Potassium acetate Sodium citrate Methenamine Oil of juniper
CARODONE (CARROLL'S) Antitussive (Carroll Chem.)	Dihydrocodeinone bitartrate 1/6 gr. Pyrilamine maleate* 30 mg. Terpin hydrate* Potassium guaiacolsulfonate* Honey Glycerin Sodium Citrate	CARROLL'S NERVINE Sedative (Carroll Chem.)	Potassium bromide* 12 gr. Sodium bromide* 12 gr. Ammonium bromide* 6 gr.
CAR-O-LAC SHELLAC SUBSTITUTE (Carroll S.&V.)		CARSINCAL CICAL Ringworm, athlete's foot (Chem. Ind.)	Fuchsin 1% Resorcin* 10% Phenol* 4% Acetone 5% Alcohol 10%
CAROLATE Therapeutant (Bartlett, F. A.)	Salicylic acid* 26.77% Urea 9.21% Copper sulfate (crystalline) 1.78%	CARSULENE OINTMENT Skin emollient (Penslar)	Carbolic acid 2% Potassium carbonate Oil of Thuja Sulfur
CARON EAU DE COLOGNE (Caron)		CARTER'S BLACK LAUNDRY INK (Carter's Ink)	Xylenol* Turpentine Dyes
CAROSANTI PERFUMES, COLOGNES, TOILET WATERS (Carosanti)		CARTER'S BLUE-BLACK WRITING FLUID (Carter's Ink)	Tannic acid Ferrous sulfate Gallic acid Sulfuric acid Cellosolve Sodium thiocyanate* Aniline dyestuff*
CAROSEL CONCENTRATE Tree disease (Bartlett,F.A.)	Helione orange* 10% 8-hydroxyquinoline sulfate 2% Malachite green 5%		
CAROTHRICIN Throat irritations (Carroll Chem.)	Tyrothricin 2 mg. Benzocaine 5 mg.	CARTER'S HECTOGRAPH INK (Carter's Ink)	Alcohol-type solvent* Dyes* Mineral acid
CARPENTER CLEANING COMPOUNDS (Carpenter)		CARTER'S HOUSEHOLD INDELIBLE INK (Carter's Ink)	Propylene glycol Pigment Synthetic resin Carboxymethylcellulose
CARPENTER-MORTON MARINE PAINT REMOVER (Carpenter-Morton)	Acetone* Toluol* Paraffin wax	DR. CARTER'S K & B TEA Cathartic (Wells,S.C.)	Senna leaves Mandrake root Aromatic herbs

*Consult Sec. II., Ingredients Index. This ingredient may be responsible for major toxic effects if poisonous amounts of this product are ingested.

Name & Use Manufacturer	Ingredients	Name & Use Manufacturer	Ingredients
CARTER'S LINIMENT Counter-irritant, rube-facient (Carter-Luff)	Camphor* Ammonia Refined spirit turpentine* Volatile oils Emulsifiers	CARYL RICHARDS PERMETTE COLD WAVE, PERMETTE COLD WAVE LANOLIN LOTION, QUICKIE COLD WAVE CREAM OIL LOTION, ROCKET SPEED WAVE CREAM WAVING LOTION (Richards, C.)	Ammonium thioglycolate with ammonia water*(pH 9.40-9.52) approx. 1-1/2-6%
CARTER'S LITTLE LIVER PILLS Choleretic, laxative (Carter Prod.)	Podophyllum resin* Curagaoaloes		
CARTER'S MUSIC INK (Carter's Ink)	Mineral acid (chromic)* Pigment Phenol		
CARTER'S OPAQUE RUBBER STAMP INKS (Carter's Ink)	Glycols Alcohols* Synthetic resins Dyes or pigments Tannic acid	CARYL RICHARDS ROCKET WAVE (dh) NEUTRALIZER, SILVER BLONDE NEUTRALIZER (Richards, C.)	Sodium bromate*approx.10-14%
CARTER'S PASTE (Carter's Ink)	Dextrine Corn syrup Sulforcited castor oil Borax Trisodium phosphate	CARYL RICHARDS ROCKET WAVE POODLE PERMANENT (Richards, C.)	Ammonium thioglycolate with ammonia water*(pH 9.4-9.52) approx. 1-1/2-6%
CARTER'S RUBBER STAMPING INK (Carter's Ink)	Propylene glycol Polyols (glycerin) Dyes or pigments	CARYL RICHARDS ROCKET WAVE (dh) WAVING LOTIONS (Richards, C.)	Ammonium thioglycolate with ammonia water*(pH 8.5-9.50) approx. 1-1/2-6%
CARTER'S SMART WEED & CAPSICUM Carmenative, rubefacient (Wells, S.C.)	Each fl. oz.: Alcohol* 65% Extr. capsicum Aromatic oils Extr. smart weed Gum camphor*	CARYL RICHARDS ROCKET WAVE WITH MILK BATH WAVING LOTIONS (Richards, C.)	Ammonium thioglycolate with ammonia water*(pH 8.5-9.52) approx.1-1/2-6%
CARTER'S STAMPING INDELIBLE INK (Carter's Ink)	Propylene glycol Butyl carbitol Resin Dyes	CARYL RICHARDS THE 400 CREME FIXATONE (Richards, C.)	Sodium bromate*approx. 10-14%
CARVER'S OINTMENT (Carver)		CARYL RICHARDS THE 400 CREME WAVING SOLUTIONS (Richards, C.)	Ammonium thioglycolate with ammonia water*(pH 9.40-9.52) approx.1-1/2-6%
CARYL RICHARDS JUST WONDERFUL CREAM WAVE LOTION (Richards, C.)	Ammonium thioglycolate with ammonia water (pH 8.5-9.42) approx. 1-1/2-6%		
CARYL RICHARDS NEW INSTA-MATIC ROCKET WAVE CREME WAVING LOTIONS (Richards, C.)	Ammonium thioglycolate with ammonia water*(pH 9.40-9.45) approx. 1-1/2-6%	CARYL RICHARDS TIKI DE PARIS NEUTRALIZER (Richards, C.)	Sodium bromate approx. 10-14%
CARYL RICHARDS PERMATONE CREME NEUTRALIZER (Richards, C.)	Sodium bromate*approx. 10-14%	CARYL RICHARDS TIKI DE PARIS WAVING LOTIONS (Richards, C.)	Ammonium thioglycolate with ammonia water*(pH 9.32-9.42) approx.1-1/2-6%
		CASA BLANCA PERFUME, TOILET WATER (Masie)	

*Consult Sec. II., Ingredients Index. This ingredient may be responsible for major toxic effects if poisonous amounts of this product are ingested.

Name & Use Manufacturer	Ingredients	Name & Use Manufacturer	Ingredients
CASCO FLEXIBLE CEMENT (Borden)	Casein-latex emulsion	CASSEBEER EAU DE COLOGNE, LAVENDER WATER, POLISH REMOVER (Cassebeer)	
CASCO HOUSEHOLD INSECTICIDE (Aerosol) (Casco)	Pyrethrins 0.25% DDT 3.00% Piperonyl butoxide 0.50% Petrolleum distillate* 11.25% Dichlorodifluoromethane (Freon 12) 42.50% Trichloromonofluoromethane (Freon 11) 42.50%	CASSILL MEN'S AFTER SHAVE LOTION, PERFUMES (Cassill)	
CASCOPHEN LT-68 Adhesive (Borden)	Phenol-resorcinol-formaldehyde resin	CASTELLANI FORMULA (Improved) For fungus infections (Gordon Labs.)	Carbolfuchsin Resorcin* Boric acid* Methyl rosaniline* Acetone-alcohol resinous base
CASCOPHEN, RS-216 & RS-240M Adhesives (Borden)	Phenol-resorcinol-formaldehyde resin	CASTELLANIS CARBO- FUCHSIN PAINT Fungicide, medical (Koehler's Lab)	Phenol* 4.5% Boric acid 1% Resorcinol* 10% Fuchsin 0.3% Acetone 5% Alcohol 10%
CASCO POWDER CASEIN GLUE (Borden)	Powdered casein glue		
CASEY'S COMPOUND (Casey, D.)	Alcohol 1-1/4%/v Potassium iodide* U.S.P. Syrup sarsaparilla compound U.S.P. Fl. extr. of glycyrrhiza Oil of sassafras Oil of anise Methyl salicylate*	CASTELLANI'S PAINT Fungicide medical (Handley)	Fuchsin Resorcinol* Acetone* Boric acid* Phenol liquefied* 5% Isopropyl alcohol* 20%
CASEY'S ERB-LAX Laxative (Casey, D.)	Extr. of cascara Aloin Podophyllin resin Extr. belladonna 1/8 gr. Oleoresin ginger Belladonna alkaloids 0.0015 gr.	CASTILLA TOOTH SOAP (Castilla)	Menthol, thymol* and sodium phosphate Soap 17-1/2%
		CASTORIA, FLETCHER'S Cathartic (Centaur- Caldwell)	Alcohol 3-1/2% Senna extract
CASHMERE BOUQUET LIPSTICK (Colgate- Palmolive)			
CASHMERE BOQUET TOILET SOAP (Colgate- Palmolive)		CASTROID EXTRACT Hemorrhoids (Sargeant)	Menthol Boric acid* Benzoic acid Sulfur lac Zinc oxide Benzocaine Sodium stearate Camphor* Salol* Balsam of fir
CASITE Oil additive (Hastings)	Light petroleum fractions* Creosote* oil		
CASITE SLUDGE SOLVENT (Graff)		CASTROID INJ. UNGUENTUM Hemorrhoids (Sargeant)	Sulfocarbolates of calcium and sodium Camphor Salol Balsam of Peru Balsam of fir Castor oil
CASMA COLOGNE WATER, PERFUME (Caswell- Massey)			
		CASUAL Home per- manent (Toni)	
CASMA TOILET WATER (Caswell-Massey)		CASWELL- MASSEY BALSAMIC OINTMENT, PERFUMES, COLOGNES, TOILET WATERS (Casswell- Massey)	

*Consult Sec. II., Ingredients Index. This ingredient may be responsible for major toxic effects if poisonous amounts of this product are ingested.

Name & Use Manufacturer	Ingredients		Name & Use Manufacturer	Ingredients	
CATEX SEED TREATER (Southern Pine Chem.)			CAVOS, CAVREX Embalming fluid (Embalmers')	Formaldehyde*	
CATTLEZE CATTLE SPRAY (Calumet Ref.)			CAWCO ANT POISON (Cawthon-Coleman)	Sodium arsenate*	2-1/2%
CAT WASH & DISINFECTANT (?) (Clayton)			C.B.L. ANTI-CHIGGER-MOSQUITO CREAM STAINLESS Insect repellent (Worth)	Dimethyl phthalate Cis-bicyclo-heptene-dicarboxylic acid dimethyl ester Butyl dimethyl dihydro gamma-pyrone carboxylate Benzocaine Citronella oil (Java)	15.375% 5.075% 4.550% 5.000% 5.000%
CAULK-O-SEAL (Calbar)					
CAULKTEX CAULKING COMPOUND (Ever-Plastics)			C.B.L. LIQUID CHIGGER-MOSQUITO Insect repellent (Worth)	Dimethyl phthalate Cis-bicyclo-heptene-dicarboxylic acid dimethyl ester Butyl dimethyl dihydro gamma-pyrone carboxylate Citronella oil* (Java) Benzocaine	21.525% 7.105% 6.370% 35.000% 5.000%
CAUSTIC BALSAM Counter-irritant (Lawrence-Williams)	Sulfonated vegetable oil Cantharides Gum euphorbia Terebene Spirit of turpentine* Camphor* Croton oil*	0.12%			
			CCC CAPTAN SPRAY Insecticide (Carbola)	Captan	50%
CAUSTIC DEHORNING PASTE Horn treatment (veterinary) (Roberts,Dr.D.)	Potassium hydroxide* Estrol absorption base	58% 10%	CCC COPPER DUST Insecticide (Carbola)	Copper*	6%
			CCC COPPER SPRAY Fungicide (Carbola)	Copper*	31%
CAVALIER BOOT CREME (Cavalier)	Vegetable waxes Beeswax Oleate soap Detergents Lanolin Turpentine*		CCC 10% DDT Insecticide (Carbola)	DDT*	10%
			CCC DDT POWDER Insecticide (Carbola)	Wettable DDT*	50%
CAVALIER COSMETICS (Isana)			CCC 3-7 DUST Insecticide (Carbola)	Copper* DDT	7% 3%
CAVALIER FINISH Paint (Atlantic V.&P.)			CCC FLEA & LOUSE KILLER (Carbola)	Rotenone Sulfur β-thiocyano ethyl esters of mixed fatty acids (10-18 carbon atoms) Sodium fluosilicate*	0.40% 15.00% 0.75% 10.00%
CAVALIER LEATHER DYES (Cavalier)	Dyestuffs Methanol and benzol* as much as 30% Shellac Vegetable oil				
			CCC FRUIT TREE SPRAY (Carbola)	DDT* Lindane Sulfur* Captan	7.00% 0.50% 33.00% 7.50%
CAVALIER NURSERY WHITE Leather whitener (Cavalier)	Titanium dioxide Detergents Vegetable wax Dowicide Casein Processed vegetable oil	0.25%	CCC 5% GARDEN DUST Insecticide (Carbola)	DDT*	5%
CAVALIER SUEDE DRESSINGS (Cavalier)	Isopropyl alcohol* 20-30% Aniline dyes*		CCC GARDEN ROTE Insecticide (Carbola)	Rotenone	0.75%
CAVALIER WHITE CLEANERS Leather cleaner (Cavalier)	Titanium dioxide Trisodium phosphate or aerosol products		CCC 25-31 GARDEN SPRAY (Carbola)	DDT Copper*	25% 31%

*Consult Sec. II., Ingredients Index. This ingredient may be responsible for major toxic effects if poisonous amounts of this product are ingested.

Name & Use Manufacturer	Ingredients		Name & Use Manufacturer	Ingredients	
CCC RAT KILLER (Carbola)	Red squill*		CEDAR FLOOR SPRAY (Pioneer)		
CCC ROSE DUST OR SPRAY (Carbola)	Rotenone	0.75%	CEDAR-GLO POLISH (Worrell)		
	Captan	7.50%			
	DDT*	5.00%	CEDAR-LUX Cedar compound (Cedar-Lux)		
	Benzene hexachloride, gamma isomer	0.50%			
	Sulfur*	20.00%	CEDAR MOTH CHIPS (Reliable Chem.)	Refined naphthalene*	97%
C.C.C. TONIC Appetite stimulant (Humphreys)	Quinine sulfate	1/5 gr.		Red cedar chips	3%
	Cinchonidine sulfate	1/4 gr.	CEDAR-NAP MOTH CRYSTALS (Reliable Chem.)	Refined naphthalene*	99-1/2%
	Berberine sulfate	1/16 gr.		Perfume oil	1/2%
	Potassium hypophosphite	2 gr.			
	Calcium hypophosphite	3 gr.	CEDAR OIL POLISH (Uncle Sam)	Mineral oil	
	Sodium hypophosphite	5 gr.		Cedar oil*	
	Thiamine hydrochloride			Perfume and dye	
C.C. & F. DROPS Antipyretic (veterinary) (Daniels, Dr. A.C.)	Solid extr. aconite root*		CEDAROLEUM ANTI-RUST COMPOUND (Bradford)		
	Solid extr. belladona root (alkaloids) each fl. oz.: 1/30 gr.				
	Solid extr. Bryonia		CETAPHEN TABLETS Analgesic (Jeffrey-Fell)	Each tablet:	
CC-413 Cathartic (Vegetrates)	Rhubarb root			Phenacetin*	2-1/2 gr.
	Base of dehydrated parsley, Irish moss, asparagus, okra, cranberry, rhubarb stalk			Caffeine	1/2 gr.
				Aspirin*	3-1/2 gr.
C & C PAINTS (Cowman-Campbell)			CETAPHIL (Ointment, Lotion) Ointment for skin irritations (Texas Pharm.)	Cetyl alcohol	
				Propylene glycol	
				Stearyl alcohol	
C.C.S. ALKALI Cleaning product (Wyandotte)	Concentrated alkali*			Sodium lauryl sulfate	
C & C UNGUENT Rubefacient, counter-irritant (Tilden)	Camphor*		CETRO-CIROSE Sedative, antitussive (Ives Cameron)	Each fl. oz.:	
	Oil of thyme			Codeine phosphate	1/2 gr.
	Menthol*			Chloroform	1-1/2 m.
	Eupinol			Alcohol	1-1/2%
	Oil of eucalyptus*			Fl. extr. of ipecac	1 m.
	Petrolatum and suet base			Glycerin	240 m.
C. & D. OIL COLORS Paints (Cook & Dunn)				Potassium guaiacolsulfonate	8 gr.
				Sodium citrate	18 gr.
C.D.R. FURNITURE CREAM (Shield-All)	Sulfonated castor oil			Citric acid	6 gr.
	Essential* such as artifical oil of citronella		CETYLIN (Ossar)	Cholesterin	
				Cetyl alcohol	
C.D.R. FURNITURE POLISH & FINISH PRESERVER (Shield-All)				Glyceryl monostearate solution	
				Corn oil	
				Butoben (Merck)	
				Methyl paraben	
CECOBEST CECODURE, CECOLAC CECOLOID, CECOLUX, CECO, CECOTEX, CECOTILE, CECOTITE, ROOF COATING, COCOTONE PAINTS (Chessman-Elliott)			CETYLON Fungicide (Fairfield)	Cetyl dimethyl benzyl ammonium chloride*	100%
			CEDAR PINE AIRTONS Deodorizer (Thayer)	Isobornyl acetate	0.75%
				Oil of cedar leaves	0.75%
				Nonionic emulsifiers	3.50%
				Quaternary ammonium	0.2%
				Antifoam silicones	
			CEE-DEE Fungicide (Fairfield)	Alkyl dimethyl benzyl ammonium chlorides*	20%
CEDACOTE Cedar compound (Cedacote)			CEFERA Food supplement (Haag)	Each tablet:	
				Ferrous sulfate* exsiccated	194 mg.
				Ascorbic acid	25 mg.

*Consult Sec. II., Ingredients Index. This ingredient may be responsible for major toxic effects if poisonous amounts of this product are ingested.

Name & Use Manufacturer	Ingredients	Name & Use Manufacturer	Ingredients
CEFERA-PLUS Food supplement (Haag)	Each tablet: Ferrous gluconate 324 mg. Ascorbic acid 30 mg. Thiamine hydrochloride 2 mg. Riboflavin 2 mg. Pyridoxine hydrochloride 0.5 mg. Nicotinamide 15 mg. Vitamin B_{12} 5 μ gm. Folic acid 0.67 mg.	CEL-TON-SA BRAND HERB TEA Cathartic (Cel-Ton-Sa)	Senna leaves
		CEL-TON-SA RE-O-LAX BRAND HERBS Cathartic (Cel-Ton-Sa)	Cascara sagrada Senna leaves
CELACETTS Laxative (Tailby)	Methyl cellulose 6 gr.	CEL-TON-SA SNOW WHITE LINIMENT Rubefacient (Cel-Ton-Sa)	Chloroform 27.36 m. Turpentine* Methyl salicylate* Oil of camphor* Oil of Mustard (synthetic) Stronger ammonia water Oleic acid Sassafras fraction of camphor oil
CELAG Bulk Laxative (Haack)	Methyl cellulose 5 gr. Magnesium hydroxide 9 gr.		
CELCURE Wood preservative (Am.Celcure)	Copper sulfate* (anhydrous) 3.84% Sodium dichromate* (anhydrous) 5.27% Acetic acid (free) 0.20%		
		CEL-TOX WOOD PRESERVATIVE (General Paint) (Calif.)	
CE-LITE PAINT (Elliott)		CEMCOAT PAINT (Sonneborn)	
CELLIUM TABLETS Laxative (Pharmex)	Sodium carboxymethyl cellulose 7.7 gr.	C.E.M DIE Insecticide (St. Lawrence)	Petroleum* Kendrin Piperonyl butoxide Pyrethrins*
CELLOMENT Adhesive (Hughes)	Nitrocellulose base Acetone* Butyl acetate Butanol*	CEMELEX Cathartic (Rossmar)	Each 60 gr.: Sodium carboxymethyl cellulose 1 gm. Dextrose
CELLO-STICK Adhesive (Varniton)	Toluene*	CEMENTROL Concrete additive (Allied Comp.)	
CELLOTHYL Laxative (Warner-Chilcott)	Methyl cellulose 0.5 gm.	CEMENTSEAL ENAMELS (Acorn Ref.)	
CELLTONE Laxative (Tutag)	Each tablet: Sodium carboxymethyl cellulose 0.5 gm.	CEM-REM Cement and concrete sealer, coating (Speco)	Silicone compounds Fish oils Processed soya resins Terpene resins Rubber copolymer resin Cement Aromatic and aliphatic solvents* Iron Chrome* Titanium Lampblack
CELLUGRAN Laxative (Tilden)	Methyl cellulose Food dextrose Powdered sugar, cocoa and vanillin		
CELLULOID STARCH (Staley)	Borax*		
CELLUTABS Laxative (Veltex)	Each tablet: Sodium carboxymethyl cellulose 0.5 gr.	CEN-DEW Dust mop wax (Central Chem.)	
CELLU-TONE SATIN PAINT (Pratt & Lambert)		CEN-DEW (Water-soluble) Polishes, waxes (Central Chem.)	
CELLZAN Laxative (Tutag)	Each tablet: Sodium carboxymethyl cellulose 7-1/2 gr. Extr. cascara sagrada 1/8 gr.	CEN-GLOW Wax (Central Chem.)	
CELOLITE ENAMELS, VARNISHES, STAINS (Sapolin)			

*Consult Sec. II., Ingredients Index. This ingredient may be responsible for major toxic effects if poisonous amounts of this product are ingested.

Name & Use Manufacturer	Ingredients	Name & Use Manufacturer	Ingredients
CEN-KLOR Disinfectant (Central Chem.)	Chlorinated compound*	CENTRAL 2, 4-D AMINE 64 Herbicide (Central Supply)	Aklanolamine salts of 2,4-dichlorophenoxyacetate monohydrate
CENTOX SPRAY Insecticide (Central Chem.)	Chlordane* Tech. piperonyl butoxide Pyrethrins	CENTRANOX PAINT (Central P.&V.)	
CENTRALOID PAINT (Central P.&V.)		CENTURY BRAND PAINT (Mound City)	
CENTRAL'S ALL-PENETRATING SEAL Polish, waxes (Central Chem.)		CENTURY PAINT & VARNISH REMOVER (Nat'l Chem.)	
CENTRAL'S BOLWHITE Toilet bowl bleach (Central Chem.)		CENTURY SCOURING POWDER (Finnell)	
CENTRAL'S C.C. CONCENTRATE Cleanser (Central Chem.)		CENUS COMPOUND RECTAL SUPPOSITORIES (Horton & Converse)	Oil of cedar* Pinus canadensis Extr. witch hazel Powdered elm Linalool Terpineol*
CENTRAL'S CEN-KLEEN, CREAMERY CLEANSER, 44 D DISH-WASHING COMPOUND, FURNITURE POLISH (Central Chem.)		CEPACOL Antibacterial solution (Merrell)	Alcohol 15% Ceepryn chloride (cetylpyridin-ium chloride) 1-4000 Phosphate buffers
		CEPACOL THROAT LOZENGES (Merrell)	Ceepryn chloride (cetylpyridini-um chloride) 1-1500 Benzyl alcohol
CENTRAL'S METAL POLISH (Central Chem.)		CEPHEB Analgesic (Superior Pharm.)	Each tablet: Acetophenetidin* 2 gr. P.E. belladonna U.S.P. 1/50 gr. Sodium salicylate* 2 gr. Gum camphor 1/8 gr. Capsicum 1/10 gr. Iodized calcium 1/3 gr.
CENTRAL'S PAINT & VARNISH REMOVER (Central Chem.)			
CENTRAL'S PIPE SOLVENT (Central Chem.)		CERATE Hemorrhoids (Boericke & Runyon)	Aesculus Hamamelis* Collinsonia Petrolatum paraffin base
CENTRAL'S PORCELAIN CLEANER, SUPER SHINO-CEN (Central Chem.)		CERESAN M SEED DISINFECTANT (and M-2X) (Du Pont)	Ethyl mercury p-toluene sulfonanilide*
CENTRAL'S 100% RUBBER BASE ENAMEL (Central Chem.)		CERESAN SEED DISINFECTANT 2% (and New Improved) (Du Pont)	Ethyl mercury chloride*
CENTRAL STA Anti-Freeze (Central Solv.)	Methanol*	CERETOL REMEDY (Manhattan Drug)	
CENTRAL'S TRAFFIC WAX LIQUID (Central Chem.)		CERFEX SPACKLING COMPOUND (United Gilson.)	Gypsum Animal glue Zinc sulfate
CENTRAL'S WAX PASTE (Central Chem.)			

*Consult Sec. II., Ingredients Index. This ingredient may be responsible for major toxic effects if poisonous amounts of this product are ingested.

- 359 -

Name & Use Manufacturer	Ingredients	Name & Use Manufacturer	Ingredients
CERICODE Antitussive (Premo)	Codeine phosphate 1 gr. Alcohol 3% Potassium guaiacol sulfonate* 8 gr. Ammonium chloride 8 gr. Chloroform 2 gr.	CERTOX INSECT SPRAY (Certox)	Petroleum distillate* Beta thiocyano ethyl esters of aliphatic acids (10-18 carbon atoms) Beta butoxy β thiocyano diethyl ether* Tech. piperonyl butoxide Pyrethrins
CERTANE VAGINAL JELLY (Vogarell)	Phenylmercuric acetate 0.02% Boric acid* Oxyquinoline sulfate Sodium sulfodioctyl succinate	CERTOX INSECT SPRAY 5% DDT PLUS PYRETHRUM (Certox)	Petroleum distillate* DDT* tech. 5% Tech. piperonyl butoxide Pyrethrins
CERTA-VIN (Certa-Vin)	Iron Ammonium Citrate Riboflavin Berberis Sarsaparilla Maganese sulfate Salicylic acid Flavoring oils Thiamine hydrochloride Gentian Bitter orange Cloves Niacin Saccharin	CERTOX INSECT SPRAY D-10 (Certox)	Petroleum distillate* DDT* tech. 5% Tech. piperonyl butoxide Pyrethrins
		CERTOX INSECT SPRAY (Certox)	DDT 1% Inert ingredients*
		CERTOX LINDANE FLY SPRAY (Certox)	Petroleum distillates* Gamma isomer of benzene hexachloride (from lindane)* Piperonyl butoxide tech. Pyrethrins
CERTIFIED PURE SHELLAC, CERTILAC (Bradshaw)		CERTOX MOTH NUGGETS (Certox)	Paradichlorobenzene* 100%
CERT-O-CIDE GRAIN FUMIGANT (Cook Chem.)	Carbon tetrachloride* 81% Carbon bisulfide 12.1% Ethylene dibromide 6.6%	CERTOX NORWAY RAT TRACKER FORMULA 25% ANTU (Certox)	ANTU* (Alpha naphthyl thiorea) 25%
CERT-O-KILL Insecticide (Planetary Chem.)	DDT (dichloro diphenyl trichloroethane) 25% Methylated naphthalene* 60%	CERTOX PROFESSIONAL MOTH SPRAY (Certox)	Petroleum distillate* Beta thiocyano ethyl esters of aliphatic acids (10-18 carbon atoms) Beta butoxy beta thiocyano di- ethyl ether* Dichloro diphenyl trichloro- ethane tech.
CERTOX Insecticide (Certox)	DDT 2%		
CERTOX 40% CHLORDANE WETTABLE POWDER Insecticide (Certox)	Tech. chlordane* 40%	CERTOX P-5 WOOD PRESERVER (Certox)	Petroleum distillate* 95.00% Pentachlorophenol* 4.40% Other chlorophenols 0.60%
CERTOX CRYSTAL MOTH SPRAY (Certox)	Carbon tetrachloride* Ethylene dichloride* Paradichlorobenzene	CERTOX P-40 WOOD PRESERVER (Certox)	Pentachlorophenol* 36.08% Other chlorophenols 4.92%
CERTOX DE-25 AQUASOL Insecticide (Certox)	Methylated aromatic petroleum deriv.* 71% DDT 25% Polyoxyethylene sorbitol esters of mixed fatty resin acids 4%	CERTOX RAT BUTTER (Certox)	Thallium sulfate* 1%
		CERTOX RAT BUTTER (contains red squill) (Certox)	Red squill powder* (fortified) 10%
CERTOX DE-50 WETTABLE POWDER Insecticide (Certox)	DDT* 50%	CERTOX RAT BUTTER (contains zinc phosphide) (Certox)	Zinc phosphide* 5%
CERTOX INSECTICIDE DUSTING POWDER (Certox)	DDT* 10%	CERTOX RAT BUTTER FORMULA ANTU (Certox)	ANTU (alpha naphthyl thiourea) 5%

*Consult Sec. II., Ingredients Index. This ingredient may be responsible for major toxic effects if poisonous amounts of this product are ingested.

Name & Use Manufacturer	Ingredients	Name & Use Manufacturer	Ingredients
CERTOX RAT GRAIN (Certox)	Red squill powder* (fortified) 10%	CHAIRMAN COLOGNE (For men) (Stanley Home)	
CERTOX R-14 MOUSE POWDER (Certox)	Dichloro diphenyl trichloro-ethane* 50%	CHAIRMAN LIQUID DEODORANT (For men) (Stanley Home)	
CERTOX ROACH & ANT POWDER (Certox)	Tech. chlordane 5%	CHAIRMAN SHAVE TALC (Stanley Home)	
CERTOX ROACH PASTE (Certox)	Phosphorus* 1.38%	CHALKBOARD FINISH (Chi-Namel)	Lampblack 2.5% Silica 7.4% Calcium carbonate 19.3% Magnesium silicate 17.8% Varnish* (naphtha) 53.0%
CERTOX ROACH POWDER (Certox)	Sodium fluoride* 95%	CHAMBERLAIN HABER PORCELAIN, TILE & MARBLE CLEANER (Chamberlain Haber)	
CERTOX SEEDS Rodenticide (Certox)	Strychnine sulfate* 0.5%	CHAMBERLAIN'S COLIC RELIEF Carminative (Standard Labs.)	Chloroform* 20 m Ether* 64 m. Camphor 0.81 gr. Capsicum 0.81 gr. Ginger 6.5 gr.
CERTOX SEEDS Rodenticide (Certox)	Thallium sulfate* 0.5%	CHAMBERLAIN'S FACE CREAM, HAND LOTION (Chamberlain Sales)	
CERTOX TERMITE LIQUID (Certox)	Orthodichlorobenzene tech. Paradichlorobenzene Trichlorobenzene*	CHAMBERLAIN STOCK DIP & DISINFECTANT (Chamberlain, F.B.)	Coal tar neutral oils* Phenols* Soap
CERTOX WARFARIN CONCENTRATE Rodenticide (Certox)	Warfarin (3-(a-acetonylbenzyl) - 4-hydroxycoumarin) 0.5%		
CETAB Fungicide (Fairfield)	Cetyl trimethyl ammonium 100% bromide*	CHAMO CREME Skin irritation (Dome)	Extr. chamomile Buffered acid cream base (pH 4.2)
CETAMIDE SOLUTION Antiseptic (Maltbie)	Cetyl trimethyl ammonium bromide 1-1000	CHAMO-POWDER Skin irritation (Dome)	Each packet: Extr. chamomile 2 gr.
CENTAMIDE TINCTURE Antiseptic (Maltbie)	Cetyl trimethyl ammonium bromide 1-500 Alcohol 50% Acetone 10%	CHAMPAGNE LATHER Toiletry (Hubere)	
CFS CAMPBELL'S FOOT SALVE (Campbell-Cook)		CHAMPION BRAND PAINTS (Champion Bronze)	
CHAFE-AID OINTMENT (Citadel)		CHAMPION CARPENTER'S CHALK (Champion Chalk)	
CHAFIX For skin irritation (Norcraft-Westware)	Spermaceti White beeswax Hydrocarbon base	CHAMPION CHALK CRAYONS (Champion Chalk)	Calcium carbonate Calcium sulfate Non-toxic colors
CHAIR-LOC Wood sweller (Chair-Loc)	Gum resin Zein (corn protein) Denatured ethyl alcohol* Triethanolamine Glycol		

*Consult Sec. II., Ingredients Index. This ingredient may be responsible for major toxic effects if poisonous amounts of this product are ingested.

Name & Use Manufacturer	Ingredients	Name & Use Manufacturer	Ingredients
CHAMPION LIQUID PLASTIC & ROOFING (Upco)		CHAPMAN CHLORDANE-4 EMULSIFIABLE CONCENTRATE Insecticide (Chapman Chem.)	Tech. chlordane* 45.2% Petroleum hydrocarbons* 49.8%
CHAMPION SPRAYON Paint (Champion Bronze)		CHAPMAN DDT-2 EMULSIFIABLE CONCENTRATE Insecticide (Champan Chem.)	DDT* 24.0% Petroleum distillate* 73.5%
CHAMPO ANTISEPTIC (Champo)		CHAPMAN DIELDRIN (497) EMULSIFIABLE CONCENTRATE Insecticide (Chapman Chem.)	Hexachloro-epoxy-octahydro-dimethano-naphthalene (from Dieldrin)* 15.40% Related compounds (from Dieldrin 2.70% Petroleum hydrocarbons 76.90%
CHANDLER'S CHICK TABLETS (Chandler)			
CHANDLER'S FAMOUS EYE SALVE (Chandler)		CHAPMAN MALATHION-5 Insecticide (Chapman Chem.)	Malathion* 55.1% Petroleum hydrocarbons 34.1%
CHANDLER'S HEALING OINTMENT & PILE SALVE (Chandler)		CHAPMAN ROACH & PEST KILLER CONCENTRATE Insecticide (Chapman Chem.)	Tech. chlordane* 20% Deodorized kerosene* 80%
CHAP-ANS Hand cream (Chap Stick)	Lanolin Camphor* Petrolatum Hexachlorophene* (bis (3,5,6-trichloro-2-hydroxyphenyl) methane)		
		CHAPMAN'S ATHLETIC LINIMENT (Chapman's)	
CHAPERONE Cat, dog repellent (Sudbury Lab.)	Oil of lemon grass* 11% Synthetic oil of mustard 0.2%	CHAPMAN'S PENTA-WR Wood preservative (Wisconsin Solv.)	Pentachlorophenol* 5.0% Petroleum hydrocarbon* 83.4% Water repellents 11.6%
CHAP-EZE Skin irritation (Binday)	Hexachlorophene* Camphor* Menthol*		
CHAP-ICE For cold sores, fever blisters (Commerce)	Hexachlorophene* Lanolin Tinct. benzoin Ammonia Benzocaine Menthol Camphor* Petrolatum	CHAPMAN'S SPECIAL OINTMENT (Chapman's)	
		CHAPMAN'S VET. LINIMENT (Chapman's)	
CHAPIN'S AROMAIRE Deodorizer (Chapin)	Denatured alcohol* 96.5% Essential oils*	CHA POLISHING CREAM (Shield-All)	
CHAPMAN ALDRIN (118) EQUIVALENT EMULSIFIABLE CONCENTRATE Insecticide (Chapman Chem.)	Hexachloro hexahydro dimethano naphthalene* 21.85% Related compounds 16.48% Petroleum hydrocarbons 54.17%	CHAP STICK Lip emollient (Chap Stick)	Petroleum Waxes Mineral oil Camphor* Hexachlorophene* (bis(3,5,6-trichloro-2-hydroxyphenyl) methane)
CHAPMAN BHC-1 EMULSIFIABLE CONCENTRATE Insecticide (Chapman Chem.)	Benzene hexachloride, gamma isomer* 11.3% Benzene hexachloride, other isomers 17.0% Methylated naphthalene* 56.7%	CHARBERT COLOGNE & COLOGNE STICK (Parfums Charbert)	

*Consult Sec. II., Ingredients Index. This ingredient may be responsible for major toxic effects if poisonous amounts of this product are ingested.

Name & Use Manufacturer	Ingredients		Name & Use Manufacturer	Ingredients	
CHARFAIN STICKS Charcoal (Am. Crayon)			CHASE'S ANT KILLER (Chase Prod.)	Sodium arsenate*	
CHARKET OIL Wood preservative (Tenn. Prod.)	Soluble hardwood tar* (higher boiling components)		CHASE'S CASCARA COMPOUND TABLETS Cathartic (Chase Chem.)	Each tablet: Cascara sagrada extr. Aloin Podophyllin* Belladonna extr.* Ginger oleoresin Glycyrrhiza	1/4 gr. 1/4 gr. 1/6 gr. 1/8 gr. 1/16 gr. 1/6 gr.
CHARLES ANTELL HAIR SPRAY (Antell)	Lanolin Alcohol*				
CHARLES ANTELL SOAP (Antell)	Lanolin Chlorophyll Hexachlorophene		CHASE'S COLD CAPSULES Analgesic, antipyretic, cathartic (Chase Chem.)	Each capsule: Acetanilid* Quinine sulfate Belladonna leaf* Camphor Podophyllin Cascara Quassia	1 gr. 1/8 gr. 1/8 gr. 1/8 gr.
CHARLES OF THE RITZ HAND- BLENDED FACE POWDER (Charles of the Ritz)			CHASE'S INSECT BOMB Insecticide (Chase Prod.)	DDT* Pyrethrins Piperonyl butoxide Beta-butoxy-beta-thiocyano diethyl ether* Petroleum	
CHARLTON VELVET LAMP BLACK (Bihn & Wolff)			CHASE'S RAT KISSES (Chase Prod.)	Red squill extr.*	
CHARM ASTRINGENT Cosmetic (Starr Sheen)			CHASKA PERFUME (Sager)		
CHARM OF YOUTH CREME COLOGNE (Wirth)			CHASOPHEN PILLS Cathartic (Chase Chem.)	Each pill: Phenolphthalein* Aloin Extr. belladonna leaves* (alkaloids 1/960 gr.) Ipecac	1/2 gr. 1/4 gr. 1/12 gr. 1/15 gr.
CHARM PAINTS, ENAMELS (Chicago Paints)					
CHARM SKIN FRESHENER (Star Sheen)			CHASSIS LUBE Automobile grease (Kendall Ref.)		
CHARO REFRIGERATOR DEODORIZER (Requa)	Activated charcoal		CHAT Machine-dish- washing detergent (Antara)		
CHASE COAL TAR OINTMENT WITH MERCURY SALICYLATE (Chase Chem.)	Each oz.: Mercury salicylate Menthol Liquid carbonis detergent	0.01 gm. 0.08 gm. 0.88 cc.	CHECKPEST C-46 CHLORDANE EMULSION CONCENTRATE Insecticide (Wood-Treating)	Tech. chlordane* Petroleum hydrocarbons*	45% 40%
CHASE COAL TAR STAINLESS SYNTHETIC OINTMENT (Chase Chem.)	Each oz.: Stainless synthetic coal tar* N.F. Zinc oxide* paste N.F.	1.418 gm. 26.932 gm.	CHECKPEST C-74 Insecticide (Wood-Treating)	Tech. chlordane*	74%
			CHECKPEST C-75 CHLORDANE EMULSION CONCENTRATE Insecticide (Wood-Treating)	Tech. chlordane* Petroleum hydrocarbons*	75% 17%
CHASE (Dr,A.W.) CO. OINT- MENT Skin irritation (Chase,Dr.A.W.)	Petrolatum Calomel* (23%) Zinc oxide Carbolic acid* Beeswax	109 gr.	CHECK PEST C-75 CHLORDANE EMULSION CONCENTRATE Insecticide (Assoc.Sales)	Tech. chlordane* Petroleum hydrocarbons*	75% 17%

*Consult Sec. II., Ingredients Index. This ingredient may be responsible for major toxic effects if poisonous amounts of this product are ingested.

Name & Use Manufacturer	Ingredients	Name & Use Manufacturer	Ingredients
CHECK PEST 25% DDT EMULSION CONCENTRATE Insecticide (Assoc.Sales)	Dichloro diphenyl trichloro-ethane 25% Xylol* 70%	CHEESEMAN PILLS (Cheeseman)	
		CHEK-ROACH POWDER (Chek)	
CHECK PEST 1.5 DIELDRIN INSECTICIDE Insecticide (Assoc.Sales)	Hexachloro epoxy octahydro dimethano naphthalene* 15.83% Related compounds 2.79% Petroleum hydrocarbons 73.38%	CHEK TABLETS (Perdue)	Chlorophyll 100 mg.
		CHEMAGRO SYSTOX SPRAY CONCENTRATE Insecticide (Chemagro)	o,o-diethyl-(2-ethyl-mercapto-ethyl) thiopho sphate* 26.2% Related organic phosphates 2.3%
CHECK PEST 11% GAMMA BHC EMULSION CONCENTRATE Insecticide (Assoc.Sales)	Gamma isomer of benzene hexachloride* 11% Other isomers of benzene hexachloride 17% Methylated naphthalenes* 35% Petroleum distillates 30%	CHEM. CORP. RID-O-WEED Herbicide (Chem.Corp.)	
CHECK PEST 2-LB ALDRIN LIQUID INSECTICIDE (Assoc.Sales)	Hexachloro-hexahydro-dimethano-naphthalene* 23.1% Related compounds 17.4% Aromatic petroleum derivative solvent* 52.0%	CHEMCRAFT Chemistry set (Porter Chem.)	
		CHEM-FROST DEFOLIANT (Pacific Coast)	Sodium and ammonium borates* Sodium chlorate*
CHECKPEST 5-LB MALATHION LIQUID FOR FLY CONTROL (Assoc.Sales)	Malathion* 57% Xylene* 33%	CHEM-FROST LIQUID DEFOLIANT (Pacific Coast)	Sodium metaborate* Sodium chlorate*
CHECK PEST OMPA SYSTEMIC INSECTICIDE SPRAY (Assoc.Sales)	Octamethyl pyrophosphoramide* 18.1% Related organic phosphates 5.2%	CHEMICAL FORMULA-TORS ALDRIN #2 Insecticide (Chem.Form.)	Hexachloro hexahydro dimethano naphthalene* 22.0% Related compounds 16.5% Aromatic hydrocarbon solvent 53.0% Emulsifier 8.5%
CHECK PEST 25% PARATHION INSECTICIDE CONCENTRATE (Assoc.Sales)	Parathion (o,o-diethyl-o-p-nitrophenyl thiophosphate* 25.0% Petroleum hydrocarbons 65.0%	CHEMICAL FORMULA-TORS BUTOXY BRUSH KILLER Herbicide (Chem.Form.)	2,4-Dichlorophenoxyacetic acid* (butoxy ethoxy propanol esters) 26.0% 2,4,5-Trichlorophenoxyacetic acid* (butoxy ethoxy propanol esters) 13.3% Emulsifier, solvents* 58.7%
CHECK PEST 40% TEPP SPRAY CONCENTRATE Insecticide (Assoc.Sales)	Tetraethyl pyrophosphate* 40.0% Other ethyl phosphates 57.5%	CHEMICAL FORMULA-TORS 5% CHLORDANE DUST Insecticide (Chem.Form.)	Tech. chlordane 5% Talc 95%
CHECK PEST TOXAPHENE Insecticide (Assoc.Sales)	Toxaphene* 60% Petroleum distillate 35%	CHEMICAL FORMULA-TORS 40% CHLORDANE EMULSION Insecticide (Chem.Form.)	Chlordane* 40.0% Methylated aromatic petroleum oil* 56.0% Aryl alkyl sulfonate emulsifier 4.0%
CHEK-PICK Veterinary (Ralston)	Pine tar oil* Tannic acid*		
CHEK-R-MYCIN Veterinary (Ralston)	Aureomycin*	CHEMICAL FORMULA-TORS COMMERCIAL BEAN DUST NO. 1 Insecticide (Chem.Form.)	Rotenone 1.0% Other cube resins 2.5% Dichloro diphenyl trichloroethane 3.0%
CHEK-R-TON Insecticide (Ralston)	Nicotine (alkaloid)*		
CHEER Detergent (Procter & Gamble)	Anionic synthetic detergent Sodium tripolyphosphate Sodium sulfate Sodium silicate		

*Consult Sec. II., Ingredients Index. This ingredient may be responsible for major toxic effects if poisonous amounts of this product are ingested.

Name & Use Manufacturer	Ingredients		Name & Use Manufacturer	Ingredients	

CHEMICAL FORMULA-TORS COMMERCIAL BEAN DUST NO. 2 Insecticide (Chem.Form.)	Rotenone
	Other cube resins
	Dichloro diphenyl trichloro-
	  ethane
		0.75%
		1.65%
		
		3.00%
			CHEMICAL FORMULA-TORS FLY & MOSQUITO AEROSOL SPRAY (Chem.Form.)	Dichloro diphenyl trichloro-
				  ethane
				Allethrin
				N-octyl bicycloheptane dicarbo-
				  ximide
				Methylated naphthalenes*
				
				Petroleum hydrocarbon*
				
				Beta butoxy beta thiocyano
				  diethyl ether
				Dichloro difluoromethane,
				  trichloro monofluoromethane
					2.00%
					0.10%
					
					0.50%
					
					5.00%
					
					11.40%
					
					1.00%
					
					80.00%

CHEMICAL FORMULA-TORS COPPER DUST Insecticide (Chem.Form.)	Basic copper sulfate* Talc	14.2% 85.8%			

CHEMICAL FORMULA-TORS COPPER 53 SPRAY Insecticide (Chem.Form.)	Basic copper sulfate* 100%
	  (copper as metallic fixed 53%)
	Inert ingredients*
			CHEMICAL FORMULA-TORS FORMULA 444 GARDEN DUST Insecticide (Chem.Form.)	Methoxychlor
				Malathion* (o,o-demethyl
				  dithiophosphate of diethyl
				  mercaptosuccinate)
				Zinc ethylene-bis (dithiocarba-
				  mate)
				Talc
					4.0%
					
					4.0%
					
					4.0%
					88.0%

CHEMICAL FORMULA-TORS DAIRY CATTLE SPRAY Insecticide (Chem.Form.)	Butoxypolypropylene glycol Pyrethins Piperonyl butoxide tech. Methoxychlor tech. Petroleum distillate*	6.2% 0.02% 0.205% 0.50% 93.06%			

CHEMICAL FORMULA-TORS 25% DDD, EMULSION CONCENTRATE Insecticide (Chem.Form.)	Dichloro diphenyl dichloro-
	  ethane
	Xylol*
	Emulsifier
		25.0%
		70.0%
		5.0%
			CHEMICAL FORMULA-TORS FRUIT & ORNAMENTAL SPRAY Insecticide (Chem.Form.)	Dichloro diphenyl trichloro-
				  ethane*
				N-trichlormethyl mercapto-4-
				  cyclohexene-1,2-dicarboximide
				Ferric dimethyl dithiocarbamate
				
				o-o-Dimethyl dithiophosphate of
				  diethyl mercapto-
				  succinate
				Sulfur
				Talc
					10.0%
					
					4.0%
					
					7.0%
					
					4.0%
					15.0%
					60.0%

CHEMICAL FORMULA-TORS 25% DDT EMULSION Insecticide (Chem.Form.)	Diphenyl dichloro trichloro- ethane* Aromatic petroleum solvent*	25.0% 75.0%			
CHEMICAL FORMULA-TORS DDT GARDEN DUST Insecticide (Chem.Form.)	Dichloro diphenyl trichloro- ethane* Talc	5.0% 95.0%	CHEMICAL FORMULA-TORS LEAD ARSENATE Insecticide (Chem.Form.)	Lead arsenate* Talc	96% 4%

CHEMICAL FORMULA-TORS 15% FERBAM DUST Insecticide, fungicide (Chem.Form.)	Ferric dimethyl dithiocarba-
	  mate
	Talc
		11.40%
		88.60%
			CHEMICAL FORMULA-TORS 1% LINDANE DUST Insecticide (Chem.Form.)	Gamma isomer of benzene
				  hexachloride
				Talc
					1%
					99%

CHEMICAL FORMULA-TORS FERBAM WETTABLE POWDER Insecticide (Chem.Form.)	Ferric dimethyl dithiocarba-
	  mate*
	Talc
		76.0%
		24.0%
			CHEMICAL FORMULA-TORS 5% MALATHION DUST Insecticide (Chem.Form.)	Malathion* (o,o-dimethyl
				  dithiophosphate of diethyl
				  mercaptosuccinate)
				Talc
					5.0%
					95.0%

			CHEMICAL FORMULA-TORS 50% MALATHION LIQUID Insecticide (Chem.Form.)	Malathion* (o,o-dimethyl
				  dithiophosphate of diethyl
				  mercaptosuccinate)
				Aromatic hydrocarbon
				  solvent*
				Emulsifier
					50.0%
					
					45.0%
					5.0%

			CHEMICAL FORMULA-TORS 1% PARATHION DUST Insecticide (Chem.Form.)	Parathion (o,o-diethyl-o,p- nitrophenyl thiophosphate* Talc	1% 99%

*Consult Sec. II., Ingredients Index. This ingredient may be responsible for major toxic effects if poisonous amounts of this product are ingested.

Name & Use Manufacturer	Ingredients
CHEMICAL FORMULATORS ROACH & ANT AEROSOL BOMB (Chem.Form.)	Tech. chlordane 2.00% Tech. piperonyl butoxide 0.115% Pyrethrins 0.046% Polymerized glycerol oleate 0.100% Petroleum distillate* 72.739% Dichlorodifluoromethane 25.000%
CHEMICAL FORMULATORS SPECIAL POTATO DUST Insecticide (Chem.Form.)	Dichloro diphenyl trichloroethane* 5.0% Fixed copper* 7.0% Talc 88.0%
CHEMICAL FORMULATORS SPECIAL TOMATO DUST Insecticide (Chem.Form.)	Rotenone 0.75% Other cube resins 1.65% Fixed copper* 7.5% Talc 90.1%
CHEMICAL FORMULATORS STRAWBERRY DUST Insecticide (Chem.Form.)	Dichloro diphenyl trichloroethane* 5.0% Chlordane tech.* 5.0% Talc 90.0%
CHEMICAL FORMULATORS 10% TDE (DDD) DUST Insecticide (Chem.Form.)	Dichloro diphenyl dichloroethane 5.0% Talc 95.0%
CHEMICAL FORMULATORS 60% TOXAPHENE CONCENTRATE Insecticide (Chem.Form.)	Toxaphene (tech. chlorinated camphene)* 60.0% Aromatic petroleum hydrocarbon solvent* 32.0% Emulsifier 8.0%
CHEMICAL FORMULATORS 50% WETTABLE DDT Insecticide (Chem.Form.)	Dichloro diphenyl trichloroethane* 50.5% Talc 50.0%
CHEMICAL FORMULATORS ZINEB BLIGHT DUST Fungicide (Chem.Form.)	Zinc ethylene-bis (dithiocarbamate) 8.0% Talc 92.0%
CHEMICAL INSECTICIDE'S CHLORDANE 20% SOLUTION (Chem.Insect.)	Chlordane tech.* 20% Petroleum distillate* 80%
CHEMICAL INSECTICIDE'S CHLORDANE 46% (Chem.Insect.)	Chlordane tech.* 46.0% Petroleum distillate* 44.5%

Name & Use Manufacturer	Ingredients
CHEMICAL INSECTICIDE'S DDT 30% EMULSIFIABLE (Chem.Insect.)	Dichloro diphenyl trichloroethane* and methylated naphthalene 98%
CHEMI-LUME LIGHTS Chemistry set (Varniton)	Fluorescein* Rhodamine B Methyl cellulose Sodium hydroxide* approx. 2.4%
CHEMIPURE ACID HARDENING FIXER (Chemipure)	Sodium thiosulfate Sodium sulfite* Potassium alum* Acetic acid*
CHEMIPURE SOLUTIONS CP-4, CP-6, CP-8 Developers (Chemipure)	Metol* Hydroquinone* Sodium sulfite Sodium carbonate Sodium metaborate* Potassium bromide*
CHEMISTS FLYPROOFING CONCENTRATE (Continental Chemistry)	DDT*
THE CHEMISTRY OF FOILLE Skin burns (Carbisulphoil)	Benzyl alcohol 4.00% Benzocaine 2.00% Oxyquinoline base 0.20% Eugenol 0.20% Sulfur 0.175%
CHEMITIZING RUST COMPOUND (Safe-Gard)	
CHEMOL RUST REMOVER (Taft)	
CHEMICAL INSECTICIDES ISOPROPYL ESTER OF 2,4-D LIQUID CONCENTRATE Herbicide (Chem.Insect.)	Isopropyl ester of 2,4-dichlorophenoxyacetic acid 44.7%
CHEMICAL INSECTICIDE'S 2,4-D SODIUM SALT 85 (Chem.Insect.)	Sodium 2,4-dichlorophenoxyacetate monohydrate* 96.8%
CHEMIC ENAMEL PAINT (U.S.Gutta)	
CHEMICO EMBALMING FLUIDS (Nat'l Sanitary)	
CHEMICO PAINTS FOR HOSPITALS (Vita-Var)	

*Consult Sec. II., Ingredients Index. This ingredient may be responsible for major toxic effects if poisonous amounts of this product are ingested.

Name & Use Manufacturer	Ingredients	Name & Use Manufacturer	Ingredients
CHEMIGLOV Laboratory hand protectant (Fisher Scient.)	Glyceryl monostearate Anhydrous lanolin Light mineral oil Levigated alumina Bentonite Talcum powder Glycerin White wax Oil of lemon Methyl paraben	CHERALTO COUGH SYRUP (Altone)	
		CHERAMY SKIN BALM Toiletry (Cheramy)	
CHEM-REM CHEMICAL RESISTANT PAINT (Speco)	Metallic pigments of chrome,* iron, aluminum, copper,* and titanium Lampblack with various hydrocarbon vehicles Resins Plasticizers Coal tar solvents*	CHERI HANCE SYRUP Antitussive (Hance)	Each fl. oz.: Chloroform 2 gr. Potassium guaiacolsulfonate 8 gr. Ammonium chloride 8 gr. Antimony and potassium tartrate 1/12 gr. Alcohol 3%
CHEM-SECT D-25 Insecticide (Chem.Insect.)	Dichloro diphenyl trichloroe-thane* and aromatic petroleum deriv.* 98% Soap of petroleum sulfonates and polyethylene glycol esters of fatty acids 2%	CHERI HANCE WITH CODEINE Antitussive (Hance)	Each fl. oz.: Codeine phosphate 1 gr. Chloroform 2 gr. Potassium guaiacolsulfonate 8 gr. Ammonium chloride 8 gr. Antimony and potassium tartrate 1/12 gr. Alcohol 3%
CHEM-WEED Herbicide	Iso-octyl ester of 2,4-dichlo-rophenoxyacetic acid* 33.7% Butoxy ethoxy propanol ester of 2,4,5-trichlorophenoxy-acetic acid* 35.3%	CHEROLA COUGH SYRUP Antitussive (Penslar)	Each fl. oz.: Syrup wild cherry bark 240 m. Syrup sanguinaria 60 m. Tartar emetic 1/4 gr. Senega 8 gr.
CHEM-WEED Herbicide (Chem.Insect.)	Butoxy ethoxy ester of 2,4-dichlorophenoxy-acetic acid* 38.8% Butoxy ethoxy propanol ester of 2,4,5-trichlorophenoxy-acetic acid* 35.3%	CHERONIA Antitussive (Veltex)	Each fl. oz.: Codeine phosphate 1 gr. Chloroform 2 m. Potassium guaiacolsulfonate 8 gr. Ammonium chloride 8 gr. Tartar emetic 1/12 gr. Wild cherry and white pine compound
CHEM-WEED Herbicide (Chem.Insect.)	Butoxy ethoxy propanol ester of 2,4-dichlorophenoxyacetic acid* 25% Butoxy ethoxy propanol ester of 2,4,5-trichlorophenoxyacetic acid* 27%	CHERRY COPOSIL FUNGICIDE (Calif.Spray)	Copper* 26%
CHEM-WEED 2,4-D Herbicide (Chem.Insect.)	Mixed isopropyl & triethyl amine salts of 2,4-dichloro-phenoxyacetic acid * 56%	CHERRY'S FAMOUS SALVE (Cherry's)	
CHEM-WEED 2,4-D WEED KILLER (Chem.Insect.)	Butoxy ethoxy propanol ester 2,4-dichlorophenoxyacetic acid* 76.0%	CHESTER - FIELD PAINTS (Roberts Paint)	
CHEM WEED 2,4,5-T Insecticide (Chem.Insect.)	2,4,5-Trichlorophenoxyacetic acid,* butoxy ethoxy propanol ester 66¢ 2,4,5-Trichlorophenoxyacetic acid*	CHESTER-FIELD RUG & UPHOLSTE-RY CLEANER (Nu-Age)	
CHENEY'S EXPECTOR-ANT (Daniel,J.)		CHESTOL Inhalant (Wisconsin Pharm.)	Guaiacol* Camphor* Methyl salicylate* Eucalyptol*
CHERACODE Sedative, expectorant (Approved)	Each fl. oz.: Codeine phosphate 1 gr.	CHEXALL DEODORANT (Quality Cosm.)	
CHERACOL-COCILLANA-STOKES EXPECTOR-ANT Antitussive (Steinmann)	Cheracol Cocillana	CHEX FOR ATHLETE'S FOOT (Howell Co.)	

*Consult Sec. II., Ingredients Index. This ingredient may be responsible for major toxic effects if poisonous amounts of this product are ingested.

Name & Use Manufacturer	Ingredients	Name & Use Manufacturer	Ingredients
CHEXIT ANTI- PERSPIRANT (Scandia)		CHILL-IT Canned refrigerant (Speco)	Cellulose derivatives Glycol blends Water-soluble dye Rust inhibitors (Nuodex 545)
CHEXIT TABLETS Antacid, adsorbent (Wander)	Aluminum hydroxide, magnesium trisilicate, calcium carbonate, and magnesium carbonate 12.04 gr.	CHIL-TONA PAINT (Chilton Paint)	
CHI-CHES- TERS Dysmenarrhea (Chichester)	Salicylamide* 3 gr. Ephedrine sulfate 1/16 gr. Para-aminobenzoic acid 1/2 gr.	CHILTON'S THROAT TABLETS Throat irritation (Chilton)	Tyrothricin 2 mg. Benzocaine 5 mg.
CHICK-EZ Sanitizer (poultry drinking water) (Wilke)	Para di-isobutyl phenoxy ethoxy ethyl dimethyl benzyl ammonium chloride 2.46%	CHIMNEY SWEEP Soot destroyer (Coughlan)	
CHICORA PAINT (Moore- Leland)		CHINACOTE PAINT (McMurtry)	
CHIEF PAINTS, ENAMELS (Chicago Paints)		CHINALINE PAINT (U.S.Gutta)	
CHIEF TWO MOON BITTER OIL, COUGH ELIXIR, HERB HOUSEHOLD OINTMENT, LINIMENT, MEDICATED CREAM, RECTAL OINTMENT (Chief Two Moon)		CHI-NAMEL ALL PURPOSE ALUMINUM PAINT (Chi-Namel)	Aluminum standard paste 15.6% Varnish* (see naphtha) 81.9% Drier 2.5%
		CHI-NA-VAR SPAR VARNISH (Chi-Namel)	China wood oil* 35.9 Phenolic resin 13.8 Petroleum thinner* 47.9 Dipentene 1.9 Drier 0.5
		CHINOSOL Skin anti- septic (Jewell Pharm.)	Each tablet: Oxyquinoline sulfate 3/5 gr.
CHIFFON FLAKES Soap (Armour)	Sodium and potassium salts of fatty acids (pure coconut oil and tallow) Glycerine	CHIONACEA Cathartic (Nelson Baker)	Each fl. oz.: Tinct. Chionanthus 180 m. Tinct. Echinacea 20 m. Lappa 16 gr. Taraxacum 16 gr. Glycyrrhiza 24 gr. Euonymus 8 gr. Syrup senna 120 m. Solution sodium phosphate 24 m.
CHIGGER-TOX (Dermal)	Soft soap U.S.P. Benzocaine Benzyl benzoate Aromatic alcohol base* 48%		
CHILAX Laxative (Chicago Pharm.)	Each tablet: Phenolphthalein* 1 gr. Sugar and flavor 4 gr.	CHI-ONA- PAINT (Chilton Paint)	
CHILCO PAINT (Chilton Paint)		CHIPEC Intestinal irritation (Chicago Pharm.)	Each oz.: Pectin 10 gr. Kaolin 100 gr. Belladonna tinct.* 10 m. Sodium benzoate 1 gr.
CHILDREN'S 217 TABLETS Analgesic (Frosst,C.E.)	Aspirin* 56 mg. Acetophenetidin* 40 mg. Caffeine citrate 8 mg.		
CHILDREN'S TONI Permanent wave (Toni)		CHIP FIX Household appliance repair (Glidden Co.)	
CHILDS SODA ACID EXTINGUISHER (Am.-La France)		CHIPMAN 20% ALDRIN Insecticide (Chipman, Ltd.)	Tech. aldrin* 20.0%

*Consult Sec. II., Ingredients Index. This ingredient may be responsible for major toxic effects if poisonous amounts of this product are ingested.

Name & Use Manufacturer	Ingredients		Name & Use Manufacturer	Ingredients	
CHIPMAN ALDRIN 2-1/2% - DDT 5% DUST Insecticide (Chipman Chem.)	Hexachloro hexahydro dimethano naphthalene* Related compounds DDT*	2.38% 0.40% 5.00%	CHIPMAN BRUSH KILLER 76 Herbicide (Chipman, Ltd.)	Iso-octyl ester 2,4-dichloro-phenoxyacetic acid* (2,4-D acid equiv. 38.4 oz./imp. gal.) Iso-octyl ester 2,4,5-trichloro phenoxyacetic acid* (2,4,5-T acid equiv. 38.4 oz./imp. gal.)	
CHIPMAN ALDRIN 2-1/2%-DDT 5%-SULPHUR 40% DUST Insecticide (Chipman Chem.)	Hexachloro hexahydro dimethano naphthalene* Related compounds DDT* Sulfur*	2.38% 0.40% 5.00% 40.00%	CHIPMAN BUNT CURE Nonmercurial seed disinfec-tant (Chipman, Ltd.)	Hexachlorobenzene*	40%
CHIPMAN 2-1/2% ALDRIN DUST Insecticide (Chipman Chem.)	Hexachloro hexahydro dimethano naphthalene* Related compounds	2.38% 0.40%	CHIPMAN CALCIUM ARSENATE Insecticide (Chipman Chem.)	Tricalcium arsenate*	70%
CHIPMAN 5% ALDRIN DUST Insecticide (Chipman, Ltd)	Aldrin* tech.	5.0%	CHIPMAN CAL-SUL 50-50 DUST Insecticide (Chipman Chem.)	Tricalcium arsenate* Sulfur	35.00% 49.00%
CHIPMAN 5% ALDRIN GRANULAR Insecticide (Chipman, Ltd)	Aldrin*	5%	CHIPMAN 7-1/2% CAPTAN DUST Fungicide (Chipman, Ltd.)	Captan	7.5%
CHIPMAN 20% ALDRIN EMULSIFIA-BLE CONCENTRATE Insecticide (Chipman, Ltd.)	Aldrin*	20%	CHIPMAN CAPTAN 50W Fungicide (Chipman, Ltd.)	Captan	50%
CHIPMAN ALDRIN 2L Insecticide (Chipman Chem.)	Hexachloro hexahydro dimethano naphthalene* Related compounds Aromatic petroleum deriv.*	22.0% 3.7% 65.0%	CHIPMAN CHLORAX 40 Herbicide (Chipman Chem.)	Sodium chlorate* Sodium metaborate*	40.0% 58.0%
CHIPMAN ALDRIN 25% SPRAY POWDER Insecticide (Chipman Chem.)	Hexachloro hexahydro dimethano naphthalene* Related compounds	23.8% 4.0%	CHIPMAN CHLORAX LIQUID Herbicide (Chipman Chem.)	Sodium chlorate* Sodium metaborate* anhydrous	18.20% 10.00%
CHIPMAN ARAMITE 4% DUST Insecticide (Chipman Chem.)	2-(p-tert-butylphenoxy) isopropyl-2-chloroethyl sulfite	4.00%	CHIPMAN 5% CHLORDANE DUST Insecticide (Chipman Chem.)	Tech. chlordane	5%
CHIPMAN ARAMITE 15% SPRAY POWDER Insecticide (Chipman Chem.)	2-(p-tert-butylphenoxy) isopropyl-2-chloroethyl sulfite*	15.00%	CHIPMAN 10% CHLORDANE DUST Insecticide (Chipman Chem.)	Tech. chlordane*	10%
CHIPMAN BORAX DUST Fungicide (Chipman, Ltd.)	Impalpable borax (sodium tetraborate)* Celite, pyrophyllite Boron equivalent	50% 50% 5.7%	CHIPMAN CHLORDANE 8L Insecticide (Chipman Chem.)	Tech. chlordane* Petroleum distillate*	73.70% 20.00%
CHIPMAN BASIC COPPER FUNGICIDE (Chipman Chem.)	Basic copper sulfate*	53.00%	CHIPMAN 50% CHLORDANE SPRAY POWDER Insecticide (Chipman Chem.)	Tech. chlordane*	50%
			CHIPMAN CHLOREA Herbicide (Chipman Chem.)	Sodium chlorate* Sodium metaborate* 3-(p-chlorophenyl)-1, 1-dimethyl urea	40.0% 57.0% 1.0%

*Consult Sec. II., Ingredients Index. This ingredient may be responsible for major toxic effects if poisonous amounts of this product are ingested.

- 369 -

Name & Use Manufacturer	Ingredients		Name & Use Manufacturer	Ingredients	
CHIPMAN CIPC-4L Herbicide (Chipman Chem.)	Isopropyl-n-(3-chlorophenyl)- carbamate*	47%	CHIPMAN DDT 3L Insecticide (Chipman Chem.)	DDT* Aromatic petroleum deriv.*	34.6% 41.0%
CHIPMAN CONCENTRA- TED BORASCU Herbicide (Chipman, Ltd.)	Sodium borate*		CHIPMAN 10% DDT-1% PARATHION DUST Insecticide (Chipman Chem.)	DDT Parathion*	10.00% 1.00%
CHIPMAN COPPER SULPHATE Fungicide (Chipman, Ltd.)	Copper sulfate*	99%	CHIPMAN 5% DDT-1/2% PARATHION- 50% SULFUR DUST Insecticide, fungicide (Chipman Chem.)	DDT* Parathion* Sulfur*	5.00% 0.50% 50.00%
CHIPMAN CUCURBIT 3-5 DUST Insecticide, fungicide (Chipman, Ltd.)	Methoxychlor tech. Fixed copper*	3% 5%	CHIPMAN 50% DDT SPRAY POWDER Insecticide (Chipman Chem.)	DDT*	50%
CHIPMAN 50% DDD Insecticide (Chipman, Ltd.)	DDD* (dichloro diphenyl dichloroethane)	50.0%	CHIPMAN 5% DDT-50% SULFUR DUST Insecticide, fungicide (Chipman Chem.)	DDT* Sulfur*	5.00% 50.00%
CHIPMAN 7-1/2 % DDD DUST Insecticide (Chipman, Ltd)	DDD (dichloro diphenyl dichloroethane)	7-1/2%			
CHIPMAN 5% DDD 75% SULFUR DUST Insecticide (Chipman Chem.)	DDD Sulfur*	5.00% 75.00%	CHIPMAN DIELDRIN- DDT 1-5L Insecticide (Chipman Chem.)	DDT Hexachloro epoxy octahydro- endo, exo-dimethano naphthalene Related compounds Aromatic petroleum deriv.*	24.2% 4.1% 0.7% 65.0%
CHIPMAN 50% DDT Insecticide (Chipman, Ltd.)	DDT*	50.0%	CHIPMAN 2-1/2% DIELDRIN- 10% DDT- 40% SULFUR DUST Insecticide (Chipman Chem.)	Hexachloro epoxy octahydro- endo, exo-dimethano naphthalene* Related compounds DDT* Sulfur*	2.13% 0.37% 10.00% 40.00%
CHIPMAN 3% DDT DUST Insecticide (Chipman, Ltd.)	DDT	3%			
CHIPMAN 5% DDT DUST Insecticide (Chipman, Ltd.)	DDT*	5%	CHIPMAN 2-1/2% DIELDRIN- 40% SULFUR DUST Insecticide (Chipman Chem.)	Hexachloro epoxy octahydro- endo, exo-dimethano naphthalene* Related compounds Sulfur*	2.13% 0.37% 40.00%
CHIPMAN 7-1/2 % DDT DUST Insecticide (Chipman, Ltd.)	DDT	7-1/2%			
CHIPMAN 10% DDT DUST Insecticide (Chipman Chem.)	DDT*	10%	CHIPMAN DIELDRIN 15L Insecticide (Chipman Chem.)	Hexachloro epoxy octahydro- endo, exo-dimethano naphthalene* Related compounds Aromatic petroleum deriv.*	16.0% 2.8% 72.0%
CHIPMAN 25% DDT EMULSIFIA- BLE CONC- ENTRATE Insecticide (Chipman, Ltd.)	DDT*	25.0%	CHIPMAN DIELDRIN W75 Insecticide (Chipman Chem.)	Hexachloro epoxy octahydro- endo, exo-dimethano naphthalene* Related compounds	63.75% 11.25%
CHIPMAN DDT 2L Insecticide (Chipman Chem.)	DDT* Aromatic petroleum deriv.*	24.8% 68.0%	CHIPMAN ENDRIN 16L Insecticide (Chipman Chem.)	Hexachloro epoxy octahydro- endo, endo-dimethano naphthalene* Aromatic petroleum deriv.*	19.9% 71.0%

---

*Consult Sec. II., Ingredients Index. This ingredient may be responsible for major toxic effects if poisonous amounts of this product are ingested.

Name & Use Manufacturer	Ingredients		Name & Use Manufacturer	Ingredients	
CHIPMAN 1% ENDRIN DUST Insecticide (Chipman, Ltd.)	Endrin*	1%	CHIPMAN 2-1/2% HEPTACHLOR DUST Insecticide (Chipman Chem.)	Heptachlor* Related compounds	2.50% 0.97%
CHIPMAN 2% ENDRIN DUST Insecticide (Chipman Chem.)	Hexachloro epoxy octahydro-endo, endo-dimethano naphthalene*	2.0%	CHIPMAN HI-TEST ARSENATE Insecticide (Chipman Chem.)	Di-ortho (acid) lead arsenate*	98.00%
CHIPMAN FERBAM 76 Fungicide (Chipman Chem.)	Ferbam* (ferric dimethyl dithiocarbamate)	76%	CHIPMAN IPC 3L Herbicide (Chipman Chem.)	Isopropyl n-phenyl carbamate	36.52%
CHIPMAN FERBAM PLANT BED DUST Fungicide (Chipman, Ltd.)	Ferbam (ferric dimethyl dithio-carbamate)	10.0%	CHIPMAN LEAD ARSENATE Insecticide (Chipman, Ltd.)	Arsenic*	19.5%
CHIPMAN FRUIT SET LIQUID (Oil type) Preharvest control (Chipman Chem.)	Alpha naphthalene acetic acid	0.80%	CHIPMAN LIME-SULPHUR SOLUTION Insecticide, fungicide (Chipman, Ltd.)	Calcium polysulfide*-sulfide sulfur	23%
CHIPMAN FRUIT SET LIQUID (Regular type) Preharvest control (Chipman Chem.)	Alpha naphthalene acetic acid	6.70%	CHIPMAN 25% LINDANE Insecticide (Chipman, Ltd.)	Gamma isomer of benzene hexachloride (from lindane)*	25%
CHIPMAN FUNGICIDE DUST SPECIAL (Chipman Chem.)	Copper*	14%	CHIPMAN 1% LINDANE DUST Insecticide (Chipman, Ltd.)	Gamma isomer of benzene hexachloride (from lindane)	1%
CHIPMAN GENERAL Herbicide (Chipman Chem.)	Dinitro-o-secbutylphenol*	55.0%	CHIPMAN 2% LINDANE DUST Insecticide (Chipman Chem.)	Gamma isomer of benzene hexachloride* (from lindane)	2.0%
CHIPMAN GRAIN FUMIGANT (Chipman Chem.)	Ethylene dichloride* Carbon tetrachloride* Ethylene dibromide Sulfur dioxide	65.0% 27.0% 5.0% 3.0%	CHIPMAN LINDANE 2L Insecticide (Chipman Chem.)	Gamma isomer of benzene hexachloride* (from lindane) Aromatic petroleum deriv.*	23.50% 29.00%
CHIPMAN GRAPE DUST SPECIAL Fungicide (Chipman Chem.)	Tribasic copper sulfate Sulfur*	2.00% 70.00%	CHIPMAN LINDANE W75 Insecticide (Chipman Chem.)	Gamma isomer of benzene hexachloride* (from lindane)	75.00%
CHIPMAN HEPTACHLOR 2L Insecticide (Chipman Chem.)	Heptachlor* Related compounds Aromatic petroleum deriv.*	22.3% 8.7% 62.0%	CHIPMAN 25% LINDANE WETTABLE POWDER Insecticide (Chipman, Ltd.)	Gamma isomer of benzene hexachloride* (from lindane)	25%
CHIPMAN 2-1/2% HEPTACHLOR-10% DDT-40% SULFUR DUST Insecticide (Chipman Chem.)	Heptachlor Related compounds DDT* Sulfur*	2.50% 0.97% 10.00% 40.00%	CHIPMAN LOUSE POWDER (Chipman, Ltd.)	Rotenone Sulfur*	0.5% 20.0%
			CHIPMAN LOW VOLATILE BRUSH KILLER NO. 2 Herbicide (Chipman Chem.)	2,4-Dichlorophenoxyacetic acid* (propylene glycol butyl ether esters) 2,4,5-Trichlorophenoxyacetic acid* (propylene glycol butyl ether esters)	34.80% 33.00%

Name & Use Manufacturer	Ingredients	
CHIPMAN 4% MALATHION DUST Insecticide (Chipman, Ltd.)	Malathion*	4%
CHIPMAN 5% MALATHION DUST Insecticide (Chipman Chem.)	Malathion*	5.0%
CHIPMAN 50% MALATHION EMULSIFIA-BLE CONCENTRATE Insecticide (Chipman, Ltd.)	Malathion*	50%
CHIPMAN MALATHION 4L Insecticide (Chipman Chem.)	Malathion Aromatic petroleum deriv. solvent*	47.00% 43.00%
CHIPMAN MALATHION 5L Insecticide (Chipman Chem.)	Malathion Aromatic petroleum deriv. solvent*	56.4% 31.0%
CHIPMAN 4% MALATHION-50% SULFUR DUST Insecticide (Chipman Chem.)	Malathion* Sulfur*	4.0% 50.0%
CHIPMAN 25% MALATHION W.P. Insecticide (Chipman, Ltd.)	Malathion*	25%
CHIPMAN MERCURIAL APPLE SPRAY Fungicide (Chipman, Ltd.)	Phenyl mercuriacetate*	2.5%
CHIPMAN METHOXONE-CHLORAX LIQUID Herbicide (Chipman Chem.)	Sodium chlorate* Sodium metaborate* 2-Methyl-4-chlorophenoxy-acetic acid	16.30% 9.10% 0.20%
CHIPMAN 50% METHOXY-CHLOR Insecticide (Chipman, Ltd.)	Methoxychlor tech.*	50%
CHIPMAN M-H AMINE 30 Herbicide (Chipman, Ltd.)	Maleic hydrazide*	30%
CHIPMAN MICROFINE SULPHUR 95 Fungicide (Chipman, Ltd.)	Sulfur*	92%
CHIPMAN NICOTINE SULPHATE 40 Insecticide (Chipman, Ltd.)	Nicotine*	40%

Name & Use Manufacturer	Ingredients	
CHIPMAN ORGANIC 6 DUST Fungicide (Chipman, Ltd.)	Zineb (zinc ethylene bis-dithiocarbamate)	3.9%
CHIPMAN ORGANIC 6-3 DUST Insecticide, fungicide (Chipman, Ltd.)	Zineb (zinc ethylene bis-dithiocarbamate) DDT	3.0% 3.0%
CHIPMAN 15% PARATHION Insecticide (Chipman, Ltd.)	Parathion*	15%
CHIPMAN 2% PARATHION DUST Insecticide (Chipman Chem.)	Parathion*	2.00%
CHIPMAN 25% PARATHION DUST BASE Insecticide (Chipman Chem.)	Parathion*	25%
CHIPMAN 25% PARATHION EMULSIFIA-BLE Insecticide (Chipman, Ltd.)	Parathion*	25.0%
CHIPMAN PARATHION 2L Insecticide (Chipman Chem.)	Parathion* Aromatic petroleum deriv. solvent	25.00% 65.00%
CHIPMAN PARATHION 4L Insecticide (Chipman Chem.)	Parathion*	45.00%
CHIPMAN 15% PARATHION SPRAY POWDER Insecticide (Chipman Chem.)	Parathion*	15%
CHIPMAN 25% PARATHION SPRAY POWDER Insecticide (Chipman Chem.)	Parathion*	25.00%
CHIPMAN PARIS GREEN Insecticide (Chipman Chem.)	Copper aceto-arsenite*	91.70%
CHIPMAN PARIS GREEN Insecticide (Chipman, Ltd.)	Copper acetometarsenite* Arsenic Copper	96.0% 39.0% 24.0%
CHIPMAN POLYBOR-CHLORATE Herbicide (Chipman, Ltd.)	Sodium pentaborate* Sodium tetraborate* Sodium chlorate*	58% 15% 25%

*Consult Sec. II., Ingredients Index. This ingredient may be responsible for major toxic effects if poisonous amounts of this product are ingested.

Name & Use Manufacturer	Ingredients		Name & Use Manufacturer	Ingredients	
CHIPMAN POTATO DUST SPECIAL Insecticide, fungicide (Chipman Chem.)	DDT* Copper hydroxysulfate*	5.0% 7.0%	CHIPMAN 40% TOXAPHENE SPRAY POWDER Insecticide (Chipman Chem.)	Toxaphene*	40%
CHIPMAN 5% ROTENONE SPRAY POWDER Insecticide (Chipman Chem.)	Rotenone* Other cube resins	5.00% 10.00%	CHIPMAN 20% TOXAPHENE- 40% SULFUR DUST Insecticide (Chipman Chem.)	Toxaphene* Sulfur	20.00% 40.00%
CHIPMAN SODIUM ARSENATE Insecticide (Chipman Chem.)	Sodium arsenate*	94%	CHIPMAN TOX-DDT 4-2 LIQUID Insecticide (Chipman Chem.)	Toxaphene* DDT Aromatic petroleum deriv. solvent*	39.3% 19.6% 34.00%
CHIPMAN SODIUM ARSENITE Insecticide (Chipman Chem.)	Sodium arsenite* (75% arsenious oxide)	90.67%	CHIPMAN 2,4-D AMINE NO. 2 Herbicide (Chipman Chem.)	Alkanolamine salts (ethanol and isopropanol series) 2,4-dichlorophenoxyacetic acid*	65.0%
CHIPMAN SODIUM CHLORATE Herbicide (Chipman Chem.)	Sodium chlorate*	99%	CHIPMAN 2,4-D BUTYL ESTER 6 Herbicide (Chipman Chem.)	2,4-Dichlorophenoxyacetic acid* (n-butyl ester)	78.7%
CHIPMAN SODIUM TCA 90% Herbicide (Chipman Chem.)	Sodium trichloroacetate*	90%	CHIPMAN 44% 2,4-D ESTER Herbicide (Chipman Chem.)	2,4-Dichlorophenoxyacetic acid* (isopropyl ester)	44%
CHIPMAN STOCK SPRAY NO. 50 Insecticide (Chipman Chem.)	DDT* Gamma isomer of benzene hexachloride* (from lindane)	24.85% 2.15%	CHIPMAN 10% 2,4-D ESTER DUST Herbicide (Chipman Chem.)	Isopropyl ester of 2,4-dichlorophenoxyacetic acid*	10%
CHIPMAN TCA-CHLORAX LIQUID Herbicide (Chipman Chem.)	Sodium chlorate* Sodium trichloroacetate Sodium metaborate anhydrous*	12.40% 2.70% 6.70%	CHIPMAN 76% 2,4-D ESTERS Herbicide (Chipman Chem.)	2,4-Dichlorophenoxyacetic acid* (isopropyl ester) 2,4-Dichlorophenoxyacetic acid* (n-butyl ester)	37.1% 39.0%
CHIPMAN THIRAM SF 75 Seed treatment (Chipman, Ltd.)	Thiram (tetramethyl thiuramdi-sulfide)*	75%	CHIPMAN 2,4-D LOW VOLAT-ILE ESTER 4L Herbicide (Chipman Chem.)	2,4-Dichlorophenoxyacetic acid* (propylene glycol butyl ether esters)	70.50%
CHIPMAN TOBACCO INSECT DUST (Chipman, Ltd.)	DDT* Gamma isomer of benzene hexachloride (from lindane)	7.5% 1.0%	CHIPMAN 44% 2,4,5-T ESTER Herbicide (Chipman Chem.)	Isopropyl ester 2,4,5-trichlorophenoxyacetic acid*	44.32%
CHIPMAN TOMATO DUST Insecticide (Chipman Chem.)	Copper hydroxysulfate Tricalcium arsenate*	7.00% 14.00%	CHIPMAN 2,4,5-T LOW VOLATILE ESTER 4L Herbicide (Chipman Chem.)	2,4,5-Trichlorophenoxyacetic acid* (propylene glycol butyl ether esters)	65.3%
CHIPMAN 20% TOXAPHENE DUST Insecticide (Chipman Chem.)	Toxaphene*	20.00%	CHIPMAN WETTABLE LEAD & ZINC Insecticide (Chipman, Ltd.)	Sulfur Arsenic* Zinc	35.0% 4.7% 11.0%
CHIPMAN 60% TOXAPHENE LIQUID Insecticide (Chipman Chem.)	Tech. toxaphene*	60%	CHIPMAN WETTABLE SULPHUR 95 Fungicide (Chipman, Ltd.)	Sulfur*	95%

*Consult Sec. II., Ingredients Index. This ingredient may be responsible for major toxic effects if poisonous amounts of this product are ingested.

Name & Use Manufacturer	Ingredients		Name & Use Manufacturer	Ingredients	
CHIPMAN ZIRAM W.P. Fungicide (Chipman, Ltd.)	Ziram (zinc dimethyl dithiocarbamate)	76%	CHLORAZENE POWDER, AROMATIC Gargle base (Frost Labs.)	Chlorazene (Chloramine-T,N.F.) Sodium bicarbonate Sodium chloride Saccharin Eucalyptol*	5%
CHIPPEWA FLAKES, SOLID Cleaning products (Wyandotte)	Concentrated alkali*		CHLORAZENE (Powder, Tablets) Antiseptic (Frost Labs.)	Chloramine-T*	89%
CHIROGILL (Red syrup) Sedative, antitussive (Massengill)	Each 5 cc: Chloroform 21.5 mg. Wild cherry 86.5 mg. Red spruce bark 86.5 mg. Blood root (sanguinaria) 86.5 mg. Pleurisy root (asclepias) 43 mg. Lungwort 43 mg. Aromatics q.s.		CHLOR-DUST Insecticide (Commercial Chem.)	Tech. chlordane	5%
			CHLORENAN Inhalant (Radin)	Chlorobutanol* (chloroform derivative) 4-1/2 gr./fl.oz. Camphor* Menthol*	
CHIROLIN LINIMENT Rubefacient, counter-irritant (Gordon Labs.)	Thymol* Eucalyptol* Camphor* Methyl salicylate* Propylene glycol and alcohol base		CHLORESIUM OINTMENT Skin irritation (Rystan)	Chlorophyll "A" N.N.R. (non-toxic water-soluble derivative) 0.5% Hydrophilic base	
CH-IVY CERATE (Nurlburt)	Chloramine-T* 4% Benzocaine 2%		CHLORETS CHLORINE TABLETS Bleach (Gliss'n)	Calcium hypochlorite*	68%
CHLORAGESIC Rubefacient, counter-irritant (La Crosse)	Each oz.: Chloral hydrate* 10 gr. Methyl salicylate* Menthol*		CHLOR-KIL HOME & GARDEN INSECTICIDE (Durham's)	Tech. chlordane*	5%
CHLOR-AGOL Antiseptic mouth wash (Agol)	Oil of peppermint Oil of anise Boric acid* Salol Sodium benzoate Methyl salicylate* Oil of cloves Oil of thyme Menthol* Turmeric Saccharin Alcohol* 47%/v		CHLORO Insecticide (Beck, I.)	Petroleum distillate* 67% Paradichlorobenzene* 33%	
			CHLOROBEN-ZILATE 15W Insecticide (Geigy)	Ethyl 4,4'-dichlorobenzilate 15%	
			CHLOROCIDE 128 Insecticide (Thompson Chem.)	Tech. chlordane* 73% Petroleum distillate* 17%	
CHLORAJETS Breath deodorizers (Chilton Labs.)	Chlorophyll Corn and cane sugar		CHLORO (CONCEN-TRATED MOTH SPRAY (Chloro)	Petroleum distillate* 67% Paradichlorobenzene* 33%	
CHLORAMEDS COUGH LOZENGES Antitussive (Chilton Labs.)	Chlorophyll Menthol* Glycerin Corn and cane sugar				
CHLORAMINT Antiseptic mouth wash (Purepac)	Alcohol 15%/v Sodium dehydroacetate Sodium n-lauroylsarcosinate Chlorophyll derivatives Mentholized base		CHLORO-FIX TABLETS (Danmar)		
			CHLOROFORM LINIMENT Counter-irritant (Purepac)	Alcohol 45% Chloroform* approx. 30%/v.	
CHLORASAL OINTMENT Rubefacient, counter-irritant (Wisconsin Pharm.)	Chloral hydrate* 10 gr. Menthol Methyl salicylate*		CHLOROGEST TABLETS Antacid (Pharmex)	Aluminum hydroxide 4 gr. Magnesium trisilicate 6 gr. Chlorophyll 50 mg.	
CHLORASOL FUMIGANT (Carbide)	Ethylene dichloride* 70%/w Carbon tetrachloride* 30%/w				

*Consult Sec. II., Ingredients Index. This ingredient may be responsible for major toxic effects if poisonous amounts of this product are ingested.

Name & Use Manufacturer	Ingredients		Name & Use Manufacturer	Ingredients	
CHLOROGIENE DUCHETTES Vaginal douche (Purdue)	Each tablet: Chlorophyll "A" concentrated water-soluble derivatives	3 gm.	CHOOZ (Medicated gum) Antacid, digestant (Pharmaco)	Magnesium trisilicate Calcium carbonate Peppermint oil Sugar Starch Chewing gum base	
	Lactose				
CHLOROLIN DEODORANT STICK (Chlorolin)			CHROM-A-NAL PAINTS (Bownes)		
CHLOROQUINOL Photographic developer (General Photo.)			CHROMATONE PAINTS (Alumatone)		
CHLORO-SALICYLATE OINTMENT Counter-irritant (Kremers)	Chloral hydrate* Menthol* Methyl salicylate*	10 gr./oz.	CHROME FINISH ALUMINUM PAINTS (Ill. Bronze)		
CHLOROSHEEN Dry cleaning detergent (Riverside)			CHROME-GLO Polish (Speco)	Abrasives Ammonia*	
CHLOROTABS Breath freshener (Pharmex)	Blended chlorophyll	100 mg.	CHROME OINTMENT Skin irritation (Wambaugh)	Balm Gilead Lanolin base	
CHLOR PINE EMULSIFI-ABLE Insecticide, disinfectant, deodorant (Collins Feed)	Tech. chlordane* Vegetable oil soap Distilled pine oil*	25.0% 7.5% 60.0%	CHROM-NU-CLEANER (Nat'l. Chem. Labs.)		
			CHYPRE BRILLIAN-TINE, EXTRACT, TOILET WATER (Coty)		
CHLORSPRAY Insecticide, wood preser-vative (Commercial Chem.)	Tech. chlordane	65.5%	CICAL LOTION Skin emollient (Chem. Ind.)	Phenol Glycerin Zinc oxide Lime water	0.80% 1.60% 6.25% 91.35%
CHLORSPRAY Insecticide (Florida Chem.)	Chlordane* Petroleum base oil* Nonionic emulsifier	50% 40% 10%	CICAL LOTION WITH OIL Skin emollient (Chem. Ind.)	Phenol Glycerin Zinc oxide Olive oil Deodorized neatsfoot oil	0.80% 1.60% 6.25% 6.25%
CHLORTHION Insecticide (Chemagro)	o,o-Dimethyl-o-3-chloro-4-nitrophenyl thiophosphate*			Lime water	6.25% 78.85%
CHLOR-TOX 96 Insecticide (Thompson Chem.)	Technical chlorinated camphene* (toxaphene) 60% Aliphatic petroleum hydro-carbons 28%		CIDANTA Antacid (Sharpe & Dohme)	Each 100 cc.: Alcohol Aluminum hydroxide Glycine Oil of maize Magnesium citrate	0.35% 12.5 gm. 3.0 gm. 20.0 gm. 3.0 gm.
CHOCTAW Detergent (Wyandotte)	Concentrated alkali*		CIDSON INK (Davids, T.)		
CHOLAXENE Cholagogue (Jenkins)	Each tablet: Extr. nux vomica* (Strychnine 1/185 gr.) Podophyllin* Sodium glycocholate Extr. wahoo Extr. chionanthus Extr. Taraxacum Hydrastis	1/10 gr. 1/8 gr. 1/2 gr. 1/8 gr. 1/8 gr. 1/8 gr. 1/8 gr.	CIMADROX Antacid, adsorbent (Massengill)	Each tablet: Aluminum hydroxide Magnesium trisilicate Ascorbic acid (as calcium salt)	0.2 gm. 0.4 gm. 20 mg.
			CIMADROX (Powder) Antacid, adsorbent (Massengill)	Each 2 gm.: Aluminum hydroxide Magnesium trisilicate Ascorbic acid (as calcium salt) Aromatic	0.6 gm. 1.2 gm. 60 mg. q.s.
CHOLELITH Laxative (Parke, Davis)	Each pill: Acid sodium oleate Sodium salicylate* Phenolphthalein* Menthol*	1-1/2 gr. 1-1/2 gr. 1/3 gr. q.s.			

*Consult Sec. II., Ingredients Index. This ingredient may be responsible for major toxic effects if poisonous amounts of this product are ingested.

Name & Use Manufacturer	Ingredients
CINCY WALLPAPER CLEANER (Cincy)	Wheat flour Refined kerosene* oil Vegetable dye, salt and preservatives
CINDERELLA LIQUID LEATHER CREAMS (Everett & Barron)	Turpentine* Water-soluble waxes Non-toxic dye
CINDERELLA SUEDE DRESSINGS (Everett & Barron)	Isopropanol*
CINDERELLA WAX FINISHES Shoe dressings (Everett & Barron)	Turpentine* Naphtha*
CINDERELLA WHITE CLEANERS Shoe dressings (Everett & Barron)	Trisodium phosphate Titanium dioxide
CIRCART, CIRCOL Embalming fluids (Embalmers')	Formaldehyde*
CIRCUT ATHLETIC LINIMENT (Chandler)	
CIRICREME VAGINAL CREME (Gray Fox)	Triethanolamine Stearic acid Glycerin Sodium oleate Paraformaldehyde Methyl p-hydroxybenzoate Propyl p-hydroxybenzoate Perfume (rose geranium)
CIRIJEL VAGINAL JELLY (Gray Fox)	Oxyquinoline sulfate* Glycocoll Glycerin Carob gum Starch Propyl p-hydroxybenzoate Lactic acid Boric acid* Tragacanth Karaya Methyl-p-hydroxybenzoate Perfume (violet)

CIRITINE
VAGINAL
DOUCHE
SOLUTION
(Gray Fox)
	Lactic acid
	Eucalyptus*
	Zinc sulfocarbolate
	Thymol*
	Menthol*
	Boric acid*
	Sodium borate, certified dye
	  and dextrose in isotonic sodium
	  chloride base (pH 3.5 in
	  dilution of 1 tbsp. to 1 qt.
	  water)

Name & Use Manufacturer	Ingredients
CISCO 48% TECHNICAL CHLORDANE EMULSION CONCEN- TRATE Insecticide (Am. Disinfect.)	Tech. chlordane* 48% Aliphatic petroleum solvents* 42%
CISTALIC, NO. 1 Diuretic (Massengill)	Each tablet: Atropine sulfate* 0.13 mg. Boric acid 0.13 gm. Potassium bicarbonate 0.13 gm. Extr. buchu 65 mg. Extr. Triticum 65 mg. Extr. corn silk 32 mg. Extr. Hydrangea 32 mg.
CISTALIC, NO. 2 Diuretic (Massengill)	Each tablet: Atropine sulfate* .13 mg. Benzoic acid .2 gm. Sodium borate .13 gm. Extr. buchu 65 mg. Extr. Triticum 65 mg. Extr. corn silk 32 mg. Extr. Hydrangea 32 mg.
CISTALIC, NO. 3 Urinary antiseptic (Massengill)	Each tablet: Atropine sulfate 0.032 mg. Extr. Hyoscyamus* 16 mg. Methenamine 32 mg. Benzoic acid 32 mg. Salol 32 mg. Methylene blue 6.5 mg.
CITROCOL Antitussive (Briggs Lab.)	Each tsp.: Potassium citrate 2-1/2 gr. Ammonium chloride 1/2 gr. Syrup ipecac 4 m. Syrup squill 4 m.
CITRO MULSION Fungicide (Sherwin- Williams)	Petroleum oil* 80%
CITROX Skin ointment (Citrox)	Lanolin Glycerin Stearic acid Sodium benzoate Oil of lemon
CITY FUMIGATING'S LINDANE 25% WETTABLE INSECTICIDE (City Fum.)	Gamma isomer of benzene hexachloride*
C.K. DDT- PARATHION DUST 20-1 Insecticide (Crop King)	DDT 20% Parathion* (o,o-diethyl o-p- nitrophenyl thiophosphate) 1%

CK-20
DISINFECTANT
(Corn King)
	Alkyl ($C_8H_{17}-C_{18}H_{37}$)
	  dimethyl benzyl ammonium
	  chlorides*
	Sodium salt of 2-bromo-4-
	  phenylphenol

CLAIRE FAST-KILL Insecticide (Claire)	Tech. chlordane 1068 2.000% Tech. piperonyl butoxide 0.115% Pyrethrins 0.046% Polymerized glycerol oleate 0.100% Petroleum distillates* 72.739%

---

*Consult Sec. II., Ingredients Index. This ingredient may be responsible for major toxic effects if poisonous amounts of this product are ingested.

- 376 -

Name & Use Manufacturer	Ingredients	Name & Use Manufacturer	Ingredients
CLAIRE INSECT REPELLENT (Claire)	2-Ethyl hexanediol-1,3* 20.00%	CLAX-WAX & CLEANER (Internat. Chem.)	
CLAIRE ROSE & PLANT SPRAY Insecticide (Claire)	Pyrethrins 0.0255% Rotenone 0.128% Other cube extractives 0.236% Tech. piperonyl cyclonene 0.256% Petroleum hydrocarbon 0.102% Inert ingredients*	CLAYOLA MODELING CLAY (Binney & Smith)	Plastic clay Grease-type binder
CLAIR REMOVES HAIR (Carter Co.)	Strontium sulfide*	CLAYTONIA SHOE DRESSING (Sigma)	
CLARKE GYM FINISH Floor sealer (Clarke Sanding)	Tung or China wood oil blended with linseed approx. 25 gal./ 100 lb. resin Modified phenolic and ester gum resin Cobalt, lead* and manganese Mineral spirits* (49 gravity)	CLAYTON'S DOG, CAT & BIRD PREPARA- TIONS (Clayton)	
		CLAYTON'S GOITER MEDICINE For dogs (Clayton)	
CLARKE INSTANT DRYING PENETRATING FLOOR SEALER (Clarke Sanding)	Polystyrene Vegetable oil Fatty acids Epoxy resin Aromatic and aliphatic hydrocarbon* solvents Cobalt based on resin solids 0.01%	CLAYTON'S SONG RESTORER For birds (Clayton)	
CLARKE PASTE WAX MR 203 F (Clarke Sanding)	Paraffin-type waxes Carnauba wax Petroleum solvents* (mineral spirits) Oil of orange 0.01% Perfume 0.02%	CLAYTON'S TAPE WORM EXPELLER For cats and dogs (Clayton)	
CLARKE SELF-POLISH- ING WAX MR 101 & MR 100 (Clarke Sanding)	Carnauba wax Hydrocarbon waxes Morpholine approx. 1% Commercial oleic-stearic acid Borax approx. 1/4% Terpene-phenolic resins	CLEANAID (Williams Soap)	
		CLEAN-ALL (Solvit)	Complex phosphates
CLARKE SELF-POLISH- ING WAX MR 106 (Clarke Sanding)	Carnauba wax Hydrocarbon waxes Morpholine approx. 1% Commercial oleic-stearic acid Borax approx. 1/4% Terpene-phenolic resins DuPont Ludox	CLEANALL DRY CLEANER (Whittemore)	
		CLEAN BRIGHT (United Chem.)	
CLARKE SLIP-RESIS- TANT LIQUID WAX (Clarke Sanding)	Paraffin waxes Carnauba wax Coumarone-indene resins Petroleum solvents* (mineral spirits)	cLEAnegg COMPOUND (Lea)	See Lea Compound (similar to)
		CLEAN HOUSE LIQUID ROACH TRAP (Bell Trap)	
CLARKE WATER EMULSION PASTE WAX MR 104 (Clarke Sanding)	Carnauba wax Paraffin Oxidized microcrystalline wax Borax less than 1/2-3/4% Ammonia approx. 1/4% Organic amine soap of stearic acid	CLEAN-O Fabric cleaner (Packard Dressing)	
CLARK'S PILL Cathartic (Chicago Pharm.)	Extr. belladonna 1/12 gr. Aloin 1/8 gr. Strychnine sulfate* 1/150 gr. Oleoresin capsicum 1/160 gr. Ipecac 1/24 gr. Podophyllin 1/24 gr. Calomel* 1/24 gr. Extr. iris 1/24 gr. Extr. chionanthus 1/65 gr.	CLEAN-O-LITE Floor cleaner (Hillyard Sales)	
		CLEAN-O- SHINE Floor cleaner (Continental Car-Na-Var)	

*Consult Sec. II., Ingredients Index. This ingredient may be responsible for major toxic effects if poisonous amounts of this product are ingested.

Name & Use Manufacturer	Ingredients		Name & Use Manufacturer	Ingredients
CLEAN-SCENT Toilet cleaner (Sanascent)	Sodium bisulfate		CLENSOL CORROSION INHIBITOR COMPOUND (Elk)	Mercurial derivative*
CLEANSILINE Dry cleaner (Assoc. Prod.)	Petroleum ether (naphtha)*		CLENSOL DISHWASHING COMPOUND (Elk)	Caustic alkali* Alkyl aryl sulfonate*
CLEAN WALLPAPER CLEANER (Clean Prod.)	Wheat flour Salt 17% Alum 0.06% Mineral spirits 1.0% Methyl salicylate 0.02% Amacid dye 0.005%		CLENSOL DRAIN PIPE SOLVENT (Elk)	Caustic alkali* Sodium bisulfite
CLEARASIL For acne (Eastco)	Sulfur* Resorcinol*		CLENZOMATIC CLEANING COMPOUNDS (French Ren.)	
CLEARCOTE WALL PAINT (Watson- Standard)			CLEODOFLEX BOWL CLEANER (Williams Soap)	
CLEAREX GLASS CLEANER (Wilco)	Isopropanol* 15%/v Ammonia Dye Perfume		CLEOPATRA'S LOTION Toiletry (Cline)	
CLEAR-GLASS Window cleaner (Cristy)			CLEREX (Hygiene)	Carbohydrate gum Glycerin
CLEAR LAC Paint (Thopmson & Co.)			CLEVELAND CLEANER'S PAINT BRUSH, PAINT & VARNISH CLEANER (Cleveland C. P.)	
CLEARLITE DELUXE PAINT (Payson Corp.)			CLIMALENE Cleaner (Climalene)	Trisodium phosphate* crystalline 100%
CLEARTOX Wood preser- vative, insecticide (Abesto)	Pentachlorophenol*		CLIMATIZED PAINTS (Miller Paint)	
CLENESCO FARM CLEANER (Cowles)	Santomerse Triton X-100* Sodium tripolyphosphate*		CLIMAX WALLPAPER CLEANER (Cleveland C. & P.)	
CLENESCO SANITIZER (Cowles)	Quaternary ammonium compound* Alkyl-dimethyl-benzyl ammonium chloride Sodium carbonates Sodium bicarbonates Sodium tripolyphosphate approx. 60%		CLIMEPROOF PAINT (Van Sickle)	
			CLING FAST ROOF & METAL PAINT (Davis,H.B.)	Pigment: 28.56% Iron oxide pigment Silicates Vehicle: 71.44% Varnish Ferric oxide Silicates Non volatile gilsonite-tung oil 33% Volatile petroleum thinners* 67%
CLENESCO STONE REMOVER (Cowles)	Hydroxyacetic acid Lactic acid Phosphoric acid* approx. 25% Triton X-100			
CLENESCO SUPERCLEN (Cowles)	Sodium metasilicate 25% Sodium carbonate 25% Santomerse 25% Sodium tripolyphosphate 25%		CLINICO HYGIENIC POWDER (Clinic)	Boric acid* Aluminum and potassium sulfate Menthol* Eucalyptol* Methyl salicylate Phenol* Salicylic acid* Thymol* Oxyquinoline sulfate
CLENOPINE Disinfectant (U.S.Sanitary)				

*Consult Sec. II., Ingredients Index. This ingredient may be responsible for major toxic effects if poisonous amounts of this product are ingested.

Name & Use Manufacturer	Ingredients	Name & Use Manufacturer	Ingredients
CLINITEST Urine Sugar Test (Ames Co.)	Each tablet: Anhydrous cupric sulfate 0.019 gr. Anhydrous sodium hydroxide 0.25 gm. Sodium bicarbonate Citric acid	C N DISINFECTANT (West Disinf.)	Coal tar neutral oils Soap Coal tar phenols*
CLINTON CEMENT COLORS (Clinton)	Iron oxides	COAST LABS' CORN SALVE Keratolytic (Coast)	Salicylic acid* Petrolatum base
CLIPPERCIDE DISINFEC- TANTS (King Res.)		COATASTONE FLOOR VARNISH (Johnston)	
CLIPPER SPAR ENAMELS (Fisher- Thorsen)		COAT-O-LITE Paint (Chi-Namel)	Titanium calcium 31.0% Titanium dioxide 12.2% Diatomaceous silica 5.0% Soya alkyd resin 19.6% Maleic resin 1.3% Drier 1.4% Mineral spirits 29.5%
CLO-FILL DIRECT-FLOW Antiseptic tablet (Products)	Alkyl aryl sulfonate Tetrasodium pyrophosphate* Oxyquinoline sulfate	COATSEAL FOUNDATION PAINT (Monroe Co.)	
CLOPANE HYDROCHLOR- IDE Nasal decongestant (Lilly)	Cyclopentamine hydrochloride 0.5% Phenylmercuric nitrate 1-50,000	COBERON Food supplement (La Crosse)	Each tablet: Ferrous sulfate (exsiccated) 4 gr. Copper sulfate 1/40 gr. Thiamine hydrochloride 1 mg.
CLORGRAN 5 Insecticide (Chipman Chem.)	Tech. chlordane 5.0%	CO-CA-SEAL, CO-CA-WALL Paint (Cowman- Campbell)	
CLORGRAN 10 Insecticide (Chipman Chem.)	Tech. chlordane* 10.0%	COCCIN SCARLET (Neo-Coccine) Photographic dye (Eastman)	
CLORGRAN 25 Insecticide (Chipman Chem.)	Tech. chlordane* 25.0%	COCI-ADE Fungicide for coccidiosis (veterinary) (Globe)	Sodium borate* Urea
CLOR-O-FEN Disinfectant (Rochester Germ.)	Alcohol* Soap Ortho-benzyl para-chlorophenol*	COCILO Antitussive (Druggists)	Each oz.: Chloroform 4 m. Wild lettuce Allspice Malt extr. Potassium hypophosphite Manganese hypophosphite Oil of eucalyptus Euphorbia Cocillana Wild cherry bark Calcium hypophosphite Iron hypophosphite Menthol
CLOROX Bleach (Clorox)	Sodium hypochlorite* 5.25% Sodium carbonate 0.20%		
CLOTIN Antihemorr- hagic (vet- erinary) (Gland-O-Lac)	Menadione sodium bisulfite U.S.P.		
C.M.C. TABLETS Laxative (Approved)	Each tablet: Carboxymethylcellulose sodium 0.5 gm.	COCOGREEN Soap (Pacific Chem.)	
CM FLAME RETARDANT (du Pont)	Ammonium sulfamate*	COCO-STER COMPOUND NO.196S Disinfectant (Troy Ind.)	Alkyl dimethyl benzyl ammonium chloride*
C.M.S. PULV. COMP. Antacid, adsorbent (Jewell Pharm.)	Calcium carbonate Sodium bicarbonate Colloidal kaolin Papain Magnesium carbonate Bismuth subcarbonate Diastase Oil of peppermint		

*Consult Sec. II., Ingredients Index. This ingredient may be responsible for major toxic effects if poisonous amounts of this product are ingested.

Name & Use Manufacturer	Ingredients		Name & Use Manufacturer	Ingredients	
CODACOMP Antitussive (Ethical)	Each fl. oz.: Alcohol	3%	**COLABY** Analgesic, cathartic (Massengill)	Each tablet: Acetophenetidin*	32 mg.
	Dihydrocodeinone bitartrate	1/6 gr.		Atropine sulfate	0.022 mg.
	Ephedrine sulfate	3/8 gr.		Aspirin*	32 mg.
	Potassium guaiacol sulfonate	8 gr.		Camphor monobromated*	8 mg.
	Ammonium chloride	8 gr.		Phenolphthalein	6.5 mg.
	Antimony and potassium tartrate	1/12 gr.		Methyl salicylate*	q.s.
	Syrup white pine Syrup wild cherry		**COLAGYN DOUCHE POWDER** (Smith Lab.)	Boric acid* Ammonium alum Carbolic acid*	
CODACOMP A.H. Antitussive, antihistamine (Ethical)	Each fl. oz.: Alcohol	3%		Menthol* Thymol* Eucalyptol*	
	Pyrilamine maleate	90 mg.		Aromatics	
	Dihydrocodeinone bitartrate	1/6 gr.	**COLAGYN VAGINAL**	Chinosol Lactic acid	
	Ephedrine sulfate	3/8 gr.	**JELLY** (Smith Lab.)	Boric acid* Zinc sulfocarbolate *	
	Potassium guaiacolsulfonate	8 gr.		Glycerin Gum tragacanth	
	Ammonium chloride	8 gr.			
	Antimony and potassium tartrate	1/12 gr.	**COLANA** Antitussive (Hance)	Each fl. oz.: Alcohol Tinct. Euphorbia pilulifera	5%
CODACOMP TABLETS Analgesic (Pharmex)	Salicylamide*	1-1/4 gr.			120 m.
	Phenacetin*	2-1/2 gr.		Syrup wild lettuce	120 m.
	Caffeine	1/2 gr.		Tinct. cocillana	40 m.
	Gelsemium	1/10 gr.		Syrup squill compound*	24 m.
	Codeine	100 µg.		Menthol	2/25 gr.
CODILENE Antitussive, antihistamine (Hance)	Each oz.: Codeine phosphate	2/3 gr.	**COLCH-OLATE** Arthritic pain (Walker Pharm.)	Colchicine*	1/60 gr./oz.
	Pyrilamine maleate	36.96 mg.			
	Alcohol	3%/v			
	Potassium citrate		**COLDANE** Insecticide (Columbia)	Gamma isomer of benzene hexachloride*	100%
	Ammonium chloride				
	Potassium guaiacolsulfonate				
	Citric acid		**COLDATE** Analgesic, antipyretic (Massengill)	Each tablet: Opium	1/40 gr.
	Terpin hydrate			Ipecac	1/40 gr.
	Sodium benzoate	0.1%		Acetophenetidin*	1-1/2 gr.
CODOL OINTMENT Skin burns, irritation (Premo)	Cod liver oil			Acetylsalicylic acid*	2 gr.
	Boric acid*			Camphor monobromated*	1/2 gr.
	Lanolin			Caffeine	1/8 gr.
COEXOL (Syrup) Antitussive (Massengill)	Each 5 cc.: Ethylmorphine hydrochloride (morphine derivative) 2.8 mg.		**COLDFOAM LINOLEUM CLEANER, PAINT & VARNISH CLEANER, PORCELAIN, TILE & MARBLE CLEANER** (Savogran)		
	Euphorbia				
	Wild lettuce				
	Cocillana				
	Syrup squill*				
	Tartar emetic*				
	Senega				
	Menthol				
COFFELT'S HAIR COLORING (Coffelt)			**COLDPHOR** Antipyretic, analgesic, laxative (Massengill)	Each tablet: Acetanilid*	0.13 gm.
COFF-O-DYNE Antitussive (Children) (VB)	Squill*			Atropine sulfate	0.032 mg.
	Ipecac			Quinine sulfate	32 mg.
	Ammonium chloride			Camphor*	16 mg.
	Sodium citrate			Podophyllum resin	1.6 mg.
	Potassium guaiacolsulfonate			Aloin	4 mg.
				Oleoresin Capsicum	2.1 mg.
COFSEDEINE (Syrup) Antitussive (Massengill)	Each 5 cc.: Chloroform	43 mg.	**COLE-ADE** Antibiotic for coryza (vet- erinary) (Globe)	Sulfathiazole	40%
	Codeine sulfate	2.1 mg.		Ginger	10%
	White pine compound	0.78 gm.		Gentian	40%
	Sassafras	25 mg.		Nux vomica*	10%
COFFEY'S RAT KILLER (Coffey)					

*Consult Sec. II., Ingredients Index. This ingredient may be responsible for major toxic effects if poisonous amounts of this product are ingested.

Name & Use Manufacturer	Ingredients	
COLEMANITE HIGH GRADE For boron-sensitive crops (Pacific Coast)	Boron trioxide* Calcium oxide	32.6% 33.8%
COLE'S CALPHENOL Skin ointment (Cole, J.W.)	Lanolin Hamamelis Phenol* Calendula Zinc oxide Eucalyptol*	
COLESCO CALSOMINE Paint (Sterling Paint)		
COLE'S VETERINARY SALVE (Cole, J.W.)	Petrolatum Zinc oxide* Fluid extr. witch hazel leaves Lanolin Phenol*	
COLFENE Disinfectant (U.S.Sanitary)		
COLGATE CHLOROPHYLL TOOTH PASTE (Colgate-Palmolive)		
COLGATE LATHER SHAVING CREAM (Colgate-Palmolive)		
COLGATE TOOTH PASTE (Colgate-Palmolive)		
COLIMIX (Veterinary, Liquid) Antispasmodic, carminative (Massengill)	Each fl. oz.: Camphor* Salicylic acid* Oil of turpentine* Castor oil Oleoresin Capsicum Oleoresin ginger Cotton seed oil base	1.2 gm. 1 gm. 8 cc. 16 cc. 0.15 gm. 0.15 gm.
COLIT LINIMENT (Colit)		
COLLA-MAC CEMENT (Lamac)	Neoprene type rubber Synthetic adhesive resins Non lead curing agents Aromatic and ketone type solvents*	
COLLA-MAC THINNER Cement thinner (Lamac)	Aromatic and ketone type solvents*	
COLLINS JEWELL BRAND ROSE DUST Insecticide, fungicide (Collins Feed)	Fermate (duPont ferric dimethyldithiocarbamate) Lindane Sulfur*	7.00% 1.00% 18.00%

Name & Use Manufacturer	Ingredients	
COLLINS LAWN GUARD Insecticide (Collins Feed)	Chlordane* DDT* Hexachloro epoxy octahydro dimethano naphthalene* Related compounds Magnesium sulfate Sulfur *	16.0% 15.0% 3.18% 0.57% 0.5% 13.5%
COLLOIDAL MULTI-FILM C Cotton defoliation (Colloidal)	Alkyl aryl poly oxyethylene Free fatty acids Petroleum oil*	
COLLOIDAL MULTI-FILM L Cotton defoliation (Colloidal)	Petroleum sulfonates Petroleum oil* Free and combined fatty acids	
COLLOIDAL Z-1 Cotton defoliation (Colloidal)	Petroleum sulfonates Combined fatty acids	
COLLO-SUL CREAM Skin irritation (Crookes)	Colloidal sulfur	2%
COLOCAINE Skin ointment (Creviston)	Benzocaine Stearyl alcohol Petrolatum Propylene glycol Polyoxyethylene sorbitan monooleate Methyl and propyl paraben	10%
COL-O-CAPS Analgesic, antipyretic (VB)	Acetophenetidin* Bromocamphor* Acetylsalicylic acid* Caffeine citrate Salicylates*	
COL-O-FLOR PAINT (Sewall)		
COLOGEL Laxative (Lilly)	Each 100 cc.: Alcohol Methyl cellulose	5% 9 gm.
COLOMADE HOUSE PAINT (Colorado)		
COLONIAL CLUB BAY RUM Toiletry (Nelson, Detroit)	Alcohol*	58%
COLONIAL CLUB BRUSHLESS SHAVING CREAM (Nelson, Detroit)		
COLONIAL CLUB CREME OIL HAIR DRESS-ING WITH LANOLIN (Nelson, Detroit)		

*Consult Sec. II., Ingredients Index. This ingredient may be responsible for major toxic effects if poisonous amounts of this product are ingested.

Name & Use Manufacturer	Ingredients		Name & Use Manufacturer	Ingredients	
COLONIAL CLUB DEODORANT FOR MEN (Nelson, Detroit)	Aluminum sulfate		COLONIAL DAMES DUSTING POWDER (Colonial Dames)	Talcum Zinc stearate Iron oxide	
COLONIAL CLUB HAIR TONIC (Nelson, Detroit)	Alcohol*	84%	COLONIAL DAMES FACE POWDER (Colonial Dames)	Zinc oxide Titanium dioxide Talcum Zinc stearate Iron oxide	
COLONIAL CLUB LILAC LOTION Toiletry (Nelson, Detroit)	Alcohol*	68%	COLONIAL DAMES LOTIONS & FACE CREAMS (Colonial Dames)	Lanolin Lanolin derivatives Lecithin Cetyl alcohol White mineral oil U.S.P. Beeswax Petrolatum Stearic acid Glycerol monostearate Borax Triethanolamine Perfume oil Parahydroxybenzoic acid esters	1/10-1/5%
COLONIAL CLUB SHAMPOO (Nelson, Detroit)	Alcohol*	47%			
COLONIAL CLUB SHAVING LOTION (Nelson, Detroit)	Alcohol*	51%	COLONIAL DAMES SKIN FRESHENER (Colonial Dames)	Denatured alcohol* 40 approx. 15% Brucine sulfate Tertiary butyl alcohol* Hexachlorophene	
COLONIAL DAMES BEAUTY WASH, MAKE-UP BEAUTIFIER (Colonial Dames)	Almond meal Oat meal Magnesium and calcium carbonate Perfume oils		COLONIAL PAINTS (Colonial)		
COLONIAL DAMES BUBBLE BATH (Colonial Dames)	Anionic wetting agents Sodium sulfate Perfume oil		COLONIAL, PURITAN, SILEX LUBRICAT-ING GREASE (Borne-Scrymser)		
COLONIAL DAMES COLOGNES (Colonial Dames)	Denatured alcohol* Diethyl phthalate Perfume oil	75% 1%	COLONIAL WALL FINISH (Morris Paint)		
COLONIAL DAMES CREAM MAKE-UP, EYE SHADOW, LIPSTICK, MASCARA, ROUGE (Colonial Dames)			COLOPTIN Eye wash (Massengill)	Boric acid* Glycerin Camphor water Phenylmercuric nitrate* Sodium borate* Berberine sulfate Rose water	
			COLORADO .44 BRUSH MURDER Herbicide (Chem. Corp.)	Each gallon: 2,4-Dichlorophenoxyacetic acid* 1.66 lb. 2,4,5-Trichlorophenoxyacetic acid* as esters 1.66 lb.	
COLONIAL DAMES DEPILATORIES NO. 1 (Colonial Dames)	Calcium carbonate Barium sulfide*		COLORADO .44 BUG KILLER (Chem. Corp.)	Piperonyl butoxide tech. 0.575% Pyrethrins 0.114% Petroleum oil* 99.311%	
COLONIAL DAMES DEPILATORIES NO. 2 (Colonial Dames)	Calcium carbonate Strontium sulfide*		COLORADO .44 CHLORDANE CONCENTRATE Insecticide (Chem. Corp.)	Tech. chlordane* 44% Petroleum oil 46% Polyoxyethylene sorbitol oleatelaurate 10%	
			COLORADO .44 BUTYL ESTER OF 2,4-D Herbicide (Chem. Corp.)	2,4-Dichlorophenoxyacetic acid* butyl ester	

*Consult Sec. II., Ingredients Index. This ingredient may be responsible for major toxic effects if poisonous amounts of this product are ingested.

Name & Use Manufacturer	Ingredients	
COLORADO .44 DDT EMULSION CONCEN- TRATE Insecticide (Chem. Corp.)	Tech. DDT*	25%
COLORADO .44 DDT WETT- ABLE POW- DER Insecticide (Chem. Corp.)	Tech. DDT*	50%
COLORADO .44 GARDEN SPRAY (Chem. Corp.)	Gamma isomer of benzene hexachloride (from lindane) 0.625% Inert ingredients* 99.375%	
COLORADO .44 GOLD STAR LIVESTOCK & BARN CON- CENTRATE Insecticide (Chem. Corp.)	Each gallon: Chlordane* 2.331 lb. DDT* 2.331 lb. Piperonyl butoxide Pyrethrins	
COLORADO .44 INSECTICIDE (Chem. Corp.)		
COLORADO .44 ISOPROPYL ESTER OF 2,4-D Herbicide (Chem. Corp.)	Each gallon: 2,4-Dichlorophenoxyacetic acid* 3.33 lb.	
COLORADO .44 KILZIT Insecticide (Chem. Corp.)	Petroleum oil* Tech. chlordane* B-butoxy-β'-thiocyano diethyl ether*	
COLORADO .44 OCTA-KILL Insecticide (Chem. Corp.)	Tech. chlordane	2-1/2%
COLORADO .44 RID-O-WEED Herbicide (Chem. Corp.)	Dimethylamine salt 2,4-dichlorophenoxyacetic acid* 18.1%	
COLORADO .44 SUPER 80 BUTYL ESTER OF 2,4-D Herbicide (Chem. Corp.)	Each gallon: 2,4-Dichlorophenoxyacetic acid* 6.4 lb.	
COLORADO .44 SUPERSPRAY Insecticide (Chem. Corp.)	Tech. chlordane*	76%
COLORADO .44 TOXAPHENE CONCEN- TRATE Insecticide (Chem. Corp.)	Toxaphene*	74%
COLORADO .44 2,4-D WEED KILLER LI- QUID AMINE CONCEN- TRATE (Chem. Corp.)	Each gallon: 2,4-Dichlorophenoxyacetic acid* (amine salt) 4 lb.	

Name & Use Manufacturer	Ingredients	
COLORADO WETTABLE DUST CON- CENTRATE Insecticide (Chem. Corp.)	Tech. chlordane*	40%
COLORAMA Dye (North American)	Aniline dyes* Levelling agent Wetting agent Water softener	
COLOR-CRAFT PAINTS (Alabama)		
COLORFAST OIL STAIN (Chi-Namel)		
COLORGLAZE (Semi-liquid colored wax base finish) (Horn)	Wax Color Mineral spirits*	
COLOR IT PLASTER COLOR (Alabastine)		
COLORIZER PAINTS (Vane-Calvert)		
COLOR-RAY COLORED CHALK (Am. Art Clay)		
COLOR-RAY POSTER & EASEL PAINT (Am. Art Clay)		
COLOR-SET 1004 Preharvest apple drop (Dow)	Alkanolamine salt alpha-(2,4,5-trichlorophenoxy) propionic acid*	
COLOR SPRAY Cosmetic (Occasion)		
COLORTHRU MASONRY ENAMEL (Evercrete)		
COLORTONE POWDER COLORS Crayons (Bradley, M.)		
COLORTREAD PAINT (Tremco)		
COLORWAX PLASTER COLORS (Tamms)		
COLOTONE LAXATIVE WAFERS (Colotone)	Each wafer: Powdered senna leaves* on mfg. label TV 10 gr. Powdered extr. belladonna* leaves 1/8 gr. Powdered extr. licorice and oil of anise q.s.	

*Consult Sec. II., Ingredients Index. This ingredient may be responsible for major toxic effects if poisonous amounts of this product are ingested.

Name & Use Manufacturer	Ingredients		Name & Use Manufacturer	Ingredients	
COL-O-VAR STAIN (Sewall)			COLUMBIAN DRY INSECTICIDE (Columbian)	Naphthalene* Sulfur Nicotine alkaloid*	25.0% 9.0% 00.1%
COL-O-WALL PAINT (Sewall)			COLUMBIAN STOCK DIP (Creosote Base) Insecticide (Columbian)	Coal tar neutral oil, anhydrous soap, phenols* (phenol coefficient 3 F.D.A.)	90%
COLSPAR VARNISH (Sterling Paint)					
COLSUL Colloidal sulfur cream paste (Bartlett, N.M.)	Sulfur*	48%	COLUMBIA PAINT (Phelan-Faust)		
COLUMA Antacid, adsorbent (Premo)	Aluminum hydroxide gel Peppermint		COLUMBIA PAINT (Wadsworth)		
COLUMBIA AMMONIA (Columbia)	Ammonia*		COLUMBIA ROACH POWDER (Sturtevant)	Sodium fluoride* Sodium silicofluoride	71.25% 0.75%
COLUMBIA ANTISEPTIC POWDER Skin burns, irritation (Sturtevant)	Boric acid* Carbolic acid* Zinc oxide Talc		COLUMBIA SYRUP COSICARA Antitussive (Meyer Bros.)	Alcohol Cocillana bark Euphorbia pilulifera Senega Yerba santa Extr. cascara Codeine sulfate* Squill* Wild lettuce Menthol*	3% 1/4 gr.
COLUMBIA ANT POW-DER (Sturtevant)	Tech. chlordane	5%			
COLUMBIA BRAND PRO-RUB Rubbing compound (Meyer Bros.)	Isopropyl alcohol*	70%/v	COLUSA Skin ointment (J & J)	Salicylic acid* Methyl salicylate* Carbolic acid Petroleum oil base	 1/2%
COLUMBIA BRAND SO-FLO Insecticide (Meyer Bros.)	Sodium fluoride*	95%	COLUSA ANTIBIOTIC OINTMENT Antiseptic (J & J)	Tyrothricin Benzocaine Hexachlorophene Zinc oxide Salicylic acid* Petrolatum Menthol* Glycerol monostearate Yellow beeswax Petroleum oil base	0.05% 5%
COLUMBIA CHER-CO-SED Antitussive (Meyer Bros.)	Alcohol Chloroform White pine bark Cherry bark Blood root Spikenard Codeine phosphate* Potassium guaiacolsulfonate ammonium chloride Tartar emetic* Balsam poplar buds Sassafras	3% 2 m. 1 gr.			
			COLYPTUS GOLDEN COUGH EXPECTOR-ANT (Commerce)	Honey Oil of eucalyptus* Pine tar* Creosote* Alcohol	 2.0%
COLUMBIA FLEA POW-DER (Sturtevant)	Pyrethrins Rotenone Other cube extracts Sulfur	0.5% 1.0% 1.0% 5.0%	COMATE MEDICINAL EMULSION Emollient, external (Comate)	Chloral hydrate Sodium phenolsulfonate* Sulfonated castor oil Resorcinol monoacetate	0.27%
COLUMBIA GLYCO-CIDE FOR AIR SANITATION (Columbia)	Triethylene glycol*	90%	COMATE MEDICINAL LOTION For the scalp (Comate)	Cinnamic acid Beta naphthol* Sodium sulfocarbolate* Alcohol	 37-1/2%
COLUMBIAN CATTLE-RUB OIL Insecticide (Columbian)	Petroleum oil* Dichloro diphenyl trichloro-ethane* Pine oil* Phenols* Sulfur*		COMESOL NOSE DROPS Sinus deconges-tant (Park-Adams)	Olive oil Menthol* Camphor* Oil of eucalyptus* Oil of peppermint	

*Consult Sec. II., Ingredients Index. This ingredient may be responsible for major toxic effects if poisonous amounts of this product are ingested.

Name & Use Manufacturer	Ingredients		Name & Use Manufacturer	Ingredients	
COMET MODEL AIRPLANE CEMENT Plastic cement (Comet)			COMMON SENSE COCKROACH PREPARATION (Common Sense)	Phosphorus*	2%
COMFORT POWDER (Parke, Davis)	Talc Corn starch Zinc stearate Exsiccated alum Magnesium carbonate Salicylic acid Phenol	3% 1.5% 0.3% 0.5% 0.25%	COMMON SENSE DDT DUST Insecticide (Common Sense)	DDT*	10%
COMFORT'S MILK OF MAGNESIA TOOTHPASTE (Comfort)	Glycerin C.P. Corn starch Gum tragacanth Saccharin Soap Calcium carbonate Magma		COMMON SENSE INSECT SPRAY (Common Sense)	Pyrethrum DDT Inert ingredients*	5%
COMMERCE BRAND SELF-POLISHING WAX (Butcher)	Waxes Oleic acid Morpholine Borax* Caustic soda Bleached shellac emulsified with ammonia		COMMON SENSE RAT PREPARATION (Common Sense)	Phosphorus*	2%
			COMMUNITY PAINTS (Empire Varnish)		
COMMERCE DRUG'S TOILET LANOLIN (Homogenized) (Commerce)			COMO SADDLE SOAP (Kopf)	Glycerin	
COMMERCE DRUG'S WHITE PINE & TAR COUGH SYRUP (Commerce)	Alcohol Chloroform White pine bark Wild cherry bark Aralia Poplar buds Ammonium chloride	2% 2 m.	COMPASS MARINE PAINTS (Reeder)		
COMMERCE DRUG'S ZINC OXIDE OINTMENT WITH TYROTHRICIN (Commerce)	Tyrothricin Zinc oxide Petrolatum	0.05%	COMP CLEANSER-SANITIZER-DISINFECTANT DEODORANT (Fuld)	Soap Isopropanol Ortho-benzyl para-chlorophenol	10.0% 3.0% 2.0%
COMMERCIAL CHEMICALS D.D.T. EMULSION Insecticide (Commercial Chem.)	Commercial DDT*	25%	COMPO-TEX PLASTIC PAINT (Fox)		
			COMPOSITION FLOOR SEAL (Holcomb, J.I.)	Isopropyl alcohol* Cellosolve*	
COMMERCIAL CHEMICALS GAMMA DUST 5 Insecticide (Commercial Chem.)	Gamma isomer of benzene hexachloride	0.5%	COMPOSOL (Purity)	Phenol*	
COMMERCIAL SOLVENTS BHC Insecticide (Commercial Solv.)	Gamma isomer of benzene hexachloride, * tech. granular	12-15%	COMPO THE GARDENER'S FRIEND Odorless fertilizer (Niagara Hort.)	Ammonium sulfate Super phosphate* Lime*	
			COMQUAT SANITIZER (Commercial Chem.)		
COMMERCIAL SOLVENT'S METALDEHYDE Slug baits (Insecticide) (Commercial Solv.)	Metaldehyde*		COMSTOCK'S NERVE & BONE LINIMENT (Comstock)	Terebinthina* Lini semina Pix canadensis* Ammonium hydroxide*	2 oz. 0.5 oz. 0.25 oz. 0.25 oz.

*Consult Sec. II., Ingredients Index. This ingredient may be responsible for major toxic effects if poisonous amounts of this product are ingested.

Name & Use Manufacturer	Ingredients	Name & Use Manufacturer	Ingredients
COMSTOCK'S WORM PELLETS (Comstock)	Santonin*	CONQUEROR PAINT (Jewell P.&V.)	
CONALUME PAINT (Continental Prod.)		CONQUEST Perfume (Perkins)	
CONCEN- TRATED BORASCU Herbicide (Pacific Coast)	Sodium oxide 28.0% Boron trioxide* 61.5% Equiv. anhydrous borax 89.0%	CONSERVO WOOD PRESERVA- TIVE (Cabot)	
CONCORD BRAND FUNGICIDE (Ellis Chem.)		CONSUMERS PAINT BRUSH CLEANER, WATERPROOF FILLER CEMENT (Consumer's Glue)	
CONCRETE PATCHER (United Gilson.)	Sand Cement		
CONCRETE SEAL (Holcomb)	Xylene* Cyclohexanone* Methyl isobutyl ketone*	CONSUMER'S SPECIAL HAND LOTION (Special Formula)	
CONCRE- WALTUM PAINT FOR CONCRETE (Vita-Var)		CONTAX WEED KILLER (Calif. Spray)	Dinitro ortho secondary amyl phenol* 75%
C-1 IDEAL BLACK STENCIL INK (Ideal Stencil)	Fuel oil Black carbon Stoddard solvent*	CONTENDER HOUSE PAINTS (Franklin, B.)	
CONFIDENCE BRAND LACQUERS (Southern Lacquer)		CONTI CASTILE SOAP (Williams,J.B.)	Sodium soap (primarily oleate)
CONFLICT BOUQUET CONCEN- TRATE, BOUQUET STICK, SPRAY DEODORANT (Blanchard)		CONTINENTAL HEMATINIC TABLETS Food supplement (Continental Drug)	Ferrous gluconate 5 gr. Folic acid 0.3 mg. Zinc sulfate 3.99 mg. Vitamin B12 1 mg. Copper sulfate 2.8 mg. Manganese sulfate 4.7 mg.
CONFLOREX PAINT (Claronex)		CONTINENTAL PAINT (Continental Prod.)	
CONGO EAU DE PARFUM (Harris,B.)		CONTI SHAMPOO (Williams,J.B.)	Potassium soap
CONIDE-20 Disinfectant (Gland-O-Lac)	Methyl alkyl benzyl trimethyl ammonium chloride* 20% Isopropyl alcohol 30%	CONTRA CREME Spermicide (Contra)	Phenylmercuric acetate 0.06% Triethanolamine 0.06% Glycerin 2.5% Glycol monostearate 3.5% Stearic acid 12%
CONOLINE PAINT THINNER (Continental Prod.)		CONTRAST Photographic developer (General Photo.)	
CONQUERINE Tonic (Conquerine)	Tinct. nux vomica 13/500 gr. Fluid extr. belladonna leaf 1/220 gr. Cascara Capsicum Aromatics	CONTREX (Jeffrey-Fell)	Lactic acid Oxyquinoline sulfate Glycerin Tragacanth Starch

*Consult Sec. II., Ingredients Index. This ingredient may be responsible for major toxic effects if poisonous amounts of this product are ingested.

Name & Use Manufacturer	Ingredients		Name & Use Manufacturer	Ingredients	
COOK & DUNN HARMONY HUES Paint (Cook & Dunn)			COOL-A-PED (Stanley Home)	Cetyl alcohol Orvus WA paste Butoben Essential oils Certified dye	
COOK'S CHLORDANE EMULSION CONCEN- TRATE Insecticide (Cook Chem.)	Chlordane* Aliphatic petroleum solvent*	44.4% 44.5%	COOLING LOTION NO. 867 Anti-perspi- rant (Specialists)	Glycerin Menthol* Salicylic* and benzoic acids Ethyl alcohol*	50%/v
COOK'S GAS GO TABLETS (Cook, T.)			COOL TINCTURE S.F. NO. 874 External ear canal antiseptic (Specialists)	Menthol* Acetone* Alcohol*	50%/v
COOK'S MILL SPRAY (Non- toxic) Insecticide (Cook Chem.)	Pyrethrins Piperonyl butoxide Aliphatic petroleum solv.*	0.13% 1.27% 98.60%			
COOK'S NU-WAY CORN REMOVER (Cook, T.)			CO-OP CATTLE GRUB POWDER Insecticide (Cotton)	Rotenone Sulfur*	1.6% 45%
COOK'S RAT & MOUSE KILLER (Cook, T.)			CO-OP 5% CHLORDANE DUST Insecticide (Cotton)	Tech. chlordane	5.0%
COOK'S REFINED CHLORDANE CONCEN- TRATE 20% Insecticide (Cook Chem.)	Chlordane* in oil	20%	CO-OP 6.5 COPPER DUST Fungicide (Cotton)	Tribasic copper sulfate*	6.5%
COOK'S 2% REFINED CHLORDANE SURFACE SPRAY Insecticide (Cook Chem.)	Chlordane in oil Inert ingredients*	2%	CO-OP 3-10 COTTON DUST Insecticide (Cotton)	Gamma isomer of benzene hexachloride* Other isomers of benzene hexachloride Dichloro diphenyl trichloro- ethane*	3.00% 6.00% 10.00%
COOK'S ROACH POWDER (Cook, T.)			CO-OP 3-10-40 COTTON DUST Insecticide (Cotton)	Gamma isomer of benzene hexachloride* Other isomers of benzene hexachloride DDT* Sulfur*	3.00% 6.00% 10.00% 40.00%
COOK'S SPOT MILL FUMIGANT (Cook Chem.)	Ethylene dichloride* Carbon tetrachloride* Ethylene dibromide*		CO-OP 20-40 COTTON DUST Insecticide (Cotton)	Toxaphene* Sulfur	20% 40%
COOK'S STOCK-BARN & GARDEN INSECT KILLER (Cook Chem.)	DDT Chlordane Aliphatic petroleum solv. Methylated naphthalenes*	12.5% 12.5% 34.0% 34.0%	CO-OP 3% DDT Insecticide (Cotton)	DDT	3%
			CO-OP 5% DDT Insecticide (Cotton)	DDT* Sulfur*	5% 90%
COOK'S WART REMOVER (Cook, T.)			CO-OP 5% DDT- SULPHUR DUST Insecticide (Cotton)	DDT * Sulfur*	5.0% 83.5%
CO-OL Rubefacient (Sorbol)	Menthol* Camphor thymol* Oil of turpentine* Oil of cedar leaf Oil of eucalyptus Oil of nutmeg		CO-OP 10% DDT DUST Insecticide (Cotton)	DDT*	10%

*Consult Sec. II., Ingredients Index. This ingredient may be responsible for major toxic effects if poisonous amounts of this product are ingested.

Name & Use Manufacturer	Ingredients		Name & Use Manufacturer	Ingredients	
COOPERATIVE ASSOCIATION SODIUM FLUORIDE Anthelmintic (veterinary) (Coop.Assoc.)	Sodium fluoride*	95%	COOPER'S SHEEP DIPPING POWDER Insecticide (Cooper)	Sodium arsenate Sodium thioarsenate Arsenic sulfide Arsenic trioxide* Sulfur Rotenone Other derris resins Arsenic sulfite residue	17.85% 3.81% 3.81% 11.91% 60% 1.21% 0.50% 1.91%
COOPER CREME Contraceptive (Whittaker)	Trioxymethylene U.S.P.0.04% Sodium oleate 0.67% Stearic acid 23.04% Trihydroxyethylamine 7.91% Dioctyl sodium sulfosuccinate 0.50% Hydrous aluminum silicate 2.34%		COOPER'S UNIVERSAL BALM Tonic, carminative (Myers Labs.)	Alcohol Benzoin Red pepper Cinnamon Spearmint Eucalyptus Sassafras Ginger Camphor Cloves Oils of origanum, peppermint, cajuput, pennyroyal, anise	60%
COOPER CREME GEL Contraceptive (Whittaker)	Trioxymethylene U.S.P.0.04% Sodium oleate 0.67% Carboxymethylcellulose Trihydroxyethylamine 7.91% Dioctyl sodium sulfosuccinate 0.50% Hydrous aluminum silicate 2.34%				
			COOPER-TOX LIVESTOCK DIP OR SPRAY Insecticide (Cooper)	Toxaphene*	61%
COOPER & NEPHEWS INSECTICI-DAL SKIN DRESSING (Cooper)	Rotenone 1% Other cube resins 1.5% Inert ingredients* 93.5%		CO-OP 1% PARATHION DUST Insecticide (Cotton)	Parathion*	1%
COOPER PHENOTHI-AZINE ARSENATE DRENCH Anthelmintic (veterinary) (Cooper)	Each fl. oz.: Phenothiazine 12-1/2 gm. Lead arsenate* 1/2 gm.		CO-OP SPECIAL COTTON DUST Insecticide (Cotton)	Toxaphene* (tech. chlorinated camphene) 20.0% Parathion* 1.0%	
COOPER PHENOTHI-AZINE DRENCH Anthelmintic (veterinary) (Cooper)	Each fl. oz.: Phenothiazine* 10 gm.		CO-OP 5% TDE DUST Insecticide (Cotton)	Dichloro diphenyl dichloroethane 5.00%	
COOPER PHENOTHI-AZINE DRENCH Anthelmintic (veterinary) (Cooper)	Phenothiazine* 12-1/2 gm./fl.oz.		CO-OP 10% TDE DUST Insecticide (Cotton)	Dichloro diphenyl dichloroethane 10.00%	
COOPER'S CATTLE DIP Insecticide (Cooper)	Arsenic trioxide* Soap Cresylic acid*		CO-OP 10% TOXAPHENE DUST Insecticide (Cotton)	Tech. chlorinated camphene* 10.00%	
COOPER'S CATTLE GRUB & LOUSE POWDER (Cooper)	Rotenone 1.5% Other derris resins 2%		CO-OP 20% TOXAPHENE COTTON DUST Insecticide (Cotton)	Toxaphene*	20%
COOPER'S DAIRY AND STOCK SPRAY WITH PYRENONE Insecticide (Cooper)	Mineral oil Tech. piperonyl butoxide Pyrethrins*		COPA Insecticide (Planetary Chem.)	Malathion*	2%
			COPAC (Ampules Yellow) Analgesic (Superior Pharm.)	Each ampule: Acetophenetidin* 2 gr. Aspirin* 4 gr. Caffeine alkaloid 1/4 gr.	
COOPER'S MILK OIL DIP Insecticide (Cooper)	Phenols* 16% Coal tar oils* 56% Soap 17%		COP-O-ZINK Fungicide (Tenn. Corp.)	Copper* as metallic 42% Zinc* as metallic 11%	

*Consult Sec. II., Ingredients Index. This ingredient may be responsible for major toxic effects if poisonous amounts of this product are ingested.

Name & Use Manufacturer	Ingredients		Name & Use Manufacturer	Ingredients	
COPPER BRITE POLISH (Copper Brite)			COPPERTONE SUN TAN LOTION (Douglas Labs.)	Lanolin Cocoa butter Glyceryl monostearate Stearic acid Meta homo menthyl salicylate* Triethanolamine Methyl paraben Propylene glycol	
COPPER CAPRYLATE COMPOUND OINTMENT External fungicide (medical) (C & M)	Copper caprylate Zinc caprylate Caprylic acid Salicylic acid Propylene glycol caprylates Aranol Carbowax	6% 3% 6.5% 1.7% 10%	COPPERTONE SUN TAN OIL (Douglas Labs.)	Lanolin Cocoa butter Liquid petrolatum Meta homo menthyl salicylate*	
COPPER CAPRYLATE COMPOUND SOLUTION Fungicide (external medical) (C & M)	Copper caprylate Zinc caprylate Caprylic acid Salicylic acid Propylene glycol caprylates Aranol n-Propyl alcohol*	6% 3% 5% 1.7% 35%	COPPERTONE SUN TAN OIL- AEROSOL (Douglas Labs.)	Lanolin Cocoa butter Liquid petrolatum Meta homo menthyl salicylate* Freon 11 and 12	
COPPER- CLEAN (Jaye)			COPPER-TOX Fungicide (Doggett- Pfeil)	Ammoniated copper*	3%
COPPER- CLEANER (Cop-R-Nu)			COPPERTREAT 80 CONCEN- TRATE Wood preser- vative (Wood-Treating)	Copper naphthenate* Hydrocarbon solvent*	80% 20%
COPPER HYDRO Fungicide (Chipman Chem.)	Copper* hydroxysulfate	26%	COPPO CLEAR Wood preser- vative (King Chem.)	Petroleum distillate* 85.1000% Zinc naphthenate (zinc as metal 1%) 7.7500% Tetrachlorphenol 0.0975% Coconutamine 0.0900%	
COPPER HYDRO BORDO Fungicide (Chipman Chem.)	Copper* hydroxysulfate	13%	COPPO COPPER NAPHTHENATE Wood preser- vative (King Chem.)	Petroleum distillate* Copper naphthenate	90% 10%
COPPERIN A Food supplement (Jewell Pharm.)	Each capsule: Iron Copper	32.0 mg. 1.0 mg.	COP-R-NU COPPER CLEANER (Cop-R-Nu)		
COPPERIN B FOR CHILD- REN Food supplement (Jewell Pharm.)	Each capsule: Iron Copper	32.0 mg. 0.25 mg.	COPRQURE Fungicide (Bonide)	Copper oxychloride* (copper 6%) 10.1%	
COPPERSHEEN Polish (General Printing)			COP-R-STICK Copper and brass cleaner (Embree)		
COPPERTONE NOSKOTE Sun tan oil (Douglas Labs.)	Lanolin Cocoa butter Beeswax Paraffin Amber petrolatum Meta homo menthyl salicylate*		CO-QUINA (Veltex)	Each fl. oz.: Quinine sulfate Chocolate base	10 gr.
COPPERTONE SHADE (Formely Soltek), COPPERTONE SUN TAN CREAM Sun tan creams (Douglas Labs.)	Lanolin Cocoa butter Beeswax Stearic acid Glyceryl monostearate Amber petrolatum Meta homo menthyl salicylate* Sodium borate*		CORASEM Bronchial decongestant (Massengill)	Each tablet: Atropine sulfate* Strychnine sulfate* Quinine sulfate Arsenic trioxide* Camphor*	1/600 gr. 1/240 gr. 1/10 gr. 1/240 gr. 1/4 gr.

*Consult Sec. II., Ingredients Index. This ingredient may be responsible for major toxic effects if poisonous amounts of this product are ingested.

Name & Use Manufacturer	Ingredients		Name & Use Manufacturer	Ingredients	
CO-RECTALS Hemorrhoids (Am. Druggists)	Each suppository: Extr. stramonium alkaloids	1/500 gr.	CORITENE Tonic, internal fungicide (veterinary) (Gland-O-Lac)	Arsanilic acid* Arsenic as metallic	3.26% 1.12%
	Benzocaine Phenol* Tannic acid* Zinc oxide Lanolin and cocoa butter base		CORNELL CHLORDANE RESIDUAL SPRAY Insecticide (Cornell Chem.)	Petroleum distillate* Tech. chlordane*	
	Lotion concentrate: Tinct. green soap Camphor* Menthol* Ti tree oil Butyl parahydroxy benzoate		CORNELL EQ-53 MOTHPROOFER FOR WASHABLE WOOLENS (Cornell Chem.)	Dichloro diphenyl trichloroethane*	25%
CORDAY JASMEN, MUGUET, CORDETTE EAU de TOILETTE, PERFUME (Parfums Corday)			CORNELL GRAINGARD Insecticide (Cornell Chem.)	Pyrethrins* Piperonyl butoxide	
CORDO THINNER #2027 (Cordo)	Ketones Aromatic hydrocarbons*		CORNELL HEPTACHLOR EM 2 Insecticide (Cornell Chem.)	Heptachlor* Related compounds Xylene*	23.2% 9.0% 63.0%
CORECTOR WAVE Permanent wave (Vienna)	Waving solution: Ammonium thioglycolate approx. 7-1/2% Neutralizer: Sodium bromate* (12% strength) 4 fl. oz.		CORNELL METHOXYCHLOR 25 E Insecticide (Cornell Chem.)	Methoxychlor* Xylene* Aromatic petroleum deriv. solvent	25% 63% 7%
CORELS Cathartic (Clapp, Otis)	Aloin* Ipomea Extr. belladonna* Podophyllin* Extr. cascara sagrada		CORNELL PENTA-GARD Insecticide (Cornell Chem.)	Pentachlorophenol* Petroleum distillate*	
CORENTA (Upjohn)	Each fl. oz.: Hydrastis (equiv.) 8 gr. Rhubarb (equiv.) 15 gr. Krameria (equiv.) 12 gr. Zinc sulfocarbolate 2 gr. Calcium sulfocarbolate 5 gr. Sodium sulfocarbolate 5 gr. Alcohol 23%		CORNELL PYRENONE BARN & STOCK SPRAY Insecticide (Cornell Chem.)	Tech. piperonyl butoxide 11.87% Pyrethrins 1.18% Polyoxyethylene sorbitol mixed ether ester 72.01%	
CORICIDIN PEDIATRIC MEDILETS Colds (Schering)	Each Medilet: Chlorprophenpyridamine maleate 0.75 mg. Aspirin* 80 mg. Phenacetin* 16 mg.		CORNELL PYRENONE INSECT SPRAY (Cornell Chem.)	Tech. piperonyl butoxide 1.1% Pyrethrins 0.2% Petroleum distillate* 98.7%	
CORICIDIN SYRUP For treatment of coughs, aches and pain associated with colds (Schering)	Each 5 cc.: Dihydrocodeinone bitartrate 1.67 mg. Chlorprophenpyridamine maleate 2 mg. Sodium salicylate* 225 mg. Sodium citrate 120 mg. Caffeine 30 mg. Glyceryl guaiacolate 30 mg.		CORNELL PYRENONE SPACE SPRAY Insecticide (Cornell Chem.)	Petroleum distillate* Piperonyl butoxide Pyrethrins	
CORICIDIN TABLETS Colds (Schering)	Each tablet: Chlorprophen pyridamine maleate 2 mg. Aspirin* 0.23 gm. Phenacetin* 0.16 gm. Caffeine 0.03 gm.		CORNELL TOXAPHENE E-60 Insecticide (Cornell Chem.)	Toxaphene* Petroleum distillate	60% 30%
CORIDENE Tonic, internal fungicide (veterinary) (Gland-O-Lac)	Arsanilic acid (4.73 gr. arsenic as metallic) 13.7 gr./oz. Hydrochloric acid		CORNELL'S LINIMENT (Cornell Med.)		

*Consult Sec. II., Ingredients Index. This ingredient may be responsible for major toxic effects if poisonous amounts of this product are ingested.

Name & Use Manufacturer	Ingredients
CORN KING DAIRY-CLEAN POWDER Detergent-sanitizer (Corn King)	Sodium carbonate Di-isobutyl phenoxy ethoxy ethyl dimethyl benzyl ammonium chloride monohydrate*
CORN KING FARM BIN SPRAY Insecticide (Corn King)	Petroleum distillates* 88.57% Methylated aromatic petroleum deriv.* 8.14% Methoxychlor tech. (dimethoxy diphenyl trichloroethane) 2.50% n-Octyl bicycloheptene dicarboximide 0.38% Allethrin (allyl homolog of cinerin 1) 0.04%
CORN KING FLY SPRAY CONCEN-TRATE, FLY SPRAY FOR LIVESTOCK AND STABLE (Corn King)	Petroleum distillates* Beta butoxy beta' thiocyano diethyl ether* Pine oil*
CORN KING FLY SPRAY WITH 0.5% METHOXY-CHLOR (Corn King)	Petroleum distillates* Beta butoxy beta' thiocyano diethyl ether* Pine oil* Methoxy chlor* tech. (dimethoxy diphenyl trichloroethane)
CORN KING GRAIN FUMIGANT FOR ELEVA-TORS, FOR FARM USE (Corn King)	Carbon tetrachloride* Benzene* Sulfur dioxide Ethylene dibromide*
CORN KING GRUB POWDER Insecticide (Corn King)	Rotenone 1.67% Other cube resins 3.98%
CORN KING HOG WORMER Anthelmintic (veterinary) (Corn King)	Each oz.: Copper acetoarsenite* (19 gr. arsenic trioxide) Antimonyl potassium tartrate* (8 gr. antimony trioxide) Phenothiazine 22%
CORN KING INCUBATOR FUMIGANT (Corn King)	Furfural* Formaldehyde*
CORN KING INHALANT Respiratory decongestant (veterinary) (Corn King)	Creosote Oil of eucalyptus* Oil of camphor Gum camphor* Cresol* Pine oil
CORN KING K-12 DISINFECTANT (Corn King)	Petroleum hydrocarbons* Pine oil* Soap Chloro-o-phenylphenol o-Phenylphenol Isopropyl alcohol*
CORN KING LARGE ROUNDWORM TABLETS Anthelmintic (veterinary) (Corn King)	Each tablet: Antimony potassium tartrate* (6.7 gr. antimony trioxide) Copper sulfate* 0.27 gr. Cobalt sulfate Sodium phenolsulfonate Boric acid*

Name & Use Manufacturer	Ingredients
CORN KING LOUSE POWDER (Corn King)	Piperonyl cyclonene tech. 0.63% Pyrethrins 0.06% Rotenone 0.31% Other cube extractives 0.63% Sulfur* 27.90%
CORN KING MINERAL BLOCK Mineral supplement (Corn King)	Defluorinated phosphate Phosphate Bone meal Manganese sulfate Iron oxide Irradiated yeast Cobalt carbonate Dicalcium Limestone Curacao rock phosphate Blue vitriol Potassium iodide Anise oil Molasses Calcium 25.000-20.000% Phosphorus 4.000% Iodine 0.038% Salt 20.000-30.000%
CORN KING PENTA Wood preser-vative (Corn King)	Pentachlorophenol* 4.37% Other chlorophenols 0.63% Petroleum hydrocarbons* 94.80%
CORN KING POULTRY ROOST AND ANIMAL INSECT POW-DER (Corn King)	Gamma isomer of benzene hexachloride* 5.0% Other isomers of benzene hexachloride* 28.3%
CORN KING ROOST PAINT Insecticide (Corn King)	Gamma isomer of benzene hexachloride 1.3% Other isomers of benzene hexachloride 3.2%
CORN KING SANI-CLEAN POWDER Detergent, sanitizer (Corn King)	Sodium carbonate Di-isobutyl phenoxy ethoxy ethyl dimethyl benzyl ammonium chloride* monohy-drate Tetrasodium pyrophosphate Polyethylene glycol mono-iso-octyl phenyl ether
CORN KING SULPHURIZED HOG OIL WITH 0.15% BHC Ectoparasiti-cide (veterin-ary) (Corn King)	Mineral oil Carbon disulfide* Sulfur* Gamma isomer and other isomers of benzene hexachlor-ide*
CORN KING SULPHURIZED OIL Ectoparasiti-cide (veterin-ary) (Corn King)	Mineral oil Sulfur* Carbon disulfide*
CORN KING STOCK DIP Disinfectant (Corn King)	Coal tar hydrocarbons* Tar acids Soap

*Consult Sec. II., Ingredients Index. This ingredient may be responsible for major toxic effects if poisonous amounts of this product are ingested.

Name & Use Manufacturer	Ingredients	Name & Use Manufacturer	Ingredients
CORN KING T. V. T. Poultry cannibalism (Corn King)	Oil of camphor* Powdered extr. quassia*	COROMERC, COROMERC LIQUID Fungicide (Pittsburgh Plate Glass (Corona Chem.))	n-Phenyl mercuriethylene diamine* (mercury as metallic 5.95%) 10%
CORN KING UDDER OINTMENT Udder irritation (veterinary) (Corn King)	Phenol* Oil of wintergreen* Oil of eucalyptus* Oil of turpentine* Lanolin and petrolatum base	CORONA ARAMITE CM-216 Insecticide (Pittsburgh Plate Glass (Corona Chem.))	2-(p-tert-Butylphenoxy) isopropyl-2-chloroethyl sulfite 15.0% Inert ingredients* 85.0%
CORN KING WARFARIN RATICIDE (Corn King)	Warfarin (3-(a-acetonylbenzyl)- 4-hydroxycoumarin) 0.5%	CORONA 1% BHC DUST CM-68 Insecticide (Pittsburgh Plate Glass (Corona Chem.))	Gamma isomer of benzene hexachloride* 1.00% Other isomers of benzene hexachloride* 6.50%
CORN KING 25% WATER MISCIBLE CONCEN- TRATE Insecticide (Corn King)	DDT 25% Aromatic petroleum deriv. solvent* 70%	CORONA BHC WETTABLE POWDER Insecticide (Pittsburgh Plate Glass (Corona Chem.))	Gamma isomer of tech. benzene hexachloride* 10.00% Other isomers of benzene hexachloride* 50.00%
CORN KING WETTABLE GRUB POW- DER Insecticide (Corn King)	Rotenone* 3.75% Other cube resins 7.50%		
CORN-O-CIDE FOOT TREAT (Brown-Vaughn)		CORONA BORDEAUX MIXTURE DRY CM-30 Fungicide, insecticide (Pittsburgh Plate Glass (Corona Chem.))	Metallic copper* 12.50%
CORN OFF (Corn Off)			
COROBLACK INK (Davids, T.)			
CORODAN COUGH SYRUP (Daniels, Robert)	Each fl. oz.: Alcohol 3% Codeine phosphate (opium deriv.) 1 gr. Chloroform 2 m. Potassium guaiacolsulfonate 8 gr. Ammonium chloride 8 gr. Tartar emetic* 1-12 gr.	CORONA BRUSH KILLER 24 Herbicide (Pittsburgh Plate Glass (Corona Chem.))	2,4,5-Trichlorophenoxyacetic acid* (butoxy ethoxy propanol ester) 23.3% 2,4-Dichlorophenoxyacetic acid* (butoxy ethoxy propanol ester) 49.6%
CORODANE 5% DUST Insecticide (Corona Chem.)	Tech. chlordane* 5.00%	CORONA 2,4, 5-T BRUSH KILLER Herbicide (Pittsburgh Plate Glass (Corona Chem.))	2,4,5-Trichlorophenoxyacetic acid* (butoxy ethoxy propanol ester) 70.6%
CORODEX Rust remover (Allied Prod., Ill.)	Phosphoric acid* Aniline dye		
CORODINOC Fungicide, insecticide (Pittsburgh Plate Glass (Corona Chem.))	Sodium salt of dinitro-ortho- cresol* 19% Sodium butyl naphthalene sulfonate 5% Sodium chromate 2%	CORONA 2, 4-D BUTYL ESTER WEED KILLER (Pittsburgh Plate Glass (Corona Chem.))	Butyl ester 2,4-dichloro phenoxy acetic acid* 40.0%
COROMEL Laxative, antacid (children) (Massengill)	Each tablet: Calomel (mercury deriv.) 3.2 mg. Powdered ipecac 1.3 mg. Sodium bicarbonate 32 mg. Bismuth subnitrate 65 mg. Oil of anise q.s.	CORONA 8# CHLORDANE EMULSION CONCEN- TRATE Insecticide (Pittsburgh Plate Glass (Corona Chem.))	Tech. chlordane* 75% Petroleum hydrocarbons 17%

*Consult Sec. II., Ingredients Index. This ingredient may be responsible for major toxic effects if poisonous amounts of this product are ingested.

Name & Use Manufacturer	Ingredients	Name & Use Manufacturer	Ingredients
CORONA COPPER-CARB NO. 20 Fungicide (Pittsburgh Plate Glass (CoronaChem.))	Metallic copper* (in basic copper carbonate) 20.0%	CORONA 75% DDT CONCEN-TRATE CM-575 Insecticide (Pittsburgh Plate Glass (Corona Chem.))	Dichloro diphenyl trichloro-ethane* 75.0%
CORONA COPPER-CARB NO. 50 Fungicide (Pittsburgh Plate Glass (Corona Chem.))	Metallic copper* (in basic copper carbonate) 50.00%	CORONA 10% DDT DUST Insecticide (Pittsburgh Plate Glass (Corona Chem.))	DDT* 10.00%
CORONA 26 COPPER FUNGICIDE (Pittsburgh Plate Glass (Corona Chem.))	Copper* (in copper oxysulfate) 26.00%	CORONA 25% DDT EMULSION Insecticide (Pittsburgh Plate Glass (Corona Chem.))	DDT 25% Aromatic petroleum deriv.* solvent 72%
CORONA COROMATE FUNGICIDE CM-245 (Pittsburgh Plate Glass (Corona Chem.))	Ferric dimethyl dithiocarbamate 76%	CORONA DIELDRIN 50% CM-290 Insecticide (Pittsburgh Plate Glass (Corona Chem.))	Hexachloro epoxy octahydro dimethano naphthalene* 42.6% Related compounds 7.6%
CORONA COROSUL D DUSTING SULFUR Fungicide (Pittsburth Plate Glass (Corona Chem.))	Sulfur* 90.00%	CORONA DINITRO POWDER CM-76 Insecticide (Pittsburgh Plate Glass (Corona Chem.))	Dinitro ortho cresol* 40%
CORONA COROSUL S WETTABLE SULFUR Fungicide (Pittsburgh Plate Glass (Corona Chem.))	Sulfur* 95.00%	CORONA DRY POWDERED ARSENATE OF LEAD CM-10 INSECTICIDE (Pittsburgh Plate Glass (Corona Chem.))	Lead arsenate* 98.00% Total metallic arsenic 19.5% Metallic lead 58.0%
CORONA COROTRAN OVEX CM-198 Fungicide, insecticide (Pittsburgh Plate Glass (Corona Chem.))	p-Chlorophenyl p-chlorobenzene sulfonate* 50%	CORONA DUST NO. 5 CM-158 Insecticide (Pittsburgh Plate Glass (Corona Chem.))	DDT* 5.00%
CORONA COROZATE CM-246 Fungicide (Pittsburgh Plate Glass (Corona Chem.))	Zinc dimethyl dithiocarbamate* 76%	CORONA DUST NO. 10 CM-144 Fungicide, Insecticide (Pittsburgh Plate Glass (Corona Chem.))	Zinc dimethyl dithiocarbamate 7.00%
CORONA 50% DDT CONCEN-TRATE CM-500 Insecticide (Pittsburgh Plate Glass (Corona Chem.))	Dichloro diphenyl trichloro-ethane* 50.0%	CORONA DUST NO. 12 CM-145 Fungicide Insecticide (Pittsburgh Plate Glass (Corona Chem.))	Tricalcium arsenate* 14.00% Total metallic arsenic 5.20% Zinc dimethyl dithiocarbamate 79.00%

*Consult Sec. II., Ingredients Index. This ingredient may be responsible for major toxic effects if poisonous amounts of this product are ingested.

Name & Use Manufacturer	Ingredients		Name & Use Manufacturer	Ingredients	
CORONA DUST NO. 57 CM-160 Fungicide, insecticide (Pittsburgh Plate Glass (Corona Chem.))	DDT* Metallic copper*	5.00% 7.00%	CORONA MALATHION 25% CM-285 Insecticide (Pittsburgh Plate Glass (Corona Chem.))	Malathion*	25%
CORONA DUST NO. 100 Insecticide (Pittsburgh Plate Glass (Corona Chem.))	Rotenone Other cube resins	1.00% 1.75%	CORONA 4% MALATHION DUST CM-286 Insecticide (Pittsburgh Plate Glass (Corona Chem.))	Malathion	4%
CORONA DUST NO. 720 CM-164 Fungicide, insecticide (Pittsburgh Plate Glass (Corona Chem.))	Tricalcium arsenate* 14.00% Total metallic arsenic 5.20% Metallic arsenic in water 0.15% Metallic copper in tribasic copper sulfate 7.00%		CORONA METHOXY-CHLOR CM-280 Insecticide (Pittsburgh Plate Glass (Corona Chem.))	Tech. methoxychlor*	50%
CORONA 1% ENDRIN DUST CM-507 Insecticide (Pittsburgh Plate Glass (Corona Chem.))	Endrin* (hexachloro epoxy octahydro-endo, endo-dimethano naphthalene) 1.0%		CORONA MICRONIZED DUSTING SULFUR Fungicide (Pittsburgh Plate Glass (Corona Chem.))	Sulfur*	90.00%
CORONA ENDRIN 16 INSECTICIDE CONCENTRATE CM-89 (Pittsburgh Plate Glass (Corona Chem.))	Hexachloro epoxy octahydro-endo, endo-dimethano naphthalene* 19.9% Aromatic petroleum derivatives* 71.0%		CORONA MICRONIZED SULFUR-PHYGON DUST CM-334 Fungicide (Pittsburgh Plate Glass (Corona Chem.))	Dichlone (2,3-dichloro-1,4-naphthoquinone) 0.75% Sulfur* 90.00%	
CORONA 50-50 W CM-150 Insecticide (Pittsburgh Plate Glass (Corona Chem.))	DDT*	50.00%	CORONA 53 MICRONIZED TRIBASIC COPPER SULPHATE Fungicide, Insecticide (Pittsburgh Plate Glass (Corona Chem.))	Basic copper sulfate*	98.00%
CORONA 11% GAMMA BHC EMULSION BASE CM-81 INSECTICIDE (Pittsburgh Plate Glass (Corona Chem.))	Gamma isomer of benzene hexachloride* 11% Other isomers of benzene hexachloride* 17% Methylated naphthalenes 35% Petroleum distillates* 30%		CORONA MICRONIZED WETTABLE SULFUR Fungicide (Pittsburgh Plate Glass (Corona Chem.))	Sulfur*	95.00%
CORONA 2,4-D ISOPROPYL ESTER WEED KILLER (Pittsburgh Plate Glass (Corona Chem.))	Isopropyl ester, 2,4-dichloro phenoxy acetic acid* 44.8%				

Name & Use Manufacturer	Ingredients	Name & Use Manufacturer	Ingredients
CORONA 25% PARATHION CM-84 Insecticide (Pittsburgh Plate Glass (Corona Chem.))	Parathion* (o,o-diethyl-o,p-nitrophenyl thiophosphate) 25.0% Xylene 62.5%	CORONET PERMANENT WAVING LOTION (Koehler & K.)	
		CORONET SHOE POLISH (Barr, G.)	
CORONA PHENO-LEAD CM-527 Fungicide Insecticide (Pittsburgh Plate Glass (Corona Chem.))	Phenothiazine 37.0% Lead arsenate* 56.6% Total metallic lead 34.2% Total metallic arsenic 11.5%	CORONOL EMBALMING FLUID (Undertakers)	
CORONA PHYGON-XL Fungicide (Pittsburgh Plate Glass (Corona Chem.))	Dichlone (2,3-dichloro-1,4-naphthoquinone)* 50%	CORO SDD CORONA LIQUID FUNGICIDE (Pittsburgh Plate Glass (Corona Chem.))	Sodium dimethyl dithiocarba-mate 40% Inert ingredients* 60%
CORONA 4-POUND 2, 4-D ACID AMINE WEED KILLER (Pittsburgh Plate Glass (Corona Chem.))	Dimethylamine salt 2,4-dichloro phenoxyacetic acid* 49.4%	COROSEC PERFUME & TOILET WATER (Corot)	
		COROT AFTER SHAVE, COLOGNE, LAVENDER WATER, TOILET WATER (Corot)	
CORONA POWDERED CALCIUM ARSENATE & OTHER CALCIUM COMPOUNDS Insecticide (Pittsburgh Plate Glass (Corona Chem.))	Tricalcium arsenate* 70.00% Total metallic arsenic 26.00%	COROTHION CM-244 Fungicide, Insecticide (Pittsburgh Plate Glass (Corona Chem.))	Parathion* 15.00%
CORONA TREE WOUND DRESSING (Pittsburgh Plate Glass (Paint div.))	Mercuric chloride* 0.193% Equiv. metallic mercury 0.142%	COROTHION DUST NO. 1 CM-247 Insecticide (Pittsburgh Plate Glass (Corona Chem.))	Parathion* 1.00%
CORONA WEED KILLER (Pittsburgh Plate Glass (Corona Chem.))	Butyl ester, 2,4-dichloro phenoxy acetic acid* 40.0%	CORRECTIVE JR. Cathartic, antacid (Jenkins)	Each tablet: Powdered ipecac 1/32 gr. Calomel 1/16 gr. Bismuth subnitrate 2 gr. Sodium bicarbonate 1 gr. Pancreatin 9/40 gr. Papain 9/40 gr. Pepsin 1/20 gr.
CORONA WEED KILLER CM-377 (Pittsburgh Plate Glass (Corona Chem.))	Isopropyl ester 2,4-dichloro-phenoxy acetic acid* 44.8%	CORRECTIVE MIXTURE Intestinal irritation (Massengill)	Each 5 cc.: Zinc sulfocarbolate* 10 mg. Salol 20 mg. Bismuth subsalicylate* 80 mg. Pepsin 40 mg. Carminatives, demulcents, aromatics q.s.
CORONA 75-25 W SPRAY MIXTURE CM-75 Insecticide (Pittsburgh Plate Glass (Corona Chem.))	DDT (dichloro diphenyl trichloroethane)* 75.00%		

*Consult Sec. II., Ingredients Index. This ingredient may be responsible for major toxic effects if poisonous amounts of this product are ingested.

Name & Use Manufacturer	Ingredients	
CORTAL Analgesic (Sterling Prod. Int.)	Aspirin*	0.37 gm.
	Phenacetin*	0.15 gm.
	Caffein	0.03 gm.
CORTISOL External fungicide (medical) (Cortisol)	Chlorobutanol (chloroform deriv.)	1%
	Ortho-benzyl phenol*	
	Para-benzyl phenol-benzoic acid	
	Menthol*	
	Benzocaine	
	Glycerin-isopropyl alcohol*	55%/v
CORTRIL ACETATE OPHTHALMIC OINTMENT (Pfizer Labs.)	Hydrocortisone 0.5 or 2.5%	
	Petrolatum base	
CORTRIL ACETATE TOPICAL OINTMENT Allergic dermatoses (Pfizer Labs.)	Each 1 gm.:	
	Hydrocortisone acetate	10 or 25 mg.
	Hydrophilic ointment base	
CORYZA Nasal decongestant (Jenkins)	Quinine sulfate	1/3 gr.
	Camphor*	1/3 gr.
	Extr. aconite*	1/10 gr.
	Caffeine	1/6 gr.
	Atropine sulfate	1/500 gr.
CO-SALT Salt substitute (Arlington)	Potassium chloride*	
	Ammonium chloride	
	Tricalcium phosphate*	
COSANYL Antitussive (Parke, Davis)	Each fl. oz.:	
	Dihydrocodeinone bitartrate	1/6 gr.
	Tinct. euphorbia pilulifera*	120 m.
	Syrup wild lettuce	120 m.
	Tinct. cocillana	40 m.
	Syrup squill* compound	24 m.
	Cascarin	8 gr.
	Menthol	2/25 gr.
	Alcohol	6%
COSMASUL Emollient (Cosmata)	Toilet soap base	
	Lanolin	
	Glycerin	
	Paraffin	
	Triethanolamine	
	Sodium borate	
	Colloidal sulfur	
	Granulated calcium carbonate	
	Stearic acid	
	Zinc oxide	
COSMETIC LABS. HOMOGENIZED SKIN CLEANSER (Cosmetic)	Lanolin	
	Polyol ester	
	Petrolatum	
	Wax	
	Magnesium sulfate	
COSMETINE For chapped hands, sunburn (Nelson, Detroit)		
COTTON PRODUCERS 3-5-BHC-DDT COTTON DUST Insecticide (Cotton)	Gamma isomer of benzene hexachloride*	3.00%
	Other isomers of benzene hexachloride	5.00%
	DDT*	5.00%

Name & Use Manufacturer	Ingredients	
COTTON PRODUCERS 3-5-40 BHC-DDT & SULFUR COTTON DUST Insecticide (Cotton)	Gamma isomer of hexachloro cyclohexane*	3.00%
	Other isomers of hexachloro cyclohexane	5.00%
	DDT*	5.00%
	Sulfur*	40.00%
COTTON PRODUCERS CATTLE GRUB POWDER Insecticide (Cotton)	Rotenone	1.60%
	Other cube resins	3.00%
	Sulfur*	45.00%
COTTON PRODUCERS COPPER-CRYOLITE DUST Fungicide (Cotton)	Copper* expressed as metallic	7.00%
	Cryolite	35.00%
COTTON PRODUCERS 6.5% COPPER DUST Fungicide (Cotton)	Copper* expressed as metallic	6.50%
COTTON PRODUCERS 2-1/2 to 5 COTTON DUST Insecticide (Cotton)	Hexachloro hexahydro dimethano naphthalene*	2.375%
	Related compounds	1.791%
	Dichloro diphenyl trichloroethane*	5.000%
COTTON PRODUCERS 2-1/2 to 5 to 40 COTTON DUST Insecticide (Cotton)	Hexachloro hexahydro dimethano naphthalene*	2.375%
	Related compounds	1.791%
	Dichloro diphenyl trichloroethane*	5.000%
	Sulfur*	40.000%
COTTON PRODUCERS 5% DDT DUST Insecticide (Cotton)	Dichloro diphenyl trichloroethane*	5.00%
COTTON PRODUCERS 10% DDT-74% SULPHUR COTTON & PEANUT DUST Insecticide (Cotton)	Dichloro diphenyl trichloroethane*	10%
	Sulfur*	74%
COTTON PRODUCERS 2-1/2% DDT SULPHUR DUST (Peanut Dust) Insecticide (Cotton)	Sulfur*	90.0%
	DDT	2.5%
COTTON PRODUCERS 1-1/2% DIELDRIN-5% DDT COTTON DUST Insecticide (Cotton)	Hexachloro epoxy octahydro dimethano naphthalene*	1.275%
	Related compounds (from dieldrin)	0.225%
	Dichloro diphenyl trichloroethane*	5.000%
	Sulfur*	40.000%

*Consult Sec. II., Ingredients Index. This ingredient may be responsible for major toxic effects if poisonous amounts of this product are ingested.

Name & Use Manufacturer	Ingredients		Name & Use Manufacturer	Ingredients	
COTTON PRODUCERS 2.5% HEPTACHLOR 5% DDT COTTON DUST Insecticide (Cotton)	Heptachlor Related compounds DDT (dichloro diphenyl trichloroethane)* Sulfur*	2.50% 0.97% 5.00% 40.00%	COTTON STATES 20% ALDRIN EQUIVALENT CONCEN-TRATE Insecticide (Cotton States)	Hexachloro hexahydro dimethano naphthalene* Related compounds	 18.21% 14.31%
COTTON PRODUCERS ROTENONE NO. 100 Insecticide (Cotton)	Rotenone Other cube resins	1.00% 1.80%	COTTON STATES 10G BHC WETTABLE Insecticide (Cotton States)	Gamma isomer of benzene hexachloride* Other isomers of benzene hexachloride and related compounds*	 10.00% 52.50%
COTTON PRODUCERS SABADILLA DUST NO. 10 Insecticide (Cotton)	Alkaloids of sabadilla	0.40%	COTTON STATES CHLORDANE 10% DUST Insecticide (Cotton States)	Tech. chlordane*	10.00%
COTTON PRODUCERS TOBACCO PLANT BED DUST NO. 10 Fungicide, insecticide (Cotton)	Zineb Parathion*	6.50% 1.0%	COTTON STATES CHLORDANE 45% EMULSIFI-ABLE Insecticide (Cotton States)	Tech. chlordane* Petroleum distillate*	45.00% 45.00%
COTTON PRODUCERS TOBACCO PLANT BED DUST NO. 15 Fungicide, insecticide (Cotton)	Ferbam Parathion*	11.4% 1.0%	COTTON STATES 74% CHLORDANE EMULSIFI-ABLE Insecticide (Cotton States)	Tech. chlordane* Petroleum distillate	74.00% 16.00%
COTTON PRODUCERS TOMATO DUST Insecticide (Cotton)	Copper sulfate Calcium arsenate*	13.25% 20.00%	COTTON STATES 40% CHLORDANE OIL SOLUTION Insecticide (Cotton States)	Tech. chlordane* Petroleum distillate*	40% 60%
COTTON PRODUCERS 20% TOXAPHENE COTTON DUST Insecticide (Cotton)	Toxaphene*	20.00%	COTTON STATES 40% CHLORDANE WETTABLE Insecticide (Cotton States)	Tech. chlordane*	40.00%
COTTON PRODUCERS 20-40 TOXAPHENE COTTON DUST Insecticide (Cotton)	Toxaphene* Sulfur	20.00% 40.00%	COTTON STATES COMBO COTTON DUST 3-5-40 Insecticide (Cotton States)	Gamma isomer of benzene hexachloride Other isomers of benzene hexachloride* DDT* Sulfur*	3% 22% 5% 40%
COTTON PRODUCERS 20-5 TOXAPHENE-DDT COTTON DUST Insecticide (Cotton)	Toxaphene* Dichloro diphenyl trichloro-ethane	20.00% 5.00%	COTTON STATES COMBO COTTON DUST NO. 10 (3-10-40) Insecticide (Cotton States)	Gamma isomer of benzene hexachloride* Other isomers of benzene hexachloride* DDT* Sulfur*	3% 20% 10% 40%
			COTTON STATES COTTON DUST 3-5-0 Insecticide (Cotton States)	Gamma isomer of benzene hexachloride* Other isomers of benzene hexachloride* DDT*	3% 22% 5%

*Consult Sec. II., Ingredients Index. This ingredient may be responsible for major toxic effects if poisonous amounts of this product are ingested.

- 397 -

Name & Use Manufacturer	Ingredients	Name & Use Manufacturer	Ingredients
COTTON STATES COTTON DUST 3-0-0 Insecticide (Cotton States)	Gamma isomer of benzene hexachloride* 3% Other isomers of benzene hexachloride* 22%	COTTON STATES 25% DIELDRIN WETTABLE Insecticide (Cotton States)	Hexachloro epoxy octahydro dimethano naphthalene* 25%
COTTON STATES COTTON DUST 3-10-0 Insecticide (Cotton States)	Gamma isomer of benzene hexachloride* 3% Other isomers of benzene hexachloride* 20% DDT* 10%	COTTON STATES 40% TOXAPHENE WETTABLE POWDER Insecticide (Cotton States)	Toxaphene* 40%
COTTON STATES 50% DDT WETTABLE POWDER Insecticide (Cotton States)	Dichloro diphenyl trichloroethane* 50%	COTTON STATES 201 DUST Insecticide (Cotton States)	Tech. chlorinated camphene* 20% Parathion* 1%
COTTON STATES 1-1/2% DIELDRIN Insecticide (Cotton States)	Hexachloro epoxy octahydro dimethano naphthalene* 1.27% Related compounds 0.23% DDT* 10.00%	COTTON STATES 251 DUST Insecticide (Cotton States)	Heptachlor 2.50% Related compounds 0.97% Dichloro diphenyl trichloroethane 5.00% Parathion* 1.00%
COTTON STATES 1-1/2% DIELDRIN- 10% DDT Insecticide (Cotton States)	Hexachloro epoxy octahydro dimethano naphthalene* 1.27% Related compounds 0.23% Dichloro diphenyl trichloroethane* 10.00% Sulfur* 40.00%	COTTON STATES 971 DUST Insecticide (Cotton States)	Hexachloro epoxy octahydro dimethano naphthalene* 1.27% Related compounds 0.23% Dichloro diphenyl trichloroethane 5.00% Parathion* 1.00%
COTTON STATES 2% DIELDRIN DUST Insecticide (Cotton States)	Hexachloro epoxy octahydro endo, exo-dimethano naphthalene* 1.7% Related compounds 0.3%	COTTON STATES ENDRIN EMULSIFIABLE CONCENTRATE Insecticide (Cotton States)	Hexachloro epoxy octahydro- endo, endo-dimethano naphthalene* 19.5% Petroleum hydrocarbons 70.5%
COTTON STATES 1-1/2% DIELDRIN EQUIVALENT- 5% DDT-40% SULFUR DUST Insecticide (Cotton States)	Hexachloro epoxy octahydro dimethano naphthalene* 1.27% Related compounds 0.23% Dichloro diphenyl trichloroethane* 5.00% Sulfur* 40.00%	COTTON STATES FLY SPRAY & REPELLENT Insecticide (Cotton States)	Tech. piperonyl butoxide 10.00% Pyrethrins 1.00% Petroleum distillate* 80.00%
COTTON STATES 1-1/2% DIELDRIN EQUIVALENT DUST Insecticide (Cotton States)	Hexachloro epoxy octahydro dimethano naphthalene* 1.27% Related compounds 0.23%		

*Consult Sec. II., Ingredients Index. This ingredient may be responsible for major toxic effects if poisonous amounts of this product are ingested.

Name & Use Manufacturer	Ingredients		Name & Use Manufacturer	Ingredients	
COTTON STATES 2-1/2% HEPTACHLOR 10% DDT DUST Insecticide (Cotton States)	Heptachlor* Related compounds Dichloro diphenyl trichloro- ethane*	2.50% 0.97% 10.00%	COTTON STATES TOXANE WETTABLE POWDER Insecticide (Cotton States)	Toxaphene* Gamma isomer of benzene hexachloride (from lindane)	40.00% 0.90%
COTTON STATES 2-1/2% HEPTACHLOR 5% SULFUR DUST Insecticide (Cotton States)	Heptachlor* Related compounds Dichloro diphenyl trichloro- ethane* Sulfur*	2.50% 0.97% 5.00% 40.00%	COTTON STATES TOXAPHENE 40% CONCEN- TRATE Insecticide (Cotton States)	Tech. chlorinated camphene*	40.00%
COTTON STATES LIVESTOCK SPRAY L-150 Insecticide (Cotton States)	Toxaphene* Xylene*	62.50% 32.20%	COTTON STATES TOXAPHENE 20% DUST Insecticide (Cotton States)	Tech. chlorinated camphene*	20.00%
COTTON STATES MALATHION Insecticide (Cotton States)	Malathion*	50%	COTTON STATES TOXAPHENE 20%-40% DUST Insecticide (Cotton States)	Tech. chlorinated camphene* Sulfur	20.00% 40.00%
COTTON STATES 5% MALATHION DUST Insecticide (Cotton States)	Malathion	5%	COTTON STATES VEGETABLE DUST NO. 1 Insecticide, Fungicide (Cotton States)	Parathion* Zineb	1.00% 3.9%
COTTON STATES MALATHION 25 W Insecticide (Cotton States)	Malathion*	25%	COTY FACE CREAM, FACE POWDER, HAND LOTION, LIPSTICK, ROUGE , SOLID COLOGNE, SOAP (Coty)		
COTTON STATES 1% PARATHION DUST Insecticide (Cotton States)	Parathion*	1.0%			

*Consult Sec. II., Ingredients Index. This ingredient may be responsible for major toxic effects if poisonous amounts of this product are ingested.

- 399 -

Name & Use Manufacturer	Ingredients
COTY NAIL POLISH (Coty)	
COUGH-X Antitussive (Binday)	Each oz.: Codeine phosphate 1 gr. Menthol Euphorbia pilulifera Wild lettuce Syrup, squill compound Cascarin Cocillana Alcohol 5%
COULEUR DE TON TONE COLOR Cosmetic (Orjene)	
COUNTESS MARITZA TOILET WATER (Countess)	
COURTLEY BODY POWDER (Antiseptic Deodorant), BUBBLE BATH (Hudnut, R.)	
COURTLEY'S AFTER SHAVE LOTIONS, COLOGNES, CREAM DE-ODORANT, CREAM HAIR-DRESS, DAN-DRUFF LOTION, DEODORANT COLOGNES, STIM-STIK (Courtley)	
COVAGRAY HAIR COLOR-ING (Covagray)	
COVERMARK CREAM Cosmetic (O'Leary)	
COVICONE CREAM (Abbott)	Silicone (dimethyl polysiloxane) Nitrocellulose Castor oil
COWLEY'S RAT & MOUSE POISON (Cowley, S.L.)	Arsenic trioxide* 1.75%
COW-TONE Tonic veterinary (Our Husbands)	Iron sulfate dried Nux vomica* Gentian Salt Foenugreek Bone meal Arsenic trioxide* Copper sulfate Epsom salts

Name & Use Manufacturer	Ingredients
DR. COX'S BARBED WIRE LINIMENT & ANTISEPTIC Veterinary (Hoover)	Oxyquinoline benzoate Crude oil Iodine* Turpentine* Linseed oil
DR. COX'S BLISTER FOR ANIMALS Veterinary (Hoover)	Red mercuric iodide* 1.5% Croton oil* Turpentine Compound solution of cresol Alcohol 6% Linseed oil Potassium iodide* Oil of sassafras Certified red color
COYZANS REVISED For colds (Tailby)	Each tablet: Tinct. gelsemium* 3 m. Acetophenetidin* 1 gr. Atropine sulfate 1/500 gr. Hyoscyamus* 1/8 gr. Camphor 1/10 gr.
CO-ZONE COUGH SYRUP (Dunwody)	
CP-4, CP-6, CP-8 Photographic supplies (Chemipure)	
CRAB APPLE CREAM Cosmetic (Hausman)	
CRAB GRASS FIX Herbicide (Thompson Chem.)	Potassium cyanate* 80.00%
CRAB-NOT SPECIAL Herbicide (Nott)	Potassium cyanate* 69.4% Sodium salt monohydrate 2, 4-dichlorophenoxyacetic acid* 16.6%
CRAB-NOT STANDARD Herbicide (Nott)	Potassium cyanate* 86%
CRACKSHOT Insecticide (Bell Chem. Co., Inc.)	Sodium fluoride* Borax* DDT* Cayenne pepper* Froud wheat
CRADOL Skin oint-ment (Homemakers')	Methyl benzethonium chloride*
CRAEL TAR Coal tar therapy (Edlich)	Crude coal tar* 10%
CRAFTCO CEMENT PAINT (Nat'l. Gypsum)	

*Consult Sec. II., Ingredients Index. This ingredient may be responsible for major toxic effects if poisonous amounts of this product are ingested.

- 400 -

Name & Use Manufacturer	Ingredients		Name & Use Manufacturer	Ingredients	
CRAFTINT DRAWING INK (Craftint)	Shellac Ammonia Borax* Carbon black Organic dyes		CRANE'S ANT-EX Insecticide (Crane)	Sodium arsenite*	0.18%
CRAFTINT LIQUID PORCELAIN GLAZE (Craftint)			CRANE'S ANT SPRAY (Crane)	Chlordane tech.* Inert ingredients*	2-1/2% 97-1/2%
CRAFTINT OIL COLORS (Craftint)	Vegetable oils Paint grade organic and in-organic pigments*		CRANE'S ANTU RAT KILLER (Crane)	Alpha naphthyl thiourea	5%
CRAFT MASTER FINGER PAINT SET (Palmer Paint)			CRANE'S CONCEN-TRATED INS-EX POWDER Insecticide (Crane)	Tech. chlordane*	50%
CRAFT MASTER OIL PAINTING SETS (Palmer Paint)			CRANE'S DDT SPRAY Insecticide (Crane)	Petroleum oil* DDT* Beta butoxy beta' thiocyano diethyl ether*	5%
CRAFT MASTER TOLEWARE PAINTS (Palmer Paint)			CRANE'S EARWIG KILLER Insecticide (Crane)	Tech. chlordane Gamma isomer of benzene hexachloride*	5% 1%
CRAFTONE EXTERIOR RESIN-EMULSION PAINT & PRIMES (Nat'l. Gypsum)			CRANE'S FLY-MAL Insecticide (Crane)	Malathion Xylol	1% 0.8%
CRAG COPPER ZINC CHRO-MATE FUNGI-CIDE 658 (Carbide)	Copper* Zinc Chromium*	29.6% 20.4% 9.7%	CRANE'S FLY-T-EX Insecticide (Crane)	Odorless kerosene* Gamma isomer of benzene hexachloride*	
CRAG FLY REPELLENT (Carbide)	Butoxy polypropylene glycol*	100%	CRANE'S INS-EX Insecticide (Crane)	Petroleum oil* Beta butoxy beta' thiocyano diethyl ether* Tech. chlordane	
CRAG FRUIT FUNGICIDE 341 (Carbide)	Glyodin (2-heptadecyl glyoxalidine acetate)* Isopropanol*	34%/w 66%/w	CRANE'S INS-EX POWDER Insecticide (Crane)	Sodium fluoride* Pyrethrins	75.00% 0.20%
CRAG FUNGICIDE 974 (Carbide)	3, 5-Dimethyl tetrahydro-1, 3, 5, 2H-thiadiazine-2-thione*	95%	CRANE'S LINDANE Insecticide (Crane)	Gamma isomer of benzene hexachloride (from lindane*)	99%
CRAG FUNGICIDE 974-85W (Carbide)	3, 5-Dimethyl tetrahydro-1, 3, 5, 2H-thiadiazine-2-thione*	85%/w	CRANE'S MDP Moth pre-ventative (Crane)	Magnesium silicofluoride	0.75%
CRAG HERBICIDE 1 (Carbide)	Sodium 2, 4-dichlorophenoxyethyl sulfate*	90%/w	CRANE'S MICE POISON (Crane)	Strychnine alkaloid*	0.75%
CRAG HERBICIDE DCU, 73W (Carbide)	Dichloral urea	73%/w	CRANE'S MICE POWDER (Crane)	Dichloro diphenyl trichloroethane*	50%
CRAG TURF FUNGICIDE 531 (Carbide)	Copper* Cadmium Zinc Chromium*	9.9% 4.2% 4.1% 3.2%	CRANE'S PHOSPHORUS RAT POISON (Crane)	Phosphorus	0.2%
			CRANOLENE OINTMENT (Cranolene)		

*Consult Sec. II., Ingredients Index. This ingredient may be responsible for major toxic effects if poisonous amounts of this product are ingested.

- 401 -

Name & Use Manufacturer	Ingredients	
CRAWL KILL Insecticide (Ampion)	Petroleum distillate* and tech. chlordane*	100%
CRAWL-X CONCEN-TRATE Insecticide (Gart)	Tech. chlordane*	50%
CRAYOFF Washable crayon (Crayoff)	Pure soap Vegetable pigments Stearic acid Triisopropanolamine Spermaceti wax	92%
CRAYOGRAPH Crayons (Crayon)		
CRAYOLA CRAYONS, WAX DRAW-ING CRAYON, CRAYOLET COLORED WAX CRAYON (Binney & Smith)		
CRAYONEX Crayons (Crayon)		
CREAMIN CREOSOTED EXPECTOR-ANT (Commerce)	Alcohol Chloroform Wild cherry bark White pine bark Aralia Poplar bud Sanguinaria Sassafras Ammonium chloride Creosote	2.0% 2 m.
CREA-MINT Antitussive (Hance)	Each fl. oz.: Chloroform Creosote* Sodium glycerophosphate Phosphoric acid Glycerin Terpin hydrate* Calcium glycerophosphate Ammonium chloride Oil of spearmint	1 m.
CREDOL Antitussive (Jenkins)	Each tablet: Creosote beechwood Vitamin A Vitamin D Nux vomica* Calcium glycerophosphate Sodium glycerophosphate Kaolin (colloidal) Calcium carbonate	1/4 m. 600 units 85 units 1/4 gr. 1/2 gr. 1/2 gr.
CREMACAL Analgesic cream (Hobart)	Calamine Glycerin Benzocaine Phenol Menthol	10% 5% 1% 0.5% 0.25%
CREMOSUL Antitussive (Boyle & Co.)	White pine* Beechwood creosote* Ipecac Antimony potassium tartrate* Alcohol Tar Cascara Menthol*	2%

Name & Use Manufacturer	Ingredients	
CREOBRON Antitussive (Nelson Baker)	Each fl. oz.: Creosote* Guaiacol* Syrup wild cherry Aromatics	1 m. 3-1/2 gr.
CREO-DERMA OINTMENT Anti-pruritic (Massengill)	Sulfur Coal tar distillate Bismuth subgallate Oil of lemon grass Cresol* Zinc oxide Oil of cade	15% 5% 1.5% 0.5% 2% 5.5% 1.5%
CREO-HYPO-PHOS Tonic (Penslar)	Each fl. oz.: Strychnine sulfate Tr. iron citrochloride eq. to Malt extract, non-diastatic Beechwood creosote Hypophosphites of potassium, sodium, manganese, copper sulfate Sherry wine Aromatics	1/128 gr. 1.1 gr. iron 1/60 gr.
CREOLIN 10 Disinfectant, antiseptic, deodorant (Merck)	Coal tar neutral oils Phenols* Soap	
CREO-MINT EMULSION Antitussive (James, L.)	Each oz.: Chloroform Creosote carbonate* Peppermint Saccharin Aluminum hydroxide Glycerin Tragacanth	2 m. 32 m.
CREOMULSION Antitussive (Creomulsion)	Beechwood creosote* Cascara bark Ipecac root Menthol* White pine bark Wild cherry bark Alcohol	2%
CREO-PINE COUGH SYRUP (Little Wonder)	Chloroform* Creosote* Pine tar* Alcohol	3%
CRETOX Disinfectant, Sheet Dip (Speekman)	Petroleum aromatic oil* Anhydrous soap Total phenols*	53% 22% 15%
CREPE DE CHINE PER-FUME AND COLOGNE (Millot, F.)		
CRESADOL Antitussive (Veltex)	Each fl. oz.: Chloroform Guaiacol Creosote Viosterol Menthol White pine compound Wild cherry Simple syrup	4 m.
CRESANOL Disinfectant, germicide (Whitmoyer)	Coal tar neutral oils* Soap Phenols*	

*Consult Sec. II., Ingredients Index. This ingredient may be responsible for major toxic effects if poisonous amounts of this product are ingested.

Name & Use Manufacturer	Ingredients		Name & Use Manufacturer	Ingredients	
CRESCENT AIRPLANE CEMENT (Crescent Prod.)			CRESMOL COUGH SYRUP (Sacramento)		
CRESCENT AXLE GREASE (Fiske)			CRESODINE TABLETS (Veterinary) (Strasenburgh)	Creosote* Potassium dichromate* Iodine*	2.5 mg.
CRESCENT FURNITURE POLISH (Crescent Prod.)	Oil Kerosene*		CRE-SO-FEC Disinfectant (Ralston)	Cresylic acid*	
CRESCENT (glossy glass) WINDOW CLEANER (Crescent Prod.)			CRESOL Insecticide (Speekman)	Tar acids*	97%
CRESCENT HOUSEHOLD OIL (Crescent Prod.)	Petroleum oil*		CRESOPERLS Tonic (Legendre's)	Creosote (beechwood) Activated cod liver oil Strychnine alkaloid* (strychnine phosphate 1/100 gr.)	3 m. 10 m.
CRESCENT INK ERADI- CATOR, JIC LIQUID PASTE, MUCILAGE, GLUE (Crescent Prod.)			CREST Toothpaste (Procter & Gamble)		
CRESCENT LAUNDRY MARKING INK, RUBBER STAMPING INK (Crescent Prod.)	Phenol* Glycerin		CRESTEX FINGER PAINT, WASHABLE PAINTING SETS (Palmer Show Card)		
CRESCENT RED-E-C- MENT PADDING COMPOUND Adhesive (Crescent Prod.)			CRES-TONE Disinfectant (Carpenter)	Coal tar phenols* Soap	50% 20%
			CRETE-FIX Floor re- surfacer (Horn)		
CRESCENT STIX PASTE (Crescent Prod.)			CRETE-TREAT Chemical cleaner for masonry, concrete- brick, tile (Crete-Treat)	Phosphoric acid* Isopropanol	25% 5%
CRESCENT SWEEPING COMPOUND (Crescent Prod.)	Sand Sawdust Paraffin oil		CRETE-TREAT Concrete cleaner (Glidden Co.)		
CRESCENT WATERPROOF INKS Crescent Prod.)			CREVISEAL Caulking compound (Pioneer)		
			CRISP'S DOG REMEDIES (Crisp)		
CRESENDO PERFUMES & COLOGNES (Assoc. Brands)			CRITERION PINE OIL DIS- INFECTANT (Majestic)		
			CROP KING DDT-PARA- THION 45-10 Insecticide (Crop King)	Parathion* DDT	10.0% 45.0%

*Consult Sec. II., Ingredients Index. This ingredient may be responsible for major toxic effects if poisonous amounts of this product are ingested.

- 403 -

Name & Use Manufacturer	Ingredients		Name & Use Manufacturer	Ingredients	
CROP KING DDT-SULPHUR Insecticide (Crop King)	Dichloro diphenyl trichloroethane* Sulfur		CROSBY ZINC OXIDE RESIN COMPOUND SPECIAL Dental preparation (Crosby)	Zinc oxide Pulverized resin Thymol* Thymol iodide* Paraformaldehyde*	
CROP KING DUSTING SULPHUR Insecticide (Crop King)	Sulfur*	98%	CROSS COUNTRY AMINE WEED KILLER CONTAINING 14% 2, 4-D ACID (Sears)	Triethanolamine salt of 2, 4-dichloro phenoxy acetic acid*	23.45%
CROP KING FLOWABLE PASTE DDT-50 Insecticide (Crop King)	Dichloro diphenyl trichloroethane*	50%	CROSS COUNTRY ANT KILLER (Sears)	Chlordane tech.*	10%
CROP KING PARATHION 200 COLLOIDAL Insecticide (Crop King)	Parathion (0, 0-diethyl-0-nitrophenyl thiophosphate*	21.7%	CROSS COUNTRY ANT SPRAY (Sears)	Tech. chlordane Refined petroleum distillate*	2% 98%
CROP KING PARATHION DUST 2 Insecticide (Crop King)	Parathion*	2%	CROSS COUNTRY CRAB GRASS KILLER (Sears)	Potassium cyanate*	46%
CROP KING PARATHION 25 FLOWABLE Insecticide (Crop King)	Parathion*	25%	CROSS COUNTRY FRUIT SPRAY Insecticide, fungicide (Sears)	DDT* Malathion* Captan (n-trichloro methyl thiotetrahydro phthalimide)	10.0% 5.0% 10.0%
CROP KING TEPP 50 Insecticide (Crop King)	Tetraethyl pyrophosphate* Other related organic phosphates	20% 30%	CROSS COUNTRY GARDEN SPRAY Insecticide (Sears)	Malathion* Methoxychlor, tech. Xylene*	24.0% 12.0% 52.8%
CROP KING 2, 4-D ESTER WEED KILLER 44 (Crop King)	2,4-Dichloro phenoxy acetic acid,* isopropyl ester 44%		CROSS COUNTRY GRASS & WEED KILLER (Sears)	Sodium arsenite*	30.06%
CROP KING 2, 4-D LIQUID SALT 40 Herbicide (Crop King)	2,4-Dichloro phenoxy acetic acid* (alkanolamine salt as free acid)	40%	CROSS COUNTRY INSECT DUST CONTAINING DDT (Sears)	DDT*	5%
CROP KING WETTABLE POWDER DDT-50W Insecticide (Crop King)	Dichloro diphenyl trichloroethane*	50%	CROSS COUNTRY INSECT SPRAY CONTAINING 50% DDT (Sears)	DDT*	50%
CROP KING'S ZINC SULPHATE SOLUTION For agricultural use (Crop King)	Zinc sulfate*	4 lb./gal.	CROSS COUNTRY INSECT DUST CONTAINING ROTENONE (Sears)	Rotenone Other cube extractives	0.75% 1.50%
CROQUIGNOLE WAX (Quaker)	Vanillin Oil coloring Petrolatum Paraffin		CROSS COUNTRY LAWN INSECTICIDE (Sears)	Tech. chlordane*	45.0%
CROSBY ZINC OXIDE RESIN COMPOUND PLAIN Dental preparation (Crosby)	Zinc oxide Pulverized resin Thymol* Thymol iodide*				

*Consult Sec. II., Ingredients Index. This ingredient may be responsible for major toxic effects if poisonous amounts of this product are ingested.

Name & Use Manufacturer	Ingredients		Name & Use Manufacturer	Ingredients	
CROSS COUNTRY 40% NICOTINE SULPHATE SOLUTION Insecticide (Sears)	Nicotine* (alkaloid)	40%	CROSS COUNTRY WEED KIL-LER DUST (Sears)	Dimethylamine-2, 4-dichloro phenoxy acetate	6%
CROSS COUNTRY PEST SPRAY (Sears)	DDT Xylene*	25.0% 70.4%	CROSS COUNTRY WETTABLE DUSTING SULFUR Insecticide, fungicide (Sears)	Sulfur*	95%
CROSS COUNTRY RAT-KILLER (Sears)	Warfarin (3-(a-acetonylbenzyl)- 4-hydroxycoumarin)	0.025%			
			CRO-TOX REPELLENT Seed protector (Bonide)	Water gas tar* Steam-distilled turpentine*	88.6% 7.4%
CROSS COUNTRY ROSE DUST Insecticide, fungicide (Sears)	Malathion* DDT* Captan Dinitro-(1-methyl-heptyl)- phenyl crotonate Other nitrogen derivatives (chiefly dinitro-(1-methyl- heptyl)-phenol)	4.00% 5.00% 5.00% 0.67% 0.80%	CROW-FEZ Rodenticide (Bonide)	Water gas tar* Steam-distilled turpentine*	88.6% 7.4%
			CROWN AMMONIA (Brate)	Ammonia*	
CROSS COUNTRY ROSE SPRAY Insecticide, fungicide (Sears)	DDT* Rotenone Other cube extractives Tech. piperonyl cyclonene (0.4% of 3-isoamyl-5- (methylene dioxyphenyl)-2- cyclohexenone, its 6-carbothoxy derivative and 0.1% related compounds) Ferbam (ferric dimethyl dithiocarbamate) Sulfur* Inert ingredients*	4.00% 0.25% 0.50% 0.50 7.60 15.00	CROWN-SEC SPRAY Insecticide (Moretex)	Dichloro diphenyl trichloroethane* Isobornyl thiocyanoacetate* Other related terpenes Petroleum distillate Inert ingredients*	5% 2.46% 0.54% 0.92%
			CRU-MO Antitussive (King, W.H.)	Camphor* Methyl salicylate* Eucalyptus Menthol* Oils of turpentine* Petrolatum base	
CROSS COUNTRY SPRAY FOR EVERGREENS Insecticide (Sears)	DDT* 2-(p-tert-Butylphenoxy)- isopropyl-2-chloroethyl sulfite Piperonyl cyclonene (1.04% of 3-isoamyl-5-(methylene- dioxyphenyl)-2-cyclohexenone, its 6-carbothoxy derivative, and 0.26% related compounds) Rotenone Other cube extractives Inert ingredients	10.00% 2.00% 1.30% 0.65% 1.30%	CRYOLITE DUST NO. 50 Insecticide (Sunland)	Sodium fluoaluminate*	50%
			CRYSTAL BORER RE-PELLENT Insecticide (Crystal)	Soap (anhydrous) Naphthalene*	22% 12%
CROSS COUNTRY THREE-WAY DUST Insecticide, fungicide (Sears)	Malathion* Methoxychlor tech.* Captan (n-trichloro methyl thio tetrahydro phthalimide) Sulfur	4.0% 5.0% 5.0% 5.0%	CRYSTAL CLEANER (Central Soap)		
			CRYSTAL COLOR PAINT-ING SET (Porter Chem.)		
CROSS COUNTRY THREE-WAY SPRAY Insecticide, fungicide (Sears)	Zineb (zinc ethylene bis (dithiocarbamate) Rotenone Other cube extractives Inert ingredients*	9.7% 1.5% 3.0%	CRYSTAL CRESOL SOLUTION SAPONATED N.F. Disinfectant (Crystal)	Cresol* U.S.P. Soap	
CROSS COUNTRY TOMATO DUST Insecticide, fungicide (Sears)	TDE* (dichloro diphenyl dichloroethane) Copper as metallic from tribasic copper sulfate*	5.0% 7.0%	CRYSTAL CRESYLIC DISINFECT-ANT (Crystal)	Cresylic acid* Soap	50% 25%

---

*Consult Sec. II., Ingredients Index. This ingredient may be responsible for major toxic effects if poisonous amounts of this product are ingested.

Name & Use Manufacturer	Ingredients		Name & Use Manufacturer	Ingredients	
CRYSTALITE (Texas Co.)	Water-white kerosene*		CUDDLE BEAR Bubble bath (Clark, R.)	Sodium sulfate (salt cake) Sodium alkyl aryl sulfonate Sodium alkyl lauryl sulfonate	
CRYSTAL WHITE Abrasive cleaner (Colgate-Palmolive)			CUKTOX CUKE DUST Insecticide, fungicide (Bonide)	Rotenone Other cube extractives Copper oxychloride* (copper content 7%)	1% 2% 12%
CRYSTAMINE Disinfectant (Crystal)	Alkyl tolyl methyl trimethyl ammonium chlorides* 10%		CULLIGAN CHLORINE REAGENT Culligan)	0-Toluidine dihydrochloride 1% Hydrochloric acid solution* 15%	
CRYSTAN LIQUID SOAP (Crystal)	Captan (n-trichloro methyl thiotetrahydro pthalimide) 1% Anhydrous soap Potassium soap of refined oils		CULLIGAN CUL-LET REFILL Toilet cleaner (Culligan)	1, 3-Dichloro-3, 5-dimethyl hydantoin* 95%	
CRYSTAN SOAP POWDER (Crystal)	Captan (n-trichloro methyl thiotetrahydro pthalimide) 0.34% Soap (anhydrous) 33.00%		CULLIGAN IRON #1 Iron detector (Culligan)	Hydrochloric acid* 1-1	
CRYSTAPHENE NO. 18 Germicidal soap (Crystal)	Hexachlorophene* G-11 (2, 2-methylene-bis-(3, 4, 6-trichloro phenol) Potassium vegetable oil soap		CULLIGAN IRON #2 Iron detector (Culligan)	Thioglycolic acid*	
CRYSTOL COAL TAR DISINFECT-ANT (Crystal)	Coal tar neutral oils Soap Phenols*		CULLIGAN IRON #3 Iron detector (Culligan)	Conc. ammonium hydroxide*	
CS-301 CRYSTAL GERMICIDE 10 (Crystal)	Soap Alcohol Orthobenzyl parachlorophenol* Sodium salt orthobenzyl para-chlorophenol* 21.6%		CULLIGAN STANDARD SOAP SOLUTION (Culligan)	Isopropyl alcohol* Potassium oleate Potassium hydroxide Methyl salicylate*	
CS ODORLESS DISINFECT-ANT (Crystal)	Soap Alcohol* 4- and 6-chloro-2-phenyl phenol* 22%		CUMPHOLIN Skin emollient (Bartz)	Camphor* Oleoresin of Capsicum Methyl salicylate* Oil of cajeput Oil of turpentine Croton oil Menthol*	
C-SPRAY Glass cleaner (Randall-Thomson)			CU-NO-ROT WOOD & FABRIC PRE-SERVATIVE (Lester)	Copper naphthenate* (2% metallic copper) 25%	
CUBOR DUST 75 Insecticide (Chipman Chem.)	Rotenone 0.75% Other cube resins 1.50%		CUPAIBA BLUE Genitourinary antiseptic (Massengill)	Each pill: Methylene blue 65 mg. Powdered cubeb 65 mg. Extr. kava 65 mg. Copaiba mass 32 mg. Oil of nutmeg 0.0062 cc. Oil of santal 0.0062 cc.	
CUBOR DUST 100 Insecticide (Chipman Chem.)	Rotenone 1% Other cube resins 2%		CUPID CHASER Male dog repellent (Pierpont)	Citral, associated terpenes, and alcohols* 42% Mineral oil 58%	
CUBOR SULFUR DUST 75 Insecticide (Chipman Chem.)	Rotenone 0.75% Other cube resins 1.50% Sulfur* 43.00%		CUPID CLEANING Cleaner (Chamberlain)		
CUCUMBER & WITCH-HAZEL CREAM Skin irritation (McAdams)	Phenol 0.5% Alcohol 10.0% Glycerin 10.0% Extr. witch hazel 4.0% Extr. cucumber 4.0% Perfume 1.0% Tragacanth 1.0%		CUPREX Ectoparasiticide (Merck)	Tetralin* Copper oleate* Liquid paraffin and acetone* 69%	

---

*Consult Sec. II., Ingredients Index. This ingredient may be responsible for major toxic effects if poisonous amounts of this product are ingested.

Name & Use Manufacturer	Ingredients	
CUPRICAP (copper caprylate compound ointment) External fungicide (medical) (C & M)	Copper caprylate*	6%
	Zinc caprylate	3%
	Caprylic acid	6.5%
	Salicylic acid	1.7%
	Propylene glycol caprylates	10%
	Aranol (penetrant)	
	Carbowax	
CUPRINOL BRAND CLEAR #20 Wood preservative (Cuprinol)	Zinc naphthenate	30%
	Stoddard solvent*	60%
CUPRINOL BRAND GREEN #10 Wood pre- (Cuprinol)	Copper naphthenate	30%
	Stoddard solvent*	60%
CUPRINOL BRAND WATER RE- PELLENT WOOD PRE- SERVATIVE PRIMER CLEAR #20 (Cuprinol)	Zinc naphthenate (metallic zinc 3%)	30%
	Stoddard solvent*	60%
CUPRINOL BRAND WATER RE- PELLENT WOOD PRE- SERVATIVE PRIMER GREEN #10 (Cuprinol)	Copper naphthenate (metallic copper 3%)	30%
	Stoddard solvent*	60%
CUPROCIDE YELLOW Insecticide (Rohm & Haas)	Yellow cuprous oxide*	90%
CUPROLIGNUM WOOD PRE- SERVATIVE (Rudd)		
CUPROTEX WOOD PRE- SERVATIVE (Woolsey)		
CUR-A-PED Rubefacient (feet) (Redolent)	Camphor*	
	Oil of thyme	
	Oil of wintergreen*	
	Oil of lemon	
	Stearic acid	
	Menthol*	
	Oil of pine*	
	Ethyl salicylate*	
	Glycerin	
	Potassium hydroxide*	
CUREN OINTMENT External fungicide (medical) (Thomas Chem.)	Salicylic acid*	
	Benzoic acid*	
	Zinc oxide	
	Calamine	
	Anhydrous lanolin	
	Liquid petrolatum*	
CUREX FLEA POWDER (Lethelin)	Rotenone	1.1%
	Other cube resins	1.9%

Name & Use Manufacturer	Ingredients	
CURLI-QUE PERMANENT WAVE (Myers, Louis)		
CURLOX COLD WAVE HOME KIT (Lenason)		
CURLTITE Hair spray (Dreyfuss)		
CURRAN DEODORANT BLOCKS OR URINAL DEODORANT BLOCKS (Curran)	Paradichlorobenzene*	100%
CURRAN MOTH BALLS, FLAKES (Curran)	Naphthalene*	100%
CURRAN NAPHTHA- LENE CRYSTALS Insecticide (Curran)		
CURRIER'S TABLETS Laxative (Currier's)	Sodium bicarbonate	
	Magnesium hydroxide	
	Certified food color tint	
	Bismuth subnitrate	
	Oil of peppermint	
CURTAIN CALL PERFUME, COLOGNE (Noblesse)		
CURTIS PHOTO- GRAPHIC SUPPLIES (Curtis Labs.)		
CUSHING'S OINTMENT Skin burns, irritation (Cushing)	Oil of tar*	
	Carbolic acid*	
	Rectified oil of turpentine*	
	Gum camphor*	
CUSTOM GUN BLUE (Casey Chem.)	Selenium*	
	Nitric acid*	
	Methanol	
CUTEX NAIL POLISH (Northam)	Nitrocellulose*	
	Sulfonamide type resin	
	Esters and hydrocarbons*	
CUTICURA MEDICATED LIQUID Skin antiseptic (Potter)	Each fl. oz.:	
	Chlorobutanol U.S.P.	2-1/4 gr.
	Resorcinol* U.S.P.	
	Oxyquinoline sulfate	
	Carbolic acid U.S.P.	
	Camphor* U.S.P.	
	Boric acid* U.S.P.	
	Glycerin U.S.P.	
	Alcohol	28%/v
CUTICURA OINTMENT (Potter)		

---

*Consult Sec. II., Ingredients Index. This ingredient may be responsible for major toxic effects if poisonous amounts of this product are ingested.

Name & Use Manufacturer	Ingredients		Name & Use Manufacturer	Ingredients	
CUTICURA SOAP Skin emollient (Potter)	Petrolatum unbleached Paraffin unbleached Mineral oil Beeswax		CYMENEX ANTISEPTIC DUSTING POWDER (Schmidt)	Phenol* Thymol Zinc stearate Benzoic acid Cymenol	
CUTIGIENE NIGHT CREAM (Franco)			CYPRO DUST Insecticide (Commercial Chem.)	Pyrethrum Rotenone* Piperonyl cyclonene	
CUTISENE Skin ointment (Cutisene)	Cod liver oil concentrate Pyrilamine maleate* Hexachlorophene Salicylic acid* Resorcin* Zinc oxide Lanolin Glycerin Carbolic acid Aromatics	1%	CYPRO EMULSION CONCEN- TRATE Wood pre- servative (Commercial Chem.)	Piperonyl butoxide Pyrethrins Inert ingredients*	11.87% 1.18%
CUTIZOL Foot oint- ment (Veltex)	Benzoic and salicylic acids* Zinc oxide Oil of juniper tar* Camphor* Menthol* Essential oils in petrolatum base		CYPRO MILL SPRAY Wood pre- servative (Commercial Chem.)	Piperonyl butoxide Pyrethrins Inert ingredients*	1.27% 0.13%
C.W.K. CHICKWEED KILLER (Garden Prod.)	Sodium arsenite* Potassium cyanate	47.50% 34.58%	CYSTEX Urinary antiseptic (Knox)	Each tablet: Acetophenetidin* Methenamine* Sodium salicylate* Benzoic acid	1 gr.
CYANI KIL BOMB Rodenticide (Long Mfg.)	Potassium nitrate Wood carbon Sulfur Litharge Sodium nitrate Zinc cyanide* Sodium fluosilicate* Sodium chlorate*	9.59% 2.68% 35.73% 7.32% 24.68% 4.00% 6.66% 9.34%	CYSTOLITHIA Diuretic, urinary antiseptic (Whorton)	Each fl. oz.: Methenamine* Lithium salicylate* and lithium benzoate Eupatorium,* stigmata maydis, triticum repens, and saw palmetto Alcohol	40 gr. 16 gr. 40 gr. 12%/v
CYANOGAS A-DUST, CALCIUM CYANIDE, G- FUMIGANT Fumigants (Am. Cyan.)	Calcium cyanide*		C-Z AIR-DIS Deodorant, sanitizer (Allied Home)	Isopropyl alcohol Triethylene glycol Propylene glycol Para di-isobutyl phenoxy ethoxy ethyl dimethyl benzyl ammonium chloride* Dichloro difluoro methane (Freon 12) Trichloro monofluoro methane (Freon 11) Petroleum distillate*	
CYCLAINE (veterinary) 5% STERILE SOLUTION Local anes- thetic (Sharp & Dohme)	Each 1 cc.: Hexylcaine hydrochloride Propylparaben Methylparaben	50 mg. 0.02% 0.15%			
			C-Z ALL PURPOSE SUDS QUALITY UTILITY CLEANER (Allied Home)		
CYCLEWELD C-14B, C-14 CATALYST (Cycleweld)	Diethylene triamine*		C-Z AQUA AMMONIA (Allied Home)	Ammonia* 26°	
CYCLO- THRYCIN Throat lozenges (Hance)	Each lozenge: Tyrothricin Cycloform (isobutyl-p-amino benzoate) Siptuim (benzalkonium chloride)	2 mg. 5 mg. 0.1%	C-Z ASPHALT TILE CLEANER, SEALER (Allied Home)		
CYDONOL MASSAGE LOTION Foot rube- facient (Gordon Labs.)	Hexachlorophene Isopropyl alcohol* Methyl salicylate* Benzalkonium chloride*		C-Z ASPHALT TILE WAX (Allied Home)	Carnauba wax	
CYMENEX Skin oint- ment (Schmidt)	Zinc oxide Thymol* Benzoic acid Monochlorthymol*		C-Z AUTO MIST Sanitizer, deodorizer (Allied Home)	Triethylene glycol Isopropyl alcohol Di-isobutyl phenoxy ethoxy ethyl dimethyl benzyl ammonium chloride Perfume oil	5.6% 9.0% 0.1% 0.3%

*Consult Sec. II., Ingredients Index. This ingredient may be responsible for major toxic effects if poisonous amounts of this product are ingested.

Name & Use Manufacturer	Ingredients	Name & Use Manufacturer	Ingredients
C-Z BOILER COMPOUND (Allied Home)	Sodium hydroxide*	C-Z INSECTICIDE CONCEN- TRATE (Allied Home)	Petroleum distillate* 87.500% Beta thiocyano ethyl esters* of mixed fatty acids (containing 10-18 carbon atoms) 9.378% Beta butoxy beta' thiocyano diethyl ether* 3.125%
C-Z CARBON TETRA- CHLORIDE (Allied Home)	Carbon tetrachloride*		
C-Z CHLORAFUME Deodorant (Allied Home)		C-Z INSECTICIDE CONCEN- TRATE WITH DDT (Allied Home)	Petroleum distillate* 82.497% Beta thiocyano ethyl esters* of mixed fatty acid (10-18 carbon atoms) 9.378% Beta butoxy beta' thiocyano diethyl ether* 3.125% DDT* 5.000%
C-Z CHLOROLEN Disinfectant, germicide (Allied Home)	Sodium hypochlorite* 4.2%		
C-Z CLEAN GLO Floor con- ditioner (Allied Home)		C-Z INSECT KILLER BOMB (Allied Home)	DDT 2.00% Pyrethrins 0.25% Tech. piperonyl butoxide 1.00% Methylated naphthalenes 5.00% Petroleum distillate* 11.75%
C-Z 25 CONCEN- TRATED GERMICIDE (Allied Home)	Alkyl dimethyl benzyl ammonium chlorides* 10%		
		C-Z KLEN- KLOR Bactericide, germicide (Allied Home)	Sodium hypochlorite* 3.25% Sodium phosphate approx. 92.25%
C-Z DANCENE Dance floor wax (Allied Home)			
C-Z DEODORANT BLOCS & CRYSTALS (Allied Home)	Paradichlorobenzene*	C-Z LDC 3 LIQUID HAND DISHWASHING COMPOUND (Allied Home)	
		C-Z LIGHT SPIRIT WAX (Allied Home)	Carnauba wax
C-Z DISHBRITE #1 DISH- GLEAM (Allied Home)		C-Z LIME-SOLV Detergent, lime remover (Allied Home)	
C-Z DRAIN PIPE OPENER (Allied Home)	Sodium hydroxide*	C-Z LINDANE Insecticide (Allied Home)	Gamma isomer of benzene hexachloride* (from lindane) 99% Other isomers of benzene hexachloride 1%
C-Z DUST TREAT Sanitizer, polisher (Allied Home)	Chloro-0-phenylphenol 3%		
		C-Z MARVEL- BAC CON- CENTRATED GERMICIDE (Allied Home)	Methyl dodecyl benzyl trimethyl ammonium chloride* 11%
C-Z EKONO CLEANER (Allied Home)	Vegetable oils		
C-Z FORMALITE SPRAY Deodorant (Allied Home)		C-Z MARVENE Dishwashing compound (Allied Home)	
C-Z GLASS WAX (Allied Home)		C-Z METAL POLISH (Allied Home)	
		C-Z MURIATIC ACID 18° (Allied Home)	Hydrochloric acid*
C-Z GRESOLV Detergent (Allied Home)		C-Z NOBURN GYM FINISH (Allied Home)	
C-Z GYM FINISH (Allied Home)		C-Z NO GERM DISINFECTANT (Allied Home)	Soap Isopropyl alcohol* Chloro-o-phenyl phenol* 30.475%
		C-Z NU-GLO Scrub soap (Allied Home)	Coconut and vegetable oil soaps

*Consult Sec. II., Ingredients Index. This ingredient may be responsible for major toxic effects if poisonous amounts of this product are ingested.

Name & Use Manufacturer	Ingredients		Name & Use Manufacturer	Ingredients	
CZO LOTION Skin counter-irritant (Massengill)	Each fl. oz.: Calamine Zinc oxide Glycerin and aromatics	2 gm. 2 gm. q.s.	C-Z 3X SERVICE CLEANER Toilet cleaner (Allied Home)	Hydrochloric acid*	
CZO LOTION WITH ANTI-HISTAMINE Skin counter-irritant (Massengill)	Each fl. oz.: Calamine Zinc oxide Phenyltoxylamine dihydrogen citrate Glycerin and aromatics	2 gm. 2 gm. 1% q.s.	C-Z SHINEX LIQUID WINDOW CLEANER (Allied Home)		
CZO LOTION WITH PHENOL Skin counter-irritant (Massengill)	Each fl. oz.: Carbolic acid liquefied Calamine Zinc oxide Glycerin and aromatics	0.3 cc. 2 gm. 2 gm. q.s.	C-Z SHUR SHINE FURNITURE POLISH (Allied Home)		
			C-Z SOLVENE Degreaser (Allied Home)		
CZO WITH BENZOCAINE LOTION Skin counter-irritant (Massengill)	Each fl. oz.: Calamine Zinc oxide Benzocaine Glycerin and aromatics	2 gm. 2 gm. 2% q.s.	C-Z SUPER KLOR Disinfectant, deodorant (Allied Home)	Sodium paratoluene sulfon chloramide*	16%
C-Z PAINT & VARNISH REMOVER (Allied Home)			C-Z SUPER MARVEL DIP Glass cleaner (Allied Home)		
C-Z PASTE CLEANER (Allied Home)			C-Z SUPER WAX HEAVY DUTY (Allied Home)	Carnauba wax	
C-Z PENA GYM SEALER HEAVY DUTY C-Z PENA-SEAL (Allied Home)	Tung oil Bakelite resins		C-Z TERRAZZO SEALER (Allied Home)		
C-Z PENA SOLV Solvent for steam cleaners (Allied Home)			C-Z TOILET BOWL CLEANER (Allied Home)	Bisulfate of soda*	
C-Z PERMA-SURF Surface finish (Allied Home)			C-Z VELVEEN Liquid toilet soap (Allied Home)	Cochine coconut oil Vegetable oils	
C-Z PINALENE DISINFECT-ANT (Allied Home)	Pine oil* Soap Isopropyl alchol*		C-Z WATERLESS HAND CLEANER (Allied Home)	Hexachlorophene* Lanolin	
C-Z RAT & MOUSE KILLER (Allied Home)	Warfarin (3-(a-acetonylbenzyl)-4-hydroxycoumarin) 0.025%		C-Z WAX REMOVER (Allied Home)		
C-Z SEALA-FLOR Concrete floor sealer (Allied Home)	Tung oil Bakelite resin		C-Z WHIFF WITH CHLO-ROPHYLL & X-ON Toilet bowl cleaner (Allied Home)	Hydrogen chloride* Formaldehyde	13.96% 1.00%
C-Z SELF POLISHING FLOOR WAX (Allied Home)	Carnauba wax		C-Z X-IT DEEP FAT FRY CLEANER (Allied Home)		
C-Z SEPTIC CAUSTIC CRYSTALS Toilet treat-ment (Allied Home)	Sodium hydroxide*		C-Z ZIP MECHANIC'S BORATED HAND SOAP (Allied Home)	Lanolin Borax*	

*Consult Sec. II., Ingredients Index. This ingredient may be responsible for major toxic effects if poisonous amounts of this product are ingested.

190

Name & Use Manufacturer	Ingredients
DABON AFTER SHAVE LOTION MEN-THOLATED (Cort-Livingston)	
DABON AFTER SHAVE STICK (Cort-Livingston)	
DABON BRUSHLESS SHAVING CREAM (Cort-Livingston)	
DABON DEODORANT STICK (Cort-Livingston)	
DAD LIQUID PAINT BRUSH CLEANER (Patent)	Methylene chloride* Isopropyl alcohol Xylol* Onyx (wetting agent)
DAINTY DEW CREAM COLOGNE (Maines)	
DAINTY DEW DEODORANT (Maines)	
DAINTY MAID JELLY (Dainty-Maid)	
DAINTY MAID POWDER (Dainty-Maid)	
DAINTY MAID SUPPOSI-TORIES (Dainty-Maid)	
DAIRYLAND 20% ANTU BROWN RAT KILLER (Wisconsin Pharm.)	Alpha-naphthyl-thiourea* 20%
DAIRYLAND CATTLE SPRAY Insecticide (Wisconsin Pharm.)	Petroleum distillate* Pine oil* Tech. piperonyl butoxide Pyrethrins
DAIRYLAND 40% DDT LIQUID CONC. Insecticide for water mixtures (Wisconsin Pharm.)	Tech. DDT* 40% Tech. xylene* 54%
DAIRYLAND HOUSEHOLD FLY SPRAY (Wisconsin Pharm.)	Petroleum distillate* Piperonyl butoxide Pyrethrins

Name & Use Manufacturer	Ingredients
DAIRYLAND INSECT SPRAY DDT 5% (Wisconsin Pharm.)	Petroleum distillate Xylene* DDT 5%
DAIRYLAND PREMIX RAT & MOUSE KILLER (Wisconsin Pharm.)	Warfarin (3-(a-acetonylbenzyl)-4-hydroxycoumarin)
DAIRYLAND WARFARIN RAT & MOUSE KILLER (Wisconsin Pharm.)	Warfarin (3-(a-acetonylbenzyl)-4-hydroxycoumarin) 0.5%
DAIRY STIK PAINT (Lake Chem.)	
DAIRYWHITE PAINT (Am. Marietta)	
DAGGETT & RAMSDELL BUBBLE BATH (Daggett and Ramsdell)	
DALAX PAINT (Am. Paint Co.)	
DALIDOME POWDER (formerly Dali-Sol) For wet-dressings) (Dome)	Zinc sulfate* Copper sulfate* Camphor*
DALILA LOTIONS For face, hands (Corot)	
DALILA PERFUME & TOILET WATER (Corot)	
DA-LUXE Paint (Davis Paint)	
DALY-HERRING SABADILLA DUST Insecticide (Daly-Herring)	Sabadilla seed 20.00 Sabadilla alkaloids 0.80
DAME NATURE BALM & LOTION (Dame Nature)	
DAMP CHEK Fungicide (Chek)	

*Consult Sec. II., Ingredients Index. This ingredient may be responsible for major toxic effects if poisonous amounts of this product are ingested.

Name & Use Manufacturer	Ingredients
DAMPCHEX Water- repellent wallcoater (Am. Fluresit)	
DAMPCOAT PAINT (Wilbur)	
DAMPNEY RUBBER (Dampney)	Iron oxide Aromatic petroleum Terpene (blend) Chlorinated rubber Chlorinated paraffin Chlorinated biphenyls
DAMP-SEAL MASONRY COATING (Monroe Co.)	
DAMP-TOX Fungicide (Doggett- Pfeil)	Oxyquinoline benzoate
DAMSCHIN- SKY'S HAIR OIL (Damschinsky)	Acid pyrogallic* crystals U.S.P. Cupric chloride* purified crystals U.S.P. Ferric chloride U.S.P.
DAM-TITE Maintenance material (Speco)	Silicone compound in aromatic solvent*
DAN-DEE Floor polish (Twin City)	Ethyl alcohol n-Butyl alcohol* Denatured alcohol Methyl alcohol* Gums Mineral spirits*
DAN-DEE FLOOR WAX (Twin City)	Waxes Resins Emulsifiers Morpholine Triethanolamine Ammonia* Dibutyl phthalate
DAN-DEE FURNITURE POLISH (Twin City)	Mineral oil* Ammonia* Triethanolamine Silicone
DANDER-EX For dandruff (Sisson's Pharm.)	Resorcinol* Sulfamerizine* Sulfathiazole* Sulfadiazine* Extract witch hazel Perfume
DANDER-OFF For dandruff (Hughel)	
DANDRICIDE For dandruff (Dandricide)	
DAND-RID'R For dandruff (Dand-Rid'r)	
DANDRIFUGE For dandruff (Burnham Labs.)	

Name & Use Manufacturer	Ingredients	
DANDRO-CIDE Antiseptic for dandruff (Arem)	Sulfanilamide High molecular alkyl dimethyl benzyl ammonium chlorides* Acetone	6.0 mg./cc. 7%
DANGER PERFUMES & TOILET WATERS (Parfums Ciro)		
DR. A. C. DANIELS' ANTISEPTIC DUSTING POWDER (Daniels, Dr. A. C.)	Boric acid* Zinc oxide Sulfur* Camphor* Ammonium alum Oil of pine*	
DR. A. C. DANIELS' ASTRINGENT TABLETS For intestinal irritation (veterinary) (Daniels, Dr. A. C.)	Bismuth subsalicylate* Salol Bismuth subnitrate	
DR. A. C. DANIELS' CARBO- NEGUS DIS- INFECTANT (Daniels, Dr. A. C.)	Coal tar neutral oils Coal tar phenols* Soap	
DR. A. C. DANIELS' COLLYRIUM Eye wash antiseptic (veterinary) (Daniels, Dr. A. C.)	Boric acid* Glycerin Camphor water* Rose water Salt	
DR. A. C. DANIELS' CONDITION TABLETS Tonic (veterinary) (Daniels, Dr. A. C.)	Blaud's mass Cascara sagrada Capsicum	
DR. A. C. DANIELS' COUGH SYRUP FOR DOGS & CATS Antitussive (veterinary) (Daniels, Dr. A. C.)	Chloroform White pine Wild cherry Sassafras Sanguinaria Poplar bud Aralia Pine tar	2 m./oz.
DR. A. C. DANIELS' DANILAX Liquid cathartic (veterinary) (Daniels, Dr. A. C.)	Phenolphthalein* Petrolatum	

*Consult Sec. II., Ingredients Index. This ingredient may be responsible for major toxic effects if poisonous amounts of this product are ingested.

Name & Use Manufacturer	Ingredients	Name & Use Manufacturer	Ingredients
DR. A. C. DANIELS' DANIVOM TABLETS For gastric irritation (veterinary) (Daniels, Dr. A. C.)	Cerium oxalate Bismuth subnitrate Phenol* Menthol* Benzocaine	DR. A. C. DANIELS' SKIN OINT-MENT For skin irritations (veterinary) (Daniels, Dr. A. C.)	Benzocaine Acid salicylate* Oil of wintergreen* Carbolic acid* Sulfur* Amber petrolatum
DR. A. C. DANIELS' DERMITITE For skin irritations (veterinary) (Daniels, Dr. A. C.)	Resorcinol* Sulfur* Tricresylic acid*	DR. A. C. DANIELS' TAPEWORM TABLETS Veterinary (Daniels, Dr. A. C.)	Arecoline hydrobromide* 1/8 gr./tablet
DR. A. C. DANIELS' EFFER WASH Germicide (Daniels, Dr. A. C.)	Thymol* Hydrogen peroxide* Acetanilid 3/16 gr./fl. oz.	DR. A. C. DANIELS' TONIC PILLS Veterinary (Daniels, Dr. A. C.)	Each pill: Arsenate* 1/60 gr. Quinine arsenate* 1/60 gr. Nuclein 4 m.
DR. A. C. DANIELS' GERMI POWDER Antiseptic for ear (veterinary) (Daniels, Dr. A. C.)	Boric acid* Thymol iodide*	DR. A. C. DANIELS' V-M CAPSULES Veterinary (Daniels, Dr. A. C.)	Brewers' yeast Brewers' yeast extract Dehydrated lemon juice Tricalcium phosphate
DR. A. C. DANIELS' GOLDEN LINIMENT (Daniels, Dr. A. C.)	Capsicum Oil turpentine* Oil camphor* Sassafrassy Gum camphor* Methyl salicylate* Kerosene*	DR. A. C. DANIELS' WONDER LOTION For skin injuries (Daniels, Dr. A. C.)	Extract oak bark Alcohol 15%/v
DR. A. C. DANIELS' LAXATIVE TABLETS Veterinary (Daniels, Dr. A. C.)	Aloin* Cascara sagrada Podophyllin*	DANISH BENZYL LOTION Skin antiseptic (Tilden)	Benzyl benzoate* 27%/w Water Triethanolamine stearate Glyceryl monostearate Lanolin 73%/w
DR. A. C. DANIELS' L-K TABLETS Diuretic (veterinary) (Daniels, Dr. A. C.)	Boric acid* Extract of corn silk Extract hydrangea Extract buchu Extract triticum Potassium bicarbonate Atropine sulfate 1/2000 gr.	DANTOL DANDRUFF REMOVER HAIR LOTION (Dantol)	
		D & A PAINT & VARNISH CLEANER (Nat'l. Broom)	
DR. A. C. DANIELS' NASAL BALM For nasal irritations (veterinary) (Daniels, Dr. A. C.)	Camphor* Menthol* Oil of eucalyptus* White petrolatum, lanolin and glycerine base	DAPCO DUST Insecticide (Doggett-Pfeil)	DDT* Copper*
		DAPSPRAY Insecticide (Doggett-Pfeil)	DDT* 30% Rotenone 1%
DR. A. C. DANIELS' SARCOPTIC MANGE SALVE Veterinary (Daniels, Dr. A. C.)	Water 3-1/2% Kaolin 10% Umber 1%	DAPTHION W15 Insecticide (Doggett-Pfeil)	Parathion* 1%
		DARA DEODORANT (Dara)	
		DARA SHAMPOO (Dara)	

*Consult Sec. II., Ingredients Index. This ingredient may be responsible for major toxic effects if poisonous amounts of this product are ingested.

Name & Use Manufacturer	Ingredients		Name & Use Manufacturer	Ingredients	
DARA SUN TAN LOTION WITH INSECT REPELLENT (Dara)			DASIN 4 (Natural) For colds (capsule) (Massengill)	Each capsule: Opium Ipecac Acetophenetidin* Atropine sulfate Acetylsalicylic acid* Camphor Caffeine	3.2 mg. 3.2 mg. 0.1 gm. 0.13 mg. 0.13 gm. 16 mg. 8 mg.
D'ARCY CEMENTS (D'Arcy)					
DARE-U COLOGNE & PERFUME (Old 97)			DASIN 4 (Yellow Tops) For colds (capsule) (Massengill)	Each capsule: Opium Ipecac Acetophenetidin* Atropine sulfate Acetylsalicylic acid* Camphor Caffeine	3.2 mg. 3.2 mg. 0.1 gm. 0.13 mg. 0.13 gm. 16 mg. 8 mg.
DAR-KAY FOR THE HAIR (Delancey)					
DARK-EYES- BOTTLE NO. 1 Cosmetic eye color (Dark-Eyes)	Silver nitrate* U.S.P. 4.75 parts Ammonium hydroxide* C.P. 1.30 parts Pectic vehicle		DASIN, C. S. (Green Tops) For colds (capsule) (Massengill)	Each capsule: Codeine sulfate Ipecac Acetophenetidin* Atropine sulfate Acetylsalicylic acid* Camphor Caffeine	1.6 mg. 3.2 mg. 0.1 gm. 0.13 mg. 0.13 gm. 16 mg. 8 mg.
DARK-EYES- BOTTLE NO. 2 Cosmetic eye color (Dark-Eyes)	Pyrogallol* (resublimed U.S.P.) 3.75 parts Solvent 96.25 parts		DASIN 1/4 STRENGTH (Pink- Flavored) Analgesic, antipyretic (tablet) (Massengill)	Each tablet: Opium Ipecac Acetophenetidin* Atropine sulfate Aspirin* Camphor, monobromated Caffeine	0.8 mg. 0.8 mg. 32 mg. 0.032 mg. 32 mg. 4 mg. 2.1 mg.
DARKTOWN PAINT (Chase Varnish)					
DAROL CAPSULES Analgesic, laxative (McKesson)	Each capsule: Acetanilid* 1 gr. Ext. of henbane* 1/8 gr. Cinchonidine dihydrobromide (blennostasine) 3/4 gr. Caffeine 1/4 gr. Aloin 1/16 gr. Cayenne pepper 1/4 gr. Monobromated camphor* 1 gr.		DA-TEX Paint (Davis Paint)		
			DAUBOLINE Paint acces- sory (Internat. Paint)	Mineral spirits* (or turpentine substitute)	
			DAUBOSOL Skin antiseptic (Beebe Labs.)	Phenyl mercuric nitrate in acetone 1-2000 Isopropyl alcohol* Propylene glycol*	
DAROLENE Water softener (Dacar)			DAVED CLOUDY AMMONIA (Robinson)	Ammonia*	
DAROL SYRUP Antitussive (Mckesson)	Ethyl alcohol 3%/v Each fl. oz.: Chloroform 2 gr. Cocillana 10 gr. Senaga 5 gr. Mullein leaves 4 gr. Thyme 4 gr. Tartar emetic 1/16 gr. Potassium creosote sulfonate 2-1/2 gr. Ammonium chloride 4 gr.		DAVEYITE & DAVEYKOTE Tree wound paints (Davey)		
			DAVEY'S WILL KILL Poison (Blue Ball)		
DARX PAINT & VARNISH REMOVER (cream) (Devoe)	Benzol* Denatured alcohol Acetone Paraffin Cellulosic thickening medium		DAVICOTE Paint (Davis Paint)		
DARX PAINT & VARNISH REMOVER (liquid) (Devoe)	Benzol* more than 15% Denatured alcohol Acetone Paraffin		DAVID'S SANATIVE WASH (Owens)	Lime* Sulfur*	
			DAVI MIRACLE FOAM (Davi)		

*Consult Sec. II., Ingredients Index. This ingredient may be responsible for major toxic effects if poisonous amounts of this product are ingested.

- 414 -

Name & Use Manufacturer	Ingredients		Name & Use Manufacturer	Ingredients	
DAVIS ANT POWDER (Davis, O. D.)	Gamma isomer of benzene hexachloride	1%	DAWN TOILETRIES (Noblesse)		
DAVIS' ANTU RAT KILLER (Davis, C. H.)			DAWSON FUMIGANT FORMULA 37 (Ferguson)	Ethylene dibromide* Methyl bromide*	30.0% 69.5%
DAVIS BUG-X Insecticide (Davis, O. D.)	Petroleum distillate* Gamma isomer of benzene hexachloride Xylene	98% 0.5% 1.16%	DAWSON FUMIGANT FORMULA 73 (Ferguson)	Ethylene dibromide* Methyl bromide*	70.0% 29.5%
DAVIS' COLORAMA PAINT (Davis, H. B.)	Titanium dioxide Zinc chromate* Phthalocyanine green Soya alkyd resin solution Raw linseed oil Petroleum thinners Driers	43.81% 52.38% 3.81% 66.04% 8.10% 21.65% 4.21%	DAWSON FUMIGANT FORMULA 82 (Ferguson)	Ethylene dibromide* Methyl bromide*	80.0% 19.5%
			DAXALAN OINTMENT (Dome)	Whole crude coal tar Zinc oxide Starch Hydrophilic base	2.88%
DAVIS FLY-X Insecticide (Davis, O. D.)	Mineral oil Beta-thiocyano ethyl esters of fatty acids averaging 10-18 carbon atoms B-butoxy-B-thiocyano diethyl ether	96.21% 2.86% 0.93%	DAXALAN PEDIATRIC OINTMENT (Dome)	Whole crude coal tar Zinc oxide Starch Hydrophilic base	1.44%
DAVIS' FORMULA External fungicide (medical) (Davis Pharm.)	Alcohol* Salicylic acid* Benzoic acid Resorcin*	56%	DAY-GLO WATER COLORS (Lawter)		
DAVIS LINDANE REFILL FOR ELECTRIC VAPORIZERS (Davis, O. D.)	Gamma isomer of benzene hexachloride*	99%	DAYLIGHT PAINT (Thompson & Co.)		
			DAY'S LIQUID PINE CLEANSER (Pine)	Pine oil Vegetable oil soap Lanolin	
DAVIS MOTH-X Insecticide (Davis, O. D.)	Mineral oil Beta-thiocyano ethyl esters of fatty acids averaging 10-18 carbon atoms B-butoxy-B-thiocyano diethyl ether	92.92% 5.34% 1.74%	DAZOLIN METAL POLISH (Foy)		
DAVIS POISON MOUSE KILLER (Davis, C. H.)			DAZY Air deodorizer (Drackett)		
DAVIS' RED SQUILL LIQUID & POWDER Rodenticide (Davis, C. H.)			DAZZEE Germicide (Clifton)	Sodium hypochlorite*	5.25%
			DAZZLE BLEACH (Prescott)		
DAVIS UNION REMEDY Laxative (Davis, C. T.)	Epsom salts Ext. buchu leaves Culver's root Ginger root Sarsaparilla root Wahoo bark Bitter apple Aromatic cascara Alcohol Ext. senna leaves Mandrake root Rhubarb root Gentian root Juniper berries Prickly ash bark Caramel coloring Salicylic acid*	1.08%	DAZZLE METAL POLISH (Clifton)		
			DAZZLE SOAP POLISH (Prescott)		
			DAZZLE STOVE POLISH (Prescott)		
			DC DANDRUFF CONTROL (D. C. Labs.)	Quaternary ammonium compound* Methocel	
DAVIS WAR-RAT (Davis, O. D.)	Pivalyl-1, 3-indandione	0.025%	D. & C. EXPECTOR- ANT (De Witt)		

*Consult Sec. II., Ingredients Index. This ingredient may be responsible for major toxic effects if poisonous amounts of this product are ingested.

Name & Use Manufacturer	Ingredients		Name & Use Manufacturer	Ingredients	
d-CON ANT-PRUFE (d-Con)	Chlordane*		D-DUST 5 Insecticide (Commercial Chem.)	DDT dust*	5%
d-CON CONCEN-TRATE Rodenticide (d-Con)	Warfarin*		DEAD EASY INSECTICIDE (Imperial Prod.)		
d-CON FLI-CON Insecticide (d-Con)	Malathion*		DEADLY BRAND RODENT DE-STROYERS (U.S. Rodent)	Top and bottom mix: Carbon Sulfur* Saltpeter* Dextrine Paraffin oil Body mix: Carbon Sulfur* Soda nitrate Paraffin oil	11% 37% 47.75% 3.75% 0.50% 9.334% 30.333% 53% 7.333%
d-CON MOTH-PRUFE (d-Con)	Perthane*				
d-CON MOUSE-PRUFE (d-Con)	Sodium salt of warfarin*				
			DEADRAT Rodenticide (Blue Ball)		
d-CON RAT POISON (d-Con)	Warfarin (3-a-acetonylbenzyl-4-hydroxycoumarin) 0.025%		DEAD-SHOT Insecticide (Flores)	Chloroform* U.S.P. Coal tar phenols* Coal tar neutral oils Naphthalene* Camphor* Soap Water Glycerin	12% 7.2% 6%
d-CON READY-MIX READY TO USE Rodenticide (d-Con)	Warfarin*				
d-CON ROACH-PRUFE (d-Con)	Chlordane*		DEAD SHOT VERMIFUGE Anthelmintic (Ross, S.)	Each fl. oz.: Castor oil Oil of chenopodium Oil of turpentine* Oil of bergamot Powdered senna leaves Magnesium carbonate Powdered turmeric	297 m. 28 m. 148 m. 2 m. 2 gr. 1-1/2 gr. 1/2 gr.
d-CON RODENTI-CIDES (d-Con)	Warfarin*				
d-CON WARFICIDE Rodenticide (d-Con)	Sodium salt of warfarin*		DEAM'S SKIPPER-PROOF COMPOUND Insecticide (Deam)	Potassium nitrate Sodium bicarbonate Magnesium carbonate Capsicum	
DDD CREAM Anti-pruritic (Campana)	Thymol Carbolic acid* Sodium salicylate* Glycerin Benzocaine Methyl salicylate* Benzoinated lard				
			PROF. DEAN'S KING SOOTH-ING OIL LINIMENT (Dean's)		
D.D.D. PRESCRIP-TION Anti-pruritic (Campana)	Alcohol Chloral hydrate* 7.6 gr./fl. oz. Glycerine Methyl salicylate* Phenol* F. D. & C. color Thymol* Salicylic acid* Water		DEATH KNELL Rodenticide (Long Mfg.)	Warfarin (3-(a-acetonylbenzyl)-4-hydroxycoumarin) 0.025%	
			DEATH TO GOPHERS (Rat Lunches)	Strychnine*	0.5%
			DEATH TO MICE (Rat Lunches)	Strychnine*	0.4%
D.D.D. SOAP (Campana)			DEATH TO MOLES (Rat Lunches)	Strychnine*	0.5%
DD-IDE SPRAY CONCEN-TRATE Insecticide (Bonide)	DDT* Isopropanol Dialkyl phenoxy polyethoxy ethanol	20% 1.20% 4.80%	DEBETONE PAINT (Debevoise)		
DDTOL Insecticide (Sherwin-Williams)	DDT*	50%	DEB-E-VAR PAINT (Debevoise)		

*Consult Sec. II., Ingredients Index. This ingredient may be responsible for major toxic effects if poisonous amounts of this product are ingested.

Name & Use Manufacturer	Ingredients	Name & Use Manufacturer	Ingredients
DEBONAIR FACIAL & HAIR OILS (Rochester Labs.)	Mineral oils Parawax Beeswax Petrolatum Lanolin Borax* Perfume	DED-TOX DUST #10 Insecticide (Thompson-Hayward)	DDT* 10.0%
DEBONAIR SKIN FRESHENER (Rochester Labs.)	Alcohol* Glycerin Perfume	DED-TOX OS-25 OIL SOLUBLE CONCEN-TRATE Insecticide (Thompson-Hayward)	DDT 23.5% Aromatic petroleum derivative solvent* 76.5%
DEBUTANTE FACE CREAM (Daggett & Ramsdell)		DED-TOX 50W Insecticide (Thompson-Hayward)	DDT* 50%
DEBUTANTE FACE POWDER (Daggett & Ramsdell)		DED-TOX 75W Insecticide (Thompson-Hayward)	DDT* 75%
DEBUTANTE HAND LOTION (Daggett & Ramsdell)		DED-TOX WE-25 Insecticide (Thompson-Hayward)	DDT 23.4% Aromatic petroleum derivative solvent* 71.6%
DECAB Fungicide (Fairfield)	Cetyl dimethyl benzyl ammonium chloride* 10% Stearyl dimethyl benzyl ammonium chloride* 10% Oleyl dimethyl benzyl ammonium chloride* 35% Linoleyl dimethyl benzyl ammonium chloride* 45%	DED-WEED 40 AMINE SALT Herbicide (Thompson-Hayward)	Dimethylamine salt of 2, 4-dichlorophenoxyacetic acid* 49.4%
DECALSO (Permutit)	Aluminosilicate compounds	DED-WEED AMINE-T AMINE SALT Herbicide (Thompson-Hayward)	Triethylamine salt of 2, 4, 5-trichlorophenoxyacetic acid* 56.7%
DECHOLIN (Ames Co.)	Each tablet: Dehydrocholic acid 0.25 mg.	DED-WEED 2-1 BRUSH KIL Herbicide (Thompson-Hayward)	2, 4-D (alkyl esters)* 18.6% 2, 4, 5-T (alkyl esters) 9.6%
DECILLIN POWDER (Medical) fungicide (Penslar)	Zinc undecylenate Undecylenic acid		
DECO ABC Photographic supplies (Deco)		DED-WEED FOR LAWNS Herbicide (Thompson-Hayward)	Dimethylamine salt of 2, 4-dichlorophenoxyacetic acid* 14%
DECORA Fabric painting colors (Weber, F.)		DED-WEED LV-4, LOW VOLATILE ESTER Herbicide (Thompson-Hayward)	2, 4-Dichlorophenoxyacetic acid* (isooctyl ester) 67.4%
DECORET PAINT (Fuller, W.P.)			
DECO-RITE PAINT (Sillers)		DED-WEED LV-6 BRUSH KIL, LOW VOLATILE ESTER Herbicide (Thompson-Hayward)	2, 4, 5-Trichlorophenoxyacetic acid (isooctyl ester)* 64.4%
DECOSEAL PAINT (Debevoise)			
DECUPRYL (Medical) fungicide (Crookes)	Copper undecylenate* 10% Undecylenic acid 5% Dioctyl sodium sulfosuccinate Tetrachlorethylene* Isopropanol*	DED-WEED LV-33 BRUSH KIL, LOW VOLATILE ESTER Herbicide (Thompson-Hayward)	2, 4-Dichlorophenoxyacetic acid* (isooctyl ester) 34.8% 2, 4, 5-Trichlorophenoxyacetic acid* (isooctyl ester) 32.5%

*Consult Sec. II., Ingredients Index. This ingredient may be responsible for major toxic effects if poisonous amounts of this product are ingested.

Name & Use Manufacturer	Ingredients		Name & Use Manufacturer	Ingredients	
DED-WEED M C P AMINE SALT Herbicide (Thompson-Hayward)	Dimethylamine salt of 2-methyl-4-chlorophenoxyacetic acid*	52.4%	DEE AITCH BACCO DUST (10% TDE) Insecticide (Daly-Herring)	TDE* Inert ingredients*	10%
DED-WEED ME-4 Herbicide (Thompson-Hayward)	2, 4-D* (methyl ester)	31.9%	DEE AITCH BACCO SPRAY (25% TDE Conc.) Insecticide (Daly-Herring)	TDE* Inert ingredients*	25%
DED-WEED ME-4 40% BUTYL ESTER Herbicide (Thompson-Hayward)	2, 4-Dichlorophenoxyacetic acid* (butyl ester)	40.0%	DEE AITCH CAR WASH (Daly-Herring)		
DED-WEED ME-5 46% ESTER Herbicide (Thompson-Hayward)	2, 4-Dichlorophenoxyacetic acid* (alkyl esters)	46.0%	DEE AITCH 74% CHLOR-DANE EMULSION CONC. Insecticide (Daly-Herring)	Tech. chlordane*	74.00
DED-WEED ME-6 56% BUTYL ESTER Herbicide (Thompson-Hayward)	2, 4-Dichlorophenoxyacetic acid* (butyl ester)	56.0%	DEE AITCH 7% COP.-3% DDT POTATO-TOMATO DUST Insecticide (Daly-Herring)	Copper* DDT*	7% 3%
DED-WEED ME-9 74% ESTER Herbicide (Thompson-Hayward)	2, 4-Dichlorophenoxyacetic acid* (alkyl esters)	74.0%	DEE AITCH 4% COP.-90% SULPHUR PEANUT DUST Insecticide (Daly-Herring)	Copper* Sulfur*	4% 90%
DED-WEED OS-9 74% ESTER Herbicides (Thompson-Hayward)	2, 4-Dichlorophenoxyacetic acid* (alkyl esters)	74.0%	DEE AITCH 5% DDT DOUBLE ACTION HOUSEHOLD SPRAY Insecticide (Daly-Herring)	DDT*	5%
DED-WEED 50-50 PENTYL BRUSH KIL Herbicide (Thompson-Hayward)	2, 4-Dichlorophenoxyacetic acid* (amyl (pentyl) ester) 30.2% 2, 4, 5-Trichlorophenoxyacetic acid (amyl (pentyl) ester) 29.3%		DEE AITCH 5% DDT DUST Insecticide (Daly-Herring)	DDT*	5%
DED-WEED T-5 BRUSH KIL Herbicide (Thompson-Hayward)	2, 4, 5-Trichlorophenoxyacetic acid* (alkyl esters)	43.8%	DEE AITCH 25% DDT EMULSION CONC. Insecticide (Daly-Herring)	DDT*	25%
DED-WEED T-6 BRUSH KIL Herbicide (Thompson-Hayward)	2, 4, 5-Trichlorophenoxyacetic acid* (alkyl esters)	52.7%	DEE AITCH 10% DITHANE DUST Insecticide (Daly-Herring)	Dithane Inert ingredients*	10%
			DEE AITCH 15% FERMATE DUST Insecticide (Daly-Herring)	Fermate* Inert ingredients*	15%
DEE AITCH 2.5% ALDRIN 5% DDT Insecticide (Daly-Herring)	Aldrin* DDT* Theoret. chlorine*	2.50 5.00 4.47	DEE AITCH 5% PENTA WOOD PRESERVATIVE (Daly-Herring)	Pentachlorophenol	5%
DEE AITCH ANTU RAT POISON (Daly-Herring)	Alpha naphthyl thiourea*	20%	DEE AITCH 41% PENTA WOOD PRE-SERVATIVE (Daly-Herring Co.)	Pentachlorophenol	41%

*Consult Sec. II., Ingredients Index. This ingredient may be responsible for major toxic effects if poisonous amounts of this product are ingested.

Name & Use Manufacturer	Ingredients	
DEE AITCH PINE OIL DISINFECT- ANT (Daly-Herring)	Pine oil*	
DEE AITCH 1.00% ROTE- NONE DUST Insecticide (Daly-Herring)	Rotenone Inert ingredients	1.00%
DEE AITCH 20% SAB- ADILLA DUST Insecticide (Daly-Herring)	Sabadilla*	20%
DEE AITCH 20% TOX- APHENE DUST Insecticide (Daly-Herring)	Toxaphene	20%
DEE AITCH 5% TRIBASIC COPPER SULPHATE DUST Insecticide (Daly-Herring)	Copper sulfate*	5%
DEECOP DUST #1 3-7 Insecticide, fungicide (Chipman, Ltd.)	DDT* Fixed copper*	3% 7%
DEECOP DUST #2 5-7 Insecticide, fungicide (Chipman, Ltd.)	DDT* Fixed copper*	5% 7%
DEECOP SPRAY POWDER Insecticide, fungicide (Chipman, Ltd.)	DDT Copper*	15% 30%
DEENATE 50W DDT IN- SECTICIDE (du Pont)	DDT* tech.	
DEENATE 75W DDT IN- SECTICIDE (du Pont)	DDT* tech.	
DEEPGLO PAINTING SETS (Palmer Show Card)		
DEEP HEAT MENTHO- LATUM RUB Rubefacient, counter- irritant (Mentholatum)	Lanolin Methyl salicylate* Menthol* Oil eucalyptus* Oil turpentine*	

Name & Use Manufacturer	Ingredients	
DEEPS ANTACID Antacid, adsorbent (Makers of Kal)	Magnesium trisilicate Calcium carbonate Aluminum hydroxide Papain	
DEEP-TREAT PENTA WOOD PRESERA- TIVE (King Chemical)	Pentachlorophenol* Petroleum hydrocarbons*	5.20% 94.80%
DEEP TREAT CONCEN- TRATE 1-10 Wood pre- servative, soil poisoner (King Chemical)	Pentachlorophenol* Aromatic petroleum solvents* Special solvents	40% 30% 30%
DEEP TREAT READY TO USE Wood pre- servative, soil poisoner (King Chemical)	Pentachlorophenol Aromatic petroleum solvents*	5.20% 94.8%
DEFENZ RESIDUAL INSECTICIDE (Am. Disinfect.)	Aliphatic petroleum solvent* Tech. chlordane	98% 2%
DEFIANCE TOILET WATER (Lustray)		
DE GRACO PAINTS (Detroit)		
DEGREASER Solvent (Stanley Home)	Triton Versene Perfume Dye	
DEKENS OINTMENTS (Deken's)		
DEKGRIP Paint acces- sory (Internat. Paint)	"Mineral spirits"* (or turpentine substitute)	
DEKKO- CALSOMINE PAINT (Enterprise Paint)		
DEKO PAINTS (Felton Sibley)		
DEKTOL DEVELOPER Photographic supply (Eastman)		
DELAGAR BATH PEARLS (Delagar)	Mineral oil Perfume	3%

*Consult Sec. II., Ingredients Index. This ingredient may be responsible for major toxic effects if poisonous amounts of this product are ingested.

- 419 -

Name & Use Manufacturer	Ingredients
DELCO QUALITY PAINT (Delco)	
DE LESCINSKIS PERFUMES AND TOILET WATERS (Leonid)	
DELETE Rust and stain remover (Dunaway)	
DELETE HAIR REMOVING CREAM (Jordeau)	
DELETTREZ BATH AC- CESSORIES (Assoc. Brands)	
DELETTREZ CREAM DE- ODORANT (Assoc. Brands)	
DELETTREZ SACHET (Assoc. Brands)	
DELKIL MICE SEED (Delk)	Strychnine*
DELMO-Z SPRAY Fungicide (Calif. Spray)	Metallic zinc* 50%
DE LOSTE'S POWDERS Analgesic (De Loste)	Each powder: Acetophenetidin* 4 gr. Caffeine alkaloid Bicarbonate of soda
DE-LOUSE- MOR Insecticide (Hilltop)	Refined petroleum oil Gamma isomer of benzene hexachloride* Other isomers of benzene hexachloride
DELTORE SHAMPOO (Liquid) (Deltex)	
DELUXE EMBALMING FLUID (Banner)	
DELUXE ENAMEL (Preservative)	
DELUXE PAINT (Sewall)	
DE LUXE PAINTS (Vane- Calvert)	

Name & Use Manufacturer	Ingredients
DE-LUXE PORCELAIN, TILE & MARBLE CLEANER (Blue Seal)	
DE LUXE SPOT REMOVER (Boyle- Midway)	Carbon tetrachloride* Naphtha*
DE-MOIST Air dryer (Coughlan)	
DE-MOTH (Dianol)	Ammonium silicofluoride* 2%
DEMUDYNE For skin burns and irritations (Bullock- Walker)	Benzocaine 2% Carbolic acid* 2% Phenyl mercury benzoate 1-10,000 Vehicle q.s.
DEMURE DEODORANT (Shy)	
DENCOTAR OINTMENT (Denver Chem.)	Crude coal tar* Precipitated sulfur* Menthol* Starch
DENCOTAR SHAMPOO (Denver Chem.)	Crude coal tar* Anhydrous castile soap 30% Sodium lauryl sulfate 1/2%
DENDRON For poison ivy (Valbar)	Sodiumhexa-metaphosphate*
DENETON BABY CREAM (Calvital)	Hexachlorophene Olive oil Lanolin. Vitamin A Vitamin D
DENNEX HAND CLEANING COMPOUND (Dennis)	Organic solvents of the glycol ether type Wetting agents Mineral oil Lanolin
DENTA-FLUR For cariesi (Denta-Flur)	In 3 tablets: Fluorine 1.62 mg. Magnesium 6.12 mg. Calcium 457.59 mg. Phosphorus 214.89 mg.
DENTA-JELL Oral, dental anesthetic (K-A-S)	Benzocaine 20% Glycerine
DENTA-KLENZ For cleaning teeth (Morgan Prod.)	Sodium chloride Tricalcium phosphate Tetrasodium pyrophosphate Sodium perborate*
DENTALGIA DROPS Dental anesthetic (Massengill)	Each fl. oz.: Morphine sulfate 1/4 gr. Chloral hydrate* 27 gr. Pellitory Oil clove Oil cajuput Oil peppermint Camphor* Ethyl alcohol 75%/v

*Consult Sec. II., Ingredients Index. This ingredient may be responsible for major toxic effects if poisonous amounts of this product are ingested.

Name & Use Manufacturer	Ingredients		Name & Use Manufacturer	Ingredients
DENTGLO DENTURE CLEANSER (Ft. Orange)			DENT'S TOOTH GUM (Dent)	Benzocaine Carbolic acid* Oleoresin capsicum
DENTINOL Antiseptic, germicide (Natl. Dental)	Alcohol 20% Ether 5% Essential oils and refined cresol* 75%		DENTU CREME Plate cleaner (Wernet)	
DENTINOL BONE WAX (Natl. Dental)	Alcohol 20% Ether 5% Essential oils and refined cresol* 75% Beeswax Cotton seed oil		DEOCARE DEODORANT STICK (Curlcare)	
DENTLOCK DENTURE POWDER (Ft. Orange)			DEODECIDE Deodorant (Eradico)	
DENTON'S FAMOUS SALVE (Denton)			DEODISOL DISINFECT- ANT (Undertakers)	
DENTRIX DENTAL CREAM (Van-S)	Glycerin C.P. Urea U.S.P. Tricalcium phosphate Sodium lauryl sulfate Algin Diammonium phosphate Mineral oil Flavor oil		DEODOR DEODORANT POWDER (Sharp & Dohme)	
			DEODOFOAM TOILET BOWL CLEANER (Solarine)	
DENTRIX TOOTH POWDER (Van-S)	Calcium carbonate Diammonium phosphate Magnesium carbonate Urea Sodium lauryl sulfate Flavor oil		DEO OINTMENT For colds (Davis Labs.)	Pure Australian eucalyptus oil* Oil peppermint Oil sassafras Camphor* Menthol*
DENT'S DENTAL POULTICE (Dent)	Benzocaine Oxyquinoline Thymol* Oleoresin capsicum		DEOTUSSIN COUGH REMEDY (Randolph Labs.)	Flaxseed Wild cherry Spruce gum chloroform Menthol Rock candy licorice
DENT'S EAR WAX DROPS (Dent)	Each fl. oz.: Chloral hydrate 10 gr. Fluid ext. hyoscyamus 8 m. Total alkaloids of hyoscyamus 0.003 gr. Alcohol 1.0% Carbolic acid Glycerin		DR. DE-PASS ANALGESIC COMP. (De-Pass)	
			DEPENDABLE PAINTS (Heath & Milligan)	
DENT'S EYE TREAT (Dent)	Boric acid* Sodium chloride Sodium borate* Berberine hydrochloride Camphor		DEPENDOLAC Paint (Heath & Milligan)	
DENT'S KEEP- AWAKES Stimulant (Dent)	Each tablet: Caffeine approx. as much as a cup of coffee		DERAYCO PAINTS (Devoe)	
DENT'S SLEEP-TABS (Dent)	Each tablet: Sodium bromide* 5 gr.		DERBAC TAR MEDICATED SHAMPOO Ectoparasiti- cide (Cereal)	Pine tar* Cocoanut oil
DENT'S TOOTH DROPS (Dent)	Alcohol* 53% Propylene glycol U.S.P. Oil cloves Oil cassia Cresol* Chloral hydrate* 1.5% Carbolic acid* Oleoresin capsicum		DEREKA PAINT (Debevoise)	
			DERMA-CEN Antiseptic (Central Chem.)	Hexachlorophene*

*Consult Sec. II., Ingredients Index. This ingredient may be responsible for major toxic effects if poisonous amounts of this product are ingested.

Name & Use Manufacturer	Ingredients	
DERMA CLEANSER SHAMPOO (Edison)	Hexachlorophene Alkylamine lauryl sulfate Lanolin Chlorophyll	
DERMACOL LIQUID Antiseptic for skin irritations (Drug Prod., N.Y.)	Alcohol Acid salicylic Acid boric* Bichloride of mercury Sodium benzoate Thymol* Eucalyptol* Acid hydrocyanic dilute* Glycerin	2% 0.28% 1.5% 1-2280 0.01% 1-1500
DERMACONE WAX (Embalmer's)		
DERMA-COTE PROTECTIVE HAND CREAM (Great Stuff)	Glycerine Bicarbonate of soda Castor oil Zinc oxide Silicate	
DERMACTIN LOTION Antiseptic, astringent (Richards Pharm.)	Acetone* Cetylpyridinium chloride Alcohol*	16% 1-2500 40%
DERMA DIET CREAMS (Rochester Labs.)	Mineral oils Parawax Beeswax Petrolatum Lanolin Borax Perfume	
DERMA DIET REFRESHER SHAMPOO (Rochester Labs.)	Liquid soap	
DERMADOR Skin lotion (Myers Labs.)	Alcohol Chlorobutanol Boric acid* Thymol* Menthol* Camphor* Turpentine*	60%/v 1/4 of 1%
DERMADOR EYE LOTION (Myers Labs.)	Alcohol Zinc sulfate* Boric acid*	7%
DERMAGILL OINTMENT For skin irritations, external fungicide (Massengill)	Carbolic acid* Cresol* Bismuth subgallate Zinc oxide Sulfur Oil of cade Aromatics	
DERMAK ACNE LOTION (Shaw)	Resorcin Boric acid Salicylic acid	approx. 2% approx. 1%
DERMA LIP AND EYE SEALER (Embalmer's)	Benzol* Vinyl resin	

Name & Use Manufacturer	Ingredients	
DERMA-LOTION (Prescript. Spec.)	Phenol* Amylum Menthol Camphor* Zinc oxide Boric acid* Glycerine Benzocaine Magnesium hydrox Methyl salicylate	
DERMA MEDICONE For perianal irritations (Medicone)	Anesthesin Ephedrine muriate Non-oxidizable base Oxyquinoline sulfate Ol. cadinum-ichthyol comp.	5% 0.1% q.s. 3% 1%
DER-MA-MOL For skin irritations (Penslar)	Zinc oxide* Precipitated sulfur* Chlorthymol*	
DERMA-PAX For skin irritations (Recsei)	Tri-histin* Chlorobutanol Isopropyl alcohol*	0.5% 1.0% 40% v/v
DERMAPHILL For skin irritations (Torch)	Aluminum acetate Phenol Menthol Camphor*	1% 1% 1/2% 3%
DERMA REGIS HAIR TONIC (Harris, B.)		
DERMA RUB LIQUID ANALGESIC (La-Mo)		
DERMASORCIN For acne (Lamond)	Resorcin Sulfur Propylene glycol Sorbitan mono-oleate Titanium oxide	2% 5%
DERMASSAGE Antiseptic, rubefacient (Edison)	Hexachlorophene* Oxyquinoline sulfate Menthol* Carbamide Lanolin Olive oil	
DERMASUL For acne (Lamond)	Sulfur Propylene glycol Sorbitan mono-oleate Titanium oxide	5%
DERMASULF 5% For acne (Smith, Carroll)	Polythionates	5%
DERMA-TEEN "AM" Skin Treatment (DermaTeen)	Resorcin* Salicylic acid* Alcohol*	70%
DERMA-TEEN "PM" Skin Treatment (DermaTeen)	Sulfur* Camphor Gums Zinc sulf.* Sulf. potassium Alcohol*	

*Consult Sec. II., Ingredients Index. This ingredient may be responsible for major toxic effects if poisonous amounts of this product are ingested.

- 422 -

Name & Use Manufacturer	Ingredients	
DERMA-TEEN SKIN SOAP (Derma-Teen)	Mercuric iodide*	1%
DERMATINE TONIC (La Vell)		
DERMATINT ROUGE (Franco)		
DERMATONE For acne (Chicago Pharm.)	Arsenic trioxide	0.0875%
	Ammoniated mercury*	4.0%
	Boric acid	6.66%
	Zinc oxide	4.16%
DERMATONE SALVE NO. 74 (Stanis)	Sulfur	
	Salicylic acid*	
	Menthol*	
	White pine tar	
DERMA-TOX LOTION For skin irritations (Hance)	Grindelia robusta	
	Hanaform (isobutyl p-amino benzoate)	
	Isopropyl alcohol*	
DERMATOX OINTMENT For skin irritations (Associated Prod.)	Mercury bichloride* 1/5 gr./oz.	
	Sulfur*	
	Calamine	
	Menthol*	
DERMA VIVA COMPLEX-ION LIQUID (Derma Viva)		
DERMAY OINTMENT (Medical) Fungicide (Lesbert)	Benzoic acid	
	Carbolic acid*	
	Salicylic acid*	
	Thymol	
	Menthol*	
DERMAY POWDER (Medical) Fungicide (Lesbert)	Benzoic acid	
	Boric acid*	
	Carbolic acid*	
	Salicylic acid*	
	Thymol	
	Menthol*	
DERMA-ZON Skin ointment (Excello)	Urea	
	Zinc sulfocarbolate	
	Thymol*	
	Benzocaine	
	Salicylic acid*	
	Phenol*	
DERMEX CREAM For acne (Dermex)	Salicylic acid	2%
	Menthol	1/4%
	LCD	5%
	Kaolin	
DERMEX LOTION For acne (Dermex)	Resorcin	2%
	Sulfur	3%
	Neutracolor	
	Talc.	
	Zinc oxide	
	Alcohol	
	Lavender oil	
DERMEZE For skin irritations (Premo)	Thenylpyramine hydrochloride* 2%	
	Benzocaine 2%	
	Tyrothrycin 0.25 mg./gm.	
DERMOCAINE For skin irritations (Walker Pharm.)	Bismuth subnitrate	
	Acid salicylic*	
	Zinc oxide	
	Benzocaine	
	Thuja	
	Petrolatum	
DERM-O-CREME For skin irritations (VB)	Balsam of Peru	
	Phenol*	
	Bismuth subnitrate	
	Sulfur*	
	Castor oil	
	Resorcin*	
DERMOIL For psoriasis (Lake Labs.)	Mercury* (chemically combined with soaps) 0.45%	
	Carbolic acid* 0.5%	
	Cresol 0.75%	
DERMOLATUM (Gesell)	Lanolin	
	Zinc oxide	
	Bismuth subnitrate	
	Resorcin*	
	Oil of tar rectified*	
DERMOLINE Protective for skin (Mentho-Listine)	Zinc oxide*	
	Zinc sulfocarbolate	
	Carbolic acid*	
	Magnesium sulfate	
	Glycerin	
DERMOLTE LOTION (Howard Labs.)		
DERMOTAN For skin irritations (Horton & Converse)	Zinc oxide U.S.P.	10%
	Phenol	0.44%
	Aromatic oils	
DERMOVAN Ointment for skin (Texas Pharm.)	Glyceryl monostearate (acid-emulsifying)	
	Spermaceti	
	Mineral oil	
	Glycerin	
DEROSITE Skin antiseptic (Chicago Pharm.)	Benzyl benzoate*	25%
	DDT	1%
	Benzocaine	2%
DEROX Insecticide (Am. Agric. Chem.)	Rotenone	0.75%
	Phospho dust	
DERUSTO Rust preventive, remover (Master Bronze)		
DESERT FLOWER HAND & BODY LOTION (Shulton)		
DESERT FLOWER PERFUME, COLOGNE & TOILET WATER (Shulton)		
DESERT FLOWER POWDER Cosmetic (Shulton)		

*Consult Sec. II., Ingredients Index. This ingredient may be responsible for major toxic effects if poisonous amounts of this product are ingested.

Name & Use Manufacturer	Ingredients	
DESERT FLOWER TOILET SOAP (Shulton)		
DESICCANT COMPOUND S.F. MFR. NO. 611 For skin irritations (Specialists)	Magnesium sulfate Potassium sulfate Sodium biborate* Sodium metaphosphate	
DESIR du COEUR PERFUMES (Ybry)		
DESITIN HEMOR-RHOIDAL SUPPOSI-TORIES (Desitin)	Norwegian cod liver oil Lanolin Zinc oxide Bismuth subgallate Balsam Peru Cocoa butter	
DESITIN LOTION For skin irritation (Desitin)	Norwegian cod liver oil Zinc oxide Magnesium carbonate Rose water Lime water	
DESITIN OINTMENT Anti pruritic (Destin)	Norwegian cod liver oil Zinc oxide Talcum Petrolatum Lanolin	
DESITIN POWDER Anti pruritic (Destin)	Norwegian cod liver oil Zinc oxide Talcum powder Magnesium oxide	
DES TEX DRY CLEANER (Research Des-Tex)		
DES TEX FOAM Cleaner (Research Dex-Tex)		
DESTINA MAKE-UP REMOVER (Revlon)	Polyoxyethylene ester Alcohol Glycerin Perfume	
DESTRUXOL Fungicide (Destruxol)	Nicotine* Wood creosote Crude carbolic acid Sodium cyanide*	12% 20% 2% 8%
DESTRUXOL ANTROACH CONCEN-TRATE Insecticide (Destruxol)	Tech. chlordane*	41%
DESTRUXOL ANTROACH DUST Insecticide (Destruxol)	Tech. chlordane*	5%
DESTRUXOL ANTROACH SPRAY Insecticide (Destruxol)	Tech. chlordane	2.5%

Name & Use Manufacturer	Ingredients	
DESTRUXOL CONTACT SPRAY Insecticide (Destruxol)	Nicotine* (as alkaloid) Sodium cyanide Crude carbolic acid Wood creosote Pine tar Soap	12.0% 8.0% 2.0% 20.0% 23.0% 2.2%
DESTRUXOL DDT PYRENONE Insecticide (Destruxol)	DDT Piperonylcyclohexenone Pyrethrins Pine oils Mineral oils Aromatic petroleum derivatives*	2% 3.30% 0.33% 5% 30% 20%
DESTRUXOL HOUSEHOLD INSECT SPRAY (Destruxol)	Pyrethrins Piperonyl butoxide Butoxy polypropylene glycol Petroleum distillate*	0.06% 0.58% 1.00% 97.36%
DESTRUXOL MALATHION 50% SPRAY Insecticide (Destruxol)	Malathion* Xylene*	50.0% 39.0%
DESTRUXOL ORCHID SPRAY Insecticide (Destruxol)	Petroleum hydrocarbons Nicotine*	42% 5%
DESTRUXOL PYRENONE Insecticide (Destruxol)	Petroleum distillate* Petroleum deriv. solvent* Pine oil Tech. piperonyl butoxide Pyrethrins	44.0% 19.5% 5.0% 5.0% 0.5%
DESTRUXOL PYRETOXIDE-BLIGHTROL DUST NO. 15-A Insecticide (Destruxol)	Pyrethrins Sulfur* Piperonyl cyclohexenone Copper-zinc-chromate* complex	0.60% 30% 0.6% 2%
DESTRUXOL SOW-BUG AND CUT-WORM BAIT (Destruxol)	Copper aceto-arsenite*	10.0%
DESTRUXOL SUPER EMULSION Insecticide (Destruxol)	Mineral oil Pine oil Ammonia Nicotine* (alkaloid) Soap	62.0% 5.5% 0.8% 0.6% 2.1%
DE-T-COP POTATO DUST Insecticide, fungicide (Bonide)	Dichloro diphenyl trichloroethane Copper oxychloride* (total copper content 7%)	3% 12%
DETERGEX CLEANSER (Pharmaseal)	Alkaline detergent* (conc. of 1 oz./gal. has pH of approx. 11)	
DETERGO Cleaning powder (Continental Car-Na-Var)		

Name & Use Manufacturer	Ingredients	
DETERGO OINTMENT For skin irritation (Peau Seche)	Stearic acid Lanolin Liquid carb. detergent Sodium borate* Potassium carbonate Starch Water Carbitol* Rose perfume Menthol*	
DETEX Insecticide (Liberty Chem.)	DDT*	25%
DETHDIET BRAND RED SQUILL Rodenticide (Penick)	Red squill powder*	100%
DETHMOR Rodenticide (Penick)	Warfarin (3-(a-acetonylbenzyl)-4-hydroxycoumarin)	0.5%
DETHMOR, WATER SOLUBLE Rodenticide (Penick)	Warfarin, sodium salt (sodium salt of 3-(a-acetonylbenzyl)-4-hydroxycoumarin)	0.54%
DETHOL (Improved) Insecticide (Dethol)	DDT* Tech. isobornyl thiocyanoacetate Petroleum distillates*	5.0% 93.7%
DETHOL (New) Insecticide (Dethol)	DDT n-Octyl bicycloheptene dicarboximide Beta butoxy beta thiocyano diethyl ether Allethrin (allyl homolog of cinerin 1) Methylated aromatic petroleum derivative* Petroleum distillate	2.0% 1.0% 1.0% 0.125% 5.0% 5.875%
DETTOL GERMICIDE & ANTISEPTIC (formerly DETT) (French, R. T.)	Vegetable soap Terpineol,* p-chlorosym-m-xylenol* Water Alcohol	 68% 16.4%
DEVASTATING PERFUME & COLOGNE (Parfums Anjou)		
DEVEL 1, 2 and 3 Developers (Shannon)	Metol* Hydroquinone* Sodium sulfite Potassium bromide*	
DEVOE & RAYNOLDS OIL COLORS (Devoe)		
DEW ALL SPAR VARNISH (Pierce, F. O.)		
DE WANS DEPILATORY (De Wans)		

Name & Use Manufacturer	Ingredients	
DE-WART-EM Keratolytic (human) (Ontario)	Salicylic acid* Acetic acid (99%) Trichloroacetic acid* Glycol type base*	15% 2% 7.5% 76.5%
DE-WART-EM Keratolytic (veterinary) (Ontario)	Salicylic acid* Acetic acid (99%) Trichloroacetic acid Glycol type base*	15% 1% 2% 82%
DEW DEODORANT CREAM, LIQUID OR SPRAY (Pearson Pharm.)		
DEWEED 2, 4-D Herbicide (Commercial Chem.)	Sodium salt 2,4-D*	60%
DEWEED 2,4-D LIQUID Herbicide (Commercial Chem.)	Isopropyl ester 2,4-D*	44%
DEWEED 2,4, 5-T Herbicide (Commercial Chem.)	Isopropyl ester 2,4,5-T*	43%
DEWITT AQUARIUM CEMENT (Dewitt)		
DEWITT CAULKING COMPOUND (Dewitt)		
DEWITT DRAIN PIPE & TRAP CLEANER (Dewitt)		
DEWITT METAL & WOOD COATING (Dewitt)		
DEWITT PAINT & VARNISH CLEANER (Dewitt)		
DEWITT ROOF COATING (Dewitt)		
DEWITT SOOT DESTROYER (Dewitt)		
DE WITT'S ABSORBENT RUB (De Witt)		
DE WITT'S ANABALM (De Witt)		
DE WITT'S COCONUT OIL SHAMPOO (De Witt)		

*Consult Sec. II., Ingredients Index. This ingredient may be responsible for major toxic effects if poisonous amounts of this product are ingested.

Name & Use Manufacturer	Ingredients		Name & Use Manufacturer	Ingredients	
De WITT'S FOOT POWDER (De Witt)	Boric acid* Salicylic acid* Alum Zinc stearate Chlorthymol Talcum powder Chlorophyll		DEXOL Bleach (Tidy)	Sodium perborate tetrahydrate* Crystalline sodium sesquicarbonate Fluorescent or optical dyes	20%-30% 70%-80%
De WITT'S FOR CORNS (De Witt)	Salicylic acid* Benzocaine Glacial acetic acid*		DEXOL MUCILAGE (powdered) (Am. Crayon)		
DE WITT'S GOLDEN LINIMENT (De Witt)			DEXTONE PAINT (Dexter)		
DE WITT'S HYGIENIC POWDER (De Witt)			DEXTRO- FEDRIN Nasal de- congestant (Lefcourt)	Ephedrine alkaloid* Chlorobutanol* Menthol* Dextrose	
DE WITT'S LITTLE EARLY RISERS (De Witt)			DEXTRO- FEDRIN VISCOUS Nasal de- congestant (Lefcourt)	Ephedrine alkaloid* Chlorobutanol* Menthol* Dextrose Methylcellulose	
De WITT'S OIL FOR EAR USE (De Witt)	Benzocaine Camphor* Menthol* Cajeput oil Thyme oil White oil Corn oil		D-HORN PASTE Veterinary (Wilke)	Sodium hydroxide (caustic soda 32%)* Calcium hydroxide	
De WITT'S PILLS Diuretic (De Witt)	Potash nitrate Uva ursi Buchu Methylene blue		DIA-BISMA Antacid (Penslar)	Sodium bicarbonate Magnesium carbonate Bismuth subcarbonate Magnesium oxide Calcium carbonate Diastase Ginger Oil peppermint	
DE WITT'S SANITARY FOOT POWDER (De Witt)			DIABISMUL For intestinal irritation (Tilden)	Each 100 cc.: Opium Bismuth subsalicylate Salol Zinc phenolsulfonate	48.000 mg. 1.750 gm. 0.350 gm. 0.175 gm.
DE WITT'S VAPO BALM (De Witt)			DIACOL Intestinal absorbent (Veltex)	Each fl. oz.: Milk of bismuth Kaolin Pectin Salol Camphor Aluminum hydroxide gel	7.5 cc. 3.6 gm. 0.22 gm. 0.04 gm. 0.01 gm. q.s.
DEW OILS LANOLIN HAIR DRESSING (Esamar)	Mineral oil Beeswax Glyceryl monostearate Lanolin				
DEW OILS RUM & EGG SHAMPOO (Esamar)	Detergent paste Sodium stearate Propylene glycol Powdered egg Rum Rum essence Formaldehyde	 1/10 of 1%	DIAKLOR 5-5 DUST Fungicide (Dianol)	Chlordane* TDE*	5% 5%
			DIAL SHAMPOO (Armour & Co.)	Sulfated alcohol type detergent Non-ionic detergent Hexachlorophene	 1%
DEX Nylon protector (Tidy)	Methycrol NH (50% dilution of a methacrylic resin suspension)		DIAL SOAP (Armour & Co.)	Soda salts of coconut oil Tallow Glycerin Hexacholorophene	 2%
DEXATOX Insecticide, fungicide (Hanna)	DDT* Sulfur*				
DEX FOR ATHLETES FOOT (Alveo)	Salicylic acid* Benzoic acid Tincture of benzoin compound Resorcin* Alcohol*	 68%			

*Consult Sec. II., Ingredients Index. This ingredient may be responsible for major toxic effects if poisonous amounts of this product are ingested.

Name & Use Manufacturer	Ingredients		Name & Use Manufacturer	Ingredients	
DIAMOND ALKALI CHEMICALS AMINE 4-T Herbicide (Diamond Alkali)	Triethylamine salt of 2, 4, 5-T*	57.0%	DIAMOND ALKALI CHEMICALS 4 BUTYL-D WEED KILLER (Diamond Alkali)	Butyl ester of 2, 4-D*	56.5%
DIAMOND ALKALI CHEMICALS BHC D-12 Insecticide (Diamond Alkali)	BHC, gamma isomer* BHC, other isomers*	12.0% 21.0%	DIAMOND ALKALI CHEMICALS 6 BUTYL-D WEED KILLER (Diamond Alkali)	Butyl ester of 2, 4-D*	78.0%
DIAMOND ALKALI CHEMICALS BHC-DDT D-9-15 DUST BASE CON- CENTRATE Insecticide (Diamond Alkali)	BHC, gamma isomer* BHC, other isomers* DDT	9.0% 61.0% 15.0%	DIAMOND ALKALI CHEMICALS 6 BUTYL-D (oil soluble) WEED KILLER (Diamond Alkali)	Butyl ester of 2, 4-D*	78.2%
DIAMOND ALKALI CHEMICALS BHC E-11 Insecticide (Diamond Alkali)	BHC, gamma isomer* BHC, other isomers* Xylene* Aromatic petroleum solvent*	11.4% 17.2% 25.2% 40.0%	DIAMOND ALKALI CHEMICALS 4 BUTYL-T BRUSH KILLER (Diamond Alkali)	Butyl ester of 2, 4, 5-T*	53.6%
DIAMOND ALKALI CHEMICALS BHC TECHNI- CAL 15% Insecticide (Diamond Alkali)	BHC, gamma plus other isomers*	100%	DIAMOND ALKALI CHEMICALS DDT D-50 Insecticide (Diamond Alkali)	DDT*	50.0%
DIAMOND ALKALI CHEMICALS BHC TECHNI- CAL 40% Insecticide (Diamond Alkali)	BHC, gamma plus other isomers*	100%	DIAMOND ALKALI CHEMICALS DDT D-75 Insecticide (Diamond Alkali)	DDT*	75.0%
DIAMOND ALKALI CHEMICALS BHC W-12 WETTABLE SPRAY & DUST Insecticide (Diamond Alakali)	BHC, gamma isomer* BHC, other isomers	12.0%	DIAMOND ALKALI CHEMICALS DDT E-25 Insecticide (Diamond Alkali)	DDT Aromatic petroleum solvent*	25.0% 72.0%
DIAMOND ALKALI CHEMICALS 2-2 BUTYL BRUSH KILLER (Diamond Alkali)	Butyl ester of 2, 4-D* Butyl ester of 2, 4, 5-T*	27.9% 27.2%	DIAMOND ALKALI CHEMICALS DDT S-30 Insecticide (Diamond Alkali)	DDT* Aromatic petroleum solvent*	30.0% 70.0
DIAMOND ALKALI CHEMICALS 2.67 BUTYL-D WEED KILLER (Diamond Alkali)	Butyl ester of 2, 4-D*	40.0%	DIAMOND ALKALI CHEMICALS DDT TECHNI- CAL Insecticide (Diamond Alkali)	DDT*	100.0%

*Consult Sec. II., Ingredients Index. This ingredient may be responsible for major toxic effects if poisonous amounts of this product are ingested.

Name & Use Manufacturer	Ingredients		Name & Use Manufacturer	Ingredients	
DIAMOND ALKALI CHEMICALS DDT W-75 WETTABLE POWDER Insecticide (Diamond Alkali)	DDT*	75.0%	DIAMOND ALKALI CHEMICALS ISOPROPYL ESTER BRUSH KILLER NO. 22 (Diamond Alkali)	Isopropyl ester of 2, 4-D* Isopropyl ester of 2, 4, 5-T*	26.5% 26.0%
DIAMOND ALKALI CHEMICALS DDT W-50 WETTABLE SPRAY BASE Insecticide (Diamond Alkali)	DDT*	50.0%	DIAMOND ALKALI CHEMICALS 3.34 ISOPROPYL D WEED KILLER (Diamond Alkali)	Isopropyl ester of 2, 4-D*	46.0%
DIAMOND ALKALI CHEMICALS DIAMOND 80-20 GRAIN FUMIGANT (Diamond Alkali)	Carbon tetrachloride* Carbon disulfide*	80.0% 20.0%	DIAMOND ALKALI CHEMICALS LINDANE 100% (99% GAMMA ISOMER) Insecticide (Diamond Alkali)	Gamma isomer of BHC*	99%
DIAMOND ALKALI CHEMICALS DIAMOND LV 10-20 Herbicide (Diamond Alkali)	Butoxy ethoxy propanol ester of 2, 4-D* Butoxy ethoxy propanol ester of 2, 4, 5-T*	28.0% 13.18%	DIAMOND ALKALI CHEMICALS LINDANE E-20 Insecticide (Diamond Alkali)	Gamma isomer of BHC* Aromatic petroleum solvent* Cyclohexanone	20.0% 70.0% 5.0%
DIAMOND ALKALI CHEMICALS 4# DIMETHYL AMINE D WEED KILLER (Diamond Alkali)	Dimethylamine salt of 2, 4-D*	49.0%	DIAMOND ALKALI CHEMICALS LINDANE W-25 Insecticide (Diamond Alkali)	Gamma isomer of BHC*	25.0%
DIAMOND ALKALI CHEMICALS 2-2 2-ETHYL HEXYL BRUSH KILLER (Diamond Alkali)	2-Ethyl hexyl (iso-octyl) ester of 2, 4-D* 2-Ethyl hexyl (iso-octyl) ester of 2, 4, 5-T*	34.3% 32.7%	DIAMOND ALKALI CHEMICALS LINDANE W-95 Insecticide (Diamond Alkali)	Gamma isomer of BHC*	95.0%
DIAMOND ALKALI CHEMICALS 4 2-ETHYL HEXYL D WEED KILLER (Diamond Alkali)	2-Ethyl hexyl (iso-octyl) ester of 2, 4-D*	69.2%	DIAMOND ALKALI CHEMICALS LV-22 BRUSH KILLER (Diamond Alkali)	Butoxy ethoxy propanol ester of 2, 4-D* Butoxy ethoxy propanol ester of 2, 4, 5-T*	37.8% 35.6%
DIAMOND ALKALI CHEMICALS 4 2-ETHYL HEXYL T BRUSH KILLER (Diamond Alkali)	2-Ethyl hexyl (iso-octyl) ester of 2, 4, 5-T*	64.9%	DIAMOND ALKALI CHEMICALS LV-4D Herbicide (Diamond Alkali)	Butoxy ethoxy propanol esters of 2, 4-D*	76.0%
			DIAMOND ALKALI CHEMICALS LV-4T Herbicide (Diamond Alkali)	Butoxy ethoxy propanol ester of 2, 4, 5-T*	70.6%

*Consult Sec. II., Ingredients Index. This ingredient may be responsible for major toxic effects if poisonous amounts of this produc are ingested.

Name & Use Manufacturer	Ingredients
DIAMOND ALKALI CHEMICALS M.C.P. AMINE WEED KILLER (Diamond Alkali)	Isopropyl and triethyl amine salts of M.C.P.* 57.0%
DIAMOND ALKALI CHEMICALS MITICIDE K-101 TECHNICAL (Diamond Alkali)	p-Chlorophenyl-p-chlorobenzene sulfonate* 100.0%
DIAMOND ALKALI CHEMICALS 4# MIXED AMINE-D WEED KILLER (Diamond Alkali)	Isopropyl and di-isopropyl amine salt of 2, 4-D* 56.0%
DIAMOND ALKALI CHEMICALS PREMIUM BRAND GRAIN FUMIGANT (Diamond Alkali)	Carbon tetrachloride* Carbon disulfide* Petroleum distillate Sulfur dioxide
DIAMOND ALKALI CHEMICALS TECHNICAL BUTYL ESTER OF 2, 4-D Herbicide (Diamond Alkali)	Butyl ester of 2, 4-D* 99.0%
DIAMOND ALKALI CHEMICALS TECHNICAL BUTYL-T Herbicide (Diamond Alkali)	Butyl ester of 2, 4, 5-T* 98.0%
DIAMOND ALKALI CHEMICALS TECHNICAL 2-ETHYL HEXYL D Herbicide (Diamond Alkali)	2-Ethyl hexyl (iso-octyl) ester of 2, 4-D* 97.0%
DIAMOND ALKALI CHEMICALS TECHNICAL 2-ETHYL HEXYL T Herbicide (Diamond Alkali)	2 Ethyl hexyl (iso-octyl) ester of 2, 4, 5-T* 70.6%

Name & Use Manufacturer	Ingredients
DIAMOND ALKALI CHEMICALS TECHNICAL ISOPROPYL ESTER OF 2, 4-D Herbicide (Diamond Alkali)	Isopropyl ester of 2, 4-D* 99.0%
DIAMOND ALKALI CHEMICALS 2, 4-D ACID Herbicide (Diamond Alkali)	2, 4-D* 99.0%
DIAMOND ALKALI CHEMICALS 2, 4-D AMINE WEED KILLER #6 (Diamond Alkali)	Dimethylamine salts of 2, 4-D* 70.0%
DIAMOND ALKALI CHEMICALS 2, 4, 5-T ESTER NO. 43 Herbicide (Diamond Alkali)	Isopropyl ester of 2, 4, 5-T* 43.0%
DIAMOND B PAINTS (Behlen)	
DIAMOND FLOOR & DECK ENAMEL (Felton Sibley)	
DIAMOND KOTE VARNISH (Tnemec)	
DIAMOND L BRAND DEER REPELLENT (Leckenby)	Nicotine*
DIAMOND L BRAND MILDEW & SUMMER PEACH LEAF CURL SPRAY (Leckenby)	Copper, expressed as metallic 3% Inert ingredients* 97%
DIAMOND L BRAND PEACH LEAF CURL SPRAY (Leckenby)	Copper in tribasic copper sulfate expressed as metallic* 10% Mineral oil 55%
DIAMOND L BRAND ROACH & SILVERFISH POWDER (Leckenby)	Active sodium fluoride* 95%

*Consult Sec. II., Ingredients Index. This ingredient may be responsible for major toxic effects if poisonous amounts of this product are ingested.

Name & Use Manufacturer	Ingredients		Name & Use Manufacturer	Ingredients	
DIAMOND L BRAND TREE PAINT For injured trees (Leckenby)	Anthracene oil* Pine tar*	50% 50%	DIAPARENE CHLORIDE BABY POWDER Antiseptic powder (Homemakers')	Methylbenzethonium chloride* N.N.R. Corn starch base Sodium bicarbonate	
DIAMOND L BRAND 82% 2, 4-D WEED KILLER (Leckenby)	Sodium salt 2, 4-D*	90%	DIAPARENE CHLORIDE OINTMENT Ointment for skin irritations (Homemakers')	Methylbenzethonium chloride* N.N.R.	
DIAMOND METALLIC ZINC PAINT (Thompson & Co.)			DIAPARENE CHLORIDE PRECRUSHED RINSE TABLETS (Homemakers')	Methylbenzethonium chloride* N.N.R.	
DIAMOND PAINT (Felton Sibley)			DIAPARENE PERI-ANAL Antiseptic, protective cream (Homemakers')	Methylbenzethonium chloride* N.N.R. Zinc oxide Starch Cod liver oil Casein	
DIAMOND SEAL For wood floors (Hillyard Chem.)	Stoddard solvent*		DIAPERSOL SOLUTION (Mark Labs.)		
DIAMOND WHITES Paint (Moore-Leland)			DIAPER-SWEET Diaper wash (Bu-Tay)	Sodium sesquicarbonate Sodium perborate* Sodium tripolyphosphate Bluing (alphzurine blue 2-G)	
DIA-NO For intestinal irritation (Rexall)	Each fl. oz.: Pectin N.F. Kaolin Zinc sulfocarbolate N.F.	4-1/2 gr. 90 gr. 1-1/2 gr.	DIAPER WITE (Diaperwite)		
			DIAPREX For skin irritation (Belle Moss)	Boric acid* Zinc oxide Zinc stearate Balsam Peru	
DIANOL INSECTICIDAL PAINT (Dianol)	TDE*	5%	DIAPURE For skin irritations (Columbia)	Each tablet: Para di-isobutyl phenoxy ethoxy ethyl dimethyl benzyl ammonium chloride* monohydrate (quat-ernary ammonium)	25%
DIANOL INSECT KILLING HOUSE SPRAY (Dianol)	TDE* Chlordane Beta butoxy beta' thiocyano diethyl ethers* and beta thiocyano ethyl esters of fatty acids	5% 2%	DIASAL Sodium-free salt substitute (Fougera)	Potassium chloride* Glutamic acid	
DIANOL PAINT INSECTICIDE (Dianol)	D-3 (dichloro diphenyl dichloroethane)*	50%	DIASTOS LIQUOR Digestant (Sharp & Dohme)	Each 30 cc.: Pepsin Papain Rennin Lactic acid Diluted nitrohydrochloric acid Nux vomica	0.52 gm. 0.1 gm. 50 mg. 0.03 cc. 0.3 cc. 27 mg.
DIANOL YARD SPRAY Insecticide (Dianol)	Chlordane* TDE*	25% 25%			
			DIATUSSIN Antitussive (Ames Co.)	Thyme Drosera Aqueous alcoholic menstruum alcohol content	22%
DIAPARENE CHLORIDE ANTIBAC-TERIAL POWDER Antiseptic powder (Homemakers')	Methylbenzethonium chloride N.N.R.* Corn starch base Sodium bicarbonate		DIATUSSIN SYRUP Antitussive (Ames Co.)	Ext. thyme Ext. drosera Aqueous syrup vehicle (alcohol content 5%)	
DIAPARENE CHLORIDE BABY LOTION Emollient (Homemakers')	Methylbenzethonium chloride* N.N.R.		DIAZINON FLY BAIT (Chipman, Ltd.)	Diazinon*	1%

*Consult Sec. II., Ingredients Index. This ingredient may be responsible for major toxic effects if poisonous amounts of this product are ingested.

Name & Use Manufacturer	Ingredients		Name & Use Manufacturer	Ingredients
DIAZINON LIQUID FLY KILLER (Geigy)	o, o-Diethyl-o-(isopropyl-4-methyl-pyrimidyl thio-phosphate* 25% Xylene* 70%		DICKS-PONTIUS PUTTIES (COMMERCIAL PUTTY, RELIABLE PUTTY, STRICTLY PURE PUTTY, 1012 ALUMI-NUM GLAZING COMPOUND, DP GLAZING COMPOUND) (Dicks-Pontius)	Ground limestone Asbestos fiber Talc Titanium dioxide or clay Linseed oil Soybean oil Mineral spirits 2%/w
DIBENZANE EMULSION Ectoparasiti-cide (Veltex)	Benzyl benzoate* 25% Gamma hexachlorocyclohexane 1.25% Dinitro-methoxy-cyclohexane 3%			
DIC A DOO CLEANER (Patent)	Processed corn material Trisodium phosphate Sodium metasilicate Soda ash Naphthalene* Lemon oil		DICKS-PONTIUS STEEL SASH PUTTY, CASEMENT PUTTY (Dicks-Pontius)	Lead* drier
DIC A DOO PAINT BRUSH BATH & CLEANER (Patent)	Processed corn material Tri-sodium phosphate soap Santomerse (wetting agent) Naphthalene* Sodium chromate* Borax*		DICKS-PONTIUS WHITE LEAD PUTTIES (Dicks-Pontius)	Lead carbonate*
DI CALCIUM PHOSPHATE, FEED GRADE Livestock feed (Inorganic)	Phosphorus 18% Calcium 27%		DICKS-PONTIUS WHITE WONDER SEALING COMPOUND (Dicks-Pontius)	Polyvinyl acetate Ground limestone Titanium dioxide
DICATNA Antacid tablet (Halperin)	Aluminum hydroxide gel Calcium carbonate Calcium hydroxide			
DI-CET Antiseptic powder for instruments (Sanford & Son)	Each 100 gm.: Methyl benzethonium chloride* 24.4 gm. Sodium carbonate monohydrate 48.8 gm. Sodium nitrite* 24.4 gm. Trisodium ethylenediamine tetraacetate monohydrate 2.4 gm.		DICTAN COUGH SYRUP (Boericke & Runyon)	White pine Yerba santa Grindelia Rumex Sticta pulmonaria lobelia* Bryonia* Ipecac and chloroform 1-1/2 m./fl. oz. Alcohol 8%
DICKEY'S EYE WASH (Dickey)	Berberine sulfate (neutral) Boracic acid		DIDEE SCENT DIAPER PAN DEODORANT (Curran)	Paradichlorobenzene* 100% Perfume
DR. J. A. DICKEY'S EYE WATER (Dickey Eye)			DIE-DEAD Insecticide (Die-Dead)	Petroleum solvent* Pyrin no. 20 Pyrethrins 2.5/100 cc. Pine oil* Pyrone
DICKEY'S OLD RELIABLE SALVE (Dickey)	Mercuric oxide* 1%			
DICKINSON'S WITCH HAZEL (Dickinson	Alcohol 14%		DIELGRAN 2-1/2 Insecticide (Chipman Chem.)	Hexachloro epoxy octahydro endo, exo-dimethano naphthalene* 2.13% Related compounds 0.37%
DICKS-PONTIUS GUN CAULKING COMPOUND (Dick-Pontius)	Ground limestone Asbestos fibers Talc (solid) Bodied vegetable oils Mineral spirits Cobalt dried (0.01%/w as metal) Sold in white and natural grades. White contains titanium dioxide.		DIELGRAN 5 (Chipman Chem.)	Hexachloro epoxy octahydro-endo, exo-dimethano naphthalene* 4.25% Related compounds 0.75%
			DIEL-TREET Insecticide (Planetary Chem.)	Hexachloro epoxy octahydro dimethano naphthalene* 42.5% Related compounds 7.5%

*Consult Sec. II., Ingredients Index. This ingredient may be responsible for major toxic effects if poisonous amounts of this product are ingested.

- 431 -

Name & Use Manufacturer	Ingredients		Name & Use Manufacturer	Ingredients	
DIENER FIRE EXTINGUISHER (Diener)			DIGESTIVE, JR. Digestant (Jenkins)	Each tablet: Pepsin Papain Bismuth subnitrate Ext. nux vomica Calcium phosphate Calcium carbonate Ext. cascara aromatic	1/8 gr. 1/4 gr. 1/4 gr. 1/1000 gr. 1/8 gr. 1/4 gr. 1/32 gr.
DIESTIANS (POND'S TABLETS) Tonic, antacid (Pond Pharm.)	Each tablet: Nux vomica (strychnine sulfate* 1/200 gr.) Sodium bicarbonate Gentian Rhubarb Ipecac Oil of peppermint				
			DIGESTOIDS B & R TABLETS NO. 206 A Digestant (Boericke & Runyon)	Papain Charcoal Capsicum Methyl salicylate Pepsin Sodium bicarbonate Nux vomica (strychnine content 0.0002 gr.)	1-50 gr.
DIET-TWINS Reducing aid (Pharmex)	Vitamins Minerals Sod. carboxymethylcellulose				
E. T. DIEZ ARGENTINE SOUTH AMERICAN ANT MIXTURE (Diez)	Arsenious oxide* Tartar emetic*	0.50% 2.45%	DIGESTOSAL Antacid powder (Purepac)	Sodium bicarbonate Magnesium carbonate Calcium carbonate Colloidal kaolin Magnesium oxide Bismuth subcarbonate Aluminum hydroxide Papain	
DIFFICULT STAINS (Blum)	Carbon tetrachloride* greater than 20% Chloroform* Naphtha Benzine soap				
			DIGITONE OINTMENT (Medical) Fungicide (Mertens)	Salicylic acid* Benzoic acid* Pine oil* Petrolatum	
DIFFICULT STAINS (Blum)	Petroleum naphtha* Carbon tetrachloride*	80% 5%			
DIF HAND CLEANER (Dif)	Pumice Soap (tallow and cocoa-tallow) Bentonite clay Sodium tripolyphosphate Synthetic detergent Lanolin Perfume	47% 23% 23% 5%	DIJEL Antacid, adsorbent (Lix)	Alumina hydroxide gel Kaolin Bismuth subsalicylate Magnesium hydroxide Zinc phenolsulfonate Alcohol	3%
			DILL'S ALL-OVER FLEA POWDER (Dill)	Beta thiocyano ethyl esters of aliphatic fatty acids Petroleum distillate	2.0% 3.0%
DIF METAL POLISH (Dif)	Silica Soap Ammonium oxalate Isopropanol Glycerin	34.0% 5.5% 3.0% 1.0% 2.0%			
			DIMACID Antacid (Clapp, Otis)	Magnesium carbonate Bismuth subcarbonate Calcium carbonate	
DIFUSO Insecticide (Tanglefoot)	Pyrethrins Piperonyl butoxide tech. Petroleum distillates*				
			DIMACID B Antacid (Clapp, Otis)	Magnesium carbonate Bismuth subcarbonate Calcium carbonate Magnesium glycinate	
DIF WATERLESS HAND CLEANER (Dif)	Paraffinic solvents* Nonionic surfactants Propylene glycol Edible emulsifier Aromatic solvents Lanolin	65.0% 10.0% 2.0% 1.0% 1.0% 1.0%			
			DIMITE 25% EMULSIFIABLE Insecticide (Sherwin-Williams)	Di-p-(chlorophenyl) methyl carbinol*	25%
DIGENEX VET. Fungicide (veterinary) (Wright, M.)	Digenol (2, 2'-dihydroxy-5, 5' dichloro diphenyl methane)* Isopropyl alcohol*				
			DIM-LUS Paint (Briggs-Maroney)		
DIGESTINE LIQUID & POWDER (Leslie Pharm.)			DIMPLES TOILET WATER (Vantines)		
			DIMTONE PAINT (Kurfees)		
DIGESTIVE AROMATIC Digestant (Massengill)	Each tablet: Saccharated pepsin Pancreatin Diastase Aromatic powder	0.26 gm. 32 mg. 16 mg. 16 mg.	DI-NITROL Herbicide (Sherwin-Williams)	Dinitro-ortho-cresol*	40%

*Consult Sec. II., Ingredients Index. This ingredient may be responsible for major toxic effects if poisonous amounts of this product are ingested.

- 432 -

Name & Use Manufacturer	Ingredients		Name & Use Manufacturer	Ingredients	
DINITROX Fungicide (Veith)	Dinitro-ocresol*		DIOTHANE OINTMENT Anesthetic, antiseptic (Merrell)	Diothane (diperodon) Oxyquinoline benzoate	1% 0.1%
DINNER PARTY PICK-UP (Beauty Couns.)			DIOWEED Herbicide (Bonide)	Dichlorophenoxyacetic acid* alkanolamine salt (expressed as the free acid) 10% Triethanolamine-2, 4-dichlorophenoxyacetate* 16-7%	
DIOCEL Cathartic (Dillard)	Each tablet: Methylcellulose	7-1/2 gr.			
DIOCEL COMPOUND Carthartic (Dillard)	Each tablet: Methylcellulose Extract cascara sagrada	7-1/2 gr. 1/8 gr.	DIOWEED DUST Herbicide (Bonide)	Triethanolamine salt of 2, 4-dichlorophenoxyacetic acid* 8.35%	
DIO-HIST WITH DIONIN Antitussive (Approved)	Each fl. oz.: Dionin* Thenylpyramine hydrochloride* 80 mg. Sodium citrate Ammonium chloride Antimony potassium tartrate Menthol* Aromatics Alcohol	1/4 gr. 1/24 gr. 1/24 gr. 1/24 gr. 1%	DIOXY SPOT REMOVER (Rhodes, P.)		
			DI-PARALENE CALAMINE CREAM (Abbott)	Di-paralene hydrochloride* 2% Calamine Phenol	16% 0.9%
			DIP & DISINFECT-ANT Insecticide (Hess, Dr.)	Coal tar phenols* Coal tar oils* Anhydrous soap	14% 56% 20%
DIONOL ANALGESIC OINTMENT Rubefacient, (Myers Labs.)	Menthol* Methyl salicylate* Benzoated goose grease Glyceryl monostearate Beeswax Camphor* Oil sassafras Anhydrous lanolin Petrolatum Paraffin		DIPEPSITOL Digestant, antacid (VB)	Bismuth subcarbonate Pepsin Sodium bicarbonate Cascara	
			DI-PER-X To treat diapers against diaper rash (Rockwell)	Para di-isobutyl phenoxy ethoxy ethyl dimethyl benzyl ammonium chloride* 3.5%	
DIONOL IODIZED OINTMENT Skin irritations (Myers Labs.)	Iodine (as iodized fatty acids) 1% Benzoated goose grease Anhydrous lanolin White mineral oil Petrolatum Beeswax Paraffin		DIP IT Coffee stain remover (Economics)	Sodium phosphate* Sodium silicate Sodium perborate* Synthetic wetting agent*	
DIONOL NASAL OINTMENT Nasal decongestant (Myers Labs.)	Menthol* Methyl salicylate* Camphor* Dist. ext. witch hazel		DIPIT DRY CLEANING COMPOUND (Elroy)		
DIONOL PLAIN OINTMENT For skin burns and irritations (Myers Labs.)	Benzoated goose grease Anhydrous lanolin White mineral oil Petrolatum Beeswax Paraffin		DIP IT FRENCH DRY CLEANER (Thoro)	Desiccant Cleaners' naphtha* Detergent	
			DIPPO SILVER CLEANER (Ultra Chem.)		
DIONOL PROCTOLOGIC OINTMENT For rectal irritation (Myers Labs.)	Menthol* Methyl salicylate* Dist. ext. witch hazel Anhydrous lanolin Petrolatum Paraffin Camphor* Eucalyptol* Benzoated goose grease White mineral oil Beeswax		DIPTEREX Insecticide (Chemagro)	o, o-Dimethyl-2, 2, 2-trichloro-1-hydroethyl phosphate*	
			DIPTEREX-199 Insecticide (Pittsburgh Coke)	o, o-Dimethyl-1-hydroxy-2, 2, 2-trichloroethyl phosphonate 1.0%	
			DIRENOL Diuretic (Veltex)	Each tablet: Methenamine* Uva ursi Buchu Saw palmetto Salol* Oil juniper*	1/2 gr. 1 gr. 1 gr. 1 gr. 1/2 gr. 1/2 m.
DIOTHANE HYDROCHLORIDE CREAM For skin burns and irritations (Merrell)	Diothane hydrochloride 0.1% Ceepryn chloride 0.1%				

---

*Consult Sec. II., Ingredients Index. This ingredient may be responsible for major toxic effects if poisonous amounts of this product are ingested.

Name & Use Manufacturer	Ingredients		Name & Use Manufacturer	Ingredients	
DI-RETIC PILLS Diuretic (Mayfair)	Methenamine* Uva ursi Potassium nitrate Buchu leaves Theobromine alkaloid Venice turpentine*		DITHAEROSOL Insecticide (DAO)	Tetraethyl dithionopyro-phosphate* Related phosphates Methyl chloride	4.5% 0.5% 95.0%
DIR-KLEEN General house-hold cleaner (Trylon)	Tripoly phosphate Pyrophosphate Alkyl aryl sulfonate Sodium sesquicarbonate Sodium bicarbonate D & C dye		DITHANE D-14 Fungicide (Rohm & Haas)	Nabam* (27% as hexahydrate)	19%
			DITHANE M-22 Insecticide (Rohm & Haas)	Maneb* (manganese ethylene bis (dithiocarbamate)) 70%	
DI-RONE For renal disorder (White, R. P.)	Potassium (as citrate, bicarbonate and acetate) 46.87% Hyoscyamus* Buchu Alcohol 26%		DITHIONO-VAPOR FORMULA NO. 178 Insecticide (Edco)	Tetraethyl dithionopyro-phosphate*	5%
DIRTBUSTER CAR WASH (Cannon)			DITZCO Enamel (Ditzler)	Polyhydroxy alcohols Poly-basic acids Drying oils	
DIRTEX Cleaner (Savogran)	Mild alkalis Synthetic detergent Coloring matter Diammonium phosphate		DITZ-LAC Lacquer (Ditzler)	Nitrocellulose Alkyd resins Plasticizers Hydrocarbons* (naphtha, toluol, Esters* xylol) Alcohols* Ketones	
DISHWASH (Stanley Home)	Water Alipal Ultrawet (see quaternary ammonium salts) Nonic Perfume		DIURESAL Diuretic (Veltex)	Each fl. oz.: Alcohol Methenamine Saw palmetto berries Corn silk Couch grass Sodium benzoate Sodium salicylate Buchu leaves Aromatics	7% 12 gr. 20 gr. 20 gr. 20 gr. 8 gr. 8 gr. 20 gr. q.s.
DISINFECTALL Disinfectant (Roberts, Dr. D.)	Coal tar neutral oils 50% Phenols* 25% Soap 15%				
DISKIN For skin irritations (Massengill)	Phenyl mercuric nitrate 1-5000 Zinc acetate Salicylic acid* Carbolic acid* Menthol* Glycerin		DIVERSOL Dairy utensils disinfectant (Diversey)	Sodium hypochlorite* Over 3.25% Sodium phosphate Over 91.75%	
DIS-O-FECT Disinfectant, deodorant (First National)	Pine oil soap* 90%		DIXIE LYE Drain cleaner (Pennsylv. Salt)	Sodium hydroxide*	
DISPERCIN Antacid, carminative (Univ. Nutrit.)	Calcium carbonate 2-1/2 gr. Magnesium trisilicate 1-1/2 gr. Glycine 1 gr. Magnesium superoxol 2/3 gr.		DIXIE-RUB Veterinary liniment (Dixie-Rub)	Each fl. oz.: Isopropyl alcohol* Chloroform Oils of wormwood Peppermint Thyme Cedar Methyl salicylate* Camphor* Menthol	75% 15 m.
DISPOSABLE AEROSOL INSECTICIDE (Whitmire)	Pyrethrins I and II 0.400% Allethrin 0.200% Rotenoids and other cube resins 0.067% Rotenone 0.033% n-Octyl sulfoxide of isosafrole 2.816% Related compounds 0.384% Butoxypolypropylene glycol* 4.900% Refined hydrocarbon oil* 11.200% Propellant gas 80.000%				
			DIXIERUB LINIMENT (Wood Chem.)	Menthol* Camphor gum* Eucalyptol* Pine oil*	
			DIXON'S AROMATIC CARMINATIVE COMPOUND (Kenton)	Alcohol 19% Blackberry root Extract logwood Jamaica ginger Rhubarb root	
DISSOLVO (solvent) Tar and road oil remover (du Pont)			DJER-KISS PERFUME (Nestle-Le Mur)		
DISTOL-X-CLEANSER (Nat'l. Soap)					

*Consult Sec. II., Ingredients Index. This ingredient may be responsible for major toxic effects if poisonous amounts of this product are ingested.

Name & Use Manufacturer	Ingredients		Name & Use Manufacturer	Ingredients
D-K Diuretic (Friendly Labs.)	Buchu Sodium nitrate Ext. buchu Aloes Capsicum Ext. juniper Ext. uva ursi Ext. stone root Oleoresin Potassium nitrate		DOBINAL Fungicide (medical) (Crowell)	Resorcin* Tincture of benzoin comp. Acetone Salicylic acid* Castor oil Dihydroxy dichloro diphenyl- methane*
D-K Insecticide (Dill)	Chlordane tech. 2% Piperonyl butoxide 0.075% Pyrethrins 0.015% Perfume 0.25% Water white petroleum oil 97.66%		DOB-ON SCRATCH FIX Scratch remover (Glidden Co.)	
D-K-NO-MOR CARBOLINEUM POULTRY MITE KILLER (Hilltop)	Anthracene oil carbolineum* 100%		DOC 75 BLOSSOM THINNER (Sunland)	Dinitro ortho secondary butyl phenol* 0.75%
D-K OINTMENT For skin irritation (D-K)	Salicylic acid* Benzoic acid Menthol* Thymol* Zinc oxide Precipitated sulfur Benzocaine Castor oil		DOCTOR ROPER FORMULA For fungus irritations of the skin (Sherry)	Salicylic acid* Potassium permanganate Isopropyl alcohol* 70% Oil of lavender
D-M-O Fungicide (Greever's)	Bis-(5-chloro-2-hydroxyphenyl) methane (2, 2'-methylene-bis- (4-chlorophenol); dihydrox- 5, 5'-dichloro diphenyl methane) (compound G-4) 2.50% Gamma isomer of benzene hexachloride (from lindane) 0.025%		DOCTORS DAUGHTER TABS (Daughter)	
			DOCTOR LOEBEL'S INSECTICIDE (Huntington)	
D-MOTH CRYSTALS & SPRAY Insecticide (D-Moth)			DOCTOR ROPER FORMULA Fungicide (Medical) (Sherry)	Salicylic acid* Potassium permanganate* Iso-propyl alcohol* 70% Oil of lavender flowers
DOAK TAR DISTILLATE For chronic exzematoid dermatitis (Doak)			DODD'S PILLS Diuretic (Dodds)	Theobromine sodium salicylate* Ext. buchu Phenacetin* 1 gr.
DOAK TERSUS Soapless detergent (Doak)	Igepon T-51 Sodium fluoresceine Sodium chloride Perfume		DOESKIN COLOGNE & PERFUME (Parfum L'Orle)	
DOAN'S PILLS Diuretic (Foster-Milburn)	Theobromine-sodio-salicylate Sodium salicylate* Ext. uva ursi Ext. buchu Vitamin A		DOGGETT-PFEIL AGRI-SPRAY Insecticide (Doggett-Pfeil)	DDT* 50%
DO-AWAY MOUSE BAIT (Southland)	Warfarin (3-(a-acetonylbenzyl)- 4-hydroxycoumarin) 0.025%		DOG POWDER Insecticide (Hartz)	Cube resins (rotenone)*
DO-AWAY RAT & MOUSE BAIT (Southland)	Warfarin (3-(a-acetonylbenzyl)- 4-hydroxycoumarin) 0.025%		DOG-SHUN ROPE Repellent (Breck, Jos.)	
DOBELL'S SOLUTION For mucous membrane irritations (Purepac)	Carbolic acid 1.22 gr./fl. oz.		DOG STAOFF Repellent (Niagara Hort.)	Soap Nicotine sulfate*
			DOGSTIK CEMENTS (Davids, T.)	
			DOG-TROT Repellent, veterinary (Spratts)	Oleum graminis citrati, br.

*Consult Sec. II., Ingredients Index. This ingredient may be responsible for major toxic effects if poisonous amounts of this product are ingested.

Name & Use Manufacturer	Ingredients		Name & Use Manufacturer	Ingredients	
DOG WASH & DISINFECT-ANT (Clayton)			DOMEBORO POWDER, TABS Makes a wet dressing (Dome)	Aluminum sulfate Calcium acetate Boric acid*	
DOGZIX REPELLENT (Bonide)	Bone oil*	38.9%	DOMICONE CREME Skin Protectant (Dome)	Silicone Acid mantle creme base	20%
D'OILENE SOLVENT (Mechanical)			DOMINANT RID-O-PESTS Insecticide (Dominant)	Pyrethrins* Petroleum distillate*	
DOLAN BUG KILLER ROACH SPRAY (Dolan Labs.)			DOMINO BRAND COSMETICS (Halitosine)		
DOLAN INSECTICIDE POWDER (Dolan Labs.)	DDT*	10%	DOMOGYN Vaginal douche powder (Dome)	Aluminum sulfate Calcium acetate Nonionic wetting agent Lauroyl amide of polyethylether	
DOLAN'S DU-BAR BLEACHES (Dolan, V. J.)	Strong acid and alkaline solution*		DOMOLENE For dry skin (Dome)	Glyceryl monostearate	
DOLAN'S NON-GRAIN RAISING STAIN (Dolan, V. J.)	Methanol*	over 5%	D-101 FOR DANDRUFF (Proof)	Sipon Hexachlorophene* Octylene glycol Thymol* Isopropanol*	
DOLCIN TABLETS (Antirheumatic (Dolcin)	Calcium succinate Aspirin*		DONFIELD LOTION For dry skin (Donfield)	Olive oil Lanolin Oxyquinoline sulfate Carbamide Menthol	
DOLCOMIST Insecticide (Dolge)	Aliphatic petroleum hydro-carbons Aromatic petroleum hydro-carbons* Piperonyl butoxide Pyrethrins Essential oils		DON JUAN CAKE MAKE UP (Don Juan)	Talc Titanium dioxide Certified colors Non-aniline colors Lanolin Petrolatum Mineral oil Polyethyline glycol 400 Perfume	
DOLGE ANTU DUST Rodenticide (Dolge)	Alpha naphthyl thiourea* 18.4%				
DOLGE E. W. T. AMINE TYPE 2, 4-D WEED KILLER (Dolge)	Diethanolamine 2, 4-dichlorophenoxyacetate* 49.6%		DON JUAN FACE POWDER (Don Juan)	Talc Zinc oxide Magnesium carbonate Zinc stearate Perfume Certified colors	
DOLGE RUST PREVENTING & REMOVING COMPOUND (Dolge)			DON JUAN LIQUID BRIL-LIANTINE (Don Juan)	Mineral oil Color Perfume	
DOLLARD'S BLUE RINSE, CREAMS, HAIR TONIC & LOTIONS (Aschenbach)			DON JUAN LIPSTICK (Don Juan)	Candelilla wax Petrolatum Lanolin Stearic acid Cetyl alcohol Castor oil Butyl stearate Perfume Certified colors	
DOLLY DIMPLE WAVESET (Brighto)			DON JUAN PERFUME (Don Juan)	Alcohol* 39C Perfume oils	
DOLO-SAN PINK TABLETS Analgesic (Tosan)	Aspirin* Acetophenetidin* Caffeine	3-1/2 gr. 2-1/2 gr. 1/2 gr.			

*Consult Sec. II., Ingredients Index. This ingredient may be responsible for major toxic effects if poisonous amounts of this product are ingested.

Name & Use Manufacturer	Ingredients		Name & Use Manufacturer	Ingredients	
DON JUAN ROUGE (Don Juan)	Talc Certified colors Santomerse Perfume		DOREX Deodorant (Veltex)	Each tablet: Chlorophyllins (from water-soluble fractions of chlorophyll)	100 mg.
DON JUAN SOLID BRIL-LIANTINE (Don Juan)	Paraffin Mineral oil Petrolatum Perfume		DORMA-REST Sedative (Pharmex)	Each capsule: Methapyrilene hydrochloride* 25 mg. Scopolamine aminoxide hydrobromide* 0.2 mg.	
DON JUAN TOILET WATER (Don Juan)	Alcohol* 39C Perfume oils		DORMATONE Hormone sprout in-hibitor for potatoes in storage (Am. Chemical)	Methyl ester of naphthaleneacetic acid 2.2%	
DON'T Discourages thumb sucking and nail biting (Commerce)	Aloes Oleoresin capsicum* Flexible collodion Isopropyl alcohol* 17.0%				
DONTÉ For skin irritation (Donté)	Lanolin Zinc oxide Petrolatum Boric acid* Salicylic acid*		DORMATOX OIL SPRAY Insecticide (Bonide)	Petroleum oil* 98%	
DONTÉ TABLETS Analgesic (Donté)	Each tablet: Aspirin* 3-1/2 gr. Phenacetin* 2-1/2 gr. Caffeine 1/2 gr.		DORMIN Sedative (Dormin)	Each capsule: n, n–Dimethyl-n'-(2-thenyl)-n'-(2-pyridyl)-ethylene diamine hydrochloride* 25 mg.	
DOOM For milky disease spores (Murray, E.)	Calcium carbonate Talc		DORM-ITE (Diamond L Brand) Insecticide (Leckenby)	Mineral oil 75%	
DOOM AEROSOL INSECTICIDE (Murray, E.)	Allethrin 0.10% Tech. piperonyl butoxide 0.25% Isobornyl thiocyanoacetate 0.82% Other related terpenes 0.18% DDT 2.00% Methoxychlor tech. 1.00% Petroleum distillate* 15.65%		DORMO-KOP Fungicide (Tenn. Corp.)	Copper in basic copper sulfate* 42%	
			DORMOL EMULSION Fungicide (Calif. Spray)	Petroleum oils* 80%	
DOOM (Roach) (Murray, E.)	Sodium fluoride* 90%		DOR MULSO Fungicide (Martin, C. J.)	Petroleum distillate* 97%	
DOOR-EASE Lubricant (Am. Grease Stick)	Microcrystalline waxes Carnauba wax Motor oil		DORMUTOL SLEEP CAPSULES (Pharmex)	n–Dimethyl-n-(2-thenyl-n)-(2-pyridyl)-ethylene diamine HCL* 25 mg.	
DOOSHO HYGIENIC POWDER Vaginal douche, antiseptic (K & B)	Oxyquinoline sulfate Sodium borate* Potassium Alum Sodium bicarb. Thymol Eucalyptol* Menthol* Methyl salicylate* Salicylic acid* 5% Phenol 1%		DOROTHY GRAY DAINTINESS CREAM DEODORANT (Gray, D.)		
			DOROTHY GRAY FACE POWDER (Gray, D.)	Coloring materials Perfumes Talcum base	
DOOZY-DOES-IT CLEANER (Protective)	Silicone		DOROTHY GRAY LIPSTICK (Gray, D.)	Coloring ingredients Perfumes Vegetable oils Waxes	
DOOZY-DOES-IT POLISH (Protective)	Silicone		DOROTHY GRAY PORTRAIT Face powder (Gray, D.)		
			DOROTHY GRAY SATURA Face cream (Gray, D.)		

*Consult Sec. II., Ingredients Index. This ingredient may be responsible for major toxic effects if poisonous amounts of this product are ingested.

Name & Use Manufacturer	Ingredients	Name & Use Manufacturer	Ingredients
DOROTHY GRAY SUNBURN CREAM (Gray, D.)		DOUBLE X HARDWOOD FLOOR CLEANER (Schalk)	
DOROTHY PERKINS ASTRINGENT (Perkins)		DOUCHENE Douche (Morris Drug)	
DOROTHY PERKINS COLOGNE Liquid and stick (Perkins)		DOUCHETTES Douche compound (Sevran)	Sodium borate* Sodium bicarbonate Sodium chloride Sodium perborate* F.D.C. color Tricalcium phosphates
DOROTHY PERKINS DEODORANT Cream and stick (Perkins)		DOUCHOL Douche (Great Lakes Labs.)	Boric acid* Ammonium alum Aromatics Zinc sulfate Carbolic acid* Oxyquinoline sulfate
DOROTHY PERKINS ROSE LOTION (Perkins)		DOUGH-BOY PROPHYLAC-TIC (Reese Chem.)	Calomel* (a mercury derivative) 30% Oxyquinoline benzoate
DOROTHY PERKINS SKIN FRESHENER (Perkins)		DOUGH-BOY PROPHYLAC-TIC KIT TWO TUBE (Reese Chem.)	Colored tube: 5% Sulfathiazole ointment with oxyquinoline benzoate 40 gr. White tube: 30% Calomel ointment* 62 gr.
DORVAL BURN LIQUID OR OINTMENT (Dorval)		DOUGLAS BRUSH KILLER Herbicide (Douglas Chem.)	Butoxy ethoxy propanol ester of 2, 4, 5-trichlorophenoxy-acid* 37.8% Butoxy ethoxy propanol ester of 2, 4-dichlorophenoxyacetic acetic acid* 35.6%
DORVAL CORN & CALLOUS REMOVER (Dorval)			
DOSATOLE Antitussive (Travine)	Each teasp.: Ammonium chloride 1 gr. Sodium citrate 1 gr. Chloroform 1/8 m. White tar Cherry syrup Antimony and potassium tartrate 1/256 gr. Potassium guaiacolsulfonate 2 gr.	DOUGLAS CATTLE SPRAY EMULSION CONC. Insecticide (Douglas Chem.)	Butoxypolypropylene glycol Petroleum distillate* Tech. piperonyl butoxide Pyrethrins
DOUBLE B BRUSH CLEANER (Double B.)	Benzol* 90% Acetone alcohol Naphtha	DOUGLAS 47% CHLORDANE EMULSION CONC. Insecticide (Douglas Chem.)	Tech. chlordane* 47% Deodorized kerosene* 47%
DOUBLE CHECK WATER SOFTNER (Elgin)		DOUGLAS CUTI-LENE Cleansing cream (Douglas Miller)	
DOUBLE-DANDERINE (Watkins, R.)	Alcohol 9% Alkyl di-methyl benzyl ammonium chloride*	DOUGLAS 25% DDT WATER MIX EMULSION Insecticide (Douglas Chem.)	DDT 25.0% Methylated aromatic petroleum oil* 72.5%
DOUBLE DANDERINE (Bayer)	Alkyl di-methyl benzyl ammonium chloride* Perfume Boric acid Alcohol 9%		
DOUBLEQUICK PAINT (Jewell)		DOUGLAS DIELDRIN EMULSION CONC. Insecticide (Douglas Chem.)	Hexachloro epoxy octahydro-endo, exo-dimethano naphthalene* 15.83% Related compounds 2.73% Related hydrocarbons 73.38%

*Consult Sec. II., Ingredients Index. This ingredient may be responsible for major toxic effects if poisonous amounts of this product are ingested.

Name & Use Manufacturer	Ingredients		Name & Use Manufacturer	Ingredients
DOUGLAS FARM BIN SPRAY Insecticide (Douglas Chem.)	Deodorized petroleum distillate* DDT* Beta thiocyano ethyl esters of aliphatic acids Beta butoxy beta thiocyano diethyl ether*		DOUGLAS TOXAPHENE 6 EMULSION CONC. Insecticide (Douglas Chem.)	Toxaphene* 60% Petroleum distillate 34%
DOUGLAS GRAIN FUMIGANT (Douglas Chem.)	Carbon tetrachloride* Benzene* Ethylene dibromide* Sulfur dioxide		DOUGLAS UNIVERSAL ELEVATOR & WARE- HOUSE SPRAY Insecticide (Douglas Chem.)	Deodorized petroleum oil DDT* Isobornyl thiocyano acetate Beta thiocyano ethyl esters of aliphatic fatty acids Beta butoxy beta thiocyano diethyl ether*
DOUGLAS HYGIENIC POWDER Antiseptic for personal hygiene (Douglas Miller)	Lactic acid Salicylic acid* Zinc sulfate * Thymol* Camphor* Boric acid* Lactose Phenol* Menthol * Eucalyptol *		DOUGLAS WEED KILLER (Douglas Chem.)	Butyl ester of 2, 4-dichloro- phenoxyacetic acid* 40%
			DOUGLAS WEED KILLER ESTER SOLUTION (Douglas Chem.)	Butyl ester of 2, 4-dichloro- phenoxyacetic acid* 37.61%
DOUGLAS LINDANE 20% EMULSION CONC. Insecticide (Douglas Chem.)	Lindane* 20.0% Aromatic hydrocarbons* 69.5% Aliphatic hydrocarbons 7.5%		DOUX JASMIN EXTRACT (Parfums Ciro)	
DOUGLAS RAT-KILL (Douglas Chem.)	Warfarin (3-(a-acetonylbenzyl)- 4-hydroxycoumarin) 0.025%		DOVAPS Analgesic (Tailby)	Acetophenetidin* 1-1/2 gr. Dover's powder 1/4 gr. Aspirin* 1-1/2 gr. Caffeine 1/8 gr. Monobromated camphor 1/10 gr.
DOUGLAS SPECIAL EMULSION SPRAY CONC. Insecticide (Douglas Chem.)	Pyrethrins 1.00% Piperonyl butoxide 10.00% Petroleum distillate* 73.00%		DOVERCLIFF DUSTLESS CHALK (Am. Crayon)	
DOUGLAS SUFFOKATO #1 & #2 Fumigant (Douglas Chem.)	Carbon tetrachloride* Benzene* Sulfur dioxide Ethylene dibromide*		DOVIUM CAPSULES Analgesic, antipyretic (Hance)	Each capsule: Dover powder 1/2 gr. Acetophenetidin* 1-1/2 gr. Atropine sulfate 1/500 gr. Aspirin* 2 gr. Camphor 1/4 gr. Caffeine 1/8 gr. Sodium sulfate 7-1/2 gr.
DOUGLAS TETRAFUME Fumigant (Douglas Chem.)	Carbon tetrachloride* Benzene* Sulfur dioxide Ethylene dibromide*		DOWANOL 1 Insecticide (Dow)	Ethylene glycol phenyl ether (2-phenoxyethanol)*
DOUGLAS TETRAKIL GRAIN FUMIGANT (Douglas Chem.)	Carbon tetrachloride* Benzene* Ethylene dibromide* Sulfur dioxide		DOWANOL 3 Insecticide (Dow)	Ethylene glycol p-sec-butyl- phenyl ether (2-(p-sec- butylphenoxy) ethanol)*
			DOWANOL 7 Insecticide (Dow)	Ethylene glycol methyl ether (2-methoxyethanol)*
DOUGLAS TETRAKOTE Grain pro- tectant (Douglas Chem.)	Ethylene tetrachloride* Petroleum distillate* Tech. piperonyl butoxide Pyrethrins		DOWANOL 16 Insecticide (Dow)	Diethylene glycol methyl ether (2-(2-methoxyethoxy) ethanol)*
			DOWANOL 2B Insecticide (Dow)	Propylene glycol phenyl ether (1-phenoxy-2-propanol)*
			DOWANOL 5B Insecticide (Dow)	Dipropylene glycol phenyl ether*
DOUGLAS TETRASPOT FUMIGANT (Douglas Chem.)	Carbon tetrachloride* Benzene* Ethylene dibromide* Sulfur dioxide		DOW-9B Seed pro- tectant (Dow)	2, 4, 5-Trichlorophenate *

*Consult Sec. II., Ingredients Index. This ingredient may be responsible for major toxic effects if poisonous amounts of this product are ingested.

- 439 -

Name & Use Manufacturer	Ingredients		Name & Use Manufacturer	Ingredients	
DOW ARSENATE OF LEAD Insecticide (Dow)	Arsenic* Lead		DOW DN-DUST NO. 12 Insecticide (Dow)	Dinitro-o-cyclohexylphenol Dicyclohexylamine salt*	1.5%
DOW BASIC ARSENATE OF LEAD Insecticide (Dow)	Basic arsenate of lead*	96%	DOW DN-SULFUR DUST NO. 10 Insecticide (Dow)	Dinitro-o-cyclohexylphenol Sulfur*	0.8% 92%
DOW CALCIUM ARSENATE Insecticide (Dow)	Calcium arsenate*	70%	DOW DRY LIME-SULPHUR Fungicide (Dow)	Calcium polysulfide* Sulfur Calcium thiosulfate	
DOWCLENE Spot remover (Dow)	Carbon tetrachloride*		DOW EPSOM SALT (Dow)	Magnesium sulfate	
DOW CONTACT WEED KILLER (Dow)	Dinitro ortho secondary butyl phenol*	6.2%	DOWFUME Fumigant (Dow)	Carbon tetrachloride*	85%
DOW DDT 50% DUST CON-CENTRATE Insecticide (Dow)	DDT*	50%	DOWFUME 50 Fumigant (Dow)	Ethylene dichloride* Carbon tetrachloride*	44% 56%
DOW DDT 25% EMULSIFI-ABLE Insecticide (Dow)	DDT*	25%	DOWFUME 75 Fumigant (Dow)	Ethylene dichloride* Carbon tetrachloride*	70.2% 29.8%
DOW DDT 50% WETTABLE Insecticide (Dow)	DDT*	50%	DOWFUME EB-5 Insecticide (Dow)	Ethylene dibromide Ethylene dichloride Carbon tetrachloride	7.20 29.20 63.60
DOW DHA Fungicide (Dow)	Dehydroacetic acid*		DOWFUME EB-15 Fumigant (Dow)	Ethylene dibromide* Ethylene dichloride* Carbon tetrachloride*	19.6% 20.4% 60.0%
DOW DICHLORO-ETHYL ETHER Fumigant (Dow)	Dichloroethyl ether*		DOWFUME G Fumigant (Dow)	Methyl bromide Xylene*	26% 74%
DOW FIRE EXTINGUISHER FLUID (Dow)	Carbon tetrachloride*	95%	DOWFUME MC-2 Fumigant (Dow)	Methyl bromide* Chloropicrin	98% 2%
DOWFLAKE Chemical air dryer (Dow)	Calcium chloride		DOWFUME N Fumigant (Dow)	Dichloro propene* Propane*	
DOW DN-111 Insecticide (Dow)	Dinitro-o-cyclohexylphenol* Dicyclohexylamine salt*	20%	DOWFUME W-40 Fumigant (Dow)	Ethylene dibromide*	41%
DOW DN-289 Insecticide (Dow)	Dinitro-o-sec-butylphenol* Triethanolamine salt	26%	DOWFUME W-85 Fumigant (Dow)	Ethylene dibromide*	83%
DOW DN-DRY MIX NO. 1 Insecticide (Dow)	Dinitro-o-cyclohexylphenol*	40%	DOW GAUGE FLUID R-200 (Dow)	ar-Dibromoethylbenzene* ar-Tribromoethylbenzene*	
			DOW GENERAL WEED KILLER (Dow)	Dinitro-o-sec-butyl phenol*	55%
DOW DN-DRY MIX NO. 2 Insecticide (Dow)	4, 6-Dinitro-o-cresol*	40%	DOW GRAIN FUMIGANT (80-20 Mixture) (Dow)	Carbon tetrachloride* Carbon bisulfide	83.5% 16.5%/w

Name & Use Manufacturer	Ingredients		Name & Use Manufacturer	Ingredients	
DOWICIDE 1 Fungicide (Dow)	Orthophenyl phenol*	98%	DOW MCP AMINE WEED KILLER (Dow)	Alkanolamine salts of 4-chloro-o-toloxyacetic acid*	
DOWICIDE 2 Fungicide (Dow)	2, 4, 5-Trichlorophenol*	95%	DOW METHYL BROMIDE Fumigant (Dow)	Methy bromide*	
DOWICIDE 4 Fungicide (Dow)	2-Chloro-4-phenylphenol*	88%	DOW 99 Herbicide (Dow)	Propylene glycol butyl ether esters of 2, 4-D*	
DOWICIDE 2S Fungicide (Dow)	2, 4, 6-Trichlorophenol*	90%	DOW PARATHION 15% Insecticide (Dow)	Parathion*	15%
DOWICIDE 5 Insecticide (Dow)	2-Bromo-4-phenylphenol*		DOW PARATHION 15% WETTABLE Insecticide (Dow)	Parathion*	15%
DOWICIDE 6 Fungicide (Dow)	Tetrachlorophenol*	92%			
DOWICIDE 7 Fungicide (Dow)	Pentachlorophenol* Other chlorophenols	83% 12%	DOW 9-B SEED PROTECTANT Insecticide (Dow)	Zinc, 2, 4, 5-trichloro-phenate*	50%
DOWICIDE 30 Insecticide (Dow)	Chloro-o-phenylphenol*	85%	DOW SODIUM TCA 90% Herbicide (Dow)	Sodium trichloroacetate	90%
DOWICIDE 31 Fungicide (Dow)	Chloro-o-phenylphenol*	85%	DOW SPECIAL GARDEN SPRAY Insecticide (Dow)	Lead arsenate* Copper	38% 19%
DOWICIDE A Fungicide (Dow)	o-Phenylphenol*, sodium salt		DOW SPECIAL POTATO SPRAY Insecticide (Dow)	Tricalcium arsenate* Copper	69% 7.5%
DOWICIDE F Fungicide (Dow)	2, 3, 4, 6-Tetrachlorophenol*, soidum salt	80%	DOWSPRAY 17 Insecticide (Dow)	Dinitro-o-cyclohexylphenol* Dicyclohexylamine salt	13.3%
DOWICIDE G Fungicide (Dow)	Sodium pentachlorophenate* Sodium salts of other chloro-phenols	75% 13%	DOWSPRAY DORMANT NO. 3 Insecticide (Dow)	Mineral oil Dinitro-o-cresol*	96% 4%
DOWICIDE H Fungicide (Dow)	2, 3, 4, 6-Tetrachlorophenol*, sodium salt	80%	DOWSPRAY 66 IMPROVED Herbicide (Dow)	Dinitro-o-sec-butylphenol* Mineral oil	9.1% 87.9%
DOWICIDE P Fungicide (Dow)	2, 3, 4, 6-Tetrachlorophenol*, sodium salt 6-Chloro-2-phenylphenol, sodium salt	60% 20%	DOW STANDARD ARSENATE OF LEAD Insecticide (Dow)	Standard arsenate of lead*	96%
DOWKLOR 5% DUST Insecticide (Dow)	Tech. chlordane*	5%			
DOWKLOR 40% EMULSIFI-ABLE OR WETTABLE Insecticide (Dow)	Tech. chlordane*	40%	DOW WOOD PRESERVATIVE (Dow)	Pentachlorophenol* Other chlorinated phenols	
DOW LIME-SULFUR SOLUTION Insecticide (Dow)	Calcium polysulfide* Calcium thiosulfate	30% 1.5%	DOX BRUSH CLEANER Paint brush cleaner (Reliable Paste)	Benzol* Acetone	
DOW LINDANE 25% WETTABLE Insecticide (Dow)	Gamma isomer of BHC*	25%			

*Consult Sec. II., Ingredients Index. This ingredient may be responsible for major toxic effects if poisonous amounts of this product are ingested.

Name & Use Manufacturer	Ingredients
DOX DENTIFRICE (Dox)	
DOYL Insecticide (Planetary Chem.)	DDT (dichloro diphenyl trichloroethane) 25% Petroleum aromatic solvent* 75%
DOZETS 3 Sedative (Melvin)	Each tablet: Hyoscine hydrobromide 0.0014 gr. Acetophenetidin* 2 gr. Sodium bromide* 7 gr.
D'PART CONCEN- TRATED VAPORIZING SPRAY Insecticide (Fuld)	Piperonyl butoxide Pyrethrum* Petroleum hydrocarbon*
D'PART INSECTICIDE AND FLY SPRAY (Fuld)	Piperonyl butoxide Pyrethrum* Petroleum hydrocarbon*
D'PART MILL AND SPACE SPRAYS Insecticides (Fuld)	Pyrethrins Piperonyl butoxide Petroleum hydrocarbons* Methoxychlor*
D'PART ROACH INSECTICIDE (Fuld)	Piperonyl butoxide Pyrethrum* Petroleum hydrocarbon*
D'PART VAPORIZING SPRAY Insecticide (Fuld)	Piperonyl butoxide Pyrethrum* Petroleum hydrocarbon*
D & P CABBAGE MAGGOT DESTROYER (Doggett- Pfeil)	Mercury*
D & P DUSTING SULPHUR Fungicide (Doggett- Pfeil)	Sulfur*
D & P FRUIT SPRAY Insecticide (Doggett- Pfeil)	DDT* 7.5% Rotenone 0.25% Ferbam 14% Sulfur 50%
D & P JAPELLENT Insecticide (Doggett- Pfeil)	Dichloro diphenyl trichloroethane* 45% Tech. chlordane 5%
D & P LINDANE- ARAMITE EMULSION Insecticide (Doggett- Pfeil)	Gamma isomer of benzene hexachloride* 6.00% 2-(p-tert-Butyl phenoxy) isopropyl 2-chloroethyl sulfite 5.00%
D & P LIQUID FUNGICIDE (Doggett- Pfeil)	Potassium polysulfide* 2.9% Potassium thiosulfate 2.96%

Name & Use Manufacturer	Ingredients
D & P LIQUID LIME SULPHUR Insecticide (Doggett- Pfeil)	Calcium polysulfides*
D & P PLANT SPRAY Insecticide (Doggett- Pfeil)	Nicotine* Soap
D.P.O. DRAIN CLEANER (Woodward- Wanger)	Sodium hydroxide*
D & P ROSE DUST Insecticide, fungicide (Doggett- Pfeil)	DDT* 5.00% Ferbam 7.00% Rotenone 0.75% Other cube resins 1.50% Gamma isomer of benzene hexachloride 0.50% Sulfur* 20.00%
D & P 1% ROTENONE GARDEN DUST Insecticide (Doggett- Pfeil)	Rotenone 1%
D & P SCALE OIL Insecticide (Doggett- Pfeil)	Crescylic acid* 5%
D & P TOMATO DUST Insecticide, fungicide (Doggett- Pfeil)	Copper expressed as metallic 7% Tri-calcium arsenate* 14%
D & P WEED KILLER (Doggett- Pfeil)	Sodium arsenite* (20% water soluble arsenic) 35%
DRAIN CLEAN (Woodward- Wanger)	Sodium hydroxide*
DRAINITE To clean drains (Crest Mfg.)	Sodium hydroxide*
DRAINKLEEN (Metropolitan)	Sodium hydroxide* composition
DRAIN PIPE CLEANER (Woodward- Wanger)	
DR. DRAKE'S Antitussive (Glessner)	Ipecac Castor oil Benzoic acid Camphor Glycerin Gum arabic Wild cherry Anise oil Alcohol 2-1/4%
DRAKE'S REMEDY (Caswell- Massey)	

*Consult Sec. II., Ingredients Index. This ingredient may be responsible for major toxic effects if poisonous amounts of this product are ingested.

Name & Use Manufacturer	Ingredients	Name & Use Manufacturer	Ingredients
DRAMACIN TABLETS (Formerly Travel-Aid) Motion sickness preventative (Pharmex)	n-p-Methoxybenzyl-n dimethyl-n-a-pyridyl ethylene diamine maleate* 25 mg. Hyoscine hydrobromide* 1/300 gr.	DRESKIN Hand cream (Campana)	F. D. & C. color Essential oils Glycerine Boric acid* Methyl parasept Alcohol*
DRAMEX CEMENT (Reardon Co.)		DREW'S CARBURETOR CLEANER (Drew, E. F.)	Coal tar distillates* Petroleum solvents* Corrosion inhibitors Detergents Chlorinated hydrocarbons*
DRAMEX INTERIOR WALL FINISH (Glidden Co.)		DREW'S COOLING SYSTEM CLEANSER (Drew, E. F.)	Chlorinated hydrocarbons* Detergents
DRANO Toilet bowl and drain cleaner (Drackett)	Sodium hydroxide*		
DRAWING SALVE (Pharmex)	Resin Ichthammol Petrolatum White wax	DREXEL'S WONDER SOAP Antiseptic for dandruff (Drexel)	Oxyquinoline sulfate Hexachlorophene (bis-(3, 5, 6-trichloro-2-hydroxphenl) methane)*
DRAW-ZIT Drawing salve (Hance)	Ichthammol 10% Deshler's salve 10% Sod. oxymercuri-o-nitrophenolate 0.1% Cycolform (isobutyl para-aminobenzoate) Methyl salicylate Petrolatum	DRI Aerosol spray (Blitz)	Carbon tetrachloride*
		DRI-BRITE LIQUID WAX (Boyle-Midway)	Waxes Emulsifiers Borax* Resins
D & R DRY CLEANER For dogs (D. & R.)		DRI-CLEAN DOG BATH Insecticide (Hartz, Mt.)	Rotenone* Naphthalene* Cream meal
DREFT Detergent (Procter & Gamble)	Anionic synthetic detergent Sodium tripolyphosphate Sodium silicate Sodium sulfate	DRI-CLOR Bleach (Pennsylv. Salt)	Calcium hypochlorite formulation Available chlorine* 40%
DREME CUTICLE REMOVER (Leighton)		DRI FAST Paint (Preservative)	
DREME NAIL POLISH REMOVER (Leighton)		DRI-FOOT POWDER (Dri-Foot)	Boric acid* Sodium thiosulfate Sodium carbonate Methylene blue
DREME NAIL TREATMENT (Leighton)		DRI-GLO POLISH (O-Cedar)	Petroleum naphtha* Inert silicones Wax solids
DRENE Shampoo, liquid (Procter & Gamble)	Anionic synthetic detergent Fatty acid amide Ethyl alcohol	DRIFTWOOD GLO Fire colors (Brown, E.)	
		DRIGARD Liquid masonry waterproofing (Drigard)	
DRESCOTE SHINGLE STAIN (Monroe Co.)		DRI-KIL Insecticide (Cooper)	Naphthalene* 4% Sulfur 10% Rotenone 0.1% Other cube resins 0.25%
DRESDEN FLAT WALL PAINT (Lawrence, W. W.)		DRI-KWICK Oil floor finish (Pioneer)	

*Consult Sec. II., Ingredients Index. This ingredient may be responsible for major toxic effects if poisonous amounts of this product are ingested.

Name & Use Manufacturer	Ingredients	Name & Use Manufacturer	Ingredients
DRI-MIST Spray deodorant (Lee Ltd.)		DROUT FUEL TANK ANTI-FREEZE (Casite)	
DRI-N-TITE (Liquid, Plastic & Primer) Roof coating (Horn)		DROX-A-GEL Antacid, adsorbent (Drew Pharm.)	Aluminum hydroxide 4.7 gr. Magnesium trisilicate 3.5 gr.
DRI-PIPE Waterproof adhesives (Chicago Show)		DROZD 101 ANTACID COMPOUND (C & D)	Rennin Pineapple juice Colloidal kaolin Bismuth subsalicylate* Methyl salicylate* Aromatics Pepsin Magnesium trisilicate Syn. saccharin Hydrochloric acid Dried aluminum hydroxide gel Salol* Zinc phenelsulfonate
DRIPLESS OIL Lubricant (Am. Grease)	Petroleum-bodied lubricating oil Naphtha* Sodium sulfo-naphthenate		
DRI-RUB Auto polish (Gilbert Labs.)		DROZD 101 CHILDREN'S COUGH SYRUP (C & D)	Ammonium chloride Menthol Glycerin Peppermint flavor Potassium guaiacol sulfonate Terpin hydrate Sugar syrup
DRI-SEAL Mildew-proofing compound (Dri-Seal)			
DRI-SEAL PAINTS (Materials)		DROZD 101 ELECTRIC BRAND OIL Liniment (C & D)	Gum camphor* Sassafrass Turpentine* Ammonia Oil wintergreen* Cloves Ether chloroform Alcohol* 70%
DRISKILL ANT POISON (Driskell)	Sodium arsenate* exsiccated 2.8%		
DRITZ RUGBACK Anti-skid carpet backing (Dritz)		DROZD 101 FOOT POWDER (C & D)	Salicylic acid* Boric acid* Menthol* Talcum Benzoic acid Chlorothymol* Kaolin
DRIVER FOR ANTS (Bohman)	Sodium fluoride* 70% Powdered silica 30%		
DRIVER FOR MICE (Bohman)	Sodium fluoride* 70% Powdered silica 30%	DROZD 101 OINTMENT Fungicide, (Medical) (C & D)	Salicylic acid* Benzoic acid Chlorothymol*
DRIVER RODENTICIDE (Bohman)	Sodium fluoride*		
DRIVO (Harrison's)	Quinine* Epsom salts Tr. ferric chloride	DROZD 101 RECTAL OINTMENT (C & D)	Each oz.: Hyoscyamine sulfate 0.0244 mg. Chloroform 0.2 cc. Alcohol 1.4 cc. Benzocaine Menthol* Camphor* Chloral hydrate* 130 mg.
D & R MANGE PRESCRIP-TION (D. & R.)			
DROCOLATE Antitussive (Lloyd)	Each fl. oz.: Dihydrocodeinone bitartrate 10.8 mg. Sodium citrate 1.17 gm. Citric acid 58 mg. Mentholated syrup base	DROZD 101 VAPORIZING & RUBBING OIL COMPOUND (C & D)	Menthol Camphor* Oils of eucalyptus, cajuput, origanum* Peppermint Wintergreen* Turpentine* Oleoresins of red pepper and ginger Expressed mustard* Pine*
DROUT Absorbs water in gas tank (Hastings)	Methyl alcohol* 100%		

Name & Use Manufacturer	Ingredients		Name & Use Manufacturer	Ingredients	
D & R PUPPY CAPSULES (D. & R.)			DRYGAS Solvent (Cristy)		
D & R ROOM FRESHENER (D. & R.)			DRY-KURE Herbicide (Central Supply)	Sodium pentachlorophenate* Sodium salts of other chlorophenols *	
DRUCO LIQUID CORN REMOVER (Philadelphia)	Each fl. oz.: Alcohol Ether* Collodion * Salicylic acid*	24% 331 m.	DRYLOK CEMENT PAINT (United Gilson.)	Cement Hydrated lime* Lime proof colors	
DRUMCOTE PAINT (Debevoise)			DRYLOK CEMENT SEALER (United Gilson.)	Cement Hydrated lime* Lime proof colors	
D & R WORM CAPSULES Veterinary (D. & R.)			DRY-MO Chemical air dryer (Hill Mfg.)		
DRYASEAL EMBALMING FLUID (Undertakers)			DRY-PITS LOTION Anti- perspirant (Dry-Pits)	Calcium chloride Ammonium potassium sulfate	
DRYBRIGHT WAX (Industrial Mat.)					
DRYCIDE Insecticide (Hess, Dr.)	Naphthalene * Coal tar phenols (tar acids) DDT	3.00% 0.25% 1.00%	DRY WALL ADHESIVE (Miracle)	Resinous materials Pigments Aliphatic petroleum hydrocarbon*	
DRYFAST ENAMEL (Globe Varnish)			D'SAPUR HOME DEODORANT (Lady America)		
DRY-DYP Insecticide (Miller Chem. Co.)	Naphthalene* Sodium fluoride Creosote oil Nicotine Sulfur	15.00% 1.00% 2.67% 0.03% 33.33%	D-T TABLETS Disinfectant, poultry drinking water (McClellan)	Potassium permanganate* 3 gr.	
DRY 50 INSECTICIDE (Corn King)	Naphthalene* Sulfur Creosote oil Sodium silicofluoride	35% 12% 1% 2%			

---

*Consult Sec. II., Ingredients Index. This ingredient may be responsible for major toxic effects if poisonous amounts of this product are ingested.

Name & Use Manufacturer	Ingredients
DUAL DUST NO. 5 Insecticide (Chipman Chem.)	DDT* 5.00% Copper expressed as metallic in the form of copper hydroxysulfate* 6.50%
DUAL PURPOSE DUST Insecticide (Soil Bldg.)	Rotenone Copper *
DUANE'S OINTMENT For skin burns (Dinet)	Bismuth subnitrate Zinc oxide Carbolic acid*
DUART PAINT (Maas & Waldstein)	
DU BAR BLEACHES (Dolan, V. J.)	Strong acid and alkaline solution*
DU BARRY EYEBROW PENCIL (Hudnut, R.)	
DU BARRY COLOGNE CONCENTRE (Hudnut, R.)	
DU BARRY CREAMS & LOTIONS (Hudnut, R.)	
DU BARRY DEODOR- ANTS (Hudnut, R.)	
DU BARRY EYE SHADOW (Hudnut, R.)	
DU BARRY LASH BEAUTY (Hudnut, R.)	
DU BARRY LIPSTICKS (Hudnut, R.)	
DU BARRY POWDERS (Hudnut, R.)	
DU BARRY ROUGE (Hudnut, R.)	
DU BARRY TALC SACHET (Hudnut, R.)	
DUBL ZEE SKIN LOTION (Hulett)	
DUCALITE PAINT (Dunne)	

Name & Use Manufacturer	Ingredients
DUCATONE PAINT (Dunne)	
DUCK KOTE Rust preven- tive (Thomas Co.)	Liquid wax Petroleum naphtha*
DUCO CEMENT (du Pont)	
DUCO ENAMELS (du Pont)	Soya-linseed-alkyd resin Solvent*
DUCO LACQUERS (du Pont)	
DUCO METAL PRIMER (du Pont)	Chinawood-linseed-alkyd resin Solvent*
DUCO PUTTIES (du Pont)	
DUFLEX BENZOL CEMENT (Hatch, H.)	
DUKE CREME OIL Hair cream (Stanhope)	Lanolin Mineral oil Triethanolamine emulsification agent
DUKONK Hair straighte- ner (Stanhope)	Caustic soda (sodium hydroxide)*
DULUX AUTOMOTIVE PAINTS AND PAINT PRODUCTS (du Pont)	
DUNNE'S PAINTS, ENAMELS (Dunne)	
DUOCAINE OINTMENT Antiseptic, local (Boyle & Co.)	Benzocaine Menthol* Oxyquinoline benzoate Petrolatum Chlorobutanol 0.5% Zinc oxide Boric acid*
DUOCIDE CONCEN- TRATE Rodenticide (Eastern St. Farmers')	2-Pivalyl-1, 3-indandione 0.50%

*Consult Sec. II., Ingredients Index. This ingredient may be responsible for major toxic effects if poisonous amounts of this product are ingested.

- 446 -

Name & Use Manufacturer	Ingredients	Name & Use Manufacturer	Ingredients
DUOCIDE MIXED BAIT Rodenticide (Eastern St. Farmers')	2-Pivalyl-1, 3-indandione 0.025%	DuPONT CLEANERS For hands, fabrics (du Pont)	
DUOCOAT Semi-paste flat white paint (Horn)		DuPONT INSECTICIDES, FUNGICIDES, HERBICIDES & AGRICULTURAL SUPPLIES (du Pont)	
DUOCREX Floor preservative (Horn)	Varnish Oil Resin Mineral spirits*	DuPONT PHOTOGRAPH- IC SUPPLIES (du Pont)	
DUO-DELLAY Rug and upholstery cleaner (Artloom)		DuPONT PLANT FOODS (du Pont)	
DUO DOUBLE DUTY Repels in- sects, prevents sunburn (Western Pharm.)	2-Ethylhexanediol* 20% Mono-glyceryl para-amino- benzoate 2%	DuPONT PAINTS AND POLISHES (du Pont)	
DUOLEAD PAINT (Debevoise)		DuPONT SILVER POLISH (du Pont)	
DUOLIN BODY LOTION (Huenelator)		DUPREE FEMI-TABS (Dupree)	
DUOLIN CLEANSING LOTION (Huenelator)		DUPREE RECTAL SUPPOSITOR- IES (Dupree)	
DUO-RAA-CO Embalming fluid (Embalmers')	Formaldehyde*	DUPREE VAGICONES (Dupree)	
DUO-RICH SHAMPOO (Modart)	Sodium lauryl sulfate Fatty acid esters	DURA DETE VARN Varnish (Atlantic Varnish)	
DUOSOL Cleaner (Drew, E.F.)	Coal tar distillates* Soaps Petroleum solvents* Corrosion inhibitors	DURAFAX Non-metallic floor hardener (Horn)	
DUO-SORB (Tutag)	Each tsp.: Kaolin 14.2 gr. Pectic 2/3 gr. Aluminum hydroxide gel 4 gr. Magnesium trisilicate 2 gr.	DURAFILM Paint (Lucas)	
		DURA FLINT VARNISH (Lucas)	
DUO-VAR Varnish (Breinig)		DURA-GLOSS NAIL LAQUER, PERFUMED (Lorr)	
DUPLEX AUTO POLISH (Hampton- Cross)		DURA-GLOSS NAIL POLISH (Lorr)	
DuPONT AUTOMOTIVE SUPPLIES (du Pont)		DURA-GLOSS NAIL POLISH REMOVER (Lorr)	

*Consult Sec. II., Ingredients Index. This ingredient may be responsible for major toxic effects if poisonous amounts of this product are ingested.

Name & Use Manufacturer	Ingredients		Name & Use Manufacturer	Ingredients	
DURALAC Paint (Sewall)			DURA VARNISH (Hotopf)		
DURAKO Paint (Durako)			DUREL PRESSED CRAYON (Binney & Smith)		
DURALEX Paint (Claronex)			DURELASTIC PAINT (Jewell P.&V.)		
DURALITE Liquid porcelain glaze (Webb)			DURFEE EMBALMING FLUIDS (Durfee)		
DURALITE PASTE PAINT (Bauer)			DURHAM BENECIDE DUST 10 Insecticide (Durham)	Hexachlorocyclohexane*	
DURAMANT VARNISH (Clover Leaf)			DURHAM CRYLITE DUST NO. 50 Fungicide, insecticide (Durham)	Sodium fluoaluminate*	
DURA MIX Paint (Lucas)					
DURANAMEL FINISHES (North & Judd)			DURHAM TETRATE SPRAY 50 Insecticide (Durham)	Tetraethyl pyrophosphate*	
DURA-PAINT (Paraffine)			DURHAM'S ANATHESIA MOP For throat irritation (Durham's)	Benzocaine Neutral acriflavine* Alcohol-glycerine menstrum	
DURASAN PAINT (Mound City)					
DURASET-20W Insecticide (Naugatuck)	n-Meta-tolyl phthalamic acid* 20%		DURHAM'S 1038 IM-PROVED SMEARLESS SCREW-WORM CONTROL Insecticide (Durham's)	DDT 25% Gamma isomer of benzene hexachloride (from lindane) 4.5% Aromatic petroleum solvent* 57.00%	
DURA-TEX CONCEN-TRATE Floor wax (Nat'l. Labs.)	Carnauba or carnauba-type waxes Emulsifiers				
DURATITE SURFACING PUTTY (Glidden Co.)			DURHAM'S RED ANT BALLS (Durham's)	Sodium cyanide* 97%	
DURATITE WOOD DOUGH (Glidden Co.)			DURHAM'S REUMA-RUB Liniment (Durham's)	Oil of wintergreen synthetic* Camphor* Menthol* Oil of turpentine* Acetone* Chloroform*	
DURATOP Non-metallic concrete aggregate (Horn)					
DURATOX A TERMITE CONTROL (Dorite)	Paraffin oil 76% Trichlorobenzene* 22-1/2% Paradichlorobenzene 1-1/2%		DURHAM'S ROACH & ANT BOMB (Durham's)	Tech. chlordane 2% DDT 3% Methylated naphthalenes* 7.5% Petroleum distillates* 27.5%	
DURATOX B TERMITE CONTROL (Dorite)	Petroleum distillate 76% Trichlorobenzene* 20% Oil of mirbane 2-1/2% Paradichlorobenzene 1-1/2%		DURHAM'S ROCK HARD WATER PUTTY (Glidden Co.)		

*Consult Sec. II., Ingredients Index. This ingredient may be responsible for major toxic effects if poisonous amounts of this product are ingested.

Name & Use Manufacturer	Ingredients	Name & Use Manufacturer	Ingredients
DURHAM'S SCREW-WORM BOMB (Durham's)	Gamma isomer of benzene hexachloride* (from lindane) 3.0% Pine oil* 17.5% Xylol* 12.5%	DUST-MOR LOUSE POWDER (Hilltop)	Anthracene oil (carbolineum) Sulfur Tech. methoxychlor 5% Naphthalene* Sodium fluoride* Nicotine sulfate*
DURHAM'S VEGETABLE GARDEN DUST Insecticide (Durham's)	Tech. methoxychlor 5.00% Rotenone 1.25% Other cube resins 2.50%	DUST OF AGICIDE Insecticide (Agicide)	Rotenone 0.75% Other cube resins 2.00%
DURMANCO Embalming materials (Durfee)		DUSTOX Insecticide (Agkem)	Rotenone and other cube resins 1.75%
DURMASEPTIC For skin irritations (Durma)	Acetylsalicylic acid* Methyl salicylate* Eugenol*	DUSTRITE DDT DUST NO. 30 Insecticide (Stoker)	DDT*
DUROCOTE PAINT (O'Neil)		DUTCH BRAND BICYCLE RIM CEMENT (Van Cleef)	
DUROLITE PAINT (Varcroft)		DUTCH BRAND HOUSE PAINTS (Perry & Derrick)	
DURO RUST PREVENTIVE & REMOVER COMPOUND (Woodhill)		DUTCH BRAND RUBBER CEMENT (Van Cleef)	
DUROSEAL PAINTS (Symolyn)		DUTCHESS PAINTS (Seriver)	
DUROTOX Wood preservative (Speekman)	Pentachlorophenol* 36% Other chlorophenols 4% Petroleum distillate 60%	DUTCH FUMIGANT (Whitmoyer)	Ethylene dichloride* Carbon tetrachloride*
DUR-TEX PAINT (Gable-Tite)		DUTCH KALSOMINE (Muralo)	
DU-SAN DUAL PURPOSE ANTISEPTIC & DEODOR-ANT (Lee)	Methyl dodecyl benzyl trimethyl ammonium chloride* 9% Isopropyl alcohol* 20% Pine oil 8-3/4%	DUTCH STANDARD PAINT (Harrison P. & V.)	
DUSHARME Hair cream (Dusharme)		DUTERRA Lotion, vaginal (Wyeth Labs.)	Kaolin Aluminum hydroxide gel Eucalyptol* Menthol* Thymol*
DUST-A-WAY Herbicide (Bonide)	Potassium cyanate* 4%	DUVELLE'S PERFUME, COLOGNE, TOILET-WATER (Duvelle)	Alcohol* denatured with diethyl phthalate
DUST CLOTH OIL (Stanley Home)	Deobase Polishing oil Perfume	DUX-BAK ROOF COATING (Herock)	
DUSTEX Dusting paper (Harvey Paper)	Paper stock Mineral seal oil White rose oil Wintergreen oil* Cedarwood oil*	DUXPAR VARNISH (Phelan-Faust)	

*Consult Sec. II., Ingredients Index. This ingredient may be responsible for major toxic effects if poisonous amounts of this product are ingested.

Name & Use Manufacturer	Ingredients	Name & Use Manufacturer	Ingredients
DUX-TOX Wood preservative (Forman, Ford)	Pentachlorophenol* 5%	DYNOL MOTH PROOFER (Bostwick)	Para chloraniline oleate 1.84% Para chloraniline salicylate 0.16% Paradichlorobenzene 3.00% Petroleum hydrocarbon oil* 27.50%
DUZ Soap (Procter & Gamble)	Soaps of animal and vegetable fats Sodium silicate	DYOCIDE Insecticide (Miller Chem. Co.)	Dichloro diphenyl trichloroethane* 25% Xylene* 69%
DUZIT PAINT (Mound City)		DYOCIDE AEROSOL BOMB Insecticide (Miller Chem. Co.)	DDT (dichloro diphenyl trichloroethane) 2.00% Pyrethrins 0.15% n-Octyl bicycloheptene dicarboximide 2.00% Methylated aromatic petroleum deriv.* 5.00% Essential oils 0.1% Petroleum distillate 5.75% Dichloro difluoromethane 42.5% Trichloro monofluoromethane 42.5%
DWIN INSECT KILLER (Aerosol) (Boyle-Midway)	Allethrin 0.4% Pyrethrins 0.1% Octyl sulfoxide of isosafrole 1.76% Petroleum distillates* 12.5%		
D-X Insecticide (Pratt, B.)	Rotenone* Piperonyl cyclonene Pyrethrum Vegetable oil		
D-X AERO SPRAY Insecticide (Pratt, B.)	Pyrethrum Rotenone Piperonyl cyclonene Active carrier* (see inert ingredients)	DYOCIDE DUST Insecticide (Miller Chem. Co.)	Dichloro diphenyl trichloroethane* 10%
D-X INSECT SPRAY (Pratt, B.)	Cyclonene 2.0% Pyrethrins 0.28% Rotenone 0.75% Soya bean Pine oil*	DYOCIDE WETTABLE DUST Insecticide (Miller Chem. Co.)	Dichloro diphenyl trichloroethane* 50%
D-X NICOTINE Insecticide (Pratt, B.)	Nicotine* in oil base 20%	DYOHEX B H C Insecticide (Miller Chem. Co.)	Gamma isomer of benzene hexachloride* 11% Other isomers of benzene hexachloride 16% Petroleum hydrocarbon 41% Xylene* 25%
D-X ROTENONE Insecticide (Pratt, B.)	Rotenone* in oil base		
DYANSHINE COLORED LIQUID SHOE POLISH (Barton Mfg.)	Vegetable, animal and mineral waxes Denatured ethanol* and/or isopropanol* Aniline derivatives * Oil of turpentine*	DYOHEX WETTABLE DUST Insecticide (Miller Chem. Co.)	Gamma isomer of benzene hexachloride* 12% Other isomers of benzene hexachloride 17%
DYANSHINE STAIN SHOE WAX (Paste Polish) (Barton Mfg.)	Vegetable, animal and mineral waxes Mineral spirits* and/or oil of turpentine* Aniline dyes *	DYOKLOR 45% EMULSIFIABLE Insecticide (Miller Chem. Co.)	Tech. chlordane* 45% Aliphatic petroleum solvent 49%
DYANSHINE WHITE LIQUID Shoe Polish (Barton Mfg.)	Essential oils Edible gum tech. Titanium dioxide Saponified wax Plasticizer Inorganic dispersing agent	DYOKLOR 40% WETTABLE Insecticide (Miller Chem. Co.)	Tech. chlordane* 40%
DYCOMENE Antitussive (Hance)	Each fl. oz.: Dihydrocodeinone bitartrate 10.8 mg. Pyrilamine maleate* 73.5 mg. Citric acid, propyl and methyl parasept	DYPERINSE POWDER For diapers (Fairfield)	
DYNACIDE Herbicide (Stieh)	Phenyl mercury acetate* 5% Phenyl mercury chloride* 5%	DYSEPT Liquid soap (Davies-Young)	Hexachlorophene Potassium soap of vegetable oils
DYNAHUE Alkaline detergent (Pennsylv. Salt)	Strong alkalies* (blend of sodium orthosilicate, sodium hydroxide, or sodium carbonate) Soap or detergents		

*Consult Sec. II., Ingredients Index. This ingredient may be responsible for major toxic effects if poisonous amounts of this product are ingested.

Name & Use Manufacturer	Ingredients
DYTOX 5 Insecticide (Arizona)	DDT* dust
DY-ZOFF-DRY STAIN (King Res.)	
EAGLE BRAND PAINTS (Turco)	
EAGLELINE DISINFECTANTS (Eagle Oil)	
EAGLE VAGINAL KONES (Eagle Pharm.)	

Name & Use Manufacturer	Ingredients	
EAR CHEER FOR LONG EARED DOGS Insecticide (House of Huston)	Denatured ethyl alcohol	50.00%
	1,1-Dichloro-2,2-bis-(p-chlorophenyl) ethane	0.10%
	Alkyl diethyl benzyl ammonium chloride (benzethonium chloride)	0.20%
	5-Methyl-2-isopropyl-1-phenol	0.20%

EARDRO Local anesthetic for ear (Jenkins)	Benzocaine*	2%
	Chlorobutanol*	2%
	Camphor*	8%
	Oil base	

EARLE'S HYPO-COL STOMACHIC TONIC Food supplement with iron (Earle)	Each fl. oz.:	
	Quinine hydrochloride	26.7 mg.
	Iron hypophosphite and iron citrochloride	26.9 mg.
	Calcium hypophosphite	25.3 mg.
	Potassium hypophosphite	38 mg.
	Manganese hypophosphite	25.3 mg.
	Alcohol U.S.P.	17%

EARLY AMERICAN OLD SPICE BATH SALTS (Shulton)	
EARLY AMERICAN OLD SPICE BODY SACHET, DUSTING POWDER & TALCUM POWDER (Shulton)	
EARLY AMERICAN OLD SPICE BUBBLE BATH (Shulton)	
EARLY AMERCIAN OLD SPICE PERFUME COLOGNE & TOILET WATER (Shulton)	

Name & Use Manufacturer	Ingredients	
EARLY AMERICAN OLD SPICE TOILET SOAP (Shulton)		
EAR-TICK BOMB Insecticide (Farnam)	Gamma isomer of benzene hexachloride*	3.488%
	Other isomers of benzene hexachloride	5.232%
	Xylol*	5.450%
	Pine oil*	40.330%
	Propellant gas	45.500%
EAR-TIX-TOX Insecticide (Martin, C.J.)	Gamma isomer of benzene hexachloride*	1.00%
	Other isomers of benzene hexachloride	1.78%
	Pine oil*	50.00%
	Pine tar oil*	20.00%
	Mineral oil	15.00%
	Xylol*	12.22%
EASTCO FINISHERS Paints (Eastern St. P. & V.)		
EASTER MORN PERFUME (Easter Morn)		
EASTER MORN REFRESHANT (Easter Morn)		
EASTERN STATES AEROSOL INSECTICIDE For flying insects (Easter St. Farmers')	Pyrethrins	0.25%
	DDT	2.00%
	Tech. piperonyl butoxide	0.75%
	Methylated naphthalene*	6.00%
	Petroleum distillate	6.00%
	Propellant	85.00%
EASTERN STATES B.H.C. MISCIBLE OIL Insecticide (Eastern St. Farmers')	Gamma isomer of benzene hexachloride*	11.8%
	Other isomers of benzene hexachloride	14.0%
	Aromatic derivative solvent*	69.2%
EASTERN STATES 5% CHLORDANE DUST Insecticide (Eastern St. Farmers')	Tech. chlordane	5.00%
EASTERN STATES 7% COPPER-5% DDT DUST Insecticide, fungicide (Eastern St. Farmers')	Copper (in basic copper sulfate)* expressed as metallic	7.00%
	DDT (dichloro-diphenyl-trichloroethane)*	5.00%
EASTERN STATES COPPER SULFATE Fungicide (Eastern St. Farmers')	Copper sulfate*	99%

*Consult Sec. II., Ingredients Index. This ingredient may be responsible for major toxic effects if poisonous amounts of this product are ingested.

Name & Use Manufacturer	Ingredients		Name & Use Manufacturer	Ingredients	
EASTERN STATES DAIRY SANITIZER (Eastern St. Farmers')	Alkyl tolyl methyl trimethyl ammonium chlorides*	25%/w	EASTERN STATES FARM ORCHARD SPRAY Insecticide, fungicide (Eastern St. Farmers')	Methoxychlor tech.* Captan (n-trichloro methylthio tetrahydro phthalimide) Malathion (o,o-dimethyl dithiophosphate of diethyl mercaptosuccinate)*	18.75% 12.50% 6.25%
EASTERN STATES 5% DDT DUST Insecticide (Eastern St. Farmers')	DDT (dichloro-diphenyl-trichloroethane)*	5.00%	EASTERN STATES FARM ORNAMENTAL MIX Insecticide, fungicide (Eastern St. Farmers')	Sulfur* Ferbam (ferric dimethyl dithiocarbamate) DDT* p-Chlorophenyl p-chlorobenzene sulfonate Gamma isomer of benzene hexachloride from lindane	20.00% 7.60% 5.00% 2.50% 1.00%
EASTERN STATES 10% DDT DUST Insecticide (Eastern St. Farmers')	DDT (dichloro-diphenyl-trichloroethane)*	10.00%			
EASTERN STATES 25% DDT MISCIBLE OIL Insecticide (Eastern St. Farmers')	DDT (dichloro-diphenyl-trichloroethane) Xylene*	25.00% 70.00%	EASTERN STATES 10% FERMATE DUST Fungicide (Eastern St. Farmers')	Ferbam (ferric dimethyl-dithiocarbamate)	7.40%
EASTERN STATES 50% DDT WETTABLE POWDER Insecticide (Eastern St. Farmers')	DDT (dichloro-diphenyl-trichloroethane)*	50.00%	EASTERN STATES HEPTACHLOR MISCIBLE OIL Insecticide (Eastern St. Farmers')	Heptachlor* Related compounds Aromatic petroleum derivative solvent*	22.30% 10.98% 61.72%
EASTERN STATES DORMANT SPRAY OIL Insecticide, fungicide (Eastern St. Farmers')	Petroleum oils*	97%	EASTERN STATES HORMONE DUST Fungicide (Eastern St. Farmers')	Each 50-lb. bag of inert material: Napthalene acetic acid 45 gm.	
EASTERN STATES DRY LIME SULFUR Fungicide (Eastern St. Farmers')	Calcium polysulfide* Calcium thiosulfate Sulfur	70% 5% 5%	EASTERN STATES LINDANE Insecticide (Eastern St. Farmers')	Gamma isomer of benzene hexachloride (from lindane)*	25.00%
EASTERN STATES DUSTING SULFUR Fungicide (Eastern St. Farmers')	Sulfur*	90%	EASTERN STATES LIVESTOCK SPRAY Insecticide (Eastern St. Farmers')	Butoxypolypropylene glycol Tech. piperonyl butoxide Pyrethrins Petroleum oil*	5.990% 0.289% 0.035% 93.686%
EASTERN STATES DUST NO. 34 Insecticide, Fungicide (Eastern St. Farmers')	Sulfur Lead arsenate* Dichloro-diphenyl-trichloro-ethane	66.75% 15.00% 5.00%	EASTERN STATES LOUSE, TICK & FLEA POWDER Insecticide (Eastern St. Farmers')	Gamma isomer of benzene hexachloride (from lindane) Inert ingredients:	1.00% 99.00%
EASTERN STATES FARM GARDEN DUST Insecticide, fungicide (Easter St. Farmers')	Rotenone Other cube resins Copper*	1.00% 3.00% 7.00%	EASTERN STATES 4% MALATHION DUST Insecticide (Eastern St. Farmers')	Malathion (o,o-dimethyl dithiophosphate of diethyl mercaptosuccinate)*	4.00%

---

*Consult Sec. II., Ingredients Index. This ingredient may be responsible for major toxic effects if poisonous amounts of this product are ingested.

Name & Use Manufacturer	Ingredients		Name & Use Manufacturer	Ingredients	
EASTERN STATES MANGANESE SULFATE Used with soya flour to prevent spray injury on apple foliage when liquid lime sulfur is applied (Eastern St. Farmers')	Manganese sulfate*, equiv. manganese oxide	30.5%	EASTERN STATES POWDERED LEAD ARSENATE Insecticide (Eastern St. Farmers')	Dry lead arsenate*	98.0%
	Ammonium sulfate, equiv. nitrogen	2.0%			
	Magnesium sulfate, equiv. magnesium oxide	4.38%			
EASTERN STATES METHOXY-CHLOR MISCIBLE OIL Insecticide (Eastern St. Farmers')	Methoxychlor tech.*	25.0%	EASTERN STATES 1% ROTENONE DUST Insecticide (Eastern St. Farmers')	Rotenone	1.00%
	Xylene*	63.0%		Other cube resins	3.00%
	Aromatic petroleum deriv. solvent	7.0%	EASTERN STATES SOYA FLOUR Spreader, sticker, buffer to be used with spray (Eastern St. Farmers')		
EASTERN STATES NEUTRAL COPPER DUST Fungicide (Eastern St. Farmers')	Copper* (in basic copper sulfate)	7.00%			
			EASTERN STATES SULFUR PASTE 70 Fungicide (Eastern St. Farmers')	Sulfur*	68%
EASTERN STATES NEUTRAL COPPER FUNGICIDE Fungicide (Eastern St. Farmers')	Copper* (in basic copper sulfate) expressed as metallic	53%			
			EASTERN STATES 40% TEPP Insecticide (Eastern St. Farmers')	Tetraethyl pyrophosphate*	40%
				Other organic phosphates	60%
EASTERN STATES 40% NICOTINE SPRAY Insecticide, fumigant (Eastern St. Farmers')	Nicotine,* expressed as alkaloid	40%	EASTERN STATES 10% TOXAPHENE-3% DDT DUST TF Insecticide (Eastern St. Farmers')	DDT (dichloro-diphenyl-trichloroethane)	3.00%
				Toxaphene* (tech. chlorinated camphene-chlorine content 67%-69%)	10.00%
EASTERN STATES 1% PARATHION DUST Insecticide (Eastern St. Farmers')	Parathion*	1%	EASTERN STATES 5% TOXAPHENE DUST Insecticide (Eastern St. Farmers')	Toxaphene (tech. chlorinated camphene-chlorine content 67-69%)*	5.00%
EASTERN STATES 3% PHYGON DUST Fungicide (Eastern St. Farmers')	Dichlone (2,3-dichloro-1,4-naphthoquinone)	3.00%	EASTERN STATES TOXAPHENE MISCIBLE OIL Insecticide (Eastern St. Farmers')	Toxaphene*	60.2%
				Petroleum distillates	34.8%
EASTERN STATES PHYGON WETTABLE POWDER Fungicide (Eastern St. Farmers')	Dichlone (2,3-dichloro-1, 4 naphthoquinone)*	50.00%	EASTERN STATES 2,4-D AMINE WEED KILLER Herbicide (Eastern St. Farmers')	Triethanolamine salt of 2,4-dichlorophenoxyacetic acid*	64.7%
EASTERN STATES POULTRY PESTICIDE Insecticide (Eastern St. Farmers')	Methylated aromatic petroleum derivatives*	97.00%	EASTERN STATES 2,4-D ESTER WEED KILLER Herbicide (Eastern St. Farmers')	2,4-Dichlorophenoxyacetic acid, isopropyl ester*	40.7%
	Gamma isomer of benzene hexachloride (from lindane)	1.50%			

*Consult Sec. II., Ingredients Index. This ingredient may be responsible for major toxic effects if poisonous amounts of this product are ingested.

Name & Use Manufacturer	Ingredients	Name & Use Manufacturer	Ingredients
EASTERN STATES WETTABLE SULFUR Fungicide (Eastern St. Farmers')	Sulfur* 95%	EASY GLAMUR Rug and up-holstery cleaner (Glamur)	
EASTERN STATES 10% ZERLATE-3% METHOXY-CHLOR Insecticide, fungicide (Eastern St. Farmers')	Ziram (zinc dimethyl dithio-carbamate) 7.6% Methoxychlor 3.0%	EASY GREASY Degreaser, motor cleaner (Lester)	
		EASY-OFF Oven cleaner (Boyle-Midway)	Sodium hydroxide*
EASTERN STATES ZINC SULFATE (Monohydrated) Fungicide (Eastern St. Farmers')	Zinc sulfate* 100% Metallic zinc (dry basis) 36%	EASY-ON FLOOR WAX (Empire Chem.)	
		EASY ON PAINT (Upco)	
EASTERN STATES 13% ZINEB-5% DDT DUST TF Insecticide, fungicide (Eastern St. Farmers')	DDT (dichloro diphenyl trichloroethane)* 5.00% Zinc ethylene-bis (dithiocarba-mate) 13.00%	EATON'S ATOMO-WHITE Laundry whitener (Eaton Chem.)	Alkyl aryl sulfonate Fluorescent dye
EASTERN STATES 13% ZINEB DUST TF Fungicide (Eastern St. Farmers')	Zinc ethylene-bis (dithiocarba-mate) 13.00%	EATON'S BIG FOUR STRIPPER Color remover (Eaton Chem.)	Sodium hydrosulfite* Magnesium oxide Sodium sulfate
EASTERN STATES 19.5% ZINEB DUST TF Fungicide (Eastern St. Farmers')	Zinc ethylene-bis (dithiocarba-mate) 19.50%	EATON'S DUXCOTE Water repellent (Eaton Chem.)	Aromatic solvent* Neutral waxes
EAS-U TABLETS (Harrison's)		EATON'S ECCO DYEPEN For use in garment dyeing (Eaton Chem.)	Alkyl aryl sulfonate*
EASY-AID Degreaser, oven cleaner (Coughlan)		EATON'S ECCOFORM Spotting agent (Eaton Chem.)	Aromatic and chlorinated solvents*
EASYBRIGHT STOVE POLISH (Prescott)		EATON'S ECCO KOBO Deodorant (Eaton Chem.)	Formaldehyde*
EASY-DO-WAVE Cosmetic (Easydo)		EATON'S ECCO SPOTTING PENCILS (Eaton Chem.)	Water-soluble aniline dyes*
EASY EYE-GLASS CLEANER (Bailes)		EATON'S ECCO WETSOL Spotter (Eaton Chem.)	Superfatted soap Aliphatic solvent* Glycol ethers
		EATON'S H W LIQUID SOAP (Eaton Chem.)	Sodium lauryl sulfate solution Sodium polyphosphate
		EATON'S KWICK BLEACH (Eaton Chem.)	Sodium hydrosulfite* Sodium bisulfite*

*Consult Sec. II., Ingredients Index. This ingredient may be responsible for major toxic effects if poisonous amounts of this product are ingested.

Name & Use Manufacturer	Ingredients	Name & Use Manufacturer	Ingredients
EATON'S LEATHER SOAP (Eaton Chem.)	Superfatted soap Aliphatic solvent*	EBY'S ATHLETE'S FOOT LOTION Fungicide, (Medical) (Eby)	Isopropyl alcohol* Salicylic acid* Benzoic acid* Camphor*
EATON'S NON-IONIC LEATHER SOAP Conc. for use in all dry solvents (Eaton Chem.)	Ethylene oxide deriv. of fatty acids	EBY'S CHICKEN SPRAY Decongestant, inhalant (veterinary) (Eby)	Creosote* Benzoic acid* Camphor oil* Oil of eucalyptus* Synthetic camphor* Chlorothymol*
EATON'S O G P REMOVER Oil, grease paint remover (Eaton Chem.)	Superfatted soap Aromatic,* aliphatic* and ketone solvent*	EBY'S HEAT POWDER MEDICATED For skin irritation (Eby)	Oxyquinoline benzoate* Benzoic acid* Salicylic acid* Lime sulfur* Camphor talcum*
EATON'S O S WRITING INK REMOVER (Eaton Chem.)	Tartaric acid	EBY'S POISON CORN Rodenticide (Eby)	Strychnine* 0.375% Dichloro diphenyl trichloro-ethane 0.125%
EATON'S PARAGENE Color restorer (Eaton Chem.)	Sodium hydrosulfite*	EBY'S SIMPLE PAIN TABLETS FOR HEADACHES AND COLDS (Eby)	Acetophenetidin* 2-1/2 gr. Aspirin* Caffeine
EATON'S SIZIN Water-soluble sizing (Eaton Chem.)	Vinyl acetate emulsion	EBY'S SWINE INHALANT Decongestant (veterinary) (Eby)	Creosote* Benzoic acid* Camphor oil* Oil of eucalyptus* Synthetic camphor* Chlorothymol*
EATON'S TRISOL Spotter (Eaton Chem.)	Superfatted potassium soap Aliphatic* and aromatic solvent*	EBY'S UDDER SALVE (Eby)	
EAU DENNA HAIR COLORER (Hair Specialty)		EBY'S VETERINARY POWDER (Eby)	
EAU DE TEWI TOILET WATER (Tewi)		E. C. ATHLETE'S FOOT REMEDY (E-C Co.)	
EAU MAUVE (Scandia)		ECCO Laxative (Link)	Wild cherry Epsom salts* Glycerin Nitro-hydrochloric acid 1/8 dr./oz.
EAU SUBLIME HAIR DYE (Guilmard)		ECCO ENAMELS, LACQUERS (Essex)	
EBREY EXTRACT Diuretic, bladder stimulant (Ebrey)	Fluid extract uva ursi Fluid extract buchu Fluid extract corn silk Fluid extract sabal Fluid extract cubeb Fluid extract juniper	ECCO FACE POWDER (Enterprise Chem.)	
		ECCO PERFUME (Enterprise Chem.)	

Name & Use Manufacturer	Ingredients	Name & Use Manufacturer	Ingredients
ECCO ROLLING MASSAGE LOTION (Enterprise Chem.)		ECONOMY PLUMBER CLOSET BOWL CLEANERS For drainpipes, hardwood floors, marble, porcelain, tile (Economy)	
ECHO COLOGNE (Brosis)		ECONOMY SOOT DESTROYER (Economy)	
ECKMAN'S IMPROVED FORMULA Antitussive, tonic with iron (Eckman)	Sodium ferric pyrophosphate Glycerin Extract licorice Calcium chloride Vegetable extractives Aromatic oils	ECONO-PINE Floor wax (Puritan Chem.)	
ECLIPSE BARN & ROOF PAINT (Thompson & Co.)		ECONOSTRIP PAINT STRIPPERS (Beck Eq.)	Chloroacetic acid Lactic acid
ECLIPSE BRAND PAINTS (Longman)		ECO-SPAR Paints (Maas & Waldstein)	
ECLIPSE OINTMENT Fungicide, (Medical) (Standard Medical)	Salicylic acid* 67 gr. Benzoic acid 67 gr.	ECO-VAR Paints (Maas & Waldstein)	
ECODUR SPEED PRIMERS & PAINTS (Maas & Waldstein)		EDGERLY'S PHENOTHI- AZINE Drench comp. (Edgerly)	Phenothiazine* 98.84%
ECO-LAC Paints (Maas & Waldstein)		EDIMETS For obesity (Commerce)	Methyl cellulose Benzocaine Calcium pantothenate
ECONO ARTERIAL, MEDIUM & HARD Embalming fluid (Embalmers')	Formaldehyde*	EDISON'S IMPROVED TRI-BASIC TOOTH POWDER (Edison)	Sodium lauroyl sarcoside Galactono lactone carbamide Dibasic ammonium phosphate Sodium hexa meta phosphate Chlorophyll Sodium lauryl sulfate
ECONO CAVITY Embalming fluid (Embalmers')	Formaldehyde*	EDKINS EXZEMA OINTMENT (Edkins)	
ECONO-GLOSS Floor wax (Puritan Chem.)		EDKINS WART REMOVER (Edkins)	
ECONOMY COLD WATER PAINT (Nat'l. Chem. & Mfg.)		EDNA WALLACE HOPPER FACIAL CREAMS (Whitehall)	
ECONOMY DEGREASING SOLVENT (Economy)		EDROLAX Laxative (Edrolax)	Plantago Bassorin Malt
		EDWAL ACID FIX Photographic supply (Edwal)	Ammonium thiosulfate Sodium sulfite* Acetic acid Boric acid*

*Consult Sec. II., Ingredients Index. This ingredient may be responsible for major toxic effects if poisonous amounts of this product are ingested.

- 456 -

Name & Use Manufacturer	Ingredients		Name & Use Manufacturer	Ingredients	
EDWAL-204 ACID-HYPO- ALUM FIXER Photographic supply (Edwal)	Each quart: Hypo* Sulfite (anhydrous) Acetic acid (28%)* Boric acid crystals* Potassium alum Water	8 oz. 1/2 oz. 1-1/2 oz. 1/4 oz. 1/2 oz. q.s.	EDWAL-36 DEVELOPER Photographic supply (Edwal)	Each quart: Fine-grain sulfite Edwal C.H.Q.* Edwal T.S.P. Potassium thiocyanate	1-2/3 oz. 375 gr. 135 gr. 75 gr.
EDWAL ANTI- SCRATCH FILM HARDENER (Edwal)	Aluminum chloride*		EDWAL-102 DEVELOPER Photographic supply (Edwal)	Each quart: Sulfite (Edwal)* Monazol Edwal T.S.P.* Potassium bromide	2-2/3 oz. 375 gr. 4 oz. 45 gr.
EDWAL ANTI-STATIC FILM & GLASS CLEANER (Edwal)	Ethanol* Methanol* Ammonia* Petroleum distillate* Alcohol denaturants		EDWAL-106 DEVELOPER Photographic supply (Edwal)	Each quart: Sulfite (Edwal) Sodium carbonate (anhyd.) Monazol Hydroquinone* Potassium bromide*	2-3/4 oz. 4-1/2 oz. 42 gr. 3/4 oz. 73 gr. 1/4 oz. 24 gr. 57 gr.
EDWAL-291 CHROME ALUM- BISULPHITE HARDENER Photographic supply (Edwal)	Each pint: Chrome alum* Sodium bisulfite	10 gm. 10 gm.	EDWAL-110 DEVELOPER Photographic supply (Edwal)	Each quart: Metol* C.H.Q.* (Edwal) Sulfite (Edwal) Potassium carbonate (Edwal) Orthazite	37 gr. 112 gr. 1 oz. 2 oz. 28 gr.
EDWAL-205 CHROME FIXING BATH Photographic supply (Edwal)	Solution A: Hypo* Sulfite* (anhydrous) Solution B: Chrome alum Sulfuric acid* (pure conc.)	2 lb. 2 oz. 2 oz. 1/4 oz.	EDWAL-111 DEVELOPER Photographic supply (Edwal)	Each quart: Metol* Sulfite (Edwal) Monazol C.H.Q.* Potassium carbonate (Edwal) Potassium bromide*	75 gr. 2-2/3 oz. 90 gr. 225 gr. 4 oz. 45 gr.
EDWAL CHROMIUM INTENSIFIER Photographic supply (Edwal)	A. Potassium dichromate*1 oz. B. Hydrochloric acid* C.P. 2 oz.		EDWAL-113 DEVELOPER Photographic supply (Edwal)	Each pint: Sulfite (anhydrous)* Chlorhydroquinone Sodium carbonate (anhydrous)*	128 gr. 17 gr. 128 gr.
EDWAL COLOR FILM CLEANER (anti-static, No. 2 formula) Photographic supply (Edwal)	1,1,1-Trichlorethane* Antistatic agent similar in chemical structure to synthetic detergent		EDWAL-120 DEVELOPER Photographic supply (Edwal)	Each quart: A. Catechol* (Edwal) Sulfite (Edwal) B. Potassium carbonate* (Edwal)	300 gr. 1-1/3 oz. 4 oz.
EDWAL COLOR TONERS Darkroom aids (Edwal)	Acetic acid Ethyl alcohol* Dyes* Potassium ferricyanide*		EDWAL-121 DEVELOPER Photographic supply (Edwal)	Each pint: Sulfite (Edwal) Catechol* (Edwal) Sodium carbonate (anhyd.) Potassium bromide*	375 gr. 150 gr. 1-2/3 oz. 30 gr.
EDWAL-10 DEVELOPER Photographic supply (Edwal)	Each quart: Metol* (Elon, Pictol) Fine-grain sulfite Monazol Borax*	75 gr. 3-1/3 oz. 75 gr. 150 gr.	EDWAL-126 DEVELOPER Photographic supply (Edwal)	Each quart: Edwal sulfite Amidol* (Edwal) Potassium bromide*	375 gr. 90 gr. 12 gr.
EDWAL-12 DEVELOPER Photographic supply (Edwal)	Each quart: Metol* Fine-grain sulfite Diamine-P* Monazol	90 gr. 3 oz. 150 gr. 75 gr.	EDWAL FARMER'S REDUCER Photographic supply (Edwal)	A. Potassium ferricyanide 15 gr./oz. B. Hypo* 1 oz./qt.	
EDWAL-20 DEVELOPER Photographic supply (Edwal)	Each quart: Gradol* Fine-grain sulfite Diamine-P* Monazol	75 gr. 3 oz. 150 gr. 75 gr.	EDWAL FERROTYPE POLISH Photographic supply (Edwal)	Chlorinated solvents* Ethyl and methyl alcohols Petroleum base Wax	
EDWAL-32 DEVELOPER Photographic supply (Edwal)	Each quart: Metol* Fine-grain sulfite Orthamine* Sodium bisulfite	180 gr. 3 oz. 180 gr. 150 gr.			

*Consult Sec. II., Ingredients Index. This ingredient may be responsible for major toxic effects if poisonous amounts of this product are ingested.

Name & Use Manufacturer	Ingredients	Name & Use Manufacturer	Ingredients
EDWAL FILM CLEANER Photographic supply (Edwal)	Chlorinated solvents* Ethyl and methyl alcohols Ammonia amines Synthetic phosphated aliphatic detergents	EDWAL MICROGRAIN-85 DEVELOPER Photographic supply (Edwal)	
EDWAL FILM STAIN REMOVER (Edwal)	Each quart: Solution A: Potassium permanganate* 75 gr. Solution B: Each quart: Sodium chloride 2-1/2 oz. Sulfric acid* (C.P.) 1/2 oz.	EDWAL MINICOL DEVELOPER Photographic supply (Edwal)	Similar to Edwal-32
EDWAL FORMALIN-CARBONATE HARDENER Photographic supply (Edwal)	Formalin* (37% formaldehyde) 2-1/2 dr. Sodium carbonate (anhydrous) 75 gr.	EDWAL ORTHAZITE Photographic supply (Edwal)	Benztriazole* Inorganic sulfite
EDWAL-20 HIGH ENERGY REPLENISHER Photographic supply (Edwal)	Each quart: Gradol 60 gr. Metol* 30 gr. Fine-grain sulfite 3 oz. Diamine-P* 150 gr. Monazol 75 gr.	EDWAL PERSULPH-ATE RE-DUCER Photographic supply (Edwal)	Each quart: Ammonia persulfate* 2 oz. Sulfuric acid C.P. 3/4 dr.
EDWAL HYPO-BORAX FIXER Photographic supply (Edwal)	Each pint: Borax* 320 gr. Hypo* 3 oz.	EDWAL PLATINUM TONE DEVELOPER Photographic supply (Edwal)	Similar to Edwal 111
EDWAL HYPO-CHEK Photographic supply (Edwal)	Potassium iodide* Formaldehyde*	EDWAL QUICK-FIX Photographic supply (Edwal)	Ammonium thiosulfate* Sodium sulfite Acetic acid Boric acid*
EDWAL HYPO ELIMINATOR Photographic supply (Edwal)	Each pint: Hydrogen peroxide* (3% solution) 4 fl. oz. Ammonia* (3% solution) 3-1/4 fl. oz.	EDWAL SIGNAL SHORTSTOP Photographic supply (Edwal)	Acid equal in strength to 28% acetic acid* Brom cresol purple
EDWAL KWIK-WET Photographic supply (Edwal)	Sulfonated aromatic hydrocarbon*	EDWAL THERMO-FINE DEVELOPER Photographic supply (Edwal)	Thermo-salt
EDWAL LIQUID C.H.Q. Photographic supply (Edwal)	Chlorohydroquinone* (10% solution)	EDWAL THERMO-SALT Photographic supply (Edwal)	Anhydrous sodium sulfate
EDWAL LIQUID FIX (Photographic supply (Edwal)	Ammonium thiosulfate* Sodium sulfite Acetic acid Boric acid*	EDWAL TWO-SOLUTION FARMER'S REDUCER Photographic supply (Edwal)	A. Potassium ferricyanide 1/4 oz/qt. B. Hypo* 7 oz./qt.
EDWAL LIQUID THERMOFINE REPLENISHER Photographic supply (Edwal)	Metol * Sulfite Sodium carbonate Sodium sulfate	EDWAL VELVET PAPER DEVELOPER Photographic supply (Edwal)	Similar to Edwal-110
EDWAL-MANSFIELD FOTOTINTS Photographic supply (Edwal)			

*Consult Sec. II., Ingredients Index. This ingredient may be responsible for major toxic effects if poisonous amounts of this product are ingested.

Name & Use Manufacturer	Ingredients
DR. EDWARDS OLIVE TABLETS Laxative (Olive)	Extract stramonium* Podophyllin Aloin Cascarin bitter po.
EDWARDS WOLF & COYOTE EXTERMIN-ATOR CAPSULES (Edwards)	Strychnine crystals*
EFFO-VET For skin irritation (veterinary) (Goodwinol)	Thiourea Orthophenylphenol Benzocaine
EFROMAL TABLETS Nasal decongestant (Dillard)	Phenylephrine hydrochloride 5.0 mg. Pyrilamine maleate* 12.5 mg.
EGGOL SHAMPOO (Eptol)	Granulated soap Calgon (water softener)
EGG-WHITEST PAINTS (Voltex)	
EG KLEEN Detergent sanitizer (Gland-O-Lac)	Alkyl tolyl methyl trimethyl ammonium chlorides* 57% Sodium metasilicate, pentahy-drate 15% Sodium carbonate 20%
EGYPTIAN ENAMELS (Ablon)	
EGYPTIAN LACQUERS & ENAMELS (Egyptian)	
E.H.S. SKIN CREAM For skin irritation (Internat. Biotical)	Sulfur* Zinc oxide Phenol*
8 IN 1 CANARY DIARRHEA FOOD (Eight in 1)	Poppy Carrot Thistle Lettuce Clover screenings Bismuth subnitrate 2%
8 IN 1 FOOT & LEG SALVE (Veterinary, avian) (Harold)	Petrolatum Tincture of merthiolate* Pine oil*
8 IN 1 PARAKEET BIRD WASH (Harold)	Glycerine 3.6%
8 IN 1 PARAKETT COLD RELIEF (Eight in 1)	Ammonium hydroxide Sodium bicarbonate Oil of peppermint Glycerine U. S. certified color

Name & Use Manufacturer	Ingredients
8 IN 1 PARAKEET DIARRHEA FOOD (Eight in 1)	Poppy Thistle Clover screenings Carrot Lettuce Bismuth subnitrate 2%
8 IN 1 PARAKEET INTESTIN-AID Cathartic (veterinary) (Harold)	Fluid extract of cascara sagrada Extract of gentian Cardamon seed Oil of anise Orange peel Glycerine U. S. certified color Alcohol 0.6%
8 IN 1 PARAKEET IRON & BLOOD TONIC (Eight in 1)	Iron phosphate Quinine phosphate Strychnine phosphate* Glycerine Oil of orange U. S. certified color Alcohol 1.5%
8 IN 1 PARAKEET NERVE TONIC (Harold)	Ammonium bromide* Potassium bromide* Sodium bromide* Oil of almonds Glycerine U. S. certified color Alcohol 0.8%
8 IN 1 PARAKEET TONIC & BITTERS Cathartic (veterinary) (Eight in 1)	Fluid extract of cascara Soluble cinnamon Glycerine U. S. certified color
E-JECT-O DRAIN OPENER (United Gilson.)	Sodium hydroxide* Sodium nitrate Aluminum
ELAINE NAIL POLISHES (Elaine)	
ELAM SHELLACS (Abelman)	
ELAN SHAMPOO (Morgan Prod.)	Shampoo base Lanolin
ELAN SUNTAN LOTION (Morgan Prod.)	Methyl parasept* Propyl parasept* Processed lanolin Propylene glycol Sun screen filter Perfume
ELASTIKOTE PAINTS FOR EXTERIOR SURFACES (Tropical)	
EL-BEE Specialized cleaning product (Wyandotte)	Concentrated alkali*
ELCAYA ASTRINGENT CREAM (Glazo)	

*Consult Sec. II., Ingredients Index. This ingredient may be responsible for major toxic effects if poisonous amounts of this product are ingested.

Name & Use Manufacturer	Ingredients	Name & Use Manufacturer	Ingredients
ELCAYA COLD CREAM (Glazo)		ELGETOL 30 Insecticide (Standard Ag.)	Sodium dinitro ortho cresylate* 30%
ELCAYA DRY SKIN CREAM (Glazo)		ELGETOL-318 Insecticide fungicide (Standard Ag.)	Dinitro-sec-butylphenol* triethanolamine salt 36%
ELCAYA FOUNDATION CREAM (Glazo)		ELIPIDE PAINTS (Hoboken)	
ELCAYA LIQUEFYING CLEANSING CREAM (Glazo)		ELIP TABLETS For hemorrhoids, laxative (Baldwin Labs.)	Potassium bitartrate Sulfur Rhubarb
EL DURO PAINTS (Ellis Paint)		ELIXIR ENTERICA Cathartic (Hurley)	Each fl. oz.: Senna 59 gr. Jalap* 29.5 gr. Taraxacum 11.9 gr. Rhubarb 1.4 gr.
ELECTRA ENAMEL, PAINT, VARNISH REMOVER (Baer Bros. (Paint))		ELIXIR FERROUS SULFATE Food supplement with iron (Success)	Each 2 fl. dr.: Alcohol 5%/v Ferrous sulfate U.S.P. 5 gr.
ELECTRA-SOL Dishwasher detergent (Economics)	Sodium phosphate* Sodium silicate Sodium carbonate Synthetic wetting agent*	ELIXIR NOVO- HEXAMINE (Smith, Upsher)	Each fl. dr.: Hexamethylenamine 7-1/2 gr. Acid sodium phosphate (monobasic) 7-1/2 gr. Alcohol 1%
ELECTRO- KILLER Insecticide (Koss)	Pyrethrins*	ELIXIR OF ALFALFA Tonic (Clapp, Otis)	Alfalfa Sodium and calcium glycerophosphates Aromatics Taraxacum Chiretta soluble ext. Glycerin
ELECTRO- KILLER MOTH SPRAY (Koss)	Organic thiocyanate* Nitrogen Chlorine*		
ELECTRONS PYRONITE Dishwasing compound (Electrons)		ELIXIR OF CATNEP & FENNEL Carminative (Purepac)	Alcohol 18%/v
ELEMITE 15W Insecticide (Crop King)	Elemite (2-(p-tert-butyl phenoxy) isopropyl-2- chloroethyl sulfite)* 15%	ELIZABETH ARDEN FACE CREAM (Arden)	
ELENE OF VIENNA PINE AIR FRESHENER (Elene)		ELIZABETH ARDEN HAND LOTION (Arden)	
ELENE OF VIENNA PINE BATH ESSENCE (Elene)		ELIZABETH ARDEN LIPSTICK (Arden)	
ELENE OF VIENNA PINE BODY COLOGNE (Elene)		ELIZABETH ARDEN POWDER (Arden)	
ELGETOL Insecticide, fungicide (Standard Ag.)	Sodium salt of dinitro-ortho- cresol* 19% Sodium butyl naphthalene sulfonate 5% Sodium chromate 2% Sodium chloride Sodium sulfate	ELIZABETH ROSEWELL BEAUTY MASK (Rosewell)	Purified clay Glycerin Preservative Certified color Perfume

*Consult Sec. II., Ingredients Index. This ingredient may be responsible for major toxic effects if poisonous amounts of this product are ingested.

Name & Use Manufacturer	Ingredients	Name & Use Manufacturer	Ingredients
ELIZABETH ROSEWELL CHEEK ROUGE (Rosewell)	Waxes Oils Lanolin Petrolatum Perfume Certified colors	ELIZABETH ROSEWELL SKIN FRESHENER (Rosewell)	Denatured alcohol Glycerine Antiseptic Certified color Perfume oil'
ELIZABETH ROSEWELL CLEANSING CREAM AND NITE CREAM (Rosewell)	Oils Lanolin Petrolatum Waxes Borax Preservatives Cetyl alcohol Perfume Certified colors	ELIZABETH ROSEWELL SUN TAN LOTION (Rosewell)	Vegetable oil Sun-screen oil Perfume
		ELKA HERB TABS. (Germadol)	
ELIZABETH ROSEWELL COLOGNE (Rosewell)	Denatured alcohol* Perfume oil	ELKAY'S MICE, RAT & ROACH PASTE (Rexall)	Phosphorus* 2.00%
ELIZABETH ROSEWELL DEODORANT (Rosewell)	Monostearate base Zinc oxide Titanium Aluminum chloride Aluminum sulfate	ELKAY'S WHITE SHOE POLISH & SOAP (Rexall)	
ELIZABETH ROSEWELL EYESHADOW (Rosewell)	Waxes Oils Lanolin Petrolatum Perfume oils Certified colors	ELK'S ECZEMA LOTION (Elk)	Phenol* Solvents*
ELIZABETH ROSEWELL FACE POWDER (Rosewell)	Talc (imported grade) Zinc oxide Zinc stearate Titanium Kaolin Certified colors Perfume	ELK'S FIRE-X LIQUID (Elk)	Chlorinated hydrocarbons*
		ELK'S PIC-RATE BURN OINTMENT (Elk)	Trinitrophenol*
ELIZABETH ROSEWELL HAND CREAM (Rosewell)	Glyceryl monostearate base Glycerine Propylene glycol Lanolin Preservative Certified color Perfume	ELLANAR DIP Silver cleaner (L and R)	Thiourea Sulfuric acid* Dyes Synthetic wetting agents
ELIZABETH ROSEWELL HORMONE CREAM (Rosewell)	Lanolin Petrolatum Oil Estrogenic hormones 10,000 units/oz. Perfume	ELLANAR JEWELRY CLEANER (L and R)	Ammoniated soap Ammonia* Isopropyl alcohol* Perfumes Dyes
ELIZABETH ROSEWELL LIPSTICK (Rosewell)	Waxes Oils Lanolin Perfume Certified colors	ELLANAR JEWELRY SERVICER (L and R)	Ammoniated soap Ammonia* Isopropyl alcohol* Perfumes Dyes
ELIZABETH ROSEWELL MAKE-UP- FILM (Rosewell)	Titanium Lanolin Oils Waxes Perfume Certified colors	ELLANAR SILVER GLEAM (L and R)	Water soap Mild abrasive
		ELLANAR SILVER POLISH (L and R)	Neutral water base soap Diatomaceous earth Cosmetic type mold inhibitor
ELIZABETH ROSEWELL MASCARA (Rosewell)	Glyceryl monostearate base Oil Certified colors	ELLENI ASTRINGENTS (Elleni)	
ELIZABETH ROSEWELL OLIVE OIL SHAMPOO (Rosewell)	Olive oil Cocoanut oil Potassium and sodium hydroxide Perfume oil	ELLENI BODY POWDER (Elleni)	
		ELLENI CREAMS For cleansing and softening (Elleni)	

*Consult Sec. II., Ingredients Index. This ingredient may be responsible for major toxic effects if poisonous amounts of this product are ingested.

Name & Use Manufacturer	Ingredients	Name & Use Manufacturer	Ingredients
ELLENI EMOLLIENTS & LOTIONS (Elleni)		ELMER'S WATERPROOF GLUE (formerly Cascophen) (Borden)	Resorcinol formaldehyde resinous product
ELLENI EYELID SHADOW (Elleni)		ELMO FACE CREAM (Elmo)	
ELLENI FACE POWDER (Elleni)		ELMO HAND LOTION (Elmo)	
ELLENI LIPSTICK (Elleni)		ELMS' Hair and scalp treatment (Elms,J. C.)	Ammoniated mercury chloride* 7% Mercuric oxide* 7% Mercuric chloride* 1% Paraffin oil 78.6%
ELLENI LUXURY BATH (Formula 175) (Elleni)		ELM SPRAY Insecticide (Sherwin-Williams)	DDT* 37%
ELLENI PERFUMES (Elleni)		ELM SPRAY B Insecticide (Sherwin-Williams)	DDT* 35%
ELLENI ROUGE Compact or cream (Elleni)		ELM SPRAY C Insecticide (Sherwin-Williams)	DDT* 26%
ELLIOTT'S COFEX Antitussive (Rafea)	Ammonium chloride Wild cherry Oil of eucalyptus* Creosote* Honey White pine Pine tar* Menthol* Glycerin Sugar syrup	ELMTONE POULTRY POWDER Insecticide (Elm, J.G.)	
		ELMTOX POULTRY DRINKING WATER ANTISEPTIC (Elm, J.G.)	
ELLVEE COMPOUND (Ell-Vee)	Linseed oil* Olive oil Glycerin Syrup of cherry bark Kerosene* Honey Syrup of hickory bark Syrup of mullein Sweet gum bark Pine tops	ELNO RUST PREVENTER (Cleveland Heater)	
		EL REY EXPECTOR-ANT (Corpus Christi)	
ELMER'S CONTACT CEMENT Adhesive (Borden)		EL REY LINIMENT (Corpus Christi)	
		ELROY'S RUG & UPHOL-STERY CLEANER (Elroy)	
ELMER'S GLUE ALL Acetate emulsion adhesive (Borden)	Polyvinyl acetate emulsion	ELTRON (Torch)	Eltar (non-staining crude coal tar)* 5% Modified Lassar's paste
		ELY'S CORN GETTER (Ely)	

*Consult Sec. II., Ingredients Index. This ingredient may be responsible for major toxic effects if poisonous amounts of this product are ingested.

Name & Use Manufacturer	Ingredients	Name & Use Manufacturer	Ingredients
EL ZAMBU CLEANSING CREAM (Beauty Affil.)	Beeswax Spermaceti petrolatum Mineral oil Lanolin Borax	EMPIRE CAULKING COMPOUND (Black Swan)	
EMAGRIN Analgesic, antipyretic (Clapp, Otis)	Acetophenetidin* 1 gr. Aspirin* 2 gr. Caffeine* 1/2 gr. Salicylamide* 1 gr.	EMPIRE FIRE EXTIN-GUISHER (Am.-La-France)	
EMAJEN Uterine stimulant (Jenkins)	Each tablet: Quinine sulfate* 1 gr. Extract ergot* 1 gr. Extract cotton root bark 1 gr. Extract black hellebore* 1 gr. Iron sulfate dried 1 gr. Aloin 1/8 gr.	EMPIRE PROTECTIVE PAINT (Atlantic Paint)	
EMAY SHELLACS (Abelman)		EMPIRE STATE COLOGNE (Haas)	
EMBECO CRAYONS (Bradley, M.)		EMPIRE STATE VARNISH (Empire State)	
EMBISOL POWDER Antacid powder (Drug Prod., N.Y.)	Magnesium carbonate Bismuth subcarbonate Sodium bicarbonate Papain Diastase Oleoresin ginger Saccharin Oil peppermint	EMROL OINTMENT & SUPPOSITOR-IES (Leslie Pharm.)	
EMBROCATION B Rubefacient (Clapp, Otis)	Borneol salicylate* Bryonia* Capsicum*	E. M. SCRUBBING COMPOUND (Huntington)	
		EM-24 Insecticide (Greever's)	Methoxychlor tech. 24% Methylated naphthalenes* 63% Dimethyl phthalate 10%
EMDESIL Digestant, antacid, adsorbent (Manhattan Drug)	Zinc sulfocarbolate* Salol* Pectin Pepsin Kaolin Bismuth subsalicylate* Magnesium trisilicate Oil peppermint	EMULLO LACQUER EMULSIONS Paints (Kepec)	
		EMULSEPT Germicide (Emulsol)	n-(Lauroyl colamino formyl-methyl) pyridinium chloride* (a quaternary ammonium salt) 12% aqueous concentration
EMELITE FINISHES Paints (Clover Leaf)		EMULSO Engine cleaner (Lester)	Pine oil* Petroleum solvents*
EMERAUDE LINE EXTRACT & TOILET WATER (Coty)		EMUL-TOX B65 Insecticide (Leffingwell)	Petroleum oil* 85.00%/w Rotenone 0.12% Other ether extractives of cube and/or derris 0.24%
EMERSON'S C-G Effervescent (Emerson)	Calcium gluconate Sodium bicarbonate Citric acid	EM-VAR-CO PAINTS, LACQUERS, VARNISHES (Empire State)	
EMOL J VARNISH (Masury)		EM-VAR-CO PRIMERS (Empire State)	
EMOLUOL Protective skin lotion, cream (C&M)	Ethyleneglycol stearate Methoxy-cellulose gel	ENAMELETTE Paint (Vita-Var)	

*Consult Sec. II., Ingredients Index. This ingredient may be responsible for major toxic effects if poisonous amounts of this product are ingested.

Name & Use Manufacturer	Ingredients		Name & Use Manufacturer	Ingredients	
ENAMEL #218-H (India)	Titanium oxide Melamine resin Glyceryl phthalate resin Maleated rosin Petroleum aromatic*		END-O-PEST FLY KILLER (Swift)	Terpene polychlorinates* Pyrethrins Tech. piperonyl butoxide Refined petroleum distillate*	2.50% 0.15% 1.00% 11.35%
ENAMEL H-2066 O.D. (General Paint, (Okla.))			END-O-PEST GARDEN DUST (Swift)	Rotenone Other cube resins Pyrethrins Zineb Sulfur Inert ingredients	1.00% 1.50% 0.10% 3.25% 10.00%
ENAMELYK PAINTS & VARNISHES (Morton Paint)			END-O-PEST MALATHION GARDEN SPRAY (Swift)	Malathion* Methylated naphthalene*	50.0% 39.0%
EN-AR-CO Ectoparasiticide (Nat'l. Remedy)	Fusel oil (amyl alcohol*) 75% Butyl alcohol 1-1/4% Turpentine Camphor oil Thyme oil Chlorothymol Peanut oil Cudbear 3-1/2% Capsicum Cedarwood oil Butyl alcohol		END-O-PEST ROSE DUST (Swift)	Malathion* DDT* Captan Karathane	4.5% 5.0% 7.5% 1.0%
			END-O-PEST TREE SPRAY (Swift)	2-Isopropyl-2-chloroethyl sulfite (Aramite)* D.D.D. (Rhothane)* Methoxychlor tech.* Ferbam Sulfur*	1.2% 5.0% 10.0% 10.0% 30.0%
ENATIN OIL CAPSULES For treatment of calculi (Carstens)	Volatile oils of turpentine* Juniper berries Peppermint Sulfonated vegetable oil		ENDOTHAL HARVEST AID Herbicide (Pennsylv. Salt)	Disodium endothal*	6.3%
EN AVION EXTRACT Toiletry (Caron)			END-O-WEED Herbicide (Swift)	Butoxy ethoxy propanol ester of 2,4-D*	22.4%
ENDAMP Drier-outer (Puritan Sales)			END-O-WEED CRAB GRASS KILLER (Swift)	Potassium cyanate*	60%
END-HAB LOZENGES To combat tobacco habit (Commerce)	Lobeline sulfate* Benzocaine Oils of anise, ginger and cloves Methyl salicylate* Vanillin Saccharin Sucrose		END-O-WEED LAWN WEED KILLER (Swift)	Butoxy ethoxy propanol ester of 2,4-D*	22.4%
END-O-CORN (End-O-Corn)	Petrolatum Salicylic acid*		ENDRIN WE-16 Insecticide (Thompson-Hayward)	Endrin (hexachloro epoxy octahydro-endo, endo-dimethano naphthalene)* Petroleum hydrocarbons	19.5% 70.5%
ENDOCREME ANTISEPTIC SCALP CONDITIONER (Hirestra)			ENDTOX DB-50 PHOENIX BRAND Insecticide (Arizona)	Endrin* (hexachloro epoxy octahydro-endo, endo-dimethano naphthalene)	50.00%
ENDOCREME SCALP LOTION (Hiresta)			ENTOX EC-20 Insecticide (Arizona)	Endrin (hexachloro epoxy octahydro-endo, endo-dimethano naphthalene)* Petroleum hydrocarbons	20.00% 72.00%
END-O-PEST ARC Insecticide (Swift)	Chlordane tech.* 45% Petroleum hydrocarbons* 49%				
END-O-PEST ARC ANT & LAWN INSECT DUST (Swift)	Chlordane tech.* 8.00% Beta thiocyano ethyl esters of aliphatic acids containing 10-18 carbon atoms (Lethane) 0.75% Beta butoxy beta thiocyano diethyl ether (Lethane) 0.25%		ENDURA HOME PERMANENT (Ball)		
			ENDURANCE PAINT PRODUCTS (Glidden Co.)		

*Consult Sec. II., Ingredients Index. This ingredient may be responsible for major toxic effects if poisonous amounts of this product are ingested.

Name & Use Manufacturer	Ingredients		Name & Use Manufacturer	Ingredients	
ENDURO COPPER-SULFUR MIXTURE NO. 1 Insecticide (Florida Agric.)	Copper* Sulfur*	6.4% 80%	ENERGY HOOF OIL (veterinary) (Energy)	Glycerine Tincture capsicum Tincture cantharides* Paraffin oil Lanolin	
ENDURO DINI-O-SPRAY NO. 4 Miticide (Florida Agric.)	Sulfur* DN (dinitro-o-cylohexyl-phenol)*	86.5% 2.5%	ENERJETS To combat drowsiness (Chilton Labs.)	Caffeine Sugar Butter Salt Flavoring	
ENDURO DRY CLEANING FLUID (Midwest)	Naphthol spirits Carbon tetrachloride*		ENGO Insecticide (Fort Dodge)	Tech. chlordane* Pine oil* Kerosene*	40% 10%w/w 38%w/w
ENDURO FURNITURE CREAM POLISH (Midwest)	Stearic acid Mineral oil Emulsion A oil Triethanolamine Perfume		ENNDS Deodorant (Pearson Pharm.)	Each tablet: Darotol (Pearson's brand of chlorophylline)	100 mg.
ENDURO LIQUID SELF POLISH FLOOR WAX (Midwest)	Carnauba wax Resin Oleic acid Amino methyl-propanol* Powdered borax*		ENO Antacid and laxative (Ritchie)	Tartaric acid Sodium bicarbonate	
ENDURO RUG & UPHOLSTERY SHAMPOO (Midwest)	Orvis paste Isopropyl alcohol* 26° Ammonia*		ENO FRUIT SALTS (Eno-Scott)	Sodium bicarbonate Tartaric acid	
ENDURO SPEEDY WAX CLEANER & PRESERVA-TIVE (Midwest)	Gum tragacanth Bentonite Alcohol* Mineral oil Sulfonated castor oil* Glycerine Filter cell Wintergreen* Oil		E. N. PARFUM (Bombi) ENRUMAY Anti-histamine (Tilden)	Each tablet: Pyrilamine maleate* Caffeine	25 mg. 32 mg.
ENDURO SPOT REMOVER (Midwest)	Amsco naphtha thinner Carbon tetrachloride*		ENTABS Cathartic, anti-spasmodic (Calvin)	Extract belladonna* Extract nux vomica* Eunymus Extract cascara	
ENDURO VEN-EZ-ON & PAINT CLEANER (Midwest)	26° Ammonia* Orvis paste Coloring		ENTERPRISE SATIN FINISH PAINT (Enterprise Paint)		
ENDUROX LACQUERS (Oxidermo)			ENTOMUL For intestinal irritation (Lloyd)	Each fl. oz.: Kaolin Aluminum hydroxide Pectin Lactose	28 gr. 8 gr. 4 gr. 4 gr.
ENERGINE CLEANING FLUID (Puhl)	Naphtha Carbon tetrachloride*	40% 60%	ENTOMUL WITH BELLADONNA For intestinal irritation (Lloyd)	Each fl. oz.: Belladonna* Kaolin Aluminum hydroxide Pectin Lactose	1/2 gr. 28 gr. 8 gr. 4 gr. 4 gr.
ENERGINE SHOE WHITE, CREAM & LIQUID (Phillips, C.)			ENTRE NOUS EAU DE TOILETTE (Bombi)		
			ENTUSSAMINE For throat irritation (Rhodes)	Each fl. oz.: Pyrilamine maleate* Ammonium chloride Aromatics	75 mg.
			ENUREX OINTMENT For hemorrhoids (Hance)	Phenol* Powdered nutgall Oil tar* Pine tar* Isobutyl para aminobenzoate* Petrolatum base	

---

*Consult Sec. II., Ingredients Index. This ingredient may be responsible for major toxic effects if poisonous amounts of this product are ingested.

Name & Use Manufacturer	Ingredients		Name & Use Manufacturer	Ingredients	
ENZAMOL Douche, gargle, spray (Jenkins)	Oxyquinoline sulfate* Acid boric* Acid benzoic* Menthol* Thymol* Eucalyptol* Oil of red thyme Oil of peppermint		EPITHEALIN For skin irritations (Kip, A.)	Zinc stearate Calamine Extract of calendula Naftalan Zinc oxide Starch Balsam Peru	
ENZO-CAL For skin irritation (Crookes)	Benzocaine Calamine Zinc oxide		EPTINE Antispasmodic (Nemow)	Phenobarbital* Theophylline* Ephedrine hydrochloride* Ascorbic acid	
ENZOTABS Antacid, digestant (Hartman)	Diastase of malt Magnesium trisilicate Calcium carbonate Colloidal kaolin		EPTO Fungicide (Medical) (Kaoloid)	Boric acid* Oil of wormwood Sodium thiosulfate Thymol*	
ENZYMES AROMATIC (Lilly)	Alcohol 18% Pepsin Pancreatin Aromatics		EPTOL BEAUTY CREAM (Eptol)	Stearic acid Gum karaya Gum tragacanth Sodium carbonate Borax Perfume Glycerin	
EPHEDROL WITH CODEINE Antitussive, antispasmodic (Lilly)	Codeine sulfate* 0.22 gm. Ma Huang 13.15 gm. Potassium guaiacol sulfonate 1.75 gm. Syrup squill 6.25 cc. Tolu balsam Menthol*		EPTOL CLEANSING CREAM (Eptol)	Stearic acid Gum karaya Gum tragacanth Sodium carbonate Borax Perfume Mineral oil Lanolin Glycerin	
EPHREMEL Antitussive, antispasmodic (Meyer Bros.)	Alcohol 5% Ephedrine hydrochloride* Tolu* Syrup squill Menthol*		EPTOL HAND CREAM (Eptol)	Stearic acid Gum karaya Gum tragacanth Sodium carbonate Borax Perfume Glycerin Lanolin	
EPIDERMICIDE For skin irritations, fungicide (Epidermicide)	Formalin* Thymol* Benzoic acid* Salicylic acid*				
EPIDERMICIDE FOOT POW- DER Fungicide (Medical) (Epidermicide)	Zinc stearate Boric acid* Salicylic acid* Thymol* Talc Para-formaldehyde* Benzocaine*		EQUICOLSIS Decongestant (Bullock- Walker)	Camphor* Oil of caraway* Oil of pine needles* Turpentine* Oil of amber* Oil of European pennyroyal*	
EPIDEX Fungicide (Medical) (Lefcourt)	Alcohol* 50%/v Salicylic acid* Sodium ethylmercuri- thiosalicylate* Oil of pine needles* Acetone* Sod. propionate Benzoic acid		EQUATORIAL ANTI-FOULING PAINT (Balto. Copper)		
EPIDEX VISCOUS (Lefcourt)	Alcohol* 50%/v Salicylic acid* Sodium ethylmercuri- thiosalicylate* Oil of pine needles Acetone* Sod. propionate Benzoic acid* Methyl cellulose		EQUI-DINE Antispasmodic (veterinary) (Globe)	Chloral hydrate* 14.38% Turpentine* 25.97% Camphor* 7.19% Ether* 21.37% Mineral oil 31.09%	
			ERADICO ANTPROOFER Insecticide (Eradico)	Tech. chlordane 0.50% Emulsifier and petroleum distillate* 0.30%	
			ERADICO BRAND EQ-53 Mothproofer (Eradico)	DDT* 25%	
EPINOLIN Antispasmodic (Legendre's)	Each 10 cc.: Levo-epinephrine* 0.1 gm. Chlorobutanol* 0.05 gm. Sod. bisulfite 0.01 gm. Normal saline q.s.		ERADICO CRABGRASS KILLER WITH CHLORDANE (Eradico)	Tech. chlordane 4.00% Petroleum distillate* 96.00%	

*Consult Sec. II., Ingredients Index. This ingredient may be responsible for major toxic effects if poisonous amounts of this product are ingested.

Name & Use Manufacturer	Ingredients	Name & Use Manufacturer	Ingredients
ERADICO EXTERMICIDE Insecticide (Eradico)	DDT* 5.00% B-thiocyano ethyl esters of mixed fatty acids 2.03% B-butoxy B'-thiocyano diethyl ether 0.66% Petroleum distillate* 92.31%	ERSKINE'S NYLON LINIMENT Rubefacient (Dacus)	Acetone* Menthol* Para tertiary butyl meta cresol* Oil peppermint Oil wormwood Oil spearmint
ERADICO MORTISPRA Insecticide (Eradico)	Dicyclohexylamine oleate* 2.5% Terpineol 1.0% Petroleum distillate* 96.5%	ERSKINE'S ROSE & FLORAL DUST Insecticide (Chem. Form.)	Gamma isomer of benzene hexachloride (from lindane) 1.0% Ferric dimethyl dithiocarba- mate 10.0% 325 mesh sulfur* 20.0% Rotenone 1.0% Other cube resins 1.85% Talc 66.15%
ERADICO MOTH NUGGETS (Eradico)	Paradichlorobenzene* 100%		
ERADICO RAT-A-KILL (Eradico)	Warfarin (3-(a-acetonylbenzyl)- 4-hydroxycoumarin) 0.5%	ERSKINS' AAA MISTURE For intestinal irritation (Dacus)	Alcohol 5% Zinc sulfocarbolate* Saloland bismuth subsalicylate* Pepsin Oil of wintergreen*
ERADICO RAT-BAIT (Eradico)	Warfarin (3-(a-acetonylbenzyl)- 4-hydroxycoumarin) 0.025%	ERUSTICATOR Rust remover (Pennsylv. Salt)	Hydrofluoric acid *
ERADICO ROACH POWDER (Eradico)	Pyrethrins 0.05% Petroleum hydrocarbons 0.60% Sodium fluoride* 63.00% Beta thiocyano ethyl esters of fatty acids containing 10 to 18 carbon atoms 0.18%	ERUSTOCETIC Rust remover (Pennsylv. Salt)	Fluosilicates* Acid fluorides (bifluorides)*
ERADICO ROACH- PROOFER (Eradico)	Tech. chlordane 2.00% Petroleum distillate* 98.00%	ERUSTOCIDE Rust remover (Pennsylv. Salt)	Fluosilicates* Acid fluorides (bifluorides)*
ERADO Germicide (Griffith)		ERUSTOLIN A Rust remover (Pennsylv. Salt)	Fluosilicates* Acid fluorides (bifluorides)*
ERADO SINGLE FLUID Ink eradicator (Cardinell)		ERUSTOMAX Rust remover (Pennsylv. Salt)	Fluosilicates* Acid fluorides (bifluorides)*
E-RAT-I- CATOR RAT- KILLER (Nat'l Rodent.)	Red squill powder* 10%	ERUSTO-RAY Rust remover (Pennsylv. Salt)	Fluosilicates* Acid fluorides (bifluorides)*
ERCOCIDE Herbicide (Electric)	Sodium chlorate* Sodium carbonate	ERUSTO SALTS Rust remover (Pennsylv. Salt)	Fluosilicates* Acid fluorides (bifluorides)*
ERCOPHOS Water softener and detergent additive (Electric)	Sodium hexametaphosphate*	ERUSTOSOL Rust remover (Pennsylv. Salt)	Hydrofluoric acid*
ERGOZIDE For boils and burns (Jenkins)	Ergot ext.* 10-1/2 gr. Carbolic acid* 10 gr. Balsam Peru Oil cade Zinc oxide ointment base	ESCAPADE BATH SALTS & BUBBLING BATH CRYSTALS (Shulton)	
E.R.H. COLORS, VARNISHES, PAINTS (Egan & Hausman)		ESCAPADE BODY SACHET, DUSTING POW- DER & TAL- CUM POWDER (Shulton)	
ERNSALIN ENAMEL PAINTS (Ernecke)			

*Consult Sec. II., Ingredients Index. This ingredient may be responsible for major toxic effects if poisonous amounts of this product are ingested.

Name & Use Manufacturer	Ingredients	Name & Use Manufacturer	Ingredients
ESCAPADE PERFUME, COLOGNE & TOILET WATER (Shulton)		ESCO LEAKPROOF SKIN Undertakers' and embalmers' supplies (Embalmers')	
ESCO BEAUTIFYING TINT Undertakers' and embalmers' supplies (Embalmers')	Chlorinated hydrocarbons*	ESCO LIP PASTE Undertakers' and embalmers' supplies (Embalmers')	
ESCO CREAMY COSMETIC Undertakers' and embalmers' supplies (Embalmers')		ESCO LIP TINT Undertakers' and embalmers' supplies (Embalmers')	
ESCO DRY SHAMPOO Undertakers' and embalmers' supplies (Embalmers')	Chlorinated hydrocarbons*	ESCO LIP WAX Undertakers' and embalmers' supplies (Embalmers')	
ESCO EMOLLIENT CREAM Undertakers' and embalmers' supplies (Embalmers')		ESCO LIQUID POWDER Undertakers' and embalmers' supplies (Embalmers')	
ESCO FACE POWDER Undertakers' and embalmers' supplies (Embalmers')		ESCO MASSAGE CREAM Undertakers' and embalmers' supplies (Embalmers')	
ESCO FLUID COLORING Undertakers' and embalmers' supplies (Embalmers')		ESCO SPOT-OUT Undertakers' and embalmers' supplies (Embalmers')	
ESCO GLO-DRESS POLISH (Embalmers')		ESCO THERMACOOL CREAM Undertakers' and embalmers' supplies (Embalmers')	
ESCO HAIR DYE Undertakers' and embalmers' supplies (Embalmers')		ESCO WAXINE Undertakers' and embalmers' supplies (Embalmers')	
ESCO HAND LOTION Undertakers' and embalmers' supplies (Embalmers')		ESCORT AFTER SHAVE LOTION (Stevens, W.)	
ESCO HYGIENIC SOAP Undertakers' and embalmers' supplies (Embalmers')		ESCORT DEODORANT (Stevens, W.)	
		ESCORT DRY GLOSS COLOGNE (Stevens, W.)	

*Consult Sec. II., Ingredients Index. This ingredient may be responsible for major toxic effects if poisonous amounts of this product are ingested.

- 468 -

Name & Use Manufacturer	Ingredients	Name & Use Manufacturer	Ingredients
ESCORT HAIR TONIC (Stevens, W.)		ESS-TEE-DEE HAIR TONIC (Ess-Tee-Dee)	
ESCOTT EAR & SKIN LOTION FOR DOGS (Santiseptic)	Calcium hydroxide Glycerin Menthol* Zinc oxide Phenol* Zinc phenolsulfonate*	ESTER AIR SPRAY Herbicide (Pittsburgh Coke)	Butyl esters of 2,4-dichloro-phenoxyacetic acid* 80.0%
ESKO For skin irritations (Myers Labs.)	Zinc oxide Sulfur* Oil birch tar Carbolic acid*	ESTERCIDE AERO CONCEN-TRATE Herbicide (Calif.Spray)	Isopropyl ester of 2,4-dichloro-phenoxyacetic acid* 75.3%
ESPECOL Antacid, digestant (Pfeiffer)	Bismuth subsalicylate Zinc sulfocarbolate* Methyl salicylate synthetic* Salol* Oil of peppermint	ESTERCIDE TD-2 BRUSH KILLER (Calif.Spray)	Tetrahydrofurfuryl and related pentane diol esters of 2,4-D* Tetrahydrofurfuryl and related pentane diol esters of 2,4,5-T*
ESPOTABS (Dill's) Laxative (Eastco)	Yellow phenolphthalein*	ESTERCIDE T-4 LOW-VOLATILE Herbicide (Calif.Spray)	Tetrahydrofurfuryl ester of 2,4,5-trichlorophenoxyacetic acid* 55%
ESQUIRE AFTER SHAVE STICK (Ayars)		ESTERCIDE T-4 SPECIAL Herbicide (Calif.Spray)	Isopropyl ester of 2,4,5-T* 53.7%
ESQUIRE BOOT STAIN Shoe polish (Knomark)		ESTERCIDE T-2 WEED & BRUSH KILLER (Calif.Spray)	Isopropyl ester of 2,4,5-T* 28.4%
ESQUIRE COLOGNE (Ayars)		ESTERCIDE T-245 WEED KILLER (Calif.Spray)	Isopropyl ester of 2,4,5-T*
ESQUIRE DEODORANT (Ayars)		ESTERCIDE 2.6 WEED KILLER (Calif.Spray)	Butyl ester of 2,4-dichloro-phenoxyacetic acid* 39%
ESQUIRE SHAVING LOTION (Ayars)		ESTERCIDE 3.3 WEED KILLER (Calif.Spray)	Isopropyl ester of 2,4-dichloro-phenoxyacetic acid* 46%
ESSENCE PEPSIN, LILLY (not N.F.) (Lilly)	Alcohol 15% Pepsin Rennin Wine Aromatics	ESTERCOL For skin irritation (Torch)	Mercury oleate 0.45% Phenol 0.5% Salicylic acid 3.0% Coal tar 1.2%
ESSENIC LIQUID For skin irritations, colds (Essenic)	Oil of turp.* Oil of cajeput* Oil of juniper* Petrolatum	ESTERON 44 Herbicide (Dow)	2,4-D isopropyl ester 44% 2,4-D acid* 37%
ESSENIC OINTMENT For skin irritations, colds (Essenic)	Oil of turp.* Oil of cajeput* Oil of juniper* Petrolatum Wax	ESTERON 245 Herbicide (Dow)	2,4,5-T isopropyl ester 43% 2,4,5-T acid* 37%
ESSEN KIT: JUNIOR & SENIOR After shave, Body freshener, foot freshener (Parfum L'Orle)		ESTERON BRUSH KILLER (Dow)	2,4-D ispropyl ester* 22% 2,4,5-T isopropyl ester* 21.5%
ESSEN KIT: SENIOR After shave, Body freshener, foot freshener (Parfum L'Orle)		ESTERON TEN-TEN Herbicide (Dow)	Propylene glycol butyl ether esters of 2,4-D* 70.5%

*Consult Sec. II., Ingredients Index. This ingredient may be responsible for major toxic effects if poisonous amounts of this product are ingested.

Name & Use Manufacturer	Ingredients	Name & Use Manufacturer	Ingredients
ESTER WEED KILLER D-4 (Pittsburgh Coke)	Iso-octyl ester of 2,4-dichloro-phenoxyacetic acid* 67.5%	ESTHER'S FACE CREAMS (Nat'l. Beauty)	Beeswax Mineral oil Paraffin wax Borax
ESTER WEED KILLER NO. 40 (Pittsburgh Coke)	Butyl ester of 2,4-dichloro-phenoxyacetic acid* 38.8%	ESTHER'S FACE POWDER (Nat'l. Beauty)	
ESTER WEED KILLER NO. 44 (Pittsburgh Coke)	Isopropyl ester of 2,4-dichloro-phenoxyacetic acid* 45.5%	ESTHER'S FINGER WAVE BASE (Nat'l. Beauty)	Amber petrolatum Paraffin wax
ESTES A TO Z LOZENGES Antitussive (Estes)	Benzocaine Eucalyptol* Menthol* Oil anise	ESTHER'S KIDDIE HAIR CREAM (Nat'l. Beauty)	White petrolatum Mineral oil Beeswax Lanolin Borax
ESTES CORN PLASTER Keratolytic (Estes)	Salicylic acid* 0.044% Belladonna alkoloids*	ESTHER'S LADY HAIR CREAM (Nat'l. Beauty)	White petrolatum Mineral oil Beeswax Lanolin Borax
ESTES INDIAN HERBS TABLETS Laxative (Estes)	Extract cascara sagrada Extract Indian rhubarb Aloes Oil peppermint Podophyllin* Oleoresin capsicum Aloin*	ESTHER'S LIPSTICK (Nat'l. Beauty)	
ESTES NU-RAL TABLETS Analgesic (Estes)	Acetylsalicylic acid* 5 gr. Caffeine 1/6 gr.	ESTHER'S MARCEL WAX (Nat'l. Beauty)	Amber petrolatum Paraffin
ESTES SAMARITAN SALVE (Estes)	Ichthyol Balsam peru Benzocain Oil gaultheria* Oil eucalyptus* Alum Boric acid*	ESTHERS' POMADE FOR MEN (Nat'l. Beauty)	Amber petrolatum Mineral oil Lanolin Resin
ESTES SKIN SALVE For skin irritations (Estes)	Benzocain Zinc oxide Oil of cade Glycerin Resorcinol* Salicylic acid* Sulfur precipitated*	ESTHER'S PRESSING OIL (Nat'l. Beauty)	Petrolatum Mineral oil Beeswax Rosin
ESTHER'S BRILLIAN-TINE (Nat'l. Beauty)	Mineral oil	ESTHER'S SHAMPOO TINT (Nat'l. Beauty)	
ESTHER'S COCONUT OIL SHAMPOO (Nat'l. Beauty)		ESTHER'S TAR HAIR CREAM (Nat'l. Beauty)	Tar* Mineral oil Petrolatum
ESTHER'S COLD WAVE CREAM (Nat'l. Beauty)		ESTHER'S TAR OIL Cosmetic (Nat'l. Beauty)	Tar* Crude oil* Mineral oil
ESTHER'S EYE SHADOW (Nat'l. Beauty)	Petrolatum Ceresin Spermaceti Mineral oil	ESTHER'S TAR WORKING OIL Cosmetic (Nat'l. Beauty)	Tar* Mineral oil Petrolatum
		ESTHER'S TOUCH-UP CREAM (Nat'l.Beauty)	

*Consult Sec. II., Ingredients Index. This ingredient may be responsible for major toxic effects if poisonous amounts of this product are ingested.

Name & Use Manufacturer	Ingredients	
ESTHER'S WATER-PROOFING CREAM Cosmetic (Nat'l. Beauty)	Amber petrolatum Mineral oil Beeswax Zinc stearate Calcium stearate	
ESTIVIN For hay fever (Schieffelin)	Infusion of rose petals	
ESTON AEROSOL HOUSE-HOLD INSECTICIDE (Eston)	DDT Pyrethrins Piperonyl butoxide	3% 0.2% 0.75%
ESTON M-B-C FUMIGANT Controls common storage insects (Eston)	Methyl bromide* Chloropicrin	97.6% 2.0%
ESTON METHYL BROMIDE Fumigant (Eston)	Methyl bromide	99.6%
ESTON TETRON-50 Insecticide (Eston)	Tetraethyl pyrophosphate* 20% Other ethyl phosphates 30%	
ESTRA DOUCHE POWDER (Caswell-Massey)		
ESTRA-LO HORMONE LOTION (Beauty Couns.)		
E-T-C NASAL SOLUTION (Lamb & Berlin)	Ephedrine HCl Chlorobutanol Menthol* Dextrose	1% 0.5%
ETERNOLIN Waterproof varnish (Baker P. & V.)		
ETERNOL TINT OIL SHAMPOO (Paragon Dist.)	Ammonia Alcohol Soap Oil Aromatic amine	
ETHCO CAULKING, GLAZING & PIPE JOINT COMPOUNDS (Holmes, E.T.)		
ETHIX FORMULA HAIR CREAM (Ethix)	Glyceryl esters Sorbitan esters Beeswax Petrolatum Mineral oil Sodium borate	

Name & Use Manufacturer	Ingredients	
ETHIX FORMULA SHAMPOO (Ethix)	Saponified myristic acid Lauric acid Polyamine alkalis Lanolin derivatives Propylene glycol Organic water softener	
ETHMO Skin emollient (Jeffrey-Fell)	Each avoir. oz.: Zinc oxide 9 gr. Phenol 4-1/2 gr. Ethyl aminobenzoate 7 gr. Aromatics Lano petro base q.s.	
ETHOL 90 Photographic supply (Robbins Ethol)		
ETHRA-ZINE SPOT REMOVER (Boyle & Co.)	Petroleum hydrocarbon fraction* Aromatics, low	
ETHYL CETAB Fungicide (Fairfield)	Cetyl dimethyl ethyl ammonium bromide* 100%	
ETHYL DECAB Fungicide (Fairfield)	Stearyl dimethyl ethyl am-monium bromide* 10% Cetyl dimethyl ethyl am-monium bromide* 10% Oleyl dimethyl ethyl am-monium bromide* 35% Linoleyl dimethyl ethyl ammonium bromide* 45%	
ETIQUET DEODORANT CREAM (Lehn & Fink)	Aluminum sulfate	
ETIWAN FERTILIZER (Etiwan)		
EUCA-MUL BINZ Antitussive (Binz)	Oil of eucalyptus* Glycerin Oil of peppermint Alcohol	
EUCASON Disinfectant (Advance Chem.)		
EUCLID COOL STEP CREAM, POWDER & REFRESHER (Galen)		
EUCLID NO CHAFE POWDER (Galen)		
EUGENIC CREME Vaginal cream (Diaphragm)	Stearic acid 20.00% Oleic acid 0.150% Triethanolamine 1.400% Sodium lauryl sulfate 0.025%	
EULAN CN Mothproofing agent (Antara)	Pentachloro-dihydroxy-triphenyl methane* Sodium sulfonate 88%	

*Consult Sec. II., Ingredients Index. This ingredient may be responsible for major toxic effects if poisonous amounts of this product are ingested.

Name & Use Manufacturer	Ingredients		Name & Use Manufacturer	Ingredients
EUPHORBIA & SQUILL COMPOUND SYRUP Antitussive (Sharp & Dohme)	Chloroform 0.12 gm. Tr. euphorbia 8.0 cc. Fluid ext. squill 0.2 cc. Ipecac 0.18 gm. Jamaica dogwood 1.04 gm. Menthol 8 mg.		EVANS ALL AROUND CLEANSER (Commercial Paste)	Trisodium phosphate*
EUPRAXINE ANTISEPTIC DOUCHE POWDER COMPOUND (Eupraxine)	Alum Boric acid* Phenol* Peppermint		EVANS' DEPILATORY CREAM (Myers Labs.)	Barium sulfide*
EUPRAXINE CORN & CALLUS SALVE Keratolytic (Eupraxine)	Beeswax Rosin Salicylic acid*		EVAN'S DEPILATORY CREAM (Evans Dep.)	
EUPRAXINE DARK SALVE (Eupraxine)	Ichthammol 5% Yellow petrolatum Camphor* Beeswax Eucalyptus oil*		EVAN'S DEPILATORY POWDER (Evans Dep.)	
			EVANS QUICK STICK WALL SIZE (Commercial Paste)	Vegetable glue derived from dextrine
EUPRAXINE ITCH LOTION (Eupraxine)	Zinc oxide 10% Glycerin 10% Boric acid* 10% Phenol .85%		EVANS STA-ZIT WALL SIZE (Commercial Paste)	Animal hide glue
EUPRAXINE SKIN SALVE WHITE (Eupraxine)	White petrolatum Boric acid Cornstarch Zinc oxide		EVANS WALLPAPER REMOVER (Commercial Paste)	Wetting agents
EUREKA ENAMELS & PAINTS (Otley)			EVENING IN PARIS FACE POWDER (Bourjois)	Talcum Zinc palmitate Kaolin Chalk Titanium dioxide Zinc oxide U.S.P. Magnesium carbonate U.S.P. Mineral oil Certified aniline colors Certified non-aniline lakes
EUREKA LIQUID WOOD FILLER (Lancaster Paint)				
EUREKA MICE BAIT (Allen)	Strychnine* 4/10%		EVENING STAR PERFUMES (Blanchard)	
EUREKA PAINTS (Con-Ferro)			EVENING STAR PURSE BOUQUET STICK (Blanchard)	
EUREKA-U-NO Medicine (De Soto Drug)				
EUTHANASIA SOLUTION Veterinary (Horton & Converse)	Sodium pentobarbital* 2.75 gr./cc. Propylene glycol 33%		EVENING STAR SPRAY DEODORANT (Blanchard)	
EUTHOL For throat irritations, decongestant (D-K)	Chlorobutanol (chloral derivative 0.50%) Oil eucalyptus* Menthol* Thymol* Camphor*		EVERBLACK Roof coating (Phelan-Faust)	
EVAC-U-GEN Laxative (Walker, Corp.)	Yellow phenolphthalein* Sodium salicylate* 1/4 gr. Bismuth subcarbonate 1/8 gr. Bismuth subgallate 1/8 gr.		EVER BLUM CLEANING FLUID (Blum)	Carbon tetrachloride* more than 20% Chloroform Naphtha Benzine soap

*Consult Sec. II., Ingredients Index. This ingredient may be responsible for major toxic effects if poisonous amounts of this product are ingested.

Name & Use Manufacturer	Ingredients		Name & Use Manufacturer	Ingredients
EVER BRITE PAINT (Davis Paint)			EVERSEAL SYNTHETIC AUTO ENAMEL NO. 760 (Everseal)	
EVER-DRY CREAM Deodorant (Ever-Dry)	Lorol (cetyl alcohol) Urea Aluminum sulfate Aluminum chloride Aluminum phenolsulfonate Carbitol Magnesium oxide Tegacid Beeswax Perfume		EVERTOX RED COPPER Paint (Balto. Copper)	
			EVER YOUTH HAIR COLORING (Ever-Youth)	Lead acetate* N.F. granular Sulfur Glycerin
EVER-DRY QUICK Deodorant (Ever-Dry)	Chlorhydrol Urea Carbowax Basic aluminum chloride		EVER YOUTH SHAMPOO (Ever-Youth)	Conc. liquid soap
EVER-DRY WATER RESISTANT PAINT (High Point)			EVONS ANTISEPTIC & HYGIENIC POWDER (Drexel)	Boric acid* Thymol* Salicylic acid* Eucalyptol* Phenol Potassium alum Methyl salicylate* Menthol* Oxyquinoline sulfate*
EVERFAST CEMENT (Howe & French)	Nitrocellulose type of cement Alcohols* Hydrocarbons* Ketones*			
			EVONS BABY POWDER (Evons)	Talcum Boric acid* 25%
EVERGLOW LIGHTER FLUID (Devil)			EVONS GREASELESS BABY OINTMENT (Evons)	Antiseptic oxyquinoline sulfate* Benzocaine Camphor* Eucalyptol* Carbamide Lanolin
EVER GREEN GARDEN SPRAY Insecticide (McLaughlin)	Pyrethrins* 1.4% Mineral oil 23.6 Pine oil* 45.0			
EVERGREEN PINE JELLY SOAP (Murphy Labs.)	Soap 11.35% Pine oil 8%		EVONS HYGIENIC POWDER For douche and skin irritations (Evons)	Boric acid* Alum (aluminum and potassium sulfate) Thymol* Methyl salicylate* Salicylic acid* Menthol Eucalyptol* Oxyquinoline sulfate
EVERGREEN PINE OIL DEODORANT (Murphy Labs.)	Pine oil and pine oil fraction* 64% Detergent 26% Kerosene 7%			
EVERLASTING Black roofing paints (U. S. Ref.)			EVONS RECTAL OINTMENT For rectal irritation (Evons)	Stearic acid and lanolin Tannic acid Camphor* Menthol* Eucalyptol* Benzocaine Oxyquinoline sulfate*
EVERNEW CLEANER (Snowwhite Chem.)				
EVERON HOUSE PAINT (Glidden Co.)			EXCELSIOR COLORED PENCILS (Reliance Pencil)	
EVERPURE INSECT POWDER (Altone)			EXCELSIOR LABORATORIES LAXATIVE TABLETS (Excelsior)	
EVER READY LIGHTER FLUID (Plough)			EXCELSIOR'S LAXATIVE TABLETS (Excelsior)	Powdered extract cascara sagrada* Powdered extract podophyllin Powdered senna leaves Powdered rhubarb* Powdered stillingia Powdered licorice Aloin*
EVERSEAL Plastic roofing (Everseal)				

*Consult Sec. II., Ingredients Index. This ingredient may be responsible for major toxic effects if poisonous amounts of this product are ingested.

Name & Use Manufacturer	Ingredients		Name & Use Manufacturer	Ingredients	
EXELENTO BLEACH CREAM (Exelento)			EXORA DEPILATORY (Meyer, C.)		
EXELENTO BRILLIAN-TINE (Exelento)			EXORA FACE POWDER (Meyer, C.)		
EXELENTO DEODORANT (Exelento)			EXORA FOUNDATION CREAM (Meyer, C.)		
EXELENTO GLASSINE & PRESSING OIL Hair preparation (Exelento)			EXORA MASCARILLO Cosmetic (Meyer, C.)		
			EXORA NOSE CREAM (Meyer, C.)		
EXELENTO HAIR POMADE (Exelento)			EXORA ROSEBUD LIPSTICK (Meyer, C.)		
EXELENTO SKIN OINTMENT (Exelento)			EXORA ROUGE (Meyer, C.)		
EXELENTO VANISHING CREAM (Exelento)			EXO'TAB Expectorant for children (Massengill)	Each tablet: Tartar emetic Powdered ipecac Ammonium chloride Aromatic	0.65 mg. 1.1 mg. 16 mg. q.s.
EXERIN EXPECTORANT HAAG Antitussive, antihistamine (Haag)	Each fl. oz.: Sodium citrate Pyrilamine maleate Ammonium chloride Tartar emetic Chloroform Alcohol	10 gr. 80 mg. 10 gr. 1/4 gr. 2 m. 5%	EXPECTING Lotion for expectant mothers (Athea)	Triethanolamine stearate Lanolin Petrolatum Hexadecanol Olive oil	
EXI-11 For poison ivy (De Wolf)			EXPECTORANT COMPOUND Antitussive (Energy)	Powder ammonia nitrate Powder ammonia carbonate Fluid ext. of licorice root Tincture lobelia* Glycerin Tincture aconite* Nux vomica(5-6 mg. strychnine/ oz.)*	
EXI DAN Anti-dandruff lotion (Quality Chem.)					
EX-IN-O-LITE VARNISH & ENAMEL (Thibault)			EXPECTORINE VETERINARY COUGH MIXTURE (Thoroughbred)	Alcohol Fluid ext. belladonna* White pine bark Sanguinaria Spikenard Benzocaine Menthol* Chloroform* Fluid ext. euphorbia Wild cherry Balm gilead buds Sassafras Ammonium chloride	7%/v 6 m./oz.
EX-LAX Cathartic (Ex-Lax)	Yellow phenolphthalein				
EXO CLEANSER PASTE (Silver Suds)					
EXODERM FOOT POWDER (Surbin)			EXPEDITE PAINT & VARNISH REMOVER (Pratt & Lambert)		
EXODERM OINTMENT (Surbin)			EXPELLO AIR FRESHENER (Dunaway)	Fir balsam perfume Deodorized kerosene Perfume fixative Freons 11 and 12	0.375% 79.625%
EXO FIRE EXTIN-GUISHER LIQUID (Carbona)					

*Consult Sec. II., Ingredients Index. This ingredient may be responsible for major toxic effects if poisonous amounts of this product are ingested.

- 474 -

Name & Use Manufacturer	Ingredients	Name & Use Manufacturer	Ingredients
EXPELLO EX-RAY VAPOR BRAND CRYSTALS Insecticide (Dunaway)	Paradichlorobenzene* 99.97% Essence of cedar and pine 0.03%	EXSORA Fungicide, emollient (Medical) (Exsora)	Sublimed sulfur* Boric acid*
EXPELLO HIGH TEST INSECT KILLER (Dunaway)	DDT 2.0% n-Octyl bicycloheptene dicarboximide* 2.0% Allethrin (allyl homolog of cinerin 1) 0.2% Methylated naphthalenes* 5.0% Petroleum distillates* 5.8%	EXTERMO LIQUID 5% DDT Insecticide (Rochester Germ.)	Petroleum distillate* DDT* Isobornyl thiocyanoacetate* Other related terpenes
EXPELLO INSECT REPELLENT (Dunaway)	2-Ethylhexanediol-1,3* 100%	EXTERMO ROACH POWDER (Rochester Germ.)	Sodium fluoride* DDT Pyrethrins
EXPELLO MOTH CRYSTALS (Dunaway)	Paradichlorobenzene* 99.97%	EXTERMO ROACH POWDER PLUS 10% DDT (Rochester Germ.)	Pyrethrum Sodium fluoride* DDT 10%
EXPELLO MOTH PROOFER (Dunaway)	Terpene polychlorinates (66% chlorine)* 5% Petroleum distillate* 35%	EXTO Insecticide (Dolge)	Petroleum distillate* Tech. chlordane* Related compounds
EXPELLO NO. 5 Insecticide (Dunaway)	Paradichlorobenzene* 99.97 Essence of cedar and pine 0.03	EXTOX For skin irritation (Penslar)	Sodium thiosulfate* Soap Camphor* Phenol*
EXPELLO PLANT & GARDEN SPRAY Insecticide (Dunaway)	Pyrethrins 0.025% Rotenone 0.128% Other cube extractives 0.236% Tech. piperonyl cyclonene 0.256% Petroleum distillate 0.102%	EXUDO For Ivy poison (Bullock-Walker)	Magnesium sulfate Ichthammol* Thymol iodide* Menthol* Glycerin Benzocaine Salol*
EXPELLO ROACH & ANT KILLER (Dunaway)	Tech. chlordane 2.00% Orthodichlorobenzene* 23.00% Petroleum distillate 10.00%	EXUDO A External counter-irritant (Bullock-Walker)	Calomel * 3% Salicylic acid 1/3% Magnesium sulfate Carbolic acid 1/3% Thymol 1/12% Glycerin
EXPORT CHEMICAL'S CHLORDANE CONCEN-TRATE Insecticide (Export)	Tech. chlordane* 44% Petroleum oil 46% Polyoxyethylene sorbitol oleate laurate 10%	EXZIN Antitussive (Massengill)	Each tablet: Ammonium chloride 0.13 gm. Terpin hydrate* 0.13 gm. Ext. senega* 6.5 mg. Ext. lobelia* 6.5 mg. Powd. ipecac 6.5 mg. Tartar emetic 2.2 mg.
EXRO ROACH KILLER FORMULA Insecticide (Aceto)	Tech. chlordane 2% Aliphatic petroleum solvents* 98%	EYE-GENE Eye drops (Pearson Pharm.)	Laevo alpha hydroxy beta methylamino-3-hydroxy ethylbenzene hydrochloride Sodium borate Camphor water Isotonic sodium chloride solution Thimerosal sodium ethyl mercurithio salicylate 0.001%
EX-SECT KILLS MOTHS (block) (Bordman)	Paradichlorobenzene* 100%		
EX-SECT MOTH CRYSTALS (Bordman)	Paradichlorobenzene* 100%	EYE-GLO Eye lotion (Kent Spec.)	Zinc salt of sulfanilic acid Sodium chloride Uranine Phenol Camphor water
EX-SECT MOTH NUGGETS (Bordman)	Paradichlorobenzene* 100%		

*Consult Sec. II., Ingredients Index. This ingredient may be responsible for major toxic effects if poisonous amounts of this product are ingested.

Name & Use Manufacturer	Ingredients		Name & Use Manufacturer	Ingredients	
EYELEEN Antiseptic eye lotion (Mother's)	Chlorobutanol Berberine sulfate Methyl para hydroxybenzoate Zinc sulfate Hydrogen borate		E-Z-GO HAND CLEANER (Glidden)		
EYELO Eye lotion (Rexall)	Sodium borate* Boric acid* Camphor*		EZ-IT External fungicide, (medical) (Gaddy, R.L.)	Alcohol* approx. 80%/v Acetone* Thymol* Menthol* Tinct. benzoin compound Salicylic acid U.S.P.* Glycerin	
EYE-LUBE Antiseptic lubricant for artifical eyes or contact lenses (Barnes-Hind)	Alkyl dimethyl benzyl am- monium chloride 1-10,000		E-Z KILL ROACH SPRAY (Slick Shine)	Aliphatic petroleum solvent* 98% Tech. chlordane 2%	
EYLAX EYE WASH (Eylax)	Hydrastis Camphor water Boric acid Chlorobutanol		E-Z KLEEN FLEA POWDER (Hartz Mt.)	Corn starch Cube resins 3.00%	
E-ZAKE Dental anesthetic (Hance)	Alcohol* 70%/v Chloroform 0.8%/v Cycloform Camphor* Cresote*		E-Z KORN REMOVER Keratolytic (E.Z. Chem.)	Each fl. oz.: Ether 318 min. Alcohol 21% Gl. acetic acid* Salicylic acid* Oil of turpentine* Collodion Benzocaine 2%	
EZALL Lubricating compound (Ezall)			E.Z. METAL POLISH & MARBLE CLEANER (Gateway)		
E Z CLEANER (Stanley Home)	Soap Trisodium phosphate* Stearic acid Borax* Sassafras Dowicide		E Z NASAL SPRAY Nasal decongestant (E.Z. Chem.)	Ephedrine sulfate Potassium acid phosphate Disodium phosphate	
EZE External fungicide, (medical) (Pino)	Denatured alcohol* Salicylic acid* Oil of pine*		EZ-O-DYNE Analgesic (Oliver's S-O)	Acetophenetidin* 8 gr/fl.oz. Aspirin* Citrated caffeine* Aromatic spirits of ammonia	
EZE CLEANER (Park Chem.)	Kerosene* Soap Pine oil* Abrasives		EZ-OFF Keratolytic (Corn Off)		
EZ-ER-HE- LER OIL (Denton)			E-Z-ON-NAIL NOURISH (Blatz)		
EZE-THIN BATH Dog prep. (T-N-T)			E-Z-O SOLVENT For removing adhesive tape (Barnes-Hind)	Methyl salicylate* Carbon tetrachloride*	
EZE-WAX- FLOOR WAX (Pioneer)			EZ PLASTIC CEMENT (Van Cleef)		
E Z FLO HOUSE PAINTS (Subox)			E-Z ROACH SPRAY (Slick Shine)	Aliphatic petroleum solvent* 98% Tech. chlordane 2%	
E Z GLOW WAX (Stanley Home)	Durez resin Red oil Morpholine Tergitol Carnauba wax Wax blend Triethanolamine* Ammonia*		E. Z. TABLETS Laxative (E.Z. Chem.)	Aloin* Cascarin* Podophyllin Ginger resin	
			E-Z-TAN Cosmetic (Morgan, H.)	Camphor* Phenol* Tannin Preservative Gums	

*Consult Sec. II., Ingredients Index. This ingredient may be responsible for major toxic effects if poisonous amounts of this product are ingested.

Name & Use Manufacturer	Ingredients	Name & Use Manufacturer	Ingredients
EZY-2-TAN Cosmetic (Morgan, H.)	Camphor* Phenol* Tannin Preservative Gums	FABULOUS PARFUM (Parfums Charbert)	
E-Z VOICE PASTILLES Antitussive (E.Z. Chem.)	Menthol* Eucalyptol* Oil anise Benzoic acid Benzaldehyde* Sucrose Gum arabic	FABULOY Wood finish (Pierce & Stevens)	Modified palmitic Stearic oleic Linolenic acids Phenolic ether resin Chlorinated biphenyl* Pentachlor biphenyl* Quadrochlor biphenyl* Aromatic* and aliphatic* hydrocarbons
E-Z WOOD Mending wood (Boyle-Midway)	Glue Wood fiber filler Preservative	FAESY & BESTHOFF FERTILIZER (Faesy & Besthoff)	
EZY WATERLESS CLEANER (Uncle Sam)	Soap Perfume	FAESY & BESTHOFF LIME-SULPHUR SOLUTION Insecticide (Faesy & Besthoff)	Calcium polysulfide*
FAB Detergent (Colgate-Palmolive)		FAESY & BESTHOFF MOTH-PROOFING (Faesy & Besthoff)	
FABERGE BATH PERFUME (Faberge)	Esters of higher aliphatic acids	FAESY & BESTHOFF TOBACCO DUST Insecticide (Faesy & Besthoff)	Nicotine* 1%
FABERGE BATH POWDERS & SACHET (Faberge)	French talc Zinc stearate Magnesium carbonate	FAESY & BESTHOFF WEED KILLER (Faesy & Besthoff)	Sodium arsenite* (23.1% arsenic) 34%
FABERGE PERFUME, COLONGES, MENS' LOTIONS (Faberge)	Specially denatured alcohol* (Formula #39 C)	FAIRMOUNT WEED KILLER (Rose Mfg.)	Sodium arsenite* 35.0%
FABERGE SOAP (Faberge)		FALCON JELLY Nasal decongestant (Falcon)	Menthol* Camphor* Oil of pine Chinese mint oil Oil of eucalyptus*
FABULON Floor finish (Pierce & Stevens)	Maleic alkyd polyester Modified maleic rosin ester Cellulose nitrate Chlorinated bi-phenyl Hexachlor bi-phenyl Quadrachlor bi-phenyl 2-Bi-phenyl Diphenyl phosphate Modified phthalic acid polyester Cresyl diphenyl phosphate Secondary butyl alcohol* Isopropyl alcohol* Secondary butyl acetate* Normal propyl alcohol* Normal propyl acetate*	FALGOS TABLETS Analgesic (Am. Ferment)	Acetophenetidin* 2 gr. Aspirin* Caffeine* Aluminum hydroxide Magnesium hydroxide
		FALK'S CAMFO CREME (Falk)	Camphor* Glycerin Turpentine* Ammonia*
FABULOUS COLOGNE STICK (Parfums Charbert)		FALSODENT DENTURE HOLDER (Cort-Livingston)	
FABULOUS EAU DE TOILETTE (Parfums Charbert)			

*Consult Sec. II., Ingredients Index. This ingredient may be responsible for major toxic effects if poisonous amounts of this product are ingested.

Name & Use Manufacturer	Ingredients		Name & Use Manufacturer	Ingredients	
FAME EAU de TOILETTE (Parfums Corday)			FARM BUREAU CUCUMBER DUST Fungicide, insecticide (Farm Bureau)	Rotenone Other cube resins DDT Copper expressed as metallic (in tribasic copper sulfate)*	1.00% 1.80% 3.00% 5.00%
FAME PERFUME (Parfums Corday)			FARM BUREAU 5% DDT DUST Insecticide (Farm Bureau)	DDT*	5%
FANCO POMADE (Fan Tan)					
FAN TAN BLEACH CREME (Fan Tan)			FARM BUREAU 8% DITHANE DUST Fungicide (Farm Bureau)	Zineb (zinc ethylene-bis (dithio-carbamate))	5.2%
FAN TAN COLD CREME (Fan Tan)			FARM BUREAU DUST NO. 1 Fungicide, insecticide (Farm Bureau)	Dichloro diphenyl trichloro-ethane* less than 3.0% Copper (in basic copper sulfate) expressed as metallic (copper in cuprous oxide expressed as metallic 0.70%; copper expressed as metallic 2.80%) 3.5%	
FAN TAN DEODORANT CREME (Fan Tan)					
FAN TAN FACE POWDER (Fan Tan)					
FAN TAN VANISHING CREME (Fan Tan)			FARM BUREAU DUST NO. 2 Fungicide (Farm Bureau)	Copper* (in tribasic copper sulfate) expressed as metallic 7%	
FANTASY FLOWER DROPS PERFUME (Wunderlich)			FARM BUREAU DUST NO. 3 Insecticide (Farm Bureau)	Rotenone Other cube resins DDT	1.00% 1.40% 3.00%
FANT NAIL POLISH REMOVER (Fant)			FARM BUREAU DUST NO. 4 Insecticide (Farm Bureau)	Rotenone Other cube resins	0.75% 1.40%
FANTUM BRAND ANTU Rodenticide (Slayer)	Alpha naphthyl thiourea* 92%				
FARBOIL FARBO WATER PAINT (Farboil)			FARM BUREAU DUST NO. 5 Insecticide (Farm Bureau)	Sodium fluoaluminate* 45%	
FARM-AID ANIMAL BALM (Astra)	Anhydrous lanolin U.S.P. Petrolatum U.S.P. Olive and mineral oil U.S.P. Beeswax U.S.P. Ferric phosphate U.S.P. Potassium phosphate U.S.P. Ceresin		FARM BUREAU DUST NO. 6 Fungicide, Insecticide (Farm Bureau)	Rotenone Other cube resins Copper* (in tribasic copper sulfate) expressed as metallic	0.75% 1.40% 5.00%
FARM BUREAU BEAN AND CABBAGE DUST Insecticide (Farm Bureau)	Rotenone Other cube resins DDT	1.00% 1.80% 3.00%	FARM BUREAU DUST NO. 7 Fungicide (Farm Bureau)	Sulfur* Copper*	20% 7%

*Consult Sec. II., Ingredients Index. This ingredient may be responsible for major toxic effects if poisonous amounts of this product are ingested.

- 478 -

Name & Use Manufacturer	Ingredients
FARM BUREAU DUST NO. 8 Fungicide, insecticide (Farm Bureau)	Sodium fluoaluminate* 45% Copper (in tribasic copper sulfate) expressed as metallic 7% Total fluorine 24.4%
FARM BUREAU DUST NO. 9 Insecticide (Farm Bureau)	DDT 3.00%
FARM BUREAU DUST NO. 11 Fungicide (Farm Bureau)	Ziram 7.60%
FARM BUREAU DUST NO. 13 Fungicide, insecticide (Farm Bureau)	DDT* (dichloro diphenyl trichloroethane) 5% Sulfur* 75%
FARM BUREAU DUST NO. 14 Insecticide (Farm Bureau)	Chlordane tech.* 5%
FARM BUREAU DUST NO. 15 Fungicide, insecticide (Farm Bureau)	Bis(methoxy-phenyl) trichloroethane* 3.8% Zinc dimethyl dithiocarbamate* 7.6%
FARM BUREAU DUST NO. 16 Insecticide (Farm Bureau)	Gamma isomer of benzene hexachloride 1%
FARM BUREAU DUST NO. 18 Insecticide (Farm Bureau)	Malathion (o,o-dimethyl dithiophosphate of diethyl mercaptosuccinate) 4.00%
FARM BUREAU DUST NO. 19 Insecticide (Farm Bureau)	Parathion* 1.00%
FARM BUREAU DUST NO. 20 Insecticide (Farm Bureau)	Parathion* (o,o-diethyl-p-nitrophenyl thiophosphate) 1.00% Dichloro dipheny trichloroethane 5.00%
FARM BUREAU DUST NO. 101 Fungicide, insecticide (Farm Bureau)	Dichloro diphenyl trichloroethane* 5.0% Copper* (in basic copper sulfate) expressed as metallic (copper in cuprous oxide expressed as metallic 0.70%; copper expressed as metallic 2.80%) 3.50%

Name & Use Manufacturer	Ingredients
FARM BUREAU DUST NO. 102 Fungicide, insecticide (Farm Bureau)	Copper expressed as metallic in basic copper sul. (copper expressed as metallic consisting approx. of cuprous oxide expressed as metallic 0.70%; copper (finely divided) expressed as metallic 2.80%) 3.5% Calcium arsenate* (derived from Robertson copper fungicide; total arsenate expressed as metallic 2.600%; water soluble arsenic 0.049%) 6.92%
FARM BUREAU DUST NO. 106 Fungicide, insecticide (Farm Bureau)	Dichloro dipheny trichloroethane (aerosol grade)* 3% Copper* (in tribasic copper sulfate) expressed as metallic* 5%
FARM BUREAU DUST NO. 116 Insecticide (Farm Bureau)	Gamma isomer of benzene hexachloride* 3.0% Other isomers and related products 5.2%
FARM BUREAU DUST (ZIRAM) NO. 17 Fungicide, Insecticide (Farm Bureau)	Zinc dimethyl dithiocarbamate* 7.6% Dichloro diphenyl trichloroethane (aerosol grade)* 3.0%
FARM BUREAU GENERAL PURPOSE DUST NO. 12 Fungicide, insecticide (Farm Bureau)	Rotenone 1.00% Other cube resins 1.80% Ferbam 10.00% DDT 3.00% 2(p-tert-Butylphenoxy) isopropyl 2-chloroethyl sulfite 2.00% Sulfur* 40.00%
FARM BUREAU GENERAL PURPOSE FRUIT SPRAY Fungicide, insecticide (Farm Bureau)	Methoxychlor, tech.* 15.50% Malathion* 6.25% Captan 9.50%
FARM BUREAU HOME AND LAWN DUST Insecticide (Farm Bureau)	Tech. chlordane 4.00% Gamma isomer of benzene hexachloride 0.20%
FARM BUREAU LIVESTOCK DUST Insecticide (Farm Bureau)	Rotenone* 1.67% Other cube resins 3.25%

*Consult Sec. II., Ingredients Index. This ingredient may be responsible for major toxic effects if poisonous amounts of this product are ingested.

Name & Use Manufacturer	Ingredients	Name & Use Manufacturer	Ingredients
FARM BUREAU POTATO DUST Fungicide, insecticide (Farm Bureau)	DDT* (dichloro diphenyl trichloroethane) 5.00% Copper* expressed as metallic in tri-basic copper sulfate (consisting approx. of cuprous oxide expressed as metallic 0.70%; copper (finely divided) expressed as metallic 2.80%) 3.50%	FARM & GARDEN BRAND CHLORDANE DUST OR SPRAY Insecticide (Niagara Chem.)	Chlordane* 6%
FARM BUREAU POTATO SPRAY Insecticide (Farm Bureau)	Copper* 39% DDT* 10%	FARM & GARDEN BRAND CHLORDANE DUST OR SPRAY Insecticide (Niagara Chem.)	Tech. chlordane* 5.00%
FARM BUREAU RHOTHANE DUST Insecticide (Farm Bureau)	DDT* 10%	FARM & GARDEN BRAND C-O-C-S COPODUST Fungicide (Niagara Chem.)	Copper* expressed as metallic (in the form of basic sulfates and chlorides) 6.00%
FARM BUREAU ROSE DUST Fungicide, insecticide (Farm Bureau)	Rotenone 1.00% Other cube resins 1.80% Ferbam (ferric dimethyl dithiocarbamate) 15.20% DDT* (dichloro diphenyl trichloroethane) 3.00% 2-p-Tert-butylphenoxy isopropyl 2-chloroethyl sulfite 2.00% Sulfur* 40.00%	FARM & GARDEN BRAND C-O-C-S COPOTEX Insecticide, fungicide (Niagara Chem.)	Copper expressed as metallic 6.00% Tricalcium arsenate* 17.50%
FARM BUREAU TOMATO DUST Fungicide, insecticide (Farm Bureau)	Methoxychlor* 5.00% Copper* expressed as metallic in tri-basic copper sulfate (copper expressed as metallic consisting approx. of cuprous oxide expressed as metallic 0.70%; copper (finely divided) expressed as metallic 2.80%) 3.50%	FARM & GARDEN BRAND C-O-C-S COPPER ROTENONE BEARING DUST Insecticide, fungicide (Niagara Chem.)	Rotenone .75% Other cube resins or extractives 1.50% Copper* expressed as metallic (in form of basic sulfates and chlorides) 5.00%
FARM BUREAU 5% TOXAPHENE DUST Insecticide (Farm Bureau)	Toxaphene* 5%	FARM & GARDEN BRAND C-O-C-S COPPER SPRAY Fungicide (Niagara Chem.)	Copper oxychloride sulfate*
FARM BUREAU VEGETABLE DUST Fungicide, insecticide (Farm Bureau)	Rotenone 1.00% Other cube resins 1.80% DDT* (Dichloro diphenyl trichloroethane (aerosol)) 5.00% Zineb (zinc ethylene bis(dith-iocarbamate); total zinc as metallic 1.50%) 7.60%	FARM & GARDEN BRAND C-O-C-S CUKE AND MELON DUST Insecticide, fungicide (Niagara Chem.)	Copper expressed as metallic 5.00% Tricalcium arsenate* 5.25%
FARMCRAFT HYGEN (Farmcraft Chem.)	Malathion 0.5%		
FARM & GARDEN BRAND APHID DUST OR SPRAY (Niagara Chem.)	Lindane* (gamma BHC) 1.2%		
FARM & GARDEN BRAND BORDEAUX MIXTURE Fungicide (Niagara Chem.)			

*Consult Sec. II., Ingredients Index. This ingredient may be responsible for major toxic effects if poisonous amounts of this product are ingested.

Name & Use Manufacturer	Ingredients
FARM & GARDEN BRAND C-O-C-S NEUTRAL COPPER SPRAY POWDER Fungicide (Niagara Chem.)	Copper* expressed as metallic 26.50%
FARM & GARDEN BRAND C-O-C-S POTATO DUST OR SPRAY Insecticide, fungicide (Niagara Chem.)	Copper* expressed as metallic 7.00% DDT* 7.50%
FARM & GARDEN BRAND DDT 5 DUST Insecticide (Niagara Chem.)	DDT* 5%
FARM & GARDEN BRAND DDT 50 SPRAY Insecticide (Niagara Chem.)	DDT* wettable powder 50%
FARM & GARDEN BRAND FERBAM SPRAY Fungicide (Niagara Chem.)	Ferbam (ferric dimethyldithio-carbamate) 76%
FARM & GARDEN BRAND HOUSEHOLD SPRAY Insecticide (Niagara Chem.)	DDT 3.00% Gamma isomer of benzene hexachloride (from lindane) 0.04 Pyrethrins 0.02 Piperonyl butoxide tech. 0.16 Cedar oil 0.10 Petroleum distillate* 96.68
FARM & GARDEN BRAND KOLO FRUIT TREE DUST OR SPRAY Insecticide, fungicide (Niagara Chem.)	Sulfur 52% DDT (dichloro diphenyl tri-chloroethane) 7.50% Basic lead arsenate* 15%
FARM & GARDEN BRAND LINDANE 25 EMULSION Insecticide (Niagara Chem.)	Gamma isomer of benzene hexachloride* 25.00 Xylene* 49.00
FARM & GARDEN BRAND LINDANE 25 SPRAY Insecticide (Niagara Chem.)	Gamma isomer of benzene hexachloride* 25.00%
FARM & GARDEN BRAND LOUSE POWDER Insecticide (Niagara Chem.)	Tech. BHC*
FARM & GARDEN BRAND MALATHION 50 SPRAY Insecticide (Niagara Chem.)	Malathion* (o,o-dimethyl dithio-phosphate of diethyl mercapto-succinate) 50.00% Xylene 38.00%
FARM & GARDEN BRAND METHOXY-CHLOR 50 WETTABLE POWDER Insecticide (Niagara Chem.)	Methoxychlor, tech.* 50.00%
FARM & GARDEN BRAND NEW POMO GREEN Insecticide, fungicide (Niagara Chem.)	Gamma isomer of benzene hexachloride (lindane) 1% DDT* 5% Sulfur* 62%
FARM & GARDEN BRAND SOILFUME-CAPS Soil fumigant (Niagara Chem.)	Ethylene dibromide* 100%
FARM & GARDEN BRAND SPIDER-MITE DUST OR SPRAY Insecticide (Niagara Chem.)	Aramite* (2(p-tertiary-butyl phenoxy) isopropyl 2 chloro-ethyl sulfite)
FARM & GARDEN BRAND 2,4-D WEED KILLER (Niagara Chem.)	Sodium salt of 2,4-D acid* 70%
FARM & GARDEN BRAND WETTABLE AND DUSTING SULPHUR Fungicide (Niagara Chem.)	Sulfur*

*Consult Sec. II., Ingredients Index. This ingredient may be responsible for major toxic effects if poisonous amounts of this product are ingested.

Name & Use Manufacturer	Ingredients	Name & Use Manufacturer	Ingredients
FARM & HOME WEED KILLER (Chem. Form.)	Dimethylamine salt of 2,4-dichlorophenoxyacetic acid* 49.4% Solvents* 50.6%	FASCO ALDRIN EQUIVALENT LIQUID 2 Insecticide (Florida Agric.)	Hexachloro hexahydro dimethano naphthalene* 21.85% Related compounds 16.48% Petroleum deriv. solvents 51.67%
FARM, RANCH & PADDOCK PAINT (Chi-Namel)	Titanium dioxide 17.7% Silica 20.1% Ester gum modified soya alkyd resin 19.4% Coal tar solvent* 8.9% Petroleum thinner* 32.0% Drier 1.9%	FASCO BASIC COPPER 53 Fungicide (Florida Agric.)	Copper* expressed as metallic from basic copper sulfate 53%
FARMRITE WATERGLASS (Central Chem.)		FASCO BHC LIQUID 16 Insecticide (Florida Agric.)	Gamma isomer of benzene hexachloride* 17.30% Other isomers of benzene hexachloride 19.50% Aromatic petroleum derivative solvents* 52.50%
FARNAM EAR-TICK BOMB Insecticide (Farnam)	Gamma isomer of benzene hexachloride* 3.488% Other isomers of benzene hexachloride 5.232% Xylol* 5.450% Pine oil* 40.330%	FASCO CHLORDANE BAIT 15 Insecticide (Florida Agric.)	Chlordane (octachloro-4,7-methano-tetrahydro indane) 1.5%
FARNAM GRUB SPRAY BOMB Insecticide (Farnam)	Rotenone, rotenoids and other cube resins 0.625% Ethylene glycol ether of pinene 5.625% Pine oil* 12.250% Camphor oil* 10.000% Polyisobutylphenoxypolyethoxy-ethanol 5.000% Propellent gas Isopropanol 66.500%	FASCO CHLORDANE-DDT DUST 3-5 Insecticide (Florida Agric.)	Chlordane* (octachloro-4,7-methano-tetrahydro indane) 3% Dichloro diphenyl trichloro-ethane* 5%
FARNAM METHANOX RESIDUAL FLY SPRAY CONC. (Farnam)	Aromatic petroleum solvent* 61.2% Methoxychlor tech. 23.3% Dimethyl phthalate 10.0% Piperonyl cyclonene tech. 0.5%	FASCO CHLORDANE-DDT DUST 5-5 Insecticide (Florida Agric.)	Chlordane* (octachloro-4,7-methano-tetrahydro indane) 5% Dichloro diphenyl trichloro-ethane* 5%
FARNAM SCREW-WORM BOMB Insecticide (Farnam)	Gamma isomer of benzene hexachloride (from lindane)* 1.800% Pine oil* 21.000%	FASCO CHLORDANE 5 DUST Insecticide (Florida Agric.)	Chlordane* (octachloro-4,7-methano-tetrahydro indane) 5%
FARNESIANA EXTRACT (Caron)		FASCO CHLORDANE 40 DB Insecticide (Florida Agric.)	Chlordane* (octachloro-4,7-methano-tetrahydro indane) 40%
FARR'S GRAY HAIR RESTORER (Brookline Chem.)		FASCO CHLORDANE 10 DUST Insecticide (Florida Agric.)	Chlordane* (octachloro-4, 7-methano-tetrahydro indane) 10%
FASCO ACTIVATED NICOTINE DUST NO. 4 Insecticide (Florida Agric.)	Nicotine*	FASCO CHLORDANE LIQUID 72 Insecticide (Florida Agric.)	Octachloro-4,7-methano-tetrahydro indane* 72%
FASCO ALDRIN EQUIVALENT-DDT 2-1/2 to 5 DUST Insecticide (Florida Agric.)	Aldrin*(hexachloro hexahydro dimethano naphthalene) 2-1/2% DDT* (dichloro diphenyl trichloroethane) 5%	FASCO CHLORPHENE BAIT 375 Insecticide (Florida Agric.)	Chlordane (octachloro-4,7-methano-tetrahydro indane) 1.5% Toxaphene* (chlorinated camphene) 2.25%
FASCO ALDRIN EQUIVALENT-DDT-S 2-1/2 to 5 to 40 DUST Insecticide (Florida Agric.)	Aldrin*(hexachloro hexahydro dimethano naphthalene) 2-1/2% DDT* (dichloro diphenyl trichloroethane) 5% Sulfur* 40%		

*Consult Sec. II., Ingredients Index. This ingredient may be responsible for major toxic effects if poisonous amounts of this product are ingested.

Name & Use Manufacturer	Ingredients	Name & Use Manufacturer	Ingredients
FASCO CONDITIONED SULPHUR 93 Insecticide (Florida Agric.)	Sulfur* 93%	FASCO 50% DDT DUST CONC. Insecticide (Florida Agric.)	Dichloro diphenyl trichloro-ethane* 50%
FASCO CONDITIONED SULPHUR 96 Insecticide (Florida Agric.)	Sulfur* 96%	FASCO DDT LIQUID 25 Insecticide (Florida Agric.)	Dichloro diphenyl trichloro-ethane* 25%
FASCO COPPER-DDT MIXTURE NO. 14-3 Insecticide, fungicide (Florida Agric.)	Dichloro diphenyl trichloro ethane* 3% Copper* expressed as metallic from basic copper sulfate 7.25%	FASCO 50% DDT WETTABLE Insecticide (Florida Agric.)	Dichloro diphenyl trichloro-ethane* 50%
FASCO COPPER-DDT DUST 18-5 Insecticide, fungicide (Florida Agric.)	Dichloro diphenyl trichloro-ethane* 5% Copper* expressed as metallic from basic copper sulfate 9.3%	FASCO DEE-TERP Insecticide (Florida Agric.)	Toxaphene* (chlorinated camphene) 4 lb. 1 gal. DDT (dichloro diphenyl trichloroethane) 2 lb. 1 gal.
FASCO 3-5 COTTON DUST Insecticide (Florida Agric.)	Gamma BHC* (benzene hexachloride) 3% DDT* (dichloro diphenyl trichloroethane) 5%	FASCO DEFLOCCUL-ATED LEAD ARSENATE Insecticide (Florida Agric.)	Lead arsenate* 98%
FASCO 3-5-40 COTTON DUST Insecticide (Florida Agric.)	Gamma BHC* (benzene hexachloride) 3% DDT* (dichloro diphenyl trichloroethane) 5% Sulfur* 40%	FASCO DIEL-D DUST 15-5 Insecticide (Florida Agric.)	Dieldrin* (hexachloro epoxy octahydro dimethano naphthalene) 1.275% DDT* (dichloro diphenyl trichloroethane) 5%
FASCO 3-10 COTTON DUST Insecticide (Florida Agric.)	Gamma BHC* (benzene hexachloride) 3% DDT* (dichloro diphenyl trichloroethane) 10%	FASCO DIEL-D LIQUID 6-2 Insecticide (Florida Agric.)	Dieldrin* (hexachloro epoxy octahydro dimethano naphthalene) 5.85% DDT* (dichloro diphenyl trichloroethane) 23.20%
FASCO 3-10-40 COTTON DUST Insecticide (Florida Agric.)	Gamma BHC* (benzene hexachloride) 3% DDT* (dichloro diphenyl trichloroethane) 10% Sulfur* 40%	FASCO DIEL-D-SUL DUST 15-5-40 Insecticide (Florida Agric.)	Dieldrin* (hexachloro epoxy octahydro dimethano napthalene) 1.275% DDT* (dichloro diphenyl trichloroethane) 5% Sulfur* 40%
FASCO CRYOBAM 26 DUST Insecticide (Florida Agric.)	Sodium fluoaluminate* 18% Zineb (fine ethylene-bis-(dithiocarbamate)) 4%	FASCO DIEL DUST 15 Insecticide (Florida Agric.)	Hexachloro epoxy octahydro dimethano naphthalene* (from dieldrin) 1.275% Related compounds (from dieldrin) 0.225%
FASCO DDD 50-WP Insecticide (Florida Agric.)	Dichloro diphenyl dichloro-ethane* 50%	FASCO DINI-O-SPRAY NO. 3 Insecticide (Florida Agric.)	DN* (dinitro-o-cyclohexylphenol) 2.5% Sulfur* 87.5%
FASCO 5% DDT DUST Insecticide (Florida Agric.)	Dichloro diphenyl trichloro-ethane* 5% Inert ingredients		
FASCO 10% DDT DUST Insecticide (Florida Agric.)	DDT* 10.00%		

*Consult Sec. II., Ingredients Index. This ingredient may be responsible for major toxic effects if poisonous amounts of this product are ingested.

Name & Use Manufacturer	Ingredients	Name & Use Manufacturer	Ingredients
FASCO ENDURO NEUTRAL C-Z-S 15 Insecticide, fungicide (Florida Agric.)	Copper* as metallic (basic copper sulfate) 6.3% Zinc* 6.3% Sulfur* 68%	FASCO NEUTRAL 1-F-N NO. 4 Insecticide (Florida Agric.)	Copper* (basic copper sulfate) 7.5% Zinc* 2.5% Manganese* 5% Sulfur* 64%
FASCO ENDURO NEUTRAL Z-S 3-10 Insecticide (Florida Agric.)	Sulfur* 74% Zinc* 9%	FASCO NU-TRI-COP Fungicide (Florida Agric.)	Copper* expressed as metallic from basic copper sulfate in tri basic form 46.25%
FASCO FUME EDB-40 Fumigant (Florida Agric.)	Ethylene dibromide* 40%	FASCO NU-TRI-HI-COP Fungicide (Florida Agric.)	Copper* as metallic from brown copper oxide 70%
FASCO HEPTA 25-DB Insecticide (Florida Agric.)	Heptachlor* (heptachloro tetrahydro-4,7-methano indane) 25.0% Related compounds 12.5%	FASCO PARA-BAMATE DUST 1-6 Insecticide (Florida Agric.)	Parathion*(o,o-diethyl-o,p-nitrophenyl thiophosphate) 1% Zineb (zinc ethylene bis-(dithiocarbamate)) 6%
FASCO HEPTA COTTON DUST 2-1/2 to 5 Insecticide (Florida Agric.)	Heptachlor* (heptachloro tetrahydro-4, 7-methano indane) 2-1/2% DDT (dichloro diphenyl trichloroethane)* 5%	FASCO PARATHION DUST 100 Insecticide (Florida Agric.)	Parathion* (o,o-Diethyl-o,p-nitrophenyl thiophosphate) 1%
FASCO HEPTA COTTON DUST 2-1/2%-5-40 Insecticide (Florida Agric.)	Heptachlor* (heptachloro tetrahydro-4, 7-methano indane) 2.5% DDT* (dichloro diphenyl trichloroethane) 5% Sulfur* 40%	FASCO PARATHION LIQUID 25 Insecticide (Florida Agric.)	o,o-Diethyl, o,p-nitrophenyl thiophosphate 25%
FASCO KYROMIX 20 Insecticide (Florida Agric.)	Sodium fluoaluminate* 18% Sulfur 72%	FASCO PARATHION-SULPHUR MIXTURE NO. 25-PS Insecticide (Florida Agric.)	Parathion* (o,o-Diethyl-o,p-nitrophenyl thiophosphate) 2.5% Sulfur 75%
FASCO KRYOMIX 30 Insecticide (Florida Agric.)	Sodium fluoaluminate* 27% Sulfur 63%	FASCO PARATHION 15-WP Insecticide (Florida Agric.)	Parathion* wettable (o,o-diethyl-o,p-nitrophenyl thiophosphate) 15%
FASCO NEUTRAL 1-F-N NO. 2 Insecticide (Florida Agric.)	Copper* (basic copper sulfate) 5% Zinc* 6% Manganese* 4% Sulfur* 64%		

Name & Use Manufacturer	Ingredients	Name & Use Manufacturer	Ingredients
FASCO PARZATE DUST 6-1/2 Fungicide (Florida Agric.)	Zineb (zinc ethylene-bis-(dithiocarbamate)) 6.5%	FASCO SEMINOLE NEUTRAL C-Z-S 15 Insecticide, fungicide (Florida Agric.)	Copper* as metallic (basic copper sulfate) 6.3% Zinc* 6.3% Sulfur* 69%
FASCO PARZATE-DDT DUST 6-1/2 to 5 Insecticide (Florida Agric.)	Dichloro diphenyl trichloroethane 5% Zinc ethylene bis(dithio-carbamate 6.5% Inert ingredients*	FASCO SEMINOLE NEUTRAL Z-S 3-10 Insecticide (Florida Agric.)	Sulfur* 75% Zinc* 9%
FASCO PARZATE LIQUID NABAM Fungicide (Florida Agric.)	Nabam* (disodium ethylene-bis-(dithiocarbamate)) 19%	FASCO SULPHUR-DDT DUST NO. 75-10 Insecticide (Florida Agric.)	Dichloro diphenyl trichloroethane* 10% Sulfur* 75%
FASCO P-D-Q SPRAY NO. 1 Insecticide (Florida Agric.)	Parathion* (o, o-diethyl-o, p-nitrophenyl thiophosphate) 3.75% DDD wettable (dichloro diphenyl dichloroethane) 25.0%	FASCO SULPHUR-DDT 84-5 DUST Insecticide (Florida Agric.)	Sulfur* 84% Dichloro diphenyl trichloroethane* 5%
FASCO P-D-Q SPRAY NO. 2 Insecticide (Florida Agric.)	Parathion* (o, o-diethyl, o, p-nitrophenyl thiophosphate) 3.75% DDD wettable (dichloro diphenyl dichloroethane) 37.50%	FASCO SULPHUR-DDT DUST 88-3 Insecticide (Florida Agric.)	Dichloro diphenyl trichloroethane 3% Sulfur* 88%
FASCO P-D-Q TOBACCO DUST NO. 3 Insecticide (Florida Agric.)	Parathion* (o, o-diethyl-o, p-nitrophenyl thiophosphate) 1% DDD or TDE (dichloro diphenyl dichloroethane) 5%	FASCO SUPERFINE FLOWER SULPHUR Insecticide (Florida Agric.)	Sulfur* 99.5%
FASCO P-D-Q TOBACCO PLANT BED DUST Insecticide (Florida Agric.)	Parathion* (o, o-diethyl-o, p-nitrophenyl thiophosphate) 1% DDT (dichloro diphenyl trichloroethane) 3% Zineb 6.5%	FASCO TEPP 40 Insecticide (Florida Agric.)	TEPP (tetraethyl pyrophosphate)* 40%
FASCO ROTENONE DUST 100 Insecticide (Florida Agric.)	Rotenone 1%	FASCO TERPENE BAIT 225 Insecticide (Florida Agric.)	Toxaphene* (chlorinated camphene) 2.25%
FASCO ROTENONE 4-WP Insecticide (Florida Agric.)		FASCO TERPENE DUST 10 Insecticide (Florida Agric.)	Toxaphene* (chlorinated camphene) 10%
FASCO ROTENONE-SULPHUR DUST 1-65 Insecticide (Florida Agric.)	Rotenone 1% Sulfur* 65%	FASCO TERPENE LIQUID 58 Insecticide (Florida Agric.)	Toxaphene* (chlorinated camphene 58%) 6 lbs. per gal.
FASCO ROTENONE-SULPHUR 75-S Insecticide (Florida Agric.)	Rotenone 0.75% Sulfur* 75%	FASCO TERPENE 70 LIQUID Insecticide (Florida Agric.)	Toxaphene* (chlorinated camphene 70%) 90%

*Consult Sec. II., Ingredients Index. This ingredient may be responsible for major toxic effects if poisonous amounts of this product are ingested.

Name & Use Manufacturer	Ingredients		Name & Use Manufacturer	Ingredients	
FASCO ZERLATE FUNGICIDE Fungicide (Florida Agric.)	Ziram*	70%	FATAL DOZE FOR ROACH & WATER-BUG (Bohman)	Sodium fluoride* Borax* Pyrethrins	6% 69% 0.12%
FASCO ZINEB DUST NO. 6 Fungicide (Florida Agric.)	Zineb (zinc ethylene-bis-(dithiocarbamate))	4%	FATAL DOZE INSECTICIDE (Bohman)	Pyrethrum* Borax*	
FASTCOTE Paint (Louisville Varnish)			FATAL DOZE RAT & ROACH PASTE (Bohman)	Phosphorus*	
FAST COURT GYM FINISH Floor finish (Lester)			FATAL DOZE RAT KILLER (Bohman)	Phosphorous* Warfarin (3-(a-acetonylbenzyl)-4-hydroxycoumarin)	
FAST CUT, HAND (Park Chem.)	Kerosene* Soap Pine oil* Abrasives		FATHER JOHN'S MEDICINE Tonic (Father John's)	Cod liver oil Gum arabic Glycerin Sugar Licorice Flavoring oils	
FAST CUT, WHEEL (Park Chem.)	Kerosene* Sulfonated oil* Abrasives		FATHER & SON AFTER SHAVE LOTION (M. E.)		
FASTEETH Denture adhesive (Clark-Cleveland)	Karaya (sterculia) gum, N.F. IX (pH 8.4) Oil of peppermint, U.S.P. 1%		FATHER TIME SPAR VARNISH (Perfection Paint)		
FAST-FIVE ENAMELS (Frost Paint)			FATSCO ANT POISON Insecticide (Fatsco)	Sodium arsenate*	3%
FASTRIP WALLPAPER REMOVER (United Gilson.)	Anionic wetting agent		FAULTLESS HALFTONE INK (General Printing)		
FAST WORK ANALGESIC Rubefacient, (Ellis, H. G.)	Alcohol 60% Methyl salicylate* Camphor Volatile oil of mustard* Menthol* Capsicum*		FAUNTLEROY STARCH (Home Needs)	Cornstarch Dowicide "A" Sodium chloride Dye Perfume	
FAST WORK RUB Rubefacient, (Ellis, H. G.)	Methyl salicylate* Camphor* Turpentine* Oleoresin capsicum* Menthol* Eucalyptol*		F & B ALL PURPOSE SPRAY OR DUST Insecticide, fungicide (Faesy & Besthoff)	Captan Malathion* Methoxychlor*	8.33% 4.16% 8.33%
FATAL Rodenticide (Bonide)	Warfarin (3-(a-acetonylbenzyl)-4-hydroxycoumarin) 0.025%		F & B CHLORDANE 5% DUST Insecticide (Faesy & Besthoff)	Chlordane*	5%
FATAL DOZE Insecticide (Bohman)	Lethane*		F & B CHLORDANE 72% SPRAY Insecticide (Faesy & Besthoff)	Tech. chlordane*	73.7%
FATAL DOZE FOR FLIES & MOS-QUITOES (Bohman)	Pyrethrum				

*Consult Sec. II., Ingredients Index. This ingredient may be responsible for major toxic effects if poisonous amounts of this product are ingested.

Name & Use Manufacturer	Ingredients		Name & Use Manufacturer	Ingredients	
F & B DDT 25% SPRAY Insecticide (Faesy & Besthoff)	DDT*	24.8%	F.C.X. 20-0 COTTON DUST Insecticide (Farmers)	Toxaphene*	20.00%
F & B DORMANT SPRAY Insecticide (Faesy & Besthoff)	Petroleum oil*	96%	F.C.X. CRYO-DIL 70-30 DUST Insecticide (Farmers)	Sodium fluoaluminate*	70%
F & B DRAINPIPE CLEANER-CESSPOOL SOLVENT (Faesy & Besthoff)	Sodium hydroxide*		F.C.X. 5% DDT DUST Insecticide (Farmers)	DDT*	5.00%
F & B CRAB GRASS KILLER (Faesy & Besthoff)	Potassium cyanate*	77.35%	F.C.X. 10% DDT DUST Insecticide (Farmers)	DDT*	10.00%
F & B LIME SULPHUR SOLUTION Fungicide (Faesy & Besthoff)	Calcium polysulfides* (total sulfur in solution 24.0%)	30.0%	F.C.X. FERBAM DUST NO. 10 Insecticide (Farmers)	Ferric dimethyl dithiocarbamate	11.40%
F & B MALATHION 50% SPRAY Insecticide (Faesy & Besthoff)	Malathion*	56.4%	F.C.X. 1% LINDANE DUST Insecticide (Farmers)	Gamma isomer of BHC (from lindane)	1.00%
F & B POTASSIUM CYANATE CRAB GRASS KILLER (Faesy & Besthoff)	Tech. potassium cyanate* powder	77%	F.C.X. 1-1/2% LINDANE DUST Insecticide (Farmers)	Gamma isomer of BHC (from lindane)	1.50%
F & B ROSE DUST WITH CAPTAN Insecticide, fungicide (Faesy & Besthoff)	Captan Malathion* DDT* Karathane	7.50% 5.00% 5.00% .75%	F.C.X. 5% MALATHION DUST Insecticide (Farmers)	Malathion*	5%
			F.C.X. 5% METHOXY-CHLOR Insecticide (Farmers)	Methoxychlor	5.00%
F.C.X. 7% COPPER DUST Insecticide (Farmers)	Copper as metallic*	7.00%	F.C.X. 1% PARATHION DUST Insecticide (Farmers)	Parathion*	1.00%
F.C.X. COPPER SULPHUR PEANUT DUST Insecticide (Farmers)	Copper* as metallic Sulfur*	4.00% 85.56%	F.C.X. POTATO DUST Insecticide (Farmers)	Copper* as metallic DDT*	7.00% 3.00%
F.C.X. 3-5-0 COTTON DUST Insecticide (Farmers)	Gamma isomer of BHC* DDT*	3.00% 5.00%	F.C.X. ROSE DUST Insecticide (Farmers)	Ferric dimethyl dithiocarbamate DDT* Sulfur*	7.60% 5.00% 75.00%
F.C.X. 3-5-40 COTTON DUST Insecticide (Farmers)	Gamma isomer of BHC* DDT* Sulfur*	3.00% 5.00% 40.00%	F.C.X. ROTOX NO. 75 Insecticide (Farmers)	Rotenone	0.75%
			F.C.X. ROTOX NO. 100 Insecticide (Farmers)	Rotenone	1.00%

*Consult Sec. II., Ingredients Index. This ingredient may be responsible for major toxic effects if poisonous amounts of this product are ingested.

Name & Use Manufacturer	Ingredients	
F.C.X. SABA-DIL NO. 10 Insecticide (Farmers)	Sabadilla seed*	10.00%
	Sabadilla alkaloids*	0.42%
F.C.X. SABA-DIL NO. 20 Insecticide (Farmers)	Sabadilla seed*	20.00%
	Sabadilla alkaloids*	0.80%
F.C.X. 5% TDE DUST Insecticide (Farmers)	DDD	5.00%
F.C.X. 10% TDE DUST Insecticide (Farmers)	DDD*	10.00%
F.C.X. 50% WETTABLE CHLORDANE POWDER Insecticide (Farmers)	Tech. chlordane*	50.00%
F.C.X. 6.5% ZINEB DUST Insecticide (Farmers)	Zinc ethylene-bis (dithio-carbamate)	6.50%
F & D MIXTURE Astringent for intestinal irritation (Humco)	Alcohol	33%
	Black catechu	
	Capsicum	
	Menthol	
	Camphor gum	
	Peppermint	
F.D. SHOE FUNGICIDIAL FUMIGANT (Noble)	Paraformaldehyde* (polyoxymethylene glycol)	
	Camphor*	
FEARONCE MEDICATED TAR POMADE (Fearonce)		
FEATHER BRAND PAINT (Irwin)		
FEATHERINE For birds (Clayton)		
FEBRIN Analgesic (Jenkins)	Each tablet:	
	Acetophenetidin*	1-1/2 gr.
	Acetylsalicylic acid*	2 gr.
	Caffeine*	1/4 gr.
	Camphor monobromated*	1 gr.
FEBRINETTS Antipyretic (Jenkins)	Acetophenetidin*	1/2 gr.
	Acid acetylsalicylic*	1 gr.
	Camphor monobromated	1/40 gr.
	Caffeine	1/20 gr.
FEDCO PAINTS (Federal Paint)		

Name & Use Manufacturer	Ingredients	
FEDERAL ANTI-FOULING PAINT (Federal Paint)	Cuprous oxide	4.4%
	Copper soap	18.1%
	Arsenious oxide*	9.8%
	Copper sulfate pentahydrate	7.9%
	Mercury soap	0.9%
	Copper as a metal	7.3%
	Arsenic as a metal	7.0%
	Mercury as a metal	0.3%
FEDERALETE VARNISH (Federal Varnish)		
FEDERAL HTS ANTI-FOULING PAINT (Federal Paint)	Metallic copper* pigment (copper expressed as metallic 26.4%)	29.3%
	Zinc oxide	10.3%
FEDERATED HALFTONE INK (General Printing)		
FEDREX Antispasmodic for allergies (Veltex)	Each tablet:	
	Ephedrine sulfate	1/3 gr.
	Calcium lactate	1-1/2 gr.
	Vitamin D	200 U.S.P. units
	Vitamin C	100 mg.
FEDROLIN Nasal de-congestant (Western Pharm.)	Ephedrine alkaloids	1/3%
	Mineral oil	q.s.
FEDROLIN AROMATIC Nasal de-congestant (Western Pharm.)	Ephedrine	3/4%
	Chlorthymol*	0.03%
	Aromatics	1%
	Camphor*	
	Menthol*	
	Oil peppermint	
	Eucalyptol*	
	Mineral oil	q.s.
FEDROLIN ISOTONIC Nasal de-congestant (Western Pharm.)	Ephedrine hydrochloride	1%
	Chlorobutanol (chloroform deriv.) in aromatized Ringer's solution	0.5%
FEDROLIN PLAIN Nasal de-congestant (Western Pharm.)	Ephedrine	3/4%
	Mineral oil	q.s.
FEEN-A-MINT (Medicated Gum) Cathartic (Pharmaco)	Phenolphthalein	
	Sugar	
	Starch	
	Chewing gum base	
FEE-TONE Foot de-odorant (Carolina)	Alum	
	Boric acid*	
	Tannic acid*	
	Glycerin	
	Isopropyl alcohol*	12%
FELCHOLAN Biliary disease (Fellows)	Each tablet:	
	Choline desoxycholate	32.5 mg.
	Choline cholate	32.5 mg.
	Choline salt of conjugated bile acids	130.0 mg.

*Consult Sec. II., Ingredients Index. This ingredient may be responsible for major toxic effects if poisonous amounts of this product are ingested.

Name & Use Manufacturer	Ingredients		Name & Use Manufacturer	Ingredients	
FELLO-SED Sedative (Fellows)	Each tbsp.: Chloral hydrate* Calcium bromide* Atropine sulfate Alcohol content	0.5 gm. 0.5 gm. 0.125 mg. 1%	FEMME EAU DE TOILETTE (Rochas)		
FELLOW'S COMPOUND SYRUP (Fellows)	Each 4 cc.: Strychnine hydrochloride* Quinine sulfate Calcium hydrophosphite Iron pyrophosphate Manganese hypophosphite Potassium hypophosphite Sodium hypophosphite	1 mg. 3 mg. 20 mg. 8 mg. 8 mg. 8 mg. 8 mg.	FEN ANTI- MILDEW, BACTERIA, MOLD INHIBITOR (Amalg. Chem.)	Phenyl mercuric acetate* 4.5%	
			FENCH OIL For throat irritations (Rothenberger)	Gum camphor* Methyl salicylate* Oil of turpentine* Oleoresin capsicum Oil of camphor* Essential oils	
FELSO Detergent (Fels)	Sodium alkyl aryl sulfonate*		FEND DERMATITIS CREAM (Carbisulphoil)		
FELSOL Analgesic, antitussive (Am. Felsol)	Antipyrine* Iodopyrine Citrated caffeine	0.869 gm. 0.031 gm. 0.100 gm.	DR. FENNER'S ANTISEPTIC OINTMENT For skin burns and irritations (Wells, S. C.)	Benzocaine Origanum Venice turpentine* Oil of nutmeg Sassafras Balsam of fir Special base	
FEL-SPAR Varnish (Felton Sibley)					
FELTON SIBLEY OIL RESISTANT GRAY MACHINERY PAINT #2 (Felton Sibley)	Lampblack dry Titanium dioxide Lithopone* Zinc oxide Linseed dehydrated castor oil phenolic resin varnish Cobalt metal Lead as metal Manganese as metal	0.525% 2.310% 30.900% 0.736% 65.300% 0.027% 0.240% 0.023%	DR. FENNER'S GOLDEN RELIEF Carminative and rube- facient (Wells, S. C.)	Each fl. oz.: Alcohol* Chloroform Turpentine* Gum myrrh Aromatic oils Ether Capsicum Ammonia* Gum guaiac	65% 5 m. 22 m.
FEMELLE Douche powder (Hale)	Boric acid* Lactose Menthol* Aromatics Lactic acid Sodium lauryl sulfate Eucalyptol* Certified color		FEPISEM PINK Antispasmodic for asthma (Massengill)	Each capsule: Pentobarbital sodium* Acetophenetidin* Atropine sulfate Ephedrine sulfate*	16 mg. 0.2 gm 0.43 mg. 16 mg.
			FERA FLOW PAINT (Am. Abrasive)		
FEM-HY Douche (Diefenbach)	Solution of 4-n-amyl-meta- cresol Chlorothymol Acidum lacticum Oleum lavandulae S.A.	0.2% 0.1% 1.0%	FERCALCIUM- D TABLETS (Campbell Pharm.)	Ferrous sulfate Dicalcium phosphate Vitamin D	3 gr. 5 gr. 333 U.S.P. units
FEMISOL ANTISEPTIC POWDER (Leslie Pharm.)			FERDICO AVIATION LIQUID MARINE GLUE (Ferdinand)	Resins in petroleum solvents*	
FEMME BATH OIL (Rochas)			FERDICO CANVAS CEMENT (Ferdinand)	Resins in petroleum solvents*	
FEMME de PARIS INFUSION de PARFUM (Ybry)			FERDICO CANVAS CEMENT NO. 72 (Ferdinand)	Pentachlorophenol*	
FEMME EAU DE COLOGNE AND PER- FUME (Rochas)			FERDICO CANVAS PATCHING ADHESIVE (Ferdinand)		

*Consult Sec. II., Ingredients Index. This ingredient may be responsible for major toxic effects if poisonous amounts of this product are ingested.

Name & Use Manufacturer	Ingredients	Name & Use Manufacturer	Ingredients
FERDICO DOUBLE X CEMENT NO. 40 (Ferdinand)	Pentachlorophenol*	FERDISEAL #21 Glue (Ferdinand)	Resins in alcohol solvent *
FERDICO FABRIC CEMENT (Ferdinand)		FERDISEAL LIQUID MARINE GLUE (Ferdinand)	Resins in petroleum solvents *
FERDICO FERRULE STICK NO. 151 Cement (Ferdinand)		FERDISEAL LIQUID MARINE SEALER (Ferdinand)	
FERDICO-JEFFREY'S BOAT CAULKING COMPOUND (Ferdinand)		FER-HEPATIS Food supplement with iron (Daniels, Robert)	Each tablet: Ferrous sulfate U.S.P. 3-3/5 gr. Liver desiccated 7 gr. Thiamine chloride (B1) 0.5 mg. Riboflavin (B2) 1.0 mg. Nicotinamide 5 mg.
FERDICO LINOLEUM PASTE & CEMENT (Ferdinand)	Resins	FERLICON Tonic (White, R. P.)	Alcohol 10% Liver extract 800 mg. Cascara sagrada 390 gm. Vitamin B1 1000 U.S.P. units Vitamin B2 1200 mg. Nicotinic acid 12 mg. Other B complex factors
FERDICO LIQUID WATER-PROOFING (Ferdinand)	Resins in petroleum solvents*		
FERDICO MARINE GLUE AND CEMENT NO. 450 (Ferdinand)		15% FERMATE DUST Fungicide (Cotton)	Ferbam (ferric dimethyldithio-carbamate) 11.40%
		FERMATE FERBAM FUNGICIDE (du Pont)	Ferbam (ferric dimethyldithio-carbamate)*
FERDICO PATCHING ADHESIVE #100 (Ferdinand)	Dispersion of rubber in water	FERRADOW Fungicide (Dow)	Ferbam* 76%
FERDICO PLYWOOD GLUE NO. 690 (Ferdinand)		FERRATE TABLETS Food supplement with iron, tablet (Barnes-Hind)	Each tablet: Ferrous gluconate 0.325 gm.
FERDICO PRIMER #630 Paint produce (Ferdinand)	Resins in petroleum solvent*	FERRI-FLOG Soil nutrient (Tenn. Corp.)	Metallic iron 20%
FERDICO THINNER NO. 600 Paint product (Ferdinand)	Pentachlorophenol *	FERRO-BOND VARNISHES (Con-Ferro)	
FERDICO WING DOPE Glue (Ferdinand)	Nitrocellulose solution*	FERRODEX METAL CLEANER (MacDermid)	
FERDICO XX CEMENT (Ferdinand)	Resins in petroleum solvents *	FERROLASTIC PAINTS (McDougall-Butler)	
FERDINAND'S CANOE GLUE (Ferdinand)	Asphalt Resins	FERROLIFE METAL PAINTS (Stewart Bros.)	

Name & Use Manufacturer	Ingredients		Name & Use Manufacturer	Ingredients	
FERRONEED Food supplement with iron, capsule (Hanlon)	Each capsule: Ferrous gluconate N.F. Ascorbic acid U.S.P.	5 gr. 20 mg.	F & F LOZENGES (Licorice Flavored) (F & F)	Menthol* Sodium salicylate* Eucalyptol* White pine Wild cherry Licorice	
FERROSATE Food supplement with iron, tablet (Kenmore)	Exsiccated ferrous sulfate U.S.P.		F & F SYRUP Antitussive (F & F)	Alcohol Chloroform Beechwood creosote* Eucalyptol*	1% 2-1/2 m. per oz.
FERRO-SEALS B COMPLEX Food supplement with iron, tablet (Bishop)	Each tablet: Ferrous sulfate exsiccated Vitamin B1 Vitamin B2 Nicotinic acid	3 gr. 0.33 mg. 0.66 mg. 5 mg.		Menthol* Sodium citrate Potassium guaiacol sulfonate Ammonium chloride White pine Wild cherry	
FERROTYPE PLATE POLISH Photographic supplies (Eastman)			FIBRECOR INKS (Sinclair & V.)		
FERRUBRON METAL PAINT (Ferrubron)			FIDELITY BRANDING FLUID Veterinary (Fidelity Labs.)	Sodium hydroxide* Sodium sulfide* Barium sulfide*	
FERTILIZER BORATE HIGH GRADE (Pacific Coast)	Sodium oxide* Boron trioxide* Equivalent boron	20.0% 44.8% 13.9%	FIDELITY DEHORNING PASTE Veterinary (Fidelity Labs.)	Sodium hydroxide* Calcium hydroxide	42%
FERTILIZER BORATE REGULAR (Pacific Coast)	Sodium oxide* Boron trioxide* Equivalent boron	15.0% 34.2% 10.6%	FIDELITY DRESSING OIL Veterinary (Fidelity Labs.)	Paraffin base oil Aniline oil, soluble red* Aromatic essential oils	
FESCO SEALER COATER (Felton Sibley)			FIDELITY MILK OIL DIP AND DIS- INFECTANT Insecticide (Fidelity Labs.)	Phenols* Coal tar oils* Soap	16% 56% 17%
FETEX (Southern Labs.)	Salicylic acid* Benzoic acid Coal tar* Iodine * Ether Alcohol* Acetone	70%	FIDELITY PHENO- THIAZINE TABLETS Anthelmintic (veterinary) (Fidelity Labs.)	Each tablet: Phenothiazine N.F.*	1.774 gm.
FETHERZIP POULTRY WAX (Nat'l. Wax)					
FEVER JR. Antipyretic, tablet (Jenkins)	Each tablet: Acid acetylsalicylic* Tincture aconite Tinc. belladonna Tinc. bryonia Tinc. eupatorium	1 gr. 1/8 m. 1/16 m. 1/10 m. 1/8 m.	FIDELITY PHENO- THIAZINE TABLETS Anthelmintic (veterinary, avian) (Fidelity Labs.)	Each tablet: Phenothiazine N.F.*	0.444 gm.
F & F COUGH LOZENGES (F & F)	Menthol* Beechwood creosote* Eucalyptol* Horehound White pine Wild cherry		FIDELITY SODIUM FLUORIDE (Tinted) Insecticide (Fidelity Labs.)	Sodium fluoride*	95%
F & F COUGH LOZENGES (Cherry Flavored) (F & F)	Wild cherry White pine Menthol* Eucalyptol* Balsam tolu				

*Consult Sec. II., Ingredients Index. This ingredient may be responsible for major toxic effects if poisonous amounts of this product are ingested.

- 491 -

Name & Use Manufacturer	Ingredients	Name & Use Manufacturer	Ingredients
FIDELITY SULFA- NILAMIDE TABLETS Veterinary (Fidelity Labs.)	Sulfanilamide* 60 gr.	52ND STREET PERFUME (Scandia)	
FIEBING'S ANTIQUE FINISH Leather polish (Fiebing)	Candelilla wax Castile soap Turpentine*	FILCOTONE Stain & Filler (Glidden Co.)	
		FILMRITE FILM CLEANER (Rosco)	
FIEBING'S BLACK SHOE DYE (Fiebing)	Denatured alcohol* Orthodichlorobenzene* Diethylene glycol monoethyl ether* Nigrosine	FILTRAY LOTION Sun tan lotion (Carmel)	Para-aminobenzoic acid 10% Alcohol* 59%
FIEBING'S BLACK SOLE & HEEL DRESSING (Fiebing)	Lacca Borax* Gelatine adhesive Sodium oleate Anhydrous ammonia* Terpine hydrate* Terpenes*	FINE ART TOILET SOAP (Armour)	Soda salts of coconut oil Fine tallow
		FINE-ART SCULPTORS' CLAY (Am. Art Clay)	
FIEBING'S BOOT POLISH (Fiebing)	Carnauba wax Montan wax Paraffin wax Turpentine* Mineral spirits* Silicone oil	DR. FINE'S PINK-KAPS (Rafea)	Each capsule: Acetylsalicylic acid* 3-1/2 gr. Acetophenetidin* (acetanilid derivative) 2-1/2 gr. Caffeine alkaloid 1/2 gr.
FIEBING'S CARE FOR LEATHER AND SHOES (Fiebing)	Crown wax Sodium stearate Sodium palmitate Gelatine adhesive Phenol* Glycerol Pine oil*	FINESS ALUMINUM CHLORIDE 25% Deodorant (Halsey)	Aluminum chloride 25% Urea 5%
FIEBING'S FACTORY TYPE BOOT POLISH (Fiebing)	Carnauba wax Montan wax Paraffin wax Turpentine* Mineral spirits* Silicone oil	FINESSE HAIR DRESSING FOR NEGROES (Humbert)	
		FINESSE SHAMPOO (Montenier)	Ammonium lauryl sulfate lanum Methyl cellulose
FIEBING'S IMPROVED ANTIQUE FINISH Leather polish (Fiebing)	Carnauba wax Candelilla wax Castile soap Turpentine*	FINEST OIL COLORS (Grumbacher)	
		FINEX-L REPLENISHER Photographic supply (Ansco)	
FIEBING'S PRIME NEATSFOOT OIL COM- POUND (Fiebing)	Neatsfoot oil Paraffin oil	FINISH Detergent (Economics)	Sodium phosphate* Sodium silicate Sodium hypochlorite*
		FINISH RUB (Park Chem.)	Water Kerosene* Soap Pine oil* Abrasives
FIEBING'S SADDLE SOAP (Fiebing)	Tallow Rosin Sodium carbonate Borax* Sodium hydroxide Japan wax Carnauba wax Palm oil Denatured alcohol* Oil of citronella*	FINNELL CRYSTAL CLEANER (Finnell)	
		FINNELL GLOSS-SEAL Floor wax (Finnell)	
FIENDOIL Lubricating oil (McCambridge)	Petroleum oil Sulfonated petroleum residue	FINNELL KOTE Floor wax (Finnell)	

*Consult Sec. II., Ingredients Index. This ingredient may be responsible for major toxic effects if poisonous amounts of this product are ingested.

Name & Use Manufacturer	Ingredients		Name & Use Manufacturer	Ingredients	
FINO KOTE Floor treatment (Finnell)			FIRZITE Wood sealer (U. S. Plywood)	Dry oils Resins Varnish solvents*	
FINOLA Scouring powder (Finnell)			FITCHMUL (Fitch, A.)	Alcohol Chloroform Fir balsam Venice turpentine* Hydrocyanic acid* Tartar emetic* Aromatics	12% 2 m. in each fl. oz.
FINO RUG SHAMPOO (Finnell)			FITCH'S BRILLIAN-TINES (Fitch, F. W.)		
FIREBOLD PAINT (Cheesman-Elliott)			FITCH'S DANDRUFF REMOVER SHAMPOO (Fitch, F. W.)		
FIRE STOPPER Fire extinguisher (Advance Merch.)			FITCH HAIR OILS (Grove)	Mineral oil U.S.P. Deodorized kerosene Perfume oil	
FIRST DANCE TOILET WATER (Masie)			FITCH'S IDEAL HAIR DRESSING (Fitch, F. W.)		
FIRMA-GRIP WHITE PASTE (Binney & Smith)			FITCH'S ROSE HAIR DRESSING W/LANOLIN (Fitch, F. W.)		
FIRST DATE TOILET WATER (Masie)			FITCH'S SHAMPOO (Grove)	Cocoanut oil soap Perfume oil Denatured alcohol No. 40	40%
FIRST KOTE OVER SEALER (Johnston)			FITCH'S SKIN PEP AFTER SHAVE LOTION (Fitch, F. W.)		
FIRST NATIONAL ANTISEPTIC MOUTH WASH (First National Labs.)	Eucalyptol* Thymol* Menthol* Methyl salicylate* Indigo root Boric acid* Benzoic acid		FITCH'S WAVE SET (Grove)	Gum karaya Isopropyl alcohol Perfume	1/2%
FIRST NATIONAL DIS-O-FECT Disinfectant, deodorant (First National Labs.)	Pine oil soap*	90%	FITOE FOR ATHLETES' FOOT (Whitman)	Alcohol* Salicylic acid* Glycerin Oil of peppermint	73%
			FIVE AND ONE DEODORANT (Kinreco)	Aluminum chloride*	
FIRST NATIONAL KILLS-EM INSECT SPRAY (First National Labs.)	Pyrethrum DDT*	5%	5 DROPS Counter-irritant (Swanson)	Oil of camphor* Menthol* Oil of eucalyptus* Oil of cajuput* Methyl salicylate* Gum camphor	
FIRST ON BURNS (F. O. B., Inc.)	Oxyquinoline sulfate Liquid petrolatum Rosemary oil Oil of linseed Oil of geranium		FIVE NINES Antitussive (Katco)	Alcohol Glycerin White pine bark Sanguinaria Spikenard Beechwood creosote Chloroform Wild cherry bark Balm Gilead buds Sassafras	7% 2 m/oz.
FIRWEIN Antitussive (Tilden)	Per fl. oz.: Sodium bromide White pine Wild cherry	0.55 gm.			

*Consult Sec. II., Ingredients Index. This ingredient may be responsible for major toxic effects if poisonous amounts of this product are ingested.

Name & Use Manufacturer	Ingredients	
FIVE NINES QUICK-AID CAPSULES Analgesic (Katco)	Acetophenetidin* Acetylsalicylic acid* Caffeine	
FIVE O'CLOCK PERFUME (House of Gourielli)		
508 COLOGNES (Assoc. Brands)		
5-WAY PET-KLEEN Insecticide (Bostwick)	Tech. piperonyl butoxide	0.44%
	Pyrethrins	0.044%
	Petroleum oil	0.232%
	Methylene-bis (trichlorophenol)	0.50%
FIXALL ENAMELS PAINTS, AND FINISHES (Louisville Varnish)		
FIX-ALL RUBBER CEMENT (Fix-All)		
FIXALL VARNISH (Louisville Varnish)	Oleo resinous varnish	
FIXOL Photographic supplies (FR)		
FIX SO LIQUID FABRIC MENDER (Alpha Chem.)	Natural latex	
	Sulfur	0.5%
	Zinc	less than 0.5%
	Inert ingredients*	
FIZRIN Antacid (Centaur-Caldwell)	Each packet: Aspirin* Sodium bicarbonate Sodium carbonate Citric acid	
FLACH'S DIURETIC (Flach)	Methenamine Zea mays Couch grass Sabal Senna Glycerin	
FLAG CHLORDANE DUST 3% Insecticide (Flag-Sulphur)	Chlordane*	3%
FLAG CHLORDANE DUST 5% Insecticide (Flag-Sulphur)	Chlordane*	5%
FLAG CHLORDANE DUST BASE 40% Insecticide (Flag-Sulphur)	Chlordane*	40%

Name & Use Manufacturer	Ingredients	
FLAG CHLORDANE WETTABLE BASE 40% Insecticide (Flag-Sulphur)	Chlordane*	40%
FLAG 30% CRYOLITE DUST (Flag-Sulphur)	Sodium fluoaluminate*	27%
FLAG 30% CRYOLITE-6% COPPER Insecticide (Flag-Sulphur)	Sodium fluoaluminate* Copper*	27% 6%
FLAG 30% CRYOLITE-SULPHUR DUST Insecticide (Flag-Sulphur)	Sodium fluoaluminate* Sulfur*	27% 63%
FLAG DDT DUST 3% Insecticide (Flag-Sulphur)	DDT	3%
FLAG DDT DUST 5% Insecticide (Flag-Sulphur)	DDT*	5%
FLAG DDT DUST 10% Insecticide (Flag-Sulphur)	DDT*	10%
FLAG 3% DDT-6% COP-PER DUST Insecticide (Flag-Sulphur)	DDT Copper*	3% 6%
FLAG 25% DDT EMULSION CONCEN-TRATE Insecticide (Flag-Sulphur)	DDT*	25%
FLAG 3% DDT-SULPHUR DUST Insecticide (Flag-Sulphur)	DDT Sulfur*	3% 80%
FLAG 50% DDT WETTABLE BASE Insecticide (Flag-Sulphur)	DDT*	50%
FLAG 3% DDT - 6-1/2% ZEBD DUST Insecticide (Flag-Sulphur)	DDT Zineb	3% 6.5%
FLAG 50% DUST BASE-DDT Insecticide (Flag-Sulphur)	DDT*	50%
FLAG DUSTING SULPHUR Fungicide (Flag-Sulphur)	Sulfur*	90 or 93%

*Consult Sec. II., Ingredients Index. This ingredient may be responsible for major toxic effects if poisonous amounts of this product are ingested.

Name & Use Manufacturer	Ingredients	
FLAG FLORIDA-FLO 90 OIL EMULSION Insecticide (Flag-Sulphur)	Oil	90%
FLAG 1% GAMMA DUST Insecticide (Flag-Sulphur)	Gamma isomer of BHC	1%
FLAG 6% GAMMA DUST BASE Insecticide (Flag-Sulphur)	Gamma isomer of BHC*	6%
FLAG 1% GAMMA-SULPHUR DUST Insecticide (Flag-Sulphur)	Gamma isomer of BHC Sulfur*	1% 80%
FLAG 6% GAMMA WETTABLE BASE Insecticide (Flag-Sulphur)	Gamma isomer of BHC*	6%
FLAG 1% HI-GAMMA-7.5% COPPER Insecticide (Flag-Sulphur)	Gamma BHC Copper as metallic*	1% 7.5%
FLAG 1% PARATHION DUST Insecticide (Flag-Sulphur)	Parathion*	1%
FLAG 1% PARATHION-7.5% COPPER Insecticide (Flag-Sulphur)	Copper Parathion*	7.5% 1%
FLAG 90-10 SULPHUR-MANGANESE DUST Fungicide (Flag-Sulphur)	Sulfur* Manganese	80% 2.25%
FLAG WETTABLE SULPHUR Fungicide (Flag-Sulphur)	Sulfur*	90%
FLAG X-TRA FINE WET-TABLE SULPHUR Fungicide (Flag-Sulphur)	Sulfur*	93%
FLAME-CHEK Checks flames (Chek)		
FLAMEX PAINT (Armor)		

Name & Use Manufacturer	Ingredients	
FLAOGEN Carminative, cathartic (Massengill)	Each tablet: Ext. nux vomica* Strychnine* Ext. cascara sagrada Asafetida Oleoresin ginger Oleoresin capsicum Diastase	1/4 gr. 0.018 gr. 1 gr. 1 gr. 1/26 gr. 1/64 gr. 1/20 gr.
FLASH 16 Floor and wall patch (Allied Comp.)		
FLASH HOUSE & HAND CLEANER (Flash)		
FLASHLITE CEMENT (Ruberoid)		
FLASHO LIGHTER FLUID (Norton)	Petroleum distillate*	
FLASH PROTECTIVE CREAM (Flash)		
FLASHSET WAVESET (Dreyfuss)		
FLASH SILVER POLISH (Flash)		
FLATCOTE PAINT (McMurtry)		
FLAT EFFECT PAINTS (Tibbets)		
FLATINA PAINT (Peerless Paint)		
FLATLUX ENAMEL (Patterson-Sargent)		
FLAT-RITE-ENAMEL UNDER-COATER (Sherwin-Williams)		
FLATTINE PAINT (Standard-Toch)		
FLAT TINT WALL FINISH (Kurfees)		
FLATVAR VARNISH (McDougall-Butler)		

*Consult Sec. II., Ingredients Index. This ingredient may be responsible for major toxic effects if poisonous amounts of this product are ingested.

Name & Use Manufacturer	Ingredients		Name & Use Manufacturer	Ingredients	
FLAVETTES To combat tobacco habit and obesity (Scientific)	Benzocaine Saccharin Extract of licorice Powdered ginger* Oils of anise, wintergreen synthetic*, peppermint, coriander*, cloves*	1/20 gr.	FLEA SOAP (Cooper)	Soap (anhydrous) Steam distilled pine oil Petroleum distillate Beta thiocyano ethyl esters of mixed fatty acids avg. 10 to 18 carbon atoms B-butoxy-B' thiocyano diethyl ether	80.0% 4.0% 2.0% 1.5% 0.5%
FLAVI HIST Antihistaminic, analgesic (Boyle & Co.)	Each capsule: Prophenpyridamine* Pyrilamine maleate* Lemon bioflavonoid Ascorbic acid Salicylamide* Phenacetin* Atropine sulfate Methapyrilene hydrochloride* Hesperidin complex Ephedrine sulfate Caffeine alkaloid	6.25 mg. 8.33 mg. 25.0 mg. 50.0 mg. 3.5 gr. 2.0 gr. 1/600 gr. 8.33 mg. 25.0 mg. 10.0 mg. 0.5 gr.	FLEAS-OFF Insecticide (Whitmire)	Pyrethrins I and II Rotenone Rotenoids and other cube resins Tech. piperonyl butoxide Ethylene glycol ether of pinene* Pine oil* Butoxypolypropylene glycol* Para di-isobutyl phenoxy ethoxy ethyl dimethyl benzyl ammonium chloride Isopropanol* Petroleum distillate Inert propellent gas	0.136% 0.084% 0.166% 0.375% 4.750% 2.000% 17.589% 0.200% 13.200% 1.500% 60%
FLAXSEED, MENTHOL & WILD CHERRY Antitussive (Commerce)	Alcohol Chloroform Flaxseed Menthol Wild cherry White pine Licorice Honey Glycerin	2% 2 m.	FLEA-TOX Insecticide (Rex. Res.)	Piperonyl cyclonene tech. Pyrethrins	1% 0.15%
FLEA-AID Insecticide (Klinzmoth)	DDT* (dichloro diphenyl trichloroethane)	5%	FLEE FLEA Insecticide (Selig)	DDT Rotenone Pyrethrins	2% 1% 0.017%
FLEA-CHEK Insecticide (Chek)			FLEET AIR REFRESHER Deodorizer (Bostwick)	Perfume Isopropanol* Propylene glycol Freon	
FLEAFOAM DOG SHAMPOO (Fleafoam)			FLEET ENEMA (Fleet)	Each 100 cc.: Sodium biphosphate Sodium phosphate	16 gm. 6 gm.
FLEAFOAM FLEA POWDER (Fleafoam)			FLEET HOUSEHOLD ODOR DE-ODORANT (Bostwick)		
FLEA-NOT POWDER (Nott)	Rotenone*	1%	FLEET LUX ENAMEL (Automotive)		
FLEANOX Insecticide (Wisconsin Pharm.)	DDT* Pyrethrins Sesame oil extractives Petroleum hydrocarbons	10.00% 0.08% 0.30% 3.00%	FLEEZOFF Insecticide (C.C.G.)	Tech. chlordane Pine oil Kerosene Diluent and inert ingredients*	0.312% 0.0780% 0.296% 99.314%
FLEA-OFF DOG SHAMPOO (White, H.)			FLEMEX Antitussive (Purepac)	Ephedrine hydrochloride Potassium guaiacolsulfonate Tinctures of euphorbia, pilulifera and cocillana Syrups of wild lettuce and squill compound Cascarin Menthol	3/4 gr./fl. oz.
FLEA POWDER (Greever's)	Gamma isomer of benzene hexachloride (from lindane) Methylene bis (chlorophenol) Propylene glycol Pine oil	1.00% 0.50% 1.00% 1.00%			
FLEA-RID (Klinzmoth)	DDT* (dichloro diphenyl trichlorethane)	5%	FLEMEX FOR CHILDREN Antitussive (Purepac)	Potassium citrate Syrup of wild cherry Syrup of ipecac Syrup of squills compound Fl. ext. licorice Syrup of tolu	

*Consult Sec. II., Ingredients Index. This ingredient may be responsible for major toxic effects if poisonous amounts of this product are ingested.

Name & Use Manufacturer	Ingredients	
FLEMMINGS DEODORANT AND VANISHING CREAM (Flemmings)		
FLEMMINGS SUPERIOR FACE CREAM (Flemmings)		
FLETCHER'S CASTORIA Cathartic (Centaur- Caldwell)	Alcohol Senna extract	3-1/2%
FLEURS DE ROCAILLE EXTRACT AND LOTION (Caron)		
FLEXICOTE ROOF PAINT (Thompson & Co.)		
FLEXILACQ Lacquer (Glidden Co.)		
FLEXILE MARINE PAINTS (Devoe)		
FLEXISEAL CAULKING COMPOUND (Landen)		
FLEXITONE PAINTS (Am. Paint Corp.)		
FLEXON Paint (Chi-Namel)	Titanium dioxide Lithopone Aluminum silicate Synthetic rubber	15.5% 8.4% 2.9% 24.0%
FLEX-O-VET ANTISEPTIC COAT Veterinary (Dairy Rem.)		
FLEX-O-VET ANTISEPTIC DUSTING POWDER Veterinary (Dairy Rem.)		
FLEX-O-VET ANTISEPTIC SALVE Veterinary (Dairy Rem.)		
FLEX-O-VET HOOFENE Veterinary (Dairy Rem.)		
FLEX-O-VET KINTOX POWDER Veterinary (Dairy Rem.)		

Name & Use Manufacturer	Ingredients	
FLEX-O-VET LOUSE POWDER Veterinary (Dairy Rem.)		
FLEX-O-VET MINERAL & STOMACHIC HORN TONIC Veterinary (Dairy Rem.)		
FLEX-O-VET SCOURENE Veterinary (Dairy Rem.)		
FLEX-O-VET UDDER LINIMENT Veterinary (Dairy Rem.)		
FLEX-O-VET UDDER OINTMENT (Diary Rem.)		
FLEXTEX PAINTS (Chicago Paints)		
FLEX TISSUE FILLER (Embalmers')		
FLEZIX FLEA & LICE POWDER (Bonide)	Rotenone*	1.25%
FLICK Pesticide (Garden Prod.)	Petroleum distillate* Pine oil* Citrus oil Oleic acid Rotenone and other cube resins Ethylene dichloride* 2-Amino-2-methyl-1-propanol Naphthalene* Soybean oil	
FLI-DY Insecticide (Russell, I.)	Petroleum distillates* Pine oil* Beta butoxy beta' thiocyano diethyl ether*	
FLIGHT Insecticide (Curran)	Naphthalene*	100%
FLIGHT BRAND 3-5-40 COT- TON DUST Insecticide (Carolina)	Gamma isomer of BHC* DDT* Sulfur*	3.00% 5.00% 40.00%
FLIGHT BRAND TOXAPHENE COTTON DUST Insecticide (Carolina)	Toxaphene*	20.00%
FLIGONE Insecticide (Central Chem.)	Petroleum oil* Tech. piperonyl butoxide Pyrethrins	
FLI-NO-MORE Insecticide (Auth. Brands)		

*Consult Sec. II., Ingredients Index. This ingredient may be responsible for major toxic effects if poisonous amounts of this product are ingested.

Name & Use Manufacturer	Ingredients	Name & Use Manufacturer	Ingredients
FLINTIDE FLOOR HARDENER (Bondrite)		FLIT FLY & MOSQUITO KILLER WITH AROMIN (Esso)	DDT 1.75% Gamma isomer of benzene hexachloride (from lindane) 0.075% Isobornyl thiocyanoacetate 0.82% Other related terpenes 0.18% Insecticidally active petroleum hydrocarbons* 25.00% Refined petroleum distillate* 72.175%
PROF. FLINT'S HORSE & CATTLE POWDERS (Kendall, Dr. B. J.)	Licorice Magnesium sulfate Fenugreek Gentian Sulfur flowers Potassium nitrate Anise Ginger Iron sulfate Nux vomica (strychnine 0.006%) 1/2% Dried sodium sulfate Charcoal filler 2-1/2%		
		FLIT INSECT KILLER (Esso)	DDT* 5% Isobornyl thiocyanoacetate 0.5% Other related terpenes 0.1% Aliphatic thiocyanates (esters & ethers) 0.4% Refined petroleum distillate* 94.0%
FLINT-TOP ENAMEL (Stewart Paint)			
		FLIT MOTH PROOFER (Esso)	Chlorinated terpenes (66% chlorine) 0.5% Refined petroleum distillate* 65%
FLINT WAX Auto wax (du Pont)			
FLIT AEROSOL FLY & MOSQUITO KILLER WITH AROMIN (Esso)	Petroleum hydrocarbons 1.5% Pyrethrins 0.25% DDT 2.0% Piperonyl butoxide 1.0% Aromatic petroleum distillate* 3.5% Refined petroleum distillate 6.75%	FLIT WITH 5% DDT Insecticide (Esso)	DDT* 5% Petroleum hydrocarbons* 25% Refined petroleum distillate* 70%
		FLIT WITH LINDANE Insecticide (Esso)	Gamma isomer of benzene hexachloride (from lindane) 0.10% Isobornyl thiocyanoacetate 0.61% Other related terpenes 0.14% Insecticidally active petroleum hydrocarbons* 25.00% Refined petroleum distillate* 74.15%
FLIT AEROSOL INSECT SPRAY (Esso)	Pyrethrins 0.25% DDT 2.0% Piperonyl butoxide 1.0% Aromatic petroleum distillate* 5.0% Refined petroleum distillate 6.75%		
		FLO EZE WRITING INKS (Ink)	
FLIT BUG KILLER WITH CHLORDANE (Esso)	Tech. chlordane 2.00% Pyrethrins 0.05% Gamma isomer of benzene hexachloride (from lindane) 0.05% Refined petroleum distillate* 97.90%	FLO-LAC VARNISH & STAIN (Sherwin-Williams)	
FLIT BUG KILLER WITH CHLORDANE PRESSURIZED (Esso)	Tech. chlordane 2.00% Gamma isomer of benzene hexachloride (from lindane) 0.05% Petroleum hydrocarbons* 25.00% Refined petroleum distillate* 47.95%	FLOMAR COLOGNE STICK AND DEODORANT STICK (Flomar)	
		FLO-MASTER Ink (Cushman)	
FLIT BUG KILLER FOR CRAWLING INSECTS WITH AROMIN (Esso)	Tech. chlordane 2.00% Gamma isomer of benzene hexachloride (from lindane) 0.05% Petroleum hydrocarbons* 25.00% Refined petroleum distillate* 47.95%	FLOMATIC PAINTS (Bradley, C. E.)	
		FLO-MULSION Insecticide (Sherwin-Williams)	Hydrocarbon oil* 83%
FLIT DOUBLE ACTION INSECT SPRAY (Penola)	DDT* 5.0% Isobornyl thiocyanoacetate 0.5% Other related terpenes 0.1% Aliphatic thiocyanates 0.4% Refined petroleum distillate* 94.0%	FLOODLITE ENAMELS (Stewart Paint)	
		FLOODLITE MILL WHITE Paint (Frazer)	

*Consult Sec. II., Ingredients Index. This ingredient may be responsible for major toxic effects if poisonous amounts of this product are ingested.

Name & Use Manufacturer	Ingredients
FLO ON WAX (Empire Chem.)	
FLOORENITE VARNISH (Atlantic V. & P.)	
FLOORETTE PAINT & FLOOR VARNISH (Glidden Co.)	
FLOOREX SEALER (Pacific Chem.)	
FLOOR FINISHES (Hockwald)	
FLOOR GUARD Paint (Detroit)	
FLOORLIFE Wood floor treatment (Sonneborn)	
FLOOR MASTER VARNISHES (DeSoto P. & V.)	
FLOORNAMEL PAINT (Monroe Co.)	
FLOOR-O-LITE DRESSING Floor treatment (Hillyard Chem.)	
FLOOR SEAL WOOD HARDENER (Sherwin-Williams)	
FLOOR SECURITY FLOOR SEALER (Johnston)	
FLOOR SHINE CLEANER & POLISH (Legge)	
FLOOR SWEEP (Withers)	Sand Sawdust Pale oil Dyes
FLOQUIL MARKING COLORS (Floquil)	

Name & Use Manufacturer	Ingredients
FLORA DELL FACE LOTION (Flora Dell)	
FLORA DELL HAIR POMADE (Flora Dell)	
FLORAL DUST AND SPRAY Insecticide (Thompson-Hayward)	DDT 3.0% Gamma isomer of benzene hexachloride (from lindane) 1.0% Zineb (zinc ethylene-bis (dithiocarbamate)) 3.9% 2-(p-tert-Butylphenoxy)-isopropyl-2-chloroethyl sulfite 1.5%
FLORA MIST PERFUMED DEODORANT SPRAY (Oleum)	
FLORASOL HYGIENIC POWDER (Calvital)	Lactose Boric acid* Zinc sulfate Salicylic acid* Oxyquinoline sulfate
FLORCREX Sealer (Horn)	
FLORENAMEL Paint (Glidden Co.)	
FLORET Effervescent antacid (Floret)	Sugar Sodium bicarbonate Citric and tartaric acids
FLOR-ETCHER Liquid sand-paper (Am. Fluresit)	Hydrochloric acid*
FLOREX ENAMEL (Wailes-D. H.)	
FLOREX VARNISH (Perfection Paint)	
FLOR HIDE ENAMEL (Pittsburgh Plate Glass (Paint Div.))	
FLORIDA AGRICULTURE ARAMITE-15W Insecticide (Florida Agric.)	Beta-chloroethyl-beta-(B-tertiary butyl phenoxy)-alpha-methyl-ethyl sulfite as a wettable powder 15%
FLORIDA AGRICULTURE DN DRY MIX NO. 1 Miticide (Florida Agric.)	DN* (dinitro-o-cyclohexylphenol) 40%

Name & Use Manufacturer	Ingredients	Name & Use Manufacturer	Ingredients
FLORIDA AGRICULTURE DN DRY MIX NO. 111 Miticide (Florida Agric.)	DN* (dinitro-o-cyclohexylphenol) 20%	FLORLUX ENAMEL (Patterson-Sargent)	
FLORIDA CHEMICAL CATTLE GRUB KILLER (Florida Chem.)	Rotenone 1.25% Inert talc 98.75%	FLOR-MASTER VARNISH (United Chem.)	
		FLOROZONE Disinfectant, deodorant (Florozone)	Triethylene glycol Propylene glycol Essential oils Para-di-isobutyl phenoxy ethoxy ethyl dimethyl ammonium chloride*
FLORIDA CHEMICAL HEXA-CHLORE-THANE DRENCH Insecticide (Florida Chem.)	Hexachloroethane* 45% Bentonite 5%	FLOR-PATCH COATINGS Paint product (Am. Asbestos)	
		FLORPLY NATURAL RUBBER PAINT (Forman, Ford)	
FLORIDA CHEMICAL LIVESTOCK SPRAY & DIP TYPE DDT BHC Insecticide (Florida Chem.)	DDT* 38.10% Gamma isomer of benzene hexachloride* 2.30% Other isomers of benzene hexachloride* 12.20%	FLOR-ZEAL Floor sealer (Bownes)	
		FLOTATION OIL For separation of various ores (Tenn. Prod.)	Hardwood oil fractions
FLORIDA CHEMICAL PARATHION POWDER Insecticide (Florida Chem.)	Parathion* 15%	FLOTOX DUSTING SULFUR Fungicide (Calif. Spray)	Sulfur* 90%
FLORIDA VEGETABLE DUST Fungicide, insecticide (Collins Feed)	Manzate 7.0% Lindane 1.0%	FLOTOX WETTABLE SULFUR Fungicide (Calif. Spray)	Sulfur* 95%
		FLOW CASEIN PAINT (Long Island)	
FLORIDA VOLCK FLOWABLE OIL EMULSION Insecticide (Calif. Spray)	Petroleum oils 80%	FLOWER DROPS PERFUMS (Rieger)	
FLORIENT Aerosol air deodorant (Colgate-Palmolive)		FLOWER OF THE MONTH EAUX DE PARFUM (House of Gourielli)	
FLORITE ENAMEL (Preservative)		FLOWETTE ENAMELS (Denny)	
FLORIZOL Disinfectant (U.S. Sanitary)		FLOWING KOTE PAINT (Paragon Paint)	
FLORKOTE For floors (Bownes)		FLOW KOTE RUBBER BASE WALL PAINTS (du Pont)	
FLOR-LIFE FLOOR FINISH (Lucas)			

*Consult Sec. II., Ingredients Index. This ingredient may be responsible for major toxic effects if poisonous amounts of this product are ingested.

Name & Use Manufacturer	Ingredients	Name & Use Manufacturer	Ingredients
FLOW ON PAINT (Barreled Sunlight)		FLURENE SALVE (Flurene)	Menthol* Camphor* Oil of thyme* Nutmeg* Cedar leaf* Pine needles Turpentine* Cajeput* Eucalyptol*
FLOWTILE PAINT (Everseal)			
F.L.S. ASTRINGENT LOTION Veterinary (Thoroughbred)	Gum camphor* Menthol* Methyl salicylate* Ethyl aminobenzoate Tannic acid Tincture of cantharides* Spirits of turpentine* Tincture of arnica Calcium acetate Boric acid* Glycerin Oils of peppermint, cedarwood, mirbane, wormwood, cedar-leaf, tansy and eucalyptus	FLUROSTONE Liquid floor hardener (Am. Fluresit)	
		FLUSHING PAINT (Chilton Paint)	
		FLUSH-IT Drain cleaner (Perolin)	Sodium hydroxide*
		FLUXINE FLUXES For welding, brazing and soldering (Krembs)	
FLUID CEREFOLIUS Diuretic (Walker Pharm.)	Alcohol 25% Saw palmetto fl. ext. 120 m. Corn silk tr. (50% drug) 60 m. Sandalwood fl. ext. 30 m. Methenamine 8 gr.		
FLUID ICE Deodorant, antiperspirant (DermaTeen)	Aluminum chloride	FLUXIT Spreader and wetting agent (Colloidal)	Casein Calcium hydroxide
FLU-O-CIDE Insecticide (Braun K.-H.)	Sodium fluosilicate*	FLUXO LIQUID SOLDERING FLUX (Sunshine)	Zinc chloride* Glycerin Hydrochloric acid* Sodium bichromate* Anti-foam emulsion Ultrawet
FLUORESCENT ARTISTS COLOR Paint (Ultra-Violet)	Linseed oil Zinc sulfide* Cadmium sulfide*		
FLUORESCENT BULLETIN COLOR Paint (Ultra-Violet)	Linseed oil Zinc sulfide* Cadmium sulfide* Driers Mineral spirits*	FLY & MOSQUITO REPELLENT (Calumet Ref.)	
		FLY BAIT Insecticide (Ralston)	Malathion*
FLUORESCENT CHALKS (Ultra-Violet)	Plaster of Paris Zinc sulfide* Cadmium sulfide*	FLY-B-GON INSECT SPRAY (Calif. Spray)	Gamma isomer of benzene hexachloride (from lindane)* 17.12% Aromatic petroleum derivative solvent* 30.6%
FLUORESCENT TEMPERA (Ultra-Violet)	Water-soluble resins Preservatives Dowicide A & G Various humectants Zinc sulfide* Cadmium sulfide*	FLY BOMB (Lee, G.)	Pyrethrins 0.20% Isobornyl thiocyanoacetate 1.64% Other related terpenes 0.36% Piperonyl butoxide tech. 2.00% Methoxychlor tech. 3.00% Petroleum distillates* 10.80% Methylated aromatic petroleum derivatives* 12.00%
FLUR-DRY Concrete sealer (Am. Fluresit)			
		FLY-CHEK Insecticide (Chek)	
FLURENE NOSE & THROAT DROPS (Flurene)	Ephedrine* Menthol Camphor* Eucalyptol* Pine needles White thyme	FLYDED AEROSOL INSECT KILLER (Boyle-Midway)	DDT 2.00% Allethrin 0.10% Tech. piperonyl butoxide 0.25% Beta butoxy beta thiocyano diethyl ether 1.00% Petroleum distillates* 51.65% Freon propellents

*Consult Sec. II., Ingredients Index. This ingredient may be responsible for major toxic effects if poisonous amounts of this product are ingested.

Name & Use Manufacturer	Ingredients
FLYDED INSECT SPRAY 5% DDT (Boyle- Midway)	DDT* 5% Methylated naphthalenes* 9.5% Beta butoxy beta thiocyanodiethyl ether 0.5% Essential oils 0.5% Petroleum distillates* 84.5%
FLY DOOM Insecticide (Murray, E.)	Petroleum distillate* 99.039% n-Octyl bicycloheptene dicarboximide 0.870% Allethrin 0.050% Pyrethrins 0.037% Related compounds 0.004%
FLY-DY Insecticide (Miller Chem.)	Petroleum distillate* Tech. piperonyl butoxide Pyrethrins
FLY-FOE INSECTICIDE (Johnson Oil)	
FLY FUNERAL Insecticide (McKesson)	DDT 1% Bornyl thiocyanate* 3% Cyclohexylamine 0.12% Pine oil fractions 1.50% Oil of cedarleaf 0.45% Kerosene* 93.93%
FLY JINX INSECT SPRAY (Claire)	DDT 2% Pyrethrins 0.15% Tech. piperonyl butoxide 0.8% Petroleum hydrocarbon* 27.05%
FLYKIL Insecticide (Du-Rite)	
FLY-MIST Insecticide (Agkem)	Petroleum distillate* Butoxypolypropylene glycol* Alkyl phenyl polyglycol ether Pine oil* Citrus oil* Ethylene glycol monobutyl ether Rotenoids (cube resins other than rotenone) n-Propyl isome Butylcarbityl (6-propyl-piperonyl) ether and related chemicals Pyrethrins 1 and 11
FLY-NO-MORE Insecticide (Germo)	
FLY RELIEF Cattle spray (United Chem.)	
FLYS-AWAY REPELLENT BOMB Insecticide (Farnam)	Butoxypolypropylene glycol 26.700% Pine oil* 21.806% Citrus oil* 5.450% Rotenone 0.136% Cube resins other than rotenone 0.408%
FLY SHOO REPELLENT (Germo)	
FLY SLAYER (Slayer)	Petroleum distillates* Piperonyl butoxide tech. Pyrethrins

Name & Use Manufacturer	Ingredients
FLY SPRAY (Hillyard Chem.)	Petroleum distillate* B-butoxy B'-thiocyano diethyl ether* Pyrethrins Essential oils*
FLY-TOX AEROSOL INSECT BOMB (Rex Res.)	DDT 2% Piperonyl butoxide tech. 1.6% Pyrethrins 0.2% Methylated naphthalenes* 5% Mineral hydrocarbon distillate 11.1% Butyl carbityl (6-propyl piperonyl) ether 1.28% Other related compounds 0.32%
FOAMCO CLEANER (Worrell)	
FOAMING BATH SACHET (Clark, R.)	Sodium sulfate (salt cake) Sodium alkyl aryl sulfonate Sodium alkyl lauryl sulfonate Perfume D & C color
FOAM KING CREAM SHAMPOO (Hennessy)	Sodium salt of lauryl sulfate Stearic acid Triethanolamine Perfume Detergents (either amine condensates or alkyl aryls)
FOAM-O-KLEEN Cleaner (Pioneer)	
FOAM SHAMPOO Rug and fabric cleaner (Golden Star)	
FOAMSOFF Automobile wash (Bonide)	
F. O. B. (First on Burns) Burn solution (F. O. B.)	Oxyquinoline sulfate Liquid petrolatum U.S.P. Rosemary oil U.S.P. Oil of linseed Oil of geranium
FOGARTY'S FOG DROPS (Hoyt)	
FOGGING SPRAY Insecticide (Thompson-Hayward)	DDT 10.0% Tech. chlordane 5.0% Aromatic petroleum derivative solvent* 20.0% Petroleum distillate 65.0%
FOGICIDE NO. C Insecticide (Lorenz)	Refined chlordane* Aliphatic hydrocarbons*
FOGICIDE NO. DC Insecticide (Lorenz)	Refined chlordane* DDT* Aliphatic hydrocarbons*
FOGICIDE NO. 10 Insecticide (Lorenz)	Refined chlordane* Aliphatic hydrocarbons*

*Consult Sec. II., Ingredients Index. This ingredient may be responsible for major toxic effects if poisonous amounts of this product are ingested.

Name & Use Manufacturer	Ingredients	Name & Use Manufacturer	Ingredients
FOGICIDE NO. 10-A Insecticide (Lorenz)	Agr. grade chlordane* Aliphatic hydrocarbons*	FOOT-MIST FOOT BATH (Foot-Rite)	Colloidal sulfur* Alum Salicylic acid* Menthol* Sodium borate* Sodium bicarbonate
FOGICIDE NO. 30 Insecticide (Lorenz)	DDT* liquid conc. 30% Aromatic petroleum distillate*	FOOT RELIEF Antiseptic counter-irritant (Am. Druggists)	Talcum Boric acid* Salicylic acid*
FOGICIDE NO. P Insecticide (Lorenz)	Piperonyl butoxide Pyrethrins Aliphatic hydrocarbons*	FOOT ROT TREATMENT Veterinary (Roberts, Dr. D.)	Crude phenols* 11-3/4% Saponified cresylic solution Oil of linseed q.s.
FOGICIDE NO. 120 Insecticide (Lorenz)	DDT 23.6% Agricultural chlordane 12.8% Aromatic petroleum distillate* 54.8%	FOOT-RUB FOOT MASSAGE CREAM (Foot-Rite)	Lanolin Zinc oxide Methyl salicylate* Menthol* Camphor* Oil of eucalyptus
FOG-OFF Glass cleaner (Kleer)		FORAMBA MOTH LIQUID (Cedar Odor) Insecticide (Uncle Sam)	Pyrethrum Paradichlorobenzene* Petroleum distillate*
FOILLE ANTISEPTIC FOR BURNS (Carbisulphoil)			
FOLEY'S HONEY & TAR COMPOUND FOR COUGHS DUE TO COLDS (Foley)	Pine tar* Ammonium chloride Gum arabic	FORAMBA MOTH LIQUID WITH DDT Insecticide (Uncle Sam)	Pyrethrum Paradichlorobenzene* DDT* 5% Methylated naphthalenes* Petroleum distillate*
FOLIAFUME Insecticide (Penick)	Pyrethrum Rotenone	FORBIDDEN MOMENT DEODORANT (Countess)	
FOLIUM INORGANIC FERTILIZER (Monsanto)	Phosphorus 20% Nitrogen 20% Potash 20%	FORBIDDEN MOMENT TOILET WATER (Countess)	
FOMOS Vaginal tablets (Fomos)	Each tablet: Quinol* (hydroquinone) Tartaric acid Oxyquinoline sulfate Sodium bicarbonate	FORCE'S GOPHER KILLER Rodenticide (Carajon)	Arsenic trioxide*
FOOTAIDE (Arnold's)		FOR-DEE Herbicide (Planetary Chem.)	Butyl ester of 2, 4-dichloro-phenoxyacetic acid* 40% Solvents* and emulsyfying agents 60%
FOOTHILL FLY SPRAY (Corona Foothill)	DDT*		
FOOTHILL OIL WEED KILLER (Corona Foothill)	Petroleum oil*	FOREZA Liquid analgesic counter-irritant, external (Cel-Ton-Sa)	Sodium salicylate* Potassium citrate Sodium phosphate Oil lemon Methyl salicylate* Saccharin soluble
FOOT LIFE Skin emollient (Mack's)	Acid boric* Zinc oxide Mineral jelly		
FOOTMASTER FOR ATHLETES FOOT Fungicide, (medical) (Drugmaster)	Di-isobutyl phenoxyethoxy ethyl dimethyl-benzyl ammonium chloride monohydrate* Benzoic acid Salicylic acid* Thymol* Menthol	FOREZA ANTACID POWDER Gastric antacid (Cel-Ton-Sa)	Bismuth subcarbonate Sodium bicarbonate Magnesium oxide
FOOTMASTER POWDER (Drugmaster)	Ortho and para benzyl phenol 0.25% Alkyl tolyl methyl trimethyl ammonium chlorides 0.25%		

*Consult Sec. II., Ingredients Index. This ingredient may be responsible for major toxic effects if poisonous amounts of this product are ingested.

Name & Use Manufacturer	Ingredients		Name & Use Manufacturer	Ingredients	
FOREZA COMPOUND Tonic, antispasmodic (Cel-Ton-Sa)	Thiamine hydrochloride Iron and ammonium citrate Black haw Blue cohash Black cohash False unicorn Squaw vine Wild yam Berberis Ginger Chamomile		FORMO-CEN Deodorant (Central Chem.)	Formaldehyde* N.F.	5%
			FORMSTONE-CEMENT PAINT (Lasting)		
FORMACIDE Insecticide (Hammond)	Formaldehyde dust*		FORMULA D. C. JELLY Vaginal jelly (Diaphragm)	Glycerin Chlorothymol Propyl-parasept Paraformaldehyde Lactic acid	15.838% 0.015% 0.198% 0.198%
FORM-A-GASKET (Permatex)	Isopropyl alcohol*		FORMULA J FOR FABRIC Moth proof, rot proof, mildew proof (Johnson, J. W.)	Xylol* type solution	
FORMA GERMKILL (Central City)			FORMWELL MODELING CLAY (Am. Crayon)		
FORMAJEN (Jenkins)	Each tablet: Hexamethylenamine* Sodium biphosphate Extract buchu	4 gr. 4 gr. 1 gr.	FORMYSKIN For skin, scalp irritations (Colbtrans)	Oil of cajeput* Amethol* Methyl salicylate* Oil of eucalyptus* Lavender oil* Terpineol in a base of petrolatum Stearic acid Green soap solution	
FORMALIN SOLUTION SCENTED Deodorant (Gordon Labs.)	Formalin* solution	10%			
FORMAMINT TABLETS Throat antiseptic (Standard Labs.)	Formaldehyde*		FORT DODGE DRY IN-SECTICIDE (Fort Dodge)	Naphthalene* Creosote oil	31% 1%
FORMAN GRADE 1 HOUSE PAINT (Forman, Ford)			FORT DODGE ENGO Insecticide (Fort Dodge)	Tech. chlordane* Pine oil* Kerosene*	40% 10% w/w 38% w/w
FORMANITE NO PAINT ODOR FINISH Paint (Forman, Ford)			FORT DODGE FLEA-GO Insecticide (Fort Dodge)	Oil anise Soap anhydrous	2% w/w 37.6% w/w
FOR MEN ONLY AFTER SHAVE (Liebert)			FORT DODGE FLEA-GO IMPROVED Insecticide (Fort Dodge)	Gamma isomer of benzene hexachloride from lindane Oil anise Soap anhydrous	0.80% w/w 2.00% 33.30% w/w
FOR MEN ONLY COLOGNE (Liebert)			FORT DODGE FLEA & LOUSE POWDER (Fort Dodge)	Isobornyl thiocyanoacetate Other related terpenes Rotenone Other extractives of cube	4.1% w/w 0.9% w/w 1.0% w/w 2.0% w/w
FORMFILM THINNER Lacquer thinner (Horn)			FORT DODGE FORMULA 144 TABLETS Disinfectant for drinking water of poultry (Fort Dodge)	Di-isobutyl-phenoxy-ethoxy-ethyl-di-methylbenzyl ammonium chloride monohydrate* 2 gm. (40%) w/w	
FORMFILM LACQUER Coating for plywood forms (Horn)			FORT DODGE GRUBCIDE (Fort Dodge)	Rotenone Other extractives of cube	1.66% w/w 2.00% w/w

*Consult Sec. II., Ingredients Index. This ingredient may be responsible for major toxic effects if poisonous amounts of this product are ingested.

- 504 -

Name & Use Manufacturer	Ingredients	Name & Use Manufacturer	Ingredients
FORT DODGE PARIFORT Insecticide (Fort Dodge)	Gamma isomer of benzene hexachloride (from lindane) 1% w/w	FORTY-PLUS SHAMPOO AND EUCALYPTUS OIL SHAMPOO ("42" Prod.)	
FORT DODGE PINE OIL DISINFECT-ANT (Fort Dodge)	Pine oil* 86% w/w Sulfonated castor oil 14% w/w	FORTY-PLUS LANOLIN WITH HORMONES TOUCH-UP AND THEATRICAL COLD CREMES ("42" Prod.)	
FORT DODGE QUAN-SEPT For general sanitation (Fort Dodge)	Alkyl tolyl methyl trimethyl ammonium chlorides* 10%	"42" HAIR PREPARATION (42 Prod.)	
FORT DODGE SAPONATED SOLUTION OF CRESOL Disinfectant (Fort Dodge)	Cresol* 50% Soap 32%	"42" SHAMPOO (42 Prod.)	
FORSTESIA RECTAL SALVE Astringent, sedative (Kansas City)	Horse chestnut Buckeye (aesculus) Stone root (collinsonia) Witch hazel (hamamelis) Kollesol (8-hydroxyquinoline sulfate) Forstesia (benzocaine U.S.P.)	FOSBOND Metal under-coating and finishing (Pennsylv. Salt)	
FORSTESIA RECTAL CONES Astringent, sedative (Kansas City)	Aesculus Collinsonia Hamamelis Kollesol (8-hydroxyquinoline sulfate) Forstesia (benzocaine U.S.P.)	FOSTER IBM PREPARED METAL COATING (Foster)	Petroleum asphalt* Colloidal clay
FORTOSULF (Torch)	Sulfur* precipitated 40% in petrolatum	FOSTER IBM ROOF COAT-ING & PLASTIC ROOF CEMENT (Foster)	Petroleum asphalt* Petroleum hydrocarbon solvents* Asbestos fiber Inorganic pigments*
FORTRON SYRUP (Physicians Prod.)	Ferrous gluconate 22.5 mg. Thiamine chloride (vitamin B1) 5 mg. Glycerin	FOSTER RESTALIC COATINGS (Foster)	Alkyd (polyester) resin Petroleum hydrocarbon* solvents Organic and/or inorganic pigments*
FORTY-EIGHT COLOGNE DEODORANT (Proof)	Alcohol* Propylene glycol* Carnation Dihydroxyhexachloro-diphenyl methane Pentachloro-dihydroxyphenyl methane D & C color (green sol. #1, yellow ecco fast)	FOSTER RESTALIC THINNERS (Foster)	Aliphatic and/or aromatic petroleum hydrocarbon solvents*
FORTY-PLUS BRONZE HENNA AND EQYPTIAN HENNA ("42" Prod.)		FOSTER'S 30 MINUTE CORN & CALLOUS REMOVER (Boyer Prod.)	
FORTY-PLUS CREME OIL HAIR TONIC AND COLOREZE CREME ("42" Prod.)		FOSTER'S W.C. LINI-MENT (Foster's, W. C.)	Oil origanium* Kerosene oil* Ammonia water Carbonate ammonia Castile soap Camphor gum*
FORTY-PLUS DUO CREME, AND HAIR LACQUER ("42" Prod.)		FOSTER VINYL FLOOR ENAMEL (Foster)	Vinyl polymers Organic hydrocarbon solvents* Organic and/or inorganic pigments*
FORTY-PLUS HAIR OIL TONIC ("42" Prod.)		FOUNDATION COATING Paint product (United Gilson.)	Asphalt Mineral spirits*

*Consult Sec. II., Ingredients Index. This ingredient may be responsible for major toxic effects if poisonous amounts of this product are ingested.

Name & Use Manufacturer	Ingredients		Name & Use Manufacturer	Ingredients	
FOUNTAIN FOAM POLISH & CLEANER (Omni)			4 ROSES NAIL POLISH AND POLISH REMOVER (Allied Drug)		
FOUNT-O-INK (Gregory)			4 ROSES SHAMPOO (Allied Drug)		
GORDON 480 SOLUTION For preparation of contact lens fluids (Gordon Labs.)	Methyl cellulose		FOURSALCO Antirheumatic (Jenkins)	Each tablet: Salicylic acid* Sodium bicarbonate Magnesium salicylate* Strontium salicylate* Acetophenetidin Methyl salicylate (Syn.) Pancreatin Diastase	1/2 gr. 3 gr. 2 gr. 2 gr. 1/4 gr. q.s. q.s. q.s.
4-4 AUTO POLISH (Techno-Chem.)					
FOUR HOUR DRY VARNISH (Vulcan)			FOUR SQUARE PAINT (Perfection Paint)		
FOUR-HOUR PAINTS (Stille-Young)			FOUR SQUARE PAINTS (Cheesman-Elliott)		
4-IN-1 RAINBOW TABLETS Analgesic (Approved)	Salicylamide* Phenacetin* Caffeine Tincture gelsemium	3-1/2 gr. 2-1/2 gr. 1/2 gr. 3 m.	4 STAR INSECT REPELLENT MIX & ANTI-SUNBURN CREME (Southland)	Dimethyl phthalate Butyl dimethyl dihydro gamma pyrone carboxylate 2-Ethyl hexanediol-1, 3 Dimethyl bicycloheptene dicarboxylate	92.5%
FOUR PENNY DANDRUFF SCALE REMOVER (Four Penny)			4 WAY COLD TABLETS (Beaumont)	Aspirin* Magnesium hydroxide Yellow phenolphthalein Salicylic acid* Salicylates*	
FOUR PENNY HAIR CREAM AND HAIR DRESS (Four Penny)			4 WAY RECTAL CONES For hemorrhoids (Beaumont)	Bismuth subgallate Resorcin* Camphorated phenol* Zinc oxide Benzocaine Camphor* Boric acid*	
FOUR PENNY SHAMPOO (Four Penny)					
4-QK-DRI ENAMEL (Sillers)			FOWLAX Laxative (veterinary, avian) (Gland-O-Lac)	Potassium sulfate Sodium chloride Sodium bicarbonate Anhydrous sodium sulfate	2.0% 18.0% 36.0% 44.0%
4 ROSES AFTER SHAVE LOTION (Allied Drug)	Alcohol*	50%			
4 ROSES ALMOND FRAGRANCE CREAM (Allied Drug)			FOX SUPERFUEL Fuel (Fox)	Castor oil Methanol* Nitromethane Detergent Ignitors	29% 64% 5% 1% 1%
4 ROSES DANDRUFF LOTION (Allied Drug)	Oxyquinoline benzoate Benzoic acid* Tr. capsicum Alcohol*	51%	FOY BEST BODIED ENAMELED PAINT (Foy)		
4 ROSES HAIR OIL (Allied Drug)			FRAGAZONE DEODORANT (United Chem.)		
4 ROSES HAND LOTION (Allied Drug)			FRAGRANCE ALLIANCE Cosmetic (Rubinstein)		

*Consult Sec. II., Ingredients Index. This ingredient may be responsible for major toxic effects if poisonous amounts of this product are ingested.

- 506 -

Name & Use Manufacturer	Ingredients		Name & Use Manufacturer	Ingredients	
FRA-GRANCENSE Toilet water (House of Fragrance)			FRANKLIN FLUKE KILLERS Veterinary (Franklin, O. M.)	Ea. capsule: Carbon tetrachloride* U.S.P. (chloroform derivative)	1 cc
FRAGRANT-AIRE DE-ODORANT BLOCKS (Clifton)			FRANKLIN FOOT ROT TREATMENT Veterinary (Franklin, O. M.)	Methyl violet* Carbolic acid* liquified Isopropyl alcohol Glycerin	2.5% 2.0% 7.7% 40.0%
FRAGRANT-AIRE HOUSE PERFUME (Fragrantaire)	Alcohol Natural flower oils Essential oils Synthetic aromatic chemicals		FRANKLIN HORNFLY CONTROL Insecticide (Franklin, O. M.)	DDT Butoxypolypropylene glycol Aromatic petroleum derivative solvent*	5% 5% 90%
FRALAC 4 HOUR ENAMEL (Frazer)			FRANKLIN LICE-TICK DIP OR SPRAY Insecticide (Franklin, O. M.)	DDT Gamma isomer of benzene hexachloride Other isomers of benzene hexachloride Xylene*	25% 3% 4-1/2% 62-1/2%
FRALITE WALL PAINT (Frazer)					
FRAN-KEM POWDER Fungicidal, bacteriostatic agent (Washington Labs.)	Fumaric acid Sodium benzoate	50% 50%	FRANKLIN LICE-TICK DIP OR SPRAY, WETTABLE POWDER (Formerly D-THANE) Insecticide (Franklin, O. M.)	DDT* Gamma isomer of benzene hexachloride* Other isomers of benzene hexachloride*	30.77% 3.84% 18.05%
FRANKLIN BHC 10 SPRAY OR DIP Insecticide (Franklin, O. M.)	Gamma isomer of benzene hexachloride* Other isomers of benzene hexachloride*	10% 60%	FRANKLIN LINDANE 20% Insecticide (Franklin, O. M.)	Gamma isomer of benzene hexachloride (from lindane)*	20%
FRANKLIN BLOOD STOPPER Anti-hemorrhagic (veterinary) (Franklin, O. M.)	Alum exsiccated* Iron subsulfate Tannin Iodoform* Liquor cresolis comp. Camphor	48.4% 32.3% 16.1% 0.8% 0.8% 0.8%	FRANKLIN NICOTINE 40% Insecticide (Franklin, O. M.)	Nicotine* expressed as alkaloid	40%
FRANKLIN BRAND-EM-OL Veterinary (Franklin, O. M.)	Barium sulfide* Sodium hydroxide* Turpentine	14.3% 14.3% 6.3%	FRANKLIN PINKEYE POWDER & WOUND DRESSING Veterinary (Franklin, O. M.)	Acriflavine HCl Sulfathiazole Sulfanilamide Calomel Boric acid*	1% 5% 3% 5% 86%
FRANKLIN BROWN BEAUTY SCREW-WORM KILLER (Franklin, O. M.)	Benzol* Chloroform* Diphenylamine* Furfural Cube extractives (including rotenone 0.06%) Pine oil	37.78% 15.11% 30.23% 12.60% 0.25% 4.03%	FRANKLIN PINKEYE TREATMENT & WOUND DRESSING Veterinary (Franklin, O. M.)	Sodium propionate Azosulfamide Benzyl alcohol Sodium sulfacetamide Urea Propylene glycol	5% 0.2% 4% 20% 10% 18.8%
FRANKLIN CRESOLIS Disinfectant (Franklin, O. M.)	Cresol* Soap	50% 31%	FRANKLIN PROTEC WOUND DRESSING & FLY REPELLENT Veterinary (Franklin, O. M.)	Bone oil Cresol U.S.P. Butoxypolypropylene glycol Pine oil* Sperm oil Diphenylamine Zinc oxide Pine tar oil*	20.00% 0.25% 5.00% 10.00% 4.75% 4.00% 20.00% 30.00%
FRANKLIN DIP POWDER Insecticide (Franklin, O. M.)	DDT*	50%			
FRANKLIN FLY SPRAY CONC. (Franklin, O. M.)	DDT* Aromatic petroleum derivative solvent*	25% 69%			

*Consult Sec. II., Ingredients Index. This ingredient may be responsible for major toxic effects if poisonous amounts of this product are ingested.

Name & Use Manufacturer	Ingredients	
FRANKLIN RESIDUAL SPRAY Insecticide (Franklin, O. M.)	DDT* Mineral oil	5% 95%
FRANKLIN RESIDUAL SPRAY CONC. Insecticide (Franklin, O. M.)	DDT Aromatic petroleum derivative solvent*	25% 75%
FRANKLIN 1038 SCREW-WORM CONTROL Insecticide (Franklin, O. M.)	DDT Gamma isomer of benzene hexachloride (from lindane) Xylene* range aromatic solvent	25.0% 4.5% 57.0%
FRANKLIN STIM LINIMENT Rubefacient, counter-irritant (Franklin, O. M.)	Oil wormwood (true) Menthol (synthetic) Isopropanol* 99% Oil sassafras (artificial) Acetone*	2.77% 2.40% 41.66% 3.17% 50.00%
FRANKLIN STOCK DIP & DISINFECT-ANT NO. 1 Veterinary (Franklin, O. M.)	Coal tar neutral oils* Soap Coal tar acids*	63% 17% 10%
FRANKLIN STRONG TINCTURE OF IODINE (Franklin, O. M.)	Iodine* N.F. Alcohol	7% 83%
FRASER'S SOLUTION Fungicide, (medical) (Handley)	Salicylic acid* Benzoic acid Tincture iodine* Spirits of camphor*	
FRASTO STIK PAINT (Lake Chem.)		
FRATEX ENAMELS (Frazer)		
FRATONE FLAT WALL PAINTS (Frazer)		
FRAZEX Fungicide, (medical) (Am. Druggists)	Iodine* Salicylic acid* Boric acid* Alcohol*	28%
FRAZUL (Sacramento)		
FREART Chalk (Am. Crayon)		

Name & Use Manufacturer	Ingredients	
FREEDAY Analgesic (Berjon)	Each fl. oz.: Alcohol Sodium salicylate* Extractives of life root (senecio aureus) Cramp bark virburnum opulus Blessed thistle (cnicus benedictus) Squaw vine (mitchella)	15% 10 gr. 10 gr. 10 gr. 10 gr. 10 gr.
FREEDOL For skin irritations (Freedol)	Salicylic acid* Menthol carbolic acid Tincture benzoin Glycerin Alcohol*	1/3 of 1% 40%
FREE FOAM Etherized liquid rug cleaner (Puritan Chem.)		
FREEZEN Cooling application (veterinary) (Thoroughbred)	Camphorated choral* Menthol* Ethyl aminobenzoate Oil of henbane Oil of cedar leaf* Chlorobutanol Ether Isopropyl alcohol*	
FREEZONE Anti-freeze (Wyeth Chem.)	Alcohol* Ether* Zinc chloride*	
FRE-FLO INK (Crescent Prod.)		
FRELCOTE VARNISH (Pratt & Lambert)		
FRENCH GLOSS SHOE POLISH (Whittemore)		
FRENCH LUSTRE Leather polish (French Ren.)		
FRENCH'S ANT KILLER Insecticide (French Labs.)		
FRENCH'S BIRD LICE POWDER (French, R. T.)	Piperonyl cyclonene (consists of 0.48% 3-isoamyl-5-(methylene-dioxyphenyl)-2-cyclohexanone and 0.12% of related compounds) Pyrethrins	0.6% 0.1%
FRENCH'S DOG SHAMPOO (French Labs.)		

---

*Consult Sec. II., Ingredients Index. This ingredient may be responsible for major toxic effects if poisonous amounts of this product are ingested.

- 508 -

Name & Use Manufacturer	Ingredients	Name & Use Manufacturer	Ingredients
FRENCH'S FLEA POWDER FOR DOGS (French, R. T.)	Piperonyl cyclonene 1.00% (0.8% of 3-isoamyl-5-(methylene-dioxyphenyl)-2-cyclohexenone and its 6-carbethoxy derivative and 0.2% of related compounds) Pyrethrins 0.10% Rotenone 0.50% Other cube extractives 1.00% Gamma isomer of benzene hexachloride (from lindane) 1.00%	FREO COUGH SYRUP (White, R. P.)	Each fl. oz.: Alcohol 11% Calcium creosote sulfonate 2 gr. Cherry bark 23 gr. Balm of Gilead buds 3 gr. Ammonium chloride 3 gr. Aralia 3 gr. Sodium glycerophosphate 4 gr. Chloroform 2 m. Calcium guaiacol sulfonate 1 gr. White pine bark 23 gr. Sanguinaria 4 gr. Sassafras bark 2 gr. Tartar emetic 1/36 gr. Terpin hydrate 1 gr.
FRENCH'S GERMICIDE, ANTISEPTIC (French, R. T.)	Vegetable soap Terpineol p-Chlorosym-m-xylenol* Alcohol 16.4%		
FRENCH'S HAND LOTION (French Labs.)		FREOKAPS For colds, Analgesic, laxative (White, R. P.)	Each capsule: Acetophenetidin* 2 gr. Aloin Atropine sulfate* Aspirin* Caffeine Camphor powder
FRENCH'S IRON COMPOUND FOR CAGE BIRDS (French, R. T.)	Ferrous sulfate Glycerin Extract of gentian Sodium benzoate 1/10% Citric acid		
		FRESH CREAM DEODORANT (Pharma Craft)	Aluminum chloride crystals Basic aluminum formate Urea Glycerin monostearate Petrolatum Stearic acid Spermaceti
FRENCH'S NESTLING FOOD (French, R. T.)	Bread Egg yolk Whole egg Alfalfa meal Skim milk solids Wheat germ Yeast Stabilized vegetable oil Cod liver oil concentrate Vitamin B12		
		FRESH DATED PAINTS (Sterling Varnish)	
FRENCH'S TURTLE FOOD (French, R. T.)	Shrimp meal Dried buttermilk Bugs Liver meal Oat, wheat, corn and soya bean flours	FRESH DEODORANT SOAP (Pharma Craft)	Pure dry soap 86.54% Actamer 1.56 Glycerin 0.73 Salt 0.52
FRENCH TOUCH PARFUME, EAU DE COLOGNE AND COLOGNE STICK (Parfums Charbert)		FRESHENOL SPRAY Air deodorant (Freshenol)	SDA #40 85% Fir and pine oil* blend 10%
		FRESHETTES (Holcomb)	Paradichlorobenzene*
		FRESNO DDT 5 SULPHUR 50 DUST Insecticide (Fresno Agric.)	Dichloro diphenyl trichloroethane* 5% Sulfur* 50%
FRENCO'S PAPAIN ABSOLUTE Digestant (Frenco)	Powdered papain (testing N.F. Formula VIII)	FRESNOL ANT SYRUP (Fresnol Mfg.)	Sodium arsenite* 0.29%
FRENCO'S PAPAYA TOOTH POWDER (Frenco)	Cal. carb. Mag. carb. Ivory soap powder Papain Sodium bicarb. Sodium chloride Polak's dry peppermint flavor	FRESNO MALATHION 4 SULFUR 50 DUST Insecticide (Fresno Agric.)	Malathion* 4% Sulfur* 50%
FRENCO'S PYACADO FACE CREAM (Frenco)	Avacado Mineral oils Stearic acid Glycerin Triethanolamine Dow's Tego-sept P. Paraffin Papain	FRIENDSHIP'S GARDEN DUSTING POWDER, BATH SALTS, AND TOILET WATER (Shulton)	

*Consult Sec. II., Ingredients Index. This ingredient may be responsible for major toxic effects if poisonous amounts of this product are ingested.

Name & Use Manufacturer	Ingredients	Name & Use Manufacturer	Ingredients
FRIENDSHIP'S GARDEN BODY SACHET (Shulton)		FROSLITE FINISHES Paint product (Frost Paint)	
FRIENDSHIP'S GARDEN BUBBLING BATH CRYSTALS, BATH SALTS, AND TOILET SOAPS (Shulton)		FROSNAMEL Enamel (Frost Paint)	
		FROSPAR VARNISH (Frost Paint)	
FRIENDSHIP'S GARDEN COLOGNE CONC., LIQUID PETALS, & TUBE TALCUM (Shulton)		FROST Laundry bleach (Pennsylv. Salt)	Calcium hypochlorite* 9% Alkaline cleaning ingredients
		FROSTEE Insecticide (Curran)	Paradichlorobenzene* 100%
FRIGID COAT PAINT (Wilbur)		FROSTILLA FRAGRANT LOTION (Wildroot)	
FRIGITONE (Firestone	Ethylene glycol*	FROSTLIKE PAINT (Eaglo)	
FRISKY COLOGNE & PERFUME (Wolff)		FROSTONE FLAT WALL PAINT (Frost Paint)	
FR NEGATIVE DEVELOPER (FR)		FROST'S NO RUST COMPOUND (Frost Paint)	
FROLIC BATH SOFTENER, EAU DE COLOGNE, AND PERFUME (Cheramy)		FROST'S KAPAK PAINTS (Frost Paint)	
FROLIC EAU DE TOILETTE (Cheramy)		FROSTY SNOW JUMBO FLAKES Decorative spray (U. S. Packaging)	Lucite Hydrofol base Methylene chloride Perfume Freon
FROMEX DEGREASING SOLVENT (Mechanical)		FROTEX FINISHES & SYNTHETICS (Frost Paint)	
FROPLIN CORE OILS (Frost Paint)		FR PAPER DEVELOPER Photographic supply (FR)	
FROSCOTE PAINTS (Frost Paint)			
FROSEAL PRIMERS (Frost Paint)		FR SUPER X-33 AND SUPER X-33 REPLENISHER Photographic supplies (FR)	
FROSFLAT PAINT (Frost Paint)			
FROSGLOS INTERIOR SEMI GLOSS Paint (Frost Paint)		FRUIT FIX To prevent pre-harvest fruit fall of apples and pears (Thompson Chem.)	Naphthaleneacetic acid spray*

*Consult Sec. II., Ingredients Index. This ingredient may be responsible for major toxic effects if poisonous amounts of this product are ingested.

- 510 -

Name & Use Manufacturer	Ingredients	Name & Use Manufacturer	Ingredients
FRUITONE T Fungicide (Am. Chemical)	2, 4, 5-Trichlorophenoxy propionic acid, triethanolamine salt* 5.3%	FULEX-G Insecticide (Fuller System)	Mono-, di-, and trichloronaphthalenes* Gamma isomer of BHC* Other isomers of BHC
FRUITONE T DOUBLE STRENGTH Fungicide (Am. Chemical)	2, 4, 5-Trichlorophenoxy propionic acid, triethanolamine salt* 10.4% 2, 4, 5-Trichlorophenoxy propionic acid equivalent 6.8%	FULEX NO. 400 LIQUID Insecticide (Fuller System)	Dichloronaphthalene* Monochloronaphthalene* Trichlorobenzene Naphthalene* Trichloronaphthalene *
F-S VARNISH (Felton Sibley)		FULEX SOIL TREATMENT Fungicide (Fuller System)	Monochloro, dichloro- and trichloro-naphthalene (all chlorophenols)* 40% Hydroxyquinoline sulfate 17% Gamma isomer of benzene hexachloride 2.6% Other isomers of benzene hexachloride 0.4%
F.T.E. (Fritted Trace Elements) Fertilizer (Inorganic)	Iron Manganese Copper Zinc Boron Molybdenum		
FUEL FLEX Sludge, carbon solvent (Flexoid)		FULEX SPIDER-MITE FUMIGATOR (Fuller System)	2-(tert-Butylphenoxy) isopropyl 2-chloroethyl sulfite 6.7%
FULBRITE (Fuller Brush)	Wax (colloidal dispersion in water) Resins Emulsifiers (anionic)	FULFILLMENT COLOGNE (Assoc. Brands)	
FUL COLOR LATEX FINISH Paint (Fuller, W.P.)		FUL-GLEAM (Fuller Brush)	Waxes Mineral spirits*
FUL DRESS Hair dressing (Allied Drug)		FUL-GLOSS ENAMEL (Fuller, W. P.)	
FULD LIQUID EMULSION DETERGENT FOR TOILET BOWLS (Fuld)	Hydrogen chloride* 23% Orthodichlorobenzene 2.5%	FUL-KILL ROACH & ANT KILLER (Fuller Brush)	Tech. chlordane 2.0% Pyrethrins 0.046% Tech. piperonyl butoxide 0.115% Petroleum distillates* 47.839
FULD MOTH CRYSTALS (Fuld)	Paradichlorobenzene*	FULLER BOWL CLEANER (Fuller Brush)	Sodium bisulfate Sodium chloride Sodium carbonate
FULD MOTH SPRAY (Fuld)	Oil Pyrethrum	FULLERCOL (Fuller, W. P.)	
FULEX A-D-O Fungicide (Fuller System)	Hydroxyquinoline sulfate* 25%	FULLER DOG SPRAY Insecticide (Fuller Brush)	Pyrethrins 9.025% Rotenone 0.128% Other cube extractives 0.236% Tech. piperonyl cyclonene 0.256% Petroleum distillate 0.102% Inert ingredients*
FULEX APHID SMOKE Fumigant (Fuller System)	Gamma isomer of benzene hexachloride* 5.6%	FULLER FLOOR CLEANER (Fuller Brush)	Detergents (anionic including soap and non-ionic) Phosphates and polyphosphates
FULEX-AZO BENZENE LIQUID Fumigant (Fuller System)	Azobenzene*	FULLER FURNITURE POLISH (Fuller Brush)	Mineral oil Wax
		FULLER GARBAGE CAN SPRAY (Fuller Brush)	Orthodichlorobenzene* 60% Petroleum distillate 10% Pine oil 5%
FULEX FUMIGATOR Insecticide (Fuller System)	Tech. parathion* 9% (o-o-Diethyl-o-p-nitrophenyl-thiophosphate)	FULLER GASOLINE TANK SLUSHING COMPOUND TL-284/ T-3864 (Fuller, W. P.)	

*Consult Sec. II., Ingredients Index. This ingredient may be responsible for major toxic effects if poisonous amounts of this product are ingested.

Name & Use Manufacturer	Ingredients	Name & Use Manufacturer	Ingredients
FULLERGLO WALL FINISHES (Fuller, W. P.)		FUL-SCAT INSECT RE-PELLENT (Fuller Brush)	2-Ethyl hexanediol-1, 3 20.00%
FULLER INSECTICIDE (Fuller Brush)	Allethrin 0.10% Piperonyl butoxide tech. 0.25% Isobornyl thiocyanoacetate 0.82% Other related terpenes 0.18% Petroleum distillate 1.65% Methoxychlor tech. 3.00%	FUL-SHINE CLEANER (Fuld)	Potassium soap (pH 8.5-8.8)
		FULSOL (Fuller Brush)	Anionic* and non-ionic detergents Phosphates* Polyphosphates
FULLER METAL POLISH (Fuller Brush)	Silica (300 mesh) Colloidal clay Ammonia and ammonium soaps Dispersing agent (anionic) Isopropanol* Oxalic acid less than 2%	FUL-STRIP REMOVER (Assoc. Just)	Ammoniated*
		FULTEX INDUSTRIAL FINISHES & BULLETIN COLORS (Fuller, W. P.)	
FULLER MOTH PROOFER (Fuller Brush)	Diethyl diphenyl dichloroethane 4.75% Related reaction products 0.025% Petroleum distillates* 32.0% Paradichlorobenzene 3.0%	FULTON COPPER PAINTS (Debevoise)	
FULLER PINE OIL DIS-INFECTANT (Fuller Brush)	Steam-distilled pine oil* Soap	FUL-TONE FLOOR CON-DITIONER & RESTORER (Assoc. Just)	
FULLER PLANT SPRAY Insecticide (Fuller Brush)	Pyrethrins 0.025% Rotenone 0.128% Other cube extractives 0.236% Tech. piperonyl cyclonene 0.256% Petroleum distillate 0.102% Inert ingredients*	FULTON'S CRAYON SETS (Fulton Specialty)	
FULLER'S ALL PURPOSE ADHESIVE (Fuller, H. B.)	Polyvinyl acetate emulsion	FULTON'S PLANTABBS Fertilizer (Plantabbs)	Nitrate nitrogen 7.25% Ammoniacal nitrogen 3.75% Nitrogen 11.00% Phosphoric acid 15.00% Potash, water soluble 20.00%
FULLER'S CLEAR NITRATE DOPE TL-8651 (Fuller, W. P.)		FUL-TROL BACTERIO-STATIC DUST CONTROL & FLOOR MAINTAINER (Assoc. Just)	Alkyl dimethyl benzyl ammonium chloride (contains from 8 to 18 carbon atoms) 00.25%
FULLER'S LACQUER THINNER (Fuller, W. P.)			
FULLER'S LASTIKO WALL SIZE (Fuller, H. B.)	Liquified animal glue Corn dextrines	FUME OGEN Dog repellent (Rose Mfg.)	Coal tar hydrocarbons* 5%
FULLERWEAR ENAMELS (Fuller, W. P.)		FUME RESISTING PAINT (Watson-Standard)	
FUL-LIFE FLEXIBLE FILM FLOOR FINISH (Assoc. Just)		FUME-SAFE ENAMELS (O'Brien Corp.)	
FULL-O-LITE PAINT (Egan & Hausman)		FUME TITE ENAMEL (Tropical)	
FULLUSTRE (Fuller Brush)	Wax (colloidal dispersion in water) Resins Emulsifiers (anionic)	FUMEX Plastic coatings (Horn)	

*Consult Sec. II., Ingredients Index. This ingredient may be responsible for major toxic effects if poisonous amounts of this product are ingested.

Name & Use Manufacturer	Ingredients		Name & Use Manufacturer	Ingredients	
FUMIGAS Fumigant (Speekman)	Ethylene dichloride* Carbon tetrachloride*	75% 25%	FUNGUS-BAN SOLUTION TO CONTROL FUNGUS (Wilbur)		
FUMIGAS Fumigant (Thompson-Hayward)	Carbon tetrachloride* Carbon bisulfide Sulfur dioxide	82.85% 16.40% 0.75%	FUNGUSIN LIQUID (Prophylactic) Fungicide, (medical) (Pfeiffer)	Sodium ortho-benzyl phenol* Sodium para-benzyl phenol*	
FUMO-DUST Insecticide (Stauffer)	Nicotine*				
FUMO-GAS Fumigant (Am. Fumig.)	Ethylene dichloride* Carbon tetrachloride*		FUNGUSOL EMULSION Insecticide, fungicide (Destruxol)	Mineral oil Pine oil Ammonia Nicotine* as alkaloid Copper as ammoniacal copper complex Soap	32.00% 2.00% 2.50% 3.20% 0.25% 4.50%
FUMO-SPRAY Fumigant (Am. Fumig.)	Refined hydrocarbons* Pyrethrins Lethane*				
FUNG-AIDE Fungicide, (medical) (Sunset)	Salicylic acid* Benzoic acid Benzoin Balsam tolu Orthophenylphenol* Methyl salicylate* Balsam Peru Aloe Storax Sulfonated oil Isopropyl alcohol*		FUNJOL Antiseptic for water (veterinary) (Gland-O-Lac)	Alkyl dimethyl dichloro-benzyl ammonium chloride Isopropyl alcohol	3.10% 37.90%
			FURAZOLIDONE FARM MIX FORMULA Insecticide (Hess, Dr.)	Furazolidone	1.1%
FUNGI-BORDO Fungicide (Sherwin-Williams)	Copper*	12.75%	FUR CLEANING SOLVENT 3901 (Hampden)		
FUNGI-FOE Fungicide, (medical) (Maypinks)	Acetone* Salicylic acid* Iodine* Potassium iodide* Alcohol*	67%	FUR-CLENE Fur cleaner (Haertel)		
FUNGI-REX (Greaseless) Fungicide, (medical) (Rexall)	Benzoic acid Salicylic acid* Carbolic acid* Thymol*		FURNACE CEMENT (United Gilson.)	Silicate of soda Fire clay Asbestos	
FUNGI-REX LIQUID Fungicide, (medical) (Rexall)	Thymol* Salicylic acid* Carbolic acid* Benzoic acid Glycerin		FUTSANA Fungicide, (medical) (J. P.)	Undecylenic acid Sodium propionate Digenol	
FUNGI R-I-D Fungicide, (medical) (Rid Co.)	Thymol Benzoic acid Salicylic acid Total ext. from coal tar Isopropyl alcohol*	0.01% 5% 5% 1.25% 60%	FUT-SANA LIQUID Fungicide, (medical) (J. P.)	Acid salicylic* Dimethyl ketone* Glycerol	
FUNG-O Fungicide (Wilson, Andrew)	Potassium polysulfides*		FUTURA TINTING COLORS Paints (Perfection Paint)		
FUNGOID TINCTURE Fungicide, (medical) (Pedinol)	Trimethyl ammonium penta-chlorophenate* Propionic acid Undecylenic acid Sodium propionate Isopropanol Dimethyl ketone*		FYRE-LES BRANDING FLUID (Globe)	Sodium hydroxide* Barium sulfide*	
FUNGTROGEN Fungicide (Rese Mfg.)	Copper (as metallic copper from copper sulfate)	0.80%	FYR-PRUF Stove, metal polish (Prescott)		

*Consult Sec. II., Ingredients Index. This ingredient may be responsible for major toxic effects if poisonous amounts of this product are ingested.

Name & Use Manufacturer	Ingredients		Name & Use Manufacturer	Ingredients	
GABY ANTI CHAP (Gaby Co.)			GAMMACIDE COTTON DUST NO. 2-10-40 Insecticide (Calif. Spray)	Gamma isomer of BHC* Other isomers of BHC* DDT* Sulfur*	2% 13% 10% 40%
GABY SUNTAN CREAM AND LOTION (Gaby Co.)			GAMMACIDE 2-10-50 COTTON DUST Insecticide (Calif. Spray)	Gamma isomer of BHC* Other isomers of BHC* DDT* Sulfur*	2% 2% 10% 50%
GADDY A P C TABLETS Analgesic (Gaddy, R. L.)	Each tablet: Aspirin* Acetophenetidin* Caffeine	0.23 gm. 0.15 gm. 0.032 gm.	GAMMACIDE 2-10X COT- TON DUST Insecticide (Calif. Spray)	Gamma BHC* DDT* Other isomers of BHC	2% 10% 2%
GALADEX ANTACID POWDER (Commerce)	Bismuth subcarbonate Sodium bicarbonate Bismuth subgallate Calcium carbonate Kaolin Magnesium oxide Magnesium trisilicate		GAMMACIDE 3-5 COTTON DUST Insecticide (Calif. Spray)	Gamma isomer of benzene hexachloride* Other isomers of benzene hexachloride* DDT*	3% 3% 5%
GALATEST For detecting sugar in urine (Denver Chem.)	Sodium hydroxide* Bismuth oxychloride		GAMMACIDE COTTON DUST NO. 3-5-40 (Calif. Spray)	Gamma isomer of BHC* Other isomers of BHC* DDT* Sulfur*	3% 20% 5% 40%
GALE LIQUID DAIRY CLEANER (Paulen Chem.)	Non-ionic detergent* and emulsifier (alkyl phenoxy polyoxyethylene ethanol types) Isopropyl alcohol* Organic sequestering agent		GAMMACIDE 3-5-50 COT- TON DUST Insecticide, fungicide (Calif. Spray)	Gamma BHC* Other isomers of BHC* Sulfur* DDT*	3% 12% 50% 5%
GALLOTOX Liquid seed disinfectant (Gallowhur)	Phenylmercuric acetate* solubilized	7%	GAMMACIDE 3-10 COT- TON DUST Insecticide (Calif. Spray)	Gamma BHC* Other isomers* DDT*	3% 12% 10%
GALLOWHUR DISINFECT- ANT- GERMICIDE CONCEN- TRATE (Gallowhur)	Alkyl dimethyl benzyl ammonium chloride*		GAMMACIDE 3-10-40 COT- TON DUST Insecticide (Calif. Spray)	Gamma BHC* Other isomers* DDT* Sulfur	3% 22% 10% 40%
GALLOWHUR SKAT Insect re- pellent (Gallowhur)	2-Ethyl hexanediol-1, 3* Alpha, alpha-dimethyl-alpha' carbobutoxy-dihydro gamma- pyrone* Dimethyl phthalate	20% 20% 60%	GAMMACIDE 2-8 COTTON DUST Insecticide (Calif. Spray)	DDT Gamma isomer of BHC Aromatic petroleum deriv. solvent*	21.8% 8.7% 44%
GALVANIDE Primer for metal sur- faces (Horn)			GAMMA DUST 5 Insecticide (Commercial Chem.)	Lindane (Benzene hexachloride, gamma isomer)	0.5%
GAMBLE'S TONIC Digestant (Shuptrine)	Alcohol Fld. ext. aloes Fld. ext. rhubarb Fld. ext. ipecac Tr. valerian ammoniated Pot. bicarb. Pancreatin Spt. lavender compound Tr. capsicum Spt. peppermint Glycerin	13%	GAMMAHEX DUST NO. 75 Insecticide (Sunland)	Gamma isomer of hexachlorocyclohexane	0.75%
			GAMMAHEX DUST NO. 75S Insecticide (Sunland)	Gamma isomer of hexa- chlorocyclohexane Sulfur*	0.75% 75%
GAMMACIDE COTTON DUST NO. 2-5-50 Insecticide (Calif. Spray)	Gamma isomer of BHC* Other isomers of BHC* DDT* Sulfur*	2% 13% 5% 50%	GAMMAHEX DUST NO. 100S Insecticide (Sunland)	Gamma isomer of hexa- chlorocyclohexane* Other isomers of hexa- chlorocyclohexane* Sulfur*	1.0% 2.0% 50.0%

Name & Use Manufacturer	Ingredients		Name & Use Manufacturer	Ingredients	
GAMMA SPRAY ZINEB Insecticide (Chem. Form.)	Zinc ethylene-bis- (dithiocarbamate) Talc	65.0% 35%	GARD ANTI-RUST SPRAY (Gard)	Silicones Polar compounds Petroleum and chlorinated solvents*	
GAMTOX-DDT DUST NO. 1-5 Insecticide (Calif. Spray)	Gamma isomer of BHC* Other isomers of BHC* DDT*	1% 6.7% 5%	GARDEN BUG-FIX (Thompson Chem.)	Pyrethrins Rotenone Other cube extractives Piperonyl cyclonene tech. Petroleum oil	0.025% 0.128% 0.236% 0.256% 0.102%
GAMTOX-DDT DUST NO. 2-5 Insecticide (Calif. Spray)	Gamma isomer of BHC* Other isomers of BHC* DDT*	2% 13% 5%	GARDEN DOWFUME Insecticide (Dow)	Ethylene dibromide*	41%
GAMTOX DUST NO. 1 Insecticide (Calif. Spray)	Gamma isomer of BHC* Other isomers of BHC*	1% 6.6%	GARDEN DUSTER (Chem. Corp.)		
GAMTOX DUST NO. 1.5 Insecticide (Calif. Spray)	Gamma isomer of BHC* Other isomers of BHC*	1.5% 10%	GARDEN NU FUME Soil fumigant (Collins Feed)	Ethylene dibromide*	12.8%
GAMTOX-S DUST NO. 1-75 Insecticide (Calif. Spray)	Gamma isomer of BHC* Other isomer of BHC* Sulfur*	1% 6.6% 75%	GARDEN SAV'R Insecticide (Beebe Ness)	Rotenone Other cube resins Tech. methoxychlor Beta thiocyano ethyl esters of aliphatic fatty acids averaging 10-18 carbon atoms (from Lethane 60) Zineb (zinc ethylene- bis (dithiocarbamate))	0.75% 1.20% 3.00% 0.56% 3.90%
GAMTOX DUST NO. 2 Insecticide (Calif. Spray)	Gamma isomer of BHC* Other isomers of BHC*	2% 13%			
GAMTOX DUST NO. 3 Insecticide (Calif. Spray)	Gamma isomer of BHC (from lindane)*	3%	GARDEN SPRAY (Chem. Corp.)		
GAMTOX-S DUST NO. 2-50 Insecticide (Calif. Spray)	Gamma isomer of BHC* Other isomers of BHC* Sulfur*	2% 13% 50%	GARDEN WITCH Insecticide (Interstate Med.)	Cube resins* Derris Gum Arabic Sulfur* Talcum	
GAMTOX MOSQUITO CON. SPRAY (Calif. Spray)	Gamma isomer of benzene hexachloride* Other isomers of BHC* Xylene* Other aromatic petroleum derivatives*	11.7% 11.7% 35% 35%	GARDERM CREAM (C & M)	Paraffin Beeswax Lanolin Oxyaminostearate emulsifier Butyl and propyl para- hydroxybenzoates	0.50 each
GAMTOX 1 SPRAY Insecticide (Calif. Spray)	Gamma isomer of BHC* Other isomers of BHC*	11.7% 11.7%	GARD FRESH AIR ROOM DEODORANT (Gard)		
GAMTOX 10 WETTABLE Insecticide (Calif. Spray)	Gamma isomer of benzene hexachloride* Other isomers of benzene hexachloride*	10% 10%	GARD GOLF BALL SPRAY Enamel (Gard)		
GARD AEROSOL INSECT KIL- LER BOMB (Gard)	DDT Methylated naphthalenes* Tech. piperonyl butoxide Pyrethrins Allethrin (allyl homolog of cinerin-1) Petroleum distillate*	2.000% 5.000% 1.200% 0.075% 0.075% 11.650%	GARD INSECT REPELLENT (Gard)	Dimethyl phthalate Butyl dimethyl dihydro gamma pyrone carboxylate 2-Ethylhexanediol-1, 3	19.152% 5.655% 5.193%
			GARD K-7 FOOT SPRAY Deodorizer, sanitizer (Gard)	Hexachlorophene* Dichlorophene* Isopropyl alcohol*	
GARDANE SPRAY IN- SECTICIDE 48% CHLORDANE (Bonide)	Tech. chlordane* Petroleum distillate*	48% 40%	GARD SUEDE CONDITIONER (Gard)	Silicones Petroleum and chlorinated solvents*	
			GARD WEATHER- PROOF SPRAY (Gard)	Synthetic resins Silicones Petroleum and chlorinated solvents*	

*Consult Sec. II., Ingredients Index. This ingredient may be responsible for major toxic effects if poisonous amounts of this product are ingested.

Name & Use Manufacturer	Ingredients		Name & Use Manufacturer	Ingredients	
GAS FLUX (Basflux)	Boric acid* Acetone* Alcohol*		GAVICIDE ALDRIN 2 LIQUID Insecticide (Pacific Guano)	Hexachloro hexahydro dimethano naphthalene* Related compounds Petroleum aromatic derivatives *	23.1% 17.4% 49.5%
GAS GUARD Automotive gasoline additive in fuel systms (du Pont)	Methanol*	30%	GAVICIDE CHLORDANE CONC. 40W Insecticide (Pacific Guano)	Tech. chlordane*	40%
GAS-O-CIDE Liquid gas fumigant (Midland Labs.)	Ethylene dichloride* Carbon tetrachloride*		GAVICIDE CHLORDANE 45% LIQUID Insecticide (Pacific Guano)	Tech. chlordane* Aliphatic petroleum hydrocarbons*	45% 40%
GASSUP Laxative, digestant, antacid (Gastom)	Magnesium trisilicate Magnesium superoxol Magnesium oxide Lactose Sodium bicarbonate Aromatics		GAVICIDE DDT CONC. 50W Insecticide (Pacific Guano)	DDT*	50%
GASTABS Antacid, adsorbent (Thompson Med.)	Aluminum hydroxide gel Magnesium trisilicate Calcium carbonate Magnesium carbonate Bismuth subcarbonate Magnesium oxide Oil of peppermint		GAVICIDE DDT 25% LIQUID Insecticide (Pacific Guano)	DDT Aromatic petroleum deriv.*	25.0% 71.0%
GASTRICTIVE TABLETS AND POWDER Antacid (Clapp, Otis)	Magnesia calcined Sodium bicarbonate Calcium phosphate precip. Potassium phosphate Bismuth subcarbonate Calcium carbonate precip.		GAVICIDE DE-FOL-ATE Defoliant (Pacific Guano)	Sodium chlorate*	41.5%
GASTROGEN TABLETS Antacid (Bristol-Myers)	Calcium carbonate Magnesium carbonate Oil of peppermint Oil of cinnamon Ginger extract		GAVICIDE DIELDRIN CONC. 50W Insecticide (Pacific Guano)	Hexachloro-epoxy-octohydro-dimethano naphthalene* Related compounds	42.4% 7.6%
GASTRO-MUL For upset stomach (Hance)			GAVICIDE DIELDRIN 1.5 LIQUID Insecticide (Pacific Guano)	Hexachloro epoxy octahydro dimethanonaphthalene* Related compounds Petroleum hydrocarbons	15.83% 2.79% 73.38%
GASTRONAL POWDER Adsorbent, antacid (Medical Arts)	Each avoirdupois oz.: Gastric mucin Aminoacetic acid Magnesium trisilicate Pectin (apple) Aluminum hydroxide gel U.S.P. Kaolin colloidal N.F.	10 gr. 4.5 gr. 30 gr. 2 gr. 31.25 gr. 194.50 gr.	GAVICIDE DINITRO SOLUBLE SPRAY OIL Insecticide (Pacific Guano)	Dinitro ortho-cresol* Petroleum oil*	2.44% 95.00%
GASTRO-PULVIS Antiacid powder (Crowell)	Sodium bicarbonate Calcium carbonate Magnesium carbonate Bismuth subcarbonate Menthol		GAVICIDE ENDRIN 1.6 LIQUID Insecticide (Pacific Guano)	Hexachloro epoxy octahydro-endo, endo-dimethano-naphthalene* Petroleum hydrocarbons	19.5% 70.5%
GATOR ROACH HIVES Insecticide (De Soto Chem.)	Lead arsenate* Total arsenic (as metallic) Water soluble arsenic (as metallic)	16.20% 3.50% 0.10%	GAVICIDE HEPTACHLOR 2 LIQUID Insecticide (Pacific Guano)	Heptachlor* Related compounds Petroleum distillate	23.4% 9.1% 61.5%
GAVICIDE CA DUST 70 Insecticide (Pacific Guano)	Arsenic*		GAVICIDE LIME SULFUR 29% Insecticide, fungicide (Pacific Guano)	Calcium polysulfide*	29%

Name & Use Manufacturer	Ingredients		Name & Use Manufacturer	Ingredients	
GAVICIDE LINDANE CONC. 25W Insecticide (Pacific Guano)	Gamma isomer of benzene hexachloride*	25%	GAVICIDE TOXAPHENE CONC. 40W Insecticide (Pacific Guano)	Toxaphene*	40%
GAVICIDE MALATHION 5 Insecticide (Pacific Guano)	Malathion* Aromatic petroleum deriv.*	55% 35%	GAVICIDE TOXAPHENE-DDT 4-2 Insecticide (Pacific Guano)	Toxaphene* DDT Petroleum deriv.	40.0% 20.0% 36.0%
GAVICIDE MALATHION 8 LIQUID Insecticide (Pacific Guano)	Malathion* Aromatic petroleum derivatives	80.8% 4.5%	GAVICIDE TOXAPHENE 60% LIQUID Insecticide (Pacific Guano)	Toxaphene* Petroleum distillate	60% 30%
GAVICIDE OVITRAN CONC. 50W Insecticide (Pacific Guano)	p-Chlorophenyl p-chlorobenzene sulfonate*	50%	GAVICIDE ZIRAM DUST 7.6 Fungicide (Pacific Guano)	Ziram	7.6%
GAVICIDE OVITRAN 25% LIQUID Insecticide (Pacific Guano)	p-Chlorophenyl p-chlorobenzene sulfonate* Aromatic petroleum deriv.	25% 65%	GAVIOTA SOIL ALDRIN 3 Insecticide (Pacific Guano)	Hexachloro hexahydro dimethano naphthalene* Related compounds	2.85% 2.24%
GAVICIDE PARATHION CONC. 25W Insecticide (Pacific Guano)	Parathion*	25%	GAY ADVENTURE BATH OIL (Newton, Paul)		
GAVICIDE PARATHION 25% LIQUID Insecticide (Pacific Guano)	Parathion* Petroleum distillate	25% 65%	GAY ADVENTURE COLOGNE, TOILET WATER (Newton, Paul)		
GAVICIDE PICK-QUIK LIQUID DEFOLIANT (Pacific Guano)	Magnesium chlorate* (anhydrous)	17.5%	GAY ADVENTURE SACHET (Newton, Paul)		
GAVICIDE SODIUM SALT OF MCP Herbicide (Pacific Guano)	Sodium salt of 2-methyl-4-chlorophenoxyacetic acid*	23.20%	GAY ADVENTURE TALCUM POWDER (Newton, Paul)		
GAVICIDE TEPP 50% LIQUID Insecticide (Pacific Guano)	Tetraethyl pyrophosphate* Other ethyl pyrophosphates*	20% 30%	GAY-OIL BASE TEXTURE PAINT (United Gilson.)	Fish oil Aluminum stearate Synthetic resin Mineral spirits*	
			GB COLORED PENCILS (Am. Crayon)		
GAVICIDE TERRACLOR DUST 20 Fungicide (Pacific Guano)	Penta chloronitrobenzene*	20.0%	GEBAUER'S P.M.C. SPRAY Fungicide, (medical) (Gebauer)	Phenyl mercuric chloride (1-1500) Carbowax Ethyl chloride* U.S.P.	0.066% 3.000% 96.934%
			GEBAUER'S TANNIC SPRAY For burns, poison ivy (Gebauer)	Tannic acid Chlorobutanol (chloroform deriv.) Ethyl alcohol	3.92% 1.18% 33.32%

*Consult Sec. II., Ingredients Index. This ingredient may be responsible for major toxic effects if poisonous amounts of this product are ingested.

Name & Use Manufacturer	Ingredients		Name & Use Manufacturer	Ingredients	
GECOLENE THINNER 8060 Paint product (General Paint (Okla.))			GEIGY 5% ALDRIN EQUIVALENT DUST Insecticide (Geigy)	Hexachloro hexahydro dimethano naphthalene* Related compounds	4.75% 3.58%
GEIGY AG 50 Insecticide (Geigy)	DDT	50%	GEIGY 2-1/2% ALDRIN EQUIVALENT- 50% SULPHUR DUST Insecticide (Geigy)	Hexachloro hexahydro dimethano naphthalene* Related compounds Sulfur*	2.375% 1.790% 50.000%
GEIGY ALDRIN CONC. NO. 4 Insecticide (Geigy)	Hexachloro hexahydro dimethano naphthalene* Related compounds	38.85% 29.35%	GEIGY 20% ALDRIN GRANULAR CONC. Insecticide (Geigy)	Hexachloro hexahydro dimethano naphthalene* Related compounds*	19.00% 14.32%
GEIGY 2-1/2% ALDRIN-5% DDT DUST Insecticide (Geigy)	Hexachloro hexahydro dimethano naphthalene* Related compounds DDT*	2.375% 1.790% 5.000%			
GEIGY 2-1/2% ALDRIN-10% DDT-40% SULPHUR DUST Insecticide (Geigy)	Aldrin* DDT* Sulfur* Theoret. chlorine*	2.50% 10.00% 40.00% 7.14%	GEIGY 25% ALDRIN WETTABLE POWDER Insecticide (Geigy)	Hexachloro hexahydro dimethano naphthalene* Related compounds*	23.75% 17.90%
GEIGY 2-1/2% ALDRIN DUST Insecticide (Geigy)	Hexachloro hexahydro dimethano naphthalene* Related compounds	2.375% 1.790%	GEIGY ARAMITE 15W Insecticide (Geigy)	2-(p-tert-Butylphenoxy) isopropyl 2-chloroethyl sulfite	15.0%
GEIGY ALDRIN 25E Insecticide (Geigy)	Hexachloro hexahydro dimethano naphthalene* Related compounds Xylene*	21.67% 16.34% 51.00%	GEIGY ARAMITE 25E Insecticide (Geigy)	2-(p-tert-Butylphenoxy) isopropyl 2-chloroethyl sulfite Xylene*	25.5% 65.0%
GEIGY ALDRIN EQUIVALENT 25E Insecticide (Geigy)	Aldrin* Theoret. chlorine*	21.67%	GEIGY 2% ARAMITE DUST Insecticide (Geigy)	2-(p-tert-Butylphenoxy) isopropyl 2-chloroethyl sulfite	2%
GEIGY 2-1/2% ALDRIN EQUIVALENT- 10% DDT Insecticide (Geigy)	Aldrin* DDT* Theoret. chlorine*	2.50% 10.00% 7.14%	GEIGY 3% ARAMITE DUST Insecticide (Geigy)	2-(p-tert-Butylphenoxy) isopropyl 2-chloroethyl sulfite	3%
GEIGY 2-1/2% ALDRIN EQUIVALENT- 5% DDT-40% SULPHUR DUST Insecticide (Geigy)	Hexachloro hexahydro dimethano naphthalene* Related compounds* DDT* Sulfur*	2.375% 1.790% 5.000% 40.000%	GEIGY 4% ARAMITE DUST Insecticide (Geigy)	2-(p-tert-Butylphenoxy) isopropyl 2-chloroethyl sulfite	4%
GEIGY 2-1/2% ALDRIN EQUIVALENT- 10% DDT-40% SULPHUR DUST Insecticide (Geigy)	Hexachloro hexahydro dimethano naphthalene* Related compounds* DDT* Sulfur*	2.375% 1.790% 10.000% 40.000%	GEIGY 3% ARAMITE- 15% TOX- APHENE DUST Insecticide (Geigy)	2-(p-tert-Butylphenoxy) isopropyl 2-chloroethyl sulfite	3%
			GEIGY ARSENATE OF LEAD Insecticide (Geigy)	Lead arsenate* Arsenic as metallic Water soluble arsenic Lead as metallic	98.00% 20.00% 0.50%

*Consult Sec. II., Ingredients Index. This ingredient may be responsible for major toxic effects if poisonous amounts of this product are ingested.

- 518 -

Name & Use Manufacturer	Ingredients	
GEIGY BA 50 Insecticide (Geigy)	DDT*	50%
GEIGY BA 75 Insecticide (Geigy)	DDT*	75%
GEIGY BRUSH KILLER Herbicide (Geigy)	Butyl ester of 2, 4-dichlorophenoxyacetic acid*	20%
	Butyl ester of 2, 4, 5-trichlorophenoxyacetic acid*	10%
GEIGY BRUSH KILLER NO. 22 Herbicide (Geigy)	Butyl ester of 2, 4-dichlorophenoxyacetic acid*	27.93%
	Butyl ester of 2, 4, 5-trichlorophenoxyacetic acid*	27.19%
GEIGY CALCIUM ARSENATE Insecticide (Geigy)	Tricalcium arsenate*	70%
GEIGY CHLORATE COTTON DEFOLIANT Herbicide (Geigy)	Sodium chlorate*	
GEIGY 5% CHLORDANE DUST Insecticide (Geigy)	Tech. chlordane	5%
GEIGY 10% CHLORDANE DUST (Geigy)	Tech. chlordane*	10%
GEIGY 40% CHLORDANE DUST CONC. Insecticide (Geigy)	Tech. chlordane*	40.0%
GEIGY 42% CHLORDANE EMULSIFI-ABLE Insecticide (Geigy)	Tech. chlordane	42%
	Aromatic petroleum deriv. solvent*	48%

Name & Use Manufacturer	Ingredients	
GEIGY 73% CHLORDANE EMULSIFI-ABLE Insecticide (Geigy)	Tech. chlordane*	73.0%
GEIGY 40% CHLORDANE WETTABLE POWDER Insecticide (Geigy)	Tech. chlordane*	40.0%
GEIGY 50% CHLORDANE WETTABLE POWDER Insecticide (Geigy)	Tech. chlordane*	50.0%
GEIGY CHLORO-BENZILATE 15W Insecticide (Geigy)	Ethyl 4, 4'-dichlorobenzilate	15%
GEIGY CHLORO-BENZILATE 25E Insecticide (Geigy)	Ethyl 4, 4'-dichlorobenzilate	25%
	Xylene*	70.0%
GEIGY CHLORO-BENZILATE 25W Insecticide (Geigy)	Ethyl 4, 4'-dichlorobenzilate	25%
GEIGY CHLORO I.P.C. EMULSION NO. 400 Herbicide (Geigy)	Isopropyl N-(3-chlorophenyl) carbamate*	47.1%
GEIGY 7% COPPER DUST Fungicide (Geigy)	Copper* (in basic copper sulfate) expressed as metallic	7%

Name & Use Manufacturer	Ingredients	Name & Use Manufacturer	Ingredients
GEIGY 14% COPPER DUST Fungicide (Geigy)	Copper* (in basic copper sulfate) expressed as metallic 14%	GEIGY 3-10 COTTON DUST Insecticide (Geigy)	Gamma isomer of benzene hexachloride* 3% Other isomers of benzene hexachloride* 17% DDT* 10%
GEIGY 4% COPPER-SULPHUR DUST Insecticide (Geigy)	Copper* (in basic copper sulfate) 4% Sulfur* (not less than 93% through 325 mesh screen) 82%	GEIGY 3-10-40 COTTON DUST Insecticide (Geigy)	Gamma isomer of benzene hexachloride* 3% Other isomers of benzene hexachloride* 17% DDT* 10% Sulfur * 40%
GEIGY COPPER-ZINC DUST NO. 10 Fungicide (Geigy)	Copper* (in basic copper sulfate) expressed as metallic 10% Zinc (in zinc oxysulfate) expressed as metallic 2.5%	GEIGY 10-20 COTTON SPRAY Insecticide (Geigy)	Hexachloro hexahydro dimethano naphthalene* 10.57% Related compounds 7.98% DDT 23.00% Xylene* 45.00%
GEIGY COPPER-ZINC-SULPHUR DUST Fungicide (Geigy)	Copper* (in basic copper sulfate) expressed as metallic 10.0% Sulfur* (not less than 93% through 325 mesh screen) 50.0% Zinc (in zinc oxysulfate) expressed as metallic 2.5%	GEIGY D 30 Insecticide (Geigy)	DDT 30% Aromatic petroleum deriv. solvent* 70%
		GEIGY DAIRY & STOCK SPRAY Insecticide (Geigy)	Tech. methoxychlor 1.000% "264" n-Octyl bicycloheptene dicarboximide 0.250% Pyrethrins 0.006% Allethrin 0.006% Petroleum distillates* 98.738%
GEIGY CORN EARWORM SPRAY Insecticide (Geigy)	DDT 7.7% Xylene* 20.5% Refined petroleum oil 69.0%		
GEIGY 1-5-70 COTTON DUST Insecticide (Geigy)	Gamma isomer of benzene hexachloride* 1.0% Other isomers of benzene hexachoride* 5.7% DDT* 5.0% Sulfur* 70.0%	GEIGY 5% DDT-3% ARAMITE DUST Insecticide (Geigy)	DDT* 5% 2-(p-tert-Butyl phenoxy) isopropyl 2-chloroethyl sulfite 3%
GEIGY 2-5-50 COTTON DUST Insecticide (Geigy)	Gamma isomer of benzene hexachloride* 2.0% Other isomers of benzene hexachloride* 11.3% DDT* 5.0% Sulfur* 50.0%	GEIGY 10%-DDT 3% ARAMITE DUST Insecticide (Geigy)	DDT* 10% 2-(p-tert-Butyl phenoxy) isopropyl 2-chloroethyl sulfite 3%
GEIGY 2-10-40 COTTON DUST Insecticide (Geigy)	Gamma isomer of benzene hexachloride* 2.0% Other isomers of benzene hexachloride* 11.3% DDT* 10.0% Sulfur* 40.0%	GEIGY 25% DDT-7-1/2% ARAMITE WETTABLE POWDER Insecticide (Geigy)	DDT* 25.0% 2-(p-tert-Butyl phenoxy) isopropyl 2-chloroethyl sulfite 7.5%
GEIGY 2-10-50 COTTON DUST Insecticide (Geigy)	Gamma isomer of benzene hexachloride* 2.0% Other isomers of benzene hexachloride* 11.3% DDT* 10.0% Sulfur* 50.0%	GEIGY 5% DDT-3% CHLORDANE DUST (Geigy)	DDT* 5% Tech. chlordane 3%
GEIGY 3-5 COTTON DUST Insecticide (Geigy)	Gamma isomer of BHC* 3.00% DDT* 5.00%	GEIGY 5% DDT-5% CHLORDANE DUST Insecticide (Geigy)	DDT* 5% Tech. chlordane 5%
GEIGY 3-5-40 COTTON DUST Insecticide (Geigy)	Gamma isomer of BHC* 3.00% DDT* 5.00% Sulfur * 40.00%	GEIGY 5% DDT-3% CHLORDANE-6-1/2% ZINEB DUST Insecticide (Geigy)	DDT* 5.0% Tech. chlordane 3.0% Zineb (zinc ethylene-bis (dithio carbamate)) 6.5%

*Consult Sec. II., Ingredients Index. This ingredient may be responsible for major toxic effects if poisonous amounts of this product are ingested.

Name & Use Manufacturer	Ingredients		Name & Use Manufacturer	Ingredients	
GEIGY 3% DDT-7% COPPER DUST Insecticide (Geigy)	DDT Copper* (in basic copper sulfate) expressed as metallic	3% 7%	GEIGY 5% DDT-1% OIL DUST Insecticide (Geigy)	DDT* Petroleum hydrocarbon	5% 1%
GEIGY 5%-DDT 7% COPPER DUST Insecticide (Geigy)	Copper as metallic* DDT*	7.00% 5.00%	GEIGY 5% DDT-2% OIL DUST Insecticide (Geigy)	DDT* Petroleum hydrocarbon	5% 2%
GEIGY 5% DDT-9% COPPER DUST Insecticide (Geigy)	DDT* Copper* (in basic copper sulfate) expressed as metallic	5% 9%	GEIGY 10% DDT-1% OIL DUST Insecticide (Geigy)	DDT* Petroleum hydrocarbon	10% 1%
GEIGY 6% DDT-14% COPPER DUST Insecticide (Geigy)	DDT* Copper* (in basic copper sulfate) expressed as metallic	6% 14%	GEIGY 10% DDT-2% OIL DUST Insecticide (Geigy)	DDT* Petroleum hydrocarbon	10% 2%
GEIGY 1% DDT-7% COPPER IMPREGNAT-ED DUST Insecticide (Geigy)	DDT Copper* (in basic copper sulfate) expressed as metallic Aromatic petroleum deriv. solvent*	1.0% 7.0% 2.3%	GEIGY 3% DDT-1% PARATHION DUST Insecticide (Geigy)	Parathion* DDT	1.0% 3.0%
GEIGY 3% DDT-7% COPPER IMPREGNAT-ED DUST Insecticide (Geigy)	Aromatic petroleum deriv. solvent* DDT Copper* (in basic copper sulfate) expressed as metallic	2.3% 3.0% 7.0%	GEIGY 5% DDT-1% PARATHION DUST Insecticide (Geigy)	Parathion* DDT	1.0% 5.0%
GEIGY 5% DDT-7% COPPER-50% SULPHUR DUST Insecticide (Geigy)	DDT* Copper* (in basic copper sulfate) expressed as metallic Sulfur*	5% 7% 50%	GEIGY 5% DDT-2% PARATHION DUST (Geigy)	DDT Parathion*	5% 2%
GEIGY 5% DDT-9% COPPER-50% SULPHUR DUST Insecticide (Geigy)	DDT* Copper* (in basic copper sulfate) expressed as metallic Sulfur* (not less than 93% through 325 mesh screen)	5% 9% 50%	GEIGY 3% DDT-50% SULPHUR DUST Insecticide (Geigy)	DDT Sulfur*	3% 50%
GEIGY 3% DDT IMPREGNAT-ED DUST Insecticide (Geigy)	Aromatic petroleum deriv. solvent* DDT	2.3% 3.0%	GEIGY 3% DDT-75% SULPHUR DUST Insecticide (Geigy)	DDT Sulfur*	3% 75%
GEIGY 5% DDT IM-PREGNATED DUST Insecticide (Geigy)	DDT* Aromatic petroleum deriv. solvent*	5% 2.3%	GEIGY 5% DDT-27% SULPHUR DUST Insecticide (Geigy)	DDT* Sulfur*	5% 27%
			GEIGY 5% DDT-50% SULPHUR DUST Insecticide (Geigy)	DDT* Sulfur*	5% 50%
GEIGY DDT MOSQUITO EMULSION Insecticide (Geigy)	DDT Xylene*	24.4% 65.3%	GEIGY 5% DDT-75% SULPHUR DUST Insecticide (Geigy)	DDT* Sulfur*	5% 75%

Name & Use Manufacturer	Ingredients		Name & Use Manufacturer	Ingredients	
GEIGY 10% DDT-50% SULPHUR DUST Insecticide (Geigy)	DDT* Sulfur*	10% 50%	GEIGY DIELDRIN AIRPLANE SPRAY Insecticide (Geigy)	Hexachloro epoxy octahydro dimethano naphthalene* Related compounds Xylene* Petroleum hydrocarbons	15.65% 2.76% 73.40% 8.19%
GEIGY 10-75 DDT-SULPHUR DUST Insecticide (Geigy)	DDT* Sulfur*	10% 74%	GEIGY 1-1/2% DIELDRIN- 10% DDT DUST Insecticide (Geigy)	Hexachloro epoxy octahydro dimethano naphthalene* Related compounds DDT*	1.275% 0.225% 10.000%
GEIGY 5% DDT-50% SULPHUR-1% OIL DUST Insecticide (Geigy)	DDT* Sulfur* Petroleum oil	5% 50% 1%	GEIGY 2-1/2% DIELDRIN- 5% DDT DUST Insecticide (Geigy)	Hexachloro epoxy octahydro dimethano naphthalene* Related compounds DDT*	2.125% 0.375% 5.000%
GEIGY DDT (Technical Grade) Insecticide (Geigy)	DDT*	100%	GEIGY 2-1/2% DIELDRIN- 10% DDT DUST Insecticide (Geigy)	Hexachloro epoxy octahydro dimethano naphthalene* Related compounds DDT*	2.125% 0.375% 10.000%
GEIGY 7-1/2% DDT-7-1/2% TOXAPHENE DUST Insecticide (Geigy)	DDT* Toxaphene*	7.5% 7.5%	GEIGY 1-1/2% DIELDRIN- 5% DDT-40% SULPHUR DUST Insecticide (Geigy)	Hexachloro epoxy octahydro dimethano naphthalene* Related compounds DDT* Sulfur*	1.275% 0.225% 5.00% 40.000%
GEIGY 50% DDT WETTABLE POWDER Insecticide (Geigy)	DDT*	50%	GEIGY 1-1/2% DIELDRIN-10% DDT-40% SULPHUR DUST Insecticide (Geigy)	Hexachloro-epoxy-octahydro-dimethano-naphthalene* Related compounds DDT* Sulfur*	1.275% 0.225% 10.000% 40.000%
GEIGY 5% DDT-7-1/2% ZINC-COP DUST Insecticide (Geigy)	DDT* Copper* (in basic copper sulfate) expressed as metallic Zinc (in zinc oxysulfate) expressed as metallic	5.0% 6.0% 1.5%	GEIGY 2-1/2% DIELDRIN- 5% DDT-40% SULPHUR DUST Insecticide (Geigy)	Hexachloro-epoxy-octahydro-dimethano-naphthalene Related compounds DDT* Sulfur*	0.375% 0.375% 5.000% 40.000%
GEIGY 5% DDT-6-1/2% ZINEB DUST Insecticide (Geigy)	DDT* Zineb (zinc ethylene-bis (dithiocarbamate)) Total zinc as metallic	5.0% 6.5% 1.5%	GEIGY 2-1/2% DIELDRIN- 10% DDT-40% SULPHUR DUST Insecticide (Geigy)	Hexachloro-epoxy-octahydro-dimethano-naphthalene* Related compounds DDT* Sulfur*	2.125% 0.375% 10.000% 40.000%
GEIGY DDT-ZINEB DUST NO. 16 Insecticide (Geigy)	DDT Zineb	1.0% 3.9%	GEIGY 1-1/2% DIELDRIN DUST Insecticide (Geigy)	Hexachloro epoxy-octahydro di-methano naphthalene* Related compounds	1.275% 0.225%
GEIGY DIAZINON 25W Insecticide (Geigy)	o,o-Diethyl-o(2-isopropyl-4-methyl-pyrimidyl-6) thiophosphate*	25%	GEIGY 25% DIELDRIN DUST CONC. Insecticide (Geigy)	Hexachloro epoxy octahydro dimethano naphthalene* Related compounds	21.25% 3.75%
GEIGY DIAZINON FLY KILLER (Geigy)	Diazinon (o-o-diethyl-o(2-isopropyl-4-methyl-pyrimidyl-6) thiophosphate)	1%	GEIGY 50% DIELDRIN DUST CONC. Insecticide (Geigy)	Hexachloro epoxy octahydro dimethano naphthalene* Related compounds	42.50% 7.50%
GEIGY DIELDRIN 18E Insecticide (Geigy)	Hexachloro epoxy octahydro dimethano naphthalene* Related compounds Xylene*	15.89% 2.81% 71.10%			

*Consult Sec. II., Ingredients Index. This ingredient may be responsible for major toxic effects if poisonous amounts of this product are ingested.

Name & Use Manufacturer	Ingredients		Name & Use Manufacturer	Ingredients	
GEIGY 25% DIELDRIN WETTABLE POWDER Insecticide (Geigy)	Hexachloro epoxy octahydro dimethano naphthalene* Related compounds	21.2% 3.8%	GEIGY 5-8-75 DUST Insecticide (Geigy)	DDT* Zineb Sulfur*	5.0% 5.2% 75.0%
GEIGY 50% DIELDRIN WETTABLE POWDER Insecticide (Geigy)	Hexachloro epoxy octahydro dimethano naphthalene* Related compounds	42.4% 7.6%	GEIGY 8-50 DUST Fungicide (Geigy)	Zineb Sulfur*	5.2% 50%
GEIGY DORMANT OIL EMULSION Insecticide (Geigy)	Petroleum oil*	80%	GEIGY 8-75 DUST Fungicide (Geigy)	Zineb Sulfur*	8.0% 75.0%
GEIGY DOUBLE M FLY SPRAY Insecticide (Geigy)	Malathion* Tech. methoxychlor Xylene*	23.10% 23.10% 47.20%	GEIGY 6-10 DUST CONCEN-TRATE Insecticide (Geigy)	Gamma isomer of benzene hexachloride* Other isomers of benzene hexachloride* DDT	6% 34% 10%
GEIGY 1-3-50 DUST FOR BEANS Insecticide (Geigy)	DDT Rotenone Other cube resins Sulfur*	3% 1% 2% 50%	GEIGY 9-15 DUST CONCEN-TRATE Insecticide (Geigy)	Gamma isomer of benzene hexachloride* Other isomers of benzene hexachloride* DDT	9.0% 13.5% 15.0%
GEIGY 3-5 DUST Insecticide (Geigy)	Gamma isomer of benzene hexachloride* Other isomers of benzene hexachloride* DDT*	3.0% 4.5% 5.0%	GEIGY DUSTING SULPHUR NO. 98 Fungicide (Geigy)	Sulfur* (93% through 325-mesh screen)	98%
GEIGY 3-5-40 DUST Insecticide (Geigy)	Gamma isomer of benzene hexachloride* Other isomers of benzene hexachloride* DDT* Sulfur*	3.0% 4.5% 5.0% 40.0%	GEIGY 5-6-50 DUST (With Zinc) Insecticide (Geigy)	DDT* Copper* (in basic copper sulfate) expressed as metallic Sulfur*	5.0% 6.0% 50%
GEIGY 3-10 DUST Insecticide (Geigy)	Gamma isomer of benzene hexachloride* Other isomers of benzene hexachloride* DDT*	3.0% 4.5% 10.0%	GEIGY 5-10-50 DUST (With Zinc) Insecticide (Geigy)	DDT* Copper* (in basic copper sulfate) expressed as metallic Sulfur*	5.0% 10.0% 50.0%
GEIGY 3-10-40 DUST Insecticide (Geigy)	Gamma isomer of benzene hexachloride* Other isomers of benzene hexachloride* DDT* Sulfur*	3.0% 4.5% 10.0% 40.0%	GEIGY E25 Insecticide (Geigy)	DDT* Xylene* Aromatic petroleum deriv. solvent	25% 63% 7%
GEIGY 5-6-50 DUST Insecticide (Geigy)	DDT* Copper* (in basic copper sulfate) expressed as metallic Sulfur*	5.0% 6.0% 50.0%	GEIGY E35 Insecticide (Geigy)	DDT* Xylene* Aromatic petroleum deriv. solvent	35% 54% 6%
GEIGY 5-6-75 DUST Insecticide (Geigy)	DDT* Zineb Sulfur*	5.0% 3.9% 75.0%	GEIGY ENDRIN EMULSIFI-ABLE NO. 16 Insecticide (Geigy)	Endrin (hexachloro epoxy octahydro-endo,endo-dimethano naphthalene)* Xylene* Aromatic petroleum deriv. solvent	19.6% 65.0% 7.0%
GEIGY 5-8-25 DUST Insecticide (Geigy)	DDT* Zineb Sulfur*	5.0% 5.2% 25.0%	GEIGY EQ-53 Moth-proofer (Geigy)	DDT*	25%

*Consult Sec. II., Ingredients Index. This ingredient may be responsible for major toxic effects if poisonous amounts of this product are ingested.

- 523 -

Name & Use Manufacturer	Ingredients		Name & Use Manufacturer	Ingredients	
GEIGY FERBAM 76 Fungicide (Geigy)	Ferbam	76%	GEIGY HEPTACHLOR 25W Insecticide Geigy)	Heptachlor* Related compounds*	25.00% 9.72%
GEIGY FERBAM DUST FOR TOBACCO BLUE MOLD Fungicide (Geigy)	Ferbam	11.4%	GEIGY 2-1/2% HEPTACHLOR- 5% DDT DUST Insecticide (Geigy)	Heptachlor* Related compounds DDT*	2.50% 0.97% 5.00%
GEIGY 15% FERMATE- 3% DDT DUST Insecticide (Geigy)	Ferric dimethyl dithio- carbamate DDT	11.40% 3.00%	GEIGY 2-1/2% HEPTACHLOR- 10% DDT DUST Insecticide (Geigy)	Heptachlor* Related compounds DDT*	2.50% 0.97% 10.00%
GEIGY 15% FERMATE DUST Insecticide (Geigy)	Ferric dimethyl dithio- carbamate	11.40%	GEIGY 2-1/2% HEPTACHLOR- 5% DDT-40% SULPHUR DUST Insecticide (Geigy)	Heptachlor* Related compounds DDT* Sulfur*	2.50% 0.97% 5.00% 40.00%
GEIGY 1% GAMMA BHC DUST Insecticide (Geigy)	Gamma isomer of benzene hexachloride* Other isomers of benzene hexachloride*	1.0% 5.7%	GEIGY 2-1/2% HEPTACHLOR- 10% DDT-40% SULPHUR DUST Insecticide (Geigy)	Heptachlor* Related compounds DDT* Sulfur*	2.50% 0.97% 10.00% 40.00%
GEIGY 2% GAMMA BHC DUST Insecticide (Geigy)	Gamma isomer of benzene hexachloride* Other isomers of benzene hexachloride*	2.0% 11.3%	GEIGY 1-1/2% HEPTACHLOR DUST Insecticide (Geigy)	Heptachlor Related compounds	1.50% 0.58%
GEIGY 3% GAMMA BHC DUST Insecticide (Geigy)	Gamma isomer of benzene hexachloride* Other isomers of benzene hexachloride*	3% 17%	GEIGY 2-1/2% HEPTACHLOR DUST Insecticide (Geigy)	Heptachlor* Related compounds	2.50% 0.97%
GEIGY GARDEN DUST Insecticide (Geigy)	Tech. methoxychlor Malathion* Captan (n-trichloromethylthio- tetrahydro-phthalamide)	3.0% 4.0% 88.0%	GEIGY 25% HEPTACHLOR DUST CONC. Insecticide (Geigy)	Heptachlor* Related compounds*	25.0% 9.7%
GEIGY GRUB DUST Insecticide (Geigy)	Rotenone Other cube extractives	1.6% 3.2%	GEIGY HORTI- CULTURAL OIL NO. 700 Spray additive (Geigy)	Petroleum oil*	100%
GEIGY HEPTACHLOR 2E Insecticide (Geigy)	Heptachlor* Related compounds Xylene*	23.2% 9.0% 63.0%			

*Consult Sec. II., Ingredients Index. This ingredient may be responsible for major toxic effects if poisonous amounts of this product are ingested.

Name & Use Manufacturer	Ingredients	Name & Use Manufacturer	Ingredients
GEIGY IPC EMULSION NO. 200 Herbicide (Geigy)	Isopropyl-n-phenyl carbamate 26%	GEIGY MALATHION 25W Insecticide (Geigy)	Malathion* 25%
GEIGY LINDANE Insecticide (Geigy)	Gamma isomer of benzene hexachloride* 99% Other isomers of benzene hexachloride 1%	GEIGY MALATHION-ZINEB DUST NO. 46 Insecticide (Geigy)	Malathion* 4.0% Zineb (zinc ethylene-bis (dithio-carbamate)) 3.9% Total zinc as metallic 0.92%
GEIGY LINDANE 20E Insecticide (Geigy)	Gamma isomer of benzene hexachloride* (from lindane) 20% Xylene* 75%	GEIGY MC 50 Insecticide (Geigy)	DDT* 50%
GEIGY LINDANE 25W Insecticide (Geigy)	Gamma isomer of benzene hexachloride* (from lindane) 25%	GEIGY MC 75 Insecticide (Geigy)	DDT* 75%
GEIGY LINDANE 75W Insecticide (Geigy)	Gamma isomer of benzene hexachloride* (from lindane) 75%	GEIGY MCP WEED KILLER NO. 4 Insecticide (Geigy)	Mixed isopropyl and triethyl amine salts of 2 methyl,4 chlorophenoxy acetic acid* 60.7%
GEIGY 1% LINDANE DUST Insecticide (Geigy)	Gamma isomer of benzene hexachloride (from lindane) 0.99%	GEIGY METHOXY-CHLOR 20 Insecticide (Geigy)	Methoxychlor 20% Aromatic petroleum deriv. solvent* 80%
GEIGY 1-1/2% LINDANE DUST Insecticide (Geigy)	Gamma isomer of benzene hexachloride (from lindane) 1.48%	GEIGY METHOXY-CHLOR 25E Insecticide (Geigy)	Methoxychlor 25% Xylene* 63% Aromatic petroleum deriv. solvent 7%
GEIGY LO-V BRUSH KILLER NO. 700 Herbicide (Geigy)	Butoxy polyethoxy propanol ester of 2,4,5-trichloro-phenoxyacetic acid* 70.6%	GEIGY METHOXY-CHLOR 50 Insecticide (Geigy)	Methoxychlor* 50%
GEIGY LO-V BRUSH KILLER NO. 800 Herbicide (Geigy)	Butoxy polyethoxy propanol ester of 2,4-dichloro-phenoxyacetic acid* 37.8% Butoxy polyethoxy propanol ester of 2,4,5-trichloro-phenoxyacetic acid* 35.6%	GEIGY METHOXY-CHLOR 90 (For manufac-turing purposes only) Insecticide (Geigy)	Methoxychlor* 90% Petroleum distillate 10%
GEIGY LO-V WEED KILLER NO. 600 (Geigy)	Butoxy polyethoxy propanol ester of 2,4-dichloro-phenoxyacetic acid* 76.0%	GEIGY METHOXY-CHLOR-ALLETHRIN EMULSIFI-ABLE CONC. Insecticide (Geigy)	Methoxychlor 20.00% Allethrin (allyl homolog of cinerin 1 and related compounds) 0.21% n-Octyl bicycloheptene dicarbox-imide 2.23% Petroleum distillate 8.20% Aromatic petroleum deriv. solvent* 64.85%
GEIGY M25 Insecticide (Geigy)	DDT 25% Aromatic petroleum deriv. solvent* 70%		
GEIGY MALATHION L-50 Insecticide (Geigy)	Malathion* 50.0% Petroleum solvent 36.4%	GEIGY 10% METHOXY-CHLOR DUST Insecticide (Geigy)	Methoxychlor* 10%
GEIGY 4% MALATHION-50% SULPHUR DUST Insecticide (Geigy)	Malathion* 4% Sulfur* (93% through 325-mesh screen) 50%	GEIGY METHOXY-CHLOR LOUSE POWDER (Geigy)	Methoxychlor* 10% Sulfur* (93% through 325-mesh screen) 20%

*Consult Sec. II., Ingredients Index. This ingredient may be responsible for major toxic effects if poisonous amounts of this product are ingested.

Name & Use Manufacturer	Ingredients	
GEIGY 5% METHOXY-CHLOR-1% OIL DUST Insecticide (Geigy)	Methoxychlor Petroleum oil	5% 1%
GEIGY 5% METHOXY-CHLOR-SULPHUR DUST Insecticide (Geigy)	Methoxychlor Sulfur*	5% 75%
GEIGY 5% METHOXY-CHLOR-6-1/2% ZINEB DUST Insecticide (Geigy)	Tech. methoxychlor Zineb	5.0% 6.5%
GEIGY MULTI-FILM C For use with cotton defoliant sprays (Geigy)	Alkylarylpolyoxyethylene glycols Free fatty acids Petroleum oil	
GEIGY MULTI-PURPOSE FRUIT SPRAY Insecticide (Geigy)	Tech. methoxychlor* Malathion* Captan (n-trichloromethylthio-tetrahydrophthalamide)	18.75% 6.25% 12.50%
GEIGY PARATHION 4M Insecticide (Geigy)	Parathion* Xylene	48% 41%
GEIGY PARATHION 15W Insecticide (Geigy)	Parathion*	15%
GEIGY PARATHION 25W Insecticide (Geigy)	Parathion*	25%
GEIGY PARATHION L25 Insecticide (Geigy)	Parathion* Xylene	25% 65%
GEIGY 1% PARATHION 7% COPPER DUST Insecticide (Geigy)	Parathion* Copper (in basic copper sulfate) expressed as metallic	1.0% 7.0%
GEIGY 8-1/3% PARATHION-50% DDT WETTABLE POWDER Insecticide (Geigy)	DDT Parathion*	50.0% 8.3%
GEIGY 1% PARATHION DUST Insecticide (Geigy)	Parathion*	1%

Name & Use Manufacturer	Ingredients	
GEIGY 2% PARATHION DUST Insecticide (Geigy)	Parathion*	2%
GEIGY 25% PARATHION DUST CONC. Insecticide (Geigy)	Parathion*	25%
GEIGY 1% PARATHION-75% SULPHUR DUST Insecticide (Geigy)	Parathion* Sulfur (93% through 325-mesh screen)	1% 75%
GEIGY 2% PARATHION-75% SULPHUR DUST Insecticide (Geigy)	Parathion* Sulfur	2% 75%
GEIGY PARATHION-ZINEB DUST NO. 16 Insecticide (Geigy)	Parathion* Zineb (total zinc as metallic 0.92%)	1.0% 3.9%
GEIGY PARATHION-ZINEB-SULPHUR DUST NO. 6 Insecticide (Geigy)	Parathion* Zineb Sulfur	2.0% 3.9% 75.0%
GEIGY PARIS GREEN Insecticide (Geigy)	Copper acetoarsenite* Arsenic as metallic Water soluble arsenic Copper as metallic	91.70% 40.65% 2.70% 23.00%
GEIGY PCP NO. 5 Wood preservative (Geigy)	Pentachlorophenol* Petroleum solvents*	5% 95%
GEIGY PCP NO. 10 Herbicide (Geigy)	Pentachlorophenol Aromatic petroleum deriv. solvent*	10% 88%
GEIGY PCP NO. 10 Wood preservative (Geigy)	Pentachlorophenol Aromatic petroleum solvent*	10% 70%
GEIGY PCP NO. 25 Herbicide (Geigy)	Pentachlorophenol* Pine oil Aromatic petroleum deriv. solvent*	25% 17% 50%
GEIGY PCP NO. 40 Wood preservative (Geigy)	Pentachlorophenol* Petroleum solvents*	40% 35%

*Consult Sec. II., Ingredients Index. This ingredient may be responsible for major toxic effects if poisonous amounts of this product are ingested.

Name & Use Manufacturer	Ingredients	
GEIGY POTATO VINE & WEED KILLER (Geigy)	Sodium arsenite*	40%
GEIGY 3% PURIFIED DDT DUST Insecticide (Geigy)	DDT	3%
GEIGY 3/4% ROTENONE DUST Insecticide (Geigy)	Rotenone Other cube resins	0.75% 1.50%
GEIGY 1% ROTENONE SULPHUR DUST Insecticide (Geigy)	Rotenone Other cube resins Sulfur*	1.00% 2.00% 50.00%
GEIGY 5% ROTENONE WETTABLE POWDER Insecticide (Geigy)	Rotenone* Other cube resins*	5% 10%
GEIGY S-6 Insecticide (Geigy)	DDT* Petroleum hydrocarbon*	6.9% 93.1%
GEIGY S-13 Insecticide (Geigy)	DDT Xylene* Petroleum hydrocarbon	13.6% 24.3% 62.1%
GEIGY S-34 Insecticide (Geigy)	DDT* Aromatic petroleum deriv. solvent*	34% 66%
GEIGY S-450 Insecticide (Geigy)	Petroleum oil* DDT*	95.5% 4.5%
GEIGY SP-50 Fungicide, pea treatment (Geigy)	Chloranil* (tetrachloro-benzoquinone)	48%
GEIGY SPREADER STICKER (Geigy)	Polyethylene glycol ester of mixed fatty acids Sorbitan monoleate	80% 20%
GEIGY TCA GRASS KILLER NO. 90 (Geigy)	Sodium trichloroacetate*	90%
GEIGY 5% TDE (DDD) DUST Insecticide (Geigy)	Dichloro diphenyl dichloro-ethane*	5%
GEIGY 10% TDE (DDD) DUST Insecticide (Geigy)	Dichloro diphenyl dichloro-ethane*	10%
GEIGY 50% TDE (DDD) DUST CONC. Insecticide (Geigy)	Dichloro diphenyl dichloro-ethane*	50%

Name & Use Manufacturer	Ingredients	
GEIGY 25% TDE (DDD) EMULSION CONC. Insecticide (Geigy)	Dichloro diphenyl dichloro-ethane Aromatic petroleum deriv. solvent*	25.0% 71.8%
GEIGY 5% TDE (DDD)-1% PARATHION DUST Insecticide (Geigy)	Dichloro diphenyl dichloro-ethane Parathion*	5% 1%
GEIGY 10% TDE (DDD)-1% PARATHION DUST (Geigy)	Dichloro diphenyl dichloro-ethane Parathion*	10% 1%
GEIGY 5% TDE (DDD)-50% SULPHUR DUST Insecticide (Geigy)	Dichloro diphenyl dichloro-ethane Sulfur*	5% 50%
GEIGY 5% TDE (DDD)-75% SULPHUR DUST Insecticide (Geigy)	Dichloro diphenyl dichloro-ethane Sulfur*	5% 75%
GEIGY TDE (DDD), TECHNICAL GRADE Insecticide (Geigy)	Dichloro diphenyl dichloro-ethane*	100%
GEIGY 50% TDE (DDD) WETTABLE POWDER Insecticide (Geigy)	Dichloro diphenyl dichloro-ethane*	50%
GEIGY 5-6 TOMATO DUST Insecticide (Geigy)	DDT* Zineb	5.0% 3.9%
GEIGY 15% TOXAPHENE-5% DDT 40% SULPHUR DUST Insecticide (Geigy)	Toxaphene* DDT Sulfur	15% 5% 40%
GEIGY 10% TOXAPHENE-1% PARATHION DUST Insecticide (Geigy)	Toxaphene Parathion*	10% 1%
GEIGY 2,4-D AMINE WEED KILLER (Geigy)	Mixed isopropyl and triethyl amine salts of 2,4-dichloro phenoxy acetic acid*	56%
GEIGY 2,4-D AMINE WEED KILLER NO. 40 (Geigy)	Dimethylamine salt of 2,4-dichloro phenoxy acetic acid*	49.4%

*Consult Sec. II., Ingredients Index. This ingredient may be responsible for major toxic effects if poisonous amounts of this product are ingested.

Name & Use Manufacturer	Ingredients		Name & Use Manufacturer	Ingredients	
GEIGY 2,4-D ESTER WEED KILLER (Geigy)	Butyl ester of 2,4-dichloro phenoxy acetic acid*	40%	GEMACEN Analgesic, colds (CaPhenin)	Acetophenetidin* Aspirin* Caffeine citrated Gelsemium	2 gr. 3 gr. 1/2 gr. 1/42 gr.
GEIGY 2,4-D ESTER WEED KILLER NO. 4 (Geigy)	Butyl ester of 2,4-dichloro phenoxy acetic acid*	56.44%	GEM BLUING (Gem)		
GEIGY 2,4-D ISOPROPYL ESTER NO. 333 Herbicide (Geigy)	Isopropyl ester of 2,4-dichloro phenoxy acetic acid*	44%	GEMEY COLOGNE, PERFUME (Hudnut, R.)		
			GEMEY SACHET (Hudnut, R.)		
GEIGY 2,4,5-T NO. 400 Herbicide (Geigy)	Butyl ester of 2,4,5-trichloro phenoxy acetic acid*	53.6%	GEMEY TOILET WATER (Hudnut, R.)		
GEIGY VD 50 Insecticide (Geigy)	DDT*	50%	GEMEY DUSTING POWDER, TALCUM (Hudnut, R.)		
GEIGY VD 75 Insecticide (Geigy)	DDT*	75%	GENARIS DROPS (Sacramento)		
GEIGY WETTABLE SULPHUR Insecticide (Geigy)	Sulfur* (93% through 325 mesh screen)	90%	GEN-CO CREAM (Sacramento)		
GEIGY ZINC-COP Fungicide (Geigy)	Copper* as metallic (from basic copper sulfate) Zinc* as metallic (from zinc oxysulfate)	42% 11%	GENERAL CHEMICAL AGRI-MYCIN Bactericide (General Chem.)	Streptomycin Oxytetracycline	15.0% 1.5%
GEIGY 6-1/2% ZINEB DUST Fungicide (Geigy)	Zineb	6.5%	GENERAL CHEMICAL 0-10-40 COTTON DUST Insecticide (General Chem.)	DDT* tech. Sulfur*	10% 40%
GEIGY ZINEB DUST NO. 6 Fungicide (Geigy)	Zineb	3.9%			
GEIGY ZINEB DUST NO. 8 Fungicide (Geigy)	Zineb	5.2%	GENERAL CHEMICAL 1-1/2-5 COTTON DUST Insecticide (General Chem.)	Dieldrin (hexachloro epoxy octahydro-endo, exo-dimethano naphthalene and related compounds)* DDT* tech.	1.5% 5.0%
GEIGY ZIRAM DUST NO. 10 Fungicide (Geigy)	Ziram (zinc dimethyl dithio-carbamate) Total zinc as metallic	7.4% 1.62%			
GEIGY ZIRAM 76 Fungicide (Geigy)	Ziram (zinc dimethyl dithio-carbamate) Total zinc as metallic	76% 16.25%	GENERAL CHEMICAL 1-1/2-5-1 COTTON DUST Insecticide (General Chem.)	Dieldrin (hexachloro epoxy octahydro-endo, exo-dimethano naphthalene and related compounds) DDT tech. Parathion* (o,o-diethyl-o-p-nitrophenyl thiophosphate)	1.5% 5.0% 1.0%
GELPIRIN COMPOUND Analgesic (Schuemann)	Aspirin* Acetophenetidin* Caffeine Gelsemium	3-1/2 gr. 2-1/2 gr. 1/2 gr. 1/5 gr.			
GELUSIL (Liquid) Antacid, adsorbent (Warner-Chilcott)	Each 4 cc.: Magnesium trisilicate Aluminum hydroxide	0.5 gm. 0.25 gm.	GENERAL CHEMICAL 1-1/2-10-1 COTTON DUST Insecticide (General Chem.)	Dieldrin (hexachloro epoxy octahydro-endo, exo-dimethano naphthalene and related compounds) DDT tech. Parathion* (o,o-diethyl-o-p-nitrophenyl thiophosphate)	1.5% 10% 1%

*Consult Sec. II., Ingredients Index. This ingredient may be responsible for major toxic effects if poisonous amounts of this product are ingested.

Name & Use Manufacturer	Ingredients	Name & Use Manufacturer	Ingredients
GENERAL CHEMICAL 1-1/2-10-40 COTTON DUST Insecticide (General Chem.)	Dieldrin* (hexachloro epoxy octahydro-endo, exo-dimethano naphthalene and related compounds) 1.5% DDT* tech. 10% Sulfur* 40%	GENERAL CHEMICAL 3-10-0 COTTON DUST Insecticide (General Chem.)	Gamma isomer of BHC* (benzene hexachloride) 3.0% Other isomers of BHC* (benzene hexachloride) 16.0% DDT* tech. 10.0%
GENERAL CHEMICAL 2-1/2-0-0 COTTON DUST Insecticide (General Chem.)	Heptachlor* (heptachloro-4-7-methano tetrahydroindene) 2.5% Related compounds 0.97%	GENERAL CHEMICAL 3-10-1 COTTON DUST Insecticide (General Chem.)	Gamma isomer of BHC (benzene hexachloride) 3% Other isomers of BHC (benzene hexachloride) 16% DDT tech. 10% Parathion* (o,o-diethyl-o-p-nitrophenyl thiophosphate) 1%
GENERAL CHEMICAL 2-1/2-5-0 COTTON DUST Insecticide (General Chem.)	Heptachlor* (heptachloro-4-7-methano tetrahydroindene) 2.5% Related compounds 0.97% DDT* tech. 5%	GENERAL CHEMICAL 3-10-40 COTTON DUST Insecticide (General Chem.)	Gamma isomer of BHC* (benzene hexachloride) 3.0% Other isomers of BHC* (benzene hexachloride) 16.0% DDT* tech. 10.0% Sulfur* 40.0%
GENERAL CHEMICAL 2-1/2-5-40 COTTON DUST Insecticide (General Chem.)	Heptachlor* (heptachloro-4,7-methano tetrahydroindene) 2.5% Related compounds 0.97% DDT* tech. 5% Sulfur* 40%	GENERAL CHEMICAL 5-0-0 COTTON DUST Insecticide (General Chem.)	Gamma isomer of BHC* (benzene hexachloride) 5.0% Other isomers of BHC* (benzene hexachloride) 27.0%
GENERAL CHEMICAL 2-1/2-10-40 COTTON DUST Insecticide (General Chem.)	Aldrin* (hexachloro hexahydro-endo, exo-dimethano naphthalene and related compounds) 2.8% DDT* tech. 10% Sulfur* 40%	GENERAL CHEMICAL 5-5-0 COTTON DUST Insecticide (General Chem.)	Gamma isomer of BHC* (benzene hexachloride) 5.0% Other isomers of BHC* (benzene hexachloride) 27.0% DDT* tech. 5.0%
GENERAL CHEMICAL 3-0-0 COTTON DUST Insecticide (General Chem.)	Gamma isomer of BHC* (benzene hexachloride) 3.0% Other isomers of BHC* (benzene hexachloride) 16.0%	GENERAL CHEMICAL 5-10-0 COTTON DUST Insecticide (General Chem.)	Gamma isomer of BHC* (benzene hexachloride) 5% Other isomers of BHC* (benzene hexachloride) 16% DDT* tech. 10%
GENERAL CHEMICAL 3-5-0 COTTON DUST Insecticide (General Chem.)	Gamma isomer of BHC* (benzene hexachloride) 3.0% Other isomers of BHC* (benzene hexachloride) 16.0% DDT* 5.0%	GENERAL CHEMICAL 5-10-40 COTTON DUST Insecticide (General Chem.)	Gamma isomer of BHC* (benzene hexachloride) 5% Other isomers of BHC* (benzene hexachloride) 16% DDT* tech. 10% Sulfur* 40%
GENERAL CHEMICAL 3-5-1 COTTON DUST Insecticide (General Chem.)	Gamma isomer of BHC (benzene hexachloride) 3% Other isomers of benzene hexachloride 16% DDT tech. 5% Parathion* (o,o-diethyl-o-p-nitrophenyl thiophosphate) 1%	GENERAL CHEMICAL 20-10-0 COTTON DUST Insecticide (General Chem.)	Toxaphene*(tech. chlorinated camphene, 67-69% chlorine) 20% DDT tech. 10%
GENERAL CHEMICAL 3-5-40 COTTON DUST Insecticide (General Chem.)	Gamma isomer of BHC* (benzene hexachloride) 3.0% Other isomers of BHC* (benzene hexachloride) 16.0% DDT* tech. 5.0% Sulfur* 40.0%	GENERAL CHEMICAL 20-40 COTTON DUST Insecticide (General Chem.)	Toxaphene* (tech. chlorinated camphene, 67-69% chlorine) 20% Sulfur 40%

*Consult Sec. II., Ingredients Index. This ingredient may be responsib.e for major toxic effects if poisonous amounts of this product are ingested.

- 529 -

Name & Use Manufacturer	Ingredients	Name & Use Manufacturer	Ingredients
GENERAL CHEMICAL CHLORO IPC EM-4 EMULSIFI-ABLE CONC. Herbicide (General Chem.)	Isopropyl n-(3-chlorophenyl) carbamate* 47.0%	GENERAL CHEMICAL GENITOX D-50 (50% DDT dust base) Insecticide (General Chem.)	DDT* tech. 50%
GENERAL CHEMICAL DDT, TECHNICAL (Ground or Flake) Insecticide (General Chem.)	DDT* tech. 100%	GENERAL CHEMICAL GENITOX D-75 (75% DDT dust base) (General Chem.)	DDT* tech. 75%
GENERAL CHEMICAL 10% DIELDRIN GRANULAR DUST Insecticide (General Chem.)	Dieldrin* (hexachloro epoxy octahydroendo, exo-dimethano naphthalene and related compounds) 10%	GENERAL CHEMICAL 25% HEPTACHLOR SPRAY POWDER Insecticide (General Chem.)	Heptachlor (heptachloro-4,7-methanotetrahydroindene)* 25% Related compounds 9.7%
GENERAL CHEMICAL 50% ENDRIN-DUST BASE Insecticide (General Chem.)	Endrin (hexachloroepoxy-octahydro-endo, endo-dimethanonaphthalene)* 50%	GENERAL CHEMICAL LINDANE (General Chem.)	Gamma isomer of BHC* (benzene hexachloride) 100%
GENERAL CHEMICAL E+Z-OFF LIQUID DEFOLIANT Herbicide (General Chem.)	Magnesium chlorate* 18.15%	GENERAL CHEMICAL 20% LINDANE CONC. FOR OIL DILUTION Insecticide (General Chem.)	Gamma isomer of BHC* (benzene hexachloride) 20%
GENERAL CHEMICAL FLY KILLER (General Chem.)	o,o-Dimethyl-1-hydroxy-2,2,2-trichloroethyl phosphonate 1%	GENERAL CHEMICAL LOW VOLATILE 1-1/3-2/3 BRUSH KILLER (General Chem.)	2,4-Dichloro phenoxy acetic acid, propylene glycol butyl ether esters* 25.4% 2,4,5-Trichloro phenoxy acetic acid, propylene glycol butyl ether esters* 12.0% 2,4-D acid equiv. 15.6% 2,4,5-T acid equiv. 7.8%
GENERAL CHEMICAL G-10 BHC DUST BASE Insecticide (General Chem.)	Gamma isomer of BHC* (benzene hexachloride) 10.0% Other isomers of BHC* (benzene hexachloride) 50.0%	GENERAL CHEMICAL LOW VOLATILE 2-2 BRUSH KILLER (General Chem.)	2,4-Dichloro phenoxy acetic acid, propylene glycol butyl ether esters* 34.8% 2,4,5-Trichloro phenoxy acetic acid, propylene glycol butyl ether esters* 33.0% 2,4-D acid equiv. 21.5% 2,4,5-T acid equiv. 21.5%
GENERAL CHEMICAL G-12 BHC DUST BASE Insecticide (General Chem.)	Gamma isomer of BHC* (benzene hexachloride) 12.0% Other isomers* 64.0%	GENERAL CHEMICAL LOW VOLATILE 2,4,5-T BRUSH KILLER (General Chem.)	2,4,5-Trichloro phenoxy acetic acid, propylene glycol butyl ether esters* 65.3% 2,4,5-T acid equiv. 34.7%
GENERAL CHEMICAL G-36 BENZENE HEXACHLORIDE Insecticide (General Chem.)	Gamma isomer of BHC* (benzene hexachloride) 36% Other isomers of BHC* and related compounds	GENERAL CHEMICAL 25% MALATHION-DUST BASE Insecticide (General Chem.)	Malathion (o,o-dimethyl dithio phosphate of diethyl mercapto succinate)* 25%

*Consult Sec. II., Ingredients Index. This ingredient may be responsible for major toxic effects if poisonous amounts of this product are ingested.

- 530 -

Name & Use Manufacturer	Ingredients
GENERAL CHEMICAL MCP AMINE WEED KILLER (General Chem.)	2-Methyl-4-chlorophenoxy acetic acid*, ethanol and isopropanol amine salts 69.1% 2-Methyl-4-chlorophenoxy acetic acid equiv. 30.9%
GENERAL CHEMICAL 25% PARATHION DUST BASE Insecticide (General Chem.)	Parathion (o,o-diethyl-o-p-nitrophenyl thiophosphate)* 25%
GENERAL CHEMICAL 25% PARATHION EMULSIFI-ABLE CONC. Insecticide (General Chem.)	Parathion (o,o-diethyl-o-p-nitrophenyl thiophosphate)* 25% Xylol 63%
GENERAL CHEMICAL 15% PARATHION SPRAY POWDER Insecticide (General Chem.)	Parathion (o,o-diethyl-o-p-nitrophenyl thiophosphate)* 15%
GENERAL CHEMICAL 25% PARATHION SPRAY POWDER (General Chem.)	Parathion (o,o-diethyl-o-p-nitrophenyl thiophosphate)* 25%
GENERAL CHEMICAL POTASSIUM CYANATE Herbicide (General Chem.)	Potassium cyanate* 92%
GENERAL CHEMICAL RITE-O-WAY TCA-CHLORATE Herbicide (General Chem.)	Sodium trichloroacetate 10.2% Sodium chlorate* 22.5%
GENERAL CHEMICAL 40% SODIUM ARSENITE SOLUTION (Colored) Herbicide (General Chem.)	Sodium arsenite* 40%
GENERAL CHEMICAL 50% SODIUM TCA WEED KILLER (Liquid conc.) (General Chem.)	Sodium trichloroacetate 50% Trichloroacetic acid* equiv. 44%

Name & Use Manufacturer	Ingredients
GENERAL CHEMICAL SPECIAL HIGH STRENGTH SODIUM ARSENITE SOLUTION (For potato vine killing) (General Chem.)	Sodium arsenite* 52.5%
GENERAL CHEMICAL STA-KLOR NON-SELECTIVE WEED KILLER (General Chem.)	Sodium chlorate* 40% Sodium trichloroacetate 18% Sodium pentaborate, decahydrate* 37%
GENERAL CHEMICAL TCA SODIUM SALT 90% POWDER Herbicide (General Chem.)	Sodium trichloroacetate 90% Trichloroacetic acid* equiv. 79.3%
GENERAL CHEMICAL TDE (DDD) TECH. Insecticide (General Chem.)	TDE* tech. 100%
GENERAL CHEMICAL 50% TDE (DDD) DUST BASE Insecticide (General Chem.)	TDE* (dichloro diphenyl dichloroethane) 50%
GENERAL CHEMICAL 40% TOXAPHENE DUST BASE Insecticide (General Chem.)	Toxaphene* (tech. chlorinated camphene, 67-69% chlorine) 40%
GENERAL CHEMICAL 2,4-D AMINE WEED KILLER (General Chem.)	2,4-D Acid (2,4 dichloro phenoxy acetic acid, ethanol and isopropanol amine salts)* 65% 2,4-D acid equiv. 39%
GENERAL CHEMICAL 2,4-D ESTER OIL CON-CENTRATE WEED KILLER (General Chem.)	2,4-Dichloro phenoxy acetic acid, isopropyl ester* 37.1% 2,4-Dichloro phenoxy acetic acid, n-butyl ester* 39.0% 2,4-D acid equiv. 62.2%

*Consult Sec. II., Ingredients Index. This ingredient may be responsible for major toxic effects if poisonous amounts of this product are ingested.

- 531 -

Name & Use Manufacturer	Ingredients		Name & Use Manufacturer	Ingredients	
GENERAL CHEMICAL 2,4-D LOW VOLATILE ESTER WEED KILLER (General Chem.)	2,4-D acid (2,4 dichloro phenoxy acetic acid), propylene glycol butyl ether esters* 2,4-D acid equiv.	70.8% 29.2%	GENTIA-JEL Vaginal fungicide (Westwood)	Gentian violet 0.2% Acidified water soluble polyethylene glycol base	
GENERAL MANUAL KLEANSER (Pennsylv. Salt)	Polyphosphates* Soda ash Alkyl aryl sulfonate*		GENTOLA Antacid (Drobinski)	Alcohol 4%-5% Fl. ext. rhubarb Glycerin Sodium bicarbonate Fl. ext. cascara arom. Spts. peppermint Magnesium carbonate	
GENERAL PAINT H-702 SYNTHETIC ENAMEL THINNER (General Paint (Okla.))			GEORGE'S LACQUERS (George, P. D.)		
			GEORGE'S LACQUER THINNERS (George, P. D.)		
GENERAL PETROLEUM 20% COPPER NAPHTHEN- ATE SOLUTION, GRADE 200S (General Petrol.)	Copper Metal naphthenate* Solvent*	2.0%/w 20.0%/w 80.0%/w	GEORGE'S #7546 REDUCER Paint product (George, P. D.)		
			GEORGE SUPER CLEANER Paint cleaner (Bu-Tay)		
GENERAL PETROLEUM 80% COPPER NAPHTHEN- ATE SOLUTION, GRADE 800S (General Petrol.)	Copper Metal naphthenate* Solvent *	8.0%/w 80.0%/w 20.0%/w	GERITIN Geriatric vitamin-mineral supplement (Vitec)	Each fl./oz.: Desoxyephedrine hydrochloride 2 mg. Choline dihydrogen citrate 500 mg. Inositol 100 mg. Thiamine hydrochloride 10 mg. Riboflavin 6 mg. Pyridoxine hydrochloride 0.5 mg. Vitamin B12 10 mcg. Niacinamide 50 mg. Calcium pantothenate 6 mg. Iron (as ferric ammon. citrate) 20 mg. Copper (as copper sulfate) 2 mg. Calcium (as calcium glycerophos) 40 mg. Phosphorus (as calcium gylcerophos) 30 mg. Alcohol 12% Wine	
GENERAL PHOTO- GRAPHIC SUPPLY DEVELOPERS (General Photo.)					
GENERAL PURPOSE PAINT THINNER (Indianapolis)	Mineral spirits* (flash point 105°) Paraffins Naphthenes* Aromatics	56.8% 30.6% 12.6%			
GENEVA OINTMENT (Chewalla)					
GENIE FINGER- PAINT POWDER (Binney & Smith)			GERITOL Food supplement with iron (Pharm- aceuticals)	Each fl. oz.: Thiamin (B1) 5 mg. Niacinamide 100 mg. Pyridoxine (B6) 1 mg. Methionine 100 mg. Iron 100 mg. Riboflavin (B2) 5 mg. Panthenol 4 mg. Vitamin B12 3 mcg. Choline bitartrate 100 mg. Other vitamin B complex factors as found in yeast ext.	
GENITOX D-50 (50% DDT dust base) Insecticide (General Chem.)	DDT* tech.	50%			
GENITOX D-75 (75% DDT dust base) Insecticide (General Chem.)	DDT* tech.	75%	GERITOL JUNIOR Food supplement with iron (Pharm- aceuticals)	Each fl. oz.: Vitamin A palmitate 8,000 U.S.P.units Vitamin D 800 U.S.P.units Thiamin (B1) 5 mg. Riboflavin (B2) 5 mg. Niacinamide 100 mg. Panthenol 4 mg. Pyridoxine (B6) 1 mg. Vitamin B12 3 mcg. Iron 100 mg. Other vitamin B complex factors as found in yeast ext.	

*Consult Sec. II., Ingredients Index. This ingredient may be responsible for major toxic effects if poisonous amounts of this product are ingested.

Name & Use Manufacturer	Ingredients	Name & Use Manufacturer	Ingredients
GERMALL DISINFECTANT (Uncle Sam)	Distilled tar acid oils* and soap 90%	G & G FOOT POWDER (Greene)	
GERMI-SOL Disinfectant (Roberts, Dr. D.)	Cresol* 50% Soap 23%	G & G LIGHTER FLUID (Greene)	
GERMO BOWL FLUSH (Cleaner (Germo)		G & G MACHINE OIL (Greene)	
GERMO ROACH POWDER (Germo)		G & G POISON IVY LOTION (Greene)	
GERMOTOX Disinfectant, deodorant (Pioneer)		G & G REPELLENT LOTION (Greene)	
GEIGY RAT & MOUSE BAIT (Geigy)	Warfarin ((3-a-acetonylbenzyl)- 4-hydroxycoumarin) 0.025%	G & G WHITE SHOE CLEANER (Greene)	
GEIGY ROSE DUST Insecticide (Geigy)	DDT 3.0% Malathion* 4.0% Captan (n-trichloro methyl thio tetrahydro phthalamide) 5.0% Sulfur* 25.0%	GIAGILL Antitussive (Massengill)	Each 5 cc: Dihydrocodeinone bitartrate 1.8 mg. Chloroform 21.5 mg. Sodium citrate 0.238 gm. Potassium guaiacol sulfonate 86.5 mg. Tinct. squill 0.21 cc. Aromatics q.s.
GERMOZONE Water disinfectant veterinary (Lee, G.)	Potassium permanganate* 2% Potassium chlorate* Aluminum sulfate Potassium chloride Salt	GIANT WINK ROSE SPRAY Insecticide (Copley)	Pyrethrins 0.025% Tech. piperonyl cyclonene 0.256% Rotenone 0.128% Other cube extracts 0.236% Petroleum distillate 0.102% Dichlone (2,3-dichloro-1,4- naphthoquinone) 0.120%
GERMTROL Disinfectant (Stanley Home)	Pine oil* Tall oil Potassium hydroxide* Sodium tetrapyrophosphate Dye	GILLETTE SHAVING CREAM (Gillette)	
GERSTLEY BORATE Herbicide (Pacific Coast)	Ulexite (sodium-calcium borate*) Colemanite (calcium borate*) Minimum borate 28%	G-I-M-P (Link)	Tincture iodine* Carbolic acid* Camphor* Menthol Glycerin Alcohol 5.7%
GESAROL E25 Insecticide (Geigy)	DDT 25% Xylene* 63% Aromatic petroleum deriv. solvent 7%	GINGISOL Oral antiseptic (Gingisol)	Potassium hydroxide harmless amt. Triple orange flower water Rose soluble Phenol 1% Fluorides trace Vitamin C
GETS-IT Keratolytic ("Gets-It")	Alcohol 24% Ether* 44% Salicylic acid* approx. 14% Zinc chloride approx. 20% Collodium		
GETZUM CARCO-X Fungicide Insecticide (Getzum)	Coal tar neutral oil* 60.0% Coal tar acids* 8.0% Gamma isomer of hexachloro- cyclohexane 0.5% Other isomers of hexachloro- cyclohexane 0.9%	GINO PILLS Stimulant diuretic (Gino Pill)	Podophyllin Potassium nitrate Ext. pareira Oil of juniper Aloes Methylene blue Ext. buchu
GETZUM LIQUID Herbicide (Getzum)	Arsenic trioxide* 8.1% Total arsenic, all in water soluble form expressed as metallic 6.1%		
G & G CASTILE SHAMPOO (Greene)			

*Consult Sec. II., Ingredients Index. This ingredient may be responsible for major toxic effects if poisonous amounts of this product are ingested.

Name & Use Manufacturer	Ingredients		Name & Use Manufacturer	Ingredients	
GIZMO MOUSE KILLER (Warren Chem.)	Thallium sulfate* impregnated seeds	0.3%	GLAND-O-LAC MITE SPRAY (Gland-O-Lac)	DDT* Xylenols* Coal tar oils* Xylene * Oils	5% 5.5% 12.5% 2% 75%
GIZZARD CAPSULE Veterinary (Lee, G.)	Areca nut Kamala Nicotine* as alkaloid Fuller's earth Shellac Lacquer Talcum	30% 12.3% 1.7% 13% 4% 0.7% 28%	GLAND-O-LAC ROOST- FUME Insecticide (Gland-O-Lac)	Gamma isomer BHC* Other isomers Xylene* Petroleum hydrocarbons*	1.5% 0.1% 3.5% 94.9%
G-LAC TYROTHRICIN OINTMENT Antiseptic (veterinary) (Beebe Labs.)	Tyrothricin 1-10,000 Lanolin anhydrous Petrolatum Methyl salicylate Cyclonol Paraffin Liquid petrolatum Guaiacol		GLAND-O-LAC ROOST SPREAD Insecticide (Gland-O-Lac)	Nicotine* Pyridine Petroleum hydrocarbons	9% 2.5% 88.5%
			GLASS WAX (Gold Seal)		
G-LAC VETERINARY Antibiotic (Beebe Labs.)	Tyrothricin 2 mg./cc. Mineral oil 60% Alcohol 3%		GLAZE Liquid porcelain glaze (Spearhead)		
GLAMORENE RUG & UPHOLSTERY CLEANER (Glamorene)			GLAZOL (United Gilson.)	Fish oil Lard oil	
GLAMORENE MIRACLE BRUSH BATH Cleaner (Glamorene)			GLEEM BRAND PAINTS (Balto. Paint)		
GLAMORENE WOOL RUG CLEANER (Glamorene)	Chlorinated hydrocarbons* (trichloroethylene) Non-toxic synthetic detergents		GLENDALE DEODORANT COLOGNE (House for Men)		
GLAMUR Rug, upholstery cleaner (Glamur Products,Inc.)			GLENDALE HAIR LOTION (House for Men)		
GLAND-O-LAC BROODER HOUSE DISIN- FECTANT (Gland-O-Lac)	Coal tar acids* 25% Coal tar hydrocarbons* 47% Anhydrous soap 18%		GLENWAY BUBBLE BATH PACKAGE (Glenway)	Sodium sulfate anhydrous Alkyl aryl sulfonate* D&C colors Perfume	
GLAND-O-LAC COMPOUND 5-40 (Gland-O-Lac)	Nicotine* 5% Phenothiazine 40%		GLESSCO FOR ADULTS Antitussive (Glessner)	Senega Ammonium carbonate Sodium benzyl succinate Glycerin Squill* Menthol *	
GLAND-O-LAC FOWL LARYNGO- TRACHEITIS VACCINE (Gland-O-Lac)	Dihydrostreptomycin Penicillin		G.L.F. ARAMITE 15W Insecticide (G.L.F.)	2-(p-tert-Butyl phenoxy) isopropyl-2-chloroethyl sulfite 15.00%	
GLAND-O-LAC FOWL POX VACINNE (Gland-O-Lac)	Dihydrostreptomycin Penicillin		G.L.F. 50% DDD (TDE) Insecticide (G.L.F.)	Dichloro diphenyl dichloro- ethane* 50.00%	
GLAND-O-LAC INCUBATOR FUMIGANT (Gland-O-Lac)	Furfuraldehyde* 51% Formaldehyde* (as gas) 16%		G.L.F. 25% DDT EMULSIFIABLE SPRAY Insecticide (G.L.F.)	DDT 25.00% Aromatic petroleum solvent and emulsifiers 75.00%	
GLAND-O-LAC LOUSE POWDER (Gland-O-Lac)	Orthophenylphenol* 5.50% Sulfur* 14.50%				

*Consult Sec. II., Ingredients Index. This ingredient may be responsible for major toxic effects if poisonous amounts of this product are ingested.

Name & Use Manufacturer	Ingredients	
G.L.F. 25% DDT SPECIAL CONC. SPRAY Insecticide (G.L.F.)	DDT Xylene*	25.00% 46.00%
G.L.F. 75% DDT WETTABLE POWDER Insecticide (G.L.F.)	DDT*	75.00%
G.L.F. DIELDRIN EMULSIFI-ABLE Insecticide (G.L.F.)	Hexachloro epoxy octahydro-endo, exo-dimethano naphthalene* Related compounds Petroleum hydrocarbons	15.83% 2.79% 73.38%
G.L.F. DIELDRIN WETTABLE POWDER Insecticide (G.L.F.)	Hexachloro epoxy octahydro-endo, exo-dimethano napthalene* Related compounds	42.40% 7.60%
G.L.F. 25% DILAN, EMULSIFI-ABLE Insecticide (G.L.F.)	2-Nitro-1,1-bis (p-chloro-phenyl) propane* 2-Nitro-1,1-bis (p-chloro-phenyl) butane* Related compounds	6.70% 13.30% 5.00%
G.L.F. DUAL GARDEN DUST Insecticide (G.L.F.)	Rotenone Other cube resins Copper* (from basic copper sulfate) expressed as metallic	1.00% 2.00% 7.00%
G.L.F. DUAL GARDEN SPRAY Insecticide (G.L.F.)	Tech. methoxychlor* Malathion* Captan	15.00% 5.00% 10.00%
G.L.F. DUST #1 Fungicide (G.L.F.)	Copper* (in basic copper sulfate) expressed as metallic	7.00%
G.L.F. DUST #2 Insecticide (G.L.F.)	Parathion* (o,o-diethyl-o-p-nitrophenyl thiophosphate)	2.00%
G.L.F. DUST #3 Insecticide (G.L.F.)	Copper (in basic copper sulfate) expressed as metallic Calcium arsenate* Total arsenic expressed as metallic arsenic	7.00% 14.00% 5.30%
G.L.F. DUST #4 Insecticide (G.L.F.)	Copper (in basic copper sulfate) expressed as metallic Calcium arsenate* Total arsenic expressed as metallic arsenic	7.00% 21.00% 8.00%
G.L.F. DUST #5 Insecticide (G.L.F.)	Parathion*	1.00%
G.L.F. DUST #6 Insecticide (G.L.F.)	Dieldrin* (hexachloro epoxy octahydro-endo, exo-dimethano naphthalene)	1.50%

Name & Use Manufacturer	Ingredients	
G.L.F. DUST #7 Insecticide (G.L.F.)	Calcium arsenate* Total arsenic, expressed as metallic arsenic	28.40% 10.65%
G.L.F. DUST #8 Fungicide (G.L.F.)	Parathion* Zineb	1.00% 4.55%
G.L.F. DUST #9A Insecticide (G.L.F.)	Parathion* DDT	1.00% 5.00%
G.L.F. DUST #11 Fungicide (G.L.F.)	Zineb DDT	6.50% 3.00%
G.L.F. DUST #12A Fungicide (G.L.F.)	Zineb (zinc ethylene bis (dithiocarbamate))	4.55%
G.L.F. DUST #17 Insecticide (G.L.F.)	DDT	3.00%
G.L.F. DUST #18 Fungicide (G.L.F.)	DDT Copper* (in basic copper sulfate) expressed as metallic	3.00% 7.00%
G.L.F. DUST #20 Insecticide (G.L.F.)	DDT* Copper* (in basic copper sulfate) expressed as metallic	5.00% 7.00%
G.L.F. DUST #21 Fungicide (G.L.F.)	Ziram Parathion*	7% 1%
G.L.F. DUST #22 Fungicide (G.L.F.)	Ziram (zinc dimethyl dithiocarbamate) Total zinc, expressed as metallic zinc	7.00% 1.49%
G.L.F. DUST #23 Insecticide (G.L.F.)	Ziram Calcium arsenate* Total zinc expressed as metallic zinc	7.00% 21.00% 1.49%
G.L.F. DUST #24 Insecticide) (G.L.F.)	Gamma isomer of benzene hexachloride Other isomers of benzene hexachloride	1.00% 4.00%
G.L.F. DUST #24G Insecticide (G.L.F.)	Gamma isomer of benzene hexachloride (from lindane)	1.00%

*Consult Sec. II., Ingredients Index. This ingredient may be responsible for major toxic effects if poisonous amounts of this product are ingested.

Name & Use Manufacturer	Ingredients		Name & Use Manufacturer	Ingredients	
G.L.F. DUST #25 Insecticide (G.L.F.)	Tech. chlordane*	5.00%	G.L.F. DUST #81 Insecticide (G.L.F.)	DDD Ziram	5.00% 7.00%
G.L.F. DUST #27 Insecticide (G.L.F.)	Rotenone Other cube resins	1.00% 2.00%	G.L.F. DUSTING SULPHUR Insecticide, fungicide (G.L.F.)	Elemental sulfur*	90.00%
G.L.F. DUST #29A Insecticide (G.L.F.)	Rotenone Other cube resins DDT	1.00% 2.00% 2.00%	G.L.F. ENDRIN EMULSIFI- ABLE Insecticide (G.L.F.)	Endrin (hexachloro epoxy octahydro-endo, endo- dimethano naphthalene)* Petroleum hydrocarbons	19.50% 73.00%
G.L.F. DUST #30 Insecticide (G.L.F.)	Malathion* (o,o-dimethyl dithiophosphate of diethyl mercaptosuccinate)	5.00%	G.L.F. FRUIT SPRAY Insecticide (G.L.F.)	DDT* Tech. methoxychlor* Sulfur* Ferbam	5.00% 15.00% 45.00% 7.60%
G.L.F. DUST #31 Insecticide (G.L.F.)	Malathion* Copper* (in basic copper sulfate) expressed as metallic	5.00% 7.00%	G.L.F. GARDEN DUST Insecticide (G.L.F.)	Copper* Rotenone*	
G.L.F. DUST #32 Insecticide (G.L.F.)	Malathion* Ziram	5.00% 7.00%	G.L.F HEPTACHLOR EMULSIFI- ABLE Insecticide (G.L.F.)	Heptachloro-4,7-methano tetrahydroindene* Related compounds Petroleum distillate*	23.40% 9.10% 61.40%
G.L.F. DUST #60 Insecticide (G.L.F.)	DDT*	5.00%	G.L.F. LICE POWDER (G.L.F.)	Nicotine* Sulfur	
G.L.F. DUST #73 Insecticide (G.L.F.)	Methoxychlor, tech.	5.00%	G.L.F. LINDANE EMULSIFI- ABLE CROP SPRAY Insecticide (G.L.F.)	Gamma isomer of benzene hexachloride (from lindane)* Xylene*	20.00% 54.00%
G.L.F. DUST #74 Insecticide (G.L.F.)	DDT*	10.00%			
G.L.F. DUST #78 Fungicide (G.L.F.)	Ziram Rotenone	7.00% 1.00%	G.L.F. 50% MALATHION EMULSIFI- ABLE Insecticide (G.L.F.)	Malathion* Petroleum distillate	55.00% 30.00%
G.L.F. DUST #79 Insecticide (G.L.F.)	DDD (dichloro diphenyl dichloroethane)	5.00%			
G.L.F. DUST #80 Insecticide (G.L.F.)	DDD (dichloro diphenyl dichloroethane) Copper* (in basic copper sulfate) expressed as metallic	5.00% 7.00%	G.L.F. 25% MALATHION WETTABLE POWDER Insecticide (G.L.F.)	Malathion*	25.00%

*Consult Sec. II., Ingredients Index. This ingredient may be responsible for major toxic effects if poisonous amounts of this product are ingested.

Name & Use Manufacturer	Ingredients	Name & Use Manufacturer	Ingredients
G.L.F. OIL (Emulsifiable Dormant) Insecticide (G.L.F.)	Paraffinic dormant oil* 98.50%	GLIDDEN CAULKING COMPOUND (Glidden Co.)	
G.L.F. OIL (Superior Type Dormant) Insecticide (G.L.F.)	Paraffinic dormant oil* 100.00%	GLIDDEN COLORS IN OIL (Glidden Co.)	
G.L.F. PENTA 10 WEED KILLER (G.L.F.)	Pentachlorophenol* 0.87 lb./gal. Oil formulation	GLIDDEN DOOR EASE Lubricant (Glidden Co.)	
G.L.F. 4% ROTENONE POWDER Insecticide (G.L.F.)	Rotenone 4.00% Other cube resins 8.00%	GLIDDEN HYGIENIC WALL SIZE (Glidden Co.)	
G.L.F. SULPHUR, DRY WETTABLE (Formula Four) Insecticide, fungicide (G.L.F.)	Elemental sulfur* 95.00%	GLIDDEN JAPAN DRIER (Glidden Co.)	
G.L.F. TOXAPHENE EMULSIFI- ABLE Insecticide (G.L.F.)	Toxaphene* 59.00% Aromatic petroleum deriv. solvent* 33.00%	GLIDDEN KNOT SEALER (Glidden Co.)	
G.L.F. VEG-OIL (Spreader- Sticker) (G.L.F.)	Vegetable oil 90.00% B-1956 10.00%	GLIDDEN LIQUID RED LEAD, MODIFIED Rust inhibitor (Glidden Co.)	
G.L.F. WEED KILLER E (G.L.F.)	Isopropyl ester of 2,4-D*		
G.L.F. WEED KILLER 66 IMPROVED (G.L.F.)	Triethanolamine salt of 2,4-D*		

Name & Use Manufacturer	Ingredients	Name & Use Manufacturer	Ingredients	
GLIDDEN PAINTS, ENAMELS, PRIMERS, FINISHES AND STAINS (Glidden Co.)		GLOAMA REDUCER For Gloama block printing ink (Binney & Smith)		
GLIDDEN PASTE WOOD FILLER (Glidden Co.)		GLOBALENE CARBURETOR NO. 101G AND METAL CLEANER (Troy Ind.)	Chlorinated hydrocarbons* Phenolic* bodies Volatile solvents*	
GLIDDEN RUST IN- HIBITING OIL (Glidden Co.)		GLOBE A-B-C POWDER Antiseptic, antihemor- rhagic (Globe)	Potassium alum* Ferric subsulfate Tannic acid Camphor* Iodoform Cresylic acid	20% 20% 5.5% 0.8% 0.8% 0.4%
GLIDDEN SHELLACS, LACQUERS, AND VARNISHES (Glidden Co.)		GLOBE A-C-TOL Anthelmintic (veterinary) (Globe)	Phenothiazine Nicotine (expressed as alkaloid)* Areca nut Copper sulfate Nux vomica (0.25 gr. strychnine/oz.)	50.000% 2.675% 3.000% 24.105% 5.000%
GLIDDEN WOOD BLEACH (Glidden Co.)				
GLIDER BRUSHLESS SHAVE CREAM (Williams, J. B.)	Triethanolamine soap Stearic acid Lanolin sterols Boric acid*	GLOBE A-D-A LICE POWDER (Globe)	Rotenone Other cube resins Sulfur* Petroleum oil	0.5% 1.0% 89.0% 1.0%
GLID-N BRUSH RESTORER (Glidden Co.)		GLOBE ALKALINE POWDER Veterinary (Globe)	Sodium hydroxide* Potassium guaiacol sulfonate Oil of eucalyptus Sodium sulfate Sodium carbonate Anethol Salt	32% 16% 4% 30% 5% 2% 11%
GLID-N FLOOR WAX, FURNI- TURE POLISH, LIQUID CLEANER (Glidden Co.)				
GLID-N MILDEW-X Mildew- proofing (Glidden Co.)		GLOBE ANTISEPTIC POWDER (Globe)	Boric acid* Potassium alum* Zinc oxide Camphor* Iodoform	31.25% 31.25% 6.25% 3% 0.25%
GLIM Detergent (Babbitt)		GLOBE AVA-LATE For intestinal irritation (veterinary) (Globe)	Each tablet: Zinc sulfocarbolate Copper sulfocarbolate Copper sulfate* Boric acid Sodium sulfocarbolate Mercury bichloride Milk sugar	24.39% 4.88% 24.39% 16.46% 14.63% 0.61% 4.88%
GLISS'N SHAMPOO Upholstery cleaner (Gliss'N)	Polyphosphates* Sodium carbonate Pine oil*			
GLIT Cleaner (Kano)	Alcohols*	GLOBE AVI-GLO Tonic, for intestinal irritation (veterinary) (Globe)	Each oz.: Strychnine* Nux vomica* (strychnine equiv. 0.115%) Gentian Ginger Capsicum Copper sulfate Manganese sulfate Iron sulfate	0.5 gr. 10.00% 5.00% 5.00% 5.00% 0.25% 0.25% 1.50%
GLITE Porcelain cleaner (Grissmer)				
GLOAMA BLOCK PRINTING INK (Binney & Smith)		GLOBE BARBED WIRE LINIMENT (Globe)	Turpentine* Balsam Sulfuric acid Methyl salicylate	45.21% 3.71% 1.58% 1.29%
		GLOBE BLACKHEAD FORMULA For blackhead (veterinary) (Globe)	2-Amino-5-n trothiazole*	10%

*Consult Sec. II., Ingredients Index. This ingredient may be responsible for major toxic effects if poisonous amounts of this product are ingested.

Name & Use Manufacturer	Ingredients	
GLOBE BLOAT REMEDY Veterinary (Globe)	Pelargonic acid compound	10% w/v
	Propylene glycol laurate	10% w/v
	Isopropyl alcohol*	75%/v
GLOBE BOVINE PURGATIVE & CARMINATIVE Cathartic (veterinary) (Globe)	Epsom salts Capsicum Ginger	99.16% 0.42% 0.42%
GLOBE BOWL KLENZO NO. 108 Cleaner (Troy Ind.)		
GLOBE CABLE OIL Insecticide (Globe)	DDT tech. Aromatic petroleum deriv. solvent*	25% 75%
GLOBE CALF SCOUR REMEDY For intestinal irritation (veterinary) (Globe)	Sulfathiazole* Kaolin (colloidal) Bismuth subcarbonate Pectin	15.43 gr. 80 gr. 5.2 gr. 4 gr.
GLOBE COPPER-IRON MIXTURE (Veterinary) (Globe)	Copper sulfate* Iron sulfate	50% 50%
GLOBE 50% CRESYLIC DISINFECT-ANT (Globe)	Cresylic acid* Soap	50% 28%
GLOBE DEHORNING PASTE Veterinary (Globe)	Potassium hydroxide*	
GLOBE DIP Disinfectant (veterinary) (Globe)	Coal tar neutral oils Soap Cresylic acids*	62% 17% 11%
GLOBE DOG EXPECTORANT Antitussive (veterinary) (Globe)	Potassium guaiacol sulfonate Ammonium chloride Fowler's solution	6% 5% 4%
GLOBE DOG EYE WASH (Globe)	Zinc sulfate Boric acid Butyn sulfate	0.20% 3.00% 0.50%
GLOBE DOG KAPS Anthelmintic (veterinary) (Globe)	Each capsule: Tetrachloroethylene* Arecoline hydrobromide Mineral oil	99.2% 0.4% 0.4%
GLOBE DOG SHAMPOO AND FLEA SOAP (Globe)	Orthophenylphenol* Synthetic oil sassafras Wood alcohol* Anhydrous soap	4.80% 1.05% 7.41% 26.70%

Name & Use Manufacturer	Ingredients	
GLOBE EAR CANKER EMULSION For skin irritation (veterinary) (Globe)	Pine tar* Bone oil* Cottonseed oil	48.2% 19.5% 32.3%
GLOBE EQUINE 6-DRAM BOT CAPSULES Intestinal antiseptic (veterinary) (Globe)	Carbon disulfide*	98.03%
GLOBE EQUINE 3-DRAM WORM CAPSULES Anthelmintic (veterinary) (Globe)	Carbon tetrachloride*	99.5%
GLOBE FLEA, LOUSE, AND TICK POWDER FOR DOGS (Globe)	Gamma isomer of benzene hexachloride (from lindane) Pine oil	1% 4%
GLOBE FLY REPELLENT & WOUND DRESSING Veterinary (Globe)	Pine tar* Bone oil* Pine oil* Turkey red oil (anhydrous) Ichthammol (anhydrous) Zinc oxide	38% 24% 3% 1.5% 2.4% 25%
GLOBE GRUB KILLER Insecticide (Globe)	Rotenone Other cube resins Sulfur	1.67% 3.33% 5.00%
GLOBE HOG TONIC POWDER Tonic with iron (veterinary) (Globe)	Copper sulfate* Iron sulfate Manganese sulfate Foenugreek Gentian Nux vomica* (strychnine equiv. 0.115%)	5% 9.25% 0.5% 15% 10% 10%
GLOBE HORN PAINT Dehorning compound (veterinary) (Globe)	Non-phenolic coal tar oils* Pine tar* Bone oil	38% 45% 3%
GLOBE KOLD DIP METAL CLEANER NO. 101K (Troy Ind.)	Chlorinated hydrocarbons* Phenolic* bodies Volatile solvents*	
GLOBE LICE POWDER (Globe)	Sodium fluoride* Sulfur Nicotine* (expressed as alkaloid)	28.500% 20.000% 0.225%
GLOBE LIVESTOCK SPRAY Insecticide (Globe)	Hydrocarbon oil* Isobornyl thiocyanoacetate* tech.	

*Consult Sec. II., Ingredients Index. This ingredient may be responsible for major toxic effects if poisonous amounts of this product are ingested.

Name & Use Manufacturer	Ingredients	
GLOBE MANGE REMEDY Ectoparasiticide (veterinary) (Globe)	Benzyl benzoate*	36.3%
GLOBE ODORLESS DISINFECT-ANT (Globe)	p-tert-Octyl phenoxy ethoxy ethyl di-methyl benzyl ammonium chloride*	12.5%
GLOBE PINE DISINFECT-ANT (Globe)	Pine oil* and soap	90%
GLOBE PINK DRENCH Anthelmintic (veterinary) (Globe)	Phenothiazine* Lead arsenate*	37.62% 0.75%
GLOBE PINK-EYE LIQUID For eye, skin irritation (veterinary) (Globe)	Sodium sulfacetamide* Sulfathiazole* Urea Propylene glycol Sulfanilamide* Azosulfamide* Benzyl alcohol	2% w/v
GLOBE POULTRY DISINFECT-ANT (Globe)	Para di-isobutyl phenoxy ethoxy ethyl di-methyl benzyl ammonium chloride*	12.5%
GLOBE POULTRY FLOCK WORMER Anthelmintic (veterinary, avian) (Globe)	Nicotine* (expressed as alkaloid) Phenothiazine	1.08% 11.00%
GLOBE POULTRY MINERAL TABLETS (veterinary) Tonic (Globe)	Each tablet: Copper sulfate* Iron sulfate Boric acid* Calcium lactate Starch Citric acid Manganese sulfate Acid calcium phosphate Epsom salts Acacia	2.75% 3.86% 20.92% 1.1% 64.76% 0.33% 0.33% 0.77% 3.86% 1.32%
GLOBE POULTRY SPRAY Inhalant, nasal decongestant (veterinary) (Globe)	Formaldehyde* Pine oil Oil of eucalyptus	11.25% 4.84% 2.87%
GLOBE POULTRY WORM TABLETS Anthelmintic (veterinary) (Globe)	Each tablet: Phenothiazine Kieselguhr Sugars Calcium carbonate Gelatin Nicotine* Talc Acacia Starch	36.58% 7.42% 32.03% 10.23% 0.35% 3.71% 2.37% 0.54% 6.77%
GLOBE POWDERED CUBE ROOT Insecticide (Globe)	Rotenone* Other cube resins	5% 8.75%

Name & Use Manufacturer	Ingredients	
GLOBE PURGATIVE CAPSULES Cathartic (veterinary) (Globe)	Aloin Barium chloride* Calomel Capsicum Sodium bicarbonate Jalap Colocynth Nux vomica* Ginger	51.6% 14.5% 6.5% 4.2% 7.7% 0.8% 0.8% 9.7% 4.2%
GLOBE ROOST PAINT Insecticide (Globe)	Petroleum distillate* Benzene hexachloride, gamma isomer Other isomers	97.2% 1% 1.8%
GLOBE SCREW-WORM REMEDY (U.S. Formula EQ 335) (Veterinary) (Globe)	Gamma isomer of benzene hexachloride* Pine oil*	3% 35%
GLOBE SCREW-WORM REMEDY (U.S. Formula No. 62) (Veterinary) (Globe)	Diphenylamine* Turkey red oil Benzol* Lamp black	35% 5.5% 35% 20%
GLOBE U.S. STOCK 1029 Insecticide (Globe)	Pyridine* Dibutyl phthalate	10% 13.5%
GLOBE W-A-C POWDER Tonic (vet-erinary) (Globe)	Arsenous acid* Potassium iodide Sulfur (flowers) Willow bark	1.5% 2.5% 1% 70%
GLOBE SODIUM ARSANILATE TABLETS To control swine dysentery (Globe)	Each tablet: Sodium arsanilate* (anhydrous)	1.12 gr.
GLOBE S.T. TABLETS Anthelmintic (veterinary) (Globe)	Nicotine* Copper sulfate P.E. kamala Sodium chloride Acacia Kieselguhr Talc	9.09% 38.48% 21.21% 9.09% 1.52% 3.03% 2.73%
GLOBE TETRA CAPSULES Anthelmintic (veterinary) (Globe)	Each capsule: Tetrachloroethylene*	5 cc.
GLOBE TETRA SHEEP AND GOAT DRENCH Anthelmintic (veterinary) (Globe)	Naphthalene Oil eucalyptus Tetrachloroethylene*	4.0% 1.5% 94.5%
GLOBE THIO-NITRO TABLETS Antidote for prussic acid poisoning (veterinary) (Globe)	Sodium thiosulfate* Sodium nitrite* Sodium chloride Mineral oil Color	42.86% 28.57% 28.29% 0.17% 0.11%

*Consult Sec. II., Ingredients Index. This ingredient may be responsible for major toxic effects if poisonous amounts of this product are ingested.

Name & Use Manufacturer	Ingredients		Name & Use Manufacturer	Ingredients	
GLOBE UDDER OINTMENT Emollient (veterinary) (Globe)	Guaiacol Lanolin Petrolatum Oil of eucalyptus* Beef tallow Beeswax	10% 10% 40% 5% 25% 10%	GLORIA MUCILAGE (Arabol)	Pure gum arabic solution	
GLOBE VETERINARY PURGATIVE (Globe)	Each fl. oz.: Barium chloride* Ext. colocynth Aloin Ext. belladonna root	65 gr. 1.25 gr. 5 gr. 2.08 gr.	GLORIA SUN TAN LOTION (La-Mo)		
			GLO-SHEEN FURNITURE POLISH (Watkins, J.)	Wax Silicone Naphtha*	
GLOBE VETERINARY TONIC POWDER (Globe)	Nux vomica* (strychnine equiv. 0.0575%) Arsenous acid* Iron sulfate Copper sulfate Manganese sulfate Gentian*	5% 2% 21% 1% 1% 15%	GLOSS BLACK LACQUER (George, P.D.)		
			GLOSSTEX Laundry starch (Tidy)	Carboxymethylcellulose 3% Total active formaldehyde 0.2%	
GLOBEX BLEACH NO. 109B (Troy Ind.)	Sodium hypochlorite*		GLOS-TONE, SATIN GLOSS FINISH, 837 SKY BLUE Paint (Martin-Senour)	Titanium calcium pigment 38% Titanium magnesium pigment 12% Maleic resin* Linseed-castor oil* Mineral spirits* and driers	6% 16% 28%
GLOBE ZINC-BUTYN EYE OINT-MENT (Veterinary) (Globe)	Zinc sulfate Butyn sulfate Lanolin anhydrous Petrolatum Mineral oil	0.22% 0.53% 10% 79.9% 1.03%			
GLOBE Z-O UDDER OINTMENT (Veterinary) (Globe)	Zinc oxide 20% in a bland ointment base		GLOSTORA Hair dressing (Sterling Prod. Div.)		
GLO-CEN Wax (Central Chem.)			GLOVER'S IMPERIAL FLEA KILLER (Glover, H. C.)	Rotenone* Pyrethrins Sulfur* Cube resins	1.00% 0.40% 20.00% 2.0%
GLO-CIDE Insecticide (Globe)	Hydrocarbon oil* DDT* tech.	95% 5%	GLOVER'S IMPERIAL HAIR DRESS (Glover, H. C.)		
GLO-CIDE 25 Insecticide (Globe)	DDT tech. Methylated aromatic petroleum solvent*	25% 50.05%	GLOVER'S IMPERIAL KENNEL & FLEA SOAP (Glover, H. C.)	Anhydrous soap (palm, coconut, olive oils) 62.15% Pine tar 14.2% Petroleum 8.85% Glycerin 3.5% Sulfur 2.8%	
GLO-COAT Floor polish (Johnson, S.C.)	Synthetic resins Petroleum and vegetable waxes Emulsifying agents				
GLO-DANE 45 (Globe)	Tech. chlordane* Aliphatic petroleum oil*	45.5% 43.3%	GLOVER'S IMPERIAL MEDICATED SOAP (Glover, H. C.)	Anhydrous soap Oil of pine tar Colloidal sulfur Crude petroleum Glycerin	
GLO-N-6 POWDER For nicotinic acid deficiency in swine (Globe)	Niacin (nicotinic acid) 1.10%		GLOVER'S IMPERIAL SCRATCH POWDER Insecticide (Glover, H. C.)	Lindane DDT Chloranil Boric acid Essential oil	1.00% 0.50% 5.00% 3.00% 0.20%
GLOOSTER HARDWOOD FLOOR CLEANER (Good, J.)			GLOVER'S IMPERIAL TICK KILLER (Glover, H. C.)	DDT* Pyrethins Sulfur*	10.00% 0.50% 20.0%
GLO'PINE Disinfectant (Great Lakes Labs.)	Steam distilled pine oil* 77% Soap 13%		GLOVER'S MANGE MEDICINE (Glover, H. C.)	Crude petroleum* Refined oil of pine tar* Colloidal sulfur	90.46% 6.76% 2.43%
GLORIA-FAY COSMETICS (Gloria-Fay)			GLUCODOX (Kirkman)	Each capsule: Calcium gluconate 5.0 gr. Ferrous gluconate 2.5 gr. Pyridoxine hydrochloride U.S.P. 2.5 mg. Vitamin D 333 U.S.P. units Cobalt 0.1 mg.	

*Consult Sec. II., Ingredients Index. This ingredient may be responsible for major toxic effects if poisonous amounts of this product are ingested.

Name & Use Manufacturer	Ingredients
GLUINE WALL SIZE (Consumer's)	
GLU-PLY (Hughes)	Buna-N rubber-phenolic resin combination dissolved in acetone* or methyl ethyl ketone*
GLUTACHLOR CAPSULES (Barnes-Hind)	Each capsule: Glutamic acid hydrochloride 5 gr.
GLUTAMIC ACID HYDRO-CHLORIDE CAPSULES For hypo-chlorhydria, achlorhydria (Inorganic)	Each capsule: Glutamic acid hydrochloride 5 gr.
GLUV-KOTE HAND PRO-TECTION CREAM (Penslar)	
GLYCALOIDS (For coughs due to colds) (Koehler's)	Per oz.: Ammon. salicylate* 2 gr. Benzocaine 1-1/2 gr. Guaiacol 4 m. Methyl sal Oil anise Oil sassafras Oil eucalyptus* Oils of peppermint
GLYCAMINE AM TABLETS For peptic ulcers, hyper-acidity (Broemmel)	Hydroxy aluminum magnesium aminoacetate 0.5 gm.
GLYCOBEN Antitussive (Tilden)	Each fl. oz.: Codeine sulfate 1 gr. Chloroform 1/8 m. Antimony and potassium tartrate 2/25 gr. Potassium guaiacol sulfonate 8 gr. Ammonium chloride 8 gr. Menthol
GLYCO-CIDE FOR AIR SANITATION (Columbia)	Triethylene glycol* 90%
GLYCODOX For low blood pressure (Tailby-Nason)	Per 1000: Strychnine sulfate 0.5 mg. d-Desoxyephedrine hydrochloride 2 mg. Calcium glycerophosphate 250 mg.
GLYCOL DEOCIDE AEROSOL Deodorant, disinfectant (Uncle Sam)	Propylene glycol Triethylene glycol Quaternary ammonium chloride* Alcohol* Petroleum distillate* Perfume Freon
GLYCOLIN AIR SPRAY Deodorizer, disinfectant (Selig)	Isopropyl alcohol* Triethylene glycol Para di-isobutyl phenoxy ethoxy ethyl dimethyl benzyl ammonium chloride*

Name & Use Manufacturer	Tox-icity	Ingredients
GLYCO-SEPO For mucous surfaces (Clapp, Otis)		Borax Glycerin Wintergreen Cinnamon Thymol Sodium carbonate Oils of eucalyptus Pinus pumilio Menthol Sodium benzoate
GLYCO THYMOLINE For skin and mucosal irritations (Kress)		Alcohol 4% Sodium benzoate Menthol Borax eucalyptol Sodium bicarbonate Sodium salicylate Thymol Oil of sweet birch Glycerin Oil of pine needles
GLYCO-MIST Deodorizer, air-sanitizer (Varley)		Isopropyl alcohol* Triethylene glycol Propylene glycol Para di-isobutyl phenoxy ethoxy ethyl dimethyl benzyl ammonium chloride*
GLYCONDA (Sugar Free) Stomachic antacid (Lloyd)		Each 100 cc.: Potassium carbonate, anhydrous 0.2 gm. Rhubarb 0.2 gm. Hydrastis Berberis Cinnamon Glycerin Oil of peppermint
GLYEUTHY-MENOL FOR VAGINAL HYGIENE (Nixon)		Phenylmercuric borate 0.0175% Lactic acid Boric acid* Borax* Oxyquinoline sulfate 0.08%
GLYMUZIN For skin irritations (Pitman-Moore)		Each fl. oz.: Calamine 2.18 gm. Zinc oxide 1.94 gm. Phenol liquid 0.23 cc. Aromatic viscous diluent q.s.
GLYPEROX For topical application (Horton & Converse)		Urea peroxide 4% 8-Hydroxyquinoline 0.1% Anhydrous glycerin
GLYPTAL CHINA, GLASS & CROCKERY CEMENT (General Electric)		
GLYPTOL Spray, gargle (Tilden)		Borax* Sodium bicarbonate Thymol Pine oil* Sodium benzoate Sodium chloride Menthol Methyl salicylate*
GLYSEM ELIXIR (Colored Green) Tonic (Massengill)		Each 5 cc: Strychnine glycerophosphate 0.67 mg. Sodium glycerophosphate 86.5 mg. Calcium glycerophosphate 86.5 mg. Phosphoric acid 0.04 cc.

*Consult Sec. II., Ingredients Index. This ingredient may be responsible for major toxic effects if poisonous amounts of this product are ingested.

Name & Use Manufacturer	Ingredients		Name & Use Manufacturer	Ingredients	
GLYSUFED INHALANT Nasal de-congestant, topical (Massengill)	Ephedrine* Menthol Glycerin Lactic acid Chlorobutanol	1% 0.075% 2.5% 0.77% 0.5%	GOLDEN ARROWS LINIMENT Antiseptic, rubefacient, (Ozark)	Oil turpentine* Cresol* Carbolic acid Methyl salicylate* Oil mustard (synthetic)* Oil eucalyptus Camphor* Coal tar	
GLYTANOCAINE Analgesic, anesthetic and astringent (oral) (Pitman-Moore)	Phenol (carbolic acid) 0.5% Benzocaine hydrochloride 0.35% Sodium bisulfite 0.2% Tannic acid Aromatized glycerinated diluent		GOLDEN CHANCE COLOGNE, PERFUME, AND SACHET (Ayer)		
GLYTONE AIR SANITIZER (Fuld)	Isopropyl alcohol* Triethylene glycol Propylene glycol Alkyl tolyl methyl trimethyl ammonium chlorides* 50%		GOLDEN CHURN'S POWDER BACTERICIDE (Golden Churn)	Calcium hypochlorite* 50%	
GLYTONE-S AEROSOL SPRAY Air sanitizer, deodorant (Fuld)	Isopropanol* Triethylene glycol Propylene glycol Geraniol Phenyl acetic acetal* Alkyl tolyl methyl trimethyl ammonium chlorides* Phenyl ethyl alcohol* Citronella oil Benzyl acetate Phenylacetaldehyde Hydroxy-citronellol Sandalwood oil Methyl ionone 20%		GOLDEN GLINT HAIR RINSES (Golden Glint)	Colors (D & C, FDC) Adipic acid (pH approx. 4)	
			GOLDEN PEACOCK LOTION AND CREAMS (Golden Peacock)		
GOBO-O-SUDS Soap (Chem. Mfg. & Dist.)			GOLDEN STAR MOTHPROOF-ING (Golden Star)		
GO-FER-GAS CRYSTALS Rodenticide (Zehrung)	Chlorine*		GOLDEN STAR PAINT & VARNISH CLEANER (Golden Star)		
GOLD BEAR MALATHION FLY SPRAY (Swift)	Malathion* 50.0% Methylated naphthalenes* 39.0%		GOLDEN STAR RUG & UP-HOLSTERY CLEANER (Golden Star)		
GOLD BOND KALSOMINE, COLOR TEXTURE (Nat'l Gypsum)			GOLDEN-WEST COMPOUND Laxative (Golden-West)	Gentian root Licorice root Cascara sagrada Damiana leaves Oregon grape root Senna leaves Psyllium seed Buchu leaves Crude pepsin	
GOLD BOND MEDICATED POWDER (Gold Bond)	Menthol Methyl salicylate* Stearate of zinc Salicylic acid* Thymol Eucalyptol* Boric acid* Talc		GOLDEN-YOUTH CLEANSING CREAM (Golden-Youth)		
GOLD CROSS FOOT POWDER (Gold Bond)	Boric acid* Stearate of zinc Thymol Menthol crystals* U.S.P. Salicylic acid* Silicate of magnesium Eucalyptol		GOLDICIDE TABS Antiseptic (Pedinol)	Benzalkonium chloride* Urea	
GOLDEN ALL SOLUBLE B-75 BORAX BASE INDUSTRIAL SKIN CLEANSER (Sugar Beet)	Soap 25% Borax* formulation 75%		GOLD MEDAL ANTACID POWDER (Pfeiffer)	Magnesium carbonate Calcium carbonate Soda bicarbonate Bismuth subcarbonate Colloidal kaolin Diastase of malt Oil of peppermint	

*Consult Sec. II., Ingredients Index. This ingredient may be responsible for major toxic effects if poisonous amounts of this product are ingested.

Name & Use Manufacturer	Ingredients	Name & Use Manufacturer	Ingredients
GOLD MEDAL CREAM ANALGESIC Rubefacient, counter-irritant (Pfeiffer)	Menthol Oleoresin of red pepper Oil of cajuput Camphor* Expressed oil of mustard* Oil of wintergreen*	GON Stain remover (Tilette)	
		GOOD-AIRE Deodorizer (Bridgeport)	Aromatic and essential oils* Petroleum distillate* Freons
GOLD MEDAL 20 HAARLEM OIL CAPSULES Diuretic (Gold Medal)	Sulfuretted oils of turpentine* and linseed Oil of peppermint	GOOD-RITE N.I.X. Herbicide (Goodrich, B. F.)	Sodium isopropyl xanthate* 91%
GOLD MEDAL LIQUID ANALGESIC Rubefacient (Pfeiffer)	Alcohol* 70% Cayenne pepper Methyl salicylate syn.* Menthol Camphor* Oil of peppermint Thymol Eucalyptol*	GOOD-RITE NO-NIB'L RABBIT RE-PELLENT (Goodrich, B. F.)	Zinc dithiocarbamate-amine complex 23%
		GOOD-RITE OKTONE WEED KILLER (Goodrich, B. F.)	Octachlorocyclohexenone* 90% Related chlorinated compounds 10%
GOLD MEDAL TEETHING LOTION (Pfeiffer)	Alcohol 12% Benzocaine Sodium borate* Sodium salicylate* Menthol Sodium benzoate Clove oil Oil of dwarf pine needles Witch hazel	GOOD-RITE SDD LIQUID FUNGICIDE (Goodrich, B. F.)	Sodium dimethyl dithio carbamate 40%
GOLD MEDAL WHITE LINIMENT (Pfeiffer)	Camphor* Turpentine* Ammonia Methyl salicylate* Oils of origanum and sassafras Soap	GOOD-RITE Z.I.P. DEER & RABBIT REPELLENT (Goodrich, B. F.)	Zinc dithiocarbamate-amine complex 30% Polyethylene polysulfide 10%
GOLD METAL CRAYON SETS (Transogram)		GOOD'S HARDWOOD FLOOR CLEANER (Good, James)	
GOLD METAL LIQUID POLISH (Gisler Polish)		GOODWINOL Ectoparasiticide (Goodwinol)	Rotenone* Orthophenylphenol*
GOLD POLO SPUR TOILET WATER AND AFTER SHAVE (Parfum L'Orle)		GOPHER DEATH (Fort Dodge)	Strychnine* alkaloid 0.5%
		GOPHER SCENT Rodenticide (Woods)	Strychnine alkaloid* 0.29%
GOLD SEAL GLASS WAX (Gold Seal)		GORDON'S ANALGESIC CREAM Rubefacient (Gordon Labs.)	Menthol* Camphor* Methyl salicylate* syn. Oil of eucalyptus Vitamin E
GOLD SEAL WOOD CREAM Furniture polish (Gold Seal)		GORDON'S BASIC LOTION For skin irritation (Gordon Labs.)	Zinc oxide Talc Magma bentonite
GOLD & WHITE TABLETS Laxative (Magay)	Each gold tablet: Asafetida 1 gr. Ext. nux vomica (1/60 gr. strychnine) 1/4 gr. Ginger 3/4 gr. Capsicum 1/8 gr. Ext. cascara sagrada 1 gr. Each white tablet: Magnesium carbonate 2 gr. Aromatics q.s. Calcium carbonate 3-1/2 gr. Bismuth subnitrate 1/2 gr.	GORDON'S DRY SKIN CREME For skin irritations (Gordon Labs.)	Cholesterols Lubricating oils

---

*Consult Sec. II., Ingredients Index. This ingredient may be responsible for major toxic effects if poisonous amounts of this product are ingested.

Name & Use Manufacturer	Ingredients		Name & Use Manufacturer	Ingredients	
GORDON'S G-4 FUNGICIDAL SOLUTION (Medical) (Gordon Labs.)	Undecylenic acid G-4 Penetrating oil base Isopropyl alcohol*	10% 1%	GOURIELLI ACTIVE OZONE SHAVE STICK AND FRESH-ENING LOTION (House of Gourielli)		
GORDON'S G-4 FUNGI-CIDAL TALC (Medical) (Gordon Labs.)	Compound G-4 Boric acid* Talc		GOURIELLI ROUGE (House of Gourielli)		
GORDON'S LIQUID TALC Astringent for feet (Gordon Labs.)	Menthol Isopropyl alcohol* Talc Bentonite magma F.D.A. color		GOWEN'S 2-1/2% ALDRIN EQUIVALENT COTTON DUST WITH 5% DDT AND 40% SULPHUR Insecticide (Howerton)	Hexachloro hexahydro dimethano naphthalene* Related compounds DDT* Sulfur as elemental*	2.375% 1.791% 5.000% 40.000%
GORDON SOCKET RINSE For irrigation of the orbital cavity after enucleation (Gordon Labs.)	Benzalkonium chloride* Sodium borate* Boric acid* Camphor*				
			GOWEN'S 20% CHLORINATED CAMPHENE COTTON DUST Insecticide (Howerton)	Toxaphene* (tech. chlorinated camphene, chlorine content 67%-69%) Sulfur as elemental	20% 40%
GORDON'S UNDECYLENIC ACID OINT-MENT (Gordon Labs.)	Undecylenic acid* Polyethylene glycol*				
GORDON'S UNDECYLENIC ACID TINCTURE (Gordon Labs.)	Undecylenic acid* Alcohol		GOWEN'S COTTON DUST 3-5-0 Insecticide (Howerton)	Gamma isomer of BHC* DDT*	3.00% 5.00%
GORHAM SILVER POLISH, CREAM FORM (Gorham)			GOWEN'S 3-5-40 COTTON DUST Insecticide (Howerton)	Gamma isomer of hexa-chlorocyclohexane* Other isomers of hexa-chlorocyclohexane* DDT* Sulfur* as elemental	3.00% 15.00% 5.00% 40.00%
GORHAM SILVER-SMITHS POLISH, LIQUID FORM (Gorham)			GOWEN'S 3-5-40 COTTON DUST WITH 40% SULPHUR Insecticide (Howerton)	Gamma isomer of hexa-chlorocyclohexane* Other isomers of hexa-chlorocyclohexane* DDT* Sulfur* as elemental	3.00% 15.00% 5.00% 40.00%
GORJUS HAIR DRESSING (Lotshaw)	Lanolin		GOWEN'S 5% DDT DUST Insecticide (Howerton)	DDT*	5.00%
GOTHAM AMBER HAIR OILS (Purepac)			GOWEN'S 10% DDT DUST Insecticide (Howerton)	DDT*	10.00%
GOTHAM MARKING & CHECKING CRAYONS (Binney & Smith)			GOWEN'S DITHANE DUST Fungicide (Howerton)	Zineb (zinc ethylene-bis (dithiocarbamate))	6.0%
GOTTLIEB'S KIL-MOR Insecticide (Gottlieb)	Tech. piperonyl butoxide Pyrethrins Dichloro diphenyl trichloroethane* Petroleum oil*	0.188% 0.075% 5.000% 94.737%	GOWEN'S 15% FERMATE DUST Insecticide (Howerton)	Ferric dimethyl dithio-carbamate	11.40%
GOTTLIEB'S MOTH KILLER Insecticide (Gottlieb)	Paradichlorobenzene*	100%	GOWEN'S 15% FERMATE DUST WITH 3% DDT Insecticide (Howerton)	Ferbam (ferric dimethyl dithiocarbamate) DDT	11.4% 3.0%

*Consult Sec. II., Ingredients Index. This ingredient may be responsible for major toxic effects if poisonous amounts of this product are ingested.

Name & Use Manufacturer	Ingredients		Name & Use Manufacturer	Ingredients	
GOWAN'S PREPARA-TION Inhalant, for colds (Gowan)	Menthol Turpentine* Carbolic acid* Camphor* Coal tar Methyl salicylate* Stearic acid		GRANDEE TOILET WATER, PERFUME (De Grasse)		
GOWEN'S 10% RHOTHANE DUST Insecticide (Howerton)	Dichloro diphenyl dichloroethane	10%	GRANDPA'S WONDER PINE TAR TOILET SOAP (Grandpa)	Vegetable pine tar*	
GOWEN'S 20% TOXAPHENE COTTON DUST Insecticide (Howerton)	Toxaphene* Sulfur	20.00% 40.00%	GRAND SLAM SHAMPOO (Carter Co.)	Sulfonated castor oil Mineral oil Sodium lauryl sulfate Hydrogenated vegetable oil	
GOWEN'S TOXAPHENE DUST 20-0 Insecticide (Howerton)	Toxaphene*	20.00%	GRANNIE'S SALVE For colds (Quality Dist.)	Mutton suet Oil pine* Menthol Oil eucalyptus* Camphor*	
G & O WEED & POISON IVY KILLER (Goulard)	Sodium arsenite* Sodium chloride	36.40% 5.00%	GRANNY'S OLD FASHIONED COUGH SYRUP (Royal Mfg.)	Alcohol Chloroform Extracts of white pine Wild cherry Aralia Poplar buds Sassafras Blood root Ipecac Lobelia Squill Euphorbia Menthol	8%/v 3 m./fl. oz.
GRAHAM'S DERMATOX OINTMENT For skin irritations (Assoc.)	Mercury bichloride* Sulfur Calamine Menthol				
GRAINFUME MB Grain fumigant (Selig)	Carbon tetrachloride* Ethylene dichloride* Ethylene dibromide*		GRANT'S MODELING CLAY (Grant)		
GRAIN-O-CIDE Liquid gas fumigant (Midland Labs.)	Carbon tetrachloride* Ethylene dichloride* Ethylene dibromide*		GRAPE FIX For increasing the size of grapes (Thompson Chem.)	Diethanolamine salt of para chlorophenoxy acetic acid*	7.75%
GRAMERCY COLD CREAM (Fisher Scient.)	Spermaceti wax White beeswax Mineral oil Borax (about 0.5%) White ceresin wax Perfume		GRAPHIC LT Photographic supplies (Graphic)		
GRAMERCY SKIN LOTION (Fisher Scient.)	Stearic acid Mineral oil Anhydrous lanolin Cetyl alcohol Quince seed Triethanolamine Perfume Ponceau red		GRAPHITE PAINT PIGMENT (Pacific Graphite)	Carbon Silica Alumina Iron oxide	35-85% 5-20% 8-20% 0-3%
			GRASS-N-WEED KILLER (Bonide)	Sodium pentaborate* Sodium tetraborate* Sodium chlorate*	58% 15% 25%
GRAMERCY SUN TAN LOTION (Fisher Scient.)	Stearic acid Mineral oil Anhydrous lanolin Cetyl alcohol Quince seed Triethanolamine Perfume Ponceau red Menthyl salicylate		GRAYLENE FOOT BATH POWDER (Graylene)		
			GRAY'S COMPOUND Tonic (Purdue)	Gentian Dandelion Sherry wine Glycerin Phosphoric acid Tr. cardamon comp. Alcohol	11%/v
GRAMICIDIN TROCHES For throat irritations (Premo)	Gramicidin* Benzocaine	0.25 mg. 5 mg.	GREAN-RUB Liniment (Grean-Rub)	Methyl salicylate* Camphor* Eucalyptus* Menthol*	

Name & Use Manufacturer	Ingredients	
GREASE-CHEK (Chek)		
GREASOLVE (Holcomb)	Caustic soda*	
GREAT STUFF HAND CLEANER (Great Stuff)		
GREAT WESTERN AEROSOL INSECT BOMB (Great Western)		
GREAT WESTERN FLEA, ROACH AND ANT POWDERS (Great Western)		
GREAT WESTERN PYRETHRUM & DDT 10% POWDER Insecticide (Great Western)	Pyrethrum DDT*	10%
GREDAG LUBRICANTS General lubricant (Gredag)	Refined mineral oil Soap Electric furnace graphite	
GREENBRIER SHAVING LOTION (Daggett & Ramsdell)		
GREEN CROSS ALDRIN 5% DUST Soil insecticide (Green Cross)	Tech. aldrin*	5%
GREEN CROSS ALDRIN 20% Insecticide (Green Cross)	Tech. aldrin*	
GREEN CROSS ALDRIN 20% EMULSIFI-ABLE CON-CENTRATE Insecticide (Green Cross)	Tech. aldrin*	2 lb./imp. gal.
GREEN CROSS AMINE 80 WEED KILLER (Green Cross)	2, 4-D* acid equiv.	80 oz./imp. gal.
GREEN CROSS ANIMAL INSECT POWDER (Green Cross)	Rotenone Methoxychlor	0.5% 1%

Name & Use Manufacturer	Ingredients	
GREEN CROSS ARSENATE OF LEAD Insecticide spray powder (Green Cross)	Arsenic*	19.5%
GREEN CROSS BASI-COP Insecticide (Green Cross)	Copper* (tri-basic copper sulfate)	52%
GREEN CROSS BASI-COP 3% DDT DUST Fungicide, insecticide (Green Cross)	DDT Copper*	3% 7%
GREEN CROSS BORDEAUX MIXTURE Fungicide (Green Cross)	Copper*	12.5%
GREEN CROSS BUG KILLER Insecticide (Green Cross)	Arsenic*	2%
GREEN CROSS CALCIUM ARSENATE Insecticide (Green Cross)	Arsenic*	26%
GREEN CROSS 40% CHLORDANE Insecticide (Green Cross)	Tech. chlordane*	40%
GREEN CROSS 5% CHLORDANE DUST Insecticide (Green Cross)	Tech. chlordane*	5%
GREEN CROSS COUCH GRASS KILLER Herbicide (Green Cross)	Trichloroacetic acid* equiv.	79%
GREEN CROSS COMMERCIAL WEED KILLER 96 (Green Cross)	2, 4-Dichlorophenoxyacetic acid* equiv.	96 oz./gal.
GREEN CROSS CRAG-1 Herbicide (Green Cross)	Sodium 2, 4-dichlorophenoxyethyl sulfate*	90%
GREEN CROSS CRAG 341 Fungicide (Green Cross)	Glyodin (2-heptadecyl glyoxalidine acetate)*	34%/w
GREEN CROSS 7-1/2% DDT AEROPLANE DUST Insecticide (Green Cross)	DDT*	7-1/2%

*Consult Sec. II., Ingredients Index. This ingredient may be responsible for major toxic effects if poisonous amounts of this product are ingested.

Name & Use Manufacturer	Ingredients	
GREEN CROSS 5% DDT-7% BASI COP DUST Fungicide, insecticide (Green Cross)	DDT* Copper*	5% 7%
GREEN CROSS 14% DDT BASI-COP SPRAY POWDER Fungicide, insecticide (Green Cross)	DDT* Copper*	14% 36%
GREEN CROSS DDT-5% COPPER DUST Fungicide, insecticide (Green Cross)	DDT Copper*	3% 5%
GREEN CROSS 3% DDT-7% COPPER DUST Fungicide, insecticide (Green Cross)	DDT Copper*	3% 7%
GREEN CROSS 50% DDD WETTABLE POWDER Insecticide (Green Cross)	DDD*	50%
GREEN CROSS 3% DDT-9% COPPER DUST Fungicide, insecticide (Green Cross)	DDT Copper*	3% 9%
GREEN CROSS 3% DDT DUST Insecticide (Green Cross)	DDT	3%
GREEN CROSS 25% DDT EMULSION Insecticide (Green Cross)	DDT*	25%
GREEN CROSS 5% DDT IN FUEL OIL Insecticide (Green Cross)	DDT*	5%
GREEN CROSS 10% DDT IN-SECT POWDER (Green Cross)	DDT* Pyrethrins Tech. piperonyl cyclonene Rotenone	10% 0.05% 0.5% 0.25%
GREEN CROSS 10% DDT SOLUTION Insecticide (Green Cross)	DDT*	10%
GREEN CROSS 3% DDT-6% THIOGREEN DUST Fungicide, insecticide (Green Cross)	DDT Thiogreen Zineb	3% 6% 3.9%

Name & Use Manufacturer	Ingredients	
GREEN CROSS 50% DDT WETTABLE POWDER Insecticide (Green Cross)	DDT*	50%
GREEN CROSS DRY LIME SULPHUR Fungicide, insecticide (Green Cross)	Sulfide sulfur* Total sulfur	40% 63%
GREEN CROSS ERAD Fungicide (Green Cross)	Phenyl mercuric acetate* Mercury equiv.	10% 6%
GREEN CROSS FLOWER SPRAY Insecticide (Green Cross)	DDT Malathion*	12% 25%
GREEN CROSS FLY BAIT Insecticide (Green Cross)	Malathion	1%
GREEN CROSS FLY-CHARMER Insecticide (Green Cross)	o, o-Dimethyl 1-hydroxy-2, 2, 2-trichloroethyl phosphonate*	2.0%
GREEN CROSS GARDEN GUARD Insecticide (Green Cross)	Rotenone	0.7%
GREEN CROSS 2-1/2% HEPTACHLOR DUST Insecticide (Green Cross)	Heptachlor*	2-1/2%
GREEN CROSS HEPTACHLOR EMULSIFI-ABLE CON-CENTRATE Insecticide (Green Cross)	Heptachlor*	2 lb./gal.
GREEN CROSS 25% HEPTACHLOR WETTABLE POWDER Insecticide (Green Cross)	Heptachlor*	25%
GREEN CROSS HOUSEHOLD SPRAY Insecticide (Green Cross)	Lindane Sulfoxide Beta butoxy beta' thiocyano diethyl ether Inert ingredients*	0.5% 0.15% 0.75%
GREEN CROSS INSECT BOMB (Green Cross)	DDT Beta butoxy beta' thiocyano diethyl ether Piperonyl butoxide Pyrethrins	2% 1% 0.5% 0.1%
GREEN CROSS KARBAM BLACK DUST Fungicide (Green Cross)	Ferric dimethyl dithio-carbamate	7%

*Consult Sec. II., Ingredients Index. This ingredient may be responsible for major toxic effects if poisonous amounts of this product are ingested.

Name & Use Manufacturer	Ingredients		Name & Use Manufacturer	Ingredients	
GREEN CROSS 10% LINDANE EMULSION CONCENTRATE Insecticide (Green Cross)	Gamma isomer of benzene hexachloride*	10%	GREEN CROSS 50% METHOXYCHLOR WETTABLE POWDER Insecticide (Green Cross)	Methoxychlor*	50%
GREEN CROSS 50% LINDANE SEED DRESSING Insecticide (Green Cross)	Gamma isomer of benzene hexachloride*	50%	GREEN CROSS 3% METHOXYCHLOR- 6% THIOGREEN DUST Fungicide, insecticide (Green Cross)	Methoxychlor Zineb	3% 3.9%
GREEN CROSS 25% LINDANE WETTABLE POWDER Insecticide (Green Cross)	Gamma isomer of benzene hexachloride*	25%	GREEN CROSS MOTH BOMB (Green Cross)	Lindane DDT	1% 2%
GREEN CROSS LIVESTOCK BOMB Insecticide (Green Cross)	Beta butoxy beta' thiocyano diethyl ether Pyrethrins Piperonyl butoxide Methoxychlor	1% 0.1% 1.0% 1.5%	GREEN CROSS MULSOLD WETTABLE SULPHUR Fungicide (Green Cross)	Sulfur* (micronized)	95%
GREEN CROSS 25% MALATHION Insecticide (Green Cross)	Malathion*	25%	GREEN CROSS NNOR GARDEN SPRAY Insecticide (Green Cross)	N.N.O.R. solidified at 65°F.	
GREEN CROSS MALATHION BARN SPRAY Insecticide (Green Cross)	Malathion DDT Inert ingredients*	1.2% 0.6%	GREEN CROSS POTATO DUST Insecticide, fungicide (Green Cross)	DDT* Copper dust*	3% 7%
GREEN CROSS MALATHION 4% DUST Insecticide (Green Cross)	Malathion*	4%	GREEN CROSS RAT & MOUSE BAIT (Green Cross)	2 Pivalyl-1, 3-indandione	0.025%
GREEN CROSS 50% MALATHION EMULSION Insecticide (Green Cross)	Malathion* o, o-dimethyl dithiophosphate (of diethyl mercaptosuccinate)	50%	GREEN CROSS RAT & MOUSE KILLER (Green Cross)	Sodium salt of 2-pivalyl-1, 3-indandione	0.14%
GREEN CROSS MCP AMINE 64 WEED KILLER (Green Cross)	2-Methyl-4-chlorophenoxyacetic acid* equiv.	64 oz./imp. gal.	GREEN CROSS ROSE DUST Fungicide, insecticide (Green Cross)	Tech. DDT* Rotenone Ferbam	5% 0.75% 7%
GREEN CROSS MCP SODIUM SALT 48 WEED KILLER (Green Cross)	2-Methyl-4-chlorophenoxyacetic acid* equiv.	48 oz./imp. gal.	GREEN CROSS ROTENONE 5% Insecticide (Green Cross)	Rotenone*	5%
GREEN CROSS MERLANE Insecticide, fungicide (Green Cross)	Phenyl mercury acetate Ethyl mercuric chloride Gamma isomer of BHC (lindane)*	2.86% 0.4% 40.00%	GREEN CROSS SLUG BAIT Insecticide (Green Cross)	Metaldehyde Arsenic*	2% 1.2%
GREEN CROSS 3% METHOXYCHLOR DUST Insecticide (Green Cross)	Methoxychlor	3%	GREEN CROSS TCA Herbicide (Green Cross)	Trichloroacetic acid* equiv.	79%
			GREEN CROSS TCA 90% SODIUM Herbicide (Green Cross)	Trichloroacetic acid* equiv.	79%

*Consult Sec. II., Ingredients Index. This ingredient may be responsible for major toxic effects if poisonous amounts of this product are ingested.

Name & Use Manufacturer	Ingredients		Name & Use Manufacturer	Ingredients	
GREEN CROSS 10% TECHNICAL CHLORDANE DUST Insecticide (Green Cross)	Tech. chlordane*	10%	GREEN LIGHT CHLORDANE DDT LIVE-STOCK SPRAY CONC. Insecticide (Klauss-White)	DDT Tech. chlordane Methylated aromatic petroleum solvent*	26.5% 24.5% 33.2%
GREEN CROSS 40% TECHNICAL CHLORDANE Insecticide (Green Cross)	Tech. chlordane*	40%	GREEN LIGHT 5% CHLORDANE DUST Insecticide (Klauss-White)	Tech. chlordane*	5%
GREEN CROSS 6% THIOGREEN DUST Fungicide (Green Cross)	Zineb	3.9%	GREEN LIGHT 10% CHLORDANE DUST Insecticide (Klauss-White)	Tech. chlordane*	10%
GREEN CROSS TOMATO DUST Fungicide, insecticide (Green Cross)	Copper Arsenic*	7% 4.6%	GREEN LIGHT CHLORDANE HOUSEHOLD INSECTICIDE (Klauss-White)	Tech. chlordane Allethrin (allyl homolog of cinerin-1) Related compounds Di-n-propyl maleate-isosafrole condensate Butoxy ethanol Petroleum distillate*	2.5000% 0.0452% 0.0149% 0.2260% 0.4520% 96.7619%
GREEN CROSS TOXAPHENE 50% EMULSION Insecticide (Green Cross)	Toxaphene* (chlorinated camphene)	50%	GREEN LIGHT 10% CHLORDANE MANY PURPOSE DUST Insecticide (Klauss-White)	Tech. chlordane*	10%
GREEN CROSS WEED KILLER 64 (Green Cross)	Iso-octyl ester of 2,4-D acid* equiv.	64 oz./imp. gal.	GREEN LIGHT 5% CHLORDANE OIL CONCENTRATE Insecticide (Klauss-White)	Tech. chlordane*	5%
GREEN-DEVIL DUST Insecticide (Pearson & Co.)	Malathion*	5%			
GREEN-DEVIL FLY BAIT (Pearson & Co.)	Malathion	1.25%	GREEN LIGHT 20% CHLORDANE OIL CONCENTRATE Insecticide (Klauss-White)	Tech. chlordane*	20%
GREEN-DEVIL WETTABLE POWDER Insecticide (Pearson & Co.)	Malathion*	25%	GREEN LIGHT 40% CHLORDANE WETTABLE POWDER Insecticide (Klauss-White)	Tech. chlordane*	40%
GREEN DOPE (Fuller, W.P.)					
GREENE'S MINERAL PASTE (Wright, J.)	Diatomaceous earth Soap Soda ash		GREEN LIGHT 74% CHLORDANE EMULSIFIABLE CONCENTRATE Insecticide (Klauss-White)	Tech. chlordane* Petroleum hydrocarbons	74% 10.2%
GREEN FROST FOOT LOTION Rubefacient, fungicide (medical) (Excello)	Urea Zinc sulfocarbolate Benzocaine Dichlorophene* Menthol* Camphor*		GREEN LIGHT DAIRY SPRAY CONC. Insecticide (Klauss-White)	Methoxychlor tech. Methylated naphthalene* Petroleum hydrocarbons Emulsifiers	21.18% 67.04% 2.35% 9.43%
GREENLEAF DUST OR SPRAY Insecticide, fungicide (Black Panther)	Rotenone Other cube extractives Copper* (in basic copper sulfate) expressed as metallic Sodium isopropyl naphthalene sulfonate	0.75% 1.50% 7.00% 0.50%	GREEN LIGHT DORMANT & SUMMER OIL SPRAY Insecticide (Klauss-White)	Petroleum oils*	97%

*Consult Sec. II., Ingredients Index. This ingredient may be responsible for major toxic effects if poisonous amounts of this product are ingested.

Name & Use Manufacturer	Ingredients		Name & Use Manufacturer	Ingredients	
GREEN LIGHT 5-5 DUST Insecticide (Klauss-White)	Tech. chlordane* DDT*	5% 5%	GREEN PANTHER SUPER DUST OR SPRAY Insecticide (Black Panther)	Rotenone Other cube extractives Copper* (in basic copper sulfate) expressed as metallic Sodium isopropyl naphthalene sulfonate	1.00% 1.50% 7.00% 0.50%
GREEN LIGHT FLEA & TICK POWDER FOR DOGS Insecticide (Klauss-White)	Tech. chlordane Rotenone* Other cube resins*	2.5% 1.5% 3.0%	GREEN PINE DISINFECT- ANT DE- ODORANT CLEANSER (House of Huston)	Pine oil* Anhydrous soap	75.00% 15.00%
GREEN LIGHT FLOWER & SHRUBBERY DUST Insecticide (Klauss-White)	DDT* Gamma isomer of benzene hexachloride (from lindane) Ferbam Sulfur*	5.00% 1.50% 7.00% 50.00%	GREEN'S AUGUST FLOWER Antacid (Myers Labs.)	Alcohol Sodium bicarbonate Socotrine aloes Oil peppermint Capsicum	7-1/2%
GREEN LIGHT FLOWER & SHRUBBERY SPRAY Insecticide (Klauss-White)	DDT Malathion* Xylene*	23.5% 23.5% 44.0%	GREEN SEAL WATERPROOF ADHESIVE (Lino-Paste)		
GREEN LIGHT FLY SPRAY CONCEN- TRATE (Klauss-White)	Malathion* Xylene*	60% 32%	GREEN SPOT GARDEN DUST Insecticide (Mayo)	Malathion* Methoxychlor* Captan Tribasic copper sulfate*	4% 4% 4% 12%
GREEN LIGHT LIVESTOCK SPRAY Insecticide (Klauss-White)	Gamma isomer of benzene hexachloride Other isomers of benzene hexachloride Toxaphene* Petroleum hydrocarbons	1.38% 2.62% 40.20% 47.20%	GREEN THUMB Plant food (Heinl's)		
			GREENTOX GARDEN SPRAY Insecticide (Bonide)	Polymethylated naphthalenes* Polyethylene glycol monoiso- octyl phenyl ether Cube resins including rotenone	
GREEN LIGHT PEACH & PECAN TREE SPRAY Insecticide (Klauss-White)	Tech. toxaphene* Sulfur* Zinc sulfate*	16% 40% 20%	GREENTOX ROTENONE GARDEN SPRAY Insecticide (Bonide)	Rotenone* Other extractives	2.25% 4.5%
GREEN LIGHT RAT & MOUSE BAIT (Klauss-White)	Warfarin (3-(a-acetonylbenzyl)- 4-hydroxycoumarin) 0.025%		GREENWICH LYE (Pennsylv. Salt)	Sodium hydroxide*	
GREEN LIGHT READY-TO- USE BUG BAIT Insecticide (Klauss-White)	Gamma isomer of benzene hexachloride (from lindane) 0.3%		GRE-SOLVENT Hand cleaner (Utility)		
GREEN LIGHT SNAIL & SLUG BAIT (Klauss-White)	Hexachloro epoxy octahydro dimethano naphthalene 0.412% Related compounds 0.088% Metaldehyde* 3.000%		GREEVER'S AMI-NO- WEED Herbicide (Greever's)	Ethanol amine 2, 4- dichlorophenoxyacetate* as triethanolamine salt	67%
GREEN LIGHT VEGETABLE GARDEN DUST Insecticide (Klauss-White)	Tech. methoxychlor Rotenone Other cube resins	5.00% 1.25%	GREEVER'S ANTISEPTIC Udder ointment (Greever's)	Dihydroxydichlorodiphenyl methane 2.00% Isopropyl myristate Oil of pine* Phenol* Refined wool fat Palmitate Oil of eucalyptus* Camphor* Petrolatum	
GREENOL CONDITIONER (Calif. Spray)	Tetra sodium pyrophosphate 10%				
GREENOL LIQUID FUNGICIDE Fungicide (Calif. Spray)	Copper oleate* Petroleum oils Ethylene glycol oleic esters	15% 12% 35%	GREEVER'S ASTRINGENT POWDER (Greever's)	Catechu N.F. Copper sulfate* Zinc sulfocarbolate N.F. Activated charcoal Fenugreek	35% 5%

Name & Use Manufacturer	Ingredients	
GREEVER'S BUG DUST Insecticide (Greever's)	Rotenone Other cube resins Dusting sulfur	0.75% 1.50% 10.00%
GREEVER'S CHLORDANE (Greever's)	Tech. chlordane* Petroleum solvent	45% 45%
GREEVER'S CHLORDANE WETTABLE POWDER 50% Insecticide (Greever's)	Tech. chlordane*	50%
GREEVER'S COAL TAR STOCK DIP AND DIS- INFECTANT Insecticide (Greever's)	Neutral tar oils Soap Phenols*	63% 21% 10%
GREEVER'S ESTERWEED Herbicide (Greever's)	Isopropyl 2, 4-dichloro- phenoxyacetate*	46.0%
GREEVER'S FLEA POWDER FOR DOGS (Greever's)	Gamma isomer of benzene hexachloride (from lindane) 1.00% Methylene-bis-chlorophenol* 0.50% Propylene glycol Pine oil	 1.00% 1.00%
GREEVER'S GRUB POWDER Insecticide (Greever's)	Rotenone* Cube resins and extractives Sulfur	1.67% 3.33% 10.00%
GREEVER'S HORN PAINT (Veterinary) (Greever's)	Oil coal tar refined Steam distilled pine oil* Phenol (carbolic acid)* 3%	
GREEVER'S INSECT SPRAY CON- CENTRATE (Greever's)	Dichloro diphenyl trichloroethane* Inert ingredients*	25% 75%
GREEVER'S LINDANE 20% Insecticide (Greever's)	Gamma isomer of benzene hexachloride (from lindane)* 20% Xylene* Methylated naphthalene* 55%	 20%
GREEVER'S 25% LINDANE WETTABLE POWDER Insecticide (Greever's)	Gamma isomer of benzene hexachloride (lindane)* 25%	
GREEVER'S MALATHION 50 Insecticide (Greever's)	Malathion* Methylated naphthalenes*	50% 44%
GREEVER'S PHENO- THIAZINE DRENCH POWDER Insecticide (Greever's)	Phenothiazine* N.F. Lorol alcohol Polyvinyl alcohol Algin, cumarin	98.84% 0.5% 0.4% 1.16%

Name & Use Manufacturer	Ingredients	
GREEVER'S PHENO- THIAZINE- LEAD ARSENATE BOLUSES (Greever's)	Phenothiazine Lead arsenate*	12.5 gm. 0.5 gm.
GREEVER'S POULTRY LOUSE POWDER (Greever's)	Tech. piperonyl cyclonene 0.625% Pyrethrins Rotenone Other cube extractives Sulfur	 0.0625% 0.3125% 0.625% 10.00%
GREEVER'S ROSE DUST Insecticide (Greever's)	Lindane Ferric dimethyldithio- carbamate (fermate) Lead arsenate* Sulfur	0.04% 5.0% 8.0% 75.0%
GREEVER'S ROTENONE RESIN CON- CENTRATE Insecticide (Greever's)	Rotenone* Other cube resins* Inert ingredients*	5% 15% 80%
GREEVER'S SODIUM FLUORIDE Insecticide (Greever's)	Sodium fluoride*	95%
GREEVER'S SUSPENSION OF PHENO- THIAZINE Insecticide (Greever's)	Phenothiazine* with bentonite 12.5 gm.	
GREEVER'S SUSPENSION OF PHENO- THIAZINE WITH LEAD ARSENATE Insecticide (Greever's)	Each oz.: Phenothiazine Lead arsenate*	 12.5 gm. 0.5 gm.
GREEVER'S TRIPLE ACTION ROACH AND ANT POWDER (Greever's)	Tech. chlordane* DDT* (dichloro diphenyl trichloroethane)	5% 10%
GREEVER'S TRIPLE STRENGTH INSECT SPRAY (Greever's)	Dichloro diphenyl tri- chloroethane Gamma isomer of benzene hexachloride (from lindane) 0.05% Beta butoxy beta' thiocyano diethyl ether B-thiocyanoethyl esters of mixed fatty acids averaging 10-18 carbon atoms Petroleum distillate*	2.50% 0.39% 1.21% 95.85%
GREEVER'S VET. ANTI- SEPTIC POWDER (Greever's)	Sulfanilamide Zinc oxide Activated charcoal Alum Iodoform* Boric acid* Zinc stearate	5%
GREEVER'S WARFARIN BAIT Rodenticide (Greever's)	Warfarin (3-(a-acetonylbenzyl)- 4-hydroxycoumarin) 0.025%	

*Consult Sec. II., Ingredients Index. This ingredient may be responsible for major toxic effects if poisonous amounts of this product are ingested.

Name & Use Manufacturer	Ingredients		Name & Use Manufacturer	Ingredients	
GRESNAMEL FLOOR ENAMEL (Monroe Co.)			GROVE'S COLD TABLETS (Bromo Quinine) (Grove)	Each tablet: Acetophenetidin* Extract belladonna (1.25% total alkaloids) Extract hyoscyamus (0.155% total alkaloids) Quinine hydrobromide Caffeine Yellow phenolphthalein Oleoresin capsicum	1-3/4 gr. 1/50 gr. 1/16 gr. 3/8 gr.
GREYBAC Antacid (Greyson)	Alcohol 5% Each 5 cc. Bismuth and ammonium citrate U.S.P. IX				
GRIFFIN ALLWITE White shoe polish (Griffin)			GROVE'S TASTELESS CHILL TONIC For malaria (Grove)	Cinchonine-cinchonidine Reduced iron Sugar syrup	
GRIFFIN BOOT STAIN Shoe polish (paste) (Griffin)			GROWER FORMULA Insecticide (Phoenix)	Nicotine* dust	
GRIFFIN SHOE DRESSINGS (Griffin)			GRUB-CHECK Insecticide (Doggett-Pfeil)	DDT* Chlordane* Organic fertilizer materials	
GRIFFIN WAX SHOE POLISH (Liquid) (Griffin)			GRUB FIX Insecticide (Thompson Chem.)	Rotenone* Other cube resins Tech. piperonyl cyclonene Pine oil* Ethylene glycol ether of pinene Petroleum distillate* Emulsifier Terpene alcohol	1.2% 1.8% 0.2% 20.0% 3.5% 40.3% 16% 17%
GRIP-TITE ADHESIVE (Lino-Paste)					
GRISWOLD SALVE (Sisson Drug)	Oleate of lead* Powdered red lead Olive oil				
GRISWOLD'S FAMILY SALVE & PLASTER Antiseptic, keratolytic (Griswold Salve)	Olive oil Rosin Oleate of lead*		GRUBTOX Insecticide (Agkem)	Petroleum distillate* Pine oil* Citrus oils Alkyl phenoxypolyethylene glycol Rotenone Other cube resins Ethylene dichloride* Naphthalene* Soy bean oil	
GRISWOLD'S HAIR OIL (Griswold)			GRUBTOX LIVESTOCK INSECTICIDE CONC. (Agkem)	Petroleum distillate* Pine oils* Citrus oils Alkyl phenoxypolyethylene glycol Rotenone* Other cube resins Ethylene dichloride* Naphthalene* Soy bean oil	
GRISWOLD'S HAZEL CREAM (Griswold Med.)					
GROUP OVER Antiseptic (Burrel-Dugger)	Iodo-phenol Iodine* Phenol (carbolic acid)* Potassium iodide* Camphor* Oil eucalyptus* Mineral oil	7/100 gr. 1/5 gr.	GTA ANT BANE Insecticide (Athelstan)	Thallium sulfate	0.05%
			GTA BAIT FOR BIRD PESTS (Athelstan)	Thallium sulfate*	1.10%
GROVE'S COLD TABLETS (Grove)	Acetophenetidin* Extract belladonna (1.25% total alkaloids) Extract hyoscyamus (0.155% total alkaloids) Podophyllin Oleoresin capsicum Caffeine Extract colocynth Extract aloes	3 gr. 1/50 gr. 1/16 gr.	GTA BAIT (Rats, Mice, Roaches, Water Bugs) (Athelstan)	Thallium sulfate*	2.89%
			GTA BAIT FOR SILVERFISH (Athelstan)	Thallium sulfate*	3%

*Consult Sec. II., Ingredients Index. This ingredient may be responsible for major toxic effects if poisonous amounts of this product are ingested.

Name & Use Manufacturer	Ingredients		Name & Use Manufacturer	Ingredients	
GTA BAT REPELLENT (Athelstan)	Paradichlorobenzene*		GUDE'S PEPTO- MANGAN Iron tonic (Breitenbach)	Each daily dose (6 tablets): Iron Manganese Vitamin B	120 mg. 15 mg. 666 U.S.P. units
GTA FLY-BAIT SPRAY Insecticide (Athelstan)	o, o-Dimethyl dithiophosphate of diethyl mercaptosuccinate 1.45% Xylene* 1.36% Inert ingredients* 97.19%		DR. GUILD'S GREEN MOUNTAIN ASTHMATIC CIGARETTES Antispasmodic for asthma (Guild)	Stramonium* Belladonna* Total alkaloids per cig. 0.06-0.08 gr. U.S.P. Potassium nitrate N.F. VIII	
GTA FLY PROOFING SPRAY Insecticide (Athelstan)	Gamma isomer of benzene hexachloride 1% Emulsifying agents and inert ingredients* 99%		DR. GUILD'S GREEN MOUNTAIN ASTHMATIC COMPOUND Antispasmodic for asthma (Guild)	Stramonium* Belladonna* Total alkaloids 0.20%-0.34% Potassium nitrate N.F. VIII	
GTA RESIDUAL SPRAY Insecticide (Athelstan)	Octachloro-4, 7-methanotetra- hydroindane and related active compounds 2% Inert ingredients* 98%				
GTA RESIDUAL SPRAY CON- CENTRATE WM25 Insecticide (Athelstan)	DDT*		GUITARE NON-SMEAR LIPSTICK (Guitare)		
GTA RESIDUAL SPRAY CON- CENTRATE CE Insecticide (Athelstan)	Octachloro-4, 7-methano tetrahydroindane* 11.4% Related active compounds 7.6% Inert ingredients* 81%		GULF LIGHTER FLUID (Gulf)	Petroleum naphthas*	
GUAIACOL AMMONIUM (Liquid) Antitussive (veterinary) (Massengill)	Potassium guaiacolsulfonate 10% Ammonium chloride 15% Glycerinated base q.s.		GULF LIVESTOCK SPRAY Insecticide (Gulf)	Pyrethrins Piperonyl butoxide Inert ingredients*	0.07% 0.19%
GUAIASEPTONE (Liquid) (veterinary) (Strasenburgh)	Creosote* Cresol* Guaiacol Camphor* Oil of camphor Oil of eucalyptus* Methyl salicylate*		GULF ROACH & ANT KILLER (Gulf)	Pyrethrins Petroleum distillate* Tech. chlordane	0.19% 97.81% 2%
GUARANTEE CORN REMEDY Keratolytic (Guarantee)	Salicylic acid*		GULF SPOT REMOVER Rug and upholstery cleaner (Gulf)		
GUARDS COLD TABLETS (Whitehall)	Aspirin* Quinine sulfate Ephedrine sulfate Magnesium trisilicate Caffeine Salicylic acid* Salicylates*		GULFSPRAY AEROSOL BOMB Insecticide (Gulf)	Pyrethrins Piperonyl butoxide Methoxychlor	0.25% 1% 2%

*Consult Sec. II., Ingredients Index. This ingredient may be responsible for major toxic effects if poisonous amounts of this product are ingested.

Name & Use Manufacturer	Ingredients		Name & Use Manufacturer	Ingredients	
GULFSPRAY CONCEN-TRATE AEROSOL INSECTICIDE (Gulf)	Pyrethrins Tech. piperonyl butoxide Petroleum distillate*	0.95% 0.67% 98.38%	GURNEY'S LINIMENT Rubefacient, (Standard Medical)	Turpentine* Oil origanum* Oil sassafras* Oil of spike*	
GULFSPRAY ROACH & ANT KILLER (Gulf)	Pyrethrins Tech. chlordane Oil	0.19% 2%	G & W ASPIRIN SUPPOSI-TORIES Analgesic (G. & W.)	Each suppository: Acid acetylsalicylic*	3-5 gr.
GULFSPRAY SPECIAL Insecticide (Gulf)	Pyrethrins Piperonyl butoxide Inert ingredients*	0.25% 0.20%	G & W ASPIRIN SUPPOSI-TORIES Analgesic (G. & W.)	Each suppository: Acid acetylsalicylic*	10 gr.
GULF STATES 6% CHLOR-DANE Insecticide (Pearson & Co.)	Tech. chlordane*	6%	GWENOID For skin irritations (Sargeant)	Boric acid* Calamine Chlorothymol* Zinc oxide Sulfur prec. Benzoic acid	
GULF STATES 10% CHLOR-DANE Insecticide (Pearson & Co.)	Tech. chlordane*	10%	G & W EYE BATH (G. & W.)	Butyl ester para hydroxy benzoic acid Boric acid (C.P. soluble acid) Sodium borate	
GULF STATES 40% CHLOR-DANE Insecticide (Pearson & Co.)	Tech. chlordane*	40%	GXI LIQUID HAND SOAP (Lester)	Hexachlorophene	
GULF STATES 50% CHLOR-DANE Insecticide (Pearson & Co.)	Tech. chlordane*	50%	GY-BAMATE 76 Fungicide (Geigy)	Ferbam*	76%
GULF STATES 5% ROTENONE Insecticide (Pearson & Co.)	Rotenone* Other cube resins*	5.00% 10.00%	GY-BEN 9 DUST CON-CENTRATE Insecticide (Geigy)	Gamma isomer of benzene hexachloride* Other isomers of benzene hexachloride*	9% 51%
GUMEZE Dental anesthetic (Velvet)	Menthol* Thymol* Benzocaine Benzalkonium chloride*		GY-BEN EMULSIFI-ABLE NO. 100 Insecticide (Geigy)	Gamma isomer of benzene hexachloride* Other isomers of benzene hexachloride Xylene*	11.8% 14.5% 59.0%
GUM MEL Liquid teeth-ing lotion (VB)	Ethylaminobenzoate Chlorobutanol Hexahydrothymol Alcohol	 2%	GY-BEN EMULSIFI-ABLE NO. 120 Insecticide (Geigy)	Gamma isomer of benzene hexachloride* Other isomers of benzene hexachloride Xylene*	13.74% 20.61% 51.50%
GUNSLICK SHOT GUN & RIFLE GREASE (Outers)			GY-BEN 10W Insecticide (Geigy)	Gamma isomer of benzene hexachloride* Other isomers of benzene hexachloride*	10.0% 17.9%
			GY-BEN 12W Insecticide (Geigy)	Gamma isomer of benzene hexachloride* Other isomers of benzene hexachloride	12% 36%

*Consult Sec. II., Ingredients Index. This ingredient may be responsible for major toxic effects if poisonous amounts of this product are ingested.

- 555 -

Name & Use Manufacturer	Ingredients		Name & Use Manufacturer	Ingredients	
GY-BEN WETTABLE POWDER Insecticide (Geigy)	Gamma isomer of benzene hexachloride* Other isomers of benzene hexachloride*	6% 34%	GYPSOLENE SKIN LOTION (Reed Labs.)		
GY-BEN 12 WETTABLE POWDER Insecticide (Geigy)	Gamma isomer of benzene hexachloride* Other isomers of benzene hexachloride*	12% 68%	GYPSY CREAM For skin irritations (Rexall)	Zinc oxide Carbolic acid* Camphor* Glycerin Lime water	
GY-COP 53 Fungicide (Geigy)	Copper*	53%	GYPSY FIRE POWDER Colored flame for the hearth (Gypsy)	Copper chloride* dried crystals Coke dust Sawdust	10%
GY-PHENE 40-20 COT-TON SPRAY Insecticide (Geigy)	Toxaphene* DDT* Aromatic petroleum deriv. solvent*	40% 20% 30%	GYPSY GIFT Rubefacient, (McCam-bridge)	Alcohol* Potassium iodide* Sodium salicylate* Fluid extract of gentian compound	30%
GY-PHENE E40 Insecticide (Geigy)	Toxaphene* Aromatic petroleum deriv. solvent*	42.0% 50.0%	GY-TET 20 Insecticide (Geigy)	Tetraethyl pyrophosphate* Other related organic phosphate esters	20% 30%
GY-PHENE E60 Insecticide (Geigy)	Toxaphene*	57.50%	GY-TET 40 Insecticide (Geigy)	Tetraethyl pyrophosphate* Other related organic phosphate esters	40% 60%
GY-PHENE E80 Insecticide (Geigy)	Toxaphene* Aromatic petroleum deriv. solvent*	69.3% 20.0%	GY-TRETE 595 Seed dis-infectant (Geigy)	Phenyl mercury acetate* Ethyl mercury acetate Total mercury as metallic	5.00% 0.95% 3.64%
GY-PHENE 20 Insecticide (Geigy)	Toxaphene*	20%	GY-ZIP AEROSOL INSECT KILLER (Geigy)	Tech. methoxychlor Tech. piperonyl butoxide Pyrethrins Petroleum distillate Methylated naphthalenes*	2% 1% 0.25% 4% 7.75%
GY-PHENE 20-S Insecticide (Geigy)	Toxaphene* Sulfur	20.00% 40.00%			
GY-PHENE 40W Insecticide (Geigy)	Toxaphene*	40%			

*Consult Sec. II., Ingredients Index. This ingredient may be responsible for major toxic effects if poisonous amounts of this product are ingested.

- 556 -

Name & Use Manufacturer	Ingredients		Name & Use Manufacturer	Ingredients	
HAARLEM OIL CAPSULES (Royal Mfg.)	Sulfurated oil of turpentine*	5 m.	HAIRLAC (Nestle-Le Mur)		
HAAS HAND LOTION CLEAR (Haas)			HAIR-O-GOLD (Goodman)	Hydrogen peroxide*	6%
			HAIR PETROLE (Noonan)		
HAAS QUININE HAIR LOTION (Haas)			DR. B. W. HAIR'S FORMULA Asthmatic bronchial decongestant (Hair, Dr. B. W.)	Alcohol Potassium iodide* Wine base	17% 27.343 gr.
HABER'S HAIR COLORING (Haber)			DR. B. W. HAIR'S LAXATIVE PILLS (Hair, Dr. B.W.)	Ext. nux vomica* (strychnine 1/400 gr.) 1/30 gr. Aloin* Podophyllin Resin jalap Oleoresin capsicum	
HACIN Antihistamine analgesic (Haag)	Each tablet: Pyrilamine maleate Salicylamide* Phenacetin* Caffeine alkaloid	25 mg. 3-1/2 gr. 2-1/2 gr. 1/2 gr.			
HACKOLITE PAINT FINISHES (Hack)			HAIR TEX (Hairtex)	Liquid petrolatum Peanut oil Anhydrous lanolin Sesame oil Beeswax Phenol Rose oil Solid petrolatum	40% 5% 10% 2% 5% 0.05% 0.05% 27%
HADACOL Dietary supplement (Le Blanc)	4 Tbsp.: Vitamin B1 Vitamin B2 Vitamin B6 Niacinamide Pantothenic acid Iron Calcium Manganese Phosphorous	6 mg. 4 mg. 2 mg. 40 mg. 4 mg. 106 mg. 250 mg. 90 mg. 250 mg.	HAIR WAVING SHAMPOO (Marlene's)		
			HAKES OINTMENT For colds (Hakes)	Camphor* Oils of eucalyptus* Cloves Menthol* Turpentine* Thyme	
HAER- DRESS ENGLISH HAIR TONIC (Castilla)	Alcohol (preservative) Denatured alcohol* Castor oil* Citrus oils	12% 84%	HALAZONE TABLETS (Abbott)	Each tablet: Halazone (p-n,n-dichloro- sulfamidobenzoic* acid 4 mg. Sodium borate* Sodium chloride	
HA-FE Nasal decongestant (Prescript.Lab.)	Ephedrine sulfate* Procaine borate Chlorobutanol Special menstruum	1.0%w/v. 0.5%w/v. 0.5%w/v. q.s.			
			HALENE PROTECTIVE LOTION (Halperin)	Lanolin Cetyl alcohol	
HA-FE HIST For colds (Prescript. Lab.)	Each tablet: Pyranisamine maleate Aspirin* Phenacetin* Caffeine alkaloid	10 mg. 3-1/2 gr. 2-1/2 gr. 1/2 gr.	DR. HALE'S HOUSEHOLD OINTMENT (Kenyon)	Alcohol Petrolatum Oil origanum Oil eucalyptus* Tincture myrrh Camphor* gum	1.8%
HAINES NERVINE (Sacramento)					
H. A. INK ERADICATOR (H. A.)			HALEY'S M-O Antacid, laxative (Phillips, C.)	Milk of magnesia Mineral oil	
HAIR-A-GAIN HAIR & SCALP SHAMPOO (George, G.O.)			HALITOSINE ANTISEPTIC (Halitosine)		
HAIR DRES (Goodman)	Gum tragacanth Water Perfume Certified color		HALITOSINE DENTRIFRICE (Halitosine)		

*Consult Sec. II., Ingredients Index. This ingredient may be responsible for major toxic effects if poisonous amounts of this product are ingested.

Name & Use Manufacturer	Ingredients		Name & Use Manufacturer	Ingredients	
HALL'S EXPECTORANT COMPOUND Antitussive (E.Z. Chem.)	Ammonium chloride Creosote* Glycerin Wild cherry Cane sugar Alcohol	1/2%	HAMMOND'S ROTENONE BEARING DUST NO. 75 Insecticide (Hammond)	Rotenone	0.75%
HALL'S NASAL OINTMENT (Cheney)			HAMMOND'S TOMATO DUST Insecticide (Hammond)	Calcium arsenate* Fixed copper	
HALOCOL Antitussive (Blue Cross)	Each fluid ounce: Chloroform* Cod. phos.* Pot. guaiac. sulf. Ammon. chlor. Tartar emetic*	2 gr. 1 gr. 8 gr. 8 gr. 1/12 gr.	HAMMOND WEED KILLER Herbicide (Hammond)	Sodium arsenate* 4 lbs./gal.	
HALOID ACID FIXING POWDER (Haloid)	Sodium acid sulfite* Sodium thiosulfate		HANABILE COMPOUND Bile salts and diastase compound (Hance)	Bile salts Ext. cascara Ext. nux vomica Oleoresin capsicum Strychnine	1 gr. 1/2 gr. 1/16 gr. 1/40 gr. 0.0046 gr.
HALOL STEAM INHALANT (Blair)	Benzoin* Menthol* Oils eucalyptus* Pine needles		HANA-CAPS Cold tablets (Hance	Acetophenetidin* Salicylamide* Camph. monobrom. Caffeine Phenolphthalein Atropine sulfate Quinine sulfate	1-1/4 gr. 1 gr. 1/4 gr 1/4 gr. 1/5 gr. 1/1000 gr. 1/4 gr.
HALO SHAMPOO (Colgate - Palmolive)					
HALZ LOZENGES (Supreme Pharm.)	Each lozenge: Hexylresorcinol* Benzocaine	2.4 mg. 5 mg.	HANACIDE Ectoparasiti- cide (Hance)	Cupric oleate* Oleic acid Mineral seal oil	
HAMAMELIS DISTILLED EXTRACT (Clapp, Otis)	Witch hazel Alcohol	14%	HANACOLE-A TABLETS Analgesic for colds (Hance)	Acetophenetidin* Atropine sulfate Caffeine Aloin Pwd. capsicum Podophyllin Camphor	2-1/2 gr. 1/2000 gr.
HAMAMELIS SALVOL s330 (Clapp, Otis)	Witch hazel		HANATAB TABLETS Analgesic (Hance)	Acetylsalicylic acid* Caffeine	5 gr. 1/4 gr.
HAMAMELIS & STRAMONIUM COMPOUND For hemmorrhoids and rectal irritation (Lilly)	Each 100 gm.: Benzocaine Camphor* Tannic acid Ext. belladonna* Ext. stramonium leaves* Witch hazel leaves	1 gm. 4 gm. 3 gm. 1 gm. 3 gm. 50 gm.	HANCE ANALGESIC BALM Rubefacient (Hance)	Methyl salicylate* Menthol* Camphor* Lanolin Petrolatum	
HAMMOND'S CUBE POW- DER Insecticide (Hammond)	Rotenone*		HANCE ANTACID POWDER (Hance)	Bismuth subcarbonate Magnesium carbonate Calcium carbonate Oil peppermint Magnesium trisilicate Diastase	
HAMMOND'S DO-DI LAWN WEED KILLER 2,4-D Herbicide (Hammond)	2,4-D*		HANCE ANTISEPTOL (Hance)	Alcohol Oil eucalyptus* Thymol* Menthol* Boric acid* Benzoic acid*	25%/v
HAMMOND'S GRAPE & ROSE DUST Insecticide (Hammond)	Copper* Sulfur*		HANCE A. P. C. CAPSULES Analgesic for colds (Hance)	Each capsule: Acetophenetidin* Caffeine Aspirin*	2-1/2 gr. 1/2 gr. 3-1/2 gr.
HAMMOND'S LINIMENT (Wells, S.C.)	Turpentine* Linseed oil Sulfuric acid*				

*Consult Sec. II., Ingredients Index. This ingredient may be responsible for major toxic effects if poisonous amounts of this product are ingested.

Name & Use Manufacturer	Ingredients		Name & Use Manufacturer	Ingredients	
HANCE BABY SYRUP Antitussive (Hance)	Alcohol Fl. ext. ipecac* Fl. ext. squill* Cherry bark	1-1/2%/v	HANCE DOUCHE POWDER For feminine hygiene (Hance)	Sodium borate* Sodium chloride Boric acid* Zinc sulfate* Carbolic acid* Alum Oil eucalyptus* Methyl salicylate*	
HANCE BEEF, IRON & WINE Tonic (Hance)	Alcohol Sherry wine Beef peptone Iron and ammonium citrate Sodium citrate Soda benzoate Aromatics	15%	HANCE IMPROVED RECTONE Rectal suppositories (Hance)	Benzocaine Bismuth subgallate Resorcinol Balsam peru Zinc oxide Boric acid*	2 gr. 2.25% 1.75% 3% 11% 18%*
HANCE BLUE OINTMENT Ectoparasiti- cide (Hance)	Unguentum hydrargyri* mite U.S.P.		HANCE LARKSPUR LOTION Ectoparasiti- cide (Hance)	Larkspur alkaloids* Acetic acid Acetone Alcohol	
HANCE BROWN LOZENGES For throat irritations (Hance)	Each lozenge: Extract licorice Benzoic acid Camphor Oil anise Tartar emetic Powdered sugar	2 gr. 1/20 gr. 1/20 gr. 1/20 m. 1/40 gr. q.s.	HANCE LAVENDER RUBBING ALCOHOL COMPOUND (Hance)	Absolute alcohol* Oil lavender	70%
HANCE BROWN LOZENGES & AMMONIUM MURIATE For throat irritations (Hance)	Each lozenge: Tartar emetic Mur. ammonia Extract licorice Benzoic acid Camphor Oil anise Powdered sugar	1/40 gr. 3 gr. 2 gr. 1/20 gr. 1/20 gr. 1/20 mn. q.s.	HANCE LAXATIVE SYRUP OF FIGS & SENNA (Hance)	Figs Senna F. E. cascara Rochelle salts Alcohol	6%/v
HANCE CREAM CAMPHOR LINIMENT (Hance)	Camphor* Stronger ammonia water* Ammonium carbonate Turpentine* Castile soap Oil origanum		HANCE LIQUID ANALGESIC BALM (Hance)	Alcohol Menthol* Camphor* Methyl salicylate*	55%
HANCE CREOSOTE EMULSION Antitussive (Hance)	Alcohol Pine tar Licorice Ipecac Spikenard Sassafras Camphor Eucalyptol Creosote Cascara White pine Wild cherry Sanguinaria Poplar bud Menthol Aromatics	3-5%/v.	HANCE MOUTH WASH ASTRINGENT (Hance)	Alcohol Zinc chloride* Formaldehyde* Oil cinnamon Menthol Oil cloves	5%
			HANCE NOSE DROPS Nasal decongestant (Hance)	Alcohol Chlorobutanol* Sodium citrate Menthol Camphor	2%/v 0.5%
			HANCE RECTAL OINTMENT For relief of simple hemorrhoids (Hance)	Powdered opium (0.1575 gr. anhydrous morphine) Phenol* Powdered nutgall Oil tar* Oil pine tar*	1-1/2 gr./oz.
HANCE DIURETIC COMPOUND Diuretic (Hance)	Uva ursi Buchu Methenamine Sodium citrate Saw palmetto Couch grass Potassium acetate Oil of juniper		HANCE RUBBING ALCOHOL COMPOUND WITH SEPTIUM (Hance)	Absolute alcohol* Septium* Alkyl dimethyl benzyl ammonium chloride*	70%/v
HANCE DIURETIC PILLS Diuretic (Hance)	Asparagus Buchu Oil juniper Uva ursi Corn silk Licorice		HANCE SUN-TAN CREME (Hance)	Isobutyl-p-aminobenzoate Lanolin	

---

*Consult Sec. II., Ingredients Index. This ingredient may be responsible for major toxic effects if poisonous amounts of this product are ingested.

Name & Use Manufacturer	Ingredients		Name & Use Manufacturer	Ingredients	
HANCE SYRUP OF TAR Antitussive (Hance)	Each fl. oz.: Alcohol Vitamin A conc. Menthol White pine bark Balm of Gilead buds Spikenard root Cudbear Aromatic flavors Chloroform Vitamin D. conc. Pine tar Wild cherry bark Sanguinaria Sassafras Sugar	1% 4 m.	DR. HAND'S COLIC MIXTURE (Hand)	Each fl. oz. Alcohol Ether Potassium bicarbonate Aromatic spirits of ammonia Tr. tolu Fl. ext. catnip	4% 3.27 m.
HANCE TERPIN HYDRATE & CODEINE ELIXIR Sedative, expectorant (Hance)	Each fl. oz.: Alcohol Codeine	39-44% 9/10 gr.	DR. HAND'S COUGH MEDICINE (Hand)	Alcohol Sodium bromide* Alkaloids of hyoscyamus 0.0009 gr. Fl. ext. sanguinaria Fl. ext. ipecac* Tr. tolu Menthol*	4% 6 gr.
HANCE WHITE PINE & TAR COM- POUND Antitussive (Hance)	Chloroform	4 m./fl.oz.	DR. HAND'S PLEASANT PHYSIC (Hand)	Each fl. oz.: Alcohol Fl. ext. cascara Fl. ext. licorice	6%
HANCE WINTER- GREEN ISOPROPYL ALCOHOL COMPOUND (Hance)	Isopropyl alcohol* Oil wintergreen*	90%/v	DR. HAND'S TEETHING LOTION (Hand)	Alcohol Tr. pelitory Witch hazel Oil sassafras* Oil cloves* Menthol*	11%
HANCE WINTER- GREEN RUBBING ALCOHOL COMPOUND (Hance)	Absolute alcohol* Oil wintergreen*	70%/v	HAN-D WATERLESS HAND CLEANER (Great Stuff)	Lanolin Red oil Lecithin Deo-base	
HANDICALK (Gibson)			HANDY DAN Liquid masking tape (Rearden)		
HANDIGLAZE Caulking compound (Gibson)			HANDY DANDY HAND SOAP & PASTE (Tilton)		
HANDI-LUBE Lubricating grease (Cities)			HANDY FLUX (Handy)	Potassium acid fluoride* Potassium tetraborate* Boric acid*	
HANDLEY CARBOL FUCHSIN Fungicide, (medical) (Handley)	Rosaniline and parosaniline hydrochloride* Resorcinol* Dimethyl ketone* Boric acid* Phenol* Isopropyl alcohol*	approx. 4.5% 20%	HANDY FLUX FOR ALUMINUM BRONZE (Handy)	Potassium acid fluoride* Potassium tetraborate* Boric acid*	
			HANDY LIQUID FLUX (Handy)	Potassium acid fluoride* Potassium tetraborate* Boric acid*	
DR. HAND'S ASTRINGENT MIXTURE For intestinal irritations (Hand)	Alcohol Ext. cranesbill Fl. ext. blackberry root Fl. ext. ginger Aromatic sulfuric acid* Camphor* Oil cinnamon Oil cloves* Oil cajuput*	4%	HANDY SCRATCH REMOVER (Golden Star)		
			HANDYVAR INSULATING VARNISH (Martindale)		
			HANORUB Counter- irritant (Hance)	Goose grease Oil mustard (syn.) Methyl salicylate (Syn.)* Menthol* Lanolin Petrolatum Cora flave Paraffin	

*Consult Sec. II., Ingredients Index. This ingredient may be responsible for major toxic effects if poisonous amounts of this product are ingested.

- 560 -

Name & Use Manufacturer	Ingredients		Name & Use Manufacturer	Ingredients	
HANSLICK Hand soap (Solar)			HAPPY FEET CORN REMEDY Keratolytic (Ozark)	Absolute alcohol Ether* Salicylic acid* Glacial acetic acid* Pyroxylin Castor oil Turpentine	22%/v 213 gr./fl.oz.
HANSON 47% CHLORDANE EMULSION CONCEN- TRATE Insecticide (Hanson, H.)	Tech. chlordane* Petroleum hydrocarbon*	47% 43%			
HANSON 50% CHLORDANE WETTABLE POWDER Insecticide (Hanson H.)	Tech. chlordane*	50%	HAPPY JACK EAR CANKER POWDER (Happy Jack)	Zinc oxide Boric acid* Iodoform*	
			HAPPY JACK FLEA-TICK POWDER FOR DOGS Insecticide (Happy Jack)	Gamma isomer of benzene hexachloride (from lindane) Dichlorophene tech.	1% 2%
HANSON 25% DDT EMULSION CONCEN- TRATE Insecticide (Hanson, H.)	DDT* Aromatic oil*	25% 70%			
HANSON DYNITRO CONTACT WEED KILLER Herbicide (Hanson, H.)	Dinitro-sec-butyl phenol* Pet. oil	6.2% 80.4%	HAPPY JACK MANGE MEDICINE (Veterinary) (Happy Jack)	Vegetable oils Sulfur Fish oil Turpentine* Pine tar oil* Carbolic acid* Collodial clay	5%
HANSON DYNITRO SELECTIVE WEED KILLER Herbicide (Hanson, H.)	Ammonium dinitro-sec- butyl phenate*	13.7%	HAPPY JACK SKIN BALM For skin irritation (veterinary) (Happy Jack)	2-Mercaptobenzothiazole* Isopropyl alcohol	1.5% 1.5%
HANSON LIVESTOCK SPRAY Insecticide (Hanson, H.)	Petroleum distillate* Piperonyl butoxide		HAPPY JACK TAPE WORM TABLETS FOR DOGS (Happy Jack)	Each tablet: 2,2' Dihydroxy-5,5' dichloro- diphenylmethane*	16 gr.
HANSON ODORLESS TYPE DAIRY FLY SPRAY Insecticide (Hanson, H.)	Petroleum distillate* Tech. piperonyl butoxide Pyrethrins	99.72% 0.25% 0.03%	HAPPY JACK WORM CAPSULES FOR DOGS (Happy Jack)	n-Butyl chloride*	
HANSON MAGIC CORN SALVE Keratolytic (Hanson, W.T.)	Benzoate Beeswax Salicylic acid*	20% 20% 30%	HAPPY RETURN TOILET WATER (Masie)		
			HARALSON'S MIXTURE Carminative, digestant (Haralson)	Each fl. oz.: Pepsin U.S.P. Bismuth subgallate Alcohol	16 gr. 41 gr. 15%
HAP ANTISEPTIC TREAT FOR HAIR & SCALP (Snow White)	Dihydroxy hexachloro diphenyl methane* Camphor* Lanolin Vegetable oil Petrolatum base		HARCOLIN ENAMELS & LACQUERS (Murphy Paint)		
HAPPY BUNNY EASTER EGG COLORS (Halwell)	Coal tar Lactose U.S.P. Dextrose		HARCOTE Paints, varnish (Murphy Paint)		
			HARDCOTE ENAMEL, VARNISH (McDougall- Butler)		

*Consult Sec. II., Ingredients Index. This ingredient may be responsible for major toxic effects if poisonous amounts of this product are ingested.

Name & Use Manufacturer	Ingredients		Name & Use Manufacturer	Ingredients	
HARD GLOSS GLO-COAT Floor polish (Johnson, S.C.)	Natural and synthetic resins Petroleum waxes Emulsifying agents		HARROP- TINTS, LIGHT REFLECTIONS (Harrop)		
HARDY'S MEDICATED LOTION For acne (Hardy)	Potassa sulfurated Zinc sulfate*		HARSHAW COPPER NAPHTHEN- ATE Fungicide (Harshaw)		
HARRIET HUBBARD AYER ASTRINGENT, COLOGNE, DEODORANT (Ayer)			HARSHAW COPPER NAPHTHEN- ATE LIQUID 8% Wood preser- vative (Harshaw)	Naphthenic acid Copper hydrate* Mineral spirits*	
HARRIET HUBBARD AYER FACE CREAM (Ayer)			HARVAMINE Bronchial antispasmodic (Harvey, G.F.)	Each tablet: Phenyltoloxamine* (2-benzyl- phenyl beta dimethylamino ethyl dihydrogen citrate) 50 mg.	
HARRIET HUBBARD AYER HAND LOTION (Ayer)			HARVEY'S EMBROCA- TION Veterinary (Kopf)	Croton oil* Ethyl alcohol 80% Methyl alcohol 8%	
HARRIET HUBBARD AYER POWDER (Ayer)			HARWOOD'S DIURETIC PILLS (Commerce)	Pot. nitrate* Ext. uva ursi Powd. scoparius Buchu Juniper oil* Hypophosphites*	
HARRIET HUBBARD AYER SKIN PREPARATIONS (Ayer)			HARWOOD'S PIN WORM REMEDY (Commerce)	Enteric coated gentian violet*	
HARRIS ASTHMA REMEDY (Hubbard, C.)			HASTINGS WEAR REDUCER For engines (Hastings)	Light petroleum oil Barium* salts Zinc dithiophosphate* Sulfur Phosphorus*	
HARRIS FAMOUS ROACH TABLETS Insecticide (Harris, P.F.)	Boric acid* 40%		HAUG A.Q.A. TABLETS Analgesic, antipyretic (Haug)	Each tablet: Acetophenetidin* 3 gr. Aspirin (acetylsalicylic acid)* 3 gr. Quinine sulfate 1/3 gr. Caffeine alkaloid 1/4 gr.	
HARRIS HAIR TONIC (Harris Hair)			HAEUSERLAC SHELLAC SUBSTITUTE (Haeuser)		
HARRIS HOUSE PAINTS (Murphy Paint)			HAEUSER LIQUID SHELLAC (Haeuser)		
HARRISON OIL COLORS (du Pont)					
HARRIS' ROACH TABLETS Insecticide (Harris Prod.)	Boric acid* 40.00%		HAUSMAN'S MEXICAN OIL BRAND (Hausman)	Alcohol* 66% Rhubarb Cardamon Capsicum Star anise Camphor* Peppermint Glycerin	

*Consult Sec. II., Ingredients Index. This ingredient may be responsible for major toxic effects if poisonous amounts of this product are ingested.

Name & Use Manufacturer	Ingredients	
HAVILAND DUST NO. 1 Insecticide (Haviland Prod.)	DDT Yellow cuprocide*	3% 6%
HAVILAND DUST NO. 1C Insecticide (Haviland Prod.)	DDT Tribasic copper*	3% 1.5%
HAVILAND DUST NO. 1D Insecticide (Haviland Prod.)	DDT Zineb	3% 6%
HAVILAND DUST NO. 2 Insecticide (Haviland Prod.)	DDT	3%
HAVILAND DUST NO. 2C Insecticide (Haviland Prod.)	Chlordane	2%
HAVILAND DUST NO. 3 Insecticide (Haviland Prod.)	DDT	3%
HAVILAND DUST NO. 4 Insecticide (Haviland Prod.)	Yellow cuprocide*	6%
HAVILAND DUST NO. 4C Insecticide (Haviland Prod.)	Tribasic copper*	13.5%
HAVILAND DUST NO. 4D Insecticide (Haviland Prod.)	Zineb	6%
HAVILAND DUST NO. 5 Insecticide (Haviland Prod.)	DDT*	5%
HAVILAND DUST NO. 5C Insecticide (Haviland Prod.)	Chlordane	5%
HAVILAND DUST NO. 10 Insecticide (Haviland Prod.)	DDT*	10%
HAVILAND DUST NO. 10D Insecticide (Haviland Prod.)	DDT*	10%
HAVILAND DUST NO. 12 Insecticide (Haviland Prod.)	Tribasic copper*	13.5%

Name & Use Manufacturer	Ingredients	
HAVILAND DUST NO.12C Insecticide (Haviland Prod.)	DDT Tribasic copper*	3% 13.5%
HAVILAND DUST NO. 15 Insecticide (Haviland Prod.)	DDT Yellow cuprocide* Sulfur	3% 6% 30%
HAVILAND DUST NO. 15C Insecticide (Haviland Prod.)	DDT Tribasic copper* Sulfur*	3% 13.5% 30%
HAVILAND DUST NO. 15D Insecticide (Haviland Prod.)	DDT Zineb	3% 6%
HAVILAND DUST NO.16C Insecticide (Haviland Prod.)	Pyrethrins Piperonyl cyclonene Tribasic copper* Sulfur*	0.04% 0.5% 13.5% 30%
HAVILAND DUST NO. 16D Insecticide (Haviland Prod.)	Pyrethrins Piperonyl cyclonene Zineb	0.04% 0.5% 6%
HAVILAND DUST NO. 17 Insecticide (Haviland Prod.)	Calcium arsenate*	10%
HAVILAND DUST NO. 17C Insecticide (Haviland Prod.)	Pyrethrins Piperonyl cyclonene Tribasic copper*	0.04% 0.5% 13.5%
HAVILAND DUST NO. 18 Insecticide (Haviland Prod.)	DDT Yellow cuprocide*	3% 6%
HAVILAND DUST NO. 18C Insecticide (Haviland Prod.)	DDT Tribasic copper*	3% 13.5%
HAVILAND DUST NO. 19 Insecticide (Haviland Prod.)	DDT	3%
HAVILAND DUST NO. 21 Insecticide (Haviland Prod.)	DDT	3%
HAVILAND DUST NO. 21P Insecticide (Haviland Prod.)	Pyrethrins Piperonyl cyclonene	0.04% 0.5%
HAVILAND DUST NO. 23 Insecticide (Haviland Prod.)	DDT Yellow cuprocide* Sulfur*	3% 6% 30%

*Consult Sec. II., Ingredients Index. This ingredient may be responsible for major toxic effects if poisonous amounts of this product are ingested.

Name & Use Manufacturer	Ingredients		Name & Use Manufacturer	Ingredients	
HAVILAND DUST NO. 23C Insecticide (Haviland Prod.)	DDT Tribasic copper* Sulfur*	3% 13.5% 30%	HAVILAND DUST NO. 34 Insecticide (Haviland Prod.)	Tribasic copper*	19%
HAVILAND DUST NO. 23D Insecticide (Haviland Prod.)	DDT* Zineb	3% 6%	HAVILAND DUST NO. 35 Insecticide (Haviland Prod.)	Calcium arsenate* Yellow cuprocide	10% 6%
HAVILAND DUST NO. 25OR Insecticide (Haviland Prod.)	Rotenone	2.5%	HAVILAND DUST NO. 36 Insecticide (Haviland Prod.)	TDE Zineb	3% 6%
HAVILAND DUST NO. 30 Insecticide (Haviland Prod.)	Calcium arsenate* Yellow cuprocide	20% 6%	HAVILAND DUST NO. 36K Insecticide (Haviland Prod.)	TDE Ziram*	3% 10%
HAVILAND DUST NO. 30C Insecticide (Haviland Prod.)	Calcium arsenate* Tribasic copper	20% 13.5%	HAVILAND DUST NO. 37 Insecticide (Haviland Prod.)	Calcium arsenate	20%
HAVILAND DUST NO. 30D Insecticide (Haviland Prod.)	Calcium arsenate* Zineb	20% 6%	HAVILAND DUST NO. 37R Insecticide (Haviland Prod.)	TDE	3%
HAVILAND DUST NO. 30K Insecticide (Haviland Prod.)	Calcium arsenate* Ziram	20% 10%	HAVILAND DUST NO. 38 Insecticide (Haviland Prod.)	TDE Tribasic copper *	3% 13.5%
HAVILAND DUST NO. 31D Insecticide (Haviland Prod.)	Zineb	6%	HAVILAND DUST NO. 39 Insecticide (Haviland Prod.)	TDE Yellow cuprocide*	3% 6%
HAVILAND DUST NO. 31K Insecticide (Haviland Prod.)	Ziram*	10%	HAVILAND DUST NO. 40 Insecticide (Haviland Prod.)	DDT* Yellow cuprocide* Sulfur*	5% 6% 30%
HAVILAND DUST NO. 32 Insecticide (Haviland Prod.)	Calcium arsenate* Tribasic copper	10% 13.5%	HAVILAND DUST NO. 44R Insecticide (Haviland Prod.)	TDE	5%
HAVILAND DUST NO. 32D Insecticide (Haviland Prod.)	Calcium arsenate* Zineb	10% 6%	HAVILAND DUST NO. 47 Insecticide (Haviland Prod.)	Piperonyl cyclonene Rotenone	0.50% 0.125%
HAVILAND DUST NO. 32K Insecticide (Haviland Prod.)	Calcium arsenate* Ziram	10% 10%	HAVILAND DUST NO. 50 Insecticide (Haviland Prod.)	DDT	3%
HAVILAND DUST NO. 33 Insecticide (Haviland Prod.)	DDT Tribasic copper*	3% 13.5%	HAVILAND DUST NO. 50R Insecticide (Haviland Prod.)	Rotenone	0.50%

Name & Use Manufacturer	Ingredients	
HAVILAND DUST NO. 60 Insecticide (Haviland Prod.)	Rotenone Yellow cuprocide*	0.75% 6%
HAVILAND DUST NO. 61 Insecticide (Haviland Prod.)	Yellow cuprocide*	6%
HAVILAND DUST NO. 70C Insecticide (Haviland Prod.)	Tribasic copper* Sulfur*	13.5% 30%
HAVILAND DUST NO. 70D Insecticide (Haviland Prod.)	Zineb	6%
HAVILAND DUST NO. 75 Insecticide (Haviland Prod.)	Rotenone	0.75%
HAVILAND DUST NO. 75R Insecticide (Haviland Prod.)	Rotenone	0.75%
HAVILAND DUST NO. 80 Insecticide (Haviland Prod.)	DDT Yellow cuprocide*	3% 6%
HAVILAND DUST NO. 86 Insecticide (Haviland Prod.)	Yellow cuprocide*	6%
HAVILAND DUST NO. 87 Insecticide (Haviland Prod.)	Piperonyl cyclonene Rotenone Pyrethrins	0.50% 0.25% 0.05%
HAVILAND DUST NO. 100R Insecticide (Haviland Prod.)	Rotenone	1%
HAVILAND DUST NO. 156 Insecticide (Haviland Prod.)	Calcium arsenate* Yellow cuprocide	5% 6%
HAVILAND DUST NO. 156C Insecticide (Haviland Prod.)	Calcium arsenate* Tribasic copper	5% 13.5%
HAVILAND DUST NO. 166 Insecticide (Haviland Prod.)	Yellow cuprocide*	6%

Name & Use Manufacturer	Ingredients	
HAVILAND DUST NO. 166C Insecticide (Haviland Prod.)	Tribasic copper*	13.5%
HAVILAND DUST NO. 176 Insecticide (Haviland Prod.)	Calcium arsenate* Yellow cuprocide	10% 6%
HAVILAND DUST NO. 176C Insecticide (Haviland Prod.)	Calcium arsenate* Tribasic copper	10% 13.5%
HAVILAND DUST NO. 235 Insecticide (Haviland Prod.)	DDT* Yellow cuprocide* Sulfur*	5% 6% 30%
HAVILAND DUST NO. 235D Insecticide (Haviland Prod.)	DDT* Zineb	5% 6%
HAVILAND DUST NO. 235DS Insecticide (Haviland Prod.)	DDT* Zineb Sulfur*	5% 6% 30%
HAVILAND DUST NO. 370 Insecticide (Haviland Prod.)	Calcium arsenate*	10%
HAVILAND DUST DS Insecticide (Haviland Prod.)	Zineb Sulfur*	6% 30%
HAVILAND ENAMEL (Chi-Namel)	Titanium dioxide Soya bean oil Resin Drier and mineral spirits*	31.6% 19.5% 12.3% 36.6%
HAVILAND SPRAY NO. 1 Insecticide, fungicide (Haviland Prod.)	DDT* Tribasic copper*	12.5% 66%
HAVILAND SPRAY NO. 4R Insecticide (Haviland Prod.)	Rotenone	4%
HAVILAND SPRAY NO. 5 Fungicide (Haviland Prod.)	Tribasic copper	80%

*Consult Sec. II., Ingredients Index. This ingredient may be responsible for major toxic effects if poisonous amounts of this product are ingested.

Name & Use Manufacturer	Ingredients		Name & Use Manufacturer	Ingredients	
HAVILAND SPRAY NO. 5D Insecticide (Haviland Prod.)	Zineb	100%	HAVILAND SPRAY NO. 21 Insecticide (Haviland Prod.)	DDT Tribasic copper*	12.5% 66%
HAVILAND SPRAY NO. 5L Insecticide (Haviland Prod.)	DDT* in oil	5%	HAVILAND SPRAY NO. 22 Insecticide (Haviland Prod.)	DDT Tribasic copper* Sulfur	6.25% 33% 50%
HAVILAND SPRAY NO. 5LS Insecticide (Haviland Prod.)	DDT* Organic thiocyanates	5% 1%	HAVILAND SPRAY NO. 24 Insecticide (Haviland Prod.)	DDT* Zineb	25% 50%
HAVILAND SPRAY NO. 5R Insecticide (Haviland Prod.)	Rotenone	5%	HAVILAND SPRAY NO. 25 Insecticide (Haviland Prod.)	Zineb	
HAVILAND SPRAY NO. 6 Insecticide (Haviland Prod.)	Pyrethrins Piperonyl cyclonene	0.28% 2.66%	HAVILAND SPRAY NO. 25D Insecticide (Haviland Prod.)	DDT* emulsion conc.	25%
HAVILAND SPRAY NO. 10 Insecticide (Haviland Prod.)	DDT* Zineb	25% 50%	HAVILAND SPRAY NO. 25E Insecticide (Haviland Prod.)	DDT* emulsifiable	25%
HAVILAND SPRAY NO. 12 Insecticide (Haviland Prod.)	DDT Tribasic copper*	12.5% 66.6%	HAVILAND SPRAY NO. 25S Insecticide (Haviland Prod.)	DDT* emulsifiable	25%
HAVILAND SPRAY NO. 14 Insecticide (Haviland Prod.)	Tribasic copper* Sulfur	33% 50%	HAVILAND SPRAY NO. 25D & D14 Insecticide (Haviland Prod.)	DDT* emulsion Nabam*	25%
HAVILAND SPRAY NO. 14D Fungicide (Haviland Prod.)	Nabam*	100%	HAVILAND SPRAY NO. 30 Insecticide (Haviland Prod.)	Tribasic copper Calcium arsenate*	44% 44%
HAVILAND SPRAY NO. 15 Insecticide (Haviland Prod.)	DDT Tribasic copper*	6.25% 33%	HAVILAND SPRAY NO. 30L Insecticide (Haviland Prod.)	DDT* in oil	30%
HAVILAND SPRAY NO. 15P Insecticide (Haviland Prod.)	Pyrethrins Tribasic copper* Piperonyl cyclonene Sulfur	0.09% 28.5% 0.8% 42%	HAVILAND SPRAY NO. 32K Insecticide (Haviland Prod.)	Calcium arsenate* Ziram	66% 33%
HAVILAND SPRAY NO. 19 Insecticide (Haviland Prod.)	DDT Tribasic copper*	12.5% 66%	HAVILAND SPRAY NO. 35 Insecticide (Haviland Prod.)	DDT Tribasic copper*	15% 60%
HAVILAND SPRAY NO. 20 Insecticide (Haviland Prod.)	Tribasic copper Calcium arsenate*	44% 44%			

*Consult Sec. II., Ingredients Index. This ingredient may be responsible for major toxic effects if poisonous amounts of this product are ingested.

- 566 -

Name & Use Manufacturer	Ingredients		Name & Use Manufacturer	Ingredients	
HAVILAND SPRAY NO. 40CE Insecticide (Haviland Prod.)	Chlordane emulsifiable 40%		HAWK SYRUP (Commerce)	Alcohol Chloroform Menthol White pine bark Wild cherry bark Spikenard Balm of Gilead buds Bloodroot Sassafras bark Eucalyptus Tolu	2% 2 m.
HAVILAND SPRAY NO. 45 Insecticide (Haviland Prod.)	DDT Tribasic copper*	15% 60%	HAWLEY'S ANTISEPTIC SOLUTION (Karrer)	Tarola* Phenol Alcohol* Oil lavender Oil ricini	less than 1%
HAVILAND SPRAY NO. 46 Insecticide (Haviland Prod.)	Rotenone Tribasic copper*	2% 40%	HAWLEY'S CORN SALVE (Hawley)		
HAVILAND SPRAY NO. 50W Insecticide (Haviland Prod.)	DDT* wettable	50%	HAYNER'S DEAD-SURE FLY KILLER & INSECTI-CIDE (Hayner)	Petroleum distillate* Tech. chlordane* Pyrethrins	
HAVILAND SPRAY NO. 70P Insecticide (Haviland Prod.)	Pyrethrins Zineb Piperonyl cyclonene	0.21% 25% 2%	HAYR APPLICATION FOR SCALP & HAIR (Hayr)		
HAVILAND SPRAY NO. 78Z Insecticide (Haviland Prod.)	Zineb	100%	HAY'S HAIR COLORING (Kraupner & K.)		
HAVOLINE LUBRICATING GREASE (Indian Ref.)			HAYSMA Respiratory antispasmotic (Haysma)	Acetanilid* Ephedrine HCl* Aspirin* Caffeine	1 gr.
HAWICK AFTER SHAVE LOTION (House of Hawick)			HAZE GRAY PAINT (George, P.D.)		
HAWICK AFTER SHAVE STICK (House of Hawick)			HAZEL BISHOP COMPLEXION GLOW (Bishop, H.)	Liquid solution of dyes	
HAWICK BRUSHLESS SHAVING CREAM (House of Hawick)			HAZEL BISHOP LONG LASTING LIPSTICK (Bishop, H.)	Waxes Solvents Dyes	
HAWICK COLOGNE (House of Hawick)			HAZEL BISHOP NAIL POLISH (Bishop, H.)	Acetone* Nitro-cellulose Coloring matter	
HAWICK DEODORANT (House of Hawick)			H-C HAIR COLOR (Odell)		
			H & C VAGINAL SUPPOSITOR-IES (Horton & Converse)	Ichthyol Boroglyceride Gelatin	5% 5% q.s.

---

*Consult Sec. II., Ingredients Index. This ingredient may be responsible for major toxic effects if poisonous amounts of this product are ingested.

Name & Use Manufacturer	Ingredients		Name & Use Manufacturer	Ingredients	
HD ATMOSPHERE DEODORANT, DISINFEC- TANT & MOP SOLUTION (Haines)			HEATHER CAKE ROUGE (Whitehall)		
H & D INSTANT AIR DEODORANT (Haines)			HEATHER LIQUID CREME ROUGE (Whitehall)		
HEAITOL CARBOLATED OINTMENT (Commerce)	Benzocaine Carbolic acid* Menthol* Thymol* Camphor* Zinc oxide Sulfur * Oils of eucalyptus* Tar Juniper tar* Extract of witch hazel		HEATHER SHAMPOO (House of Ross)	Triethanolamine* Mirapon RK-conc. Dupanol WAT Neroli Tergitol Antaron 125	
			HEAT-REM HEAT RESISTANT PAINT (Speco)	Chrome* Iron Aluminum Copper* Titanium Hydrocarbon vehicle Resins Plasticizers Coal tar solvents*	
HEAITOL RECTAL OINTMENT (Commerce)	Benzocaine Carbolic acid* Menthol* Thymol* Zinc oxide Boric acid* Tannic acid Sulfur Oils of eucalyptus* Tar and juniper tar* Extracts of witch hazel and nutgall		HEAVEN SENT COLOGNE STICK, EAU de TOILETTE, AND PERFUME (Rubinstein)		
			HEAVEN SENT DEODORANT CREAM (Rubinstein)		
HEAL A BURN OINTMENT (Royal Mfg.)	Zinc oxide Benzocaine Carbolic acid	3/4%	HEAVEN SENT SACHET POWDER (Rubinstein)		
HEALITOL For skin (Larkin)	Carbolic acid* Aluminum hydrate Balsam Peru Ichthy-tar Zinc oxide Beeswax Petrolatum base Sassafras oil Thyme oil Eucalyptol*	1%	HEAVY BODIED FLOOR CLEANER (Klean-Strip)		
			HEBOL Fungicide (medical) (Boldt)	Acid salicylic* Acid benzoic* Acetone* Alcohol	37%
HEAPWHITE ENAMEL (Hancock P.&V.)			HECK DEODORANT (Halitosine)		
HEARN'S SALVE For skin burns and irritations (Hearn)	Menthol* Camphor* Oil of sassafras Oil of citronella Oil of pine* Phenol* Distilled extract witch hazel Purified talc. Petrolatum Bismuth subnitrate		HEED DEODORANT (Pharma- Craft)	Aluminum chlorhydroxide complex Aluminum chloride Urea Perfume	
			HEET Rubefacient, (Whitehall)	Alcohol* Capsicum Chloroform Methyl salicylate* Camphor*	53% 85 m./fl.oz.
HEATABS For excessive perspiration (Boyle & Co.)	Each tablet: Sodium chloride Sucrose Thiamine mononitrate Ascorbic acid	7 gr. 3 gr. 0.05 mg. 1.5 mg.	HEL For skin burns and irritations (Ellis, H.G.)	Paraffin Soft petrolatum Liquid petrolatum Cera alba Vanillin Methyl salicylate* Saccharin	
HEAT-COTE ALUMINUM PAINT (Debevoise)					

*Consult Sec. II., Ingredients Index. This ingredient may be responsible for major toxic effects if poisonous amounts of this product are ingested.

Name & Use Manufacturer	Ingredients	Name & Use Manufacturer	Ingredients
HEL Veterinary (Ellis, H.G.)	Paraffin Soft petrolatum Liquid petrolatum Cera alba Vanillin Methyl salicylate* Phenyl salicylate*	HELENA RUBINSTEIN TOILET WATERS (Rubinstein)	
HELENA RUBINSTEIN COLOR SHEEN, GOLD TONE, NATURAL & SILVER TONE (Rubinstein)		HELENA RUBINSTEIN WAKE-UP CREAM (Rubinstein)	
		HELEN AYARS COLOGNES (Ayars)	
HELENA RUBINSTEIN COLOR TINT RINSE (Rubinstein)		HELEN AYARS DA-TONE FOUNDATION (Ayars)	
HELENA RUBINSTEIN COVERTONE (Rubinstein)		HELEN AYARS DEODORANT (Ayars)	
HELENA RUBINSTEIN FACE CREAM (Rubinstein)		HELEN AYARS PERFUME (Ayars)	
HELENA RUBINSTEIN LIPSTICK (Rubinstein)		HELEN AYARS SKIN FRESHNER (Ayars)	
HELENA RUBINSTEIN NAIL POLISH REMOVER (Rubinstein)		HELEN AYARS WATER SOFTENER (Ayars)	
HELENA RUBINSTEIN PERFUME SPRAY DEODORANT (Rubinstein)		HELENE CURTIS COLD WAVE NEUTRAL- IZERS (Curtis, H.)	Bromates* Or Hydrogen peroxide*
HELENA RUBINSTEIN POWDER (Rubinstein)		HELENE CURTIS COLD WAVE SOLUTIONS (Curtis, H.)	Thioglycollic acid* (pH 9.4)
HELENA RUBINSTEIN ROUGE (Rubinstein)		HELENE CURTIS LANOLIN DISCOVERY HAIR CON- DITIONER (Curtis, H.)	Lanolin
HELENA RUBINSTEIN SILK-SCREEN FOR DRY SKIN (Rubinstein)		HELENE CURTIS SHAMPOOS (Curtis, H.)	Sodium or triethanolamine salts of lauryl alcohol sulfate
HELENA RUBINSTEIN SKIN LOTIONS (Rubinstein)		HELENE CURTIS SPRAY NET (Curtis, H.)	Esters of abietic acid (bleached shellac acids)
HELENA RUBINSTEIN SUN & WINDPROOF CREAM (Rubinstein)		HELEN NEUSHAFER NAIL POLISHES, REMOVERS AND FOUNDATIONS (Neushafer)	

*Consult Sec. II., Ingredients Index. This ingredient may be responsible for major toxic effects if poisonous amounts of this product are ingested.

Name & Use Manufacturer	Ingredients	Name & Use Manufacturer	Ingredients
HELIO COLOGNE, PERFUME, AND TOILET WATER (Caswell-Massey)		HELPALAK 1 Laxative (Hepa)	Extract of cascara sagrada Extract of podophyllum Magnesium sulfate Bile salts compound Extract of senna Myrtillin Extract of malt Extract of alfalfa Extract of spinach Sodium benzoate Glycerin Saccharin
HELICO HAIR LACQUER (Caswell-Massey)			
HELLWIG ALUMINUM PAINT (Hellwig)	Aluminum paste Lacquers	HEMATONE B Dietary supplement with iron (Chicago Pharm.)	Each oz.: Strychnine hypophosphite* 0.027 gr. Nux vomica* tincture 1.328 m. Hypophosphites of sodium calcium, manganese Ferrous gluconate Calcium hypophosphate Potassium citrate Hypophosphorus acid Berberine sulfate* Phosphates Sulfates Chlorides of potassium & sodium Vitamin B_1 2.25 mg.
HELLWIG GAS & OIL LINE COMPOUND (Hellwig)	Denatured alcohol* Powdered graphite Black strap		
HELLWIG GRAPHITE RUST REMOVER (Hellwig)	Gas* Crude oil* Kerosene* Blending oils		
		HEMCAPS For hemorrhoids (Marlo)	Yellow dock Horse chestnut Witch hazel Stoneroot
HELMINEX MINOR ELEMENT DRENCH LIQUID (Veterinary) (Florida Chem.)	Each fl. oz.: Phenothiazine 0.25 gm. Copper 0.0019% Iron elemental 0.0121 Cobalt elemental 0.0008 Manganese elemental 0.0072 Zinc elemental 0.0014 Boron elemental 0.0013 Bentonite 5.0000	HEMEX RECTAL OINTMENT For hemorrhoids (Vogarell)	Benzocaine Zinc oxide Boric acid* Bismuth subgallate Resorcin*
		HEMOLATE Dietary supplement with iron (Approved)	Each capsule: Ferrous sulfate (dried) U.S.P. 2-1/10 gr. Liver concentrate 3 gr. Thiamine hydrochloride U.S.P. 333 units
HELMINEX PHENOTHI-AZINE DRENCH (Veterinary) (Florida Chem.)	Each fl. oz.: Phenothiazine* 12 gm. Bentonite 5%		
		HEM-O-RAL For hemorrhoids (oral preparation) (Surf)	Sulfur Oil of peppermint Ext. hamamelis Mineral oil U.S.P.
HELMINEX WETTABLE POWDER (Veterinary) (Florida Chem.)	Phenothiazine* 99% Wetting agent 1%		
		HEMORR-AID For hemorrhoids (Hemorr-Aid)	Copper sulfate* Calcium chloride Iron citrate Sodium chloride Zinc sulfate* Potassium alum sulfate
HELM'S ALL-PURPOSE CREAM (Helm Goat)	Gum tragacanth Bay rum Boric acid Powdered soap Borax Glyco stearate Mineral oil Sodium benzoate Powdered goat's milk Perfume		
		HENASPHEN PULVOID (Green) Analgesic, antipyretic (Drug Prod., N.Y.)	Acetophenetidin* 0.13 gm. Powd. ext. hyoscyamus* 11 mg. Total hyoscyamus alkaloids 0.01 mg. Aspirin* 0.13 gm. Caffeine alkaloid 16 mg. Powd. ext. gelsemium 2.2 mg.
HELPALAX 0, 2,3 Laxative (Hepa)	Extract of podophyllum Extract of cascara sagrada Magnesium sulfate Extract of senna Bile salts compound Extract of malt Extract of alfalfa Extract of spinach Sodium benzoate Glycerin Saccharin	HENLAN HAIR TRAINER (Henlan)	Gum tragacanth Gum karaya Sodium borate Sonoquol Perfume Methyl parasept Propyl parasept Glycerin Tween

*Consult Sec. II., Ingredients Index. This ingredient may be responsible for major toxic effects if poisonous amounts of this product are ingested.

Name & Use Manufacturer	Ingredients	Name & Use Manufacturer	Ingredients
HENNEN'S FOOT POWDER (Hennen)		HEP AEROSOL INSECT KILLER (Bostwick)	Methoxychlor, tech. 1.0% Allethrin* 0.10% n-Octyl bicycloheptene dicarb- oximide 0.166% Isobornyl thiocyano acetate 0.82% Related terpenes 0.18% DDT 3.00% Petroleum distillate 5.434% Methylated naphthalene* 9.30%
HENNEN'S LIQUID DENTIFRICE (Hennen)			
HENNEN'S LOTIONS (Hennen)			
HENNEN'S MOUTH RINSE (Hennen)		HEPTAGRAN 2-1/2 Insecticide (Chipman Chem.)	Heptachlor* 2.50% Related compounds 0.97%
HENRI BENDEL BABY OIL, BATH OILS (Bendel)		HEPTAGRAN 20 Insecticide (Chipman Chem.)	Heptachlor* 20% Related compounds 7.8%
HENRI BENDEL BRILLIAN-TINE (Bendel)		HEPTOX EC-24 Insecticide (Arizona)	Heptachlor* 24.00% Related compounds 9.50% Petroleum hydrocarbons* 61.50%
HENRI BENDEL BRUSHLESS SHAVING CREAM (Bendel)		HEP 2-5 For intestinal and liver irritation (veterinary) (Corn King)	2-Amino-5-nitrothiazole* 47.5%
HENRI BENDEL LAUNDEL Laundering preparation (Bendel)		HERBAL SKIN LOTION (Rubinstein)	
		HERBATE AMINE 20 Herbicide (Chipman Ltd.)	Dimethyl amine salt of 2,4-D* 12% 2,4-D acid equiv. 20 oz./imp. gal.
HENRI BENDEL LOTIONS, ASTRINGENT, TOILET WATERS, AND PERFUME (Bendel)		HERBATE AMINE 80 Herbicide (Chipman Ltd.)	Dimethylamine salt of 2,4-D acid* 2,4-D acid equiv. 80 oz./imp. gal.
		HERBATE ESTER 64 Herbicide (Chipman Ltd.)	Mixed ester formulation of iso-butyl ester and normal butyl ester of 2,4-D acid* 2,4-D acid equiv. 64 oz./imp. gal.
HENRI BENDEL SHOE CREAM (Bendel)		HERBATE ESTER 76 Herbicide (Chipman Ltd.)	Iso-octyl ester of 2,4-D acid* 2,4-D acid equiv. 76 oz./imp.gal.
HEN-ROIB TABLETS (Leonhardt)	Aloin Podophyllin Henbane Stillingia Witch hazel Turpentine*, Atropine sulfate* Oleoresin capsicum Horse chestnut Stoneroot	HERBATE ESTER 96 Herbicide (Chipman Ltd.)	Mixed ester formulation of iso-butyl ester and normal butyl ester of 2,4-D acid* 2,4-D acid equiv. 96 oz./imp. gal.
HENRY ROSENFELD SPRAY DEODORANT (Rosenfeld)		HERB DOCTOR COMPOUND Laxative (McKewen)	Alcohol 16% Senna Frangula Bitter orange peel Sarsaparilla Aloin* F.E. cascara Gentian* Licorice
HENTZEN'S ENAMELS (Wisconsin Paint)		HERBEX G.O.S. SHAMPOO (Parker Herbex)	Glycerinated soap solution

*Consult Sec. II., Ingredients Index. This ingredient may be responsible for major toxic effects if poisonous amounts of this product are ingested.

Name & Use Manufacturer	Ingredients	Name & Use Manufacturer	Ingredients
HERBEX HAIR CONDITIONER NO. 3 (Parker Herbex)	Glycerin Sulfonated castor oil* Chloral hydrate (deriv. of chloral) 0.221 gm./fl.oz. Alcohol 0.03%/v	HERCULES INK RE-MOVER (Kohnstamm)	Alcohol Potassium oleate Oil of mirbane*
HERBEX HAIR & SCALP FRESHENER NO. 1 (Parker Herbex)	Alcohol 14.76%/v Mullein ext. Jaborandi ext. Stoneroot ext. Figwort herb ext. Soap bark ext.	HERCULES TOXAPHENE Insecticide (Hercules)	Chlorinated camphene* containing 67-69% chlorine
		HEREFORD CRESYLIC OINTMENT (Swamp)	Wood creosote 0.374% Wood rosin U.S.P. 0.219% Raw cottonseed oil 0.129% Sodium hydroxide 0.074%
HERBEX HAIR & SCALP FRESHENER NO. 2 (Parker Herbex)	Alcohol 14.76%/v Nux vomica ext. 0.008 gm./fl.oz. Strychnine* alkaloid 0.6 mg./fl.oz. Colocynth ext. Capsicum* ext.	HERE'S HOUR AFTER SHAVE LOTION AND COLOGNE (House of Guorielli)	
HERBEX HAIR SOFTENER (Parker Herbex)	Turkey red oil Sodium carbonate Glycerin	HERMESOL External germicide, fungicide (Kahlenberg)	Colloidal mercury bioleate* 2.5%
HERBEX SHAMPOO (Parker Herbex)	Mild soap solution	HERO FIRE EXTIN-GUISHER (Bostwich)	Carbon tetrachloride* Carbon dioxide
HERBEX S.P. PINK OINTMENT For dandruff (Parker Herbex)	Thymol* Sulfur* Salicylic acid*	HERPICIDE HAIR TONIC (Herpicide)	
HERBEX S.P. YELLOW OINTMENT Hairdressing, conditioner (Parker Herbex)	Sulfur* Salicylic acid* CP glycerin Petroleum base	HERP'S CALA-DERM SKIN LOTION (Herp)	
		HERP'S SUN TAN LOTIONS (Herp)	
HERBEX TRIPLE X Hair conditioner (Parker Herbex)	Chloral hydrate (deriv. of chloral) 0.11 gm./fl.oz. Alcohol 36.64%/v Jaborandi ext. Colocynth ext. Capsicum ext. Mullein ext. Glycerin	HERSHEY'S SOAP FLAKES (Hershey)	
		HERSHEY SOAP (Hershey)	Cocoa butter Coconut oil Caustic soda
		HERSHKOWITZ CHALKS (Hershkowitz)	
HERBEX WHITE OINTMENT Hairdressing (Parker Herbex)	Beeswax Ceresin Cetyl alcohol	HERSHKOWITZ CRAYONS (Hershkowitz)	
		HE-SHE Antiseptic vaginal suppositories (Helm)	Oxyquinoline benzoate Acidum boricum* Acidum salicylicum* Oil of theobroma
HERB FARM SPRAYMIST DEODORANT (Herb Farm)			
HERB FARM TOILET WATERS, PERFUMES, ASTRINGENT LOTIONS (Herb Farm)		HESKOR OINTMENT-CRAFT For skin irritation (Bullock-Walker)	Resorcinol* 8% Zinc oxide Balsam Peru Bismuth subnitrate Oil of cade
HERBOLD LOTION (Herbold)		HESPERIDIN WITH C CAPSULES (West-Ward)	Each capsule: Hesperidin 100 mg. Ascorbic acid 100 mg.

*Consult Sec. II., Ingredients Index. This ingredient may be responsible for major toxic effects if poisonous amounts of this product are ingested.

Name & Use Manufacturer	Ingredients	Name & Use Manufacturer	Ingredients
DR. HESS BENZENE HEXACHLORIDE WETTABLE 12% GAMMA ISOMER Insecticide (Hess, Dr.)	Gamma isomer of benzene hexachloride* 12% Other isomers of benzene hexachloride* 63%	DR. HESS POULTRY INHALANT (Hess, Dr.)	Pine oil Oil of eucalyptus* Oil of camphor* Guaiacol Beachwood creosote* Castor oil soap
DR. HESS CADMIUM HOG WORMER (Hess, Dr.)	Cadmium anthranilate 4.4%	DR. HESS POWDERED LOUSE KILLER (Hess, Dr.)	Rotenone 0.5% Other cube extractives 1.0%
DR. HESS CATTLE GRUB KILLER (Hess, Dr.)	Rotenone 1.5% Other cube extractives 3.0%	HESSPRAY NEW OIL TYPE FOR LIVESTOCK Insecticide (Hess, Dr.)	Petroleum distillate* 99.11% Pine oil 0.56% Tech. piperonyl butoxide 0.30% Pyrethrins 0.03%
DR. HESS CHICK & POULTRY TABLETS (Hess, Dr.)	Borax* 35.6% Boric acid* 34.2% Potassium permanganate* 16.0%	DR. HESS PTZ DRENCH Anthelmentic (veterinary) (Hess, Dr.)	Each fl. oz.: Phenothiazine (drench grade) 12.5 gm. Lead arsenate* (spray grade) 0.5 gm.
DR. HESS CORYZA TABLETS Poultry remedy (Hess, Dr.)	Each tablet: Sodium sulfathiazole* 30 gr.	DR. HESS PTZ PASTURE MIX (Hess, Dr.)	Salt Defluorinated phosphate Phenothiazine Bone black Molasses Copper sulfate 0.20% Cobalt carbonate Potassium iodide
HESS DANDRUFF REMOVER SHAMPOO (Hess Hair)	Alcohol* 47% Coconut oil soap Color Perfume		
DR. HESS 50% DDT WETTABLE POWDER Insecticide (Hess, Dr.)	DDT 50%	DR. HESS PTZ PELLETS WITH LEAD ARSENATE (veterinary) (Hess, Dr.)	Each pellet: Phenothiazine (drench grade) 7.5 gm. Lead arsenate* (spray grade) 0.3 gm.
DR. HESS DIP & DISINFECTANT (Hess, Dr.)	Coal tar phenols* (tar acids) 16% Neutral coal tar oils* 52% Anhydrous soap 22%	DR. HESS PTZ POWDER (veterinary) (Hess, Dr.)	Phenothiazine* 98% Phenothiazine deriv. 1.10% Lauryl alcohol 0.50% Polyvinyl alcohol 0.35% Coumarin 0.05%
HESS HAIRMILK Hair preparation (Hess Hair)	Alcohol 25% Lead* Glycerin Sulfur Perfume	DR. HESS ROOST PAINT SIX MITE SPRAY Insecticide (Hess, Dr.)	Mineral oil 97% Gamma isomer of benzene hexachloride 1% Other isomers of benzene hexachloride 2%
HESS HAIR-KREAM Hair dressing (Hess Hair)	Lanolin Mineral oil Glyco B Perfume	DR. HESS SCREW-WORM KILLER (Liquid) (Hess, Dr.)	Benzol* 53% Diphenylamine 35%
DR. HESS HOUSE SPRAY Insecticide (Hess, Dr.)	Petroleum distillate* 99.72% Tech. piperonyl butoxide 0.25% Pyrethrins 0.03%	DR. HESS SCREW-WORM SMEAR EQ 335 (Hess, Dr.)	Gamma isomer of benzene hexachloride* (from lindane) 3% Pine oil* 35%
HESSKLOR EMULSIFIABLE CHLORDANE Insecticide (Hess, Dr.)	Tech. chlordane * 45% Aliphatic petroleum hydrocarbons* 45%	DR.HESS SKP For scours (veterinary) (Hess, Dr.)	Isopropyl alcohol 2.5% Kaolin Pectin Sulfathiazole Ox bile
DR. HESS MEDICATED POWDER (veterinary) (Hess, Dr.)	Talc Boric acid Zinc oxide Alum Magnesium carbonate Copper sulfate	DR. HESS SQX Insecticide (Hess, Dr.)	Sodium sulfaquinoxaline 11.0%

*Consult Sec. II., Ingredients Index. This ingredient may be responsible for major toxic effects if poisonous amounts of this product are ingested.

Name & Use Manufacturer	Ingredients	Name & Use Manufacturer	Ingredients
DR. HESS STOCK SPRAY (Concentrated) Insecticide (Hess, Dr.)	Isobornyl thiocyanoacetate* 41.0% Other active terpenes 9.0% Methoxychlor 6.5%	HEX-ANE For liver flukes (veterinary) (Texas Pheno.)	Hexachloroethane* 40.94%
DR. HESS UDDER OINTMENT (Hess, Dr.)	Petrolatum Lanolin Camphor* Methyl salicylate* Eucalyptus oil* Oxyquinoline benzoate	HEXASOL Cathartic (Bell Chem. Co., Inc.)	Sodium phosphate Sodium bicarbonate Sodium chloride Sodium sulfate Tartaric acid Saccharin
DR. HESS WATER SOLUBLE RAT & MOUSE KILLER (Hess, Dr.)	Sodium salt of 2-pivalyl-1, 3-indandione 0.14%	HEXA-TETRA-TOX Insecticide, fungicide (Hanna)	TEPP (tetraethyl pyrophosphate)*
DR. HESS WEED KILLER (Hess, Dr.)	2,4-D alkanolamine salts* 22.75%	HEXOL GERMICIDE (Hexol)	Steam distilled white pine oil* 70% Neutral soap 12-14%
HESS WITCH HAZEL CREAM (Hess, E.E.)		HEXOLIN Antiseptic lotion (La Crosse)	Hexachlorophene 1% Lanolin Xerol "B" borax* Mineral oil
HEX Cleaner (Pioneer)		HEXON Insecticide (Whitmoyer)	Petroleum oils Xylene* Gamma isomer of benzene hexachloride* (from lindane)
HEXADOW DUST CONCENTRATE Insecticide (Dow)	Gamma isomer of BHC*10% Other isomers* 53%	HEXORAL H & C Antiseptic (Horton & Converse)	Glycerin-aqueous solution of hexylresorcinol U.S.P. 1-1000 (0.1%)
HEXADOW-WETTABLE Insecticide (Dow)	Gamma isomer of benzene hexachloride* 10%/w	HEX-PHEN Fungicide, antiseptic, (medical) (Russell, A.)	Dichlorophene Hydroalcoholic base of natural balsamic resins Ethyl alcohol 15% Isopropyl alcohol* 65%
HEXADOW WETTABLE POWDER Insecticide (Dow)	Gamma isomer of BHC*10% Other isomers 53%	HEXYLTAN JELLY For skin burns (Sharp & Dohme)	Hexylresorcinol 0.1% Tannic acid 5% Water soluble jelly base
HEX-A-FLUKE For liver flukes (veterinary) (Franklin, O. M.)	Hexachloroethane* 38.4% Bentonite and water 61.6%	H. & H. CLEANERS (H. and H.)	
		H.H. INK ERADICATOR (Collins-Benton)	Solution #1: Pine liquid* Fruit citrate Solution #2: Sodium hydroxide Chlorine*
HEXA-GLO CATTLE DRENCH For liver flukes (Globe)	Hexachloroethane* 36.78%		
		H.H.H., TOMLINSON'S LINIMENT (Aschenbach)	
HEXAGUM (Tailby-Nason)	Each tablet: Lymiodin (iodized lime containing 15% total iodine)* 1/3 gr. Paraform 1/20 gr. Benzocaine 1/8 gr. Extract gelsemium 1/20 gr. Menthol Red gum Oil anise	HI-A-LIN VARNISHES (Reliance Varnish)	
		HIAWATHA PAINTS (Chicago Paints)	
HEXAMO Spotting compound (Riverside)		HI-BALL PAINTS (Walker, Norris)	

*Consult Sec. II., Ingredients Index. This ingredient may be responsible for major toxic effects if poisonous amounts of this product are ingested.

Name & Use Manufacturer	Ingredients	Name & Use Manufacturer	Ingredients
HI-CURL HAIR LACQUER Hair preparation (Nestle-Le Mur)		HIKE Antiseptic (Hike)	Phenol* (carbolic acid) Boric acid* Menthol* Camphor* Oil of thyme Glycerin Alcohol 4%
HIDE-IT DUO CREAM Make-up base (Clark-Millner)		HI-KO Disinfectant, deodorant (Hillyard Chem.)	Sodium hypochlorite* 3.6%
HIDE-KOTE Semi Paste Paint (Kurfees)		HIL-BRITE Soap and wax (Hillyard Chem.)	
HIDES-ALL-PAINT (Preservative)	.	HILCO CLEANER Powdered cleaner (Hillyard Chem.)	Alkali*
HIDE-X Skin conditioner (veterinary) (Lehman Bros.)	Mineral oil Lanolin	HILCO CLEANING COMPOUND (Hill Mfg. Co.)	
HIDE-X PINE OIL DEODORIZING DISINFECTANT (Lehman Bros.)	Steam distilled pine oil* 80% Soap 10%	HILCO LUSTRE Floor preparation (Hillyard Chem.)	
HIDEX WALL PAINT (Watson-Standard)		HIL-CRETE THINNER (Hillyard Chem.)	Organic solvent
HIE PIN CURL HOME PERMANENT (L. & S.)		HILD BRAND FLOOR WAX (Hild)	
HIGGINS AMERICAN DRAWING INKS (Higgins Ink)		HILD RUG & UPHOLSTERY SHAMPOO (Hild)	
HIGGINS PASTES (Higgins Ink)		HILEX HEAVY DUTY DRY BLEACH (Hilex)	Dichlorodimethyl hydantoin* 9% Avail. chlorine 5.25%/w
HIGGINS WRITING INK (Higgins Ink)		HILEX KROMA X FINE FABRICS BLEACH (Hilex)	Sodium perborate*
HIGH FLASH PRIMER (Dampney)	Zinc chromate* Diatomaceous earth Butanol* Naphtha* Phosphoric acid Polyvinyl butyral	HILEX LIQUID BLEACH (Hilex)	Sodium hypochlorite* 5.25%
HIGHLIGHTS HAIRINSE (Ogilvie)		HIL-FINISH Floor finish (Hillyard Chem.)	Organic solvents
HIGH STANDARD VARNISHES (Thresher)		HIL-GLO Wood finish (Hillyard Chem.)	
HI-GLO ENAMELS AND LACQUERS (Western States)			

*Consult Sec. II., Ingredients Index. This ingredient may be responsible for major toxic effects if poisonous amounts of this product are ingested.

Name & Use Manufacturer	Ingredients		Name & Use Manufacturer	Ingredients	
HI-LITE (Simoniz)			HILLSHIRE DOWN PURE OIL (Perfumed) (Hillshire)		
HI-LITE WHITE PAINT (Kuhn Paint)			HILLSHIRE DOWN QUINCY HAND LOTION (Hillshire)	Quince Glycerin Rose water	
HIL-KOTE Liquid wax (Hillyard Chem.)	Stoddard solvent*		HILLSHIRE DOWN SPECIAL LOTION FOR SENSITIVE SKIN (Hillshire)	Goat's milk whey Thymol	
HILLMAN'S D COMPOUND Antispasmodic analgesic (Hillman)	Ephedrine hydrochloride* Acetylsalicylic acid* Caffeine citrate Oil of peppermint Lactose				
HILL R-S LOTION NO. 1 Drying antiseptic (Hill Labs. (Fla.))	Resorcin* 4% Sulfur 8% Zinc oxide 20%		HILLTOP FINISHED VAPO-MOR SPRAY Respiratory decongestant (veterinary, avian) (Hilltop)	Camphor* Guaiacol Cresol* Formaldehyde* Mineral oil Methyl salicylate* Oil of eucalyptus* Oil of anise Deodorized kerosene	
HILL'S CASCARA QUININE COLD TABLETS (Whitehall)	Acetophenetidin* 2 gr. Cascara sagrada Quinine sulfate Aloin Aspirin* Ephedrine sulfate		HILLTOP K-M Antiseptic for drinking water (veterinary) (Hilltop)	Alkyl toly methyl trimethyl ammonium chloride* (quaternary amm. compound*) 3.3% Sodium sulfate (Glauber's salts) Potassium acetate Magnesium sulfate (Epsom salts) Potassium chlorate*	
HILL'S HAIR DYE (Century)					
HILLSHIRE DOWN AFTER SHAVE LOTION (Hillshire)	Whey of goat's milk Witch hazel		HILLTOP MOR-EEN POWDER Anthelmintic (veterinary, avian) (Hilltop)	Phenothiazine 25% Copper sulfate* 20% Nicotine sulfate* 1% Kamala Tobacco powder Nux vomica* 9% Guaiacol Iron sulfate Capsicum Areca nut Iron oxide Sulfur Oil of anise Mineral oil	
HILLSHIRE DOWN CASTILE SHAMPOO (Hillshire)	Soap Olive oil Vegetable oils				
HILLSHIRE DOWN CLEANSING CREAM (Hillshire)	Curds of goat's milk Lanolin Mineral oil				
HILLSHIRE DOWN FOUNDATION CREAM, SPECIAL CREAM FOR SENSITIVE SKIN (Hillshire)	Curds of goat's milk Zinc-oxide Lanolin Petrolatum		HILLTOP SODIUM FLUORIDE (Tinted) Vermifuge (veterinary) (Hilltop)	Sodium fluoride* 95.5% Sodium silicofluoride 1.5%	
HILLSHIRE DOWN KOMPLEX MASK Cosmetic (Hillshire)	Mercurized wax*		HILLTOP VAPOR SPRAY CONCEN-TRATE For respiratory ailments (veterinary) (Hilltop)	Methyl phenol* Methyl salicylate* Oil of camphor* Mineral oil	
HILLSHIRE DOWN M B OIL Hair conditioner (Hillshire)	Castor oil Olive oil		HILLYARD'S ASPHALT TILE SEALER (Hillyard Chem.)	Alcohol*	
HILLSHIRE DOWN MILK BATH (Hillshire)	Dehydrated goat's milk				

*Consult Sec. II., Ingredients Index. This ingredient may be responsible for major toxic effects if poisonous amounts of this product are ingested.

Name & Use Manufacturer	Ingredients		Name & Use Manufacturer	Ingredients	
HILLYARD'S BKL VARNISH REMOVER (Hillyard Chem.)			HILLYARD'S PINE DISINFECTANT DEODORIZER (Hillyard Chem.)	Pine oil* soap	90%
HILLYARD'S CAUSTIC CHEMICAL Disinfectant, germicide (Hillyard Chem.)	Sodium hydroxide*		HILLYARD'S RUG SHAMPOO, PINE CLEANER (Hillyard Chem.)	Soap	
HILLYARD'S DANCE SPANGLES Floor finish (crystals) (Hillyard Chem.)	Alkali*		HILLYARD'S SAN-O-FECT Disinfectant, fungicide (Hillyard Chem.)	Sodium orthophenyl phenate* Soap	15% 2.5%
HILLYARD'S DISHWASHING AND BOILER COMPOUNDS; WATER SOFT-ENER; PORCELAIN, RUBBER AND DAIRY CLEANERS (Hillyard Chem.)	Alkali*		HILLYARD'S SODIUM HYPOCHLOR-ITE SOLUTION Disinfectant, deodorant (Hillyard Chem.)	Sodium hypochlorite	3.6%
HILLYARD'S SODIUM HYPO-CHLORITE SOLUTION Disinfectant, deodorant (Hillyard Chem.)	Sodium hypochlorite 3.6%		HILLYARD'S SPECIAL SOLVENT #8564 (Hillyard Chem.)	Organic solvents	
HILLYARD'S #784 FLOOR POLISH (Hillyard Chem.)	Soap Wax		HILLYARD'S WAXES, POLISHES, SEALERS, AND DRESSINGS FOR FLOORS AND FURNITURE (Hillyard Chem.)	Stoddard solvent* (or other organic solvents)	
HILLYARD'S H-101 Germicide, disinfectant, antiseptic (Hillyard Chem.)	Para di-isobutyl phenoxy ethoxy ethyl di-methyl benzyl ammonium chloride 2.5%		HIL-MIST FLOOR DRESSING Polish (Hillyard Chem.)	Organic solvents*	
HILLYARD'S I-KLENZE; POWDERED BOWL CLEANER; FORMULA NO. 777 (Hillyard Chem.)	Acid*		HILO DIP For fleas, lice in dogs (Hilo)	Rotenone Other cube resins Pine oil* Triethanolamine oleate Sulfonated castor oil	1% 2% 71% 9% 5%
HILLYARD'S INSECTI-ANNI POWDER Insecticide (Hillyard Chem.)	Petroleum distillate pyrethrins 3.3% Pyrethrum flowers other than pyrethins 96.7%		HILO DOG SPRAY Insecticide (Hilo)	Pyrethrins Cube ext. Petroleum dist. Rotenone Tech. piperonyl cyclonene Ethyl alcohol Butoxy polypropylene glycol	0.025% 0.236% 0.102% 0.128% 0.256% 24.253% 15.000%
HILLYARD'S KURL-OFF Remover (Hillyard Chem.)	Chlorinated hydrocarbon		HILO DRY BATH Flea exterminator (Hilo)	Piperonyl butoxide Pyrethrins*	

*Consult Sec. II., Ingredients Index. This ingredient may be responsible for major toxic effects if poisonous amounts of this product are ingested.

Name & Use Manufacturer	Ingredients		Name & Use Manufacturer	Ingredients	
HILO FLEA & FUNGUS POWDER (Hilo)	Rotenone Other cube resins Dichlorophene Hexachlorophene	1.2% 2.4% 0.5% 0.5%	HINKLE'S TABLETS Laxative (McKesson)	Extract of belladonna* leaf 0.008 gm. Podaphyllin Aloin* Ext. of cascara sagrada Oleoresin of ginger	
HILO KILTIX Tick exterminator (Hilo)	Tech. chlordane Gamma isomer of benzene hexachloride Pine oil* Petroleum distillate*	8% 1% 20% 51%	HINKLE'S TABLETS Laxative (Purepac)		

HILO OINTMENT For skin irritations (veterinary) (Hilo)	Petrolatum
	Mineral oil
	Derris resins
	Lanolin
	Camphor oil*
			"H" INSECT BOMB (Airsol Co.)	Petroleum distillates* 71.138%
				Tech. chlordane "1068" 3.000%
				Beta butoxy beta' thiocyano
				  diethyl ether 0.500%
				Allethrin (allyl homolog of
				  cinerin 1) 0.040%
				Pyrethrins 0.006%
				n-Octyl bicycloheptene dicarbox-
				  imide 0.200%
				Iso-octylphenoxypolyethoxy-
				  ethanol (Triton) 0.100%
				Phenyl mercuric lactate
				   0.016%	

HILO ROTENONE FLEA POWDER (Hilo)	Rotenone	1.20%			
HILO TICK & FLEA SPRAY (Hilo)	Tech. chlordane Petroleum distillate*	2% 98%	HINZE AMBROSIA AFTER SHAVE LOTION (Hinze)		
HILO TICK OINTMENT (Hilo)	Tech. chlordane	2%	DR. HIRSCH HAIR COLORING (Assoc. Brands)		
HILO TICK POWDER (Hilo)	Tech. chlordane Gamma isomer of benzene hexachloride	1.0% 0.5%	DR. HIRSCH HAIR PREPARATIONS (Assoc. Brands)		
HIL-SWEEP (Improved) Mop cleaner (Hillyard Chem.)	Organic solvents		HIRSUTUS (Barker, W.J.)	Sage Tansy Celandine Alcohol 35% Diethyl phthalate approx. 2-1/2%	
HIL-TEX Masonry seal (Hillyard Chem.)			"HIS" AFTER SHAVE LOTIONS (House for Men)		

HIL-TONE Floor wax (Hillyard Chem.)			HISDRIN TABLETS Antihistamine (Massengill)	Each tablet:
				Semikon hydrochloride (Metha-
				  pyrilene hydrochloride*)
				   50 mg.
				Semoxydrine hydrochloride
				  (methamphetamine hydro-
				  chloride) 2.5 mg.	

HIMROD'S POWDER Bronchial antispasmodic (Himrod)	Stramonium* (alkaloids total 0.185%) Saltpetre* Anise oil Cedar oil				
HINDERCORN SALVE (Hiscox)			HI-SEAS MARINE PAINTS (Yoder)		
HIND'S HONEY & ALMOND CREAM (Lehn & Fink)			HI-SPEED DRY CLEANING COMPOUND (Dural)		
HINKLE'S HANDY EASTER EGG COLORS (Hinkle)					
HINKLE'S PILLS N.F. Laxative (Massengill)	Each pill: Ext. belladonna* Aloin Oleoresin ginger Ext. cascara sagrada Podophyllum resin Glycyrrhiza	1/8 gr. 1/4 gr. 1/16 gr. 1/4 gr. 1/6 gr. 1/6 gr.	HISTACOMP Antihistaminic, analgesic (Approved)	Each tablet: Pyranisamine maleate 25 mg. Acetylsalicylic acid* 3-1/2 gr. Phenacetin* 2-1/2 gr. Caffeine alkaloid 1/2 gr.	

*Consult Sec. II., Ingredients Index. This ingredient may be responsible for major toxic effects if poisonous amounts of this product are ingested.

Name & Use Manufacturer	Ingredients	Name & Use Manufacturer	Ingredients
HISTACOMP SYRUP Anti-histaminic (Approved)	Each fl. oz.: Thenylpyramine hydrochloride 80 mg. Sodium citrate Ammonium chloride Antimony potassium tartrate 1/24 gr. Menthol Aromatics	HISTAPRIN COUGH SYRUP Antihistamine (Pharmex)	Pyrilamine maleate* Ammonium chloride Sodium citrate Antimony potassium tartrate* Menthol* Aromatics Alcohol
HISTA-GUAIATONE COUGH SYRUP Antitussive (Horton & Converse)	Pyrilamine maleate* 10 mg. Sodium monobenzyl succinate 80 mg. Potassium guaiacol sulfonate 80 mg. Ammonium chloride 80 mg. Antimony and potassium tartrate* 1 mg. Chloroform 20 mg. Menthol 1 mg. Dextrose, sucrose and propylene glycol 8%	HISTAPYRAN COMPOUND Antihistamine (Horton & Converse)	Histapyran 25 mg. Aspirin* 0.23 gm. Phenacetin* 0.16 gm. Caffeine alk. 30 mg.
		HISTAPYRAN H & C Antihistamine (Horton & Converse)	Pyrilamine maleate (n-p-methoxybenzyl-n-n'-dimethyl-n-a-pyridyl ethylene amine maleate)* 25 mg.
HISTA-KOL Antihistamine colds (Allied Drug)	Each tablet: Pyrilamine maleate* 25 mg.	HISTEEN TABLETS Antihistamine, colds, hay fever (Kenton)	Each tablet: Acetophenetidin* 1 gr. Racephedrine sulfate* Aspirin* Camphor monobromated*
HISTALON Antihistamine, colds, hay fever (Hance)	Each tablet: Pyranisamine maleate* (n-p-methoxybenzyl-n,n'-dimethyl-n-a,-pyridyl-ethylene-diamine maleate) 25 mg.	HISTOBALM Antihistamine lotion (Carroll Chem.)	Pyrilamine maleate 3/4% Calamine Camphor* Menthol* Alcohol 1-1/2%
HISTANA Antihistamine (Approved)	Each tablet: Pyranisamine maleate* 25 mg.	HIST-O-PLUS Antihistamine, analgesic (Anahist)	Thonzylamine hydrochloride 25 mg. Aspirin* 2.5 gr. Phenacetin* 2.5 gr. Caffeine 0.5 gr.
HISTA NEPHRIN Nasal antihistaminic decongestant (Approved)	Phenylephrine HCl U.S.P. 1/2 % Thenylpyramine HCl 0.25% Benzalkonium chloride 1-5000	HISTOSEP-S For enterohepatitis (veterinary, avian) (Whitmoyer)	2-Amino-5-nitrothiazole* 45%
HISTA-PAC Antihistamine, analgesic, colds (Hance)	Each tablet: Pyranisamine maleate* 25 mg. Salicylamide* 1-1/2 gr. Acetophenetidin* 2-1/2 gr. Caffeine 1/2 gr.	HISTOSTAT For blackhead infection (veterinary, avian) (Salsbury's)	4-Nitrophenylarsenic acid* 25%
HISTAPACO TABLETS Antihistamine, colds (Horton & Converse)	Histapyran (pyrilamine maleate)* Phenacetin 0.12 gm. Aspirin* 0.2 gm. Caffeine alkaloid 30 mg. Quinine sulfate 30 mg.	HI-TONE PAINTS (Gates Paint)	
HISTAPHEN CAPSULES AND TABLETS (Chase Chem.)	Each capsule or tablet: Pyranisamine maleate 25 mg. Aspirin* 227 mg. Acetophenetidin* 162 mg. Caffeine 32 mg.	H.L. FEMININE HYGIENE POWDER (Henry Labs.)	Alum Eucalyptus* Thymol* Carica papaya Citric acid Boric acid* Sodium salicylate* Zinc sulfate* Lactose Carbolic acid*
HISTAPHEN COUGH SYRUP WITH ANTI-HISTAMINE (Chase Chem.)	Each 4 cc.: Thenylpyramine maleate* 12.5 mg. Sodium citrate 40.0 mg. Ammonium chloride 40.0 mg. Cetyldimethylbenzylammonium chloride* 0.4 mg.	H.L.R. (Howell Co.)	
		HOBO MEDICINE Diuretic (Hobo)	Galium herb Salicylic acid* Sodium benzoate Glycerin
HISTAPRIN COLD TABLETS Antihistamine (Pharmex)	Pyrilamine maleate 25 mg. Aspirin* 3-1/2 gr. Phenacetin* 2-1/2 gr. Caffeine 1/2 gr.	HOBSON'S BLACK-BERRY ROOT & GINGER For intestinal irritation (Standard Labs.)	Cinnamon Allspice Cardamon Cloves Alcohol 10%

*Consult Sec. II., Ingredients Index. This ingredient may be responsible for major toxic effects if poisonous amounts of this product are ingested.

Name & Use Manufacturer	Ingredients		Name & Use Manufacturer	Ingredients	
HOBSON'S CORN HUSKERS LOTION For skin irritations (Standard Labs.)	Tragacanth Glycerin Alcohol	5-3/4%	HOFER POULTRY SPRAY (Hofer)	Cresolis compound Eucalyptus* Menthol Creosote U.S.P.* Formaldehyde* Denatured alcohol	
HOBSON'S DERMA ZEMO OINTMENT For skin irritations (Standard Labs.)	Boric acid* Benzocaine Phenyl mercuric benzoate Pine tar* Zinc oxide	400 p.p.m.	HOFF'S GOODLAX TABLETS Laxative (Goodrich Drug)	Cascara Aloin* Podophyllin Gentian* Ginger	
			HOFF'S LINIMENT (Goodrich Drug)	Ammonia* Camphor* Turpentine* Castile soap	
HOBSON'S LARKSPUR & SABADILLA LOTION Ectoparasiticide (Standard Labs.)	Alkaloids from larkspur and sabadilla seeds Essential oils	0.15% 0.20%	HOG OIL WORMER Anthelmintic (veterinary) (Lee, G.)	Creosols Oil chenopodium Chloroform* Oil cajeput White mineral oil U.S.P. Paraffin oil	0.1% 3.7% 3.5% 0.3%
HOBSON'S POISON IVY LOTION (Standard Labs.)	Alcohol Aluminum hydroxide Boric acid* Borax*	29%	HOGOYL Insecticide (veterinary) (Hess, Dr.)	Hydrocarbon oils* Methyl naphthalenes* Coal tar phenols (tar acids) Gamma isomer of benzene hexachloride Other isomers of benzene hexachloride	96.23% 3.50% 0.12% 0.05% 0.10%
HOBSON'S RAT & ROACH PASTE (Standard Labs.)	Phosphorus*	2-1/2%			
			HOG SARCOPTIC MANGE OIL (veterinary) (Hilltop)	Crude petroleum oil* (containing 0.25%-0.5% sulfur) Creosote oil* Gamma isomer of benzene hexachloride	0.1%
HOBS SULPHUR FUMIGATOR (Hobs)	Sulfur*	100%			
HOCKWALD'S DDT Insecticide (Hockwald)	DDT*		HOLCOMB'S BOWL CLEANER (Holcomb)	Sodium bisulfate	
HOCKWALD'S HOKSOL Insecticide (Hockwald)	Chlorine*		HOLCOMB'S GYM FINISH PENETRATING SEAL (Holcomb)	Mineral spirits* High flash naphtha*	
HOCKWALD'S LIVESTOCK SPRAY Insecticide (Hockwald)	DDT*		HOLCOMB'S HEXACHLORO-PHENE LIQUID SOAP, 0.5% (Holcomb)	2,2'-Methylenebis-3,4,6-trichlorophenol	
HOCKWALD'S SOAP & DISINFECTANT (Hockwald)			HOLCOMB'S LO-BAX Cleaner (Holcomb)	Calcium hypochlorite*	
HOFER CAUSTIC PASTE Dehorning paste (Hofer)	Sodium hydroxide*		HOLCOMB'S PENETRATING SEAL (Holcomb)	Mineral spirits* High flash naphtha*	
			HOLCOMB'S WINDOW CLEANER (Holcomb)	Dioxan*	
HOFER LINIMENT (veterinary) (Hofer)	Synthetic oil of wintergreen* Oil of rosemary Camphor* Alcohol* Soap		HOLDENT Denture adhesive (Morgan Prod.)	Gum karaya Sodium borate	
			HOLDFAST PASTE (Scriptex)		

*Consult Sec. II., Ingredients Index. This ingredient may be responsible for major toxic effects if poisonous amounts of this product are ingested.

- 580 -

Name & Use Manufacturer	Ingredients	Name & Use Manufacturer	Ingredients
HOLDFAST RUBBER CEMENT (Holdfast)		HOMEOPATHIC RHUS TOX 3X PILLS (Washington Hom.)	Rhus toxicodendron
HOLDTU PASTE (Am. Crayon)		HOME ORCHARD SPRAY Insecticide (Imperial Chem.)	Ferbam (ferric dimethyl dithiocarbamate) 14.25% Sulfur 15.00% Tech. methoxychlor* 10.00% 2,2-Bis (p-methoxyphenyl)- 1,1-i-trichloroethane 8.85% Other isomers and related compounds 1.15% Dichloro diphenyl dichloro- ethane* 10.00% 2-(p-Tert-butylphenoxy) isopripyl 2-chloroethyl sulfite* 1.50%
HOLIDAY 100 TO 1 CONCEN- TRATE Insecticide (Collins Feed)	Tech. chlordane* 40% Piperonyl butoxide 0.10% Total pyrethrins 0.01% Petroleum solvents* 49.89%		
HOLIDAY SCREEN PAINT Insecticide (Collins Feed)	Tech. chlordane* Pyrenone 50-5 New mown hay Fly repellent (Crag) Dieldrin tech. flake* Sovacide 544C	HOME TERMITE CONCEN- TRATE Insecticide (Chem. Form.)	Gamma isomer of benzene hexachloride 0.30% Other isomers of benzene hexachloride 1.70% Dichloro diphenyl trichloro- ethane 3.00% Chlordane tech.* 47.00% Alkyl aryl sulfonate emulsifier 4.0% Petroleum solvent* 44.00%
HOLLANDEX SILICONE OINTMENT For skin irritations (Holland Rantos)	Silicones (dimethylpolysiloxane) Norwegian cod liver oil Zinc oxide Hexachlorophene Improved lanolin		
HOLLAND PAINTS & ENAMELS (Arnesto)		HOME TONE COLORS Paint (Colonial Works)	
HOLLANETE ENAMELS (Phelan- Faust)		HONEYSUCKLE HAND BALM (Assoc. Brands)	
HOLMES FLEA LOTION (Holmes, E.S.)	Isobornyl thiocyanoacetete 0.86% Other active terpenes 0.19%	HOOD AMMONIA (Hood	Ammonia* 5-10%
HOLMES FLEA POWDER (Holmes, E.S.)	Isobornyl thiocyanoacetate 3.28% Other related terpenes 0.72% Octachloro-4,7-methanotetra- hydroindane 0.60% Other related compounds 0.40%	HOOD BLEACH DISINFECTANT, 33 BLEACH, MOONSHINE BLEACH (Hood)	Sodium hypochlorite* 5-1/4%/w Sodium chloride 5-1/4%/w Sodium hydroxide and/or sodium carbonate 0.2-0.3%
HOLMES PINE SHAMPOO Insecticide (Holmes, E.S.)	Anhydrous soap 21.80% Pine oil 3.20%	HOOD E-Z LIQUID STARCH (Hood)	Pure starch Preservative less than 0.1%
HOLMES SULPHO SHAMPOO Insecticide (Holmes, E.S.)	Anhydrous soap 20% Calcium polysulfide 1.5% Calcium thiosulfate 0.15%	HOOD'S HAIR COLOR PREP. (Dolle)	
HOME CRAFT PAINTS (Harris Standard)		HOOFOILIN (veterinary) (Thoroughbred)	Cod liver oil Lanolin Oil of turpentine* Pine Neatsfoot oil Beeswax Cedarwood Pine tar*
HOME-KRAFT ENAMELS & STAINS (McQuade, J.)		HOOSIER STA Anti-freeze (Hoosier)	Methanol*
HOMELAWN CRABGRASS KILLER (Northrup)	Phenyl mercuric acetate* 2.50%	HOOVER POWDERS For headache, neuralgia (Fuller, C.F.)	One powder(10 gr.): Acetanilid* 2-1/2 gr. Caffeine (alkaloid) 1/2 gr. Sodium bicarbonate Celery

*Consult Sec. II., Ingredients Index. This ingredient may be responsible for major toxic effects if poisonous amounts of this product are ingested.

Name & Use Manufacturer	Ingredients		Name & Use Manufacturer	Ingredients	
HOPALONG CASSIDY HAIR TRAINER (Assoc. Brands)			HOPKINS GARDEN DUST Insecticide (Hopkins Agric.)	Pyrethrins Petroleum distillate	0.20% 2.00%
HOPE DENTURE ADHESIVE (Whitehall)			HOPKINS GRAIN FUMIGANT NO. 4 Insecticide, fumigant (Hopkins Agric.)	Ethylene dichloride* Carbon tetrachloride*	70.2% 29.8%
HOPKINS 2.5% ALDRIN DUST Insecticide (Hopkins Agric.)	Hexachloro hexahydro dimethano naphthalene* Related compounds	2.4% 0.4%	HOPKINS 25% LINDANE WETTABLE POWDER Insecticide (Hopkins Agric.)	Gamma isomer of benzene hexachloride* (from lindane)	25.0%
HOPKINS ALDRIN EQUIVALENT EMULSION Insecticide (Hopkins Agric.)	Hexachloro-hexahydro- dimethano-naphthalene* Related compounds Petroleum hydrocarbons	23.10% 17.37% 52.03%	HOPKINS MALATHION BAIT FLY KILLER Insecticide (Hopkins Agric.)	Malathion*	2%
HOPKINS 20% ALDRIN GRANULES Insecticide (Hopkins Agric.)	Hexachloro hexahydro dimethano-naphthalene* Related compounds	19.0% 3.2%	HOPKINS MALATHION 5% DUST Insecticide (Hopkins Agric.)	Malathion* (o,o-dimethyl dithiophosphate of diethyl mercaptosuccinate)	5.00%
HOPKINS 5% CHLORDANE DUST Insecticide (Hopkins Agric.)	Tech. chlordane	5.0%	HOPKINS MALATHION SPRAY CONCEN- TRATE FOR FLY CONTROL (Hopkins Agric.)	Malathion* (o,o-dimethyl dithiophosphate of diethyl mercaptosuccinate) Xylene*	49.5% 42.5%
HOPKINS CHLORDANE EMULSION Insecticide (Hopkins Agric.)	Chlordane tech.* Petroleum distillate*	45.0% 47.0%			
HOPKINS 5% DDT DUST Insecticide (Hopkins Agric.)	DDT (dichloro diphenyl trichloroethane)*	5.0%	HOPKINS MALATHION 25% WETTABLE POWDER Insecticide (Hopkins Agric.)	Malathion* (o,o-dimethyl dithiophosphate of diethyl mercaptosuccinate)	25.00%
HOPKINS 50% DDT WETTABLE POWDER Insecticide (Hopkins Agric.)	DDT (dichloro diphenyl trichloroethane)*	50%	HOPKINS MH-40 QUACK GRASS HERBICIDE & GROWTH INHIBITOR (Hopkins Agric.)	Sodium salt of 1,2-dihydro- pyridazine-3, 6-dione	48.3%
HOPKINS DIELDRIN 50% WETTABLE POWDER Insecticide (Hopkins Agric.)	Hexachloro epoxy octahydro dimethano naphthalene* Related compounds	42.5% 7.5%	HOPKINS ONION DUST Insecticide (Hopkins Agric.)	Parathion* Copper	1.00% 5.565%
HOPKINS ENDRIN EMULSIFI- ABLE CONCEN- TRATE Insecticide (Hopkins Agric.)	Endrin* (hexachloroepoxy- octahydro-endo-dimethano naphthalene) Petroleum hydrocarbons	19.5% 73.0%	HOPKINS 25% PARATHION EMULSION Insecticide (Hopkins Agric.)	Parathion* (o,o-diethyl-o-p- nitrophenyl thiophosphate) Xylene	25% 65%

*Consult Sec. II., Ingredients Index. This ingredient may be responsible for major toxic effects if poisonous amounts of this product are ingested.

Name & Use Manufacturer	Ingredients	Name & Use Manufacturer	Ingredients
HOPKINS POTATO DUST 3-7 Insecticide (Hopkins Agric.)	DDT (dichloro diphenyl trichloroethane) 3.0% Copper* (in cuprous and cupric oxide) expressed as metallic 7.0%	HOPKINS WARFARIN RAT & MOUSE KILLER (Hopkins Agric.)	Warfarin (3-(a-acetonylbenzyl)- 4-hydroxycoumarin) 0.25%
HOPKINS POTATO DUST CO 57 Insecticide (Hopkins Agric.)	DDT (dichloro diphenyl trichloroethane)* 3.0% Copper* (in basic copper sulfate) expressed as metallic 7.0%	HOPKINS WARFARIN REDI-MIX PELLETS RAT & MOUSE KILLER (Hopkins Agric.)	Warfarin 0.025%
HOPKINS PYRETHRIN DUST Insecticide (Hopkins Agric.)	Pyrethrins 0.20% Petroleum distillate 2.00%	HORICUM, Fungicide (Hammond)	Liquid lime sulfur*
HOPKINS PYRETHRIN PLUS COPPER DUST Insecticide (Hopkins Agric.)	Pyrethrins 0.15% Petroleum distillate 1.50% Copper*(basic copper sulfate) expressed as metallic 7.00%	HORNEX Dehorning Paste Veterinary (Holt)	Potassium hydroxide* 45% Bentonite Ointment base
HOPKINS 1-1/2% ROTENONE Insecticide (Hopkins Agric.)	Rotenone (as derived from cube) 1.5% Other cube extractives 2.4%	HORN, HORNBRITE, HORNGLAZE Cleaners, wax (Horn)	
HOPKINS ROTENONE PLUS COPPER DUST Insecticide (Hopkins Agric.)	Rotenone 0.75% Other cube extractives 1.25% Copper*(basic copper sulfate) expressed as metallic 5.00%	HORN, HORNSPAR PAINTS, ENAMELS, UNDERCOATS (Horn)	
HOPKINS TOMATO DUST Fungicide (Hopkins Agric.)	Copper*(basic copper sulfate) expressed as metallic 7.0%	HORSE SHOE BRAND ENAMEL, PAINT (Mound City)	
HOPKINS TOMATO SPRAY Fungicide (Hopkins Agric.)	Copper*(in basic copper sulfate) expressed as metallic 50.15%	HORSE SHOE LYE (Babbitt)	Sodium hydroxide* Sodium carbonate
HOPKINS TOOTHACHE LIQUID (Hopkins Prod.)	Alcohol 36% Oil of cloves* U.S.P. Creosote* U.S.P.	DR. HORTON'S EU-CA OINTMENT Skin ointment (Evert's)	Petrolatum Lanolin Zinc oxide Wax Oil eucalyptus* Menthol* Thymol* 1/3 gr.
HOPKINS TOXAPHENE EMULSION NO. 6 Insecticide (Hopkins Agric.)	Toxaphene* (tech. chlorinated camphene, 67-69% chlorine content) 60.2% Petroleum distillates 33.8% Modified phthalic glycol alkyd resin 1.0%	HORTON'S EUTHANASIA SOLUTION (Veterinary) (Horton & Converse)	Sodium pentobarbital* 2.75 gr./cc. Propylene glycol 33%
HOPKINS WARFARIN 0.5% CON- CENTRATE RAT & MOUSE KILLER (Hopkins Agric.)	Warfarin (3(a-acetonylbenzyl)- 4-hydroxycoumarin) 0.5%	HOSE MIX'T FRUIT & VEGETABLE GARDEN SPRAY PELLETS Insecticide (Internat. Res.)	Tech. methoxychlor* 15% Malathion* 6.25% Captan 15.00% Sodium alkyl benzene sulfonate 15%
		HOT SHOT 3-10-40 Insecticide (Port)	DDT* (dichloro diphenyl trichloroethane) 10% Gamma isomer of benzene hexachloride* 3% Other isomers of benzene hexachloride 5.2% Sulfur*(93% passing 325-mesh screen) 40.0%

*Consult Sec. II., Ingredients Index. This ingredient may be responsible for major toxic effects if poisonous amounts of this product are ingested.

Name & Use Manufacturer	Ingredients	Name & Use Manufacturer	Ingredients
HOT SPOT ELECTRIC BRAND LINIMENT (Katco)	Ether* (alcohol deriv.) 28 m. Oil mustard syn. 1/10 m./fl.oz. Oil thyme Turpentine* Refined petroleum Saxoline oil Oleoresin capsicum	HOWES FABRIC CEMENT (Howes)	
HOT SPOT PENN WALL SIZE (Miner- Hillard)		HQZ CASTILE SHAMPOO (H.Q.Z.)	Coco-castile liquid soap Trisodium phosphate Lavender D & C green
HOT SPRINGS BRAND IMPROVED SARSAPARILLA COMPOUND Tonic (Allied Drug)	Potassium iodide* Iron sulfate U.S.P. Extract of gentian* Aloin*. Epsom salt U.S.P.	HQZ FOOT OIL (H.Q.Z.)	Olive oil Apricot kernel oil NF mineral oil (95 vis.) Menthol* Thymol* Perfume
		HQZ HAIR LUSTRE (H.Q.Z.)	Olive oil NF mineral oil (95 vis.) Menthol Perfume
HOUSE FOR MEN GLENDALE COLOGNE (House for Men)		HQZ HAIR OIL (H.Q.Z.)	Olive oil Apricot kernel oil NF mineral oil (95 vis.) Menthol* Thymol* D & C oil soluble chlorophyll green Perfume
HOUSEHOLD BUG KILLER Insecticide (Chem. Corp.)		H & R COUGH SYRUP WITH PINE TAR & HONEY (Allied Drug)	Chloroform 3 m/fl. oz. White pine bark* Wild cherry bark Aralia Balm of Gilead buds Sanguinaria Creosote*
HOUSEHOLD ODOR DEODORANT (Korex)			
HOUSEHOLD OIL (Kendall Ref.)		H.S.G. EYEBROW PENCILS, EYEBROW CRAYONS (Gompes, H.)	
HOUSE OF BRISTOL HARDWOOD FLOOR CLEANER (House of Bristol)		H.S.G. FACE CREAM, CLEANSING & OVERNIGHT CREAM (Gompes, H.)	
HOUSE OF BRISTOL PAINT AND VARNISH CLEANER (House of Bristol)		H.S.G. FACE POWDER (Gompes, H.)	
HOUSE OF LOWELL BUBBLE BATH (House of Lowell)	Anionic detergent* Nonionic detergent* Methyl parahydroxy benzoate Perfume compound	H.S.G. LIPSTICK, ROUGE, MASCARA, EYE SHADOW (Gompes, H.)	
		HUBBARD BLIGHT CONTROL DUST Fungicide (Rogers & Hubbard)	Copper* expressed as metallic 7.00%
HOUSE OF LOWELL FRAGRANCE FOR HAIR AND BODY (House of Lowell)	Lanolin Propylene glycol monostearate Glycerin monostearate Diglyco stearate Cetyl alcohol Silicone Hexachlorophene Isopropyl myristate Palmitate Veegum Glycerin Triethanolamine Perfume compound	HUBBARD CABBAGE MAGGOT DUST Insecticide (Rogers & Hubbard)	Mercurous chloride* 3.90%

*Consult Sec. II., Ingredients Index. This ingredient may be responsible for major toxic effects if poisonous amounts of this product are ingested.

- 584 -

Name & Use Manufacturer	Ingredients	
HUBBARD DITHANE Z-78 DUST Fungicide (Rogers & Hubbard)	Zineb	3.90%
HUBBARD DOUBLE DUTY DUST Fungicide, Insecticide (Rogers & Hubbard)	Rotenone Other cube resins Yellow cuprous oxide	0.75% 1.20% 4.50%
HUBBARD FRUIT SPRAY Fungicide, insecticide (Rogers & Hubbard)	Sulfur* Tech. chlordane* Dichloro diphenyl dichloro- ethane Ferric dimethyl dithiocarbamate	33.30% 6.50% 6.50% 5.00%
HUBBARD LINDANE 25% WETTABLE Insecticide (Rogers & Hubbard)	Gamma isomer of benzene hexachloride*	25.00%
HUBBARD MITE KILLER Insecticide (Rogers & Hubbard)	2-(p-tert-Butylphenoxy) isopropyl 2-chloroethyl sulfite*	15.00%
HUBBARD NO. 10 FERMATE DUST Fungicide (Rogers & Hubbard)	Ferric dimethyl dithiocarbamate	7.60%
HUBBARD 10 POWDER Insecticide (Rogers & Hubbard)	Dichloro diphenyl trichloro- ethane*	10%
DR. HUBBARD'S VEGETABLE GERMICIDE Wound antiseptic (Hubbard, J.)	Alcohol* Mixture of thymol*, origanum, oil cajeput, oil lavender, oil rosemary, oil pine*	85% 10%
HUBBARD VEGETABLE SPRAY-DUST Fungicide, insecticide (Rogers & Hubbard)	Tech. piperonyl cyclonene Pyrethrins Rotenone Other cube extractives Zineb Inert ingredients* (presumed to be petroleum distillates)	1.05% 0.10% 0.50% 1.05% 5.30% 92.00%
HUBBARD ZERLATE DUST Fungicide (Rogers & Hubbard)	Ziram*	11.40%
HUBCO COATINGS, PAINTS (Boston Putty)		

Name & Use Manufacturer	Ingredients	
NO. 5 HUBKLOR DUST Insecticide (Rogers & Hubbard)	Tech. chlordane*	5%
HUBROTE DUST Insecticide (Rogers & Hubbard)	Rotenone Other cube resins	1.00% 1.60%
HU-CASE Powdered casein glue (Hughes)	Casein Lime Sodium fluoride* Trisodium phosphate Sodium oxalate* Sodium sulfite	
HUDSON LYE (Babbitt)	Sodium carbonate Sodium hydroxide*	
HUGHES CEMENT #4024 (Hughes)	Synthetic resin base Methanol*	
HUGHES CEMENT #4024-A (Hughes)	Synthetic resin base Denatured alcohol*	
HUM Detergent (Theobald)	Alkyl aryl sodium sulfonate	
HUM-I-DRI Maintenance material (Speco)	Chloride salts of aluminum, potassium and calcium Sodium tripolyphosphate	
HUMPHREYS 1 Antipyretic (homeopathic) (Humphreys)	Aconite American hellebore White bryony Belladonna	3x 2x 3x 3x
HUMPHREYS 3 Analgesic, sedative (homeopathic) (Humphreys)	Chamomile Calcium phosphate Coffee Belladonna	3x 12x 3x 3x
HUMPHREYS 4 For diarrhea (homeopathic) (Humphreys)	China Ipecac Calcium carbonate Hahn Chamomile	3x 3x 12x 3x
HUMPHREYS 7 Antitussive (homeopathic) (Humphreys)	Belladonna Phosphorus Sponge White bryony	3x 6x 2x 3x
HUMPHREYS 8 Facial neuralgia (homeopathic) (Humphreys)	Mezereon Belladonna Aconite Magnesium phosphate	2x 3x 3x 12x
HUMPHREYS 9 Analgesic (homeopathic) (Humphreys)	Blood root Blue flag Yellow jessamine St. Ignatius' bean	3x 3x 3x 6x
HUMPHREYS 10 Digestant (homeopathic) (Humphreys)	Nux vomica China Golden seal Club moss	2x 2x 3x 3x

*Consult Sec. II., Ingredients Index. This ingredient may be responsible for major toxic effects if poisonous amounts of this product are ingested.

Name & Use Manufacturer	Ingredients		Name & Use Manufacturer	Ingredients	
HUMPHREYS 11 For menstrual irregularity (homeopathic) (Humphreys)	Black cohosh Wind flower Sepia	3x 3x 3x	HUMPHREYS 31 For menstrual pain (Humphreys)	High bush cranberry Belladonna Black cohosh Yellow jessamine	3x 3x 3x 3x
HUMPHREYS 13 For spasmodic croup (homeopathic) (Humphreys)	Sponge Aconite Crude calcium sulfide	2x 3x 12x	HUMPHREYS 32 For discomforts during menopause (Humphreys)	Black cohosh Sepia Lachesis	3x 6x 12x
HUMPHREYS 14 For skin (homeopathic) (Humphreys)	Honey bee Ivy Coal oil Crude calcium sulfide	3x 6x 3x 6x	HUMPHREYS 34 For throat irritations (Humphreys)	Honey bee Belladonna Poke Lachesis	3x 3x 3x 8x
HUMPHREYS 15 For rheumatic pains (homeopathic) (Humphreys)	Ivy Meadow saffron Hahnemann's causticum White bryony	6x 6x 3x 3x	HUMPHREYS 40 Insomnia (Humphreys)	Chamomile Coffee Henbane	3x 3x 3x
HUMPHREYS 17 For hemorrhoids (homeopathic) (Humphreys)	Stone-root Horse chestnut Witch hazel Sulfur	3x 3x 3x 6x	HUMPHREYS 44 Analgesic (Humphreys)	Each tablet: Acetophenetidin* Aspirin* Caffeine*	3 gr.
HUMPHREYS 18 For eye irritations (Humphreys)	Eyebright Honey bee Wind flower	3x 3x 3x	HUMPHREYS 55 Antacid (Humphreys)	Magnesium hydroxide Aluminum hydroxide	1.25 gr. 0.625 gr.
HUMPHREYS 19 Nasal decongestant (Humphreys)	Arsenious oxide Wind flower Potassium iodide Cevadilla	3x 3x 2x 3x	HUMPHREYS 60 Antihistamine (Humphreys)	Each tablet: Pyrilamine maleate*	25 mg.
HUMPHREYS 21 Asthmatic antispasmodic (Humphreys)	Ipecac Indian tobacco Arsenious oxide	3x 3x 3x	HUMPHREYS 77 For colds (Humphreys)	Arsenious oxide Yellow jessamine Onion Aconite	3x 3x 3x 3x
HUMPHREYS 24 Tonic tablets (Humphreys)	Each tablet: Calcium glycerophosphate 0.7 gr. Sodium glycerophosphate 0.7 gr. Thiamine hydrochloride 111 U.S.P.units		HUMPHREYS 99 Laxative (Humphreys)	Each tablet: Phenolphthalein*	0.375 gr.
			HUMPHREYS OINTMENT (Humphreys)	Camphor* Witch hazel extract Pyroligneous acid Oil of rosemary	
HUMPHREYS 26 For simple nausea, vomiting (Humphreys)	Antimonous sulfide Poison nut Ipecac	3x 3x 3x	HUMPHREYS RECTAL SUPPOSITOR- IES For hemorrhoids (Humphreys)	Hamamelis (witch hazel) 1-1/2 gr. Collinsonia Benzocaine Aesculus Cocoa butter base	1-1/2 gr. 1/4 gr. 1-1/2 gr.
HUMPHREYS 27 For simple disorders of the urinary tract (Humphreys)	Pipsissewa Oil of turpentine Club moss Barberry	3x 3x 3x 3x	HUNT-CO DRY CLEANING SOAP PASTE (Huntington)		
HUMPHREYS 28 For nervous conditions (Humphreys)	Yellow jessamine Picric acid China Potassium phosphate	3x 6x 2x 3x	HUNTER'S 5% ANTU BROWN RAT BAITS (Hunter)	Alpha naphthyl thiourea	5%
HUMPHREYS 29 For fever blisters, nursing sore mouth (Humphreys)	Sodium chloride Wild indigo Sodium pyroborate	4x 3x 2x	HUNTERS' INSECT SPRAY (Hunter)	Refined petroleum oil Piperonyl butoxide ((butyl carbityl) (6 propyl piperonyl) ether) and related compounds Pyrethrins	
			HUNTER'S MOLE KILLER (Hunter)	Strychnine sulfate*	0.5%
HUMPHREYS 30 For bedwettings, simple bladder irritations (Humphreys)	Spanish fly Mercuric chloride Causticum hahnemann Scouring rush	6x 3x 3x 3x	HUNTER'S MOUSE KILLER SEED (Hunter)	Strychnine alkaloid*	0.38%

---

*Consult Sec. II., Ingredients Index. This ingredient may be responsible for major toxic effects if poisonous amounts of this product are ingested.

Name & Use Manufacturer	Ingredients	Name & Use Manufacturer	Ingredients
HUNTER'S 10% RED SQUILL RAT BAITS (Hunter)	Red squill powder* 10%	HYAMINE 10-X Fungicide (Rohm & Haas)	Di-isobutyl cresoxy ethoxy ethyl dimethyl benzyl ammonium chloride* 98.8%
HUNTER'S WARFARIN RAT & MOUSE MIX (Hunter)	Warfarin (3-(a-acetonylbenzyl)- 4-hydroxycoumarin) 0.025%	HYAMINE 1622 Fungicide (Rohm & Haas)	Para di-isobutyl phenoxy ethoxy ethyl dimethyl benzyl ammonium chloride* 98.8%
HUNTER'S WATER SOLUBLE WARFARIN Rodenticide (Hunter)	Sodium salt of warfarin (sodium salt of 3(a-acetonyl- benzyl)-4-hydroxycoumarin) 0.54%	HYAMINE 2389 (50% Aqueous) Fungicide (Rohm & Haas)	Alkyl tolyl methyl trimethyl ammonium chlorides* 50%
HUNT'S LIGHTNING OIL LINIMENT Rubefacient (Allied Drug)	Kerosene* Capsicum extractive Camphor* Methyl salicylate*, syn. Allyl isothiocyanate*	HYAMINE 3104 Fungicide (Rohm & Haas)	Dimethyl didodecenyl ammonium chloride* 60-70% Isopropyl alcohol
HUNT'S SALVE For skin irritations (Allied Drug)	Carbolic acid* Sulfur* Petrolatum	HYANILID OINTMENT Fungicide (medical) (Peau Seche)	Salicyl Anilide* in carbowax 5%
HU-REZ #7 (Hughes)	Polyvinyl acetate emulsion- type adhesive	HY-BEAUTE HAIR DRESSING, SLIK (Pomade) (Hy-Beaute)	
HURRY-UP BLACK ENAMEL (Lawrence, W. W.)		HY-BEAUTE SMOKELESS PRESSING OIL (Hy-Beaute)	
HUSH CREAM DEODORANT (Hush)		HYBEPHEN ELIXIR Antispasmodic, visceral sedative (Massengill)	Each 5 cc.: Phenobarbital* 15 mg. Tinc. belladonna 0.3 cc. Tinc. hyoscyamus 1 cc. Thiamine hydrochloride 3 mg.
HUSK DRESSING Antiseptic dressing (Bullock- Walker)	Calomel 1.1% Carbolic acid 1/2% Resorcinol Zinc oxide Oil of cade Salicylic acid 1/4% Benzocaine Bismuth subnitrate Balsam Peru Phenyl mercury benzoate 1-10,000	HYCO 10 ODORLESS DISINFECTANT (Hockwald)	
		HYDALL, JAY ARR WALL AND ROOF COATING (Roberts Paint)	
HUXII Fungicide (medical) (Bullock- Walker)	Each ounce: Calomel* 5 gr. Salicylic acid* 29-1/6 gr. Carbolic acid 2.3 gr. Ammonium alum Ammoniated mercury* 2.50 gr. Benzoic acid 21-7/8 gr. Thymol* Sulfur	HYDALL PAINTS (Roberts Paint)	
		HYDRACREME (Newton, Paul)	
HVC (Hayden's Viburnum Compound) (New York Pharm.)	Alcohol* 48% Viburnum opulus Dioscorea Prickly ash berries	HYDRISINOL CREME Water washable base for ointment, mas- sage or shaving cream (Pedinol)	Sulfated hydrogenated castor oil N.F.*
H & W PURE PAINT (Louisville Paint)		HYDRO CIDE Disinfectant (Corn King)	Di-isobutyl phenoxy ethyl dimethyl benzyl ammonium chloride* 3.4%

*Consult Sec. II., Ingredients Index. This ingredient may be responsible for major toxic effects if poisonous amounts of this product are ingested.

Name & Use Manufacturer	Ingredients	Name & Use Manufacturer	Ingredients
HYDRO FIRE EXTIN-GUISHER (Am.-La France)		HY-ER GLOSS ENAMEL (McDougall-Butler)	
HYDROGEL Adsorbent, antacid (Success)	Alumina	HYG-A-TABS (Hyg-A-Tabs)	
HYDROL Insecticide (Whitmoyer)	Petroleum oil* Cresylic acid* (consisting of ortho, meta and para cresols, ethyl phenol, xylenol and higher molecular weight phenols)	HYGENA ANTISEPTIC POWDER (Hygena)	All U.S.P.: Powdered sodium bicarbonate Powdered sodium borax* Powdered sodium perborate* Powdered zinc sulfate* Camphor* Peppermint Menthol* Eucalyptol* Thymol*
HYDROLAMINS For anal irritations (Lewal Pharm.)	Lactalbumin hydrolysate 10% Methionine Cystine Polyethylene glycol 1500		
HYDROLEUM (Pratt, B.)	Methyl salicylate* Menthol* Turpentine* Sulfonated mustard seed oil White mineral oil	HYGENOL Vaginal douche (Veltex)	Boric acid* Zinc sulfate* Salicylic and carbolic* acids Eucalyptol* Menthol* Thymol* Methyl salicylate*
HYDROPEL OINTMENT (C & M)	Silicone Paraffinated starch Butyl and propyl parahydroxy-benzoates 0.50% each Petrolatum	HYGETTE Astringent powder (Western Pharm.)	Boric acid* 75% Alum potassium 16% Zinc sulfate 7% Aromatics q.s.
HYDROPHILIC OINTMENT (Chase Chem.)	Stearyl alcohol White petrolatum Glycerin Sodium lauryl sulfate Preservatives	HYGIEIA DUSTLESS CHALK, FORSYTE CHALK, CRAYON (Am. Crayon)	
HYDROSAL OINTMENT For skin irritations (Hydrosal)	Colloidal aluminum acetate Bland emollient base	HYGIENIC SOAP 403 (Beauty Couns.)	
HYDRO-SEAL SILICONE WATER REPELLENT For masonary walls (Hydrotex)	Solvent* (presumed to be petroleum distillates) Silicone conc. approx. 5%	HY-GLO-LAC LACQUER (Midcontinent)	
		HY-G POWDER (Sacramento)	
HYDROSIL, Adsorbent, antacid (Success)	Magnesium trisilicate 0.5 gm. Aluminum hydroxide 0.25 gm.	HYGRADE HOUSE PAINT (Monroe Co.)	
HYDRO TABS Disinfectant (Corie King)	Di-isobutyl phenoxy ethoxy ethyl dimethyl benzyl ammonium chloride mono-hydrate* 20.3%	HY-GRADE LOTION Hand Lotion (Smith, C.D.)	Glycerin Camphor* Ammonia water* 2%
HYDROTONE PAINTS (Sterling Paint)		HY-GRO Plant food (Hy-Gro)	Nitrogen 13% Phosphoric acid 26% Potash 13%
		HY-GRO FOR ORCHIDS Plant food (Hy-Gro)	Nitrogen 18% Phosphoric acid 18% Potash 18%
HYDROTOX Fungicide (medical) (Mayer)	Hexachlorophene Precipitated sulfur* Salicylic acid* Undecylenic acid	HY-GRO ROSE & FLOWER Insecticide, fungicide (Hy-Gro)	Rotenone 1.00% Cube resins 2.00% Ferbam 8.75% Sulfur* 59.00% Gamma isomer of benzene hexachloride (from lindane) 1.00%
HYDRYL (Torch)	Wool hydrolysate		

---

*Consult Sec. II., Ingredients Index. This ingredient may be responsible for major toxic effects if poisonous amounts of this product are ingested.

Name & Use Manufacturer	Ingredients	
HY-KLAS PAINT PRODUCTS (Merchants & Mfrs.)		
HYKOSTAR DISINFECTANT (Gerson-Stewart)		
HY-KRESOL Deodorant, disinfectant (Smith, H.V.)	Cresylic acid*	50%
	Soap	30%
HY-LIFE WORMER SALT FOR SHEEP (Hy-Life)		
HY-LO Insecticide (Sweeney, W.R.)	Pyrethrins	0.5%
HYMOSA Artirheumatic (Walker Pharm.)	Alcohol	18-1/2%
	Sodium salicylate*	16 gr.
	Sodium citrate	8 gr.
	Potassium iodide*	4 gr.
	Caffein citrate	1/2 gr.
	Cimicifuga tr.	48 m.
	Colchicum fl. ext.	5 gr.
	Colchicine	1/60 gr.
HYMO-SALVA Counter-irritant, local analgesic (Walker Pharm.)	Methyl salicylate*	
	Menthol*	
	Camphor*	
	Capsicum*	
	Lanolin	
	Cocoa butter	
	Petrolatum	
HYNE VAGINAL SUPPOSITOR-IES (Myers Labs.)	Ammonium alum	
	Boric acid*	
	Cocoa butter	
	Salicylic acid*	
	Stearic acid	
	Thymol*	
	Oxyquinoline sulfate*	
HYO CARBONATES Antacid, intestinal sedative (Jewell Pharm.)	Each capsule:	
	Ext. hyoscyamus N.F.* 0.21 gr.	
	Calcium carbonate	
	Bismuth subcarbonate	
	Magnesium carbonate	
	Diastase	
HYO CARBONATES WITH BELLADONNA Antacid, intestinal sedative (Jewell Pharm.)	Each capsule:	
	Ext. hyoscyamus N.F.* 0.14 gr.	
	Ext belladonna U.S.P.* 0.07 gr.	
	Calcium carbonate	
	Bismuth subcarbonate	
	Magnesium carbonate	
	Diastase	
HY-PHEN Analgesic (Hy-Phen)	Acetophenetedin*	2-1/2 gr.
	Aspirin*	3 gr.
	Caffeine alkaloid	1/4 gr.
HYPO-CHEK Photographic supply (Edwal)	Potassium iodide*	
	Formaldehyde*	

Name & Use Manufacturer	Ingredients	
HYPONEX PLANT FOOD (Hydroponic)	Total nitrogen	7%
	Nitrate nitrogen	5.80%
	Ammoniacal nitrogen	1.20%
	Phosphoric acid	6%
	Water soluble potash	19%
	Chlorine	0.05%
HY-TONER PAINTS Paint (Roberts Paint)		
HYTRON DISINFECTANT & SANITIZER (Keystone Plast.)	Para di-isobutyl phenoxy ethoxy ethyl dimethyl benzyl ammonium chloride mono-hydrate*	20%
HY-TROUS LIQUID FERTILIZER (Hy-Trous)	Nitrogen	4%
	Phosphoric acid	8%
	Potash	4%
	Chlorine	1%
IATOL External fungicide (Medical) (Bullock-Walker)	Ammoniated mercury*	7%
	Zinc oxide	10%
	Hydrogenated vegetable fat and beeswax	q.s.
I BATH Eye wash (McKesson)	Ethyl alcohol	0.07%/v
	Hydrastine hydrochloride	
	Berberine hydrochloride	
	Camphor	
	Boric acid	
	Salt	
	Copper sulfate	
IBI MULTIPLE TRACE ELEMENTS Food supplement (Inorganic)	Each tablet:	
	Manganese sulfate	170 mg.
	Copper sulfate	3 mg.
	Zinc sulfate	1 mg.
	Copper sulfate	1 mg.
	Cobalt sulfate	3 mg.
	Iron sulfate	10 mg.
	Lecithin	
IBI (With Iron) Food supplement (Inorganic)	Each tablet:	
	Manganese lactate	260 mg.
	Iron lactate	8 mg.
	Copper lactate	2 mg.
	Magnesium lactate	70 mg.
	Cobalt lactate	4 mg.
	Zinc sulfate monohydrate	1 mg.
I. C. DEGREASER (Ultra Chem.)		
ICELIKE FLOOR ENAMEL (Moore, B.)		
ICE-MINT Rubefacient, foot (United Sales)	Camphor gum	
	Menthol*	
	Lanolin	
	Essential oils of peppermint, eucalyptus*, thyme and camphor*	
ICE REM Maintenance material (Speco)	Chloride salts of aluminum, potassium and calcium	
	Sodium tripolyphosphate	

Name & Use Manufacturer	Ingredients		Name & Use Manufacturer	Ingredients	
IC FINISH WAX (Interna. Chem.)			IDEAL CREAM SILVER POLISH (Golden Star)		
ICHTHYOL OINTMENT Skin irritation (Schering)	Ichthammol N.F.		IDEAL LIGHTER FLUID (Hollingshead)	VM & P naphtha* almost 100%	
ICHTHYSALLE OINTMENT 10% Antiseptic, counter-irritant (Horton & Converse)	Ichthammol N.F. Petrolatum Wool fat	10%	IDO GO DEODORANT (Auth. Brands)		
			IDOL Skin burns, irritation (Bullock-Walker)	Cod liver oil Benzocaine Chlorothymol*	
ICR BRAND Insecticide (Insect)	DDT*	5%	I DROPS Eye drops (McKesson)	Alcohol Hydrastine hydrochloride Berberine hydrochloride Camphor Boric acid Salt Copper sulfate	0.07%/v
IDEAL ANTISEPTIC (Assoc. Prod.)	Thymol* Eucalyptol* Boric acid* Menthol* Methyl salicylate* Benzoic acid*				
			I-FIX Eye preparation (Sacramento)		
IDEAL BRAND BROWN COPPER OXIDE Fungicide (Florida Agric.)	Copper* expressed as metallic 75%		I.G. (Ising Germicide) (Ising)		
			I-HEAL-U-CYANIDE SORE HEALER Burns (Wambaugh)	Picric acid* Lanolin base	
IDEAL BRAND COPPER A MIXTURE NO. 14 Fungicide (Florida Agric.)	Copper* expressed as metallic (from copper oxychloride) 6.2%		I-KLEEN Eye hygiene (K-A-S)	Antipyrine Boric acid Aqua camphorae Alkalizer	
IDEAL BRAND DUSTING SULPHUR Insecticide (Florida Agric.)	Sulfur*	93%	I.K.O. GARDEN SPRAY Insecticide (Kirchner)		
IDEAL BRAND LIME SULPHUR SOLUTION Insecticide (Florida Agric.)	Calcium polysulfides* Calcium thiosulfate	28.50% 1.50%	ILLBRONZE ALUMINUM POWDERS GOLD & COLORED Paints (Ill. Bronze)		
			ILLUSION CREME COLOGNE (Lura-Glo)		
IDEAL BRAND OIL-EMULSION CONCEN-TRATE Insecticide (Florida Agric.)	Petroleum oil*	84%	IMADYL UNCTION (Roche) Antirheumatic (Hoffmann-La Roche)	Histamine dihydrochloride* 1% Acetyl-glycol-salicylic ester 5% Methyl salicylate* 15% Menthol (Not U.S.P.) 10% Thymol 1%	
IDEAL BRAND SULPHUR-MANGANESE-DDT DUST NO. 83-5-3 Insecticide (Florida Agric.)	DDT (Dichloro diphenyl trichloroethane) Sulfur* Manganese	3% 83% 1.12%	IMDRIN Antirheumatic (Rhodes Pharm)	Panithal (salicylamide*) Potassium salicylate* Acetophenetidin* Caffeine Ascorbic acid	

*Consult Sec. II., Ingredients Index. This ingredient may be responsible for major toxic effects if poisonous amounts of this product are ingested.

Name & Use Manufacturer	Ingredients	
IMDRIN RUB Rubefacient, (Rhodes Pharm.)	Methyl salicylate* Oil of turpentine* Isopropyl alcohol Oil of camphor* Extr. capsicum	5%/v
IMMAC LOTION DEODORANT (Whitehall)	Alcohol	38%
IMPERIAL 24% ALDRIN EQUIVALENT EMULSIFI-ABLE CON-CENTRATE Insecticide (Imperial Chem.)	Hexachloro hexahydro dimethano naphthalene* Related compounds Xylene and methylated naphthalenes	21.66% 16.34% 52.00%
IMPERIAL BRUSH CLEANER (Wilson-Imperial)		
IMPERIAL BUG DUST Insecticide (Imperial Chem.)	Rotenone Other cube resins Cuprous oxide Beta thiocyano ethyl esters of aliphatic fatty acids (10-18 carbon atoms from Lethane 60) Sulfur	0.75% 1.87% 4.60% 0.75% 5.00%
IMPERIAL CATTLE GRUB DUST Insecticide (Imperial Chem.)	Rotenone Other cube resins Inert ingredients	1.67% 2.00% 96.33%
IMPERIAL CHALKS (Imperial Cray.)		
IMPERIAL CHLORDANE EMULSION CONCEN-TRATE Insecticide (Imperial Chem.)	Tech. chlordane* Aliphatic petroleum hydro-carbons*	45% 45%
IMPERIAL CLEANING FLUID (Hubbard Co.)	Petroleum*	
IMPERIAL CLEANSER Hand cleanser (Imperial Prod.)		
IMPERIAL COMPOUND, POWDER Cleanser (Imperial Prod.)		
IMPERIAL DAIRY & STOCK FLY SPRAY (Imperial Chem.)	Petroleum distillate Beta butoxy beta' thiocyano diethyl ether (Lethane 384)* Pyrethrins	

Name & Use Manufacturer	Ingredients	
IMPERIAL DRY INSECTICIDE (Imperial Chem.)	Naphthalene crude* Sulfur Creosote oil	22.5% 17.5% 1.0%
IMPERIAL HALFTONE INKS (General Printing)		
IMPERIAL LOTION Skin, scalp irritation (Bourland)	Each fl. oz.: Chloral hydrate* Alcohol Carbolic acid* Salicylic acid* Picric acid* Benzoic acid Synthetic oil of wintergreen* Glycerin	10 gr. 40%
IMPERIAL MULTI-PURPOSE BUG DUST (Imperial Chem.)	Rotenone Other cube resins Cuprous oxide Beta thiocyano ethyl esters of aliphatic fatty acids (10-18 carbon atoms from Lethane 60) Sulfur Inert ingredients	0.75% 1.87% 4.60% 0.75% 5.00%
IMPERIAL MULTI-PURPOSE HOME ORCHARD SPRAY Insecticide (Imperial Chem.)	Ferbam Sulfur* Tech. methoxychlor* (2,2-bis(p-methoxy phenyl)-1,1,1-trichloroethane 8.85%) Other isomers and related compounds DDD* 2-(p-tert-Butylphenoxy) isopropyl-2-chloroethyl sulfite	14.25% 15.00% 10.00% 1.15% 10.00% 1.50%
IMPERIAL MULTI-PURPOSE HOUSEHOLD INSECTICIDE (Imperial Chem.)	Petroleum distillates* Tech. chlordane 1068 Tech. piperonyl butoxide Pyrethrins	97.839% 2.000% 0.115% 0.046%
IMPERIAL PAINTS, COATINGS, ETC. (Imperial Floor.)		
IMPERIAL RAPID BRUSH CLEANER, ROLLER CLEANER & WATER RINSABLE REMOVER (Wilson-Imperial)		
IMPERIAL RED SPIDER DUST (Imperial Chem.)	Rotenone Cube resins Sulfur*	0.80% 1.00% 78.12%

*Consult Sec. II., Ingredients Index. This ingredient may be responsible for major toxic effects if poisonous amounts of this product are ingested.

Name & Use Manufacturer	Ingredients		Name & Use Manufacturer	Ingredients	
IMPERIAL RESIDUAL HOUSEHOLD INSECTICIDE (Imperial Chem.)	Petroleum distillates* Tech. chlordane 1068 Tech. piperonyl butoxide Pyrethrins	97.839% 2.000% 0.115% 0.046%	IMPROVED WAX OFF Wax remover (Glidden Co.)		
IMPERIAL RUSSE ESSENCE Toiletry (Assoc. Brands)			IMPROVED WONDER POWDER Cleanser (Puritan Chem.)		
			IMP PAINTS (Indust. Marine)		
IMPERIAL SODIUM FLUORIDE INSECTICIDES (Imperial Chem.)	Sodium fluoride*	90%	IMP SOOT DESTROYER (Foard)		
			IMRA Depilatory (Union Pharm.)	Calcium thioglycolate*	
IMPERIAL STANDARD DRY INSECTICIDE (Imperial Chem.)	Naphthalene* crude Sulfur Creosote oil	22.5% 17.5% 1.0%	IMUN IVY Allergen (Bullard)	Pure alcoholic* extr. rhus toxicodendron	
			IMUN OAK Allergen (Bullard)	Pure alcoholic extr. rhus diversiloba	
IMPERIAL SUPER SPOTTER (Hubbard Co.)			INCO GAS WELDING & BRAZING FLUX (Internat. Nickel)	Boric acid*	
IMPERIAL WARFARIN CONCEN- TRATE Rodenticide (Imperial Chem.)	Warfarin (3-(a-acetonylbenzyl)- 4-hydroxycoumarin) 0.5%				
			INCO 2 & 3 GAS WELDING FLUX (Internat. Nickel)	Fluorides* of alkaline and alkaline earth metals	
IMPERIAL WARFARIN READY MIX Rodenticide (Imperial Chem.)	Warfarin (3-(a-acetonylbenzyl)- 4-hydroxycoumarin) 0.025%		INCOLASTIC ROOF PAINT (Inter- Coastal)		
IMPERVO VARNISH (Moore, B.)			INCO PAINTS (Inter- Coastal)		
IMP-O TILE CLEANER (Imperial Prod.)			INCOTIN (Iodise)	Isopropyl alcohol* Methyl salicylate* Menthol* Camphor Capsicum Alcoholic soap base	23-1/2% 15% 15%
IMPROVED MECCA- LACS Cathartic (Foster- Dack)	Each pill: Extr. colocynth compound Extr. jalap Podophyllin* Leptandrin Extr. hyoscyamus* Extr. gentian* Oil peppermint Total alkaloids	0.065 gm. 0.0325 gm. 0.016 gm. 0.016 gm. 0.016 gm. q.s. q.s. 1/2600 gr.	INDELIBLO EXTERIOR COLD WATER PAINTS (Muralo)		
IMPROVED PRULEZE TABLETS Cathartic (Preston Labs.)	Methyl cellulose Prune concentrate Acetophenolisatin	400 mg. 100 mg. 2 mg.	INDEX READY MIXED PAINT (Bridges, Smith)		
IMPROVED TRI-BASIC TOOTH POWDER (Edison)	Sodium lauroyl sarcoside Galactono-lactone-carbamide Dibasic ammonium phosphate Sodium hexametaphosphate Chlorophyll sodium lauryl sulfate		INDIANAPOLIS FURNITURE POLISH (Indianapolis)	Petroleum naphtha* Tergital 4 (sodium alkyl sulfate)* Diglycol laurate Sassafras oil* Methylcellulose	

*Consult Sec. II., Ingredients Index. This ingredient may be responsible for major toxic effects if poisonous amounts of this product are ingested.

Name & Use Manufacturer	Ingredients
INDIANAPOLIS LACQUER THINNER (Indianapolis)	Butyl acetate Butyl alcohol Toluene* Xylene*
INDIANAPOLIS ODORLESS PAINT THINNER (Indianapolis)	Petroleum solvent*
INDIAN HEAD GASKET SHELLAC COMPOUND, HYDRAULIC BRAKE FLUID (Permatex)	Isopropyl alcohol*
INDIAN HERBS TABLETS Laxative (Estes)	Extr. cascara sagrada Extr. Indian rhubarb Aloes Oil of peppermint Podophyllin Oleoresin capsicum Aloin
INDIAN SAGE POMADE (Fearonce)	
INDICATOR STOP BATH, CONCEN-TRATED Photographic supply (Eastman)	
INDO LANOLINE SCALP CREAM (Fearonce)	
INDORLITE ENAMEL PAINT (Colonial Works)	
INDURO ENAMELS (Pratt Paint)	
INDUSTRIAL ALKALI, FLAKE Cleanser (Wyandotte)	Conc. alkali*
INDUSTRIAL MATERIALS COAL TAR DISIN-FECTANT (Indust. Mat.)	Coal tar neutral oils, soap, and phenols* 90%
INDUSTRIAL TERMITE LIQUID (Indust. Mat.)	Mineral oil Cresylic acid*
INECTO A Hair coloring (Sales)	Aminobenzene* Hydroxybenzene*

Name & Use Manufacturer	Ingredients
INECTO B Hair coloring (Sales)	Hydrogen peroxide* 20%
INFECTIOUS SCOUR TREATMENT Intestinal irritation (veterinary) (Franklin, O.M.)	Each fl. oz.: Sulfaguanidine* 15 gr. Sulfathiazole* 10 gr. Sulfamerazine* 5 gr. Kaolin 80 gr. Pectin 150 5 gr. Bismuth subcarbonate 5 gr. Methyl parahydroxybenzoate 0.18%
INFERNITE PAINTS (Sterling Varnish)	
INFRARUB Analgesic (Whitehall)	Methyl nicotinate Histamine dihydrochloride* Glycol monosalicylate* Capsicum oleoresin*
INFUCO CHLORDANE SPRAY Insecticide (Winru)	Tech. chlordane 2% Petroleum distillate* 98%
INFUCO 80-20 GRAIN FUMIGANT (Winru)	Carbon tetrachloride* 83.5% Carbon bisulfide* 16.5%
IN-2555 FUNGICIDE, IN-5499 FUNGICIDE (Du Pont)	Phenyl mercury oleate*
INFUSO SILVER POLISH (Lord)	
INGRAM SHAVING CREAM (Bristol-Myers)	Sodium and potassium stearates Coconut oil Glycerin or sorbitol Borax* Sodium chloride
INGRAM'S IQU For athlete's foot, super-ficial burns, insect bites (Willox)	Isopropyl alcohol* 49-1/2% Glycerin Creosote* Gum camphor*
INHALE-IT Decongestant (Binday)	Camphor* Menthol* Oil of eucalyptus*
INHALER FORTHANE Nasal de-congestant (Lilly)	Each inhaler: Methylhexamine* 250 mg. Menthol 32 mg. Aromatics q.s.
INHALER TUAMINE (Tuamino-heptane) Nasal decongestant (Lilly)	Each inhaler: 2-Amino-heptane* 325 mg. Menthol 32 mg. Aromatics q.s.

*Consult Sec. II., Ingredients Index. This ingredient may be responsible for major toxic effects if poisonous amounts of this product are ingested.

Name & Use Manufacturer	Ingredients		Name & Use Manufacturer	Ingredients	
INHIBITE PAINT (Debevoise)			INORGANIC BIOELEMENTS MONO CAL- CIUM PHOSPHATE STOCK FOOD GRADE (Inorganic Bioelements Inc.)	Calcium Phosphorus	17-18% 24%
INHISTON Antihistaminic (Union Pharm.)	Prophenpyridamine*				
INHISTON-APC Analgesic, antihistaminic (Union Pharm.)	Prophenpyridamine maleate* Aspirin* Acetophenetidin* Caffeine		INORGANIC BIOELEMENTS SOYA LECITHIN Dietary supplement (Inorganic)	Each tbsp.: Choline Inositol Phosphorus	250 mg. 250 mg. 225 mg.
INHISTON THROAT LOZENGE Antihistaminic (Union Pharm.)	Prophenpyridamine maleate* Acetophenetidin* Terpin hydrate Propesin		INOROUT VARNISH & ENAMEL (Wadsworth)		
INJECT-R- MYCIN Veterinary (Ralston)	Dihydrostreptomycin sulfate Penicillin G potassium Procaine penicillin G		INOSAN DROPS FOR HAY FEVER (Tablax)		
INK-OUT SINGLE FLUID Ink eradicator (Cardinell)			INOTON OINTMENT (Fougera)	Ammonium sulfoichthyolate* Extr. hamamelis Zinc oxide Sodium borate*	
INNER-AID LAXATIVE (Inner-Aid)	Aloe Sodium sulfate Cascara sagrada Buckthorn Senna Sodium phosphate		INRAY COUNTER- IRRITANT RUB (Vogarell)	Methyl salicylate* U.S.P. Menthol Oil of mustard Lanolin	
INNER CLEAN HERBAL LAXATIVE (Innerclean)	Agar Frangula Senna Psyllium seed		INSANCO DISINFEC- TANTS (Interstate San.)		
INNER-TONE Tonic (Inner-Tone)	Iron and ammonium citrate Riboflavin Stillingia Manganese sulfate Vitamin B6 Hydrochloric acid Caramel Niacin Thiamine hydrochloride Gentian Berberis Pantothenic acid Oil of orange Salicylic acid Saccharin		INSECOTE Insecticide (Holcomb)	Chlordane* DDT*	
			INSECT FOE Insect repellent (Pfeiffer)	Dimethyl phthalate 90.8% cis-Bicyclo-(2,2,1)-5-heptene- 2,3-dicarboxylic acid, dimethyl ester 4.6% Butyl dimethyl dihydro gamma pyrone carboxylate 4.6%	
INNIS, SPEIDEN LARVACIDE Fumigant (Innis)	Chloropicrin*(trichloro nitro methane)		INSECTISAN-5 Insecticide (Ampion)	Petroleum distillate Dichloro diphenyl trichloro- ethane* Isobornyl thiocyanoacetate* Other active terpenes	
INNIS, SPEIDEN LARVACIDE- 15 MIX Fumigant (Innis)	Chlorpicrin* 15% Carbon tetrachloride* 84.4%		INSECT-O BLITZ Insecticide (Blitz)	Terpene polychlorinates* (66% chlorine) 2.0% Tech. piperonyl butoxide 0.5% Pyrethrins 0.2% Petroleum distillates* 17.3%	
			INSECTOL INSECTICIDES (Clifton)		
			INSECT-OUT REPELLENT (Warren Chem.)	Dimethyl phthalate 60% Indolin 20% Ethyl hexanediol* 20%	

*Consult Sec. II., Ingredients Index. This ingredient may be responsible for major toxic effects if poisonous amounts of this product are ingested.

Name & Use Manufacturer	Ingredients		Name & Use Manufacturer	Ingredients	
INSECT SLAYER (Slayer)	Petroleum hydrocarbons* Chlordane* Pyrethrins*		INSTANT PAINT & VARNISH REMOVER (Chi-Namel)	Benzol*	more than 15%
INSECT SLAYER EMULCHLOR (Slayer)	Tech. chlordane* 46.00% Petroleum hydrocarbons* 43.50%		INSTANT VIGORO Fertilizer (Swift)	Nitrogen 19% Phosphoric acid 28% Potash 14%	
INSECT SLAYER MILL SPRAY (& Concentrate) (Slayer)	Petroleum distillates* Piperonyl butoxide tech. Pyrethrins		INSTANT WIPE General purpose cleaner (Lewal Ind.)		
INSECT SLAYER MOTH-PROOFER (Slayer)	Petroleum hydrocarbons* DDT* Gamma isomer of benzene hexachloride (from lindane)*		INSURED HOUSE PAINT (Warren Paint)		
INSECT SPRA DUST .75 ROTENONE Insecticide (Bonide)	Rotenone 0.75% Other cube resins 1.50% Inert ingredients 97.75%		INTERCLUB RACING BRONZE COPPER PAINT (Internat. Paint)	Copper bronze powder Pine tar* Denatured alcohol*	
INSEKIL 100 Insecticide (Holcomb)	Pyrethrins* Piperonyl butoxide Methoxychlor*		INTERCOTE CASEIN PASTE PAINT (Nat'l Chem. & Mfg.)		
INSILITE PAINT (Glidden Co.)			INTERLAC PAINT (Internat. Paint)	Mineral spirits Xylol*	
INSL-X PAINTS (Insl-X)			INTERLUX ENAMELS (Internat. Paint)	Mineral spirits* Pigments*	
INSOLA PRIMER For metallic coating Paint (Acorn Ref.)			INTERNATIONAL HOG POWDER (Internat. Stock)	Wormseed Quassia Epsom salts Areca nuts* Glauber's salt Iron sulfate	
INSO WITE COLD WATER PAINT (Tamms)			INTERNATIONAL POULTRY POWDER (Internat. Stock)	Kamala Gentian 1% Wormseed Capsicum* Areca nuts* Nux vomica* 2% Oil of Chenopodium 2% Powdered tobacco* Manganese sulfate Powdered sulfur*	
INSTANT BARBO NO. 1, 2, 3 Hair dyes (Barbo)	Coal tar product				
INSTANT CLEAN GLASS WASHER (Hoag-Farmer)					
INSTANT DIP (Lewal Ind.)			INTERNATIONAL SILVER POLISH (Internat.)		
INSTANT FELS NAPHTHA Soap powder (Fels)					
INSTANT NON-INFLAMM-ABLE PAINT & VARNISH REMOVER (Chi-Namel)	Chlorinated hydrocarbon*				

*Consult Sec. II., Ingredients Index. This ingredient may be responsible for major toxic effects if poisonous amounts of this product are ingested.

- 595 -

Name & Use Manufacturer	Ingredients	Name & Use Manufacturer	Ingredients
INTERNATIONAL STOCK TONIC (Internat. Stock)	Nux vomica* 1.50% Gentian Quassia Sodium nitrate Charcoal Calcium phosphate Salt Irradiated yeast Dried whey solubles Fish liver and glandular meal Calumba Foenugreek Soda bicarbonate Copperas Steam bone meal Calcium carbonate Potassium iodide Soybean oil meal Dried milk by-products Niacin Riboflavin Thiamine Choline Pantothenic acid	IODENT Toothpaste (Iodent)	
		IODEX Antiseptic ointment (Menley & James)	Mono-iodo-oleic acid*
		IODEX CUM METHYL SALICYLATE Counter-irritant, antiseptic (Menley & James)	Mono-iodo-oleic acid* Oil of wintergreen* (synthetic) Petrolatum base
INTEROL (Morgan Prod.)	Mineral oil	IODIZED OINTMENT, STAINLESS, N.F. Antiseptic, counter-irritant (Massengill)	Iodine* 5%
INTERSTATE LOUSE POWDER (Interstate Med.)	Pyrethrum* Cube resin of derris Talcum	IODOBOR Antiseptic (Iodobor)	Iodine-boric acid powder*
INTER-TOX WOOD PRE-SERVATIVE (Internat. Paint)	Petroleum distillate* 67.4% Copper naphthenate* (copper as metal 3%) 30.4%	IODO-NUCLEOID (Dinet)	Iodine* 21.5%
INTESTINAL CORRECTIVE (Jenkins)	Each tablet: Calomel* 1/50 gr. Zinc sulfocarbolate 1/16 gr. Salol* 1/8 gr. Bismuth subnitrate 1/2 gr. Magnesium carbonate 1/2 gr. Pancreatin 1/8 gr. Papain 1/16 gr. Oil of anise q.s.	I-ODORAL MEDICATED POWDER For skin (I-Odoral)	Talcum Boric acid* Methyl salicylate* Salicylic acid* Zinc oxide Calomel* 1% Thymol-iodide*
IN-TES-TROL Intestinal medication (veterinary) (Pratt Food)	Methylrosanilin (gentian violet)* Lactic acid Ferrous sulfate (Copperas) Copper sulfate* (hydrated) 11% Zinc sulfate* Isopropyl alcohol 10%/v	I-ODORAL OINTMENT For skin (Royal Pharm.)	Calomel* 5% Zinc oxide Thymol-iodide* Petrolatum
		I-ODORAL SKIN EASE BALM (I-Odoral)	Methyl salicylate* Camphor* Menthol Oil of eucalyptus*
INTRADERM TYROTHRICIN SOLUTION For skin (Wallace)	Each ml.: Tyrothricin U.S.P. 1.0 mg. Sodium ethyl mercuri thiosalicylate 1-40,000	IODOSYL 6% Antiseptic ointment (Nelson Barker)	Iodine* Salicylic acid*
INTRIGUE EAU DE TOILETTE (Blanchard)		IONCOP Tonic (Massengill)	Each fl. oz.: Strychnine sulfate* 32 mg. Copper acetate* 8 mg. Cobalt sulfate* 32 mg. Tinct. gentian 6 cc. Tinct. iron citrochloride 4.8 cc.
INVISIBLE RAINCHEK Water-proofing agent (Protection)	Inert water-repellent ingredients or solids Petroleum solvents*	IOPHENE Nasal spray, gargle (Meyer Bros.)	Phenol* Iodine* Menthol* Sodium bicarbonate
IODASE Iodine remover (Greenville)	Sodium thiosulfate*	I-O-SAL Fungicide (medical) (Atlas Labs.)	Alcohol* 87% Iodine* 1% Potassium iodide 2% Salicylic acid* 5%

*Consult Sec. II., Ingredients Index. This ingredient may be responsible for major toxic effects if poisonous amounts of this product are ingested.

Name & Use Manufacturer	Ingredients		Name & Use Manufacturer	Ingredients	
IOSALEX Ointment (Pitman- Moore)	Iodine* Oleic acid and methyl salicylate*	5% 10%	I.P.T 1% GAMMA B.H. C. DUST Insecticide (Thomas, I.)	Gamma isomer of benzene hexachloride* Other isomers of benzene hexachloride Inert ingredients	1.0% 6.6% 92.4%
IOSALINE Rubefacient, colds bites (Iosaline)	Alcohol * Menthol* Methyl salicylate* Iodine salt* Alcohol base	70%	I.P.T. 1% LINDANE-6% DITHANE Z-78 Fungicide, insecticide (Thomas, I.)	Gamma isomer of benzene hexachloride* lindane 1.0% Zineb Inert ingredients	3.9% 95.1%
IOSEPTIC Antiseptic (Jenkins)	Iodine* Methyl salicylate (synthetic) Eucalyptus oil	5% 7-1/2% 1%	I.P.T. LINDANE DUST Insecticide (Thomas, I.)	Gamma isomer of benzene hexachloride* lindane 1% Inert ingredients*	99%
IPANA TOOTH PASTE (Bristol- Myers)	Dicalcium phosphate Glycerin or sorbitol Gum Sodium lauryl sulfate Sodium benzoate Saccharin		I.P.T. 10% MARLATE Insecticide (Thomas, I.)	Methoxychlor tech. Inert ingredients	5% 95%
IPA OINTMENT For skin (I.P.A.)	Ammoniated mercury* 5% Benzocaine Resorcin Carbolic acid 1/2% Benzoinated petroleum base Zinc oxide Bismuth subnitrate Carmine coloring		I.P.T. POTATO DUST Fungicide, insecticide (Thomas,I.)	Copper* (copper sulfate) as metallic) DDT Inert ingredients	7.00% 3.00% 90.00%
			I.P.T. 40% RYANIA DUST Insecticide (Thomas, I.)	Powdered stem of Ryania speciosa*	40%
I.P.T. BEAN DUST (With C.P.R.S) Insecticide (Thomas, I.)	Tech. piperonyl cyclonene 0.50% Pyrethrins 0.05% Rotenone 0.25% Other cube extractives 0.50% Sulfur* 25.00% Inert ingredients 73.70%		I.P.T. TOMATO DUST Insecticide (Thomas, I.)	Tricalcium arsenate* 14.00% Copper (copper sulfate) as metallic 7.00% Arsenic (as metallic) 5.20% Arsenic (water-soluble as metallic) 0.49%	
I.P.T. 5% CHLORDANE DUST Insecticide (Thomas, I.)	Tech. chlordane* Inert ingredients	5.0% 95.0%	I.P.T. TOMATO DUST (Special) Insecticide (Thomas, I.)	Tricalcium arsenate* 14.00% Zinc dimethyldithiocarbamate 7.00% Arsenate (as metallic) 5.20% Arsenic (as metallic) 0.49%	
I.P.T CORN DUST Insecticide (Thomas, I.)	DDD Inert ingredients	5.00% 95.00%	I.P.T. TOMATO HORNWORM DUST Insecticide (Thomas, I.)	Tricalcium arsenate* 20.00% Copper aceto-arsenite 0.85% Copper (basic copper sulfate)* 7.00% Arsenic (as metallic) 5.20% Arsenic (water-soluble as metallic) 0.49%	
I.P.T. C.P.R. ZINEB DUST Fungicide, insecticide (Thomas, I.)	Zinc ethylene bisdithio- carbamate (Metallic zinc content 0.92%) 3.90% Tech. piperonyl cyclonene 0.50% Pyrethrins 0.05% Rotenone 0.25% Other cube extractives 0.50% Inert ingredients 94.80%		I.P.T. TOMATO INSECT DUST (Thomas, I.)	Tricalcium arsenate* 14.00% Arsenic (as metallic) 5.20% Arsenic (water-soluble as metallic) 0.49%	
I.P.T. 5% DDT DUST Insecticide (Thomas, I.)	Dichloro diphenyl trichloro- ethane* 5.00% Inert ingredients 95.00%		I.P.T. 10% TOXAPHENE DUST Insecticide (Thomas, I.)	Toxaphene* (tech. chlorinated camphene 10%	
I.P.T. DITHANE DUST WITH DDT Fungicide, insecticide (Thomas, I.)	Zinc ethylene bisditho- carbamate (metallic zinc content 0.92%) 3.9% Dichloro diphenyl trichloro- ethane 3.0%		I.P.T. TRUCK & GARDEN DUST Insecticide (Thomas, I.)	Tech. piperonyl cyclonene 0.50% Pyrethrins 0.05% Rotenone 0.25% Other cube extractives 0.50% Inert ingredients 98.70%	
I.P.T. DITHANE RHOTHANE DUST Fungicide, insecticide (Thomas, I.)	Zinc ethylene-bis (dithio- carbamate) 3.9% Dichloro diphenyl dichloro- ethane 5% Inert ingredients 91.1%		I.P.T Z DUST Fungicide (Thomas,I.)	Zinc dimethyl dithio carbamate* 7.00% Inert ingredients 93.00%	

*Consult Sec. II., Ingredients Index. This ingredient may be responsible for major toxic effects if poisonous amounts of this product are ingested.

- 597 -

Name & Use Manufacturer	Ingredients	Name & Use Manufacturer	Ingredients
IQUISINE Iron tonic, stimulant (Massengill)	Each 5 cc.: Quinine sulfate 40 mg. Strychnine phosphate* 1.3 mg. Tinct. iron citrochloride 0.5 cc.	**IRTEX** For skin irritation (Premo)	Acid salicylic* Acid benzoic Benzocaine Sulfur* Carbolic acid* Lanolin Petrolatum
IRECOTINE CONCEN- TRATE (Liquid) Veterinary (Strasenburgh)	Arecoline hydrobromide Copper sulfate Nicotine sulfate* Iron sulfate Manganese citrate	**I-SEDRIN PLAIN** Nasal decongestant (Lilly)	Ephedrine alkaloid* 1% Gluconic acid Chlorobutanol (chloroform deriv.) 0.5% Dextrose
IREX Iron tonic (Friendly Labs.)	Ferric chloride*	**ISLAND MIST COLOGNE DEODORANT** (Tattoo)	
IREX TABS Dietary supplement (Friendly Labs.)	Yeast Ferrous carbonate Thiamine chloride Copper peptonate*	**ISO-PAR** Ointment Counter- irritant (Medical Chem. Inc.)	Iso-par (coparaffinate) (14% isoparaffinic acids) 17% Cetyl alcohol Beeswax Titanium dioxide Lanolin Petrolatum
IR HAIR REMOVING LOTION (Jordeau)		**ISOPHRIN** Nasal decongestant (Broemmel)	Isophrin (phenylephrine) hydrochloride* 0.25%
IROCITE HULL PAINT (Internat. Rust.)		**ISOPTO FRIN** Ophthalmic solution (Alcon)	Phenylephrine hydrochloride 1/8% Methyl cellulose base
IRON CLAD PAINTS (Moore, B.)		**ISOTHAN Q-15** Fungicide (Onyx)	Lauryl isoquinolinium bromide* 20%
IRON-GARD SYSTEM METAL PAINTS & PRIMERS (Detroit)		**ISOTOX 20 CONCEN- TRATE** Insecticide (Calif. Spray)	Lindane* 20%
IRON GLUE (McCormick)	Protein 50%		
IRONIZED YEAST Dietary supplement (Centaur- Caldwell)	Adult dose (6 tablets): Ferrous sulfate* 5.25 gr. Vitamin B1 2.25 mg.	**ISOTOX DAIRY SPRAY** Insecticide (Calif. Spray)	Lindane * 25%
IRON KOTE BLACK ENAMEL (Johnston)		**ISOTOX-DDT 1-5 DUST** Insecticide (Calif. Spray)	Lindane* 1% DDT* 5%
IRONSIDE PAINT (Thompson & Co.)		**ISOTOX-DDT 1.5-5 DUST** Insecticide (Calif. Spray)	DDT* 5% Lindane* 1.5%
IROQUOIS WHITE PAINT (McDougall- Butler)		**ISOTOX DUST NO. 1** Insecticide (Calif. Spray)	Lindane* 1% Inert ingredients
		ISOTOX DUST NO. 1.5 Insecticide (Calif. Spray)	Lindane* 1.5% Inert ingredients
IRRIGOL Douche powder (Alkalol)	Sodium sulfocarbolate Sodium bicarbonate Sodium borate* Salt Thymol* Eucalyptol* Menthol*	**ISOTOX DUST NO. 2** Insecticide (Calif. Spray)	Lindane* 2% Inert ingredients

*Consult Sec. II., Ingredients Index. This ingredient may be responsible for major toxic effects if poisonous amounts of this product are ingested.

Name & Use Manufacturer	Ingredients		Name & Use Manufacturer	Ingredients	
ISOTOX GARDEN DUST Insecticide (Calif. Spray)	Lindane*	1.5%	ISOTOX-S 2-50 DUST Insecticide (Calif. Spray)	Lindane* Sulfur*	2% 50%
ISOTOX 5 GRANULAR Insecticide (Calif. Spray)	Lindane*	5%	ISOTOX 25 SEED TREATER (Calif. Spray)	Lindane* Captan (n-trichloro methyl mercapto-4-cyclohexene-1, 2-dicarboximide)	25% 12.5%
ISOTOX-K 1-5 DUST Insecticide, fungicide (Calif. Spray)	Gamma isomer of benzene hexachloride (from lindane) 1% Copper* expressed as metallic 5%		ISOTOX 75 SEED TREATER (Calif. Spray)	Lindane*	75%
ISOTOX-K 1-25 DUST Insecticide, fungicide (Calif. Spray)	Lindane Copper* Zinc*	1% 4.5% 4.5%	ISOTOX SPERGON 1 SEED TREATER (Calif. Spray)	Lindane* Tetrachloro parabenzoquinone*	10.5% 82%
ISOTOX-K 1.5-6.8 DUST Insecticide, fungicide (Calif. Spray)	Lindane* Copper*	1.5% 6.8%	ISOTOX- SPERGON 2 SEED TREATER (Calif. Spray)	Lindane* Tetrachloro parabenzoquinone*	30% 57%
ISOTOX-K 1-7 DUST Insecticide, fungicide (Calif. Spray)	Lindane Copper*	1% 7%	ISOTOX 1 SPRAY Insecticide (Calif. Spray)	Lindane Aromatic petroleum deriv. solvent*	12.9% 80.3%
ISOTOX-K DUST NO. 10-68 Insecticide, fungicide (Calif. Spray)	Gamma isomer of benzene hexachloride (from lindane) 1.0% Copper* (as metallic) 6.8%		ISOTOX SPRAY NO. 200 Insecticide (Calif. Spray)	Lindane*	20%
ISOTOX LINDANE SPRAY Insecticide (Calif. Spray)	Aromatic petroleum deriv. solvent* 83.9%* Lindane 12.9%		ISOTOX TRANS- PLANTER SOLUTION (Calif. Spray)	Lindane*	5%
ISOTOX LINDANE SPRAY WETTABLE Insecticide (Calif. Spray)	Lindane*	12.5%	ISOTOX WETTABLE NO. 25 Insecticide (Calif. Spray)	Lindane*	25%
ISOTOX LIQUID DAIRY SPRAY Insecticide (Calif. Spray)	Lindane*	20%	ISOTOX- ZINEB 1.5-3. 25 DUST Insecticide, fungicide (Calif. Spray)	Lindane Zineb (zinc ethylene bis-dithiocarbamate (as metallic) Inert ingredients*	1.5% 3.25% 0.77%
ISOTOX 50 PASTE SEED TREATER (Calif. Spray)	Lindane*	50%	ISOTOX- ZINEB 1.5-4 DUST Insecticide, fungicide (Calif. Spray)	Lindane Zineb (zinc ethylene-bis-dithiocarbamate* Inert ingredients	1.5% 4%
ISOTOX PMA SEED TREATER (Calif. Spray)	Lindane* 45% Phenyl mercuric acetate* 1.68% Mercury (as elemental) 1.0%		ISOTOX- ZINEB 1-6 DUST Insecticide, fungicide (Calif. Spray)	Lindane Zineb (zinc ethylene-bis-dithiocarbamate* Inert ingredients	1% 6%
ISOTOX-S DUST NO. 1-50 Insecticide (Calif. Spray)	Sulfur* Lindane	50% 1%	ISOTOX- ZINEB-S 1-3.25-25 DUST Insecticide, fungicide (Calif. Spray)	Lindane Zineb Sulfur* Inert ingredients	1% 3.25% 25%
ISOTOX-S DUST NO. 1.5-50 Insecticide (Calif. Spray)	Sulfur* Lindane*	50% 1.5%			

*Consult Sec. II., Ingredients Index. This ingredient may be responsible for major toxic effects if poisonous amounts of this product are ingested.

Name & Use Manufacturer	Ingredients	Name & Use Manufacturer	Ingredients
ITALIAN BALM Skin softener (Campana)	Essential oils* Alcohol Phenol* Benzoic acid* Gum tragacanth Glycerin Sorbitol	IVANHOE HAIR STAY (Fearonce)	
ITALINA Laxative (Floret)	Phenolphthalein* Cane sugar Milk sugar Sodium bicarbonate Tartaric acid Citric acid	IVAR MEN'S AFTER SHAVE LOTION, EAU DE COLOGNE (Assoc. Brands)	
ITCH-A-WAY Dog, cat remedy (Jamaica)		IVCO PAINTS (Impervious)	
ITCH-ME-NOT Fungicide, keratolytic (medical) (Sorbol)	Alcohol* 86% Benzocaine Tannic acid Camphor* Phenol* Benzoic acid Salicylic acid*	IVORY BAR, FLAKES, SNOW Soap (Procter & Gamble)	Animal and vegetable fats
ITCH-STICK Itch reliever (Evans Dep.)		IVORY KOTE WALL PAINT (Johnston)	
ITCH-TONE (Delancey)		IVY-CHEK For skin irritations (Rexall)	Alcohol 21% Sol. chloride of iron Dimeric alkylated aryl (poly- ether alcohol 2%
ITCH WITCH FOR YOUR DOG Fungicide, ectoparasiti- cide (vet- erinary) (House of Huston)	Bis-(5-chloro-2-hydroxyphenyl)- methane 1.00% Gamma isomer of benzene hexachloride (from lindane) 0.10% Sodium carboxy methylcellulose 0.50% Isopropanol* 45.50%	IVYCIDE Counter- irritant (Russell, A.)	Zirconium oxide 8% Hexachlorophene 0.5%
I-TONE EYE DROPS (Purepac)	Antipyrine 0.4% Boric acid* Borax* Ephedrine sulfate 0.1% Camphor*	IVY-KIL Herbicide (Lethelin)	Isooctyl ester 2,4-dichloro phenoxy acetic acid* 7.68% Isooctyl ester 2,4,5-trichloro phenoxy acetic acid* 7.32%
I-TONE EYE LOTION (Purepac)	Antipyrine 0.4% Boric acid* Borax*	IVY-MAN For poison ivy, oak (Pedrick)	Grindelia Camphor* Calamine Eucalyptus oil* Oxyquinoline sulfate* Lobelia* Menthol* Zinc oxide* Aluminum silicate
IT SHOE CREAM & KID LOTION (It)		IVY-OFF (Ivy-Off)	
ITSO INSECT KILLER (Red Label) (Capitol Chem.)	Petroleum distillate* (Ultrasene) Tech. piperonyl butoxide Pyrethrins Gamma isomer of benzene hexachloride (from lindane)*	IVY-X For poison ivy, oak (Binday)	Tannic acid* Phenol 1/2% Sodium thiosulfate
ITSO INSECT KILLER (Yellow Label) (Capitol Chem.)	Petroleum distillate* Tech. piperonyl butoxide Pyrethrins*	IVY-X TABLETS Antipruritic (Prescript. Pharm.)	Pyranisamine maleate* 25 mg.
IT STICK SUEDE CLEANER (It)		I.W.P. WATER- PROOFING MATERIAL (Imperial Floor.)	
		I.X. FLEXIBLE GLUE (Gane)	

*Consult Sec. II., Ingredients Index. This ingredient may be responsible for major toxic effects if poisonous amounts of this product are ingested.

Name & Use Manufacturer	Ingredients	Name & Use Manufacturer	Ingredients
IXL LIGHTER FLUID (Hollingshead)	VM & P naphtha* almost 100%	JACK WILSON PELLETIZED IPC-10 Herbicide (Wilson, Jack)	Isopropyl-n-phenyl carbamate* 10%
IZAL COAL TAR DISINFECTANT (Kennedy)	Phenol* 40%	JACK WILSON 2,4-D AMINE WEED KILLER (Wilson, Jack)	Alkanolamine salts 2,4-dichloro-phenoxyacetic acid*
IZOL Eye irritations (Thomas, W.G.)	Boric acid* Chlorobutanol* Camphor water Zinc sulfate* Salt	JACK WILSON 2,4-D LIQUID WEED KILLER (Wilson, Jack)	Isopropanolamine salts 2,4-dichlorophenoxyacetic acid*
JAC-FROST CREAMERY ENAMELS (Frost Paint)		JACK WILSON 2,4,5-T WEED KILLER (Wilson, Jack)	Isopropyl ester 2,4,5-trichloro-phenoxyacetic acid*
JACK CARBON SOLVENT COMPOUNDS (Zip Abr.)		JACK WILSON WEED KILLER 99 (Wilson, Jack)	Trichloroacetic acid* Aromatic oil* Pentachlorophenol*
JACK RABBIT SEMI-PASTE REMOVER (Davis, H.B.)	Benzol* Wax Acetone	JACK WILSON WESTERN 2,4-D WEED KILLER (Wilson, Jack)	Sodium salt 2,4-D monohydrate*
JACKS DRASOL Drain cleaner (Jacks)	Sodium hydroxide*	JA-GO-DA FACE CREAM (Mentho-Listine)	Ammoniated mercury* 5%
JACKSON'S SCALP CREAM Rubefacient (Jackson, E.B.)	Mutton tallow Sulfur* Turpentine* Oil eucalyptus* Petrolatum Tinct. cantharides* Perfume	JANICE COSMETICS (Allan)	
JACKS SEPTIK TANK CLEANER (Jacks)	Sodium hydroxide*	JANNEY BEST PAINTS & ENAMELS (Janney)	
JACK WILSON EMULSIFIABLE IPC 24 Herbicide (Wilson, Jack)	Isopropyl-n-phenyl carbamate* 24%	JANNEY BEST VARNISHES (Janney)	
JACK WILSON IPC CONCEN-TRATE Herbicide (Wilson Jack)	Isopropyl-n-phenyl carbamate* 41%	JAPALAC ALUMINUM READY MIXED Paint (Glidden Co.)	
JACK WILSON PELLETIZED CHLORO IPC-10 Herbicide (Wilson, Jack)	Isopropyl-n-(3-chlorophenyl) carbamate* 10%	JAPALAC ENAMELS, VARNISHES, STAINS (Glidden Co.)	

---

*Consult Sec. II., Ingredients Index. This ingredient may be responsible for major toxic effects if poisonous amounts of this product are ingested.

Name & Use Manufacturer	Ingredients	Name & Use Manufacturer	Ingredients
JAPALAC GRAINING COMPOUND (Glidden)		JAY DRY COLORS, OIL COLORS (Jaye)	
JAPANESE FURNITURE POLISH (Techno Chem.)		JAYE PATCHING CEMENT, PLASTIC CEMENT, ROOFING CEMENT (Jaye)	
JAPELIENT Insecticide (Doggett- Pfeil)	DDT* Chlordane*	JAYNE'S P-W VERMIFUGE (Centaur- Caldwell)	Gentian violet*
JAPIDE Insecticide (Bonide)	Dichloro diphenyl trichloro-ethane* 44% Tech. chlordane 6%	J.B. OIL LINIMENT (Bretocol)	
JAPONEX Insecticide (Hydroponic)		JEALOUSY BOUQUET CONCEN-TRATE, BOUQUET STICK, BRILLIAN-TINE, DEODOR-ANT, PER-FUME & SACHET (Blanchard)	
JARMANS SCALP TREATMENT (Lester Drug)	Castor oil Capsicum Cantharides* Resorcin* Aromatic oils Alcohol		
JASMIN DE CORSE LINE EXTRACT (Coty)			
JASON CHALK CRAYONS (Hershkowitz)		JEAN GAIL APPLE BLOSSOM PERFUMES (Gail)	
JATAMANSI HAIR DRESSING (Washington Hom.)		JEANNE MAURAY LOTIONS, COLOGNES, DEODORANT CREAM, NAIL POLISH, POWDER (Howell Co.)	
JAUNTY COLOGNE & PERFUME (Miahati)			
JAVARE HAIR TONIC (Coulter)		JEAN NOLAN HAND CREAM (Nelson, Detroit)	
JAVELIN COLOGNE, PERFUME, TOILET WATER (Duvelle)	Denatured alcohol* (denatured with diethyl phthalate)	JEBCOLAC ENAMELS, VARNISHES (Bauer, J.E.)	
JAYBRA HAIR RINSE (Jaybra)		JEFFERY'S #1 and #7 Glues (Ferdinand)	Resins in solid form
JAYBRA HAIR STRAIGHT-ENER (Jaybra)		JEFFERY'S C QUALITY Glue (Ferdinand)	Resins Alcohol
JAY CLAY CHALK (Hershkowitz)		JEFFERY'S MARINE GLUES (Ferdinand)	
JAYE CAULKING COMPOUND (Jaye)		JEFFERY'S #2 SHIP GLUE (Ferdinand)	Asphalt Resins in solid form

*Consult Sec. II., Ingredients Index. This ingredient may be responsible for major toxic effects if poisonous amounts of this product are ingested.

Name & Use Manufacturer	Ingredients	Name & Use Manufacturer	Ingredients
JEMS CLAY CHALK (Hershkowitz)		JET AIROSOL Insecticide (Airosol)	DDT* Petroleum* Pyrethrins* Piperonyl butoxide tech.
JENKINS ANTACID SPECIAL NO. 1 (Jenkins)	Each tablet: Magnesium carbonate 3 gr. Calcium carbonate 2 gr. Bismuth subcarbonate 1 gr. Cerium oxalate 1/2 gr.	JET CONCEN-TRATED RESIDUAL MILL SPRAY Insecticide (Adco)	Petroleum distillate* (Butyl carbityl) (6-propyl piperonyl) ether and related compounds Pyrethrins*
JENKINS ANTACID SPECIAL NO. 2 (Jenkins)	Each tablet: Magnesium carbonate 3 gr. Calcium carbonate 2 gr. Bismuth subcarbonate 1 gr. Cerium oxalate 1/2 gr. Atropine sulfate 1/1000 gr.	JET EAU de TOILETTE, JET FOR JENTLEMEN, PERFUME (Parfums Corday)	
JENKINS COLD AND FEVER TABLETS (Jenkins)	Each tablet: Tinct. eupatorium* 1/4 m. Tinct. gelsemium* 1/4 m. Tinct. aconite* 1/4 m. Tinct. bryonia 1/4 m. Camphor monobromated* 1/10 gr.	JET INSECT KILLER (Airosol)	Petroleum distillates* 97.638% Tech. chlordane 1068 2.000% Allethrin (allyl homolog of cinerin 1) 0.046% n-Octyl bicycloheptene di-carboximide 0.200% iso-Octyl phenoxy polyethoxy ethanol 0.100% Phenyl mercuric lactate 0.016%
JENKINS TONIC ELIXIR Nerve tonic (Jenkins)	Iron glycerophosphate 4 gr. Calcium glycerophosphate 4 gr. Sodium glycerophosphate 4 gr. Quinine glycerophosphate* 1 gr. Strychnine phosphate* 1/10 gr.	JET LIGHTER FUEL (Dryco)	
JERGENS LOTION Hand cream (Jergens)		JET POWDER INSECT KILLER (Airsol)	Dichloro diphenyl trichloro-ethane 2.00% Pyrethrins 0.02% Allethrin (allyl homolog of cinerin 1) 0.08% Beta butoxy beta thiocyano diethyl ether 1.00% n-Octyl bicycloheptene dicarboximide 0.50% Methylated aromatic petroleum deriv.* 7.00% Petroleum distillates 9.40%
JERIS ANTISEPTIC HAIR TONIC (Jeris)	8-Hydroxyquinoline* Resorcinol monoacetate* Tinct. capsicum Fixed and volatile oils* Ethyl alcohol		
JERMAX, JERMAX MEDICATION Vaginal douche (Clo-Fill)	Oxyquinoline* sulfate Lactic acid Borosalicylic acid* Thymol*	JET NO. 711 Carburetor, metal cleaner (Troy Ind.)	Chlorinated hydrocarbons* Phenolic bodies* Volatile solvents
JERMAX QDC TABLET FORMULA Douche solution (Clo-Fill)	Sodium laurylsulfate Eucalyptol* Thymol* Chlorophyllins Oxyquinoline benzoate*	JEWEL'S DRAIN CLEANER (Jewel Tea)	Sodium hydroxide*
JERMAX VDC TABLETS Douche solution (Clo-Fill)	Alkyl aryl sulfonate* Tetrasodium pyrophosphate* Oxyquinoline sulfate*	JEWEL'S BOWL CLEANER & DEODORANT (Jewel Tea)	Soda bisulfate*
JERSEY BALM Rubefacient, (Reed, L.L.)	Oil of wormwood Oil of sassafras* Oil of wintergreen* (synthetic) Oil of peppermint Oil of cedarwood Linseed oil	JEWEL WAX POLISH & FLOOR CLEANER (Fromeyer)	
JESTADE Antacid (Burrough)	Small tablets: Sodium bicarbonate Capsicum Hydrastis Large tablets: Bismuth subnitrate Magnesium carbonate Pepsin Ginger Diastase	JIFFIX Photo developer (Mallinckrodt)	Ammonium thiosulfate*
		JIFFY CORN PLASTERS (J. R. Co.)	Salicylic acid* Extract belladonna alkaloids 0.044%

*Consult Sec. II., Ingredients Index. This ingredient may be responsible for major toxic effects if poisonous amounts of this product are ingested.

Name & Use Manufacturer	Ingredients		Name & Use Manufacturer	Ingredients	
JIFFY FOOT POWDER (J. R. Co.)	Eucalyptus oil* Boric acid powder* Zinc stearate		JOCKEY CLUB PERFUMES, COLOGNES, TOILET WATER (Caswell- Massey)		
JIFFY LINOLEUM RENEWER (Felton Sibley)			JOCUR WAVESETS (Whitehall)		
JIFFY-NAMEL ENAMELS (Felton Sibley)			JODIRENAN Inhalent (Radin)	Epinephrine Iodine* Sodium iodide* Glycerin	
JIFFY PAINT & VARNISH CLEANER (Miner- Hillard)			JOGEN HAIR DRESSING (Crescent Pharm.)		
JIFFY SPOT REMOVER (Zanol)			JOHNSON BROMIDE LIQUID Photographic developer (General Photo.)		
JIFFY TYPE- WRITER TYPE CLEANER (Gies)			JOHNSON'S ANT KILLER (J. A. K.)	Sodium arsenate* Lead arsenate*	1.3% 1.4%
JIFFY-WAY EGG CLEANER (Jiffy-Way)			JOHNSON'S BABY LOTION (Johnson & Johnson)	Mineral oil Lanolin Hexachlorophene (dihydroxy hexachloro diphenyl methane)	
JIGGER Astringent (insect bites) (Standard Medicines)	Alcohol Ether* Creosote* Carbolic acid* Coal oil* Chloroform* Oil of cloves Tinct. capsicum Oil of mirbane*	3.2% 15.6% 15.6%	JOHNSON'S BABY OIL (Johnson & Johnson)	Mineral oil Refined lanolin	
			JOHNSON'S BABY POWDER (Johnson & Johnson)	Italian talc	
JIM DANDY STOVE & TORCH FUEL (Modern Metal)			JOHNSON'S BABY SHAMPOO (Johnson & Johnson)		
JIM WADE FOOT MEDICINE (Wade)	Salicylic acid* Sucrose octaacetate Acetone* Alcohol*	 66%	JOHNSON'S BEAUTIFLOR Floor finisher (Johnson, S.C.)	Petroleum naphtha* Animal, vegetable and petroleum waxes	
JITTER BUG INSECT REPELLENT (Sayman)	Hydrogenated rotenone and other cube resins Terpeniol Secondary terpene alcohols* Inert ingredients*	 0.375% 7.500% 14.000% 78.125%	JOHNSON'S CAR-PLATE Automobile polish (Johnson, S.C.)	Petroleum naphtha* Petroleum waxes Silicone fluid	
J-K HAIR TONIC (Kirby's Mineral)			JOHNSON'S CAR-PLATE CLEANER Automobile cleaner (Johnson, S.C.)	Petroleum and vegetable oils* Powdered abrasives Petroleum naphtha*	
JNT Silver polish (J. N. T.)			JOHNSON'S CHROME CLEANER (Johnson, S.C.)	Petroleum oils* Powdered abrasives Alcohol solvents* Naphtha*	
J-O BUG LIQUID (Opitz)	DDT*				

*Consult Sec. II., Ingredients Index. This ingredient may be responsible for major toxic effects if poisonous amounts of this product are ingested.

Name & Use Manufacturer	Ingredients
JOHNSON'S CLEANER (Johnson's)	
JOHNSON'S CREAM WAX (Johnson, S.C.)	Petroleum naphtha* Petroleum waxes*
JOHNSON'S DEEP GLOSS CARNU Automobile polish (Johnson, S.C.)	Petroleum and vegetable oils Petroleum wax Powdered abrasives Petroleum naphtha*
JOHNSON'S FOOT SOAP (Gill, T.)	Borax* Iodine* Bran
JOHNSON'S GLO-COAT Floor polish (Johnson, S.C.)	Synthetic resins Petroleum and vegetable waxes Emulsifying agents*
JOHNSON'S HARD GLOSS GLO-COAT Floor polish (Johnson, S.C.)	Natural and synthetic resins Petroleum waxes Emulsifying agents*
JOHNSON'S HEAVY-DUTY CLEANER (Johnson, S.C.)	Powdered abrasives Petroleum oils* Alcohol solvents* Naphtha*
JOHNSON'S JUBILEE KITCHEN WAX (Johnson, S.C.)	Petroleum naphtha* Emulsifying agents* Petroleum waxes*
JOHNSON'S MAGIC LIQUID (Johnson Prod.)	
JOHNSON'S NO. 6088 Rubefacient, counter- irritant (Johnson, Matt.)	Each fl. oz.: Alcohol 5% Sodium salicylate* 40 gr. Potassium iodide 5 gr.
JOHNSON'S PASTE WAX (Johnson, S.C.)	Petroleum naphtha* Animal, vegetable and petroleum waxes
JOHNSON'S PRIDE Furniture polish (Johnson, S.C.)	Petroleum naphtha* Silicone fluid Petroleum waxes
JOHNSON'S SALVE For hemorrhoid irritation (Bodeker)	Petrolatum Beeswax Powdered camphor* Menthol* Spirits of gum turpentine* Resin Pine tar* Fluid extr. balm of Gilead buds
JOHNSTON'S SUPER NO- ROACH Insecticide (Johnston, Gaston)	Malathion*

Name & Use Manufacturer	Ingredients	
JOHN SUNSHINE PIPE JOINT COMPOUND, SPUD CEMENT (Sunshine)		
JOIE de VIVRE PERFUMES (Ybry)		
J-O INSECT POWDER (Opitz)	Pyrethrins*	
JOINT CEMENT (United Gilson.)	Casein Soya protein Hydrated lime* Soda ash* Inert fillers*	
JO-LAR PORCELAIN CEMENT (Johnson Prod.)		
JOLY LOTION For skin irritations, burns (Joly)	Chlorobutanol 0.5% Camphor* Isopropyl alcohol 10%/v Menthol* Oil of eucalyptus*	
JONCAIRE AIR SPRAY, PERFUME, TOILET WATER (Joncaire)		
JON JEL DEODORANT (Airline)		
JORDEAU COLOGNE DEODORANT (Jordeau)		
J-O ROACH- RAT PASTE (Opitz)	Phosphorus*	
JOT CREAMS, DOUBLE- PURPOSE ASTRINGENT, FACE POWDER, BLEMISH CORRECT, HAIR GROOM, LOTIONS, PRE- SCRIPTION FOR BRITTLE NAILS, FOR DANDRUFF, SHAMPOOS (Galen)		
JOY Detergent (Procter & Gamble)	Anionic synthetic detergent Aqueous ethyl alcohol Fatty acid amide	
JOYCE SHOE POLISH (Barr, G.)		

*Consult Sec. II., Ingredients Index. This ingredient may be responsible for major toxic effects if poisonous amounts of this product are ingested.

Name & Use Manufacturer	Ingredients		Name & Use Manufacturer	Ingredients	
JOY SOLVENT (Joy)	Trichlorethylene*		JUV-A-TON Tonic, food supplement (veterinary) (Lee)	Arsanilic acid * White mineral oil Bacitracin Vitamin B12 Niacin Manganese sulfate Potassium iodide* Rock phosphate Penicillin G Riboflavin Iron oxide Copper sulfate* Calcium sulfate Malted wheat bran and shorts	1% 1.8%
JOYTAN SUN CREME (Mother's)	Esters of anthranilic and salicylic acids*				
J.R. FOR ATHLETE'S FOOT (J. R. Pharm.)	Salicylic acid* Benzoic acid* Tannic acid * Phenol	1%			
J-R LIQUIDINE #4 Dietary supplement (Jamol)	Each 100 cc.: Iodine approx. 0.4 cc. Sodium iodide approx. 0.2 cc. Potassium iodide approx. 0.2 cc. Ammonium iodide approx. 0.2 cc.		KABA Cathartic (Battle Creek)	Karaya gum Dextrin Vegetable extracts Lactose Brewers yeast	
J-R ROMA-NOL For skin irritations (Jamol)	Iodine, free * Potassium iodide*	0.8% 1.2%	KABINITE PAINTS (Am. Paint Corp.)		
JU-BERRY TABLETS Diuretic (Richards Bros.)	Concentrated extr. buchu, squill*, juniper, kava, cubeb Potassium nitrate Methylene blue Caffein		KABNET WAX (Harrison, A. S.)		
JUBILEE KITCHEN WAX (Johnson, S.C.)	Petroleum naphtha* Emulsifying agents Petroleum waxes		KABROK CEMENT (Nat'l Gypsum)		
JUMBO JUNIOR Bubble bath (Clark, R.)	Sodium sulfate Sodium alkyl aryl sulfonate* Sodium alkyl lauryl sulfonate*		KACTUS KOTE PAINT (Door-O-Western)		
JUNIOR CHEST RUB (Binday)	Camphor* Oil of eucalyptus* Menthol*		KADENTOL MOUTH WASH For irritations of mouth and throat (Mentho-Listine)	Phenol* Sodium benzoate Zinc sulfocarbolate Menthol* Eucalyptol* Boric acid* Alum Oil spearmint Thymol* Alcohol	
JUNO CLEANERS, DISIN-FECTANTS (Linco)					
JUST DISINFECTANT, DEODORANT (Assoc. Just)	Soap Orthobenzylparachlorophenol Isopropanol	14.0% 3.0% 3.0%	KAMOID PAINTS (Univ. Paint)		
JUSTRITE CHALKS & CRAYONS (Am. Art Clay)			KADMOLAC LACQUERS (Univ. Paint)		
JUST RITE HAIR DRESSING (Bailes)			KADOL External fungicide, astringent, medical (Kadol)	Oil of cade * Oxide of zinc Petrolatum base Salicylic acid* Bismuth subnitrate	
JUST WONDERFUL CREME WAVE LOTION (Richards, C.)	Ammonium thioglycolate with ammonia water* (pH 8.5-9.42) approx. 1-1/2-6%		KA-DON (Berjon)	Bismuth subsalicylate* Salol Zinc phenolsulfonate*	
JUVARE AFTER SHAVE LOTION, COLOGNE (Coulter)			KALASEP LOTION For skin irritations (Lyons, I.L.)	Zinc oxide* Calomine Bentonite Lime Water Carbolic acid* Camphor* Menthol* Thymol*	

Name & Use Manufacturer	Ingredients
KA-LAX TABS Laxative (Sacramento)	
KALUDURA CALSOMINE Paint (Sterling Paint)	
KALER COLD WAVES Hair preparation (Koehler & K.)	
KALEX Insecticide (Agkem)	Rotenone and other cube resins 0.75% Yellow copper oxide*
KALF-KARE Antibiotic and vitamin B12 supplement, veterinary (Dairy Assoc.)	Chlortetracycline (Aureomycin) hydrochloride 2.3 gr./lb. Vitamin B12 1.5 mg./lb.
KALINATE LIQUID AND TABLETS (Allied Prod. Mo.)	Each 5 cc. or each tablet: Potassium gluconate (normal potassium salt of d-gluconic acid) 0.5 gr.
KALITE 75 Insecticide (Agkem)	Rotenone and other cube resins* 0.75% Inert ingredients*
KALITE 100 Insecticide (Agkem)	Rotenone 1% Other cube resins 20%
KALO BRAND PAINTS (Longman)	
KALOL Oral and nasal antiseptic (Jenkins)	Boric acid* Sodium biborate Sodium chloride Menthol* Thymol* Oil of eucalyptus* Methyl salicylate*(syn.) Carbolic acid*
KAL-O-MIN Lotion for skin irritations (Drugmaster)	Each fl. oz.: Calamine 40 gr. Zinc oxide 20 gr. Propylene glycol 20 m. Carbolic acid 4 m.
KAL-O-MIN PLUS LOTION For skin irritations (Drugmaster)	Calamine Camphor* Methyl salicylate* Bentonite Benzocaine Propylene glycol Di-isobutyl phenoxy ethoxy ethyl dimethyl benzyl ammonium chloride*
KALON CREAM Embalming cosmetic (Dodge)	
KALO PAINT (Fisher-Thorsen)	

Name & Use Manufacturer	Ingredients
KALPEC VETERINARY For intestinal irritations (Wyeth Labs.)	Adsorbent, demulcent alumina gel Kaolin Pectin
KALSITEX PIGMENTS (Franklin Mineral)	
KALSKOTE Paint (Central P. & V.)	
KALSOKOATER Paint product (Waterproof)	
KALSO-LITE Calcimine (Tamms)	
KALSOVAL COLD WATER PAINT (Bownes)	
KALVELAX LAXATIVE TABLETS (Makers of Kal)	Powdered senna leaves Dehydrated fig Dehydrated prune Oil of orange Peppermint flavoring
KAL-ZOO (see Parsons Kal-Zoo)	
KAMADROX JEL Antacid, adsorbent (Massengill)	Each 5 cc.: Magnesium trisilicate 0.65 gm. Aluminum hydroxide gel, dried 0.32 gm. Aromatics q.s.
KAMADROX AND KAMADROX POWDER Antacid, adsorbent (Massengill)	Magnesium trisilicate 50% Dried aluminum hydroxide gel 25% Colloidal kaolin 25% Saccharin Aromatics
KAMADROX TABLETS Antacid, adsorbent (Massengill)	Magnesium trisilicate 4 gr. Colloidal kaolin 2 gr. Aluminum hydroxide 2 gr.
KAM CAPSULES (Friendly Labs.)	Each capsule: Haarlem oil (sulfurated linseed oil and turpentine*) 5 m.
KAMO MILE SHAMPOO (Germadol)	
KA-NA-BA PASTE WAX FINISH Spirit wax (Clean Surface)	Carnauba wax Naphtha*
KA-NA-BA WATER EMULSION Self-shining wax (Clean Surface)	Carnauba wax

*Consult Sec. II., Ingredients Index. This ingredient may be responsible for major toxic effects if poisonous amounts of this product are ingested.

Name & Use Manufacturer	Ingredients		Name & Use Manufacturer	Ingredients	
KANE DEODORANT (Grove)	Alcohol Aluminum chlorhydroxide complex*	7-1/2%	KAO-STREP Veterinary (Wyeth Labs.)	Each level tsp.: Dihydrostreptomycin base (as sulfate) Kaolin Pectin Hydrated alumina powder	0.075 gm. 1.50 gm. 0.135 gm. 0.210 gm.
KA-NO-MOR CAPSULES Analgesic (Luebert)	Aspirin* Phenacetin* Caffeine				
KANT KLOG PIPE & TRAP CLEANER (Robbins, G.)	Sodium hydroxide*		KAPAK Enamels (Frost Paint)		
			KAPECTIN For intestinal irritation (Approved)	Kaolin Pectin	90 gr. 2 gr.
KANT-LIN RAT PASTE Rodenticide (Velodent)			KAPEX HAIR TONIC (Winsale)		
KANT-MAR PAINT (Boehmer)			KAPONTABS Veterinary, avian (McClellan)	Each tablet: Diethylstilbestrol	15 mg.
KANTROLL DRAWINGS CRAYONS (Am. Crayon)			KAPSULATE Fertilizer (Summers)	Each 6 gr. capsule: Sodium selenate*	5.0%
KAOCASIL Adsorbent, for intestinal irritations (Jenkins)	Kaolin colloidal Calcium carbonate Magnesium trisilicate Bismuth subgallate Papain Atropine sulfate	1 gr. 1-1/2 gr. 1 gr. 1/4 gr. 1/8 gr. 1/2000 gr.	KARAJEL PLAIN Cathartic (Welin-Sater)	Karaya gum	
KAO-COP Adsorbent, antacid, for intestinal irritation (Cole)	Powdered opium Ext. krameria Kaolin heavy Copper phenol sulfonate Camphor monobromated Calcium carbonate (heavy) Pectin Oil peppermint and cinnamon flavor	1/20 gr. 4/5 gr. 8 gr. 1/15 gr. 1/10 gr. 2 gr. 1/4 gr.	KARALOSE Laxative (Thompson, Wm. T.)	Karaya gum Cascara Papain	
			KARATHANE WD Fungicide (Rohm & Haas)	Dinitro (1-methyl heptyl) phenyl crotonate* Related nitro phenols and derivatives	22.5% 2.5%
KAOGESTIN Adsorbent for gastric irritation (Daniels, Robert)	Bismuth subsalicylate Salol Methyl salicylate* synthetic Benzocaine Pectin Colloidal kaolin		KARBON KING Carbon remover (Lester)	Mild alkali Emulsifier Chlorinated solvents*	
			KARBAM BLACK Fungicide (Sherwin-Williams)	Ferbam*	76%
KAO-GESTOL For gastric irritation (Veltex)	Bismuth subcarbonate Kaolin Salol Zinc sulfocarbolate Methyl salicylate* Oil of peppermint		KARBAM WHITE Fungicide (Sherwin-Williams)	Ziram*	6%
KAOMIN (Kaolin bismuth compound) For gastric and intestinal irritations (Lilly)	Bismuth subcarbonate Kaolin Magnesium hydroxide Sucrose Vegetable mucilage Vanillin	100 parts 280 parts 60 parts 180 parts 20 parts 0.6 parts	KARBON OFF DRAIN PIPE & TRAP CLEANER (Diamond Chem.)		
			KARE #33 Floor wax (Windsor Wax)	Gamma isomer of benzene hexachloride Inactive ingredients*	0.5% 99.5%
KAOPATCH (formerly Patch's Kaolin & Mineral Oil) (Patch)	Colloidal kaolin Mineral oil Irish moss	12% 40%	KARGLO AUTO GLAZE Polish (Speco)	Gum trag.* Alcohol*	

Name & Use Manufacturer	Ingredients	Name & Use Manufacturer	Ingredients
KARIMAR HAIR TINT (Noramex)		KAY FORMULA 301 Cosmetic (Kay)	Alcohol* 40% Titanium dioxide Zinc oxide Menthol* Glycerin
KARITH CLEANING FLUID (Karith)	Apcothiner (refined naphtha* base) Shellacol* (alcohol) Ether* Chloroform*	KAYLEK OINTMENT For skin irritations, fungicide, medical (K & B)	Salicylic benzoic acid* 3% Crude coal tar 2% Inert ingredients*
KARKOTE Paint (Vita-Var)			
K-ARMAND'S QUICK SHOT OINTMENT For skin irritations (K-Armand)	Menthol Salicylic acid* Zinc oxide Sulfur ppt.* Phenol* Boric acid* Beta naphthol*	KAYLOID Adsorbent (Kaoloid)	Kaolin Dried brewers yeast Oil of peppermint Hemicellulose gums Aluminum hydroxide Butoben (preservative)
KARNAK PILE OINTMENT (Karnak)		KAYNENE FOR DOGS For skin irritations (veterinary) (Horton & Converse)	Purified hydrocarbon* from coal tar Iodized oil base
KARN'S NU SALVE (Falk)	Pine gum* Rosin Beef fat Beeswax Linseed oil	KAY-SEN For skin irritations (Stenton)	Mercury salicylate* 1/3 gr./oz. Acid salicylic* Resorcin Coal tar
KAS-MO SALVE Local anesthetic, antiseptic (Kas-Mo)	Copper acetate* Solid ext. of stramonium Rosin	KAZ For vaporizers (Kaz)	Methyl salicylate* U.S.P. Oil of eucalyptus* U.S.P. Oil of peppermint U.S.P. Oil of lavender U.S.P. Menthol* U.S.P. Camphor* U.S.P. Light mineral oil U.S.P. Yellow AB
KATHY STICK COLOGNE (General Prod.)			
KATONIC Veterinary (Daniels, Dr. A.C.)	Potassium phosphate Cascarilla Tincture of catnip Glycerine Alcohol 15%	KAZON For skin irritations (B & B)	Menthol* Camphor* Carbolic acid* Milk of sulfur Zinc oxide Calamine Salicylic acid*
KATONIC IRON TONIC Veterinary (Daniels, Dr. A.C.)	Iron pyrophosphate soluble Infusion cascarilla Infusion catnip	K-BIOTIC Anti-hemorrhagic (veterinary, avian) (Vineland)	Oxytetracycline hydrochloride 106.0 gm. Menadione sodium bisulfite 8.0 gm. Vitamin B12 activity 4243 gm.
KAT-POWDER Insecticide (Texas Pheno.)	Tech. piperonyl cyclonene 0.625% Pyrethrins 0.062%	K. B. X FLAKE Cleaning product (Wyandotte)	Conc. alkali*
KAUKIT Paint product (Sonneborn)		KCD-1 FORMULA CD-1 Detergent (Klenzade)	Alkyl dimethyl benzyl ammonium chloride* 2%
K-A-U-R-I PAINTS (Brooklyn, P. & V.)		KCD-3 FORMULA CD-3 Detergent (Klenzade)	Alkyl dimethyl ethyl benzyl ammonium chloride* 2%
KAUROZARE PAINTS (Buckeye P. & V.)		K CREME LOTION For hands, skin (K)	Lanolin Stearic acid Glycerin or propylene glycol Camphor* Ammonia* Potassium hydroxide Perfume

*Consult Sec. II., Ingredients Index. This ingredient may be responsible for major toxic effects if poisonous amounts of this product are ingested.

Name & Use Manufacturer	Ingredients	Name & Use Manufacturer	Ingredients
KDS KLENZADE DETERGENT SANITIZER FORMULA KDS-1 Germicidal detergent (Klenzade)	Para di-isobutyl phenoxy ethoxy ethyl dimethyl benzyl ammonium chloride* 10.7%	KELLY'S INSECT SPRAY (Solvit)	DDT* 5% Tech chlordane (1.2% of octachloro-4,7-methanotetra-hydroindane and 0.8% of related compounds) 2% Petroleum oil* 93%
KD THE ALL PURPOSE DISINFECTANT (Klinzmoth)	Coal tar acids * 27% Coal tar hydrocarbons* 44% Soap 19%	KELLY'S INSECT SPRAY VAPORIZER CONC. (Solvit)	Piperonyl butoxide tech.* (1.016% of butyl carbityl (6-propyl piperonyl ether) and 0.254% of related compounds) 1.27% Pyrethrins 0.13% Petroleum oil* 98.60%
KEEL For irritations of the lips (Carolina)	Alum Boric acid* Camphor* Glycerin Isopropyl alcohol 11% Oil of cloves Sodium borate* Tincture of benzoin Zinc sulfate*	KELLY'S REDI-MIX WARFARIN RAT & MOUSE KILLER (Solvit)	Warfarin (3-(a-acetonylbenzyl)-4-hydroxycoumarin) 0.25%
KEEP-DRI Chemical air dryer (Hill Mfg.)		KELNEED (Hanlon)	Pacific kelp C.T. 5 gr. Mineral supplement with trace elements
KEEPKAN PAINT BRUSH CLEANER (Howe Co.)		KELSEY Rectal suppositories (Gesell)	Nux vomica (strychnine 0.025 gr. average) Stramonium (alkaloids 0.0016 gr. average) Ichthammol Benzocaine
KEK BOILER CLEANER & STEAM CONDITIONER (Kenite)		KELSEY OINTMENT (Gesell)	Zinc oxide Menthol* Carbolic acid* Petrolatum Waxes
KEK PROTECTIVE HAND CREAM (Horton & Converse)		KELVINATOR CLEANER & WAX (Nash Kelvin.)	
KELLEY'S ANT KILLER (Kelley)	Chlordane 5%	KEL-ZYME For skin irritations of allergies (Kahlenberg)	Each capsule: 0.33 gm. Trypsin 1/125
KELLOGG'S ANT BOMB & INSECT KILLER (Kellogg's)	Pyrethrins I and II 0.200% Tech. piperonyl butoxide (butyl-carbityl) (6-propyl-piperonyl) ether and related compounds 0.500% Rotenone, rotenoids and other cube resins 0.200% Butoxypolypropylene glycol 8.000 % Ethylene glycol ether of pinene 1.800% Mineral oil refined 29.300%	KEM-GLO FLAT WALL PAINT (Lawrence, W.W.)	
		KEM-O-DRY (Detrex)	Perchlorethylene*
		KEM PAINT & VARNISH CLEANER (Hill Mfg.)	
KELLOG'S ANT PASTE (Kellog's)	Arsenious oxide* 5.5%	KEMP'S BALSAM Antitussive (Kemp & Lane)	Each fl. oz.: Chloroform 6-2/5 m. Fluid of squills and senega Tartar emetic* Oil of tar Sodium citrate Sodium salicylate*
KELLOGG'S ANT SPRAY & INSECTICIDE (Kellogg's)	Tech. chlordane 2% Petroleum distillate* 98%		
KELLY'S GERMICIDE Germicide, sanitizer, fungicide (Solvit)	Methyl dodecyl benzyl tri-methyl ammonium chloride* 10%	KEMP'S SHEEEP BRANDING LIQUID (Cooper)	
		KEMTEX CLEANER (MacDermid)	

*Consult Sec. II., Ingredients Index. This ingredient may be responsible for major toxic effects if poisonous amounts of this product are ingested.

Name & Use Manufacturer	Ingredients	Name & Use Manufacturer	Ingredients
KEMTONE PAINT (Lawrence, W.W.)		KENT AFTER SHAVE STICK (Wright)	
KEM-TONE WATER PAINTS (Rogers Paint)		KENT BRICK COAT Paint (Cheesman-Elliott)	
KEM-TOX TERMITE CONTROL (Phelan-Faust)		KENTHOL (Kondon)	Menthol* Camphor* Phenol* Oil of eucalyptus* Mutton tallow
KENBRIC SOOT REMOVER (Kenite)	Zinc chloride*	KENT KAPS Veterinary capsules (Kent Spec.)	Gelatin Garlic
KENCEL C-9 Laxative (Kendall,C.B.)	Each tablet: Sodium carboxymethylcellulose 0.50 gm. Extract ox bile U.S.P. 0.03 gm.	KENT'S DENTAL PLATE POWDER (Kent Co.)	Magnesium silicate Calcium carbonate Sodium perborate* Chloramine Aromatic oils*
KENDALL'S Counter-irritant liniment (veterinary) (Kendall, Dr. B.J.)	Turpentine* Alcohol 44% Oil of cade Iodine* Thymol* Oil of cloves	KENT'S FOOT POWDER (Kent Co.)	Boric acid* Salicylic acid* Ammonium alum Oxyquinoline sulfate Magnesium oxide
KENDALL'S Liniment, counter-irritant, (Kendall, Dr. B.J.)	Camphor* Ether 9.3%/v. Turpentine* Alcohol 42% Oil of cade Iodine* Thymol* Oil of cloves*	KENT'S FORMULA A Douche powder (Kent Co.)	Sodium bicarbonate Sodium perborate* Chloramine* Calcium carbonate
KENDEX WATER-PROOF COMPOUND (Kendall Ref.)		KENT'S SPECIAL FORMULA FOR MOUTH & THROAT HYGIENE (Kent Co.)	Sodium bicarbonate Sodium perborate* Chloramine* Aromatic oils*
KENITE JOINT COMPOUND (Kenite)		KENT'S SPECIAL FORMULA 2 Antiseptic for mouth and throat (Kent Co.)	Sodium bicarbonate Sodium perborate* Chloramine* Aromatic oils*
KENO CAPS Anthelmintic (veterinary) (Globe)	Each capsule: Oil chenopodium* 56.13% Arecoline hydrobromide 0.47% Aloin* 14.15% Magnesium carbonate 23.59% Calcium carbonate 5.66%	KENWOOD HAIR OIL (Griswold Med.)	
KENOO CLEANING COMPOUND (Keystone Chem.)		KENWOR PAINT (Boehmer)	
		KENYCAS Paint (Central P. & V.)	
KENSINGTON SOAP (Hewitt)	Tallow Cocoanut oil Sodium hydroxide	KERAMIX TILE BLEACH (Hillyard Chem.)	Hydrochloric acid*
KENSOL PETROL. SOLVENT (Kendall Ref.)		KER-A-TOC CUTICLE REMOVER (La Vell)	

*Consult Sec. II., Ingredients Index. This ingredient may be responsible for major toxic effects if poisonous amounts of this product are ingested.

Name & Use Manufacturer	Ingredients	Name & Use Manufacturer	Ingredients
KERATOGEN Fungicide, medical (Franklin Labs.)	Acid salicylic* Acid benzoic* Menthol crystals* Methyl para hydroxybenzoate Benzocaine	KETOKIL NO. 18 Insecticide (Cotton States)	Hexachloro hexahydro dimethano naphthalene* 22.5% Related compounds 17.0% Xylene* 36.5% Petroleum distillate 14.0%
KERBEX To curb appetite (Veland)	Sodium methyl cellulose Dextrose	KETOKIL NO. 42 Insecticide (Cotton States)	Tech. chlorinated camphene* 40.00% Dichloro diphenyl trichloro- ethane 20.00% Xylene* 23.0% Petroleum oil 0.05%
KERECO PAINTS & VARNISH (Keystone Ref.)		KETOKIL NO. 47 Insecticide (Cotton States)	Heptachlor* 23.55% Related compounds 9.15% Petroleum distillate 62.30%
KERODEX 51 Barrier cream (Ayerst)	Methyl paraben 0.19% Sodium pentachlorophenate 0.07%	KETOKIL NO. 97 Insecticide (Cotton States)	Hexachloro epoxy octahydro dimethano naphthalene* 15.80% Related compounds 2.85% Petroleum hydrocarbons 73.90%
KERODEX 71 Water repellent (Ayerst)	Methyl paraben 0.11% Propyl paraben 0.08%	KETOKIL NO. 278 Insecticide (Cotton States)	Methoxychlor tech. 27.8% Xylene* 68.0%
KEROS VAGINAL TABLETS (Keros)	Hydroquinone* Oxyquinoline sulfate* Tartaric acid Sodium bicarbonate	K-E-Y DISINFECTANT (Baxter)	
KESTER SOLDERING FLUX (Kester)	Inorganic halides*	KEY GRAPHITE PASTE (Key)	Blackstrap molasses approx. 50% Amorphous graphite approx. 50% Sodium pentachlorphenate less than 1/2 of 1%
KESTER SOLDERING PASTE (Kester)	Inorganic chloride Conc. zinc halide* Petrolatum	KEY PAINT (Eagle P.&V.)	
KESTER SOLDERING SALTS (Kester)	Zinc halide* Other inorganic salts	KEYS ASTRINGENT POWDER (E.Z. Chem.)	
KESTON For gastric irritation (McKesson)	Aluminum hydroxide Bismuth subsalicylate Salol Oil of anise Oil of cassia	KEYS NOSE DROPS (E.Z. Chem.)	Chlorobutanol* (chloroform deriv.) 4 gr./fl.oz. Ephedrine* Chlorothymol camphor 3/4 of 1% Menthol* Cinnamic aldehyde Oleic acid Liquid petrolatum
KETOKIL NO. 2 Insecticide (Cotton States)	DDT (dichloro diphenyl trichloroethane) 25% Xylene* 65%	KEYS PERFECTED NOSE DROPS (E.Z. Chem.)	Chlorobutanol* (chloroform deriv.) 4 gr./fl.oz. Ephedrine* 3/4 of 1% Chlorothymol Camphor* Menthol* Cinnamic aldehyde Oleic acid Liquid petrolatum
KETOKIL NO. 3-0 Insecticide (Cotton States)	Gamma isomer of benzene hexachloride* 13.50% Other related isomers of benzene hexachloride 20.40% Xylene* 42.00%		
KETOKIL NO. 3-5 Insecticide (Cotton States)	Gamma isomer of benzene hexachloride 9.87% Other related isomers of benzene hexachloride 14.81% Dichloro diphenyl trichloro ethane 16.45% Xylene* 37.30%	KEY'S POWDER Hygienic powder (E.Z. Chem.)	Carbolic acid* Boric acid* Zinc sulfate* Salicylic acid* Thymol* Menthol* Eucalyptol*
KETOKIL NO. 6 Insecticide (Cotton States)	Toxaphene* 60% Petroleum distillate 23%		

Name & Use Manufacturer	Ingredients	Name & Use Manufacturer	Ingredients
KEYSTONA PAINT (Keystone P. & V.)		KIDMETICS CHILDREN'S TOILET PREP. (Assoc. Brands)	
KEYSTONE DISINFECTANT (Keystone Chem.)		KIDMETICS SMOOTH SKIN LOTION (Assoc. Brands)	
KEYSTONE LAMP BLACK (Bihn & Wolff)		KILARVA MOTH PREVENTIVE (Libby Oil)	
KEYSTONE METAL POLISH (Imperial Prod.)		KIL BALM RAT AND MOUSE POISON (Kil Balm)	Arsenic trioxide* (metallic arsenic as water soluble 1.72%) 2.25%
KEYSTONE MOTH-PROOFING (Keystone Chem.)		KILBRUSH 8-16 ESTER Herbicide (Bonide)	Butyl 2,4,5-trichlorophenoxy-acetate 9.8% Butyl 2,4-dichlorophenoxy-acetate* 20.0%
KEYSTONE OIL COLORS (Keystone V.)		KILBURN For skin irritations (Assoc. Prod.)	Carbolic acid* Camphor* Boric acid* Menthol* Oil cloves*
KEYSTONE SLIKUP ODORLESS RAPID-DRYING ENAMEL (Keystone P. & V.)		KILBURN SKIN CREAM (Peoples)	Phenol* Menthol* Camphor* Potassium stearate Boric acid* Orthochlorophenol* Oils of lavender, cloves, bergamot, persic, cassia, seranium and citronella
K-4 POWDER FOR ATHLETE'S FOOT (Litle)	Salicylic acid* Chlorothymol* Boric acid* Magnesium silicate 87-1/2%	KILCHLOR Insecticide (Kilgore Seed)	Chlordane*
KHAIR FOR THE HAIR Dandruff remover (Mann, Leo)	Resorcinal mono acetate* Castor oil* deriv. Aliphatic esters and glycols Cholesterol Mineral pomade wax Parahydroxy benzoic acid* Aromatics* Isopropanol* Ethyl alcohol	KILCIDE Insecticide (Kilgore Seed)	DDT*
		KILDIRT Soap (United Chem.)	
KIDDIE COUGH SYRUP Antitussive (Hance)	Cocillana Euphorbia Horehound Squill Licorice Sanquinaria nitrate Senega Wild lettuce leaves Menthol Honey with aromatics	KILFLEA POWDER (Clayton)	
		KILGAM Insecticide (Kilgore Seed)	Lindane*
KIDDIE NOSE DROPS (Hance)	Alcohol 2%/v Chlorobutanol 0.5% Menthol* Ephedrine sulfate 1/2% Sodium citrate Camphor*	KILHEX Insecticide (Kilgore Seed)	Gamma isomer BHC*
KIDDO Diuretic (Duffy)	Buchu Potassium acetate Corn silk Formin Juniper berries Sabal Sandalwood	KIL INSECTICIDE (Kenyon)	Petroleum hydrocarbons* Tech. chlordane* Isobornyl thiocyanoacetate* and other related terpenes Tech. piperonyl butoxide Pyrethrins

*Consult Sec. II., Ingredients Index. This ingredient may be responsible for major toxic effects if poisonous amounts of this product are ingested.

Name & Use Manufacturer	Ingredients		Name & Use Manufacturer	Ingredients	
KILLALL BRAND ROACH & RAT PASTE (Pfeiffer)	Phosphorus *	3%	KILLER BLITEX (D-5 T-5) Insecticide, fungicide (Agsco)	DDT* Copper* expressed as metallic	5.0% 5.0%
KILLALL INSECTICIDE POWDER (Pfeiffer)	DDT* Pyrethrins Sesamin conc.	10.00 0.08 0.30	KILLER BLITEX D-5 T-7 Insecticide, fungicide (Agsco)	DDT* Tribasic copper sulfate*	
KILL BRAND INSECTICIDE POWDER (Pfeiffer)	DDT* Petroleum hydrocarbons Pyrethrins	10.00% 2.70% 0.08%	KILLER DUST CH-5 Insecticide (Agsco)	Chlordane*	5%
KILLDUST SWEEPING COMPOUND (Internat. Sisal)			KILLER DUST D-5 and D-10 Insecticide (Agsco)	DDT*	5% and 10%
KILLEMOL INSECT DUST (Sentinel Chem.)	Pyrethrum Inert ingredients		KILLER DUST D-5 ZS-4 Insecticide (Agsco)	DDT * Zinc sulfate*	5% 4%
KILL-EM-QUICK BED BUG LIQUID (Elk)	Phenol* Aliphatic hydrocarbons*		KILLER DUST Tox-10 Insecticide (Agsco)	Toxaphene*	10.0%
KIL-EM-QUICK RATICIDE (Elk)	Squill*powdered		KILLER MILLER'S JAYGOL Insecticide (Nat'l Jaygol)	Boric acid* Tech. piperonyl cyclonene Pyrethrins	68.900% 0.020% 0.010%
KIL-EM-QUICK ROACH POWDER (Elk)	Fluorides*		KILL-KO 10% CHLORDANE DUST Insecticide (Rigo)	Tech. chlordane*	10%
KILLER BLITEX D-3 C-5 Insecticide, fungicide (Agsco)	DDT* Copper*		KILL-KO 25% DDT CONC. Insecticide (Rigo)	DDT Polymethyl naphthalenes* Petroleum oil Beta-thiocyano b' butoxy-diethyl ether	25.00% 55.00% 14.18% 1.07%
KILLER BLITEX D-3 Di-6 Insecticide, fungicide (Agsco)	DDT* Zineb		KILL-KO FLEA & INSECT POWDER 10% DDT (Rigo)	DDT* Beta beta dithiocyano diethyl ether	10% 0.50%
KILLER BLITEX D-3 T-7 Insecticide, fungicide (Agsco)	DDT* Tribasic copper sulfate*		KILL-KO FLORAL DUST Insecticide, fungicide (Rigo)	Rotenone Other cube resins Beta thiocyano ethyl esters of mixed fatty acids containing 10 to 18 carbon atoms Sulfur* Zineb (zinc ethylene-bis(dithiocarbonate) DDT (dithloro diphenyl trichloroethane)	1.00% 2.00% 0.37% 20.00% 3.13% 3.00%
KILLER DUST D-4 TOX-5 Insecticide (Agsco)	DDT* Toxaphene*	4% 5%			
KILLER BLITEX D-5 C-5 Insecticide, fungicide (Agsco)	DDT* Copper*		KILL-KO FLY BAIT Insecticide (Rigo)	Malathion	2.00%
KILLER BLITEX D-5 DI-6 Insecticide, fungicide (Agsco)	DDT* Zineb		KILL-KO FLY KILLER MALATHION (Rigo)	Malathion* Aromatic petroleum distillate*	50% 45%

*Consult Sec. II., Ingredients Index. This ingredient may be responsible for major toxic effects if poisonous amounts of this product are ingested.

- 614 -

Name & Use Manufacturer	Ingredients		Name & Use Manufacturer	Ingredients	
KILL-KO 3 in 1 GARDEN DUST Insecticide (Rigo)	Rotenone	0.75%	KILL QUICK Ectoparasiti- cide (Sterling Prod. Div.)	Mineral oil	83.04%
	Other cube resins	1.50%		Camphor*	11.93%
	Yellow cuprous oxide*(expressed as metallic copper)	4.00%		Carbolic acid* (phenol)	4.65%
				Oil of bay	0.20%
	Beta thiocyano ethyl esters of aliphatic fatty acids	0.75%		Oil of lavender	0.18%
KILL-KO INSECT SPRAY Insecticide (Rigo)	Tech. chlordane	2.50%	KILL RAT (Manco)		
	Beta thiocyanoethyl esters of aliphatic acids	1.01%	KILLSECT Insecticide (Warren Ref.)	Thanite	2%
	Beta thiocyano B'butoxy diethyl ether	0.33%		DDT*	5%
				Odorless kerosene*	93%
	Pyrethrins	0.047%			
	Tech. piperonyl butoxide	0.118%	KILL-TOX DRY-FOLATE NO. 2 Herbicide (Veith)	Aromatic oils*	
	Petroleum distillate*	95.995%		Pentachlorophenol*	
				Other chlorophenols*	
KILL-KO KATTLE SPRAY Insecticide (Rigo)	Piperonyl butoxide	0.30%			
	Pyrethrins	0.03%	KILL WEED DUST IE-5 (Agsco)	2,4-D ester	5%
	Petroleum distillate*	99.67%			
KILL-KO LINDANE EMULSIFI- ABLE CONC. Insecticide (Rigo)	Gamma isomer of benzene hexachloride* (from lindane)	13.0%	KILL WEED DUST S-4 (Agsco)	2,4-D sodium salt*	
				2,4-D acid*	4%
	Aromatic petroleum solvent*	83.0%	KILMICE (Mice Seed) (Nott)	Strychnine sulfate*	0.75%
KILL-KO QUICK KILL INSECT KILLER (Rigo)	Piperonyl butoxide	0.30%			
	Pyrethrins	0.03%	KIL-MOE Insecticide (Halaby)	Petroleum hydrocarbons*	
	Beta butoxy beta' thiocyano diethyl ether	1.50%		Piperonyl butoxide	
				Pyrethrins	
	DDT	0.50%		Perfumes	
	Petroleum distillate*	96.78%			
KILL-KO 25% RHOTHANE EMULSIFI- ABLE CONC. Insecticide (Rigo)	Dichloro diphenyl dichloro- ethane, tech. (Rhothane d-3)	25.0%	KIL-O-FLY (Interstate Med.)	Pyrocide booster	
				#10 base oil*	
				Perfume	
	Aromatic petroleum deriv. sol*	71.8%	KILPAIN KREAM Liniment (Richards Bros.)	Stearic acid	
				Oil thyme*	
KILL-KO ROACH & ANT KILLER Insecticide (Rigo)	Petroleum distillate*	94.52%		Camphor*	
	Tech. chlordane	2.50%		Chloroform*	
	Beta thiocyano ethyl esters of aliphatic acids	1.79%		Soap	
				Turpentine*	
	Beta butoxy beta thiocyano diethyl ether	1.19%		Capsicum*	
				Ammonia*	
KILL-KO SCREW- WORM KILLER (Rigo)	Benzol*	72%	KIL-PEL CONC. FLY SPRAY (Wilke)	DDT*	4%
	Carbon tetrachloride*	17%		Beta butoxy beta thiocyano diethyl ether*	16%
	Pine tar oil	11%		Petroleum distillates*	80%
KILL-KO SUPER STRENGTH 5% DDT Insecticide (Rigo)	DDT*	5.00%	KILPHENE Insecticide (Kilgore Seed)	Toxaphene*	
	Beta thiocyano ethyl esters of aliphatic acids containing 10-18 carbon atoms	2.03%	KILPHOS Insecticide (Kilgore Seed)	Parathion*	
	Beta thiocyano beta butoxy diethylether	0.67%			
KILL-KOTE INSECTICIDE (Yates & Smart)			KILRITE Insecticide (U. S. Sanitary)		
KILL MOR FLY SPRAY (Hilltop)	Malathion*	49.5%	KILSPRAY Insecticide (Kilgore Seed)	Pyrethrins*	
	Xylene*	42.5%		DDT*	
KILL-OGEN Insecticide (Rose Mfg.)	Pyrethrins	0.025%	KIL-SPRAY AEROSOL INSECTICIDE (Uncle Sam)	DDT*	
	Rotenone	0.128%		Pyrethrum	
	Other cube extractives	0.236%		Lethane*	
	Tech. piperonyl cyclonene	0.256%		Piperonyl butoxide	
	Petroleum distillate	0.102%		Freon	
	Inert ingredients*	99.253%			

*Consult Sec. II., Ingredients Index. This ingredient may be responsible for major toxic effects if poisonous amounts of this produc are ingested.

Name & Use Manufacturer	Ingredients		Name & Use Manufacturer	Ingredients	
KILTHOX Insecticide (Kilgore Seed)	Methoxychlor*		KING DDT DUST Insecticide (King Calcium)	DDT	3.0%
KILTICK D CATTLE DIP Insecticide (Sherwin-Williams)	Sodium arsenite* Sodium cresylate Soap	32.4% 11.1% 11.1%	KING 5% DDT DUST Insecticide (King Calcium)	DDT*	5%
KIL-VE Ectoparasiti-cide (Victoria)	Alkaloids of sabadilla Picrotoxin from fishberries Inert ingredients*	0.04% 0.06% 99.9%	KING 7-1/2% DDT DUST Insecticide (King Calcium)	DDT*	7-1/2%
KILZIT Insecticide (Chem. Corp.)			KING DITHANE DUST Fungicide (King Calcium)	Zineb (zinc ethylene-bis (dithio-carbamate)) (Dithane Z-78 contains 65% zineb) Inert ingredients	3.9%
KILZUM Insecticide (A-Penn.)	Pyrethrins DDT* Piperonyl butoxide Petroleum Methylated naphthalene*				
KIMO Disinfectant (Robbins, G.)	Diisobutylphenoxyethoxy ethyl dimethyl benzyl ammonium chloride*	10%	KING 7% FIXED COPPER DUST Fungicide (King Calcium)	Copper*	7%
KIN-AM-EL VARNISH STAIN (Perfection Paint)			KING FLOWER DUST Insecticide, fungicide (King Calcium)	DDT* Gamma isomer of BHC (from lindane) Malathion* Zineb (from X Dithane Z-78) Sulfur* Dinitro capryl phenyl crotonate* (from x Karathane)	5.0% 0.5% 3.0% 3.9% 30.0% 0.2%
KINDERTONE CRAYON (Nat'l Crayon)					
KINDL KAVAL KOLOR KINDLER Fire kindler (Kindl)			KING FRUIT TREE DUST OR SPRAY Insecticide, fungicide (King Calcium)	Malathion* Methoxychlor Zineb (from x Dithane Z-78) Sulfur*	4.0% 3.0% 6.5% 40.0%
KINDOGRAPH CRAYONS (Am. Crayon)					
KING BUG KILLER Insecticide (King Calcium)	Arsenic	2.4%	KING GLADIOLUS DUST Insecticide, fungicide (King Calcium)	DDT* Gamma isomer of BHC* (from lindane) Malathion* Zineb (from x Dithane Z-78) Dinitro capryl phenyl crotonate* (from x Karathane) Sulfur*	5.0% 5.0% 3.0% 3.9% 0.2% 30.0%
KING CHLORDANE DUST Insecticide (King Calcium)	Tech. chlordane*	5.0%			
			KING-KOOLANT Cutting oils (Rex Oil)		
KING DDT & COPPER DUST Insecticide, fungicide (King Calcium)	DDT Copper*	3.0% 7.0%	KING MALATHION DUST Insecticide (King Calcium)	Malathion*	4.0%
KING DDT, DITHANE & SULPHUR DUST Insecticide, fungicide (King Calcium)	DDT Zineb (zinc ethylene-bis (dithio-carbamate)) (Dithane Z-78 contains 65% zineb) Sulfur	3.0% 3.9% 10.0%	KING-OF-ALL BOWL KLEENER (King Mfg.)	Sodium bisulfate*	

Name & Use Manufacturer	Ingredients		Name & Use Manufacturer	Ingredients	
KING-OF-ALL DRAIN PIPE, GREASE TRAP AND SEWER & SEPTIC TANK KLEENERS (King Mfg.)	Sodium hydroxide* (caustic soda)		KING VEGETABLE DUST Insecticide, fungicide (King Calcium)	DDT* Malathion* Zineb (from x Dithane Z-78) Maneb (from x Dithane M-22) Sulfur*	5.0% 4.0% 2.0% 2.0% 20.0%
KING ORGANIC FUNGICIDE WITH DDT (King Calcium)	Zineb (zinc ethylene bisdithio-carbamate) DDT	3.9% 3.0%	KING VINO-DUST Insecticide, Fungicide (King Calcium)	Rotenone Malathion* Zineb (from x Dithane Z-78) Maneb (from x Dithane M-22) Sulfur	0.7% 4.0% 2.0% 2.0% 10.0%
KING POTATO BLIGHT DUST Fungicide (King Calcium)	Zineb Sulfur Inert ingredients	3.9% 10.0%	KING WARBLE FLY SPRAY POWDER (King Calcium)	Rotenone* Inert ingredients	5%
KING POTATO DUST Insecticide, fungicide (King Calcium)	DDT* Zineb (from Dithane Z-78)	5.0% 3.9%	KIOLITE PAINT (Debevoise)		
KING ROSE DUST Insecticide, fungicide (King Calcium)	Rotenone DDT* Gamma isomer of BHC (from lindane) Dinitro capryl phenyl crotonate* (from x Karathane) Zineb (from x Dithane Z-78) Sulfur*	1.0% 3.0% 0.5% 0.2% 3.9% 30.0%	KIP For skin injuries (Kip, Inc.)	Oils of spearmint and bay Methyl salicylate* Salicylic acid* Lanolin Zinc oxide Phenol Orthohydroxyphenyl mercuric chloride	0.44% 0.056%
KING ROTENONE DUST Insecticide (King Calcium)	Rotenone Inert ingredients	1%	KIP ANTISEPTIC OIL For burns, cuts (Kip, Inc.)	Benzocaine Oils of bergamot, bay, spearmint, castor bean, thyme Methyl salicylate* Acid salicylic* Mercurated phenol (1-10,000 parts)	2%
KING ROTENONE & DITHANE DUST Insecticide, fungicide (King Calcium)	Rotenone Zineb (zinc ethylene-bis (dithio-carbamate))(Dithane Z-78) contains 65% zineb) Inert ingredients	1% 3.9%	KIP PILE BALM For rectal irritation (Kip, Inc.)	Snow white petrolatum Lanolin Bay Thyme Castor Benzocaine Zinc oxide Oil of wintergreen syn.* Spearmint Bergamot Sesame Orthohydroxyphenyl mercuric chloride (less than 1-20,000)	3%
KINGS MEN SHAVING AND AFTER SHAVE LOTION (Kings Men)			KIP TANNIC For burns (Kip, Inc.)	Tannic acid Salicylic acid* Oil of bay Glycerin Chlorothymol* Methyl salicylate* Oil of spearmint Carbolic acid	5% 1/2 of 1%
KINGS MEN COLOGNE AND DEODORANT (Kings Men)					
KING TOBACCO DUST Insecticide, fungicide (King Calcium)	DDD or TDE (Rhothane)	7.5%	KIRBY'S BALMA OINTMENT (Kirby's Mineral)		
			KIRBY'S BREATH DEODORANT (Kirby's Mineral)		
KING TOMATO DUST Insecticide, fungicide (King Calcium)	DDD or TDE (from Rhothane) Maneb (from Dithane M-22)	5.0% 4.2%	KIRBY'S CORN SOLVENT (Kirby's Mineral)		

*Consult Sec. II., Ingredients Index. This ingredient may be responsible for major toxic effects if poisonous amounts of this product are ingested.

Name & Use Manufacturer	Ingredients		Name & Use Manufacturer	Ingredients	
KIRKMAN SOAPS & DETERGENTS (Colgate-Palmolive)			KLEANBOL Cleaner (United Chem.)		
KIRK'S AMERICAN FAMILY BAR LAUNDRY SOAP (Procter & Gamble)			KLEAN GLOW Cleaner (United Chem.)		
KIRN'S TEA Diuretic, laxative (Brant)	Senna Buchu leaves Uva ursi Berberis Sarsparilla Ginger Safflower Licorice root Anise		KLEAN KLAY Modeling clay (Art Chem.)	Powdered kaolloid clay Powdered gypsum Petrolatum Wax Castor oil	
			KLEANKOTE PAINT (Standard-Toch)		
KIRSCH LOTION For irritations of the lips (Assoc. Prod.)	Alcohol* Camphor* Menthol* Oxyquinoline sulfate*	85%/v	KLEAN KROP WEED KILLER (Thompson-Hayward)	Isopropyl n-(3-chlorophenyl)-carbamate* 46.5%	
S. B. KITCHEL'S LINIMENT (Wells, E.B.)	Sal soda Saltpetre* Pure copperas Nutgalls Potassium carbonate Aqua ammonia*		KLEAN-STRIP FLOOR CLEANER (Klean-Strip)		
			KLEAN-STRIP PAINT & VARNISH CLEANER (Klean-Strip)		
KITCHEN KLENZER (Fitzpatrick)	Powdered mineral abrasive Phosphates* Alkaline detergent* Perfume		KLEANU FURNITURE POLISH (Manhattan Kreole)		
KITCHEN POLICE K.P. 200 Cleanser (Pioneer)			KLEANU SUEDE DRESS Shoe polish (Manhattan Kreole)		
KITCHEN QUEEN Cleaner (Apex Chem.)	Trisodium phosphate* Sodium carbonate Sodium bicarbonate Complex sodium phosphates Pine oil* Butyl cellosolve Alkyl aryl sulfonate* Wetting agents		KLEANWELL MOUTH WASH Astringent deodorant (Am. Druggists)	Zinc chloride* Oil peppermint Oil cinnamon Formaldehyde*	
			KLEENABOLE (U. S. Sanitary)		
KITCH-N-TINT HIGHT GLOSS INTERIOR WALL PAINT (Chi-Namel)	Titanium calcium 30.0 Titanium dioxide 11.9 Soya alkyd resin 24.6 Maleic resin 3.5 Mineral spirits* 28.0 Drier 2.0		KLEEN-A-BRUSH Cleaner (Sheffield Bronze)		
KITERLINE TABLETS Veterinary (Clayton)			KLEEN A SKIN FOOTEZE Foot lotion (Kleen-A-Skin)	Ac. salicyl* Ac. benz. Menthol* Formalin* Alum. chloride Methyl salicyl.* Alcohol 50% Vegetable oil	
KITTY CARE FLEA POWDER (House of Huston)	Tech. piperonyl cyclonene 0.635% Pyrethrins 0.625% Rotenone 0.3125% Other cube resins 0.625%				
			KLEEN-BRITE Floor compound (Peerless Chem.)		
KIWI BOOT STAIN Shoe polish (Kiwi)					

*Consult Sec. II., Ingredients Index. This ingredient may be responsible for major toxic effects if poisonous amounts of this product are ingested.

Name & Use Manufacturer	Ingredients	Name & Use Manufacturer	Ingredients
KLEEN-CEAL FLOOR COATINGS Floor finishers (McGuire)		KLEEN STIK Rubber cement (Craftint)	
KLEENDRAIN Cleaner (U. S. Sanitary)		KLEEN SPOT CLEANING FLUID (Uncle Sam)	Carbon tetrachloride* Naphtha
KLEEN-EZE Floor cleaner (Peerless Chem.)		KLEENSWEET HOUSEHOLD ODOR DEODORANT (Liquid)	
KLEEN-EZY Cleaner (Teen)		KLEENTEX FABRIC CLEANER (U. S. Spec.)	
KLEEN GLASS Cleaner (Uncle Sam)	Isopropanol* Cellosolve Dye	KLEENUP FLOWABLE OIL EMULSION Insecticide, fungicide (Calif. Spray)	Petroleum oils* 80%
KLEENGRIP TYPE CLEANER (Hampshire)			
KLEEN-KLOZ DRY CLEANER (Dyrud)	Paraffin hydrocarbons*	KLEENUP READY-MIX DORMANT OIL SPRAY Insecticide, fungicide (Calif. Spray)	Petroleum oils* 98%
KLEEN-KOW Insecticide (Rockland)	Petroleum distillate* Steam distilled pine oil* Beta butoxy beta thiocyano diethyl ether* Tech. methoxychlor* Pyrethrins*		
		KLEENUP READY-MIX OIL SPRAY Insecticide (Calif. Spray)	Petroleum oils* 97%
KLEEN-KOW STAINLESS FLY-SPRAY (Rockland)	Petroleum distillate* Beta butoxy beta' thiocyano diethyl ether* Steam distilled pine oil* DDT 0.5% Pyrethrins*	KLEEN-ZALL Cleaning powder (Peerless Chem.)	
KLEEN MIST Deodorant, sanitizer (Allied Home)	Isopropyl alcohol* Triethylene glycol Para di-isobutyl phenoxy ethoxy ethyl dimethyl benzyl ammonium chloride*	KLEENZEM Cleaner (General P. & V.)	
		KLEER-A-KOLD For colds (B & S)	Menthol Camphor* Oils of wintergreen, pine and eucalyptus*
KLEENOL KLEENER (Triple-X)			
KLEENO SPOT REMOVER (D-Moth)		KLEER BRITE Dish cleaner (Paul, J.C.)	Triton -X-100* (alkylated aryl poly-ether alcohol) Ultra wet - 60 L* water
KLEEN-O- TYPE Type cleaner (Gulf States)	Carbon tetrachloride*	KLEEREX For skin blemishes (Kleerex)	Alcohol 25% Prepared calamine Spirit camphor* Phenol* Zinc oxide Resorcin Sulfur precipitate Distilled extract witch hazel
KLEEN PIKE DISINFECTANT (Howell Co.)			
KLEEN-RITE CLEANER Upholstery, rug cleaner (System)			
		KLEER GLASS CLEANER (Kleer)	
KLEEN-R- KREME Hand cleaner (Engine)		KLEERITE Ink (Am. Writing)	

*Consult Sec. II., Ingredients Index. This ingredient may be responsible for major toxic effects if poisonous amounts of this product are ingested.

Name & Use Manufacturer	Ingredients	Name & Use Manufacturer	Ingredients
KLEER-MOR LC-0 Detergent (Klenzade)		KLENZADE BRITE-KLENZ FORMULA HC-19 Detergent (Klenzade)	Caustic soda*
KLEER-MOR LC 99 LIQUID Detergent (Klenzade)		KLENZADE CAR WASH COMPOUND HC-3 Detergent (Klenzade)	
KLEER-STICK-ADHESIVES (Am. Writing)		KLENZADE CATTLE SPRAY FORMULA INS-20 Insecticide (Klenzade)	Piperonyl butoxide tech. 0.25% Pyrethrins 0.03% Petroleum oil* 99.72%
KLEE SEALANT Waterproof striping compound (Am. Fluresit)		KLENZADE CBS CLEANER FORMULA HC-66 Hand cleaner (Klenzade)	
KLEENZWELL OUT-INK ERADICATOR (Am. Writing)			
KLENSA Paint (Standard-Toch)		KLENZADE CHLORINATED PIPELINE CLEANER (Klenzade)	Sodium hypochlorite*
K-LENS-M ANTI-FOGGING LIQUID AND K-LENS-M CLEANER For lenses (Wilkins)	Isopropanol* Wetting agent	KLENZADE CLEANERS Detergent (Klenzade)	
KLENZADE ALUMINUM CLEANER FORMULA HC-70 (Klenzade)		KLENZADE DETERGENT BRICKS FORMULA NO. 3 (Klenzade)	Acid phosphates*
KLENZADE ANTI-FOAM EMULSION FORMULA LC-31 (Klenzade)	Silicone product	KLENZADE DETERGENT SANITIZER FORMULA KDS-3 Germicidal detergent (Klenzade)	Alkyl dimethyl benzyl ammonium chloride* 7.7%
KLENZADE BAKERY PAN-KLEEN FORMULA HC-30 (Klenzade)	Wetting agents* Polyphosphates* Detergent* ingredients Potassium dichromate* 2%	KLENZADE FLASH-KLEEN FORMULA HC-12 Dairy cleaner (Klenzade)	Caustic soda*
KLENZADE BILD-MOR FORMULA HC-12 Soap builder (Klenzade)	Caustic soda	KLENZADE FLY SPRAY FORMULA INS-10 (Klenzade)	Piperonyl butoxide tech. 0.50% Pyrethrins 0.06% Petroleum oil* 99.44%
KLENZADE BOTTLE WASH COMPOUND FORMULA HC-2 (Klenzade)		KLENZADE HARD WATER TREAT-MENT A FORMULA WT-11 (Klenzade)	Polyphosphate* compound
KLENZADE BOWL KLEENER (Klenzade)	Hydrochloric acid* over 10%	KLENZADE HC-8 CLEANER (Klenzade)	Sodium hypochlorite*

*Consult Sec. II., Ingredients Index. This ingredient may be responsible for major toxic effects if poisonous amounts of this product are ingested.

Name & Use Manufacturer	Ingredients	Name & Use Manufacturer	Ingredients
KLENZADE KCD-1 FORMULA CD-1 Detergent (Klenzade)	Alkyl dimethyl benzyl ammonium chloride* 2%	KLENZADE O-R CLEANING SYSTEM FORMULA O-R-1 Cleanser, short time pasteurizer (Klenzade)	Caustic soda*
KLENZADE KCD-3 FORMULA CD-3 Detergent (Klenzade)	Alkyl dimethyl ethyl benzyl ammonium chloride* 2%	KLENZADE O-R ORGANIC ACID DETERGENT FORMULA O-R-3 (Klenzade)	Organic acids*
KLENZADE KLEEN-SHEL POWDER FORMULA KS-1 Sanitizing detergent (Klenzade)	Para di-isobutyl phenoxy ethoxy ethyl dimethyl benzyl ammonium chloride* 5.0% Sodium carbonate 35.0%	KLENZADE PICK-EASY Detergent for poultry scalding vats (Klenzade)	
KLENZADE KLEER-BRITE FORMULA HC-29 Bottle washing alkali (Klenzade)	Sodium hydroxide over 10%	KLENZADE PIPELINE CLEANER FORMULA PL-1 Detergent (Klenzade)	Sodium hydroxide* over 10%
KLENZADE KLENZ-KLOR FORMULA X-3 For dairy & food plant cleaning (Klenzade)	Sodium hypochlorite* 3.25% Sodium phosphate* (expressed as $Na_3PO_4 \cdot 12H_2O$)	KLENZADE PIPELINE CLEANER FORMULA PL-3 Detergent (Klenzade)	Organic acids*
KLENZADE K-Q-10 FORMULA S-10 Sanitizer (Klenzade)	Methyldodecylbenzyl trimethyl ammonium chloride* 10%	KLENZADE RESIDUAL SPRAY FORMULA INS-30 Insecticide (Klenzade)	Methoxychlor tech. 3.00% Gamma isomer of benzene hexachloride (from lindane) 0.50% Pyrethrins 0.04% Piperonyl butoxide tech. 0.33% Petroleum oil* 86.13%
KLENZADE LAUNDERETTE COMPOUND Detergent (Klenzade)		KLENZADE ROACH SPRAY FORMULA INS-40 Insecticide (Klenzade)	Piperonyl butoxide tech. 0.714% Pyrethrins 0.088% Petroleum oil* 99.198%
KLENZADE MALATHION SPRAY FORMULA INS-50 Insecticide (Klenzade)	Malathion* 49.5% Xylene* 42.5%	KLENZADE SOFT FLOOR CLEANER FORMULA 1M-2 (Klenzade)	
KLENZADE MECHANICAL DISHWASH COMPOUND Detergent (Klenzade)	Sodium hypochlorite*	KLENZADE SPECIAL ALKALI FORMULA HC-41 Cleanser (Klenzade)	Caustic soda*
KLENZADE MECHANICAL DISHWASH COMPOUND FORMULA HC-44 Detergent (Klenzade)	Caustic soda*	KLENZADE STAINLESS STEEL DEEP FRY CLEANER FORMULA OR-1 (Klenzade)	Sodium hydroxide* over 10%

*Consult Sec. II., Ingredients Index. This ingredient may be responsible for major toxic effects if poisonous amounts of this product are ingested.

Name & Use Manufacturer	Ingredients	Name & Use Manufacturer	Ingredients
KLENZADE STER-KLEEN FORMULA LC-112 Detergent (Klenzade)	Organic acids*	KLIC AUTO WAX (Chem. Mfg. & Dist.)	
KLENZADE X-4 LIQUID BACTERICIDE (Klenzade)	Sodium hypochlorite* 6.4%	KLIK LIQUID CLEANER (Cardinell)	
KLENZADE X-15 Laundry bleach (Klenzade)	Chlorine* 15%	KLIK MEDICATED CREAM For skin burns, irritations (Miscible)	Ethyl aminobenzoate Camphor* Thymol* Stearate base Zinc oxide Menthol* Oils of clove and eucalyptus*
KLENZADE XY-12 CHLORINE DISINFEC- TANT & GERMICIDE (Klenzade)	Chlorine* 10.0%	KLIK NOSE DROPS For infants and children (Miscible)	Ephedrine* Chlorobutanol* Menthol* Isotonic aqueous solution
KLENZ EYE WASH (Rafea)	Sod. propionate Boric acid* Rose camphor water Glycerin Zephiran chloride* Borax* Sod. chloride Distilled ext. witch hazel Berberine sulf.*	KLING-TITE DRY Plant hormone (Calif. Spray)	Alpha naphthalene acetic acid 1.6% Inert ingredients*
		KLING-TITE 50 Insecticide (Calif. Spray)	Alpha naphthalene acetic acid 1.35% Inert ingredients*
KLENZIN POWDER Douche, wash or gargle (Jenkins)	Acid boric* Powdered alum Oxyquinoline sulfate Thymol* Menthol* Oil of eucalyptus* Carbolic acid	KLING-TITE 800 Plant hormone (Calif. Spray)	Alpha naphthalene acetic acid* 21%
		KLINK DRY CLEANING FLUID (Klink)	Carbon tetrachloride* Salvasol #3
KLENZO ANTISEPTIC Mouth wash (Rexall)	Alcohol 25% Zinc chloride* Benzoic acid Ammonium chloride Citric acid Menthol* Oil cloves* Cinnamic aldehyde Methyl salicylate* Alcohol	KLINK LIPSTICK STAIN REMOVER (Klink)	Butyl cellosolve (ethylene glycol monobutyl ether) Carbon tetrachloride* Chloroform* Alcohol
		KLINZMOTH CRYSTALS Insecticide (Klinzmoth)	Paradichlorobenzene*
KLERACID Laundry detergent (Wyandotte)	Fluorides*	KLINZMOTH LARVA-RID (Klinzmoth)	DDT 5% Paradichlorobenzene Naphthalene*
KLERE-SEAL (Pecora)		KLINZMOTH LUMPS Insecticide (Klinzmoth)	Paradichlorobenzene*
KLERRO Detergent (Physicians & Hosp.)		KLINZMOTH MOTH BALLS AND FLAKES (Klinzmoth)	Naphthalene* Paradichlorobenzene
KLETTEN- WURZEL HAAR OEL Hair prepara- tion (Germadol)		KLIX CLEANER (Garland)	
KLEX PAINT BRUSH CLEANER (Patty Remover)			

Name & Use Manufacturer	Ingredients		Name & Use Manufacturer	Ingredients	
KLIX DOG TREAT (French, R.T.)	Liver meal Cooked wheat cereal Rendered animal fat Cooked corn cereal Cheese whet and rinds Wheat germ Fish meal Fish solubles Cooked potato Tomato pomace Irradiated yeast Salt Bone meal Oxytetracycline feed supplement Certified food color Butylated hydroxy anisole Propyl gallate Citric acid	1/2% 1% 1% 0.1% 0.05% 0.0018% 0.0005% 0.0004%	KM KWIK-MIST Insecticide (Knapp)	DDT (dichloro diphenyl tri-chloroethane) n-Octyl bicycloheptene dicarboximide Allethrin (allyl homolog of cinerin 1) Beta butoxy beta thiocyano diethyl ether Methylated aromatic petroleum deriv.* Petroleum distillate Freon-12* (dichloro difluoro methane) Freon-11* (trichloro monofluoro methane)	2.00% 0.50% 0.10% 1.00% 7.20% 9.20% 40.00% 40.00%
KLONDIKE BRONZE POWDERS Paint product (Baer Bros. (Bronze))			KM MAGIK-MIST Insecticide (Knapp)	Pyrethrins Allethrins (allyl homolog of cinerin 1) Sesame oil extractives (inc. 0.5% Sesamin) Dichloro diphenyl trichloro-ethane Methoxychlor tech. Methylated aromatic petroleum deriv.* Petroleum distillates Inert ingredients	0.2% 0.1% 0.3% 2.0% 2.0% 12.2% 8.2% 75.0%
KLOREX Disinfectant for poultry drinking water (Whitmoyer)	Calcium hypochlorite* 56%		KM MAGIK-RID DOG SPRAY Insecticide (Knapp)	Pyrethrins Inert ingredients*	0.20%
KLORO For bromidroses and halitosis (Preston Labs.)	Chlorophyllins 100 mg.		KM REPEL-A-MIST Insecticide (Knapp)	2-Ethyl hexanediol-1,3 Inert ingredients*	20% 80%
KLORO-CEN Disinfectant (Central Chem.)	Chlorine* 70% Concentrated calcium hypochlorite*		KNICKER-BOCKER FLAT PAINT (Pierce, F.O.)		
KLOROCOL SYRUP (Chase Chem.)	Alcohol Each fl. oz.: Chloroform Potassium guaiacol sulf. Ammonium chloride Tartar emetic Syrup of white pine and wild cherry bark	3%/v 2 m. 8 gr. 8 gr. 1/12 gr.	KNIFER'S PREPARATION Antitussive (McMurray)	Tincture nux vomica* Strychnine alkaloids* 13-200 gr. Creosote* Tincture gentian compound* Glycerin	
KLORONOL Nasal decongestant (Sumlar)	Alcohol Ephedrine sulfate* Potassium bicarbonate Borax* Eucalyptol* Chlorobutanol Epinephrine hydrochloride Thymol* Methyl salicylate*	2% 0.5%	KNOCK-EM-STIFF FLEA POWDER (Knock-Em)		
K LOTION For hands & skin (K)	Glycerin or propylene glycol Camphor* Ammonia* Perfume		KNOK-EM-KOLD (Outdoor Fly Spray) (Nourse Oil)	Pyrin P-B* Pine oil* Lethane*	
KLUTCH Denture powder (Klutch)			KNO KLOG DRAIN PIPE SOLVENT (Univ. Ref.)		
			KNO-RUN To prevent stocking runs (Weartest)	Benzol* 17%	
			KNO-SAND Paint & varnish remover (Hillyard Chem.)	Chlorinated hydrocarbon*	

*Consult Sec. II., Ingredients Index. This ingredient may be responsible for major toxic effects if poisonous amounts of this product are ingested.

Name & Use Manufacturer	Ingredients		Name & Use Manufacturer	Ingredients
KNOTTY WOOD FINISH (Chi-Namel)	Pigment: Magnesium carbonate 100.0% Vehicle: Soya alkyd resin 35.4% Ester gum 4.1% Mineral spirits* 56.6% Drier 3.9%		KODAK CHEMICAL PHOTO-GRAPHIC SUPPLIES (Eastman)	Bleaches, desensitizers, developers, fixers, hardeners, intensifiers, lacquers, lacquer thinners, replenishers, re-touching fluids, solutions, spotting colors, toners
KNOX-OUT DUAL USE GARDEN DUST Insecticide (Pennsylv. Salt)	DDT 3% Copper as metallic 5% Sodium aluminum fluoride* 42%		KODAK GLACIAL ACETIC ACID Photographic supply (Eastman)	Glacial acetic acid*
KNOX-OUT INSECTICIDE POWDER (Pennsylv. Salt)	DDT* 10%		KÓ DEODORANT (Pittsburgh Plate Glass (Corona Chem.))	
KNOX-OUT INSECT SPRAY (Pennsylv. Salt)	DDT (dichloro diphenyl tri-chloroethane)* 5.0% Pyrethins 0.02% Crude sesame oil extractives 0.08% Methylated naphthalenes* 6.00% Petroleum oil* 88.90%		KOENIG'S NERVINE (Koenig)	
			KOFREDENE SYRUP Abbott)	Each fl. oz.: Chloroform 2 m. Ammonium chloride 10 gr. Tartar emetic 1/16 gr. Syrup ipecac 12 m. Menthol Honey Flavors Syrup q.s.
KNOX-OUT INSECT SPRAY DOUBLE USE (Pennsylv. Salt)	DDT* 5.00% Pyrethrins 0.02% Crude sesame oil extractives 0.08% Methylated naphthalenes* 6.00% Petroleum oil* 88.90%		KOHLER ONE NIGHT CORN SALVE Keratolytic (Kohler Mfg.)	Salicylic acid*
KNOX-OUT MULTI-PURPOSE AEROSOL INSECTICIDE (Pennsylv. Salt)	DDT 3.00% Pyrethrins 0.10% Allethrin 0.15% Piperonyl butoxide 0.75% Petroleum distillate 2.25% Methylated naphthalenes* 8.75%		KOHLER POWDERS Analgesic (Kohler Mfg.)	Acetophenetidin* 5 gr Caffeine
KNOX OUT ROACHES (Pennsylv. Salt)	DDT (dichloro diphenyl tri-chloroethane) 4.0% Tech. chlordane* (1.2% of octachloro-4,7-methano-tetrahydroindane and 0.8% of related compounds) 2.0% Methylated naphthalenes* 5.0% Petroleum oil* 89.0%		KOHLURA MASCARA (Mehron)	Castor oil Perfume Lamp black Stearic acid Beeswax Carnauba wax Olive oil Mineral oil Triethanolamine
KNOX-RUST (Bownes)			K.O. (Kill Odor) LIQUID B.O.R. 600 Deodorant (Pioneer)	
KOAGAMIN Parenteral blood coagulant (Chatham)	Oxalic acid 0.5% Malonic acid 0.25% Phenol 0.25%		KOJENE antiseptic (Kojene)	Oxyquinoline sulfate* Benzoic acid*
KOCOSCOPE Soap (U. S. Sanitary)			KOJENE OINTMENT Skin ointment (Kojene)	Oxyquinoline sulfate*
KODAK ACETIC ACID 28% Photographic supply (Eastman)	Acetic acid 28%		KO-KO Concentrated liquid soap (Adco)	Concentrated cocoanut oil Synthetic soap

*Consult Sec. II., Ingredients Index. This ingredient may be responsible for major toxic effects if poisonous amounts of this product are ingested.

- 624 -

Name & Use Manufacturer	Ingredients	Name & Use Manufacturer	Ingredients
KOLAGEN Tonic (Tosan)	Iron ammonium citrate Maganese chloride Brucine sulfate Caffeine Alcohol	KOMBO KIT NEUTRAL-IZER Hair straight-ener neutral-izer (Stanhope)	Potassium bromate*
KOLANA SYRUP Antitussive, for colds (Nelson Baker)	Tincture of euphorbia Tincture of cocillana Syrup of squill compound Syrup of wild lettuce Menthol Ext. of cascara	KOMBO KIT SHAMPOO STRAIGHTEN-ING LOTION (Stanhope)	Ammonium thioglycolate*
KOLD-E COMPOUND (Am. Pharm.)		KOME-GLO Sanitizing liquid, veterin-ary (Globe)	Para di-isobutyl phenoxy ethoxy ethyl dimethyl benzyl ammonium chloride* 2.5%
KOLINAL Lipotropic (Medical Arts)	Choline bitartrate 30 gm. Bataine bitartrate 30 gm. Inositol 5 gm. Di-methionine 7 gm. Yeast extraction and liver fraction (q.s.) 100 gm. Citrus flavor q.s.	KOMONOL SYNTHETIC DETERGENT (Minnesota)	
KOLLESOL Antiseptic (Kansas City)	8-Hydroxy-quinoline sulfate*	KCMPO HEAVY DUTY WAX (Kompolite)	
KOLON-TABS Cathartic (Univ. Nurit.)	Sodium carboxymethylcellulose 0.5 gm.	KOMPO LIQUID CLEANER Floor cleaner (Kompolite)	
KOLOR BRITE MARTIN-SENOUR ALL PURPOSE ENAMEL (97 White) (Martin-Senour)	Pigment: Titanium calcium pigment* 43% Titanium dioxide 57% Vehicle: Synthetic varnish* 89% Mineral spirits* 11%	KONCEAL HAIR COLORING (Germadol)	
KOLOR-ROX CEMENT FLOOR STAIN (Tamms)		KONDON'S JELLY WITH EPHEDRINE (Kondon)	Menthol* Oil eucalyptus* Phenol* Camphor* Ephedrine* Alkaloid
KOLPEX TAR OINTMENTS (Dome)		KONDON'S NASAL JELLY (Kondon)	Menthol* Oil eucalyptus* Phenol* Camphor*
KOLPIX A & KOLPIX D Skin ointment (Dome)	Whole crude coal tar 2% Acid mantle creme* base	KONDON'S NOSE & THROAT DROPS (Kondon)	Menthol* Camphor* Oil eucalyptus* Oil peppermint Phenol*
KOLPOSINE Douche, liquid (Optimus)	Aluminum ammonium sulfate Boric acid* Phenol* less than 3% Menthol Glycerin	KONGOLENE HAIR STRAIGHT-ENER (Kongo)	
KOLTAROL Disinfectant (Huggins)	Anhydrous soap 18% Tar acid oil (to a maximum of 20% phenol*) 72%	KON KOTE PAINT (Gable-Tite)	
KOLYNOS TOOTH-PASTES (Whitehall)		KONTROL DENTAL STAIN REMOVER (Allen, Mark)	Neutral salt hendecenoic acid Calcium phosphate Aromatics
KOMAC PAINTS (Kohler-McLister)		KONTROL TOOTH-PASTE (Allen, Mark)	

*Consult Sec. II., Ingredients Index. This ingredient may be responsible for major toxic effects if poisonous amounts of this product are ingested.

Name & Use Manufacturer	Ingredients		Name & Use Manufacturer	Ingredients	
KOPERTOX Fungicide (medicinal) (Kopertox)	Copper naphthenate*		KOPPERS PARANAP BALLS Insecticide (Koppers)	Refined naphthalene* Paradichlorobenzene	98% 2%
KOP-KARB Fungicide (Thompson-Hayward)	Copper carbonate* (expressed as metallic copper) 20%		KOPPERS SNOWFLAKE VAPORIZER Insecticide (Koppers)	Refined naphthalene*	100%
KOPPERS CAMPHORETTE BLOCKS Insecticide (Koppers)	Refined naphthalene* Perfume oils	99-1/2% 1/2 %	KOPPERS TOILET BOWL ODORIZER (Reliable Chem.)	Paradichlorobenzene*	
KOPPERS CEDAR MOTH CHIPS (Koppers)	Refined naphthalene* Red cedar chips	97% 3%	KO RAKE Antitussive, for colds (T-Lax)	Chloroform 6 m. Ext. cascara sagrada aromatic and white pine compound* Ammonium chloride Sodium citrate Sodium salicylate* Menthol* Oil of peppermint	
KOPPERS CEDAR-NAP MOTH CRYSTALS (Koppers)	Refined naphthalene* Perfume oils	99.5% 0.5%			
KOPPERS MOTH BALL BLOCK (Koppers)	Refined naphthalene*	100%	KORE GERMICIDAL DETERGENT (King Res.)		
KOPPERS MOTH BALLS (Koppers)	Refined naphthalene*	100%	KOREX COPPER CLEANER (Korex)	Acid*-based preparation with high percentage of abrasive	
KOPPERS MOTH CAKE AND MOTH SQUARES (Koppers)	Refined naphthalene* Perfume oils	99.5% .5%	KOREX OVEN CLEANER (Korex)	Highly alkaline with caustic* base	
KOPPERS MOTH FLAKES (Koppers)	Refined naphthalene*	100%	KOREX STOVE CLEANER (Korex)	High percentage of abrasive	
KOPPERS MOTH OCTONS (Koppers)	Refined naphthalene*	100%	KORJENA (Myers Labs.)	Phenolphthalein* Sodium choleinate Calcium iodide*	
KOPPERS MOTHALENE VAPORIZER Insecticide (Koppers)	Paradichlorobenzene*	100%	KORKO PAINTS (Smith-Corwin)		
KOPPERSOL Fungicide (Destruxol)	Mineral oil Vegetable oil Ammonia* Copper as metallic*	35% 2% 2.5% 0.7%	KOROMEX CREAM Vaginal cream (Holland-Rantos)	Boric acid 2.0% Oxyquinoline benzoate 0.02% Phenylmercuric acetate 0.02% Stearic acid Cetyl alcohol Glycerin Perfume	
KOPPERS PARADI-CHLORO-BENZENE Insecticide (Koppers)	Paradichlorobenzene*	100%	KOSELANO COMPOUND Antitussive (Blue Cross)	Menthol euphorbia* Wild lettuce Cascarin Pilulifera Syrup squill comp.* Cocillana	
KOPPERS PARADI-CHLORO-BENZENE VAPORIZER Insecticide (Koppers)	Paradichlorobenzene*	100%	KOTALKO LIQUID (Kotalko)	Lanolin Mineral oil Oleoresin capsicum Perfume Camphor* deriv.	
			KOTALKO OINTMENT (Kotalko)	Sulfur* Petrolatum Lanolin Castor oil* Oleoresin capsicum Camphor* deriv.	

---

*Consult Sec. II., Ingredients Index. This ingredient may be responsible for major toxic effects if poisonous amounts of this product are ingested.

Name & Use Manufacturer	Ingredients		Name & Use Manufacturer	Ingredients	
KOTALKO SOAP (Kotalko)	Pine tar* Ichthyol Sulfur* Sodium soaps of coconut and palm oil fatty acids		KP PINE OIL (Klinzmoth)	Steam distilled pine oil* Soap	75% 15%
KOTOFOM LINOLEUM CLEANER (My-Ko)			K-P LIQUID For intestinal irritation (veterinary) (Beebe Labs.)	Sulfathiazole Pectin Aluminum hydroxide Bentonite Sodium benzoate Glycerin Peppermint oil Amaranth #2 F.D.	1.76% 0.75% 2.00% 3.00% 0.50% 1.00% 0.02% 0.01%
KOTOFOM PAINT & VARNISH CLEANER (My-Ko)					
KOTOFOM RUG, UPHOLSTERY CLEANER (My-Ko)			K-P POWDER For intestinal irritation (veterinary) (Beebe Labs.)	Sulfathiazole* Pectin Aluminum hydroxide Bentonite Sodium lauryl sulfate* Peppermint	
KOVA ALL ENAMEL (Nat'l Paint)			KRAB Herbicide (Bonide)	Potassium cyanate*	75%
KOVER BEST PAINT (Republic)			KRAB-DETH Ectoparasiticide (Wisconsin Pharm.)	Alkaloids of larkspur seed Isopropyl alcohol*	0.04% 50%
KOVERFLOR Paint (Standard-Toch)			KRAB-FOIL (Sacramento)		
			KRAKNO Paints (Johnston)		
KOVER KAL, KOVEROIL, KOVERWALL, KOVERWELL PAINTS (Bauer)			KRANK'S SHAVING CREAM (Consolid. Royal)		
KOW-KARE Iron tonic (veterinary) (Dairy Assoc.)	Dried iron sulfate Epsom salts Gentian root Colombo Nux vomica (3/20 gr. strychnine* per oz.) Ginger Cayenne pepper Potassium iodide* Cobalt carbonate* Vitamins A and D Manganese* sulfate Bone meal		KRASHÉ BEAUTIFYING NIGHT CREAM (Grellva)		
			KRASHÉ CREAMS (Grellva)		
			KRASHÉ FIRMSKIN LOTION (Grellva)		
KOZINE For colds (Veltex)	Each tablet: Acetanilid* Ext. belladonna Ext. cascara sagrada Aloin* Oleoresin capsicum	3/4 gr. 1/20 gr.	KRASHÉ SHAVING AID & SKIN SMOOTHER & CLEANSER (Grellva)		
K-PAC OINTMENT Rubefacient (Kory)	Histamine dihydrochloride* Glyceryl monostearate Spermaceti Sodium lauryl sulfate	1/2% 23% 8% 1%	K-R COMPOUND (Park Chem.)	Kerosene* Soap Pine oil* Abrasives	
K.P.G. 9 Grease-oil remover, deodorizer (Pioneer)			KRAWLTOX Insecticide (Warren Ref.)	DDT Thanite Odorless kerosene*	1% 3% 96%
K.P. INSECTICIDE (Schaeffer Mfg.)			KREAM KUT-KOTE REMOVER Paint and varnish (Day, James B.)	Benzol* Methyl acetate*	

*Consult Sec. II., Ingredients Index. This ingredient may be responsible for major toxic effects if poisonous amounts of this product are ingested.

Name & Use Manufacturer	Ingredients
KRE-A-TOR Antitussive (Oliver's S-O)	Chloroform 5 m. per fl. oz. Creosote* Squill* Oil tar* Oil eucalyptus* Camphor* Aromatic spirit of ammonia Glycerin Aromatic elixir Alcohol 20%
KRE-COTE PAINTS (Keystone Ref.)	
KREEN Motor tonic (Kano)	Petroleum solvents* Other oils
KREITZER'S SALVE (Aschenbach)	
KREML HAIR TONIC (Williams, J.B.)	Alcohol 19% Phenylcarboxylate Acetyl methyl pyrandione Methyl dodecyl benzyl trimethyl ammonium chloride* Essential oils Mineral oil base
KREML CORRECTIVE For dandruff (Williams, J.B.)	Alcohol 25% Dihydroxy dichloro diphenyl methane* Benzalkonium chloride*
KREML CREAM HAIR DRESSING (Williams, J.B.)	Amine soap Lanolin Mineral oil
KRE-O-DOR Cleanser (Plunkett)	Coal tar neutral oils* Soap Phenols*
KRE-O-KOTE STAIN Paint product (Stewart Paint)	
KREOLE KORN KURE (Howell Co.)	
KREOLE SHOE POLISH (Manhattan Kreole)	
KREOSEM ELIXIR Antitussive (Massengill)	Each 5 cc.: Ethylmorphine hyd. (morphine deriv.) 2.8 mg. Ammonium chloride 86.5 mg. Terpin hydrate 43 mg. Potassium guaiacolsulfonate 43 mg. Tartar emetic 2.8 mg. Sodium glycerophosphate 21.5 mg. Potassium glycerophosphate 21.5 mg.
KREOSEPTIC PRESERVA-TIVES Paints (Sweeney, W.H.)	

Name & Use Manufacturer	Ingredients
KRESOLA DISINFECTANT (Tilden)	Cresylic acid* 50.1% Soap 24.9%
KRESO-TOL Antiseptic (Diefenbach)	Solution of 4-n-amyl-meta-cresol 0.2% Chlorothymol 0.1%
KRESYLINOL Disinfectant (Corn King)	Cresylic acid* Soap Glycerin
KRIEGER'S OINTMENT (Krieger)	Mercuric nitrate* ointment 24% Benzocaine Zinc oxide Petroleum base
KRILIUM For soil treatment (Monsanto)	Synthetic polyelectrolyte: Hydrolized acrylonitrile* or a vinyl acetate-maleic anhydride resin
KRINOL For burns (Sedarex)	Zinc oxide Calamine Camphor* Tincture benzoin compound Salicylic acid* Paraffin Coal tar creosote Hydrocarbon oil* White petrolatum
KRIPTIN Anti-histamine tablets (Whitehall)	Pyrilamine maleate* 25 mg.
KROIL Penetrating oil (Kano)	Petroleum solvents* Other oils
K-R-O KILLS RATS (K-R-O)	Red squill* powder (fortified) 100%
K-R-O READY MIXED WARFARIN DOUBLE STRENGTH RAT & MOUSE KILLER (K-R-O)	Warfarin (3-(a-acetonylbenzyl)-4-hydroxycoumarin) 0.05%
K-R-O READY MIXED WARFARIN RAT & MOUSE KILLER (K-R-O)	Warfarin (3-(a-acetonylbenzyl)-4-hydroxycoumarin) 0.025%
KROSHEEN Hair pomade (Kroy)	Lanolin Mineral oil Petrolatum Cetyl alcohol Perfume
K-R-O WARFARIN Rodenticide (K-R-O)	Warfarin 0.50
K-R-O WARFARIN RAT & MOUSE KILLER (K-R-O)	Warfarin (3-(a-acetonylbenzyl)-4-hydroxycoumarin) 0.5%

*Consult Sec. II., Ingredients Index. This ingredient may be responsible for major toxic effects if poisonous amounts of this product are ingested.

Name & Use Manufacturer	Ingredients	Name & Use Manufacturer	Ingredients
KROMAX Paint (Atlantic V. & P.)		KUMFOOT ICY FOOT CREAM (Commerce)	Digenol* Hexachlorophene Menthol Thymol* Camphor* Eucalyptus*
KROMELAX Cathartic (Weldona)	Cascarin		
		KUNKEL'S WORM SYRUP (Aschenbach)	
KROME-LITE Paint (Elliott)			
		KURAMINE Herbicide (Dow)	Alkanolamine salt of 2-(2,4,5-trichlorophenoxy) propionic acid*
KROY WEN Ointment (Manhattan Drug)	Carbolic acid* 2% Camphor tar* Eucalyptus* Boric acid* Zinc oxide Sulfur* Thymol* Menthol* Witch hazel Benzocaine	KURB TABLETS Analgesic (Kimberly)	Acetophenetidin* Aspirin* Caffeine
		KURE-A-LEKE Roof coating (Stelwagon)	
KROY WEN RECTAL SUPPOSI-TORIES (Manhattan Drug)	Benzocaine Ext. of witch hazel bark Ichthynate Pine tar* Tannin*	KURESEMA SKIN CREAM (Assoc. Brands)	
KRYLON SPRAY COATINGS (Krylon)	Acrylic resins Alkyd resins Cellulose lacquers Freon Toluol*	KURLENE Eyelash pomade (Kurlash)	Cholesterol (pure crystals) Balsam Peru U.S.P. 1X White petrolatum U.S.P. and amber petrolatum U.S.P.
KRYOCIDE Insecticide (Florida Agric.)	Sodium fluoaluminate 90%	KURLSET Hair preparation (Noonan)	
KUBECIDE GARDEN DUSTER Fungicide, insecticide (Miller Chem.)	Rotenone 0.75% Other cube resins 1.20% Beta thiocyano ethyl esters of aliphatic fatty acids (average 10-18 carbon atoms) 0.56% Zineb 3.90% Inert ingredients 93.59%	KURON Herbicide (Dow)	2-(2,4,5-Trichlorophenoxy) propionic acid* Esters of mono-, di-, and tri-propylene glycol monobutyl ethers
KUDYMERN FORMULA 111 Antitussive (Kudymern)	Chloroform 2 m./fl. oz. Wild cherry bark Poplar buds Yerba santa Menthol* Glycerin White pine bark Blood root Spikenard Eucalyptol* Creosote*	KU-RU TABLETS Analgesic (Harrison's)	Aspirin* Acetophenetidin* Caffeine
		KUT-KOTE PAINT & VARNISH REMOVER (Day)	Methylene chloride*
KUHN'S MEDICIDE Rubefacient, (Kuhn Med.)	Alcohol 12% Sodium salicylate* Amino acetic acid	KUT-KOTE REMOVER (Day)	Benzol* Acetone*
		KUTOL WALLPAPER CLEANER (Cincy)	Wheat flour Refined kerosene* Vegetable dye Salt Preservative
KUHN'S CLIMATIZED PAINT (Kuhn Paint)		KUT-OL WITH LANOLIN Cuticle softener, stain remover (Creative Cosm.)	
KUMFOOT Foot powder (Commerce)	Chlorophyll Hexachlorophene Tincture benzoin* Balsam peru Menthol* Thymol* Camphor* Starch Zinc oxide Boric acid*	KUTZIT PAINT & VARNISH REMOVER (Savogran)	Toluol* Benzol* Methanol Acetone

*Consult Sec. II., Ingredients Index. This ingredient may be responsible for major toxic effects if poisonous amounts of this product are ingested.

Name & Use Manufacturer	Ingredients	Name & Use Manufacturer	Ingredients	
KUV-ER-ALL PAINT (Armor)		LACCO BRAND APPLE BAIT Insecticide (Los Angeles Chem.)	Sodium fluosilicate*	4.5%
KWICKILL Insecticide (Easterday)		LACCO BRAND BASIC LEAD ARSENATE Insecticide (Los Angeles Chem.)	Basic lead arsenate*	96%
KWIKEEZE BRUSH CLEANER (Glidden Co.)		LACCO BRAND BLACK MAGIC SULPHUR Insecticide (Los Angeles Chem.)	Sulfur*	92%
KWIKEEZE LIQUID PAINT BRUSH CLEANER (Savogran)	Toluol* Xylol* Methanol Acetone	LACCO BRAND CALCIUM ARSENATE Insecticide (Los Angeles Chem.)	Calcium arsenate*	80%
KWIK-FYRE Fire kindler (Kwick-Fyre)		LACCO BRAND CARBON BI-SULPHIDE Fumigant (Los Angeles Chem.)	Carbon bisulfide*	
KWIK GLASS WASHER (Hoag-Farmer)				
KWIKGLOSS (General Printing)				
KWIK-KILL BAIT Insecticide (Pearson & Co.)	Calcium arsenate* 5.00% Metaldehyde* 2.00% Arsenic expressed as metallic 1.88 Water-soluble arsenic 0.035	LACCO BRAND CHLORDANE CONC. Insecticide (Los Angeles Chem.)	Tech. chlordane*	20%
KWIK-LITE LIGHTER FLUID (Boyle-Midway)	Naphtha*	LACCO BRAND CREOSOTE A.W.P.A. Fungicide (Los Angeles Chem.)	Creosote*	97%
KWIK PAINT & VARNISH CLEANER (Chem. Prod.)		LACCO BRAND DORMANT EMULSION Insecticide (Los Angeles Chem.)	Petroleum oils*	85%
KWIK-RUB (Leslie Pharm.)				
KWIK WAX (Chandler)				
KWIK WASH (Park Chem.)	Alkyl aryl sulfates* Sodium sulfate	LACCO BRAND DUST NO. 6-30 Fungicide (Los Angeles Chem.)	Copper*	15%
KWIK-WET Darkroom aid (Edwal)	Sulfonated aromatic hydrocarbon*			
K & W WATERLESS SOAP (K & W)	Cottonseed fatty acid Kerosene* Aqueous ammonia* Caustic potash* Essential oil* Lanolin	LACCO BRAND DUST NO. 6-50 Fungicide (Los Angeles Chem.)	Copper*	25%
LABCO DRY CLEAN LOTION Veterinary (Labco)		LACCO BRAND DUST NO. 10 Insecticide (Los Angeles Chem.)	Nicotine*	3.6%
LABCO GERMICIDE Veterinary (Labco)				

*Consult Sec. II., Ingredients Index. This ingredient may be responsible for major toxic effects if poisonous amounts of this product are ingested.

Name & Use Manufacturer	Ingredients		Name & Use Manufacturer	Ingredients	
LACCO BRAND DUST NO. 10-F Insecticide (Los Angeles Chem.)	Nicotine*	3.6%	LACCO BRAND LIQUID LIME SULPHUR Insecticide (Los Angeles Chem.)	Calcium polysulfide* Calcium thiosulfate	29% 2%
LACCO BRAND DUST NO. 86-S Insecticide (Los Angeles Chem.)	Lead arsenate* Copper Sulfur	44.% 5% 24%	LACCO BRAND MAGIC SULPHUR Insecticide (Los Angeles Chem.)	Sulfur*	98%
LACCO BRAND DUST NO. 98-S Insecticide (Los Angeles Chem.)	Tricalcium arsenate* Copper Sulfur	35% 7.5% 24%	LACCO BRAND MEDIUM EMULSION Insecticide (Los Angeles Chem.)	Petroleum oils*	83%
LACCO BRAND EMULSIVE COPPER NAPHTHEN-ATE SOLUTION Fungicide (Los Angeles Chem.)	Copper naphthenate Petroleum oils*	3% 88%	LACCO BRAND PARIS GREEN Insecticide (Los Angeles Chem.)	Copper aceto-arsenite*	90%
LACCO BRAND FLYZAWAY Insecticide (Los Angeles Chem.)	DDT* Petroleum oils*	5% 94%	LACCO BRAND POISONED BAIT Insecticide (Los Angeles Chem.)	Calcium arsenate	5%
LACCO BRAND FLYZGONE Insecticide (Los Angeles Chem.)	Piperonyl butoxide DDT* Pyrethrins Petroleum oil*	0.27% 5% 0.03% 94.7%	LACCO BRAND POISONED BARLEY Rodenticide (Los Angeles Chem.)	Strychnine alkaloid	0.23%
LACCO BRAND GRUB-TOX Insecticide (Los Angeles Chem.)	Rotenone Additional extractives Sulfur*	2.5% 7.5% 50%	LACCO BRAND SAND-O-FLY Insecticide (Los Angeles Chem.)	Piperonyl butoxide Pyrethrins* Petroleum oil*	
LACCO BRAND HEAVY MEDIUM EMULSION Insecticide (Los Angeles Chem.)	Petroleum oils*	83%	LACCO BRAND SECTONE Insecticide (Los Angeles Chem.)	Rotenone Other extractives Phenothiazine Pyridine Fish oil soap	0.55% 1.65% 5% 2% 12%
LACCO BRAND INSECTO Insecticide (Los Angeles Chem.)	Pyrethrins Petroleum oil Fish oil soap Phenothiazine Pyridine Inert ingredients*	0.2% 11.3% 12% 5% 2%	LACCO BRAND SHEEP DIP Insecticide (Los Angeles Chem.)	Total phenols* Aromatic oils Anhydrous soap	15% 53% 22%
LACCO BRAND KALI-DUST Insecticide (Los Angeles Chem.)	Calcium arsenate*	35%	LACCO BRAND SPRAY BLUESTONE Fungicide (Los Angeles Chem.)	Copper sulfate pentahydrate*	94.3%
LACCO BRAND LIGHT MEDIUM EMULSION Insecticide (Los Angeles Chem.)	Petroleum oils*	83%			

*Consult Sec. II., Ingredients Index. This ingredient may be responsible for major toxic effects if poisonous amounts of this product are ingested.

Name & Use Manufacturer	Ingredients		Name & Use Manufacturer	Ingredients
LACCO BRAND STANDARD LEAD ARSENATE Insecticide (Los Angeles Chem.)	Lead arsenate*	93.6%	LADCO SYRUP OF MAMOU Antitussive (Louisiana)	White pine* compound Infusion of mamou roots Glycerin Syrup Menthol* Tar* Honey Chloroform*
LACCO BRAND WETTABLE SULPHUR Insecticide (Los Angeles Chem.)	Sulfur*	95%	LADY BEVERLY CREME MAKE-UP (Enterprise Chem.)	
LACCO BRAND ZINC-ORDO Fungicide (Los Angeles Chem.)	Zinc*	20%	LADY BEVERLY ESTROGENIC HORMONE SKIN CREAM (Enterprise Chem.)	
LACO GENUINE CASTILE SHAMPOO (Laco)			LADY BEVERLY FACE POWDER (Enterprise Chem.)	
LAC-R-TINT (Hubere)				
LACTIKOL CREME Vaginal cream (Durex)	p-Tri-isopropyl phenoxy polyethoxy ethanol 1.25% Sodium lauryl sulfate 0.6% Glycerin 8.0% Glyceryl mono fatty esters Stearic acid Lactic acid Sodium chloride		LADY ESQUIRE DUPLEX CREAM Shoe polish (Knomark)	
LACTIKOL VAGINAL JELLY (Durex)	Lactic acid 1.5% Oxyquinoline sulfate 0.05 Glyceryl monoricinoleate 1.0% p-Tri-isopropyl phenoxy polyethoxy ethanol 1.25% Sodium lauryl sulfate 0.2% Glycerin Carbohydrate gum base		LADY GENE DEODORANT DOUCHE TABS (Scott Jay)	
			LADY LENNOX HAIR COLORING (Lady Lennox)	
LACTIVES Laxative (Clapp, Otis)	Aloin* 1/7 gr. Resin of jalap 1/8 gr. Resin scammony 1/7 gr. Resin of podopyllum 1/8 gr. Ext. nux moschata 1/25 gr. Phenolphthalein 1/2 gr.		LADY LENNOX STAIN REMOVER (Lady Lennox)	
LACTO DEXTRIN For favorable intestinal flora (Battle Creek)	Lactose Dextrins Tricalcium phosphate Flavoring		LADY WILDROOT CREAM HAIR DRESSING (Wildroot)	
LACTOSE DEXTRINS For favorable intestinal flora (Battle Creek)	Lactose 48.0% Dextrine 33.0% Maltose 16.0% Dry lemon juice 0.5% Moisture 2.5%		LADY WILDROOT WAVE (Wildroot)	
LA DANA HAIR RINSE (La Dana)				
LADCO PINE OIL DISINFECTANT (Louisiana)	Pine oil* soap			

Name & Use Manufacturer	Ingredients		Name & Use Manufacturer	Ingredients	
LA FETE DES ROSES (Caron)			LA-MO HOSPITAL DOUCHE POWDER (La-Mo)		
L.A. FORMULA Laxative (Burton, Parsons)	Plantago ovata Lactose Dextrose		LA MONA TOILET WATER (Assoc. Brands)		
LA FRANCE Bluing detergent (Baker, F.)	Alkyl aryl sulfonate* Sodium sulfate* Sodium phosphates* Blue and fluorescent dyes		L'AMOUR TOUJOUR PERFUME (Ybry)		
LA FRE PERFUME (La Fre)			LA MYRA SKIN SALVE (Auto-Loks)		
LAGAL Laxitive (Wallace)	Sodium alginate Calcium alginate		LANACADE OINTMENT (Solway- Annan)	Oil of cade* Sulfur* Resorcin* Ointment base Bismuth subnitrate Thymol iodide* Zinc oxide	
L'AIMANT LINE TOILET WATER & EXTRACT (Coty)					
LAKE CHEMICAL C. T.B.C.S. 53 Insecticide (Lake Chem.)	Copper as metallic* 53.00%		LANACAINE For skin irritations (Vogarell)	Benzocaine Chlorthymol* Phenylmercuric acetate 0.02% Zinc oxide Sodium sulfo dioctyl succinate Vitamin D2 resorcin 2000 U.S.P. units	
LAKEROL PASTILLES Antiussive (Ahlgrens)	Gum arabic Sugar Licorice Menthol* Eucalyptol*		LANALLURE CREME SET For hair (Ogilvie)		
LALOTIN 1 Lascoff's lotio instanta (Lascoff)	Zinc sulfate*		LANE'S TEA Cathartic (Kemp & Lane)	Alexandria senna Anise and fennel seed Coriander seed Licorice root	
LALOTIN 2 Lascoff's lotio instanta (Lascoff)	Polysulfides*		LANEX FOR PILES For hemorrhoids (Carma)	Lanolin Menthol* Petrolatum Alum Camphor* Phenol* Salicylic acid* Cocoa butter	
LAMAC'O CEMENT Re-soling adhesive (Lamac)	Acetone Aromatic solvents* Nitrated cotton base				
LAMAC'O THINNER Cement thinner (Lamac)	C.P. acetone*		LANIKOL OINTMENT For skin irritations (Lanikol)	Salicylic acid* Bismuth subnitrate Thymol iodide* Zinc oxide Ichthammol Lanolin	
LAMBERTS IRISH REDUCINE Veterinary (Kopf)	Pine tar*		LANITOL Detergent (Arkansas)	Alkyl aryl sulfonates*	
			LANOIL TINT (Hubere)		
LAMO Skin emollient (Nason)	Lanolin Cold cream		LANOL Scalp emollient (Hance)	Lanolin Boric acid* Cholesterol	
			LANOLAVE Body rub, and lotion (Lanolave)	Lanolin Wintergreen* Rubbing alcohol* Ethyl alcohol* 70%	

*Consult Sec. II., Ingredients Index. This ingredient may be responsible for major toxic effects if poisonous amounts of this product are ingested.

Name & Use Manufacturer	Ingredients	Name & Use Manufacturer	Ingredients
LANOLE EMOLLIENT (Connors)	Stearic acid Lanolin (anhydrous) Lanolin (concentrate) Wax Mineral oil Butoben Colonial bouquet Triethanolamine	LANOLIN PLUS SUNTAN LOTION (Consolid. Cosm.)	Lanolin U.S.P. Fatty esters Emulsifiers Sun screening agent Perfume Certified coloring
LANOLIN DISCOVERY Spray net (Curtis, H.)		LANORA HAIR DRESSING (Noramex)	
LANOLIN PLUS BODY LOTION (Consolid. Cosm.)	U.S.P. lanolin Fatty alcohols Fatty esters Refined oils Glycerin Perfume Certified coloring	LANO-SCALP SHAMPOO (Glen-Star)	
		LANO-SET HAIR SET (Ogilvie)	
LANOLIN PLUS CLEANSING CREAM FOR DRY SKIN (Consolid. Cosm.)	Lanolin U.S.P. Mineral oil Waxes Perfume Polyhydric glycol	LAN-O-SHEEN GLASS CLEANER (Lan-O-Sheen)	Isopropanol* Naphthalene* Beta meta umbelliferone AZO red Ethylene diamine tetra-acetate U.S.P. sassafras*
LANOLIN PLUS FOR THE HAIR (Consolid. Cosm.)	U.S.P. lanolin Fatty esters Refined oils Certified coloring Perfume	LAN-O-SHEEN SOAP POWDER (Lan-O-Sheen)	High titer soap Sodium phosphates* Sodium sulfate Pine oil* Lanolin U.S.P. Fatty acid Ethylene oxide condensate Oil of sassafras* U.S.P.
LANOLIN PLUS HAND LOTION (Consolid. Cosm.)	Vegetable and mineral oils U.S.P. lanolin Fatty esters Certified coloring Perfume	LANO SUN SCREEN LOTION (Lura-Glo)	
LANOLIN PLUS LIPSTICK (Consolid. Cosm.)	Vegetable Mineral oils Waxes Lanolin U.S.P. Propylene glycol Perfume Certified coloring	LANOTAN SUNTAN CREAM (Peau D'Or)	Stearic acid Glyeryl monostearate Mineral oil Heliophan Triethanolamine Perfume Vitamin D 2 Sunarome OMMO Lanolin
LANOLIN PLUS LIQUID (Consolid. Cosm.)	Lanolin U.S.P. Mineral oil U.S.P. Liquid fatty esters Certified coloring Perfume	LANTEEN JELLY (Breon)	Sodium benzoate U.S.P.* Glycerol U.S.P. Chlorothymol N.F.* Tragacanth U.S.P. Ricinoleic acid Hexylresorcinol U.S.P.
LANOLIN PLUS LIQUID CLEANSER (Consolid. Cosm.)	U.S.P. lanolin Fatty esters Refined oils Perfume	LANTEEN YELLOW POWDER For douche (Breon)	Chlorothymol* Menthol* Lactose Methyl salicylate* Oil of cassia Lactic acid (pH approx. 3.8)
LANOLIN PLUS LIQUID MAKE-UP (Consolid. Cosm.)	Titanium dioxide Inert inorganic pigments Fatty esters Waxes Oils Water Perfume	LANTU RODENTICIDE (Laconia)	Alpha naphthyl thiourea
		LAN-II For hair and scalp (Commerce)	Lanolin Hexachlorophene* Sodium undecylenate* Sodium caprylate
LANOLIN PLUS SHAMPOO (Consolid. Cosm.)	Lauryl alcohol Sulfate salts Soap Fatty esters Lanolin U.S.P. Perfume Certified coloring	LAPACTIC PILLS Laxative (Sharp & Dohme)	Aloin* 15 mg. Ipecac 4 mg. Ext. belladonna (equiv. to 0.06 mg. total alkaloids) 5 mg.

---

*Consult Sec. II., Ingredients Index. This ingredient may be responsible for major toxic effects if poisonous amounts of this product are ingested.

Name & Use Manufacturer	Ingredients
LAPEPTOL 240 (Elixir) Proteolytic digestant (Massengill)	Pepsin 24 gr. per fl. oz. Lactic acid Hydrochloric acid* Aromatics q.s.
LAPODO Astringent for skin irritations (Sargeant)	Boric acid* Benzoic acid* Camphor* Menthol* Balsam of fir Salol Chlorthymol*
L'ARDENTE NUIT EAU de TOILETTE & PERFUME (Parfums Corday)	
LARIEUSE HAIR PREPARATIONS (Godefroy)	
LARIEUSE SHAMPOO (Godefroy)	
LARIEUSE STAIN REMOVER (Godefroy)	
LARIOBEN Oral antiseptic (Marvell)	Benzyl alcohol 2%/v Iodine in organic combination* Potassium iodide* Liquefied carbolic acid 0.39% Tannic acid* Sodium chloride Glycerin Oil cinnamon Oil peppermint Flavor
LARKIN ANALGESIC BALM Rubefacient (Larkin)	Methyl salicylate* Balsam Peru Menthol* Lanolin Beeswax
LARKIN MENTO KANFO For skin irritations (Larkin)	Camphor* Boric acid* Oil of pine* White wax Menthol* Eucalyptol* Methyl salicylate* Petrolatum
LA ROSE COLOGNES AND PERFUMES (Rochas)	
LA ROSE JACQUEMINOT TOILET WATER AND EXTRACT (Coty)	

Name & Use Manufacturer	Ingredients
LARSON'S ADHESIVE BALM SPRAY Pre-tape dressing (Larson)	Benzalkonium chloride 0.184% Hexachlorophene 0.699% Dichlorophene 0.517% Film base 38.6% Dichloro difluoro methane* 39.0% Monofluoro trichloro methane* 21.0%
LARSON'S FOOT NOTE Astrigent, fungicide (medical) (Larson)	Hexachlorophene* Dichlorophene* Menthol*
LARSON'S MIST INSECT REPELLENT (Larson)	Ethylhexanediol* 33-1/3%
LARVABROME-20 Insecticide (Larvacide)	Methyl bromide* 80% Chloropicrin* 20%
LARVACIDE Fungicide (Larvacide)	Chloropicrin (trichloronitro-methane)
LARVACIDE AEROSOL Insecticide (Larvacide)	Chloropicrin* 50%/w Methyl chloride* 50%/w
LARVACIDE EDB Fungicide (Larvacide)	Chloropicrin* 95% Ethylene dibromide 5%
LARVATOX Insecticide (Speekman)	Zinc fluosilicate* 10.00% Poly amino poly carbocylic acid 0.50% Alkylphenyl ester of polyethylene glycol 0.25%
LARVEX Insecticide (Zonite)	Fluoride* Sodium aluminum silicofluoride*
LA SANADORA For muscular aches (Romero)	Alcohol* 33% Camphor* Oil peppermint Oil sassafras* Ammonia Cayenne pepper Caramel Ethyl alcohol
LASCO-PLEX Dietary supplement (Lascoff)	Each capsule: Thiamine hydrochloride 3 mg. Riboflavin 3 mg. Pyridoxine hydrochloride 0.25 mg. Calcium pantothenate 5 mg. Niacinamide 20 mg. Whole liver powder 50 mg.
LASSAR'S PASTE (Allied Dist.)	Petrolatum Zinc oxide Starch
LASTIDECK LIQUID ROOFING (United Gilson.)	Asphalt* Inert fillers Mineral spirits*

*Consult Sec. II., Ingredients Index. This ingredient may be responsible for major toxic effects if poisonous amounts of this product are ingested.

Name & Use Manufacturer	Ingredients	Name & Use Manufacturer	Ingredients
LASTIKALK Caulking compound (Lastik)		LA VALLIERE PERFUMES, COLOGNES, TOILET WATER (Specialty)	
LASTIKO WALL SIZE Paint product (Fuller, H.B.)	Liquified animal glue Corn dextrines	LA VALLIERE VIOLET BATH SALTS (Specialty)	
LASTIK ROOFING CEMENT (Lastik)		LAVANDOR For toilet and bath (Marto)	Alcohol* 92%
LAUDRIN SYRUP Anti-histaminic, antitussive (Kip, A.)	Each fl. oz.: Pyrilamine maleate* 90 mg. Ephedrine hydrochloride* 60 mg. Potassium guaiacol sulfonate 20 gr. Menthol* Aromatics	LAVASEPTINE Douche (Kip, A.)	Zinc sulfate* 6% Phenol 1/10% Thymol* Methyl salicylate* Boric acid granules* Potassium alum 1% Sodium salicylate 1% Eucalyptol* Menthol*
LAUNDRI-BRITE FORMULA HC-40 Detergent (Klenzade)		LA VERE HAIR RINSE (La Dana)	
LAUND-R-PAX WITH & WITHOUT PAXCIDE Cleaner (Packwood)	Silicate and phosphate* Alkaline salts Sulfonated powdered detergents* Bleach agents Phenolic bactericidal agent*	LAVIDERM A-D OINTMENT For skin irritations (Pastol)	Pure cod liver oil Burow's solution Zinc oxide White petrolatum Water washable base
LAUNDRY GEMS Laundry blue (Seibert)	Granulated borax* Trisodium phosphate Granular tripolyphosphate Pure soap 92% Dye Denatured alcohol	LAVIDERM FUNGICIDAL SOLUTION Fungicide (medical) (Pastol)	Dichloro dihydroxy diphenyl methane* Triethano undecylenate Salicylanilide* Aromatized isopropyl alcohol* 75%
LAURO-BORACIC Eye bath (Clapp, Otis)	Borax Sodium chloride Camphor water Cherry laurel water Boric acid Berberine hydrochloride Rose water	LAVIDERM MEDICATED POWDER For foot irritations (Pastol)	Dichloro dihydroxy diphenyl methane* Trioxymethylene* Chlorothymol* Zinc peroxide Boric acid* Absorbent aromatized base
LAUTRIC Vaginitis (Gynecological)	Alcohol sulfates*	LAVIDERM WITH POLY-SULPHIDES For skin irritation (Pastol)	Zinc sulfate* solution Hexachlorophene solution #1 Polysulfide* solution #2
LAUXEIN Coating resin, adhesive (Monsanto)	Casein Soybean adhesives	LAVO LINOLEUM CLEANER (Lavo)	
LAUXITE Coating resin, adhesive (Monsanto)	Urea Phenolic melamine and resorcinol resins	LAVO PAINT & VARNISH CLEANER (Lavo)	
LAVA Soap (Procter & Gamble)	Inert inorganic abrasive Vegetable fat Glycerin	LAVO PORCELAIN, TILE & MARBLE CLEANER (Lavo)	
LA VALLIERE DEODORANT SPRAY (Specialty)			

*Consult Sec. II., Ingredients Index. This ingredient may be responsible for major toxic effects if poisonous amounts of this product are ingested.

Name & Use Manufacturer	Ingredients	Name & Use Manufacturer	Ingredients
LAVOPTIK EYE LOTION (Lavoptik)	Boric acid* Hydrastine hydrochloride Camphor* Sodium chloride	LAXATIVE JR. (Jenkins)	Each tablet: Senna 1/4 gr. Ext. cascara sweet 3/8 gr. Phenolphthalein 1/2 gr. Ext. nux vomica 1/1000 gr. Strychnine 0.00007 gr.
LAVORIS Mouthwash and gargle (Lavoris)	Zinc chloride 0.2% Formaldehyde 0.02% Menthol Insoluble saccharin Oil of cassia Oil of cloves Ethyl alcohol 5%	LAXA-TRATE Laxative (Vegetrates)	Cut senna leaves Peeled Russian licorice Aniseed Peppermint leaves Juniper berries Uva ursi leaves Lavender flowers
LAVO RUG, UPHOLSTERY CLEANER (Lavo)		LAXCEL Laxative (Battle Creek)	Psyllium gum (mucilaginous) Karaya gum (mucilaginous) Wheat germ Maltose Milk sugar Dextrine Powdered lemon juice
LAVOTEX Skin cleanser (Torch)	Hexachlorophene (G-11) 1% Sulfated detergent* Vegetable oil		
LAWN-A-GEN Insecticide, fungicide (Dextruxol)	Dichlorethyl ether* 70.00% Copper chloride dihydrate 2.68%	LAXETTS Laxative (Jenkins)	Each tablet: Phenaphthalein 1/4 gr. Ext. cascara 1/4 gr. Aloin* 1/8 gr. Podophyllin 1/8 gr. Atropine sulfate* 1/1000 gr. Powdered ipecac 1/32 gr. Ext. nux vomica* (strychnine 0.0046 gr.) 1/16 gr.
LAWN BOOSTER Water soluble lawn nutrient (Collins Feed)			
LAWN GUARD Insecticide (Collins Feed)	Chlordane* 20.00% Hexachloro epoxy octahydro dimethano naphthalene 10.50% Related compounds 1.86% Petroleum hydrocarbons 45.00% DDT 15.00%	LAXMO Cathartic (Battle Creek)	Phenolphthalein Heavy mineral oil
		LAXO Laxative (Battle Creek)	Blond psyllium seeds
LAX Veterinary (Anchor Serum)	Magnesium hydroxide 272.4 gm. Sodium phosphate dibasic 64.7 gm. Citric acid 3.41 gm.	LAXOL Laxative (White, A.)	Castor oil* 99.5% Flavoring and sweetening 0.5%
LAXACARTHIC Laxative (Yates Drug)	Atropine sulfate* 1/500 gr. Emetin 1/1000 gr. Capsicine 1/250 gr. Podophyllin 1/8 gr. Aloin* 1/5 gr.	LAXOM Laxative (Hance)	Yellow phenolphthalein 1-1/4 gr. Magnesium sulfate Citric acid Sugar Calc. carb. Calc. stearate Confectioners glaze Powdered gum Arabic
LAX-A-GEL (Baker, J.)			
LAXAGILL Cathartic (Massengill)	Castor oil* 96% Saccharin Aromatized and colored ruby		
LAXA-PIRIN For colds (Laxa-Pirin)	Each tablet: Acetophenetidin* 1 gr. Aspirin* Ext. cascara Caffeine* Aloin* Pd. capsicum Podophyllin		
LAXATION Laxative (Bodkin)	Senna California fruit Sodium benzoate 1/10 of 1%		

*Consult Sec. II., Ingredients Index. This ingredient may be responsible for major toxic effects if poisonous amounts of this product are ingested.

Name & Use Manufacturer	Ingredients	Name & Use Manufacturer	Ingredients
LAXONA COMPOUND Laxative (Cel-Ton-Sa)	Buckthorn Cascara sagrada Senna Aloe* Ginger Fennel Quassia Mandrake Iron and amm. citrate Oil spearmint Calamus Coriander Burdock* Salicylic and benzoic acid* Saccharin soluble Wahoo Anise Gentian Licorice Oil cassia Methyl salicylate* Butternut Colocynth Uva ursi Wild cherry Sarsaparilla Buchu Juniper berries Carmel	**LAYMON'S SHAVING LOTION** (World's Prods.)	
		LAZARIN Ointment (Lazarin)	Zinc oxide Starch Olive oil Petrolatum
		LAZY LIVER PILLS Laxative (Gino Pill)	Podophyllin Aloin* Gamboge* Culver's root Blue flag
		LEA COMPOUND (All grades) (Lea)	Aluminum oxide or other abrasive Glue Sassafras*
LAXWELL (Arend)		**LEAFOX ZINC OXIDE** Fungicide (New Jersey)	Zinc oxide*
LAYMON'S ASPIRIN (World's Prods.)	Aspirin*	**LEAF SHINE** For polishing and shining the leaves of plants (Destruxol)	
LAYMON'S CLEANSING, COLD, HAND, VANISHING CREAM (World's Prods.)		**LEAF LINIMENT** (Leaf Oil)	Oil of cassia Spruce Cedar Cloves* Birch Turpentine* Tinct. of fleabane Alcohol
LAYMON'S CREAM DEODORANT (World's Prods.)		**LEAROK** (All grades) Buffing or polishing medium (Lea)	Abrasives Greases Waxes Fatty acids
LAYMON'S FACE POWDER (World's Prods.)		**LEAVENS** Asthmatic antispasmodic (Leavens)	Each fl. oz.: Potassium iodide* 40 gr. Alkaloids of belladonna root 0.0425 gr. Sodium bromide 3 gr. Sarsaparilla Syrup Alcohol
LAYMON'S HAND LOTION (World's Prods.)		**LEBANON ALDRIN EMULSIFI-ABLE** Insecticide (Lebanon)	Hexachloro hexahydro dimethano naphthalene* 22.9% Related compounds 17.3% Petroleum hydrocarbons 7.5%
LAYMON'S LIPSTICK (World's Prods.)		**LEBANON AMINE 40, 2,4-D WEED KILLER** Herbicide (Lebanon)	2,4-D dimethylamine 64% 2,4-D acid* 41%
LAYMON'S NAIL POLISH REMOVER (World's Prods.)		**LEBANON ARISOD WEED & GRASS KILLER** Herbicide (Lebanon)	Sodium arsenite* 30.06%
LAYMON'S ROUGE (World's Prods.)			

*Consult Sec. II., Ingredients Index. This ingredient may be responsible for major toxic effects if poisonous amounts of this product are ingested.

Name & Use Manufacturer	Ingredients	
LEBANON ARSENATE OF LEAD Insecticide (Lebanon)	Lead arsenate* Arsenic as metallic Water soluble arsenic Lead as metallic	96.00 19.60 0.50 58.00
LEBANON BAIT KILLS MICE & RATS Rodenticide (Lebanon)	Warfarin (3-(a-acetonyl benzyl)-4-hydroxycoumarin)	0.025%
LEBANON BASIC COPPER 53% FUNGICIDE (Lebanon)	Copper*	53.0%
LEBANON BHC W-10 Insecticide (Lebanon)	Wettable powder benzene hexachloride*	
LEBANON BOR-DOX COPPER FUNGICIDE (Lebanon)	Copper*	12.75%
LEBANON BRUSH KILLER Herbicide (Lebanon)	Tetrahydro furfuryl ester of 2,4-dichlorophenoxy acetic acid* Tetrahydro furfuryl ester of 2,4,5-trichlorophenoxy acetic acid*	21.4% 10.3%
LEBANON COTTON DUST 3-5-0 Insecticide (Lebanon)	Gamma isomer of benzene hexachloride* DDT*	3.00% 5.00%
LEBANON DAIRY CATTLE FLY SPRAY Insecticide (Lebanon)	Tech. piperonyl butoxide Pyrethrins Mineral oil	0.2895% 0.036% 99.6745%
LEBANON DDT 5 DUST Insecticide (Lebanon)	DDT*	5.00%
LEBANON DDT 10 DUST Insecticide (Lebanon)	DDT*	10.00%
LEBANON DDT EMULSION CONC. Insecticide (Lebanon)	DDT Aromatic petroleum deriv. solvent*	25.00% 70.00%
LEBANON DDT 50% WETTABLE POWDER Insecticide (Lebanon)	DDT*	50.00%
LEBANON 34% DDT XYLENE SPRAY Insecticide (Lebanon)	DDT* Xylene*	34.00% 61.00%
LEBANON DI-COP POTATO SPRAY Insecticide (Lebanon)	DDT Copper*	8.25% 66%
LEBANON DI-COP POTATO-TOMATO DUST Fungicide, insecticide (Lebanon)	DDT Copper*	3.0% 7.0%
LEBANON 50% DIELDRIN WETTABLE POWDER Insecticide (Lebanon)	Hexachloro epoxy octahydro-endo, exo-dimethano naphthalene* Related compounds	42.5% 7.5%
LEBANON DI-NITROL WETTABLE POWDER FOR DORMANT SPRAYING Insecticide (Lebanon)	Dinitro ortho cresol*	40%
LEBANON DRY LIME SULFUR Fungicide (Lebanon)	Calcium polysulfides*	
LEBANON DUST F-15 Insecticides (Lebanon)	Ferric dimethyl dithiocarbamate Inert ingredients	11.40%
LEBANON DUSTING SULFUR Fungicide (Lebanon)	Sulfur*	
LEBANON EGG PRESERVA-TIVE (Lebanon)	Sodium silicate*	
LEBANON ESTER 2,4-D WEED KILLER Herbicide (Lebanon)	2,4-D ester 2,4-D acid*	39% 35.2%
LEBANON ESTER 44 2,4-D WEED KILLER Herbicide (Lebanon)	2,4-D isopropyl ester*	44.0%
LEBANON 76% FERBAM Fungicide (Lebanon)	Ferbam*	76%
LEBANON FLOTATION SULFUR PASTE Fungicide (Lebanon)	Sulfur*	40%

*Consult Sec. II., Ingredients Index. This ingredient may be responsible for major toxic effects if poisonous amounts of this product are ingested.

Name & Use Manufacturer	Ingredients		Name & Use Manufacturer	Ingredients	
LEBANON FRUIT SPRAY OR DUST Insecticide, fungicide (Lebanon)	Gamma isomer of benzene hexachloride (from lindane)* 2.50% DDT* 5.00% Ferbam 3.80% Sulfur* 25.00%		LEBANON MALATHION GARDEN SPRAY Insecticide (Lebanon)	Malathion* 50.0% Xylol* 42.4%	
LEBANON GARDEN DUST Insecticide, fungicide (Lebanon)	Malathion* 4.0% Methoxychlor tech. 5.0% Captan 5.0% Sulfur 5.0%		LEBANON MALATHION 25% WETTABLE SPRAY POWDER Insecticide (Lebanon)	Malathion* 25%	
LEBANON HEPTACHLOR 25% WETTABLE POWDER Insecticide (Lebanon)	Heptachlor* 25.0% Related compounds 9.72%		LEBANON ORNAMENTAL DUST Insecticide, fungicide (Lebanon)	2-(p-tert-Butyl phenoxy) isopropyl-2-chloroethyl sulfite 2.00% Captan 5.00% Gamma isomer of benzene hexachloride (from lindane) 1.00% Inert ingredients	
LEBANON IMPROVED ROSE DUST OR SPRAY Insecticide (Lebanon)	Gamma isomer of benzene hexachloride (from lindane) 1.25% 2-(p-tert-Butyl phenoxy) isopropyl-2-chloroethyl sulfite 2.00% DDT* 5.00% Ferbam 7.50% Sulfur* 25.00%		LEBANON ORNAMENTAL SPRAY Insecticide (Lebanon)	2-(p-tert-Butyl phenoxy) isopropyl-2-chloroethyl sulfite 5.70% Captan 25.00% Gamma isomer of benzene hexachloride (from lindane)* 6.50%	
LEBANON IMPROVED WEEDETH Herbicide (Lebanon)	2-ethylhexyl ester of 2,4-dichlorophenoxy acetic acid* 9.48% 2-ethylhexyl ester of 2,4,5-trichloro phenoxy acetic acid 4.53%		LEBANON PARATHION 25% EMULSIFIABLE Insecticide (Lebanon)	Parathion* 25.2% Xylol 66.8%	
LEBANON INSECT & ROACH SPRAY (Lebanon)	Petroleum distillates* Tech. chlordane* Beta butoxy beta thiocyano diethyl ether*		LEBANON P.C. CRABGRASS KILLER (Lebanon)	Potassium cyanate* 46%	
LEBANON JAPANESE BETTLE SPRAY (Lebanon)	DDT* 25.00% Tech. chlordane* 20.00%		LEBANON RO-DUST 100 Insecticide (Lebanon)	Rotenone 1.00% Other active cube resins 2.00% Inert ingredients	
LEBANON KLOR-DUST INSECTICIDE (Lebanon)	Tech. chlordane* 5.00%		LEBANON RO-DUST 301 Insecticide (Lebanon)	Rotenone 1% DDT 3%	
LEBANON KLOR-SPRAY Insecticide (Lebanon)	Tech. chlordane* 46%		LEBANON RO-SPRAY 400 Insecticide (Lebanon)	Rotenone* 4%	
LEBANON KLOR-SPRAY Insecticide (Lebanon)	Tech. chlordane* 40%		LEBANON 0.75% ROTENONE GARDEN DUST Insecticide (Lebanon)	Rotenone 0.75% Other active cube resins 1.50% Sulfur 10.00%	
LEBANON LIME SULPHUR SOLUTION Insecticide, fungicide (Lebanon)	Calcium polysulfide* 29.00%		LEBANON 3-D 50% WETTABLE POWDER Insecticide (Lebanon)	Dichloro diphenyl dichloro ethane* 50.0%	
LEBANON 25% LINDANE WETTABLE POWDER Insecticide (Lebanon)	Gamma isomer of benzene hexachloride* 25.0%		LEBANON TOMATO BLIGHT DUST Fungicide (Lebanon)	Metallic copper* 7%	

*Consult Sec. II., Ingredients Index. This ingredient may be responsible for major toxic effects if poisonous amounts of this product are ingested.

Name & Use Manufacturer	Ingredients	
LEBANON TOXAPHENE 60% EMULSION CONC. Insecticide (Lebanon)	Petroleum distillate Toxaphene*	35.00% 60.00%
LEBANON WETTABLE SULPHUR FUNGICIDE (Lebanon)	Sulfur*	95.0%
LEBANON ZINC SULPHATE (Powdered monohydrated) Fungicide (Lebanon)	Zinc*	36%
LECILAN (Horton & Converse)	Lanolin Lecithin	
LECI-TRATE Dietary supplement (Vegetrates)	Cephalin Soybean oil Lecithin-choline Sugars sterol glucosides Inositol phosphatides	29.2% 4.0% 29.2% 5.2% 31.4%
LE DEMAQUILLANT (Caron)		
LEECH HOUSEHOLD CEMENTS (Leech)	Nitro cellulose base Acetone* Dineltone Toluol*	
LEECH LIQUID SOLDER (Leech)	Plastic cement Aluminum powder	
LEECH PATCH (Latex) CEMENT (Leech)	Natural latex Ammonia*	
LEECH PLASTIC RESIN WOOD GLUE (Leech)	Resins	
LEECH PORCELAIN FINISH Paint (Leech)		
LEECH WEATHER- STRIP CEMENT (Leech)	Rubber base Ketone* solvents	
LEEMULSION For colds (veterinary) (Lee, G.)	Eucalyptus oil* Camphor* Anethole Cresols* Paraffin oil Creosote* N.F. Carvacrol Methyl salicylate* Chloroform* Linseed oil	2-1/2%

Name & Use Manufacturer	Ingredients	
LEE RUBBER CEMENT (Lee R. & T.)	Rubber Naphtha*	
LEE'S CALF SCOUR MEDICINE (veterinary) (Lee, G.)	Sulfathiazole Colloidal kaolin Bismuth subcarbonate Pectin Methyl parahydroxybenzoate	3.38% 17.5% 1.14% 0.9% 0.18%
LEE'S CREOSOTE DIP PHENOL COEFFICIENT 5 Insecticide (Lee, G.)	Tar acid* Hydrocarbons* Anhydrous resin soap	20% 56% 15%
LEE'S DAIRY FLY SPRAY Insecticide (Lee, G.)	Piperonyl butoxide tech.* Pyrethrins Petroleum oil*	0.510% 0.051 99.439
LEE'S DOG WORMER CAPSULES Anthelmintic (veterinary) (Lee, G.)	Each capsule: Tetrachlorethylene* Arecoline hydrobromide Mineral oil	99.2% 0.4% 0.4%
LEE'S DRI RUB Insecticide (Lee, G.)	Naphthalene* Creosote oil Micro-mesh sulfur	19% 1% 15%
LEE'S EAR CANKER OINTMENT Veterinary (Lee, G.)	Methyl dodecyl benzyl trimethyl ammonium chloride Gamma isomer of benzene hexachloride (from lindane) Pine oil* Petrolatum tech.	1% 0.25% 30% 68.75%
LEE'S E.Q. 3-35 Insecticide (Lee, G.)	Gamma isomer of benzene hexachloride (from lindane)* Pine oil* Mineral oil Colloidal silica	3% 35%
LEE'S FLOCK WORMER Anthelmintic (veterinary, avian) (Lee, G.)	Nicotine* Sodium sulfate tech. Molasses Phenothiazine Absorbent clay Malted grain products	2.5% 25%
LEE'S LINDANE SPRAY Insecticide (Lee, G.)	Gamma isomer of benzene hexachloride (from lindane)* Aromatic petroleum deriv. solvent*	12.9% 83.9%
LEE'S LIQUID FLEA KILLER (Lee, G.)	Rotenone Other cube resins Allethrin Paradichlorobenzene Petroleum hydrocarbons* Isopropyl alcohol*	0.55% 1.40% 0.05% 2% 76% 20%

*Consult Sec. II., Ingredients Index. This ingredient may be responsible for major toxic effects if poisonous amounts of this product are ingested.

Name & Use Manufacturer	Ingredients		Name & Use Manufacturer	Ingredients	
LEE'S LOUSE POWDER (Lee, G.)	Micronized sulfur* DDT tech. dichloro diphenyl trichloroethane Talc	46% 1% 53%	LEE'S WOUND DRESSING & FLY REPELLENT (veterinary) (Lee, G.)	Pine oil Bone oil anhydrous Pine tar* Sulfonated bitumen anhydrous Turkey red oil Zinc oxide	3% 22% 35% 5% 2% 25%
LEE'S MANGE REMEDY Ectoparasiti- cide (vet- erinary) (Lee, G.)	Benzyl benzoate* Gamma isomer of benzene hexachloride (from lindane) Isopropyl alcohol* Emulsifying oil base	35.95% 0.05% 45% 19%	LEF'S OIL LINIMENT (Auth. Brands)		
LEE'S MIST HANDY AEROSOL BOMB Insecticide (Lee, G.)	Menthol* Camphor* Oil of eucalyptus* Carvacrol Creosote* N.F. White mineral oil Inert propellant*	 25% 75%	LEF'S OINTMENT (Auth. Brands)		
LEE'S MITE KILLER (Lee, G.)	Coal tar phenols* Coal tar neutral oils* Petroleum oils* Trichlorobenzenes*	8% 15% 72% 5%	DR. LEGEAR'S ANT & ROACH KILLER (Le Gear)	Tech. chlordane* Petroleum distillate*	33.8% 60.2%
LEE'S PERCH PAINT Insecticide (Lee, G.)	Phenols Nicotine alkaloid*	8.5% 5%	DR. LEGEAR'S 50% CRESYLIC SOLUTION Disinfectant (Le Gear)	Cresylic acid* Soap Glycerin	
LEE'S NO. 62 SCREW- WORM SMEAR Veterinary (Lee, G.)	Diphenylamine Benzol* Turkey red oil Lamp black	35% 35% 5.5% 20%	DR. LEGEAR'S 50% DDT WETTABLE POWDER Insecticide (Le Gear)	DDT*	50%
LEE'S PICKPASTE For cannibalism in poultry (Lee, G.)	Picolines* Petrolatum amber tech. Pine tar oil* Wood rosin		DR. LEGEAR'S DIP & DISINFECTANT Animal remedy (Le Gear)	Coal tar hydrocarbons* Soap Coal tar acids*	64% 15% 11%
LEE'S SULFA- MERAZINE VET. To reduce infections of animals and poultry where accurate diagnosis is established. (Lee, G.)	Sodium sulfamerazine 13.0%		DR. LEGEAR'S DRY INSECTICIDE For lice on livestock (Le Gear)	DDT Creosote oil* Sulfur*	1.25% 2.50% 24.75%
			DR. LEGEAR'S EQ 335 SCREW- WORM REMEDY (Le Gear)	Gamma isomer of benzene hexachloride(from lindane)* Pine oil*	 3% 35%
LEE'S SULFA- QUINOXALINE For coccidiosis (veterinary, avian) (Lee, G.)	Sodium sulfaquinoxaline 3.44 gr./100 cc. Sodium hydroxide		DR. LEGEAR'S FLEA & TICK POWDER (Le Gear)	DDT* Pyrethrins	10% 0.5%

LEE'S
UDDER
CREAM
For udder
irritations
(Lee, G.)
	Lanolin
	Cetyl alcohol
	Methyl salicylate*
	Para di-isobutyl phenoxy ethoxy
	  ethyl dimethyl benzyl
	  ammonium chloride*
	Petrolatum
	Camphor*
	Menthol*
			DR. LEGEAR'S
			FLY SPRAY
			KILLS
			(Le Gear)
				Mineral oil
				Tech. piperonyl butoxide
				Pyrethrins* 1 and 2	

			DR. LEGEAR'S GRUB DUST (Le Gear)	Total cube resins Inert ingredients	4.33%

---

*Consult Sec. II., Ingredients Index. This ingredient may be responsible for major toxic effects if poisonous amounts of this product are ingested.

- 642 -

Name & Use Manufacturer	Ingredients		Name & Use Manufacturer	Ingredients	
DR. LEGEAR'S HOUSEHOLD INSECT SPRAY (Le Gear)	Tech. chlordane Pyrethrins 1 and 2 Tech. piperonyl butoxide Petroleum distillate*	2.00% 0.03% 0.25% 97.72%	LEHMAN AQUARIUM CEMENT (Lehman Bros.)		
DR. LEGEAR'S INSECT POWDER (Le Gear)	Pyrethrins	0.5%	LEHMAN SHINGLE STAINS & FINISHES (Lehman Bros.)	Lead	1%
DR. LEGEAR'S KILL-GERM Disinfectant (Le Gear)	Isopropyl alcohol* Vegetable oil soap o-Benzyl p-chlorophenol* Sodium lauryl sulfate o-Phenyl phenol Essential oils	10% 7% 4.5% 2% 0.75% 0.50%	LEHMAN TRIM PAINTS (Lehman Bros.)	Lead	1%
DR. LEGEAR'S LOUSE POWDER (Le Gear)	Gamma isomer of benzene hexachloride (from lindane) 	1.00%	LEHMAN VARNISHES (Lehman Bros.)	Lead	less than 1%
DR. LEGEAR'S MANGE MEDICINE For dogs (Le Gear)	Triethanolamine and potassium soaps Pine tar oil Juniper tar Oil of turpentine Isopropyl alcohol	11.40% 5.60% 2.10% 2.20% 3.90%	LEKOTORIA HERB TEA (Myers Labs.)	Senna Elder flowers Fennel Sarsaparilla Sassafras* Uva ursi Chamomile Centaury Triticum Aniseed	
DR. LEGEAR'S MANGE TREATMENT Animal remedy (Le Gear)	Tech. chlordane* Petroleum distillate*	33.8% 60.2%	LEKOTORIA SOLID HOT LINIMENT (Myers Labs.)	Oleoresin capsicum Camphor* Ocotea cymbarum Petrolatum base Methyl salicylate* Oils of turpentine* Origanum imitation	
DR. LEGEAR'S NEW LOUSE POWDER (Le Gear)	Gamma isomer of benzene hexachloride (from lindane) Inert ingredients	1%	LEKTROLITE FLUID (Lektrolite)		
DR. LEGEAR'S ROOST PAINT WITH LINDANE Insecticide (Le Gear)	Lindane Petroleum distillates* 	1.25% 98.75%	LEMBROSE Rubefacient (Wheth Labs.)	Methacholine chloride Menthol Thymol Eucalyptol Methyl salicylate*	0.25% 5.5% 0.1% 1% 11%
DR. LEGEAR'S SCREW WORM KILLER Animal remedy (Le Gear)	Chloroform* Tar acids* Coal tar hydrocarbons Soap	23% 9% 40% 20%	LEMCKE'S DIP-N-RINSE Chemical cleaner for silver (Bellaire)		
DR. LEGEAR'S SCREW-WORM SMEAR Animal remedy (Le Gear)	Chloroform tech.* Cresote oil* Potassium and triethanolamine oleates	15.6% 6.5% 7.5%	LEM-O-GLO TABLETS (Alladin Labs.)	Citric acid Boric acid*	50% 45%
LE GUI PERFUME, COLOGNE, TOILET-WATER (Duvelle)	Alcohol* Di-ethyl-phthalate		LEMON OIL COMPANY'S STANDARD INSECTICIDE (Miller Chem. & Fert.)	Dry soap Essential oils Terpenes Nicotine*	7.0% 1.5% 2.0% 1.6%
LEGULO Ointment for skin irritations (Legulo)	Benzocaine Zinc oxide Juniper tar U.S.P.* Ointment base Resorcinol* Bismuth subnitrate Rosin		LENATE Analgesic antiseptic (external) (Maurry)	Menthol U.S.P. Strong iodine tinct. N.F. Phenol* U.S.P. Guaiacol N.F. Alcohol Glycerin U.S.P.	0.55% 3.1% 2.75% 1.5% 5%
LEGULO-SAL Effervescent (Legulo)	Sodium bicarbonate Potassium carbonate Citric acid		LENEVA LENITIVE LOTION Skin (Leneva)	Oils distillates* Belladonna* Birch Cassia Cedar Cloves* Fleabane Spruce Turpentine* Alcohol*	 83%

*Consult Sec. II., Ingredients Index. This ingredient may be responsible for major toxic effects if poisonous amounts of this product are ingested.

Name & Use Manufacturer	Ingredients		Name & Use Manufacturer	Ingredients	
LENK LIQUID SOLDERING FLUX (Lenk)	Hydrochloric acid*		LEPAGE'S LIQUID SOLDER (Le Page's)	Solvent* cement Nitrocellulose base	
LENK PERFECT TORCH FUEL (Lenk)	Denatured alcohol*		LEPAGE'S MIRACLE MENDER Adhesive (Le Page's)		
LENOIR'S LOTION For skin irritations, fungicide (Cawthon-Coleman)	Alcohol* 84.44% Acetanilide* 12.15 gr./oz.		LEPAGE'S WALL SIZE (Le Page's)	Corn dextrine Yellow corn paste powder	
			LE PAGE'S WHITE GLUE (Le Page's)	Polyvinyl acetate emulsion Solvent*	
LENSAL Fungicide (medicinal) (Buzze's)	Alcohol* 50% Benzoic acid* Salicylic acid*		LE PRINCE PERFUMES, HAND LOTION, & TOILET WATER (Le Prince)		
LENZO EYE GLASS CLEANER (Curley)			LERGENEX CAPSULES Asthmatic analgesic (Marion Pharm.)	Ext. stramonium* 1/40 gr. Phenacetin* 1/2 gr. Ephedrine sulfate* 1/4 gr. Aminophylline* Pot. chloride*	
LEONARDI WORM SYRUP Anthelmintic (Leonardi)	Oleum chenopodi* 1.00 cc. Flxt. spigelia marilandica 8.40 cc. Flxt. sennae 5.60 cc.		LE SAGER PERFUME & TOILET WATER (Sager)		
LEONARD PIPE SEAL (Leonard)	Vegetable drying oils Petroleum wax Titanium dioxide Calcium carbonate		LESCO DRY CLEANING COMPOUND (Scott, L.E.)		
LEONARD PLASTIC STIK (Leonard)	Vegetable drying oils Petroleum wax Titanium dioxide Calcium carbonate		LESCO RUST PREV. & REMOVER COMPOUND (Scott, L.E.)		
LEOPARD SPOT REMOVER (Carbona)			LESLIE ELECTRIC CLEANSER (Leslie & Co.)	Carbon tetrachloride* Benzine	
LEPAGE'S AEROPLANE GLUE (Le Page's)	Solvent* cement Cellulose acetate		LESLIE SEBORRHOEA COMP.& LOTION (Leslie & Co.)	Salicylic acid* Cologne spirits Alcohol*	
LEPAGE'S CASEIN GLUE (Le Page's)	Animal base (casein)		LESLIE'S HEALING & DRAWING SALVES (Leslie Pharm.)		
LEPAGE'S GOLD METAL MUCILAGE (Le Page's)	Vegetable base (gum arabic)				
LEPAGE'S GRIPSPREADER MUCILAGE (Le Page's)	Vegetable base (gum arabic)		LES POIS DE SENTEUR DE CHEZ MOI (Caron)		
LEPAGE'S LIQUID GLUE (Le Page's)	Animal or vegetable base				
LEPAGE'S LIQUID PLASTIC MENDER (Le Page's)	Solvent* cement Ethylene dichloride*		LES-SLIP FLOOR GLOSS Self-polish wax (Lester)	Wax Colloidal silica	

*Consult Sec. II., Ingredients Index. This ingredient may be responsible for major toxic effects if poisonous amounts of this product are ingested.

- 644 -

Name & Use Manufacturer	Ingredients
LESTER W. HANNA'S H.M.-204 GENERAL PURPOSE INSECTICIDE & FUNGICIDE (Hanna)	Basic copper arsenate* 13.65% Sulfur 46.35% DDT 5%
LESTOIL Solvent soap (Adell)	Sulfonated alcohol type detergent* base
L'ESTRONA HORMONE CREAM For complexions (Andre)	Estrogenic hormones 10,000 I.U./oz.
LESWEED Herbicide (Lester)	Isopropanol amine salts of 2,4-dichlorophenoxy acetic acid* 16.3%
LETO'S FOR THE GUMS (Leto)	Copper sulfate* Iodine* Potassium iodide*
LEUCO-DERM OINTMENT For skin irritations (Mann Chem.)	Pine tar* Zinc oxide Starch Benzoic acid* Petrolatum
LE VERTIGE EXTRACT & TOILET WATER (Coty)	
LEVIS EAR CANKER OINTMENT Veterinary (Levis)	Bismuth oxyiodide* Thymol iodide* Boric acid
LEVIS FLEA POWDER Insecticide (Levis)	Rotenone 1.25% Pyrethrins 0.14% Other cube resins 1.25% Inert ingredients
LEV-L-ASTIC Underlayment and patching compound (Allied Comp.)	
LEWIS & BENNETTS' MULEY MAKER Dehorning fluid (Hatch, Ora)	Sodium hydroxide* Potassium hydroxide*
LEWIS LYE (Pennsylv. Salt)	Sodium hydroxide* 96.00% Sodium carbonate 00.75%
LEXATOL EYE CONC. (Pearson Pharm.)	
LEXOL LEATHER CONDITIONER (Martin Dennis)	

Name & Use Manufacturer	Ingredients
LEXTOX Insecticide (Lester)	Pyrethrums synergist
L'HEUR TOILET WATER & PERFUME (Volay)	
L'HORIZON BLEU #10 COLOGNE (World's Prods.)	
LIBIDO PERFUME, COLOGNES, & TOILET WATER (Parfum L'Orle)	
LIBRADOL MILD Antiphlogistic, local analgesic (Lloyd)	Camphor* Oils of eucalyptus* Cajuput Camphor Glucose Propylene glycol Magnesium carbonate Citric acid
LICK HAIR & SCALP PREPARATION (Lick)	Benzalkonium chloride*
LI-COR-CO Antitussive (Drobinski)	Alcohol less than 3% Licorice Oil anise Glycerin Ephedrine sulfate*
LIDO WAVE SET Hair preparation (Morris Drug)	
LIEN CARBON TETRA CHLORIDE Cleanser (Lien)	Carbon tetrachloride*
LIEN 656 CHINA STAIN REMOVER LIQUID (Lien)	Sodium hypochlorite* 8.0%
LIEN 10% CHLORDANE DUST Insecticide (Lien Chem.)	Chlordane*
LIEN 250 CHLOROLIEN Bactericide, cleanser (Lien)	Sodium hypochlorite* over 3.25% Sodium phosphate* over 91.75% Sodium chloride under 5.00%
LIEN 254 CLIEN CHLORO Cleanser for glassware, dishes, silverware and cooking utensils (Lien)	Sodium hypochlorite* 8%

*Consult Sec. II., Ingredients Index. This ingredient may be responsible for major toxic effects if poisonous amounts of this product are ingested.

Name & Use Manufacturer	Ingredients	Name & Use Manufacturer	Ingredients
LIEN DAIRY CATTLE & LIVESTOCK SPRAY Insecticide (Lien)	Butoxy polypropylene glycol* 52.95% Piperonyl butoxide tech. 7.49% Pyrethrins 0.75% Petroleum distillate* 23.84% Polyoxyethylene sorbitol oleatelaurate 14.97%	LIFEBUOY HEALTH SOAP WITH "PURALIN" (Lever)	
LIEN 25% DDT Insecticide (Lien)	DDT (dichloro diphenyl trichloroethane) tech. 25% Methylated naphthalene* 70%	LIFEBUOY SHAVING CREAM (Lever)	
LIEN 25% DDT EMULSION SPRAY CONCEN-TRATE Insecticide (Lien)	Dichloro diphenyl trichloro-ethane 25% Methylated naphthalene* 70%	LIFE O'WOOD POLISH (Instant)	Paraffin-mineral oil 55% Emulsifying oil 2-3/4% Isopropanol 91% 4-1/4% Silicone oil 1/4%
LIEN 5% DDT RESIDUAL COMPOUND 406 Insecticide (Lien)	Petroleum hydrocarbons* DDT* (dichloro diphenyl trichloroethane)	LIFE PROT-EGG SHAMPOO (Prot-Egg)	Saponified proteins and distilled fatty acid 20% Soluble proteins of fresh eggs and their natural serum 10%
LIEN DELUXE 408 Insecticide (Lien)	Petroleum distillate* Piperonyl butoxide tech. Pyrethrins	LIFESPAN COCOANUT OIL SHAMPOO For dogs and cats (Nat'l. Canine)	Pure conc. cocoanut oil
LIEN 159 DRAIN PIPE OPENER (Lien)	Potassium hydroxide*	LIFESPAN EAROL Veterinary (Nat'l. Canine)	Propylene glycol Sulfathiazole* Sulfanilimide* Urea
LIEN INSECTICIDE POWDER (Lien)	Sodium fluoride* 50% Exhausted pyrethrum flowers 50%	LIFESPAN I-F POWDER Insecticide, fungicide (Nat'l. Canine)	Rotenone 1% Other cube resins 2% Sulfur 10% Tetrachloro para benzoquinone* 10%
LIEN MET-L-CLIEN For degreasing metal parts (Lien)	Sodium hydroxide*	LIFESPAN RINSE DIP FLY & TICK SPRAY Insecticide (Nat'l. Canine)	Gamma isomer of benzene hexachloride (from lindane) 10% Polyethylene oxide sorbitan oleate emulsifier 5% Methylated naphthalene* 85%
LIEN MOTHICIDE Insecticide (Lien)	Petroleum hydrocarbons* Beta butoxy beta' thiocyano diethyl ether* Dichloro diphenyl trichloro-ethane* Pyrethrins*	LIFESPAN SKIN LOTION For dogs and cats (Nat'l. Canine)	Vegetable oil Sulfur Deodorized kerosene* Oil of turpentine* Calcium caseinate
LIEN MURIATIC ACID (Lien)	Hydrochloric acid*	LIGHTHOUSE Abrasive cleaner (Armour & Co.)	
LIEN NO. 156 TOILET BOWL CLEANER (Lien)	Hydrochloric acid*	LIGHTNING AEROSOL INSECT BOMB (Perrigo)	DDT 3.0% Tech. piperonyl butoxide 0.5% Pyrethrins 0.20% Petroleum distillate 8.30% Methylated naphthalene* 8.00% Propellents 80.00%
LIEN 592 WASTE TREATMENT Accelerates digestion of garbage and sewage solids (Lien)	Orthodichlorobenzene* 80.0%	LIGHTNING FLY KILLER (Perrigo)	Dichloro diphenyl trichloro-ethane* tech. 5.000% Piperonyl butoxide tech. 0.110% Pyrethrins 0.044% Petroleum distillates* 94.846%

*Consult Sec. II., Ingredients Index. This ingredient may be responsible for major toxic effects if poisonous amounts of this product are ingested.

- 646 -

LIGHTNING MOTOR DESLUDGER
For car motors
(Solvent)

LIGHTNING NITRO SOLVENT
(Solvent)

LIGHTNING RADIATOR FLUSH
For car radiators
(Solvent)

LIGHTNING RUST SOLVENT
(Solvent)

LIGHTNING SCALE SPRAY
Insecticide
(World Spray)

Petroleum oil*

LIGHTNING SHOE DYE
(Whittemore)

LIGHTNING TUNE-UP
For car motors
(Solvent)

LIGNASAN
Fungicide
(du Pont)

Ethyl mercury phosphate*

LIGNASAN X
Fungicide
(du Pont)

Ethyl mercury phosphate*

LIK-ZIT SPOT REMOVER
(Johnson Prod.)

LILAFECT 5 DISENFECTANT
(Peck's)

Soap
Terpineol
4-Chloro-2-phenyl phenol*
6-Chloro-2-phenyl phenol*

LILLY ACETANILID, BROMIDE & PHENACETIN COMPOUND
Alalgesic, oral solution
(Lilly)

Each 100 cc.:
Acetanilid*   2.2 gm.
Sodium bromide*   4.4 gm.
Acetophenetidin (Phenacetin)   0.875 gm.
Caffeine   0.44 gm.
Alcohol*   45%

LILLY ANALGESIC BALM OINTMENT
Rubefacient,
(Lilly)

Menthol*   15%
Methyl salicylate*   15%

LILLY A.S.A. COMPOUND
Antipyretic, analgesic, antirheumatic
(Lilly)

Each pulvule:
Acetophenetidin*   0.16 gm.
Acetylsalicylic acid*   0.227 gm.
Caffeine   0.0325 gm.

LILLY CALOMEL, RHUBARB & COLOCYNTH COMPOUND
Cathartic
(Lilly)

Calomel*   0.13 gm.
Ext. rhubarb N.F.   0.029 gm.
Ext. colocynth   0.005 gm.
Myrrh   0.026 gm.
Resin scammony   0.06 gm.
Eugenol   0.006 cc.
Oil peppermint   0.0018 cc.
Aloe*   0.103 gm.

LILLY CASCARA COMPOUND N.F.
(Hinkle's Pills)
Cathartic
(Lilly)

Ext. cascara   0.016 gm.
Aloin*   0.016 gm.
Podophyllin   0.01 gm.
Ext. belladonna*   0.008 gm.
Oleoresin ginger   0.004 gm.

LILLY CASCARA COMPOUND WITH STRYCHNINE
Cathartic
(Lilly)

Ext. cascara   0.016 gm.
Aloin*   0.016 gm.
Podophyllin   0.011 gm.
Ext. belladonna*   0.008 gm.
Strychnine sulfate*   0.0011 gm.
Oleoresin ginger   0.004 gm.

LILLY CATHARTIC COMPOUND
(Mild mercurous chloride compound N.F.)
(Lilly)

Ext. colocynth compound   0.08 gm.
Calomel*   0.06 gm.
Resin jalap   0.02 gm.
Gamboge*   0.015 gm.

LILLY CATHARTIC, IMPROVED
(Lilly)

Ext. colocynth compound   0.065 gm.
Ext. jalap   0.0325 gm.
Podophyllin   0.016 gm.
Leptandrin   0.016 gm.
Ext. hyoscyamus*   0.016 gm.
Ext. gentian
Oil peppermint

LILLY CATNIP & FENNEL COMPOUND
(Lilly)

Each 100 cc:
Alcohol   25%
Catnip   3.3 gm.
Fennel   8.75 gm.
Sodium bicarbonate   1 gm.
Carminatives

LILLY EPHEDRINE COMPOUND
Nasal decongestant
(Lilly)

Ephedrine*   1% w/v
Menthol
Camphor
Oil of thyme
Vegetable oil

LILLY EPHEDRINE JELLY
(not N.F.)
(Lilly)

Ephedrine sulfate*   1%
Propylene glycol
Merthiolate

LILLY EPHEDRINE
(Plain)
Nasal decongestant
(Lilly)

Ephedrine*   1% w/v
Cinnamic aldehyde
Benzaldehyde
Aromatized vegetable oil

---

*Consult Sec. II., Ingredients Index. This ingredient may be responsible for major toxic effects if poisonous amounts of this product are ingested.

Name & Use Manufacturer	Ingredients		Name & Use Manufacturer	Ingredients	
LILLY EPHEDRINE SULFATE (Lilly)	Alcohol Ephedrine sulfate*	12% 0.44 gm.	LILLY TERPIN HYDRATE & CREOSOTE COMPOUND (Lilly)	Each 100 cc.: Alcohol Chloroform Creosote Terpin hydrate Calcium glycerophosphate Sodium glycerophosphate	30% 0.21 cc. 0.42 cc. 0.44 gm. 0.875 gm. 0.875 gm.
LILLY FERROUS GLUCONATE Dietary supplement with iron (Lilly)	Alcohol Ferrous gluconate 6 gm./100 cc.	7%			
			LILLY WHITE PINE & AMMONIUM CHLORIDE COMPOUND (Lilly)	Alcohol Chloroform White pine bark Wild cherry Sanguinaria Balm Gilead buds Spikenard Sassafras* Ammonium chloride	7% 0.42 cc. 8.5 gm. 8.5 gm. 0.8 gm. 1 gm. 1 gm. 1 gm. 1.75 gm.
LILLY GLYCERO-PHOSPHATES COMPOUND, N.F. (Lilly)	Each 100 cc.: Alcohol Calcium glycerophosphate 1.6 gm. Sodium glycerophosphate 3.5 gm. Iron glycerophosphate 0.3 gm. Manganese glycerophosphate 0.2 gm. Quinine hydrochloride 0.0875 gm. Strychnine nitrate* 0.0125 gm.	11%			
			LILLY WHITE PINE COMPOUND (Lilly)	Alcohol Chloroform White pine bark Wild cherry Sanguinaria Balm Gilead buds Spikenard Sassafras*	7% 0.42 cc. 8.5 gm. 8.5 gm. 0.8 gm. 1 gm. 1 gm. 1 gm.
LILLY IRON, QUININE & STRYCHNINE N.F. (Lilly)	Each 100 cc.: Alcohol Tincture ferric citrochloride 12.5 cc. Quinine hydrochloride 0.8 gm. Strychnine sulfate* 0.0175 gm.	24%			
			LILLY ZINC OXIDE PASTE WITH SALICYLIC ACID N.F. (Lilly)	Each 100 gm.: Salicylic acid* Zinc oxide Starch White petrolatum	2 gm. 24.5 gm. 24.5 gm. 49 gm.
LILLY IRON, QUININE & STRYCHNINE. PHOSPHATES N.F. (Lilly)	Each 100 cc.: Alcohol Iron phosphate Quinine phosphate Strychnine phosphate* 0.025 gm.	23% 3.5 gm. 0.5 gm.			
			LILLY ZINC SULFATE COMPOUND N.F. (Lilly)	Salicylic acid Phenol Eucalyptol Menthol Thymol Zinc sulfate* Boric acid*	0.5 gm. 0.1 gm. 0.1 gm. 0.1 gm. 0.1 gm. 12.5 gm. 86.6 gm.
LILLY LACTATED PEPSIN (Lilly)	Alcohol Elixir lactated pepsin N.F.	15%			
LILLY MENTHOLATED EXPECTORANT (Lilly)	Alcohol, each 100 cc.: 2% Lobelia* 0.985 gm. Ipecac 0.44 gm. Sanguinaria 0.77 gm. Ammonium chloride 1.75 gm. Menthol and tolu balsam q.s.		LILT HOME PERMANENT WAVE (Procter & Gamble)	Waving lotion: Monoethanolamine thioglycolate (dilute solution) Neutralizer powder: Sodium perborate* Citric acid	
			LILT PARTY CURL Home permanent (Procter & Gamble)		
LILLY PEPSIN, BISMUTH & STRYCHNINE (Lilly)	Alcohol Strychnine* Elix. pepsin and bismuth q.s.	10% 0.0125 gm.			
LILLY'S ANT CUPS (Sturtevant)	Sodium arsenate*	3%	LILY CREAM (Ohio Valley)	Gum tragacanth No. 1 Formaldehyde solution Glycerin U.S.P. Alcohol S.D. No. 40 Tincture benzoin U.S.P. Synfleur M cologne Antiseptic solution N.F.	0.80 oz. 0.04 oz. 22.4 oz. 9.0 oz. 0.26 oz. 0.03 oz. 1.6 oz.
LILLY'S ANT TRAPS (Sturtevant)	Thallium sulfate Inert ingredients*	0.1%			
LILLY'S WARFARIN FOR RATS & MICE (Sturtevant)	Warfarin (3-(a-acetonylbenzyl)-4-hydroxycoumarin) 0.025%		LILY WHITE SHOE CLEANER (Rex Home)		
LILLY TERPIN HYDRATE & CODEINE N.F. (Lilly)	Alcohol Codeine alkaloid Terpin hydrate	42% 0.2 gm. 1.7 gm.	LIMICOL Antihistamine, oral (Cel-Ton-Sa)	Pyranisamine maleate*	25 mg.

Name & Use Manufacturer	Ingredients		Name & Use Manufacturer	Ingredients	
LIMB'RTONE Rubefacient, (Veterinary) (Troy Chem.)	Isopropyl alcohol* Oil wormwood Iodine* Camphor* Ammonia*		LIN (Emulsion) KILLS ANTS (Noble)	Gamma isomer of benzene hexachloride (from lindane) 0.5%	
LINCIDE Insecticide (Thompson Chem.)	Gamma isomer of benzene hexachloride (from lindane)* 5% Petroleum distillate* 85%		L'INFINI EXTRACT (Caron)		
LINCIDE 20 Insecticide (Thompson Chem.)	Gamma isomer of benzene hexachloride (from lindane)* 20% Aromatic hydrocarbon (xylene)* 70%		LINGERLENE HAIR BLACK (Kongo)		
LINCO (Linco)	Sodium hypochlorite*		LININGILL LINIMENT Rubefacient (Massengill)	Ethyl alcohol* 68% Camphor* Oil sassafras* Oil peppermint Oil turpentine* Oil white thyme Methyl salicylate*	
LINCOLN PINE SCENT DISINFEC- TANT (Baird & M.)	Pine oil* Vegetable oil soap		LIN INSECT POWDER Insecticide (Noble)	Gamma isomer of benzene hexachloride (from lindane) 1%	
LINCTUS COMPOUND Antitussive, sedative (Sharp & Dohme)	Alcohol 0.75% Codeine sulfate* 30 mg. Chloroform* 0.12 gm. Fl. ext. ipecac 0.12 cc. Fl. ext. squill* 0.12 cc. Phosphoric acid 1.0 cc.		LINIT BRAND LIQUID STARCH (Corn Prod.)	Sodium chloride Coloring material Fermentation preservative	
LIND Insecticide (Greever's)	Gamma isomer of benzene hexachloride* (from lindane) 3% Dichloro diphenyl trichloro- ethane* 12.5%		LINITE Antiseptic (Naylor)	Carbolic acid* Dihydroxy dichloro diphenyl- methane* Oil turpentine* Camphor* Chlorortho-phenylphenol* Croton oil*	
LINDANOX Insecticide (Farnam)	Gamma isomer of benzene hexachloride* (from lindane) 12.2% Aromatic petroleum deriv. solvent* 84.6%		LIN KILL ROACHES (Noble)	Petroleum distillate Gamma isomer of benzene hexachloride (from lindane)*	
LINDEX DUST #10 Insecticide (Thompson- Hayward)	Gamma isomer of benzene hexachloride (from lindane) 1.0% Inert ingredients		LINK'S OINTMENT Skin irritations (Link)	Calomel* 3.75% Carbolic acid* 2% Zinc oxide Camphor* Menthol*	
LINDEX MILL SPRAY Insecticide (Thompson- Hayward)	Gamma isomer of benzene hexachloride (from lindane) 20.0% Aromatic petroleum deriv. solvent* 35.0%		LINNET POISON Rodenticide (Santa Clara)	Strychnine alkaloid* 0.6%	
LINDEX SPRAY Insecticide (Thompson- Hayward)	Gamma isomer of benzene hexachloride (from lindane) 0.10% Tech. piperonyl butoxide 0.25% Pyrethrins 0.025% Petroleum distillate* 99.625%		LIN-O-DYNE LINIMENT (Veltex)	Chlorobutanol* (chloroform derivative) 0.8 gr. Benzyl alcohol 0.375% Oils of wormwood and sassafras Eucalyptol* Thymol* Menthol* Acetone*	
LINDEX 25W Insecticide (Thompson- Hayward)	Gamma isomer of benzene hexachloride (from lindane) * 25%		LINOIL Fungicide (medical) (Sutton Laboratories)	Acid salicylic* Acid benzoic* Sulfurated balsam base	
LINDEX WE 125 Insecticide (Thompson- Hawyard)	Gamma isomer of benzene hexachloride* (from lindane) ⚹ 12.5% Xylol* 82.5%		LINOLEIC & LINOLENIC ACIDS Skin ointment (Chicago Pharm.)	Linoleic acid Linolenic acid	

*Consult Sec. II., Ingredients Index. This ingredient may be responsible for major toxic effects if poisonous amounts of this product are ingested.

- 649 -

Name & Use Manufacturer	Ingredients		Name & Use Manufacturer	Ingredients	
LINO-PASTE RUBBER CEMENT (Lino-Paste)			LIPO-VEE SYRUP (Harvey Labs.)	Each tsp.: Thiamine HCl Riboflavin Pyridoxine HCl Niacinamide d-l-Methionine Inositol Choline bitartrate Butoben	5 mg. 2 mg. 0.5 mg. 50 mg. 50 mg. 100 mg. 100 mg. 0.2%
LINO-PASTE WATERPROOF FILLER CEMENT (Lino-Paste)					
LIN-O-SPRAY Insecticide (Gland-O-Lac)	Gamma isomer of benzene hexachloride* (from lindane) 12.9% Tech. xylene* 83.9%		LIQUALGINE 3 Antipyretic, analgesic (Whorton)	Each fl. dr.: Acetylsalicylic acid* Salicylic acid Alcohol*	5 gr. trace 50%/v
			LIQUA-VITA FERTILIZER (Am. Liquid)		
LINTON CREAM Vaginal (Linton, McIntosh)	Paraformaldehyde 0.1% Triethanolamine 0.9% Potassium carbonate 0.2% Paraffin 2.0% Stearic acid 22.0%		LIQUIBALM ANALGESIC (Pharmart)	Menthol Camphor* Methyl salicylate*	2-1/2% 5% 10%
LINTON JELLY Vaginal (Linton, McIntosh)	Lactic acid 1.5% Boric acid* 4.0% Glycerin 7.7% Starch 8.0% Gum karaya 1.33%		LIQUID CHIN STRAP Facial preparation (Assoc. Brands)		
LINTON'S LEAD PENCILS (Linton Pencil)	Pencil lead: Wax Clay Graphite Finish: Lacquer Eraser: Natural rubber G.R.S. Sulfur Factice Titanium		LIQUIDINE (Jamol)	Total iodine* content 0.25%	
			LIQUID NOXFISH For control of rough fish (Penick)	Rotenone* Other cube extractives*	5% 15%
LIN-X CLEAR GLOSS Varnish (Sherwin-Williams)	Ester gum-linseed-alkyd resin 50% Mineral spirits* 50%		LIQUID STITCH Run stopper (Porter Mfg.)		
LIN-X HARDWOOD FLOOR & LINOLEUM CLEANER (Acme Q. P.)			LIQUID-TAR-PAPER Insecticide (Noble)	Pine wood oils* Paradichlorobenzene*	
			LIQUID VENEER Wood preserver (Liquid)		
LIN-X VARNISH (Sherwin-Williams)	Linseed-alkyd-ester gum Mineral spirits* 50%		LIQUID WRENCH Rust preventative, remover (Radiator)	Aromatic solvents* Petroleum oils Colloidal graphite Pyridine Mercaptans	
LIOB Counter-irritant salve (Am. Druggists)	Ichthammol Oil eucalyptus* Methylparaben Petrolatum Rosin Lanolin base		LIQUI-RID DRINKING WATER WORMER (Hess, Dr.)	Piperazine base 5.05 gm./fl.oz.	
LIPOIODINE Organic iodide (Ciba)	Each tablet: Ethyl di-iodobrassidate* (41% iodine) 0.2916 gm.		LIQUI-SEAL (Varniton)	Acetone* Toluene* Plastic	
LIPOSORB Internal, for skin disorders (Haack)	Polyoxy sorbitan monooleate 200 gm. Lecithin-soya 200 mg. Fish liver oil 100 mg.		LIQUOR SEDANS Uterine sedative (Parke, Davis)	Each ounce: Black haw Jamica dogwood Hydrastis Aromatics Alcohol	60 gr. 30 gr. 30 m. 28%

Name & Use Manufacturer	Ingredients	Name & Use Manufacturer	Ingredients
L.I.R.B.M. For iron deficiency anemias (Armour Labs.)	Each fl. oz.: Liver fraction 1 (N.F.) 1.25 gm. Ferric ammonium citrate 2.17 gm. Alcohol 12%	LITTLE LADY CUTICLE OIL (Pessl)	
LIRO CAPSULES Analgesic (Partola)	Each capsule: Acetylsalicylic acid* 7-3/4 gr. Caffeine Inactive lactose	LITTLE LADY DOLL COLOGNE (Pessl)	
LISTERINE ANTISEPTIC (Lambert)	Thymol* Eucalyptol* Methyl salicylate* Benzoic acid Boric acid* Alcohol 25%	LITTLE LADY FACE POWDER (Pessl)	
LISTERINE ANTIZYME TOOTH PASTE (Lambert)	Alumina hydrate Titanium dioxide Sodium lauryl sulfate Irish moss extractive Saccharin Sodium oxalate Glycerin Sorbitol Oils of spearmint, peppermint and menthol	LITTLE LADY HAND LOTION (Pessl)	
		LITTLE LADY LIP POMADE (Pessl)	
LISTERINE TOOTH PASTE (Lambert)	Calcium sulfate Alumina hydrate Titanium dioxide Sodium lauryl sulfoacetate Irish moss extractive Saccharin Glycerin Sorbitol Methyl salicylate	LITTLE LADY NAIL POLISH (Pessl)	
		LITTLE LADY NAIL POLISH REMOVER (Pessl)	
		LITTLE LADY TOILET SOAP (Pessl)	
LITE-AIRE Deodorizer (Washington Barber)	Formaldehyde* Glycerin Volatile oils	LITTLE LADY TOILET WATER (Pessl)	
LITTLE BEAR LIQUID FABRIC CEMENT (Little Bear)	Benzol*	LITTLE RED WORM BULLETS Dog preparation (Clayton)	
LITTLE BO-PEEP AMMONIA (Puhl)		LITTLE TOTS BABY OIL (Allied Drug)	Lanolin Mineral oil
LITTLE BOY BLUE BLUING (Puhl)		LITTLE WONDER DRAIN PIPE & TRAP CLEANER (Durst Mfg.)	
LITTLE DOC CLEANING COMPOUND (Schaffner)			
LITTLE DOC PAINT BRUSH CLEANER (Schaffner)		LITTLE WONDER DRAIN PIPE & TRAP RUST PREV. (Durst Mfg.)	
LITTLE DOC RUG & UPHOLSTERY CLEANER (Schaffner)		LITTLE WONDER RUST PREVENTING COMPOUND (Durst Mfg.)	
LITTLE LADY BUBBLE BATH (Pessl)		LITTLE WONDER STOMACH MEDICINE (Little Wonder)	Rhubarb Bismuth Aquacalcis

*Consult Sec. II., Ingredients Index. This ingredient may be responsible for major toxic effects if poisonous amounts of this product are ingested.

Name & Use Manufacturer	Ingredients		Name & Use Manufacturer	Ingredients	
LITTLE WORKERS PILLS Veterinary (Howell Co.)			LOCK'S MEDICINAL BALM Skin ointment	Camphor* Oil eucalyptus* Oxyquinoline sulfate* Lanolin Menthol*	
LIVITAMIN WITH IRON (Liquid) (Massengill)	Each 30 cc.: Iron peptonized Manganese citrate Thiamine hydrochloride Riboflavin Vitamin B$_{12}$ Niacinamide (nicotinamide) Pyridoxine hydrochloride Pantothenic acid Liver fraction Rice bran Inositol Choline	0.42 gm. 0.158 gm. 10 gm. 10 mg. 10 mg. 50 mg. 1 mg. 5 mg. 2 gm. 1 gm. 30 mg. 60 mg.	LOCK'S MEDICINAL FOOT & BODY POWDER Fungicide (medical) (Twitty)	Hydroxy-quinoline sulfate* Aluminum silicate Magnesium silicate Boric acid* Salicylic acid*	
			LOCOROL Vaginal jelly (Peck & Sterba)	Potassium oxyquinoline sulfate* Boric‡ acetic and tartaric acids Glycerin in vegetable gum base	
LIX Antitussive (Lix)	White pine* Tar* Ammonium chloride Wild cherry Bloodroot Chloroform Alcohol	3/4 m. 0.5%	LODORANTE AFTER SHAVE (Parfum L'Orle)		
LIX-MOTH Insecticide (Winsale)			LODORANTE COLOGNES, PERFUMES, DEODORANT CREAM (Parfum L'Orle)		
LIX-RUST METALLIC PAINT (Phelen-Faust)			L-O LOTION Cosmetic for skin irritation (Hill Labs. (Fla.))	Lanolinized zinc oxide 15% Cream base	
L-K-T HAIR TONIC (Kirby's Mineral)			DR. LONDON'S PRESCRIPTION Antacid, carminative (London's)	Bismuth subnitrate Aromatic cascara sagrada Milk of magnesia Chloroform Aromatic syrup rhubarb Alcohol 4.0%/v	
L-L-M'S GIBSONS (Lyons, J.)	Linseed Licorice Menthol Sugars Gelatine		LONG AID BLACK HAIR DYE (Keystone Labs.)	Paraphenyldiamine Resorcinol* Isopropyl alcohol* Hydrogen peroxide*	
LLOYD BROS. TINCTURE OF POISON IVY For poison ivy dermatitis (Lloyd)	Rhus toxicodendron*		LONG AID HOT OIL TREATMENT (Keystone Labs.)	Petrolatum Lanolin Mineral oil Oil of bergamot	
LOBANA BODY RUB (Ulmer)	Stearic acid Lanolin Mentholated base		LONG AID POMADE (Keystone Labs.)	Petroleum jelly Lanolin Hexachlorophene 2/10% Perfume oil Isopropyl myristate	
LOCK EASE GRAPHITED LOCK FLUID Lubricant (Am. Grease)	Lubricating oil* Naphtha solvent* Colloidal graphite Lead naphthenate*		LONG AID SHAMPOO (Keystone Labs.)	Triethanolamine Lauryl sulfate Ninol AA62 Water softener Sequestrene Perfume oil	
LOCKHEED Hydraulic brake fluid (Wagner)			LONG AID SULPHUR POMADE TREATMENT (Keystone Labs.)	Petrolatum Lanolin Oil of tar rect. Wettable sulfur Salicylic acid* Isobornyl acetate*	
LOCK'S CORN CALLOUS REMOVER (Twitty)	Salicylic acid* Ethyl alcohol Ether*	20% 60%/v			

*Consult Sec. II., Ingredients Index. This ingredient may be responsible for major toxic effects if poisonous amounts of this product are ingested.

Name & Use Manufacturer	Ingredients	Name & Use Manufacturer	Ingredients
LONG LIFE PAINT BRUSH CLEANER (Day-Kingsley)		LORODO DEODORANT & ANTI-PERSPIRANT (Parfum L'Orle)	
LONGO RAPID HAIR COLORING (Longo)		LOROPHYN JELLY N.N.R. (Eaton Labs.)	Phenylmercuric acetate 0.05% Polyethylene glycol of mono-iso-octyl phenyl ether 0.3% Methylparaben 0.05% Sodium borate 3%
LOOKASINE Vaginal douche powder (Nat'l. Drug)	Acid boric* 80.5% Zinc sulfate, exsic. 4% Zinc phenolsulfonate 2.5% Potassium alum 9% Sodium salicylate 2.5%	LOROPHYN SUPPOSI-TORIES N.N.R. (Eaton Labs.)	Each suppository: Phenylmercuric acetate 0.4 mg. Methyl benzethonium chloride Methylparaben
LOOSITE Solvent (Petroleum)	Aromatic solvent*	LORR CREAM (Lorr)	
L'OPERA FRANCAIS PERFUME (Specialty)		LORTONA MEDICATED CREAM (Myers Labs.)	Phenol* Camphor* Eucalyptol* Cloves Menthol*
LORATE Vaginal douche powder (Standard Labs.)	Sodium borate* perhydrate Sodium bicarbonate Sodium chloride Castile soap Menthol*	LOTION BASE-CASTILL (Thomas & Thompson)	Carboxymethylcellulose Triethanolamine Butoben Aqua
L'ORIGAN LINE TOILET WATER & EXTRACT (Coty)		LOTION HISTADYL (Thenylpyra-mine, Lilly) For skin irritations of allergy (Lilly)	Each 100 cc.: Histadyl* 2 gm. Zinc oxide 16 gm.
LORENZ ACTIVATED PYRETHRUM KNOCKDOWN CONCEN-TRATE Insecticide (Lorenz)	Aliphatic hydrocarbons* Piperonyl butoxide Pyrethrins*	LOTION SURFADIL (Cyclomethy-caine & Thenylpyra-mine, Lilly) For skin irritations of allergy (Lilly)	Each 100 cc.: Histadyl* 2 gm. Surfacaine 0.5 gm. Titanium dioxide 5 gm.
LORENZ BHC 1# E.C. Insecticide (Lorenz)	Benzene hexachloride* Aromatic hydrocarbons* Emulsifier		
LORENZ COLLOIDAL CHLORDANE CONCEN-TRATE (Water soluble) Insecticide (Lorenz)	Chlordane tech.* Alkylated aryl polyether alcohol	LOTOCREME Rubefacient (Abbott)	Lanolin Olive oil Glycerin Menthol* Methylparaben U.S.P. Borax
LORENZ 25% DDT EMULSI-FIABLE CON-CENTRATE Insecticide (Lorenz)	DDT* Aromatic hydrocarbons* Emulsifier	LOTSHAW HAIR DRESS FOR MEN (Lotshaw)	Lanolin Mineral oil Stearic acid composition
		LOTSHAW'S PELLENT Repellent (Lotshaw)	Repellent 448 40%/w 2 Phenyl cyclohexanol 28%/w 2-cyclohexyl cylohexanol* 12%
LORENZ TOXAPHENE 60% CONC. Insecticide (Lorenz)	Toxaphene* Kerosene Emulsifier	LOVALON HAIR RINSE (Marcus-Lesoine)	Citric Coloring
		LOVE LACE COLOGNES & PERFUMES (Quality Cosm.)	
LORENZ WATER EMULSIFI-ABLE CHLORDANE CONC. 46% Insecticide (Lorenz)	Chlordane* No. 1 fuel oil* Emulsifier	LOVELY LADY LOTION (Herp)	

*Consult Sec. II., Ingredients Index. This ingredient may be responsible for major toxic effects if poisonous amounts of this product are ingested.

- 653 -

Name & Use Manufacturer	Ingredients	Name & Use Manufacturer	Ingredients
LOVER'S MOON JOCKEY CLUB PERFUME (Ashworth)		LT FLUX (Handy)	Potassium acid fluoride* Potassium tetraborate* Boric acid*
LOVER'S MOON LIPSTICK (Ashworth)		LUBAFAX Surgical lubricant (Burroughs-Wellcome)	o-Chloromercuriphenol 0.02%
LOVER'S MOON MEN'S POMADE (Ashworth)		LUBEX Laxative (Haysma)	Semi-solid hydrocarbons Petrolatum Sulfur
LOVESTER Herbicide (Planetary Chem.)	Butoxy ethoxy propanol ester of 2, 4, 5-trichlorophenoxy-acetic acid* 70.6%	LUBRACIL Cathartic (Vitec)	Methyl cellulose Sodium carboxymethylcellulose
LOW-DEE Herbicide (Planetary Chem.)	Butoxy ethoxy propanol ester of 2, 4-dichlorophenoxyacetic acid* 75.6% Solvents and emulsifying agents 24.4%	LUBRIDERM For skin irritations (Texas Pharm.)	Cholesterin Sorbitol Cetyl alcohol Mineral oil U.S.P. Oxycholesterin
LOWELL HAND CREAM (House of Lowell)	Stearic acid Oleic acid Isopropylmyristate Isopropylpalmitate Cetyl alcohol Lanolin Oxy-cholesterin Witch hazel Propylene glycol Glycerin Ammonia water Borax Methylpara hydroxy benzoate Sodium alginate Perfume compound	LUCA CEMENT-CHINA, CROCKERY. GLASS, MODEL AIRPLANE (Luca)	
		LUCAS KALSOMINE Paint (Lucas)	
		LUCIDE A-20 Household insecticide semi-concentrate (Pest Control Equip.)	Chlordane* emulsion 19%
LOWELL LIQUID DEODORANT (House of Lowell)	Para diisobutyl cresoxy ethoxy ethyl dimethyl benzyl ammonium chloride monohydrate* Aluminum chlor hydroxy complex Glycerin Alcohol Perfume compound	LUCIDE D-25 Insecticide (Pest Control Equip.)	Dichloro diphenyl trichloroethane 25% Aromatic petroleum deriv. sol.* 70%
LOWILA CAKE Soapless, non-irritant efficient skin cleanser (Westwood)	Sodium lauryl sulfoacetate Corn dextrin base	LUCIDE EIGHT Insecticide (Pest Control Equip.)	Petroleum distillates* 22% Chlordane tech.* 72%
LOWILA LIQUID Household cleanser, soapless detergent (Westwood)	Aryl alkyl sulfonate*	LUCIDE LM-10 Insecticide (Pest Control Equip.)	Methylated aromatic petroleum deriv.* 80.0% Gamma isomer of benzene hexachloride* (from lindane) 10.0% Polyoxyethylene sorbitolesters of mixed fatty and resin acids 10.0%
LP INDUSTRIAL SPRAY Insecticide (Larvacide)	Piperonyl botoxide Pyrethrins* Inert ingredients*	LUCIDE M-65 Insecticide (Pest Control Equip.)	Chlordane tech.* 65% Petroleum distillates* 15%
L S A LOTION For skin irritations (Hill Labs. (Fla.))	Each 3 oz.: Zinc oxide 6 gm. Lead subacetate* 7-1/2 gm. Glycerin Lime water Jell base	LUCIDE S-60 Insecticide (Pest Control Equip.)	Tech. chlordane*, refined 60.3%

*Consult Sec. II., Ingredients Index. This ingredient may be responsible for major toxic effects if poisonous amounts of this product are ingested.

- 654 -

Name & Use Manufacturer	Ingredients		Name & Use Manufacturer	Ingredients	
LUCIDIN EYE DROPS (Pearson Pharm.)			LURA-GLO HAND LOTION (Lura-Glo)		
LUCKY LEAF 15% FERMATE DUST Insecticide (Black Panther)	Ferric dimethyl dithio-carbamate*	11.40%	LURA-GLO NAIL POLISH REMOVER (Lura-Glo)		
LUCKY STAR COLOGNE (Lucky Star)			LURIN Antacid (Myers Labs.)	Aluminum hydroxide gel	
LUCKY TIGER OINTMENT Hair, health aid (Lucky Tiger)	Sulfur* Oxyquinoline* Methyl salicylate* Balsam Peru Camphor* Menthol oil of eucalyptus*		LURON WITH LANOLIN Hand cleaner (Pacific Coast)	Borax* Powdered toilet soap Lanolin Rose bouquet perfume	
LUCKY TIGER SPECIAL FORMULA WITHOUT OIL Health aid (Lucky Tiger)	Alcohol Sodium salicylate* Oxyquinoline phosphate*	50%	LUSTER LOY HAIR TONIC (Kirby's)		
			LUSTERO Detergent (Olson Prod.)		
LUCKY TIGER 3 PURPOSE HAIR TONIC Health aid (Lucky Tiger)	Alcohol Sodium salicylate* Oxyquinolinephosphate*	55%	LUSTERTEX VEGETABLE OIL SHAMPOO FOR PETS (Magitex)	Coconut oil soap	
LUKOREX POWDER Douche powder (Horton & Converse)	Sodium perborate* Sodium bicarbonate Menthol* Thymol* Methyl salicylate* Eucalyptol* Alum Boric acid*		LUST-O-WITE Porcelain bowl cleaner (Hillyard Chem.)	Sodium bisulfite	
			LUSTRAY E-Z BLEACH (Lustray)		
LUMAG Antacid (Friendly Labs.)	Magnesium trisilicate Dried aluminum hydroxide gel Flavoring		LUSTRAY TOILET WATER (Lustray)		
LUMASATE POWDER For wet dressings in skin irritations (Hill Labs.)	Calcium acetate Aluminum sulfate Aluminum subacetate		LUSTRE-AMBER BRILLANTINE (H.Q.Z.)	Mineral oil D and C yellow oil soluble Oriental bouquet	
			LUSTRE-CREME HAIR DRESSING (Colgate-Palmolive)	Moisture Mineral oil Lanolin and non-ionic detergents Cationic detergent* Perfume and preservative	50% 3-10%
LUMBRICIDE (Syrup) Anthelmintic (Massengill)	Each 5 cc.: Santonin Spigelia Frangula Senna Aromatics	10 mg. 0.16 gm. 80 mg. 80 mg. q.s.	LUSTRE-CREME SHAMPOO (Colgate-Palmolive)	Moisture Sodium lauryl sulfate Lanolin Sodium chloride Potassium stearate Fatty acid-triethanolamine condensate Perfume and preservative	65%
LUMIGEL Antacid (Veltex)	Aluminum hydroxide gel U.S.P.				
LUMINALL CONCRETE FLOOR PAINT (Nat'l. Chem. & Mfg.)			LUSTRE-ROSE HAIR OIL (H.Q.Z.)	Mineral oil (95 vis.) D and C red color Oil soluble rose perfume	
			LUSTREX Molding powder (Monsanto)	Styrene	
LUMINOUS LURE PERFUME, COLOGNE, DEODORANT & FRESHENER (Riker)			LUSTREX Coating resin & adhesive (Monsanto)	Vinyl butyral	

*Consult Sec. II., Ingredients Index. This ingredient may be responsible for major toxic effects if poisonous amounts of this product are ingested.

Name & Use Manufacturer	Ingredients
LUSTRO WALLPAPER CLEANER (Cincy)	Wheat flour Kerosene oil* Vegetable dye Salt Preservatives
LUX Toilet soap (Lever)	
LUX FLAKES Soap flakes (Lever)	
LUX LIQUID (Lever)	
LUZIER'S HAND BALM (Luzier's)	
LV 2, 4, 5-T BRUSH KILLER (Agric. Proc.)	Butoxy ethoxy propanol ester of 2, 4, 5-trichloro phenoxy acetic acid 73.00%
LYCOBOROL Skin astringent (Tampa)	Bismuth Boric acid* Magnesium silicate Lycopodium and starch
LYCONS CONCEN- TRATED LYE (Babbitt)	Sodium hydroxide* 94% Sodium carbonate 2%
LYDIA E. PINKHAM'S LAXATIVE (Pinkham)	Each tablet: Senna Phenolphthalein 1/4 gr. Cascara Ext. belladonna* 1/16 gr.
LYDIA E. PINKHAM'S TABLETS Uterine sedative (Pinkham)	Iron Pleurisy root Ext. of Jamaica dogwood Licorice
LYDIA E. PINKHAM'S VEGETABLE COMPOUND Uterine sedative (Pinkham)	Alcohol 13-1/2% Black cohosh Life root plant Dandelion Jamaica dogwood Gentian Vitamin B1 Pleurisy root Chamomile Licorice True and false unicorn

Name & Use Manufacturer	Ingredients	
LYGEL VAGINAL JELLY (Lehn & Fink)	Benzalkonium chloride	0.10%
	Lactic acid	0.25%
	p-Chloro-sym.-m-xylenol	0.05%
	p-tert-Amylphenol	0.05%
	Glycerol	15.00%
	Gum tragacanth	2.50%
	Pectin	1.00%
	Perfume oil	0.10%
	Water, q.s.	100.00%
LYGENES VAGINAL SUPPOSI- TORIES (Lehn & Fink)	Zinc sulfocarbolate	0.50%
	Hydroxyquinoline benzoate	0.30%
	p-Chloro-sym.-m-xylenol	0.05%
	p-tert-Amylphenol	0.05%
	Boric acid	0.10%
	Beeswax, white	5.00%
	Corn starch	9.00%
	Perfume	0.20%
	Cocoa butter	84.80%
LYKETTE LIQUID DEODORANT (Iodent)	Aluminum chlorhydroxide complex	
LYK-NU KOTE-O-WAX POLISH (Lyk-Nu)		
LYNN'S FLEA POWDER (Pfeiffer)	Rotenone	1.00%
	Pyrethrins	0.07%
LYNSOL Shellac thinner, alcohol, stove fuel, printing press cleaner (Clark-Lurton)	Methanol*	5%
	Alcohol	90%
LYON OINTMENT (Lyon)	Cresylic acid* Sodium hydroxide* Wood resin Tallow	
DR. LYONS DENTIFRICE (Watkins, R.)		
LYSOL BRAND DISINFECT- ANT (Lehn & Fink)	Soap Orthohydroxydiphenyl Propylene glycol Cresylic acid (xylenol fraction) less than 2% Alcohol 7.2%/v	

---

*Consult Sec. II., Ingredients Index. This ingredient may be responsible for major toxic effects if poisonous amounts of this product are ingested.

Name & Use Manufacturer	Ingredients		Name & Use Manufacturer	Ingredients	
MAALOX Antacid (Rorer)	Magnesium hydroxide Aluminum hydroxide		M.A.C. VETERINARY (Carter-Luff)	Mercuric chloride Mercurous chloride* Potassium chloride Potassium iodide* Silver iodide* Volatile oils Iodo-terpene	
MAAS' CLEANER & WATER SOFTENER (Maas, A. G.)	Tri sodium phosphate*		MACY'S WALL & WOOD- WORK CLEANER (Macy's)		
MAAS' DRAIN PIPE OPENER (Maas, A. G.)	Sodium hydroxide*		MADAM C. J. WALKER HAIR & SCALP PREPARATION (Walker, Mme.)	Copper sulfate* Precipitated sulfur*	
MACCO VARNISHES & DRIERS (Macneal)					
MACKIE'S PINE SKRUB KLEEN Cleanser, deodorant (Standard Wood)	Oil of pine* Soap		MADAM C. J. WALKER SKIN BRIGHTENER (Walker, Mme.)	Ammoniated mercury* Bismuth subnitrate	5%
MACKIE'S PINEXO Disinfectant, cleanser, deodorant (Standard Wood)	Pine oil* Anhydrous soap	80% 10%	MADAM C. J. WALKER TEMPLE SALVE (Walker, Mme.)	Precipitated sulfur* Petrolatum	
MACLEAN'S CHLORDANE 72% EMULSI- FIABLE CONC. Insecticide (MacLean)	Tech. chlordane*	72%	MADAME FRIEDA TOSAN COMPOUND For menstrual difficulties (Tosan)	Each fl. oz.: Alcohol Gentian Unicorn Jamaica dogwood Dandelion Thiamine HCl Black cohosh Life and pleurisy root Licorice Chamomile	13-1/2% 2 mg.
MACLEAN'S I-P-F Fumigant (MacLean)	Isopropyl alcohol Ethylene dibromide* Ethyl acetate Propylene oxide Methyl formate* Methylene chloride* Chloroform*		MADAME OLGA BLEMISH LOTION DEODORANT, COLOGNES, ASTRINGENTS (Pataky)		
MACLEAN'S LINDANE EMULSIFI- ABLE CONC. Insecticide (MacLean)	Gamma isomer of benzene hex- achloride (from lindane)* Aromatic petroleum deriv. solvent*	13.1% 81.9%	MADAM LA FORD'S DEPILATORY POWDER (La Ford)		
MACLEAN'S SOIL FUMIGANT (MacLean)	Ethylene dibromide*	20%	MADAM LA FORD'S SKIN LOTION (La Ford)		
MACLEAN'S S-T-D SPECIAL Insecticide (MacLean)	Ethylene dibromide* DDT* Tech. chlordane*		MADAM LINDSAY HAIR DRESSING (Exelento)		
MACO BRAND MARINE PAINTS (Marine Coatings)			MAESTRO CLEANER & POLISH (Lusterine)		

*Consult Sec. II., Ingredients Index. This ingredient may be responsible for major toxic effects if poisonous amounts of this product are ingested.

- 657 -

Name & Use Manufacturer	Ingredients		Name & Use Manufacturer	Ingredients	
MAGAY'S GOLD & WHITE TABLETS For flatulence (Magay)	Each gold tablet: Ginger	3/4 gr.	MAGIC FLOOR WAX (Slick Shine)		
	Capsicum	1/8 gr.			
	Ext. cascara sagrada	1 gr.	MAGIC FOAM RUG & UP-HOLSTERY CLEANER (Wiggs)	Castile soap	
	Asafetida	1 gr.		1, 1, 1-Trichloroethane	3/4 of 1%
	Ext. nux vomica* (1/60 gr. strychnine)	1/4 gr.		Tetrasodium salt of ethylene Diamine-tetra-acetic acid	
	Each white tablet:			Ammonia*	
	Calcium carbonate	3-1/2 gr.			
	Bismuth subnitrate	1/2 gr.	MAGIC FUT EZ (Magic Fut-Ez)	Sodium anhydrous	15%
	Magnesium carbonate	2 gr.		Sulfate of magnesia	35%
	Aromatics	q.s.		Sodium salicylate*	20%
				Phosphate	15%
MAGIC Piston seal (Magic Seal)				Processed oils	10%
				Essence of pine	5%
MAGIC ANT-KILLER (Barton Chem.)	Sodium arsenate*	2%	MAGIC GUN BLUER (Casey Chem.)	Selenium*	
	Cane sugar			Nitric acid*	
	Honey			Gun Blue	
	Benzoate of soda			Methanol	
	Tartaric acid	1/2 of 1%			
MAGIC BRAND BUG KILLER Insecticide (Allied Drug)	Petroleum distillates*	97.723%	MAGIC HOODOO INSECTICIDES & RODENTI-CIDES (Stumpf's)		
	Tech. chlordane	2.000%			
	Polyoxyethylene sorbitol hexaoleate	0.100%			
	Tech. piperonyl butoxide	0.115%	MAGIC INSECT REPELLANT (Quality Dist.)	Dimethyl phthalate*	100%
	Pyrethrins	0.046%			
	Phenyl mercuric lactate	0.016%	MAGIC INSECT SPRAY WITH CHLORDANE (Allied Drug)		
MAGIC BRAND OLD FASHIONED WHITE LINIMENT Rubefacient (Allied Drug)	Stronger ammonia water*				
	Ammonium chloride*				
	Gum camphor*		MAGIC IRON CEMENT & CRYSTAL CLEAR CEMENT (Glidden Co.)		
	Spirits of turpentine*				
	Oil of pine*				
	Kerosene*				
	Oleic acid				
MAGIC BRAND QUICK RELIEF COUGH SYRUP (Allied Drug)	Alcohol	2%	MAGI-CLEANER RUG & UP-HOLSTERY CLEANER (Magicleaner)		
	Chloroform	2 m./fl. oz.			
	Menthol				
	Glycerin				
	Syrup wild cherry				
	Syrup tolu		MAGIC LINIMENT Rubefacient (McNeil)	Spirits turpentine*	
	Capsicum			Acetic acid*	
MAGIC BRAND RAT & MOUSE KILLER (Allied Drug)	Arsenic trioxide*	2.6%			
MAGIC BRAND ROACH & INSECT KILLER (Allied Drug)	Tech. chlordane	2.0%/w	MAGIC REMEDY ALTERATIVE COMPOUND Rubefacient (McNeil)	Sodium salicylate*	
	B-butoxy, B' thiocyanodiethyl ether	0.3%/w		Potassium iodide*	
	B-thiocyanoethyl esters of aliphatic acids containing 10-18 carbon atoms	0.9%/w		Epsom salt	
				Extract gentian	
	Petroleum distillate*	96.8%/w			
MAGIC BRAND STOCK SPRAY Insecticide (Allied Drug)	B-butoxy, B' thiocyanodiethyl ether	1.6%/w	MAGIC RUG CLEANER (Gateway)		
	Pine oil	2.1%/w			
	Cresol	1.1%/w	MAGIC SHAVING POWDER Depilatory (Shaving Powder)	Barium sulfide*	
	Paradichlorobenzene	0.4%/w		Calcium hydroxide	
	Petroleum base oil*	94.8%/w			
MAGIC CEMENTS (Magic Iron)					
MAGIC COAT OF MAGIC COLOR (Alabama)					

Name & Use Manufacturer	Ingredients		Name & Use Manufacturer	Ingredients	
MAGIC SHOE DYE & POLISH (Ideal Paste)			MAGITEX BUBBLE BATH SHAMPOO FOR DOGS & CATS (Magitex)	Pine oil* Pyrethrins Isopropyl alcohol* Glycerin Isobornyl thiocyanoacetate* Other related terpenes	
MAGIC SILVER & PEWTER POLISH (Magic Polish)			MAGITRACK MOUSE DUST (Lethelin)	DDT*	50%
MAGIC STOCK SPRAY WITH DDT 1/2% Insecticide (Allied Drug)			MAGNEX Antacid powder (McKesson)	Bismuth subcarbonate Precipitated calcium carbonate Sodium bicarbonate Colloidal kaolin Magnesium trisilicate Aromatic flavoring oils	
MAGIC TOUCH CREAM MAKE-UP (Campana)	Butyl myristate Mineral oil Carnauba wax Lanolin Cellolyn 102 Propyl parasept Talc Titanium dioxide Iron oxides		MAGRON Vegetable maturant (Dow)	Magnesium chlorate*	
MAGIC WALLPAPER GREASE SPOT REMOVER (Glidden Co.)			MAG-SUL EPSOM SALTS TABLETS Cathartic (Dillard)	Each tablet: Epsom salts (magnesium sulfate) 18 gr.	
MAGIC WAND ODORLESS AIR DE-ODORANT (Interstate San.)			MAHDEEN FOR DANDRUFF (Mahdeen)		
MAGIC WASHER Granulated soap (Iowa)	Sodium phosphates*		MAID-EASY COFFEE STAIN REMOVER (Powder) (Maid-Easy)	Alkali* Phosphates Active oxygen Active synthetic detergent (pH 2%) solution at 25°C. is 11.05 Carbonates Silicates	
MAGIC WASHING & CLEANING COMPOUND (Togstad)			MAID-EASY MULTI-CLEANER (Powder) (Maid-Easy)	Alkali* Phosphates Active oxygen Active synthetic detergent (pH 2%) solution at 25°C. is 9.0 Carbonates	
MAGIC WAX SHOE POLISH (White) (Ideal Paste)			MAID-EASY WOW METAL CLEANER (Maid-Easy)	Tartaric acid Citric acid Silica Synthetic detergent Gums Glycols	
MAGIC WONDER ANT POISON (Quality Dist.)	Sodium arsenate*	2%	MAID OF HONOR AEROSOL IN-SECTICIDE For crawling insects (Sears)	Tech. chlordane* Tech. piperonyl butoxide* Pyrethrins Polymerized glycerol oleate Petroleum distillates* Dichlorodifluoromethane	
MAGI-KIL Ant trap poison (Lethelin)	Thallium Sulfate* Metallic thallium	1.0% 0.80%			
MAGIKIL ANT & ROACH DUST (Lethelin)	Chlordane*	5%			
MAGIKIL JELLY ANT BAIT (Lethelin)	Thallium sulfate*	1%			
MAGIKIL ANT DUST (Lethelin)	Chlordane*	5%			

*Consult Sec. II., Ingredients Index. This ingredient may be responsible for major toxic effects if poisonous amounts of this product are ingested.

- 659 -

Name & Use Manufacturer	Ingredients		Name & Use Manufacturer	Ingredients	
MAID OF HONOR AEROSOL IN- SECTICIDE For flying insects (Sears)	DDT* Pyrethrins* Tech. piperonyl butoxide* Petroleum hydrocarbons* Freon propellent		MALABAR- SUNNYHILL FOR SOILS BELOW pH 6.8 Multiple trace elements for fertilizer applications (Inorganic)	Sulfates: manganese, copper, zinc, cobalt Borax Sodium molybdenate Potassium iodide	
MAID OF HONOR CREAM WAX Furniture polish (Sears)			MALACIDE Insecticide (Bonide)	Malathion*	50%/w
MAID OF HONOR OIL Furniture polish (Sears)			MALADROX Antacid (Physicians Prod.)	Hydroxy-aluminum-magnesium aminoacetate 0.5 gm./tablet	
MAID'S NOSE SPRAY (Flower City Labs.)	Acidum boricum Menthol* Atropine sulfate*		MALANOX RESIDUAL BAIT SPRAY CONC. Insecticide (Farnam)	Malathion* Aromatic petroleum deriv. solvent*	50% 45%
MAIN LINE PAINTS (Gagnon- Haskell)			MALATHIDE Insecticide (Thompson Chem.)	Malathion* Aromatic petroleum deriv. solvent*	50% 39%
MAINTENEX Cleaner (Horn)			MALCONONE (Maltbie)	Each fl. oz.: Alcohol Dihydrocodeinone bitartrate Ephedrine hydrochloride* Sodium citrate Benzoic acid Menthol	5% 1/6 gr. 1 gr. 22 gr. 1/10 of 1%
MAINTENITE Cleaner for rubber floors (Continental Car-Na-Var)					
MAJIC-ADE Tonic, carminative (Humco)	Alcohol* Camphor* Capsicum Menthol Alcohol Chloroform* Peppermint Black catechu Ammonia methyl salicylate*	33% 3 m.	MALEX WOOD SEALERS (101, 102) (Malex)		
			MAL FOOT & SHOE DE- ODORANT (Victor)		
MAJOR'S CEMENT (Plough)	Nitrocellulose Ketones* Alcohols*		MALITHOX EMULSIFI- ABLE CON- CENTRATE Insecticide (Bonide)	Malathion*	50%/w
MAJOR'S CEMENT (China, Glass Crockery) (Plough)	Flake glue Camphor* Denatured alcohol* Zinc oxide		MALLINC- KRODT CALO-CLOR Fungicide (Mallinckrodt)	Mercurous chloride Mercuric chloride*	60% 30%
MAJOR'S CEMENT (Furniture) (Plough)			MALLINC- KRODT CALOGREEN Fungicide (Mallinckrodt)	Mercurous chloride*	90%
MAJOR VARNISH (Perfection Paint)			MALLINC- KRODT CORROSIVE SUBLIMATE Fungicide (Mallinckrodt)	Mercuric chloride*	
MAJUL PAINT & ENAMEL (Hardig)					

---

*Consult Sec. II., Ingredients Index. This ingredient may be responsible for major toxic effects if poisonous amounts of this product are ingested.

Name & Use Manufacturer	Ingredients		Name & Use Manufacturer	Ingredients	
MALLINC-KRODT PHOTO PURIFIED PICTOL (Mallinckrodt)	Monomethyl para aminophenol sulfate*		MANDRAKE BITTERS Digestant (Richard Drug)	Mandrake root Cape aloes Anise seed Glycerin Oil sweet orange Quassia chips Gentian root Orange peel sweet Coriander seed Tartaric acid Salicylic acid Caramel	
MALLINC-KRODT ROACH KILLER (Mallinckrodt)	Sodium fluoride*	95%			
MALTBIE'S ANALGESIC-IODAHL Rubefacient (Maltbie)	Iodine* Methyl salicylate* Menthol Camphor*	1% 15% 5% 2%	MANICARE (For Nails) Manicure preparation (Allcock)	Oil (persic) Sugar Perfume Glycerin Sodium hydroxide* Potassium hydroxide* Stearic acid Triethanolamine Dye	
MALTBIE'S METHYL SALICYLATE & COLCHICINE (Maltbie)	Each perle: Methyl salicylate* Colchicine*	3 m. 1/250 gr.			
			MANNING'S POWDER For skin irritations (Manning)	Salicylic acid* Zinc oxide Talcum Boric acid* Zinc stearate	
MALTOL Aromatic (Dow)	3-Hydroxy-2-methyl-1, 4-pyrone*				
MALUCIDIN PREPARA-TION Skin fungicide (veterinary) (Nat'l. Canine)	Parfentjev's yeast fraction Soap Alcohol	3%/v	MANOLINE For skin irritations (Gilbert, B. S.)	Alcohol Gum tragacanth Orris root Oil of lavender Oil of orange Rose geranium Cloves Citronella Glycerin Gum benzoin Nutmeg Oil of bergamot Oil of lemon Rosemary Cassia	12%
MAMORA CEMENTS: CHINA, CROCKERY, GLASS, PLASTIC Furniture model airplane (Van Stan)					
MAMZELL DRY CLEANER (Sapo)			MAN-O-WAR BLOOD TONIC HEMATINIC FOR HORSES (Man-O-War)	Gentian Iron Cobalt*	
MANDELIC ACID & AMMONIUM CHLORIDE For urinary tract infections (Lilly)	Each enseal: Mandelic acid* (as monoethanolamine mandelate) 5 gr. Ammonium chloride 3-1/2 gr.		MAN-O-WAR POLTIS POWDER Counter-irritant (veterinary) (Man-O-War)	Bentonite Aromatic oils	
MANDEX Fungicide (Collins Feed)	Manganese ethylene bisdithiocarbamate Dinitro capryl phenyl crotonate*	52.50% 10.00%	MAN-O-WAR VET. GALL LOTION For skin irritations (Man-O-War)	Gentian violet* Formalin* Pine oil*	
MANDEX CUCUMBER DUST WITH LINDANE Insecticide, fungicide (Collins Feed)	Manzate (manganese ethylene-bis (dithiocarbamate))* 6.3% Mildex (dinitro capryl phenyl crotonate)* 0.75% Lindane G.l.* 1.00%		MAN-O-WAR VETERINARY SALVE Antiseptic (Man-O-War)	Thymol iodide* Thymol* Phenol* Alum*	
MANDO DEPILATORY (LeFevre, J.)			MAN-ZAN For rectal irritations (De Witt)	Benzocaine* Tannic acid* Carbolic acid*	1%

*Consult Sec. II., Ingredients Index. This ingredient may be responsible for major toxic effects if poisonous amounts of this product are ingested.

- 661 -

Name & Use Manufacturer	Ingredients		Name & Use Manufacturer	Ingredients	
MANZATE FUNGICIDE (du Pont)	Manganese ethylene-bis (dithiocarbamate)*		MARCELLE FACE POWDER (Marcelle)	Talcum Titanium dioxide Zinc stearate Calcium carbonate Magnesium carbonate Kaolin Mineral oil Purified inorganic pigments and insoluble lake colors Synthetic perfume	
MANZATE 8%-PARATHION 1% (Port Brand) Fungicide (Port)	Manganese ethylene-bis (dithiocarbamate) Parathion*	5.6% 1.0%			
MANZATE 8% (Port Brand) Fungicide (Port)	Manganese ethylene-bis (dithiocarbamate)	5.6%	MARCELLE FACE POWDER (with 4% Sulfur) (Marcelle)	Talcum Titanium dioxide Zinc stearate Calcium carbonate Magnesium carbonate Kaolin Mineral oil Purified inorganic pigments and insoluble lake colors Synthetic perfume Sulfur	4%
MARATONE Hair pomade (Marion Pharm.)	Lanolin Oils Resorcin monoacetate* Pilocarpine* Quinine* Sulfur* Cholesterin Lead acetate*				
MARBLEX MODELING CLAY (Am. Art Clay)			MARCELLE FOUNDATION LOTION FOR DRY & NORMAL SKIN (Marcelle)	Vegetable oil Isopropyl esters of fatty acid blend Glyceryl esters of fatty acid blend Purified lecithin p-Hydroxy methylbenzoate Propenyl methyl guaethol Titanium dioxide Talc Iron oxide colors Synthetic perfume	
MAR-BORERCIDE Insecticide (Martin, C. J.)	Ethylene dichloride*	50%			
MARCELLE ASTRINGENT (Marcelle)	Tincture of benzoin Ethyl alcohol Certified cosmetic color Synthetic perfume		MARCELLE FOUNDATION LOTION FOR OILY SKIN (Marcelle)	Zinc oxide Talc Glycerin Kaolin Bentonite Titanium dioxide Ethyl alcohol Inorganic cosmetic colors Synthetic perfume p-Hydroxy methylbenzoate	
MARCELLE CLEANSING COLD CREAM (Marcelle)	Beeswax Mineral oil Spermaceti Cetyl alcohol Borax Synthetic perfume Glyceryl esters of fatty acid blend p-Hydroxymethylbenzoate				
MARCELLE DEODORANT (Marcelle)	Glycerin Spermaceti Modified glyceryl esters of fatty acid blend Aluminum chlorhydroxide complex Inorganic colloid gel p-Hydroxymethylbenzoate Titanium dioxide Synthetic perfume		MARCELLE HAND CREAM (Marcelle)	Modified glyceryl esters of fatty acid blend Glycerin Petrolatum Mineral oil Stearyl alcohol Spermaceti Potash emulsion of stearic acid p-Hydroxy methylbenzoate p-Hydroxy propylbenzoate Certified cosmetic color Synthetic perfume	
MARCELLE DRY ROUGE (Marcelle)	Talcum Calcium carbonate Kaolin Zinc oxide Certified lake colors Synthetic perfume		MARCELLE LIP & FACIAL ROUGE (Marcelle)	Glyceryl monostearate Castor oil Oxycholesterin absorption base Mineral oil Petrolatum Ozokerite Certified cosmetic colors Synthetic perfume	
MARCELLE DUSTING POWDER & TALCUM POWDER (Marcelle)	Talcum Zinc stearate Synthetic perfume		MARCELLE LIPSTICK (Marcelle)	Glyceryl monostearate Castor oil Oxycholesterin absorption base Candelilla wax Certified cosmetic colors Synthetic perfume	
MARCELLE EYE SHADOW (Marcelle)	Petrolatum Ozokerite Mineral oil Zinc oxide Mineral colors Synthetic perfume		MARCELLE LIQUEFYING CREAM (Anhydrous) (Marcelle)	Mineral oil Ceresin Petrolatum Paraffin Synthetic perfume	

*Consult Sec. II., Ingredients Index. This ingredient may be responsible for major toxic effects if poisonous amounts of this product are ingested.

Name & Use Manufacturer	Ingredients	Name & Use Manufacturer	Ingredients
MARCELLE MASCARA (Cream) (Marcelle)	Beeswax Ceresin Glyceryl monostearate Pure white petrolatum p-Hydroxy propylbenzoate p-Hydroxy methylbenzoate Non-ionic emulsifiers Iron oxide pigments Carbon	MARCHAND'S CREME SHAMPOO (Marchand)	Sodium lauryl sulfate approx. 7% Amide type surfactants approx. 13% Ethylene diamine tetra-acetic acid approx. 1%
MARCELLE MILD ASTRINGENT LOTION (Marcelle)	Aluminum chloride Glycerin Ethyl alcohol Synthetic perfume	MARCHAND'S GOLDEN HAIR WASH (Marchand)	Liquid: Hydrogen peroxide* 6% Powder per 4 gm. envelope: Sodium ammonium phosphate Sodium carbonate Sodium lauryl sulfate
MARCELLE SHAMPOO (Marcelle)	Potassium soaps of cocoanut and olive oils Glycerin Certified cosmetic color Synthetic perfume Chelating agent	MARCHAND'S HAIR CON-DITIONING RINSE (Marchand)	Mineral oil approx. 8% Cationic surfactants* approx. 2.5%
MARCELLE SKIN LUBRI-CATING CREAM (Marcelle)	Ceresin Petrolatum Mineral oil Zinc oxide Cholesterol Cetyl alcohol Paraffin Certified cosmetic color Synthetic perfume	MARCHAND'S HAIR RINSE (Colored)	Each 2-gm. envelope: Certified coloring 0.002-0.03 gm. Citric acid or a mixture of sulfamic and boric acids*
MARCELLE SKIN LUBRI-CATING OIL (Marcelle)	Mineral oil Cetyl alcohol Certified cosmetic color Synthetic perfume	MARCHAND'S HYDROGEN PEROXIDE (Marchand)	Hydrogen peroxide* 4%
		MARCHITA PERFUME (Joyce)	
MARCELLE SPECIAL FOUNDATION CREAM FOR DRY SKIN (Marcelle)	Mineral oil Modified glyceryl esters of fatty acid blend Diethylene glycol monoethyl ether p-Hydroxy methylbenzoate Stearyl alcohol Spermaceti Titanium dioxide Glycerin Propylene glycol Certified cosmetic color Synthetic perfume p-Hydroxy propylbenzoate	MAR-CHLOR DUST Insecticide (Mar-Prods.)	Tech. chlordane* 5%
		MAR-CHLOR 46-E Insecticide (Mar-Prods.)	Chlordane tech.* 46% Petroleum distillate* 44.5%
		MAREZINE BRAND CYCLIZINE TABLETS For motion sickness (Burroughs-Wellcome)	Cyclizine hydrochloride* 50 mg./tablet
MARCELLE SPECIAL FOUNDATION CREAM FOR OILY SKIN (Marcelle)	Potassium stearate Sodium stearate Stearic acid Glycerin p-Hydroxy methylbenzoate Synthetic perfume	MAR-FRIN Rodenticide (Martin, C. J.)	Warfarin (3-(a-acetonylbenzyl)-4-hydroxycoumarin) 0.025%
MARCELLE SPECIAL SKIN LOTION (Marcelle)	Triethanolamine emulsion of stearic acid Diethylene glycol monoethyl ether Mineral oil Cetyl alcohol p-Hydroxy methylbenzoate Methyl-cellulose Synthetic perfume	MAR-FRIN WARFARIN RAT & MOUSE KILLER (Martin, C. J.)	Warfarin (3-(a-acetonylbenzyl)-4-hydroxycoumarin) 0.5%
		MARGON WOOD PUTTY (United Gilson.)	Gypsum Dextrine
MARCELLE TALCUM POWDER (with 5% Sulfur) (Marcelle)	Talcum Zinc stearate Synthetic perfume Sulfur 5%	MARIE ANTOINETTE SHAMPOO (Heifler & Heifler)	
MARCELLE WAVING & CURLING FLUID (Marcelle)	Quince seed extract Ethyl alcohol Benzoic acid Synthetic perfume	MARIE BRIL-LIANTINE (Dewey)	Mineral oil

*Consult Sec. II., Ingredients Index. This ingredient may be responsible for major toxic effects if poisonous amounts of this product are ingested.

Name & Use Manufacturer	Ingredients		Name & Use Manufacturer	Ingredients	
MARIE CAMPAU NAIL POLISH REMOVER (Campau)			MARINE PAINTS (Chi-Namel)	Carbon black Linseed alkyd resin Mineral spirits* Drier	6.4% 43.0% 43.1% 7.5%
MARIE CAMPAU WAVE SET (Campau)			MARIVONNE CREME SHAMPOO, PERFUME (Enterprise Chem.)		
MARIE NAIL POLISH REMOVER (Dewey)	Acetone* Amyl acetate* Ethyl acetate*		MARIVONNE MASSAGE LOTION (Enterprise Chem.)		
MARIE POWDERED HENNA Hair rinse (Dewey)	Powdered henna		MARK-4 ANTISEPTIC OINTMENT SOLUTION MOUTH WASH (Mark Labs.)		
MARIE SHAMPOO (Dewey)	Cocoanut castile soap		MARKLEY'S LOTION (C & M)	Salicylic acid* Solution of coal tar Camphor water* Alcohol (isopropyl)*	1.5% 3.0% 10.0%
MARIETA'S CHINA, CROCK, GLASS CEMENT (Marieta)			MARKWELL CHECKING CRAYON (Markwell)		
MARIE WAVE SET (Dewey)	Karaya gum		MARKWELL METAL & MARKING INK (Markwell)		
MARIGOLD BORATED TALCUM (Boericke & Runyon)	Boric acid* Calendula flower extract		MARLATE 50 METHOXY-CHLOR INSECTICIDE (du Pont)	Tech. methoxychlor*	50%
MARIGOLD WALLPAPER CLEANER (Imperial Paper)	Edible pastry flour Carbonates of sodium and calcium Chlorides of sodium and calcium Pine Oil		MARLATE 2MR, 24% TECHNICAL METH-OXYCHLOR INSECTICIDE (du Pont)	Tech. methoxychlor*	2 lb./gal.
MARIN COUNTY EARWIG BAIT (Marin)	Sodium fluosilicate	0.75%	MAR-LIN PERCH PAINT Insecticide (Martin, C. J.)	Petroleum hydrocarbons* Pine oil* Gamma isomer of benzene hexachloride (from lindane)*	
MARIN COUNTY POISON GRAIN Rodenticide (Marin)	Strychnine* expressed as alkaloid	0.25%			
MARIN COUNTY RAT BAIT (Marin)	Alcohol extractives of red squill* Inert ingredients*	5% 95%	MARLO AFTER SHAVE LOTION & SKIN FRESHENER (Marlo)	Alcohol* Menthol* Perfume	
MARIN COUNTY SODIUM FLUOSILICATE Insecticide (Marin)	Sodium fluosilicate*	95%			
MARIN COUNTY WARFARIN RAT BAIT (Marin)	Warfarin (compound 42)	0.025%	MARLO ANTISEPTIC SOLUTION Mouth wash (Marlo)	Alcohol	25%
MARIN COUNTY ZINC PHOSPHIDE POISON GRAIN Rodenticide (Marin)	Zinc phosphide	0.5%	MARLO COAL TAR DIS-INFECTANT (Marlo)		
MARINE BRAND NO. 80 Cement (Ferdinand)	Resins in alcohol solvent*		MARLO DISINFECT-ANT (Marlo)		

*Consult Sec. II., Ingredients Index. This ingredient may be responsible for major toxic effects if poisonous amounts of this product are ingested.

Name & Use Manufacturer	Ingredients	Name & Use Manufacturer	Ingredients
MARLO GOLDEN HAIR WASH (Marlo)	20 Vol. (6%) peroxide*	MARSHALL'S POMADE Tint for gray hair (Gray's)	Lead acetate* Ppt. sulfur* Lanolin Glycol Lard Mixture petroleum hydrocarbons
MARLO INFLAM- MABLE DRY CLEANER (Marlo)	Stoddard solvent*	MAR- TERMINO TERMITE CONTROL (Martin, C. J.)	Tech. chlordane* 74% Petroleum hydrocarbons 20%
MARLO LIGHTER FLUID (Marlo)		MARTINI TEMPERA, MADDER, ALIZARINE Art supplies (Nobema)	
MARLO LILAC LOTION (Marlo)	Alcohol* Perfume	MARTIN'S ANTI-PICK For poultry cannibalism (Martin, C. J.)	
MAR-O-VEL OIL Rubefacient (Mar-O-Vel)	Oil red thyme Oil eucalyptus* Oil sassafras* Spirits turpentine* Menthol* Gum camphor* Raw linseed oil	MARTIN'S BENZOL Screw-worm control (veterinary) (Martin, C. J.)	U.S. formula #62 Benzol content
MAR-O-VEL OINTMENT (Mar-O-Vel)	Oil eucalyptus Oil wintergreen* Oil turpentine* Gum camphor* Menthol crystals* Chlorophyll White petrolatum	MARTIN'S 17% BHC-33% DDT DIP SPRAY Insecticide (Martin, C. J.)	DDT* 33% BHC* 2% Other isomers of benzene hexachloride 15%
MAR-PENTA Wood pre- servative (Martin, C. J.)	Pentachlorophenol* 5% Pine oil 5% Petroleum distillate* 74%	MARTIN'S BHC WET- TABLE POWDER (Martin, C. J.)	Gamma isomer of benzene hexachloride 6% Other isomers of benzene hexachloride* 40%
MAR-PERMA WOOD PRE- SERVER (Martin, C. J.)	Petroleum distillate* Pentachlorophenol* Other chlorophenols*	MARTIN'S BLOOD CLOTTER For wounds (veterinary) (Martin, C. J.)	Alum, dried ammonium U.S.P.* 48.5% Ferric subsulfate po. 32.3% Acid tannic U.S.P.* 15.0% Saponated solution of cresol U.S.P.* 1.6% Camphor U.S.P. po. syn.* 0.8% Oil eucalyptus U.S.P. 0.8% Oxyquinoline sulfate* 1.0%
MRS. MARPLE'S SALVE (Aschenbach)			
MAR-QUINSOL For coccidiosis (veterinary, avian) (Martin, C. J.)	Sulfaquinoxaline sodium 3.44 gm./100 cc.		
MARRIOTT'S OINTMENT Counter- irritant for skin irritations (Marriott)	Camphor* Gum turpentine* Lead oleate*	MARTIN'S CANINE CAPS Anthelmintic (veterinary) (Martin, C. J.)	Tetrachlorethylene* 97.68% Arecoline hydrobromide 0.39% Ethyl cellulose 1.51% Mineral oil 0.42%
MARROW'S MAR-O-OIL SUPER FOAMY TYPE SHAMPOO (Marrow's)		MARTIN'S CARBOLIN OIL ROOST PAINT OR SPRAY Insecticide (Martin, C. J.)	Petroleum distillate* Anthracene oil*
MARSHALL'S CAMPHOR CREAM (Goodrich- Gamble)	Camphor* Turpentine* Glycerin	MARTIN'S CATTLE DRENCH Anthelmintic (veterinary) (Martin, C. J.)	Phenothiazine* 30% Bentonite

*Consult Sec. II., Ingredients Index. This ingredient may be responsible for major toxic effects if poisonous amounts of this product are ingested.

Name & Use Manufacturer	Ingredients		Name & Use Manufacturer	Ingredients	
MARTIN'S COW TONIC Veterinary (Martin, C. J.)	Nux vomica inc. strychnine* Columbo Spearmint Calcium carbonate Iron oxide Cupric sulfate Cobalt sulfate Quassia Potassium phosphate Sodium chloride Potassium carbonate Manganese sulfate Zinc sulfate	1.4%	MARTIN'S DEHORNING PROTECTIVE DRESSING (Martin, C. J.)	Coal tar* Pine tar* Bone oil	
			MARTIN'S DOG SHAMPOO (Martin, C. J.)	Coconut oil base	
			MARTIN'S DOR MULSO Fungicide (Martin, C. J.)	Petroleum distillate*	97%
MARTIN'S CREOSOTE DIP Disinfectant, deodorizer, cleanser (veterinary) (Martin, C. J.)	Coal tar neutral oils* Soap Phenols*		MARTIN'S EAR-TIX-TOX Insecticide (Martin, C. J.)	Gamma isomer of benzene hexachloride* Other isomers of benzene hexachloride Pine oil* Pine tar oil* Mineral oil Xylol*	1.00% 1.78% 50.00% 20.00% 15.00% 12.22%
MARTIN'S CUBE POWDER Insecticide (Martin, C. J.)	Rotenone* Other cube resins	5% 10%	MARTIN'S EYE CREAM (Assoc. Brands)		
MARTIN'S DAIRY & GARDEN SPRAY Insecticide (Martin, C. J.)	Methoxychlor* tech.	50%	MARTIN'S FLEA POWDER Insecticide (Martin, C. J.)	Cube resins Nicotine*	1.35% 0.5%
MARTIN'S DDT-BHC WETTABLE POWDER Insecticide (Martin, C. J.)	DDT* BHC* Other isomers of benzene hexachloride	25.0% 3.0% 22.0%	MARTIN'S FUMA-GRAIN Fungicide (Martin, C. J.)	Carbon tetrachloride* Ethylene dichloride*	25% 75%
MARTIN'S 35% DDT CONC. Insecticide (Martin, C. J.)	DDT* Aromatic hydrocarbons*	35% 51%	MARTIN'S GRUB DUST Insecticide (Martin, C. J.)	Rotenone* Other cube resins	1.67% 3.33%
MARTIN'S 25% DDT EMULSO Insecticide (Martin, C. J.)	DDT Aromatic petroleum deriv. solvent*	25% 73%	MARTIN'S HEXACHLORO-ETHANE For liver flukes (veterinary) (Martin, C. J.)	Hexachloroethane* Bentonite and water	38.4%
MARTIN'S 5% DDT HOUSEHOLD SPRAY Insecticide (Martin, C. J.)	DDT* Isobornyl thiocyanoacetate Other related terpenes Petroleum distillate	5%	MARTIN'S LAMP BLACK (Martin, L.)	Carbon, non-toxic	
MARTIN'S 10% DDT POWDER Insecticide (Martin, C. J.)	DDT*	10%	MARTIN'S LINIMENT (Martin, C. J.)	Pine oil* Sassafras* Methyl salicylate* Isopropyl alcohol* Soap Oil camphor* Turpentine* Ammonia water*	
MARTIN'S 10% DDT RESIDUAL SPRAY Insecticide (Martin, C. J.)	Petroleum distillate Dimethylbenzene* (xylene) DDT		MARTIN'S LIVESTOCK SPRAY Insecticide (Martin, C. J.)	Petroleum distillate* Isobornyl thiocyanoacetate Related terpenes	
MARTIN'S 50% DDT WETTABLE POWDER Insecticide (Martin, C. J.)	DDT*	50%	MARTIN'S 50% MALATHION EMULSIFI-ABLE CON-CENTRATE Insecticide (Waltham)	Malathion* Xylol*	50% 42.4%

*Consult Sec. II., Ingredients Index. This ingredient may be responsible for major toxic effects if poisonous amounts of this product are ingested.

Name & Use Manufacturer	Ingredients	
MARTIN'S MALATHION 50% FLY KILLER (Martin, C. J.)	Malathion*	50.0%
	Xylol	42.4%
MARTIN'S MAR-CHLOR Insecticide (Martin, C. J.)	Tech. chlordane*	45%
	Petroleum hydrocarbon*	45%
MARTIN'S MAR-CHLOR 5% DUST Insecticide (Martin, C. J.)	Tech. chlordane*	5%
MARTIN'S MAR-CHLOR 10% DUST Insecticide (Martin, C. J.)	Tech. chlordane*	10%
MARTIN'S MAR-CHLOR 40% WETTABLE Insecticide (Martin, C. J.)	Tech. chlordane*	40%
MARTIN'S MAR-DANE 1883 SCREW-WORM CONTROL Ectoparasiticide, insecticide (Martin, C. J.)	Gamma isomer of benzene hexachloride (from lindane)	3%
	Pine oil	35%
	Benzol*	35%
MARTIN'S MAR-DANE 10% LINDANE Insecticide (Martin, C. J.)	Gamma isomer of benzene hexachloride*	10%
	Aromatic petroleum deriv. solvent*	70%
MARTIN'S MAR-DANE 25% LINDANE Insecticide (Martin, C. J.)	Gamma isomer of benzene hexachloride (from lindane)*	25%
MARTIN'S M & S CREOSOTE OIL Wood preservative (Martin, C. J.)	Creosote oil*	
MARTIN'S MULTI-PURPOSE GARDEN DUST Insecticide (Martin, C. J.)	Zineb	6.00%
	Methoxychlor tech.	5.00%
	Rotenone	0.75%
	Other cube resins	1.50%
MARTIN'S PHENO-THIAZINE DRENCH Anthelmintic (veterinary) (Martin, C. J.)	Sodium arsenate*	0.770%
	Phenothiazine*	37.527%
	F. D. & C. colors	0.094%

Name & Use Manufacturer	Ingredients	
MARTIN'S PHENO-THIAZINE LIQUID SUS-PENSION DRENCH Anthelmintic (veterinary)	Phenothiazine*	12.5 gm./fl. oz.
	Bentonite	
MARTIN'S PHENO-THIAZINE POWDER Anthelmintic (veterinary) (Martin, C. J.)	Phenothiazine*	100%
MARTIN'S PINE TAR OIL Antiseptic for wounds (veterinary) (Martin, C. J.)	Pine tar oil*	
MARTIN'S PINK EYE POWDER (veterinary) (Martin, C. J.)	Sulfanilamide*	
	Sulfathiazole*	
	Sulfathiazole sodium*	
	Mercurous chloride*	
	Neoprontosil*	
	Aspirin*	
	Boric acid*	
MARTIN'S PLANT SPRAY Insecticide (Martin, C. J.)	Petroleum distillate*	
	Ethylene glycol ether of pinene*	
	Oleic acid	
	Pine oil	
	Hydrogenated rotenone*	
	Other cube resins	
	2-Amino-2-methyl-1-propanol	
	Citrus oil	
	Pyrethrins I and II	
MARTIN'S POULTRY INHALANT Respiratory decongestant (veterinary, avian) (Martin, C. J.)	Pine oil*	
	Oil of eucalyptus*	
	Beechwood creosote*	
	Camphor*	
	Guaiacol	
	Menthol*	
	Soap	
MARTIN'S POULTRY TABLETS (Martin, C. J.)	Zinc sulfocarbolate	
	Sodium sulfocarbolate	
	Calcium sulfocarbolate	
	Copper sulfate*	
	Powdered boric acid*	
MARTIN'S POWDER Insecticide (Waltham)	DDT*	10.00%
	Pyrethrins	0.2%
MARTIN'S PURE ANTHRACENE OIL Insecticide (Martin, C. J.)	Anthracene oil*	
MARTIN'S PURE BONE OIL Fly repellent (Martin, C. J.)		

*Consult Sec. II., Ingredients Index. This ingredient may be responsible for major toxic effects if poisonous amounts of this product are ingested.

Name & Use Manufacturer	Ingredients		Name & Use Manufacturer	Ingredients	
MARTIN'S PYRENONE EMULSIFI-ABLE CON-CENTRATE Insecticide (Waltham)	Tech. piperonyl butoxide* Pyrethrins Polyoxyethylene sorbital mixed ether ester Petroleum oil*	11.87% 1.18% 14.94% 72.01%	MARTIN'S SMEAR 70 Fly-repellent wound dressing (veterinary) (Martin, C. J.)	Pine tar oil* Rosin Petrolatum Bone oil Gamma isomer of benzene hexachloride (from lindane)*	
MARTIN'S PYRENONE INSECTICIDE (Waltham)	Tech. piperonyl butoxide Pyrethrins Petroleum oil*	1.59% 0.16% 98.25%	MARTIN'S SODIUM FLUORIDE Insecticide (Martin, C. J.)	Sodium fluoride*	90-95%
MARTIN'S QUAMM DIS-INFECTANT (Martin, C. J.)	Para di-isobutyl phenoxy ethoxy ethyl dimethyl benzyl ammonium chloride* 10%		MARTIN'S SPECIAL PHENO-THIAZINE DRENCH Anthelmintic (veterinary) (Martin, C. J.)	Sodium arsenate* Phenothiazine* F. D. & C. colors	0.770% 37.527% 0.094%
MARTIN'S RAT STOP (Martin, C. J.)	Thallium sulfate*	1%			
MARTIN'S RESIDUAL SPRAY Insecticide (Waltham)	DDT* Deodorized hydrocarbon solvents*	5% 95%	MARTIN'S SPECIAL WORM POWDER Anthelmintic (veterinary) (Martin, C. J.)	Tobacco powder* Pumpkin seed Sodium bicarbonate Sodium sulfate ex. Iron sulfate Quassia Arsenic trioxide* Aromatics	0.375%
MARTIN'S ROTENONE & SULPHUR DIP Insecticide (Martin, C. J.)	Rotenone Other cube resins Sulfur*	0.5% 1.0% 83.7%			
MARTIN'S 20% SABADILLA DUST Insecticide (Martin, C. J.)	Sabadilla alkaloids*	0.8%	MARTIN'S STOCK 1029 Insecticide (Martin, C. J.)	Pyridine* Dibutyl phthalate	
MARTIN'S SCOUR MEDICINE For intestinal irritation (veterinary) (Martin, C. J.)	Bismuth subgallate Copper sulfate* Calcium Sodium & zinc phenolsulfonates* Bentonite Calcium carbonate Extract stramonium* (32.23-38.27 mg. alkaloids of stramonium per 100 gm.)		MARTIN'S STOCK TONIC (Veterinary) (Martin, C. J.)	Nux vomica* (equiv. 0.0175% strychine) Capsicum Columbo Iron sulfate Magnesium sulfate Sodium sulfate Salt Calcium carbonate Iron oxide Potassium iodide Manganese sulfate Quassia Spearmint Sodium bicarbonate Copper sulfate* Salt Magnesium sulfate Sodium sulphate Superphosphate Magnesium carbonate Cobalt sulfate* Zinc sulfate*	
MARTIN'S SCREW-WORM BOMB Insecticide (Martin, C. J.)	Gamma isomer of benzene hexachloride* Pine oil*	1.72% 20.10%			
MARTIN'S SCREW-WORM KILLER Insecticide (Martin, C. J.)	Benzol* Pine oil* Diphenylamine* Rosin soap				
MARTIN'S SCREW-WORM SMEAR U. S. FORMULA NO. 62 Insecticide (Martin, C. J.)	Diphenylamine* Benzol* Turkey red oil	35.0% 35.0% 7.5%	MARTIN'S SULFA-REA POWDER Antiseptic powder (veterinary) (Martin, C. J.)	Urea Sulfanilamide* Sulfathiazole* Calcium phosphate	
			MARTIN'S SULFA-SOL For colds (veterinary, avian) (Martin, C. J.)	Sodium sulfathiazone 12.5 gm./100 cc.	
MARTIN'S SHEEP MARKING PAINT (Martin, C. J.)			MARTIN'S SULFA-THIAZOLE BOLUS For infections (veterinary) (Martin, C. J.)	Sulfathiazole U.S.P.*	240 gr.

Name & Use Manufacturer	Ingredients		Name & Use Manufacturer	Ingredients	
MARTIN'S TABLETS Cathartic (veterinary) (Martin Herb)	Ext. rhubarb* Aloes* Sodium bicarbonate Podophyllin* Oil cardamom Ext. belladonna*	1/8 gr.	MARVEL CLEANSER & WATER SOFTENER (Central Chem.)		
MARTIN'S TETRA- CHLORE- THYLENE OIL Anthelmintic (veterinary) (Martin, C. J.)	Tetrachlorethylene* Oil eucalyptus Naphthalene	94.5% 1.5% 4.0%	MARVELLA RUG & UP- HOLSTERY CLEANER (Keystone Chem.)		
MARTIN'S UDDER LOTION For udder irritation (veterinary) (Martin, C. J.)	Camphor* Creosote* Guaiacol Oil eucalyptus Menthol Aromatic oil base	1.50% 1.50% 1.00% 1.00% 0.05% 94.95%	MARVEL MYSTERY OIL Cylinder lubricant (Emerol)		
MARTIN'S U. S.-E. Q. 335 Screw-worm remedy for calves (Martin, C. J.)	Mineral oil Pine oil* Gamma isomer of benzene hexachloride* (from lindane)	42% 35% 3%	MARVEL'S HAIR & SCALP CON- DITIONER (Marvel)		
MARTIN'S UTERINE BOLUS For infections (veterinary) (Martin, C. J.)	Sulfanilamide* Sulfathiazole* Urea Corn starch Amaranth color	33 gr. 5 gr. 207 gr.	MARVEL SPRAY Insecticide (Rose Mfg.)	Rotenone Other cube resins Mannitan monolaurate Pine oil	0.90% 1.90% 30.00% 5.00%
MARTIN'S WARFARIN BAIT FOR RATS & MICE (Waltham)	Warfarin (3-(a-acetonylbenzyl)- 4-hydroxycoumarin)	0.025	MARY ETTA NAIL POLISH REMOVER (Dattilo)		
			MARY JOHNSON HAIR COLOR- ING (Newbro)		
MARTIN'S WHITE FLY REPELLENT For wounds (veterinary) (Martin, C. J.)	Fish oil Mineral oil Petrolatum Pine oil Diphenylamine	25.0% 20.0% 6.6% 6.7% 6.7%	MARY T. GOLDMAN QUICK HAIR COLOR PREPARATION (A) (Goldman, M.)	Ammoniacal silver nitrate solution*	
MARTIN- SENOUR FLOOR & TRIM ENAMEL (Martin- Senour)	Pigment: Calcium titanium pigment Magnesium silicate Lamp black Varnish vehicle: Non-volatile (linseed maleic resin) Volatile (mineral spirits* and driers)	30% 70%	MARY T. GOLDMAN QUICK HAIR COLOR PREPARATION (B) (Goldman, M.)	Pyrogallic acid* Sodium sulfite solution	
MARTIN- SENOUR VARNISH 08000 (Martin- Senour)	Non-volatile (tung-linseed oil phenolic resin) Volatile (mineral spirits* and driers)	50% 50%	MASEDA FOOT POWDER Skin fungicide (medicinal) (Massengill)	Phenylmercuric nitrate (mercury prep.) Oxyquinoline sulfate* Boric acid* Salicylic acid* Zinc stearate Aromatics	1-5,000
MARTY'S GLASS CLEANER (Dyrud)	Denatured alcohol*		MASON'S HAIR DYE (Mason)		
MARVEL CLEANING FLUID (Barco Chem.)	Carbon tetrachloride*		MASON'S OLIV CREME (Aschenbach)		

*Consult Sec. II., Ingredients Index. This ingredient may be responsible for major toxic effects if poisonous amounts of this product are ingested.

- 669 -

Name & Use Manufacturer	Ingredients		Name & Use Manufacturer	Ingredients	
MASSENGILL'S ANALGESIC BALM, NO. 2 Rubefacient (Massengill)	Methyl salicylate* Menthol* (synthetic) Camphor* Eugenol* Oil eucalyptus*		MASSENGILL'S CASCARA COMPOUND Laxative (Massengill)	Each tablet: Ext. belladonna* Ext. cascara sagrada Aloin* Podophyllum resin Oleoresin ginger	8 mg. 16 mg. 16 mg. 11 mg. 4 mg.
MASSENGILL'S ANALGESIC BALM, NO. 3 Rubefacient (Massengill)	Chloral hydrate* Methyl salicylate* Camphor* Menthol* (synthetic) Essential oils*	0.6 gm./oz.	MASSENGILL'S CATHARTIC COMP. N.F. (Massengill)	Each tablet: Calomel (mercury deriv.)* Ext. colocynth compound* Resin of jalap Powd. gamboge	65 mg. 80 mg. 21.5 mg. 16 mg.
MASSENGILL'S ANTACID POWDER (Massengill)	Magnesium carbonate Sodium bicarbonate Calcium carbonate, prec. Oil peppermint	40% 40% 20% q.s.	MASSENGILL'S COLLYRIUM (Liquid) For eye irritations (Massengill)	Berberine sulfate* Boric acid* Zinc sulfate*	
MASSENGILL'S ANTHEL-MINTIC LIQUID (Swine) (Massengill)	Each 100 cc.: Chloroform* Oil chenopodium Oil anise Oil camphor * Castor oil*	6.25 cc. 4.6 cc. 2.08 cc. 2.08 cc. 85.00 cc.	MASSENGILL'S CORRECTIVE MIXTURE For intestinal irritation (Massengill)	Each 5 cc.: Zinc sulfocarbolate Salol Bismuth subsalicylate Pepsin (1-3000) Carminatives, demulcents, aromatics	10 mg. 20 mg. 80 mg. 40 mg. q.s.
MASSENGILL'S BABY OINTMENT For skin irritations (Massengill)	Aluminum hydrate Zinc oxide Boric acid* Tinct. benzoin comp. Carbolic acid*	0.2%	MASSENGILL'S CORRECTIVE MIXTURE & PAREGORIC (Pink) Astringent, carminative (Massengill)	Each 5 cc.: Paregoric (tinct. opium camphorated)* Zinc sulfocarbolate* Salol* Bismuth subsalicylate Pepsin Carminatives, demulcents, aromatics	0.6 cc. 11 mg. 21.5 mg. 86.5 mg. 43 mg. q.s.
MASSENGILL'S BENZOCAINE & PICRIC ACID Local anesthetic, antiseptic (Massengill)	Benzocaine Picric acid*	1% 1/4%			
			MASSENGILL'S CREME LINIMENT (White) rubefacient (Massengill)	Each fl. oz.: Soap Ammonium carbonate Camphor* Oil turpentine* Strong sol. of ammonia* Oil white thyme	1.4 gm. 1.4 gm. 0.72 gm. 5 cc. 0.5 cc. 0.28 cc.
MASSENGILL'S BENZOIN COMPOUND U.S.P. (Tincture) Decongestant, protective, inhalant (Massengill)	Benzoin Aloe Storax Balsam tolu Alcohol*	10% 2% 8% 4%	MASSENGILL'S CRESOL DIS-INFECTANT (Liquid) (Massengill)	Cresol* U.S.P. Vegetable oil soap base	46-52%
MASSENGILL'S BROWN COMPOUND WITH AMMONIUM CHLORIDE Antitussive (Massengill)	Each tablet: Ext. glycyrrhiza Benzoic acid Camphor Tartar emetic* Ammonium chloride Oil anise	0.12 gm. 1.95 mg. 1.95 mg. 0.97 mg. 65 mg. 0.0018 cc.	MASSENGILL'S DIGESTIVE MIXTURE (Massengill)	Each 5 cc.: Pepsin (1-3000) Pancreatin Diastase of malt Caffeine Oil celery Lactic & hydrochloric acids	43 mg. 43 mg. 11 mg. q.s. q.s.
MASSENGILL'S CALOMEL, RHUBARB & COLOCYNTH COMPOUND (Pink) Laxative (Massengill)	Each capsule: Calomel (mercury deriv.)* Rhubarb Aloe* Myrrh Colocynth ext. Ipomea resin	2 gr. 7/8 gr. 1-1/2 gr. 2/5 gr. 1/13 gr. 7/8 gr.	MASSENGILL'S HEMOR-RHOIDAL CONSTRICTOR Rectal suppositories (Massengill)	Each suppository: Ext. belladonna* Bismuth oxyiodide Ephedrine sulfate* Cocoa butter mass Zinc oxide Bismuth subcarbonate Phenacaine hydrochloride*	0.7% 7% 0.14% q.s. 14% 7% 0.7%
MASSENGILL'S CAMPHOR SPIRIT, N.F. Antispasmodic, sedative, carminative (Massengill)	Each 100 cc.: Camphor*	9-11 gm.	MASSENGILL'S IMITATION VANILLA FLAVOR (Massengill)	Ethyl alcohol Vanillin Coumarin* Sugar Alcohol Caramel	12%/v

*Consult Sec. II., Ingredients Index. This ingredient may be responsible for major toxic effects if poisonous amounts of this product are ingested.

- 670 -

Name & Use Manufacturer	Ingredients		Name & Use Manufacturer	Ingredients	
MASSENGILL'S LAXATIVE NO. 5 (Massengill)	Each pill: Strychnine* Ext. belladonna* Aloin* Powd. ipecac Phenolphthalein	0.80 mg. 5.4 mg. 16 mg. 4.8 mg. 32 mg.	MASSENGILL'S POWDER Vaginal douche, oral and skin antiseptic (Massengill)	Boric acid* Ammonium alum Berberine salt* Phenol* Menthol isomers* Thymol* Eucalyptol* Methyl salicylate*	
MASSENGILL'S LAXATIVE NO. 6 (Massengill)	Each tablet: Ext. belladonna* Aloin* Ext. cascara sagrada Podophyllum resin Phenolphthalein	8 mg. 16 mg. 16 mg. 16 mg. 32 mg.	MASSENGILL'S QUININE SULFATE CAPSULES (5 Gr.; 0.3 Gm.) Antiperiodic, anti-malarial (Massengill)	Quinine sulfate*	
MASSENGILL'S LAXATIVE NO. 7 (Massengill)	Each tablet: Ext. belladonna* Strychnine sulfate* Ext. cascara sagrada Aloin* Podophyllum resin Oleoresin ginger	8 mg. 0.54 mg. 16 mg. 16 mg. 11 mg. 4 mg.	MASSENGILL'S SOLIDIFIED LINIMENT Counter- irritant (Massengill)	Oleoresin capsicum Oil croton* Oil mustard* Camphor* Oil cajuput Oil turpentine*	
MASSENGILL'S LIQUID DRESSING For skin burns, ir- ritations (Massengill)	Scarlet red (Biebrich) Camphor* Eucalyptol* Carbolic acid* Mineral oil Menthol* Thymol* Salol* Oil tar		MASSENGILL'S TANNIC ACID JELLY & BENZOCAINE For burns (Massengill)	Tannic acid Phenylmercuric nitrate mercury preparation Benzocaine Aromatics	7% 1-20,000 1%
MASSENGILL'S LOCAL ANALGESIC LIQUID (Massengill)	Chloral hydrate* 1.75 gm./100 cc. Menthol* Oil caraway Benzocaine Methyl salicylate*		MASSENGILL'S TEAT OINTMENT Veterinary (Massengill)	Oil of thuja Scarlet red Zinc oxide ointment base	
MASSENGILL'S LUBRICATING JELLY (Massengill)	Phenylmercuric nitrate* (mercury prep.) Boric acid Glycerin Vegetable products	1-5,000	MASSENGILL'S TERPIN HYDRATE & CODEINE N.F. (Elixir) Antitussive (Massengill)	Each 5 cc.: Codeine Terpin hydrate	10 mg. 85 mg.
MASSENGILL'S MAGNESIUM TRISILICATE (7-1/2 Gr.) Antacid (Massengill)	Each tablet: Magnesium trisilicate Oil peppermint	0.5 gm. q.s.	MASSENGILL TERPIN HYDRATE & CODEINE (Pink) Expectorant, antitussive (Massengill)	Each lozenge: Codeine sulfate Terpin hydrate	5 mg. 50 mg.
MASSENGILL'S MERCURY AMMONIATED OINTMENT U.S.P. Ectoparisiti- cide, antiseptic (Massengill)	Ammoniated mercury* 4.5-5.5%		MASSENGILL'S VERMIFUGE (Veterinary) (Massengill)	Each tablet: Calomel* Santonin* Arecoline hydrobromide* Powd. areca nut Sodium bicarbonate	8 mg. 8 mg. 6.5 mg. 32 mg. 65 mg.
MASSENGILL'S METHYL SALICYLATE (20%) OINTMENT Rubefacient (Massengill)	Methyl salicylate* (syn.)	20%	MASTER BRAND 3-5 COTTON DUST Insecticide (Stevens Ind.)	Gamma isomer of BHC* DDT*	3.00% 5.00%
MASSENGILL'S PINE OIL (Medicinal) Antiseptic, deodorant (Massengill)	Pinus palustris* Phenol* coefficient	3.5-4.0	MASTER CAULK Caulking compound (Calbar)		
			MASTER LIQUID HOG MEDICINE For intestinal irritation (veterinary) (Master Labs.)	Sodium arsanilate* Sodium nicotinate* Sodium hydroxide Extract of licorice Oil of anise	2.1% 0.63% 3.0%

*Consult Sec. II., Ingredients Index. This ingredient may be responsible for major toxic effects if poisonous amounts of this product are ingested.

Name & Use Manufacturer	Ingredients		Name & Use Manufacturer	Ingredients	
MASTERMIXED VARNISH REMOVER (Sears)	Benzol* Acetone* Alcohol (methyl)* Wax (paraffin)		MATHIESON BHC-DDT COTTON EMULSIFI- ABLE CONC. Insecticide (Olin Mathieson)	Methylated aromatic petroleum deriv.* DDT* Gamma isomer of benzene hexachloride Other isomers of benzene hexachloride	50.0% 18.0% 10.8% 16.2%
MASTERPIECE OIL PAINT- ING SET (Palmer Paint)					
MATCHLESS OIL HAIR TONIC & SULPHUR CREAM (House of Marshall)			MATHIESON BHC 1 LB. EMULSIFI- ABLE CONC. Insecticide (Olin Mathieson)	Methylated aromatic petroleum deriv.* Gamma isomer of benzene hexachloride Other isomers of benzene hexachloride*	67.5% 11.0% 16.5%
MATERNA CREAM For skin (Dumas- Wilson)	Lanolin Cocoa butter		MATHIESON BHC 1.2 LB. EMULSIFI- ABLE CONC. Insecticide (Olin Mathieson)	Methylated aromatic petroleum deriv.* Gamma isomer of benzene hexachloride Other isomers of benzene hexachloride	61.8% 13.3% 19.9%
MATHIESON AGRICUL- TURAL DUSTING SULPHUR Insecticide, fungicide (Olin Mathieson)	Sulfur*　　　　93%		MATHIESON BHC 12% WETTABLE POWDER Insecticide (Olin Mathieson)	Gamma isomer of benzene hexachloride* Other isomers of benzene hexachloride	12.0% 28.6%
MATHIESON ALDRIN 2-1/2% DUST Insecticide (Olin Mathieson)	Hexachloro hexahydro dimethano naphthalene* 　　　　　2.38% Related compounds　0.43%		MATHIESON BUTYL ESTER 22 BRUSH KILLER Herbicide (Olin Mathieson)	Butyl ester of 2, 4-dichloro phenoxy acetic acid*　27.2% Butyl ester of 2, 4, 5- trichloro phenoxy acetic acid*　　　　　26.5%	
MATHIESON ALDRIN 2 LB. EMULSIFI- ABLE CONC. Insecticide (Olin Mathieson)	Hexachloro hexahydro dimethano naphthalene* 　　　　　23.03% Related compounds　3.90% Methylated aromatic petroleum deriv.*　35.00% Petroleum distillates　34.07%		MATHIESON BUTYL ESTER D4 WEED KILLER (Olin Mathieson)	Butyl ester of 2, 4-dichloro phenoxy acetic acid*　56.3%	
MATHIESON ALDRIN 5% GRANULES Insecticide (Olin Mathieson)	Hexachloro hexahydro dimethano naphthalene* 　　　　　4.75% Related compounds　0.87%		MATHIESON BUTYL ESTER D6 WEED KILLER (Olin Mathieson)	Butyl ester of 2, 4-dichloro phenoxy acetic acid*　78.0%	
MATHIESON ALDRIN 2-1/2%- SULPHUR 40% DUST Insecticide (Olin Mathieson)	Hexachloro hexahydro dimethano naphthalene* 　　　　　2.4% Related compounds　0.4% Sulfur*(93% through 325 mesh)　　　　40.0%		MATHIESON BUTYL ESTER D267 WEED KILLER (Olin Mathieson)	Butyl ester of 2, 4-dichloro phenoxy acetic acid*　40%	
MATHIESON ALDRIN 25% WETTABLE POWDER Insecticide (Olin Mathieson)	Hexachloro hexahydro dimethano naphthalene* 　　　　　23.750% Related compounds　4.340%		MATHIESON BUTYL ESTER T4 BRUSH KILLER Herbicide (Olin Mathieson)	Butyl ester of 2, 4, 5- trichloro phenoxy acetic acid*　　　　　53.6%	
MATHIESON AMINE 40 WEED KILLER (Olin Mathieson)	Di-methyl amine salt of 2, 4- dichloro phenoxyacetic acid* 　　　　　49.4%		MATHIESON CHLORDANE 5% DUST Insecticide (Olin Mathieson)	Tech. chlordane*　　5%	

Name & Use Manufacturer	Ingredients	
MATHIESON CHLORDANE 10% DUST Insecticide (Olin Mathieson)	Tech. chlordane*	10%
MATHIESON CHLORDANE 4-LB. EMULSIFI- ABLE CONC. Insecticide (Olin Mathieson)	Tech. chlordane* Petroleum distillates*	45.25% 50.75%
MATHIESON CHLORDANE 8 LB. EMULSIFI- ABLE CONC. Insecticide (Olin Mathieson)	Tech. chlordane* Petroleum distillates	73.6% 22.4%
MATHIESON CHLORDANE 40% WET- TABLE POWDER Insecticide (Olin Mathieson)	Tech. chlordane*	40.0%
MATHIESON CHLORO-IPC EMULSIFI- ABLE CONC. Herbicide (Olin Mathieson)	Isopropyl n-(3-chlorophenyl) carbamate*	48%
MATHIESON COPPER 5% DUST Fungicide (Olin Mathieson)	Copper*as metallic (from tri-basic copper sulfate)	5%
MATHIESON 2.5-5-0 COTTON DUST Insecticide (Olin Mathieson)	Hexachloro hexahydro dimethano naphthalene* Related compounds DDT*	2.4% 0.4% 5.000%
MATHIESON 2-10-40 COTTON DUST Insecticide (Olin Mathieson)	Gamma isomer of benzene hexachloride* Other isomers of benzene hexachloride DDT* Sulfur*	2% 11.6% 10% 40%
MATHIESON 3-5 COTTON DUST Insecticide (Olin Mathieson)	Gamma isomer of benzene hexachloride* Other isomers of benzene hexachloride DDT*	3% 4.5% 5%
MATHIESON 3-5-40 COTTON DUST Insecticide (Olin Mathieson)	Gamma isomer of benzene hexachloride* Other isomers of benzene hexachloride DDT* Sulfur*	3% 4.5% 5% 40%

Name & Use Manufacturer	Ingredients	
MATHIESON 3-10-40 COTTON DUST Fungicide (Olin Mathieson)	Gamma isomer of benzene hexachloride* Other isomers of benzene hexachloride DDT* Sulfur*	3.00% 4.50% 10.00% 40.00%
MATHIESON 50-50 COTTON DUST Insecticide (Olin Mathieson)	Tricalcium arsenate* Sulfur	35% 50%
MATHIESON CUCUMBER DUST NO. 113 Fungicide (Olin Mathieson)	Sodium fluoaluminate* Copper as metallic (from tribasic copper sulfate) Nicotine alkaloids*	33.00% 6.00% 1.25%
MATHIESON CUCUMBER DUST NO. 102 Insecticide, fungicide (Olin Mathieson)	Sodium fluoaluminate* Copper as metallic	33% 6%
MATHIESON 3% DDT-7% COPPER POTATO DUST Insecticide, fungicide (Olin Mathieson)	DDT Copper as metallic (from tribasic copper sulfate)*	3% 7%
MATHIESON DDT 5% DUST Insecticide (Olin Mathieson)	Dichloro diphenyl trichloroethane*	5.00%
MATHIESON DDT 10% DUST Insecticide (Olin Mathieson)	DDT*	10%
MATHIESON DDT 25% EMULSIFI- ABLE CONC. Insecticide (Olin Mathieson)	DDT Methylated aromatic petroleum deriv.*	25% 70%
MATHIESON DDT 10%- SULPHUR 75% Insecticide (Olin Mathieson)	DDT* Sulfur (93% through 325 mesh)*	10% 75%
MATHIESON DDT-SULPHUR PEANUT DUST Insecticide, fungicide (Olin Mathieson)	Sulfur* (95% through 325-mesh screen) DDT*	83% 5%

*Consult Sec. II., Ingredients Index. This ingredient may be responsible for major toxic effects if poisonous amounts of this product are ingested.

- 673 -

Name & Use Manufacturer	Ingredients		Name & Use Manufacturer	Ingredients	
MATHIESON DDT 50% WETTABLE POWDER Insecticide (Olin Mathieson)	DDT*	50%	MATHIESON DIELDRIN 2-1/2% - DDT 5% - SULPHUR 40% DUST Insecticide (Olin Mathieson)	Hexachloro epoxy octahydro dimethano naphthalene* Related compounds DDT* Sulfur*	2.125% 0.375% 5.000% 40.000%
MATHIESON DDT 75% WETTABLE POWDER Insecticide (Olin Mathieson)	DDT*	75%	MATHIESON DIELDRIN 2-1/2% - DDT 10% - SULPHUR 40% DUST Insecticide (Olin Mathieson)	Hexachloro epoxy octahydro dimethano naphthalene* Related compounds DDT* Sulfur*(93% through 325 mesh)	2.125% 0.375% 10.000% 40.000%
MATHIESON DDT 5% - ZINEB 3.9% DUST Insecticide, fungicide (Olin Mathieson)	DDT* Zineb (zinc ethylene bis- (dithiocarbamate); 0.92% total zinc as metallic)	5.0% 3.9%	MATHIESON DIELDRIN 1-1/2% DUST Insecticide (Olin Mathieson)	Hexachloro epoxy octahydro dimethano naphthalene* Related compounds	1.275% 0.225%
MATHIESON DIELDRIN 1-1/2% - DDT 5% DUST Insecticide (Olin Mathieson)	Hexachloro epoxy octahydro dimethano naphthalene* Related compounds DDT*	1.275% 0.225% 5.000%	MATHIESON DIELDRIN 2% DUST Insecticide (Olin Mathieson)	Hexachloro epoxy octahydro- endo, exo-dimethano naphthalene* Related compounds	1.7% 0.3%
MATHIESON DIELDRIN 1-1/2% - DDT 10% DUST Insecticide (Olin Mathieson)	Hexachloro epoxy octahydro dimethano naphthalene* Related compounds DDT*	1.275% 0.225% 10.000%	MATHIESON DIELDRIN 2-1/2% DUST Insecticide (Olin Mathieson)	Hexachloro epoxy octahydro dimethano naphthalene* Related compounds	2.125% 0.375%
MATHIESON DIELDRIN 2-1/2% - DDT 5% DUST Insecticide (Olin Mathieson)	Hexachloro epoxy octahydro dimethano naphthalene* Related compounds DDT*	2.125% 0.375% 5.000%	MATHIESON DIELDRIN 5% GRANULES Insecticide (Olin Mathieson)	Hexachloro epoxy octahydro- endo, exo-dimethano naphthalene* Related compounds	4.3% 0.7%
MATHIESON DIELDRIN 2-1/2% - DDT 10% DUST Insecticide (Olin Mathieson)	Hexachloro epoxy octahydro dimethano naphthalene* Related compounds DDT*	2.125% 0.375% 10.000%	MATHIESON DIELDRIN 10% GRANULES Insecticides (Olin Mathieson)	Hexachloro epoxy octahydro- endo, exo-dimethano naphthalene* Related compounds	8.5% 1.5%
MATHIESON DIELDRIN 1-1/2% - DDT 5% - SULPHUR 40% DUST (Olin Mathieson)	Hexachloro epoxy octahydro dimethano naphthalene* Related compounds DDT* Sulfur*(93% through 325 mesh)	1.275% 0.225% 5.000% 53.500%	MATHIESON DIELDRIN 1.5 LB. EMULSIFI- ABLE CONC. Insecticide (Olin Mathieson)	Hexachloro epoxy octahydro dimethano naphthalene* Related compounds Methylated aromatic petroleum deriv.*	15.16% 2.68% 77.16%
MATHIESON DIELDRIN 1-1/2% - DDT 10% - SULPHUR 40% DUST Insecticide (Olin Mathieson)	Hexachloro epoxy octahydro dimethano naphthalene* Related compounds DDT* Sulfur*(93% through 325 mesh)	1.275% 0.225% 10.000% 40.000%	MATHIESON DIELDRIN 1-1/2% - SULPHUR 40% DUST Insecticide (Olin Mathieson)	Hexachloro epoxy octahydro dimethano naphthalene* Related compounds Sulfur*(93% through 325 mesh)	1.275% 0.225% 40.000%
			MATHIESON DIELDRIN 2-1/2% - SULPHUR 40% DUST Insecticide (Olin Mathieson)	Hexachloro epoxy octahydro dimethano naphthalene* Related compounds Sulfur*(93% through 325 mesh)	2.125% 0.375% 40.000%

Name & Use Manufacturer	Ingredients	
MATHIESON ENDRIN 1.5% DUST Insecticide (Olin Mathieson)	Endrin (hexachloro epoxy octahydro-endo, endo-dimethano naphthalene)*	1.5%
MATHIESON ENDRIN 2% DUST Insecticide (Olin Mathieson)	Endrin (hexachloro epoxy octahydro-endo, endo-dimethano naphthalene)*	2%
MATHIESON ENDRIN 1.6 LB. EMULSIFI-ABLE CONC. Insecticide (Olin Mathieson)	Endrin (hexachloro epoxy octahydro-endo, endo-dimethano naphthalene)* Methylated aromatic petroleum deriv.*	18.48% 75.52%
MATHIESON ENDRIN 1-1/2%-SULPHUR 40% DUST Insecticide (Olin Mathieson)	Endrin (hexachloro epoxy octahydro-endo, endo-dimethano naphthalene)* Sulfur*(93% through 325 mesh)	1.5% 40.0%
MATHIESON ENDRIN 2%-SULPHUR 40% DUST Insecticide (Olin Mathieson)	Endrin (hexachloro epoxy octahydro-endo, endo-dimethano naphthalene)* Sulfur*(93% through 325 mesh)	2% 40%
MATHIESON FERBAM 76% Fungicide (Olin Mathieson)	Ferbam (ferric dimethyl dithiocarbamate)*	76%
MATHIESON FERBAM-DDT DUST Insecticide, fungicide (Olin Mathieson)	Ferbam (ferric dimethyl dithiocarbamate) DDT	11.40% 3.00%
MATHIESON FUNGICIDAL SULPHUR WETTABLE (Olin Mathieson)	Sulfur*	95%
MATHIESON GARDEN DUST Insecticide, fungicide (Olin Mathieson)	Piperonyl cyclonene tech. Pyrethrins Rotenone Other cube extractives Copper as metallic (from tri basic copper sulfate)*	0.50% 0.05% 0.25% 0.50% 5.00%
MATHIESON HEPTACHLOR 2-1/2%-DDT 5% DUST Insecticide (Olin Mathieson)	Heptachlor* Related compounds DDT*	2.50% 0.97% 5.00%

Name & Use Manufacturer	Ingredients	
MATHIESON HEPTACHLOR 2-1/2%-DDT 10% DUST Insecticide (Olin Mathieson)	Heptachlor* Related compounds DDT*	2.50% 0.97% 10.00%
MATHIESON HEPTACHLOR 2-1/2% DDT 5%-SULPHUR 40% DUST Insecticide (Olin Mathieson)	Heptachlor* Related compounds DDT* Sulfur*(93% through 325 mesh)	2.50% 0.97% 5.00% 40.00%
MATHIESON HEPTACHLOR 2-1/2%-DDT 10%-SULPHUR 40% DUST Insecticide (Olin Mathieson)	Heptachlor * Related compounds DDT* Sulfur*(93% through 325 mesh)	2.50% 0.97% 10.00% 40.00%
MATHIESON HEPTACHLOR 2-1/2% DUST Insecticide (Olin Mathieson)	Heptachlor* Related compounds	2.50% 0.97%
MATHIESON HEPTACHLOR 5% GRANULES Insecticide (Olin Mathieson)	Heptachlor* Related compounds	5.00% 1.95%
MATHIESON HEPTACHLOR 2 LB. EMULSIFI-ABLE CONC. Insecticide (Olin Mathieson)	Heptachlor* Related compounds Methylated aromatic petroleum deriv.*	22.2% 10.9% 62.4%
MATHIESON HEPTACHLOR 2-1/2%-SULPHUR 40% DUST Insecticide (Olin Mathieson)	Heptachlor* Related compounds Sulfur*(93% through 325 mesh)	2.50% 0.97% 40.00%
MATHIESON HEPTACHLOR 25% WET-TABLE POWDER Insecticide (Olin Mathieson)	Heptachlor* Related compounds	25.00% 9.72%
MATHIESON HTH-15 Rodenticide (Olin Mathieson)	Available chlorine*	15%
MATHIESON ISOPROPYL ESTER D334 WEED KILLER (Olin Mathieson)	Isopropyl ester of 2, 4-dichlorophenoxyacetic acid*	44%

*Consult Sec. II., Ingredients Index. This ingredient may be responsible for major toxic effects if poisonous amounts of this product are ingested.

Name & Use Manufacturer	Ingredients	Name & Use Manufacturer	Ingredients
MATHIESON LINDANE CUCUMBER & MELON DUST Insecticide, fungicide (Olin Mathieson)	Gamma isomer of benzene hexachloride (from lindane) 1.5% Copper*as metallic (from tri-basic copper sulfate) 5.0%	MATHIESON MALATHION 50% EMULSI-FIABLE CONC. Insecticide (Olin Mathieson)	Malathion* 50% Methylated aromatic petroleum deriv.* 45%
MATHIESON LINDANE 1% DUST COMPOSITION Insecticide (Olin Mathieson)	Gamma isomer of benzene hexachloride (from lindane) 1%	MATHIESON MALATHION 5 LB. EMULSIFI-ABLE CONC. Insecticide (Olin Mathieson)	Malathion* 55% Methylated aromatic petroleum deriv.* 39%
MATHIESON LINDANE 1.5% DUST COMPOSITION Insecticide (Olin Mathieson)	Gamma isomer of benzene hexachloride (from lindane) 1.5%	MATHIESON MALATHION 25% WET-TABLE POWDER Insecticide (Olin Mathieson)	Malathion* 25%
MATHIESON LINDANE 20% EMULSIFI-ABLE CONC. Insecticide (Olin Mathieson)	Gamma isomer of benzene hexachloride (from lindane)* 20.0% Methylated aromatic petroleum deriv.* 32.5%	MATHIESON MC1 GRAIN FUMIGANT (Olin Mathieson)	Ethylene dichloride* 70.2% Carbon tetrachloride* 29.8%
MATHIESON LOBAX SPECIAL Chlorine sanitizing agent (Olin Mathieson)	Calcium hypochlorite* 50%	MATHIESON MC3 GRAIN STORAGE FUMIGANT (Olin Mathieson)	Ethylene dichloride* 65% Carbon tetrachloride* 27% Ethylene dibromide 5% Sulfur dioxide 3%
MATHIESON LV ESTER 22 BRUSH KILLER (Low Volatile) Herbicide (Olin Mathieson)	Butoxy ethoxy propanol ester of 2, 4-dichloro phenoxy acetic acid* 37.8% Butoxy ethoxy propanol ester of 2, 4, 5-trichloro phenoxy acetic acid* 35.6%	MATHIESON MC5 GRAIN FUMIGANT (Olin Mathieson)	Ethylene dibromide* 8% Ethylene dichloride* 65% Carbon tetrachloride* 27%
MATHIESON LV ESTER D4 WEED KILLER (Low Volatile) (Olin Mathieson)	Butoxy ethoxy propanol ester of 2, 4-dichloro phenoxy acetic acid* 76%	MATHIESON MELON & CUCUMBER DUST 123 Insecticide, fungicide (Olin Mathieson)	Bis (methoxyphenyl) trichloroethane 3.5% Copper as metallic (from tri-basic copper sulfate)* 5.0%
MATHIESON LV ESTER T4 BRUSH KILLER (Low Volatile) Herbicide (Olin Mathieson)	Butoxy ethoxy propanol ester of 2, 4, 5-trichloro phenoxy acetic acid* 70.6%	MATHIESON MELON DUST 116 Insecticide (Olin Mathieson)	Sodium fluoaluminate* 33.00% Copper as metallic 6.00%
MATHIESON MALATHION 4% DUST Insecticide (Olin Mathieson)	Malathion* 4%	MATHIESON MILL MACHINERY FUMIGANT (Olin Mathieson)	Ethylene dibromide* 20.4% Ethylene dichloride* 19.6% Carbon tetrachloride* 60%
		MATHIESON NICOTINE 3% DUST Insecticide (Olin Mathieson)	Nicotine alkaloid* 3.00%

*Consult Sec. II., Ingredients Index. This ingredient may be responsible for major toxic effects if poisonous amounts of this product are ingested.

- 676 -

Name & Use Manufacturer	Ingredients	
MATHIESON OMAZENE 50% W.P. Fungicide (Olin Mathieson)	Copper dihydrazinium sulfate*	50%
MATHIESON PARATHION 1% - COPPER 5.3% DUST Insecticide, fungicide (Olin Mathieson)	Parathion* Copper (in basic copper sulfate) expressed as metallic	1.0% 5.3%
MATHIESON PARATHION 1% - DDT 10% DUST Insecticide (Olin Mathieson)	Parathion* DDT	1.0% 10.0%
MATHIESON PARATHION 2% - DDT 5% Insecticide (Olin Mathieson)	Parathion* DDT	2.0% 5.0%
MATHIESON PARATHION 1% DUST COMPOSITION Insecticide (Olin Mathieson)	Parathion*	1%
MATHIESON PARATHION 2% DUST Insecticide (Olin Mathieson)	Parathion*	2%
MATHIESON PARATHION 2 LB. EMULSIFI-ABLE CONC. Insecticide (Olin Mathieson)	Parathion* Methylated aromatic petroleum deriv.	24.25% 72.75%
MATHIESON PARATHION 1% - SULPHUR 40% DUST Insecticide (Olin Mathieson)	Parathion* Sulfur	1% 40%
MATHIESON PARATHION 2% - SULPHUR 40% DUST Insecticide, fungicide (Olin Mathieson)	Parathion* Sulfur	2% 40%
MATHIESON PARATHION 15% WET-TABLE POWDER Insecticide (Olin Mathieson)	Parathion*	15%

Name & Use Manufacturer	Ingredients	
MATHIESON PARATHION 1% - ZINEB 3.9% DUST Insecticide, fungicide (Olin Mathieson)	Parathion* Zineb (zinc ethylene-bis(dithiocarbamate); total zinc as metallic	1.0% 0.92% 3.9%
MATHIESON PCP 9.5% EMULSIFI-ABLE CONC. Herbicide (Olin Mathieson)	Pentachlorophenol* Aromatic petroleum deriv. solvent*	9.50% 88.50%
MATHIESON PEANUT DUST Insecticide, fungicide (Olin Mathieson)	Copper* as metallic Sulfur*	4% 89%
MATHIESON 5-7 POTATO & TOMATO DUST Insecticide, fungicide (Olin Mathieson)	DDT* Copper as metallic (from tribasic copper sulfate) *	5% 7%
MATHIESON 5% RHOTHANE (TDE) DUST Insecticide (Olin Mathieson)	Dichloro diphenyl dichloroethane	5%
MATHIESON ROTENONE 3/4% DUST Insecticide (Olin Mathieson)	Rotenone Other cube resins	0.75% 1.50%
MATHIESON ROTENONE 1% DUST Insecticide (Olin Mathieson)	Rotenone Other cube resins	1% 2%
MATHIESON ROTENONE 5% WET-TABLE POWDER Insecticide (Olin Mathieson)	Rotenone* Other cube resins	5% 8%
MATHIESON TDE (DDD) 3% DUST Insecticide (Olin Mathieson)	DDD	3.00%
MATHIESON TDE (DDD) 5% DUST Insecticide (Olin Mathieson)	Dichloro diphenyl dichloroethane	5.00%

---

*Consult Sec. II., Ingredients Index. This ingredient may be responsible for major toxic effects if poisonous amounts of this product are ingested.

- 677 -

Name & Use Manufacturer	Ingredients	
MATHIESON TDE (DDD) 10% DUST Insecticide (Olin Mathieson)	Dichloro diphenyl dichloroethane*	10%
MATHIESON TDE (DDD) 25% EMULSI-FIABLE CONC. Insecticide (Olin Mathieson)	Dichloro diphenyl dichloroethane Aromatic petroleum deriv. solvent*	25.0% 72.0%
MATHIESON TDE (DDD) 5% - SULPHUR 50% DUST Insecticide (Olin Mathieson)	Dichloro diphenyl dichloroethane* Sulfur*(93% through 325 mesh)	5% 50%
MATHIESON TDE (DDD) 50% WET-TABLE POWDER Insecticide (Olin Mathieson)	Dichloro diphenyl dichloroethane*	50%
MATHIESON TDE (DDD) 5% - ZINEB 3.9% TOMATO DUST Insecticide, fungicide (Olin Mathieson)	Dichloro diphenyl dichloroethane Zineb (zinc ethylene-bis(dithiocarbamate); total zinc as metallic 0.92%)	5.0% 3.9%
MATHIESON TEPP-40 Insecticide (Olin Mathieson)	Tetraethyl pyrophosphate* Other related organic phosphates	40% 60%
MATHIESON TERRACLOR 75% W.P. Fungicide (Olin Mathieson)	Pentachloronitrobenzene*	75%
MATHIESON TOBACCO DUST: 10% RHOTHANE (TDE)-1% PARATHION (Olin Mathieson)	Dichloro diphenyl dichloroethane Parathion*	10% 1%
MATHIESON TOXAPHENE-DDT EMULSIFI-ABLE CONC. Insecticide (Olin Mathieson)	Toxaphene* DDT Xylene *	40.70% 20.35% 34.95%
MATHIESON TOXAPHENE 40% DUST BASE Insecticide (Olin Mathieson)	Chlorinated camphene*	40%

Name & Use Manufacturer	Ingredients	
MATHIESON TOXAPHENE 6 LB. EMULSIFI-ABLE CONC. Insecticide (Olin Mathieson)	Toxaphene* (tech. chlorinated camphene; chlorine content 67-69%) Petroleum distillates	60.40% 37.85%
MATHIESON TOXAPHENE-SULPHUR DUST Insecticide (Olin Mathieson)	Toxaphene* Sulfur	20% 40%
MATHIESON TOXAPHENE 40% WET-TABLE POWDER Insecticide (Olin Mathieson)	Toxaphene* (tech. chlorinated camphene; chlorine content 67-69%)	40%
MATHIESON VEGETABLE DUST NO. 82X Fungicide (Olin Mathieson)	Copper (from tribasic copper sulfate) Sodium fluoaluminate*	7.00% 42.00%
MATHIESON ZINEB 3.9% DUST Fungicide (Olin Mathieson)	Zineb (zinc ethylene-bis(dithiocarbamate); total zinc as metallic 0.92%)	3.9%
MA-TONE For malaria (Oliver's S-O)	Quinine sulfate* Iron sulfate Potassium nitrate*	
MATRILIN TABLETS (New England Pharm.)	Magnesium trisilicate Dried aluminum hydroxide Collodial kaolin	4 gr. 2 gr. 2 gr.
MATSA For skin irritations (Whitney)	Mercury ammoniated* Mercury salicylate* Resorcin Coal tar solution N.F.	4% 4%
MATTHEW'S AIR FRESHENER, SUNTAN SPRAY, DEODORANT SPRAY (Matthew)		
MAURRY'S FUNGICIDE Skin fungicide (medical) (Maurry)	4-Nitro anhydrohydroxy mercuri orthocresol* Coal tar U.S.P.* Quillaja N.F. Benzoin U.S.P. Certified F.D.C. dye Isopropyl alcohol*	2.22 gm. 0.74 gm. 2.96 gm. q.s. 80-85%
MAX FACTOR FACE CREAM (Factor)	Mineral oil Beeswax Borax Perfume	about 1%

*Consult Sec. II., Ingredients Index. This ingredient may be responsible for major toxic effects if poisonous amounts of this product are ingested.

- 678 -

Name & Use Manufacturer	Ingredients		Name & Use Manufacturer	Ingredients	
MAX FACTOR FACE POWDER (Factor)	Talc Kaolin Zinc stearate Zinc oxide Magnesium carbonate Colors (iron oxides, organic lakes) Perfume		MAXWELL ROSE DUST Insecticide (Maxwell)	Ferric dimethyl dithio- carbamate DDT* Sulfur*	7.60% 5.00% 70.00%
MAX FACTOR HAND LOTION (Factor)	Triethanolamine 1% Stearic acid Lanolin Isopropyl palmitate Quince-seed mucilage Perfume		MAXWELL 1% ROTENONE DUST Insecticide (Maxwell)	Rotenone Sulfur	1.00% 15.00%
			MAXWELL 20% SABADILLA DUST Insecticide (Maxwell)	Sabadilla alkaloids	0.80%
MAX FACTOR LIPSTICK (Factor)	Castor oil (preserved with small trace of ditertiarybutyl hydroquinone) Lanolin Carnauba wax Mineral oil Hydrocarbon waxes Color (lakes) Indelible colors Candelilla wax Perfume		MAXWELL 10% TDE DUST Insecticide (Maxwell)	DDD	10.00%
			MAXWELL 20% TOXAPHENE DUST Insecticide (Maxwell)	Toxaphene*	20.00%
MAXINE TOILET SOAP (Swift)	Neutral tallow and coconut oil soap Titanium dioxide Perfume oil		MAYA Insect repellent (McKesson)	Dimethyl carbobutoxy dihydro pyrone* Dimethyl phthalate Oil of cedarleaf	40.0% 58.5% 1.5%
MAXWELL 5% COPPER DUST Insecticide (Maxwell)	Copper* as metallic 5.00%		MAYBELLINE EYEBROW PENCIL (Maybelline Co.)		
MAXWELL 3-5-0 COTTON DUST Insecticide (Maxwell)	Gamma isomer of BHC *3.00% DDT* 5.00%		MAYBELLINE MASCARA (Maybelline Co.)		
MAXWELL 70-30 CRYOLITE DUST Insecticide (Maxwell)	Sodium fluoaluminate* 63.00%		MAYER'S OINTMENT For skin irritations (Lloyd)	Vegetable oils Turpentine* Red lead* Camphor* Beeswax	
MAXWELL M5 5% DDT DUST Insecticide (Maxwell)	DDT* 5.00 %		MAYNARD BEAUTIFUL LADY HAND CREAM (Maynard)	Glycerin Mineral oil Olive oil Stearic acid Glyceryl monostearate Perfume Color (certified food)	
MAXWELL 10% DITHANE DUST Insecticide (Maxwell)	Zinc ethylene-bis(dithio- carbamate) 6.50%		MAYOR'S HAIR DYE (Mayor Co.)		
MAXWELL 15% FERMATE DUST Insecticide (Maxwell)	Ferric dimethyl dithio- carbamate 11.40%		MAYPINKS Carminative, antacid (Maypinks)	Po. extract cascara Zinc valerinate Soda bicarbonate Calcined magnesia Papaya Oil of peppermint	
MAXWELL 1% PARATHION DUST Insecticide (Maxwell)	Parathion* 1.00%		MAYR'S Laxative (Berosol)	Cottonseed oil Saccharin Oil of anise Epsom salts Licorice powder Ginger Sodium phosphate U.S.P.	
MAXWELL 10% PARZATE DUST Insecticide (Maxwell)	Zinc ethylene-bis(dithio- carbamate) 6.50%		MAZON OINTMENT (Belmont)		

*Consult Sec. II., Ingredients Index. This ingredient may be responsible for major toxic effects if poisonous amounts of this product are ingested.

Name & Use Manufacturer	Ingredients		Name & Use Manufacturer	Ingredients	
M B A DOUCHE POWDER (APCO)	Magnesium sulfate Boric acid* Alum Menthol* Thymol* Methyl salicylate* Citric acid (sufficient to adjust pH to 3.5)		McCLELLAN'S EYELID OINTMENT Veterinary (McClellan)	Yellow oxide of mercury* Petroleum base*	1.0%
M.B. READY MIXED PAINT (Eagle P. & V.)			McCLELLAN'S FLEA KILLER (McClellan)	Sulfur DDT Beta beta' dithiocyano diethyl ether Nicotine* expressed as alkaloid	20.0% 5.0% 0.6% 0.1%
McCAMBRIDGE BLUE OINTMENT (McCambridge)	Mercury* (elemental) Petrolatum Beeswax		McCLELLAN'S FLEA POWDER WITH PYRETHRIN (McClellan)	Sulfur* Pyrethrins	35.00% 0.24%
McCLELLAN'S ANT POWDER (McClellan)	Sodium fluoride* Pyrethrins	65.00% 0.22%	McCLELLAN'S FLEA POWDER WITH ROTENONE (McClellan)	Cube resins Rotenone*	4% 2%
McCLELLAN'S ANT SPRAY (McClellan)	Tech. chlordane	2.5%			
McCLELLAN'S CHLORDANE SPRAY Insecticide (McClellan)	Petroleum distillate* Tech. chlordane* Pine oil Tech. piperonyl butoxide Pyrethrins	56.0% 25.0% 5.0% 1.8% 12.0%	McCLELLAN'S FLY-FITE Insecticide (McClellan)	Petroleum distillate* B-thiocyano ethyl esters of mixed fatty acids averaging 10-18 carbon atoms B-butoxy B' thiocyano diethyl ether	96.00% 3.00% 1.00%
McCLELLAN'S COMPOUND LICE POWDER (McClellan)	Sulfur DDT Sodium fluoride Cresylic acid Nicotine* expressed as alkaloid	51.5% 5.0% 4.5% 1.5% 0.1%	McCLELLAN'S FLY-FITE WITH 5% DDT Insecticide (McClellan)	Lethane* DDT*	3% 5%
McCLELLAN'S DE-DUS-TREX NO. 5 LIQUID BARN SPRAY Insecticide (McClellan)	Petroleum distillate* DDT* B-thiocyano ethyl esters of mixed fatty acids averaging 10-18 carbon atoms B-butoxy B' thiocyano diethyl ether	92.36% 5.00% 1.99% 0.65%	McCLELLAN'S FUMIGATOR (McClellan)	Formaldehyde*	37%
			McCLELLAN'S INHALANT Respiratory decongestant (veterinary, avian) (McClellan)	Mineral oil Pine oil* Oil of camphor* Oil of eucalyptus Menthol* Thymol*	
McCLELLAN'S DE-DUS-TREX NO. 50 Insecticide (McClellan)	DDT*, wettable	50%	McCLELLAN'S KILS-A-WEEVIL Insecticide (McClellan)	Petroleum distillate Carbon tetrachloride* B-thiocyano ethyl esters of mixed fatty acids averaging 10-18 carbon atoms B-butoxy B' thiocyano diethyl ether	75.70% 20.00% 3.25% 1.05%
McCLELLAN'S DISINFECT-ANT DIP Insecticide (McClellan)	Coal tar neutral oil* Anhydrous soap Cresylic acid*	57% 17% 16%			
McCLELLAN'S DOG SHAMPOO (McClellan)	Soap		McCLELLAN'S KREOSOL DISINFECT-ANT DIP Veterinary (McClellan)	Coal tar neutral oil* Anhydrous soap Cresylic acid*	57% 17% 16%
McCLELLAN'S D-T TABLETS Disinfectant, poultry drink-ing water (McClellan)	Potassium permanganate* 3 gr.		McCLELLAN'S LIN-SMEAR Ectoparasiti-cide, insecticide (McClellan)	Gamma isomer of benzene hexachloride (from lindane)* Pine oil	3% 35%
McCLELLAN'S R-O TABLETS Disinfectant, poultry drink-ing water (McClellan)	Potassium permanganate* 3 gr.		McCLELLAN'S LIQUID I. C. SULFA For poultry drinking water (McClellan)	Each 100 cc.: Sulfathiazole sodium* Sodium sulfate	12.5 gm.

Name & Use Manufacturer	Ingredients	
McCLELLAN'S MOTH FATE BLOCK Insecticide (McClellan)	Paradichlorobenzene*	99%
McCELLAN'S NICOTINE SULPHATE SOLUTION Insecticide (McCellan)	Nicotine (as alkaloid)*	40%
McCLELLAN'S O-X-ZEL Disinfectant, deodorizer, cleanser (McClellan)	Cresylic acid* Anhydrous soap	50% 25%
McCLELLAN'S PINK EYE POWDER Veterinary (McClellan)	Sulfanilamide U.S.P.* Sulfathiazole U.S.P.* Boric acid U.S.P.* Phenacaine hydrochloride N.F.	77% 20% 2% 1%
McCLELLAN'S POCCO POWDER For internal infections (veterinary, avian) (McClellan)	Sulfanilamide* (with sodium citrate) Sulfur Powdered anise Calcium carbonate	20%
McCLELLAN'S POULTRY HOUSE SPRAY Insecticide (McClellan)	Coal tar creosote* Cresylic acid	92% 5%
McCLELLAN'S RAT DEATH LIQUID (McClellan)	Sodium arsenite*	5%
McCLELLAN'S RAT-WAR (McClellan)	Warfarin	0.5%
McCLELLAN'S RED MITE & LICE KILLER (McClellan)	Petroleum distillate Coal tar oils Cresylic acid Nicotine*expressed as alkaloid*	44.44% 43.94% 5.49% 5.71%
McCLELLAN'S REX LIQUID SPECIAL Disinfectant, poultry drink- ing water (McClellan)	Diisobutyl phenoxy ethoxy ethyl dimethyl benzyl ammonium chloride*	1.25%
McCLELLAN'S ROACH POWDER (McClellan)	Sodium fluoride* Pyrethrins	58.00% 0.22%
McCLELLAN'S ROOST PAINT Insecticide (McClellan)	Coal tar neutral oil Nicotine* expressed as alkaloid Pyridine	20.0% 10.0% 7.5%
McCLELLAN'S SCREW- WORM KILLER Insecticide (McClellan)	Benzol* Pine oil Petroleum distillate Sulfonated castor oil Diphenylamine	25% 23% 23% 18% 2%

Name & Use Manufacturer	Ingredients	
McCLELLAN'S SHEEP DIP (McClellan)	Cresylic acid* Coal tar neutral oil*	16% 57%
McCLELLAN'S SODIUM FLUORIDE (McClellan)	Sodium fluoride*	95.00%
McCLELLAN'S STOCK COMPOUND Veterinary (McClellan)	Calcium Phosphorus Sodium Iron Vitamin A Vitamin D Copper Cobalt Iodine Manganese Zinc Magnesium Thiamine hydrochloride Riboflavin Niacin Pyridozine hydrochloride Calcium pantothenate	99 gm. 20 gm. 120 gm. 300 mg. 35,000 units 2,250 units 20 mg. 2 mg. 2 mg. 20 mg. 22 mg. 20 mg. 25 mg. 40 mg. 130 mg. 3 mg. 40 mg.
McCLELLAN'S STOCK FLY KILL (McClellan)	Petroleum distillate* Pine oil B-butoxy B' thiocyano diethyl ether Naphthalene*	90.18% 4.00% 3.82% 2.00%
McCLELLAN'S SULFA SKOUR For intestinal irritation (veterinary) (McClellan)	Sulfaguanidine U.S.P. Ginger Lactose	
McCLELLAN'S SUL-NOX- AQUINE For coccidiosis (veterinary, avian) (McClellan)	Sulfaquinoxaline sodium 3.44 gm./100 cc.	
McCLELLAN'S SULZO POWDER For wounds (veterinary) (McClellan)	Sulfanilamide Sulfathiazole Zinc oxide Bentonite Pyrophyllite	3% 2%
McCLELLAN'S TABLETS Disinfectant (poultry use) (McClellan)	Potassium permanganate* 3 gr. Montimorillonite, ferrous sulfate, and potassium dichromate* 12 gr.	
McCLELLAN'S TOE PICK For poultry (McClellan)	Pine tar Pine oil Pyridine Oil of citronella Petroleum jelly Coloring	
McCLELLAN'S UDDER BALM For udder irritation (veterinary) (McClellan)	Lanolin Petroleum jelly Turpentine Phenol	
McCLELLAN'S WHITE UDDER CREAM Veterinary (McClellan)	Allyl isothiocyanate* Orthophenylphenol sodium* Zinc oxide Sulfonated castor oil	

*Consult Sec. II., Ingredients Index. This ingredient may be responsible for major toxic effects if poisonous amounts of this product are ingested.

Name & Use Manufacturer	Ingredients		Name & Use Manufacturer	Ingredients	
McCORMICK FOG IN-SEKTOSPRAY Insecticide (McCormick)	Pyrethrins Piperonyl butoxide tech. Petroleum distillate*	0.60% 0.12% 99.28%	McKESSON'S COLD SORE LOTION (McKesson)	Ethyl alcohol* Benzyl alcohol* t-Amyl phenol* s-Octyl phenol* n-Heptyl phenol* Camphor* Synthetic gum benzoin Benzoic acid Methyl salicylate*	70%/v 5%/v
McCORMICK IRON GLUE (McCormick)					
McCORMICK LIVESTOCK & BARN SPRAY Insecticide (McCormick)	Pyrethrins Piperonyl butoxide tech. Polyoxyethlene sorbitol oleate-laurate Petroleum distillate*	1.15% 11.50% 14.90% 72.45%	McKESSON'S COPPER-IRON COMPOUND Food supplement (McKesson)	Each tablet: Copper Iron	 1/4 mg. 4 mg.
McCORMICK PYRETHROL INDUSTRIAL SPRAY Insecticide (McCormick)	Pyrethrins Tech. piperonyl butoxide Petroleum distillate*	0.29% 2.33% 97.38%	McKESSON'S COUGH SYRUP WITH WHITE PINE TAR (McKesson)	Ethyl alcohol Chloroform White pine bark Wild cherry bark Spikenard root Blood root Balm of Gilead buds Rectified oil of tar	5%/v 3.0 m./fl. oz.
McCORMICK PYRETHRUM-PIPERONYL BUTOXIDE EMULSION CONC. Insecticide (McCormick)	Pyrethrins Piperonyl butoxide tech. Polyoxyethylene sorbitol oleate-laurate Petroleum distillate*	1.15% 11.50% 14.90% 72.45%	McKESSON'S EFFER-VESCENT SODIUM PHOSPHATE U.S.P. Effervescent laxative (McKesson)		
McELROY'S LOTION Eye antiseptic (Assoc. Prod.)	Boric acid Sodium borate Sodium chloride Camphor Antipyrine	 0.4%	McKESSON'S ELIXIR OF CATNEP & FENNEL Carminative, antacid (McKesson)	Ethyl alcohol	18%/v
McKESSON'S ALBA-GAR PLAIN Laxitive (McKesson)	Mineral oil		McKESSON'S GLYCERIN SUPPOSITORIES For infants (McKesson)	Glycerin	95%
McKESSON'S ALBAGAR WITH PHENOL-PHTHALEIN Laxative (McKesson)	Each tsp.: Phenolphthalein Mineral oil	 3/4 gr.	McKESSON'S LIQUID CORN REMEDY (McKesson)	Pyroxylin Acetone* Salicylic acid* Castor oil	
McKESSON'S ANTIBIOTIC ZINC OXIDE OINTMENT For wounds (McKesson)	Zinc oxide Tyrothricin	 0.05%	McKESSON'S MAGNEX POWDER Antacid (McKesson)	Bismuth subcarbonate Precipitated calcium carbonate Sodium bicarbonate Colloidal kaolin Magnesium trisilicate Aromatic flavoring oils	
McKESSON'S BABY COUGH SYRUP Antitussive (McKesson)	Each fl. oz.: Ethyl alcohol Tolu balsam Euphorbia Cocillana Blood root Senega	 0.5%/v 1.5 gr. 9.6 gr. 15.3 gr. 2.0 gr. 5.75 gr.	McKESSON'S MAGNEX TABLETS Antacid (McKesson)	Aluminum hydroxide gel Magnesium trisilicate Kaolin Calcium carbonate Bismuth subcarbonate Oils of peppermint	
McKESSON'S BLAUD'S PILLS N.F. (McKesson)	Ferrous carbonate* 60 mg./pill		McKESSON'S NAVAP Inhalant (McKesson)	Ethyl alcohol* 4-Beta-ethyl hexyl phenol* Eucalyptol* Menthol* Thymol* Camphor* Aromatics	75%/v 0.63%
McKESSON'S CITRATED CARBONATES EFFER-VESCENT Antacid (McKesson)	Sodium bicarbonate Potassium bicarbonate Calcium lactate Sodium chloride Sodium phosphate Cream of tartar Magnesium sulfate Citric acid Tartaric acid				

*Consult Sec. II., Ingredients Index. This ingredient may be responsible for major toxic effects if poisonous amounts of this product are ingested.

Name & Use Manufacturer	Ingredients	
McKESSON'S NEO AQUA DRIN (McKesson)	Each lozenge: Tyrothricin Benzocaine	2 mg. 10 mg.
McKESSON'S OCTOFEN POWDER Skin fungicide (medical) (McKesson)	8-Hydroxyquinoline benzoate Aluminum phenolsulfonate	2.0% 1.0%
McKESSON'S POISON IVY CREAM (McKesson)	Zirconium oxide (carbonated hydrous zirconia) Benzocaine Pyrilamine maleate* Polyvinyl pyrolidone	4%
McKESSON'S RUBBING ALCOHOL COMPOUND (McKesson)	Alcohol	70%/v
McKESSON'S SEIDLITZ POWDERS N.F. Laxative (McKesson)		
McKESSON'S SODIUM FLUORIDE Insecticide (McKesson)	Sodium fluoride*	90.00%
McKESSON'S SOLUTION #59 Antiseptic mouthwash (McKesson)	Ethyl alcohol Eucalyptol * Eucalyptus oil * Menthol * Oil of thyme Methyl salicylate * Benzoic acid Boric acid *	25%/v
McKESSON'S SPECIAL BEXEL FORMULA Dietary food supplement (McKesson)	Each capsule: Ferrous sulfate*	200 mg.
McKESSON'S THROAT GARGLE (McKesson)	Each fl. oz.: Ethyl alcohol (4%/v) Carbolic acid Tannic acid Formaldehyde Glycerin	20 m. 0.05 gr.
MC MOTH & DEODORANT CRYSTALS Insecticide (Fuld)	Paradichlorobenzene*	
McQUADE'S VELVET CREAM Vanishing cream (McQuade Drug)		
M. C. QUALITY LACQUERS (Morris Paint)		
MC-3 CLEANSER (Pennsylv. Salt)	Polyphosphate* Soda ash* Sodium bicarbonate Alkyl aryl sulfonate *	

Name & Use Manufacturer	Ingredients	
M-D-C RECTAL OINTMENT For rectal irritations (Manhattan Drug)	Benzocaine Carbolic acid* Tar Camphor* Zinc oxide Eucalyptus * Sulfur Boric acid* Balsam Peru Menthol (not U.S.P.) *	1%
MEADOW SWEET PERFUME & TOILET WATER (Thornton, R.)		
MECCA COMPOUND OINTMENT For skin burns (Foster-Dack)	Olive oil Cottonseed oil Stearine Petrolatum Camphor* Carbolic acid* Boracic acid* Zinc oxide Sodium benzoate	
MECCALINE RECTAL OINTMENT (Foster-Dack)	Camphor* Carbolic acid* Menthol* Balsam capivi Turpentine* Boracic acid* Zinc oxide Olive oil Cotton seed oil Petrolatum Stearine Sodium benzoate	
MECCO CONCRETE MENDER (Curtis Mfg.)	Sand Cement	
MECCO FURNACE CEMENT (Curtis Mfg.)	Silicate of soda Pulverized silica Clay Asbestos fiber	
MECCO PATCHING PLASTER (Curtis Mfg.)	Plaster of Paris Whiting Clay Vegetable adhesive	
MECCO PIPE JOINT CEMENT (Curtis Mfg.)	Whiting Oil Clay	
MECCO PLASTIC FILLER (Curtis Mfg.)	Plaster Glue Whiting Color (yellow ochre) Adhesive	
MECCO SPATULING COMPOUND (Curtis Mfg.)	Plaster of Paris Whiting Clay Zinc sulfate Adhesives	approx. 3/4 of 1% approx. 3%
MECCO STOVE LINING (Curtis Mfg.)	Clay Silica sand Asbestos fiber Salt	approx. 1-1/2%
M.E.C. ECZEMA (Arend)		

*Consult Sec. II., Ingredients Index. This ingredient may be responsible for major toxic effects if poisonous amounts of this product are ingested.

Name & Use Manufacturer	Ingredients	Name & Use Manufacturer	Ingredients
MECHANO-KILL Insecticide (Slayer)	Gamma isomer of benzene hexachloride (from lindane)* 99%	MEDI-KOOL-PAK (veterinary) (Thoroughbred)	Camphor* Aluminum sulfate Spts. turpentine* Tannic acid Methyl salicylate* Boric acid* Eucalyptus oil * Myrbane oil Cedarleaf and tansy Menthol Tinct. of cantharides * Calcium acetate Tinct. arnica Ethyl aminobenzoate Peppermint oil Cedarwood oil Wormwood oil
M-E CLEANERS COFFEE URN, MIRA TEX PLASTIC, SHORT CUT SPARK (Maid-Easy)	Alkali* Phosphates Active oxygen Active synthetic detergent Carbonates Silicates		
MECOB LOZENGES WITH BENZOCAINE Antitussive (Halperin)	Each tablet: Benzocaine 1/1000 gr. Menthol 1/35 gr. Oil anise 1/40 m. Benzoic acid 1/12 gr. Eucalyptol 1/16 m. Sugar and diluent q.s.	MEDI-KOOL-TITENER Veterinary leg tightener (Thoroughbred)	Gum camphor* Methyl salicylate* Tannic acid* Spts. turpentine* Oil peppermint Oil myrbane Oil cedarleaf Oil eucalyptus * Menthol* Ethyl aminobenzoate Tinct. cantharides* Tinct. arnica Oil cedarwood Oil wormwood Oil tansy
M. E. C. RHEUMATIC (Arend)			
M. E. C. ROMAN COLD CREAM (Arend)			
M. E. C. STOMACH TABLETS (Arend)		MEDLIN Mildew control (Noble)	Trioxymethylene* (paraformaldehyde) Camphor*
MEDI-CALGON Detergent (Calgon)	Sodium hexametaphosphate*	MEDOSOL EXTRA LIGHT Herbicide (Shell Oil)	Petroleum emulsions
MEDICONE DRESSING Antiseptic skin cream (Medicone)	Benzocaine Cod liver oil Petrolatum Hydroxyquinoline* Zinc oxide Lanolin	MEI-LING TOILET WATER (Nissy)	Denatured alcohol* Essential oils *
MEDIGEN For the appetite (Naylor)	Nux vomica* (strychnine 1/2 gr./oz.) Gentian Colombo Cinchona Galangal	MEJORAL TABLETS Analgesic (Ross)	Aspirin* Caffeine
MEDIGUM (Medicated Chewing Gum) (Pharmaco)	Terpin hydrate* Propyl p-aminobenzoate Ammoniated glycyrrhizin Sugar Starch Chewing gum base	MELCALOSE TABLETS Cathartic (Whitehall)	Carboxy methyl cellulose
MEDI-KOFF Antitussive (Phenacedol)	Each fl. oz.: Ammonium chloride Ephedrine sulfate* 1 gr. Fldext. lobelia Tr. opium camphorated* 60 m. Chloroform 2 m. Syr. white pine comp. Sodium citrate Fldext. ipecac Fldext. hyoscyamus Mixture glycyrrhiza comp. Tar	MEL-LIC HANCE Antitussive (Hance)	Cocillana Euphorbia Horehound Squill Licorice Sanguinaria nitrate Menthol Honey with aromatics
		MELLO GLO BEAUTY CREAMS (Am. Ind.)	
		MELLO-GLO FACE POWDERS (Am. Ind.)	

*Consult Sec. II., Ingredients Index. This ingredient may be responsible for major toxic effects if poisonous amounts of this product are ingested.

Name & Use Manufacturer	Ingredients		Name & Use Manufacturer	Ingredients	
MELO-PAK Skin pack (Alberto-C.)	Dried milk Dried yeast Purified clay		MENDEN- HALL'S MALARIA TONIC WITH ARSENIC For chills and fever (Myers Labs.)	Alcohol Quinine sulfate* Fowler's solution of arsenic* U.S.P. Glycerin Licorice Yerba santa	1-1/2%
MEL-O-WAX Leather cleaner (Mel-O-Wax)	Carnauba wax Edible oils Triethanolamine				
MEL-PIX Antitussive (Wisconsin Pharm.)	Squill* Senega Honey Ammon. chloride Oil of tar Acid benzoic Camphor * Oil of anise Alcohol Tartar emetic * Caramel		MENDEN- HALL'S NUMBER 40 Cathartic (Myers Labs.)	Potassium iodide* Poke root Prickley ash Mandrake	
			MENDEN- HALL'S TONIC For malaria chill and fever (Myers Labs.)	Quinine sulfate U.S.P. Glycerin Licorice Yerba santa Alcohol	1-1/2%
MELSAN FUNGICIDE (du Pont)	Ethyl mercury phosphate* Sodium pentachlorophenate *		MENNEN BABY MAGIC Baby oil (Mennen)	Glyceryl monostearate Lanolin Hyamine 10X Glycerin D. & C. red #19 Perfume	
MELTONE Solvents (Am. Lacquer)					

MEMA
Disinfectant
(Chipman
  Chem.)
	Methoxy ethyl mercury
	  acetate* 11.4%
			MENNEN
			BABY MAGIC
			CREAM
			(Mennen)
				Glyceryl monostearate
				Glycerin
				Hyamine 10X
				Cetyl alcohol
				F. D. & C. red #4
				Mineral oil
				Perfume	

MEM BUBBLE BATH (Mem)	Detergents Perfume oil compounds Solvent (carbitol) *				
MEM COLOGNES FOR MEN (Mem)	Ethyl alcohol Perfume oil compounds		MENNEN BABY OIL (Mennen)	Lanolin Perfume Mineral oil	
MEM SHAVE & SHOWER Soap (Mem)			MENNEN BABY OIL (Unscented) (Mennen)	Lanolin Mineral oil	
MEM SHAVE'N' SHAMPOO, AFTER SHAVE, DEODORANT, COLOGNE, TALCUM STICKS (Mem)			MENNEN BABY POWDER (Mennen)	Magnesium stearate Perfume Talc	
			MENNEN BABY SOAP (Mennen)	Glycerin Boric acid Sodium, coconut and tallow soap Perfume	
MEM SHAVING CREAMS, BATH OIL, AFTER- SHAVE LOTION, DEODORANT (Mem)			MENNEN BATH TALC (With De- odorant) FOR MEN (Mennen)	Magnesium stearate Boric acid Perfume Talc	
			MENNEN BRUSHLESS CREAM (Mennen)	Stearic acid Potassium hydroxide Methyl parasept Glycerin Mineral oil Lanamine Perfume	
MENACAPS Analgesic for dysmenorrhea (Halperin)	Each capsule: Acetylsalicylic acid* 2-1/2 gr. Acetophenetidin* 1 gr. Caffeine citrate 1/2 gr. Ephedrine sulfate* 1/8 gr. Atropine sulfate 1/2000 gr. Lactose				
			MENNEN DEODORANT FOR MEN (Mennen)	Aluminum chloride Aluminum chlorhydroxide complex Propylene glycol Hyamine Alcohol SD #40 Perfume	
MENDACO Antitussive, antispasmodic (Knox)	Each tablet: Potassium iodide* 2-1/4 gr. Extract lobelia*				

*Consult Sec. II., Ingredients Index. This ingredient may be responsible for major toxic effects if poisonous amounts of this product are ingested.

Name & Use Manufacturer	Ingredients		Name & Use Manufacturer	Ingredients	
MENNEN FOAM SHAVE (Menthol Iced) (Mennen)	Coconut fatty acids Stearic acid Triethanolamine Glycerin Perfume Menthol		MENTHA RUB ANALGESIC BALM WITH LANOLIN (Commerce)	Lanolin Menthol* Methyl salicylate*	
MENNEN FOAM SHAVE (Regular) (Mennen)	Coconut fatty acids Stearic acid Triethanolamine Glycerin Perfume		MENTHOFAX Rubefacient (Burroughs-Wellcome)	Methyl salicylate* Menthol Eucalyptol Camphor Ointment base	40% 6% 3% 1%
MENNEN HAIR CREAM FOR MEN (Mennen)	Mineral oil Lanolin Menthol parasept Glycerin Stearic acid Oleic acid Triethanolamine Glyceryl monostearate D. & C. brown #1 Perfume		MENTHOLATUM Rubefacient, nasal, de-congestant (Mentholatum)	Menthol* Camphor* Boric acid* Petrolatum Oil sweet birch Oil pine * Oil eucalyptus*	
MENNEN LATHER SHAVE (Menthol Iced)	Glycerin Coconut oil Stearic acid Liquid caustic potash Liquid caustic soda Menthol Alcohol Perfume		MENTHOLIN Rubefacient (APCO)	Alcohol Methyl salicylate* Chloroform* Hard soap Camphor gum Menthol	35% 30% 20% 3% 2.2% 0.8%
MENNEN LATHER SHAVE (Plain) (Mennen)	Glycerin Coconut oil Stearic acid Liquid caustic potash Liquid caustic soda Perfume		MENTHO-TERPENOL Local analgesic (Tailby)	Chloroform* Menthol* Camphor* Capsicum Turpentine Aromatic oils Lubricating base	
MENNEN QUINSANA Skin fungicide (medical) (Mennen)	Hydroxyquinoline* Magnesium stearate Boric acid*		MENTO KANFO For skin irritations (Larkin)	Camphor* Boric acid* Oil of pine* White wax Menthol* Eucalyptol* Methyl salicylate* Petrolatum	
MENNEN SHAMPOO (Mennen)	Lanolin Hexachlorophene		MENTOS MEDICATED BEARD SOFTENER (Mentos)	Boric acid* Menthol* Benzocaine* Ammonium carbonate Peppermint Isopropyl alcohol	4%
MENNEN SKIN BALM (Mennen)	Boric acid Zinc stearate Menthol Alcohol Glycerin Perfume Tragacanth		MENTOS MEDICATED LANA-CREAM Emollient (Mentos)	Lanolin Boric acid* Benzyl benzoate* Menthyl-Paraben	
MENNEN SKIN BRACER (Mennen)	Alcohol Menthol Perfume Certified dyes (F. D. & C.)		MENTOS MEDICATED SHAMPOO (Mentos)	Boric acid* Sodium borax* Sodium carbonate Ammonium carbonate	
MENNEN SKIN MAGIC Hand lotion (Mennen)			MENTOS SCALP & SKIN MEDICINE (Mentos)	Sulfur Ammonium carbonate Sodium carbonate Boric acid* Sodium borax* Isopropyl alcohol	1-1/2%
MENNEN TALCUM FOR MEN (Mennen)	Boric acid Titanium dioxide Ochre Umber Perfume Talc		MEN-ZO-LIN Keratolytic (Men-Zo-Lin)	Salicylic acid*	
MENTHAGILL PROTECTIVE EMOLLIENT (Massengill)	Boric acid Glycerin Magnesium sulfate Sodium benzoate Menthol Tragacanth Aromatics		MEPHOSAL CAPSULES Antirheumatic, antispasmodic (Crookes)	Mephenesin* Sodium salicylate*	250 mg. 250 mg.

Name & Use Manufacturer	Ingredients		Name & Use Manufacturer	Ingredients
MEPHOSAL (Elixir) Antirheumatic (Crookes)	Each 4 cc.: Mephenesin* 400 mg. Sodium salicylate* 400 mg. Homatropine methylbromide 2.5 mg.		MERGAMMA C Seed treatment (Chipman Ltd.)	Gamma isomer of benzene hexachloride BHC (from lindane)* 40% Phenyl mercury acetate* 2.82% Total mercury equivalent 2%
MEPHOSAL TABLETS WITH HMB Antirheumatic (Crookes)	Mephenesin* 125 mg. Sodium salicylate* 125 mg. Homatropine methylbromide 1.25 mg.		MERITOL-METOL Photographic developer (General Photo.)	
MERBELS Antacid (Bell Labs.)	Bismuth subgallate Magnesium oxide Sodium bicarbonate Bismuth subcarbonate Magnesium carbonate		MERIX CHEMICAL AIR DRYER (Merix)	
MERCIREX (MERCY-REX) OINTMENT Emollient (Mercirex)	Mercury-zinc iodide* 0.1% Mercurous chloride 0.5% Acetanilid 0.6% Phenol* 0.4% Menthol* Zinc oxide		MERIX MILDEW-PROOFING COMPOUND (Merix)	
MERCK SODIUM FLUORIDE TINTED Insecticide (Merck)	Sodium fluoride* 95.00% Sodium silicofluoride 1.50%		MERKIN PAINT & ENAMEL (Merkin)	
MERCK STRYCHNINE Rodenticide (Merck)	Strychnine*		MER-KU-TOL (Davis Wholesale)	Spirits turpentine* Camphor* Methyl salicylate*
MERCODOL COUGH SYRUP (Merrell)	Each fl. oz.: Mercodinone 10 mg. Nethamine hydrochloride* 100 mg. Sodium citrate 1.2 gm. Alcohol 5%		MER-Q-REE MILDEW PREVENTIVE (Rust-Oleum)	Phenyl mercury salt of cyclopentane carboxylic acid* 10% Mercury naphthenate* 10%
MERC-O-DUST P Seed disinfectant (Seed-Treet)	Mercury pentanedione* 2.00%		DR. MERRICK'S SCRATCHEX Veterinary (Westchester)	Gamma isomer of benzene hexachloride (from lindane) 1.00% Hexachlorophene (2-2-methylenebis-(3,4,6-trichlorophenol) Mercaptobenzothiazole 1.50% Boric acid 3.00% Propylene glycol 3.00% Essential oil 0.20%
MERCOLIZED WAX CREAM (Dearborn Supply)	Borax Beeswax, ozokerite wax Paraffin Zinc oxide 2% Ammoniated mercury* 2-1/2% Mineral oil		DR. MERRICK'S SULFODENE (Veterinary) (Brookfield)	2-Mercaptobenzo thiazole 1-1/2% Isopropyl alcohol 1.65%/w
MERCREOL For skin irritations (Texas Pharm.)	Oleate of mercury* 1/2% Cresol* 3/4% Cotton seed oil Sesame oil Mineral oil U.S.P.		MERRY MAID RUG & UP-HOLSTERY CLEANER (Ultra Chem.)	
MERCURIDE SUPPOSI-TORIES (Kenmore)	Mercurochrome* 2% Hydro-glyceride base		MERRY WAR HIGH TEST POWDERED LYE (Babbit)	Sodium hydroxide* 94% Sodium carbonate 2%
MERCURO CHROME Antiseptic for cuts (Purepac)	Merbromin (dibromoxymercuri-fluorescein sodium)		MERTOK For skin irritations (Hance)	Acetanilid* 3-1/8 gr./oz. Mild mercurous chloride 15.63 gr./oz. Phenol* Salicylic acid* Zinc oxide Methyl salicylate* Phenol sodique
MERGAMMA Insecticide (Chipman Chem.)	Gamma isomer of benzene hexachloride* 40.00% Other isomers of benzene hexachloride and related compounds 2.00% Phenyl mercury urea 1.93%		M-E SHORT CUT (Powder) Cleaner (Maid-Easy)	Alkali Phosphates* Active oxygen Active synthetic detergent* (pH of 2% solution at 25°C. is 9.5) Carbonates

*Consult Sec. II., Ingredients Index. This ingredient may be responsible for major toxic effects if poisonous amounts of this product are ingested.

Name & Use Manufacturer	Ingredients	Name & Use Manufacturer	Ingredients
M-E SPARK (Powder) Cleaner (Maid-Easy)	Alkali Phosphates* Active oxygen Active synthetic detergent* (pH of 2% solution at 25ºC. is 11.05) Carbonates Silicates	METAPHEN Antiseptic (Abbott)	Benzyl alcohol 3% Metaphen*(organic mercurial) in an alkalinized solution
		METAPHEN TINCTURE, 1-200 (Nitro-mersol Tinc-ture) (Abbott)	Metaphen* 500 mg./100 cc. of an alkalinized solvent con-sisting of: Alcohol* 50% Acetone* 10%
META CHLOR CHLORINE TABLETS Disinfectant, sanitizer (Gliss'n)	Calcium hypochlorite* 68%		
		METEOR BRAND ZINC SULFATE CRYSTALS (Calif. Spray)	Zinc sulfate* crystals 99.5% Zinc expressed as metallic 22.80%
METACIDE 50 Insecticide (Pittsburgh Coke)	Parathion (o, o-diethyl o-p-nitrophenyl thiophosphate)* 10.0% o, o-Dimethyl o-p-nitrophenyl thiophosphate* 40.0% Emulsifier 50.0%	METEOR EAU DE TOILETTE Perfume (Coty)	
METAFOS Water softener (Rumford)	Phosphorus pentoxide* 67% Sodium oxide* 32.5%	METHALGEN Counter-irritant, analgesic (Schuemann)	Camphor* Menthol* Methyl salicylate* Cream base
METAG AGRICUL-TURAL BAIT (Pellets) Insecticide (Calif. Spray)	Calcium arsenate* 5.16% Metaldehyde 1.50%	METHANOX Insecticide (Farnam)	Methoxychlor tech. 23.3% Dimethyl phthalate 10.0% Aromatic petroleum solvent* 61.7%
METAG XX AGRIC. BAIT (Pellet) Insecticide (Calif. Spray)	Calcium arsenate* 5.16% Metaldehyde 3%	METHILOSE TABLETS Laxative (Horton & Converse)	Methylcellulose 0.5 gm.
METAKOL VAGINAL JELLY (Durex)	Triisopropyl-phenoxy-polyethoxy-ethanol 1.25% Sodium lauryl sulfate Boric acid Glycerin 7% Vegetable gum base Sodium chloride	METHODINE TABLETS Laxative (Preston Labs.)	Methylcellulose 2-1/2 gr. Dextro amphetamine sulfate* 5 gr. Dicalcium phosphate 1-1/2 gr.
		METH-O-LIN Rubefacient (Maltbie)	Methyl salicylate* Camphor* Menthol* Emulsion base
METALDEHYDE Slug baits (Insecticide) (Commercial Solv.)	Metaldehyde*		
		METHOXONE Herbicide (Chipman Chem.)	Sodium salt of 2-methyl-4-chlorophenoxy acetic acid* 23.20%
METALGLAS Cleaner (Belvidere)			
METALLITE PAINTS & FINISHES (Glidden Co.)		METHOXONE -AMINE 64 Herbicide (Chipman Ltd.)	Triethanolamine formulation of 2-methyl-4-chloro-phenoxyacetic acid* (MCP) MCP acid equiv. 64 oz.
METAL LUSTER (Holcomb)	Denatured alcohol Oxalic acid* Aqueous ammonia	METHOXONE -ESTER 80 Herbicide (Chipman Ltd.)	Butyl ester formulation of 2-methyl-4-chloro-phenoxyacetic acid* (MCP) MCP acid equiv. 80 oz.
METAL TREAT CONCEN-TRATE Rust pre-ventative (Klean-Strip)		METHOXONE -SODIUM 48 Herbicide (Chipman Ltd.)	Sodium salt formulation of 2-methyl-4-chloro-phenoxyacetic acid (MCP)* MCP acid equiv. 48 oz.
		MET-L-CLIEN For degreasing metal parts (Lien)	Sodium hydroxide*
METALUX (Uncle Sam)	Soap Silica Perfume Alkali Dye	METROSAN CREME Vaginal creme (Diaphragm)	Stearic acid Triethanolamine Oleic acid Sodium lauryl sulfur

Name & Use Manufacturer	Ingredients		Name & Use Manufacturer	Ingredients	
METROSAN VAGINAL JELLY (Diaphragm)	Lactic acid Aluminum subacetate Benzoic acid Chlorothymol Glycerine		MEYER'S MIX POWDER Insecticide (Meyer, T.)	Pyrethrins Sodium fluoride*	0.12% 69.12%
MEX FLOOR CLEANER & BLEACH (United Gilson.)	Trisodium phosphate* Sodium perborate*		MEYER'S PUTZ CREAM METAL POLISH (Am. Metal)	Infusorial earth Silica Oleic acid (red oil) Oxalic acid* Ammonia* Pine oil*	
MEXICAN POTTERY CLAY (Am. Art)			MEYER SUXALMID Analgesic, antipyretic (Meyer & Co.)	Each tablet: Salicylamide* Acetophenetidin* Potassium para-amino benzoate	5 gr. 1 gr. 4 gr.
MEXSANA For skin irritations (Plough)	Camphor* Corn starch Zinc oxide Oil of eucalyptus* Kaolin Hexachlorophene		MEYER SYRUP ALMEHIST Antihistamine, decongestant (Meyer)	Each 5 cc.: Pyrilamine maleate Hyoscine hydrobromic acid Hyoscyamine hydrobromic acid	25 mg. 0.008 mg. 0.040 mg.
MEYER ALMETUSSIN Antitussive (Meyer)	Each 5 cc.: Codeine phosphate* Pyrilamine maleate* Potassium guaiacolsulfonate Hyoscine hydrobromic acid Hyoscyamine hydrobromic acid Chloroform* Alcohol Menthol	10.9 mg. 13.5 mg. 169 mg. 0.005 mg. 0.025 mg. 0.333 m. 10% 0.62 mg.	MFR NO. 928 MEDICATED SHAMPOO S.F. For dandruff (Specialists)	Sodium thiosulfate Potassium sulfate Triethanolamine Benzalkonium chloride* Sodium metaphosphate	
			M-G FOOT OIL Liniment (Gustafson)	Oils of flaxseed, cedar, pine,* and olive Mineral oil	
MEYER BROTHERS CARBO-CRESOL DIS-INFECTANT (Meyer Bros.)	Coal tar neutral oils* Soap Phenols*		MGK ALDRIN 2 LB. EMULSIFI-ABLE CON-CENTRATE Insecticide (McLaughlin)	Hexachloro hexahydro dimethano naphthalene* Related compounds Petroleum distillate	25.46% 4.32% 60.22%
MEYER BROTHERS MY-RUB Rubbing alcohol compound (Meyer Bros.)	Alcohol*	70%/v	MGK ALLETHRIN CONC. 2.5% Insecticide (McLaughlin)	Petroleum distillate* Allethrin*(allyl homolog of cinerin-1) Related compounds	97.28% 2.50% 0.22%
MEYER'S BEATSALL CRYSTALS Fumigant, insecticide (Meyer, T.)	Paradichlorobenzene*	100%	MGK ALLETHRIN CONC. 20% Insecticide (McLaughlin)	Petroleum distillate* Allethrin*(allyl homolog of cinerin-1) Related compounds	78.25% 20.00% 1.75%
MEYER'S BEATSALL FOG SPRAY Insecticide (Meyer, T.)	Petroleum distillate* Tech. piperonyl butoxide Pyrethrins	98.206% 1.496% 0.298%	MGK ALLETHRIN CONC. 90% Insecticide (McLaughlin)	Allethrin* (allyl homolog of cinerin-1) Related compounds Petroleum distillate	90%
MEYER'S CHLORDANE EMULSION CONCEN-TRATE Insecticide (Meyer, T.)	Chlordane tech.* Petroleum distillate	50% 5%	MGK CHLORDANE 20% OIL-CONC. Insecticide (McLaughlin)	Chlordane*	20%
MEYER'S LINDANE SPRAY Insecticide (Meyer, T.)	Gamma isomer of benzene hexachloride (from lindane) Petroleum distillate*	0.5% 99.5%	MGK CONC. NO. 1129 Insecticide (McLaughlin)	DDT Tech. chlordane n-Octyl bicycloheptene dicarboximide Allethrin Methylated aromatic petroleum deriv.*	25.0% 12.0% 2.0% 0.2% 56.8%

Name & Use Manufacturer	Ingredients	
MGK CONC. NO. 1426 Insecticide (McLaughlin)	DDT	25.0%
	Heptachlor (heptachloro tetrahydro-4, 7-methanoindene)	3.2%
	Related compounds	1.3%
	n-Octyl bicycloheptene dicarboximide	2.0%
	Allethrin	0.2%
	Methylated aromatic petroleum deriv.*	64.3%
MGK DIELDRIN 1.5 LB. EMULSIFI-ABLE CONC. Insecticide (McLaughlin)	Hexachloro epoxy octahydro dimethano naphthalene*	16.93%
	Related compounds	0.17%
	Methylated aromatic petroleum deriv.*	74.90%
MGK EMULSIFI-ABLE CHLORDANE CONC. 40% (PCO) Insecticide (McLaughlin)	Oil	54%
	Chlordane*	40%
MGK FARM SPRAY 4 LB. CHLORDANE CONC. Insecticide (McLaughlin)	Chlordane*	45%
	Oil	48%
MGK FARM SPRAY 8 LB. CHLORDANE CONC. Insecticide (McLaughlin)	Chlordane*	74%
	Oil	18%
MGK FARM SPRAY 4 LB. TOXAPHENE CONC. Insecticide (McLaughlin)	Toxaphene*	44%
	Oil	46%
MGK FARM SPRAY 6 LB. TOXAPHENE CONC. Insecticide (McLaughlin)	Toxaphene*	60.3%
	Oil	36.1%
MGK HEPTACHLOR 2 LB. EMULSIFI-ABLE CONC. Insecticide (McLaughlin)	Heptachlor*	23.41%
	Related compounds	9.10%
	Methylated aromatic petroleum deriv.*	61.36%
MGK INSECT LOOSENER Insecticide (McLaughlin)	Oil*	36%
	Pyrethrins*	9%
MGK MOUSE & RAT KILLER (McLaughlin)	2-Pivalyl-1, 3-indandione*	0.025%
MGK PYROCIDE BOOSTER CONC. Insecticide (McLaughlin)	Petroleum distillate*	94.75%
	Tech. piperonyl butoxide*	3.75%
	Pyrethrins	1.50%

Name & Use Manufacturer	Ingredients	
MGK ROACH CONCEN-TRATE 933 Insecticide (McLaughlin)	n-Octyl bicycloheptene dicarboximide*	5.0%
	Pyrethrins	1.5%
	Tech. piperonyl butoxide*	3.0%
	Petroleum distillate*	90.5%
M-G THOROBRED OIL (Gustafson)	Oils of flaxseed, olive, pine* and cedar Mineral oil	
MH-30 Insecticide (Naugatuck)	Maleic hydrazide* (1, 2-dihydro pyridazine-3, 6-dione)	30%
MH-40 Insecticide (Naugatuck)	Maleic hydrazide* (1, 2-dihydro pyridazine-3, 6-dione)	40%
M & H COLD CAPSULES (Fountain)	Tr. belladonna*	M ss
	Caffeine alkaloid	gr. i
	Phenacetin*	gr. ii ss
	ASA talis caps.	gr. iii
M & H PAINT BRUSH CLEANER (M & H)		
MH TECHNICAL Insecticide (Naugatuck)	Maleic hydrazide (1, 2-dihydro pyridazine-3, 6-dione)*	97%
MICE DOOM PELLETS (Murray, E.)	Strychnine*	0.21%
MICO Skin fungicide (medical) (H. S.)	Salicylic acid*	
	Benzoic acid*	
	Gum thus	
	Chlorobutanol*	
	Acetone*	
	Ethyl acetate	
	Alcohol	31%
MICRODOL REPLEN-ISHERS & DEVELOPERS Photographic supplies (Eastman)		
MICRO-FLOTOX DUSTING SULFUR Fungicide (Calif. Spray)	Sulfur*	90%
MICRO-FLOTOX WETTABLE SULFUR Fungicide (Calif. Spray)	Sulfur*	95%
MICROGEL Fungicide (Tenn. Corp.)	Copper* as metallic	51%
MICROIL Lubricant (Kano)	Refined petroleum oil*	
MICRO NU-COP Fungicide (Faesy & Besthoff)	Copper*	53%

*Consult Sec. II., Ingredients Index. This ingredient may be responsible for major toxic effects if poisonous amounts of this product are ingested.

Name & Use Manufacturer	Ingredients	
MICROZINE OINTMENT 5% (Horton & Converse)	Microcrystalline sulfadiazine*	
MICULES Anthelmintic (Veterinary, avian) (Gland-O-Lac)	Nicotine* Phenothiazine	2.5% 21.42%
MIDLAND GAS-O-CIDE Liquid gas fumigant (Midland Labs.)	Ethylene dichloride* Carbon tetrachloride*	
MIDLAND GRAIN-O-CIDE Liquid gas fumigant (Midland Labs.)	Carbon tetrachloride* Ethylene dichloride* Ethylene dibromide*	
MIDLAND INSECT-O-LOH 68 Insecticide (Midland Labs.)	Tech. chlordane Pyrethrins I and II Sesamin Refined mineral oil	2.50% 0.05% 0.19% 97.26%
MIDLAND LIN-O-CIDE Insecticide (Midland Labs.)	Refined mineral oil Aromatic petroleum deriv.* Methoxychlor tech.* Gamma isomer of benzene hexachloride* (from lindane)	
MIDLAND MILL-O-CIDE CONCEN-TRATE Insecticide (Midland Labs.)	Refined mineral oil B-butoxy-B' thiocyanodiethyl ether* Methyl salicylate* Pyrethrins I and II Sesamin	
MIDLAND MILL-O-CIDE FORMULA B-9 Insecticide (Midland Labs.)	Tech. piperonyl butoxide* Refined mineral oil Methyl salicylate* Pyrethrins I and II	
MIDLAND MILL-O-CIDE FORMULA P-5 Insecticide (Midland Labs.)	Refined mineral oil B-butoxy-B' thiocyanodiethyl ether* Methyl salicylate* Sesamin Pyrethrins I and II	
MIDLAND ML-10 Germicide (Midland Labs.)	Para di-isobutyl phenoxy ethoxy ethyl dimethyl benzyl ammonium chloride* 10.0%	
MIDLAND NEO GERMOLYPTUS Germicide (Midland Labs.)	Isopropyl alcohol* Soap Ortho benzyl para-chlorophenol* Glycerin	
MIDLAND PINE DISINFECT-ANT 5 (Midland Labs.)	Pine oil* Soap	

Name & Use Manufacturer	Ingredients	
MIDLAND WARE-O-CIDE CONCEN-TRATE Insecticide (Midland Labs.)	Refined mineral oil Tech. chlordane* (octa chloro-4, 7-methano tetrahydro indane and related compounds) Methylated aromatic petroleum deriv.* Sesamin oil extractives Pyrethrins Methyl salicylate*	
MIDOL Analgesic (Centaur-Caldwell)	Acetaphenetidin* Aspirin Cinnamylephedrine* Caffeine	3 gr.
MI-D-STROY Insecticide (Lehman Bros.)	Petroleum distillate* Sesame oil extractives Pyrethrins	
MIGATON COMPOUND Tonic (San Pedro)	Iron Calcium Sherry wine base Creosote Manganese Thiamine hydrochloride malt Guaiacol	
MIGATON SYRUP Antitussive (San Pedro)	Methyl ethyl amino phenyl propanol hydrochloride* F.E. ipecac Ammonium chloride Menthol*	
MIGHTY MENDER GLUE (Mighty)		
MIGRAGEN For colds (Halperin)	Each tablet: Acetophenetidin* Camphor Podophyllin Aloin Atropine sulfate Quinine sulfate	0.12 gm. 15 mg. 1.5 mg. 4 mg. 0.03 mg. 30 mg.
MIKE SULPHUR Insecticide (Dow)	Sulfur*	95.00%
MIKET CAPSULES Anthelmintic (veterinary, avian) (Gland-O-Lac)	Nicotine* Phenothiazine	0.9 gr. 7.5 gr.
MILAM COMPOUND Tonic (Owen)	Vitamins Iron Alcohol Strychnine Iron ammonium citrate Yeast concentrate	10% 1-100 gr./oz.
MILBURN CAPSULES For colds (E. Z. Chem.)	Acetophenetidin* Podophyllin Colocynth Scammony Cardamon Aloes* Ginger Gentian Aspirin*	
MILDEW CHEK Fungicide (Chek)		

*Consult Sec. II., Ingredients Index. This ingredient may be responsible for major toxic effects if poisonous amounts of this product are ingested.

Name & Use Manufacturer	Ingredients		Name & Use Manufacturer	Ingredients	
MILDEX Fungicide (Larvacide)	Dinitro (1-methyl heptyl) phenyl crotonate*	22.5%	MILKY WAY DRY DIP Insecticide (Interstate Med.)	Naphthalene* Sulfur Creosote oil* Sodium silicofluoride* Talcum	
	Other nitro phenols and deriv., chiefly dinitro (1-methyl heptyl) phenol*	2.5%			
MILDOOM Fungicide (Sapolin)	Di-(phenylmercuric) dodecenyl succinate*	11.6%	MILL CRAYONS (Imperial Cray.)		
MILD SILVER PROTEIN (Ophthalmic Ointment) Antiseptic, astringent for eyes (Massengill)	Mild silver protein Lanolin White petrolatum	10% q.s. q.s.	MILLER #2 ALDRIN EMULSION Insecticide (Miller Chem. & Fert.)	Hexachloro hexahydro dimethano naphthalene* Related compounds Petroleum hydrocarbons	23.10% 4.68% 69.22%
MILD SKIN ASTRINGENT (Assoc. Brands)			MILLER 2-1/2% ALDRIN EQUIVALENT DUST Insecticide (Miller Chem. & Fert.)	Hexachloro hexahydro dimethano naphthalene* Related compounds	2.37% 0.41%
MIL-DU-RID Mildewproofing compound (Ultra Chem.)			MILLER 25% ALDRIN EQUIVALENT WETTABLE POWDER Insecticide (Miller Chem. & Fert.)	Hexachloro hexahydro dimethano naphthalene* Related compounds	23.8% 4.68%
MILES NERVINE Sedative (Miles)	Each tablet: Sodium bromide* Potassium bromide* Ammonium bromide* Citric acid Sodium bicarbonate	4.5 gr. 4.5 gr. 0.5 gr. 22.5 gr. 27.25 gr.			
MILEX CREME (Milex)	Glycerol ester of ricinoleic acid Sodium lauryl sulfate Oxyquinoline sulfate Stearic acid Methyl parasept Glycerin Glyceryl monostearate Polyethylene monostearate Lactic acid (pH 4.5)	0.50% 0.60% 0.02% 15.00% 0.10% 6.31% 2.07% 0.50%	MILLER ALUMINUM SULFATE Soil acidifier (Miller Chem. & Fert.)	Aluminum sulfate	
			MILLER ARAMITE-15W Insecticide (Miller Chem. & Fert.)	2 (p-tert-Butyl phenoxy) isopropyl 2-chloroethyl sulfite	15%
MILEX P400 DOUCHE POWDER (Milex)	Salicylic acid Phenol Eucalyptol Menthol Thymol Perfume Zinc sulfate* Boric acid*	0.05% 0.01% 0.01% 0.01% 0.01% 0.005% 12.5% 86.59%	MILLER ARSENATE OF LEAD (Powdered) Insecticide (Miller Chem. & Fert.)	Arsenate of lead*	97.00%
MILKINOL Laxative (Kremers)	Liquid petrolatum Flavoring Emulsifier		MILLER BEAN & VEGETABLE DUST Insecticide (Miller Chem. & Fert.)	Rotenone Other extractives (cube) DDT Sulfur*	0.50% 1.25% 1.00% 25.00%
MILK OF MAGNESIA TOOTHPASTE (Comfort)	Glycerin C.P. Corn starch Gum tragacanth Saccharin Soap Calcium carbonate Magma		MILLER BENZENE HEXA- CHLORIDE #10 Insecticide (Miller Chem. & Fert.)	Gamma isomer of benzene hexachloride* Other isomers of benzene hexachloride	10% 15%
MILKY WAY DIP Insecticide (Interstate Med.)	Phenols or tar acids* Neutral coal tar oils* Rosin soap		MILLER 1/2% BENZENE HEXA- CHLORIDE DUST Insecticide (Miller Chem. & Fert.)	Gamma isomer of benzene hexachloride Other isomers of benzene hexachloride	1/2% 2-1/2%

*Consult Sec. II., Ingredients Index. This ingredient may be responsible for major toxic effects if poisonous amounts of this product are ingested.

- 692 -

Name & Use Manufacturer	Ingredients	
MILLER BLUE MOLD DUST Fungicide (Miller Chem. & Fert.)	Ferbam*	10.5%
MILLER BORDEAUX MIXTURE Fungicide (Miller Chem. & Fert.)	Copper* (as metallic)	12.75%
MILLER CALCIUM CASEINATE SPREADER White wash (Miller Chem. & Fert.)	Calcium caseinate	
MILLER 2% CHLORDANE Insecticide (Miller Chem. & Fert.)	Tech. chlordane Petroleum distillates*	2% 98%
MILLER 46 CHLORDANE Insecticide (Miller Chem. & Fert.)	Tech. chlordane* Methyl naphthalenes*	46% 52%
MILLER 5% CHLORDANE DUST Insecticide (Miller Chem. & Fert.)	Tech. chlordane*	5%
MILLER 40% CHLORDANE WETTABLE POWDER Insecticide (Miller Chem. & Fert.)	Tech. chlordane*	40%
MILLER COMMERCIAL FLOUR OF SULPHUR Insecticide (Miller Chem. & Fert.)	Sulfur*	99-1/2%
MILLER CORN EAR WORM & BORER SPRAY (Miller Chem. & Fert.)	DDT tech.* Mineral oil Methyl naphthalenes*	7.4% 74.0% 15.8%
MILLER CORN EAR WORM & BORER SPRAY #2 (Miller Chem. & Fert.)	DDT tech. Mineral oil Methyl naphthalenes*	12.5% 50.5% 34.5%
MILLER CPR DUST CONTAINING CYCLONENE PYRETHRINS & ROTENONE Insecticide (Miller Chem. & Fert.)	Tech. piperonyl cyclonene Pyrethrins Rotenone Other cube extractives	0.50% 0.05% 0.25% 0.50%

Name & Use Manufacturer	Ingredients	
MILLER CUCUMBER-MELON DUST Insecticide (Miller Chem. & Fert.)	Rotenone Other extractives (cube) Zineb	1.00% 3.50% 3.90%
MILLER DDD (TDE) 5% DUST Insecticide (Miller Chem. & Fert.)	Dichloro diphenyl dichloroethane tech.	5%
MILLER DDD (TDE) DUST 5-7 Insecticide (Miller Chem. & Fert.)	Dichloro diphenyl dichloroethane tech. Copper*(basic copper sulfate) as metallic	5% 7%
MILLER DDD (TDE) 10% DUST Insecticide (Miller Chem. & Fert.)	Dichloro diphenyl dichloroethane tech.	10%
MILLER 5% DDD-6% DITHANE DUST Insecticide (Miller Chem. & Fert.)	Dichloro diphenyl dichloroethane tech. Zineb	5% 3.9%
MILLER 3% DDT-6% CRAG 658 POTATO-TOMATO DUST Insecticide, fungicide (Miller Chem. & Fert.)	Copper-zinc-chromate complex* DDT tech. Methyl naphthalenes*	5.7% 3.0% 2.0%
MILLER 3% DDT-6% DITHANE DUST Insecticide (Miller Chem. & Fert.)	DDT tech. Zineb Methyl naphthalenes*	3.0% 3.9% 2.0%
MILLER 25% DDT LIQUID Insecticide (Miller Chem. & Fert.)	DDT Aromatic petroleum deriv. solvent	25% 70%
MILLER 3% DDT-1% PARATHION DUST Insecticide (Miller Chem. & Fert.)	DDT tech. Parathion*	3% 1%
MILLER 5% DDT-1% PARATHION DUST (Miller Chem. & Fert.)	DDT tech. Parathion*	5% 1%
MILLER 5% DDT-1-1/2% PARATHION DUST Insecticide (Miller Chem. & Fert.)	DDT tech. Parathion*	5% 1-1/2%

*Consult Sec. II., Ingredients Index. This ingredient may be responsible for major toxic effects if poisonous amounts of this product are ingested.

Name & Use Manufacturer	Ingredients		Name & Use Manufacturer	Ingredients	
MILLER 10% DDT-2% PARATHION DUST Insecticide (Miller Chem. & Fert.)	DDT tech. Parathion*	10% 2%	MILLER DIELDRIN 50% WETTABLE POWDER Insecticide (Miller Chem. & Fert.)	Hexachloro epoxy octahydro-endo, exo-dimethano naphthalene* Related compounds	42.6% 7.4%
MILLER 3% DDT-1% PARATHION-50% SULPHUR DUST Insecticide (Miller Chem. & Fert.)	DDT tech. Parathion* Sulfur	3% 1% 50%	MILLER 6% DITHANE Z-78 DUST Fungicide (Miller Chem. & Fert.)	Zineb	3.9%
MILLER 5% DDT-1% PARATHION-50% SULPHUR DUST Insecticide (Miller Chem. & Fert.)	DDT tech. Parathion* Sulfur	5% 1% 50%	MILLER DRY LIME SULPHUR Fungicide (Miller Chem. & Fert.)	Calcium polysulfide* Calcium thiosulfate Sulfur	70% 5% 10%
MILLER 3% DDT-50% SULPHUR DUST Insecticide (Miller Chem. & Fert.)	DDT Sulfur*	3% 50%	MILLER DUO COPPER Fungicide (Miller Chem. & Fert.)	Basic copper sulfate* (as metallic)	53%
MILLER 5% DDT-50% SULPHUR DUST Insecticide (Miller Chem. & Fert.)	DDT* Sulfur*	5% 50%	MILLER DUO COPPER DUST Fungicide (Miller Chem. & Fert.)	Copper*(basic copper sulfate) as metallic	7.0%
MILLER D-3-1 DUST CONTAINING 3% DDT INCLUDING 1% IMPREGNATED DDT Insecticide (Miller Chem. & Fert.)	DDT Methyl naphthalenes*	3% 2%	MILLER DUST CONTAINING ROTENONE 1.00% Insecticide (Miller Chem. & Fert.)	Rotenone Other extractives (cube)	1.00% 2.00%
MILLER D-5-1 DUST CONTAINING 5% DDT INCLUDING 1% IMPREGNATED DDT Insecticide (Miller Chem. & Fert.)	DDT tech.* Methyl naphthalenes*	5% 2%	MILLER 1% ENDRIN DUST Insecticide (Miller Chem. & Fert.)	Endrin (hexachloro epoxy octahydro-endo, endo-dimethano naphthalene)*	1%
MILLER 1-1/2% DIELDRIN DUST Insecticide (Miller Chem. & Fert.)	Hexachloro epoxy octahydro-endo, exo-dimethano naphthalene* Related compounds	1.28% 0.22%	MILLER 1.6 ENDRIN LIQUID (Emulsifiable) Insecticide (Miller Chem. & Fert.)	Endrin (hexachloro epoxy octahydro-endo, endo-dimethano naphthalene)* Petroleum hydrocarbons	19.5% 77.5%
MILLER DIELDRIN 25 WETTABLE POWDER Insecticide (Miller Chem. & Fert.)	Hexachloro epoxy octahydro dimethano naphthalene* Related compounds	21.25% 3.75%	MILLER FERBAM FUNGICIDE Fungicide (Miller Chem. & Fert.)	Ferbam (ferric dimethyl dithiocarbamate)*	76%
			MILLER FLOW-TOX Insecticide (Miller Chem. & Fert.)	Parathion*	50%
			MILLER FLY-AWAY Insect repellent (Miller Chem. & Fert.)	Pyrethrins Butoxy polypropylene glycol*	0.6% 89.4%
			MILLER FLY-A-WAY AEROSOL Insecticide (Miller Chem. & Fert.)	Pyrethrins Piperonyl butoxide tech. Petroleum distillates	0.25% 2.00% 9.75%

*Consult Sec. II., Ingredients Index. This ingredient may be responsible for major toxic effects if poisonous amounts of this product are ingested.

- 694 -

Name & Use Manufacturer	Ingredients	
MILLER FLY-AWAY DAIRY SPRAY CONC. Repellent (Miller Chem. & Fert.)	Butoxy polypropylene glycol*	53.29%
	Piperonyl butoxide tech.	5.38%
	Pyrethrins	0.54%
	Petroleum distillate*	25.72%
MILLER FLY BAIT Insecticide (Miller Chem. & Fert.)	Malathion (o, o-dimethyl dithiophosphate of diethyl mercapto succinate)	1.00%
MILLER FREE FLOWING SULPHUR SMOKE Fungicide (Miller Chem. & Fert.)	Sulfur*	95%
MILLER FRUIT SPRAY OR DUST Insecticide (Miller Chem. & Fert.)	Captan	8.0%
	Malathion*	4.0%
	Methoxychlor tech*	8.0%
MILLERFUME Insecticide, fungicide (Miller Chem. & Fert.)	Carbon tetrachloride*	25%
	Ethylene dichloride*	75%
MILLER 1-1/2% GAMMA BHC DUST Insecticide (Miller Chem. & Fert.)	Gamma isomer of benzene hexachloride*	1-1/2%
	Other isomers of benzene hexachloride	8-1/2%
MILLER 11% GAMMA BHC EMULSION Insecticide (Miller Chem. & Fert.)	Gamma isomer of benzene hexachloride*	11.0%
	Other isomers of benzene hexachloride and related compounds	17.0%
	Methylated naphthalenes*	48.5%
	Xylene*	16.5%
MILLER GARDEN DUST OR SPRAY Insecticide (Miller Chem. & Fert.)	Malathion*	5.0%
	Methoxychlor tech.*	5.0%
	Zineb	3.9%
MILLER HEPTACHLOR NO. 2 LIQUID (Emulsifiable) Insecticide (Miller Chem. & Fert.)	Heptachlor*	23.41%
	Related compounds	9.10%
	Petroleum distillate	61.36%
MILLER HORMONE BEAN DUST Insecticide (Miller Chem. & Fert.)	Rotenone	1.00%
	DDT	1.00%
	Other extractives (cube)	2.50%
	Sulfur*	25.00%

Name & Use Manufacturer	Ingredients	
MILLER HORN WORM TOMATO DUST Insecticide (Miller Chem. & Fert.)	Copper acetoarsenite	1.8%
	Arsenic expressed as metallic arsenic	0.8%
	Total arsenic expressed as arsenic trioxide	1%
	Other metallic copper from Paris green	1/2%
	Tricalcium arsenate from calcium arsenate*	21.0%
	Copper (basic copper sulfate) as metallic	7.0%
MILLER HOUSEHOLD DUST Insecticide (Miller Chem. & Fert.)	DDT*	10%
MILLER HOUSEHOLD SPRAY Insecticide (Miller Chem. & Fert.)	DDT*	5%
	Kerosene*	85%
	Aromatics	10%
MILLER HYTOX INSECT DUST Insecticide (Miller Chem. & Fert.)	Malathion*	4%
MILLER HY-TOX INSECT SPRAY Insecticide (Miller Chem. & Fert.)	Malathion*	25%
	Methoxychlor*	25%
MILLER HY-TOX SULPHUR FOR DUSTING OR SPRAYING Fungicide (Miller Chem. & Fert.)	Elemental sulfur*	95%
MILLER 1% IMPREGNATED DDT & 6% CRAG 658 DUST Insecticide, fungicide (Miller Chem. & Fert.)	Copper-zinc-chromate* complex	5.7%
	DDT tech.	1.0%
	Methyl naphthalenes*	2.0%
MILLER 1% IMPREGNATED DDT & 6% DITHANE DUST Fungicide (Miller Chem. & Fert.)	DDT tech.	1.0%
	Zineb	3.9%
	Methyl naphthalenes*	2.0%
MILLER KILL-ALL Herbicide (Miller Chem. & Fert.)	Sodium arsenite*	40%
MILLER KILMITE DUST Insecticide (Miller Chem. & Fert.)	Tetraethyl pyrophosphate*	1%
	Other ethyl phosphates	1.50%

Name & Use Manufacturer	Ingredients		Name & Use Manufacturer	Ingredients	
MILLER KILMITE-P Insecticide (Miller Chem. & Fert.)	Tetraethyl pyrophosphate*	20%	MILLER LIQUID 55 MALATHION Insecticide (Miller Chem. & Fert.)	Malathion*	55%
	Other ethyl phosphates	30%			
MILLER KILMITE-40 (40% TEPP) Insecticide (Miller Chem. & Fert.)	Tetraethyl pyrophosphate*	40%	MILLER LIQUID 25 PARATHION Insecticide (Miller Chem. & Fert.)	Parathion*	25%
	Other ethyl phosphates	60%		Xylene	70%
MILLER K SOLUBLE 33 (For Blending) Insecticide (Miller Chem. & Fert.)	DDT*	33%	MILLER LIQUID PHENYL MERCURY Fungicide (Miller Chem. & Fert.)	Phenyl mercuric acetate*	10.00%
MILLER LATE BEAN DUST-XR Insecticide (Miller Chem. & Fert.)	Rotenone	1.00%	MILLER LIQUID 30 RESIDUAL SPRAY CON-TAINING 30% DDT Insecticide (Miller Chem. & Fert.)	DDT*	30%
	DDT	3.00%		Methyl naphthalenes*	65%
	Other extractives (cube)	1.25%			
	Sulfur*	50.00%			
MILLER LIME SULPHUR SOLUTION Insecticide (Miller Chem. & Fert.)	Calcium polysulfide*	29%	MILLER LIQUID TUBACIDE ROTENONE CONC. Insecticide (Miller Chem. & Fert.)	Rotenone*	2%
				Other extractives (cube)	4%
MILLER LINDANE Insecticide (Miller Chem. & Fert.)	Gamma isomer of benzene hexachloride*	25%			
MILLER 1% LINDANE DUST Insecticide (Miller Chem. & Fert.)	Gamma isomer of benzene hexachloride (from lindane)	1%	MILLER LIQUID WEEDAWAY Herbicide (Miller Chem. & Fert.)	Dimethyl amine salt of 2, 4-dichlorophenoxy-acetic acid*	49.8%
MILLER 1-1/2% LINDANE DUST Insecticide (Miller Chem. & Fert.)	Gamma isomer of benzene hexachloride (from lindane)*	1-1/2%	MILLER 25% MALATHION Insecticide (Miller Chem. & Fert.)	Malathion*	25%
MILLER 20% LINDANE EMULSION Insecticide (Miller Chem. & Fert.)	Gamma isomer of benzene hexachloride*	20%	MILLER M-58 DUST Insecticide (Miller Chem. & Fert.)	Rotenone	0.75%
	Petroleum hydrocarbons	74%		Metallic copper*	7%
MILLER LINDANE INDUSTRIAL SPRAY Insecticide (Miller Chem. & Fert.)	Gamma isomer of benzene hexachloride (from lindane)	0.50%	MILLER 5% METH-OXYCHLOR DUST Insecticide (Miller Chem. & Fert.)	Methoxychlor*	5%
	Petroleum oils*	99.50%			
MILLER LIQUID 1.5 DIELDRIN Insecticide (Miller Chem. & Fert.)	Hexachloro epoxy octahydro dimethano naphthalene*	15.83%	MILLER MICO SULPHUR Fungicide (Miller Chem. & Fert.)	Sulfur*	95%
	Related compounds	2.79%			
	Petroleum hydrocarbons	73.38%	MILLER MISCIBLE SUMMER OIL Insecticide (Miller Chem. & Fert.)	Petroleum oil*	97%

*Consult Sec. II., Ingredients Index. This ingredient may be responsible for major toxic effects if poisonous amounts of this product are ingested.

- 696 -

Name & Use Manufacturer	Ingredients	
MILLER NICOTINE SULPHATE 40% Insecticide (Miller Chem. & Fert.)	6 Nicotine*	40%
MILLER NU-FILM STICKER & SPREADER (Miller Chem. & Fert.)		
MILLER NU-SET 2,4,5-Tp HORMONE SPRAY Fungicide (Miller Chem. & Fert.)	2,4,5-T*	
MILLER NU-TONE CONCEN-TRATED Fungicide (Miller Chem. & Fert.)	Naphthalene acetic acid*	1 gm./fl. oz.
MILLER ORTAZOL POWDER Insecticide (Miller Chem. & Fert.)	Dinitro-ortho-cresol*	40%
MILLER ORTHODI-CHLORO-BENZENE Fungicide (Miller Chem. & Fert.)	Orthodichlorobenzene*	100%
MILLER PARADI-CHLORO-BENZENE MOTH CRYSTALS (Miller Chem. & Fert.)	Paradichlorobenzene*	100%
MILLER 1% PARATHION-7% COPPER DUST Insecticide (Miller Chem. & Fert.)	Parathion* Copper (basic copper sulfate) as metallic	1% 7%
MILLER 1% PARATHION-6% DITHANE DUST Insecticide (Miller Chem. & Fert.)	Parathion* Zineb	1% 3.9%
MILLER 1% PARATHION DUST Insecticide (Miller Chem. & Fert.)	Parathion*	1%
MILLER 2% PARATHION DUST Insecticide (Miller Chem. & Fert.)	Parathion*	2%
MILLER 1% PARATHION-50% SULPHUR DUST Insecticide (Miller Chem. & Fert.)	Parathion* Sulfur	1% 50%
MILLER 15% PARATHION WETTABLE POWDER Insecticide (Miller Chem. & Fert.)	Parathion*	15%
MILLER PARIS GREEN Insecticide (Miller Chem. & Fert.)	Copper aceto arsenite*	90%
MILLER P-C WEED KILLER FOR CRAB-GRASS & CHICKWEED Herbicide (Miller Chem. & Fert.)	Potassium cyanate*	76%
MILLER PEANUT DUST Insecticide (Miller Chem. & Fert.)	DDT tech. Sulfur*	1% 90%
MILLER 40% PENTA-CHLORO-PHENOL WOOD PRE-SERVATIVE (Miller Chem. & Fert.)	Tech. pentachlorophenol*	40%
MILLER PHENYL MERCURY POWDER Fungicide (Miller Chem. & Fert.)	Phenyl mercuric acetate*	10.00%
MILLER POTATO DUST D-5-C-7 Insecticide (Miller Chem. & Fert.)	DDT* Copper*(basic copper sulfate) as metallic	5% 7%
MILLER POWDERED ARSENATE OF CALCIUM Insecticide (Miller Chem. & Fert.)	Tri-calcium arsenate*	70.0%
MILLER RAT-A-WAY Rodenticide (Miller Chem. & Fert.)	3-(a-Phenyl-b-acetyl ethyl) 4-hydroxycoumarin	0.5%

*Consult Sec. II., Ingredients Index. This ingredient may be responsible for major toxic effects if poisonous amounts of this product are ingested.

Name & Use Manufacturer	Ingredients		Name & Use Manufacturer	Ingredients	
MILLER RAT-A-WAY BAIT Rodenticide (Miller Chem. & Fert.)	3-(Alpha-acetonylbenzyl)-4-hydroxycoumarin	0.025%	MILLER 40% TOXAPHENE CONTAINING WETTABLE POWDER 40% TOXAPHENE Insecticide (Miller Chem. & Fert.)	Toxaphene* (tech. chlorinated camphene)	40%
MILLER ROSE-DUST OR SPRAY Insecticide (Miller Chem. & Fert.)	Malathion* DDT Captan Sulfur*	4.0% 4.0% 7.0% 40.0%	MILLER 10% TOXAPHENE DUST Insecticide (Miller Chem. & Fert.)	Toxaphene*	10%
MILLER SCALE-TOX Insecticide (Miller Chem. & Fert.)	Petroleum oil*	97%	MILLER 20% TOXAPHENE DUST Insecticide (Miller Chem. & Fert.)	Toxaphene*	20%
MILLER SPRAY MATERIAL CONTAINING 4% ROTENONE Insecticide (Miller Chem. & Fert.)	Rotenone* Other extractives (cube)	4.0% 9.0%	MILLER TOXAPHENE EMULSION #60 Insecticide (Miller Chem. & Fert.)	Toxaphene* (tech. chlorinated camphene) Petroleum distillates Iso-octyl phenoxy polyethoxy ethanol	60.2% 29.8% 10.0%
MILLER STRAWBERRY DUST Insecticide (Miller Chem. & Fert.)	DDT Sulfur *	3% 75%	MILLER TU-BA-CIDE CONTAINING ROTENONE 1.00% Insecticide (Miller Chem. & Fert.)	Rotenone Other extractives (cube) Sulfur*	1.00% 2.50% 25.00%
MILLER SUPERIOR NU-OIL Insecticide (Miller Chem. & Fert.)	Petroleum oil*	97-1/2%	MILLER V-75 DUST CONTAINING ROTENONE 0.75% Insecticide (Miller Chem. & Fert.)	Rotenone Other extractives (cube)	0.75% 1.50%
MILLER 3-WAY DUST 4% MALATHION-3% DDT-50% SULPHUR Insecticide (Miller Chem. & Fert.)	Malathion* DDT Sulfur*	4% 3% 50%			
MILLER TOBACCO WORM & APHID DUST Insecticide (Miller Chem. & Fert.)	TDE (dichloro diphenyl dichloroethane) Parathion*	5% 1%	MILLER VEG-SET (CLPA) HORMONE SPRAY Fungicide (Miller Chem. & Fert.)	Each 4 fl. oz.: Parachloro phenoxy acetic acid*	2 gm.
MILLER TOMATO DUST Insecticide (Miller Chem. & Fert.)	Copper (basic copper sulfate) as metallic Tri-calcium arsenate*	7.0% 13.3%	MILLER WEEDAWAY Herbicide (Miller Chem. & Fert.)	Chloro IPC #4 (isopropyl-n-(3-chlorophenyl) carbamate)*	45.8%
MILLER TOMATO DUST D-1-C-7 Insecticide (Miller Chem. & Fert.)	DDT tech. Copper*(basic copper sulfate) as metallic Methyl naphthalenes*	1% 7% 2%	MILLER WEEDAWAY BRUSH-KILLER Herbicide (Miller Chem. & Fert.)	2, 4, 5-T Ester* 2, 4-D Ester*	9% 18%
MILLER TOMATO POTATO & CELERY DUST OR SPRAY Insecticide, fungicide (Miller Chem. & Fert.)	Copper*(basic copper sulfate) as metallic DDT tech.	7% 3%	MILLER WEEDAWAY CHLORO IPC #4 Herbicide (Miller Chem. & Fert.)	Isopropyl n (3-chlorophenyl) carbamate*	45.8%

*Consult Sec. II., Ingredients Index. This ingredient may be responsible for major toxic effects if poisonous amounts of this product are ingested.

Name & Use Manufacturer	Ingredients		Name & Use Manufacturer	Ingredients	
MILLER WEEVIL-TOX Fungicide (Miller Chem. & Fert.)	Carbon bisulfide*	100%	MILLER'S 5% CHLORDANE DUST Insecticide (Miller Chem. Co.)	Tech. chlordane*	5%
MILLER WETTABLE POWDER 50% DDT Insecticide (Miller Chem. & Fert.)	DDT*	50%	MILLER'S CRABGRASS KILLER Herbicide (Miller Chem. Co.)	Potassium cyanate*	78%
MILLER 10% ZERLATE DUST Fungicide (Miller Chem. & Fert.)	Ziram (zinc dimethyl dithio carbamate)* Zinc expressed as metallic	7% 1.49%	MILLER'S CRESYLIC Disinfectant (Miller Chem. Co.)	Cresylic acid* and soap 75%	
MILLER ZERLATE TOMATO DUST Insecticide, fungicide (Miller Chem. & Fert.)	Ziram (zinc dimethyl dithio carbamate) Tri-calcium arsenate*	7.0% 13.3%	MILLER'S DAIRY FLY SPRAY Insecticide (Miller Chem. Co.)	Petroleum distillate* n-Octyl bicycloheptene dicarboximide Tech. methoxyclor* Allethrin (allyl homolog of cinerin-1 and related compounds)* Pyrethrins	
MILLER 6.5% ZINEB DUST Fungicide (Miller Chem. & Fert.)	Zineb	6.5%	MILLER'S 5% DDT DUST Insecticide (Miller Chem. Co.)	Dichloro diphenyl trichloroethane*	5%
MILLERHAUS' COMPOUND TABLETS Cathartic (Cel-Ton-Sa)	Aloin* Aloe* Extract of cascara sagrada		MILLER'S 25% DDT EMULSI- FIABLE Insecticide (Milller Chem. Co.)	Dichloro diphenyl trichloroethane* Petroleum hydrocarbons*	25% 70%
MILLERHAUS' FAMOUS LINIMENT Rubefacient, counter- irritant (Cel-Ton-Sa)	Oil eucalyptus* Turpentine* Oil mustard (syn.) Methyl salicylate (syn.)* Oil sassafras (imitation)* Pine oil* Camphor* Refined kerosene* Certified color		MILLER'S 1.5# DIELDRIN EMULSIFI- ABLE Insecticide (Miller Chem. Co.)	Methylated aromatic petroleum deriv.* Hexachloro epoxy octahydro dimethano naphthalene* Related compounds	77.54% 14.84% 2.62%
MILLER'S 2# ALDRIN EQUIVALENT Insecticide (Miller Chem. Co.)	Hexachloro hexahydro dimethano naphthalene*21.9% Related compounds 16.5% Petroleum distillates 51.6%		MILLER'S DRY-DYP Insecticide (Miller Chem. Co.)	Naphthalene* Sodium fluoride* Creosote oil Nicotine Sulfur	15.00% 1.00% 2.67% 0.03% 33.33%
MILLER'S 2#-2# BRUSH KILLER Herbicide (Miller Chem. Co.)	Butyl ester of 2,4-dichloro phenoxy acetic acid* 28.4% Butyl ester of 2,4,5-trichloro phenoxy acetic acid* 27.6% Aromatic petroleum solvent* 38.0%		MILLER'S DUSTING SULPHUR Fungicide (Miller Chem. Co.)	Sulfur*	90%
MILLER'S 10-20 BRUSH KILLER Herbicide (Miller Chem. Co.)	Butyl ester of 2,4,5-trichloro phenoxy acetic acid* 10% Butyl ester of 2,4-dichloro phenoxy acetic acid* 20% Aromatic petroleum solvent* 60%		MILLER'S 4# ESTER Herbicide (Miller Chem. Co.)	Butyl ester of 2,4-dichloro phenoxy acetic acid* 57.3%	
MILLER'S CHLORDANE 45% Insecticide (Miller Chem. Co.)	Tech. chlordane* 45% Aliphatic petroleum solvent* 49%		MILLER'S 6# ESTER Herbicide (Miller Chem. Co.)	Butyl ester of 2,4-dichloro phenoxy acetic acid* 78.3%	
			MILLER'S FORMALDE- HYDE Fungicide (Miller Chem. Co.)	Formaldehyde* 37% Methyl alcohol less than 15%	

*Consult Sec. II., Ingredients Index. This ingredient may be responsible for major toxic effects if poisonous amounts of this product are ingested.

Name & Use Manufacturer	Ingredients		Name & Use Manufacturer	Ingredients	
MILLER'S 2# HEPTACHLOR Insecticide (Miller Chem. Co.)	Heptachlor* Related compounds Petroleum distillate	22.6% 8.8% 62.6%	MILLER'S SODIUM FLUORIDE (Nile Blue) Insecticide (Miller Chem. Co.)	Sodium fluoride*	95%
MILLER'S ISOPROPYL ESTER 44 Herbicide (Miller Chem. Co.)	Isopropyl ester of 2,4-dichloro phenoxy acetic acid*	45.5%	MILLER'S STOCK DIP & DISIN-FECTANT Insecticide (Miller Chem. Co.)	Active Ingredients: Coal tar neutral oils* Soap Phenols*	90%
MILLER'S LO VOL BRUSH KILLER Herbicide (Miller Chem. Co.)	Iso-octyl ester of 2,4,5-trichloro phenoxy acetic acid* Iso-octyl ester of 2,4-dichloro phenoxy acetic acid*	31.7% 36.15%	MILLER'S 2,4,5-T ESTER 46 Herbicide (Miller Chem. Co.)	Butyl ester of 2,4,5-trichlorophenoxy acetic acid Aromatic petroleum solvent*	46% 48%
MILLER'S LO VOL 4# 2,4-D ESTER Herbicide (Miller Chem. Co.)	Iso-octyl ester of 2,4-dichloro phenoxy acetic acid*	67.2%	MILLER'S UNIVERSAL BALM Tonic, counter-irritant (Myers Labs.)	Alcohol* Red pepper Cinnamon Spearmint Cajeput Pennyroyal Camphor* Cloves Oils of origanum Eucalyptus* Sassafras* Cinnamon	59%
MILLER'S LO VOL 2,4,5-T ESTER Herbicide (Miller Chem. Co.)	Iso-octyl ester of 2,4,5-trichloro phenoxy acetic acid*	62.6%			
MILLER'S MALATHION 50 Insecticide (Miller Chem. Co.)	Malathion* Methylated aromatic petroleum deriv.*	55% 39%	MILLION DOLLAR HAND CLEANER (Glisten)		
MILLER'S MOTH CRYSTALS Insecticide (Miller Chem. Co.)	Paradichlorobenzene*	100%	MILO MODELIT PLASTIC MODELING MATERIAL (Am. Crayon)		
MILLER'S ONE-PAK FRUIT SPRAY Fungicide, insecticide (Miller Chem. Co.)	DDT (dichloro diphenyl trichloroethane) Arsenate of lead* Ferbam Total arsenic expressed as metallic Water-soluble arsenic expressed as metallic	7.5% 24.5% 11.4% 4.87% 0.125%	MILORGANITE Fertilizer (Sewerage) MILTON BRADLEY CRAYONS (Bradley, M.)		
MILLER'S PINE ODOR DISINFECT-ANT Disinfectant (Miller Chem. Co.)	Active Ingredients: Vegetable oil soap Steam distilled pine oil* Isopropyl alcohol* Orthophenylphenol* Chloro-2-phenylphenol*	20%	MINERAL BLOCK (Formula L-B 33) Avian (Lehman Bros.)	Minerals Lime Eggshell Cuttle bone Salt Iron oxide	
MILLER'S ROSE DUST Fungicide, insecticide (Miller Chem. Co.)	Ferbam (ferric dimethyl dithiocarbamate) Sulfur* DDT* Rotenone Other cube resins	7% 15% 5% 1% 2%	MINER'S COLD CREAM & CLEANSING CREAM (Miner's Inc.)	Beeswax Ceresin wax Lanolin Borax* Perfume oils less than 1/2 of 1%	
MILLER'S 1.67% ROTENONE CATTLE GRUB DUST Insecticide (Miller Chem. Co.)	Rotenone Other cube resins Pyrophyllite	1.67% 3.00% 95.33%	MINER'S STICK COLOGNES, DEODORANT STICKS (Miner's Inc.)	Denatured alcohol Hexachlorophene less than 1/2 of 1% Perfume oils less than 5% Stearic acid Sodium hydroxide less than 1%	

*Consult Sec. II., Ingredients Index. This ingredient may be responsible for major toxic effects if poisonous amounts of this product are ingested.

Name & Use Manufacturer	Ingredients		Name & Use Manufacturer	Ingredients	
MINIMAX INSECTICIDE (Am. Disinfect.)	Aliphatic petroleum solvent* DDT*	95% 5%	MIRASECT (Lorenz)	Chlordane DDT Pyrenone 20 Aliphatic hydrocarbons*	2% 2% 5%
MINIPOO DRY SHAMPOO (Cosmetic)	Magnesium silicate Powdered soap Perfume		MIRIFIK HARDWOOD FLOOR CLEANER (Lavo)		
MINIT-RUB Rubefacient (Bristol Myers)	Lanolin Camphor Menthol* Oil of eucalyptus* Methyl salicylate*		MISCIBLE TAR (Misicible)	Crude coal tar*	80%
MIN-R-RUB Analgesic balm, counter-irritant (Sanders)	Methyl salicylate* Menthol* Camphor* Lanolin Petrolatum		MISRY Antirheumatic (General Vitamin)	Salicylamide* Calcium succinate Para-amino benzoic acid Vitamin D	3 gr. 1250 units
MINTGLO Rubefacient (Larson)	Oil of peppermint Methyl salicylate U.S.P.*		MISSION BRAND ALDRIN 2.5-0-0 DUST Insecticide (Hayes-Sammons)	Hexachloro hexahydro-endo, exo-dimethano naphthalene* Related compounds	2.38% 0.40%
MINTO-PAYES Digestant, antacid (Tailby)	Selected jamaica ginger Sodium bicarbonate Bismuth subsalicylate Bismuth subgallate Papain Magnesium trisilicate Mint		MISSION BRAND ALDRIN 2.5-0-40 DUST Insecticide (Hayes-Sammons)	Hexachloro hexahydro-endo, exo-dimethano naphthalene* Related compounds Sulfur* (93-325 mesh)	2.38% 0.40% 41.80%
MIRACLE ADHESIVE (Glidden Co.)			MISSION BRAND ALDRIN 2.5-5-0 DUST Insecticide (Hayes-Sammons)	Hexachloro hexahydro-endo, exo-dimethano naphthalene* Related compounds DDT (dichloro diphenyl trichloroethane)*	2.38% 0.40% 5.00%
MIRACLE ANCHOR ADHESIVE CERAMIC TILE CEMENTS, FLOOR ADHESIVE, TUB-CAULK (Miracle)	Resinous material Pigments Aliphatic petroleum hydrocarbon*		MISSION BRAND ALDRIN 2.5-5-40 DUST Insecticide (Hayes-Sammons)	Hexachloro hexahydro-endo, exo-dimethano naphthalene* Related compounds DDT (dichloro diphenyl trichloroethane)* Sulfur (93-325 mesh)*	2.38% 0.40% 5.00% 41.80%
MIRACLE FOAM Rug and upholstery cleaner (Burton)			MISSION BRAND ALDRIN 2.5-10-0 DUST Insecticide (Hayes-Sammons)	Hexachloro hexahydro-endo, exo-dimethano naphthalene* Related compounds DDT (dichloro diphenyl trichloroethane)* Sulfur (93-325 mesh)*	2.38% 0.40% 10.00% 41.80%
MIRACLE #41 PLASTIK CEMENT (Miracle)	MEK Cyclohexenone* Vinyl resins				
MIRACLE R-MIR-DEK, MIRACLE SLIP-NOT Non-slip floor coating (Miracle)	Abrasive Petroleum solvents* Phenolic base varnish		MISSION BRAND ALDRIN 2 LB. WATER EMULSIFI-ABLE Insecticide (Hayes-Sammons)	Hexachloro hexahydro-endo, exo-dimethano naphthalene* Related compounds Petroleum hydrocarbon	23.04% 3.68% 51.60%
MIRACLE 23 SKIDOO (formerly Miraclene) Waterless handcleaner (Miracle)	Petroleum solvents* Glycerol monostearate Sodium tetra decyl sulfate Propylene glycol Lanal Oil mirbane*		MISSION BRAND BHC 1-DDT 5-0 DUST Insecticide (Hayes-Sammons)	Gamma isomer of benzene hexachloride Other isomers of benzene hexachloride DDT (dichloro diphenyl trichloroethane)*	1.0% 5.7% 5.0%
MIRACLE WALLPAPER CLEANER (Kristee)					

*Consult Sec. II., Ingredients Index. This ingredient may be responsible for major toxic effects if poisonous amounts of this product are ingested.

Name & Use Manufacturer	Ingredients
MISSION BRAND BHC 1-DDT 5-40 DUST Insecticide (Hayes-Sammons)	Gamma isomer of benzene hexachloride 1.0% Other isomers of benzene hexachloride 5.7% DDT (dichloro diphenyl trichloroethane)* 5.0% Sulfur*(93-325 mesh) 41.8%
MISSION BRAND BHC 2-DDT 10-0 DUST Insecticide (Hayes-Sammons)	Gamma isomer of benzene hexachloride* 2.0% Other isomers of benzene hexachloride 11.3% DDT (dichloro diphenyl trichloroethane)* 10.0%
MISSION BRAND BHC 2-DDT 10-40 DUST Insecticide (Hayes-Sammons)	Gamma isomers of benzene hexachloride* 2.0% Other isomers of benzene hexachloride 11.3% DDT (dichloro diphenyl trichloroethane)* 10.0% Sulfur*(93-325 mesh) 41.8%
MISSION BRAND BHC 3-DDT 5-0 DUST Insecticide (Hayes-Sammons)	Gamma isomer of benzene hexachloride* 3.0% Other isomers of benzene hexachloride* 17.0% DDT (dichloro diphenyl trichloroethane)* 5.0%
MISSION BRAND BHC 3-DDT 5-40 DUST Insecticide (Hayes-Sammons)	Gamma isomer of benzene hexachloride* 3.0% Other isomers of benzene hexachloride* 17.0% DDT (dichloro diphenyl trichloroethane)* 5.0% Sulfur*(93-325 mesh) 41.9%
MISSION BRAND BHC 3-DDT 10-0 DUST Insecticide (Hayes-Sammons)	Gamma isomer of benzene hexachloride* 3.0% Other isomers of benzene hexachloride* 17.0% DDT (dichloro diphenyl trichloroethane)* 10.0%
MISSION BRAND BHC 3-DDT 10-40 DUST Insecticide (Hayes-Sammons)	Gamma isomer of benzene hexachloride* 3.0% Other isomers of benzene hexachloride* 17.0% DDT (dichloro diphenyl trichloroethane)* 10.0% Sulfur*(93-325 mesh) 41.8%
MISSION BRAND BHC 5-DDT 5-40 DUST Insecticide (Hayes-Sammons)	Gamma isomer of benzene hexachloride* 5.0% Other isomers of benzene hexachloride* 28.3% DDT (dichloro diphenyl trichloroethane)* 5.0% Sulfur*(93-325 mesh) 41.8%
MISSION BRAND BHC 5-DDT 10-0 DUST Insecticide (Hayes-Sammons)	Gamma isomer of benzene hexachloride* 5.0% Other isomers of benzene hexachloride* 28.3% DDT (dichloro diphenyl trichloroethane)* 10.0%
MISSION BRAND BHC 5-DDT 10-40 DUST Insecticide (Hayes-Sammons)	Gamma isomer of benzene hexachloride* 5.0% Other isomers of benzene hexachloride* 28.3% DDT* (dichloro diphenyl trichloroethane)* 10.0% Sulfur*(93-325 mesh) 41.8%
MISSION BRAND BHC-DDT (3-5) WATER EMULSIFIABLE Insecticide (Hayes-Sammons)	Gamma isomer of benzene hexachloride* 9.46% Other isomers of benzene hexachloride* 16.81% Dichloro diphenyl trichloroethane* 15.75% Petroleum hydrocarbon* 52.98%
MISSION BRAND BHC 3-0-0 DUST Insecticide (Hayes-Sammons)	Gamma isomer of benzene hexachloride* 3.0% Other isomers of benzene hexachloride* 17.0%
MISSION BRAND BHC 3-0-40 DUST Insecticide (Hayes-Sammons)	Gamma isomer of benzene hexachloride* 3.0% Other isomers of benzene hexachloride 17.0% Sulfur*(93-325 mesh) 41.8%
MISSION BRAND BHC 5-0-0 DUST Insecticide (Hayes-Sammons)	Gamma isomer of benzene hexachloride* 5.0% Other isomers of benzene hexachloride* 28.3%
MISSION BRAND BHC 5-0-40 DUST Insecticide (Hayes-Sammons)	Gamma isomer of benzene hexachloride* 5.0% Other isomers of benzene hexachloride* 28.3% Sulfur*(93-325 mesh) 41.8%
MISSION BRAND BHC 5-5-0 DUST Insecticide (Hayes-Sammons)	Gamma isomer of benzene hexachloride* 5.0% Other isomers of benzene hexachloride* 28.3% DDT (dichloro diphenyl trichloroethane)* 5.0%
MISSION BRAND BHC GAMMA WATER EMULSIFIABLE Insecticide (Hayes-Sammons)	Gamma isomer of benzene hexachloride* 12.9% Other isomers of benzene hexachloride* 23.0% Petroleum hydrocarbon* 59.1%
MISSION BRAND BHC 2-METHOXYCHLORO 5-0 DUST Insecticide (Hayes-Sammons)	Gamma isomer of benzene hexachloride* 2.00% Other isomers of benzene hexachloride* 11.30% Methoxychlor tech. 5.00% Petroleum hydrocarbon 0.02%
MISSION BRAND CALCIUM ARSENATE 50-PARATHION 1 DUST Insecticide (Hayes-Sammons)	Tri-calcium arsenate (neutral)* 35.0% Parathion (o, o-diethyl-o, p-nitrophenyl thiophosphate)* 1.0%

*Consult Sec. II., Ingredients Index. This ingredient may be responsible for major toxic effects if poisonous amounts of this product are ingested.

- 702 -

Name & Use Manufacturer	Ingredients		Name & Use Manufacturer	Ingredients	
MISSION BRAND CALCIUM ARSENATE- SULPHUR MIXTURE 50-50 Insecticide (Hayes- Sammons)	Tri-calcium arsenate* Sulfur (93-325 mesh)	35.0% 49.0%	MISSION BRAND DDT 5-0 DUST Insecticide (Hayes- Sammons)	DDT* (dichloro diphenyl trichloroethane)	5.0%
MISSION BRAND CENTINELA DUST Insecticide (Hayes- Sammons)	Heptachlor (heptachlor-4, 7- methano tetrahydroindene) Related compounds Dichloro diphenyl trichloroethane Parathion* (o,o-diethyl-o, p- nitrophenyl thiophosphate)	5.00% 1.94% 5.00% 1.00%	MISSION BRAND DDT 5-40 DUST Insecticide (Hayes- Sammons)	DDT (dichloro diphenyl trichloroethane)* Sulfur*(93-325 mesh)	5.0% 41.8%
MISSION BRAND CHLORDANE 5% DUST Insecticide (Hayes- Sammons)	Tech. chlordane* Related compounds	5.0% 2.0%	MISSION BRAND DDT 5-82 DUST Insecticide (Hayes- Sammons)	DDT* (dichloro diphenyl trichloroethane) Sulfur*(93-325 mesh)	5.0% 82.0%
MISSION BRAND CHLORDANE 10% DUST Insecticide (Hayes- Sammons)	Tech. chlordane*	10.0%	MISSION BRAND DDT 10-0 DUST Insecticide (Hayes- Sammons)	DDT (dichloro diphenyl trichloroethane)*	10.0%
MISSION BRAND CHLORDANE 3.44 LB. WATER EMULSIFI- ABLE Insecticide (Hayes- Sammons)	Tech. chlordane* Petroleum hydrocarbon	40.0% 53.0%	MISSION BRAND DDT 10-40 DUST Insecticide (Hayes- Sammons)	DDT (dichloro diphenyl trichloroethane)* Sulfur*(93-325 mesh)	10.0% 41.8%
MISSION BRAND CHLORDANE 40% WET- TABLE POWDER Insecticide (Hayes- Sammons)	Tech. chlordane*	40.0%	MISSION BRAND DDT 20-0 DUST Insecticide (Hayes- Sammons)	DDT (dichloro diphenyl trichloroethane)*	20.0%
MISSION BRAND CHLORDANE 8 LB. WATER EMULSIFI- ABLE Insecticide (Hayes- Sammons)	Tech. chlordane* Petroleum hydrocarbon	72.82% 26.48%	MISSION BRAND DDT 2 LB. WATER EMULSIFI- ABLE Insecticide (Hayes- Sammon)	Dichloro diphenyl trichloroethane* Petroleum hydrocarbon*	23.6% 71.4%
			MISSION BRAND DDT 3 LB. WATER EMULSIFI- ABLE Insecticide (Hayes- Sammons)	Dichloro diphenyl trichloroethane* Petroleum hydrocarbon*	33.7% 61.3%
MISSION BRAND 5 COPPER DUST Insecticide (Hayes- Sammons)	DDD (dichloro diphenyl dichloroethane)* Copper*(in basic copper sulfate) expressed as metallic	5.0% 5.3%	MISSION BRAND DDT 50% WETTABLE CONCEN- TRATE Insecticide (Hayes- Sammons)	Dichloro diphenyl trichloroethane*	50%

*Consult Sec. II., Ingredients Index. This ingredient may be responsible for major toxic effects if poisonous amounts of this product are ingested.

- 703 -

Name & Use Manufacturer	Ingredients	
MISSION BRAND DIELDRIN 2.5-DDT 5-0 Insecticide (Hayes-Sammons)	Hexachloro epoxy octahydro-endo, exo-dimethano naphthalene*	2.12%
	Related compounds	0.38%
	DDT (dichloro diphenyl trichloroethane)	5.00%
MISSION BRAND DIELDRIN 1.5-DDT 10-0 DUST Insecticide (Hayes-Sammons)	Hexachloro epoxy octahydro-endo, exo-dimethano naphthalene*	1.28%
	Related compounds	0.22%
	DDT (dichloro diphenyl trichloroethane)*	10.00%
MISSION BRAND DIELDRIN 2.5-DDT 0-40 DUST Insecticide (Hayes-Sammons)	Hexachloro epoxy octahydro-endo, exo-dimethano naphthalene*	2.12%
	Related compounds	0.38%
	Sulfur (93-325 mesh)*	41.80%
MISSION BRAND DIELDRIN 2.5-DDT 5-40 DUST Insecticide (Hayes-Sammons)	Hexachloro epoxy octahydro-endo, exo-dimethano naphthalene*	2.12%
	Related compounds	0.38%
	Dichloro diphenyl trichloroethane*	5.00%
	Sulfur (93-325 mesh)*	41.80%
MISSION BRAND DIELDRIN 2.5-DDT 10-0 DUST Insecticide (Hayes-Sammons)	Hexachloro epoxy octahydro-endo, exo-dimethano naphthalene*	2.12%
	Related compounds	0.38%
	Dichloro diphenyl trichloroethane*	10.00%
MISSION BRAND DIELDRIN 2.5-DDT 10-40 DUST Insecticide (Hayes-Sammons)	Hexachloro epoxy octahydro-endo, exo-dimethano naphthalene*	2.12%
	Related compounds	0.38%
	Dichloro diphenyl trichloroethane*	10.00%
	Sulfur (93-325 mesh)*	40.00%
MISSION BRAND DIELDRIN-DDT 1.5 WATER EMULSIFIABLE Insecticide (Hayes-Sammons)	Hexachloro epoxy octahydro dimethano naphthalene*	4.70%
	Related compounds	0.71%
	Dichloro diphenyl trichloroethane*	23.53%
	Petroleum hydrocarbon*	65.96%
MISSION BRAND DIELDRIN 1.5 WATER EMULSIFIABLE Insecticide (Hayes-Sammons)	Hexochloro epoxy octahydro dimethano naphthalene*	15.12%
	Related compounds	2.67%
	Petroleum hydrocarbons	77.21%
MISSION BRAND DIELDRIN-DDT 1-3 WATER EMULSIFIABLE Insecticide (Hayes-Sammons)	Hexachloro epoxy octahydro dimethano naphthalene*	7.56%
	Related compounds	1.34%
	Dichloro diphenyl trichloroethane*	26.44%
	Petroleum hydrocarbon*	50.56%
MISSION BRAND DIELDRIN 1.5-0-0 DUST Insecticide (Hayes-Sammons)	Hexachloro epoxy octahydro-endo, exo-dimethano naphthalene*	1.28%
	Related compounds	0.22%
MISSION BRAND DIELDRIN 1.5-0-40 DUST Insecticide (Hayes-Sammons)	Hexachloro epoxy octahydro-endo, exo-dimethano naphthalene*	1.28%
	Related compounds	0.22%
	Sulfur*(93-325 mesh)	41.80%
MISSION BRAND DIELDRIN 1.5-5-0 DUST Insecticide (Hayes-Sammons)	Hexachloro epoxy octahydro-endo, exo-dimethano naphthalene*	1.28%
	Related compounds	0.22%
	DDT (dichloro diphenyl trichloroethane)*	5.00%
MISSION BRAND DIELDRIN 1.5-5-40 DUST Insecticide (Hayes-Sammons)	Hexachloro epoxy octahydro-endo, exo-dimethano naphthalene*	1.28%
	Related compounds	0.22%
	DDT (dichloro diphenyl trichloroethane)*	5.00%
	Sulfur*(93-325 mesh)	41.80%
MISSION BRAND DIELDRIN 1.5-10-40 DUST Insecticide (Hayes-Sammons)	Hexachloro epoxy octahydro-endo, exo-dimethano naphthalene*	1.28%
	Related compounds	0.22%
	DDT (dichloro diphenyl trichloroethane)*	10.00%
	Sulfur (93-325 mesh)*	41.80%
MISSION BRAND DIELDRIN 2.5-0-0 DUST Insecticide (Hayes-Sammons)	Hexachloro epoxy octahydro-endo, exo-dimethano naphthalene*	2.12%
	Related compounds	0.38%
MISSION BRAND DIELDRIN 50% WETTABLE POWDER Insecticide (Hayes-Sammons)	Hexachloro epoxy octahydro dimethano naphthalene*	42.4%
	Related compounds	7.6%
MISSION BRAND 5-0-40 DUST Insecticide (Hayes-Sammons)	Gamma isomer of benzene hexachloride*	5.0%
	Other isomers of benzene hexachloride*	28.3%
	Sulfur*(93-325 mesh)	41.8%

*Consult Sec. II., Ingredients Index. This ingredient may be responsible for major toxic effects if poisonous amounts of this product are ingested.

- 704 -

Name & Use Manufacturer	Ingredients		
MISSION BRAND DYNATOX COTTON DUST Insecticide (Hayes-Sammons)	o, o-Diethyl-o, p-nitrophenyl thiophosphate* Hexachloro epoxy octahydro-endo, exo-dimethano naphthalene Related compounds Dichloro diphenyl trichloroethane	1.00% 1.28% 0.22% 10.00%	
MISSION BRAND DYNATOX COTTON SPRAY EMULSIFI-ABLE CONC. SPRAY Insecticide (Hayes-Sammons)	o, o-Dimethyl-o, p-nitrophenyl thiophosphate* Heptachloro tetrahydro-4, 7 methanoindene Dichloro diphenyl dichloroethane Petroleum hydrocarbon (xylene range)	6.25% 10.00% 18.75% 58.00%	
MISSION BRAND ENDRIN 1.6 LB. EMULSIFI-ABLE CONC. Insecticide (Hayes-Sammons)	Hexachloro epoxy octahydro-endo, endo-dimethano naphthalene* Petroleum hydrocarbons	19.5% 70.5%	
MISSION BRAND FUNGICIDE NO. 6 (Hayes-Sammons)	Zineb (zinc ethylene bis (dithiocarbamate) 3.9%		
MISSION BRAND FUNGICIDE NO. 8 (Hayes-Sammons)	Zineb (zinc ethylene bis (dithiocarbamate) 5.2%		
MISSION BRAND 12% GAMMA WETTABLE POWDER Insecticide (Hayes-Sammons)	Gamma isomer of benzene hexachloride* Other isomers of benzene hexachloride	12.0% 21.3%	
MISSION BRAND HEPTACHLOR 2.5-DDT 5-0 DUST Insecticide (Hayes-Sammons)	Heptachlor*(heptachloro-4, 7-methano tetrahydro indene) Related compounds DDT (dichloro diphenyl trichloroethane*	2.50% 0.97% 5.00%	
MISSION BRAND HEPTACHLOR 5-DDT 5-0 DUST Insecticide (Hayes-Sammons)	Heptachlor*(heptachloro-4, 7-methano tetrahydro indene) Related compounds DDT (dichloro diphenyl trichloroethane)*	5.00% 1.94% 5.00%	
MISSION BRAND HEPTACHLOR 5-DDT 10-0 DUST Insecticide (Hayes-Sammons)	Heptachlor*(heptachloro-4, 7-methano tetrahydro indene) Related compounds DDT (dichloro diphenyl trichloroethane)*	5.00% 1.94% 10.00%	
MISSION BRAND HEPTACHLOR 5-DDT 10-40 DUST Insecticide (Hayes-Sammons)	Heptachlor* (heltachloro-4, 7-methano tetrahydro indene) Related compounds DDT (dichloro diphenyl trichloroethane)* Sulfur*(93-325 mesh)	5.00% 1.94% 10.00% 40.00%	
MISSION BRAND HEPTACHLOR 2.5-0-0 DUST Insecticide (Hayes-Sammons)	Heptachlor*(heptachloro-4, 7-methano tetrahydro indene) Related compounds	2.50% 0.97%	
MISSION BRAND HEPTACHLOR 2.5-0-40 DUST Insecticide (Hayes-Sammons)	Heptachlor (heptachloro-4, 7-methano tetrahydro indene)* Related compounds Sulfur*(93-325 mesh)	2.50% 0.97% 41.80%	
MISSION BRAND HEPTACHLOR 2.5-5-40 DUST Insecticide (Hayes-Sammons)	Heptachlor*(heptachloro-4, 7-methano tetrahydro indene) Related compounds Dichloro diphenyl trichloroethane* Sulfur*(93-325 mesh)	2.50% 0.97% 5.00% 41.80%	
MISSION BRAND HEPTACHLOR 2.5-10-0 DUST Insecticide (Hayes-Sammons)	Heptachlor*(heptachloro-4, 7-methano tetrahydro indene) Related compounds Dichloro diphenyl trichloroethane*	2.50% 0.97% 10.00%	
MISSION BRAND HEPTACHLOR 2.5-10-40 DUST Insecticide (Hayes-Sammons)	Heptachlor*(heptachloro-4, 7-methano tetrahydro indene) Related compounds DDT (dichloro diphenyl trichloroethane)* Sulfur*(93-325 mesh)	2.50% 0.97% 10.00% 41.80%	
MISSION BRAND HEPTACHLOR 5-0-0 DUST Insecticide (Hayes-Sammons)	Heptachlor*(heptachloro-4, 7-methano tetrahydro indene) Related compounds	5.00% 1.94%	
MISSION BRAND HEPTACHLOR 5-0-40 DUST Insecticide (Hayes-Sammons)	Heptachlor*(heptachloro-4, 7-methano tetrahydro indene) Related compounds Sulfur* (93-325 mesh)	5.00% 1.94% 40.00%	
MISSION BRAND HEPTACHLOR 5-5-40 DUST Insecticide (Hayes-Sammons)	Heptachlor*(heptachloro-4, 7-methano tetrahydro indene) Related compounds DDT (dichloro diphenyl trichloroethane)* Sulfur*(93-325 mesh)	5.00% 1.94% 5.00% 41.80%	
MISSION BRAND HEPTACHLOR 2 LB. EMULSIFI-ABLE CONC. Insecticide (Hayes-Sammons)	Heptachlor* Related compounds Petroleum hydrocarbon	23.41% 9.10% 61.36%	

*Consult Sec. II., Ingredients Index. This ingredient may be responsible for major toxic effects if poisonous amounts of this product are ingested.

Name & Use Manufacturer	Ingredients	Name & Use Manufacturer	Ingredients
MISSION BRAND KARATHANE 1-PARATHION 1-DUST Insecticide (Hayes-Sammons)	Karathane (dinitro capryl phenyl crotonate) 1.0% Parathion (o, o-diethyl-o, p-nitrophenyl thiophosphate)* 1.0%	MISSION BRAND METHYL PARATHION 2 LB. WATER EMULSIFI- ABLE Insecticide (Hayes-Sammons)	Methyl parathion (o, o-dimethyl-o, p-nitrophenyl thiophosphate)* 25.00% Petroleum hydrocarbon (xylene range) 68.00%
MISSION BRAND KILL-TOX DUST Insecticide (Hayes-Sammons)	Toxaphene* (tech. chlorinated camphene (chlorine content 67-69%)) 12.0% DDT (dichloro diphenyl trichloroethane) 8.0%	MISSION BRAND PARATHION 1-DDT 5 DUST Insecticide (Hayes-Sammons)	Parathion (o, o-diethyl-o, p-nitrophenyl thiophosphate)* 1.0% DDT (dichloro diphenyl trichloroethane) 5.0%
MISSION BRAND KILL-TOX WATER EMULSIFI- ABLE Insecticide (Hayes-Sammons)	Toxaphene* (tech. chlorinated camphene (chlorine content 67-69%)) 39.7% Dichloro diphenyl trichloroethane 19.9% Petroleum hydrocarbon 33.1%	MISSION BRAND PARATHION 1-DDT 10 DUST Insecticide (Hayes-Sammons)	Parathion (o, o-diethyl o, p-nitrophenyl thiophosphate)* 1.0% DDT (dichloro diphenyl trichloroethane) 10.0%
MISSION BRAND LINDANE 1% DUST Insecticide (Hayes-Sammons)	Gamma isomer of benzene hexachloride 1.0%	MISSION BRAND PARATHION 1 DUST Insecticide (Hayes-Sammons)	Parathion (o, o-diethyl-o, p-nitrophenyl thiophosphate)* 1.0%
MISSION BRAND LINDANE 2% DUST Insecticide (Hayes-Sammons)	Gamma isomer of benzene hexachloride* 2.0%	MISSION BRAND PARATHION 2 DUST Insecticide (Hayes-Sammons)	Parathion (o, o-diethyl-o, p-nitrophenyl thiophosphate)* 2.0%
MISSION BRAND LINDANE 1.7 LB. WATER EMULSIFI- ABLE Insecticide (Hayes-Sammons)	Gamma isomer of benzene hexachloride (from lindane)* 20.0% Petroleum hydrocarbon 75.0%	MISSION BRAND PARATHION 2 SULPHUR DUST Insecticide (Hayes-Sammons)	Parathion (o, o-diethyl-o, p-nitrophenyl thiophosphate)* 2.0% Sulfur (93-325 mesh) 41.8%
MISSION BRAND MALATHION 25% WET- TABLE POWDER Insecticide (Hayes-Sammons)	Malathion*(ortho-ortho dimethyl dithiophosphate of diethyl mercapto succinate) 25%	MISSION BRAND PARATHION 2 LB. WATER EMULSIFI- ABLE Insecticide (Hayes-Sammons)	Parathion (o, o-diethyl-o, p-nitrophenyl thiophosphate)* 25% Petroleum hydrocarbon 68%
MISSION BRAND MALA-TOX 5 LB. WATER EMULSIFI- ABLE Insecticide (Hayes-Sammons)	Malathion (o, o-dimethyl dithiophosphate of diethyl mercapto succinate)* 50.0% Petroleum hydrocarbon 42.0%	MISSION BRAND POWER TOX INSECTICIDE (Hayes-Sammons)	Toxaphene (tech. chlorinated camphene (chlorine content 67-69%)) 60.0% Parathion (o, o-diethyl-o, p-nitrophenyl thiophosphate)* 8.0% Petroleum hydrocarbon 24.7%
MISSION BRAND METHYL PARATHION 1.5 DUST Insecticide (Hayes-Sammons)	Methyl parathion*(o, dimethyl-o, p-nitrophenyl thiophosphate) 1.50%	MISSION BRAND RHOTHANE 5-COPPER- SULPHUR DUST Insecticide (Hayes-Sammons)	DDD (dichloro diphenyl dichloroethane) 5.0% Copper*(in basic copper sulfate) expressed as metallic 5.3% Sulfur*(93-325 mesh) 41.8%

*Consult Sec. II., Ingredients Index. This ingredient may be responsible for major toxic effects if poisonous amounts of this product are ingested.

Name & Use Manufacturer	Ingredients		Name & Use Manufacturer	Ingredients
MISSION BRAND RHOTHANE 5 DUST Insecticide (Hayes-Sammons)	DDD (dichloro diphenyl dichloroethane) 5.0%		MISSION BRAND TOXAPHENE 6 LB. WATER EMULSIFI-ABLE Insecticide (Hayes-Sammons)	Toxaphene* tech. chlorinated camphene (chlorine content 67-69%)) 60.0% Petroleum hydrocarbon 32.7%
MISSION BRAND RHOTHANE 10% DUST Insecticide (Hayes-Sammons)	DDD (dichloro diphenyl dichloroethane) 10.0%		MISSION BRAND TOXAPHENE 8 LB. WATER EMULSIFI-ABLE Insecticide (Hayes-Sammons)	Toxaphene* (tech. chlorinated camphene (chlorine content 67-69%)) 72.0% Petroleum hydrocarbon 20.7%
MISSION BRAND RHOTHANE 5-SULPHUR DUST Insecticide (Hayes-Sammons)	DDD (dichloro diphenyl dichloroethane) 5.0% Sulfur*(93-325 mesh) 41.8%		MISSION BRAND TOXAPHENE 40% WET-TABLE POWDER Insecticide (Hayes-Sammons)	Tech. chlorinated camphene* 40.00%
MISSION BRAND TOXAPHENE 20-DDT 5-0 DUST Insecticide (Hayes-Sammons)	Toxaphene* (tech. chlorinated camphene (chlorine content 67-69%)) 20.0% Dichloro diphenyl trichloroethane 5.0%		MISSION BRAND VAPOTOX 40% (Hayes-Sammons)	Tetraethyl pyrophosphate* 40% Other ethyl phosphates 60%
MISSION BRAND TOXAPHENE 10-0 DUST Insecticide (Hayes-Sammons)	Toxaphene* (tech chlorinated camphene (chlorine content 67-69%)) 10.0%		MISS TWINKLE DUSTING POWDER & TALCUM (Wright & Glenn)	Talc Magnesium carbonate Zinc stearate Perfume
MISSION BRAND TOXAPHENE 10-40 DUST Insecticide (Hayes-Sammons)	Toxaphene* (tech. chlorinated camphene (chlorine content 67-69%)) 10.0% Sulfur*(93-325 mesh) 41.8%		MISS TWINKLE HAND LOTION (Wright & Glenn)	Stearic acid Lanolin Liquid petrolatum Glycerin Propylene glycol monostearate Triethanolamine Methyl cellulose
MISSION BRAND TOXAPHENE 20-0 DUST Insecticide (Hayes-Sammons)	Toxaphene* (tech. chlorinated camphene (chlorine content 67-69%)) 20.0%		MISS TWINKLE NAIL POLISH (Glenmore)	Nitrocellulose Dibutyl phthalate Camphor* Toluol* Denatured alcohol Ethyl acetate Butyl acetate Certified org. pigments and dyes
MISSION BRAND TOXAPHENE 20-40 DUST Insecticide (Hayes-Sammons)	Toxaphene* (tech. chlorinated camphene (chlorine content 67-69%)) 20.0% Sulfur (93-325 mesh) 41.8%		MISTACIDE INSECT KILLER WITH DDT Insecticide (Am. Aerosol)	DDT 3.00% Pyrethrins 0.15% Piperonyl butoxide 1.20% Methylated naphthalenes* 10.00% Mineral oil 5.65%
MISSION BRAND TOXAPHENE 20-PARATHION 1 DUST Insecticide (Hayes-Sammons)	Toxaphene* (tech. chlorinated camphene (chlorine content 67-69%)) 20.0% Parathion (o, o-diethyl-o, p-nitrophenyl thiophosphate)* 1.0%		MIST-A-POLISH Polish (Victory Chem.)	
MISSION BRAND TOXAPHENE 20-PARATHION 2 DUST Insecticide (Hayes-Sammons)	Toxaphene* (tech. chlorinated camphene (chlorine content 67-69%)) 20.0% Parathion (o, o-diethyl-o, p-nitrophenyl thiophosphate)* 2.0%			

*Consult Sec. II., Ingredients Index. This ingredient may be responsible for major toxic effects if poisonous amounts of this product are ingested.

Name & Use Manufacturer	Ingredients	Name & Use Manufacturer	Ingredients
MIST-BLO 26-C Insecticide (Chem. Insect.)	Methylated naphthalene* Dichloro diphenyl trichloro-ethane* Petroleum distillate Rotenone Other rotenone extractives	MITEE SOIL PIPE CEMENT, SOLDERING PASTE, CUTTING OIL, PIPE JOINT COMPOUND (Sunshine)	
MISTI SHAMPOO (Research Spec.)	Amine fatty acid condensate 14% Unsaturated fatty acid amine 4% Perfume 1%	MITETOX Insecticide (Bonide)	p-Chlorophenyl phenyl sulfone* 20% Related diaryl sulfones 5%
MISTLETOE PERFUME, COLOGNE, TOILET-WATER (Duvelle)	Alcohol (denatured with di-ethyl-phthalate)*	MITE-EX Insecticide (Crane)	Tech. piperonyl butoxide 0.50% Pyrethrins 0.05% Deodorized base oil* 99.45%
MISTOL MIST Nasal de-congestant spray (Plough)	Neo-synephrine (brand of phenylephrine HCl) 0.25% Pyrilamine maleate 0.2%	MITEY SPRAY Insecticide (Gland-O-Lac)	DDT * 5.0% Ortho, meta, and para xylenols* 5.5% Coal tar neutral oils 12.5% Xylene * 2.0% Petroleum hydrocarbons* 75.0%
MISTOL NOSE DROPS Nasal de-congestant (Plough)	Chlorobutanol (chloral deriv. 4 gr./fl. oz. Camphor * Menthol* Eucalyptol* Light mineral oil	MIXIRO Dietary supple-ment (Durst, S. F.)	Each tablet: Ferrous gluconate N.F.* 100 mg. Ferrous sulfate exsic. U.S.P.* 100 mg. Iron reduced electrolytic N.F.* 200 mg. Copper gluconate 7.5 mg. Vitamin B12 1.5 mg.
MISTOL WITH EPHEDRINE Nasal de-congestant (Plough)	Ephedrine* Camphor* Menthol* Eucalyptol* Mineral oil		
MISTRESS OF THE NIGHT PERFUME (Thornton, R.)		MIXTURE BISMUTH & SALOL COMPOUND WITH PAREGORIC (Lilly)	Opium, powdered 0.05 gm. Tinct. opium, camphorated* 12.5 cc. Bismuth subsalicylate 0.35 gm. Salol* 0.35 gm. Zinc sulfocarbolate 0.175 gm. Oil wintergreen* q.s.
MISTRESS OF THE NIGHT TOILET WATER (Thornton, R.)		MIZPAH (Kessler)	Watercress Anise Sage Licorice Non-alcoholic solution
MIST-X Insecticide (United National)	DDT (dichloro diphenyl trichloroethane) 2.00% Allethrin (allyl homolog of cinerin) 0.10% n-Octyl bicycloheptene di-carboximide 0.50% Petroleum hydrocarbon*16.40% Beta butoxy beta thiocyano diethyl ether 1.00%	M-K AFTER SHAVE LOTION (Kirby's Mineral)	
MITALENE For washing cages, perches (Spratts)	Alcohol 6.80%	ML-10 Germicide (Midland Labs.)	Para di-isobutyl phenoxy ethyl dimethyl benzyl ammonium chloride* 10.0%
MITCHAM LAVENDER WATER (Caswell-Massey)		MOAVA OINTMENT For skin irritation (Internat. Labs.)	Zinc oxide Bismuth subnitrate Eucalyptus oil* Benzocaine Boric acid* Sulfur precipitate * Salicylic acid*
MITEE BOILER CLEANER (Sunshine)	Soda ash* Trisodium phosphate*	MOAVA RECTAL SUPPOSI-TORIES (Internat. Labs.)	Tannic acid* Balsam of Peru Oxide of zinc Carbolic acid* Benzocaine Cocoa butter base
MITEE BOILER SEALER (Sunshine)			

Name & Use Manufacturer	Ingredients		Name & Use Manufacturer	Ingredients	
MOBIL FREEZONE Anti-freeze, automotive (Socony)	Methanol* anti-freeze		MOIST-CHEX Liquid vapor barrier (Am. Fluresit)		
MOBIL HYDRAULIC BRAKE FLUID (Socony)	Glycols* Polyglycols Glycol ethers Higher alcohols* Castor oil		MOISTURE MAGIC HAND CREAM (Sofskin)	Stearic acid Potassium stearate Butyl stearate Polyethylene deriv. of lanolin Cholesterol Wool wax alcohols Mineral oil Glycerin Propylene glycol Floral perfume oil D. & C. red Methyl paraben U.S.P.	
MOBIL PERMAZONE Anit-freeze (Socony)	Ethylene glycol* anti-freeze				
MOBO ANTI-FREEZE COMPOUND (Stanley, J.)			MOLA MOSQUITO LOTION Repellent (Caswell-Massey)		
MODART CREME COLD WAVE Neutralizer (Modart)	Sodium bromate*		MOLE DEATH Rodenticide (Fort Dodge)	Strychnine alkaloid*	0.5%
MODART CREME COLD WAVE Waving solution (Modart)	Ammonium thioglycollate*		M-O-LENE RUG & UP-HOLSTERY CLEANER (d-Con)		
MODART CREME HAIRDRESS (Modart)	Mineral oil Lanolin Atlas powders Sorbitol oleates or laurates		MOLE-NOTS Rodenticide (Nott)	Strychnine sulfate*	0.75%
MODART CREME RINSE (Modart)	Quaternary* (Triton-400)		MOL-FERATE (Prenatal Dietary supplement) (Tutag)	Each tablet: Dicalcium phosphate (anhy.) 750 mg. Ferrous sulfate 3 gr. Sodium molybdate 3 mg. Vitamin B1 0.5 mg. Vitamin B2 0.5 mg. Vitamin C 20 mg. Vitamin D 400 U.S.P.	
MODART CREME SHAMPOO (Modart)	Sodium lauryl sulfate Fatty acid esters				
MODENE Paint & varnish cleaner (Bownes)			MOLITE MOLE KILLER Pesticide (Garden Prod.)	Saltpeter 30.00% Arsenic sulfide* 25.00% Barium nitrate* 20.00% Sulfur 8.00% Sodium sulfate 5.00% Rosin 2.00% Sawdust 5.00% Clay 3.00% Dextrine 2.00%	
MODERN ROACH KONTROL Insecticide (Arlenge)					
MODIFIED-B Cream for skin irritations (Saravil)	Tars Benzocaine Menthol* Mercury oleate* 1% Salicylic acid* Camphor*		MOLLE BRUSHLESS SHAVE CREAM (Centaur-Caldwell)	Emollient oils	
DR. MOFFETT'S TEETHINA POWDERS Cathartic (Moffett, C. J.)	Each pwd.: Calomel* (mercury 1/18 gr. deriv. with bismuth subnitrate) Sodium citrate Cassia* Calcium carbonate		MOLOGEN Rodenticide (Rose Mfg.)	Ricine*	0.3%
			MONA LISA TOILET WATER (Ritornelle)		
MO-GO Rodenticide (Linck)	Thallium sulfate* 1%		MON AMI PERFUMES (Ybry)		

*Consult Sec. II., Ingredients Index. This ingredient may be responsible for major toxic effects if poisonous amounts of this product are ingested.

Name & Use Manufacturer	Ingredients		Name & Use Manufacturer	Ingredients
MONARCH PAINT (Martin-Senour)	Pigment: 63% Titanium magnesium pigment Titanium dioxide Titanium calcium pigment Zinc oxide White lead basic sulfate Vehicle: 37% Non-volatile (linseed oil) Volatile (heat-bodied linseed oil)		MONSANTO M C P TECHNICAL Herbicide (Monsanto)	2-Methyl-4-chlorophenoxyacetic acid* Other methyl chlorophenoxyacetic acids
MONARCH POWDER COLOR Art material (Weber Costello)			MONSANTO 2, 4, 5-TRI-CHLORO-PHENOXY-ACETIC ACID Herbicide (Monsanto)	2, 4, 5-T*
MONA ROSA CREAM Cosmetic (Rameau)			MONSANTO 2, 4-DI-CHLORO-PHENOXY-ACETIC ACID Herbicide (Monsanto)	2, 4-D*
MONAX Vaginal antiseptic, trichomonacide (Medical Arts)	Boric acid* 26.5000% Citric acid 0.5000% Sodium caprylate 0.3125% Zinc caprylate 0.0033% Cinnamic acid 0.0011% Menthol 0.0011% Oil of lavender 0.6250% Duponal 2.000% Mag. carbonate 1.000% Lactose 69.0570%		MONSANTO 2, 4-D ISOPROPYL ESTER Herbicide (Monsanto)	Isopropyl ester of 2, 4-D*
			MONSANTO 2, 4, 5-T ISOPROPYL ESTER Herbicide (Monsanto)	Isopropyl ester of 2, 4, 5-T*
MONDY-BLACK ENAMEL (Olo)			MONTAGE TOILET WATER (Countess)	
MONITE DRY POWDER MOTH-PROOFING (Adco)	DDT* 67% Methoxychlor tech. 10%		MONTE CARLO HIGH SPEED LANOLIN COLD WAVE Neutralizer (Vienna)	Potassium bromate* 12 gm.
MONIZETS Antiseptic, antitussive (Reese Chem.)	Each lozenge: Methyl paraben 10 mg. Propyl paraben 2.5 mg. Tyrothricin 2 mg. Benzocaine 6.5 mg. Benzyl alcohol 0.06 m.		MONTE CARLO HIGH SPEED LANOLIN COLD WAVE Waving solution (Vienna)	Ammonium thioglycolate* approx. 7-1/2%
MONOBASE Hydrophilic, washable ointment (Torch)			MONTECATINI BRAND SALTS Cathartic (Banfi)	Sodium sulfate
MONOCOP 26 Fungicide (Chipman Ltd.)	Monohydrate copper sulfate and hydrated spray lime Copper* 9%		MONTE CHRISTO SILVER TINT Hair tint (Monte Christo)	
MONOCOP 35 Fungicide (Chipman Ltd.)	Monohydrate copper sulfate and hydrated spray lime Copper* 12%		MONTGOMERY'S HAIR RESTORER (Aschanbach)	
MONOGRAM AFTER SHAVE & COLOGNE (L. & K.)			MONTOX LIVESTOCK SPRAY Insecticide (Commercial Chem.)	Oil* Piperonyl butoxide* Pyrethrins
MONOSULPH (Nopco)	Sulfated castor oil			
MONOZOL (Aircraft-M.)	Vinylcarbazole*			
MONSANTO FOLIUM (Inorganic Fertilizer) (Monsanto)	Nitrogen 20% Phosphorus 20% Potash 20%			

*Consult Sec. II., Ingredients Index. This ingredient may be responsible for major toxic effects if poisonous amounts of this product are ingested.

- 710 -

Name & Use Manufacturer	Ingredients
MOONBEAM PERFUME (Noblesse)	
MOON DROPS Facial treatment (Revlon)	
MOORE'S EMERALD OIL Rubefacient (Internat. Labs.)	Chlorthymol camphor U.S.P.* Carbolic acid U.S.P.* Wintergreen syn. U.S.P.* Eucalyptol U.S.P. Oil of eucalyptus U.S.P.* Essential oil of camphor*
MOONLIGHT & LACE COLOGNE; MOONLIGHT PERFUME; MOONLIGHT MIST EAU DE PARFUM, MAKE-UP LOTION (Assoc. Brands)	
MOORE'S ANTISPETIC FOOT POWDER (Moore Mfg.)	French chalk Boric acid* Salicylic acid*
MOORE'S 4T5 BARN PAINT (Moore, B.)	
MOORE'S CARBOLIZED SALVE Skin antiseptic (Moore Mfg.)	Phenol* Vaseline
MOORE'S CUTICLE SALVE For skin irritation (Moore Mfg.)	Vaseline Zinc oxide Corn starch Salicylic acid powder*
MOORE'S DEPILATORY POWDER (Moore Mfg.)	Barium sulfide* Zinc oxide Starch powder
MOORE'S ECZEMA LOTION For skin irritations (Moore Mfg.)	Zinc oxide Calamine Glycerin Alcohol* Phenol*
MOORE'S ECZEMA SALVE #42 For skin irritations (Moore Mfg.)	Pilocarpus* Powd. sulfur* Vaseline
MOORE'S FACE LOTION (Moore Mfg.)	Sulfate of zinc* Sulfurate of potassium H_2O
MOORE'S GENUINE HAIR POMADE For scalp irritations (Moore Mfg.)	Pilocarpus* Powd. sulfur* Vaseline

Name & Use Manufacturer	Ingredients	
MOORE'S GENUINE HAIR TONIC (Moore Mfg.)	Sage Boxwood bark Borax Alcohol	4-1/6%
MOORE'S OIL COLORS (Moore, B.)		
MOORE'S PEDICURE OIL Rubefacient for feet (Moore Mfg.)	Castor oil Salicylic acid powder* Alcohol	18%
MORALINE CREAM HAIR TONICS (Plough Sales Corp.)		
MORDETH Insecticide (Moretex)	Isobornyl thiocyanoacetate* Other related terpenes Petroleum distillate*	4.1% 0.9% 95.0%
MORETEX CHLOR-TOX SPRAY Insecticide (Moretex)	Tech. chlordane Isobornyl thiocyanoacetate Other related terpenes Petroleum distillate*	2.00% 2.46% 0.54% 95.00%
MORGAN EYE LOTION (Morgan Prod.)	Sodium chloride Boric acid Sodium borate Zinc sulfate Camphor	
MORGAN'S POMADE (Heifler & Heifler)		
MORLOTAN OINTMENT For skin burns and irritations (Drug Prod., N.Y.)	Cod liver oil Urea Oxyquinoline benzoate Benzocaine Lanolin base	approx. 53% 10% 0.1% 2%
MOR-O LIQUID For control of coccidiosis in chickens (Hilltop)	Sodium arsanilate* Quebracho liquid extract* Sodium hydroxide	
MOR-O TABLETS For control of coccidiosis in chickens (Hilltop)	Sodium arsanilate*	2.28 gr.
MORRIS' ANTISEPTIC (Goode-Cage)	Alcohol	62%
DR. MORSE'S INDIAN ROOT PILLS (Comstock)	Aloes* Mandrake Gamboge* Chillies Jalap	
MORTITE TAPE Caulk (Mortell, J.)	Wax Polybutene Petroleum sulfonate less than 5% Titanium dioxide Chrysotile asbestos	

*Consult Sec. II., Ingredients Index. This ingredient may be responsible for major toxic effects if poisonous amounts of this product are ingested.

Name & Use Manufacturer	Ingredients		Name & Use Manufacturer	Ingredients	
MORTON'S MIXTURE For intestinal irritation (Oliver's S-O)	Bismuth Milk of magnesia Chalk Salol* Camphor* Ginger Rhubarb	30 gr./oz. 2 fl. dr./oz.	MOTH-CHEK Insecticide (Chek)		
MORUGUENT Rectal suppositories (Massengill)	Each suppository: Cod liver oil concentrate Cocoa butter base		MOTH DED Insecticide (Boyle-Midway)	DDT tech.* Petroleum solvent* Pyrenone BM 1-8 Oil cedar-leaf tech. Alpha neutroleum Spray base oil (petroleum distillate)	
MORUGUENT OINTMENT For skin burns and wounds (Massengill)	Cod liver oil concentrate		MOTHER GRAY'S SWEET POWDERS Cathartic (United Sales)	Each powder: Calomel*(mercurous chloride) Mandrake Licorice Sulfur * Slippery elm Bicarbonate of soda Anise Sugar	11/100 gr.
MORUGUENT (Ophthalmic Ointment) (Massengill)	Cod liver oil concentrate				
MORUSAN (Ointment) For skin burns and wounds (Massengill)	Cod liver oil concentrate Benzocaine	2%	MOTHER'S FRIEND Rubefacient (S.S.S. Co.)	Alcohol* Winter pressed cottonseed oil Soft liquid soap Camphor* Menthol*	6-1/2%
MORUTOIN OINTMENT For skin ulcers (Massengill)	Cod liver oil concentrate Allantoin	1%	MOTH-EX Insecticide (Crane)	Deodorized base oil Paradichlorobenzene* Tech. chlordane*	
MOSAN Fumigant, disinfectant (Moretex)	Alkyl dimethyl benzyl ammonium chloride*	10%	MOTH-GAS CEDARIZED SPRAY Insecticide (Lewy)	Petroleum distillate* Essential oils* (camphor terpenes and cedar oil) Sesame oil extractives (including sesamin) Pyrethrins	
MOSCO Keratolytic (Moss Co.)	Salicylic acid*		MOTH-GAS LIQUID FROST (Lewy)	Paradichlorobenzene* Trichloroethylene*	
MOS-KEE-TOL Mosquito repellent (Penslar)	Dimethyl phthalate	100%			
MOSQUE DEODORANT (Caswell-Massey)			MOTH-GAS VAPORIZER Insecticide (Lewy)	Paradichlorobenzene*	100%
MOSQUITONE STICK Insect repellent (McKesson)	Dimethyl phthalate Ethyl hexanediol*	13.4% 18.0%	MOTH GETTER Insecticide (Stumpf's)		
MOSQUITROL Insecticide (Ampion)	DDT* Rotenone Other cube resins Pyrethrins Sesame oil extract	25% 0.05% 0.100% 0.009% 0.003%	MOTH JINX MOTH PROOFER Insecticide (Claire)	Orthohydroxy benzoyl-p-chloranilide oleate (tech.) Paradichlorobenzene Petroleum hydrocarbon*	2% 2% 46%
MOTH-A-WAY Insecticide (Ellis, H. G.)	Aluminum chloride Sodium silicate Sodium fluoride Active constituents	0.02% 0.13% 0.84% 0.99%	MOTH-KIL Insecticide (Chek)		
			MOTHMASTER Mothproofing (Sani-Wax)		
MOTHBAN MOTH KILLER Insecticide (Standard Oil)	DDT Methoxychlor tech. Pyrethrins Tech. piperonyl butoxide Methylated naphthalene* Petroleum oil	2% 2% 0.25% 1% 5.75% 19%	MOTH NOK-R Insecticide (Pro-Tex-All)	Oil Paradichlorobenzene* Dicyclohexylamine oleate*	

*Consult Sec. II., Ingredients Index. This ingredient may be responsible for major toxic effects if poisonous amounts of this product are ingested.

Name & Use Manufacturer	Ingredients		Name & Use Manufacturer	Ingredients	
MOTH-O BLITZ (Aerosol) Insecticide (Blitz)	Para chloraniline oleate Para chloraniline salicylate Paradichlorobenzene* Petroleum hydrocarbon*	1.84% 0.16% 2.00% 46.00%	MOYER GERMICIDAL TABLETS Antiseptic (Moyer)	Benzethonium chloride (p-(2-methyl-4, 4-dimethyl) pentane-2 (phenoxy-ethoxy-ethyl) dimethyl benzyl ammonium chloride monohydrate*) refined	12.2%
MOTH OCTONS INSECTICIDE (Reliable Chem.)	Refined naphthalene*	100%	M.P.C. WASHING FLUID (Mezzacon)	Sodium hypochlorite*	
MOTH PROOFER CONCENTRATE Insecticide (Stanley Home)	Orthodichlorobenzene* Methoxychlor* Perfume Freon		M-Q-R ATHLETIC FOOT REMEDY (McPhail)		
MOTH SQUARES Insecticide (Reliable Chem.)	Refined naphthalene* Perfume oils	99-1/2% 1/2%	MR. & MRS. COLOGNE STICKS (Mem)		
MOUCHE EAU DE TOILETTE, EAU DE COLOGNE, AND PERFUME (Rochas)			M. S. A. Skin antiseptic (James, L.)	Methyl salicylate* Salicylic acid* Acetone* Pyoktanin	
MOUSE-CHEK Rodenticide (Chek)			M-S-A FEND... CREAMS & LOTIONS Skin protectives (Mine)		
MOUSE DEATH Rodenticide (Fort Dodge)	Strychnine sulfate*	0.4%	M-S-A FEND-PC CREAM Antiperspirant (Mine)		
MOUSE-NOTS (Mice Seed) Rodenticide (Nott)	Strychnine sulfate*	0.75%	M-S-A FEND-X CREAM Skin conditioner (Mine)		
MOUSE SEED Rodenticide (Reardon, W.)	Strychnine*	0.4%	M-S-A SALT & DEXTROSE COMBINATION TABLETS (Mine)	Salt (sodium chloride) Dextrose	70% 30%
MOUSE SLAYER Rodenticide (Chem. & Ext.)	Thallium sulfate*	1%	M-60 Insecticide (Am. Aerosol)	DDT Tech. methoxychlor Isobornyl thiocyano acetate* Other related terpenes n-Octyl bicycloheptene dicarboximide Allethrin (allyl homolog of cinerin 1) Petroleum distillate Aromatic petroleum deriv.*	3.0% 1.0% 0.82% 0.18% 0.166% 0.10% 2.734% 12.00%
MOUSSELINE PERFUME REGULAR MODEL AND COLOGNE (Rochas)					
MOUSTACHE AFTER-SHAVE LOTION, EAU DE TOILETTE, AND EXTRACT (Rochas)			M-2 OINTMENT For skin irritations (Mace)	Menthol Starch Salicylic acid* Lanolin Camphor* Zinc oxide Hexachlorophene*	
MOUTH REFRESHER (Stanley Home)	Water Propylene glycol N.F. Essential oils* Saccharin soluble U.S.P. Formaldehyde U.S.P. Hydrochloric acid C.P. conc. Certified dye		MUCARA PLAIN Cathartic (Ives-Cameron)	Karaya gum granules	

*Consult Sec. II., Ingredients Index. This ingredient may be responsible for major toxic effects if poisonous amounts of this product are ingested.

- 713 -

Name & Use Manufacturer	Ingredients		Name & Use Manufacturer	Ingredients	
MU-COL HYGIENIC POWDER Oral, nasal, antiseptic (Mu-col)	Sodium borate* Boric acid* Menthol* Eucalyptol* Sodium chloride Sodium bicarbonate Thymol* Methyl salicylate*		MULLOIDS Hemorrhoidal suppositories (Rowland)	Powdered ext. belladonna Istrain nut gall Ephedrine* Ichthammol Acid boric* Powdered ext. strammonium Benzocaine Silver iodide* Zinc oxide Cocoa butter	
MUFTI DRY CLEANING COMPOUND (Plough)	Naphtha gas* Alcohol* Ether* Turpentine*		MULLOINT (Medicated Ointment) (Rowland)	Bismuth subcarbonate Zinc oxide Phenol less than 1/2 of 1% Oil linseed Boric acid* Benzocaine	
MUFTI LIGHTER FLUID (Plough)	Naphtha (special)*		MULSOID SULFUR Fungicide (Sherwin-Williams)	Sulfur* 93%	
MUFTI RUG CLEANER & SPOT REMOVER (Plough)			MULTICAINE OINTMENT Anesthetic antiseptic (Barfred)	n-Butyl para-amino benzoate 1% Hypnocaine (n-propanol para-amino benzyl carboxylate) 1% Benzyl alcohol 1%	
MUFTI SHOE WHITE (Plough)			MULTICIDE EMULSION SPRAY CONC. (25%) Insecticide (McLaughlin)	DDT 25% Methylated petroleum* 50% Xylol* 21%	
MUGUET DES BOIS EXTRACT & TOILET WATER (Coty)			MULTICIDE EMULSION SPRAY CONC. (30%) Insecticide (McLaughlin)	DDT 30% Xylol* 49%	
MULE-HIDE ROOFING CEMENT (Lehon)			MULTICIDE 50 Insecticide (McLaughlin)	DDT* 50%	
MULE KICK DRAIN PIPE CLEANER (Sexauer)			MULTICIDE 50W Insecticide (McLaughlin)	DDT* (wettable) 50%	
MUL-EN-OL ANTISEPTIC (Specialty)			MULTICIDE OIL-SOLUBLE SPRAY CONC. Insecticide (McLaughlin)	Methylated petroleum* DDT 24% Xylol*	
MUL-LEVES Scalp preparation (Gray's)	Extract mullein leaves Boric acid* Sodium benzoate*				
MUL-LEVES EYELASH POMADE (Gray's)	Extract mullein leaves Lanolin Petroleum		MULTI FILM Fungicide (Colloidal)	Zinc*	
MUL-LEVES POMADE FOR THE HAIR (Gray's)	Extract mullein leaves Lanolin Petrolatum Perfume		MULTI-KILL Insecticide (Martin, C.J.)	Petroleum distillate* DDT* Tech. chlordane* Pyrethrins	
MUL-LEVES SHAMPOO (Gray's)	Extract mullein leaves Medicinal soft soap Oil of lavender Alcohol		MULTITINT ENAMEL (Seidlitz)	Titanium dioxide Titanium calcium Titanium magnesium Diatomonous silica Calcium carbonate	
MULLIKIN'S VERMIFUGE Anthelmintic (veterinary) (Parker, W.)	American wormseed oil* Castor oil				

Name & Use Manufacturer	Ingredients		Name & Use Manufacturer	Ingredients	
MULTITOX Insecticide, fungicide (Hanna)	DDT* Malathion* Captan		MURRAY & LANMAN'S FLORIDA WATER Toiletries (Lanman)		
MULTI-TOX L Insecticide (Thompson Chem.)	Gamma isomer of benzene hexachloride 1.25% DDT (dichloro diphenyl trichloroethane) 25% Xylene* 63.75%		MUSCO RUBBING OIL Counter- irritant (Assoc. Prod.)	Turpentine oil* Camphor* Kerosene* Methyl salicylate* Menthol* Light mineral oil	
MULTI-TOX-T Insecticide (Thompson Chem.)	Toxaphene* 24.6% DDT 24.6% Xylene* 40.8%		MUSCO-RUB LINIMENT (Triangle)	Gum camphor* Light mineral oil Kerosene* Oil of sassafras* Oil of cassia Oil of wintergreen* Oil of cajuput Turpentine*	
MUM Deodorant (cosmetic) (Bristol- Myers)	Hydrogenated fatty oils Hydrocarbons Zinc oxide Zinc stearate Beeswax Hexachlorophene Perfume				
MURALITE Calcitine, kalsomine (Ewing)			MUSE LINE EXTRACT & TOILET WATER (Coty)		
MURALO, MURAL- TONE WATER COLORS (Muralo)			MUS-L-EZE Liniment (Globe)	Oil of wormwood Potassium iodide* Menthol* Oil of peppermint Alcohol* 79.62%/v Acetone*	
MURALO WALL SIZE (Muralo)			MUSTARINE Counter- irritant (Wells, S. C.)	Oleoresin capsicum Turpentine* Camphor* Menthol* Various oils Petrolatum base	
MURINE FOR YOUR EYES Eyewash (Murine)	Potassium bicarbonate Potassium borate Berberine hydrochloride Boric acid Glycerin Hydrastine hydrochloride Merthiolate (Thimerosal, Lilly) 0.001%		MUSTEROLE Counter- irritant (Musterole)	Oil mustard* Camphor* Menthol* Methyl salicylate* Glycol monosalicylate	
MURPHY'S OIL SOAP Cleaner (Murphy- Phoenix)	Vegetable oil soap		MUTOSCOPE FORMULA #1 Insecticide (Internat. Muto.)	Tech. DDT* Xylene* SAE 20 or 30 oil Kerosene	6 lb. 2 gal. 1 gal. 2 gal.
			MUTOSCOPE FORMULA #2 Insecticide (Internat. Mutoscope)	Tech. DDT* Xylene* Agricultural oil	6 lb. 2 gal. 3 gal.

*Consult Sec. II., Ingredients Index. This ingredient may be responsible for major toxic effects if poisonous amounts of this product are ingested.

Name & Use Manufacturer	Ingredients		Name & Use Manufacturer	Ingredients
MUTOSCOPE FORMULA #3 Insecticide (Internat. Muto.)	Tech. DDT* Sovacide F or Velsical AR 50-60 or 70	5 lb. 5 gal.	MY FOLLY PERFUME, COLOGNE, TOILET- WATER (Duvelle)	Alcohol denatured with di- ethyl-phthalate
MUTOSCOPE FORMULA #4 Insecticide (Internat. Muto.)	Tech. DDT* Sun-solvent 1547 Triton X-100 Water to make	5 lb. 1 gal. 4 oz. 5 gal.	MY FRENCH COUSIN COLOGNE & PERFUME (Wolff)	
MWK #102 ALUMINUM (Dampney)	Volatiles: V. M. & P. naphtha* Xylol* Non-volatiles: Ester gum Cumar Tung Linseed	48.4% 51.6%	MYKEL TOOTH POWDER (Kent Co.)	
			MY-KNIGHT HAIR POMADE & SPECIAL HAIR DRESSING (Purex Prod.)	Petroleum jelly U.S.P. Perfume oils Olive oil U.S.P.
M & W LACQUERS & ENAMELS (Maas & Waldstein)			MY-KOSOL Dietary sup- plement (veterinary, avian) (McClellan)	Copper* Iodine* Cobalt* Potassium Manganese Hydrochloric acid
MY-ALGINE Rubefacient (My-Algine)	Methyl salicylate* Menthol* Oil of mustard* Camphor* Turpentine* Greaseless liniment			
			MYNA Glass cleaner (Zonite)	
MYANESOL For spastic and neurological disorders (Frankay)	Mephenesin* (3-o-toloxy- 2-propanediol)		MYOPONE OINTMENT Topical ointment for myositis (Drug Prod., N.Y.)	Solvent-extracted wheat germ oil
MYCOMIST Fungicidal deodorant spray for shoes (Gordon)	Chlorophyll Formalin* Benzalkonium chloride* Perfume		MYOPONE RECTAL SUPPOSI- TORIES For anorectal irritations (Drug Prod., N.Y.)	d-Alpha-tocopheryl acetate 5 mg. Wheat germ oil (with vitamin E) 0.6 gm.
MYCOZANE Skin fungicide, (medical) (Veltex)	Zinc undecylenate* 20% Undecylenic acid* 5% Vesanisal 5% Salicylic and benzoic acids* Hydroquinone Lavender		MYOPONE VAGINAL SUPPOSI- TORIES For vulvovagi- nal irritations (Drug Prod., N.Y.)	Wheat germ oil (with vitamin E) Alpha tocopherol
MY FANCY COLOGNE & PERFUME (Miahati)				

*Consult Sec. II., Ingredients Index. This ingredient may be responsible for major toxic effects if poisonous amounts of this product are ingested.

- 716 -

Name & Use Manufacturer	Ingredients		Name & Use Manufacturer	Ingredients	
MY-PINE DISINFECT- ANT (Meyer Bros.)	Steam-distilled pine oil* Soap		MYSTIKIL ROACH POWDER (Lethelin)	Boric acid* Pyrethrum	70%
MY PRESCRIPTION Antacid (Crockenberg)	Bismuth subnitrate Ammonium citrate		MYSTIKIL ROSE DUST Insecticide, fungicide (Lethelin)	Gamma isomer of benzene hexachloride DDT* Zineb (zinc ethylene bis(dithio carbamate)) Sulfur*	1% 5% 3.9% 20.0%
MYRO PORCELAIN, TILE & MARBLE CLEANER (My-Ko)			MYSTIKIL TERMITE EMULSION, MTE (Concentrate) Insecticide (Lethelin)	Chlordane*	72.3%
MY-RUB Rubbing alcohol compound (Meyer Bros.)	Alcohol*	70%/v	MYTEE BOND FISHING ROD CEMENT (Slomons)		
MYSTACIN Antibiotic and antihistaminic cream (Nemow)	Mercury oleate* Digidex (2, 2'-dihydroxy- 3, 5, 6, 3', 5', 6'-hexa- chlorodiphenyl methane) Benzocaine Pyrilamine maleate* Tyrothricin Cresol* Coal tar	0.4% 0.05%	MYTINIC Dietary supple- ment (Bristol Labs.)	Each fl. oz.: Ferric ammonium citrate, green, N.F. Thiamine hydrochloride Riboflavin Niacinamide Liver fraction 1 N.F. Vitamin B12 Sodium benzoate	667 mg. 10 mg. 4 mg. 100 mg. 1 gm. 20 gm. 0.1%
MYSTERIOUS ROACH KILLER OUTFITS; MYSTERIOUS ROACH POWDER (Lethelin)	Pyrethrum DDT* Boric acid*	0.225% 10.000% 53.000%	MYTINIC TABLETS Dietary supple- ment (Bristol Labs.)	Each tablet: Dried ferrous sulfate Liver fraction 2 N.F. Thiamine HCl Riboflavin Niacinamide Pyridoxine HCl Calcium pantothenate Ascorbic acid Vitamin B12	225.0 mg. 330.0 mg. 3.3 mg. 1.3 mg. 10.00 mg. 0.5 mg. 2.0 mg. 50.0 mg. 5 gm.
MYSTIC CREAM Cosmetic (Whitehall)	Sodium potassium stearate and palmitate Glycerin Unguent base Oxycholestrins				
MYSTIC DRI QUICK Dry cleaning compound (Mystic Foam)			MY-T-MITE HARTZ MOUNTAIN POWDER Insecticide (Hartz)	Rotenone	0.50%
MYSTIC FOAM, MYSTIC ZIP Cleaners (Mystic Foam)					
MYSTIC FRESH UP RUG & UP- HOLSTERY CLEANER (Mystic Foam)					
MYSTIC HAND CREAM (Whitehall)					
MYSTIC HAND LOTION (Whitehall)					

*Consult Sec. II., Ingredients Index. This ingredient may be responsible for major toxic effects if poisonous amounts of this product are ingested.

Name & Use Manufacturer	Ingredients	
NACCANOL Photographic supplies (Nat'l. Chem.)		
NA-CHURS LIQUID FERTILIZER (Na-Churs)	Nitrogen Phosphoric acid Potash	7% 14% 7%
NA-CHURS LIQUID FERTILIZER 10-20-10 (Na-Churs)	Nitrogen Phosphorus Potash	10% 20% 10%
NACO ALDRIN 118 COTTON DUST 2.5-5-40 Insecticide (Davison)	Aldrin* DDT* Sulfur* Theoret. chlorine*	2.50% 5.00% 40.00% 4.47%
NACO ALDRIN 118 DUST 2.5-5.0 Insecticide (Davison)	Aldrin* DDT* Theoret. chlorine*	2.50% 5.00% 4.47%
NACO BENNY-HEX COTTON DUST Insecticide (Davison)	Gamma BHC* Other isomers DDT*	3% 5% 5%
NACO BENNY-HEX COTTON DUST WITH SULPHUR Insecticide (Davison)	Gamma BHC* Other isomers DDT* Sulfur*	3% 5% 5% 40%
NACO BHC CONC. NO. 120 Insecticide (Davison)	Gamma BHC* Other isomers	12% 21%
NACO 10% DDT Insecticide (Davison)	DDT*	10.00%
NACO 5% DDT DUST Insecticide (Davison)	DDT*	5.00%
NACO 50% DDT DUST BASE CONC. Insecticide (Davison)	Tech. DDT*	50%
NACO 50% DDT WETTABLE CONC. Insecticide (Davison)	Tech. DDT*	50%
NACO 10% DITHANE Z-78 Insecticide (Davison)	Zinc ethylene bisdithio- carbamate	6.50%
NACO 15% FERMATE DUST Insecticide (Davison)	Ferric dimethyl dithiocarbamate	11.40%

Name & Use Manufacturer	Ingredients	
NACO 1% PARATHION DUST Insecticide (Davison)	Parathion*	1.00%
NACO 15% PARATHION WETTABLE POWDER Insecticide (Davison)	Parathion*	15%
NACO 25% PARATHION WETTABLE POWDER Insecticide (Davison)	Parathion*	25%
NACO 20% TOXAPHENE COTTON DUST Insecticide (Davison)	Toxaphene*	20%
NACO 20% TOXAPHENE COTTON DUST WITH SULPHUR Insecticide (Davison)	Sulfur Toxaphene*	40% 20%
NACO 40% TOXAPHENE DUST BASE CONC. & WETTABLE CONC. Insecticide (Davison)	Toxaphene*	40%
NACOR Antitussive (Nacor)	Alcohol Potassium iodide Ammonium chloride	6% 30 gr.
NACOR KAPS Antitussive (Nacor)	Potassium iodide* Ammonium chloride	1-7/8 gr.
NACORLAX TABLETS Cathartic (Nacor)	Ext. belladonna Total alkaloids Ext. cascara aloin*	1/1280 gr.
NACREM Nasal decongestant cream (Jenkins)	Ammonium chloride Menthol* Methyl salicylate* (syn.) Camphor* Oil eucalyptus*	1.5% q.s. q.s. q.s. q.s.
NACTION TABLETS (Van-S)	Methyl cellulose	
NACTO FABRIC CLEANER (Nacto)		
NACTO GREES-WASH (Nacto)		
NACTO TAR REMOVER (Nacto)		

*Consult Sec. II., Ingredients Index. This ingredient may be responsible for major toxic effects if poisonous amounts of this product are ingested.

Name & Use Manufacturer	Ingredients	
NACTO WATERLESS HAND CLEANER (Nacto)		
NADINOLA BLEACHING CREAM (Nat'l. Toilet)	Ammoniated mercury* Bismuth subnitrate Zinc oxide	5%
NADISAL Analgesic, antipyretic (Lilly)	Alcohol Sodium salicylate* Aromatics	5% 7.5 gm./100 cc.
NAFTEX For skin irritations (Lascoff)	Refined fractions of petroleum Aliphatic hydrocarbons Aromatic and naphthenic hydrocarbons*	
N'AIMEZ QUE MOI EXTRACT Cosmetic (Caron)		
NAIRN SELF POLISHING WAX (Congoleum-Nairn)		
NA-KLOR 40 D DUST BASE CONC. Insecticide (Davison)	Chlordane*	40%
NA-KLOR 40 W WETTABLE CONC. Insecticide (Davison)	Chlordane*	40%
N-ALCOS-O Counter-irritant (Bullock-Walker)	Methyl salicylate* Menthol* Turpentine* Thymol* Camphor* Zinc oxide	
NAPHTHA MINERAL SPIRITS (Western Rosin)		
NAPKO DRY CLEANER (Kumfort)		
NAP-LENE MOTH BLOCK Insecticide (Relible-Chem.)	Naphthalene*	
NAP-OL OINTMENT For nipples during nursing (Superior Pharm.)	Bismuth subnitrate Castor oil Lanolin anhydrous Ceresin wax Balsam Peru Tr. benzoin compound	30% 30% 32% 4% 3% 1%

Name & Use Manufacturer	Ingredients	
NAPRYLATE POWDER & OINTMENT Skin fungicide (medical) (Strasenburgh)	Sodium caprylate Zinc caprylate	10% 5%
NAPTOX (Naphthenate preservative) Fungicide (Speekman)	Copper* naphthenate Petroleum distillate*	20% 80%
NARADA RHEUMATIC TABLETS (Denver Radium)		
NARAKON Nasal decongestant (Baybank)	Benzalkonium chloride* Allantoin	
NARAKON WITH DESOXY-EPHEDRINE Nasal decongestant (Baybank)	Desoxyephedrine hydrochloride* Benzalkonium chloride* Allantoin	1%
NARCISSE BLEU PERFUME SOAP (Corot)		
NARCISSE PERFUME, TOILET WATER & COLOGNE (Corot)		
NARCISSE NOIR EXTRACT (Caron)		
NARTON Tonic (veterinary, avian) (Gland-O-Lac)	Sodium arsanilate* Procaine penicillin Manganese sulfate Aureomycin hydrochloride Vitamin B12 Nux vomica* Cobalt sulfate Wild mustard Quassia Copper sulfate Areca nut Gentian Foenugreek Anise oil Diatomaceous earth Antibiotic adsorbents Soya bean meal	1.50% 120 mg./lb. 0.33% 250 mg./lb. 430 mg per lb. 11.25% 2.7%
NASAL-AID JELLY Nasal decongestant (Massengill)	Ephedrine sulfate* Sodium chloride Oil cinnamon Menthol* Boric acid* Carbolic acid* Chlorobutanol	1% 3/4%

---

*Consult Sec. II., Ingredients Index. This ingredient may be responsible for major toxic effects if poisonous amounts of this product are ingested.

Name & Use Manufacturer	Ingredients	Name & Use Manufacturer	Ingredients
NASDRO NO. 3 WITH EPHEDRINE (Aqueous) Nose and throat drops and spray (Jenkins)	Ephedrine sulfate* 1% Chlorobutanol with menthol* 0.5% Camphor* Oil eucalyptus* Thymol* Oil red thyme	NATURE-FRESH To preserve flavor and stop browning in freezing and home canning (Approved)	Cevitamic acid (vitamin C)
NASDRO NO. 4 WITH EPHEDRINE (Aqueous) Nose and throat drops or spray (Jenkins)	Ephedrine sulfate* 3% Chlorobutanol with menthol* 0.5% Camphor* Oil eucalyptus Thymol* Oil red thyme	NAUGATUCK ALANAP-1 Herbicide (Naugatuck)	n-1-Naphthyl phthalamic acid* 90%
NASOMIST Antihistamine nasal decongestant (Dumas-Wilson)	Pyrilamine maleate* 0.5% Ephedrine HCl* 0.5% Chlorobutanol (chloral deriv.) 0.5% Camphor* q.s. Menthol* q.s. Dextrose q.s.	NAUGATUCK ALANAP-3 Herbicide (Naugatuck)	n-1-Naphthyl phthalamic acid* 22%
NASPRIN WITH GELSEMIUM Analgesic (Tailby)	Acetophenetidin* 2 gr. Aspirin* 3 gr. Caffeine* 1/8 gr. Tincture gelsemium 2 m.	NAUGATUCK ALANAP TECHNICAL Insecticide (Naugatuck)	n-1-Naphthyl phthalamic acid* 95%
NATCOL HAIR LOTION (Laser)		NAUGATUCK ARAMITE TECHNICAL Insecticide (Naugatuck)	2-(p-tert-Butylphenoxy) isopropyl 2-chloroethyl sulfite 90%
NATEX Tonic laxative (McKewen)	Alcohol 16% Aloin Frangula Bitter orange peel Sarsaparilla Senna F.E. cascara Gentian Licorice	NAUGATUCK ARAMITE 15W Insecticide (Nagatuck)	2-(p-tert-Butylphenoxy) isopropyl 2-chloroethyl sulfite 15%
		NAUGATUCK THIRAM 50 DUST (Naugatuck)	Thiram* (tetramethyl thiuram disulfide) 50%
		NAUGATUCK THIRAM TECHNICAL (Naugatuck)	Thiram* (tetramethyl thiuram disulfide) 97%
NATONE NOSE DROPS Nasal decongestant (Boyle & Co.)	Ephedrine sulfate* 1% Chlorobutanol 0.5% Aqueous-isotonic mentholated solution	NAUGATUCK THIRAM 75W (Naugatuck)	Thiram* (tetramethyl thiuram disulfide) 75%
		NAUGETS (Naugatuck)	Thiram* (tetramethyl thiuram disulfide) 75%
NATPIRIN Analgesic (Schiff)	Sodium salicylate* 7.5 gr. Kelp from Pacific sea kelp Calcium carbonate Oil wintergreen natural*	NAVAL STORES GUM SPIRITS OF TURPENTINE (Naval Stores)	Alpha-pinene* 2/3 Beta-pinene* 1/3
NATRIPHENE DISIN-FECTANT (Natriphene)	Sodium salt of 2-hydroxy diphenyl* 100%	NAVAP Inhalant (McKesson)	Ethyl alcohol* 75%/v 4-Beta-ethyl hexyl phenol* 0.63% Eucalyptol Menthol Thymol Camphor* Aromatics
NATRIPHENE FUNGICIDE (Natriphene)	Sodium salt of 2 hydroxy diphenyl,* medical grade 100%		
NATROSE TABLETS Dietary suplement (Horton & Converse)	Sodium chloride U.S.P. 7 gr. Dextrose 3 gr.	DR. NAYLOR'S ANTISEPTIC DRES (Naylor)	Carbolic acid* Picric acid* Oils of castor, thyme, thuja and clove

*Consult Sec. II., Ingredients Index. This ingredient may be responsible for major toxic effects if poisonous amounts of this product are ingested.

- 720 -

Name & Use Manufacturer	Ingredients		Name & Use Manufacturer	Ingredients	
DR. NAYLOR'S ANTISEPTIC DUSTING POWDER (Naylor)	Chlorothymol* Thymol iodide* Tannic acid* Boric acid*		NEATAMINE LOTION Lotion for hands and body (Ghem. Ind.)	Neatsfoot oil Alcohol	5-1/2%
DR. NAYLOR'S BLU-KOTE Antiseptic for wounds (Naylor)	Acriflavine gentian violet Sodium propionate Urea Glycerin Isopropyl alcohol* 30%		NEATSOL BASE Ointment base for skin irritations (Chem. Ind.)	Neatsfoot oil	
DR. NAYLOR'S DEHORNING PASTE Veterinary (Naylor)	Caustic soda* Calcium hydroxide Glycerin		NECRONO (Hess, Dr.)	Nitrofurazone* Magnesium aluminum silicate	
DR. NAYLOR'S DIRENE (Naylor)	Bismuth subnitrate Kaolin Aluminum hydroxide Magnesium oxide Zinc phenolsulfonate Catechu Calcium carbonate precip.		NEECE ANTISEPTIC (Earle)	Alcohol* 80-83% Camphor* Menthol* Methyl salicylate* Resorcin* Benzocaine Wormwood	
DR. NAYLOR'S LOUSE & GRUB POWDER (Naylor)	Rotenone* 1.67% Other cube extractives 3.33% Pyrethrins 0.11% Dusting sulfur* 12%		NEET CREAM ODORLESS HAIR REMOVER (Whitehall)	Calcium thioglycolate*	
DR. NAYLOR'S MEDICATED TEAT DILATORS (Naylor)	Sulfathiazole Methyl violet* Antiseptic ointment: Oxyquinoline* Menthol Eucalyptol* Camphor* Oils of thyme, clove, thuja, pine* Petrolatum Lanolin		NEET ODORLESS LOTION Hair remover (Whitehall)	Calcium thioglycolate*	
DR. NAYLOR'S STOP-A-LEAK For cows' teats that leak milk (Naylor)	Iodine* Alcohol 20%/v Monesia Ethyl acetate		NELATOL (Haslam)	Syrup of ipecac* Syrup of squill* Syrup of tolu Honey	
DR. NAYLOR'S UDDER BALM Antiseptic ointment (veterinary) (Naylor)	Oxyquinoline* Menthol* Oils of thyme, clove, thuja, pine* Petrolatum Eucalyptol* Camphor* Lanolin		NELCO LACQUERS, ENAMELS, COATINGS (New Eng. Lacquer)		
			NELSON'S ANTACID MIXTURE (Nelson Baker)	Carbonates of sodium, magnesium and calcium	
DR. NAYLOR'S UDDER LINIMENT (Naylor)	Thymol* Methyl salicylate* Oil pine* Oil wormwood* Menthol* Camphor* Oil thuja		NELSON'S DOUCHOL Dusting powder or cleansing douche (Great Lakes Labs.)	Boric acid* Ammonium alum Oxyquinoline sulfate Zinc sulfate* Carbolic acid* Aromatics	
N & B LINIMENT (Erie)	Art. oil sassafras* Oil eucalyptus* Synthetic oil wintergreen* Capsicum		NELSON'S SHAVING LOTION (Nelson, Detroit)	Alcohol* 54%	
NEATAMINE CREAM Skin cleanser (Chem. Ind.)	Neatsfoot oil Triethanolamine		NEMAGON Soil fumigant (Shell Chem.)	1,2-Dibromo-3-chloropropane* 97.0% Related brominated and/or chlorinated C_3 hydrocarbons 2.0%	

Name & Use Manufacturer	Ingredients	
NEMARON Dietary supplement with iron (Veltex)	Each capsule: Vitamin B12 Liver fraction no. 2 Folic acid Ferrous gluconate Stomach activating powder	25 μg. 200 mg. 0.67 mg. 300 mg. 100 mg.
NEMA WORM CAPSULES Anthelmintic (veterinary) (Parke, Davis)	Tetrachlorethylene*	
NEMEX SOIL FUMIGANT (Larvacide)	Ethylene dibromide*	23%
NEMEX 42 SOIL FUMIGANT (Larvacide)	Ethylene dibromide*	42%
NEMOW TABLETS Analgesic for menstruation (Nemow)	Each tablet: Acetophenetidin* Phenylpropanol amine hydrochloride* (propadrine' hydrochloride) Aspirin*	2 gr.
NEO-A-FIL Hypo-allergenic sunscreening prep. (Texas Pharm.)	Digalloyl trioleate	3%
NEO-AQUA-DRIN Throat lozenges (McKesson)	Each lozenge: Tyrothricin Benzocaine	2 mg. 10 mg.
NEO-AQUA-DRIN Antibiotic nasal decongestant (McKesson)	Ephedrine* as lactate Gramicidin Sodium mercuric thiosalicylate	1% 0.004% 0.004%
NEOBASE BRAND GREASELESS OINTMENT BASE (Burroughs-Wellcome)	Mineral oil Emulsifying agents Preservative	
NEO BISCALOX (Jeffrey-Fell)	Anesthesin* Cerium oxalate* Bismuth subcarbonate Magnesium carb levis Aromatics	1 4 gr. 1 gr. 2 gr. 4 gr. q.s.
NEOBOVININE 20 Dietary supplement (Wyeth Labs.)	Each 100 cc.: Ferric ammonium citrate Defibrinated beef blood Liver fraction 1, N.F.	0.68 gm. 56 gm. 7.6 gm.
NEO-BROM DEPPS Nerve sedative (Atlas Drug)	Each oz.: Sodium bromide* Potassium bromide* Ammonium bromide* Tr. adonis Vitamin B1	40 gr. 40 gr. 32 gr. 16 m. 320 I.U.

Name & Use Manufacturer	Ingredients	
NEOCAL For skin irritations (Wisconsin Pharm.)	Calamine Zinc oxide Phenol* Neocalamine Glycerin Bentonite	
NEO CARON CREME For skin burns (Jeffrey-Fell)	Each fl. oz.: Linseed oil Lime water Ethyl amino benzoate	q.s. q.s. 1/2 of 1%
NEO-COL TABLETS (Sacramento)		
NEOCURTASAL Seasoning agent for salt-free diet (Winthrop)	Potassium chloride Ammonium chloride Potassium formate Calcium formate Magnesium citrate Potassium iodide	0.01%
NEO-DERMATOLE Local anesthetic skin lotion (Tone)	Camphor* Benzocaine Aluminum acetate Resorcinol Distilled coal tar Menthol* Carbolic acid* Zinc oxide Alcohol	5% 1% 10%
NEO-DEX BABY POWDER (Wright, M.)	Hexachlorophene Tincture of benzoin Balsam of Peru Zinc oxide Camphor Starch Menthol Thymol Talc	
NEO-DEX OINTMENT For diaper rash (Wright, M.)	Hexachlorophene Benzocaine Cod liver oil Olive oil Tinct. benzoin compound Calamine Zinc oxide	
NEO-FERINE Intranasal decongestant (Success)	Sodium chloride Sodium benzoate Sodium bisulfite Neo-ferine brand of ephedrine* lactate	0.5% 0.1% 0.1%
NEOFRIN 1% (Rafea)	Synthetic salts of ephedrine* and epinephrine* Sod. benzoate Sod. chloride Sod. bisulfite	0.1% 0.8% 0.1%
NEOL Respiratory decongestant (veterinary, avian) (Gland-O-Lac)	Oils of thyme N.F. 6 and eucalyptus* Beechwood creosote* Chlororthophenylphenol* Liquid petrolatum Chlorophyll	0.05%
NEOMARK LOTION For dandruff and skin irritations (C & M)	Salicylic acid* Betanaphthol Castor oil Isopropanol* Solution of coal tar* Resorcin monoacetate* Camphor water*	2% 1% 5% 2% 2.5%

Name & Use Manufacturer	Ingredients	Name & Use Manufacturer	Ingredients
NEON TUBE PAINT (Clantz)		NEOTAR OINTMENT For skin irritations (Lascoff)	Empyreumatic oil of juniper*
NEO-PHEN CAPSULES (Sacramento)		NEO-THRYCEX (Children's) Nose drops (Wright, M.)	Tyrothricin 0.01% Menthol
NEOPHRIN ANTIHISTA-MINE NASAL DECONGES-TANT (Horton & Converse)	Phenylephrine hydrochloride 0.25% Pyrilamine maleate 0.5% Chlorobutanol 0.2% Menthol 0.1% Camphor 0.1%	NEO-THRYCEX ISOTONIC ANTIBIOTIC Nose drops (Wright, M.)	Tyrothricin 0.02% Ephedrine hydrochloride* Menthol
NEO-SAL Sedative (Western Pharm.)	Each tsp.: Sodium bromide* 11 gr. Potassium bromide* 3 gr. Strontium bromide* 1 gr. Neo-Sal, as citrates of sodium, potassium and magnesium Calcium lactate and sodium bicarbonate	NEOTRAN Acaricide (Dow)	Bis (parachlorophenoxy) methane*
		NEOTRAN, WETTABLE Insecticide (Florida Agric.)	Bis (p-chlorophenoxy) methane* as a dry wettable powder formerly known as K-1875) 40%
NEO-SAL Effervescent antacid, diuretic (Western Pharm.)	Sodium citrate 19 gr. Potassium citrate 9 gr. Calcium lactate 5 gr. Magnesium citrate 1 gr. Sodium bicarbonate 10 gr.	NEOTROL Nasal decongestant (Hance)	Phenylephrine HCl 0.25% Pyrilamine maleate 0.2% Cetalkonium chloride 0.05% Tyrothricin 0.03% Phenyl mercuric acetate 1-50,000
NEO-SAL WITH ANALGESIC COMPOUND (Western Pharm.)	Aspirin* 6.40 gr. Acetophenetidin* 3.20 gr. Caffeine alkaloid* 0.06 gr. Neo-Sal: as citrates of sodium, potassium and magnesium Calcium lactate and sodium bicarbonate	NEPHRON INHALANT (Nephron)	Synthetic epinephrine (racemic)* 2.9% Chlorobutanol (chloroform deriv.) 0.5%
NEO-SEPTINE For skin irritations (Leavens Prods.)	Benzoic acid* Glycerin Oil peppermint Saccharin Sodium borate* Tr. vanallin co. Boric acid* Menthol* Phenol* Oil cloves Tinc. cudbear	NEPTUNE LUBRICATING GREASE (Fiske)	
		NERVINE Sedative (Hance)	Each fl. oz.: Sodium bromide* 12 gr. Potassium bromide* 12 gr. Ammonium bromide* 6 gr.
NEOSORB TABLETS & LIQUID Antacid, adsorbent (Haack)	Each tablet: Aluminum hydroxide gel (dried) 0.26 gm. Magnesium trisilicate 0.45 gm. Methylcellulose (a mucin like colloid) 0.065 gm. Liquid: 1 tbsp. is equiv. to 2 Neosorb tablets	NERVTABS Sedative (Manhattan Drug)	Each tablet: Pot. bromide* 3 gr. Sod. bromide* 3 gr. Ammon. bromide* 1-1/2 gr. Passiflora 2 gr. Gelsemium 1/4 gr. Hyoscyamus 1/4 gr.
NEOSPAZ Antispasmodic, sedative, antacid tablet (Continental Drug)	Phenobarbital* 1/4 gr. Hyoscyamine sulfate* Charcoal activated Aluminum hydroxide Atropine sulfate* Hyoscine hydrogen bromide* Magnesium trisilicate	NESS' 5% CHLORDANE DUST Insecticide (Beebe Ness)	Chlordane tech.* 5%
		NESTLE-LE MUR HAIR RINSES, COLORS, LACQUERS (Nestle-Le Mur)	
NEO-SULF OINTMENT (Thomas & Thompson)	Oil of rose geranium Deod. oil G.D. 4440 Vlemincks solution* Tragacanth Glycerin Zinc sulfate *	NETHACOL (Merrell)	Each fl. oz.: Alcohol 5% Nethamine hydrochloride 65 mg. F.E. ipecac 0.06 cc. Ammonium chloride 0.65 gm. Menthol 8 mg.

*Consult Sec. II., Ingredients Index. This ingredient may be responsible for major toxic effects if poisonous amounts of this product are ingested.

Name & Use Manufacturer	Ingredients
NETTLE HAIR TONIC (Germadol)	
NEUDUST Insecticide (Bonide)	Dichloro diphenyl trichloro-ethane* 5%/w
NEURABALM Liniment, antiseptic (external) (S.S.S.)	Alcohol 54% Chloroform* 24 m./fl. oz. Methyl salicylate* Chloroform* Alcohol S.D. 27 Oil of eucalyptus* Camphor* Menthol Chlorothymol* Acetone* Oil of cajeput* Benzocaine
NEUROINE Sedative (Link)	Each fl. oz.: Bromide of soda* approx. 47gr. Alcohol 16-2/3% Extract of lettuce Celery seed Passion flower
NEU-TONE ALKYD FLAT ENAMEL FOR WALLS AND WOODWORK 666 CHARTREUSE (Martin-Senour)	Pigment: 60% Titanium calcium pigment Titanium dioxide Calcium carbonate Silica and silicates Vehicle: 40% Alkyd resin varnish* Mineral spirits* and driers
NEU-TONE FLAT OIL FINISH (Martin-Senour)	
NEUTOX Insecticide (Bonide)	Dichloro diphenyl trichloro-ethane* 50%/w
NEUTRA Neutral wet spotter, penetrant, lubricant (Adco)	
NEUTRACID Antacid, adsorbent (Internat. Labs.)	Calcium tribasic phosphate Colloidal kaolin Magnesium tribasic phosphate Calcium and magnesium carbonate
NEUTRALIZE For eye burns (Bullard)	Monobasic potassium phosphate Dibasic sodium phosphate Chlorobutanol 0.25%
NEUTROX (Vick)	Sodium perborate*(U.S.P. dehydrated) 32.3% Mono-calcium phosphate* 32.3% Tri-calcium phosphate* 24.6% Basic magnesium carbonate 10.8%
NEVA-ROT Wood preservative (Glidden Co.)	

Name & Use Manufacturer	Ingredients
NEV-A-RUST Paint product (Glidden Co.)	
NEVASCO BRAND PRODUCTS AF-1-DI NO. 1 Fungicide (Nevasco)	Petroleum oil* Dichloro ethyl ether* Soap, anhydrous
NEVER FREEZE Anti-freeze compound (Mirrorlike)	
NEVERLEAK TIRE FLUID For tire leaks (Liquid)	
NEV'R CREEP BICYCLE RIM CEMENT (Van Cleef)	
NEVR-DULL MAGIC CREME WAX (Basch)	
NEWCASTLE DISEASE VACCINE LIVE VIRUS Veterinary, avian (Gland-O-Lac)	Antibiotics*: Dihydrostreptomycin* Penicillin
NEW ERA SHOE POLISH Shoe polish (Whittemore)	
NEW NAP CARPET CLEANER CONC. (Rex Home)	
NEWPORT PERFUME & COLOGNE (Caswell-Massey)	
NEWPORT TOILET WATER (Caswell-Massey)	
NEWS Detergent (Purex Corp.)	Alkyl aryl sulfonate* Polyphosphates Sulfates
NEW-SKIN Antiseptic covering (Newskin)	Alcohol 8.7% Pyroxylin solution* Oil of cloves 8-Hydroxyquinoline*

*Consult Sec. II., Ingredients Index. This ingredient may be responsible for major toxic effects if poisonous amounts of this product are ingested.

- 724 -

Name & Use Manufacturer	Ingredients	
NEWTON'S CPR DUST Insecticide (Newton Chem.)	Rotenone Piperonyl cyclonene Pyrethrins Other cube resins	0.25% 0.5% 0.05% 0.40%
NEWTON'S 6% DITHANE DUST Fungicide (Newton Chem.)	Zineb	3.9%
NEWTON'S 6% DITHANE-3% DDT DUST Insecticide (Newton Chem.)	Zineb (zinc ethylene bis-(dithiocarbamate)) DDT	3.9% 3%
NEWTON'S 7-1 DUST Insecticide (Newton Chem.)	Copper* as basic copper sulfate DDT	7% 1%
NEWTON'S 50-3 DUST Insecticide (Newton Chem.)	DDT Sulfur*	3% 50%
NEWTON'S DUST NO. 3, 5, & 10 Insecticide (Newton Chem.)	DDT* 3%, 5%, and 10%	
NEWTON'S 10% MARLATE DUST Insecticide (Newton Chem.)	Methoxychlor	10%
NEWTON'S 3% & 5% NICOTINE DUST Insecticide (Newton Chem.)	Nicotine* alkaloid 3% and 5%	
NEWTON'S 5% RHOTHANE-7% COPPER DUST Insecticide (Newton Chem.)	TDE Copper* as basic copper sulfate	5% 7%
NEWTON'S 5% RHOTHANE DUST Insecticide (Newton Chem.)	TDE	5%
NEWTON'S 3/4% ROTENONE DUST Insecticide (Newton Chem.)	Rotenone* Other cube resins	0.75% 1.2%
NEWTON'S 1% ROTENONE DUST Insecticide (Newton Chem.)	Rotenone* Other cube resins	1% 1.6%

Name & Use Manufacturer	Ingredients	
NEWTON'S 1% ROTENONE-50% SULFUR-3% DDT DUST Insecticide (Newton Chem.)	Rotenone Other cube resins Sulfur* DDT	1% 1.8% 50% 3%
NEWTON'S SPECIAL DUST (6% Dithane-5% Rhothane) Insecticide (Newton Chem.)	Zineb TDE	3.9% 5%
NEWTON'S TRI-BASIC COPPER NO. 7 DUST Fungicide (Newton Chem.)	Metallic copper* (from basic copper sulfate) 7%	
NEWTON'S TRI-BASIC 7-3 DUST Insecticide (Newton Chem.)	Copper* as basic copper sulfate DDT	7% 3%
NEWTON'S TRI-BASIC 7-5 DUST Insecticide (Newton Chem.)	Copper* as basic copper sulfate DDT*	7% 5%
NEWTON'S TRI-BASIC 7-20 DUST Insecticide (Newton Chem.)	Copper as basic copper sulfate Calcium arsenate*	7% 13.8%
NEWTON'S VETERINARY COMPOUND For indigestion (Newton Horse)	Stramonium seed Arsenous acid Tartar emetic* Calcium hydroxide Iron oxide (ferric) Red pepper	1.8% 0.9% 2.4% 64.0%
NEY CREAM DEODORANT (Evans, G.)		
NEY LIQUID DEODORANT (Myers Labs.)	Alcohol* Aluminum chloride Camphor*	49%
nf-180 TABLETS Bacteriostatic (veterinary) (Hess, Dr.)	Furazolidone (n-(5-nitro-2-furfurylidene)-3-amino-2-oxazolidone)* 50 mg.	
N-44 Photographic supplies (Nat'l. Chem. Co.)		
NIAGARA ALDRIN EQUIVALENT 10 DUST Insecticide (Niagara Chem.)	Hexachloro-hexahydro-dimethano naphthalene* Related compounds	9.40% 7.16%

*Consult Sec. II., Ingredients Index. This ingredient may be responsible for major toxic effects if poisonous amounts of this product are ingested.

Name & Use Manufacturer	Ingredients	Name & Use Manufacturer	Ingredients
NIAGARA ALDRIN MISCIBLE Insecticide (Niagara Chem.)	Hexachloro hexahydro dimethano naphthalene* 22.09% Related compounds 16.66% Xylene* 53.00%	NIAGARA BHC-NIATOX- SULPHUR 2- 10-50 DUST Insecticide (Niagara Chem.)	Gamma isomer of benzene hexachloride* 2% Other isomers of benzene hexachloride 11% DDT* 10% Sulfur* 50%
NIAGARA AM SOL Herbicide (Niagara Chem.)	2,4-D acid* (amine salt) 4 lb.	NIAGARA BHC-1 NIATOX-5 SULPHUR DUST Insecticide (Niagara Chem.)	Gamma isomer of benzene hexachloride* 3% Other isomers of benzene hexachloride 5.55% DDT* 5% Sulfur* 40%
NIAGARA BASIC COPPER SULPHATE Fungicide (Niagara Chem.)	Copper* expressed as metallic 53.50%	NIAGARA BHC 1.0 PEACH DUST Fungicide (Niagara Chem.)	Gamma isomer of benzene hexachloride* 1% Other isomers of benzene hexachloride 5.55% Sulfur* 52.80%
NIAGARA BASIC LEAD ARSENATE Insecticide (Niagara Chem.)	Basic powdered arsenate of lead* 96%	NIAGARA BHC 10 SPRAY Insecticide (Niagara Chem.)	Gamma isomer of benzene hexachloride* 10.00% Other isomers of benzene hexachloride* 55.57%
NIAGARA BASIC ZINC SULPHATE Fungicide (Niagara Chem.)	Zinc* as metallic 50%	NIAGARA BHC SPRAY & DIP Insecticide (Niagara Chem.)	Tech. BHC*
NIAGARA BHC CROP SPRAY Insecticide (Niagara Chem.)	Tech. BHC*	NIAGARA BHC 2 SULPHUR DUST Insecticide (Niagara Chem.)	Gamma isomer of benzene hexachloride* 2% Other isomers of benzene hexachloride 11.11% Sulfur* 50%
NIAGARA BHC 1.0 DUST Insecticide (Niagara Chem.)	Gamma isomer of benzene hexachloride* 1% Other isomers of benzene hexachloride 6.67%	NIAGARA BHC 3 SULPHUR DUST Insecticide (Niagara Chem.)	Gamma isomer of benzene hexachloride* 3% Other isomers of benzene hexachloride 16.66% Sulfur* 40%
NIAGARA BHC 1.2 DUST Insecticide (Niagara Chem.)	Gamma isomer of benzene hexachloride* 1.20% Other isomers of benzene hexachloride 6.66%	NIAGARA BLUEBERRY DUST 50-10- 40 Insecticide (Niagara Chem.)	Tricalcium arsenate* 35% Monohydrated copper sulfate 10%
NIAGARA BHC 1.5 DUST Insecticide (Niagara Chem.)	Gamma isomer of benzene hexachloride* 1.50% Other isomers of benzene hexachloride 8.33%	NIAGARA BRAND LAUNDRY STARCH (Corn Prod.)	Boric acid* 5% Calcium chloride less than 1/10 of 1% Deactivated enzyme 1/2 of 1%
NIAGARA BHC MISCIBLE Insecticide (Niagara Chem.)	Gamma isomer of benzene hexachloride* 11.60% Other isomers of benzene hexachloride 15.58% Xylene* 54.50%	NIAGARA CALCIUM ARSENATE Insecticide (Niagara Chem.)	Calcium arsenate*
NIAGARA BHC 1- NIATOX 5 DUST Insecticide (Niagara Chem.)	Gamma isomer of benzene hexachloride* 1% Other isomers of benzene hexachloride 5.55% DDT* 5%	NIAGARA CARBAMATE Fungicide (Niagara Chem.)	Ferbam* 76%
NIAGARA BHC-NIATOX- SULPHUR 2- 5-50 DUST Insecticide (Niagara Chem.)	Gamma isomer of benzene hexachloride* 2% Other isomers of benzene hexachloride 12% DDT* 5% Sulfur* 50%		

*Consult Sec. II., Ingredients Index. This ingredient may be responsible for major toxic effects if poisonous amounts of this product are ingested.

- 726 -

Name & Use Manufacturer	Ingredients		Name & Use Manufacturer	Ingredients	
NIAGARA CARBAMATE APPLE NIATOX 5 DUST Insecticide (Niagara Chem.)	Standard lead arsenate* Ferbam DDT	15% 7% 5%	NIAGARA CHLORKIL 10 DUST Insecticide (Niagara Chem.)	Tech. chlordane*	10%
NIAGARA CARBAMATE DUST Fungicide (Niagara Chem.)	Ferbam	7%	NIAGARA CHLORKIL 72 MISCIBLE Insecticide (Niagara Chem.)	Chlordane*	8 lb./gal.
NIAGARA CARBAMATE DUST FOR TOBACCO Fungicide (Niagara Chem.)	Ferbam	11.40%	NIAGARA CHLORKIL 25 SPRAY Insecticide (Niagara Chem.)	Tech. chlordane*	25%
NIAGARA CARBAMATE KOLODUST Fungicide (Niagara Chem.)	Ferric dimethyl dithiocarbamate Sulfur*	3% 41.50%	NIAGARA CHLORKIL 40 SPRAY Insecticide (Niagara Chem.)	Chlordane*	40%
NIAGARA CARBAMATE NIATOX 5 DUST Insecticide (Niagara Chem.)	Ferbam DDT*	7% 5%	NIAGARA CHLORO I.P.C. MISCIBLE Herbicide (Niagara Chem.)	Isopropyl n(3-chlorophenyl) carbamate*.	47.00%
NIAGARA CARBAMATE PHOSKIL DUST Insecticide (Niagara Chem.)	Sulfur Ferbam Parathion*	10% 6.60% 1.00%	NIAGARA C-O-C-S BHC 1 DUST Insecticide (Niagara Chem.)	Copper* expressed as metallic 5% Gamma isomer of benzene hexachloride* 1% Other isomers of benzene hexachloride 5.55%	
NIAGARA CHELATE OF IRON To correct iron deficiency in soil (Niagara Chem.)	Iron as metallic	9.0%	NIAGARA C-O-C-S BHC 1.2 DUST Insecticide (Niagara Chem.)	Gamma isomer of benzene hexachloride* 1.20% Other isomers of benzene hexachloride 8% Copper* expressed as metallic 6%	
NIAGARA CHLORDANE 5 DUST Insecticide (Niagara Chem.)	Tech. chlordane*	5%	NIAGARA C-O-C-S 7 CHLORKIL 5 DUST Fungicide (Niagara Chem.)	Copper* expressed as metallic 7% Chlordane* 5%	
NIAGARA CHLORINATED CAMPHENE DUST Insecticide (Niagara Chem.)	Chlorinated camphene* Sulfur*	20% 40%	NIAGARA C-O-C-S COPODUST Fungicide (Niagara Chem.)	Copper* expressed as metallic (copper oxychloride sulfate) 6%	
NIAGARA CHLORKIL 5 DUST Insecticide (Niagara Chem.)	Tech. chlordane*	5%	NIAGARA C-O-C-S COPODUST SPECIAL Fungicide (Niagara Chem.)	Copper* expressed as metallic 6%	
			NIAGARA C-O-C-S COPOTEX Insecticide (Niagara Chem.)	Copper oxychloride sulfate Calcium arsenate*	

*Consult Sec. II., Ingredients Index. This ingredient may be responsible for major toxic effects if poisonous amounts of this product are ingested.

Name & Use Manufacturer	Ingredients	Name & Use Manufacturer	Ingredients
NIAGARA C-O-C-S COPOTEX, EXTRA STRENGTH Insecticide (Niagara Chem.)	Copper expressed as metallic 12% Tricalcium arsenate* 28%	NIAGARA C-O-C-S METHOXCIDE 5 DUST Insecticide (Niagara Chem.)	Copper* expressed as metallic 6% Methoxychlor tech. 5%
NIAGARA C-O-C-S COPOTROL DUST Insecticide (Niagara Chem.)	Tricalcium arsenate* 14% Copper expressed as metallic 6%	NIAGARA C-O-C-S NIATOX DUST Insecticide (Niagara Chem.)	DDT 2% Copper oxychloride*
NIAGARA C-O-C-S COPOZIM DUST Fungicide (Niagara Chem.)	Copper* expressed as metallic 6%	NIAGARA C-O-C-S NIATOX 3 DUST Insecticide (Niagara Chem.)	DDT 3% Copper* expressed as metallic 6%
NIAGARA C-O-C-S COPOZIM LINDANE 0.75 DUST Insecticide (Niagara Chem.)	Copper* expressed as metallic 6% Gamma isomer of benzene hexachloride 0.75%	NIAGARA C-O-C-S NIATOX 3-10 DUST Insecticide (Niagara Chem.)	Copper expressed as metallic 3% DDT* 10%
NIAGARA C-O-C-S COPOZIM SPRAY Insecticide (Niagara Chem.)	Copper* expressed as metallic 33.30%	NIAGARA C-O-C-S NIATOX 5 DUST Insecticide (Niagara Chem.)	DDT* 5% Copper oxychloride sulfate*
NIAGARA C-O-C-S DDD 5 DUST Insecticide, fungicide (Niagara Chem.)	Copper* expressed as metallic 6% DDD* 5%	NIAGARA C-O-C-S NIATOX 6-10 DUST Insecticide (Niagara Chem.)	Copper* expressed as metallic 6% DDT* 10%
NIAGARA C-O-C-S DUST FOR GRAPES Fungicide (Niagara Chem.)	Copper* expressed as metallic 6%	NIAGARA C-O-C-S 7-NIATOX 5 DUST Insecticide (Niagara Chem.)	Copper* expressed as metallic 7% DDT* 5%
NIAGARA C-O-C-S KOLOKILL Insecticide (Niagara Chem.)	Sulfur 48% Standard lead arsenate* 15% Copper expressed as metallic 5%	NIAGARA C-O-C-S NIATOX DUST, EXTRA STRENGTH Insecticide (Niagara Chem.)	DDT* 9% Copper* expressed as metallic 18%
NIAGARA C-O-C-S LINDANE 1 DUST Insecticide (Niagara Chem.)	Copper* expressed as metallic 6% Gamma isomer of benzene hexachloride* 1%	NIAGARA C-O-C-S NIATOX GRAPE DUST Insecticide fungicide (Niagara Chem.)	Copper* expressed as metallic 7.00% DDT* 5.00%
NIAGARA C-O-C-S METHOXCIDE 3 DUST Insecticide (Niagara Chem.)	Copper* expressed as metallic 5% Methoxychlor tech. 3%	NIAGARA C-O-C-S NIATOX 5 KOLODUST Insecticide (Niagara Chem.)	Sulfur* 53% DDT* 5% Copper* expressed as metallic 3.50%

*Consult Sec. II., Ingredients Index. This ingredient may be responsible for major toxic effects if poisonous amounts of this product are ingested.

Name & Use Manufacturer	Ingredients		Name & Use Manufacturer	Ingredients	
NIAGARA C-O-C-S PHOSKIL 1 DUST Insecticide (Niagara Chem.)	Copper expressed as metallic Parathion*	6% 1%	NIAGARA COPODUST Fungicide (Niagara Chem.)	Monohydrated copper sulfate*	20%
NIAGARA C-O-C-S 7 PHOSKIL 2 DUST Fungicide (Niagara Chem.)	Copper expressed as metallic Parathion*	7% 2%	NIAGARA COPOITE Insecticide (Niagara Chem.)	Monohydrated copper sulfate Lead arsenate*	15% 15%
NIAGARA C-O-C-S QUIK-KILL COPOTEX Insecticide (Niagara Chem.)	Copper expressed as metallic Tricalcium arsenate* Calcium arsenite	5.27% 22.05% 1.93%	NIAGARA COPOTEX Insecticide (Niagara Chem.)	Monohydrated copper sulfate Tri-calcium arsenate*	20% 17.50%
NIAGARA C-O-C-S ROTENONE-BEARING DUST Insecticide (Niagara Chem.)	Copper* expressed as metallic Rotenone* Other cube resins or extractives	5% 0.75% 0.75%	NIAGARA COPOZIM DDD 3 SPRAY Insecticide (Niagara Chem.)	Copper* expressed as metallic DDT* Sulfur*	19.8% 15% 5.6%
NIAGARA C-O-C-S SPRAY 65 Fungicide (Niagara Chem.)	Copper* expressed as metallic	34%	NIAGARA COPOZIM EMULSO Insecticide (Niagara Chem.)	Petroleum oils* Copper* expressed as metallic	48.50% 3.30%
NIAGARA C-O-C-S SULPHUR DUST NO. 5 Fungicide (Niagara Chem.)	Sulfur* Copper oxychloride sulfate*	82.50% 8.93%	NIAGARA COPOZIM NIATOX 3 SPRAY Insecticide (Niagara Chem.)	Copper* expressed as metallic DDT*	19.8% 15.0%
NIAGARA C-O-C-S SULPHUR NIATOX 6-50-5 DUST Insecticide (Niagara Chem.)	Sulfur* DDT* Copper* expressed as metallic	50% 5% 6%	NIAGARA COPPER-BEARING DUST Fungicide (Niagara Chem.)	Monohydrated copper sulfate*	15%
NIAGARA C-O-C-S SULPHUR NIATOX 6-50-10 DUST Insecticide (Niagara Chem.)	Copper* expressed as metallic Sulfur* DDT*	6% 50% 10%	NIAGARA COPPER BHC 1 DUST Insecticide (Niagara Chem.)	Basic copper sulfate* Gamma isomer of benzene hexachloride* Other isomers of benzene hexachloride	9.43% 1% 5.55%
NIAGARA COMMERCIAL BRUSH KILLER Herbicide (Niagara Chem.)	2,4,5-Trichloro phenoxy acetic acid,* butoxy ethanol ester 2,4-Dichloro phenoxy acetic acid,* butoxy ethanol ester	29.60% 30.90%	NIAGARA COPPER COMPOUND NO. 53 Fungicide (Niagara Chem.)	Basic copper sulfate*	53%
			NIAGARA COPPER 7 DUST Fungicide (Niagara Chem.)	Copper* expressed as metallic	7%
NIAGARA COMMERCIAL FLOUR SULPHUR Fungicide (Niagara Chem.)	Sulfur*	99.5%	NIAGARA COPPER-LEAD-NIATOX 5 DUST Insecticide (Niagara Chem.)	Monohydrated copper sulfate Standard lead arsenate* DDT	15% 15% 5%

*Consult Sec. II., Ingredients Index. This ingredient may be responsible for major toxic effects if poisonous amounts of this product are ingested.

Name & Use Manufacturer	Ingredients		Name & Use Manufacturer	Ingredients	
NIAGARA COPPER NIATOX 3 DUST Insecticide (Niagara Chem.)	DDT Copper* expressed as metallic	3% 7%	NIAGARA D-B TREATED BLUESTONE Fungicide (Niagara Chem.)	Copper sulfate* crystals	88%
NIAGARA COPPER NIATOX 5 DUST Insecticide (Niagara Chem.)	DDT* Copper* expressed as metallic	5% 7%	NIAGARA DDD 5 COPPER 7 DUST Insecticide (Niagara Chem.)	DDD Copper*	5% 7%
NIAGARA COPPER NIATOX GRAPE DUST Insecticide (Niagara Chem.)	DDT* Copper* expressed as metallic	5% 7%	NIAGARA DDD 5 DUST Insecticide (Niagara Chem.)	DDD	5%
NIAGARA COPPER 2.5 ROTENONE-BEARING 0.75 DUST Insecticide (Niagara Chem.)	Copper* expressed as metallic Rotenone* Other cube resins or extractive	2.5% 0.75% 0.75%	NIAGARA DDD DUST FOR TOBACCO Insecticide (Niagara Chem.)	DDD	10%
NIAGARA COPPER ROTENONE-BEARING DUST Insecticide (Niagara Chem.)	Copper* expressed as metallic Rotenone* Other cube resins or extractives	6% 0.75% 0.75%	NIAGARA DDD 25 MISCIBLE Insecticide (Niagara Chem.)	Dichloro diphenyl dichloro-ethane (DDD) Xylene*	25.00% 70.50%
NIAGARA COPPER 7 SULPHUR DUST Insecticide (Niagara Chem.)	Sulfur* Copper* expressed as metallic	30% 7%	NIAGARA DDD PHOSKIL 5-2 DUST Insecticide (Niagara Chem.)	DDT Parathion*	5.00% 2.00%
NIAGARA 3-10-0 COTTON DUST Insecticide (Niagara Chem.)	Gamma isomer of benzene hexachloride* Other isomers of benzene hexachloride DDT*	3% 18% 10%	NIAGARA DDD TEPP 5-1.0 DUST Insecticide (Niagara Chem.)	DDD Tetraethyl pyrophosphate* Other ethyl phosphates	5% 1% 2%
NIAGARA 3-10-40 COTTON DUST Insecticide (Niagara Chem.)	Gamma isomer of benzene hexachloride* Other isomers of benzene hexachloride* DDT* Sulfur*	3% 20% 10% 40%	NIAGARA DDD 50 WETT-ABLE POWDER Insecticide (Niagara Chem.)	DDD (dichloro diphenyl dichloroethane)*	50%
NIAGARA CR 50 DUST Insecticide (Niagara Chem.)	Sodium fluoaluminate*	45%	NIAGARA DDT Insecticide (Niagara Chem.)	DDT*	100%
NIAGARA CUCURBIT DUST Insecticide (Niagara Chem.)	Copper expressed as metallic Tricalcium arsenate*	5% 5.25%	NIAGARA DDT 4.5 LIQUI MIST Insecticide (Niagara Chem.)	DDT* Petroleum oils*	4.5% 95.50%
			NIAGARA D-6 DUST MIXTURE Fungicide (Niagara Chem.)	Monohydrated copper sulfate*	20%
			NIAGARA D-18 DUST MIXTURE Insecticide (Niagara Chem.)	Monohydrated copper sulfate Tri-calcium arsenate*	20% 17.50%

*Consult Sec. II., Ingredients Index. This ingredient may be responsible for major toxic effects if poisonous amounts of this product are ingested.

Name & Use Manufacturer	Ingredients	Name & Use Manufacturer	Ingredients
NIAGARA D-20 DUST MIXTURE Insecticide (Niagara Chem.)	Monohydrated copper sulfate 20% Tri-calcium arsenate* 14%	NIAGARA DIELDRIN 50 WETTABLE POWDER Insecticide (Niagara Chem.)	Hexachloro epoxy octahydro dimethano naphthalene* (from dieldrin) 42.50% Related compounds (from dieldrin) 7.50%
NIAGARA D-25 DUST MIXTURE Fungicide (Niagara Chem.)	Monohydrated copper sulfate* 25%	NIAGARA DINITRO DRY Insecticide (Niagara Chem.)	Dinitro ortho cresol* 40%
NIAGARA DIELDRIN 1.5 DUST Insecticide (Niagara Chem.)	Hexachloro epoxy octahydro dimethano naphthalene* 1.275% Related compounds 0.225%	NIAGARA DN DORMANT QUICK-MIX HEAVY Insecticide (Niagara Chem.)	Petroleum oil* 97% Dinitro-o-cyclo-hexylphenol* 2%
NIAGARA DIELDRIN MISCIBLE Insecticide (Niagara Chem.)	Hexachloro epoxy octahydro dimethano naphthalene* 14.45% Related compounds 2.55% Polymethylated naphthalenes* 75.00%	NIAGARA DN SUMMER SPRAY Insecticide (Niagara Chem.)	Dinitro-o-cyclohexylphenol dicyclohexylamine salt* 20%
NIAGARA DIELDRIN 1.5 MISCIBLE Insecticide (Niagara Chem.)	Hexachloro epoxy octahydro dimethano naphthalene* 15.83% Related compounds 2.79% Xylene* 73.38%	NIAGARA DORMANT FLOWABLE EMULSION Insecticide (Niagara Chem.)	Petroleum oil* 80%
NIAGARA DIELDRIN 1.5-NIATOX 5 DUST Insecticide (Niagara Chem.)	Hexachloro epoxy octahydro dimethano naphthalene*(from dieldrin) 1.275% Related compounds (from dieldrin) 0.225% DDT* 5.000%	NIAGARA DORMANT QUIK-MIX HEAVY Insecticide (Niagara Chem.)	Petroleum oil* 98%
NIAGARA DIELDRIN 1.5-NIATOX 10 DUST Insecticide (Niagara Chem.)	Hexachloro epoxy octahydro dimethano naphthalene* (from dieldrin) 1.275% Related compounds (from dieldrin) 0.225% DDT* 10.000%	NIAGARA DRY LIME SULPHUR Insecticide (Niagara Chem.)	Calcium polysulfide* 70% Calcium thiosulfate 5% Free sulfur 5%
NIAGARA DIELDRIN 1.5-NIATOX 5-SULPHUR 40 DUST Insecticide (Niagara Chem.)	Hexachloro epoxy octahydro dimethano naphthalene* (from dieldrin) 1.275% Related compounds (from dieldrin) 0.225% DDT* 5% Sulfur* 40%	NIAGARA 20-5-75 DUST Insecticide (Niagara Chem.)	Standard lead arsenate* 20% Sulfur 5%
NIAGARA DIELDRIN 1.5-NIATOX 10-SULPHUR 40 DUST Insecticide (Niagara Chem.)	Hexachloro epoxy octahydro dimethano naphthalene* (from dieldrin) 1.275% Related compounds (from dieldrin) 0.225% Sulfur* 40.00%	NIAGARA DUST 300 Fungicide (Niagara Chem.)	Sulfur* 57% Petroleum oil 5%
		NIAGARA DUST 302 Fungicide (Niagara Chem.)	Sulfur 52% Lead arsenate* 10% Petroleum oil 5%
NIAGARA DIELDRIN 2.5-NIATOX 10-SULPHUR 40 DUST Insecticide (Niagara Chem.)	Hexachloro epoxy octahydro dimethano naphthalene* (from dieldrin) 2.125% Related compounds (from dieldrin) 0.375% DDT* 10% Sulfur* 40%	NIAGARA DUST 533 Fungicide (Niagara Chem.)	Sulfur 52% Lead arsenate* (basic) 14% Petroleum oil 5%
		NIAGARA 7 DUST FOR TOMATOES Fungicide (Niagara Chem.)	Manganese ethylene bis-(dithiocarbamate) 4.90%

*Consult Sec. II., Ingredients Index. This ingredient may be responsible for major toxic effects if poisonous amounts of this product are ingested.

Name & Use Manufacturer	Ingredients		Name & Use Manufacturer	Ingredients	
NIAGARA DUSTING SULPHUR Insecticide (Niagara Chem.)	Sulfur*	98%	NIAGARA GRANULAR 2% ALDRIN DUST Insecticide (Niagara Chem.)	Hexachloro hexahydro dimethano naphthalene* Related compounds	1.90% 1.43%
NIAGARA EAR-TICK-OIL Insecticide (Niagara Chem.)	Gamma isomer of benzene hexachloride Other isomers of benzene hexachloride	0.72% 4.75%	NIAGARA GRANULAR 5% ALDRIN DUST Insecticide (Niagara Chem.)	Hexachloro hexahydro dimethano naphthalene* Related compounds	4.75% 3.58%
NIAGARA EMULSO Insecticide (Niagara Chem.)	Petroleum oil emulsion*	83%	NIAGARA HEPTACHLOR 1.5 DUST Insecticide (Niagara Chem.)	Heptachlor* Related compounds	1.50% 0.58%
NIAGARA EMULSO 90 Insecticide (Niagara Chem.)	Petroleum oils*	89%	NIAGARA HEPTACHLOR 2.0 MISCIBLE Insecticide (Niagara Chem.)	Heptachlor* Related compounds Petroleum distillate	23.41% 9.10% 61.36%
NIAGARA ENDRIN 2 DUST Insecticide (Niagara Chem.)	Endrin*(hexachloro epoxy octahydro-endo,endo-dimethano naphthalene)	2%	NIAGARA HOOKER PARACIDE Insecticide (Niagara Chem.)	Paradichlorbenzene*	100%
NIAGARA ESTASOL Herbicide (Niagara Chem.)	2,4-D Acid*(isopropyl ester) 3.34 lb. per gal.		NIAGARA HORTICUL-TURAL'S ROSE DUST Insecticide (Niagara Chem.)	Sulfur Arsenic* Nicotine*	80% 1% 2%
NIAGARA ETHYLENE DICHLORIDE EMULSION Insecticide (Niagara Chem.)	Ethylene dichloride*	88%	NIAGARA HOUSEHOLD SPRAY BHC Insecticide (Niagara Chem.)	Gamma isomer of BHC DDT Organic thiocyanate	0.75% 0.50% 0.50%
NIAGARA FARM BRUSH KILLER Herbicide (Niagara Chem.)	2,4,5-Trichlorophenoxyacetic acid, butoxy ethanol ester* 2,4-Dichlorophenoxyacetic acid,* butoxy ethanol ester	10.80% 22.60%	NIAGARA IPC 25 MISCIBLE Herbicide (Niagara Chem.)	Isopropyl n-phenyl carbamate	25%
NIAGARA FERBAM TOBACCO DUST Fungicide (Niagara Chem.)	Ferbam	11.40%	NIAGARA KOLO 100 Fungicide, insecticide (Niagara Chem.)	Sulfur* Phygon (2,3-dichloro-1, 4-napthoquinone)	75.40% 3.50%
NIAGARA 9 GAMMA BHC DUST BASE Insecticide (Niagara Chem.)	Gamma isomer of benzene hexachloride* Other isomers of benzene hexachloride*	9.00% 50.00%	NIAGARA KOLO APPLE NIATOX 5 DUST Insecticide (Niagara Chem.)	DDT Lead arsenate* Sulfur	5% 15% 10%
NIAGARA GRANULAR 25% ALDRIN BASE Insecticide (Niagara Chem.)	Hexachloro hexahydro dimethano naphthalene* Related compounds	23.750% 17.915%	NIAGARA KOLOBEAN SPRAY Fungicide (Niagara Chem.)	Sulfur* Copper* expressed as metallic	50% 3.09%

Name & Use Manufacturer	Ingredients
NIAGARA KOLO BHC 4.8 COTTON DUST Insecticide (Niagara Chem.)	Gamma isomer of benzene hexachloride* 4.80% Other isomers of benzene hexachloride* 32% Sulfur* 17.20%
NIAGARA KOLO BHC 1.0 DUST Insecticide (Niagara Chem.)	Gamma isomer of benzene hexachloride* 1% Other isomers of benzene hexachloride 5.55% Sulfur* 41%
NIAGARA KOLO 30-BHC 1.0 DUST Insecticide (Niagara Chem.)	Gamma isomer of benzene hexachloride 1% Other isomers of benzene hexachloride 5.55% Sulfur 9%
NIAGARA KOLO BHC 3 DUST Insecticide (Niagara Chem.)	Gamma isomer of benzene hexachloride* 3% Other isomers of benzene hexachloride* 16.66% Sulfur* 52.25%
NIAGARA KOLO BHC 3-NIATOX 5 PEACH DUST Insecticide (Niagara Chem.)	Gamma isomer of benzene hexachloride* 3% Other isomers of benzene hexachloride* 18% DDT* 5% Sulfur* 40% Petroleum distillate 1%
NIAGARA KOLO BHC PEACH SPRAY Insecticide (Niagara Chem.)	Gamma isomer of benzene hexachloride* 3% Other isomers of benzene hexachloride* 20% Sulfur* 15%
NIAGARA KOLO CARBAMATE Fungicide (Niagara Chem.)	Ferbam* Fused bentonite sulfur
NIAGARA KOLO CARBAMATE 200 Insecticide (Niagara Chem.)	Ferbam 10.80% Sulfur* 69%
NIAGARA KOLOCIDE Livestock spray (Niagara Chem.)	DDT* 32.60% Gamma isomer of benzene hexachloride* 3.50% Sulfur 4.60%
NIAGARA KOLO C-O-C-S NIATOX 5 DUST Insecticide (Niagara Chem.)	Sulfur 10% Copper* expressed as metallic 6% DDT* 5%
NIAGARA KOLOCOP BHC 1.5 DUST Insecticide (Niagara Chem.)	Sulfur* 30% Copper* expressed as metallic 6% Gamma isomer of benzene hexachloride* 1.5% Other isomers of benzene hexachloride* 10%
NIAGARA KOLOCOP DDD 5 DUST Insecticide (Niagara Chem.)	Sulfur* 30% Copper* expressed as metallic 6% DDD 5.0%
NIAGARA KOLOCOP DUST Insecticide (Niagara Chem.)	Copper* expressed as metallic 6% Sulfur* 60%
NIAGARA KOLOCOP NIATOX 3 DUST Insecticide (Niagara Chem.)	Sulfur* 30% Copper* expressed as metallic 6% DDT 3%
NIAGARA KOLO 2-10-40 COTTON DUST Insecticide (Niagara Chem.)	Gamma isomer of benzene hexachloride* 2% Other isomers of benzene hexachloride 11.11% DDT* 10% Sulfur* 40%
NIAGARA KOLO 3-10-40 COTTON DUST Insecticide (Niagara Chem.)	Gamma isomer of benzene hexachloride* 3% Other isomers of benzene hexachloride 16.66 DDT* 10% Sulfur* 38%
NIAGARA KOLO DIELDRIN 1.5-NIATOX 5-SULPHUR 40 DUST Insecticide (Niagara Chem.)	Hexachloro epoxy octahydro dimethano naphthalene* 1.275% Related compounds (from dieldrin) 0.225% DDT* 5% Sulfur* 40%
NIAGARA KOLODUST Insecticide, fungicide (Niagara Chem.)	Sulfur* 84%
NIAGARA KOLODUST-100 Fungicide (Niagara Chem.)	Sulfur* 83.16% Phygon 0.50%
NIAGARA KOLODUST BHC 75-1 DUST Insecticide (Niagara Chem.)	Sulfur* 63% Gamma isomer of benzene hexachloride* 1% Other isomers of benzene hexachloride 6.66%
NIAGARA KOLODUST BL 30 DUST Insecticide (Niagara Chem.)	Sulfur 56.25% Basic lead arsenate* 30%

*Consult Sec. II., Ingredients Index. This ingredient may be responsible for major toxic effects if poisonous amounts of this product are ingested.

Name & Use Manufacturer	Ingredients		Name & Use Manufacturer	Ingredients	
NIAGARA KOLODUST CA 25-75 DUST Insecticide (Niagara Chem.)	Sulfur Tri calcium arsenate*	20% 51%	NIAGARA KOLODUST METHOXCIDE 5 DUST Fungicide (Niagara Chem.)	Sulfur* Methoxychlor tech.	74% 5%
NIAGARA KOLODUST C-O-C-S DIELDRIN 50-6-1.5 DUST Insecticide (Niagara Chem.)	Sulfur* Copper* as metallic Hexachloro epoxy octahydro dimethano naphthalene* Related compounds	42% 6% 1.27% 0.23%	NIAGARA KOLODUST METHOXCIDE 75-5 DUST Insecticide (Niagara Chem.)	Sulfur* Methoxychlor	63% 5%
NIAGARA KOLODUST C-O-C-S 50-6 DUST Fungicide (Niagara Chem.)	Copper* expressed as metallic Sulfur*	6% 42%	NIAGARA KOLODUST METHOXCIDE 85-5 DUST Insecticide (Niagara Chem.)	Sulfur* Methoxychlor	71% 5%
NIAGARA KOLODUST C-O-C-S NIATOX 50-6-5 DUST Insecticide (Niagara Chem.)	Sulfur* Copper* expressed as metallic DDT*	42% 6% 5%	NIAGARA KOLODUST NIAGARATRAN 50-7.5 DUST Insecticide (Niagara Chem.)	Sulfur* p-Chlorophenyl p-chlorobenzene sulfonate*	42% 7.5%
NIAGARA KOLODUST DDD 30-5 DUST Insecticide (Niagara Chem.)	Sulfur* DDD	25% 5%	NIAGARA KOLODUST NIATOX CHLORDANE 50-5-3 DUST Fungicide (Niagara Chem.)	Sulfur* DDT* Tech. chlordane*	42% 5% 3%
NIAGARA KOLODUST DDD 75-5 DUST Insecticide (Niagara Chem.)	DDD Sulfur*	5% 63%	NIAGARA KOLODUST NIATOX 5 DUST Insecticide (Niagara Chem.)	DDT* Sulfur*	5% 67.50%
NIAGARA KOLODUST DIELDRIN 75-1.5 DUST Insecticide (Niagara Chem.)	Sulfur* Hexachloro epoxy octahydro dimethano naphthalene* Related compounds	63% 1.27% 0.23%	NIAGARA KOLODUST NIATOX 10 DUST Insecticide (Niagara Chem.)	DDT* Sulfur*	10% 64.60%
NIAGARA KOLODUST EXTRA Fungicide (Niagara Chem.)	Sulfur*	69%	NIAGARA KOLODUST NIATOX 50-5 DUST Insecticide (Niagara Chem.)	DDT* Sulfur*	5% 42%
NIAGARA KOLODUST MALATHION 25-4 DUST Insecticide (Niagara Chem.)	Malathion* Sulfur*	4% 21%	NIAGARA KOLODUST NIATOX 50-10 DUST Insecticide (Niagara Chem.)	Sulfur* DDT*	42% 10%
NIAGARA KOLODUST MALATHION 50-4 DUST Insecticide (Niagara Chem.)	Malathion* Sulfur*	4% 42%	NIAGARA KOLODUST NIATOX 75-5 DUST Insecticide (Niagara Chem.)	Sulfur* DDT*	63% 5%

*Consult Sec. II., Ingredients Index. This ingredient may be responsible for major toxic effects if poisonous amounts of this product are ingested.

Name & Use Manufacturer	Ingredients	
NIAGARA KOLODUST NIATOX 75-10 DUST Insecticide (Niagara Chem.)	DDT* Sulfur*	10% 66%
NIAGARA KOLODUST NIATOX PHOSKIL 50-5-.5 DUST Insecticide (Niagara Chem.)	Sulfur DDT Parathion*	45% 5% 0.50%
NIAGARA KOLODUST NIATOX PHOSKIL 50-5-1 DUST Insecticide (Niagara Chem.)	Sulfur DDT Parathion*	45% 5% 1%
NIAGARA KOLODUST NIATOX TOXAKIL 50-5-10 DUST Insecticide (Niagara Chem.)	Sulfur * DDT* Toxaphene*	42% 5% 10%
NIAGARA KOLODUST PHOSKIL 1 DUST Insecticide, fungicide (Niagara Chem.)	Sulfur Parathion*	77% 1%
NIAGARA KOLODUST 100-PHOSKIL 1 DUST Insecticide (Niagara Chem.)	Sulfur Parathion* 2,3-Dichloro-1,4-naphthoquinone	76.12% 1% 0.50%
NIAGARA KOLODUST 100-PHOSKIL 1.5 DUST Insecticide (Niagara Chem.)	Sulfur Parathion* 2,3-Dichloro-1,4-naphthoquinone	73.20% 1.50% 0.50%
NIAGARA KOLODUST-PHOSKIL 75-2 DUST Insecticide (Niagara Chem.)	Parathion* Sulfur	2% 63%
NIAGARA KOLODUST-PHOSKIL 90-2 DUST Insecticide (Niagara Chem.)	Parathion* Sulfur	2.00% 75.00%

Name & Use Manufacturer	Ingredients	
NIAGARA KOLODUST-TEPP 35-1.0 DUST Insecticide (Niagara Chem.)	Sulfur Tetraethyl pyrophosphate* Other ethyl phosphates	30% 1% 2%
NIAGARA KOLODUST-TOXAKIL 50-10 DUST Insecticide (Niagara Chem.)	Sulfur Toxaphene*	42% 10%
NIAGARA KOLODUST XTRA Fungicide (Niagara Chem.)	Fused bentonite sulfur dust*	
NIAGARA KOLODUST XTRA DUST OR SPRAY Fungicide (Niagara Chem.)	Fused bentonite sulfur dust*	
NIAGARA KOLODUST-ZEC 75-8 DUST Insecticide (Niagara Chem.)	Zineb Sulfur*	8% 63%
NIAGARA KOLODUST ZINEB 80-3.25 DUST Fungicide (Niagara Chem.)	Zineb Sulfur*	3.25% 67.20%
NIAGARA KOLO-EX 90 DUST Insecticide (Niagara Chem.)	Sulfur*	27%
NIAGARA KOLOFOG Fungicide (Niagara Chem.)	Fused bentonite sulfur*	
NIAGARA KOLOFOG WETTEX Insecticide (Niagara Chem.)	Fused bentonite sulfur*	
NIAGARA KOLOFRUIT PHOSKIL 1 DUST Insecticide (Niagara Chem.)	Parathion* Lead arsenate* Sulfur	1% 15% 10%
NIAGARA KOLOITE Insecticide (Niagara Chem.)	Sulfur Basic lead arsenate*	60% 10%

*Consult Sec. II., Ingredients Index. This ingredient may be responsible for major toxic effects if poisonous amounts of this product are ingested.

Name & Use Manufacturer	Ingredients	
NIAGARA KOLOKIL Insecticide (Niagara Chem.)	Fused bentonite sulfur Lead arsenate*	15%
NIAGARA KOLOKIL NIATOX 5 DUST Insecticide (Niagara Chem.)	DDT Standard lead arsenate* Sulfur	5% 15% 61%
NIAGARA KOLOKIL NIATOX 10 DUST Insecticide (Niagara Chem.)	Sulfur Standard lead arsenate* DDT	51.65% 15% 10%
NIAGARA KOLOKIL SPECIAL Insecticide (Niagara Chem.)	Fused bentonite sulfur Lead arsenate*	25%
NIAGARA KOLO MALATHION CARBAMATE DUST Insecticide, fungicide (Niagara Chem.)	Sulfur* Malathion* Ferbam*	60.20% 4.00% 7.00%
NIAGARA KOLO M-550 DUST Insecticide (Niagara Chem.)	Standard lead arsenate* Sulfur	30% 20%
NIAGARA KOLO M-555 DUST Insecticide (Niagara Chem.)	Standard lead arsenate* Sulfur	20% 25%
NIAGARA KOLOMENTAL 753-NIATOX 5 DUST Insecticide (Niagara Chem.)	Sulfur* Copper* expressed as metallic DDT*	30% 6% 5%
NIAGARA KOLO M-555 NIATOX 5 DUST Insecticide (Niagara Chem.)	DDT Lead arsenate* Sulfur	5% 20% 26%
NIAGARA KOLO-NIATOX 5-BHC 1.5 DUST Insecticide (Niagara Chem.)	Sulfur* Gamma isomer of benzene hexachloride* Other isomers of benzene hexachloride DDT*	50% 1.50% 10% 5%

Name & Use Manufacturer	Ingredients	
NIAGARA KOLO NIATOX 5 DUST Insecticide (Niagara Chem.)	DDT* Sulfur*	5% 10%
NIAGARA KOLO NIATOX 10 DUST Insecticide (Niagara Chem.)	DDT* Sulfur*	10% 10%
NIAGARA KOLO NIATOX 3-PHOSKIL 1 DUST Insecticide (Niagara Chem.)	Sulfur Parathion* DDT	65.90% 1% 3%
NIAGARA KOLO NIATOX 5-PHOSKIL 1.5 DUST Insecticide (Niagara Chem.)	Sulfur Parathion* DDT	30% 1.5% 5%
NIAGARA KOLONOX Insecticide (Niagara Chem.)	DDT* Gamma isomer of benzene hexachloride Other isomers of benzene hexachloride Sulfur	27.00% 1.08% 7.20% 8.10%
NIAGARA KOLO-PEACH Insecticide (Niagara Chem.)	Sulfur Standard lead arsenate*	66% 5%
NIAGARA KOLO PHOSKIL 1 DUST Insecticide (Niagara Chem.)	Sulfur Parathion* Petroleum oil	10% 1% 2%
NIAGARA KOLO PHOSKIL 1.5 DUST Insecticide (Niagara Chem.)	Sulfur Parathion* Petroleum distillate	10% 1.50% 2%
NIAGARA KOLO PHOSKIL DUST 15 Insecticide (Niagara Chem.)	Sulfur Parathion*	69.25% 1.50%
NIAGARA KOLO PHOSKIL 1-NIATOX 3 DUST Insecticide (Niagara Chem.)	Parathion* DDT Sulfur	1% 3% 10%

---

*Consult Sec. II., Ingredients Index. This ingredient may be responsible for major toxic effects if poisonous amounts of this product are ingested.

Name & Use Manufacturer	Ingredients	
NIAGARA KOLO PHOSKIL PEACH SPRAY Insecticide (Niagara Chem.)	Parathion* Sulfur	3% 52.60%
NIAGARA KOLO PHOSKIL 2 SPRAY Insecticide (Niagara Chem.)	Sulfur Parathion*	53% 3%
NIAGARA KOLO PHYGON 1 DUST Fungicide (Niagara Chem.)	Sulfur* 2,3-Dichloro-1,4 naphthoquinone*	30% 1.0%
NIAGARA KOLO PHYGON SPRAY Fungicide (Niagara Chem.)	Sulfur* Dichlone*	15.5% 7.5%
NIAGARA KOLO RANGE CATTLE SPRAY Insecticide (Niagara Chem.)	Gamma isomer of benzene hexachloride* Other isomers of benzene hexachloride* DDT* Sulfur	1.60% 8.90% 26.70% 6%
NIAGARA KOLO ROTENONE - BEARING DUST Insecticide (Niagara Chem.)	Rotenone Fused bentonite sulfur*	0.75%
NIAGARA KOLO ROTENONE- BEARING 1.0 DUST Insecticide (Niagara Chem.)	Sulfur* Rotenone Other cube resins or extractive	29% 1% 1%
NIAGARA KOLO ROTENONE- BEARING 1-NIATOX 3 DUST Insecticide (Niagara Chem.)	Sulfur* Rotenone Other cube resins or extractives DDT	40% 1% 1% 3%
NIAGARA KOLO ROTENONE SPECIAL DUST Insecticide (Niagara Chem.)	Rotenone Other cube resins or extractives Sulfur*	0.85% 0.85% 29%

Name & Use Manufacturer	Ingredients	
NIAGARA KOLOROTE SULPHUR ROTENONE- BEARING DUST 75 Insecticide (Niagara Chem.)	Rotenone Other cube resins or extractives Sulfur*	0.75% 0.75% 56.50%
NIAGARA KOLOSPRAY Fungicide (Niagara Chem.)	Fused bentonite sulfur*	
NIAGARA KOLO STRAW- BERRY DUST Insecticide, fungicide (Niagara Chem.)	DDT* Tech. chlordane* Sulfur*	5% 5% 50%
NIAGARA KOLOTEX Fungicide (Niagara Chem.)	Sulfur Standard lead arsenate*	73.70% 10%
NIAGARA KOLO THREE-N-ONE COTTON DUST Insecticide (Niagara Chem.)	Gamma isomer of benzene hexachloride* Other isomers of benzene hexachloride DDT* Sulfur*	3% 16.66% 5% 33.70%
NIAGARA KOLO TOXAKIL 5 DUST Insecticide (Niagara Chem.)	Sulfur* Toxaphene*	60% 5%
NIAGARA KOLOTOX DUST Fungicide (Niagara Chem.)	Sulfur Lead arsenate*	72% 5%
NIAGARA KOLOZIM NIATOX 5 DUST Insecticide (Niagara Chem.)	Sulfur* DDT*	67.50% 5%
NIAGARA KOLOZIM PHOSKIL DUST 15 Insecticide (Niagara Chem.)	Sulfur Parathion*	67.5% 1.5%
NIAGARA KOLOZINC Fungicide (Niagara Chem.)	Fused bentonite sulfur Zinc sulfate*	
NIAGARA L-10 DUST Insecticide (Niagara Chem.)	Standard lead arsenate*	10%

*Consult Sec. II., Ingredients Index. This ingredient may be responsible for major toxic effects if poisonous amounts of this product are ingested.

Name & Use Manufacturer	Ingredients		Name & Use Manufacturer	Ingredients	
NIAGARA L-15 DUST Insecticide (Niagara Chem.)	Standard lead arsenate*	14.40%	NIAGARA LINDANE 25 SPRAY Insecticide (Niagara Chem.)	Lindane*	25%
NIAGARA L-40 DUST Insecticide (Niagara Chem.)	Standard lead arsenate*	38.40%	NIAGARA LINDANE 75 SPRAY Insecticide (Niagara Chem.)	Gamma isomer of benzene hexachloride*	75%
NIAGARA LEAD KOLOZINC Insecticide (Niagara Chem.)	Fused bentonite sulfur Lead arsenate* Zinc sulfate		NIAGARA LIQUID NIATOX 25 Insecticide (Niagara Chem.)	DDT Polymethylated naphthalenes Xylene*	25% 23% 45.50%
NIAGARA LEAD KOLOZINC NO. 2 Insecticide (Niagara Chem.)	Sulfur Lead arsenate*	42% 16.10%	NIAGARA LIQUID NIATOX 35 SOLUTION Insecticide (Niagara Chem.)	DDT* Polymethylated naphthalenes	35% 65%
NIAGARA LIME SULPHUR SOLUTION Fungicide (Niagara Chem.)	Calcium polysulfide*	29%	NIAGARA LIQUID NIATOX 33 SPRAY Insecticide (Niagara Chem.)	DDT* 2.81 lbs. per gal. Xylene* base	
NIAGARA LINDANE 25 CONC. Insecticide (Niagara Chem.)	Gamma isomer of benzene hexachloride* Xylene	25% 54%	NIAGARA LIQUI-MIST DORMANT Fungicide (Niagara Chem.)	Petroleum oil*	99%
NIAGARA LINDANE 1 DUST Insecticide (Niagara Chem.)	Gamma isomer of benzene hexachloride	1%	NIAGARA LIQUI-STIK CONC. Insecticide (Niagara Chem.)	Naphthalene acetic acid*	5.70%
NIAGARA LINDANE 1.5 DUST Insecticide (Niagara Chem.)	Gamma isomer of benzene hexachloride*	1.50%	NIAGARA LO-ESTASOL Herbicide (Niagara Chem.)	2,4-Dichlorophenoxyacetic acid,* butoxyethanol ester	62.40%
NIAGARA LINDANE 25 EMULSION Insecticide (Niagara Chem.)	Lindane* (water miscible)	25%	NIAGARA MALTHION 4 DUST Insecticide (Niagara Chem.)	Malathion*	4%
NIAGARA LINDANE 20 MISCIBLE Insecticide (Niagara Chem.)	Gamma isomer of benzene hexachloride* Xylene*	20% 54.50%	NIAGARA MALATHION MISCIBLE Insecticide (Niagara Chem.)	Malathion* Xylene*	46.20% 43%
NIAGARA LINDANE 25 MISCIBLE Insecticide (Niagara Chem.)	Gamma isomer of benzene hexachloride* Xylene*	25% 49%	NIAGARA MALATHION 25 SPRAY Insecticide (Niagara Chem.)	Malathion*	25%

*Consult Sec. II., Ingredients Index. This ingredient may be responsible for major toxic effects if poisonous amounts of this product are ingested.

- 738 -

Name & Use Manufacturer	Ingredients	Name & Use Manufacturer	Ingredients
NIAGARA MALATHION 25 WETTABLE Insecticide (Niagara Chem.)	Malathion* 25%	NIAGARA NABAM SOLUTION Insecticide (Niagara Chem)	Nabam* (disodium ethylene bis-dithio-carbamate) 19%
NIAGARA M C P (Amine Weed Killer) Herbicide (Niagara Chem.)	Diethanolamine salt of chlorotoloxyacetic acid* 49.50%	NIAGARA N-3 DUST Insecticide (Niagara Chem.)	Nicotine* expressed as alkaloid 1%
NIAGARA METACIDE 50 Insecticide (Niagara Chem.)	Parathion* 10.00% o,o-Dimethyl o-p-nitrophenyl thiophosphate 40.00%	NIAGARA N-5 DUST Insecticide (Niagara Chem.)	Nicotine* expressed as alkaloid 1.75%
NIAGARA METHOXCIDE 5 DUST Insecticide (Niagara Chem.)	Methoxychlor tech. 5%	NIAGARA N-10 DUST Insecticide (Niagara Chem.)	Nicotine* expressed as alkaloid 3.70%
NIAGARA METHOXCIDE 15 DUST Insecticide (Niagara Chem.)	Methoxychlor* 15%	NIAGARA NEU-CAL X BHC 1 DUST Insecticide (Niagara Chem.)	Tricalcium arsenate* 69% Gamma isomer of benzene hexachloride 1% Other isomers of benzene hexachloride 6%
NIAGARA METHOXCIDE MISCIBLE Insecticide (Niagara Chem.)	Methoxychlor tech. 24% Methylated naphthalenes* 63% Dimethyl phthalate 10%	NIAGARA NEU-ROTE Insecticide (Niagara Chem.)	Rotenone* Pyrethrum
NIAGARA METHOXCIDE 50 WETTABLE Insecticide (Niagara Chem.)	Methoxychlor* tech. 50%	NIAGARA NEW POMO GREEN Insecticide (Niagara Chem.)	Gamma isomer of benzene hexachloride 1%
NIAGARA MISCIBLE OIL Insecticide (Niagara Chem.)	Petroleum oils* 97.97%	NIAGARA NF-10 DUST Insecticide (Niagara Chem.)	Nicotine* expressed as alkaloid 3.70%
NIAGARA 70-10-20 MIXTURE Fungicide, insecticide (Niagara Chem.)	Sulfur 67% Lead arsenate* 10%	NIAGARA NIAGARA-MITE-DIELDRIN 3-1.5 DUST Insecticide (Niagara Chem.)	2-(p-tert-Butyl phenoxy) isopropyl-2-chloroethyl sulfite 3% Hexachloro epoxy octahydro dimethano naphthalene* 1.27% Related compounds 0.23%
NIAGARA 80-10-10 MIXTURE Insecticide (Niagara Chem.)	Sulfur 77% Standard lead arsenate* 10%	NIAGARA NIAGARA-MITE 2 DUST Insecticide (Niagara Chem.)	2-(p-tert-Butyl phenoxy) isopropyl-2-chloroethyl sulfite 2%
NIAGARA MONO COPPER-SULPHUR 20-10 DUST Fungicide (Niagara Chem.)	Monohydrated copper* sulfate 20% Sulfur 10%	NIAGARA NIAGARA-MITE 3 DUST Insecticide (Niagara Chem.)	2-(p-tert-Butyl phenoxy) isopropyl-2-chloroethyl sulfite (from Aramite) 3%

*Consult Sec. II., Ingredients Index. This ingredient may be responsible for major toxic effects if poisonous amounts of this product are ingested.

Name & Use Manufacturer	Ingredients		Name & Use Manufacturer	Ingredients	
NIAGARA NIAGARA-MITE-KOLODUST 2-40 DUST Insecticide (Niagara Chem.)	2-(p-tert-Butyl phenoxy) isopropyl-2-chloroethyl sulfite	2%	NIAGARA NIAGARA-MITE-PHOSKIL 3-1 DUST Insecticide (Niagara Chem.)	2-(p-tert-Butyl phenoxy) isopropyl-2-chloroethyl sulfite	3%
	Sulfur*	33%		Parathion*	1%
NIAGARA NIAGARA-MITE-KOLODUST 3-25 DUST Insecticide (Niagara Chem.)	2-(p-tert-Butyl phenoxy) isopropyl-2-chloroethyl sulfite	3%	NIAGARA NIAGRA-MITE-PHOSKIL 3-2 DUST Insecticide (Niagara Chem.)	2-(p-tert-Butyl phenoxy) isopropyl-2-chloroethyl sulfite	3%
	Sulfur*	21%		Parathion*	2%
NIAGARA NIAGARA-MITE-KOLODUST 3-50 DUST Insecticide (Niagara Chem.)	2-(p-tert-Butyl phenoxy) isopropyl-2-chloroethyl sulfite		NIAGARA NIAGARA-MITE-NIATOX-PHOSKIL 3-10-1 DUST Insecticide (Niagara Chem.)	2-(p-tert-Butyl phenoxy) isopropyl-2-chloroethyl sulfite	3%
	Sulfur*	42%		DDT	10%
				Parathion*	1%
NIAGARA NIAGARA-MITE MISCIBLE Insecticide (Niagara Chem.)	2-(p-tert-Butyl phenoxy) isopropyl-2-chloroethyl sulfite	30.40%	NIAGARA NIAGARA-MITE SPRAY Insecticide (Niagara Chem.)	2-(p-tert-Butyl phenoxy) isopropyl-2-chloroethyl sulfite* (from Aramite)	15%
	Xylene*	61.00%			
NIAGARA NIAGARA-MITE 25 MISCIBLE Insecticide (Niagara Chem.)	2-(p-tert-Butyl phenoxy) isopropyl-2-chloroethyl sulfite	25%	NIAGARA NIAGARA-MITE-TOXAKIL 3-10 DUST Insecticide (Niagara Chem.)	2(p-tert-Butyl phenoxy) isopropyl-2-chloroethyl sulfite	3%
				Toxaphene*	10%
NIAGARA NIAGARA-MITE-NIATOX 2-5 DUST Insecticide (Niagara Chem.)	2-(p-tert-Butyl phenoxy) isopropyl-2-chloroethyl sulfite	2%	NIAGARA NIAGARATHAL Herbicide (Niagara Chem.)	Disodium 3,6-endoxo hexahydro phthalate*	
	DDT*	5%			
NIAGARA NIAGARA-MITE-NIATOX 3-5 DUST Insecticide (Niagara Chem.)	2-(p-tert-Butyl phenoxy) isopropyl-2-chloroethyl sulfite	3%	NIAGARA NIAGARATHAL-DF DUST Insecticide (Niagara Chem.)	Disodium 3,6-endoxo hexahydro phthalate*	3.20%
	DDT*	5%		Petroleum distillate	1.50%
NIAGARA NIAGARA-MITE-NIATOX 4-10 DUST Insecticide (Niagara Chem.)	2-(p-tert-Butyl phenoxy) isopropyl-2-chloroethyl sulfite	4%	NIAGARA NIAGARATHAL-DF LIQUID Defoliant (Niagara Chem.)	Disodium 3,6-endoxo hexahydro phthalate* (Endothal)	6.3%
	DDT*	10%			
NIAGARA NIAGARA-MITE-NIATOX-KOLODUST 3-5-40 DUST Insecticide (Niagara Chem.)	2-(p-tert-Butyl phenoxy) isopropyl-2-chloroethyl sulfite	3%	NIAGARA NIAGARATHAL-DF SPRAY Insecticide (Niagara Chem.)	Disodium 3,6-endoxo hexahydro phthalate*	6.30%
	DDT*	5%			
	Sulfur*	33%	NIAGARA NIAGARATRAN 7.5 DUST Insecticide (Niagara Chem.)	p-Chloro phenyl p-chloro benzene sulfonate*	7.50%

*Consult Sec. II., Ingredients Index. This ingredient may be responsible for major toxic effects if poisonous amounts of this product are ingested.

Name & Use Manufacturer	Ingredients		Name & Use Manufacturer	Ingredients	
NIAGARA NIAGARATRAN 50 SPRAY Insecticide (Niagara Chem.)	p-Chlorophenyl p-chlorobenzene sulfonate*	50%	NIAGARA NIATOX 20 DUST Insecticide (Niagara Chem.)	DDT*	20%
NIAGARA NIATOX 5-BHC 1.5 DUST Insecticide (Niagara Chem.)	DDT* Gamma isomer of benzene hexachloride* Other isomers of benzene hexachloride	5% 1.50% 9%	NIAGARA NIATOX 50 DUST BASE Insecticide (Niagara Chem.)	DDT*	50%
NIAGARA NIATOX-BHC 5-0.5 DUST Insecticide (Niagara Chem.)	DDT* Gamma isomer of benzene hexachloride Other isomers of benzene hexachloride	5% 0.50% 3.33%	NIAGARA NIATOX 1.5 DUST IMPREGNATED Insecticide (Niagara Chem.)	DDT Polymethylated naphthalenes*	1.50% 2.70%
NIAGARA NIATOX 10-BHC 2 DUST Insecticide (Niagara Chem.)	Gamma isomer of benzene hexachloride* Other isomers of benzene hexachloride DDT*	2% 11.11% 10%	NIAGARA NIATOX 3-LINDANE 1.5 DUST Insecticide (Niagara Chem.)	DDT Gamma isomer of benzene hexachloride*	3% 1.50%
NIAGARA NIATOX 10-BHC 2 SULPHUR DUST Insecticide (Niagara Chem.)	DDT* Gamma isomer of benzene hexachloride* Other isomers of benzene hexachloride Sulfur*	10% 2% 11.11% 40%	NIAGARA NIATOX 25 MISCIBLE Insecticide (Niagara Chem.)	DDT Xylene*	25% 70%
NIAGARA NIATOX 2 DUST Insecticide (Niagara Chem.)	DDT	2%	NIAGARA NIATOX 3-PHOSKIL 1 DUST Insecticide (Niagara Chem.)	DDT Parathion*	3% 1%
NIAGARA NIATOX 3 DUST Insecticide (Niagara Chem.)	DDT	3%	NIAGARA NIATOX 3-PHOSKIL 1.5 DUST Insecticide (Niagara Chem.)	DDT Parathion*	3% 1.50%
NIAGARA NIATOX 5 DUST Insecticide (Niagara Chem.)	DDT*	5%	NIAGARA NIATOX 5-PHOSKIL 1.5 DUST Insecticide (Niagara Chem.)	DDT Parathion*	5% 1.5%
NIAGARA 302 NIATOX 5 DUST Insecticide (Niagara Chem.)	DDT Standard lead arsenate* Sulfur	5% 10% 49%	NIAGARA NIATOX-PHOSKIL 5-2 DUST Insecticide (Niagara Chem.)	DDT Parathion*	5% 2%
NIAGARA 533 NIATOX 5 DUST Insecticide (Niagara Chem.)	DDT Basic lead arsenate* Sulfur	5% 14% 49%	NIAGARA NIATOX-PHOSKIL 10-1 DUST Insecticide (Niagara Chem.)	Parathion* DDT	1% 10%
NIAGARA NIATOX 10 DUST Insecticide (Niagara Chem.)	DDT*	10%			

*Consult Sec. II., Ingredients Index. This ingredient may be responsible for major toxic effects if poisonous amounts of this product are ingested.

Name & Use Manufacturer	Ingredients	
NIAGARA NIATOX-PHOSKIL 10-2 DUST Insecticide (Niagara Chem.)	Parathion*	2%
	DDT	10%
NIAGARA NIATOX-PHOSKIL 20-2 DUST Insecticide (Niagara Chem.)	DDT	20%
	Parathion*	2%
NIAGARA NIATOX-PHOSKIL 25-1.5 DUST Insecticide (Niagara Chem.)	DDT	25%
	Parathion*	1.50%
NIAGARA NIATOX-PHOSKIL 35-2 DUST Insecticide (Niagara Chem.)	DDT	35%
	Parathion*	2%
NIAGARA NIATOX 50 SPRAY Insecticide (Niagara Chem.)	DDT*	50.00%
NIAGARA NIATOX 20-SULPHUR 50 DUST Insecticide (Niagara Chem.)	DDT*	20%
	Sulfur*	50%
NIAGARA NIATOX-TEPP 5-1.0 DUST Insecticide (Niagara Chem.)	DDT	5%
	Tetraethyl pyrophosphate*	1%
	Other ethyl phosphates*	2%
NIAGARA NIATOX-TEPP 10-1.0 DUST Insecticide (Niagara Chem.)	DDT	10%
	Tetraethyl pyrophosphate*	1%
	Other ethyl phosphates	2%
NIAGARA NIATOX-TEPP 20-1.0 DUST Insecticide (Niagara Chem.)	DDT	20%
	Tetraethyl pyrophosphate*	1%
	Other ethyl phosphates	2%
NIAGARA NIATOX-TOXAKIL 5-15 DUST Insecticide (Niagara Chem.)	DDT*	5%
	Toxaphene*	15%
NIAGARA NIATOX 20 TOXAPHENE MISCIBLE Insecticide (Niagara Chem.)	Toxaphene*	40%
	DDT	20%
	Xylene*	30%
NIAGARA NIATOX 50 WETTABLE Insecticide (Niagara Chem.)	DDT*	50%
NIAGARA NIATOX 75 WETTABLE POWDER Insecticide (Niagara Chem.)	DDT*	75%
NIAGARA NIATOX 5 ZINC DUST Insecticide (Niagara Chem.)	DDT*	5%
NIAGARA NICOTINE SULPHATE 40 Insecticide (Niagara Chem.)	Nicotine* expressed as alkaloid	40%
NIAGARA PAC Fungicide (Niagara Chem.)	Peracetic acid*	40%
NIAGARA PA DUST Insecticide (Niagara Chem.)	Nicotine sulfate*	4%
NIAGARA PARIS GREEN Insecticide (Niagara Chem.)	Cupric acetoarsenite*	85%
NIAGARA PEACH KOLODUST Fungicide (Niagara Chem.)	Sulfur*	79.9%
	2,3-Dichloro-1,4-naphthoquinone	0.5%
NIAGARA PEACH KOLOFORM Fungicide (Niagara Chem.)	Sulfur*	53%
	2,3-Dichloro-1,4-naphthoquinone	1.25%
NIAGARA PENINSULAR OIL EMULSION Insecticide (Niagara Chem.)	Petroleum oil* emulsion	83%

*Consult Sec. II., Ingredients Index. This ingredient may be responsible for major toxic effects if poisonous amounts of this product are ingested.

- 742 -

Name & Use Manufacturer	Ingredients		Name & Use Manufacturer	Ingredients	
NIAGARA PHENO- LEAD Insecticide (Niagara Chem.)	Lead arsenate* Thiodipheny lamine (pheno- thiazine)	56.76% 36.00%	NIAGARA PHOSKIL 1- NIATOX 10 DUST Insecticide (Niagara Chem.)	DDT Parathion*	10% 1%
NIAGARA PHOSKIL. CARBAMATE KOLODUST Insecticide (Niagara Chem.)	Ferbam Parathion* Sulfur	3% 1% 41.50%	NIAGARA PHOSKIL 2-NIATOX 5 DUST Insecticide (Niagara Chem.)	DDT Parathion*	5% 2%
NIAGARA PHOSKIL 1-COPPER 7 DUST Insecticide, fungicide (Niagara Chem.)	Copper expressed as metallic 7% Parathion* 1%		NIAGARA PHOSKIL 2- NIATOX 10 DUST Insecticide (Niagara Chem.)	DDT Parathion*	10% 2%
NIAGARA PHOSKIL 1 DUST Insecticide (Niagara Chem.)	Parathion*	1%	NIAGARA PHOSKIL 1 PEACH DUST Insecticide (Niagara Chem.)	Sulfur Parathion* Petroleum distillate	70% 1% 2%
NIAGARA PHOSKIL 2.0 DUST Insecticide (Niagara Chem.)	Parathion*	2%	NIAGARA PHOSKIL 1.5 PEACH DUST Insecticide (Niagara Chem.)	Parathion*	1.50%
NIAGARA PHOSKIL 1 DUST SPECIAL Insecticide (Niagara Chem.)	Parathion*	1%	NIAGARA PHOSKIL SOLUTION Insecticide (Niagara Chem.)	Parathion* Xylene	46% 45%
NIAGARA PHOSKIL KOLOSPRAY Insecticide, fungicide (Niagara Chem.)	Sulfur Parathion*	67.70% 4.00%	NIAGARA PHOSKIL SPRAY Insecticide (Niagara Chem.)	Parathion*	15%
NIAGARA PHOSKIL 25 MISCIBLE Insecticide (Niagara Chem.)	Parathion* Xylene	25.00% 69.00%	NIAGARA PHOSKIL 25 SPRAY Insecticide (Niagara Chem.)	Parathion*	25%
NIAGARA PHOSKIL 1-NIATOX 3 DUST Insecticide, fungicide (Niagara Chem.)	DDT Parathion*	3.00% 1.00%	NIAGARA PHYGON Fungicide (Niagara Chem.)	2,3-Dichloro-1, 4-naphthoquinone* 50%	
NIAGARA PHOSKIL 1-NIATOX 5 DUST Insecticide (Niagara Chem.)	DDT Parathion*	5% 1%	NIAGARA PHYGON DUST Fungicide (Niagara Chem.)	2,3-Dichloro-1, 4-naphthoquinone 4.00%	
			NIAGARA PHYGON 3 DUST Fungicide (Niagara Chem.)	2,3-Dichloro-1, 4-naphthoquinone 3%	

*Consult Sec. II., Ingredients Index. This ingredient may be responsible for major toxic effects if poisonous amounts of this product are ingested.

Name & Use Manufacturer	Ingredients		Name & Use Manufacturer	Ingredients	
NIAGARA PHYGON NIATOX 5 APPLE DUST Insecticide, fungicide (Niagara Chem.)	2,3-Dichloro-1, 4-napthoquinone Standard lead arsenate* DDT	4% 15% 5%	NIAGARA RO-KILL 75 DUST Insecticide (Niagara Chem.)	Rotenone Other cube extractives	0.75% 1.50%
NIAGARA PINK KOLODUST Fungicide (Niagara Chem.)	Sulfur*	83%	NIAGARA RO-KILL 100 DUST Insecticide (Niagara Chem.)	Rotenone Other cube extractives	1% 2%
NIAGARA POMO-GREEN WITH NICOTINE Insecticide (Niagara Chem.)	Sulfur Basic lead arsenate* Nicotine*	60% 9.5% 2%	NIAGARA RO-KIL SPRAY Insecticide (Niagara Chem.)	Rotenone* Other cube resins or extractives	5% 5%
NIAGARA POTATO DUST 7-20 Insecticide (Niagara Chem.)	Tri-calcium arsenate* 14% Copper expressed as metallic 7%		NIAGARA RO-KIL- TEPP 75-1.0 DUST Insecticide (Niagara Chem.)	Tetraethyl pyrophosphate* 1% Other ethyl phosphates 2% Rotenone 0.75% Other cube extractives 1.50%	
NIAGARA POTA-TOX Insecticide (Niagara Chem.)	Copper expressed as metallic 6.50% Tri-calcium arsenate* 60%		NIAGARA ROTENONE- BEARING 2.5 BLUEBERRY DUST Insecticide (Niagara Chem.)	Rotenone* Other cube resins or extractives 2.50%	2.50%
NIAGARA POWDERED BLUESTONE Fungicide (Niagara Chem.)	Copper sulfate*	90.35%	NIAGARA ROTENONE- BEARING NIATOX 3 DUST Insecticide (Niagara Chem.)	Sulfur* DDT Rotenone Other cube resins or extractives 0.50%	40% 3% 0.50%
NIAGARA PYRENONE GRAIN PROTECTANT Insecticide (Niagara Chem.)	Tech. piperonyl butoxide 0.80% Pyrethrins 0.05%		NIAGARA ROTENONE- BEARING DUST Insecticide (Niagara Chem.)	Rotenone Other cube resins or extractive 0.75%	0.75%
NIAGARA PYRENONE STOCK SPRAY Insecticide (Niagara Chem.)	Pyrethrins 0.05% Piperonyl butoxide tech. 0.53% Mineral oil 99.42%		NIAGARA ROTENONE- BEARING DUST Insecticide (Niagara Chem.)	Rotenone Other cube resins or extractive 1%	1%
NIAGARA QUIK-KILL COPOTEX Insecticide (Niagara Chem.)	Monohydrated copper sulfate 15% Tri-calcium arsenate* 22.05% Calcium arsenite 1.93%		NIAGARA ROTENONE- BEARING DUST Insecticide (Niagara Chem.)	Rotenone* Other cube resins or extractive 2%	2%
NIAGARA QUIK-KILL POISON Insecticide (Niagara Chem.)	Calcium arsenate* Calcium arsenite*		NIAGARA ROTOX LIGHT MEDIUM Insecticide (Niagara Chem.)	Petroleum oil* Rotenone	99.30% 0.05%
NIAGARA RICE DESICCANT Fungicide (Niagara Chem.)	Sodium chlorate*	40%			

*Consult Sec. II., Ingredients Index. This ingredient may be responsible for major toxic effects if poisonous amounts of this product are ingested.

Name & Use Manufacturer	Ingredients	
NIAGARA SHADE TOBACCO DUST Insecticide (Niagara Chem.)	DDD Parathion*	10% 1%
NIAGARA SHADE TOBACCO DUST 10-0-0 Fungicide (Niagara Chem.)	Zineb	6.50%
NIAGARA SHADE TOBACCO DUST 10-1-10D Insecticide (Niagara Chem.)	DDD Parathion* Zineb	10% 1% 6.50%
NIAGARA SHADE TOBACCO DUST 1-10T (Niagara Chem.)	DDT Parathion*	10% 1%
NIAGARA SHADE TOBACCO DUST 10-1-10T Insecticide (Niagara Chem.)	DDT Parathion* Zineb	10% 1% 6.50%
NIAGARA SODIUM TCA Herbicide (Niagara Chem.)	Sodium trichloroacetate*	90%
NIAGARA SODIUM TCA SOLUTION Herbicide (Niagara Chem.)	Sodium trichloroacetate*	47%
NIAGARA SOILFUME 60-40 Soil fumigant (Niagara Chem.)	Ethylene dibromide*	41%
NIAGARA SOILFUME 85 Fungicide (Niagara Chem.)	Ethylene dibromide*	83%
NIAGARA SOILFUME 40 MISCIBLE Insecticide (Niagara Chem.)	Ethylene dibromide*	40%

Name & Use Manufacturer	Ingredients	
NIAGARA SOILFUME 75 MISCIBLE Insecticide (Niagara Chem.)	Ethylene dibromide*	75%
NIAGARA SOIL SULPHUR GRANULAR Insecticide (Niagara Chem.)	Sulfur*	99.5%
NIAGARA SOIL TREATER NO. 3 Insecticide (Niagara Chem.)	Hexachloro hexahydro dimethano naphthalene* Related compounds	2.85% 2.15%
NIAGARA SPECIAL DUST FOR VEGETABLES Fungicide (Niagara Chem.)	Sulfur* Copper* expressed as metallic Petroleum distillate	25% 6.30% 1%
NIAGARA SPECIAL DUST MIXTURE Insecticide (Niagara Chem.)	Tricalcium arsenate*	28%
NIAGARA SPECIAL MIXTURE Insecticide (Niagara Chem.)	Standard lead arsenate* Sulfur	20% 5.50%
NIAGARA SPERGON 5 DUST Fungicide (Niagara Chem.)	Chloranil*	4.80%
NIAGARA SPERGON 10 DUST Fungicide (Niagara Chem.)	Tetrachloro parabenzo quinone*	10%
NIAGARA SPERGON 5-TOXAKIL 10 DUST Insecticide (Niagara Chem.)	Chloranil Toxaphene*	4.80% 10%
NIAGARA SPOR BRAND SUPERFINE DUSTING SULPHUR Insecticide (Niagara Chem.)	Sulfur*	99.50%
NIAGARA STANDARD LEAD ARSENATE Insecticide (Niagara Chem.)	Standard lead arsenate*	96.00%

*Consult Sec. II., Ingredients Index. This ingredient may be responsible for major toxic effects if poisonous amounts of this product are ingested.

Name & Use Manufacturer	Ingredients		Name & Use Manufacturer	Ingredients	
NIAGARA-STIK Fungicide (Niagara Chem.)	Naphthalene acetic acid* sodium salt	3.55%	NIAGARA SULPHUR-COPPER PEANUT DUST Fungicide (Niagara Chem.)	Copper* expressed as metallic Sulfur*	3.40% 88.50%
NIAGARA-STIK DUST (Double Strength) Fungicide (Niagara Chem.)	Naphthalene acetic acid	0.2%	NIAGARA SULPHUR-CR-MALATHON 40-40-4 DUST Insecticide (Niagara Chem.)	Sulfur Sodium fluoaluminate* Malathion	40% 36% 4%
NIAGARA-STIK DUST (Triple Strength) Fungicide (Niagara Chem.)	Naphthalene acetic acid	0.3%	NIAGARA SULPHUR DDD 25-5 DUST Insecticide (Niagara Chem.)	Sulfur* DDD	25% 5%
NIAGARA-STIK XTRA Fungicide (Niagara Chem.)	Naphthalene acetic acid* sodium salt	4%	NIAGARA SULPHUR-DDD 50-10 DUST Insecticide (Niagara Chem.)	Sulfur* DDD	50% 10%
NIAGARA SULFOBRITE Insecticide (Niagara Chem.)	Sulfur*	90%	NIAGARA SULPHUR-DDD 75-5 DUST Insecticide (Niagara Chem.)	DDT* Sulfur*	5% 75%
NIAGARA SULPHUR-BHC 50-1 DUST Insecticide (Niagara Chem.)	Sulfur* Gamma isomer of benzene hexachloride Other isomers of benzene hexachloride	50.00% 1.00% 6.66%	NIAGARA SULPHUR-DIELDRIN 50-1.5 DUST Insecticide (Niagara Chem.)	Sulfur* Hexachloro epoxy octahydro dimethano naphthalene* Related compounds	50% 1.27% 0.23%
NIAGARA SULPHUR-BHC 60-2 DUST Insecticide (Niagara Chem.)	Sulfur* Gamma isomer of benzene hexachloride* Other isomers of benzene hexachloride	60% 2% 12%	NIAGARA SULPHUR-LINDANE C-Z DUST Insecticide (Niagara Chem.)	Gamma isomer of benzene hexachloride Copper* expressed as metallic Zinc* expressed as metallic Sulfur*	1% 4.50% 4.50% 50%
NIAGARA SULPHUR-BL 70-30 DUST Insecticide (Niagara Chem.)	Sulfur Basic lead arsenate*	63.40% 30%	NIAGARA SULPHUR-NIAGARATHAN 50-7.5 DUST Insecticide (Niagara Chem.)	Sulfur* p-Chlorophenyl p-chloro benzene sulfonate*	50% 7.50%
NIAGARA SULPHUR-CA 25-75 DUST Insecticide (Niagara Chem.)	Sulfur Tri-calcium arsenate*	23% 51%	NIAGARA SULPHUR-NIATOX-CHLORDANE 60-5-2 DUST Insecticide (Niagara Chem.)	Sulfur* DDT* Chlordane	60% 5% 2%
NIAGARA SULPHUR-CA 50-50 DUST Insecticide (Niagara Chem.)	Sulfur Tri-calcium arsenate*	47.60% 35%	NIAGARA SULPHUR-NIATOX 5 DUST Insecticide (Niagara Chem.)	DDT* Sulfur*	5% 67.5%
NIAGARA SULPHUR-CALCIUM DUST 33 Insecticide (Niagara Chem.)	Sulfur Tri-calcium arsenate*	60% 23.10%			
NIAGARA SULPHUR-COPPER DUST FOR PEANUTS Insecticide (Niagara Chem.)	Sulfur* Copper* expressed as metallic	84.40% 4%			

*Consult Sec. II., Ingredients Index. This ingredient may be responsible for major toxic effects if poisonous amounts of this product are ingested.

Name & Use Manufacturer	Ingredients		Name & Use Manufacturer	Ingredients	
NIAGARA SULPHUR-NIATOX 10 DUST Insecticide (Niagara Chem.)	Sulfur* DDT*	72.8% 10%	NIAGARA SULPHUR-PARATHION SPRAY Insecticide (Niagara Chem.)	Sulfur Parathion*	50% 3%
NIAGARA SULPHUR-NIATOX 50-3 DUST Insecticide (Niagara Chem.)	DDT Sulfur*	3% 50%	NIAGARA SULPHUR-PHOSKIL 50-2 DUST Insecticide (Niagara Chem.)	Parathion* Sulfur	2% 50%
NIAGARA SULPHUR-NIATOX 50-10 DUST Insecticide (Niagara Chem.)	DDT* Sulfur*	10% 50%	NIAGARA SULPHUR-PHOSKIL 1-NIATOX 3 DUST Insecticide (Niagara Chem.)	Sulfur Parathion* DDT	50% 1% 3%
NIAGARA SULPHUR-NIATOX 75-5 DUST Insecticide (Niagara Chem.)	Sulfur* DDT*	73% 5%	NIAGARA SULPHUR ROTENONE-BEARING DUST Insecticide (Niagara Chem.)	Rotenone Other cube resins or extractives Sulfur*	0.75% 0.75% 25.00%
NIAGARA SULPHUR-NIATOX 85-5 DUST Insecticide (Niagara Chem.)	DDT* Sulfur*	5% 85%	NIAGARA SULPHUR ROTENONE-BEARING DUST Insecticide (Niagara Chem.)	Sulfur* Rotenone Other cube resins or extractives	23% 1% 1%
NIAGARA SULPHUR-NIATOX-PHOSKIL 50-5-0.5 DUST Insecticide (Niagara Chem.)	Sulfur DDT Parathion*	50% 5% 0.50%	NIAGARA SULPHUR ROTENONE-BEARING 1-NIATOX 2 DUST Insecticide (Niagara Chem.)	Rotenone Other cube resins or extractives Sulfur* DDT	1% 1% 25% 2%
NIAGARA SULPHUR-NIATOX-PHOSKIL 50-10-1 DUST Insecticide (Niagara Chem.)	Sulfur DDT Parathion*	50% 10% 1%	NIAGARA SULPHUR ROTENONE-BEARING 1-NIATOX 3 DUST Insecticide (Niagara Chem.)	Sulfur* Rotenone Other cube resins or extractives DDT	40% 1% 1% 1%
NIAGARA SULPHUR-NIATOX-PHOSKIL 50-10-2 DUST Insecticide (Niagara Chem.)	Sulfur DDT Parathion*	50% 10% 2%	NIAGARA SULPHUR-TOXAKIL 60-10 DUST Insecticide (Niagara Chem.)	Sulfur* Toxaphene*	60% 10%
NIAGARA SULPHUR-NIATOX-ZEC 25-5-5 DUST Insecticide (Niagara Chem.)	Sulfur* DDT* Zineb	25% 5% 3.25%	NIAGARA SULPHUR-ZEC 75-5 DUST Fungicide (Niagara Chem.)	Sulfur* Zineb	75% 3.25%

*Consult Sec. II., Ingredients Index. This ingredient may be responsible for major toxic effects if poisonous amounts of this product are ingested.

- 747 -

Name & Use Manufacturer	Ingredients	Name & Use Manufacturer	Ingredients
NIAGARA SUMMER FLOWABLE EMULSION (Light-medium) Insecticide (Niagara Chem.)	Petroleum oil* 80%	NIAGARA TEPP 20 Insecticide (Niagara Chem.)	Tetra ethyl pyrophosphate* 20.00% Other ethyl phosphates 30.00%
NIAGARA SUMMER QUIK-MIX-LIGHT MEDIUM Insecticide (Niagara Chem.)	Petroleum oil* 98.00%	NIAGARA TEPP DUST Insecticide (Niagara Chem.)	Tetraethyl pyrophosphate* 1.15% Other ethyl phosphates 1.85%
NIAGARA SUPERFINE CONDITIONED DUSTING SULPHUR Fungicide (Niagara Chem.)	Sulfur* 93%	NIAGARA TEPP 1.0 DUST Insecticide (Niagara Chem.)	Tetraethyl pyrophosphate* 1% Other ethyl phosphates 2%
NIAGARA SUPERFINE DUSTING SULPHUR Fungicide (Niagara Chem.)	Sulfur* 99.5%	NIAGARA TEPP NIATOX 3 DUST Insecticide (Niagara Chem.)	Tetraethyl pyrophosphate* 1.15% Other ethyl phosphates 1.85% DDT 3%
NIAGARA SUSPENSO LEAD ARSENATE Insecticide (Niagara Chem.)	Standard lead arsenate* 96%	NIAGARA TEPP NIATOX 5 DUST Insecticide (Niagara Chem.)	Tetraethyl pyrophosphate* 1.15% Other ethyl phosphates 1.85% DDT 5%
NIAGARA SYSTOX SPRAY CONCEN-TRATE Insecticide (Niagara Chem.)	o,o-Diethyl-o-2-(ethylmercapto)-ethyl thiophosphate* 21.20% Related organic phosphates 1.80%	NIAGARA THREE-N-ONE COTTON DUST Insecticide (Niagara Chem.)	Gamma isomer of benzene hexachloride* 3% Other isomers of benzene hexachloride* 16.66% DDT* 5% Sulfur* 40%
NIAGARA TCA WEED KILLER (Niagara Chem.)	Sodium trichloroacetate* 90%	NIAGARA TOBACCO DUST 1-10 Insecticide (Niagara Chem.)	DDD 10% Parathion* 1%
NIAGARA TECHNICAL BENZENE HEXACHLORIDE Insecticide (Niagara Chem.)	Gamma BHC* 12.5%	NIAGARA TOBACCO DUST 10D Insecticide (Niagara Chem.)	DDT* 10%
NIAGARA TECHNICAL GRADE DDT Insecticide (Niagara Chem.)	DDT*	NIAGARA TOMATO DUST Insecticide, fungicide (Niagara Chem.)	Copper expressed as metallic 7% Tri-calcium arsenate* 14%
NIAGARA TEPP Insecticide (Niagara Chem.)	Tetraethyl pyrophosphate* 40% Other related organic phosphate esters 60%	NIAGARA TOMATO PLANT DUST 15 Insecticide (Niagara Chem.)	Tri-calcium arsenate* 10.50% Copper, expressed as metallic 7%
		NIAGARA TOXAKIL 5 DUST Insecticide (Niagara Chem.)	Toxaphene* 5%

*Consult Sec. II., Ingredients Index. This ingredient may be responsible for major toxic effects if poisonous amounts of this product are ingested.

- 748 -

Name & Use Manufacturer	Ingredients	
NIAGARA TOXAKIL 10 DUST Insecticide (Niagara Chem.)	Toxaphene*	10%
NIAGARA TOXAKIL 20 DUST Insecticide (Niagara Chem.)	Toxaphene*	20%
NIAGARA TOXAKIL MISCIBLE Insecticide (Niagara Chem.)	Toxaphene*	6 lb./gal.
NIAGARA TOXAKIL PHOSKIL 10-2 DUST Insecticide (Niagara Chem.)	Toxaphene Parathion*	10% 2%
NIAGARA TOXAKIL 10-SULPHUR 40 DUST Insecticide (Niagara Chem.)	Tech. chlorinated camphene* 10% Sulfur* 40%	
NIAGARA TOXAKIL 20-SULPHUR 40 DUST Insecticide (Niagara Chem.)	Tech. chlorinated camphene* 20% Sulfur 40%	
NIAGARA TOXAKIL 40 WETTABLE POWDER Insecticide (Niagara Chem.)	Toxaphene*	40%
NIAGARA TOXAPHENE 10 DUST Insecticide (Niagara Chem.)	Toxaphene*	10%
NIAGARA TOXAPHENE 20 DUST Insecticide (Niagara Chem.)	Toxaphene*	20%
NIAGARA TOXAPHENE MISCIBLE Insecticide (Niagara Chem.)	Toxaphene* Petroleum distillate	60% 28.50%

Name & Use Manufacturer	Ingredients	
NIAGARA TRIONA LIGHT SOLUBLE, LIGHT MEDIUM SOLUBLE, MEDIUM SOLUBLE, HEAVY MEDIUM SOLUBLE & HEAVY SOLUBLE Insecticide (Niagara Chem.)	Petroleum oil*	99.3%
NIAGARA TRIONA MEDIUM, LIGHT MEDIUM HEAVY MEDIUM EMULSION Insecticide (Niagara Chem.)	Petroleum oil*	80%
NIAGARA TRIUMPH Insecticide (Niagara Chem.)	Petroleum oil* Cresylic acid* Soap Fish oil	79% 4.5% 4% 2.5%
NIAGARA 2,4,5-T Herbicide (Niagara Chem.)	2,4,5-Trichlorophenoxyacetic acid,* butoxy ethanol ester 58.50%	
NIAGARA 2,4,5-TA Fungicide (Niagara Chem.)	2,4,5-Trichlorophenoxyacetic acid* equiv. 242 gm./gal.	
NIAGARA TWO-N-ONE COTTON DUST Insecticide (Niagara Chem.)	Gamma isomer of benzene hexachloride* 3.00% DDT* 5.00%	
NIAGARA TWO-N-ONE COTTON SPRAY Insecticide (Niagara Chem.)	Gamma isomer of benzene hexachloride 7.20% Other isomers of benzene hexachloride 10.80% DDT 12.00% Xylene* 64.00%	
NIAGARA TWO-N-ONE COTTON SPRAY (Double Strength) Insecticide (Niagara Chem.)	Gamma isomer of benzene hexachloride* 12.40% Other isomers of benzene hexachloride 15.10% DDT 20.70% Xylene* 31.20%	
NIAGARA VANCIDE 51 SEED TREATMENT Fungicide (Niagara Chem.)	Sodium salt of dimethyl-dithiocarbamic acid* Sodium salt of 2-mercapto-benzothiazole* 30%	

*Consult Sec. II., Ingredients Index. This ingredient may be responsible for major toxic effects if poisonous amounts of this product are ingested.

Name & Use Manufacturer	Ingredients		Name & Use Manufacturer	Ingredients	
NIAGARA VANCIDE Z-65 Insecticide (Niagara Chem.)	Zinc salt of dimethyldithio-carbamic acid* Zinc salt of 2-mercapto-benzothiazole*	65%	NIAGARA ZINC-KOLO-BHC-SPRAY Fungicide (Niagara Chem.)	Sulfur* Gamma isomer of benzene hexachloride* Other isomers of benzene hexachloride Zinc* expressed as metallic	28.90% 1.60% 8.89% 9.24%
NIAGARA VITIDUST Insecticide (Niagara Chem.)	Monohydrated copper sulfate Lead arsenate*	11% 15%	NIAGARA ZINC KOLOCOP SPRAY 63 Fungicide (Niagara Chem.)	Sulfur* Copper* expressed as metallic	63.70% 4.79%
NIAGARA WETTABLE SULPHUR Insecticide (Niagara Chem.)	Sulfur*	95%	NIAGARA ZINC KOLOFORM Insecticide (Niagara Chem.)	Sulfur*	50%
NIAGARA Z-C DUST Fungicide (Niagara Chem.)	Ziram*	7%	NIAGARA ZINC KOLO PHOSKIL 1.5 SPRAY Insecticide (Niagara Chem.)	Sulfur Parathion*	42.50% 1.70%
NIAGARA Z-C KOLODUST Fungicide (Niagara Chem.)	Sulfur* Ziram*	77.10% 5%	NIAGARA ZINC KOLO PHOSKIL 2 SPRAY Insecticide (Niagara Chem.)	Sulfur Parathion*	41.30% 2.30%
NIAGARA Z-C NIATOX 3 DUST Insecticide (Niagara Chem.)	Ziram* DDT*	7% 3%	NIAGARA ZINC KOLO WETTEX Insecticide (Niagara Chem.)	Fused bentonite sulfur Zinc sulfate Lead arsenate*	
NIAGARA Z-C PHOSKIL 1 DUST Insecticide (Niagara Chem.)	Ziram Parathion*	7% 1%	NIAGARA ZINC SULFUR PARATHION SPRAY Insecticide (Niagara Chem.)	Sulfur Parathion*	50% 3%
NIAGARA Z-C SPRAY Fungicide (Niagara Chem.)	Ziram*	70%	NIAGARA ZINEB 6.5-DDD 5 DUST Insecticide (Niagara Chem.)	Zineb DDD	6.5% 5%
NIAGARA ZINC C-O-C-S SPRAY 252 Fungicide (Niagara Chem.)	Copper* expressed as metallic Zinc* expressed as metallic	28.30% 24%	NIAGARA ZINEB DIELDRIN 1.5 DUST Insecticide (Niagara Chem.)	Zineb Hexachloro epoxy octahydro dimethano naphthalene* Related compounds	4.550% 1.275% 0.225%
NIAGARA ZINC COPPER EMULSO Insecticide (Niagara Chem.)	Petroleum* oils Copper* expressed as metallic	49.80% 3.33%	NIAGARA ZINEB 6.5 DUST Fungicide (Niagara Chem.)	Zineb	6.5%
NIAGARA ZINC EMULSO Insecticide (Niagara Chem.)	Petroleum oils*	63.30%	NIAGARA ZINEB 13 DUST Fungicide (Niagara Chem.)	Zineb	13%

*Consult Sec. II., Ingredients Index. This ingredient may be responsible for major toxic effects if poisonous amounts of this product are ingested.

Name & Use Manufacturer	Ingredients	
NIAGARA ZINEB 13.5 DUST FOR TOBACCO Fungicide (Niagara Chem.)	Zineb	13.50%
NIAGARA ZINEB 16.25 DUST FOR TOBACCO Fungicide (Niagara Chem.)	Zineb	16.25%
NIAGARA ZINEB LINDANE 1 DUST Insecticide (Niagara Chem.)	Zineb Gamma isomer of benzene hexachloride*	4.55% 1%
NIAGARA ZINEB 4 LINDANE 1 DUST Insecticide (Niagara Chem.)	Zineb Gamma isomer of benzene hexachloride*	4% 1%
NIAGARA ZINEB 4-LINDANE 0.75 DUST Insecticide (Niagara Chem.)	Zineb Gamma isomer of benzene hexachloride	4% 0.75%
NIAGARA ZINEB NIATOX 5 DUST Insecticide (Niagara Chem.)	Zineb DDT*	4.55% 5%
NIAGARA ZINEB 4-NIATOX 10 DUST Insecticide (Niagara Chem.)	Zineb DDT*	4% 10%
NIAGARA ZINEB 16.25-NIATOX 5 DUST Insecticide (Niagara Chem.)	Zineb DDT*	16.25% 5%
NIAGARA ZINEB PHOSKIL 1 DUST Insecticide, fungicide (Niagara Chem.)	Zineb Parathion*	4.55% 1.00%
NIAGARA ZINEB 4 PHOSKIL 1 DUST Insecticide (Niagara Chem.)	Zineb Parathion*	4% 1%

Name & Use Manufacturer	Ingredients	
NIAGARA ZINEB 13 PHOSKIL 1-NIATOX 5 DUST Insecticide (Niagara Chem.)	Parathion* DDT Zineb	1% 5% 13%
NIAGARA ZINEB 16.25 & 13.5-PHOSKIL 1-NIATOX 5 DUST Insecticide, fungicide (Niagara Chem.)	Zineb Parathion* DDT	13.5% 1.0% 5.0%
NIAGARA ZINEB SULPHUR DIELDRIN 1.5 DUST Insecticide, fungicide (Niagara Chem.)	Zineb Sulfur* Hexachloro epoxy octahydro dimethano naphthalene (from Dieldrin)*	4.55% 30.00% 1.275%
NIAGARA ZINEB SULPHUR DUST Fungicide (Niagara Chem.)	Zineb Sulfur*	4.55% 30%
NIAGARA ZINEB SULPHUR NIATOX 5 DUST Insecticide, fungicide (Niagara Chem.)	Zineb DDT* Sulfur*	4.55% 5.00% 30.00%
NIAGARA ZINEB SULPHUR PHOSKIL 1 DUST Insecticide, fungicide (Niagara Chem.)	Zineb Sulfur Parathion*	4.55% 30.00% 1.00%
NIAGARA ZIRAM 10 DUST Fungicide (Niagara Chem.)	Ziram*	10%
NIAGARA ZIRAM-PHOSKIL 10-1 DUST Insecticide (Niagara Chem.)	Ziram Parathion*	10% 1%
NIAGARA Z M SPRAY Fungicide (Niagara Chem.)	Zinc* expressed as metallic 18.5% Manganese* expressed as metallic 7.0%	
NIAGROL Insecticide (Niagara Chem.)	Petroleum oil*	83%
NIAGROL 90 Insecticide (Niagara Chem.)	Petroleum oils*	90%
NIAGROL QUICK-MIX Insecticide (Niagara Chem.)	Petroleum oils*	97%

*Consult Sec. II., Ingredients Index. This ingredient may be responsible for major toxic effects if poisonous amounts of this product are ingested.

Name & Use Manufacturer	Ingredients		Name & Use Manufacturer	Ingredients	
NICHOLS DRY CLEANER (Norton)	V.M. & P. naphtha* Denatured alcohol Tech. grade chloroform*		NICOTINE KRUMBLES Anthelmintic (veterinary, avian) (Mc Clellan)	Phenothiazine Nicotine* (as alkaloid) Gentian, ginger and iron sulfate	30.00% 5.00% 65.00%
NICHOLS TRIANGLE BRAND COPPER SULPHATE, BASIC Fungicide (Phelps)	Metallic copper* 53%		NICOTINE PYROX Insecticide (Am. Agric. Chem.)	Nicotine* Arsenate* Copper	
NIC-KA-MAL (Adult) Anthelmintic (veterinary, avian) (Mc Clellan)	Each tablet: Nicotine* (as alkaloid) 45 mg. Phenothiazine 450 mg.		NICOTINE SULPHATE SOLUTION Insecticide (McClellan)	Nicotine (as alkaloid)* 40%	
NIC-KA-MAL (Pullet) Anthelmintic (veterinary, avian) (Mc Clellan)	Each tablet: Nicotine* (as alkaloid) 33 mg. Phenothiazine 330 mg.		NICOZINE Poultry remedy (Hess, Dr.)	Phenothiazine (drench grade) Nicotine*	20% 4%
NICKELETTE Chromium finish plating compound (Tilette)	Silver nitrate Cyanide*		NICOZINE TABS Insecticide (Hess, Dr.)	Phenothiazine Nicotine*	20.0% 3.5%
NICKEL-ITCH OINTMENT For skin irritations (Wambaugh)	Zinc oxide Calamine Glycerin Phenol* Petrolatum base		NICSOLAN Skin fungicide (medical) (Vogel)	Nickel sulfate Salicylic acid* Aerosol OT Isopropanol*	1% 1/4% 1% 50%
NICMIX (Salsbury's)	Nicotine (as alkaloid)* 5.5%		NIKA POWDER Anthelmentic (veterinary, avian) (Corn King)	Nicotine (as alkaloid)* 5.0%	
NICOCIDE NO. 10 Insecticide (Calif. Spray)	Nicotine alkaloid* 3.6%		NILS VERMIN EMULSION Ectoparasiticide (Miscible)	Benzyl benzoate* Triethanolamine oleate	
NICO-FUME PRESSURE FUMIGATOR Insecticide (Diamond Black)	Nicotine* (expressed as alkaloid) 14%		NIM Skin fungicide (medical) (Elars)	Alcohol Benzoic acid* Phenol* Salicylic acid* Thymol* Para di-isobutyl phenoxy ethoxy ethyl dimethyl benzyl ammonium chloride* monohydrate	47.5%
NICO-FUME LIQUID Insecticide (Diamond Black)	Nicotine* expressed as alkaloid 40%		99 Herbicide (Dow)	Propylene glycol butyl ether esters of 2, 4-D*	
NICO-MIX Anthelmintic (veterinary, avian) (Gland-O-Lac)	Nicotine* 5%		999 FOR COLDS (Howell Co.)		
NICO-MULSION Insecticide (Sherwin-Williams)	Nicotine alkaloid* 3% Petroleum oil 80%		910 VARNISH (O'Brien Corp.)		
NICONA GARDEN EMULSION Herbicide (Shell Oil)	Petroleum oil*		NIP DISINFECTANT PINE OIL (Howell Bros.)		
NICO-STOP To combat tobacco habit (Nico-Stop)	Sulfate of lobeline* (inflata)		NIP FURNITURE POLISH Cream, wax (Howell Bros.)		

*Consult Sec. II., Ingredients Index. This ingredient may be responsible for major toxic effects if poisonous amounts of this product are ingested.

Name & Use Manufacturer	Ingredients

NIP-ON
Insecticide
(Chamberlain Haber)
	Cube resins other than
	  rotenone 0.10%
	Mineral oil 3.4%
	Fenchyl thiocyanoacetate
	     0.75%
	Pyrethrins 10%
	Sodium silicofluoride* 70%

NIP WAX- SOAP CLEANER (Howell Bros.)	
NITE-BRITE LUMINOUS PAINT (United Gilson.)	Alkyd resin Phosphorescent zinc sulfide* pigment
NITRALLIUM TABLETS For the symptomatic relief of arterial hypertension (Bishop)	Each tablet: Sodium nitrite* 1/3 gr.

NITRO-BLEND
Tonic
(veterinary)
(Salsbury's)
	3-Nitro-4-hydroxyphenylarsonic
	  acid (corresponds to 300 mg.
	  arsenic trioxide* per gm.)
	    80%

NITROL VAPAROL SPRAY Insecticide (Calif. Spray)	Petroleum oils * 97% Dinitro-orthocresol* 1.8%
NITRO READY-MIX- OIL SPRAY Insecticide (Calif. Spray)	Petroleum oils * 95% Dinitro ortho cresol* 2.44%

NITROSAL
Veterinary drug for coccidiosis in chickens and turkeys, and preventing bluecomb in turkeys
(Salsbury's)
	n^4-Acetyl-n^1-(4-nitrophenyl)
	  sulfanilamide) 30%
	3-Nitro-4-hydroxyphenylarsonic
	  acid* 9%

NITRO-SEAL Cement (Varniton)	Acetone* Toluene*

NITROX SPRAY
CONCENTRATE
Insecticide
(Pittsburgh Coke)
	Methyl parathion* (o,o-dimethyl-
	  o-p-nitrophenyl thiophosphate)
	    25.3%
	Aromatic petroleum hydrocar-
	  bons 64.7%

NIX DEODORANT CREAM (Nix)	
NIX DOG REPELLENT (Knock-Em)	

Name & Use Manufacturer	Ingredients
NIX-NAP Stimulant (Commerce)	Caffeine alkaloid* Extract kola* Vitamin B1
NIXON CREME (Nixon)	Glycerin Propylene glycol monostearate Triethanolamine Stearic acid Phenylmercuric borate 0.0175% Oxyquinoline sulfate 0.08%
N.J.F. HEMORRHOID- AL SUP- POSITORIES (G. & W.)	Bismuth subgallas Resorcinol Balsam Peru Zinc oxide Aethylis aminobenzoas Oleum theobromatis
N.J. SOLVENT #1 ALTER- NATE (Western Rosin)	
N-L CONCENTRATE General purpose cleaning product (Nat'l. Lab.)	Synthetic detergents * Complex phosphates pH approx. 10
NNOR GARDEN SPRAY Insecticide (Atlas)	Rotenone 1% Tech. mannitan monolaurate 97.1%
NOAH'S PITCH Roofing cement (Carey)	
NOBACCO To combat tobacco habit (Approved)	Each lozenge: Lobeline sulfate* 1/64 gr. Dextrose 3 gr. Oil of peppermint
NOBEMA AIR BRUSH COLORS (Nobema)	
NOBEMA AMERICAN MADE VINE CHAR- COAL STICKS Artists's supply (Nobema)	
NOBEMA ARTISTS' COLORS, INKS, VAR- NISHES (Nobema)	
NOBESITY Medication (Davin)	
NOBLESSE SKIN FRESHENER (Noblesse)	
NO BUGS M'LADY Insecticidal paper (Paper Prod.)	

*Consult Sec. II., Ingredients Index. This ingredient may be responsible for major toxic effects if poisonous amounts of this product are ingested.

Name & Use Manufacturer	Ingredients	Name & Use Manufacturer	Ingredients
NO-CHAFE CREAM For diaper rash (Binday)	Aluminum acetate Zinc oxide Starch Lanolin White petrolatum	NOLVASAN Disinfectant (Fort Dodge)	Bis-p-cholorphenyldiguanido-hexane dihydrochloride* in three forms: Solution 5% Ointment 1% Effervescent tablet 1 gm.
NOCTIL Water conditioner (Rumford)	Water-softener Sodium tripolyphosphate Mild buffering alkalis, sodium carbonate and bicarbonate	NOMAR PLUS (Fuller Brush)	Wax Silicone oil Mineral spirits*
NO DOZ AWAKENERS Stimulant (Harrison)	Caffeine*	NOMETA TABLETS Vaginal suppository (New Idea)	Thymol* Boric acid* Powder ammonium alum*
NODS Sedative (Carroll Chem.)	Methapyrilene hydrochloride* 25 mg.	NOMO OINTMENT For rectal irritation (Crowell)	Benzocaine* Eucalyptus* Boric acid* Benzoated mutton tallow Oil chaulmoogra* Olive oil Zinc oxide Aluminum acetate
NOEL COLOGNE & EAU DE COLOGNE (Noblesse)			
NO EXCUSE FOR ODORS SPRAY DEODORANT (Rexclif)	Liquid formaldehyde* U.S.P. 2.5% Isopropyl alcohol* Propylene glycol Triethylene glycol Aromatic oils	NON-GRAIN RAISING STAIN (Dolan, V.J.)	Methanol* over 5%
		NO-NIB'L Repellent (Larvacide)	Amine compound of zinc Dimethyl dithiocarbamate* Polyethylene polysulfide
NO FLAMEO Fire re-tardant coating (Sudbury Lab.)		NONSPI Deodorant (Standard Lab.)	Aluminum chlorhydroxide complex Benzalkonium chloride*
NO-GRIT Sweeping compound (Pioneer Mfg.)		NONTOX LIVESTOCK SPRAY Insecticide (Commercial Chem.)	Pyrethrins* Piperonyl butoxide
NO-HAL Mouth deodorant (Branower)	Thymol* Menthol* Tannic acid*	NOONAN'S DANDRUFF REMOVER (Noonan)	
NO-ITCH (Bailes)		NOONAN'S LEMON SPECIAL WAVE SETS (Noonan)	
NOKORODE SOLDERING PASTE (Dunton)	Water solution of zinc* and ammonium chloride* salts Petrolatum carrier	NOONAN'S RINSE FOR HAIR (Noonan)	
NO-KOTIN To combat tobacco habit (Walker Pharm.)	Lobeline sulfate* 1/16 gr.	NOPCO 1440 (Nopco)	Sulfonated pine oil*
NOLA SOAPS (Iowa)	Tallow Coconut oil	NO-PIK To discourage cannibalism in poultry (Gland-O-Lac)	Oil of mustard* Scarlet lake Oethene Oleoresin of capsicum
NOLEX, DERMATOL-OGIC LOTION To prevent sunburn, windburn (Kahlenberg)	Neatsfoot oil Homo menthyl salicylate* Triethanolamine oleate	NORCOHOL RUBBING ALCOHOL COMPOUND (Norwich)	Each 100 gal. of ethyl alcohol: Acetone* 8 gal. Methyl isobutyl ketone* 1.5 gal. Sucrose octa acetate

*Consult Sec. II., Ingredients Index. This ingredient may be responsible for major toxic effects if poisonous amounts of this product are ingested.

Name & Use Manufacturer	Ingredients	Name & Use Manufacturer	Ingredients
NORDEX MEDICATED SKIN CREAM (Norwich)	Dianestol (oil eucalyptus*, phenol*, eugenol*, menthol*, camphor* and white thyme)	NO-RUB FLOOR WAX (Wilbert)	Carnauba wax Synthetic resins Morpholine Oleic acid (red oil) (Ammonia)
NOREEN COLOR HAIR RINSE (Noreen)	Mildly acidic substances Stable coal tar dyes	NO-RUST Rust pre-servative and remover, compound (Frost Paint)	
NOREEN CREME SHAMPOO (Noreen)	Duponol (synthetic detergent) Sodium citrate Sodium hydroxide Sulfonated castor oil Perfume Sodium stearate	NORUSTO RUST PRE-VENTING COMPOUND (Fiske)	
NOREEN PROFES-SIONAL SHAMPOO (Beauty Prod.)	Duponol (synthetic detergent) Sodium citrate Sodium hydroxide Sulfonated castor oil Perfume Chlorophyll	NORWICH BABY COUGH SYRUP (Norwich)	Alcohol 1.875% Extractives from balsam tolu and horehound Ammonium chloride Sodium citrate
NOREEN SHAMPOO (Noreen)	Duponol (synthetic detergent) Sodium citrate Sodium hydroxide Sulfonated castor oil Perfume	NORWICH POISON IVY LOTION (Norwich)	Tannic acid Aluminum sulfocarbolate Dianestol (phenol, camphor, menthol, eugenol, oil of eucalyptus, and oil thyme) Isopropyl alcohol* 31.99%
NORFOLK'S CLIMATIZED HOUSE PAINT (Norfolk)		NORWOOD'S AFTER SHAVE LOTION (Curley)	
NORFORMS Antiseptic vaginal suppositories (Norwich)	Each suppository: Phenylmercuric acetate 0.006 gr. Methylbenzethonium chloride Methylparaben	NOSE LAX Cathartic Veterinary (hairball remedy) (Vermex)	Phenolphthalein* 25%
NORGLUCON Food supplement (Approved)	Each capsule: Liver fraction 2 455 mg. Ferrous gluconate N.F. 170 mg. Vitamin B1 0.20 mg. Vitamin B2 0.05 mg. Vitamin B12 conc. 1 mcg. Other B-complex factors	NOS-KOL Nasal decongestant (Allied Drug)	Petroleum distillate* Menthol* Camphor* Methyl salicylate* Oil of eucalyptus* Oil of cassia Phenol*
NO-RINSE SHAMPOO (No-Rinse)	Duponol Stearic acid Lanolin Propylene glycol Perfume	NO-SO-TO Skin fungicide (medical) (Carr's)	Benzoic and salicylic acids* Resorcinol Sol. coal tar N.F. Tr. merthiolate (sodium mercuri thiosalicylate, Lilly) 0.0008% Alcohol* 61%
NORITO Analgesic (Norito)	Aspirin (acetyl salicylic acid)* Calcium salicylate* Caffeine	NOSTALGIA BATH OIL (Monteil)	Perfume oils Lauric, myristic and palmitic acid alkyl esters
NORITO-PLUS Analgesic antirheumatic (Norito)	Salicylamide* Sodium salicylate caffeine alkaloid*	NOSTALGIA COLOGNE (Monteil)	Perfume oil less than 10% Denatured alcohol* (ethanol); denaturant: diethyl phthalate
NORMADOL REPLENISHER Photographic supplies (Ansco)		NOSTALGIA DUSTING POWDER (Monteil)	Talc Perfume oil
NOROLAR PLAIN Laxative (Norwich)	Heavy mineral oil emulsified	NOSTALGIA PERFUME (Monteil)	Perfume oils 15 to 30% Ethyl alcohol*
NO RO Insecticide (Meyer, T.T.)	Tech. chlordane 2% Petroleum distillate* 98%	NO STANE NAIL POLISH REMOVER (Ball)	

*Consult Sec. II., Ingredients Index. This ingredient may be responsible for major toxic effects if poisonous amounts of this product are ingested.

Name & Use Manufacturer	Ingredients		Name & Use Manufacturer	Ingredients	
NO STINKY GARBAGE CAN DEODORIZER (Dioptron)	Paradichlorobenzene* Pine oil Essential oils and aromatics	93.00% 1.50% 0.50%	NOXACORN Keratolytic (Noxacorn)	Alcohol Castor oil Iodine* Camphor Salicylic acid* Collodion (ether 79 m.) Benzocaine	21%
NOTOXIDE (Peroxide) (Sales)	Hydrogen peroxide*	20 vol.	NOX-AKE (Sacramento)		
NOTT'S ARTOX Herbicide (Nott)	Disodium monomethyl arsonate* Arsenic as metallic	31.5% 12.75%	NOXEM BUG JUICE Insecticide (Noxem)		
NOTT'S RAT-TU Rodenticide (Nott)	ANTU (alpha naphthyl thiourea)*	25%	NOXEM CORN REMEDY (Am. Pharm.)		
NOTT'S ROACH POWDER Insecticide (Nott)	Sodium fluoride* DDT Sodium silico fluoride	85% 10% 0.5%	NOXEM DRY CLEANER POWDER (Noxem)		
NOTT'S SEL-TOX Herbicide (Nott)	Phenyl mercury monoethanol ammonium acetate*	2.30%	NOXEM MOTH & FLY SPRAY Insecticide (Noxem)		
NOTT'S 2,4-D Herbicide (Nott)	2, 4-D*	16.6%	NOXEM MOTH MIST & POWDER Insecticide (Noxem)		
NOURISHINE FOR GRAY HAIR (Nourishine)			NOXEM ROACH, ANT, FLEA & PLANT BUG POWDER (Noxem)		
NOVADOL TABLETS Analgesic (Harvey Labs.)	Each tablet: Dover's powder Acetophenetidin* Aspirin* Camphor monobromated	1/4 gr. 2 gr. 2 gr. 1/4 gr.	NOXEM WHITENER POWDER (Noxem)		
NOVERM (Strand)	Tetralin* Copper* oleate Liquid paraffin Acetone*		NOX-I-DENE For dandruff (Gross)	Denatured alcohol* 50% Essential oils Potassium bicarbonate U.S.P. Acid arsenious* U.S.P. 0.45% Terpineol* Fluid extract soap bark Menthol* Vanillin Glycerin	
NOVETT Urinary stimulant (Partola)	Each tablet: Tincture nux vomica Tincture belladonna Tincture cubeb Tincture cascarilla Tincture rhubarb aromatic	1 m. 1 m.			
			NOXIT TABLETS Analgesic (Cel-Ton-Sa)	Acetophenetidin* Aspirin* Caffeine*	2-1/2 gr.
NO-VEX OINTMENT Skin fungicide (medical) (Falls)	Salicylic acid* Benzoic acid* Boric acid* Methaform*		NOX-IVY For poison ivy (Noxzema)	Isopropyl alcohol* Extract of jewel weed	17%
NOVO-HEXAMINE ELIXIR (Smith Upsher)	Each fl. dr.: Hexamethylenamine* Acid sodium phosphate (monobasic) Alcohol	7-1/2 gr. 7-1/2 gr. 1%	NOXON Metal polish (Noxon)	Dilute ammonium oxalate* in an excess of ammonia*(pH 8.4)	
			NOX-RAT BRAND Rodenticide (Collins Feed)	Warfarin (3-(a-acetonylbenzyl)- 4-hydroxycoumarin) 0.025%	
NO WASH PAINT REMOVER (Wilson-Imperial)	Toluol* Alcohol Acetone		NOX-RUSTS' RUST PRE-VENTIVE & REMOVER COMPOUND (Nox-Rust)		

---

*Consult Sec. II., Ingredients Index. This ingredient may be responsible for major toxic effects if poisonous amounts of this product are ingested.

Name & Use Manufacturer	Ingredients		Name & Use Manufacturer	Ingredients	
NOX-TOX Insecticide (Carpenter)	Petroleum distillate* DDT* Piperonyl butoxide tech. Pyrethrins	94.72% 5.00% 0.25% 0.03%	NUBILAX Laxative, bile stimulant (Hobart)	Dehydrocholic acid P. E. cascara sagrada	0.12 gm. 0.12 gm.
NOXZEMA FACE AND SHAVE CREAM (Noxzema)	Stearic acid base Phenol Menthol* Camphor* Oil of eucalyptus* Oil of clove Lime water	1/2%	NU-DA FURNITURE POLISH (Indianapolis)	Petroleum naphtha* Tergitol 4 (sodium alkyl sulfate wetting agent) Diglycol laurate Sassafras oil* Methyl cellulose	
NOXZEMA GREASELESS SUNTAN LOTION (Noxzema)			NU-DA GENERAL PURPOSE PAINT THINNER (Indianapolis)	Mineral spirits* (flash point 105°): Paraffins Naphthenes* Aromatics	56.8% 30.6% 12.6%
NOZAIN CREAM For skin irritations (Noxzema)	Cycloform (isobutyl para- amino benzoate) Carbolic acid less than 1/2% Menthol* Camphor* Oil of clove Oil of eucalyptus* Lime water		NU-DA LACQUER THINNER (Indianapolis)	Butyl acetate Butyl alcohol Toluene* Xylene*	
N-P READY MIX OIL SPRAY Insecticide (Calif. Spray)	Petroleum oils*	97%	NU-DA ODORLESS PAINT THINNER (Indianapolis)	Specially refined odorless petroleum solvent* (flash point 124°)	
NP-27 Skin fungicide (medical) (Norwich)	Orthochloro mercuriphenol Benzoic acid* Salicylic acid* Propylparaben* Isopropyl alcohol*	0.022% 50%	NU-DA PAINT AND VARNISH REMOVER (Indianapolis)	Benzene* Solox (proprietary, denatured ethyl alcohol solvent) C.P. acetone* Paraffin wax	
N S K OINTMENT For skin irritations (York Labs.)	Zinc carbonate Salicylic acid* Boric acid* Lanolin Petrolatum		NUDECK ROOF CEMENT & COATING (United Gilson)	Asphalt Mineral spirits*	
N S K RECTAL SUPPOSI- TORIES For hemorrhoids (York Labs.)	Zinc carbonate Salicylic acid* Boric acid* Cocoa butter Wax		NUDIT DEPILATORY CREAM (Rubinstein)		
N S K VAGINAL SUPPOSI- TORIES (York Labs.)	Zinc carbonate Salicylic acid* Boric acid* Cocoa butter White wax		NU-EZE FOOT BALM Ointment (Cel-Ton-Sa)	Benzoic acid* Salicylic acid* Camphor* Menthol* Oil eucalyptus* Methyl salicylate* Thymol* Witch hazel Isopropyl alcohol	0.75%
N-TIFEBRIN Vet. astringent (Thoroughbred)	Lead acetate* Aluminum sulfate		NU FINISH (Holcomb)	Stoddard solvent*	
N-2 IDEAL STENCIL INK (Ideal Stencil)	Stoddard solvent* Fuel oil* Black dye		NU-GLO PAINT & VARNISH CLEANER (Radiant)		
NTZ NASAL SPRAY (Winthrop)	Neo-synephrine* Hcl Thenfadil HCl Zephiran chloride 1-5000	0.5% 0.1%	NU-GLO SILICONE POLISH (Uncle Sam)	Waxes Silicones Mineral spirits*	
NuAIR SPACE DEODORIZER (Lester Labs.)	Ammonia Formaldehyde*		NUHIDE HOUSE PAINT (United Gilson.)	Titanium Lead* Zinc Linseed oil Mineral spirits*	
NU-AP For skin irritations (Dermateen)	Metadihydroxybenzol Oxybenzoic acid Alcohol		NUIT DE NOEL EXTRACT Toiletries (Caron)		

Name & Use Manufacturer	Ingredients	Name & Use Manufacturer	Ingredients
NUJOL Laxative (Plough)	Heavy mineral oil	NUNILE SUPER 7 Hair and scalp conditioner (Peerless Prod.)	Super lanolin (adepa lanal) Super sulfur*
NU-KLEEN LIQUID DAIRY CLEANER (Klenzade)	Organic acids*	NU-PAX (Somnyl)	Passiflores P.E. Anthemis P.E. Xalyl (valeryl diethamide)
NU-LEAF BLACK FUNGICIDE (Calif. Spray)	Ferbam* 76%	NUPERCAINAL CREAM For skin burns (Ciba)	Dibucaine (n, n-diethyl-n' (alpha butoxy cinchoninyl)- ethylene diamine)* 1/2% Acetone sodium bisulfite 1/2%
NU-LEAF 15 DUST Insecticide (Calif. Spray)	Ferric dimethyl dithiocarbamate 11.40%	NUPERCAINAL OINTMENT Local anes- thetic, for skin irritations (Ciba)	Dibucaine (n, n-diethyl-n' (alpha butoxy cinchonyl)- ethylene diamine)* 1% Acetone sodium bisulfite 1/2%
NULLO CHLOROPHYLL TABLETS Bromidrosis, halitosis (DePree)	Water soluble chlorophyllins	NU-PLATE SILVER CREAM (Nordicson)	
NU-LOOK Cleaner (Embree)	Pumice Synthetic detergents Alkaline phosphates Silicates	NUPORALS Lozenge, local anesthetic for mouth and throat (Ciba)	Dibucaine hydrochloride (n, n- diethyl-n' (alpha butoxy cinchoninyl) ethylene diamine hydrochloride)* 1 mg.
NUMBER SIX PER- FUME COLOGNE (Caswell- Massey)		NURAN Analgesic (La Salle)	Each tablet: Acetophenetidin* 2 gr. Camphor monobromated 1/2 gr. Aspirin* Caffeine* anhydrous
NUMBER SIX TOILET WATER (Caswell- Massey)		NUREXFORM STANDARD LEAD ARSENATE Insecticide (du Pont)	Lead arsenate*
NUMBER 2 OIL Solvent, paint and varnish remover, brush cleaner, insecticide, wood pre- server (Tenn. Prod.)	Lower boiling hardwood oil* fractions	NUROOF Roof coating (Acorn Ref.)	
NUMOROIDAL SUPPOSI- TORIES For hemorrhoids (Hobart)	Ephedrine hydrochloride* 0.22% Benzocaine 5.00%	NUROPATHIC DROPS Counter-irri- tant (internal and external) (Osgood)	Alcohol* 86% Capsicum Lobelia* Camphor* Oils of spearmint Cassia Spruce Wormwood
NUMOTIZINE Rubefacient (Hobart)	Each 100 gm.: Guaiacol 0.260 gm. Beechwood creosote 1.302 gm. Methyl salicylate 0.260 gm. Sol. formaldehyde 0.260 gm. Polyols 51.000 gm. Aluminum silicate 46.888 gm. Carmine 0.030 gm.	NUROSYCHOL Sedative (Jonjeems)	Bromide salts* 120 gr./fl. oz.
NUMOTIZINE COUGH SYRUP Antitussive (Hobart)	Each fl. oz.: Glyceryl guaiacolate 0.324 gm. Ammonium chloride 0.324 gm. Sodium citrate 1.296 gm. Menthol 2.6 mg. Dioctyl sodium sulfosuccinate 1-20,000	NUROTABS (Chase Chem.)	Each tablet: Calcium succinate 2 gr. Aspirin* 2 gr. Acetophenetidin* 1 gr. Caffeine alkaloid* 1/4 gr. Thiamine HCl (vit. B1) 1 mg.
		NU-SHINE Wax (Central Chem.)	

Name & Use Manufacturer	Ingredients	Name & Use Manufacturer	Ingredients
NUTAP PATCHING CEMENT (Lino-Paste)		NU-Z Fungicide (Tenn. Corp.)	Zinc* as metallic 52%
NU-TONE AIR DEODORIZER (Nu-Tone)		NUZINE OINTMENT For anorectal irritations (Hobart)	Guaiacol 1.66% Oxyquinoline sulfate 0.42% Zinc oxide 2.50% Glycerin C.P. 1.66% Lanum (anhyd.) 43.76% White petrolatum 50.00%
NUTRA-CEL Cathartic (Makers of Kal.)	Carboxymethylcellulose		
NUTRELS (Multiple trace elements for livestock feeding (Inorganic)	Manganese,* copper,* cobalt,* zinc,* magnesium, iron in sulfate form	NYCOL Antiseptic (Nycol)	Nitric acid* Camphor* Lanolin Witchhazel
		NYKO-CRUMS For poultry nutrition (Corn King)	D-activated animal sterol (source vit. D 3) 30,000 A.O.A.C. units Riboflavin (vitamin B2) 83 mg. Niacin 416 mg. Pantothenic acid 115 mg. Manganese sulfate Copper sulfate (blue vitriol) Iron sulfate (copperas) Potassium iodide Dicalcium phosphate Defluorinated phosphate Sodium chloride Calcium carbonate (limestone)
NUTRINE HEMATINIC COMPOUND Food supplement (Randolph Labs.)	Each 2 fl. oz.: Iron and ammonium citrate 6 gr. Vitamin B2 20 mg. Vitamin B12 12 mg. Tricholine citrate 24 mg. Vitamin B1 12 gr. Vitamin B6 1 mg. Niacinamide 40 mg. Folic acid 4 mg.		

NUTRITIONAL SPRAY Fungicide, miticide (Collins Feed)	Zinc sulfate* 19.5%
	Copper A. compound:
	Tetra copper* calcium
	oxychloride 7.9%
	Copper* expressed as metallic
	   3.5%
	Manganese sulfate 3.5%
	Sulfur* 28.0%
	Neotran 3.5%
		NYLMERATE ANTISEPTIC SOLUTION CONC. Douche (Holland-Rantos)	Phenylmercuric acetate*
			   0.2%
			Buffered solvent of alcohol
			   50%
			Acetone* 10%
			pH 4.9

		NYLMERATE JELLY Vaginal antiseptic (Holland-Rantos)	Phenylmercuric acetate 0.02% Boric acid 1.0% Gum tragacanth base (pH 4.0)
NUTRI TONIC PERMANENT SOLUTION (Neutralizer Powder) (Beauté)	Potassium bromide* 70% Salt and reducing hydrolysis in mildly acid solution 30%	NYMORE For throat irritations (Durst, S. F.)	Tyrothricin 1 mg. Benzocaine 5 mg.

NUTRI TONIC PERMANENT SOLUTION (Waving Solution) (Beauté)	Ammonium thioglycollate
	   about 7.5%
	Nonionic emulsifiers
	   about 5.0%
	Lanolin and lanolin deriv.
	   0.5%
	Mineral oil and deriv.
	   about 5.0%
	pH 9
		N-Z CREAM Skin creme (Lascoff)	Naftex (saponaceous mixture of
			aliphatic hydrocarbons* with
			some aromatic and naphthenic
			hydrocarbons*)
			Zinc oxide U.S.P.

NUVETTE SHAMPOO For fabrics (W-B Chem.)	Sodium-n-methyl-n-oleyl taurate		
NUVITONE HAIR TONIC (Winsale)			
NU-WAY WAX Polish (Macklanburg-Duncan)	Naphtha* (Stoddard solvent) Oleic acid Paraffin Corvus oil Trigamine Silican		
NU-WHITE FURNITURE POLISH (Central Chem.)			

*Consult Sec. II., Ingredients Index. This ingredient may be responsible for major toxic effects if poisonous amounts of this product are ingested.

Name & Use Manufacturer	Ingredients		Name & Use Manufacturer	Ingredients
OAKES ARROYO BRAND 10% CHLORDANE DUST Insecticide (Oakes)	Chlordane*	10%	OBEGYNE Douche powder (Dayton Labs.)	Essential oils and aromatics Boric acid* Ammon. alum Magnesium sulfate Zinc sulfate* Sodium bicarbonate
OAKES ARROYO BRAND COPPER DUST Fungicide (Oakes)	Basic copper sulfate*	10%	O'BRIEN ASPHALT PAINT (O'Brien Corp.)	
OAKES ARROYO BRAND 10% DDT DUST Insecticide (Oakes)	DDT* Sulfur*	10% 40%	O'BRIEN WALL SIZE (O'Brien Corp.)	
OAKES ARROYO BRAND 10% DDT-COP-SUL DUST Insecticide (Oakes)	DDT* Basic copper sulfate* Sulfur*	10% 10% 40%	OBTUNDIA CALAMINE CREAM For skin irritations (Clapp, Otis)	Meta-cresolated camphor* Eugenol* Thymol iodide* Essential oil of pine* Calamine Limewater Anethol Geraniol Balsam of Peru Zinc oxide Glycerin Magma of bentonite
OAKES ARROYO BRAND 3-10-40 DUST Insecticide (Oakes)	DDT* Gamma isomer of benzene hexachloride* Other isomers of benzene hexachloride and inert Sulfur*	10% 3% 47% 40%	OBTUNDIA CALAMINE LOTION For skin irritations (Clapp, Otis)	Meta-cresolated camphor* Eugenol* Thymol iodide* Balsam of Peru Zinc oxide Glycerin Magma of bentonite Anethol Geraniol Essential oil of pine* Calamine Lime water
OAKES ARROYO BRAND T & O SUPER DUST Insecticide (Oakes)	Toxaphene* DDT Sulfur	20.00% 10.00% 30.00%		
OAKES ARROYO BRAND 20-TOX-SUL DUST Insecticide (Oakes)	Toxaphene* Sulfur	20% 40%	OBTUNDIA CREAM For skin burns (Clapp, Otis)	Meta-cresolated camphor* Eugenol* Thymol iodide* Essential oil of pine* Anethol Geraniol Balsam of Peru Calendula
OAKES ARROYO BRAND 20-TOX-TALC DUST (Oakes)	Toxaphene*	20%	OBTUNDIA EPHEDRINE INHALANT For nasal irritation (Clapp, Otis)	Meta-cresolated camphor* Eugenol Thymol iodide* Ephedrine* Anethol Geraniol Essential oil of pine*
OAKES ARROYO BRAND TWO & ONE DUST Insecticide (Oakes)	Toxaphene* DDT Sulfur	15.00% 7.50% 40.00%	OBTUNDIA GLYCO BORON VAGIOBULBS For vaginal irritation (Clapp, Otis)	Meta-cresolated camphor* Eugenol* Thymol iodide* Essential oil of pine* Anethol Geraniol Balsam of Peru
OAKITE CLEANSER (Oakite)	Alkaline salts (essentially phosphates and carbonates) Synthetic surface active agents		OBTUNDIA INHALANT PLAIN For nasal irritation (Clapp, Otis)	Meta-cresolated camphor* Eugenol Thymol iodide* Anethol Geraniol Essential oil of pine*
OBAY PRESTO SPRAY DEODORANT (Pharma-Craft)				
OBCELLOID LACQUERS (O'Brien Corp.)				

*Consult Sec. II., Ingredients Index. This ingredient may be responsible for major toxic effects if poisonous amounts of this product are ingested.

Name & Use Manufacturer	Ingredients		Name & Use Manufacturer	Ingredients	
OBTUNDIA LINIMENT Local analgesic (Clapp, Otis)	Meta-cresolated camphor* Eugenol* Thymol iodide* Essential oil of pine* Oil of peppermint Oil of turpentine Oil of mustard syn. Anethol Geraniol Balsam of Peru Methyl salicylate* Oil of eucalyptus* Oil of thyme Oil of camphor*		OCAS NASAL CREAM Nasal decongestant (Clapp, Otis)	Oil pinus sylvestris Oil thyme Camphor-menthol* Oil thuja Oil pine needles* Oil pinus pumilio Oil eucalyptus* White petrolatum jelly	
			OCCO-EX For round worms in hogs (Oelwein)	Chenopodium* Chloroform Castor oil Oil of anise F. D. & C. red no. 32 (coloring, inert)	5.75% 1.89% 0.118%
OBTUNDIA NASAL CREAM For nasal irritation (Clapp, Otis)	Meta-cresolated camphor* Eugenol* Thymol iodide* White petroleum jelly Anethol Geraniol Essential oil of pine*		OCCO GOLDEN OIL For sarcoptic mange of hogs (Oelwein)	Cresylic acid* Mineral oil Glycerin	1.00% 98.75%
OBTUNDIA NON-OILY INHALANT For colds (Clapp, Otis)	Meta-cresolated camphor* Thymol iodide* Geraniol Essential oil of pine*		OCCO-LENE Deodorant for hogs (Oelwein)	Nicotine* Sulfur Naphthalene	0.14% 1.75% 30.00%
OBTUNDIA SALICYLIC ACID CORN APPLICATION Keratolytic (Clapp, Otis)	Alcohol 29% Salicylic acid* Anethol Geraniol Ether* 50% Meta-cresolated camphor* Eugenol* Essential oil of pine*		OCCO-NOX For round worms and nodular worms in hogs (Oelwein)	Phenothiazine Pomegranate bark Areca nut American wormseed Senna leaves Capsicum Anise Fennel seed Copper sulfate* Bentonite Iron sulfate Iron oxide	30% 3% 5% 1%
OBTUNDIA SODIUM CHLORIDE & BIBORATE GARGLE TABLETS (Clapp, Otis)	Sodium chloride Obtundia surface anesthetic Meta-cresolated camphor* Eugenol* Thymol iodide* Sodium biborate Anethol Geraniol Essential oil of pine*		OCCO TON-EX For round worms in poultry (Oelwein)	Nicotine sulfate* American Wormseed Copper sulfate Areca nut Bentonite Ginger Senna leaves Pomegranate bark Iron oxide Capsicum Fennel Columbo Anise Iron sulfate Sodium nitrate	8.75% 1.8% 1.6% 6.6% 25%
OBTUNDIA SURFACE ANESTHETIC Local (Clapp, Otis)	Meta-cresolated camphor* Eugenol* Essential oil of pine* Anethol Geraniol				
OBTUNDO-BULBS Analgesic (Clapp, Otis)	Aesculus horse chestnuts Hamamelis green leaves Meta-cresolated camphor* Eugenol* Thymol iodide* Essential oil of pine* Fresh nuts Twigs Anethol Geraniol Balsam of Peru		OCEANA MARINE PAINT (Standard-Toch)		
			O'CEDAR ALL PURPOSE POLISH (O-Cedar)	Mineral seal oil	
OBTUNDOR-RHOID For hemorrhoids (Clapp, Otis)	Aesculus astringent Meta-cresolated camphor* Anethol Geraniol Balsam of Peru Hamamelis green leaves & twigs Eugenol* Thymol iodide* Essential oil of pine*		O'CEDAR DRI-GLO POLISH (O-Cedar)	Petroleum naphtha* Inert silicones Wax solids	
			O'CEDAR NO-RUBBING CREAM POLISH (O-Cedar)	Mineral seal oil low concentration emulsifiers	
OCAS ANTI-HISTAMINIC Oral (Clapp, Otis)	Pyrilamine maleate* 25 mg.		O'CEDAR PERMA-MOTH OCTALENE (Compound 118) Insecticide (O-Cedar)	Magnesium silicofluoride* Ethanolamine silicofluoride*	

*Consult Sec. II., Ingredients Index. This ingredient may be responsible for major toxic effects if poisonous amounts of this product are ingested.

Name & Use Manufacturer	Ingredients	Name & Use Manufacturer	Ingredients
O'CEDAR RUG CLEANER (O-Cedar)	Synthetic detergents*	OCULINE EYE DROPS (Oculine)	Boric acid Menthol Rose water Methylparaben Zinc sulfate Borax Camphor Oil of peppermint
O'CEDAR TOUCH-UP FURNITURE POLISH (O-Cedar)	Mineral seal oil Petroleum naphtha* Asphaltic material Perfumes		
OCTAB Fungicide (Fairfield)	Octadecyl dimethyl benzyl ammonium chloride* 85% Oleyl dimethyl benzyl ammonium chloride 15%	OCULINE EYE PADS (Oculine)	Boric acid Menthol Camphor Zinc sulfate Oil of peppermint Borax Methylparaben Rose water Glycerin
OCTAGON Bar laundry soap (Colgate-Palmolive)			
OCTAVAPOR-10 FORMULA NO. 225 Insecticide (Edco)	Octamethyl pyrophosphoramide* 7% Related compounds 3%	OCULINE EYE SALVE (Oculine)	Boric acid Zinc sulfate Menthol Borax Camphor Oil of peppermint White vasoline Lanolin
OCTIMET Fungicide (Fairfield)	Octadecyl dimethyl ethyl ammonium bromide* 85% Octadecenyl dimethyl ethyl ammonium bromide 15%	OCUSOL EYE DROPS (Norwich)	Boric acid Borax Dist. ext. witch hazel Berberine sulfate Sodium chloride Rose and camphor water Glycerin Ephedrine hydrochloride 0.1%
OCTOFEN For athlete's foot (McKesson)	8-Hydroxyquinoline benzoate*		
OCTOGEN Rubefacient (Octogen)	Essential oils of eucalyptus,* pine needles, turpentine, hemlock, cedar leaves and thyme Methyl salicylate* Volatile crystals of camphor* and menthol Coloring matter	OCUSOL EYE LOTION (Norwich)	Boric acid Sodium chloride Dist. ext. witch hazel Berberine sulfate Borax Rose and camphor water Glycerin
OCU-BATH Eye lotion (Wright, M.)	Sodium propionate Boric acid Rose water Dist. ext. witch hazel Berberine sulfate Borax Sodium chloride Camphor water Glycerin Benzalkonium chloride	ODER CHEK Deodorant (Watkins, J.)	Iso-propanol* Formaldehyde* Perfume
		ODOL Mouth wash (Odol)	Alcohol 80%
		ODORALL Insecticide (Dill)	Paradichlorobenzene*
OCU DROP Eye drops (Commerce)	Sodium propionate Boric acid Rose water Dist. ext. witch hazel Berberine sulfate Borax Sodium chloride Camphor water Glycerin Benzalkonium chloride	ODOR-BLITZ AEROSOL Deodorizer (Blitz)	
		ODOR CHEK Deodorizer (Chek)	
		ODORCIDE Deodorant (Beecham)	
OCULINE Eye bath (Oculine)	Boric acid Menthol Rose water Methylparaben Zinc sulfate Borax Camphor Oil of peppermint	ODOR CRYSTALS Insecticide (Holcomb)	Paradichlorobenzene*
		ODOREX AEROSOL DEODORANT Deodorizer (Kilgore Chem.)	Lauryl methacrylate 4% Deodorized kerosene* 6% Freon 90%

*Consult Sec. II., Ingredients Index. This ingredient may be responsible for major toxic effects if poisonous amounts of this product are ingested.

Name & Use Manufacturer	Ingredients	Name & Use Manufacturer	Ingredients
ODOR-LESS DAMPCOAT ENAMEL (Wilbur)		OF THEE I SING DEODORANT & EAU DE COLOGNE (Parfums Charbert)	
ODOR-MASTER WAFER Deodorant (Edco)	Water-soluble chlorophyll Precipitated calcium carbonate 1% p-Formaldehyde Methyl cellulose Certified food colors	OGEN CORN EAR WORM DROPS (Rose Mfg.)	Mineral oil Dichloroethyl ether*
ODOR-NEVER Deodorant (Odor-Never)		OGILVIE SISTERS CUTICAL CREAM (Ogilvie)	
ODORONO CREAM Deodorant (Northam)	Glyceryl monostearate Polyhydric alcohols	OGILVIE SISTERS HAND CREAM (Ogilvie)	
ODORONO ICE Deodorant (Northam)	Alcohol solution of aluminum chloride Waxes	OGILVIE SISTERS SHAMPOOS, LOTIONS, OILS, RINSES (Ogilvie)	
ODORONO REGULAR & INSTANT (Liquid) (Northam)			
ODORONO SPRAY Deodorant (Northam)	Water-alcohol solution of aluminum chlorhydroxide	OGILVIE SISTERS SPECIAL OINTMENT (Ogilvie)	Cade oil* Sulfur* Acid salicylic* Methyl salicylate*
ODOROT-LESS Wood preservative (Planetary Chem.)	Pentachlorophenol* 5% Petroleum distillate* 74% Methylated rosin 10% Paraffin 1%	O G S ODORLESS GERMICIDE-SANITIZER (Alkem)	Alkyl tolyl methyl trimethyl ammonium chlorides* 10% and 25%
ODOR OUT LIQUID AIR DEODORANT (Puritan Chem.)		O G V MEN'S CONCEN-TRATED SCALP LOTION (Ogilvie)	Tannic acid* Glycerin Propylene glycol Cantharides* Benzoin Nutgalls Phenol* Alcohol 7.5%
ODOR-SOLV DEODORANTS (Du-Rite)			
ODORZONE MIST INSEC-TICIDE (Nat'l. Sanitary)		O G V MEN'S HAIR LOTION For dry hair, dandruff (Ogilvie)	Tannic acid* Glycerin Propylene glycol Cantharides* Benzoin Nutgalls Alcohol 7.5%
OFF-EZY CORN RE-MOVER Keratolytic (Comm.)	Benzocaine Flexible collodion* Salicylic acid*	O G V MEN'S HAIR LOTION For oily hair, dandruff (Ogilvie)	Pine tar oil* Witch hazel Extract of juniper berries Alcohol 8%
OFFICE PAX Skin cleaner (Packwood)	Borax* Powdered soap Phosphate-type salts Emollients		
OFLYO LIQUID SPRAY Insecticide (Adco)	Petroleum distillate* Tech. piperonyl butoxide Pyrethrins*	O G V MEN'S SCALP POMADE & HAIR DRESS-ING (Ogilvie)	
OF THEE I SING AFTER SHAVE LO-TION (Parfums Charbert)		O G V MEN'S SPECIAL HAIR LOTION (Ogilvie)	Salicylic acid* Tannic acid* Glycerin Tincture of cantharides* Alcohol 10%

*Consult Sec. II., Ingredients Index. This ingredient may be responsible for major toxic effects if poisonous amounts of this product are ingested.

Name & Use Manufacturer	Ingredients	Name & Use Manufacturer	Ingredients
O G V MEN'S SPECIAL OINTMENT (Ogilvie)	Cade oil* Sulfur* Salicylic acid* Methyl salicylate*	OJACO MILL WHITE PAINTS (Johnson)	
OH BOY FURNITURE POLISH (U. S. Sanitary)		O-JOY PILLS Urinary stimulant (T-Lax)	Methenamine Uva ursi Buchu Saw palmetto Salol Oil juniper*
O-H COW'S RELIEF OINTMENT Counter-irritant (veterinary) (Our Husbands)	Pine oil* Eucalyptol* Common soft soap Menthol* Petrolatum	O-KAY CEMENT PAINT (Stucco)	
OHIO ANTI-FREEZE COMPOUND (Ohio Solv.)		OK CEMENT (Glass, Crockery & China) (Tip Top)	Cement Butanol* Acetone*
O-H LOUSE POWDER (Our Husbands)	Pyrethum Po. (1/2 of 1% pyrethrin) 10% Sodium fluoride* 20% Naphthalene 1-1/4% Powdered sabadilla seed 10% Sulfur 20%	OK CHEMICAL DRY CLEAN-ING FLUID (Blum)	Carbon tetrachloride* greater than 20% Chloroform Naphtha* 70% Benzine soap
OIL-DRI NON SLIP PAINT (Oil-Dri)		O.K. CLEAR CEMENT (Tip Top)	Cellulose nitrate Acetone*
OILEX NAIL POLISH RE-MOVER (Darling)		OK HEADACHE REMEDY (Houston)	
OIL OF INDIA MOSQUITO REPELLENT (Oil of India)		OK LIQUID SOLDER (Tip Top)	Cellulose nitrate Acetone*
OIL-O-SOL (Mosso's) Antiseptic for wet dressing (Mosso)	Linseed oil Turpentine* Camphor* Oils of sassafras*spearmint and eucalyptus*	OK MODEL AIRPLANE CEMENT (Tip Top)	Clear cement Butanol* Citric acid Acetone*
OILZUM LUBRICATING GREASE (White & Bagley)	Oil-soap type lubricating grease	OK TYPEWRITER OIL (Cardinell)	
OILZUM MOTOR, HYDRAULIC & GEAR OILS (White & Bagley)		OLALA For tired liver, kidneys, stomach, bowels (Richards (Bros.)	Wahoo Sarsaparilla Sassafras* Prickly ash Queen's root Mandrake Clover Aloes* Salicylic acid 1/2% Sugar Burdock Rhubarb Yellow dock Lobelia Dandelion Wild cherry Skunk cabbage Wintergreen* Rochelle salt 1% Water
OINT-EASE Rubefacient (Pope)	Eucalyptus oil* Camphor* Menthol* Methyl salicylate* Oil of turpentine* Acid salicylic* Petrolatum		
OINTMENT-CRAFT CREAM OB TYPE Skin emollient (Bullock-Walker)	Cocoa butter Lanolin	OLCO DISINFEC-TANTS (Oliver Chem.)	
		OLCOCIDE INSECT SPRAY (Oliver Chem.)	Petroleum distillates* Tech. chlordane* Pyrethrins

*Consult Sec. II., Ingredients Index. This ingredient may be responsible for major toxic effects if poisonous amounts of this product are ingested.

- 764 -

Name & Use Manufacturer	Ingredients		Name & Use Manufacturer	Ingredients
OLCO COMPLETE INSECT SPRAY (Oliver Chem.)	Petroleum oil* 98.60% Piperonyl butoxide tech. 1.27% Pyrethrins 0.13%		OLD DUTCH CLEANSER (Purex Corp.)	Siliceous abrasive
OLCO HY-POWER IN-SECT SPRAY (Oliver Chem.)	Petroleum distillates* Tech. piperonyl butoxide Pyrethrins		OLD DUTCH FLOOR WAX (Banner Mfg.)	
OLCO INDUSTRIAL INSECT SPRAY (Oliver (Chem.)	Petroleum oil* 99.27% Piperonyl butoxide tech. 0.66% Pyrethrins 0.07%		OLD DUTCH PAINTS & ENAMELS (Aladdin)	
			OLD EAGLE HOUSE PAINTS (Vanguard)	
OLCO 50% MALATHION EMULSIFI-ABLE CON-CENTRATE Insecticide (Oliver Chem.)	Malathion* 50% Xylol* 42.4%		OLD ENGLISH PAINT OIL (du Pont)	
			OLD ENGLISH PASTE WAX (Boyle-Midway)	Waxes Petroleum naphtha* Turpentine*
OLCO NEW INSECT SPRAY (Oliver Chem.)	Petroleum oil* 98.60% Piperonyl butoxide tech. 1.00% Pyrethrins 0.40%		OLD ENGLISH RED OIL POLISH (Boyle-Midway)	Petroleum polishing oil* Oil of cedarwood* Turpentine*
OLCO POWDERED INSECTICIDE (Oliver Chem.)	Sodium fluoride* 61.75% Dichloro diphenyl trichloro-ethane 10.00% Pyrethrins 0.20%		OLD ENGLISH SELF POLISH-ING DRI BRITE (Boyle-Midway)	Vegetable and/or mineral waxes Emulsifiers of the fatty acid amine type Borax Resins
OLCO RESIDUAL INSECTICIDE (Oliver Chem.)	Beta butoxy beta' thiocyano diethyl ether* 0.75% Beta thiocyano ethyl esters of mixed fatty acids* 2.25% DDT* 5% Oil 92%		OLD EUROPE PINE BATH OIL EAU DE COLOGNE & LAVENDER WATER (Masie)	
OLCO SPECIAL MILL SPRAY Insecticide (Oliver Chem.)	Petroleum oil* 98.80% Piperonyl butoxide tech. 1.00% Pyrethrins 0.20%		OLD FAITHFUL LIGHTER FLUID (Hollingshead)	V M & P naphtha* almost 100%
OLD BELMONT HOTEL ENGLISH HAIR TONIC (Castilla)	Denatured alcohol* 84% Castor oil Citrus oils		OLD FASHIONED GARDEN COLOGNE & PERFUME (Ybry)	
OLD CHELSEA QUICK ENAMEL (Johnston)			OLD-FASHIONED LINIMENT (Olliffe)	Chloroform* oz.* xxv Methyl salicylate* oz. iv, dr. iii Salicylic acid* oz. ii, dr. iv Tincture iodine* oz. ii, dr. iv Oleum sinapis vol. dr. iv Fluidextract capsicum oz. iii Benzocaine oz. i.z. Linimentum saponis q.s. ad gal. i Tr. amaranth q.s. for coloring
OLD COLONIAL EAU DE COLOGNE (Delex)				
OLD COLONIAL ENAMELS & VARNISHES (DeSoto)				
OLD COLONY PAINT PRODUCTS (Old Colony)				

*Consult Sec. II., Ingredients Index. This ingredient may be responsible for major toxic effects if poisonous amounts of this product are ingested.

- 765 -

Name & Use Manufacturer	Ingredients	Name & Use Manufacturer	Ingredients
OLD HICKORY OINTMENT For itching of ringworm, acne, athletes foot, piles, etc. (Old Hickory)	Zinc oxide Camphor* Calomel* 1.23% Petrolatum Salicylic acid* Menthol Carbolic acid* 3.75 oz.	OLD STYLE COPPER PAINTS (Kirby)	
OLD HONESTY PREPARED PAINT FOR WOOD (Vita-Var)		OLD TRAPPER ANTU 20 Rodenticide (Stanley Ind.)	Alpha naphthyl thiourea*
OLD MARINERS SPAR VAR-NISH & DECK ENAMELS (Federal Paint)		OLD TRAPPER ANTU GRAIN Rodenticide (Stanley Ind.)	Alpha naphthyl thiourea*
		OLD TRAPPER GOPHER KILLER (Stanley Ind.)	Strychnine*
OLD MASTER PAINTS, VARNISHES & ENAMELS (DeSoto)		OLD TRAPPER HOTEL POWDER Insecticide (Stanley Ind.)	DDT*
OLD MASTERS ENAMEL & PASTE WHITE (Breinig)		OLD TRAPPER MOLE KILLER (Stanley Ind.)	Strychnine*
OLD 97 ANTISEPTIC (Old 97)		OLD TRAPPER POISONED GRAIN FOR RATS (Stanley Ind.)	Strychnine*
OLD NOBILITY LAVENDER (Noblesse)			
OLD RELIABLE DYE (French Ren.)		OLD TRAPPER RAT KRUNCHES (Stanley Ind.)	Red squill*
OLD SALEM WHITE PAINT (Pettit)		OLD TRAPPER WEED NOX (Stanley Ind.)	2, 4-D*
OLD SPICE AFTER SHAVE LOTION (Shulton)		OLD VIRGINIA WHITE PAINT (Cabot)	
		OLD ZANZIBAR FINISH FOR ALL SURFACES (Rudd)	
OLD SPICE COLOGNE & TOILET WATER (Shulton)		OLEEN DANDRUFF TREATMENT SHAMPOO (Curley)	
OLD SPICE DEODORANT CREAM & STICK (Shulton)		O-LE-IDE Rubefacient (Oleide)	Oil of wintergreen* Camphor* Capsicum Menthol* Iodine*
OLD SPICE MEN'S COLOGNE (Shulton)		O-LE-IDE SPRAY Nasal decongestant (Oleide)	Iodine* Camphor* Oil cinnamon Menthol* Thymol* Oil eucalyptus*
OLD SPICE SHAVE CREAM & STICK (Shulton)		OLEON Dishwashing detergent (Lester Labs.)	
OLD SPICE TALCUMS (Shulton)		OLEPHINE LIQUID SOAPS (Aix Olein)	

*Consult Sec. II., Ingredients Index. This ingredient may be responsible for major toxic effects if poisonous amounts of this product are ingested.

Name & Use Manufacturer	Ingredients	Name & Use Manufacturer	Ingredients
OLEPHINE TAR RE- MOVERS (Aix Olein)		OLO-SEAL WALL SIZE (Passonno)	
OLIO O'LITE RESIN ENAMEL PAINT (O'Brien Corp.)		OLO WALL & ROOF COATING (Passonno)	
OLIVE CREAM POMADE (Fearonce)		OLYMPIC CAMPHOR ICE (Woltra)	Camphor* Petrolatum Paraffin
OLIVENA LIQUID SOAP (U. S. Sanitary)		OMAR WALLPAPER CLEANER (Omar)	
O-LIV-ER SALTS Cathartic, antacid (Oliver's S-O)	Epsom salts Sodium bicarbonate Calcium carbonate	O-M DEODORANT WAFERS (Edco)	Water-soluble chlorophyll Calcium carbonate Paraformaldehyde 1% Methyl cellulose
OLIVER'S POISON IVY LOTION (Oliver's S-O)	Zinc sulfate* Sugar of lead* Potassium permanganate*	OMEGA CHALKBOARD CHALK IN COLOR (Weber Costello)	
OLIVER'S RED HOT BRAND LINIMENT Rubefacient (Oliver's S-O)	Chloroform 5 m./fl. oz. Camphor* Capsicum Oil origanum Oil cedar* Kerosene*	OMEGA OIL Rubefacient (Omega)	Chloroform 39 m./fl. oz. Isopropyl alcohol* 48% Methyl salicylate* Mineral oil
OLIVER'S TOILET CREAM (Favorite) Skin emollient (Oliver's S-O)		OMNICIDE Insecticide (Superior Chem.)	Oil* Pyrethrum
OLIVO BRUSHLESS CREAM (Olivo)	Stearic acid Cocoanut oil Boric acid* Potassium carbonate Ammonia	OMNICIDE BB Insecticide (Superior Chem.)	Pyrethrum DDT*
		OMNICIDE C Insecticide (Superior Chem.)	Pyrethrum Chlordane*
OLIVO HAIR POMADE (Olivo)	Petrolatum	OMPA SPRAY CONCEN- TRATE NO. 803 Insecticide (Stauffer)	Octamethyl pyrophosphoramide* 59.3% Related organic phosphates* 16.9%
OLIVO HAIR TONIC (Olivo)	Alcohol Castor oil Glycerin		
OLIVO SHAMPOO (Olivo)	Cocoanut fatty acid Lanolin Oleic acid Potassium pyro phosphorite	ONALIM ANTISEPTIC SOLUTION (Onalim)	Dihydroxy dichloro diphenyl- methane 0.4% Phenol 0.1% Alcohol 14%
OLO CAULKING COMPOUND (Passonno)		ONCE ONLY MOTH PROOFER (Hermann)	
OLO OIL COLORS (Passonno)		ONCE OVER FLAT WALL FINISH (Stacoat)	
OLO PAINTS & ENAMELS (Olo)		ONCE OVER POLISH (Kleer)	
OLO ROOFING CEMENT (Passonno)		ONE-COAT FLAT WASH- ABLE WALL PAINT (Foy)	

*Consult Sec. II., Ingredients Index. This ingredient may be responsible for major toxic effects if poisonous amounts of this product are ingested.

Name & Use Manufacturer	Ingredients		Name & Use Manufacturer	Ingredients	
ONECONAMEL ENAMEL (Paragon Paint)			ONE-SHOT DUST NO. 20 (Tobacco & Cotton) Insecticide (Cotton)	Endrin (hexachloro epoxy octahydro-endo, endo-dimethano naphthalene)*	2.0%
111 BALM Rubefacient (Kudymern)	Menthol* Camphor* Guaiacol Methyl salicylate* Beechwood creosote Oil of wormwood		ONE SHOT LIGHTER FLUID (Tubed)	V. M. & P. naphtha* Rubber solvent naphtha*	
ONE-HUNDRED-PERCENT HOUSE PAINT (Parr Paint)			ONE-SHOT 5% MALATHION DUST Insecticide (Cotton)	Malathion*	5.0%
100% PURE HOUSE PAINT (General Paint)			ONE-SPOT FLEA KILLER (One-Spot)	Rotenone* Other derris or cube extractives*	1% 2%
"100" ROTENONE Insecticide (Chem. Form.)	Rotenone Other cube resins Talc	1.00% 2.50% 96.50%	$1000.00 GUARANTEED ANT-BANE (Heller)	Sodium fluoride* Tech. chlordane*	50% 2%
O-NE-KO PAINTS, ENAMELS, STAINS (Tredennick)			$1000.00 GUARANTEED ROACH KILLER (Heller)	Boric acid* Tech. chlordane	51.0% 0.2%
ONE KOTE SATIN LATEX PAINT (Louisville Paint)			1, 2, 3 PAINT SET (Palmer Paint)		
ONE 19 FLOOR VARNISH (Tropical)			ONEXIT White liquid cleaner (Hillyard Chem.)	Alkali*	
101 LIQUID BLEACH (Gardiner Mfg.)	Sodium hypochlorite*	5.25%	ONEX-SEAL SPECIAL, NATURAL, REGULAR, SUPER, WHITE Blended floor seal and polish (Hillyard Chem.)	Stoddard solvent*	
101 LIQUID DETERGENT (Gardiner Mfg.)	Sodium alkyl aryl sulfonate Lauric diethanolamine A nonionic of the nonyl phenol ethylene oxide condensate type Ethyl alcohol				
ONE-PAK FRUIT SPRAY Fungicide, insecticide (Miller Chem.)	DDT (dichloro diphenyl trichloroethane) Arsenate of lead* Ferbam Total arsenic expressed as metallic arsenic Water-soluble arsenic expressed as metallic	7.5% 24.5% 11.4% 4.87% 0.125%	ONLYCOAT FLAT WALL PAINT (Deer-O)		
			ONLY ORIGINAL SOOT DESTROYER (Saginaw)		
ONE-SHOT DUST NO. 5 Insecticide (Cotton)	Parathion* Dichloro diphenyl dichloroethane	1% 5%	O-N MEN-THO-SOTE For colds (Owen)	Alcohol 1-M beechwood creosote Wild cherry syrup Horehound Ammonium chloride	5%
ONE-SHOT DUST NO. 10 Insecticide (Cotton)	Parathion* Dichloro diphenyl dichloroethane	1% 10%		Menthol 2-M chloroform White pine syrup Ext. ipecac Sanguinaria Cascara Syrup base	
ONE-SHOT DUST NO. 15 Insecticide (Cotton)	Endrin (hexachloro epoxy octahydro-endo, endo-dimethano naphthalene)*	1.5%			

*Consult Sec. II., Ingredients Index. This ingredient may be responsible for major toxic effects if poisonous amounts of this product are ingested.

Name & Use Manufacturer	Ingredients		Name & Use Manufacturer	Ingredients	
O-N MILAM FOOT POWDER (Owen)	Powdered alum Menthol Boric acid* Zinc stearate Carbolic acid Camphor* Talc Starch Para tertiary butyl meta cresol*		OPHTHALMIC ISOPHRIN SOLUTION For eye disorders (Broemmel)	Isophrin hydrochloride (brand of phenylephrine hydrochloride) aqueous solution, approx. isotonic with tears	1/8%
ONOX Fungicide (medical) (Onox)	Zinc chloride* Sodium chloride Sodium nitrate Sodium silicofluoride* Boric acid*		O-PRO-TEX Fungicide (medical) (Stewart-Simmons)	Alcohol* Benzoic acid Acetone Copper nitrate*	
O-N SKIN ITCH ANTISEPTIC Fungicide (medical) (Owen)	Salicylic acid-resorcin* Benzoic acid* q.s. Alcohol		OPTAURAL Local analgesic and deconges-tant for ear (Optimus)	Atropine sulfate* Benzocaine Antipyrine* Glycerin q.s. and 1/2 fl. oz.	1/40 gr. 2 gr. 8 gr.
ONTHANK'S PAINT & VARNISH CLEANER (Onthank)			OP-THAL-ZIN Ophthalmic solution (Alcon)	Zinc sulfate Chlorobutanol Benzalkonium chloride	0.25%
ON THE NOSE Tonic, dis-temper, preventive, (veterinary) (Vermex)	Metallic mercury* 15%		OPT-I-BATH Eye bath (Premo)	Boric acid Sodium borate Potassium chloride Methyl paraben	0.1%
ONYCHOMYCE-TIN Fungicide, emol-lient, (medical) (Gordon Labs.)	Undecylenic acid 25% Compound G-4 1% Penetrating oil base*		OPTIC DROP Eye lotion (Romero)	1 oz. each: Chlorbutanol (chloroform deriv.) 1 gr. Sulfate zinc* Berberine hydrochloride Boracic acid* Potassium borate* Glycerin Distilled water	
ON YOUR TOES FOOT LOTION (Randolph-Tenney)			OPTICLEAN EYE DROPS (Ohio Pharm.)	Hydrastis Boric acid Chlorobutanol (chloroform derivative 0.25%)	
OPALATE DUST NO. 10 Fungicide (Calif. Spray)	Ziram* 7.6%		OPTIMO BRAND POWDERED CUBE OR DERRIS ROOT 5% ROTENONE Insecticide (Penick)		
OPALATE WHITE FUNGICIDE (Calif. Spray)	Ziram* 76%		OPTONE DUO For eyes (Ohio Pharm.)	Boric acid U.S.P. Camphor U.S.P. Berberine sulfate N.F. & O. Sodium borate U.S.P. Sodium chloride U.S.P. Chlorbutanol 0.25%	
OPAL FURNITURE POLISH (Louisiana)	Kerosene* Pale paraffin oil Red oil color Synthetic peach oil		OPTREX EYE DROPS (Chemdrug)	Sodium borate Boric acid Zinc sulfate* Salicylic acid* Comfrey root Tormentil Antipyrene 0.2% Witch hazel Alcohol 3%/v	
OPALON Laminating and molding material, base for various plastics (Monsanto)	Polyvinyl chloride Dry powder resin		ORADEX (Wright, M.)	Tyrothrycin 1 mg. Benzocaine 10 mg.	
OPEEKO HOUSEHOLD INSECTICIDE (Oleum)			ORA-JEL Dental analgesic (Commerce)	Benzocaine*	
OPENUP Plumbing cleaner (Ampion)	Sodium hydroxide*		ORAL HYGIENE Antiseptic (Massengill)	Each fl. oz.: Eucalyptol 0.03 cc. Methyl salicylate syn. 0.017 cc. Boric acid* 0.72 gm. Benzoic acid 32 mg. Menthol 12.2 mg. Thymol 26.3 mg.	

*Consult Sec. II., Ingredients Index. This ingredient may be responsible for major toxic effects if poisonous amounts of this product are ingested.

Name & Use Manufacturer	Ingredients	
ORANGE LAC SHELLAC SUBSTITUTE (Thompson & Co.)		
ORASTIN For colds (Commerce)	Pyrilamine maleate Salicylamide* Phenacetin* Caffeine Vitamin C	
ORAVAX TABLETS Oral bacterial vaccine (Merrell)	Killed bacteria and their water-soluble antigens	
ORBISCIDE CUBE POWDER Insecticide (Orbis)	Rotenone*	4 or 5%
ORBISCIDE CUBE RESIN Insecticide (Orbis)	Rotenone*	
ORBISCIDE DERRIS POWDER Insecticide (Orbis)	Rotenone*	4 or 5%
ORBISCIDE DERRIS RESIN Insecticide (Orbis)	Rotenone*	
ORBISCIDE EMULSIFI- ABLE ROTENONE CONC. Insecticide (Orbis)	Rotenone	1.5%
ORBISCIDE ROTENONE- CARBON TETRACHLO- RIDE SOLVATE Insecticide (Orbis)	Rotenone* Carbon tetrachloride*	
ORBISCIDE ROTENONE CRYSTALS C.P. Insecticide (Orbis)	Rotenone*	
ORBISCIDE 5% & 10% ROTENONE OIL CONC. Insecticide (Orbis)	Rotenone*	5% and 10%
ORBISCIDE ROTENONE* TECH. 90/95% Insecticide (Orbis)	Rotenone*	
OR-BLOS ORANGE BLOSSOM PERFUME (Or-Blos)		

Name & Use Manufacturer	Ingredients	
ORBOLENE EYE LOTION (Orbolene)	Alcohol Ephedrine hydrochloride* Carbolic acid Boric acid* Glycerin	0.0039%
ORCHARD BRAND ALDRIN EM-2 EMULSI- FIABLE CONC. Insecticide (General Chem.)	Aldrin* (hexachloro hexahydro-endo, exo- dimethano naphthalene) Related compounds	23.5% 3.9%
ORCHARD BRAND 20% ALDRIN GRANULAR DUST CONC. Insecticide (General Chem.)	Aldrin* (hexachloro hexahydro-endo, exo- dimethano naphthalene) Related compounds	19.0% 3.2%
ORCHARD BRAND 25% ALDRIN WETTABLE SPRAY POWDER Insecticide (General Chem.)	Aldrin* (hexachloro hexahydro-endo, exo- dimethano naphthalene) Related compounds	23.8% 4.0%
ORCHARD BRAND 3% ARAMITE DUST Insecticide (General Chem.)	2-(p-tert-Butylphenoxy) isopropyl 2-chloroethyl sulfite	3%
ORCHARD BRAND ARAMITE EM-2 EMULSI- FIABLE CONC. Insecticide (General Chem.)	2(p-tert-Butylphenoxy) isopropyl 2-chloroethyl- sulfite Xylol*	25.8% 66.0%
ORCHARD BRAND 15% ARAMITE WETTABLE SPRAY POWDER Insecticide (General Chem.)	2-(p-tert-Butylphenoxy) isopropyl 2-chloroethyl- sulfite	15%
ORCHARD BRAND ASTRINGENT LEAD ARSENATE Insecticide (General Chem.)	Lead arsenate*	97.0%
ORCHARD BRAND BASIC LEAD ARSENATE POWDERED Insecticide (General Chem.)	Basic lead arsenate*	97.0%

*Consult Sec. II., Ingredients Index. This ingredient may be responsible for major toxic effects if poisonous amounts of this product are ingested.

Name & Use Manufacturer	Ingredients
ORCHARD BRAND BHC EM-1 EMULSI-FIABLE OIL-SOLUBLE CONC. Insecticide (General Chem.)	Gamma isomer of benzene hexachloride* 11.8% Other isomers of benzene hexachloride 18.0% Xylol* 59.0%
ORCHARD BRAND CALCIUM ARSENATE POWDERED (With Other Calcium Compounds) Insecticide (General Chem.)	Calcium arsenate* 69.2%
ORCHARD BRAND 40% CHLORDANE DUST BASE Insecticide (General Chem.)	Tech. chlordane* and related compounds 40%
ORCHARD BRAND CHLORDANE EM-8 EMULSI-FIABLE CONC. Insecticide (General Chem.)	Tech. chlordane* and related compounds 73.1% Petroleum distillate 18.0%
ORCHARD BRAND 40% CHLORDANE SPRAY POWDER Insecticide (General Chem.)	Tech. chlordane* and related compounds 40%
ORCHARD BRAND 1-1/2 COTTON DUST Insecticide (General Chem.)	Dieldrin* (hexachloro epoxy octahydro-endo, exo-dimethano naphthalene) and related compounds 1.5%
ORCHARD BRAND 1-1/2—5—0 COTTON DUST Insecticide (General Chem.)	Dieldrin* (hexachloro epoxy octahydro-endo, exo-dimethano naphthalene) and related compounds 1.5% DDT* Tech. 5.0% Sulfur* 40.0%
ORCHARD BRAND 1-1/2—10—0 COTTON DUST Insecticide (General Chem.)	Dieldrin* (hexachloro epoxy octahydro-endo, exo-dimethano naphthalene) and related compounds 1.5% DDT* tech. 10.0%

Name & Use Manufacturer	Ingredients
ORCHARD BRAND 2-1/2 COTTON DUST Insecticide (General Chem.)	Aldrin* (hexachloro hexahydro-endo, exo-dimethano naphthalene and related compounds 2.8%
ORCHARD BRAND 2-1/2—5 COTTON DUST Insecticide (General Chem.)	Aldrin* (hexachloro hexahydro-endo, exo-dimethano naphthalene) and related compounds 2.8% DDT tech. 5.0%
ORCHARD BRAND 2-1/2—5—40 COTTON DUST Insecticide (General Chem.)	Aldrin* (hexachloro hexahydro-endo, exo-dimethano naphthalene) and related compounds 2.8% DDT tech. 5.0% Sulfur 40.0%
ORCHARD BRAND 2-1/2—10—0 COTTON DUST Insecticide (General Chem.)	Aldrin* (hexachloro epoxy octahydro- endo, exo-dimethano naphthalene) and related compounds 2.8% DDT tech. 10.0%
ORCHARD BRAND 20—5 COTTON DUST Insecticide (General Chem.)	Tech. chlorinated camphene* 20% DDT tech. 5%
ORCHARD BRAND 3—5 COTTON SPRAY EMULSI-FIABLE CONC. Insecticide (General Chem.)	Gamma isomer of benzene hexachloride 8.8% Other isomers of benzene hexachloride 14.3% DDT tech. 14.7% Xylene* 53.5%
ORCHARD BRAND DDT EM-2 EMULSI-FIABLE CONC. Insecticide (General Chem.)	DDT 25.0% Aromatic petroleum deriv. solvent* 72.0%
ORCHARD BRAND DIELDRIN EM-1-1/2 EMULSI-FIABLE CONC. Insecticide (General Chem.)	Dieldrin* (hexachloro epoxy octahydro-endo, exo-dimethano naphthalene) and related compounds 18.7% Xylol* 71.1%

*Consult Sec. II., Ingredients Index. This ingredient may be responsible for major toxic effects if poisonous amounts of this product are ingested.

Name & Use Manufacturer	Ingredients	Name & Use Manufacturer	Ingredients
ORCHARD BRAND 50% DIELDRIN SPRAY POWDER Insecticide (General Chem.)	Dieldrin* (hexachloro epoxy octahydro-endo, exo-dimethano naphthalene) and related compounds 50.0%	ORCHARD BRAND G-12 BHC SPRAY POWDER Insecticide (General Chem.)	Gamma isomer of benzene hexachloride* 12.0% Other isomers of benzene hexachloride* 60.0%
ORCHARD BRAND "75" DUST Insecticide (General Chem.)	Rotenone 0.75% Other cube resins* 1.50%	ORCHARD BRAND GENICOP (Micro-Particle) SPRAY POWDER Insecticide, fungicide (General Chem.)	DDT* tech. 25.0% Basic copper sulfate* 38.0%
ORCHARD BRAND EM 5—25 PARATHION-DDT EMULSI-FIABLE Insecticide (General Chem.)	Parathion*(o, o-diethyl-o-p-nitrophenyl thiophosphate) 5% DDT tech. 25% Aromatic petroleum deriv. 65.5%	ORCHARD BRAND GENITE EM-923 MITICIDE EMULSI-FIABLE CONC. (General Chem.)	2, 4-Dichlorophenyl ester of benzene sulfonic acid* 50% Aromatic petroleum deriv. solvent* 46%
ORCHARD BRAND 1% ENDRIN DUST Insecticide (General Chem.)	Endrin* (hexachloro epoxy octahydro-endo, endo-dimethano naphthalene) 1%	ORCHARD BRAND GENITOX S-50 (50% DDT Wettable Spray Powder) Insecticide (General Chem.)	DDT* tech. 50%
ORCHARD BRAND 1-1/2% ENDRIN DUST Insecticide (General Chem.)	Endrin* (hexachloro epoxy octahydro-endo, endo-dimethano naphthalene) 1.5%	ORCHARD BRAND GENITOX S-75 (75% DDT Wettable Spray Powder) Insecticide (General Chem.)	DDT* tech. 75%
ORCHARD BRAND 2% ENDRIN DUST Insecticide (General Chem.)	Endrin* (hexachloro epoxy octahydro-endo, endo-dimethano naphthalene) 2%	ORCHARD BRAND HEPTACHLOR EM-2 Insecticide (General Chem.)	Heptachlor*(heptachloro 4, 7-methano tetrahydro indene) 23.4% Related compounds 9.1% Xylene* 60.0%
ORCHARD BRAND ENDRIN EM-1.6 EMULSI-FIABLE CONC. Insecticide (General Chem.)	Endrin* (hexachloro epoxy octahydro-endo, endo-dimethano naphthalene) 19.8% Xylol* 72.5%	ORCHARD BRAND LIME SULFUR SOLUTION Fungicide (General Chem.)	Calcium polysulfide* 29%
ORCHARD BRAND FERBAM Fungicide (General Chem.)	Ferbam*(ferric dimethyl dithiocarbamate) 76%	ORCHARD BRAND 20% LINDANE EMULSI-FIABLE CONC. Insecticide (General Chem.)	Gamma isomer of benzene hexachloride* 20% Xylol* 56% Cyclohexanone 5.5%
ORCHARD BRAND G-10 BHC SPRAY POWDER Insecticide (General Chem.)	Gamma isomer of benzene hexachloride* 10.0% Other isomers of benzene hexachloride* 50.0%		

*Consult Sec. II., Ingredients Index. This ingredient may be responsible for major toxic effects if poisonous amounts of this product are ingested.

Name & Use Manufacturer	Ingredients	Name & Use Manufacturer	Ingredients
ORCHARD BRAND 25% LINDANE SPRAY POWDER & SEED TREATER Insecticide (General Chem.)	Gamma isomer of benzene hexachloride* 25%	ORCHARD BRAND 25% MALATHION WETTABLE SPRAY POWDER Insecticide (General Chem.)	Malathion*(o, o-dimethyl dithio phosphate of diethylmercapto succinate) 25%
ORCHARD BRAND 75% LINDANE WETTABLE POWDER Insecticide (General Chem.)	Gamma isomer of benzene hexachloride (from lindane)* 75%	ORCHARD BRAND MERCURY SPRAY FOR SCAB ON APPLES (General Chem.)	Phenylmercuric acetate* 10%
ORCHARD BRAND 3—5 LIQUID Insecticide (General Chem.)	Gamma isomer of benzene hexachloride* 13.6% Other isomers of benzene hexachloride 1.2% DDT tech. 22.6% Xylene* 56.5%	ORCHARD BRAND METHOXY-CHLOR EM-2 EMULSI-FIABLE CONC. Insecticide (General Chem.)	Methoxychlor*(2, 2' bis-(p-methoxy phenyl)- 1, 1, 1-trichloroethane)-tech. 25% Xylene* 63% Aromatic petroleum deriv. solvent 7%
ORCHARD BRAND LOW VOLATILE 1-1/3—2/3 BRUSH KILLER (General Chem.)	2, 4-Dichloro phenoxy acetic acid, iso-octyl ester* 24.5% 2, 4, 5-Trichloro phenoxy acetic acid, iso-octyl ester* 11.7% 2, 4-D acid equiv. 16.3% 2, 4, 5-T acid equiv. 8.1%	ORCHARD BRAND 50% METHOXY-CHLOR WETTABLE SPRAY POWDER Insecticide (General Chem.)	Methoxychlor*(2, 2' bis-(p-methoxy phenyl)-1, 1, 1 trichloroethano) tech. 50%
ORCHARD BRAND LOW VOLATILE 2—2 BRUSH KILLER (General Chem.)	2, 4-Dichlorophenoxy acetic acid, iso-octyl ester* 33.7% 2, 4, 5-Trichloro phenoxy acetic acid, iso-octyl ester* 32.1% 2, 4-D acid equiv. 22.3% 2, 4, 5-T acid equiv. 22.3%	ORCHARD BRAND (Micro-) DRITOMIC SULFUR Fungicide (General Chem.)	Sulfur* 95%
ORCHARD BRAND LOW VOLATILE 2, 4, 5-T BRUSH KILLER (General Chem.)	2, 4, 5-Trichloro phenoxy acetic acid, iso-octyl ester* 63.2% 2, 4, 5-T acid equiv. 36.8%	ORCHARD BRAND NICOTINE SULFATE SOLUTION Insecticide (General Chem.)	Nicotine as alkaloid* 40%
ORCHARD BRAND MALATHION EM-5 EMULSI-FIABLE CONC. Insecticide (General Chem.)	Malathion*(o, o-dimethyl dithio phosphate of diethyl mercapto succinate) 55.9% Aromatic petroleum deriv.* 33.5%	ORCHARD BRAND 50% OVEX WETTABLE POWDER MITICIDE (General Chem.)	Ovex*(p-chlorophenyl-p-chlorobenzene sulfonate) 50%
ORCHARD BRAND MALATHION 50% EMUL-SIFIABLE CONC. Insecticide (General Chem.)	Malathion*(o, o-dimethyl dithio phosphate of diethyl mercapto succinate) 50.0% Xylol* 40.8%	ORCHARD BRAND 1% PARATHION COTTON DUST Insecticide (General Chem.)	Parathion*(o, o-diethyl-o-p-nitrophenyl thiophosphate) 1%

*Consult Sec. II., Ingredients Index. This ingredient may be responsible for major toxic effects if poisonous amounts of this product are ingested.

Name & Use Manufacturer	Ingredients	Name & Use Manufacturer	Ingredients
ORCHARD BRAND 2% PARATHION COTTON DUST Insecticide (General Chem.)	Parathion* (o, o-diethyl-o-p-nitrophenyl thiophosphate) 2%	ORCHARD BRAND STASET (General Chem.)	Alpha-(2, 4, 5-trichlorophenoxy) propionic acid, triethanol-amine salt* 10.6%
ORCHARD BRAND PARATHION EM-4 EMULSI-FIABLE CONC. Insecticide (General Chem.)	Parathion* (o, o-diethyl-o-p-nitrophenyl thiophosphate) 46.5% Aromatic petroleum deriv. or xylol 43.0%	ORCHARD BRAND 25% TDE (DDD) EMULSI-FIABLE SPRAY CONC. Insecticide (General Chem.)	TDE (dichloro diphenyl dichloroethane) Tech. 25% Aromatic petroleum deriv.* 69.5%
ORCHARD BRAND PARIS GREEN COPPER ACETO-ARSENITE Insecticide (General Chem.)	Copper acetoarsenite* 91.7%	ORCHARD BRAND 50% TDE (DDD) SPRAY POWDER Insecticide (General Chem.)	TDE* (dichloro diphenyl dichloroethane) tech. 50%
ORCHARD BRAND SOIL L.S. SOLUTION (Lime-Sulfur. Solution for Treating Soil) Fungicide (General Chem.)	Calcium polysulfide* 29%	ORCHARD BRAND 20% TEPP Insecticide (General Chem.)	Tetraethyl pyrophosphate* 20% Other organic phosphates* 30%
ORCHARD BRAND 400 SPRAY Insecticide (General Chem.)	Rotenone* 4.0% Other cube resins* 9.0%	ORCHARD BRAND 40% TEPP Insecticide (General Chem.)	Tetraethyl pyrophosphate 40% Other organic phosphates 60%
ORCHARD BRAND 340 SPRAYCOP Fungicide (General Chem.)	Basic copper sulfate equiv. to metallic copper* 34%	ORCHARD BRAND 20% TOXAPHENE COTTON DUST Insecticide (General Chem.)	Toxaphene* (tech. chlorinated camphene, 67-69% chlorine) 20%
ORCHARD BRAND 530 SPRAYCOP Fungicide (General Chem.)	Basic copper sulfate equiv. to metallic copper* 53.0%	ORCHARD BRAND TOXAPHENE EM-6 EMULSIFI-ABLE CONC. Insecticide (General Chem.)	Toxaphene* (tech. chlorinated camphene, 67-69% chlorine) 60% Petroleum distillate 29%
ORCHARD BRAND STAFAST (General Chem.)	Alpha naphthalene acetic acid 3.5% Alkylaryl sodium sulfonates 9.0%	ORCHARD BRAND TOXAPHENE EM-8 EMULSI-FIABLE CONC. Insecticide (General Chem.)	Toxaphene* (tech. chlorinated camphene, 67-69% chlorine) 72% Petroleum distillate 17%
ORCHARD BRAND STANDARD LEAD ARSENATE (Powdered) Insecticide (General Chem.)	Lead arsenate* 97.0%	ORCHARD BRAND 40% TOXAPHENE SPRAY POWDER Insecticide (General Chem.)	Toxaphene* (tech. chlorinated camphene, 67-69% chlorine) 40%

*Consult Sec. II., Ingredients Index. This ingredient may be responsible for major toxic effects if poisonous amounts of this product are ingested.

Name & Use Manufacturer	Ingredients	Name & Use Manufacturer	Ingredients
ORCHARD BRAND TRIBASIC BORDEAUX POWDER Fungicide (General Chem.)	Basic copper sulfate* equiv. to metallic copper 12.7%	ORIOLE BRAND VARNISH, SHELLAC & PINE TAR (Corner)	
ORCHARD BRAND 2, 4-D AMINE WEED KILLER (General Chem.)	2, 4-Dichloro phenoxyacetic acid, dimethylamine salt* 49.4% 2, 4-D acid equiv. 41.0%	ORJENE TOILET WATER (Orjene)	
		O-R-95 SURFACE ANESTHETIC THROAT TABLETS (Medico-Chem.)	2-Butyloxyquinoline Carboxylic acid 4-Diethyl ethylenediamide 2, 8 - Diamine 10-Methylacridinium chloride 2, 8 - Diaminoacridine hydrochloride
ORCHARD BRAND 2, 4-D BUTYL ESTER WEED KILLER (General Chem.)	2, 4-Dichlorophenoxyacetic acid, butyl ester* 40% 2,4-D acid equiv. 31.9%	ORNOLACK PAINT FOR ORNAMENTAL IRON (Vita-Var)	
ORCHARD BRAND 2,4-D ESTER WEED KILLER (General Chem.)	2, 4-Dichloro phenoxyacetic acid, isopropyl ester* 44% 2, 4-D acid equiv. 37%	OROCAIN Throat swab, gargle (K-A-S)	Tannic acid* Glycerin Benzocaine Iodine*
		OROGESIC EAR DROPS (K-A-S)	Phenyl dimethyl pyrazolon* 5% Ethyl aminobenzoate* 1%
ORCHARD BRAND 2, 4-D LOW VOLATILE ESTER WEED KILLER (General Chem.)	2, 4-Dichloro phenoxyacetic acid, iso-octyl ester* 67.8% 2, 4-D acid equiv. 32.2%	OROLINE ALUMINUM PAINT & BRONZE POWDERS (Crescent Brand)	
		OROTHRICIN MOUTH WASH For throat irritations (Rexall)	Tyrothricin Propylene glycol Oil of spearmint Methyl salicylate* Oil of cloves* Cetyl trimethyl ammonium bromide* Octadecyl dimethyl ethyl ammonium bromide* Alcohol 9%/v
ORCHARD BRAND ZIRAM Fungicide (General Chem.)	Ziram*(zinc dimethyl dithio carbamate) 76%		
ORCHIDEE BLUE EAU de TOILETTE (Parfums Corday)		OROVIN For hay fever and rose fever (K-A-S)	Boric acid Ethyl aminobenzoate Ephedrine sulfate* Aqua rosa
ORCHIDEE BLUE PERFUME (Parfums Corday)		OROX Nasal decon-gestant (K-A-S)	Ephedrine sulfate* 1% Benzocaine Sodium chloride
OR ET NOIR EXTRACT (Caron)		ORTHAZITE LIQUID Darkroom aid (Edwal)	Benztriazole* Inorganic sulfite*
ORIENTAL HAIR TONIC (Lanman)		ORTHENE 3D 5 DUST Insecticide (Calif. Spray)	TDE 5%
ORIENTAL INK (Davids)		ORTHENE 3D 10 DUST Insecticide (Calif. Spray)	DDD 10.00

*Consult Sec. II., Ingredients Index. This ingredient may be responsible for major toxic effects if poisonous amounts of this product are ingested.

Name & Use Manufacturer	Ingredients	
ORTHENE 3D-K 5-7 DUST Insecticide, fungicide (Calif. Spray)	DDD Copper*	5% 7%
ORTHENE 3D-S DUST NO. 5-25 Insecticide (Calif. Spray)	TDE Sulfur*	5% 25%
ORTHENE 3D-S DUST NO. 5-50 Insecticide (Calif. Spray)	TDE Sulfur*	5% 50%
ORTHENE 3D-S 5-75 DUST Insecticide (Calif. Spray)	DDD Sulfur*	5% 75%
ORTHENE 3D 2 SPRAY Insecticide (Calif. Spray)	TDE*	25%
ORTHENE 3D 50 WETTABLE Insecticide (Calif. Spray)	DDT*	50%
ORTHENE 3D ZINEB 5-6 DUST Insecticide, fungicide (Calif. Spray)	DDD Zineb (zinc ethylene bis-dithiocarbamate)	5% 6%
ORTHENE 3D-ZINEB-S 5-3.25-25 DUST Insecticide, fungicide (Calif. Spray)	Dichloro diphenyl dichloro-ethane Zineb (zinc ethylene bis-dithiocarbamate) Sulfur* Zinc expressed as metallic	5.00% 3.25% 25.00% 0.77%
ORTHO ADHESIVE FLOWABLE Fungicide (Calif. Spray)	Petroleum oils* Ammonium caseinate Anhydrous soap Condensation product of ethylene oxide and alkylated cresol	80% 0.3% 0.7% 0.1%
ORTHO AERO BUTYL CONCENTRATE Herbicide (Calif. Spray)	n-Butyl ester of 2,4-dichloro phenoxyacetic acid*	76%
ORTHO A-K BAIT Insecticide (Calif. Spray)	Tech. chlordane Toxaphene*	1% 3%
ORTHO ALDRIN-DDT 2.5-5 DUST Insecticide (Calif. Spray)	Hexachloro hexahydro dimethano naphthalene* Related compounds Dichloro diphenyl trichloro-ethane	2.38% 0.40% 5.00%
ORTHO ALDRIN 2.5-5 DDT DUST Insecticide (Calif. Spray)	Aldrin* DDT* Theoret. chlorine*	2.50% 5.00% 4.47%
ORTHO ALDRIN-DDT 2.5-10 DUST Insecticide, fungicide (Calif. Spray)	Aldrin* DDT*	2.5% 10%
ORTHO ALDRIN-DDT-S 2.5-5-40 DUST Insecticide, fungicide (Calif. Spray)	Aldrin* DDT* Sulfur*	2.5% 5% 40%
ORTHO ALDRIN-DDT-S 2.5-10-40 DUST Insecticide, fungicide (Calif. Spray)	Aldrin* DDT* Sulfur*	2.5% 10% 40%
ORTHO ALDRIN 2.5 DUST Insecticide (Calif. Spray)	Aldrin*	2.5%
ORTHO ALDRIN 3 DUST Insecticide (Calif. Spray)	Aldrin*	3%
ORTHO ALDRIN 2.5 GRANULAR Insecticide (Calif. Spray)	Aldrin*	2.5%
ORTHO ALDRIN 2 SPRAY Insecticide (Calif. Spray)	Hexachloro hexahydro dimethano naphthalene* Related compounds Aromatic petroleum deriv. solvent*	23.0% 3.9% 67.0%
ORTHO ALDRIN 20 WETTABLE Insecticide (Calif. Spray)	Hexachloro hexahydro dimethano naphthalene*	20.%
ORTHO ALDRIN 25 WETTABLE Insecticide (Calif. Spray)	Aldrin*	25%
ORTHO ANT & MOTH SPRAY (Calif. Spray)	Chlordane	2.5%
ORTHO ANT POWDER (Calif. Spray)	Lindane Tech. chlordane	0.5% 2.5%
ORTHO AQUATIC SOLVENT (Calif. Spray)	Aromatic petroleum distillates*	95%
ORTHO AQUATIC WEED KILLER (Calif. Spray)	Oils*	95%
ORTHO AQUATIC WEED KILLER NO. 60 (Calif. Spray)	Oil*	95%

*Consult Sec. II., Ingredients Index. This ingredient may be responsible for major toxic effects if poisonous amounts of this product are ingested.

Name & Use Manufacturer	Ingredients		Name & Use Manufacturer	Ingredients	
ORTHO BASIC LEAD ARSENATE Insecticide (Calif. Spray)	Basic lead arsenate*	96%	ORTHO 3-CHLORO 1PC EMULSIVE Herbicide (Calif. Spray)	Isopropyl-n-(3-chlorophenyl) carbamate*	46%
ORTHO BENTOX DUSTING SULFUR Insecticide, fungicide (Calif. Spray)	Sulfur*	85%	ORTHOCIDE-DDT 5-5 DUST Insecticide (Calif. Spray)	Captan DDT*	5% 5%
ORTHO BHC WETTABLE Insecticide (Calif. Spray)	Gamma isomer of benzene hexachloride* Other isomers of benzene hexachloride*	6% 24%	ORTHOCIDE 5 DUST Insecticide (Calif. Spray)	Captan	5%
ORTHO BLENDING SULFUR Fungicide (Calif. Spray)	Sulfur*	98%	ORTHOCIDE 7.5 DUST Insecticide (Calif. Spray)	Captan	7.5%
ORTHO BRAND PARADI-CHLORO-BENZENE (PDB) Soil fumigant (Calif. Spray)	Paradichlorobenzene*	99%	ORTHOCIDE 10 DUST Insecticide (Calif. Spray)	Captan	10%
			ORTHOCIDE 20 DUST Insecticide (Calif. Spray)	Captan	20%
ORTHO CALCIUM ARSENATE Insecticide (Calif. Spray)	Calcium arsenate*	70%	ORTHOCIDE GARDEN FUNGICIDE (Calif. Spray)	Captan	50%
ORTHO CATTLE GRUB SPRAY OR DUST Insecticide (Calif. Spray)	Rotenone from cube* Other cube resins	5% 5%	ORTHOCIDE-MITE 10-3 DUST Insecticide, fungicide (Calif. Spray)	Captan Aramite	10% 3%
ORTHO C-B WEED KILLER (Calif. Spray)	Sodium chlorate* Sodium pentaborate* Sodium tetraborate	40% 31% 7%	ORTHOCIDE PERSISTOPHOS 5-5-1 DUST Insecticide (Calif. Spray)	Captan DDT Parathion*	5% 5% 1%
ORTHO CDA SPECIAL Adjuvant (Calif. Spray)	Oils* Surface active agents	95% 4%	ORTHOCIDE-S 5-30 DUST Insecticide, fungicide (Calif. Spray)	Captan Sulfur*	5% 30%
ORTHO C-1 DEFOLIANT & WEED KILLER (Calif. Spray)	Sodium chlorate* Sodium pentaborate* Sodium tetraborate*		ORTHOCIDE-S 5-40 DUST Insecticide, fungicide (Calif. Spray)	Captan Sulfur*	5% 40%
ORTHO C-40 DUST Insecticide (Calif. Spray)	Sodium fluoaluminate*	36%	ORTHOCIDE-S 10-50 DUST Fungicide (Calif. Spray)	Captan Sulfur*	10% 50%
ORTHO C-50 DUST Insecticide (Calif. Spray)	Sodium fluoaluminate*	45%	ORTHOCIDE 75 SEED PROTECTANT (Calif. Spray)	Captan	75%
ORTHO CHIGGER & TICK POWDER (Calif. Spray)	Gamma isomer of benzene hexachloride (from lindane)	1%	ORTHOCIDE VAPOPHOS 5-1 DUST Insecticide (Calif. Spray)	Captan (n-trichloro methyl mercapto-4-cyclohexene-1,-2-dicarboximide) Parathion* (o,o-diethyl-o-p-nitrophenyl thiophosphate)	5% 1%

Name & Use Manufacturer	Ingredients		Name & Use Manufacturer	Ingredients	
ORTHOCIDE-VAPOPHOS 5-1.5 DUST Insecticide, fungicide (Calif. Spray)	Captan Parathion*	5% 1.5%	ORTHO DIELDRIN-DDT-S 1.5-5-40 DUST Insecticide, fungicide (Calif. Spray)	Dieldrin* Related compounds DDT* Sulfur*	1.27% 0.23% 5% 40%
ORTHOCIDE-VAPOTONE 5-66 DUST Insecticide, fungicide (Calif. Spray)	TEPP* Other ethyl phosphates Captan	1% 1.5% 5%	ORTHO DIELDRIN-DDT-S 1.5-10-40 DUST Insecticide, fungicide (Calif. Spray)	Dieldrin* DDT* Sulfur*	1.5% 10% 40%
ORTHOCIDE 50 WETT-ABLE Fungicide (Calif. Spray)	Captan (n-trichloro methyl mercapto-4-cyclohexene-1, 2-dicarboximide) 50%		ORTHO DIELDRIN-DDT S 1.5-5-50 DUST Insecticide, fungicide (Calif. Spray)	Dieldrin* DDT* Sulfur*	1.5% 5% 50%
ORTHO CITRUS LEAF FEED (Calif. Spray)	Nitrogen Available phosphoric acid* Zinc* Manganese	25% 10% 4% 1.4%	ORTHO DIELDRIN-DDT-S 2.5-10-40 DUST Insecticide, fungicide (Calif. Spray)	Dieldrin* DDT* Sulfur*	2.5% 10% 40%
ORTHO-COP 53 Fungicide (Calif. Spray)	Copper*	53%			
ORTHO COPPER FUNGICIDE 53 (Calif. Spray)	Basic copper sulfate*	98%	ORTHO DIELDRIN-3D-S 1.5-5-50 DUST Insecticide (Calif. Spray)	Dieldrin* DDD Sulfur*	1.5% 5% 50%
ORTHO 3-5 COTTON SPRAY Insecticide (Calif. Spray)	DDT* Gamma isomer of benzene hexachloride* Other isomers of benzene hexachloride	21.8% 13.1% 1.4%	ORTHO DIELDRIN 1.5 DUST Insecticide (Calif. Spray)	Dieldrin*	1.5%
ORTHO CRAB GRASS KILLER (Calif. Spray)	Phenyl mercuric acetate*	0.74%	ORTHO DIELDRIN 2 DUST Insecticide (Calif. Spray)	Hexachloro epoxy octahydro-dimethano naphthalene (from Dieldrin)* Related compounds (from Dieldrin)	1.70% 0.30%
ORTHO CREME Vaginal cream (Ortho)	Ricinoleic acid Boric acid Sodium lauryl sulfate	0.75% 2.00% 0.28%	ORTHO DIELDRIN 10 GRANULES Insecticide (Calif. Spray)	Dieldrin*	10%
ORTHO C-S 50-47 DUST Insecticide (Calif. Spray)	Sodium fluoaluminate* Sulfur	45% 44%			
ORTHO C-S 70-25 DUST Insecticide, fungicide (Calif. Spray)	Sodium fluoaluminate* Sulfur Fluorine expressed as elemental	63.0% 23.4% 34.2%	ORTHO DIELDRIN-S 1.5-50 DUST Insecticide, fungicide (Calif. Spray)	Dieldrin* Sulfur*	1.5% 50%
ORTHO C-70 DUST Insecticide (Calif. Spray)	Sodium fluoaluminate*	63%	ORTHO DIELDRIN-S 2.5-40 DUST Insecticide (Calif. Spray)	Dieldrin* Sulfur*	2.5% 40%
ORTHO DIELDRIN-DDT 1.5-5 DUST Insecticide (Calif. Spray)	Dieldrin* DDT*	1.5% 5%			
ORTHO DIELDRIN-DDT 1.5-10 DUST Insecticide (Calif. Spray)	Dieldrin* DDT*	1.5% 10%	ORTHO DIELDRIN 1.5 SPRAY Insecticide (Calif. Spray)	Dieldrin* Related compounds (from Dieldrin)	15.8% 2.8%

Name & Use Manufacturer	Ingredients		Name & Use Manufacturer	Ingredients	
ORTHO DIELDRIN 50 WETTABLE Insecticide (Calif. Spray)	Dieldrin*	42.5%	ORTHO FLY KILLER M (Calif. Spray)	Malathion*	29.2%
	Related compounds (from Dieldrin)	7.5%		Gamma isomer of benzene hexachloride*(from lindane)	10.0%
				Aromatic petroleum deriv. solvent*	42.8%
ORTHO DILAN 8 CONCEN- TRATE Insecticide (Calif. Spray)	2-Nitro-1, 1-bis-(p-chloro- phenyl) propane	21.3%	ORTHO FLY SPRAY (Calif. Spray)	Pyrethrins	0.05%
	2-Nitro-1, 1-bis-(p-chloro- phenyl) butane*	42.7%		Piperonyl butoxide tech.	0.50%
	Related compounds	16.0%		Isobornyl thiocyanoacetate	0.25%
	Xylene*	20.0%		Other related terpenes	0.05%
ORTHO DILAN 1.5 DUST Insecticide (Calif. Spray)	2-Nitro-1, 1-bis-(p-chloro- phenyl) propane	0.4%		Methoxychlor tech.	0.50%
	2-Nitro-1, 1-bis-(p-chloro- phenyl) butane	0.8%		Petroleum distillate*	98.65%
	Related compounds	0.3%	ORTHO-GRO DRY FERTILIZER (Calif. Spray)	Total organic nitrogen	7%
ORTHO DILAN 2 EMULSIVE Insecticide (Calif. Spray)	2-Nitro-1, 1-bis-(p-chloro- phenyl) propane*	6.7%		Available phosphoric acid	9%
	2-Nitro-1, 1-bis-(p-chloro- phenyl) butane*	13.3%		Soluble potash	5%
	Related compounds	5%	ORTHO-GRO LIQUID FERTILIZER (Calif. Spray)	Total nitrogen (organic)	10%
ORTHO DILAN 25 WETTABLE Insecticide (Calif. Spray)	2-Nitro-1, 1-bis-(p-chloro- phenyl) propane*	6.7%		Available phosphoric acid	5%
	2-Nitro-1, 1-bis-(p-chloro- phenyl) butane*	13.3%		Soluble potash	5%
	Related compounds	5%	ORTHO-GRO LIQUID PLANT FOOD (Calif. Spray)	Total organic nitrogen	10%
ORTHO D-S 30-70 DUST Fungicide (Calif. Spray)	Basic lead arsenate*	28%		Available phosphoric acid	5%
	Sulfur*	68%		Soluble potash	5%
ORTHO DUSTING SULFUR Fungicide (Calif. Spray)	Sulfur*	98%	ORTHO G-S 60-40 DUST Insecticide (Calif. Spray)	Calcium arsenate*	40%
				Sulfur	37.3%
ORTHO 30 DUSTING SULFUR Insecticide, fungicide (Calif. Spray)	Sulfur*	30%	ORTHO-GYNOL Vaginal jelly (Ortho)	p-Di-isobutyl phenoxypoly- ethoxy ethanol	1.00%
				Ricinoleic acid	0.7%
				Boric acid	3.00%
ORTHO 60 DUSTING SULFUR Insecticide, fungicide (Calif. Spray)	Sulfur*	60%	ORTHO HEALTHY HERD WETTABLE POWDER Insecticide (Calif. Spray)	DDT*	45.0%
				Gamma isomer of benzene hexachloride	2.5%
				Other isomers of benzene hexachloride	2.5%
ORTHO EARWIG BAIT (Calif. Spray)	Sodium fluosilicate*	5%	ORTHO HEPTACHLOR 1.5 DUST Insecticide (Calif. Spray)	Heptachlor	1.5%
ORTHO EGG WASH Egg cleaner (Calif. Spray)	Dodecyl dimethyl benzyl ammonium chloride*	15%	ORTHO HEPTACHLOR 2.5 DUST Insecticide (Calif. Spray)	Heptachlor*	2.5%
				Related compounds	0.97%
ORTHO EMULSIFIER NO. 5 Adjuvant (Calif. Spray)	Polyethylene glycol monoiso- octylphenyl ether	35%	ORTHO HEPTACHLOR 2 SPRAY Insecticide (Calif. Spray)	Heptachlor*	23.4%
	Polyethylene glycol dioleate	57%		Related compounds	9.1%
				Aromatic petroleum deriv. solvent	61.4%
ORTHO EQ335 Insecticide (Calif. Spray)	Gamma isomer of benzene hexachloride (from lindane)*	3%	ORTHO HEPTACHLOR 25 WETTABLE Insecticide (Calif. Spray)	Heptachlor* (4,7-methano tetra- hydroindene)	25%
	Pine oil*	35%		Related compounds	9.72%
ORTHO FLY KILLER DRY BAIT (Calif. Spray)	Malathion*	2%			

*Consult Sec. II., Ingredients Index. This ingredient may be responsible for major toxic effects if poisonous amounts of this product are ingested.

Name & Use Manufacturer	Ingredients		Name & Use Manufacturer	Ingredients	
ORTHO HOME ORCHARD SPRAY Insecticide (Calif. Spray)	Ferbam DDT* DDD Gamma isomer of benzene hexachloride*(from lindane) Aramite (2-(p-tert-butylphenoxy)-isopropyl-2-chloro-ethyl sulfite)	12.25% 8.00% 8.00% 2.00% 4.25%	ORTHO-K-S DUST 25-50 Fungicide (Calif. Spray)	Zinc* Copper* Sulfur*	4.5% 4.5% 50%
			ORTHO-K 35 DUST Fungicide (Calif. Spray)	Metallic copper* Metallic zinc*	6.3% 6.3%
ORTHO HYDRATED LIME Dilutent (Calif. Spray)	Calcium hydroxide*	90%	ORTHO KLEEN STOCK SPRAY Insecticide (Calif. Spray)	Gamma isomer of benzene hexachloride (from lindane) Toxaphene* Aromatic petroleum deriv. solvent*	1.7% 42.8% 46.0%
ORTHO IMPROVED ISOTOX GARDEN SPRAY M Insecticide (Calif. Spray)	Gamma isomer of benzene hexachloride (from lindane) Malathion DDD Methyl isobutyl ketone Aromatic petroleum deriv. solvent*	5.0% 12.5% 5.0% 15.0% 56.5%	ORTHO-KLOR 1.5 BAIT Insecticide (Calif. Spray)	Chlordane	1.5%
			ORTHO-KLOR 44 CHLORDANE SPRAY Insecticide (Calif. Spray)	Tech. chlordane* Petroleum distillate*	44% 42%
ORTHO INSTANT BLUESTONE Fungicide (Calif. Spray)	Cupric sulfate pentahydrate*	90%	ORTHO-KLOR DUST NO. 5 Insecticide (Calif. Spray)	Inert ingredients Chlordane*	5%
ORTHO IPC 15 DUST Herbicide (Calif. Spray)	Isopropyl-n-phenyl carbamate	15%	ORTHO-KLOR DUST NO. 10 Insecticide (Calif. Spray)	Chlordane*	10%
ORTHO IPC 2 EMULSIVE Herbicide (Calif. Spray)	Isopropyl-n-phenyl carbamate	26%	ORTHO-KLOR 8 SPRAY Insecticide (Calif. Spray)	Tech. chlordane*	72%
ORTHO IPC 15 G (Granular) Herbicide (Calif. Spray)	Isopropyl-n-phenyl carbamate	15%	ORTHO-KLOR WETTABLE NO. 40 Insecticide (Calif. Spray)	Chlordane*	40%
ORTHO IPC 50 WETTABLE Herbicide (Calif. Spray)	Isopropyl-n-phenyl carbamate*	50%	ORTHO-KO 5 DUST Fungicide (Calif. Spray)	Copper*	5%
ORTHO-K 5 DUST Fungicide (Calif. Spray)	Copper*	5%	ORTHO-KO 6.7 DUST Fungicide (Calif. Spray)	Copper*	6.7%
ORTHO-K 6.8 DUST Fungicide (Calif. Spray)	Metallic copper*	6.8%	ORTHO-KO 10 DUST Fungicide (Calif. Spray)	Copper*	10%
ORTHO-K 7 DUST Fungicide (Calif. Spray)	Copper*	7%	ORTHO-KO-S 5-50 DUST Fungicide (Calif. Spray)	Copper* Sulfur*	5% 50%
ORTHO-K 20 DUST Fungicide (Calif. Spray)	Metallic copper* Metallic zinc*	3.6% 3.6%	ORTHO-K-S 25-15 DUST Insecticide, fungicide (Calif. Spray)	Copper* Zinc* Sulfur	4.5% 4.5% 15%
ORTHO-K 25 DUST Fungicide (Calif. Spray)	Copper* Zinc*	4.5% 4.5%	ORTHO-K-S 25-30 DUST Insecticide, fungicide (Calif. Spray)	Copper* Zinc* Sulfur*	4.5% 4.5% 30%

*Consult Sec. II., Ingredients Index. This ingredient may be responsible for major toxic effects if poisonous amounts of this product are ingested.

Name & Use Manufacturer	Ingredients	
ORTHO-K-S 35-30 DUST Insecticide, fungicide (Calif. Spray)	Copper*	6.3%
	Zinc*	6.3%
	Sulfur *	30%
ORTHO LAWN GROOM Insecticide (Calif. Spray)	2,4-D	1%
	Gamma isomer of benzene hexachloride	0.25%
ORTHOL-D SOLUBLE OIL Insecticide (Calif. Spray)	Petroleum oil*	96%
ORTHO L 10 DUST Insecticide (Calif. Spray)	Lead arsenate*	10%
ORTHO L 40 DUST Insecticide (Calif. Spray)	Standard lead arsenate*	40%
ORTHO LEAF FEED Plant food (Calif. Spray)	Nitrogen (organic, derived from urea)	30.0%
	Zinc*(expressed as metallic)	4.0%
	Manganese (expressed as metallic)	1.4%
ORTHO LIME-SULPHUR SOLUTION Fungicide (Calif. Spray)	Calcium polysulfide*	29%
ORTHO LINDANE 95 Insecticide (Calif. Spray)	Lindane*	95%
ORTHO LINDANE 100 Insecticide (Calif. Spray)	Gamma isomer of benzene hexachloride*(from lindane)	100%
ORTHO L-K 40-25 DUST Insecticide (Calif. Spray)	Lead arsenate*	38.0%
	Copper	4.5%
	Zinc	4.5%
ORTHOL-K FLOWABLE HEAVY EMULSION Insecticide (Calif. Spray)	Petroleum oils*	83%
ORTHOL-K FLOWABLE, HEAVY-MEDIUM Insecticide (Calif. Spray)	Petroleum oils*	80%
ORTHOL-K FLOWABLE, LIGHT Insecticide (Calif. Spray)	Petroleum oils*	80%
ORTHOL-K FLOWABLE, LIGHT-MEDIUM Insecticide (Calif. Spray)	Petroleum oils*	80%
ORTHOL-K FLOWABLE, LIGHT-MEDIUM N.W. Insecticide (Calif. Spray)	Petroleum oils*	80%
ORTHOL-K FLOWABLE, LIGHT N.W. Insecticide (Calif. Spray)	Petroleum oils*	80%
ORTHOL-K FLOWABLE, MEDIUM Insecticide (Calif. Spray)	Petroleum oils*	80%
ORTHOL-K READY-MIX HEAVY-MEDIUM Insecticide (Calif. Spray)	Petroleum oils*	98%
ORTHOL-K READY-MIX, LIGHT-MEDIUM Insecticide (Calif. Spray)	Petroleum oils*	98%
ORTHOL-K READY-MIX, MEDIUM Insecticide (Calif. Spray)	Petroleum oils*	99%
ORTHO LOUSE & TICK POWDER (Calif. Spray)	Gamma isomer of benzene hexachloride (from lindane)	1.00%
ORTHO MALATHION-C 4-36 DUST Insecticide (Calif. Spray)	Malathion (o,o-dimethyl dithio phosphate of diethyl mercapto succinate)	4%
	Sodium fluoaluminate*	36%
ORTHO MALATHION-C-S 4-36-40 DUST Insecticide (Calif. Spray)	Malathion (o,o-dimethyl dithio phosphate of diethyl mercapto succinate)	4%
	Sodium fluoaluminate*	36%
	Sulfur	40%
ORTHO MALATHION-3D 4-5 DUST Insecticide (Calif. Spray)	Malathion*	4%
	DDD	5%
ORTHO MALATHION 4 DUST Insecticide (Calif. Spray)	Malathion*	4%
ORTHO MALATHION 5 DUST Insecticide (Calif. Spray)	Malathion*(o,o-dimethyl dithio phosphate of diethyl mercapto succinate)	5%
ORTHO MALATHION-S 4-25 DUST Insecticide, fungicide (Calif. Spray)	Malathion*	4%
	Sulfur*	25%

*Consult Sec. II., Ingredients Index. This ingredient may be responsible for major toxic effects if poisonous amounts of this product are ingested.

Name & Use Manufacturer	Ingredients	
ORTHO MALATHION-S 4-30 DUST Insecticide, fungicide (Calif. Spray)	Malathion* Sulfur*	4% 30%
ORTHO MALATHION-S 4-50 DUST Insecticide, fungicide (Calif. Spray)	Malathion* Sulfur*	4% 50%
ORTHO MALATHION 5 SPRAY Insecticide (Calif. Spray)	Malathion* Aromatic petroleum deriv. solvents*	55.7% 30.2%
ORTHO MALATHION 50 SPRAY Insecticide (Calif. Spray)	Malathion* Aromatic petroleum deriv. solvent*	50% 39%
ORTHO MALATHION 25 WETTABLE Insecticide (Calif. Spray)	Malathion*	25%
ORTHO MC DEFOLIANT (Calif. Spray)	Magnesium chlorate hexahydrate*	58%
ORTHO MCP 4 WEED KILLER (Calif. Spray)	Diethanolamine salt of 2-methyl-4-chloro phenoxy acetic acid* 2-Methyl-4-chloro phenoxy acetic acid equivalent*	52% 42.6%
ORTHO METACIDE 50 SPRAY Insecticide (Calif. Spray)	Parathion* o,o-Dimethyl-o-p-nitrophenyl thio-phosphate*	10% 40%
ORTHO MH-30 SPRAY Insecticide (Calif. Spray)	Diethanolamine salt of 1,2-dihydro pyridazine-3,6-dione*(equiv. to 30% maleic hydrazide)	58%
ORTHO-MITE 3D 3-5 DUST Insecticide, fungicide (Calif. Spray)	Aramite DDD	3% 5%
ORTHO-MITE 3D 4-5 DUST Insecticide (Calif. Spray)	Aramite Dichloro diphenyl dichloro-ethane	4% 5%
ORTHO-MITE-DIELDRIN 3-1.5 DUST Insecticide (Calif. Spray)	Aramite Dieldrin*	3% 1.5%
ORTHO-MITE 2 DUST Insecticide (Calif. Spray)	2-(p-tert-Butylphenoxy) isopropyl-2-chloroethyl sulfite	2%
ORTHO-MITE 3 DUST Insecticide (Calif. Spray)	2-(p-tert-Butylphenoxy) isopropyl-2-chloroethyl sulfite	3%
ORTHO-MITE 4 DUST Insecticide (Calif. Spray)	2-(p-tert-Butylphenoxy) isopropyl-2-chloroethyl sulfite	4%
ORTHO-MITE 2 EMULSION Insecticide (Calif. Spray)	2-(p-tert-Butylphenoxy) isopropyl-2-chloroethyl sulfite*	25%
ORTHO-MITE-MALATHION 3-4 DUST Insecticide (Calif. Spray)	2-(p-tert-Butylphenoxy) isopropyl-2-chloroethyl sulfite Malathion*(o,o-dimethyl dithiophosphate of diethyl mercapto succinate)	3% 4%
ORTHO-MITE-MALATHION-S 3-4-20 DUST Insecticide (Calif. Spray)	Aramite Malathion* Sulfur*	3% 4% 20%
ORTHO-MITE-S 3-20 DUST Insecticide, fungicide (Calif. Spray)	Aramite Sulfur*	3% 20%
ORTHO-MITE-S 3-30 DUST Insecticide, fungicide (Calif. Spray)	Aramite Sulfur*	3% 30%
ORTHO-MITE-S 3-50 DUST Insecticide, fungicide (Calif. Spray)	Aramite Sulfur*	3% 50%
ORTHO-MITE-S 4-20 DUST Insecticide, fungicide (Calif. Spray)	Aramite Sulfur*	4% 20%
ORTHO-MITE-S 4-30 DUST Insecticide, fungicide (Calif. Spray)	Aramite Sulfur*	4% 30%
ORTHO-MITE-S 4-50 DUST Insecticide, fungicide (Calif. Spray)	Aramite Sulfur*	4% 50%
ORTHO-MITE SPRAY Insecticide (Calif. Spray)	2-(p-tert-Butylphenoxy) isopropyl-2-chloroethyl sulfite*	25%
ORTHO-MITE 15 WETTABLE Insecticide (Calif. Spray)	2-(p-tert-Butylphenoxy) isopropyl-2-chloroethyl sulfite*	15%
ORTHO MULTI-FILM C Spreader and activator for use with cotton defoliant sprays (Calif. Spray)	Alkyl aryl polyoxyethylene glycols Petroleum oil Free fatty acids	

*Consult Sec. II., Ingredients Index. This ingredient may be responsible for major toxic effects if poisonous amounts of this product are ingested.

Name & Use Manufacturer	Ingredients	
ORTHO MULTI-FILM L Spreader and deposit builder for agricultural sprays (Calif. Spray)	Petroleum sulfonates Petroleum oil* Free and combined fatty acids	
ORTHO NABAM LIQUID SPRAY Fungicide (Calif. Spray)	Nabam*	19%
ORTHO N 5 DUST Insecticide (Calif. Spray)	Nicotine alkaloid*	1.8%
ORTHO N-P 90 OIL EMULSION Insecticide (Calif. Spray)	Oils*	90%
ORTHO 0-20 DUST Fungicide (Calif. Spray)	Cupric sulfate monohydrate*	20%
ORTHO 2.5-10-90 PEANUT DUST Insecticide, fungicide (Calif. Spray)	DDT Copper* expressed as metallic Sulfur*	2.5% 3.4% 80.7%
ORTHO 2.5-90 PEANUT DUST Insecticide, fungicide (Calif. Spray)	DDT Sulfur*	2.5% 80.7%
ORTHO 10-90 PEANUT DUST Fungicide (Calif. Spray)	Copper expressed as metallic* Sulfur*	3.4% 80.7%
ORTHO P-G BAIT (Meal) Insecticide (Calif. Spray)	Cupric aceto-arsenite*	3.2%
ORTHOPHOS 1 DUST Insecticide (Calif. Spray)	Parathion*	1%
ORTHOPHOS 4 SPRAY Insecticide (Calif. Spray)	Parathion*	42%
ORTHO POWDERED BORDEAUX MIXTURE Fungicide (Calif. Spray)	Copper*	12.7%

Name & Use Manufacturer	Ingredients	
ORTHO PYRENONE 63 SPRAY Insecticide (Calif. Spray)	Piperonyl butoxide Pyrethrins Polyethylene glycol oleic ester Oil*	10.7% 0.53% 10.5% 78.27%
ORTHORIX FOLIAGE SPRAY Insecticide, fungicide (Calif. Spray)	Calcium polysulfides* Polyethylene glycol monoiso- octyl phenyl ether	26% 10%
ORTHORIX SPRAY Fungicide (Calif. Spray)	Calcium polysulfides*	26%
ORTHO ROOST PAINT Insecticide (Calif. Spray)	Lindane*	1.5%
ORTHO ROSE DUST Insecticide (Calif. Spray)	Lindane Captan DDT* Ferbam Sulfur*	1.0% 7.5% 5.0% 3.5% 40.0%
ORTHO-SAN POWDER Deodorizer, sanitizer (Calif. Spray)	Dodecyl dimethyl benzyl ammonium chloride*	
ORTHO 1038 SCREW-WORM CONTROL (Calif. Spray)	DDT Lindane Aromatic petroleum deriv. solvent*	25.0% 4.5% 57.0%
ORTHO SEED GUARD DRY Insecticide, fungicide (Calif. Spray)	Gamma isomer of benzene hexachloride*(from lindane) Captan (n-trichloro methyl mercapto-4-cyclo hexene-1, 2-dicarboximide)	25% 25%
ORTHO SEED GUARD WETTABLE Insecticide, fungicide (Calif. Spray)	Lindane* Captan	16.5% 50%
ORTHO SEPTIC SEEP To correct soils for seepage (Calif. Spray)	Calcium polysulfides* Iso-octyl phenoxy polyethoxy ethanol	26% 10%
ORTHOSIL Detergent (Pennsylv. Salt)	Sodium orthosilicate	
ORTHO 10 SLUG DUST Insecticide (Calif. Spray)	Metaldehyde*	10%
ORTHO SODIUM TCA 90% Herbicide (Calif. Spray)	Sodium trichloroacetate*	90%

*Consult Sec. II., Ingredients Index. This ingredient may be responsible for major toxic effects if poisonous amounts of this product are ingested.

Name & Use Manufacturer	Ingredients	Name & Use Manufacturer	Ingredients
ORTHO SPINDLWET To increase efficiency of mechanical cotton pickers (Calif. Spray)		ORTHOTRAN 5 DUST Insecticide (Calif. Spray)	p-Chlorophenyl p-chloro-benzene sulfonate 5%
ORTHO-SPRAY LIME Dilutent (Calif. Spray)	Calcium hydroxide* 90%	ORTHOTRAN 7.5 DUST Insecticide, fungicide (Calif. Spray)	p-Chlorophenyl p-chloro-benzene sulfonate 7.5%
ORTHO STANDARD LEAD ARSENATE Insecticide (Calif. Spray)	Standard lead arsenate* 95%	ORTHOTRAN 10 DUST Insecticide (Calif. Spray)	p-Chlorophenyl-p-chloro-benzene sulfonate 10%
ORTHO STREPTO-MYCIN 0.024 DUST Fungicide (Calif. Spray)	Streptomycin 0.024%	ORTHOTRAN 1.5 EMULSIVE Insecticide (Calif. Spray)	p-Chlorophenyl p-chloro-benzene sulfonate* 18.7%
ORTHO SUB-SOIL (Calif. Spray)	Calcium polysulfide* 29%	ORTHOTRAN-S 5-50 DUST Insecticide, fungicide (Calif. Spray)	p-Chlorophenyl-p-chloro-benzene sulfonate 5% Sulfur* 50%
ORTHO TACK WASH Fungicide (Calif. Spray)	Captan (n-trichloromethyl mercapto-4-cyclohexene-1, 2-dicarboximide) 45%	ORTHOTRAN-S 7.5-20 DUST Insecticide, fungicide (Calif. Spray)	p-Chlorophenyl p-chloro-benzene sulfonate 7.5% Sulfur* 20%
ORTHO TANK MIX OIL Insecticide (Calif. Spray)	Petroleum oils* 100%	ORTHOTRAN-S 7.5-50 DUST Insecticide, fungicide (Calif. Spray)	p-Chlorophenyl p-chloro-benzene sulfonate 7.5% Sulfur* 50%
ORTHO TEPP 40 SPRAY Insecticide (Calif. Spray)	TEPP*(tetraethyl pyrophosphate) 40% Other ethyl phosphates* 60%	ORTHOTRAN-S 10-50 DUST Insecticide, fungicide (Calif. Spray)	p-Chlorophenyl p-chloro-benzene sulfonate 10% Sulfur* 50%
ORTHO-TIL 40 POWDER Soil conditioner (Calif. Spray)	Hydrolyzed polyacrylonitrile* 40%	ORTHOTRAN 50 WETTABLE Insecticide (Calif. Spray)	p-Chlorophenyl-p-chloro-benzene sulfonate* 50%
ORTHO-TIL SOLUBLE CHEMICAL SOIL CONDITIONER (Calif. Spray)	Hydrolyzed polymer of acrylonitrile* 83%	ORTHO 2,4-D BRUSH KILLER (Calif. Spray)	Isopropyl ester of 2,4,5-T* 15.4%
ORTHO 7-20 TOMATO DUST Insecticide, fungicide (Calif. Spray)	Copper 7% Calcium arsenate* 20%	ORTHO VEGETABLE DUST Insecticide (Calif. Spray)	Captan 5.00% Methoxychlor tech. 5.00% Rotenone from cube 0.75% Other resins from cube 0.75%
ORTHO-TOX 5 DUST Insecticide (Calif. Spray)	Methoxychlor 5%	ORTHO VOLCK ISOTOX SPRAY Insecticide (Calif. Spray)	Petroleum oils* 80% Gamma isomer of benzene hexachloride (from lindane) 1% DDT 2% Aromatic petroleum deriv. solvent* 10%
ORTHOTOX 50 WETTABLE Insecticide (Calif. Spray)	Methoxychlor* 50%	ORTHO VOLCK OIL SPRAY Insecticide (Calif. Spray)	Petroleum oils* 97.00%
ORTHOTRAN 3D 7.5-5 DUST Insecticide (Calif. Spray)	p-Chlorophenyl-p-chloro-benzene sulfonate 7.5% TDE 5%	ORTHO WEEVIL BAIT (Meal) (Calif. Spray)	Sodium fluosilicate* 4.75%
		ORTHO WEEVIL BAIT (Pelleted) (Calif. Spray)	Sodium fluosilicate* 4.75%

*Consult Sec. II., Ingredients Index. This ingredient may be responsible for major toxic effects if poisonous amounts of this product are ingested.

Name & Use Manufacturer	Ingredients	
ORTHO W-41 LIQUID CORROSION INHIBITOR (Calif. Spray)	Arsenic compound*	
ORTHO ZINC COPPER FUNGICIDE (Calif. Spray)	Copper* Zinc*	4% 20%
ORTHO ZINEB 3.25 DUST Fungicide (Calif. Spray)	Zineb	3.25%
ORTHO ZINEB 4 DUST Fungicide (Calif. Spray)	Zineb	4%
ORTHO ZINEB 6 DUST Fungicide (Calif. Spray)	Zineb	6%
ORTHO ZINEB ONION DUST Insecticide, fungicide (Calif. Spray)	Zineb Sulfur Parathion*	4% 30% 1%
ORTHO ZINEB-s 3.25-15 DUST Fungicide (Calif. Spray)	Zineb Sulfur*	3.25% 15%
ORTHO ZINEB-S 3.25-25 DUST Fungicide (Calif. Spray)	Zineb Sulfur*	3.25% 25%
ORTHO ZINEB WETTABLE Fungicide (Calif. Spray)	Zineb	65%
ORTHO Z-M DEFICIENCY SPRAY NO. 20-7 For agricultural use (Calif. Spray)	Zinc* Manganese	20% 7%
ORZENE Insecticide (Selig)	Orthodichlorobenzene*	100%
O.S. Detergent (Wyandotte)	Concentrated alkali*	
OSAGE RUB HAIR TONIC (Assoc. Brands)		
O'SHELLAC (Advance Paint)		
OSO-TITE CEMENT (Rubbercraft)		

Name & Use Manufacturer	Ingredients	
OTALGAN For otitis media (Otalgan)	Boric acid Benzocaine Propylene glycol Glycerin	2% 2%
OUR FAVORITE GOLD ENAMEL (Sapolin)		
OURINE For removal of hardened ear wax (Aurine)	Glycerin Tincture belladonna (belladonna alkaloids 0.0002 gr./fl. oz.) Boric acid* Chamomile Plantain Hydrastis Procaine hydrochloride Camphor* Extract witch hazel Aromatic oils	
OUR-OWN AERO-HOPPER SPRAY Insecticide (Calif. Farm)	Petroleum oil* DDT	98% 2%
OUR-OWN AERO-SPRA-OIL Insecticide (Calif. Farm)	Petroleum oil*	98%
OUR-OWN BASIC COPPER SULPHATE Fungicide (Calif. Farm)	Copper*	52%
OUR-OWN BLIGHT DUST NO. 5-15 Fungicide (Calif. Farm)	Zineb Sulfur*	3% 15%
OUR-OWN CAS DUST 50-50 Insecticide (Calif. Farm)	Calcium arsenate* Sulfur	35% 48.6%
OUR-OWN CHLORDANE DUST 5 Insecticide (Calif. Farm)	Chlordane*	5%
OUR-OWN CHLORDANE EMULSION Insecticide (Calif. Farm)	Chlordane*	45%

Name & Use Manufacturer	Ingredients	
OUR-OWN DDT-CUPER-SULFUR DUST 5-5-25 Insecticide (Calif. Farm)	DDT* Cuprous oxide Sulfur*	5% 4.5% 24%
OUR-OWN DDT-CUPER-SULFUR DUST 5-5-50 Insecticide (Calif. Farm)	DDT* Cuprous oxide Sulfur*	5% 4.5% 49%
OUR-OWN DDT DUST NO. 5 Insecticide (Calif. Farm)	DDT*	5%
OUR-OWN DDT LIQUID CONC. Insecticide (Calif. Farm)	DDT Xylene*	25% 55%
OUR-OWN DDT-S DUST NO. 4-85 Insecticide (Calif. Farm)	DDT* Sulfur*	4% 82.6%
OUR-OWN DDT-S DUST NO. 5-50 Insecticide (Calif. Farm)	DDT* Sulfur*	5% 48.6%
OUR-OWN DDT-S DUST NO. 5-85 Insecticide (Calif. Farm)	DDT* Sulfur	5% 82.6%
OUR-OWN DORMANT EMULSION FLOWABLE Insecticide (Calif. Farm)	Petroleum oil*	80%
OUR-OWN DORMANT OIL EMULSIVE (Calif. Farm)	Petroleum oil*	98%
OUR-OWN D-S DUST 30-70 Insecticide (Calif. Farm)	Basic lead arsenate* Sulfur	28% 67.8%
OUR-OWN G-S DUST NO. 10 Insecticide (Calif. Farm)	Gamma isomer of benzene hexachloride Other isomers of benzene hexachloride Sulfur*	1% 2.5% 70%
OUR-OWN K DUST 40 Insecticide (Calif. Farm)	Sodium fluoaluminate*	36%
OUR-OWN K DUST 50 Insecticide (Calif. Farm)	Sodium fluoaluminate*	45%
OUR-OWN K-S DUST 40-25 Insecticide (Calif. Farm)	Sodium fluoaluminate* Sulfur	36% 24.3%
OUR-OWN K-S DUST 50-25 Insecticide (Calif. Farm)	Sodium fluoaluminate* Sulfur	45% 24.3%
OUR-OWN NICOTINE DUST 10A & 10B Insecticide (Calif. Farm)	Nicotine alkaloid*	3.6%
OUR OWN PAINTS (Con-Ferro)		
OUR-OWN SOLUBLE COPPER Fungicide (Calif. Farm)	Copper*	3%
OUR-OWN SUMMER EMULSION, HEAVY-MEDIUM, LIGHT, & LIGHT-MEDIUM Insecticide (Calif. Farm)	Petroleum oil*	80%
OUR-OWN SUMMER EMULSIVE, LIGHT, LIGHT-MEDIUM, & MEDIUM Insecticide (Calif. Farm)	Petroleum oil*	99%
OUR-OWN TETRAPHOS SPRAY 50 Insecticide (Calif. Farm)	Tetraethyl pyrophosphate* Other organic phosphates*	20% 30%
OUR-OWN Z-DDT DUST 5-5 Insecticide (Calif. Farm)	Zineb DDT*	3% 5%
OUR-OWN Z-DDT-S DUST 5-5-50 Insecticide (Calif. Farm)	Zineb DDT* Sulfur*	3% 5% 50%
OUR PET FLEA POWDER (Blue Ball)		
OUR PET MANGE REMEDY (Blue Ball)		

Name & Use Manufacturer	Ingredients	Name & Use Manufacturer	Ingredients
OUT Bowl and porcelain cleaner (Assoc. Just)	Hydrogen chloride* 8.50% Orthodichlorobenzene 2.25%	OVUMIX Anthelmintic, tonic (vet-erinary, avian) (Whitmoyer)	Areca nuts Tobacco dust Nicotine alkaloid* Nux vomica 8% Strychnine* 40 gr./oz. Ginger Anise Copper sulfate Gentian Mustard Ferrous sulfate Foenugreek
OUTBOARD OIL Non-detergent (Kendall Ref.)			
OUTDOOR FRIEND INSECT REPELLENT (Allied Home)	Dimethyl phthalate 12.76% 2-Ethylhexanediol-1,3* 3.47% Butyl dimethyl dihydro gamma pyrone carboxylate* 3.77%	OXA CASGO Antacid (Statler)	Calcium carbonate Bismuth subnitrate Magnesium carbonate Saccharin Oil peppermint
OUTGRO For ingrown nails (Whitehall)	Chlorobutanol* 28 gr./fl. oz. Tannic acid* Alcohol* 44%	OXILAC LACQUERS (Oxidermo)	
OUT-RITE INK ERADICATOR (Stafford)		OXALIN PAINTS (Bell Chem. Co., Inc.)	
OUTSO-LITE COLD WATER PAINT (Tamms)		OXIDERMO PAINTS, LACQUERS (Oxidermo)	
OVENLUBE High temperature lubricant (Kano)	Graphited base Blended oils	OXINE DUSTING POWDER Deodorant, bacteriostatic (Borocyl)	Boridiorthotic oxybenzoic acid Zinc* Sodium borate* Sodium perborate* Boric acid* Benzoic acid* Ammoniated alum Purified talcum
OVER-AWL BRAND PAINTS (Liebich)			
OVERTON'S HIGH-BROWN BLEACH OINTMENT Cosmetic (Overton)	Ammoniated mercury* 5%	OXINOL (Eastern Pharm.)	Magnesium carbonate Lactose Saccharin Sodium bicarbonate Bismuth subcarbonate Essential oils*
OVERTON'S RO-ZOL BLEACH Face bleach (Overton)	Ammoniated mercury* 5%	OXIPHEN ORANGE Cathartic (Pitman-Moore)	Each tablet: Sodium glycocholate 16.2 mg. Sodium taurocholate 16.2 mg. Phenolphthalein 32.4 mg. Extract cascara 32.4 mg. Aloin* 8.8 mg.
OVEX 50-W Insecticide (Stauffer)	p-Chlorophenyl-p-chloro-benzene sulfonate* 50%	OXIUM Aluminum brightner (Lester Labs.)	Acids*
OVOFERRIN Tonic (Barnes, A.C.)	Elementary iron 64 mg./tbsp Alcohol 8%/v Colloidal iron	OX LINE PAINTS & VARNISHES (Lehman Bros. Corp.)	
OVOTOX SPRAY Fungicide, insecticide, ovicide (Bonide)	p-Chlorophenyl-p-chloro-benzene sulfonate* 12.5% Dichloro diphenyl trichloro-ethane* 12.5% Gamma isomer of benzene hexachloride* 3.125% Ferbam 10.18%	OX-LINE ONE COAT FUME PROOF HOUSE PAINT (Lehman Bros. Corp.)	Lead less than 1%
OVOTRAN (Dow)	p-Chlorophenyl-p-chloro-benzene sulfonate*	OX-LINE TINTING SYSTEM Paints in tubes (Lehman Bros. Corp.)	1, 2, 3, 4: Lead more than 1%

*Consult Sec. II., Ingredients Index. This ingredient may be responsible for major toxic effects if poisonous amounts of this product are ingested.

Name & Use Manufacturer	Ingredients	Name & Use Manufacturer	Ingredients
OX-O-DECK FLOOR PAINTS (Lehman Bros. Corp.)	Contain less than 1% lead with the exception of Vermilion and Tile Green	OZARK MINERAL-HERB MIXTURE Laxative (Ozark)	Aloe* Cascara sagrada (sacred bark) Life everlasting herb Iron and ammonium citrate* Sodium bicarbonate Epsom salts Boneset herb Queen of meadow herb Licorice root Ferrous sulfate*
OX-O-FLOW ONE COAT FLAT PAINTS (Lehman Bros. Corp.)	Contain less than 1% lead with the exception of Pale Yellow and Chartreuse	OZARK MT. LAXATIVE COMPOUND (Ozark)	Aloe* Epsom salts Queen of meadow herb Licorice root Ferrous sulfate* Sodium bicarbonate Cascara sagrada (sacred bark) Boneset herb Life everlasting herb Iron and ammonium citrate*
OX-O-GLOSS ENAMELS (Lehman Bros. Corp.)	Contain less than 1% lead with the exception of Pale Yellow and Chartreuse		
OX-O-SHEEN SEMI-GLOSS Paints (Lehman Bros. Corp.)	Contain less than 1% lead with the exception of Pale Yellow and Chartreuse	OZARK RUBBING OIL Counter-irritant (Ozark)	Oil turpentine* Cresol* Carbolic acid* Methyl salicylate* Oil mustard (synthetic) Oil eucalyptus* Camphor* Kerosene*
OX-O-SPAR QUICK DRYING ENAMELS (Lehman Bros. Corp.)	Only Canary Yellow, Burnt Orange and Shutter Green contain any amount of lead	OZARK SALVE (Black balm) (Ozark)	Methyl salicylate* Oil eucalyptus* Oil pine* Kerosene * Carbolic acid and camphor (combined as camphorated phenol)*
OX-O-TONE ALKYD FLAT Paints (Lehman Bros. Corp.)	Contain less than 1% lead with the exception of Pale Yellow and Chartreuse		
OXYDOL Detergent (Procter & Gamble)	Anionic synthetic detergent* Sodium tripolyphosphate Sodium sulfate Sodium silicate Sodium perborate*	OZ CREAM POLISH (Behlen)	
		OZEX Insecticide (Woodlets)	Pyrethrin* Methoxychlor* Piperonyl butoxide
OXYFUME FUMIGANT (Carbide)	Ethylene dichloride* 81%/w Ethylene oxide 19%/w	OZIUM Air sanitizer (Woodlets)	Triethylene glycol 10% Propylene glycol 10%
OXYLIN ANTISEPTIC OINTMENT For skin (Evons)	Oxyquinoline sulfate Ethyl amino benzoate Urea Menthol Camphor* Eucalyptol* Lanolin Aromatics*	OZON ALBUTONE SKIN LOTION (Assoc. Brands)	
		OZO-NAPHTHOL DISINFECTANT (White, H.)	
O-X-ZEL Disinfectant, deodorizer, cleanser (McClellan)	Cresylic acid* 50% Anhydrous soap 25%	OZON COCOA BUTTER ODEUR CREAM (Assoc. Brands)	
		OZON DEODORANT CREAM (Assoc. Brands)	
OZARK MINERAL CRYSTALS Cathartic (Ozark)	Sodium sulfate Magnesium sulfate Sodium salicylate Iron and ammonium citrate* Methyl salicylate*	OZONE ENAMELS (Chase Varnish)	

---

*Consult Sec. II., Ingredients Index. This ingredient may be responsible for major toxic effects if poisonous amounts of this product are ingested.

Name & Use Manufacturer	Ingredients		Name & Use Manufacturer	Ingredients	
OZON LEMON ASTRINGENT CREAM (Assoc. Brands)			PABCO PAINTS, VARNISH, ENAMELS, PABCOAT MASONARY & SHAKE PAINT, PABCOTE ROOF COATING (Pabco)		
OZON MANICOTE DYE & STAIN REMOVER (Assoc. Brands)			PABILAX Cathartic (Veltex)	Each tablet: Papain Bile salts Extr. cascara sagrada Phenolphthalein, yellow* Extr. nux vomica* Oleoresin capsicum	1 gr. 1 gr. 1/2 gr. 1/2 gr. 1/16 gr. 1/40 gr.
OZON NAIL POLISH REMOVER (Assoc. Brands)					
OZON WAVE SET (Assoc. Brands)			PABISAL TABLETS Antirheumatic (Veltex)	Each tablet: Sodium salicylate U.S.P.* Para-aminobenzoic acid sodium	5 gr. 5 gr.
PABACINE Analgesic (Dillard)	Each tablet: Sodium salicylate* Para-aminobenzoic acid Ascorbic acid	0.25 gm. 0.25 gm. 20 mg.	PABST'S OKAY SPECIAL (Myers Labs.)	Balsam copaiba Oil of copaiba Uva ursi Juniper berries Sweet spirit of niter Oil of sandalwood Cubeb Buchu Matico	
PABACINE WITH COLCHICINE Analgesic (gout) (Dillard)	Each tablet: Sodium salicylate* Para-aminobenzoic acid Ascorbic acid Colchicine*	0.25 gm. 0.25 gm. 60.00 mg. 0.25 mg.			
			P-A-C COMPOUND, CAPSULES Analgesic (Upjohn)	Each capsule: Acetophenetidin* Acetylsalicylic acid* Caffeine	2-1/2 gr. 3-1/2 gr. 1/2 gr.
PABASALATE Analgesic (Approved)	Each tablet: Sodium salicylate* Para-aminobenzoic acid	0.3 gm. 0.3 gm.			
PABASALIC Analgesic (Gotham)	Each tablet: Sodium salicylate* Sodium para-aminobenzoic acid Ascorbic acid	0.3 gm. 0.3 gm. 10 mg.	P-A-C COMPOUND, HALF- STRENGTH, TABLETS Analgesic (Upjohn)	Each tablet: Acetophenetidin* Acetylsalicylic acid* Caffeine	1-1/4 gr. 1 3/4 gr. 1/4 gr.
PABA- SALICYLATE Analgesic (West-Ward)	Each tablet: Sodium salicylate* Para-aminobenzoic acid	0.3 gm. 0.3 gm.	PACER PAINT (Pysol)		
PABA- SALICYLATE TABLETS- SODIUM- FREE E. C. PINK Analgesic (West-Ward)	Each tablet: Ammonium salicylate* Potassium para-aminobenzoate	5 gr. 5 gr.	PACIFIC LUBRICATING FLAKE GRAPHITE (Pacific Graphite)	Carbon Silica	70-98% 0-0.5%
			PACIFISEAL ASBESTOS ROOF CEMENT (Pacific Paint)		
PABA- SALICYLATE WITH C Analgesic (West-Ward)	Each tablet: Sodium salicylate* Para-aminobenzoic acid Ascorbic acid	0.3 gm. 0.3 gm. 60 mg.			
PABASOD TABLETS Antirheumatic (Preston Labs.)	Each tablet: Sodium salicylate* Sodium para-aminobenzoate	5 gr. 5 gr.	PACKARD OIL COLORS (Packard Paint)		
PABASONE Antirheumatic (Pinex)	Sodium salicylate* Para-aminobenzoic acid Ascorbic acid	5 gr. 5 gr. 20 mg.	PACKER'S SHAMPOO (Packer's)		

---

*Consult Sec. II., Ingredients Index. This ingredient may be responsible for major toxic effects if poisonous amounts of this product are ingested.

Name & Use Manufacturer	Ingredients	Name & Use Manufacturer	Ingredients
PACOPHINE (Syrup) Sedative, antitussive (Massengill)	Each 5 cc.: Chloroform 21.5 mg. Morphine sulfate* 2.7 mg. Potassium guaiacolsulfonate 86.5 mg. Ammonium chloride 86.5 mg. Tartar emetic* 0.9 mg. White pine bark Wild cherry base	PAGLO SCALP OINTMENT (Paglo)	Resorcin Salicylic acid* Benzoic acid Hydroquinone* Oxyquinoline* Precipitated sulfur
PACQUIN'S ANTI- DETERGENT CREAM (Pacquin)	Glycerin Sorbitol Lanolin Cholesterols Methyl-and propylparaben less than 1%	PAIL-PRIDE DEODORANT Repellent, deodorizer (San-A-Lizer)	Naphthalene* 85% Methyl salicylate 5%
PACQUIN'S DRY SKIN CREAM, HAND CREAM (Pacquin)	Stearic acid Glycerin Sorbitol Ammonium hydroxide Sodium metabisulfite less than 1%	PAINALLAY Antiseptic (Mouth, throat) (Glessner)	Boric acid* Glycerin Saccharin Cresol* Oil of peppermint Zinc chloride*
PACQUIN'S SILK'N SATIN LOTION (Pacquin)	Stearic acid Sorbitol Triethanolamine Dihydroxyacetic acid 0.08% Cetyl alcohol	PAIN EXPELLER (Richter)	Alcohol* 49% Capsicum Ammonia Camphor* Soap Essential oils*
PAD KOTE Astringent, external (veterinary) (Happy Jack)	Cod liver oil Juniper tar Balsam Peru Tannic acid* Turpentine less than 2% Gentian violet* Brilliant green Phenol less than 1% Alcohol isopropyl* 60%	PAIN-EZE LINIMENT Rubefacient (Binday)	Menthol* Camphor* Methyl salicylate*
		PAIN-EZ-ER HOT DROPS (Denton)	
PADROPHYLL TABLETS Asthmatic antispasmodic (Sharp & Dohme)	Propadrine phenyl propanolamine hydrochloride* 30 mg. Theophylline* 0.12 gm.	PAIN-EZE TABLETS Analgesic (Binday)	Aspirin* Caffeine Phenacetin* 2-1/2 gr.
PAGE'S CAPSULES Diuretic (Page, E.R.)	Oil of Erigeron Methyl salicylate*	PAINOL Rubefacient (Boericke & Runyon)	Alcohol 47%/v Methyl salicylate* Menthol Arnica Capsicum Camphor*
PAGE'S INHALERS (Consolid. Chem.)	Stramonium leaves* Chestnut leaves Tea leaves Gum benzoin Kola nuts	PAINTALL QUALITY PAINT (Van Sickle)	
PAGE'S LAXATIVE PILLS (Page, E.R.)	Extr. cascara sagrada	PAINTER'S FRIEND PAINTS (Porter Paint)	
PAGE'S OINTMENT (rectal) (Page, E. R.)	Tannic acid* Carbolic acid* Menthol (synthetic)* Zinc oxide Benzocaine Amber petrolatum	PAINTER'S FRIEND PAINTS, PAINT BRUSH CLEANER, PAINT & VARNISH CLEANER, PORCELAIN, TILE, ETC. CLEANERS, SOAP & PASTE (Cleveland C. & P.)	
PAGE'S OINTMENT FOR ATHLETES FOOT (Assoc. Prod.)	Salicylic acid* Benzoic acid* Petrolatum and lanolin base		
PAGE'S TABLETS Diuretic (Page, E.R.)	Oil of Erigeron Methyl salicylate*	PAINTMASTER PAINTS (Lasting)	

*Consult Sec. II., Ingredients Index. This ingredient may be responsible for major toxic effects if poisonous amounts of this product are ingested.

Name & Use Manufacturer	Ingredients		Name & Use Manufacturer	Ingredients	
PAINT OFF BRUSH TYPE PAINT & VARNISH REMOVER (Beck Eq.)	Mixed amines Methylene chloride*		PALM BEACH FOOT-STICK & STICK DEODORANT (Collins, M.)	Alcohol* Hexachlorophene Perfume oils	70%
PAINT-RITE CRAYONS (Nat'l Crayon)			PALMER DRY ART COLORS, POSTER & SHOW CARD COLOR SETS (Palmer Show Card)		
PAINT-TEX Plastic paint (Lasting)					
PAISLEY CHINA, CROCKERY, GLASS, FABRIC, MODEL AIRPLANE, RUBBER & PLASTIC CEMENTS (Paisley)			PALMER OVERGLAZE (Palmer Paint)		
			PALMER POSTER PAINTS (Palmer Paint)		
P.A.L. Antiseptic, fungicide (medical) (Passaic)	Isopropyl alcohol* 88% Salicylic acid* Para-propyl-aminobenzoate* Menthol Para-tertiary-butyl-meta-cresol Chloral hydrate 3% Benzoic acid Thymol* Iodoform*		PALMER'S ANTISEPTIC LOTION (Palmer, S.)	Bichloride of mercury* 0.18% Alcohol 70%/v Turpentine* Sweet almond oil Balsam of Peru Oil of bitter almonds Oil of cloves*	
P.A.L. For poison ivy and oak (Passaic)	Isopropyl alcohol* 35% Stabilized ferric chloride Para-propyl-amino benzoate hydrochloride* Urea		DR. FRED PALMER'S SKIN DELIGHT SOAP (Galenol)		
PALATONE Aromatic specialty (Dow)	3-Hydroxy-2-methyl-1,4-pyrone*		DR. PALMER'S SKIN WHITENER (Galenol)	Ammoniated mercury* 3% Petrolatum Lanolin	
PALBROMA Sedative (Clapp, Otis)	Alcohol 5%/v Potassium bromide* 20 gr. Sodium bromide* 20 gr. Ammonium bromide* 20 gr. Tinct. Hyoscyamus (total alkaloids 0.00016 gr.) 4 m. Tinct. stramonium (total alkaloids 0.0012 gr.) 4 m. Sodium glycerophosphate 2 gr. Calcium glycerophosphate 1 gr.		PALMETTS Counter-irritant (genito-urinary) (Jenkins)	Each tablet: Extr. saw palmetto 1 gr. Extr. zea 1/4 gr. Extr. couch grass 1/4 gr. Sodium benzoate 1/2 gr. Oil sandalwood q.s.	
			PALMO-DIONIN SYRUP Antitussive (Upjohn)	Dionin (morphine deriv.) 1/4 gr. Ammonium chloride 8 gr. Alcohol 11% Sabal Eucalyptus Tolu balsam Glycerin Aromatics	
PAL DOG FLEA POWDER (House of Huston)	DDT* 5.0% Gamma isomer of benzene hexachloride (from lindane)* 1.0% Pyrethrins 0.25%		PALMOLIVE LATHER SHAVING CREAM (Colgate-Palmolive)		
PALISADES PAINTS (Hoboken)					
PALM BEACH DEODORANT & AFTER SHAVE STICKS FOR MEN (Collins, M.)	Alcohol* 70% Hexachlorophene Perfume oils		PALMOLIVE TOILET SOAP (Colgate-Palmolive)		

*Consult Sec. II., Ingredients Index. This ingredient may be responsible for major toxic effects if poisonous amounts of this product are ingested.

Name & Use Manufacturer	Ingredients
PALMOSAN Genito- urinary disease (Jenkins)	Each tablet: Extr. saw palmetto 2 gr. Extr. zea 1/2 gr. Extr. couch grass 1/2 gr. Sodium benzoate 1 gr. Oil sandalwood q.s.
PALO ALTO PERFUME (Ybry)	
PALVO Tonic, cathartic (Spicer)	Fl. extr.: Cimicifuga Viburnum prunifolium Aletris Caulophyllum Viburnum opulus Hydrastis Mitchella repens Cascara sagrada
PALVO POWDER Vaginal douche (Spicer)	Menthol* Glycerine Boric acid* Phenol* Thymol* Eucalyptol* Zinc sulfate*
PAN-AID Skin antiseptic (Mother's)	Carbamide Chlorhydrol Alkenyl aryl ethyl amido chloride Chlorobutanol* Alkyl morpholinium ethosulfate Alkyl dimethyl benzyl ammonium bromide*
PANAMA WHITE SHOE CLEANER (Penslar)	
PANAMIDES #205 Antibacterial (Vitec)	Sulfadiazine* 0.150 gm. Sulfamerazine* 0.100 gm. Sulfacetamide* 0.150 gm. Sulfamethazine* 0.100 gm.
PAN APPLE SPRAY Insecticide (Talyor)	Lead arsenate*

PANCROTOL
Biliary
stimulant,
antispasmodic
(Calvital)
	Dehydrocholic acid 1/2 gr.
	Bile salts 1-1/2 gr.
	Pancreatin U.S.P 4-1/2 gr.
	Atropine sulfate 0.0097 mg.
	Hyoscyamine sulfate*
	  0.0518 mg.
	Hyoscine hydrobromide
	  0.0033 mg.

PAN-DERMA SKIN LOTION (Pan Derma)	Ethyl aminobenzoate (benzocaine)* Phenol* Menthol* Camphor* Zinc tannate
PANDURA ENAMEL & PAINT (Mound City)	
PANITE RESIN GLUE (Le Page's)	Urea formaldehyde

Name & Use Manufacturer	Ingredients

PANO-DRENCH
4
Soil drench
(Panogen)
	Cyano-(methylmercuri)-
	  guanidine (mercury equiv.
	  0.4%) * 0.6%

PANODRIN
Seed
disinfectant
(Panogen)
	Each gal:
	  Methyl mercury dicyandiamide
	  0.4%
	Hexachloro hexahydro-endo,
	  exo-dimethano naphthalene*
	  24.4%
	Related compounds 4.1%
	Aldrin* 2.4 lb./gal.

PANOGEN 15 LIQUID SEED DISINFECTANT (Panogen)	Methyl mercury dicyandiamide* 2.2%
PANOGEN 42 LIQUID SEED DISINFECTANT (Panogen)	Methyl mercury dicyandiamide* 6.3%
PANORAM 75 Seed disinfectant (Panogen)	Thiram (tetramethyl thiuram disulfide*) 75%

PANORAM D-31
Insecticide,
fungicide
(Panogen)
	Thiram (tetramethyl thiuram
	  disulfide*) 56.2%
	Hexachloro-epoxy-octahydro-
	  endo, exo-dimethano-
	  naphthalene* (dieldrin equiv.
	  18.8%) 16.0%
	Related compounds 2.8%

PAN PEACH SPRAY NO. 3 Insecticide (Taylor)	Sulfur* 40.35% Zinc* 10%

PAN PLANT
SPRAY
Insecticide
(Woolfolk)
	Lead arsenate* 9.00%
	Sulfur 28.00%
	Copper (basic sulfate) as
	  metallic 10.00%
	Zinc (basic sulfate) as metallic
	  4.00%
	Nicotine alkaloid* 2.80%
	Arsenic as metallic 1.76%
	Water-soluble arsenic
	  0.10%
	Lead* as metallic 5.20%

PAN SAYF TINWARE STERILIZING DETERGENT (Griffith)	
PANTACOL Antihistaminic, antitussive (Commerce)	Dihydrocodeinone bitartrate* Pyrilamine maleate* Potassium guaiacolsulfonate Sodium citrate Antimony and potassium tartrate* Propyl and methyl parasept
PANTHERMIC 777 Photographic agent (Harvey Photo.)	
PANYON PERFUME (De Grasse)	

*Consult Sec. II., Ingredients Index. This ingredient may be responsible for major toxic effects if poisonous amounts of this product are ingested.

Name & Use Manufacturer	Ingredients
PAOCIN Intestinal adsorbent (Massengill)	Each 15 cc.: Colloidal kaolin 90 gr. Pectin 2 gr. Aromatics q.s.
PAOCIN TABLETS Intestinal adsorbent (Massengill)	Each tablet: Colloidal kaolin 0.63 gm. Pectin 16 mg. Aromatics q.s.

PAPA CARIA
Antacid,
digestant
(Jenkins)
	Magnesium carbonate
	   100 gr.
	Calcium carbonate 50 gr.
	Sodium bicarbonate 120 gr.
	Bismuth subnitrate 50 gr,
	Cerium oxalate 25 gr.
	Magnesium trisilicate
	   70 gr.
	Powdered ginger 4 gr.
	Papain 11 gr.
	Pancreatin 5-1/2 gr.
	Aromatics

PAPAIN COMPOUND Digestant (Hance)	Each tablet: Papain 3/4 gr. Charcoal 1/3 gr. Sodium bicarbonate 4 gr. Oil of wintergreen* q.s.

PAPE'S COLD
COMPOUND
Antipyretic,
analgesic
(Sterling Prod.
Div.)
	Each tablet:
	Acetanilid* 1 gr.
	Extr. belladonna U.S.P.
	  (total alkaloids 3/20,000 gr.)
	   2/250 gr.)
	Phenolphthalein
	Gum turpentine

PAPESIA
COMPOUND
Antacid,
(cathartic)
carminative
(Tailby)
	Tailby-Nason's Milk of
	  Magnesia (with papain, ginger,
	  peppermint)

PAPSO-GENS Antacid, digestant (Richards Bros.)	Papain Gentian Willow charcoal Peppermint Ginger Soda
PAPSOMAX Antacid, digestant (Papsomax)	Aluminum hydroxide U.S.P. Magnesium carbonate U.S.P. Sodium bicarbonate U.S.P. Calcium carbonate U.S.P. Papain Chinese rhubarb U.S.P. Oil of peppermint
PAP TABS Digestant (motion sickness) (Frenco Labs.)	Papain Bismuth Subnitrate Sodium carbonate Calcium carbonate Magnesium carbonate Magnesium hydroxide Cerium oxalate Saccharin sodium Kaolin Peppermint
PAP TEA Tonic, digestant (Frenco Labs.)	Green papaya leaf
PAQUA Water paste paint (Moore, B.)	

Name & Use Manufacturer	Ingredients
PARA-BACO Fungicide (Solvay)	Paradichlorobenzene* 99.5-100%
PARABIS Paraciticide, internal (veterinary) (Dow)	Diphenol*
PARABOND CHLORINATED RUBBER PAINTS (Bondrite)	
PARACIDE Insecticide (Hooker)	Paradichlorobenzene* 100%
PARACIDE OINTMENT (Durham's)	Methyl salicylate* Menthol crystals* Flower of sulfur* Benzoinated lard Gum camphor* Oil of tar*
PARACYL TABLETS Antirheumatic (Pharmex)	Sodium para-aminobenzoic acid Salicylamide*
PARADE (Newport)	Alkyl aryl sulfonate* Sodium pyro- and polyphosphates* Sodium sulfate Carboxymethylcellulose
PARA- DEODORANT BLOCKS Deodorizer (Reliable Chem.)	Paradichlorobenzene*
PARADERM SKIN LOTION (Research Spec.)	Mineral oil Stearyl alcohol Glycerin Cetyl alcohol Essential oils*(pH approx. 6.7)
PARADI Insecticide (Hooker)	Paradichlorobenzene* 100%
PARADISE BOWL DEODORANT, LIQUID DETERGENT, DEODORANT BLOCKS (Paradise Prod.)	
PARADISE MOTH CRYSTALS, BALLS, NUGGETS, SPRAY (Paradise Prod.)	
PARADOW Insecticide (Dow)	Paradichlorobenzene*

*Consult Sec. II., Ingredients Index. This ingredient may be responsible for major toxic effects if poisonous amounts of this product are ingested.

Name & Use Manufacturer	Ingredients	Name & Use Manufacturer	Ingredients
PARAEROSOL Insecticide (Dao)	o,o-Diethyl-o-p-nitrophenyl thiophosphate* 10.0% Methyl chloride 90.0%	PARANAY Lubricating oil (McAlester)	Refined oil*
PARAEUSAL For nose & throat (Paraeusal)		PAR & WHITE MAGIC SOAP (Newport)	Anhydrous soap Sodium pyrophosphate Sodium silicate Sodium carbonate
PARAFILM RUBBER BASE ENAMELS (Upco)		PARA NUGGETS & CRYSTALS Insecticide (Uncle Sam)	Paradichlorobenzene* 100%
PARAFLOW 400 Insecticide (Stauffer)	Parathion*(o,o-diethyl-o-p-nitrophenyl thiophosphate 42%	PARAPLI RUBBER BASE PAINT (Parr Paint)	
PARAFORMOL PASTE Topical anesthetic (Crosby)	Paraformaldehyde* Calcium sulfate Metycaine thymol* Fibrous petrolatum base Trioxymethylene	PARAPLY SHELLAC SUBSTITUTE (Foundry)	
PARAGON OIL BLEACH, NEUTRAL Cosmetic (Paragon)	Ammoniacal alcoholic aqueous soap-oil emulsion	PARA-PURE Insecticide (Reefer-Galler)	Paradichlorobenzene*
PARAGON PEROXIDE (Paragon)	Hydrogen peroxide* 20%/v	PARASAL COLORED WOOD COATING Paint (Parker Paint)	
PARA-JEL Analgesic (dental) (Approved)	Benzocaine Cetyl-dimethyl-benzyl ammonium chloride*	PARASMA TABLETS Asthmatic antispasmodic (Raymond, C.)	Each tablet: Ephedrine hydrochloride* 1/8 gr. Aminophylline 1 gr. Sodium bromide* 3 gr.
PARALUX RUBBER BASE FLOOR PAINT (Allentown)		PARASOLV PAINT THINNER & CLEANER (Foundry)	
PARA-MOTH Insecticide (Kelley)	Paradichlorobenzene*	PARASPAR VARNISH (Paragon Paint)	
PARA MOTH CAKES UNBOXED & BOXED (Uncle Sam)	Paradichlorobenzene* 100%	PARATRAN 1-5 DUST Insecticide (Calif. Spray)	Parathion* 1% p-Chlorophenyl-p-chlorobenzene sulfonate 5%
PARAMOUNT BRAND INKS (Frye)		PARATRAN 2-7.5 DUST Insecticide (Calif. Spray)	Parathion* 2.0% p-Chlorophenyl-p-chlorobenzene sulfonate 7.5%
PARAMOUNT COLD CREAM Cosmetic (Premo)		PARA-ZENE AIR CLEANER Deodorizer (Reliable Chem.)	Paradichlorobenzene* 100%
PARA NAP BALLS & FLAKES Insecticide (Reliable Chem.)	Refined naphthalene* 98% Paradichlorobenzene 2%	PARDNER SHAMPOO (Vantines)	
PARANATE Respiratory disease (veterinary) (Salsbury's)	Para-aminobenzoic acid 50.0%	P.A.R. DUST 20-50S Insecticide (Sunland)	Parathion* 2% Sulfur 50%

*Consult Sec. II., Ingredients Index. This ingredient may be responsible for major toxic effects if poisonous amounts of this product are ingested.

- 794 -

Name & Use Manufacturer	Ingredients	Name & Use Manufacturer	Ingredients
PARFAIT WHITE GLOSS ENAMEL (Union Paint)		PARKO CHROME CLEANER (Park Chem.)	Ammonia Ammonium oxalate*
PARFUM ODESANT (Richelieu)		PARKO FABRIC CLEANER (Park Chem.)	Aromatic hydrocarbons* Chlorinated hydrocarbons*
PARFUM SEC (Noblesse)		PARKO FINISH RUB (Park Chem.)	Kerosene* Soap Pine oil*
PARIS LINE EXTRACT & TOILET WATER (Coty)		PARKO FIRE EXTIN- GUISHER FLUID (Park Chem.)	Chlorinated hydrocarbons*
PARISPRAY Deodorizer (House of Gabler)	Formaldehyde*	PARKO GASKET CEMENTS (Park Chem.)	Alcohols Aromatic hydrocarbons* Resins
PARKE DAVIS ANTACID TABLETS (Parke, Davis)	Dried aluminum hydroxide gel Magnesium carbonate Calcium carbonate Taka-diastase (Aspergillus oryzae enzymes) Peppermint	PARKO GLOSS POLISH AND CLEANER (Park Chem.)	Alcohol* or paraformaldehyde*
PARKE DAVIS GERMICIDAL DETERGENT (Parke, Davis)	Phemerol (benzethonium chloride*) 2-1/2% Alcohol 5%	PARKO HYDRAULIC BRAKE FLUID (Standard, S. A.E. Moderate Duty, S.A.E. Heavy Duty) (Park Chem.)	Alcohols* Ethers* Glycols* Castor oil or polyglycol
PARKE DAVIS MEDICATED THROAT DISCS (Parke, Davis)	Each disc: Chloroform 1/2 m. Capsicum Peppermint Anise Cubeb Licorice Linseed	PARKO LIQUID POLISHES (Park Chem.)	Alcohol* or paraformaldehyde*
PARKER FINGER PAINT SET (Parker Bros.)		PARKO MIRACLE METAL SOLVENT (Park Chem.)	Ketones* Aromatic hydrocarbons*
PARKER'S BRAND PAINT, PUTTY (Parker, I.)		PARKO PENETRATING OIL (Park Chem.)	Aromatic solvents*
PARKER'S PERFECT POLISH (Parker, C.W.)		PARKO POLISHING PASTE (Park Chem.)	Kerosene*
PARKO ANTI-STATIC PLASTIC POLISH (Park Chem.)	Paraformaldehyde*	PARKO POLISH NO. 4-BL (Pexiglas) (Park Chem.)	Paraformaldehyde*
PARKO BRAKE FLUIDS (Park Chem.)	Alcohols* Ethers* Glycols* Castor oil or polyglycol	PARKO RADIATOR CLEANER & RUST PREVENTER (Park Chem.)	Oxalic acid* or sodium bisulfate*
PARKO BUFFING LIQUID (Park Chem.)	Proprietary solvent*	PARKO RADIATOR STOP LEAK (Park Chem.)	Proprietary solvent*

*Consult Sec. II., Ingredients Index. This ingredient may be responsible for major toxic effects if poisonous amounts of this product are ingested.

Name & Use Manufacturer	Ingredients	Name & Use Manufacturer	Ingredients
PARKO RUBBER LUBRICANT (Park Chem.)	Isopropyl alcohol*	PARRA-PHENIQUE For skin (Polk, C.)	Hydrastis Camphor* Witch hazel Zinc oxide Phenol*
PARKO SILICONE REMOVER (Park Chem.)	Aromatic hydrocarbons* Chlorinated hydrocarbons*	DR. PARRISH GLOSSHEEN OINTMENT, HAIR & SCALP FORMULA, HOT OIL TREATMENT, LANOLIN CREAM SHAMPOO, PRESSING COMPOUND (Gordon Thomas)	
PARKO SUPER-DRI (Park Chem.)	Ethyl or isopropyl alcohol*		
PARKO SUPER SOLVENT CLEANER (Park Chem.)	Cresylic acid* Chlorinated hydrocarbons*		
PARKO TANK-O-LENE, TANK SOLV. Solvents (Park Chem.)	Cresylic acid* Chlorinated hydrocarbons*	PARSONS 50% BENZENE HEXACHLORIDE POWDER INSECTICIDE WETTABLE (Parsons Chem.)	Gamma isomer of hexachloro-cyclohexane* 6% Other isomers of hexachloro-cyclohexane* 44%
PARKO TAR REMOVER (Park Chem.)	Xylene* Chlorinated hydrocarbons*		
PARKO TIRE PAINT (Park Chem.)	Aliphatic solvents* Rubber Plasticizers* Pigments	PARSONS BORDEAUX MIXTURE Insecticide, fungicide (Parsons Chem.)	Metallic copper*
PARKO WHITE SIDEWALL CLEANER (Park Chem.)	Soap Alkali salts* Abrasive	PARSONS BROODER SPRAY Insecticide (Parsons Chem.)	Steam-distilled pine oils* Soap
PARKO WINDSHIELD WASHER SOLVENT (Park Chem.)	Ethyl or isopropyl alcohol*		
PARK & TILFORD PERFUME, COLOGNE, DEODORANT (Park & Tilford)		PARSONS CAD-I-CIDE Anthelmintic (veterinary) (Parsons Chem.)	Cadmium oxide* 1.5%
PAR LIGHT SATIN FINISH FLAT WALL PAINT (Parr Paint)		PARSONS CAL-C-NATE Insecticide (Parsons Chem.)	Calcium arsenate*
PARNAMEL PAINTS (Paramount)		PARSONS CHEMICAL SEWER CLEANER CRYSTALS (Parsons Chem.)	Potassium hydroxide* 100%
PAR-O-FLEX METAL PAINT (Parr Paint)			
PARON PLASTIC RUBBER PAINT (Rudd)		PARSONS CHLORDANE DUST, POWDER INSECTICIDE (Parsons Chem.)	Chlordane* tech. 5%
PAR-O-SAN, DR. SALSBURY'S Antiseptic, deodorizer (Salsbury's)	Ortho-hydroxy-diphenyl* 10% Pine oil* 74% Soap 8%	PARSONS CHLORDANE OIL SPRAY Insecticide (Parsons Chem.)	Chlordane tech. 2%

Name & Use Manufacturer	Ingredients		Name & Use Manufacturer	Ingredients	
PARSONS CHLORDANE WETTABLE POWDER INSECTICIDE (Parsons Chem.)	Tech. chlordane*	40%	PARSONS KAL-ZOO EMULSION MALATHION CONCEN-TRATE 50% Insecticide (Parsons Chem.)	Malathion* Xylol*	50.0% 42.4%
PARSONS CRAB GRASS KILLER (Parsons Chem.)	Tech. chlordane*		PARSONS KAL-ZOO FUMIGANT (Parsons Chem.)	Ethylene dichloride* Carbon tetrachloride*	
PARSONS CUCUMBER DUST Insecticide (Parsons Chem.)	Methoxychlor*		PARSONS KAL-ZOO INSECTICIDE DUST (Parsons Chem.)	DDT Copper*	3% 6%
PARSONS DRY LIME SULPHUR Fungicide (Parsons Chem.)	Calcium polysulfides* Calcium thiosulfate Sulfur*		PARSONS KAL-ZOO MALATHION 25% WETTABLE POWDER INSECTICIDE (Parsons Chem.)	Malathion*	25%
PARSONS FLY-DI INSECT SPRAY (Parsons Chem.)	Pyrethrins* Petroleum distillate*		PARSONS KAL-ZOO SPECIAL EMULSION INSECTICIDE 25% DDT (Parsons Chem.)	DDT*	25%
PARSONS FRUIT TREE SPRAY Insecticide, fungicide (Parsons Chem.)	Sulfur* Ferbam Methoxychlor tech. Malathion* tech. Phenothiazine	33.000% 5.000% 8.800% 4.900% 0.005%	PARSONS KAL-ZOO SPECIAL INSECTICIDE 5% D.D.T. FORTIFIED (Parsons Chem.)	DDT* Thiocyanates Refined mineral oils	5.00% 2.25% 92.75%
PARSONS GENUINE FAMILY AMMONIA (Brate)	Ammonia*				
PARSONS INSECTICIDE DUST (Parsons Chem.)	Rotenone Derris powder	0.75% 15%	PARSONS KAL-ZOO SPECIAL INSECTICIDE 5% D.D.T. NON-FORTIFIED (Parsons Chem.)	DDT*	5%
PARSONS KAL-ZOO AND & ROACH INSECTICIDE DUST (Parsons Chem.)	Chlordane* tech.(octachloro-4, 7-methano-tetrahydroindane 1.2%, related compounds 0.8%) 5%		PARSONS KAL-ZOO 50% WETTABLE POWDER Insecticide (Parsons Chem.)	DDT*	50%
PARSONS KAL-ZOO DAIRY BARN SPRAY Insecticide (Parsons Chem.)	Lindane*		PARSONS KILANE CONTACT SPRAY Insecticide (Parsons Chem.)	Isobornyl thiocyanoacetate* Chlordane* Pyrethrins* Oils Ethylhexanediol*	
PARSONS KAL-ZOO DUST 3% D.D.T. Insecticide (Parsons Chem.)	DDT	3%	PARSONS LETHO-DUST Insecticide (Parsons Chem.)	Beta-thiocyanoethyl esters of aliphatic fatty acids Sulfur Nicotine* Calcium arsenate* Copper	

*Consult Sec. II., Ingredients Index. This ingredient may be responsible for major toxic effects if poisonous amounts of this product are ingested.

Name & Use Manufacturer	Ingredients		Name & Use Manufacturer	Ingredients	
PARSONS LETHOGAS FUMIGANT (Parsons Chem.)	Dichloroethane* Carbon tetrachloride* Orthodichlorobenzene Ethylene dibromide Paradichlorobenzene Tetrachlorethylene Propylene dichloride Paratoluene sulfonchloramide Pentachloroethane	69.1867% 28.795% 1.005% 1.0015% 0.005% 0.004% 0.003% 0.0002% 0.0001%	PARSONS POTATO SPRAY MIXTURE Insecticide (Parsons Chem.)	DDT* Copper*	16% 6.7%
PARSONS LINDANE WETTABLE SPRAY POWDER NO. 25 Insecticide (Parsons Chem.)	Gamma isomer of benzene hexachloride* (from lindane) 12-1/2%		PARSONS POTATO SPRAY WETTABLE POWDER Insecticide (Parsons Chem.)	DDT* Copper* Zinc sulfate*	6% 3%
PARSONS LOUSE DUST (Parsons Chem.)	Naphthalene* Sulfur* (325 mesh) Coal tar neutral oils* Rotenone Other derris resins	7.500% 5.500% 5.000% 0.125% 0.005%	PARSONS PRE-FUMIGANT WEEVIL SPRAY (Parsons Chem.)	Isobornyl thiocyanoacetate* Chlordane* Pyrethrins* Oils Ethylhexanediol*	
PARSONS METHOXY- CHLOR 50% WETTABLE INSECTICIDE (Parsons Chem.)	Methoxychlor* tech. 50%		PARSONS SEED SAVER CROW REPELLENT (Parsons Chem.)	Coal tar neutral oil* Benzene* Coal tar acids* Pine oil* Linseed oil Fish oil Turpentine Wood creosote oil* Petroleum distillate* Soap	
PARSONS MOSQUITO YARD SPRAY (Parsons Chem.)	Methoxychlor* tech. 2-Ethylhexanediol-1,3 B-butoxy B-thiocyanodiethyl ether Pyrethrins*				
PARSONS MOTH CRYSTALS (Parsons Chem.)	Paradichlorobenzene*		PARSONS SEED SAVER DUST (Parsons Chem.)	p-tert-Octylphenoxy ethoxy ethyl dimethyl benzyl ammonium mercuric chlorides* 5.15% Trioxymethylene 0.01% Mercuric chloride 0.01%	
PARSONS PARASOTE (Parsons Chem.)	Refined creosote oils*		PARSONS SEED SAVER LIQUID CONCEN- TRATE (Parsons Chem.)	Sodium and mercury salts polyamino polycarboxylic acids* 74.88% Metallic mercury 7.6%	
PARSONS PARATHION DUST (Wettable) Insecticide (Parsons Chem.)	Parathion* 15%		PARSONS SEWER ROOT KILLER (Parsons Chem.)	Copper sulfate* 99%	
PARSONS PAR-DIP NO. 6 DISINFECTANT (Parsons Chem.)	Coal tar hydrocarbons* Soap Phenols*		PARSONS SMUT-OFF SOLUTION Fungicide (Parsons Chem.)	Formaldehyde* Mercury*	
PARSONS PINE-O-LIN DISINFECTANT (Parsons Chem.)	Steam-distilled pine oil* 77% Soap 13%		PARSONS SODIUM FLUORIDE Anthelmintic (veterinary) (Parsons Chem.)	Sodium fluoride* 97%	
PARSONS POTATO DUST Insecticide (Parsons Chem.)	Metallic copper (cuprous oxide) 6% DDT (dichloro diphenyl trichloroethane) 3% Zinc sulfate*		PARSONS SODIUM TCA WEED KILLER (Parsons Chem.)	Sodium trichloroacetate* (trichloroacetic acid equiv. 61.7%) 90%	

*Consult Sec. II., Ingredients Index. This ingredient may be responsible for major toxic effects if poisonous amounts of this product are ingested.

Name & Use Manufacturer	Ingredients	Name & Use Manufacturer	Ingredients
PARSONS STANDARD LEAD ARSENATE Insecticide (Parsons Chem.)	Lead arsenate* 96%	PARSONS 2,4-D WEED KILLER NO. 40 (Parsons Chem.)	Dimethylamine salt 2,4- dichlorophenoxy acetic acid* 49.8%
PARSONS SUDSY AMMONIA (Parsons Ammonia)	Ammonia* 5.02%	PARSONS 2,4,5-T BRUSH KILLER Herbicide (Parsons Chem.)	2,4,5-Trichlorophenoxy acetic acid* 43.6%
PARSONS 3-WAY DUST Insecticide (Parsons Chem.)	Active ingredients: 9.01% Sulfur (300 mesh) Beta thiocyano ethyl esters of aliphatic fatty acids 54.5% Petroleum distillates 45.5% Rotenone and derris resins Cupric oxide Inert ingredients: 90.99% Kaolinite powder 78.00% Derris powder other than derris resins 11.74% Magnesium carbonate 1.25%	PARSONS WARFARIN BAIT RAT KILLER (Parsons Chem.)	Warfarin (3-(a-acetonylbenzyl)- 4-hydroxycoumarin) 0.025%
PARSONS TO-DOT COW-SPRAY Insecticide (Parsons Chem.)	Mineral oils Pine oil* Thiocyanates Beta dithiocyano diethyl ether* Pyrethrins*	PARSONS WORMICIDE TABLETS Anthelmintic (dog, puppy) (Parsons Chem.)	Arecoline hydrobromide*
PARSONS TOMATO DUST Insecticide (Parsons Chem.)	Methoxychlor tech. (44% 2,2-bis- (p-methoxyphenyl)-1,1,1- trichloroethane and 6% other isomers end reaction products) 5%	PARSONS WORMICIDE TABLETS Anthelmintic (hog) (Parsons Chem.)	Chenopodium Calomel* Nux vomica* Digitalis* Copper sulfate* Iron oxide Nicotine sulfate* Pyrethrum 40%
PARSONS 20TH CENTURY BACTERICIDE (Parsons Chem.)	p-tert-Oxtyl phenoxy ethoxy ethyl dimethyl benzyl ammonium chloride*	PARSONS WORMICIDE TABLETS Anthelmintic (sheep) (Parsons Chem.)	Kamala Nicotine sulfate* Turpentine Monohydrated copper sulfate* Carbon tetrachloride*
PARSONS 2,4-D WEED KILLER (Parsons Chem.)	Dimethylamine salt 2,4- dichlorophenoxy acetic acid* 24.9%	PARTAGLOSS ENAMEL (McDougall- Butler)	
PARSONS 2,4-D WEED KILLER (Isopropyl Ester) (Parsons Chem.)	Isopropyl ester 2,4- dichlorophenoxy acetic acid* 44%	PARTISTIC ENAMEL (Parr Paint)	

Name & Use Manufacturer	Ingredients	
PARTO CARPANTEA Antitussive (Partola)	Horehound Licorice root Mullen leaves Orris root Mullen flowers Coltsfoot leaves Anise Chamomile Saffron Red poppy flowers	
PARTO CORN Keratolytic (Partola)	Each oz.: Alcohol Ether* Chlorobutanol* Menthol Salicylic acid* Collodion	21% 205 gr. 4-1/2 gr.
PARTO COUGH SYRUP (Partola)	Each fl. oz.: Chloroform Pyrilamine maleate* Monosodium citrate Ammonium chloride Aromatics	1-1/2 m. q.s.
PARTOCYL Skin ointment (Partola)	Resorcinol Benzocaine Tinct. benzoin Balsam Peru Lac sulfur Menthol crystals* Boric acid* Zinc oxide	
PARTO DYNE Rubefacient (Partola)	Chlorobutanol* Ether* Chloroform* Methyl salicylate* Tinct. camphor* Aqua ammonia Tinct. Capsicum Oil of sassafras* Oil of cloves* Oil of turpentine*	3.4 gr. 88 m. 62 m.
PARTO ELZAWATER HAIR DYE (Partola)	Lead acetate* Sulfur precipitated* Glycerin Bay rum	
PARTO EYE LOTION (Partola)	Each fl. oz.: Chlorobutanol Zinc sulfate Ammonium chloride Waters of peppermint, rose Camphor Sodium borate Boric acid Glycerin	1-1/7 gr.
PARTOFORM Throat lozenges (Partola)	Fl. extr. coltsfoot Oil of peppermint Powdered extr. Glycyrrhiza Oil of anise Cubeb oleoresin Fl. extr. Capsicum Balsam tolu	
PARTO GLORY TONIC (Partola)	Each fl. dr.: Strychnine* Quinine* Potassium hypophosphite Manganese hypophosphite Hypophosphorus acid Sucrose Caramel coloring Sodium bromide Calcium hypophosphite Sodium hypophosphite Iron hypophosphite Sodium citrate Glycerin	1/160 gr. 1.7 gr.
PARTOHERB Diuretic, laxative (Partola)	Gentian root Cubeb berries Uva ursi leaves Juniper berries Rhubarb root Wormwood Centaury herb Licorice root	
PARTOLA LAXATIVE (Partola)	Each tablet: Phenolphthalein Sucrose Oil of peppermint	
PARTOLIN FOR HAIR & SCALP (Partola)	Alcohol*	20%/v
PARTOLIN POWDER Soap (Partola)		
PARTOPILE Hemorrhoids (Partola)	Tannic acid* Menthol* Eucalyptol* Hydrocarbon oil*	
PARTO RUB Counter-irritant (muscular) (Partola)	Chlorobutanol* Tinct. iodine* Tinct. Capsicum Methyl salicylate* Oil of mustard Soap liniment Oil of turpentine* Aqua ammonia Spirit camphor*	3.4 gr.
PARTOSTRINGE Astringent (diarrhea) (Partola)	Bismuth subnitrate Kino Mercury*(with chalk) Aromatic powder Sodium bicarbonate Camphor	
PARTOSWEAT Astringent (feet) (Partola)	Alcohol* Aluminum chloride Camphor* Solution formaldehyde*	45%/v
PARTOWILL Digestant (Partola)	Powdered pepsin U.S.P. 12% Lactose U.S.P. 24% Sodium bicarbonate U.S.P. 32% Powdered cubebs U.S.P. 32%	
PARTOWORM Anthelmintic (Partola)	Santonin* Calomel*	
PARVALAC ENAMEL, PARVANERE FLOOR ENAMEL (Parr Paint)		
PAR-X ROACH & INSECT POWDER (Surbin)		
PARZATE DUST Fungicide (Thomas, I.)	Zinc ethylene bis (dithiocarbamate) (metallic zinc 0.92%) 3.9%	

*Consult Sec. II., Ingredients Index. This ingredient may be responsible for major toxic effects if poisonous amounts of this product are ingested.

Name & Use Manufacturer	Ingredients	Name & Use Manufacturer	Ingredients
PARZATE LIQUID NABAM FUNGICIDE (du Pont)	Disodium ethylene bis (dithio carbamate)*	PATEX RUST REMOVER (Patek)	Ammonium fluoride* Hydrogen fluoride*
PARZATE ZINEB FUNGICIDE (du Pont)	Zinc ethylene bis (dithio-carbamate)	PATINA VENETIAN BLIND LINOLEUM CLEANER (Jackson of London)	
PASADENA PERFUME, COLOGNE, TOILET-WATER (Duvelle)	Denatured alcohol* (with diethylphthalate)	PATIO PAINTS (Zymolyte)	
		PATONE HAIR TONIC (Capatone)	
PASIDERM Rubefacient (Supreme Pharm.)	Zinc oxide Calamine Benzocaine Phenol* Menthol* Camphor*	PATRICIAN POLISH (Concentrate) For furniture, plastics, glass, metals, china, leathers, painted or lacquered surfaces, washable wall paper, etc. (Protective)	
PASTELLE FLAT PAINTS (Moore-Leland)			
PASTELLO FLAT WALL PAINT (Upco)		PATRICK'S AFTER SHAVE (Patrick's)	
PASTICK LIQUID GLUE (Scriptex)		PATTERNSEAL Sealing material (Tamms)	
PASTOXINE Rodenticide (Astor)	Red squill* powder (fortified) 30%	PATTERSON'S BLUE RIBBON AMMONIA (Patterson Labs.)	Ammonia*
PASTURITE Cleaner (Wyandotte)	Sodium chromate*		
PATCH'S GADOMENT Skin ointment (Patch)	Cod liver oil 70% Carbolic acid 0.375% Fl. extr. benzoic and zinc oxide	PATTERSON'S DRAIN PIPE OPENER (Patterson Labs.)	
PATCH'S KONDREMUL (Plain) Cathartic (Patch)	Mineral oil Irish moss (Chondrus crispus)	PATTERSON'S FOOT BATH SPECIAL Fungicide (medical) (Patterson Labs.)	Sodium hypochlorite* 4%
PATCH'S KONDREMUL WITH CASCARA Laxative (Patch)	Mineral oil Extr. cascara Irish moss (Chondrus crispus)	PATTERSON'S GERMICIDAL SOLUTION (Patterson Labs.)	Alkyl-dimethyl-benzyl ammonium chloride* Coconut oil
PATCH'S KONDREMUL WITH PHENOL-PHTHALEIN Cathartic (Patch)	Mineral oil Phenolphthalein Irish moss (Chondrus crispus)	PATTERSON'S HYPO-CHLORITE BACILLICIDE (Patterson Labs.)	Sodium hypochlorite* 4%
PATEXOL ACTIVATED Spot remover (Patek)	DIBK MIBK Orthodichlorobenzene* Methylene dichloride*	PATTERSON'S HYPO-CHLORITE BREWERY SPECIAL Disinfectant (Patterson Labs.)	Sodium hypochlorite* 6%

*Consult Sec. II., Ingredients Index. This ingredient may be responsible for major toxic effects if poisonous amounts of this product are ingested.

Name & Use Manufacturer	Ingredients		Name & Use Manufacturer	Ingredients	
PATTERSON'S INSECT SPRAY (Patterson Labs.)			PAUL NEWTON STOP STICK Deodorant (Newton, P.)		
PATTERSON'S ISOPROPYL RUBBING ALCOHOL COMPOUND (Patterson's Labs.)	Isopropyl alcohol*	70%/v	PAWNEE ANT EXTERMI- NATORS (Pawnee)		
PATTERSON'S MOTH PROOF SOLUTION (Patterson Labs.)			PAX Sedative (Carroll Chem.)	Sodium bromide* Potassium bromide* Ammonium bromide* Belladonna leaf Cypripedium	3 gr. 2 gr. 2 gr. 1/3 gr. 1-1/2 gr.
PATTERSON'S POOL HYPO- CHLORITE (Patterson Labs.)			PAX-ALL GENERAL PURPOSE CLEANER (Packwood)	Alkaline salts*	
PATTERSON'S STANDARD BLEACH (Patterson Labs.)			PAX ALUMINUM ETCH F (Packwood)	Alkaline detergent salts* Detergent	
PATTERSON'S SUPER- BACILLICIDE (Patterson Labs.)	Sodium hypochlorite*	12%	PAX ALUMINUM ETCH X (Packwood)	Alkaline salts* Caustic soda* Detergent	
PATTERSON'S SUPERCHLOR BLEACH (Patterson Labs.)	Sodium hypochlorite*	5.25%	PAX BIG-CAT LIQUID METAL CLEANER (Packwood)	Detergent Petroleum type solvents* Pine oil*	
PATTERSON'S SUPERCHLOR POWDER Disinfectant (Patterson Labs.)	Available chlorine	4%	PAX BO-PEEP Skin cleanser (Packwood)	Borax* Soap	
			PAX CAR WASH SUPREME (Packwood)	Detergent mixture* Detergent salts * Soil-suspending agents	
PATTERSON'S SUPERCHLOR SOLUTION Sanitizer (Patterson Labs.)	Sodium hypochlorite*	4%	PAX CM-118 Skin cleanser (Packwood)	Alkaline salts*	
PATTERSON'S WINDOWLITE GLASS POLISH (Patterson Labs.)			PAX CORN-TEX REGULAR Skin cleanser (Packwood)		
			PAX CORN-TEX (with minimum of 5% lanolin) Skin cleanser (Packwood)	Lanolin*	5%
PAULDERMA Skin ointment (Paul Labs.)	Anesthesin (benzocaine)* Calamine Methyl para-hydroxybenzoate Sulfur Benzoic acid Lanolin Salicylic acid*		PAX CORN-TEX WITH PAX- LANO-SAV EMOLLIENT Skin cleanser (Packwood)	Lanolin Other bland emollient oils	
PAULDERMA SOAP (Paul Labs.)	Lanolin		PAX DICTATOR SUPREME & REGULAR Skin cleanser (Packwood)	Alkaline salts* Lanolin	
PAUL NEWTON SHAVING CREAM & LOTION (Newton, P.)			PAX F-54 FLOOR CLEANING COMPOUND (Packwood)	Alkaline salts* Detergents *	

*Consult Sec. II., Ingredients Index. This ingredient may be responsible for major toxic effects if poisonous amounts of this product are ingested.

- 802 -

Name & Use Manufacturer	Ingredients	Name & Use Manufacturer	Ingredients
PAX FORMULA TL-13 ALL PURPOSE LIQUID CLEANER (Packwood)	Liquid detergents*	PAX LIQUID DISHWASH (Packwood)	Liquid detergents*
PAX FORMULA T-22 WITH SUPER WETTING ACTION Skin cleanser (Packwood)	Sulfonated detergent*	PAX LIQUID SOAPS (Regular & Antiseptic) (Packwood)	Potash soaps of refined coconut and vegetable oils 15-40% Bacteriostatic agent 2%
PAX HECTO INK CLEANSING CREAM (Packwood)	Glycol type solvents Mineral adsorbent Alcohols Lanolin	PAX MECHANICS Skin cleanser (Packwood)	Pumice and vegetable scrubbers Water-softening agents
PAX HEL-CAT LIQUID METAL CLEANER (Packwood)	Phenolic acids * Petroleum solvents* Alkaline type liquid detergents *	PAX NO. 11, NO. 25, NO. 31 Metal cleaners (Packwood)	Alkaline salts* Surface active agents
		PAX NO. 21 Metal cleaner (Packwood)	Polyphosphates* Silicates Surface active agents*
PAX HI-SUDS WITH & WITHOUT BACTERICIDE Cleaner (Packwood)	Synthetic detergents* Phosphate and silicate type alkaline salts Phenolic type bactericidal agent*	PAX NO. 26 GENERAL PURPOSE CLEANER (Packwood)	Polyphosphate and silicate type salts* Surface active agents*
PAX HY-SPEED Skin cleanser (Packwood)	Lanolin Water-softening agents	PAX-100 Skin cleanser (Packwood)	Borax* Powdered soap
PAXIDE TYPE B Insecticide (Biocerta)	Tech. piperonyl butoxide 1% Pyrethrins 0.3% Oil* 98.7%	PAX PACKING HOUSE CLEANER (Packwood)	Alkaline salts* Detergent*
PAXIDE TYPE R Insecticide (Biocerta)	Pyrethrins 0.5% Oil* 99.5%	PAX PAINT STRIPPER (Packwood)	Chlorinated hydrocarbons* Petroleum distillates Synthetic detergent emulsifiers Corrosion inhibitors Evaporation-retarding agents
PAXIDE (Type S) Insecticide (Biocerta)	Pyrethrins 0.48% Sesame oil extractive 0.9% Odorless petroleum oil distillate* 98.62%	PAX RADIOLOGI-CAL SKIN DECONTAM-INANT-202 LIQUID (Packwood)	Liquid detergents Sequestering,* chelating* and complexing agents* Hexachlorophene
PAX LANOLIN LOTION Hand lotion (Packwood)	Anhydrous lanolin 5%		
PAX-LANO-SAV HEAVY DUTY GRANULATED SKIN CLEANSER (Packwood)	Sterilized Pax duramen-meal Lanolin Other bland emollient oils Water-softening agents Antiseptic	PAX RADIOLOGI-CAL SKIN DECONTAM-INANT-203 (Powdered All Soluble-204) (Powdered Organic Scrubber) (Packwood)	Sequestering,* chelating* and complexing* agents Bithionol (Actamer)
PAX LIQUID DETERGENT FLOOR CLEANER (with & without Disinfectant & Super Concentrate) (Packwood)	Liquid detergents * Sequestering agents Water-softening agents	PAX REPEATER Skin cleanser (Packwood)	Pumice and vegetable scrubbers Water-softening salts
		PAX RUST REMOVER (Packwood)	Phosphoric acid* Liquid metal-cleaning detergents
		PAX SANITIZER TABLETS (Packwood)	Chloramine* type material

*Consult Sec. II., Ingredients Index. This ingredient may be responsible for major toxic effects if poisonous amounts of this product are ingested.

Name & Use Manufacturer	Ingredients	Name & Use Manufacturer	Ingredients
PAX SILICONE LOTION & CREAM (Packwood)	Silicone (dimethyl polysiloxane) 10%	PAYONS MAGIC PAINTING CRAYONS (Am.)	
PAX SPECIAL Skin cleanser (Packwood)	Cornmeal and woodflour meal scrubber Water-softening agents	PAYSON-LITE INTERIOR GLOSS Paint (Payson Corp.)	
PAX SUDSLESS- FOR MACHINE DISHWASHING WITH & WITHOUT BACTERICIDE (Packwood)	Silicate and phosphate type salts* Quaternary ammonium* bactericidal agents	PAYSON'S INDELIBLE INK (Payson's Indel.)	
PAX SULPHONATED OIL LIQUID SKIN CLEANSER (Packwood)	Sulfonated vegetable oil Liquid petrolatum Sulfonated detergent Lanolin Lecithin	PAZE ANTACID TABLETS (Vegetrates)	Pepsin Calcium carbonate Dried malt diastase Celery Magnesium trisilicate Papain Dehydrated asparagus Okra
PAX SUPER-X Skin cleanser (Packwood)	Cornmeal and woodflour meal scrubbers Water-softening agents	PAZO Hemorrhoids (Grove)	Zinc oxide Ephedrine sulfate* Eucalyptus oil* Petrolatum Benzocaine Camphorated phenol* Lanolin
PAX SUPREME LIQUID HAND CLEANER (Concentrate or Extra) (with or without Hexachlorophene) (Packwood)	Liquid surface active agents* Hexachlorophene	PAZO PILE OINTMENT (Grove)	Bismuth subgallate Camphorated phenol* Zinc oxide Lanolin Resorcin Balsam Peru Camphor* Petrolatum
PAX TANK CAR CLEANER (Packwood)	Alkaline type salts * Powdered surface active agent *		
PAX-3-X POWDERED METAL CLEANER (Packwood)	Alkaline salts* Free caustic soda* Surface active agents *	PAZO PILE SUPPOSI- TORIES (Grove)	Zinc oxide Ephedrine sulfate* Resorcinol monoacetate Cocoa butter base Benzocaine Camphorated phenol* Eucalyptus oil *
PAX TOM-CAT LIQUID METAL CLEANER (Packwood)	Solvents* Surface active agents *	PCC THE WATER SOFTENING CLEANSER (Pioneer)	
PAX T-22 WITH SUPER WETTING ACTION Skin cleanser (Packwood)	Cornmeal and cornmeal deriv. type scrubbers Synthetic wetting agent	P.C. 80 Herbicide (Garden Prod.)	Potassium cyanate* 80%
PAX WATERLESS SKIN CLEANER (Extra Heavy Duty) (Packwood)	Aliphatic hydrocarbons* Cyclic compounds*	P.C.E. MULTI- PURPOSE CONCEN- TRATE Insecticide (Pest Control Equip.)	Petroleum distillates* n-Octyl bicycloheptene dicarboximide* Tech. piperonyl butoxide Pyrethrins
PAX WAX STRIPPER (Packwood)	Soap Detergents* Alkaline salts* Sequestering agents	P.D.R. MIGRAINE Headache remedy (Keenan)	Calcium lactate 389 mg. Potassium chloride 259 mg. Niacinamide 12 mg.
PAYA-PEPSOL Digestant, tonic (Pitman- Moore)	Each fl. oz.: Extr. nux vomica 5 m. Pepsin 8 gr. Papain 1-1/2 gr. Rennin 3/4 gr. Lactic acid 1/2 m. Nitro-hydrochloric acid (dilute) 5 m.	PEACOCK ENAMELS (Bishop- Conklin)	

*Consult Sec. II., Ingredients Index. This ingredient may be responsible for major toxic effects if poisonous amounts of this product are ingested.

Name & Use Manufacturer	Ingredients	
PEAK (Commercial Solv.)	Ethylene glycol type*	
PEARL POLISH Stove, metal polish (Pearl Prod.)		
PEARL PORCELAIN, TILE & MARBLE CLEANER (Pearl Polishes)		
PEARLS IN WINE ROUGE, NITE CREAM, LIPSTICK, DRY SKIN CREME, COMBINATION CREAM, COMPACT MAKEUP, HAND CREAM & LOTION, BATH TALC, SPRAY DE-ODORANT, PARFUM, FACE POWDER, SHAMPOO, DEODORANT, COLOGNE (Armand)		
PEARSON'S AZALEA PETAL BLIGHT DUST Fungicide (Pearson & Co.)	Zineb	3.25%
PEARSON'S 5% CHLORDANE DUST Insecticide (Pearson & Co.)	Tech. chlordane*	5%
PEARSON'S 62-1/2% CHLORDANE EMULSIFIABLE CONCENTRATE Insecticide (Pearson & Co.)	Tech. chlordane* Aliphatic petroleum hydrocarbons	62.5% 22.5%
PEARSON'S 20% CHLORDANE OIL CON-CENTRATE Insecticide (Pearson & Co.)	Tech. chlordane* Petroleum hydrocarbon*	20% 80%
PEARSON'S 25% DDT EMULSION CONCENTRATE Insecticide (Pearson & Co.)	DDT Aromatic petroleum deriv. solvent*	25.0% 71.8%
PEARSON'S 50% DDT WETTABLE POWDER Insecticide (Pearson & Co.)	Dichloro diphenyl trichloroethane*	50%

Name & Use Manufacturer	Ingredients	
PEARSON'S ROSE DUST & ROSE SPRAY Fungicide, insecticide (Pearson & Co.)	Sulfur* Copper (as metallic) Dichloro diphenyl tri-chloroethane* Rotenone Other cube resins	20.00% 3.70% 5.00% 0.75% 1.50%
PEARSON'S ROTENONE .75% Insecticide (Pearson & Co.)	Rotenone Other cube resins	0.75% 1.5%
PEARSON'S SUPPOSI-TORIES (Lester Drug)	Ephedrine sulfate* Benzocaine Oxyquinoline sulfate* Zinc oxide Bismuth subgallate Balsam Peru Cocoa butter	
PEARSON'S TOMATO DUST Fungicide, insecticide (Pearson & Co.)	Zineb Dichloro diphenyl dichloroethane	3.9% 3.0%
PEARSON'S ZEBRA DUST Insecticide, fungicide (Pearson & Co.)	Rotenone Other cube resins* Zineb	1.00% 2.00% 3.25%
PEAU FRAICHE Toiletry (Caron)		
PEAU SECHE CREAM & SOAP, LIQUID SKIN GROOM Hypoallergenic cosmetic (Peau Seche)		
PECALIN Adsorbent (Veltex)	Each fl. oz.: Kaolin Pectin	90 gr. 2 gr.
PECHEUR PERFUMES, EAU DE TOILETTE, BATH ESSENCE (Parfums Pecheur)		
PECK'S GERMICIDAL RINSE (Peck's)	Para-diisobutyl phenoxy ethoxy ethyl dimethyl benzoyl ammonium chloride*	10%
PECK'S HYSOL CRESOL COMPOUND Germicide, deodorizer (Peck's)	Cresylic acid* Soap	
PECK'S LIQUOR CRESOLIS COMPOUND Germicide, deodorizer (Peck's)	Cresol* U.S.P. Soap	

*Consult Sec. II., Ingredients Index. This ingredient may be responsible for major toxic effects if poisonous amounts of this product are ingested.

Name & Use Manufacturer	Ingredients		Name & Use Manufacturer	Ingredients	
PECORA ADHESIVES, PUTTIES, COATINGS, ALUMINUM PAINTS, ENAMELS (Pecora)			PECTORAL (Ayer's) Antitussive (Watkins, R.)	Each oz.: Alcohol Chloroform Terpin hydrate Benzaldehyde Wild cherry White pine Ipecac	16-1/2% 2 m.
PECORA ARCHITEC- TURAL CALKING COMPOUND (Pecora)	Asbestos fiber Titanium calcium pigment Calcium carbonate Vegetable mineral thinner Vegetable oils Lead * Cobalt * Manganese *	5%	PECTORRHEA Adsorbent (Daniels, Robert)	Each fl. oz.: Colloidal kaolin Pectin Aromatics	180 gr. 4 gr. q.s.
			PECTROL PLAIN Laxative (Horton & Converse)	Mineral oil Pectin Methylcellulose Benzoic acid	50%/v 0.1%
PECORA FURNACE CEMENT (Pecora)	Clay Silicon dioxide Silicate of soda Asbestos fiber Carbon black		PECTROL WITH CASCARA Laxative (Horton & Converse)	Cascara sagrada aromatic Mineral oil Pectin Methylcellulose Benzoic acid	1 dr. 50%/v 0.1%
PECORA TILE MASTICS (Pecora)	China clay Titanium calcium pigment Magnesium silicate Calcium carbonate Vegetable oil Lead* Mineral thinner Phenyl mercurial oleate	12%	PECTROL WITH PHENOL- PHTHALEIN Cathartic (Horton & Converse)	Benzoic acid Mineral oil Pectin Methyl cellulose	0.1% 50%/v
PECTAGORIC For diarrhea (Carroll Chem.)	Paregoric* Kaolin Pectin	1 fl. dr. 87.5 gr. 2.5 gr.	PED Skin fungicide (medical) (G. & W.)	Formaldehyde* Gum camphor Acetone U.S.P. Mercury bichloride* Petrohol	1 gr. 110 m.
PECTALMAG Antacid, adsorbent (Barlow- Maney)	Aluminum hydroxide gel U.S.P. Magnesium trisilicate Kaolin Pectin	5 gr. 5 gr. 5 gr. 1 gr.	PED Skin fungicide (medical) (Penslar)	Benzoic acid* Salicylic acid* Chlorthymol	
PECTINAL Antacid, absorbent (Tailby)	Hyoscyamine sulfate Atropine sulfate Hyoscine hydrobromide Colloidal kaolin Bismuth subgallate Pectin	1/1250 gr. 1/6700 gr. 1/20,000 gr. 5 gr. 1 gr. 1/4 gr.	PEDATONE ATHLETE'S FOOT CREAM (Commerce)	Digenol (2, 2' dihydroxy 5, 5' dichloro diphenyl methane)* Undecylenic acid Sodium propionate	
PECTODYNE Antitussive, sedative (Claflin)	Each oz.: Alcohol Wild cherry Sanguinaria Ammonium chloride Chloroform White pine Spikenard Sugar syrup	2-1/2% 2 m.	PEDATONE ATHLETE'S FOOT LIQUID (Commerce)	Digenol (2, 2' dihydroxy 5, 5' dichloro diphenyl methane)* Undecylenic acid Tannic acid * Boric acid* Isopropyl alcohol* Benzoic acid Salicylic acid* Glycerin	65%
PECTO-KAPS Antacid (Kenmore)	Each capsule: Citrus pectin	7-1/2 gr.	PEDATONE ATHLETE'S FOOT POWDER (Commerce)	Undecylenic acid Sodium propionate Digenol (2, 2' dihydroxy 5, 5' dichloro diphenyl methane)*	
PECTOKATE Antacid (Pharmex)	Kaolin Pectin		PE-DES CREME Rubefacient (foot) (Georges)	Anhydrous lanolin Methyl salicylate* Camphor* White petrolatum Cersine wax	1% 3% 6%
PECTOPINE Antitussive (infant) (Tailby)	Ipecac Squill Senega Tolu Coltsfoot Pineapple flavor		PEDES FOOT BALM (Arlenge)		

*Consult Sec. II., Ingredients Index. This ingredient may be responsible for major toxic effects if poisonous amounts of this product are ingested.

- 806 -

Name & Use Manufacturer	Ingredients		Name & Use Manufacturer	Ingredients	
PED-EX OINTMENT Rubefacient (foot) (Ped-Ex)	Lanolin Thymol* Peppermint oil Glyceryl monostearate Spermaceti Menthol* Camphor* Eucalyptus oil * Glycerin		PEERLESS ANT CAPS Insecticide (Blue Ball)		
PEDICADE OINTMENT Skin fungicide (medical) (Binday)	Zinc undecylenate* Dihydroxy dichloro diphenyl methane * Undecylenic acid*		PEERLESS CAULKING COMPOUND, & ROOFING CEMENT (Weaver-Wall)		
PEDIGREE DEODORANT COLOGNE & STICK (Mem)			PEERLESS ENAMEL, PAINT, ROOF COATING (Akron)		
PEDIGREE PAINT (George, P.D.)			PEERLESS ROACH CAPS AND PASTE (Blue Ball)		
PEDI-MED FOOT BATH (Medi-Ped)	Magnesium sulfate Sodium bicarbonate Boric acid* Oil of thyme Menthol * Oil of pine * (Alkyl) benzine sulfonate		PEERLESS SCREW WORM KILLER (Peerless Co.)	Chloroform tech.* Naphthalene U.S.P.*	14.2% 3.8%
			PEE VEE LACQUER REMOVER (Riverside)		
PEDINOL DERMAL POWDER Antiseptic, fungicide, deodorant (medical) (Pedinol)	Goldicide Undecylenic acid * Benzoic acid * Boric acid* Zinc borate * Sodium propionate Salicylic acid* Menthol * Bentonite		PEGGY NEWTON BATH OIL & BUBBLE BATH (Newton, P.)		
PED-I-RUB (Ped-I-Rub)	Alcohol 8% Methyl salicylate* Menthol* Camphor* Tragacanth		PEGGY NEWTON CREAM CON- DITIONER, NIGHT CREAM, HAND CREAM & FOOT CREAM (Newton, P.)		
PED-LO Counter- irritant (foot) (Imperial Pharm.)	Salicylic acid* Menthol * Chloral hydrate Benzoic acid * Formaldehyde*		PEGGY NEWTON DE- ODORANTS, CREAM & SOLID (Newton, P.)		
PEDOGENE Skin fungicide (medical) (Hance)	Each oz.: Benzoic acid * Thymol iodide* Methyl salicylate* Salicylic acid* Camphor* Cycloform Ether 21-2/3 m.		PEGGY NEWTON LIPSTICK (Newton, P.)		
PEDOGENE CREME Fungicide (medical) (Hance)	Undecylenic acid* 5% Zinc undecylenate* 20% Cycloform* 2%		PEGGY NEWTON LIQUID LEG SHAVE (Newton, P.)		
PED-O-REM Astringent (foot) (Sacramento)			PEGGY NEWTON MAKE-UP BASE (Newton, P.)		
PED-X Ectoparasiticide (Gart)	Benzyl benzoate 68% Benzocaine 12% Dichloro diphenyl trichloroethane* 6%		PEGGY NEWTON MAKE-UP CLEANSER (Newton, P.)		

*Consult Sec. II., Ingredients Index. This ingredient may be responsible for major toxic effects if poisonous amounts of this product are ingested.

Name & Use Manufacturer	Ingredients		Name & Use Manufacturer	Ingredients	
PEGGY NEWTON MASCARA (Newton, P.)			PELCO DITHANE DUST 10% Insecticide (Peele)	Zinc ethylene bisdithio-carbamate	6.50%
PEGGY NEWTON NAIL POLISH (Newton, P.)			PELCO 15% FERMATE DUST Insecticide (Peele)	Ferric dimethyl dithio-carbamate	11.40%
PEGGY NEWTON "O" Complexion grains (Newton, P.)			PELCO TOBACCO DUST 10% TDE Insecticide (Peele)	DDD	10.00%
PEGGY NEWTON ROUGE (World's Prods.)			PELCO 20% TOXAPHENE DUST Insecticide (Peele)	Toxaphene*	20.00%
PEGGY NEWTON SKIN FRESHENER (Newton, P.)			PELDANE TABLETS Insecticide (Peters)	Gamma isomer of benzene hexachloride (from lindane)*	100%
PEGGY NEWTON STARDUST Face powder (Newton, P.)			PEN-A-SHEEN FLOOR FINISH (O'Brien Corp.)		
PEGGY NEWTON TOILET SOAP (Newton, P.)			PENATHOL Fungicide, (medical) deodorant (Milburn)	Salicylic acid* Benzoic acid Thymol Tricresol* Acetone in alcohol *	
PEGGY NEWTON VELVASHEEN Liquid shampoo (Newton, P.)			PENCO ARAMITE W-15 Insecticide (Pennsylv.)	Aramite	15%
PEGGY SAGE FAIRHAND LOTION, POLISH REMOVER (Sage, P.)			PENCO BHC D-12 Insecticide (Pennsylv. Salt)	Gamma isomer of benzene hexachloride* Other isomers of benzene hexachloride*	12% 18%
PEKAL Antacid (Falcon)	Kaolin Magnesium trisilicate Lactose Karaya Pectin Powdered skim milk	20% 15% 20% 15% 10% 20%	PENCO BHC-DDT EMULSION 3-5 Insecticide (Pennsylv. Salt)	DDT* Gamma isomer of benzene hexachloride* Other isomers of benzene hexachloride	14.5% 8.7% 8.7%
PEKTAMOL TABLETS Antacid, adsorbent (Pektamol)	Aluminum hydroxide Kaolin Zinc phenolsulfonate Methyl salicylate * Magnesium trisilicate Bismuth sub-salicylate Salol*		PENCO BHC E-11 Insecticide (Pennsylv. Salt)	Gamma isomer of benzene hexachloride* Other isomers of benzene hexachloride*	11% 11%
PELCO 3-5 COTTON DUST Insecticide (Peele)	Gamma isomer of benzene hexachloride* DDT*	3.00% 5.00%	PENCO BHC TECHNICAL Insecticide (Pennsylv. Salt)	Gamma isomer of benzene hexachloride*	36%
PELCO 3-5-40 COTTON DUST Insecticide (Peele)	Gamma isomer of benzene hexachloride* DDT* Sulfur*	3.00% 5.00 % 40.00%	PENCO BHC W-12 Insecticide (Pennsylv. Salt)	Gamma isomer of benzene hexachloride* Other isomers of benzene hexachloride	12% 12%
PELCO 5% DDT DUST Insecticide (Peele)	DDT*	5.00%			

*Consult Sec. II., Ingredients Index. This ingredient may be responsible for major toxic effects if poisonous amounts of this product are ingested.

Name & Use Manufacturer	Ingredients		Name & Use Manufacturer	Ingredients	
PENCO CALCIUM ARSENATE Insecticide (Pennsylv. Salt)	Tricalcium arsenate*	70%	PENCO DDT D-50 Insecticide (Pennsylv. Salt)	DDT*tech.	50%
PENCO COPPER-SULFUR-DDT DUST Insecticide, fungicide (Pennsylv. Salt)	Copper* Sulfur* DDT	3.4% 81.1% 2.5%	PENCO 5% DDT DUST Insecticide (Pennsylv. Salt)	DDT*	5%
			PENCO 10% DDT DUST Insecticide (Pennsylv. Salt)	DDT*	10%
PENCO 2-10-40 COTTON DUST Insecticide (Pennsylv. Salt)	Gamma isomer of benzene hexachloride * Other isomers of benzene hexachloride DDT * Sulfur*	2% 2% 10% 40%	PENCO DDT EMULSION 25 Insecticide (Pennsylv. Salt)	DDT*	25%
PENCO 2-1/2 - 5 - 0 COTTON DUST Insecticide (Pennsylv. Salt)	Aldrin* DDT	2.5% 5%	PENCO DDT EMULSION 34 Insecticide (Pennsylv. Salt)	DDT*	34%
PENCO 2-1/2 - 10 - 0 COTTON DUST Insecticide (Pennsylv. Salt)	Aldrin * DDT	2.5% 10%	PENCO DDT-SULFUR 5-80 Insecticide, fungicide (Pennsylv. Salt)	DDT* Sulfur*	5% 80%
PENCO 3-5-0 COTTON DUST Insecticide (Pennsylv. Salt)	Gamma isomer of benzene hexachloride* Other isomers of benzene hexachloride DDT*	3% 3% 5%	PENCO DDT-SULFUR 10-75 Insecticide, fungicide (Pennsylv. Salt)	DDT* Sulfur*	10% 74%
PENCO 3-5-40 COTTON DUST Insecticide (Pennsylv. Salt)	Gamma isomer of benzene hexachloride* Other isomers of benzene hexachloride DDT* Sulfur*	3% 3% 5% 40%	PENCO 10-40 DDT-SULFUR DUST Insecticide, fungicide (Pennsylv. Salt)	DDT* Sulfur*	10% 40%
PENCO 3-10-0 COTTON DUST Insecticide (Pennsylv. Salt)	Gamma isomer of benzene hexachloride* Other isomers of benzene hexachloride DDT*	3% 3% 10%	PENCO DDT W-50 Insecticide (Pennsylv. Salt)	DDT*	50%
PENCO 3-10-40 COTTON DUST Insecticide (Pennsylv. Salt)	Gamma isomer of benzene hexachloride* Other isomers of benzene hexachloride DDT* Sulfur*	3% 3% 10% 40%	PENCO DE-FOL-ATE Herbicide (Pennsylv. Salt)	Magnesium chlorate hexahydrate*	
PENCO 20-0 COTTON DUST Insecticide (Pennsylv. Salt)	Toxaphene*	20%	PENCO 1-1/2% DIELDRIN DUST Insecticide (Pennsylv. Salt)	Dieldrin*	1.5%
PENCO 20-40 COTTON DUST Insecticide (Pennsylv. Salt)	Toxaphene* Sulfur	20% 40%	PENCO 1-1/2 - 5 - 0 DIELDRIN DUST Insecticide (Pennsylv Salt)	Dieldrin* DDT*	1.5% 5%
PENCO DDT-COPPER-SULFUR 5-4-75 Insecticide, fungicide (Pennsylv. Salt)	DDT* Copper* Sulfur*	5% 3.4% 75%			

*Consult Sec. II., Ingredients Index. This ingredient may be responsible for major toxic effects if poisonous amounts of this product are ingested.

Name & Use Manufacturer	Ingredients	
PENCO 2-1/2 - 5 - 0 DIELDRIN DUST Insecticide (Pennsylv. Salt)	Dieldrin* DDT	2.5% 5%
PENCO 2-1/2 - 5 - 40 DIELDRIN DUST Insecticide (Pennsylv. Salt)	Dieldrin* DDT Sulfur	2.5% 5% 40%
PENCO DIELDRIN E-1-1/2 Insecticide (Pennsylv. Salt)	Dieldrin*	18.6%
PENCO DIMITE E-2 Insecticide (Pennsylv. Salt)	Di (p-chlorophenyl) methyl carbinol*	25%
PENCO D-PHOS 37-5 Insecticide (Pennsylv. Salt)	DDT Parathion*	37.5% 5%
PENCO D-PHOS 38-6 Insecticide (Pennsylv. Salt)	DDT Parathion*	38% 6.25%
PENCO EMULSION CONCEN- TRATE Insecticide (Pennsylv. Salt)	DDT*	25%
PENCO EMULSION CONCEN- TRATE Insecticide (Pennsylv. Salt)	DDT*	34%
PENCO ENDOTHAL DEFOLIANT S-4069 ENDOTHAL DESICCANT, ENDOTHAL HARVEST AID Herbicides (Pennsylv. Salt)	Disodium endothal*	6.3%
PENCO ENDOTHAL WEED KILLER S-3003 (Pennsylv. Salt)	Disodium endothal*	19.2%
PENCO ENDRIN EMULSION 16 Insecticide (Pennsylv. Salt)	Endrin*	19.5%

Name & Use Manufacturer	Ingredients	
PENCO FERBAM Fungicide (Pennsylv. Salt)	Ferbam*	76%
PENCO KRYOCIDE Insecticide (Pennsylv. Salt)	Sodium fluoaluminate*	90%
PENCO 1% LINDANE DUST Insecticide (Pennsylv. Salt)	Lindane	1%
PENCO LINDANE E-20 Insecticide (Pennsylv. Salt)	Lindane*	20%
PENCO LINDANE- MERCURY 37-1 Insecticide, fungicide (Pennsylv. Salt)	Lindane* Phenyl mercuric ammonium acetate*	37% 1.75%
PENCO LINDANE W-25 Insecticide (Pennsylv. Salt)	Lindane*	25%
PENCO LINDANE W-75 Insecticide (Pennsylv. Salt)	Lindane*	75%
PENCO MALATHION E-8 Insecticide (Pennsylv. Salt)	Malathion*	80%
PENCO MALATHION E-50 Insecticide (Pennsylv. Salt)	Malathion*	50%
PENCO MALATHION W-25 Insecticide (Pennsylv. Salt)	Malathion*	25%
PENCO 1% PARATHION DUST Insecticide (Pennsylv. Salt)	Parathion*	1%
PENCO PARATHION W-15 Insecticide (Pennsylv. Salt)	Parathion*	15%

*Consult Sec. II., Ingredients Index. This ingredient may be responsible for major toxic effects if poisonous amounts of this product are ingested.

Name & Use Manufacturer	Ingredients	Name & Use Manufacturer	Ingredients
PENCO PARATHION W-25 Insecticide (Pennsylv. Salt)	Parathion* 25%	PENDANE 10% EMULSIFI-ABLE Insecticide (Penick)	Gamma isomer of benzene hexachloride (from lindane) 10% Polyethylene oxide sorbitan oleate emulsifier 5% Methylated naphthalene* 85%
PENCO PENCAL Insecticide (Pennsylv. Salt)	Tricalcium arsenate* 70%	PENDANE 20% EMULSIFI-ABLE Insecticide (Penick)	Gamma isomer of benzene hexachloride* (from lindane) 20% Polyethylene oxide sorbitan oleate emulsifier 5% Cyclohexanone 10% Methylated naphthalene* 65%
PENCO PENITE 6X Herbicide (Pennsylv. Salt)	Sodium arsenite* 71.5%	PENDANE (Lindane) Insecticide (Penick)	Gamma isomer of benzene hexachloride* 99% Other isomers of benzene hexachloride 1%
PENCO PENITE 35 Herbicide (Pennsylv. Salt)	Sodium arsenite* 46.5%	PENDANE 10% SOLUTION Insecticide (Penick)	Gamma isomer of benzene hexachloride (from lindane) 10% Methylated naphthalene* 90%
PENCO PENTRETE Fungicide (Pennsylv. Salt)	Phenyl mercuric ammonium acetate* 7%	PENDANE 20% SOLUTION Insecticide (Penick)	Gamma isomer of benzene hexachloride (from lindane)* 20% Methylated naphthalene* 70% Cyclohexanone 10%
PENCO SODIUM CHLORATE Herbicide (Pennsylv. Salt)	Sodium chlorate* 99%	PENDANE 25% WETTABLE POWDER Insecticide (Penick)	Gamma isomer of benzene hexachloride* (from lindane) 25%
PENCO SUPER-SEVENTY Insecticide (Pennsylv. Salt)	Sodium fluoaluminate* 72%	PENE-SEAL Floor sealer (Merkin)	
PENCO SYTAM Insecticide (Pennsylv. Salt)	Octamethyl pyrophosphoramide (OMPA)* 42% Related organic phosphates 15%	PENETRATING LINIMENT (Little Wonder)	Chloroform* 30% Camphor* and soap 70%
PENCO TOXAPHENE D-40 Insecticide (Pennsylv. Salt)	Toxaphene* 40%	PENETREX Paint product (Glidden Co.)	
PENCO TOXAPHENE DDT E2-1 Insecticide (Pennsylv. Salt)	Toxaphene* 40% DDT 20%	PENETREX WOOD FLOOR PRESERVA-TIVES (Bondrite)	
PENCO TOXAPHENE E-6 Insecticide (Pennsylv. Salt)	Toxaphene* 60.4%	PENETROID Wood floor sealer (Lawrence, W.W.)	
		PENETRO INHALER (Plough)	Camphor* Menthol Thymol Methyl salicylate*
		PENETRO NOSE DROPS (Plough)	Ephedrine* Menthol Camphor* Eucalyptol*
PENCO TOXAPHENE W-40 Insecticide (Pennsylv. Salt)	Toxaphene* 40%	PENETRO QUICK ACT-ING RUB Chest rubefacient, (Plough)	Methyl salicylate* Turpentine* Menthol* Camphor* Thymol* Pine oil*

*Consult Sec. II., Ingredients Index. This ingredient may be responsible for major toxic effects if poisonous amounts of this product are ingested.

Name & Use Manufacturer	Ingredients	
PEN-FLO-SEAL FLOOR SEALER (Sewall)		
PEN-GESIC Analgesic (Penslar)	Menthol Methyl salicylate* Alcohol*	70%
PENICK ALLETHRIN TECHNICAL Insecticide (Penick)	Allethrin*(allyl homolog of cinerin 1) Related compounds	
PENICK ANTU Rodenticide (Penick)	Alpha-naphthyl thiourea*	92%
PENICK 20% ANTU POWDER Rodenticide (Penick)	Alpha-naphthyl thiourea* tech.	20%
PENICK 25% AND 30% DDT EMULSIFI-ABLE & SOLUTION Insecticides (Penick)	DDT*	
PENICK DDT 50% WET-TABLE POWDER Insecticide (Penick)	DDT*	50%
PENICK DIELDRIN 1.5 EMULSION Insecticide (Penick)	Hexachloro epoxy octahydro-endo, exo-dimethano naphthalene* Related compounds Petroleum hydrocarbons	15.98% 2.82% 76.20%
PENICK EMULSIFI-ABLE ROTENONE 5% W/W Insecticide (Penick)	Rotenone Other cube extractives Methylated naphthalene*	5% 15% 50%
PENICKLOR BRAND TECHNICAL CHLORDANE REFINED Insecticide (Penick)	Tech. chlordane*	100%
PENICKLOR 46% EMULSI-FIABLE W/W Insecticide (Penick)	Chlordane tech.* Petroleum distillate*	46% 47%
PENICKLOR 50% EMULSI-FIABLE W/W Insecticide (Penick)	Chlordane tech.* Petroleum distillate	50% 5%
PENICKLOR 62% EMULSI-FIABLE-STABLE Insecticide (Penick)	Chlordane tech.*	62%

Name & Use Manufacturer	Ingredients	
PENICKLOR 73-1/2% EMULSIFI-ABLE Insecticide (Penick)	Chlordane*	73.5%
PENICKLOR 20% OIL SOLUTION W/W Insecticide (Penick)	Chlordane tech.* Petroleum distillate*	20% 80%
PENICKLOR 50% WET-TABLE POWDER Insecticide (Penick)	Chlordane*	50%
PENICK MALATHION 90% CON-CENTRATE Insecticide (Penick)	Malathion* Xylol	90% 10%
PENICK MALATHION E-5 Insecticide (Penick)	Malathion* Xylol*	57% 35%
PENICK 50% MALATHION EMULSIFI-ABLE CON-CENTRATE Insecticide (Penick)	Malathion * Xylol*	50% 42.4%
PENICK MALATHION 30% OIL SOLUTION Insecticide (Penick)	Malathion*	30%
PENICK MALATHION 25% WET-TABLE POWDER Insecticide (Penick)	Malathion *	25%
PENICK POWDERED CUBE ROOT Insecticide (Penick)	Rotenone* Other cube resins	
PENICK POWDERED SABADILLA 50% CALCINED Insecticide (Penick)	Alkaloids of sabadilla seed	3%
PENICK POWDERED SABADILLA INSECTICIDE (Penick)	Sabadilla*	

*Consult Sec. II., Ingredients Index. This ingredient may be responsible for major toxic effects if poisonous amounts of this product are ingested.

Name & Use Manufacturer	Ingredients	
PENICK POWDERED SABADILLA & SULFUR 33/67 Insecticide (Penick)	Sabadilla* Sulfur*	33% 67%
PENICK POWDERED SABADILLA & SULPHUR 50/50 Insecticide (Penick)	Sabadilla* Sulfur*	50% 50%
PENICK PURIFIED PYRETHRUM OLEORESIN Insecticide (Penick)	Pyrethrins* Petroleum distillate*	20% 80%
PENICK PYRETHRUM POWDER Insecticide (Penick)	Pyrethrins	0.9%
PENICK SULFOXIDE PYREXCEL 20 Insecticide (Penick)	Petroleum distillate* 2-Butoxy ethanol n-Octyl sulfoxide of isosafrole Pyrethrins* Compounds related to sulfoxide	
PENICK 40% SULFOXIDE SOLUTION Insecticide (Penick)	n-Octyl sulfoxide of isosafrole* Butoxypolypropylene glycol 2-Butoxy ethanol Compounds related to sulfoxide	
PENITE 35 Herbicide (Commercial Chem.)	Arsenic*	26.5%
PENNACAP Fungicide (Collins Feed)	Pentachloro nitrobenzene* 36.00% n-Trichloro methyl mercapto-4-cyclohexene-1, 2-dicarboximide* 25.00%	
PENN-A-SEAL PENETRATING FLOOR VARNISH (Sweeney, W. H.)		
PENN CHAMP DRY CLEANING COMPOUND (Penn-Champ)		
PENNCLEAN (Pennsylv. Salt)	Phosphoric acid *	
PENN-DRAKE SELF-POLISHING WAX (Pennsylv. Ref.)		
PENN-DRAKE SPOT REMOVER, PETROLATUM DRY CLEANER (Pennsylv. Ref.)		

Name & Use Manufacturer	Ingredients	
PENNEX LIGHTER FLUID (Pennex)		
PENNSALT CLEANER 30 (Pennsylv. Salt)	Silicated alkali	
PENNSALT 20-0 COTTON DUST Insecticide (Pennsylv. Salt)	Toxaphene*	20.00%
PENN-TONE Paste paint (Penn Crete)		
PEN-O-FLOOR Floor treatment (Breinig)		
PEN-O-LIN Rubefacient (Penslar)	Oil of wormwood Oil of sassafras * Menthol* Oil of tansy Acetone*	
PEN-O-LITE VARNISHES (Sterling Varnish)		
PEN-O-SEAL Floor sealer (Felton Sibley)		
PENOTRITE SOLVENTS (General Solv.)		
PENSAL B, M, O, W Detergents (Pennsylv. Salt)	Sodium orthosilicate Sodium hydroxide* or sodium carbonate	
PEN-SAN Vaginal antiseptic (Penslar)	Phenol* Boric acid* Zinc sulfate * Oxyquinoline sulfate Thymol Eucalyptol * Salicylic acid Menthol	1% 0.5%
PENSLAR A-P-C CAPSULES Analgesic (Penslar)	Each capsule: Acetophenetidin* Caffeine Aspirin*	2-1/2 gr.
PENSLAR BLUE OINTMENT Ectoparasiticide (Penslar)	Mercury*	10%
PENSLAR DENTAL PLATE CLEANER (Penslar)	Sodium perborate* Trisodium phosphate*	
PENSLAR EYE BATH (Penslar)	Sodium borate C.P. Sodium chloride C.P. Camphor water U.S.P.	

*Consult Sec. II., Ingredients Index. This ingredient may be responsible for major toxic effects if poisonous amounts of this product are ingested.

Name & Use Manufacturer	Ingredients		Name & Use Manufacturer	Ingredients	
PENSLAR EYE TONE (Penslar)	Boric acid C.P. Camphor Copper sulfate C.P. Zinc sulfate C.P. Berberine sulfate		PENTA PRESERVA- TIVE Wood pre- servative (Commercial Chem.)	Pentachlorophenol* Petroleum hydrocarbons*	5% 95%
PENSLAR HAND CREAM (Penslar)			PENTA PRESERVA- TIVE, CONC. Wood pre- servative (Commercial Chem.)	Pentachlorophenol*	40%
PENSLAR INHALIT DROPS Nasal de- congestant (Penslar)	Ephedrine* Camphor* Menthol Pine needle oils Eucalyptus *	1%			
PENSLAR L. C. COLD CAPSULES WITH LAXATIVE (Penslar)	Acetophenetidin* Camphor Asafetida Capsicum Aloin	3 gr.	PENTA-SEAL Wood pre- servative (Barber)	Pentachlorophenol* Pine oil Petroleum solvents *	21.6% 4.2% 40.5%
			PENTA- WEEDICIDE Herbicide (Thompson Chem.)	Pentachlorophenol* Butyl 2, 4-dichlorophenoxy acetate	40% 10%
PENSLAR MENTHO- LATED BRUSHLESS SHAVING CREAM (Penslar)			PENTA WOOD PRESERVA- TIVE 10-1 CONCEN- TRATE (Protection)	Pentachlorophenol*	40.0%
PENSLAR NOSE DROPS Nasal de- congestant (Penslar)	Ephedrine* Camphor* Menthol Oil of pine needles Eucalyptus *	1%	PENTA-WR Water- repellent wood preservative (Commercial Chem.)	Pentachlorophenol* Petroleum hydrocarbons*	18% 57%
PENTA- BROMIDES Sedative (Merrell)	Each fl. oz.: Sodium bromide* Ammonium bromide* Potassium bromide* Calcium bromide Lithium bromide	4.16 gm. 1.30 gm. 1.30 gm. 0.78 gm. 0.25 gm.	PENTECH Insecticide (Pennsylv. Salt)	Tech. DDT*	
PENTA-CHLOR Insecticide (Central Solv.)	Pentachlorophenol*	5%	PENTIDE Wood preservative (Bonide)	Pentachlorophenol* Other chlorophenols Petroleum hydrocarbons*	4.4% 0.6% 91.63%
PENTAGILL (Green) Analgesic, antipyretic (Massengill)	Opium Ipecac Acetophenetidin* Acetylsalicylic acid* Camphor* Caffeine	1.6 mg. 1.6 mg. 0.1 gm. 0.1 gm. 16 mg. 8 mg.	PENTOL Disinfectant, germicide (Horton & Converse)	Soap p-(Alpha, alpha dimethyl propyl) phenol* Pine oil	37% 8.3% 1%
PENTAGILL (Orange) Analgesic, antipyretic (Massengill)	Each capsule: Opium Ipecac Dover powder Acetophenetidin* Acetylsalicylic acid* Camphor Caffeine	1.6 mg. 1.6 mg. 0.1 gm. 0.1 gm. 16 mg. 16 mg.	PENTREX Rust pre- ventative remover (Claronex)		
			PEN-TRIN Liniment (veterinary) (Thoroughbred)	Camphor* Menthol * Oil of wormwood Turpentine* Peppermint Cedarwood Mirbane Cedarleaf Tansy Cantharides*	
PENTA MR Wood pre- servative (Thompson- Hayward)	Pentachlorophenol* Petroleum distillate* Polymerized resin acids	5.0% 84.5% 5.0%			
PENTA NASAL OINTMENT (Fountain)	Ephedrine hydrochloride* Bismuth subcarbonate Metycaine* (Lilly) Aquaphor Lanolin Petrolatum	1% 1/2% 10%	PENTRONOL WOOD TREATMENT Wood pre- servative (Pioneer)		

*Consult Sec. II., Ingredients Index. This ingredient may be responsible for major toxic effects if poisonous amounts of this product are ingested.

Name & Use Manufacturer	Ingredients	
PENTROX FLOOR SEALER (Advance Chem.)		
PEOPLES IMPORTED BAY RUM (Peoples)	Each fl. oz.: Alcohol* Tartar emetic*	50%/v 1/4 gr.
PEPPI-BARR LINIMENT (Solid) (Sintos)	Methyl salicylate* Menthol Oils of thyme, cajuput, pine-needle, turpentine, rosemary, peppermint Alcohol*	75%/w
PEPSINIC SELTZER Antacid (Pepsinic)	Sodium bicarbonate Tartaric acid	
PEPSODENT ANTISEPTIC (Pepsodent)	Chlorthymol Boric,* malic, citric acids Alcohol	26%
PEPSOMAL Digestant (Chase Chem.)	Bismuth subsalicylate Salol* Zinc sulfocarbolate Methyl salicylate*	
PEPTEX Dairy cleaner (Diversey)		
PEP-TI-KON FORMULA Food supplement (Berjon)	Each fl. oz.: Ferrous gluconate (105.0 mg. iron) Thiamine hydrochloride Riboflavin Niacinamide Manganese citrate Zinc chloride	14.0 gr 3.0 mg. 3.0 mg. 10.0 mg. 0.5 gr. 0.07 gr.
PEPTOACID Digestant (Jamol)	Hydrochloric acid Pepsin	1%
PEPTO-BISMOL Digestant (Norwich)	Bismuth subsalicylate Salol Zinc phenosulfonate Methyl salicylate	
PEPTONIZED VEHICLE ELIXIR (Massengill)	Each fl. oz.: Ethyl alcohol Lactated pepsin powder Lactic acid Hydrochloric acid	10%/v 40 gr.
PEQUOD PAINTS, ENAMELS, STAINS (Tredennick)		
PERBORASAL COMPOUND Antiseptic (oral, nasal) (Haug)	Sodium perborate* Sodium chloride Sodium bicarbonate	
PERCHLORON Bleach (Pennsylv. Salt)	Calcium hypochlorite* (available chlorine)	70%

Name & Use Manufacturer	Ingredients	
PERCY MEDICINE Antacid (Merrick)	Bismuth subnitrate Rhubarb syrup Lime water Alcohol	5%
PERFACOTE PAINTS & ENAMELS (Arnesto)		
PERFECTION FURNITURE POLISH (Avon Prod.)		
PERFECTION LINOLEUM CLEANER (Bartley)		
PERFECTION PAINT & VARNISH CLEANER (Bartley)		
PERFECTION PAINTS, VARNISHES, ENAMELS (Yarnell)		
PERFECTION PORCELAIN, TILE & MARBLE CLEANER (Bartley)		
PERFECTION RUG & UP-HOLSTERY CLEANER (Bartley)		
PERFECTION SHOE POLISH (Avon Prod.)		
PERFECTION SILVER POLISH (Avon Prod.)		
PERFECTO HOUSE PAINT (Phelan-Faust)		
PERFECTSEAL ROOF COAT-ING (Merkin)		
PERFEKTION Paint, varnish (Pratt Paint)		
PERFEX Cleaner (Tidy House)	Crystalline trisodium phosphate* Crystalline sodium sesquicarbonate Anhydrous sodium tripolyphosphate	60% 35% 5%
PERFEX BRAND PAINTS (Balto. Paint)		

*Consult Sec. II., Ingredients Index. This ingredient may be responsible for major toxic effects if poisonous amounts of this product are ingested.

Name & Use Manufacturer	Ingredients	Name & Use Manufacturer	Ingredients
PER-FEX-ION VARNISHES (Thresher)		PERMA-STA Anti-freeze (Western Solvent)	Ethylene glycol* 90% Borax
PERFEX PAINT (Vane-Calvert)		PERMA STARCH Laundry starch (Milner)	
PERFUMED CRYSTALS Deodorizer (Stanley Home)	Paradichlorobenzene * Perfume	PERMATEX AVIATION FORM-A-GASKET (Permatex)	Isopropyl alcohol*
PERIODON Periodontal therapy (Barnes-Hind)	Urea peroxide* Sodium lauryl sulfate*	PERMATEX BLOCK & HEAD SEALER (Permatex)	Silicate of soda
PERMA-BOND PAINTS (Sec Mfg.)		PERMATEX COOLING SYSTEM CLEANER & CONDITIONER (Permatex)	Oxalic acid*
PERM-A-CLOR NA (Detrex)	Trichlorethylene*		
PERMAGARD DEFOLIANT CONCEN-TRATE (Thompson-Hayward)	Pentachlorophenol* 44.0% Aromatic petroleum deriv. solvent * 19.0%	PERMATEX DOUBLE ACTION RADIATOR CEMENT (Permatex)	Potassium dichromate*
PERMA-GLOSS Waxes, polishes (Central Chem.)		PERMATEX FABRIC CLEANER (Permatex)	Carbon tetrachloride*
PERM-A-KLEEN (Detrex)	Perchlorethylene*	PERMATEX FORM-A-GASKET NO. 1 (Permatex)	Isopropyl alcohol*
PERMA-KROME ALUMINUM PAINTS (Greenwood)		PERMATEX GLASS SEALER (Permatex)	Toluol*
PERMA-LASTIC ACID RESISTING PAINT (Sterling Varnish)		PERMATEX LIQUID RADIATOR CLEANER (Permatex)	Muriatic acid*
PERMALIN LINOLEUM VARNISH (Hays-Taylor)		PERMATEX LIQUID RADIATOR SEALER (Permatex)	Isopropyl alcohol *
PERMA-NAIL POLISH REMOVER (Perma-Nail)		PERMATEX PIPE JOINT COMPOUND (Permatex)	Isopropyl alcohol*
PERMA RID INSECT SURFACE SPRAY (Ray-Claw)	Tech. chlordane 2-1/2% Aliphatic petroleum hydrocarbons 6%	PERMATEX RUBBER LUBRICANT (Permatex)	Polyglycol
PERMA-STA Anti-freeze compound (Amsco)	Glycol base*	PERMATEX TAROFF (Permatex)	Chlorinated solvent*
PERMA STA Anti-freeze (Central Solv.)	Glycol *	PERMATONE FLAT PAINTS (Graves)	
PERMA STA Anti-freeze (Hoosier)	Glycol *		

*Consult Sec. II., Ingredients Index. This ingredient may be responsible for major toxic effects if poisonous amounts of this product are ingested.

Name & Use Manufacturer	Ingredients		Name & Use Manufacturer	Ingredients	
PERMA- VENEER ENAMELS, VARNISHES, FLOOR FINISHERS (Standard Ind.)			PER-MO MOTH- PROOFING LIQUID (Per-Mo)	Sodium arsenite* (as arsenious oxide)	1.00%
PERMAWOOD WOOD PRE- SERVATIVE READY TO USE 1-A (Admiralty)	Pentachlorophenol*		PERMO MOTH- PROOFING SPRAY (Uncle Sam)		
PERMAX Insecticide (Dolge)	Aliphatic petroleum hydro- carbons Aromatic petroleum hydro- carbons* Dichloro diphenyl tri- chloroethane* Pyrethrins		PERMONEX VARNISH (Thompson & Co.)		
			PERMOPLAST MODELING CLAY (Am. Art Clay)		
PERMAX-WL Insecticide (Dolge)	Aliphatic petroleum hydrocarbons* Aromatic petroleum hydrocarbons* Gamma isomer of benzene hexachloride* Sesame oil extractives Pyrethrins		PER-MO-PRO Insecticide (M.B.C.)	Sodium fluosilicate*	
			PER-MO RAT & MICE LIQUID (Per-Mo)	Sodium arsenite*	2.27%
PERM-E- LASTIC CAULKING COMPOUND (Perfection Model)			PER-MO RAT PASTE (Per-Mo)	Extractives of red squill*	10.2%
PERMEX INK PASTE (Am. Crayon)			PERMO-SEAL & NO-TAR- KOTE ASBESTOS FIBRE LIQUID CEMENT (Pioneer)		
PERMITE Wood pre- servative (Speekman)	Pentachlorophenol* 4.5% Other chlorophenols 0.5% Petroleum distillate* 95.0%		PERMO SEAL ROOF CEMENTS (Pioneer)		
PER-MO BITS KILLS RATS (Per-Mo)	Extractives of red squill* 5.1%		PERMOVITE EXTERIOR TRIM Paint (Hancock P. & V.)		
PER-MO BROWN RAT KILLER CONTAINS ANTU (Per-Mo)	ANTU 4%		PER-MO WARFARIN KILLS RATS AND MICE (Per-Mo)	3-(a-Phenyl-b-acetyl ethyl)- 4-hydroxycoumarin 0.025%	
PERMODIP Wood pre- servative (King, E. & F.)	Pentachlorophenol* 5% Petroleum derivatives (mainly mineral spirits)		PERMUTIT Q (Permutit)	Sulfonated polystyrene*	
PERMO FINISHES Paint (Superior Paint)			PERRY DAVIS LINIMENT (Davis & Lawrence)	Capsicum Gums Guaiac Myrrh Camphor* Oil of spruce Alcohol* 51%	
PERMOLITE ENAMELS (Superior Paint)			PERSIAN HAIR OIL (Peerless Barber)	Mineral oil Vegetable coloring Synthetic perfume oil	
PER-MO MOTH- PROOFING LIQUID (Per-Mo)	Magnesium silicofluoride* 1.25%				

---

*Consult Sec. II., Ingredients Index. This ingredient may be responsible for major toxic effects if poisonous amounts of this product are ingested.

Name & Use Manufacturer	Ingredients	
PERSISTO C-S 5-45-40 DUST Insecticide, fungicide (Calif. Spray)	DDT Cryolite * Sulfur	5% 45% 40%
PERSISTO C-S 10-35-40 DUST Insecticide, fungicide (Calif. Spray)	DDT* Cryolite * Sulfur*	10% 35% 40%
PERSISTO 3 DUST Insecticide (Calif. Spray)	DDT	3%
PERSISTO 5 DUST Insecticide (Calif. Spray)	DDT*	5%
PERSISTO 10 DUST Insecticide (Calif. Spray)	DDT*	10%
PERSISTO DUST NO. 20 Insecticide (Calif. Spray)	DDT*	20%
PERSISTO DUST NO. 25 Insecticide (Calif. Spray)	DDT*	25%
PERSISTO DUST NO. 35 Insecticide (Calif. Spray)	DDT*	35%
PERSISTO FLOTOX 5-50 DUST Insecticide (Calif. Spray)	DDT* Sulfur*	5% 50%
PERSISTO FLOTOX 5-75 DUST Insecticide, fungicide (Calif. Spray)	DDT* Sulfur*	5% 75%
PERSISTO FLOTOX 10-50 DUST Insecticide, fungicide (Calif. Spray)	DDT* Sulfur*	10% 50%
PERSISTO-K 1-7 DUST Insecticide, fungicide (Calif. Spray)	DDT Copper* Oil	1% 7% 1.5%
PERSISTO-K 3-6.8 DUST Insecticide (Calif. Spray)	DDT Copper*	3% 6.8%
PERSISTO-K 3-7 DUST Insecticide, fungicide (Calif. Spray)	DDT Copper*	3% 7%
PERSISTO-K 5-7 DUST Insecticide, fungicide (Calif. Spray)	DDT* Copper*	5% 7%
PERSISTO-K 5-25 DUST Insecticide, fungicide (Calif. Spray)	DDT * Copper * Zinc * Zinc Coposil	5% 4.5% 4.5% 25%
PERSISTO-K 5-35 DUST Insecticide, fungicide (Calif. Spray)	DDT * Copper as metallic* Zinc as metallic* Zinc Coposil	5% 6.3% 6.3% 35%
PERSISTO-K 20-15 DUST Insecticide (Calif. Spray)	DDT * Copper	20% 2.7%
PERSISTO- KLOR 10-5 DUST Insecticide (Calif. Spray)	DDT * Tech. chlordane* (3% octachloro-4, 7-methano tetrahydroindane, 2% related compounds)	10% 5%
PERSISTO- KLOR-S 5-4-50 DUST Insecticide, fungicide (Calif. Spray)	DDT * Chlordane Sulfur *	5% 4% 50%
PERSISTO-K-O 5-6.7 DUST Insecticide, fungicide (Calif. Spray)	DDT * Copper *	5% 6.7%
PERSISTO K-O 5-8 DUST Insecticide (Calif. Spray)	DDT* Copper*	5% 8%
PERSISTOL 25 EMULSIVE Insecticide (Calif. Spray)	DDT *	25%
PERSISTOL 4.5 VAPO DUST Insecticide (Calif. Spray)	DDT * Oil *	4.5% 89%
PERSISTOL VAPO-DUST NO. 24 Insecticide (Calif. Spray)	Dichloro diphenyl tri- chloroethane Petroleum oils*	2.4% 96.0%
PERSISTO- MALATHION 5-5 DUST Insecticide (Calif. Spray)	DDT* Malathion *	5% 5%
PERSISTO 50 MICRO CON- CENTRATE Insecticide (Calif. Spray)	DDT *	50%
PERSISTO 75 MICRO CON- CENTRATE Insecticide (Calif. Spray)	DDT *	75%

*Consult Sec. II., Ingredients Index. This ingredient may be responsible for major toxic effects if poisonous amounts of this product are ingested.

Name & Use Manufacturer	Ingredients	
PERSISTO- MITE 3-3 DUST Insecticide (Calif. Spray)	DDT Aramite	3% 3%
PERSISTO- MITE 5-3 DUST Insecticide (Calif. Spray)	DDT * Aramite	5% 3%
PERSISTO- MITE 5-4 DUST Insecticide (Calif. Spray)	DDT * Aramite	5% 4%
PERSISTO- MITE 10-3 DUST Insecticide (Calif. Spray)	DDT * Aramite	10% 3%
PERSISTO- MITE 20-3 DUST Insecticide (Calif. Spray)	DDT * Aramite	20% 3%
PERSISTO- MITE 25-3 DUST Insecticide (Calif. Spray)	DDT * Aramite	25% 3%
PERSISTOPHOS 3-1 DUST Insecticide (Calif. Spray)	DDT Parathion *	3% 1%
PERSISTOPHOS 3-2 DUST Insecticide (Calif. Spray)	DDT Parathion *	3% 2%
PERSISTOPHOS 5-1 DUST Insecticide (Calif. Spray)	DDT Parathion *	5% 1%
PERSISTOPHOS 5-2 DUST Insecticide (Calif. Spray)	DDT Parathion*	5% 2%
PERSISTOPHOS 10-1 DUST Insecticide (Calif. Spray)	DDT Parathion *	10% 1%
PERSISTOPHOS 10-2 DUST Insecticide (Calif. Spray)	DDT Parathion *	10% 2%
PERSISTOPHOS 20-2 DUST Insecticide (Calif. Spray)	DDT Parathion *	20% 2%
PERSISTOPHOS 25-2 DUST Insecticide (Calif. Spray)	DDT Parathion *	25% 2%
PERSISTOPHOS 30-2 DUST Insecticide (Calif. Spray)	DDT Parathion *	30% 2%

Name & Use Manufacturer	Ingredients	
PERSISTO- PHOS-K 5-1-25 DUST Insecticide (Calif. Spray)	DDT Parathion * Zinc Coposil Copper as metallic	5% 1% 25% 4.5%
PERSISTO- PHOS-K 5-2-25 DUST Insecticide, fungicide (Calif. Spray)	Dichloro diphenyl tri- chloroethane Parathion* Copper as metallic	5.0% 2.0% 4.5%
PERSISTO- PHOS-KO 5-1-5 DUST Insecticide, fungicide (Calif. Spray)	Dichloro diphenyl tri- chloroethane Parathion* Copper as metallic	5% 1% 5%
PERSISTO- PHOS-KO 5-2-5 DUST Insecticide (Calif. Spray)	Dichloro diphenyl tri- chloroethane Parathion* Copper as metallic	5% 2% 5%
PERSISTO- PHOS KO-S 5-1-5-10 DUST Insecticide (Calif. Spray)	Dichloro diphenyl tri- chloroethane Parathion* Copper as metallic Sulfur	5% 1% 5% 10%
PERSISTO- PHOS-S 3-1-50 DUST Insecticide (Calif. Spray)	DDT Parathion * Sulfur	3% 1% 50%
PERSISTO- PHOS-S 5-1-25 DUST Insecticide (Calif. Spray)	DDT Parathion * Sulfur	5% 1% 25%
PERSISTO- PHOS-S 5-1-50 DUST Insecticide (Calif. Spray)	DDT Parathion* Sulfur	5% 1% 50%
PERSISTO- PHOS-S 5-1.5-25 DUST Insecticide (Calif. Spray)	DDT Parathion* Sulfur	5% 1.5% 25%
PERSISTO- PHOS-S 5-2-25 DUST Insecticide (Calif. Spray)	DDT Parathion * Sulfur	5% 2% 25%
PERSISTO- PHOS-S 5-2-50 DUST Insecticide (Calif. Spray)	DDT Parathion * Sulfur	5% 2% 50%
PERSISTOPHOS 25-5 SPRAY Insecticide (Calif. Spray)	DDT Parathion*	25% 5%
PERSISTOPHOS 30-10 WET- TABLE Insecticide (Calif. Spray)	DDT Parathion*	30% 10%

*Consult Sec. II., Ingredients Index. This ingredient may be responsible for major toxic effects if poisonous amounts of this product are ingested.

Name & Use Manufacturer	Ingredients		Name & Use Manufacturer	Ingredients	
PERSISTOPHOS 33-5 WET-TABLE Insecticide (Calif. Spray)	DDT Parathion *	33% 5%	PERSISTO-S 10-25 DUST Insecticide, fungicide (Calif. Spray)	DDT * Sulfur *	10% 25%
PERSISTOPHOS 38-6 WET-TABLE Insecticide (Calif. Spray)	DDT Parathion*	38% 6%	PERSISTO-S 10-50 DUST Insecticide (Calif. Spray)	DDT * Sulfur *	10% 50%
PERSISTOPHOS 38-9 WET-TABLE Insecticide (Calif. Spray)	DDT Parathion *	38% 9%	PERSISTO-S 10-75 DUST Insecticide, fungicide (Calif. Spray)	DDT * Sulfur *	10% 75%
PERSISTOPHOS 40-5 WET-TABLE Insecticide (Calif. Spray)	DDT Parathion*	40% 5%	PERSISTO S-K 5-25-25 DUST Insecticide (Calif. Spray)	DDT * Sulfur* Zinc * Copper *	5% 25% 4.5% 4.5%
PERSISTOPHOS ZINEB-S 5-1-3.25-15 DUST Insecticide, fungicide (Calif. Spray)	DDT Parathion * Zineb (zinc as metallic 0.77%) Sulfur	5% 1% 3.25% 15%	PERSISTO S-K 5-50-25 DUST Insecticide (Calif. Spray)	DDT* Sulfur * Copper * Zinc	5% 50% 4.5% 4.5%
PERSISTO-R 2-1 DUST Insecticide (Calif. Spray)	DDT Rotenone	2% 1%	PERSISTO S-KO 5-25-5 DUST Insecticide, fungicide (Calif. Spray)	DDT * Sulfur * Copper*	5% 25% 5%
PERSISTO-S 2-80 DUST Insecticide (Calif. Spray)	DDT Sulfur *	2% 80%	PERSISTO S-KO 5-50-5 DUST Insecticide, fungicide (Calif. Spray)	DDT * Sulfur* Copper *	5% 50% 5%
PERSISTO-S 2-90 DUST Insecticide, fungicide (Calif. Spray)	DDT Sulfur *	2% 90%	PERSISTO-TRAN-S 4-5-75 DUST Insecticide (Calif. Spray)	DDT Orthotran Sulfur*	4% 5% 75%
PERSISTO-S 3-75 DUST Insecticide, fungicide (Calif. Spray)	DDT Sulfur *	3% 75%	PERSISTO 50 WETTABLE Insecticide (Calif. Spray)	DDT *	50%
PERSISTO-S 4-75 DUST Insecticide (Calif. Spray)	DDT Sulfur *	4% 75%	PERSISTO-Y 5-8 DUST Insecticide, fungicide (Calif. Spray)	DDT * Copper as metallic *	5% 6.4%
PERSISTO-S 5-25 DUST Insecticide (Calif. Spray)	DDT * Sulfur *	5% 25%	PERSISTO ZINEB 1-4 DUST (Impregnated) Insecticide, fungicide (Calif. Spray)	DDT Zineb	1% 4%
PERSISTO-S 5-50 DUST Insecticide (Calif. Spray)	DDT * Sulfur *	5% 50%	PERSISTO ZINEB 5-3.25 DUST Insecticide, fungicide (Calif. Spray)	DDT* Zineb	5% 3.25%
PERSISTO-S 5-75 DUST Insecticide (Calif. Spray)	DDT* Sulfur *	5% 75%	PERSISTO ZINEB 5-4 DUST Insecticide, fungicide (Calif. Spray)	DDT * Zineb	5% 4%
PERSISTO-S 5-80 DUST Insecticide (Calif. Spray)	DDT * Sulfur *	5% 80%			

*Consult Sec. II., Ingredients Index. This ingredient may be responsible for major toxic effects if poisonous amounts of this product are ingested.

Name & Use Manufacturer	Ingredients	
PERSISTO ZINEB-S 5-3.25-25 DUST Insecticide, fungicide (Calif. Spray)	DDT * Zineb Sulfur *	5% 3.25% 25%
PERSISTO ZINEB-S 5-5.2-50 DUST Insecticide, fungicide (Calif. Spray)	DDT * Zineb Sulfur *	5% 5.2% 50%
PERSULAN ANTISEPTIC SHAMPOO (Drake Labs.)		
PERSULAN OINTMENT (Drake Labs.)		
PER-SYN- AMEL SYNTHETICS Paint products (Thresher)		
PERTENAL Hypertension (Crookes)	Veratrum viride ext.* Mannitol hexanitrate Homatropine methylbromide Phenobarbital*	100 mg. 30 mg. 2.5 mg. 15 mg.
PERTEX Dairy cleaner (Diversey)		
PERTHANE TECHNICAL Fungicide (Rohm & Haas)	Diethyl diphenyl dichloroethane* Related reaction products	95% 5%
PERTHANE 50% WP Fungicide (Rohm & Haas)	Diethyl diphenyl dichloroethane* Related reaction products	47.5% 2.5%
PERTOXIN FUMIGANT (Whitmoyer)	Ethylene dichloride* Carbon tetrachloride* Propylene dichloride	
PERTOXIN SPRAY Insecticide (Whitmoyer)	Petroleum oil Carbon tetrachloride* Tech. piperonyl butoxide Pyrethrins	
PERTUSSIN Antitussive (Seeck)	Extr. thyme Ethyl alcohol	 9%
PE-RU-NA Antitussive (Consolid. Royal)	Alcohol Potassium iodide Iron citrate Ammonium citrate Extr. gentian Extr. boniset Extr. cascara sagrada Oleoresin ginger	15%
PERZON LOTION Rubefacient (Vital)	Ferric oxides Ferric chloride* Zinc oxide Calcium oxide Benzocaine Carbolic acid* Aluminum ammonium sulfate *	 0.5%

Name & Use Manufacturer	Ingredients	
PESGEL INSECT REPELLENT (Jay's)		
PESTAWAY INSECT SPRAY (Uncle Sam)	DDT* Pyrethrum Petroleum distillate*	5%
PEST-B-GON 2 SPRAY Insecticide (Calif. Spray)	DDT Aromatic petroleum deriv. solvent*	25.0% 72.1%
PEST-B-GON WETTABLE- DDT 50% Insecticide (Calif. Spray)	DDT*	50.00%
PEST CONTROL HEXACHLOR 47 Insecticide (Pest Control Prod.)	Tech. chlordane*	47%
PESTENE INSECTICIDE POWDER (Uncle Sam)	DDT*	10%
PESTENE INSECT SPRAY (Uncle Sam)	DDT* Pyrethrum Petroleum distillate*	5%
PEST-HEX Insecticide (Blue Ridge)	n-Trichloromethyl thio- tetrahydro phthalamide 2-(p-tert-Butylphenoxy) isopropyl 2-chloroethyl sulfite	 2.5% 2.25%
PESTMASTER DUTCH ELM SPRAY Insecticide (Michigan)	DDT Xylene* Oil	25%
PESTMASTER EASY- EMULSIFYING CONCEN- TRATE 25% DDT Insecticide (Michigan)	DDT* Oil	25%
PESTMASTER METHYL BROMIDE Fumigant (Michigan)	Methyl bromide*	100%
PESTMASTER METHYL BROMIDE WITH CHLOROPI- CRIN WARN- ING AGENT Fumigant (Michigan)	Methyl bromide* Chloropicrin	98% 2%
PESTMASTER SOIL FUMI- GANT-1 (Michigan)	Methyl bromide* Chloropicrin	98% 2%

---

*Consult Sec. II., Ingredients Index. This ingredient may be responsible for major toxic effects if poisonous amounts of this product are ingested.

Name & Use Manufacturer	Ingredients		Name & Use Manufacturer	Ingredients	
PESTMASTER WETTABLE POWDER 50% DDT Insecticide (Michigan)	DDT*	50%	DR. PETER'S GOMOZO Cathartic (Fahrney)	Alcohol Senna Fennel Mandrake root Peppermint Spearmint Sarsparilla Sassafras Hyssap Bussed thistle Dittany Ground ivy Johnswort Lemon balm sage Spikenard Yarroii	14%
PESTMASTER WETTABLE POWDER 75% DDT Insecticide (Michigan)	DDT*	75%			
PESTRON PESTICIDE (Pest Control Prod.)	Gamma isomer of benzene hexachloride* (from lindane)	99%	PETERSON'S OINTMENT (Peterson)	Carbolic acid* Camphor* Tannic acid* Zinc oxide Beeswax Balsam of fir Oil of lavender Petrolatum	
PESTROY 25% DDT CON- CENTRATE Insecticide (Acme Q.)	DDT concentrate Xylene*	25%			
PESTROY 25% DDT CON- CENTRATE Insecticide (Sherwin- Williams)	DDT Xylene*	25% 65%	PETIKET CHLOROPHYLL DEODORANT FOR PETS (U. S. Chem.)		
PESTROY DDT LIQUID COATING & INSECT POWDER (Lucas)	DDT*		PETKLENE FOR DOGS Cleanser, deodorant, flea killer (Levis)	Pine oil * Soap	80% 10%
PESTROY PRE- EMERGENCE WEED KILLER (Sherwin- Williams)	Diethyl xanthogen disulfide*	58%	PETROFOL Cathartic (Rexall)	Mineral oil	
			PETROGALAR Cathartic (Wyeth Labs.)	Mineral oil	65%
PEST WAX Insecticide (Chemurgic)	DDT*		PETROGEN IODIZED Rubefacient (Wyeth Labs.)	Iodized ammonium oleate Total iodine* Alcohol	10% 7%
PETADERM Fungicide (veterinary) (Levis)	Sodium caprylate*	20%	PETROHOL Rubefacient (Enjay)	Isopropyl alcohol*	91-99%/v
PET-D-TICK Insecticide (Martin, C. J.)	Gamma isomer of benzene hexachloride (from lindane) Rotenone Other cube resins Pine oil	0.05% 1.00% 2.00% 3.00%	PETROHOL ISOPROPYL ALCOHOL COMPOUND N.F. Rubefacient (Allied Drug)	Isopropyl alcohol*	70%
PET-EEZ ANTISEPTIC POWDER (Ridd Lab.)	Iodine* Boric acid*		PETROPINE PAINT THINNER (Reliable Paste)	Mineral spirits Toluol * Benzol *	
PETER PUTTER'S SPOT REMOVER Wall paper cleaner (Glidden Co.)			PETRO- SYLLIUM NO. 2 WITH PHENOL- PHTHALEIN Cathartic (Whitehall)	Each fl. oz.: Phenolphthalein Mineral oil Psyllium jelly	3-3/4 gr.

Name & Use Manufacturer	Ingredients	
PETROZOIN NIPPLE OINTMENT (Petrozoin)	Alcohol Gum benzoin Aloes Stryax Balsam tolu Pure petrolatum	11-1/2%
PETRYN IMPROVED Spot remover (Patek)	Decalin* Paracymene	
PETSELANE DEODORANT (Pearson Pharm.)		
PET SPECIAL CLEANSER (Solvay)	Carbonates Silicates Phosphates*	
DR. PETTIT'S AMERICAN EYE SALVE (Howard Bros.)	Mercury ammoniated* Boric acid* Camphor* Zinc oxide	8.75 gr.
DR. PETTIT'S AMERICAN EYE WATER (Howard Bros.)	Potassium alum Boric acid Camphor Glycerin Salt	
DR. PETTIT'S RECTAL SALVE (Howard Bros.)	Mercury ammoniated* Calomel* Boric acid* Camphor* Zinc oxide	8.75 gr. 5.83 gr.
PETZOL Ectoparasiticide (veterinary) (Levis)	Benzyl benzoate Benzyl alcohol	25% 2%
PEXOL GRAHAM'S Antitussive (Assoc. Prod.)	Chloroform White pine Wild cherry Spikenard Poplar buds Sanguinaria Sassafras * Irish moss Menthol * Oil of tar * Oil of eucalyptus * Ammonium chloride Glycerin Honey	3 m./fl. oz.
PEXOLINE PINOLENE & THREECO, FOURCO, FIVECO, SIXCO PINE OIL DISINFECTANTS (Peck's)	Steam-distilled pine oil * Soap	
PEX O PINE 5 DISINFECTANT (Peck's)	Soap Steam-distilled pine oil * 4-Chloro-2-phenyl phenol* 6-Chloro-2-phenyl phenol*	
PFANSTIEHL 20 BACTERICIDE (Pfanstiehl)	Para-di-isobutyl phenoxy ethoxy ethyl dimethyl benzyl ammonium chloride monohydrate* 20%/w	

Name & Use Manufacturer	Ingredients	
PFEIFFER'S BEEF, IRON & WINE Food supplement (Pfeiffer)	Alcohol Beef peptone Iron ammonium citrate	18%
PFEIFFER'S WHITE PINE & TAR MENTHOLATED Antitussive (Pfeiffer)	Ammonium chloride Glycerin Sugar syrup Chloroform	4 m./fl. oz.
P-51 FAST KILL INSECT SPRAY WITH DDT (Tru-Pine)	DDT Allethrin n-Octyl bicycloheptene dicarboximide Methylated naphthalenes* Petroleum hydrocarbon* Beta butoxy beta thiocyano diethyl ether	2.00% 0.10% 0.50% 5.00% 11.40% 1.00%
P. F. OINTMENT (Casmith)	Phenol Nutgalls Quinine Petrolatum Beeswax	
P-40 Insecticide (Plant Prod.)	Sodium selenate*	2%
P-F RECTAL OINTMENT (Casmith)		
PFUNDER'S TABLETS FOR HYPERACID STOMACHS (Grove)	Bismuth subcarbonate Sodium bicarbonate Magnesium hydroxide Calcium carbonate	
P & G BAR LAUNDRY SOAP (Procter & Gamble)		
PHAGENE POWDER Vaginal douche (Dumas-Wilson)	Citric acid Lactose Papain Methyl salicylate* Eucalyptol* Menthol* Chlorothymol * Chlorophyll	
PHALEN'S PAINTS, ENAMELS, VARNISHES (Phelan-Faust)		
PHARMALAX LAXATIVE SUPPOSITORIES (Pharmacia)	Each suppository: Sodium bicarbonate Potassium bitartrate	0.6 gm. 0.9 gm.
PHARMEX CHILDREN'S ASPIRIN (Pharmex)	Aspirin* Raspberry flavoring	1/4 gr.
PHARMEX CHILDREN'S COLD TABLETS (Pharmex)	Aspirin* Acetophenetidin* Caffeine	1-1/2 gr. 1 gr. 1/10 gr.

*Consult Sec. II., Ingredients Index. This ingredient may be responsible for major toxic effects if poisonous amounts of this product are ingested.

Name & Use Manufacturer	Ingredients		Name & Use Manufacturer	Ingredients	
PHARMEX CHILDREN'S NOSE DROPS (Pharmex)	Phenylephrine hydrochloride*	1/4%	pH DERMACAP Cradle cap (Fredenburgh- Hecht)	Peptone-gluconic acid buffer pH 3.5 Chlorothymol Benzoic acid	0.1% 1.2%
PHARMEX COLD SORE LOTION (Pharmex)	Benzoin * Storax Tolu Camphor* Alcohol*		pH DERMAGUENT Antiseptic skin ointment (Fredenburgh- Hecht)	Gluconic acid buffer pH 3.5 Benzoic acid Chlorothymol Zinc phenolsulfonate	0.2% 0.1% 1%
PHARMEX CORN RE- MOVER (Pharmex)	Salicylic acid* Flexible collodion*		PHELAC BRUSHING LACQUER (Phelan- Faust)		
PHARMEX DIURETIC PILLS-GREEN (Pharmex)	Asparagus Uva ursi Buchu Corn silk Oil of juniper Licorice		PHELITE INDUSTRIAL WHITE Paint (Phelan- Faust)		
PHARMEX GLYCERINE SUPPOSI- TORIES (Pharmex)	Glycerin U.S.P.	95%	PHELUXE PAINTS, ENAMELS, LACQUERS, VARNISHES (Phelan-		
PHARMEX INHALER (Pharmex)	Amphetamine* Mustard Menthol * Camphor* Eucalyptol*	250 mg.	Faust) PHE-MER- CAINE (Yellow) Counter- irritant (throat)	Each tablet: Phe-Mer-Nite (mercury* preparation) Benzocaine Menthol* Eucalyptol *	0.16 mg. 4 mg.
PHARMEX LIQUID ANALGESIC (Pharmex)	Gum camphor* Methyl salicylate* Turpentine Oil of sassafras * Alcohol		(Massengill)	Pinene * Eugenol * Methyl salicylate (synthetic)* Oil of lemon	
PHARMEX MEDICATED SALVE (Pharmex)	Oil linseed Petrolatum Zinc oxide Starch Phenol* Boric acid*		PHE-MER-NITE Vaginal sup- positories (Massengill)	Phe-Mer-Nite (phenylmercuric nitrate) Glycero-gelatin base	
PHARMEX RECTAL COMBINATION PACKAGE Suppositories, ointment (Pharmex)	Istrian nutgalls Zinc oxide Benzocaine		PHE-MER-NITE NO. 2 OINT- MENT Skin fungicide (medical) (Massengill)	Phe-Mer-Nite (mercury preparation)	1-1500
PHARMEX RECTAL SUPPOSI- TORIES (Pharmex)	Bismuth subgallate Bismuth oxyiodide Peru balsam Resorcin* Zinc oxide Boric acid*		PHE-MER-NITE (Pink) Throat Lozenge (Massengill)	Each tablet: Phe-Mer-Nite (phenylmercuric nitrate) Benzocaine Menthol* Eucalyptol * Pinene *	1/200 gr. 1/16 gr.
PHARMEX TEETHING LOTION (Pharmex)	Benzocaine Iodine* Alcohol*			Eugenol * Methyl salicylate (synthetic)*	
PHARMEX TOOTHACHE OUTFIT (Pharmex)	Oil of cloves* Oil of casia Benzocaine Iodine* Petrohol		PHE-MER-NITE SPERMICIDAL Vaginal sup- positories (Massengill)	Phe-Mer-Nite (phenylmercuric nitrate) Cocoa butter base	
PHARMEX WART REMOVER (Pharmex)	Ricinic acid Castor oil Isopropyl alcohol*				
PHASTA LIQUID PASTE (Stafford)					

*Consult Sec. II., Ingredients Index. This ingredient may be responsible for major toxic effects if poisonous amounts of this product are ingested.

Name & Use Manufacturer	Ingredients		Name & Use Manufacturer	Ingredients	
PHENACIDE WE-60 Insecticide (Thompson-Hayward)	Toxaphene* Petroleum distillate	60.0% 34.0%	PHENO Dietary supplement (avian) (Gland-O-Lac)	Calcium phenolsulfonate* Sodium phenolsulfonate* Zinc phenolsulfonate* Dextrose Sodium sulfate Boric acid*	6.25% 3.85% 15.9%
PHENASEPTOL Disinfectant, deodorant (Burrough)	Tar acids* Coal tar hydrocarbon oils* Soap		PHENO AID Counter-irritant (skin) (Wisconsin Pharm.)	Camphor* Carbolic acid* Eucalyptol *	
PHENATIN Analgesic (Jenkins)	Each tablet: Acetophenetidin* Acetylsalicylic acid* Caffeine Camphor monobromated*	3 gr. 4 gr. 1/2 gr. 1-1/2 gr.	PHENO-BOLUS Anthelmintic (veterinary) (Martin, C. J.)	Phenothiazine* Cornstarch	12.5 gm. 1 gm.
PHEN-NIC POWDER Insecticide (Greever's)	Phenothiazine Nicotine (as alkaloid)*	33.33% 2.5%	PHENO-BROMIDE COMPOUND Analgesic, sedative (Jeffrey-Fell)	Each oz.: Phenobarbital* Sodium bromide Potassium bromide Ammonium bromide Extr. belladonna Extr. hyoscyamus Aromatic Alcohol	1 gr. 20 gr. 20 gr. 20 gr. 1/8 gr. 1/8 gr. q.s. 3-3/4%
PHEN-NIC TABLETS Insecticide (Greever's)	Phenothiazine Nicotine (as alkaloid)* Kaolin	7.75 gr. 50 gr. 3.00 gr.
PHEN-I-CIDE Insecticide (Interstate Med.)	Phenothiazine* Phenolphthalein* Ground oil cake		PHENO-CASALATE Biliary stimulant, cathartic (Clapp, Otis)	Extr. nux vomica* Copper arsenite Bile, dried and partially purified Phenolphthalein Extr. cascara Capsicum	1/16 gr. 1/1000 gr. 1 gr. 1/2 gr. 1/2 gr. 1/100 gr.
PHENIDONE Photo developing agent (Ringwood)		
PHENIKA POULTRY WORM PILLS Anthelmintic (veterinary, avian) (Martin, C. J.)	Phenothiazine Nicotine sulfate* Powdered extr. kamala Shellac Calcium carbonate Gelatin Acacia Castor oil Calcium pyrophosphate Talcum Stearic acid	25.30% 3.25% 6.84%	PHENO-CHENAL KRUMBLES FOR HOGS Anthelmintic (veterinary) (McClellan)	Phenothiazine* Aloes * Epsom salts American wormseed oil (containing ascardiol) Magnesium carbonate	60% 6% 10% 2% 22%
			PHENO-COSAN Counter-irritant (skin) (Whitney)	Mercury ammoniated* Sulfur* Coal tar solution* Mercury salicylate* Resorcin	0.3% 0.3%
PHENIKA WORMER Anthelmintic (veterinary) (Martin, C. J.)	Each fl. oz.: Phenothiazine Nicotine sulfate* Kamala	12.5 gr. 0.5 gr. 1.5 gr.	PHENO-FLAVINE EYE DROPS (Altone)		
PHENIKA WORM POWDER Anthelmintic (veterinary) (Martin, C. J.)	Phenothiazine Kamala Nicotine sulfate*	12.5 gm. 1.5 gm. 0.5 gm.	PHENOLAX WAFERS Laxative (Upjohn)	Phenolphthalein Sugar Aromatics	1 gr.
PHE-NI-ZENE (Granules) Anthelmintic (veterinary, avian) (Corn King)	Nicotine* Phenothiazine		PHENOL-PHTHALEIN PETROGALAR Laxative (Wyeth)	Phenolphthalein Mineral oil	0.3% 65%
PHE-NI-ZENE (Tablets) Anthelmintic (veterinary, avian) (Corn King)	Nicotine* (as alkaloid) Phenothiazine	0.75 gr. 7.5 gr.	PHENOL SODIQUE OINTMENT (Hance)	Phenol sodique* Cycloform Zinc stearate Lanolin petrolatum Resorcin Zinc peroxide Zinc oxide Glycerin	
PHENLIN-ORIS OINTMENT (Wood, J.)	Sodium phenolate* Tertiary amyl phenol* Lanolin-wax ointment		PHENO-NIC POWDER Anthelmintic (veterinary, avian) (Hilltop)	Phenothiazine Nicotine*	33-1/3% 3-1/3%

*Consult Sec. II., Ingredients Index. This ingredient may be responsible for major toxic effects if poisonous amounts of this product are ingested.

Name & Use Manufacturer	Ingredients

Name & Use Manufacturer	Ingredients	
PHENOPLAST METAL, WOOD, PLASTIC COATINGS (Phenoplast)		
PHENOPLAST WATER-PROOF COATING (Phenoplast)		
PHENOSAN Disinfectant, deodorant (Carpenter)	Isopropyl alcohol* Vegetable oil soap Orthophenylphenol* Chlor-orthophenylphenol* Essential oils*	
PHEN-OVINE Anthelmintic (veterinary) (Globe)	Phenothiazine*	37.62%
PHENRIN Analgesic (Pinkham)	Each tablet: Phenacetin* Aspirin* Caffeine	2.50 gr.
PHENSAL GRAY Analgesic (Pitman-Morre)	Each tablet: Acetophenetidin* Acetylsalicylic acid* Extr. gelsemium Caffeine	2 gr. 4 gr. 1/4 gr. 3 m.
PHENYLDRINE NOSE DROPS & SOLUTION (Pharmex)	Phenylephrine hydrochloride* Antihistamine*	1/4% 0.1%
PHEOCAL PASTE (P.C.P. Paste) (Torch)	Phenol* Calomel* Lassar's paste	1% 3% q.s.
PHE-O-NIK POWDER Anthelmintic (veterinary, avian) (Texas Pheno.)	Phenothiazine N.F. Nicotine* (as alkaloid)	33.33% 3.33%
PHE-O-NIK TABLETS Anthelmintic (veterinary, avian) (Texas Pheno.)	Each tablet: Phenothiazine Nicotine*	7.4 gr. 0.8 gr.
pH HAIR PREPARATION (Fredenburgh-Hecht)	Peptone-gluconic acid buffer pH 3.5 Chlorthymol Benzoic acid	0.05% 0.2%
PHILADELPHIA WEED KILLER (West Disinf.)	Coal tar neutral oil* Soap Higher homologs of phenol Cresols* Phenol*	
PHIL-COTE PAINTS (Harris Stand.)		
PHILLIPS CORONA OINTMENT (Corona Mfg.)	Lanolin Concentrated lanolin deriv. Petrolatum Beeswax Borax Aromatic oil Methyl salicylate * Parachlormercuriphenol 1/1500%	
PHILLIPS MILK OF MAGNESIA DENTIFRICE (Phillips, C.)		
PHISODERM (and for Dry Skin & Scalp) Detergent (Winthrop)	Entsufon Lanolin Cholesterols Petrolatum	
PHISOHEX Detergent, antiseptic (Winthrop)	Entsufon (sodium octyl-phenoxyethoxyethyl ether sulfonate) Lanolin Petrolatum Hexachlorophene	3%/w
PHLOGO PHLOGESTIC POWDER (Veterinary) (Thoroughbred)	Thymol* Oil of peppermint Boric acid* Bentonite Methyl salicylate* Oil of eucalyptus * Kaolin	
PHLO HECTO CREAM Ink remover (Chem. Spec.)		
PHLO NEUTRAL SKIN PROTECTOR (Chem. Spec.)	Lanolin Silicone fortified	
PHLO WATERLESS CLEANER (Chem. Spec.)		
PHOENIX BRAND ADTOX 2.5 Insecticide (Arizona)	Hexachloro hexahydro dimethano naphthalene*	2.375%
PHOENIX BRAND ARATOX 3 Insecticide (Arizona)	2-(p-tert-Butylphenoxy) isopropyl-2-chloroethyl sulfite (Aramite)	3.00%
PHOENIX BRAND BENTOX 1 AND 2 Herbicide (Arizona)	Hexachlorocyclohexane*	
PHOENIX BRAND BENTOX DB-10 Insecticide (Arizona)	Gamma isomer of benzene hexachloride* Other isomers of benzene hexachloride and related compounds*	10% 15%
PHOENIX BRAND BENTOX 2 PLUS DYTOX 5 Insecticide (Arizona)	Gamma isomer of benzene hexachloride* Other isomers of benzene hexachloride Dichloro diphenyl tri-chloroethane*	2.00% 3.50% 5.00%

*Consult Sec. II., Ingredients Index. This ingredient may be responsible for major toxic effects if poisonous amounts of this product are ingested.

Name & Use Manufacturer	Ingredients		Name & Use Manufacturer	Ingredients	
PHOENIX BRAND BENTOX 2 PLUS DYTOX 5 w/SULFUR Insecticide (Arizona)	Gamma isomer of benzene hexachloride* Other isomers of benzene hexachloride Dichloro diphenyl-trichloroethane* Sulfur*	2.00% 3.50% 5.00% 50.00%	PHOENIX BRAND CAMTOX EC-60 Insecticide (Arizona)	Toxaphene*	60.00%
PHOENIX BRAND BENTOX 2 PLUS DYTOX 10 Insecticide (Arizona)	Gamma isomer of benzene hexachloride* Other isomers of benzene hexachloride Dichloro diphenyl tri-chloroethane*	2.00% 3.50% 10.00%	PHOENIX BRAND CAMTOX 10 PLUS CUPROCIDE 9 WITH 50% SULFUR Insecticide, fungicide (Arizona)	Toxaphene* Yellow cuprous oxide* Sulfur *	10.00% 9.00% 50.00%
PHOENIX BRAND BENTOX 2 WITH SULFUR Insecticide (Arizona)	Gamma isomer of benzene hexachloride* Other isomers of benzene hexachloride Sulfur*	2.00% 4.80% 50.00%	PHOENIX BRAND CAMTOX 10 PLUS DYTOX 5 Insecticide (Arizona)	Toxaphene* Dichloro diphenyl tri-chloroethane*	10.00% 5.00%
PHOENIX BRAND BENTOX 3 Insecticide (Arizona)	Gamma isomer of benzene hexachloride * Other isomers of benzene hexachloride	3.00% 5.25%	PHOENIX BRAND CAMTOX 10 PLUS DYTOX 5 w/50% SULFUR Insecticide (Arizona)	Toxaphene* DDT* Sulfur*	10.00% 5.00% 50.00%
PHOENIX BRAND BENTOX 3 PLUS DYTOX 5 Insecticide (Arizona)	Gamma isomer of benzene hexachloride* Other isomers of benzene hexachloride Dichloro diphenyl tri-chloroethane*	3.00% 5.25% 5.00%	PHOENIX BRAND CAMTOX 10 WITH SULFUR Insecticide (Arizona)	Toxaphene* Sulfur*	10.00% 50.00%
PHOENIX BRAND BENTOX 3 PLUS DYTOX 5 w/SULFUR Insecticide (Arizona)	Gamma isomer of benzene hexachloride* Other isomers of benzene hexachloride Dichloro diphenyl tri-chloroethane* Sulfur*	3.00% 5.25% 5.00% 40.00%	PHOENIX BRAND CAMTOX 15 Insecticide (Arizona)	Toxaphene*	15.00%
PHOENIX BRAND BENTOX 3 PLUS DYTOX 10 Insecticide (Arizona)	Gamma isomer of benzene hexachloride * Other isomers of benzene hexachloride Dichloro diphenyl tri-chloroethane *	3.00% 5.25% 10.00%	PHOENIX BRAND CAMTOX 15 PLUS CHLORTOX 5 Insecticide (Arizona)	Toxaphene* Tech. chlordane	15.00% 5.00%
PHOENIX BRAND BENTOX 3 PLUS DYTOX 10 WITH SULFUR Insecticide (Arizona)	Gamma isomer of benzene hexachloride* Other isomers of benzene hexachloride Dichloro diphenyl tri-chloroethane* Sulfur*	3.00% 7.20% 10.00% 40.00%	PHOENIX BRAND CAMTOX 15 PLUS DYTOX 5 Insecticide (Arizona)	Toxaphene* DDT	15.00% 5.00%
PHOENIX BRAND CAMTOX 10 Insecticide (Arizona)	Toxaphene* (tech. chlorinated camphene; chlorine content 67-69%)	10.00%	PHOENIX BRAND CAMTOX 15 PLUS DYTOX 5 PLUS ZINTOX 5 Insecticide, fungicide (Arizona)	Toxaphene* DDT Zineb (zinc ethylene-bis(dithiocarbamate)	15.00% 5.00% 5.20%
PHOENIX BRAND CAMTOX DB-40 Insecticide (Arizona)	Toxaphene*	40.0%			

*Consult Sec. II., Ingredients Index. This ingredient may be responsible for major toxic effects if poisonous amounts of this product are ingested.

Name & Use Manufacturer	Ingredients	
PHOENIX BRAND CAMTOX 15 PLUS DYTOX 5 WITH 40% SULFUR Insecticide (Arizona)	Toxaphene*	15.00%
	DDT	5.00%
	Other isomers of dichloro diphenyl trichloroethane	1.25%
	Sulfur	40.00%
PHOENIX BRAND CAMTOX 15 PLUS DYTOX 10 Insecticide (Arizona)	Toxaphene*	15.00%
	DDT	10.00%
PHOENIX BRAND CAMTOX 15 WITH 50% SULFUR Insecticide (Arizona)	Toxaphene*	15.00%
	Sulfur	50.00%
PHOENIX BRAND CAMTOX 20 Insecticide (Arizona)	Toxaphene* (tech. chlorinated camphene; chlorine content 67-69%)	20.00%
PHOENIX BRAND CAMTOX 20 PLUS DYTOX 5 Insecticide (Arizona)	Toxaphene*	20.00%
	DDT	5.00%
PHOENIX BRAND CAMTOX 20 WITH SULFUR Insecticide (Arizona)	Toxaphene*	20.00%
	Sulfur	40.00%
PHOENIX BRAND CHLORTOX DB-25 Insecticide (Arizona)	Tech. chlordane*	25.00%
PHOENIX BRAND CHLORTOX EC-40 Insecticide (Arizona)	Tech. chlordane*	44.2%
PHOENIX BRAND CHLORTOX 5 Insecticide (Arizona)	Tech. chlordane* (3% octachloro-4, 7-methano tetrahydroindane and 2% related compounds)	5.00%
PHOENIX BRAND CHLORTOX 5 PLUS DYTOX 5 Insecticide (Arizona)	Tech. chlordane*	5.00%
	Dichloro diphenyl tri-chloroethane*	5.00%
PHOENIX BRAND CHLORTOX 5 PLUS DYTOX 10 Insecticide (Arizona)	Tech. chlordane*	5.00%
	Dichloro diphenyl tri-chloroethane*	10.00%

Name & Use Manufacturer	Ingredients	
PHOENIX BRAND CUPROCIDE 9 Fungicide (Arizona)	Yellow cuprous oxide* (copper as metallic 8.00%)	9.00%
PHOENIX BRAND DIELTOX 2 Insecticide (Arizona)	Hexachloro epoxy octahydro dimethano naphthalene*	1.70%
	Related compounds	0.30%
PHOENIX BRAND DIELTOX 2 PLUS DYTOX 5 Insecticide (Arizona)	Hexachloro epoxy octahydro-endo,exo-dimethano naphthalene (from dieldrin)*	1.70%
	Related compounds (from dieldrin)	0.30%
	Dichloro diphenyl tri-chloroethane*	5.00%
PHOENIX BRAND DIELTOX 2 PLUS DYTOX 5 WITH 50% SULPHUR Insecticide (Arizona)	Hexachloro epoxy octahydro-endo,exo-dimethano naphthalene (from dieldrin)*	1.70%
	Related compounds (from dieldrin)	0.30%
	Dichloro diphenyl tri-chloroethane*	5.00%
	Sulfur*	50.00%
PHOENIX BRAND DIELTOX 2 WITH 50% SULPHUR Insecticide (Arizona)	Hexachloro epoxy octahydro-endo,exo-dimethano naphthalene (from dieldrin)*	1.70%
	Related compounds (from dieldrin)	0.30%
	Sulfur*	50.00%
PHOENIX BRAND DIELTOX 2 WITH 80% SULPHUR Insecticide (Arizona)	Hexachloro epoxy octahydro-endo, exo-dimethano naphthalene (from dieldrin)*	1.70%
	Related compounds (from dieldrin)	0.30%
	Sulfur*	80.00%
PHOENIX BRAND DUST Insecticide (Arizona)	DDT*	
	Sulfur*	
PHOENIX BRAND DYTOX DB-50 Insecticide (Arizona)	Dichloro diphenyl tri-chloroethane*	50.0%
PHOENIX BRAND DYTOX 5 Insecticide (Arizona)	Dichloro diphenyl tri-chloroethane*	5.00%
PHOENIX BRAND DYTOX 5 PLUS KRYTOX 50 Insecticide (Arizona)	Sodium fluoaluminate* (fluorine as elemental 50.00%)	45.00%
	Dichloro diphenyl tri-chloroethane	5.00%
PHOENIX BRAND DYTOX 5 PLUS ZINTOX 5 Insecticide, fungicide (Arizona)	Dichloro diphenyl tri-chloroethane	3.75%
	Zineb (zinc ethylene-bis-(dithiocarbamate)	5.20%

*Consult Sec. II., Ingredients Index. This ingredient may be responsible for major toxic effects if poisonous amounts of this product are ingested.

Name & Use Manufacturer	Ingredients	
PHOENIX BRAND DYTOX 5 WITH SULFUR Insecticide (Arizona)	Dichloro diphenyl tri-chloroethane* Sulfur*	5.00% 50.00%
PHOENIX BRAND DYTOX 5 WITH 75% SULFUR Insecticide (Arizona)	Dichloro diphenyl tri-chloroethane* Sulfur*	5.00% 75.00%
PHOENIX BRAND DYTOX 7.5 WITH 50% SULFUR Insecticide (Arizona)	Dichloro diphenyl tri-chloroethane* Sulfur*	7.50% 50.00%
PHOENIX BRAND DYTOX 10 Insecticide (Arizona)	Dichloro diphenyl tri-chloroethane*	10.00%
PHOENIX BRAND DYTOX 10 PLUS ZINTOX 5 Insecticide, fungicide (Arizona)	Dichloro diphenyl tri-chloroethane* Zineb (zinc ethylene-bis-(dithiocarbamate)	10.00% 5.20%
PHOENIX BRAND DYTOX 10 WITH SULFUR Insecticide (Arizona)	Dichloro diphenyl tri-chloroethane* Sulfur*	10.00% 50.00%
PHOENIX BRAND DYTOX 10 WITH 70% SULFUR Insecticide (Arizona)	Dichloro diphenyl tri-chloroethane* Sulfur*	10.00% 70.00%
PHOENIX BRAND ENDTOX 2 Insecticide (Arizona)	Endrin (hexachloro epoxy octahydro-endo, endo-dimethano naphthalene)*	2.00%
PHOENIX BRAND ENTOX 2 WITH 50% SULFUR Insecticide (Arizona)	Endrin (hexachloro epoxy octahydro-endo, endo-dimethano naphthalene)* Sulfur	2.00% 50.00%
PHOENIX BRAND HEPTOX DB-25 Insecticide (Arizona)	Heptachlor (heptachloro-4, 7-methano tetrahydroindane)* Related compounds	25.00% 9.72%
PHOENIX BRAND KARATOX .75 Fungicide (Arizona)	Dinitro (1-methyl heptyl) phenyl crotonate* Other nitro phenols and derivatives, chiefly dinitro (1-methyl heptyl) phenol	0.675/w 0.075/w
PHOENIX BRAND KRYTOX 50 WITH SULFUR Insecticide (Arizona)	Sodium fluoaluminate* (fluorine as elemental 24.50%) Sulfur	45.00% 28.50%
PHOENIX BRAND KRYTOX 70 Insecticide (Arizona)	Sodium fluoaluminate* (fluorine as elemental 34.30%)	63.00%
PHOENIX BRAND MALATOX 5 Insecticide (Arizona)	Malathion*	5.00%
PHOENIX BRAND MALATOX DB-25 Insecticide (Arizona)	Malathion*	25.00%
PHOENIX BRAND MALATOX 5 & DYTOX 5 Insecticide (Arizona)	Malathion* Dichloro diphenyl tri-chloroethane*	5.00% 5.00%
PHOENIX BRAND MALATOX EC-57 Insecticide (Arizona)	Malathion* Xylene*	57.00% 32.00%
PHOENIX BRAND MALATOX EC-80 Insecticide (Arizona)	Malathion* Petroleum hydrocarbons	80.00% 4.00%
PHOENIX BRAND MALATOX 5 PLUS ZINTOX 5 Fungicide, insecticide (Arizona)	Malathion* Zineb (zinc ethylene-bis-(dithiocarbamate)	5.00% 5.20%
PHOENIX BRAND NICOTOX 10-X DRY Insecticide (Arizona)	Nicotine alkaloid*	3.60%
PHOENIX BRAND OVOTOX DB-50 Insecticide (Arizona)	p-Chlorophenyl p-chlorobenzene sulfonate*	50.00%
PHOENIX BRAND OVOTOX 7.5 Insecticide (Arizona)	p-Chlorophenyl p-chlorobenzene sulfonate*	7.50%
PHOENIX BRAND OVOTOX 10 Insecticide (Arizona)	p-Chlorophenyl p-chlorobenzene sulfonate* (Ovotran)	10.00%

*Consult Sec. II., Ingredients Index. This ingredient may be responsible for major toxic effects if poisonous amounts of this product are ingested.

Name & Use Manufacturer	Ingredients		Name & Use Manufacturer	Ingredients	
PHOENIX BRAND PARATOX 1 Insecticide (Arizona)	Parathion* (o, o-diethyl-o-p-nitro-phenyl thiophosphate)	1.00%	PHOENIX BRAND PARATOX 2 PLUS DYTOX 5 Insecticide (Arizona)	Parathion* Dichloro diphenyl tri-chloroethane	2.00% 5.00%
PHOENIX BRAND PARATOX 1 PLUS CAMTOX 15 PLUS DYTOX 5 Insecticide (Arizona)	Parathion* Toxaphene* (tech. chlorinated camphene; chlorine content 67-69%) DDT	1.00% 15.00% 5.00%	PHOENIX BRAND PARATOX 2 PLUS DYTOX 5 Insecticide (Arizona)	Parathion* Dichloro diphenyl tri-chloroethane Other isomers dichloro diphenyl trichloroethane	2.00% 3.75% 1.25%
PHOENIX BRAND PARATOX 1 PLUS CAMTOX 15 PLUS DYTOX 5 PLUS ZINTOX 5 Fungicide, insecticide (Arizona)	Parathion* Toxaphene* Dichloro diphenyl tri-chloroethane Zineb (zinc ethylene-bis-(dithiocarbamate)	1.00% 15.00% 5.00% 5.20%	PHOENIX BRAND PARATOX 2 PLUS DYTOX 10 Insecticide (Arizona)	Parathion* Dichloro diphenyl tri-chloroethane	2.00% 10.00%
			PHOENIX BRAND PARATOX 2 PLUS DYTOX 10 PLUS ZINTOX 5 Fungicide (Arizona)	Parathion* Dichloro diphenyl tri-chloroethane Zineb (zinc ethylene-bis-(dithiocarbamate)	2.00% 10.00% 5.20%
PHOENIX BRAND PARATOX 1 PLUS CAMTOX 15 PLUS DYTOX 5 WITH 40% SULFUR Insecticide (Arizona)	Parathion* Toxaphene* DDT Sulfur	1.00% 15.00% 5.00% 40.00%	PHOENIX BRAND PARATOX 2 PLUS OVOTOX 7.5 Insecticide (Arizona)	Parathion* Ovotran sulfonate (p-chlorophenyl p-chloro-benzene sulfonate)	2.00% 7.50%
PHOENIX BRAND PARATOX 1 PLUS CAMTOX 20 Insecticide (Arizona)	Parathion Toxaphene*	1.00% 20.00%	PHOENIX BRAND PARATOX 2 PLUS ZINTOX 5 Insecticide, fungicide (Arizona)	Parathion* Zineb (zinc ethylene-bis-(dithiocarbamate)	2.00% 5.20%
PHOENIX BRAND PARATOX 1 PLUS OVOTOX 7.5 Insecticide (Arizona)	Parathion* Ovotran (p-chlorophenyl p-chlorobenzene sulfonate)	1.00% 7.50%	PHOENIX BRAND PARATOX 2 PLUS ZINTOX 5 WITH 50% SULFUR Fungicide, insecticide (Arizona)	Parathion* Zineb (zinc ethylene-bis-(dithiocarbamate) Sulfur	2.00% 5.20% 50.00%
PHOENIX BRAND PARATOX 1 PLUS ZINTOX 5 Insecticide, fungicide (Arizona)	Parathion* Zineb (zinc ethylene-bis-(dithiocarbamate)	1.00% 5.20%			
PHOENIX BRAND PARATOX 2 Insecticide (Arizona)	Parathion*	2.00%	PHOENIX BRAND PARATOX 2 WITH 50% SULFUR Insecticide (Arizona)	Parathion* Sulfur	2.00% 50.00%
PHOENIX BRAND PARATOX 2 PLUS CAMTOX 15 Insecticide (Arizona)	Parathion* Toxaphene*	2.00% 15.00%	PHOENIX BRAND PARATOX 20 PLUS DYTOX 5 WITH 50% SULFUR Insecticide (Arizona)	Parathion* Dichloro diphenyl tri-chloroethane Sulfur	2.00% 5.00% 50.00%

Name & Use Manufacturer	Ingredients		Name & Use Manufacturer	Ingredients	
PHOENIX BRAND PENTA-FOLIANT (Arizona)	Pentachlorophenol* Petroleum solvents Special solvents	40.00% 35.00% 25.00%	PHYGON-XL Fungicide (Naugatuck)	Phygon (2, 3-dichloro-1, 4-naphthoquinone)* (dichlone)	50%
PHOENIX BRAND ZINTOX 5 Fungicide (Arizona)	Zineb (zinc ethylene-bis-(dithiocarbamate)	5.20%	PHYGON-XL-DDT Fungicide (Naugatuck)	Phygon (2, 3-dichloro-1, 4-naphthoquinone)* (dichlone) DDT	50% 3%
PHOENIX DUST MIXTURES MALATOX DB-25 Insecticide (Arizona)	Malathion (o, o-dimethyl dithiophosphate of diethyl mercaptosuccinate*)	25.00%	PHYGON-XL-N Fungicide (Naugatuck)	2, 3-Dichloro-1, 4-naphthoquinone* (dichlone)	50%
PHOENIX PAINTS (Adelphi)			PHYLEX Nasal spray (Professional)	Phenylephrine hydrochloride* U.S.P. Methylparaben Propylparaben Sodium bisulfite	1/4% 0.02% 0.01% 0.2%
PHOSFUME WE-25 Insecticide (Thompson-Hayward)	Parathion* Aromatic petroleum deriv. solvent	25% 70%	PHYLORINOL Oral antiseptic (Schaffer)	Iodophenol * Chlorophyll Boric acid	
PHOSPHATON Tonic (Tosan)	Alcohol Glycerophosphates Lecithin Avenine Vitamin B1	10%	PHYTEX OINTMENT Skin fungicide (medical) (Ames Drug)	Benzoic acid* Salicylic acid* Carbolic acid*	
PHOSPHO-SODA (Fleet) Antacid (Fleet)	Each 100 cc.: Sodium biphosphate Sodium phosphate	48 gm. 18 gm.	PHYTICIDE Skin fungicide (medical) (Southern Res.)	Benzoic acid* Thymol * Salicylic acid* Alcohol*	50%/v
PHOTO ACID FIXING BATH (Uricheck)			PHYTOLINE Overweight diet supplement (Walker Pharm.)	Pure phytolacca berry juice Alcohol	75% 23-1/2%
PHYGON-2D Fungicide (Naugatuck)	Phygon (dichlone: 2, 3-dichloro-1, 4-naphthoquinone)	2%	PHYTOMYCIN Fungicide (Squibb)	Streptomycin (as nitrate)	20%
PHYGON-3D Fungicide (Naugatuck)	Phygon (dichlone: 2, 3-dichloro-1, 4-naphthoquinone)	3%	PHY-TOX ANTISEPTIC OINTMENT Skin fungicide (medical) (Rae Chem.)	Salicylic acid* Benzoic acid Mercuric salicylate* Arsenic trioxide*	
PHYGON-4D Fungicide (Naugatuck)	Phygon (dichlone: 2, 3-dichloro-1, 4-naphthoquinone)	4%	PIAX PAINT (Debevoise)		
PHYGON MINT DUST Fungicide (Naugatuck)	2, 3-Dichloro-1, 4-naphthoquinone	1.5%	PICKARD 433 BRUSH KILLER Herbicide (Pickard)	Isopropyl ester 2, 4-dichloro phenoxy acetic acid* Isopropyl ester 2, 4, 5-trichloro phenoxy acetic acid* Pentachlorophenol*	15% 15% 15%
PHYGON NAUGETS Insecticide (Naugatuck)	2, 3-Dichloro-1, 4-naphthoquinone* (dichlone)	50%	PICKARD 434 BRUSH KILLER Herbicide (Pickard)	Isopropyl ester 2, 4-dichloro phenoxy acetic acid Isopropyl ester 2, 4, 5-trichloro phenoxy acetic acid Pentachlorophenol*	3.75% 3.75% 10.0%
PHYGON PASTE Fungicide (Naugatuck)	2, 3-Dichloro-1, 4-naphthoquinone*	55%	PICKERS FRIEND Hand lotion (Whayne)	Alcohol Glycerin Carbolic acid Bay rum Witch hazel	8% 0.1%
PHYGON SEED PROTECTANT (Naugatuck)	Phygon (2, 3-dichloro-1, 4-naphthoquinone)* (dichlone)	50%	PICK-GLO Poultry cannibalism control (Globe)	Oil chenopodium Paraffin oil Turkey red oil Sulfur Microcrystalline wax	2.5% 68% 1% 5.5% 23%
PHYGON TECHNICAL Insecticide (Naugatuck)	2, 3-Dichloro-1, 4-naphthoquinone* (dichlone)	95%			

*Consult Sec. II., Ingredients Index. This ingredient may be responsible for major toxic effects if poisonous amounts of this product are ingested.

Name & Use Manufacturer	Ingredients	
PICK-PASTE Poultry cannibalism control (Hess, Dr.)	Oil of chenopodium Pine oil	2.5% 1.0%
PIC-NIX Poultry cannibalism control (Hilltop)		
PICRAGOL Vaginal suppositories (Wyeth Labs.)	Silver picrate* 65 mg. or 0.13 gm. Boroglyceride-gelatin base	
PICRAGOL POWDER Vaginal antiseptic (Wyeth Labs.)	Silver picrate* Kaolin base	1%
PICRATAN OINTMENT Skin burns (Roemer)	Picric acid*	approx. 1/2%
PICRIDE Space fumigant (Dow)	Methyl bromide* Chloropicrin*	80%/w 20%
PICTOL Photo developer (Mallinckrodt)	Monomethyl-para-aminophenol sulfate*	
PICTONE Photographic agent (Mallinckrodt)		
PIEDMONT PAINT PRODUCTS (Purdum)		
PIED PIPER ANTU RAT KILLER (Pied Piper)	ANTU*	25%
PIED PIPER CHLOR-O- CIDE Insecticide (Pied Piper)	Tech. chlordane*	5%
PIED PIPER DOG SHAMPOO (Pied Piper)	Tech. chlordane*	6.5%
PIED PIPER FLEA POWDER (Pied Piper)	Lethane B71* Rhothane Dust	10% 50% 5%
PIED PIPER FLEA POWDER FOR PET BIRDS (Pied Piper)	Pyrethrins *	100%
PIED PIPER HOUSEHOLD INSECTICIDE (Pied Piper)	DDT*	
PIED PIPER INSECTICIDE (Pied Piper)	Tech. chlordane*	2%

Name & Use Manufacturer	Ingredients	
PIED PIPER KWIK-KILL MOUSE SEED (Pied Piper)	Strychnine*	0.3%
PIED PIPER MOTH CRYSTALS (Pied Piper)	Paradichlorobenzene*	95%
PIED PIPER RAT & MOUSE KILLER (Pied Piper)	Warfarin (3-(a-acetonylbenzyl)- 4-hydroxycoumarin)	0.025%
PIED PIPER ROACHOCIDE (Pied Piper)	Pyrethrins Sodium fluoride*	15% 10%
PIED PIPER RODENTICIDE (Pied Piper)	Red squill*	5%
PIED PIPER SURFACE SPRAY Insecticide (Pied Piper)	DDT*	5%
PIED PIPER WEED KILLER (Pied Piper)	2, 4-D amine salt* (2, 4- dichlorophenoxyacetic acid equiv. 32 oz./gal.)	
PIERCE S. S. COLOGNE (Pierce, S. S.)		
PIERCE OIL COLORS, PERFECT PAINT (Pierce, F. O.)		
DR. PIERCE'S A-NURIC TABLETS Diuretic, analgesic (Pierce's Prop.)	Sodium citrate Sodium salicylate* Sodium bicarbonate	
DR. PIERCE'S COMPOUND Tonic (Pierce's Prop.)	Extr. smart-weed herb Jamaica dogwood Wild yam Gum camphor Jamaica ginger	
DR. PIERCE'S FAVORITE PRESCRIPTION For menopause pain (Pierce's Prop.)	Caulophyllum Cimicifuga Berberis Black haw (Verburnum prunifoliam) Valerian	
DR. PIERCE'S GOLDEN MEDICAL DISCOVERY Tonic, gastric stimulant (Pierce's Prop.)	Gentian Berberis Sanguinaria Wild cherry bark Stone root Cascara Stillingia	
DR. PIERCE'S PLEASANT PELLETS Laxative (Pierce's Prop.)	Stramonium (alkaloid 1/6000 gr.) Podophyllin Resin Jalap Aloin	

*Consult Sec. II., Ingredients Index. This ingredient may be responsible for major toxic effects if poisonous amounts of this product are ingested.

Name & Use Manufacturer	Ingredients	
PIERRE CARTIER'S MEDICINE (Bay State)		
DR. PIERRE'S BORO-PHENO-FORM Suppositories (Pierre)	Boric acid* Salicylic acid* Methenamine* Chlorothymol* Oxyquinoline sulfate* Sodium phenolsulfonate* Lactic acid	
DR. PIERRE'S HYGEIAFORMS Douche (Pierre)	Each tablet: Acetanilid*	4 gr.
	Boric acid*	
	Beta-naphthol	1/8 gr.
	Powdered extr. henbane	1/2 gr.
	Powdered hydrastis	
	Zinc sulfate*	
DR. PIERRE'S LIVRO TONE Laxative (Pierre)	Each tablet: Extr. belladonna*	1/12 gr.
	Extr. cascara	
	Aloin *	
	Podophyllin	
	Oleoresin ginger	
DR. PIERRE'S SANGUI-NEURO Tonic (Pierre)	Each tablet: Extr. nux vomica*	1/10 gr.
	Asafetida	
	Extr. damiana	
	Extr. sumbul	
	Acid arsenous*	1/60 gr.
	Zinc phosphide	
	Ferrous carbonate	
	Extr. cascara sagrada	
PIG-NEEM Food supplement (veterinary) (Anchor Serum)	Iron	4000 ppm
	Copper	1000 ppm
	Manganese	50 ppm
	Cobalt	30 ppm
	Arsenic trioxide	20 ppm
PIKE'S CENTENNIAL SALVE Ointment (Pike, J. J.)	Methyl salicylate* Paraffin oil and wax Pure yellow beeswax Artificial oil sassafras*	
PIK-NO-MOR Poultry cannibalism control (Pratt Food)	Steam-distilled pine oil* Carbolic acid* Petrolatum base	4.5%
PILODERM Fungicide (medical) (Tarkan)	Sulfur* Salicylic acid* Oil of cade* Pilocarpine hydrochloride*	
PILOT Stove fuel (Carroll S. & V.)		
PIM Ointment (Rundle)	PCMX (parachlorometaxylenol)* Oil of cloves* Oil of sassafras * Lanolin Vanishing cream base Camphor* Oil of cajuput* Zinc oxide	
PINATINE TURPENTINE SUBSTITUTE (Baker P. & V.)		

Name & Use Manufacturer	Ingredients	
PINAUD'S AFTER SHAVE LOTION, HAIR TONIC (Nestle-Le Mur)		
PINAUD'S EAU DE QUININE HAIR TONIC (Pinaud)		
PINEASENE Deodorant cleanser (dogs) (McClellan)		
PINE-CO DISINFECTANT (Lyons, I. L.)	Pine oil*	80%
	Anhydrous soap	10%
PINE DISINFECTANT (Lester Labs.)	Pine oil* Soap	
PINEE COUGH SYRUP (Daly-Herring)		
PINEE LIVESTOCK PREPARATION (Daly-Herring)		
PINE EMULSO NO. 194 Disinfectant (Troy Ind.)	Steam-distilled pine oil* Vegetable oil Resin soap	
PINE FUME INHALANT (Am. Pharm.)		
PINE-O-CIDE Disinfectant (Hillyard Chem.)	Pine oil* and soap	96%
PINE OIL SANITIZING FLUID (Uncle Sam)	Pine oil* Soap	
PINE-OLA Disinfectant cleanser (Holcomb)	Caustic soda*	
PINE-O-LEAN CLEANER (Edison)		
PINE-OLE DISINFECTANT (Robertson)		
PINE-O-LENE PRESERVATIVES & STAINS (Moore-Leland)		

*Consult Sec. II., Ingredients Index. This ingredient may be responsible for major toxic effects if poisonous amounts of this product are ingested.

- 833 -

Name & Use Manufacturer	Ingredients	Name & Use Manufacturer	Ingredients
PINEOLEUM Nasal de-congestant (Baybank)	Menthol* Oil of cassia Pine needles Camphor* Oil of eucalyptus * Liquid petrolatum	PINEXT WOOD PRESERVA-TIVE (Southern Pine Extr.)	
PINEOLEUM WITH EPHEDRINE Nasal de-congestant (Baybank)	Menthol Oil of cassia Pine needles Ephedrine* Camphor* Oil of eucalyptus * Petrolatum	PINEY PINE DISINFECT-ANT (Martin, C. J.)	Pine oil* Soap
PINEOLEUM PINE OIL DIS-INFECTANTS (Hockwald)		PINGO STOVWAX & STOVGLAZ (Pingo)	
PINEOLL DISINFECT-ANT (Uncle Sam)		PINGO TARFREE Tar remover (Pingo)	
PINE-OL PINE Disinfectant (Germo)		PINK-A-DINE Analgesic (Etheridge)	Each fl. oz.: Phenacetin* 10 gr. Acetylsalicylic acid* Caffeine
PINE-OX-GEN GERMICIDE (Pine-Ox-Gen)		PINK DREFT Detergent (Procter & Gamble)	
PINESEPTIC HAIR LOTION (Pinetrine)	Resorcinol monoacetate N.N.R.* Beta-naphthol*	PINK GARDEN EAU DE TOILETTE (Parfums Charbert)	
PINE-SOL Disinfectant (Milner)	Steam-distilled pine oil* Isopropyl alcohol*	PINK ICE Cosmetic (Seager)	Magnesium oxide 0.042%
PINE TAR Insecticide (Florida Chem.)	Distilled pine tar from yellow pine Mixed terpenes* Resin acids	PINK MAGIC Hair rinse (Kroy)	Quaternary ammonium compound* Wetting agent Glyceryl mono stearate D & C color Perfume
PINE TREE DISINFECT-ANT (Ampion)	Pine oil* soap 90%	PINK SALVARINE DISHWASHING COMPOUND (Helder)	
PINE TREE GLOSS-CLEANER (Clifton)		PINKY NAIL POLISH REMOVER (Pinky)	
PINETRINE Rubefacient (Pinetrine)	Camphor* Menthol Oil of wintergreen* Alcohol* 50% Chloroform Turpentine* Oil of pine	PINO ALL PURPOSE SALVE Counter-irritant (Pino)	Oil pine * Camphor* Petrolatum Menthol * Methyl salicylate*
PINEX (Concentrate) (2-1/2 oz.) Antitussive (Pinex)	Alcohol 17% Chloroform* 18 m. Oil of pine tar * Potassium guaiacol sulfonate Oil of eucalyptus * Extr. grindelia Glycerin	PINO ANTISEPTIC HEALING OIL Counter-irritant (Pino)	Oil of pine* Gum camphor* Menthol*
PINEX (Prepared) (3.8 oz.) Antitussive (Pinex)	Alcohol 3% Chloroform 3 m. Potassium guaiacol sulfonate Oil of pine tar * Oil of eucalyptus * Extr. grindelia Glycerin	PINO-CEN Disinfectant (Central Chem.)	Steam-distilled pine oil* 83% Vegetable oil soap Phenol *

*Consult Sec. II., Ingredients Index. This ingredient may be responsible for major toxic effects if poisonous amounts of this product are ingested.

Name & Use Manufacturer	Ingredients
PINO HOT OIL LINIMENT (Pino)	Pine oil* Oil of wintergreen* Oil of mustard* Methyl salicylate*
PINOL ROOF COATING (Pinol)	
PINOL ROOFING CEMENT (Pinol)	
PINOL TAR MANGE SHAMPOO (veterinary) (Nat'l Prod.)	
PINOL WALL SIZE (Pinol)	
PINO PINE TAR & HONEY Antitussive (Pino)	Beechwood creosote * Menthol* Ipecac Cascarin Oil tar* Chloroform*
PI-NO-SEPTIC Antiseptic (Owl)	
PINOTOL Disinfectant (McKesson)	Pine oil* 84.8% Sulfonated vegetable oil anhydrous 6.0% Artificial oil of sassafras 0.2%
PINOZENE OINTMENT (Barlow-Maney)	Carbolic acid* 1% Zinc oxide Thymol Ichthyol Aromatic oils Aluminum acetate Menthol Camphor* Anesthesin
PINTAR DISINFECT-ANT, DE-ODORANT & CLEANSER (Robbins, G.)	Pine oil* Anhydrous soap
PINTOFF PAINT & VARNISH REMOVER (Internat. Paint)	Methylene chloride* Methanol*
PINTO PONY PAINTS (Deer-O)	
PINUS-CODEIA COMPOUND Antitussive (Stoddard)	Each fl. oz.: Codeine acetate 1 gr. Belladonna leaves 1/4 gr. (total alkaloids 0.3%) White pine bark 4 gr. Wild cherry bark 4 gr. Ipecac 1/2 gr. Terpin hydrate 1/2 gr. Magnesium sulfate 4 gr. Senna 4 gr. Glycerin

Name & Use Manufacturer	Ingredients
PINWAE PERMANENT WAVE SOLUTION (New Formula) (G. G.)	Waving solution: Thioglycolic acid* Monoethanolamine Ammonium sulfite* monohydrate Urea Cloud #104 Ammonia* Brij 35 Neutralizer: Ammonium dihydrogen phosphate Sodium bromate* Duponol M.E. or C.
PINWAE PERMANENT WAVE SOLUTION (Standard) (G. G.)	Waving solution: Monoethanolamine Thioglycolic acid* 100% Aqua ammonia* Ammonium carbonate* Nopco 1408 Neutroleum gamma Cloud #106 Neutralizer: Potassium bromate* Monosodium phosphate Trend
PINXAV Skin ointment (Bredenbeck)	Zinc and ferric oxide Aromatics Menthol Oleostearin Aluminum hydroxide Phenol 0.3% Petrolatum Lanolin
PINX PASTILLES (Baker, W. A.)	
PIONEER HEAVY DUTY CLEANER (Pioneer)	
PIONEER-HUDSON WHITE FLOOR OILS (Pioneer)	
PIONEER LEATHER SHAMPOO (Pioneer)	Neatsfoot oil Saddle soap Beeswax
PIONEER NEATSFOOT COMPOUND Leather cleaner (Pioneer)	
PIPEPLAST ENAMEL & PRIMERS (Indust. Mat.)	
PISO'S Antitussive (Piso)	Each fl. oz.: Chloroform 5 m. Ipecac Ammonium chloride Menthol
PITCAIRN VARNISHES (Pittsburgh Plate Glass)	

*Consult Sec. II., Ingredients Index. This ingredient may be responsible for major toxic effects if poisonous amounts of this product are ingested.

- 835 -

Name & Use Manufacturer	Ingredients		Name & Use Manufacturer	Ingredients	
PITTSBURGH ALDRIN 20 Insecticide (Pittsburgh Coke)	Hexahydro hexachloro dimethano naphthalene* (equiv. to 25% aldrin) Related compounds Aliphatic petroleum hydrocarbons	22.9% 17.3% 53.8%	PITTSBURGH CREOSOTE NO. 1 Wood pre- servative (Pittsburgh Plate Glass (Paint Div.))	Coal tar creosote*	98-1/2%
PITTSBURGH 60% ALDRIN EQUIVALENT SOLUTION Insecticide (Pittsburgh Coke)	Hexachloro hexahydro dimethano naphthalene* (equiv. to 60.0% aldrin) Related compounds	57.0% 43.0%	PITTSBURGH CREOSOTE NO. 2 Wood pre- servative (Pittsburgh Plate Glass (Paint Div.))	Coal tar creosote*	96-1/2%
PITTSBURGH BENZENE HEXA- CHLORIDE, TECHNICAL Insecticide (Pittsburgh Coke)	Gamma isomer of benzene hexachloride* Other isomers of benzene hexachloride*	13.5% 86.5%	PITTSBURGH DDT AL 20% Insecticide (Pittsburgh Coke)	DDT*	20%
PITTSBURGH BRUSH CLEANER (Pittsburgh Plate Glass)			PITTSBURGH 50% DDT DUST CON- CENTRATE Insecticide (Pittsburgh Coke)	DDT*	50.0%
PITTSBURGH 10-20 BRUSH KILLER Herbicide (Pittsburgh Coke)	Isooctyl ester 2, 4-dichloro- phenoxyacetic acid* Isooctyl ester 2, 4, 5-tri- chlorophenoxyacetic acid*	24.5% 11.7%	PITTSBURGH 25% DDT SPRAY CON- CENTRATE Insecticide (Pittsburgh Coke)	DDT Aromatic petroleum hydrocarbons *	25.0% 72.0%
PITTSBURGH BRUSH KILLER LO-VOL 4 Herbicide (Pittsburgh Coke)	Isooctyl ester 2, 4, 5-tri- chlorophenoxyacetic acid*	63.2%	PITTSBURGH DDT, TECH- NICAL Insecticide (Pittsburgh Coke)	DDT, tech.*	100.00%
PITTSBURGH BRUSH KILLER NO. 22 Herbicide (Pittsburgh Coke)	Isooctyl ester 2, 4-dichloro- phenoxyacetic acid* Isooctyl ester 2, 4, 5-tri- chlorophenoxyacetic acid*	33.7% 32.1%	PITTSBURGH 50% DDT WETTABLE POWDER Insecticide (Pittsburgh Coke)	DDT, tech.	50.0%
PITTSBURGH 45% CHLORDANE EMULSION CONCEN- TRATE Insecticide (Pittsburgh Coke)	Chlordane tech.* Aliphatic petroleum hydrocarbon*	45.0% 45.0%	PITTSBURGH DIELDRIN-150 Insecticide (Pittsburgh Coke)	Hexachloro epoxy-octahydro dimethano naphthalene* Related compounds Aromatic petroleum hydrocarbons*	15.8% 2.8% 76.4%
PITTSBURGH COMPOUND DRYER (Pittsburgh Plate Glass)			PITTSBURGH ESTER AIR SPRAY Herbicide (Pittsburgh Coke)	Butyl esters 2, 4-dichloro phenoxyacetic acid* (equiv. to 63.8% 2, 4-dichloro phenoxyacetic acid)	80.0%
PITTSBURGH 9-15 COTTON SPRAY CON- CENTRATE Insecticide (Pittsburgh Coke)	Gamma isomer hexachloro cyclohexane Other isomers hexachloro cyclohexane DDT Aromatic petroleum hydrocarbons *	10% 16% 16% 53%	PITTSBURGH ESTER WEED KILLER NO. 44 (Pittsburgh Coke)	Isopropyl ester 2, 4-dichloro phenoxy acetic acid* (equiv. to 38.3% 2, 4-dichloro phenoxy acetic acid)	45.5%
PITTSBURGH CRACK FILLER (Pittsburgh Plate Glass)			PITTSBURGH ESTER WEED KILLER NO. 80 (Pittsburgh Coke)	Butyl ester 2, 4-dichloro phenoxy acetic acid*	80%

*Consult Sec. II., Ingredients Index. This ingredient may be responsible for major toxic effects if poisonous amounts of this product are ingested.

Name & Use Manufacturer	Ingredients	Name & Use Manufacturer	Ingredients
PITTSBURGH ESTER WEED KILLER D-4 (Pittsburgh Coke)	Isooctyl ester 2, 4-dichloro phenoxy acetic acid* (equiv. to 45.0% 2, 4-dichloro phenoxy acetic acid) 67.8%	PITTSBURGH 20% LINDANE SPRAY CON- CENTRATE Insecticide (Pittsburgh Coke)	Gamma isomer of benzene hexachloride* 20.0% Aromatic petroleum hydrocarbons* 75.0%
PITTSBURGH FLOOR CLEANER (Pittsburgh Plate Glass)		PITTSBURGH 25% LINDANE WETTABLE POWDER Insecticide (Pittsburgh Coke)	Gamma isomer of benzene hexachloride* 25.0%
PITTSBURGH FLORHIDE FLOOR ENAMEL (Pittsburgh Plate Glass (Paint Div.))		PITTSBURGH MCP WEED KILLER (Pittsburgh Coke)	Dimethyl amine salt 2-methyl-4-chlorophenoxyacetic acid* (equiv. to 42.1% 2-methyl-4-chlorophenoxyacetic acid) 52.0%
PITTSBURGH FLUID OIL COLORS (Pittsburgh Plate Glass)		PITTSBURGH NITROX SPRAY CON- CENTRATE Insecticide (Pittsburgh Coke)	Methyl parathion* (o, o-dimethyl-o-nitrophenyl thiophosphate) 25.3% Aromatic petroleum hydrocarbons 64.7%
PITTSBURGH 10% GAMMA BHC DUST CONCEN- TRATE Insecticide (Pittsburgh Coke)	Gamma isomer of benzene hexachloride * 10.0% Other isomers of benzene hexachloride * 64.0%	PITTSBURGH 15% PARATHION WETTABLE POWDER, DUSTLESS Insecticide (Pittsburgh Coke)	Ethyl parathion* (o, o-diethyl-o-p-nitrophenylthiophosphate) 15.0%
PITTSBURGH 10% GAMMA BHC WET- TABLE POWDER Insecticide (Pittsburgh Coke)	Gamma isomer of benzene hexachloride* 10.0% Other isomers of benzene hexachloride* 64.0%	PITTSBURGH 25% PARATHION WETTABLE POWDER, DUSTLESS Insecticide (Pittsburgh Coke)	Ethyl parathion* (o, o-diethyl-o-p-nitrophenyl thiophosphate) 25.0%
PITTSBURGH GX-BHC SPRAY CON- CENTRATE Insecticide (Pittsburgh Coke)	Gamma isomer of benzene hexachloride 10.7% Other isomers of benzene hexachloride 19.9% Aromatic and aliphatic petroleum hydrocarbons* 66.4%	PITTSBURGH PARATHION 25 WM Insecticide (Pittsburgh Coke)	Parathion* (o, o-diethyl-o-p-nitrophenylthiophosphate) 25.0% Aromatic petroleum hydrocarbons 65.0%
PITTSBURGH HERBICIDE LO-VOL 6 (Pittsburgh Coke)	Isooctyl ester 2, 4, 5-trichloro phenoxy acetic acid 88.5%	PITTSBURGH SATINHIDE ENAMEL (Pittsburgh Plate Glass (Paint Div.))	
PITTSBURGH ISOOCTYL ESTER OF 2, 4-D TECHNICAL Herbicide (Pittsburgh Coke)	Isooctyl ester 2, 4-dichloro phenoxy acetic acid (equiv. to 63.0% 2, 4-dichloro phenoxy acetic acid) 95.0%	PITTSBURGH SHINGLE STAIN (Pittsburgh Plate Glass)	
PITTSBURGH ISOPROPYL ESTER OF 2, 4, 5-T TECHNICAL Herbicide (Pittsburgh Coke)	Isopropyl ester of 2, 4, 5-trichloro phenoxy acetic acid* (equiv. to 84.6% 2, 4, 5-trichloro phenoxy acetic acid) 98.5%	PITTSBURGH SODIUM PENTA- CHLORO- PHENATE TECHNICAL Herbicide (Pittsburgh Coke)	Sodium pentachlorophenate* 75% Sodium salts of other chlorophenols 13%

Name & Use Manufacturer	Ingredients	Name & Use Manufacturer	Ingredients
PITTSBURGH SODIUM SALT OF 2, 4-D MONOHY-DRATE Herbicide (Pittsburgh Coke)	Sodium salt 2, 4-dichloro phenoxy acetic acid* (equiv. to 82.0% 2, 4-dichloro phenoxy acetic acid) 96.8%	PITTSBURGH WALLHIDE (PBX) FLAT WALL PAINT, RUBBERIZED SATIN FINISH (Pittsburgh Plate Glass (Paint Div.))	
PITTSBURGH SODIUM TCA 90% Herbicide (Pittsburgh Coke)	Sodium salt trichloro acetic acid* (equiv. to 79.0% trichloro acetic acid) 90.0%	PITTSBURGH WATERSPAR ENAMEL (Pittsburgh Plate Glass (Paint Div.))	
PITTSBURGH STREAKLESS PAINT CLEANER (Pittsburgh Plate Glass)		PIVAL Rodenticide (Motomco)	2-Pivalyl-1, 3-indandione 0.5%
PITTSBURGH SUN-PROOF HOUSE PAINT (Pittsburgh Plate Glass (Paint Div.))		PIVALYN Rodenticide (Motomco)	Sodium salt of 2-pivalyl-1, 3-indandione
		PIXSOL CREAM (MacEslin)	Liquor carbonis detergens 5% Coal tar 1%
PITTSBURGH SYSTOX SPRAY CON-CENTRATE Insecticide (Pittsburgh Coke)	o, o-Diethyl-o-2-(ethylmercapto)-ethyl thiophosphate* 21.2% Related organic phosphates 1.8% Emulsifier (thiosolve) 77.0%	PLA Paint for plastics (Testor)	Short oil penta alkyd Mineral spirits* and driers Pigments* the same as Testor's Colored Dopes
PITTSBURGH SYSTOX SPRAY CON-CENTRATE Insecticide (Pittsburgh Coke)	Demeton* 26.2% Related organic phosphates 2.3% Aromatic petroleum hydrocarbons* 64.5%	PLAM-LAK LINOLEUM FINISH (Great Lakes P. & V.)	
PITTSBURGH TOXAPHENE-40 Insecticide (Pittsburgh Coke)	Tech. toxaphene* 45% Petroleum distillate 50%	PLAM VAR FINISH, PRIMER, SEALER, PAINTS, VARNISH (Great Lakes P. & V.)	
PITTSBURGH TOXAPHENE-60 Insecticide (Pittsburgh Coke)	Toxaphene* 60.0% Aliphatic petroleum hydrocarbons 30.0%	PLANACIDE Insecticide (Planetary Chem.)	Chlordane tech. 2% Deodorized kerosene* 98%
PITTSBURGH 40% TOXAPHENE WETTABLE POWDER Insecticide (Pittsburgh Coke)	Tech. toxaphene* (chlorine content 67-69%) 40%	PLAN-A-DIEL Insecticide (Planetary Chem.)	Hexachloro epoxy octahydro dimethano naphthalene* 15.83% Related compounds 2.79% Petroleum hydrocarbons 73.38%
		PLANA-THION Insecticide (Planetary Chem.)	Parathion* (o, o-diethyl-o-paranitrophenyl thiophosphate) 25% Xylol 61.6%
PITTSBURGH VARNISH (Pittsburgh Plate Glass)		PLANCELLO Cathartic (Am. Ferment)	Methyl cellulose Vitamin B1 Purified hemicellulose from Plantage loeflingii
PITTSBURGH VARNISH REMOVER (Pittsburgh Plate Glass)		PLAN-DANE Insecticide (Planetary Chem.)	Tech. chlordane* 46% Deodorized petroleum distillate * 44%

*Consult Sec. II., Ingredients Index. This ingredient may be responsible for major toxic effects if poisonous amounts of this product are ingested.

Name & Use Manufacturer	Ingredients		Name & Use Manufacturer	Ingredients	
PLAN-DEE Insecticide (Planetary Chem.)	DDT Xylene*	25% 70%	PLANETARY POP-UP Plant starter (Planetary Chem.)	Ammoniacal nitrogen Available phosphoric acid Potash	10% 52% 17%
PLANETARY B-HEX Insecticide (Planetary Chem.)	Gamma isomer of benzene hexachloride* Other isomers of benzene hexachloride Methylated naphthalene* Petroleum distillates	11% 17% 35% 30%	PLANETARY PY-FLY Insecticide (Planetary Chem.)	Piperonyl butoxide, tech. ether, and related compounds Pyrethrins Petroleum distillate* (deodorized)	0.50% 0.05% 99.45%
PLANETARY 5% CHLOR- DANE DUST Insecticide (Planetary Chem.)	Chlordane tech.*	5%	PLANETARY SPREADER (Planetary Chem.)	Alkyl aryl sulfonate	25%
PLANETARY COPPER-8 Fungicide (Planetary Chem.)	Copper-8-quinolinolate	25%	PLANETARY TCA SODIUM SALT 90% Herbicide (Planetary Chem.)	Sodium trichloroacetate*	90%
PLANETARY FARMCHLOR INSECT KILLER (Planetary Chem.)	Tech. chlordane* Petroleum hydrocarbons*	46% 44%	PLANETARY TET 200 Insecticide (Planetary Chem.)	Tetraethyl pyrophosphate* Other organic phosphates	38% 57%
PLANETARY FORMULA 913 Insecticide (Planetary Chem.)	Chlordane tech.* Petroleum distillate*	20% 80%	PLANETARY WARFARIN RAT & MOUSE BAIT (Planetary Chem.)	Warfarin (3-(a-acetonylbenzyl)- 4-hydroxycoumarin)	0.025%
PLANETARY FUMIGANT DAWSON FORMULA 82 (Planetary Chem.)	Ethylene dibromide* Methyl bromide*	80.0% 19.5%	PLANETARY X-TERMIN-S Wood pre- servative (Planetary Chem.)	Tech. pentachlorophenol* Petroleum solvent*	5% 90%
PLANETARY 50% MALATHION Insecticide (Planetary Chem.)	Malathion* Xylol *	50% 39%	PLANETIZER 6-12-6 Plant food concentrate (Planetary Chem.)	Nitrogen Phosphoric acid Potash	6% 12% 6%
PLANETARY OMPA SYSTEMIC SPRAY Insecticide (Planetary Chem.)	Octamethyl pyrophosphoramide* Related organic phosphates	18.1% 5.2%	PLANETIZER 8-8-8 Plant food concentrate (Planetary Chem.)	Nitrogen Phosphoric acid Potash	8% 8% 8%

*Consult Sec. II., Ingredients Index. This ingredient may be responsible for major toxic effects if poisonous amounts of this product are ingested.

Name & Use Manufacturer	Ingredients	
PLANETIZER 20 Plant food concentrate (Planetary Chem.)	Nitrate nitrogen	0.4%
	Ammoniacal nitrogen	0.10%
	Nitrogen	0.20%
	Phosphoric acid	0.20%
	Potash	0.20%
PLANETIZER 1735 Plant food (Planetary Chem.)	Nitrate nitrogen	0.8%
	Ammoniacal nitrogen	15.7%
	Nitrogen	17.5%
	Phosphoric acid	35.0%
	Potash	17.5%
PLAN-O-LIN Insecticide (Planetary Chem.)	Gamma isomer of benzene hexachloride*	20%
	Xylol*	56%
	Cyclohexanone	5.5%
PLAN-O-WEED Herbicide (Planetary Chem.)	Isopropyl ester 2, 4-dichloro phenoxy acetic acid	44%
	Aromatic petroleum naphtha *	51%
PLANTABBS Plant food (Plantabbs)		
PLANT BOOSTER Plant nutrient (Collins Feed)		
PLANT DDT Insecticide (Plant Prod.)	DDT *	5%
PLANT DDT 50% WET-TABLE POWDER Insecticide (Plant Prod.)	DDT *	50%
PLANT DITHIO AEROSOL BOMB Insecticide (Plant Prod.)	Tetraethyl dithiono pyrophosphate*	5%

Name & Use Manufacturer	Ingredients	
PLANTERS ALDRIN COTTON DUST Insecticide (Planters)	Hexachloro hexahydro dimethano naphthalene*	2.375%
	Related compounds	1.791%
PLANTERS 5% ALDRIN DUST Insecticide (Planters)	Hexachloro hexahydro-endo, exo-dimethano naphthalene*	4.750%
	Related compounds	0.80%
PLANTERS 20% ALDRIN DUST BASE CONCEN-TRATE Insecticide (Planters)	Hexachloro hexahydro-endo, exo-dimethano naphthalene*	19.04%
	Related compounds	3.20%
PLANTERS ALDRIN EMULSION CONCEN-TRATE Insecticide (Planters)	Hexachloro hexahydro-endo, exo-dimethano naphthalene*	23.5%
	Related compounds	4.0%
	Petroleum hydrocarbons	65.0%
PLANTERS ALDRIN EQUIVALENT-DDT COTTON DUST Insecticide (Planters)	Hexachloro hexahydro-endo, exo-dimethano naphthalene *	2.375%
	Related compounds	0.375%
	DDT	5.000%
PLANTERS 2% ALDRIN EQUIVALENT DUST Insecticide (Planters)	Hexachloro hexahydro dimethano naphthalene*	1.904%
	Related compounds	1.432%
PLANTERS BLUE MOLD DUST Insecticide (Planters)	Ferric dimethyl dithio-carbamate	11.40%
PLANTERS 10% CHLOR-DANE DUST Insecticide (Planters)	Chlordane* tech.	10.00%

*Consult Sec. II., Ingredients Index. This ingredient may be responsible for major toxic effects if poisonous amounts of this product are ingested.

- 840 -

Name & Use Manufacturer	Ingredients		Name & Use Manufacturer	Ingredients	
PLANTERS COMBINATION DUST Insecticide (Planters)	Parathion * DDT	1.00% 5.00%	PLANTERS DOUBLE DUST Insecticide (Planters)	DDT Sulfur*	3% 50%
PLANTERS COPPER-SULFUR DUST FOR PEANUTS Fungicide (Planters)	Basic copper sulfate* (expressed as metallic copper 4%) Sulfur*	7.7% 85%	PLANTERS DOUBLE STRENGTH INSECT SPRAY (Planters)	DDT*	10%
PLANTERS 3-5-0 COTTON DUST Insecticide (Planters)	Gamma isomer of benzene hexachloride * 3% Other isomers of benzene hexachloride and related compounds 5.25% DDT* 5.00%		PLANTERS 1-1/2% ENDRIN DUST Insecticide (Planters)	Endrin* (hexachloro epoxy octahydro-endo, endo-dimethano naphthalene) 1.5%	
PLANTERS 3-5-40 COTTON DUST Insecticide (Planters)	Gamma isomer of benzene hexachloride * 3% Other isomers of benzene hexachloride 5.25% DDT* 5% Sulfur* 40%		PLANTERS ENDRIN EMULSIBLE CONCEN-TRATE Insecticide (Planters)	Endrin (hexachloro epoxy octahydro-endo, endo-dimethano naphthalene) 19.5% Petroleum hydrocarbons 70.5%	
PLANTERS CUKE & MELON DUST Insecticide (Planters)	Tech. piperonyl cyclonene 0.50% Pyrethrins 0.04% Basic copper sulfate* (expressed as metallic copper 5.00%) 9.62%		PLANTERS FERMATE-DDT PLANT BED DUST Insecticide (Planters)	Ferric dimethyl dithiocarbamate 11.40% DDT 3.00%	
PLANTERS 1% DDT SULFUR DUST Insecticide (Planters)	DDT Sulfur*	1% 90%	PLANTERS 1% GAMMA ISOMER BENZENE HEXACHLORIDE DUST Insecticide (Planters)	Gamma isomer of benzene hexachloride 1.00% Other isomers of benzene hexachloride and related compounds 1.75%	
PLANTERS 5% DDT-SULFUR DUST Insecticide (Planters)	DDT* Sulfur*	5.00% 75.00%			
PLANTERS 10% DDT DUST Insecticide (Planters)	DDT*	10.00%	PLANTERS 5% HEPTACHLOR DUST Insecticide (Planters)	Heptachlor* Related compounds	5.00% 1.94%
PLANTERS 25% DDT WATER EMULSION CONCEN-TRATE Insecticide (Planters)	Methylated aromatic petroleum deriv.* 71% DDT 25% Polyoxyethylene sorbitol esters of mixed fatty and resin acids 4%		PLANTERS HEPTACHLOR EMULSION Insecticide (Planters)	Heptachlor* 23.41% Related compounds 9.10% Petroleum distillate 64.49%	
PLANTERS DEE-KOP DUST Insecticide (Planters)	DDT Copper sulfate* (basic) (expressed as metallic copper 7.00%)	3% 13.46%	PLANTERS 1% IMPREGNATED DDT DUST Insecticide (Planters)	DDT Petroleum hydrocarbons	1% 4%
PLANTERS DEE-KOP DUST NO. 5 Insecticide (Planters)	DDT* 5.00% Basic copper sulfate* (expressed as metallic copper 7.00%) 13.46%		PLANTERS JAP BEETLE KILLER (Planters)	DDT*	50%
PLANTERS DEE-KOP DUST WITH COPPER A Insecticide (Planters)	DDT 3.00% Tetra copper calcium oxy-chloride*(expressed as metallic copper 7.00%) 15.25%		PLANTERS 1% LINDANE-6% DITHANE DUST Insecticide (Planters)	Gamma isomer of benzene hexachloride (from lindane) 1.00% Zinc ethylene-bis(dithiocarbamate) 3.90% Metallic zinc content 0.92%	
			PLANTERS 4% MALATHION DUST Insecticide (Planters)	Malathion*	4.00%

*Consult Sec. II., Ingredients Index. This ingredient may be responsible for major toxic effects if poisonous amounts of this product are ingested.

- 841 -

Name & Use Manufacturer	Ingredients		Name & Use Manufacturer	Ingredients	
PLANTERS MEXICAN BEAN BEETLE DUST & GARDEN SPRAY (Planters)	Rotenone Sulfur* Other cube resins	0.75% 25% 1.5%	PLANTERS SAV-A-ROOT Insecticide (Planters)	Tech. chlordane* Xylene*	75.00% 20.00%
PLANTERS ONE PLUS SEVEN DUST Insecticide (Planters)	DDT Methylated aromatic petroleum deriv.* Basic copper sulfate* (expressed as metallic copper 7.00%)	1.00% 2.30% 13.46%	PLANTERS SEVEN KOP DUST Fungicide (Planters)	Basic copper sulfate*(7% as metallic copper)	13.46%
PLANTERS 1% PARATHION DUST Insecticide (Planters)	Parathion*	1%	PLANTERS SEVEN KOP DUST WITH COPPER A Fungicide (Planters)	Tetra copper calcium oxy-chloride* (expressed as metallic copper 7%)	15.25%
PLANTERS 2% PARATHION DUST Insecticide (Planters)	Parathion*	2%	PLANTERS SPECIAL INSECT SPRAY (Planters)	Chlordane	2%
PLANTERS PARATHION-ZINEB DUST Insecticide (Planters)	Parathion* Zinc ethylene-bis(dithio-carbamate) Metallic zinc content	1.00% 3.90% 0.92%	PLANTERS SPECIAL JAP BEETLE KILLER (Planters)	Methoxychlor*	50%
PLANTERS P C TWENTY DUST Insecticide (Planters)	Tech. piperonyl cyclonene Pyrethrins	0.5% 0.04%	PLANTERS SQUASH BUG, HARLEQUIN BUG KILLER (Planters)	Sabadilla	10%
PLANTERS PDQ BEAN & GARDEN DUST Insecticide (Planters)	Tech. piperonyl cyclonene Pyrethrins Rotenone Other cube resins Sulfur	0.37% 0.03% 0.40% 0.8% 10%	PLANTERS SQUASH BUG, HARLEQUIN BUG KILLER (Planters)	Ground sabadilla seed	20%
PLANTERS PDQ TRIPLE DUST Insecticide (Planters)	DDT Tech. piperonyl cyclonene Pyrethrins Rotenone Other cube resins Sulfur*	3% 0.37% 0.03% 0.25% 0.50% 50%	PLANTERS 10% TDE DUST Insecticide (Planters)	DDD*	10.00%
PLANTERS RAT & MOUSE BAIT (Planters)	Warfarin (3-(a-acetonylbenzyl)-4-hydroxycoumarin) 0.025%		PLANTERS 25% TDE EMULSION CONCEN-TRATE Insecticide (Planters)	Dichloro diphenyl dichloro-ethane, tech. Aromatic petroleum deriv. solvent*	25.0% 71.8%
PLANTERS 10% RHOTHANE-1% PARATHION DUST Insecticide (Planters)	TDE or DDD Parathion*	10.00% 1.00%	PLANTERS TERMITOX 75% CHLORDANE EMULSIFIABLE CONCEN-TRATE Insecticide (Planters)	Tech. chlordane* Xylene*	75.00% 20.00%
PLANTERS 10% SABADILLA DUST Insecticide (Planters)	Sabadilla alkaloids	0.4%	PLANTERS TOMATO DUST Insecticide (Planters)	Tricalcium arsenate* 14.00% Basic copper sulfate (expressed as metallic copper 5.00%) Total arsenic (as metallic 5.27%; as water-soluble arsenic 0.50%)	9.62% 8.08%
PLANTERS 20% SABADILLA DUST Insecticide (Planters)	Sabadilla alkaloids	0.8%	PLANTERS TOMATO HORNWORM DUST (Planters)	Tricalcium arsenate* Copper acetoarsenite (Paris-green) Metallic copper	14% 3.32% 7%

*Consult Sec. II., Ingredients Index. This ingredient may be responsible for major toxic effects if poisonous amounts of this product are ingested.

Name & Use Manufacturer	Ingredients
PLANTERS TOXAPHENE COTTON DUST Insecticide (Planters)	Toxaphene* (tech. chlorinated camphene) (chlorine content 67-69%) 20.00% Sulfur 40.00%
PLANTERS TOXAPHENE-DDT DUST Insecticide (Planters)	Toxaphene* (tech. chlorinated camphene) (chlorine content 67-69%) 10.00% DDT * 5.00%
PLANTERS 10% TOXAPHENE DUST Insecticide (Planters)	Toxaphene* (tech. chlorinated camphene) (chlorine content 67-69%) 10.00%
PLANTERS TOXAPHENE 6 LB. EMULSION CONCENTRATE Insecticide (Planters)	Toxaphene* (tech. chlorinated camphene) (67-69% chlorine content) 60.2% Petroleum distillates 29.8%
PLANTERS TRIPLE DUST Insecticide (Planters)	DDT 3% Rotenone 0.5% Other cube resins 1% Sulfur* 50%
PLANTERS 5% TRUK DUST Insecticide (Planters)	DDT* 5% Petroleum hydrocarbons 4%
PLANTERS 40% WETTABLE CHLORDANE Insecticide (Planters)	Tech. chlordane* 40.00%
PLANTERS WETTABLE SULFUR FOR DUSTING & SPRAYING Fungicide (Planters)	Sulfur* 95%
PLANTERS ZINEB DUST Insecticide (Planters)	Zinc ethylene-bis(dithio-carbamate) 6.50%
PLANTERS ZINEB DUST WITH DDT Insecticide (Planters)	Zinc ethylene-bis(dithio-carbamate) 3.90% Metallic zinc content 0.92% DDT 3.00%
PLANTERS ZINEB DUST WITH IMPREGNATED DDT Insecticide (Planters)	DDT 1.00% Methylated aromatic petroleum derivatives* 2.30% Zinc ethylene-bis(dithio-carbamate) 3.90% Metallic zinc content 0.92%
PLANTEX-50 ANTI TRANSPIRANT Water-loss preventer (plant) (Larvacide)	Vinyl resin 50%

Name & Use Manufacturer	Ingredients
PLANTFUME 103 SMOKE GENERATOR Insecticide (Plant Prod.)	Tetraethyl dithionopyrophosphate* 15%
PLANTGARD BUG DUSTER Insecticide (Agkem)	Rotenone 1% Rotenone extractives 2% Cuprous oxide* 5%
PLANT PLATE Insecticide (Milligan)	Sulfur* 20% DDT* 5% Rotenone 1.2% Other cube resins 2.4% Ferric dimethyl dithio-carbamate (fermate) 5.6% Beta chloro ethyl beta-(p-tertiary butyl phenoxy)-alpha methyl ethyl sulfide (aramite) 1.6% Total nitrogen 1.2% Potash 3.0%
PLANT PLATE FUNGICIDE (Milligan)	
PLANT PLATE INSECTICIDE & FUNGICIDE (Milligan)	Ferric dimethyl dithio-carbamate (ferbam) DDT* Micronized wettable sulfur Rotenone*and other cube resins (total 34.44%)
PLANT PLATE WEATHERIZED DUST Insecticide (Milligan)	Sulfur* 20% Dichloro diphenyl trichloro-ethane* 5% Ferric dimethyl dithio-carbamate 5.0% Rotenone 1.0% Other cube resins 2.0% Gamma isomer of benzene hexachloride (from lindane) 0.5%
PLANT PLATE WEATHERIZER Spray protector (Milligan)	Polyethylene polysulfide* 56%
PLANT PRODUCTS TEPP AEROSOL BOMB Insecticide (Plant Prod.)	Tetraethyl pyrophosphate* 4% Other organic phosphates 6%
PLANT SHINE Plant food (Plant Shine)	
PLANT SODIUM SELENATE Insecticide (Plant Prod.)	Sodium selenate* 99%
PLANTTHION AEROSOL BOMB Insecticide (Plant Prod.)	o,o-diethyl-o-p-nitrophenyl thiophosphate* 10%
PLANTTHION AEROSOLS Insecticide (Plant Prod.)	Parathion* 10%

*Consult Sec. II., Ingredients Index. This ingredient may be responsible for major toxic effects if poisonous amounts of this product are ingested.

Name & Use Manufacturer	Ingredients	Name & Use Manufacturer	Ingredients
PLANTTHION 2% DUST Insecticide (Plant Prod.)	Parathion* 2%	PLASTICO FURNITURE, PORCELAIN, CEMENT & WATER-PROOF FILLER (Technical Supply)	
PLANTTHION TECHNICAL Insecticide (Plant Prod.)	o,o-diethyl-o-p-nitrophenyl thiophosphate* 95%	PLASTIC PAINTS (Symolyn)	
PLANTTHION 15% WETTABLE POWDER Insecticide (Plant Prod.)	Parathion* 15%	PLASTIC STIK (Leonard)	Vegetable drying oils Petroleum wax Titanium dioxide Calcium carbonate
PLASCOTE COLD WATER PAINT (Made Rite)		PLASTIGILT POLISH (Uncle Sam)	
PLASTICATE PLASTIC CEMENT (Stewart-Lunhal)		PLASTIGLEAM WIPE ON FLOOR & LINOLEUM FINISH (Deer-O)	
PLASGON Plastic cement (Cabot)		PLASTOY MODELING CLAY (Ill. Clay)	
PLASTERKOTE PAINT (Vita-Var)		PLATELUSTRE TRANSPARENT LACQUERS & SYNTHETIC FINISHES (Maas & Waldstein)	
PLASTER PARIS, PLASTER-PATCH (United Gilson.)	Calcine gypsum	DR. PLATT'S CAL RINEX FORMULA Analgesic, antispasmodic (Fougera)	Each capsule: Extract belladonna (total alkaloids 1/1280 gr.)1/16 gr. Acetophenetidin* 1 gr. Aspirin* Each tablet: Calcium carbonate Sodium bicarbonate
PLASTER-STIK & PIPE-SEAL (Leonard)	Vegetable drying oils Petroleum wax Titanium dioxide Calcium carbonate		
PLASTEX PLASTIC COATING (Plastex)		PLEXIGLAS POLISHES (Park Chem.)	Paraformaldehyde*
PLASTEX Plastic texture paint (Reardon Co.)		PLEXITE PORCELAIN LIKE ENAMEL INTERIOR & EXTERIOR PAINT (Sundure)	
PLASTIC CAULK-PLASTIC COMPOUND (Maas & Waldstein)		PLEXTONE MULTI-COLOR ENAMELS (Maas & Waldstein)	
PLASTIC GLOSS POLISH (Uncle Sam)	Gums* Shellacs Isopropanol*	PLEZ-AIR Deodorizer (Winsale)	
PLASTICLEAR PAINT & VARNISH CLEANER, PORCELAIN, TILE, & MARBLE CLEANER, LINOLEUM & HARDWOOD CLEANER (Plasticlear)		PLI-NAMEL ENAMEL & CONCRETE SEALER (Glidden Co.)	

*Consult Sec. II., Ingredients Index. This ingredient may be responsible for major toxic effects if poisonous amounts of this product are ingested.

Name & Use Manufacturer	Ingredients		Name & Use Manufacturer	Ingredients	
PLIOBEX RUBBER BASE PAINT (Cheesman-Elliott)			P.M.C. ASTRINGENT POWDER Vaginal douche (Thomas & Thompson)	Boric acid* Alum Phenol Eucalyptus * Oil of peppermint Menthol* Thymol *	
PLIOBOND RUBBER CEMENT (U.S. Plyood)			P.M.C. DOUCHE POWDER Antiseptic (Handley)	Boric acid* Powdered alum Oil of peppermint Phenol liquefied*	
PLI-X RUBBER BASE PAINT (Sundure)			PNEUMATICA Counter-irritant (Polk, C.)	Camphor* Methyl salicylate* Capsicum Belladonna* Phenol*	
PLOW BRAND FERTILIZER (Etiwan)			POCKET GOPHER POISON (Santa Clara)	Strychnine*	90.9%
PLUG-A-LEAK Roof paint & compounds (Toch)			PODAPHEN PILLS Cathartic (Norwich)	Extr. belladonna* Phenolphthalein Aloin* Podophyllin Ipecac	1/12 gr.
PLUMITE Drain cleaner (Dearborn Chem.)	Sodium hydroxide*		POISON BARLEY Rodenticide (Lake County)	Strychnine*	
PLURAC Cleaning product (Wyandotte)	Conc. alkali*		POISONED BRAN FOR EARWIGS Insecticide (Santa Clara)	Sodium fluosilicate* 10.4% Fluorine (as elemental fluorine) 6.3%	
99 PLUS INSECTICIDE (Brilco)			POISON GRAINS FOR MICE (Robbins, G.)	Strychnine*	
PLUS PRE-SPOTTER Drycleaning spotter (Adco)			POISON IVY-OAK BOMB (Thompson Chem.)	Butoxy ethoxy propyl ester of 2,4,5-trichloro phenoxy acetic acid 8.1%	
PLUTO SPRING WATER (Pluto)	Sodium sulfate Magnesium sulfate		POISON OATS Rodenticide (Lake County)	Zinc phosphide*	
PLYMOUTH SEA FIRE Fire kindler (Plymouth)			POISON WHEAT Rodenticide (Sonoma)	Strychnine alkaloid* 0.25%	
PLYTHERM ENAMELS (Ault & Wiborg)			POKEY PUTTY (Chaulking Putty) (Houck)		
PMAS Herbicide (Cleary)	Phenyl mercuric acetate* 10%		POL Cattle remedy (Hess, Dr.)	Alcohol 21%/v Ether* 66%/v Antimony trichloride * Salicylic acid*	
PMAS 2-1/2% Herbicide, fungicide (Cleary)	Phenyl mercuric acetate* 2-1/2%		POLANA WASHING POWDER (Polana)		
PMAS 3% Antiseptic (Cleary)	Phenyl mercuric acetate* 3%		POLARCOTE FOR PAINTING OVER ASPHALT (Tremco)		
PMAS 10% Herbicide, fungicide (Cleary)	Phenyl mercuric acetate* 10%				

*Consult Sec. II., Ingredients Index. This ingredient may be responsible for major toxic effects if poisonous amounts of this product are ingested.

Name & Use Manufacturer	Ingredients	
POLAR KOTE ENAMEL (Morris Paint)		
POLAR NAPHTHALENE MOTH BALLS, RING & FLAKES (Barrett)	Naphthalene*	100%
POLAR TYPE RUST PREVENTIVES (Am. Rust)		
POLERGEX For relief of hay fever (Marion Pharm.)	Chlorbutanol	0.5%
	Benzocaine	
	Ephedrine*	
	Camphor*	
	Menthol*	
	Oil of pine needles *	
	Oil of eucalyptus *	
	Gamma propyl benzoate	
POLICE CORN REMEDY (Majestic)		
POLICE & FIREMEN'S CORN SALVE (Coast)	Salicylic acid*	
POLINEL Skin ointment (Polinel)	Zinc oxide	
	Resorcin	
	White petrolatum	
	Phenol*	
	Precipitated sulfur *	
	Starch	
	Camphor*	
	Aromatic oils	
POLISHEEN Silver polish (Protective)	Phosphoric acid *	
POLLO FURNITURE POLISH (Cedar Hill)		
POL-MER-IK BOILED LINSEED OIL (Archer-D.-M.)	Linseed oil	
	Lead	0.2%
POLO LIQUID BOILER COMPOUND (Klenzade)	Caustic soda*	
POLORIS TABLETS Dental analgesic (Poloris)	Aspirin*	3-1/2 gr.
	Acetophenetidin*	2 gr.
	Caffeine alkaloid	1/3 gr.
POLO SPUR COLOGNE LODORANTE (Parfum L'Orle)		
POLYBOR Herbicide (Pacific Coast)	Disodium octaborate tetrahydrate* (equiv. boron trioxide 66%)	98%

Name & Use Manufacturer	Ingredients	
POLYBOR-2 Boron supplement (agric.) (Pacific Coast)	Disodium octaborate tetra-hydrate*	78%
	Sodium tetraborate penta-hydrate*	20%
	(equiv. to boron trioxide 66.0% or boron 20.5%)	
POLYBOR-3 Insecticide (Pacific Coast)	Sodium polyborates*	98%
POLYBOR-CHLORATE WEED & GRASS KILLER (Pacific Coast)	Disodium octaborate tetra-hydrate*	73%
	Sodium chlorate *	25%
POLYBOR-CHLORATE 88 WEED & GRASS KILLER (Pacific Coast)	Disodium octaborate tetra-hydrate* 55% or boron trioxide	36%
	Sodium chlorate*	22%
POLYCHRO-MATIC ALPHASITE CHALKBOARD CHALK (Weber Costello)		
POLYMEROL SYNTHETIC VARNISH & INK (Wilson, W.D.)		
POLYMOL HAIR DRESSING (Farenga)		
POLYSEAM-SEAL NO. 710 Seam compound (Ferdinand)		
POLYSTAT Internal fungicide, tonic, anthelmintic (veterinary) (Salsbury's)	Acetyl-(para-nitrophenyl)-sulfanilamide	15.00%
	Dibutyltin dilaurate	10.00%
	Dinitro diphenyl sulfonyl ethylene diamine	10.00%
	3-Nitro-4-hydroxyphenylarsenic acid*(14.1 mg./gm. arsenic trioxide)	3.75%
POLYTHIONATE LOTION For acne (Smith,Upsher)	Sulfur (polythionates of sodium)*	1.5%
	Zinc oxide	
POMADA SAN PEDRO Rubefacient, (San Pedro)	Oil of eucalyptus *	
	Cajuput	
	Camphor*	
	Menthol *	
POMAGEL SKIN CLEANER (Jay's)		
POMERIO-18 Disinfectant (Shiffer's)	Potassium mercuric iodide*	2.3%

*Consult Sec. II., Ingredients Index. This ingredient may be responsible for major toxic effects if poisonous amounts of this product are ingested.

- 846 -

Name & Use Manufacturer	Ingredients	Name & Use Manufacturer	Ingredients
POMMADE HONGROISE Toiletry (Nestle-Le Mur)		PORCENITE PAINTS (Advance Paint)	
POMO HAIR POMADE (Rabin)		POROUSEAL Wall Board Sealer (Foy)	
POM-PO-LAY HAIR TONIC (Weyer)		PORT BRAND ALDRIN-DDT EMULSION Insecticide (Port)	Hexachloro hexahydro dimethano naphthalene* 10.92% Related compounds 8.24% Dichloro diphenyl trichloro-ethane 23.00%
PONARIS OIL Nasal decongestant (Jamol)	Eucalyptus oil* Cajuput oil Pine oil*	PORT BRAND ALDRIN EMULSION Insecticide (Port)	Hexachloro hexahydro dimethano naphthalene* 23.10% Related compounds 17.37%
PONCHOTEX CEMENT PAINT (Building)		PORT BRAND ALDRIN (Equiv.) 2-1/2% Insecticide (Port)	Hexachloro hexahydro dimethano naphthalene* 2.37% Related compounds 1.79% Sulfur 40.00%
POND'S ANGEL FACE MAKE-UP MIST & PAT, POND'S HAND & FACE CREAMS, LIPSTICKS, LOTIONS, POWDERS, FRESHENERS, VANISHING CREAM (Pond's Extr.)		PORT BRAND BHC-DDT EMULSION Insecticide (Port)	Benzene hexachloride* 27.44% Dichloro diphenyl trichloro-ethane 16.66%
POND'S LAXATIVE PILLS (Pond Pharm.)	Extr. belladonna* (total alkaloids 1/640 gr.) Cascarin Aloin* Podophyllin Ginger	PORT BRAND B H C EMULSION Insecticide (Port)	Benzene hexachloride* 34.55%
PONTOCAINE CREAM Skin ointment (Winthrop)	Pontocaine hydrochloride* (tetracaine HCl) 0.5% Methylparaben 0.1% Sodium bisulfite 0.1%	PORT BRAND BHC-DDT-SULFUR 3-5-40 Insecticide (Port)	Dichloro diphenyl trichloro-ethane* 5% Gamma isomer of benzene hexachloride* 3% Other isomers of benzene hexachloride 5.2% Sulfur* 40%
POOF DEODORANT BODY POWDER (Montenier)	Aluminum hydroxide U.S.P. Magnesium stearate	PORT BRAND BHC W-12% (Gamma) Insecticide (Port)	Gamma isomer of benzene hexachloride* 12% Other isomers of benzene hexachloride and related compounds* 21%
POPULAR FLOOR ENAMEL (Woolsey)		PORT BRAND CHLORDANE 5% Insecticide (Port)	Tech. chlordane * 5.0%
PORCELANITE ENAMEL (Hommel)		PORT BRAND CHLORDANE 10% Insecticide (Port)	Tech. chlordane* 10.0%
PORCELITE ENAMELS (Thomson-Porcelite)		PORT BRAND CHLORDANE EMULSION Insecticide (Port)	Tech. chlordane* 74%
PORCELPATCH ENAMEL (Hommel)		PORT BRAND COMBINATION NO. 50 CONTAINS 50% CALCIUM ARSENATE Insecticide (Port)	Tricalcium arsenate* 40.25% Sulfur 50.00% Total arsenic (as metallic) 15.5% Arsenic in water-soluble form (as metallic) 4.0%
PORCELYN ENAMEL (Sillers)			

*Consult Sec. II., Ingredients Index. This ingredient may be responsible for major toxic effects if poisonous amounts of this product are ingested.

Name & Use Manufacturer	Ingredients	Name & Use Manufacturer	Ingredients
PORT BRAND CRYOLITE 50% Insecticide (Port)	Sodium fluoaluminate* 45%	PORT BRAND DITOX NO. 2-S 1-5-40 Insecticide (Port)	Gamma isomer of benzene hexachloride 1.0% Other isomers of benzene hexachloride and related compounds 1.7% Dichloro diphenyl trichloro-ethane* 5.0% Sulfur* 40.0%
PORT BRAND DDT 5% Insecticide (Port)	Dichloro diphenyl trichloro-ethane* 5.0%		
PORT BRAND DDT 10% Insecticide (Port)	Dichloro diphenyl trichloro-ethane* 10.0%	PORT BRAND DUSTING SULFUR 93% Insecticide, fungicide (Port)	Sulfur* 93.0%
PORT BRAND DDT 25% EMULSION Insecticide (Port)	Dichloro diphenyl trichloro-ethane* 25.0%	PORT BRAND ENDRIN EMULSION Insecticide (Port)	Endrin* (hexachloro epoxy octahydro endo,endo-dimethano naphthalene) 19.5%
PORT BRAND DDT NO. 5-S Insecticide (Port)	Dichloro diphenyl trichloro-ethane* 5.0% Sulfur* 40.0%	PORT BRAND HEPTACHLOR 2-1/2% Insecticide (Port)	Heptachlor* 2.5% Related compounds 1.25%
PORT BRAND DDT NO. 20-S Insecticide (Port)	Dichloro diphenyl trichloro-ethane* 20.00% Sulfur* 40.00%	PORT BRAND HEPTACHLOR 5% Insecticide (Port)	Heptachlor* 5.00% Related compounds 2.50%
PORT BRAND DDT 10-PARATHION 1 Insecticide (Port)	Parathion* (o,o-diethyl-o-p-nitrophenyl thiophosphate) 1.0% Dichloro diphenyl trichloro-ethane 10.0%	PORT BRAND HEPTACHLOR EMULSION Insecticide (Port)	Heptachlor* 23.2% Related compounds 11.4%
PORT BRAND DDT-SULFUR 10-40 Insecticide (Port)	Dichloro diphenyl trichloro-ethane* 10.00% Sulfur* 40.00%	PORT BRAND HOP-TOX TOXAPHENE 10% Insecticide (Port)	Toxaphene* (tech. chlorinated camphene) (chlorine content 67-69%) 10.0% Sulfur* 40.0%
PORT BRAND DIELDRIN 2-1/2% Insecticide (Port)	Hexachloro epoxy octahydro dimethano naphthalene* 2.12% Related compounds 0.38%	PORT BRAND KARATHANE 1% Fungicide (Port)	Dinitro (1-methyl heptyl) phenyl crotonate* 0.90% Other nitrophenols and deriva-tives, chiefly dinitro (1-methyl heptyl) phenol 0.10%
PORT BRAND DIELDRIN-DDT 2-1/2-10 Insecticide (Port)	Hexachloro epoxy octahydro dimethano naphthalene* 2.12% Related compounds 0.38% DDT 10.00%	PORT BRAND LINDANE EMULSION Insecticide (Port)	Gamma isomer of benzene hexachloride* 20.0%
PORT BRAND DIELDRIN-DDT-SULFUR 2-1/2-10-40 Insecticide (Port)	Hexachloro epoxy octahydro dimethano naphthalane* 2.12% Related compounds 0.38% DDT 10.00% Sulfur 40.00%	PORT BRAND MALATHION EMULSION Insecticide (Port)	Malathion* (o,o-dimethyl dithio phosphate of diethyl mercapto succinate) 57%
PORT BRAND DIELDRIN EMULSION Insecticide (Port)	Dieldrin (hexachloro epoxy octahydro dimethano naphthalene*) 15.83% Related compounds 2.79%	PORT BRAND MANZATE 8% Fungicide (Port)	Manganese ethylene-bis(dithio-carbamate)*(as metallic 1.16%) 5.6%
PORT BRAND DIELDRIN SULFUR 2-1/2-40 Insecticide (Port)	Hexachloro epoxy octahydro dimethano naphthalene* 2.12% Related compounds 0.38% Sulfur 40.00%	PORT BRAND MANZATE 8%-PARATHION 1% Fungicide (Port)	Manganese ethylene-bis-(dithio-carbamate) 5.6% Parathion* 1.0%
PORT BRAND DITHANE 6% Fungicide (Port)	Dithane Z-78 (equiv. to 3.9% zinc ethylene-bis(dithio carbamate) 6.0%		

*Consult Sec. II., Ingredients Index. This ingredient may be responsible for major toxic effects if poisonous amounts of this product are ingested.

Name & Use Manufacturer	Ingredients	Name & Use Manufacturer	Ingredients
PORT BRAND METHYL PARATHION 1-1/2% Insecticide (Port)	Methyl parathion* (o,o-dimethyl-o-p-nitrophenyl thiophosphate) 1.5%	PORT BRAND RHOTHANE 10% Insecticide (Port)	Dichloro diphenyl dichloro-ethane 10%
PORT BRAND METHYL PARATHION 2-1/2% Insecticide (Port)	Methyl parathion* (o,o-dimethyl-o-p-nitrophenyl thiophosphate) 2.5%	PORT BRAND RHOTOX NO. 5 Insecticide (Port)	Dichloro diphenyl dichloro-ethane 5%
PORT BRAND METHYL PARATHION EMULSION Insecticide (Port)	Methyl parathion* 25%	PORT BRAND TAN-TOX NO. 2 3-5-0 Insecticide (Port)	Dichloro diphenyl trichloro-ethane* 5% Gamma isomer of benzene hexachloride* 3% Other isomers of benzene hexachloride and related compounds 5.2%
PORT BRAND PARATHION 1% Insecticide (Port)	Parathion*(o,o-diethyl-o-p-nitrophenyl thiophosphate) 1.0%	PORT BRAND TEPP 40% WATER MISCIBLE Insecticide (Port)	Tetraethyl pyrophosphate* 40% Other related organic phosphates (phosphorus expressed as elemental 12%) 60%
PORT BRAND PARATHION 2% Insecticide (Port)	Parathion* (o,o-diethyl-o-p-nitrophenyl thiophosphate) 2.0%	PORT BRAND TOXAPHENE 20% Insecticide (Port)	Toxaphene* (tech. chlorinated camphene) (chlorine content 67-69%) 20.0%
PORT BRAND PARATHION EMULSION Insecticide (Port)	Parathion* 25%	PORT BRAND TOXAPHENE 40% DUST BASE CONCENTRATE (Port)	Tech. chlorinated camphene* 40.00%
PORT BRAND PENTA (Pentachlorophenol 40%) DEFOLIANT & CROP DRIER Insecticide (Port)	Pentachlorophenol* 40.0%. Aromatic hydrocarbons* 43.0%	PORT BRAND TOXAPHENE-PARATHION 20-1 Insecticide (Port)	Toxaphene* (chlorine content 67-69%) 20.0% Parathion* (o,o-diethyl-o-p-nitrophenyl thiophosphate) 1.0%
PORT BRAND PORTHION-SULFUR Insecticide (Port)	Parathion* (o, o-diethyl-o-p-nitrophenyl thio-phosphate) 1.0% Sulfur 40.0%	PORT BRAND TOXAPHENE SULFUR 20-40 Insecticide (Port)	Toxaphene* (chlorine content 67-69%) 20.0% Sulfur 40.0%
PORT BRAND PORT-PHEN EMULSION Insecticide (Port)	Toxaphene* (chlorine content 67-69%) 60%	PORT CITY PAINTS & ENAMELS (Muskegon)	
PORT BRAND PORT-TOX 2-10-40 Insecticide (Port)	Dichloro diphenyl trichloro-ethane* 10.0% Gamma isomer of benzene hexachloride* 2.0% Other isomers of benzene hexachloride 3.4% Sulfur* 40.0%	PORTER PERFECT PAINT PRODUCTS (Porter Paint)	
PORT BRAND PORT-TOX NO. 2 2-10-0 Insecticide (Port)	Dichloro diphenyl trichloro-ethane* 10.0% Gamma isomer of benzene hexachloride* 2.0% Other isomers of benzene hexachloride and related compounds 3.4%	PORTER'S ANTACID (Rundle)	Each tablet: Calcium carbonate Magnesium carbonate Bismuth subnitrate
PORT BRAND RHOTHANE (DDD) EMULSION Insecticide (Port)	Rhothane* (dichloro diphenyl dichloroethane) 25.0%	DR. PORTER'S ANTISEPTIC OIL For skin (Grove)	Camphorated phenol* Camphor* Cottonseed oil Linseed oil

*Consult Sec. II., Ingredients Index. This ingredient may be responsible for major toxic effects if poisonous amounts of this product are ingested.

- 849 -

Name & Use Manufacturer	Ingredients		Name & Use Manufacturer	Ingredients	
PORTER'S A.P.C. Analgesic (Rundle)	Each tablet: Aspirin* Phenacetin* Caffeine	3-1/2 gr. 2-1/2 gr. 1/2 gr.	POSNER'S WAX Hair preparation (Posner)		
PORTER'S ASPIRIN (Rundle)	Aspirin*		POSNER'S BERGAMOT Hair conditioner (Posner)	Castor oil Olive oil Lanolin	
PORTER'S LINIMENT (Rundle)	Each fl. oz.: Ether Ammonia Capsicum Camphor* Oil of cajuput* Cloves Myrrh Galangal Safrol Ethyl alcohol*	12 m. 63%/v	POSNER'S PRESSING OIL Hair preparation (Posner)	Lanolin	
			POST AD BULLETIN COLORS & PAINTS (Glidden Co.)		
PORTER'S LINIMENT SALVE (Rundle)	Each fl. oz.: Chlorotone Camphor* Oil of cloves * Myrrh Oil of cajuput* Petrolatum Cresylic acid* Ammonia Zinc oxide Oil of sassafras * Lanolin Beeswax	4 gr.	POS-TER-ART COLORED CHALK CRAYON (Binney & Smith)		
			POSTER PASTELLO COLORED DUSTLESS CHALK (Am. Crayon)		
PORTER'S THROAT LOZENGES (Rundle)	Capsicum Clove oil* Myrrh Galangal Camphor* Safrol Cajuput oil* Chlorophyll		POTABLE- AQUA TABLETS Water sterlizer (Frost Labs.)	Tetraglycine potassium tri- iodide*	
PORTLAND PERFUME, COLOGNE, TOILET- WATER (Duvelle)	Alcohol denatured with diethyl phthalate		POTENTEX CLEANING COMPOUND (Texo)		
PORTLAN- SEMENT PAINT (Missouri)			PO-TOX Lotion for poison ivy (Commerce)	Tannic acid * Carbolic acid Isopropyl alcohol*	1% 20%
POSITOS RECTAL OINTMENT (McKesson)	Tyrothricin Benzocaine Ephedrine hydrochloride* Zinc oxide Bismuth subsalicylate Menthol	0.05% 3.3% 0.5%	POTSAL Antirheumatic (Baldwin)	Potassium bicarbonate Salicylic acid* Fl. extr. licorice Glycerin Antimony and potassium tartrate* Spirit of ethyl nitrate Alcohol	4-5%/v
POSITOS RECTAL SUPPOSI- TORIES (McKesson)	Each suppository: Gramicidin Benzocaine Ephedrine hydrochloride* Zinc oxide Bismuth subsalicylate	0.2 mg. 50 mg. 10 mg.	POTTER NURSERIES SPRAY DUST Insecticide (Chem. Form.)	o,o-Dimethyl dithiophosphate of diethyl mercaptosuccinate* 5.0% Methoxychlor tech. Ferric dimethyl dithiocarbamate 7.8% Sulfur * 15.0% Talc 67.2%	
POSLAM Skin ointment (Emergency)	Tar distillate* Sulfur Salicylic acid* Phenol* Zinc oxide Menthol Lanolin		POULAX Laxative (veterinary, avian) (Hilltop)	Epsom salts* 15% Potassium chlorate* Saltpeter Potassium dichromate*	

*Consult Sec. II., Ingredients Index. This ingredient may be responsible for major toxic effects if poisonous amounts of this product are ingested.

- 850 -

Name & Use Manufacturer	Ingredients	Name & Use Manufacturer	Ingredients
POULTRY HOUSE FUMIGANT (Hilltop)	Furfuraldehyde* 50% Formaldehyde* 18.50% Methyl alcohol 5%	PPP Rubefacient (Three P)	Fl. extr. poke root, prickly ash, and stillingia Alcohol 4.22%/v Potassium iodide * Sodium salicylate * Glycerin
POULTRYTONE Tonic (veterinary, avian) (Martin, C.J.)	Quassia Capsicum Colombo Anhydrous manganous sulfate Copper sulfate 1-1/2% Iron sulfate Nux vomica (containg 1.4% strychnine*) 1% Calcium carbonate Magnesium sulfate Calcium phosphate Magnesium carbonate Venetian red 10% Iodized salt	PRACTI-KREME SKIN PROTECTOR AND CLEANER (Chem. Spec.)	
POUR LA PRINCESSE PERFUME (House of Goureilli)		PRAEFECTA WATER LILY FERTILIZER (Tricker)	
POUR UN HOMME EXTRACT Toiletry (Caron)		PRAGMATAR OINTMENT Rubefacient (Smith, Kline & French)	Cetyl alcohol-coal tar distillate* 4% Near-colloidal sulfur 3% Salicylic acid* 3%
POVINE Nasal decongestant (Success)	Povine hydrochloride 0.1% Potassium biphosphate 0.7% Potassium chloride 0.2% Sodium phosphate 0.2% Sodium chloride 0.07% Dextrose	PRAMCYL TABS Antirheumatic (Allied Prod.)	Each tablet: Ammonium salicylate* 0.3 gm. Para-aminobenzoic acid 0.3 gm. Ascorbic acid 50 mg.
POWDER CITY PAINT PRODUCTS (Rowe)		PRANG CHARCOAL PENCILS, PASTELLO CRAYONS (Am. Crayon)	
POWDERED UTILITY CLEANER (Chemco)	Trisodium phosphate *50% Tetrasodium pyrophosphate 10% Sesquicarbonate 25% Bicarbonate of soda 12% Nytron 1% Santomerse 1.5% Triton X-100 0.5%	PRANG TEMPERA, TEXTILE COLORS, WATER COLORS, DEK-ALL THERMO SETTING COLORS, DRAWING INK (Am. Crayon)	
POWDER-ENE Rug cleaner (Von Schrader)	Petroleum naphtha* Cellulose absorbent powder Calcium Aluminum Iron Silica	PRATT'S BAG OINTMENT Antiseptic (Pratt Food)	Ortho phenyl phenol * Gum benzoin Gum turpentine* Petrolatum base
POWER'S RELIEF Asthmatic, antispasmodic (Powers)	Stramonium* (0.125-0.15% stramonium alkaloid) 50% Powdered mullein leaves Saltpeter	PRATT'S BROILER WORMER (Pratt Food)	Nicotine (alkaloid)* 5.00% Bentonite Fuller's earth
POWOW CLEANSER (West Coast)		PRATT'S CATTLE & BARN SPRAY Insecticide (Pratt Food	Beta butoxy beta' thiocyano diethyl ether 15% Methoxychlor tech. 8.00% Methylated aromatic petroleum deriv.* 55% Petroleum distillate 14%
POW-R CAPS PLANT FOOD (Daniels, Ross)			
POWRITE METAL CLEANER (Whitfield)			

*Consult Sec. II., Ingredients Index. This ingredient may be responsible for major toxic effects if poisonous amounts of this product are ingested.

Name & Use Manufacturer	Ingredients		Name & Use Manufacturer	Ingredients	
PRATT'S 50W CHLORDANE Insecticide (Pratt, B.)	Chlordane*	50%	PRATT'S 622 INSECT REPELLENT (Pratt, B.)	Indalone (alpha, alpha-dimethyl-alpha'-carbobutoxy dihydro-gamma-pyrone) Dimethyl phthalate Dimethyl carbate	
PRATT'S 5% CHLORDANE DUST Insecticide (Pratt, B.)	Tech. chlordane*	5%	PRATT'S IN-TES-TROL (veterinary, avian) (Prat Food)	Methylrosaniline (gentian violet) Copper sulfate* (hydrated) 40% Ferrous sulfate (Copperas) Zinc sulfate* Manganese sulfate Tartaric acid Calcium sulfate (native) 50%	
PRATT'S C-KA-GENE For coccidiosis (poultry) (Pratt Food)	Guaiacol* Sulfur* Copper sulfate Manganese sulfate Iron sulfate Red oxide of iron Ground limestone Vitamin D	0.2% 5.5%			
			PRATT'S LICE KILLER (Pratt Food)	Rotenone Other cube extractives Methoxychlor tech.	1.0% 1.8% 0.5%
PRATT'S COW TONIC (Pratt Food)	Nux vomica* Sodium bicarbonate Iron sulfate Manganese sulfate Calcium carbonate Irradiated yeast Fennel Salt Copper sulfate Cobalt carbonate Potassium iodide Fenugreek Red oxide of iron	10% 32% 10% 0.4%	PRATT'S 5% LINDANE SPRAY Insecticide (Pratt, B.)	Lindane* (gamma isomer of benzene hexachloride) 5%	
			PRATT'S 50% MALATHION SPRAY Insecticide (Pratt, B.)	Malathion* (o,o-dimethyl dithiophosphate of diethyl mercaptosuccinate) 50%	
PRATT'S D-X AERO SPRAY Insecticide (Pratt, B.)	Pyrethrum Rotenone * Piperonyl cyclonene Active carrier*		PRATT'S MILL-MIX POULTRY REGULATOR Tonic (vet-erinary, avian) (Pratt Food (Phila.))	Potassium iodide Iron sulfate Copper sulfate* Zinc sulfate* Manganese sulfate Oxide of iron Cobalt carbonate 200-Mesh limestone flour	
PRATT'S D-X INSECT SPRAY (Pratt, B.)	Cyclonene Pyrethrins Rotenone Soya bean Pine oil*	2.0% 0.28% 0.75%			
			PRATT'S NICOTINE SPRAY Insecticide (Pratt, B.)	Nicotine* Soya bean oil Pine oil	20%
PRATT'S FLY SPRAY (Pratt Food)	Beta butoxy beta' thiocyano diethyl ether 2.00% Beta thiocyanoethyl esters of mixed fatty acids containing 10-18 carbon atoms 0.80% Petroleum distillate* 96.95% Essential oils 0.25%		PRATT'S PARA-SCALECIDE Insecticide (Pratt, B.)	Miscible oil (scalecide) Paradichlorobenzene* 12.6%	
			PRATT'S POTASSIUM CYANATE CRAB GRASS KILLER (Pratt, B.)	Potassium cyanate* 77.35%	
PRATT'S FRUIT TREE SPRAY (Pratt, B.)	Basic lead arsenate* DDT Sulfur	14.4% 7.5% 62%			
PRATT'S GARDEN & ROSE DUST OR SPRAY Insecticide, fungicide (Pratt, B.)	Pyrethrins Piperonyl cyclonene Rotenone Other cube resins Sulfur* Copper	0.03% 0.375% 0.50% 0.75% 30% 3.4%	PRATT'S POULTRY TABLETS Drinking water antiseptic (Pratt Food)	Potassium permanganate* 30.00% Alum Salt Bentonite Calcium sulfate Parawax Calcium stearate	
PRATT'S HOG OIL Ectoparasiticide (veterinary) (Pratt Food)	Gamma isomer of benzene hexachloride 2.0% Methylated aromatic petroleum deriv.* 26.0% Petroleum distillate 67.0%		PRATT'S POULTRY WORM POWDER (Pratt Food)	Nicotine (alkaloid)* Phenothiazine	4.00% 15.00%
PRATT'S INHALANT Respiratory decongestant (veterinary, avian) (Pratt Food)	Oil of eucalyptus * Beechwood creosote * Oil of camphor * Pine oil * White mineral oil	85%			

*Consult Sec. II., Ingredients Index. This ingredient may be responsible for major toxic effects if poisonous amounts of this product are ingested.

Name & Use Manufacturer	Ingredients		Name & Use Manufacturer	Ingredients	
PRATT'S RAT & MOUSE KILLER (Pratt Food)	2-Pivalyl-1,3-indandione	0.025%	PRATT'S SWINE BUILDER Antibiotic, food suplement (Pratt Food)	Dried fermentation solubles Niacin Irradiated yeast Nux vomica* Copper sulfate Manganese sulfate Zinc sulfate* Corn distillers dried grains with solubles Dried brewers yeast Calcium pantothenate Corn distillers dried solubles Iron sulfate Potassium iodide Cobalt sulfate Soybean oil meal	2.0%
PRATT'S RED MITE SPECIAL Insecticide (Pratt Food)	Tech. chlordane (60% octachloro-4,7-methano tetrahydro indane and 40% related compounds) 0.5% Beta butoxy beta' thiocyano diethyl ether 1.0% Dichloro diphenyl trichloro-ethane* 5.0% Methylated aromatic petroleum deriv.* 10.0% Essential oils 0.25% Petroleum distillate* 83.25%				
			PRATT'S TOMATO DUST OR SPRAY Fungicide (Pratt, B.)	Copper*	7.0%
PRATT'S ROOST PAINT Ectoparasiticide (veterinary, avian) (Pratt Food)	Gamma isomer of benzene hexachloride 1.0% Other isomers of benzene hexachloride 1.0% Dichloro diphenyl trichloro-ethane 2.0% Polymethylated naphthalenes* 3.5% Petroleum oils* 92.0% Essential oils 0.5%		PRATT'S TRIPLE ACTION WORMER (veterinary, avian) (Pratt Food)	Nicotine* Phenothiazine Dihydroxy dichlorodiphenyl methane	2.20% 12.80% 15.00%
PRATT'S ROSE & FLORAL SPRAY Insecticide (Pratt, B.)	Pyrethrum Rotenone* Piperonyl cyclonene Volatile carrier*		PRATT'S VEGETABLE DUST OR SPRAY Insecticide, fungicide (Pratt, B.)	Rotenone Copper*	0.75% 7.0%
PRATT'S 3/4% ROTENONE DUST OR SPRAY Insecticide (Pratt, B.)	Rotenone	0.75%	PREACHER'S HAIR TONIC (Preachers)		
PRATT'S SCREW-WORM KILLER Insecticide (Pratt Food)	Gamma isomer of benzene hexachloride (from lindane)* 3% Pine oil* 35%		PRECEPTIN Vaginal jelly (Ortho)	Diisobutyl phenoxy polyethoxy ethanol 1.00% Ricinoleic acid 1.17%	
PRATT'S SODIUM ARSENITE WEED KILLER (Pratt, B.)	Sodium arsenite*	35%	PREDICAINE Skin ointment (Rhodes Pharm.)	Methyl benzethonium chloride Ethyl p-aminobenzoate (benzocaine) p-Chloro-m-xylenol Tyrothricin	
			PREEN Wax (Harrison, A.S.)	Natural and petroleum waxes Oil-soluble dyes Stoddard solvent* Turpentine*	
PRATT'S SULFA-QUINOXA-LINE LIQUID Coccidiosis (veterinary, avian) (Pratt Food)	Sodium sulfaquinoxaline*	3.44 gr.	PREENET Wax (Harrison, A.S.)	Natural and petroleum waxes Stearates Ammonia*	
			PREEN WALL WAX (Harrison, A.S.)	Similar to PREEN	
PRATT'S SUPERIOR DORMANT OIL Insecticide (Pratt, B.)	Emulsifiable oil	98%	PREEN WAVE SET (Julienne)		
			PRE-FAB PREFABRI-CATED HOUSE PAINT (Arco)		

*Consult Sec. II., Ingredients Index. This ingredient may be responsible for major toxic effects if poisonous amounts of this product are ingested.

Name & Use Manufacturer	Ingredients	Name & Use Manufacturer	Ingredients
PRELIM Wax (Harrison, A.S.)	Petroleum waxes Tall oil Stearates	PREMO-TOSS Antitussive (Premo)	Alcohol 9%/v Ammonium chloride 1-1/2 gr. Thenylpyramine hydrochloride* 10 mg.
PRELL Shampoo, gel or liquid (Procter & Gamble)	Anionic synthetic detergent Fatty acid amide Methyl cellulose Ethyl alcohol	PRENTILS TABLETS Analgesic (Prentil)	Acetophenetidin* 2-1/2 gr. Aspirin* 2-1/2 gr.
PREMEER POWDER Insecticide (Destruxol)	Pyrethrum powder 70% Sodium acid fluoride* 5%	PRENTISS ANTU Rodenticide (Prentiss)	Alpha naphthyl thiourea* 97.5%
PRE-MENS Premenstrual tension (Purdue)	Each tablet: Ammonium chloride 5.0 gr. Homatropine methylbromide* 0.5 mg. Caffeine alkaloid 0.5 gr. Vitamin B$_1$ (thiamine hydro- chloride) 2.0 mg. Vitamin B$_2$ (riboflavin) 1.0 mg. Vitamin B$_6$ (pyridoxine hydro- chloride) 0.5 mg. Calcium pantothenate 1.0 mg. Niacinamide 5.0 mg.	PRENTISS PYRETHRUM POWDERS Insecticide (Prentiss)	Pyrethrins 0.5-1.3%
PREMERGE (Dow)	Ethanolamine and isopropanol- amine series salts of dinitro- o-sec-butylphenol*	PRENTOX BENZENE HEXACHLORIDE POWDER (Wettable) Insecticide (Prentiss)	Gamma isomer of benzene hexachloride* 5% Other isomers of benzene hexachloride* 40%
PREMIER PAINTS (Bishop- Conklin)		PRENTOX 20% CHLORDANE CONCEN- TRATE (Oil-Soluble) Insecticide (Prentiss)	Chlordane* 20% Petroleum distillates* 80%
PREMIER VARNISHES (Louisville Varnish)		PRENTOX CHLORDANE 20% (Oil-Soluble) Insecticide (Prentiss)	Chlordane* 1.45 lb./gal.
PREMIER WATERPROOF ADHESIVE (Metal)		PRENTOX CHLORDANE 46% & 72% EMULSIFIABLE CONCEN- TRATE Insecticide (Prentiss)	Chlordane* 4 and 8 lb./gal.
PREMIUM Paints & Varnishes (Pratt Paint)		PRENTOX CHLORDANE 62% EMULSIFIABLE CONCEN- TRATE Insecticide (Prentiss)	Chlordane* 6.3 lb./gal.
PREMO C.R.C. TABLETS Cathartic (Premo)	Calomel* 2 gr. Extr. colocynth* Aloes * Rhubarb U.S.P. Resin scammony Myrrh	PRENTOX 50% CHLORDANE POWDER Insecticide (Prentiss)	Chlordane*
PREMOPHEN Laxative (Premo)	Extr. belladonna leaves * 1/12 gr. Phenolpthalein 1/2 gr. Aloin * 1/4 gr. Ipecac 1/15 gr.	PRENTOX CHLORDANE TECH. AG & REFINED Insecticide (Prentiss)	Chlordane*
PREMO SYRUP EUCILLANA COMPOUND Antitussive (Premo)	Ethyl morphine hydrochloride* 1/4 gr. Alcohol 6% Cocillana 4 m. Extr. euphorbia pilulifera 120 m. Syrup squill compound 24 m. Syrup wild lettuce 120 m. Cascarin 1 gr. Menthol 2/25 gr.	PRENTOX CHLORDANE 40% & 50% WETTABLE POWDERS Insecticide (Prentiss)	Chlordane* 40 and 50%

*Consult Sec. II., Ingredients Index. This ingredient may be responsible for major toxic effects if poisonous amounts of this product are ingested.

Name & Use Manufacturer	Ingredients		Name & Use Manufacturer	Ingredients	
PRENTOX CUBE POWDER Insecticide (Prentiss)	Ground cube root Rotenone*and other active resins	90% 4-6%	PRENTOX 25% LINDANE WETTABLE Insecticide (Prentiss)	Lindane*	25%
PRENTOX CUBE RESINS Insecticide (Prentiss)	Rotenone*	30-45%	PRENTOX MICRO MESH 50% & 75% DDT DUST CONCEN- TRATE Insecticide (Prentiss)	DDT*	50 and 75%
PRENTOX 25% DDT EMULSIFIABLE CONCEN- TRATE Insecticide (Prentiss)	DDT*	25%	PRENTOX MICRO MESH 50% to 75% DDT WETTABLE POWDER Insecticide (Prentiss)	DDT*	50 and 75%
PRENTOX 50% DDT MICRO-MESH DRY POWDER (Clay Base) Insecticide (Prentiss)	DDT*	50%			
PRENTOX 50% DDT MICRO- MESH DRY POWDER (Pyrophyllite Base) Insecticide (Prentiss)	DDT*	50%	PRENTOX 20% OIL & EMULSIFIABLE CONCEN- TRATE Insecticide (Prentiss)	Lindane*	1.78 and 1.74 lb./gal.
			PRENTOX PHENO- THIAZINE DRENCH POWDER (Veterinary) (Prentiss)	Phenothiazine N.F.*	99%
PRENTOX 30% DDT OIL SOLUBLE CONCEN- TRATE Insecticide (Prentiss)	DDT*	30%	PRENTOX PHENO- THIAZINE* N.F. Anthelmintic (veterinary) (Prentiss)	Phenothiazine*	
PRENTOX 10% DDT POWDER Insecticide (Prentiss)	DDT*	10%	PRENTOX PYRETHRUM CONCEN- TRATE NO. 20 Insecticide (Prentiss)	Pyrethrins Oil *	2.4% 97.6%
PRENTOX 50% DDT TRACKING POWDER Rodenticide (Prentiss)	DDT*	50%	PRENTOX PYRETHRUM CONCEN- TRATE #100 Insecticide (Prentiss)	Pyrethrins * Inert ingredients	11.8%
PRENTOX 25% DDT WATER MISCIBLE Insecticide (Prentiss)	DDT Methyl naphthalenes *	25% 70%	PRENTOX ROACH POWDER (Prentiss)	Pyrethrins Chlordane	0.4% 2%
PRENTOX 95% LINDANE Insecticide (Prentiss)	Lindane *	95%	PRENTOX SABADILLA 50% DUST CONCEN- TRATE Insecticide (Prentiss)	Alkaloids of sabadilla*	2.0%
PRENTOX LINDANE TECH. Insecticide (Prentiss)	Gamma isomer of benzene hexachloride*	99%	PRENTOX 500 SERIES OF CON- CENTRATE Insecticide (Prentiss)	Pyrethrum or allethrin Piperonyl butoxide with or with- out DDT* Inert ingredients*	

*Consult Sec. II., Ingredients Index. This ingredient may be responsible for major toxic effects if poisonous amounts of this product are ingested.

Name & Use Manufacturer	Ingredients	
PRENTOX STABILIZED RED SQUILL Rodenticide (Prentiss)	Fortified red squill*	equiv. to 100%
PRENTOX TECHNICAL GRADE DDT Insecticide (Prentiss)	DDT*	
PRENTOX TOXAPHENE CONCENTRATE Insecticide (Prentiss)	Toxaphene*	40%
PRENTOX 5% WETTABLE CUBE POWDER Insecticide (Prentiss)	Rotenone*	5%
PREPARAKOTE PRIMER-SURFACERS Automotive finish (du Pont)		
PREPARATION H CONTAINS BIO-DYNE (Suppositories & ointment) Hemorrhoid relief (Whitehall)	Live yeast cell deriv. (skin respiratory factor) 2,000 units/oz. Shark liver oil 3.0% Phenyl mercuric nitrate 1:10,000	
PREPARATION NO. B 2851 (Myers Labs.)	Potassium iodide* Fl. extr. cimicifuga (black cohash) Sodium salicylate* Ascorbic acid	
PREPARATION NO. 77 SHIPPING MEDICINE Conditioner (veterinary) (Thoroughbred)	Ether* 8%/v Salol * Eucalyptol * Oil of eucalyptus * Oil of peppermint Olive oil Fl. ext. belladonna (0.0108 gr./ fl. oz. alkaloids) Linseed oil	
PREP BRUSHLESS CREAM (Allen, Mark)	(Same as Prep shaving cream)	
PREP-COAT ENAMEL UNDERCOAT (Lasting)		
PREPICK MICRO-SCOPIC Fungicide (Bartlett, N.M.)	Sulfur* 99%	
PREP SHAVE LOTION (Allen, Mark)	S.D. alcohol* #40 Menthol*	

Name & Use Manufacturer	Ingredients	
PREP SHAVING CREAM (Allen, Mark)	Saponified stearic acid Free stearic acid Mineral oil Glycerin Menthol, thymol, camphor, and phenol (less than 1/4%) approx. 1.1%	
PREP-SOL SOLVENT (du Pont)		
PRESCO BABY CREAM (Prescrip. Spec.)	Zinci carbonas 1.5 gm. Oxycholesterin 3.0 gm. Ung. aq. ros. 15.0 gm. Petrolatum 30.0 gm.	
PRESCO CARMINATIVE (Prescript. Spec.)	Calcium carbonate 2.5 gm. Syrup rhei 2.5 cc. Aqua gaultheriae 30.0 cc.	
PRESCO CRADLE CAP OINTMENT (Prescript. Spec.)	Sulfur* Resorcin Oxycholesterin Petrolatum	
PRESCO NOSE DROPS (Prescript. Spec.)	Phenylephrine 0.25% Sodium chloride 0.5% Sodium benzoate Sodium bisulfite Methylparaben Propylparaben	
PRESCO NURSERY OIL (Prescript. Spec.)	Olive and vegetable oils	
PRESCRIPTION CREAM LOTION Cosmetic (LaFayette)	Homogenized lanolin Aethol Urea Almond oil Mineral oil Benzoic acid	
PRESCRIPTION TWENTY-FIVE (Buschemeyer's) Analgesic (Heywood Labs.)	Methenamine* Pipsissewa Cimicifuga Magnesia carbonate Uva ursi Sodium acid phosphate* Sodium salicylate*	
PRESERVALL Wood preservative (Van Sickle)		
PRESERVAR VARNISH (Martin Varnish)		
PRESERVO Water-mildew-proofing (cotton duck) (Robeson)	Copper naphthenate 8% Di-(phenyl mercury) dodecenyl succinate* Zinc naphthenate (if colored fabric) 8%	
PRESIDENT PAINTS & VARNISHES (Harrison P. & V.)		

*Consult Sec. II., Ingredients Index. This ingredient may be responsible for major toxic effects if poisonous amounts of this product are ingested.

- 856 -

Name & Use Manufacturer	Ingredients	Name & Use Manufacturer	Ingredients
PRESSURIZED ROACH SPRAY (Holcomb)	Chlordane* Pyrethrins Piperonyl butoxide	PRETONE HARDWOOD FLOOR CLEANER, PAINT & VARNISH CLEANER, PORCELAIN, TILE & MARBLE CLEANER (Pretone)	
PRESSURIZED YARN TREAT (Holcomb)	Stoddard solvent*		
PRESTO CLOSET BOWL CLEANER (Chamberlain Haber)		PRE-VENT-RUST (Stull, A.J.)	
PRESTO CORN CURE (Olliffe)	Salicylic acid* Alcohol Carbolic acid Flexible collodion Acetone Benzocaine	PREWEED Herbicide (Wilson, Jack)	Isopropyl-n-(3-chlorophenyl)-carbamate* 47%
PRESTO DRAIN PIPE CLEANER (Chamberlain Haber)		PRIDE Furniture polish (Johnson, S.C.)	Petroleum naphtha* Silicone fluid Petroleum waxes
PRES-TO FABRIC CEMENT (Dural)		PRIMATENE Asthmatic, antispasmodic (Whitehall)	Theophylline * Ephedrine hydrochloride* Phenobarbital 1/8 gr.
PRESTO-NAMEL ENAMEL (Perry & Derrick)		PRIMATROL House paint primer (Kurfees)	
PRESTONE Anti freeze (Nat'l Carbon)	Ethylene glycol *	PRIM CREAM SPRAY OR STICK DEODORANT (Daggett & Ramsdell)	
PRESTON'S POISON IVY REMEDY (Preston Drug)		PRIMECOTE WOOD PRIMER (White Co.)	Pigment: Titanium dioxide 43.69% Titanium calcium pigment 19.07% Basic silicate white lead* 17.05% Magnesium silicate 22.84% Vehicle: Refined linseed oil 29.10% Heat-treated fish oil 10.00% Varnish 32.46% Mineral spirits and driers* 28.44%
PRESTO PORCELAIN, TILE & MARBLE CLEANING COMPOUND (Chamberlain Haber)			
PRES-TO RUBBER CEMENT (Dural)		PRIMEKOTER (Pioneer)	
PRESTO SARCOPTIC MANGE REMEDY (Presto)	Linseed oil Diethyl ether* Mineral oil Turpentine*	PRIMOX LACQUER SEALER (Oxidermo)	
		PRIMOX METAL PAINT (Cheesman-Elliott)	
PRESTO SPOT REMOVER (Gobberdiel)		PRIMROSE HOUSE ALL-PURPOSE CREAM Face cream (Daggett & Ramsdell)	

*Consult Sec. II., Ingredients Index. This ingredient may be responsible for major toxic effects if poisonous amounts of this product are ingested.

Name & Use Manufacturer	Ingredients
PRIMROSE HOUSE BUBBLE BATH (Daggett & Ramsdell)	
PRIMROSE HOUSE COLOGNE & TOILET WATER (Daggett & Ramsdell)	
PRIMROSE HOUSE CREAM SHAMPOO (Daggett & Ramsdell)	
PRIMROSE HOUSE FACE POWDER (Daggett & Ramsdell)	
PRIMROSE HOUSE HAND LOTION (Daggett & Ramsdell)	
PRIMROSE HOUSE LIPSTICK (Daggett & Ramsdell)	
PRIMROSE HOUSE MAKE-UP BASE (Daggett & Ramsdell)	
PRIMROSE HOUSE SHAMPOO (Liquid) (Daggett & Ramsdell)	
PRINCE MATCHA-BELLI PERFUMES & COLOGNES (Prince)	Aldehydes* Amyl salicylate* Benzyl alcohol Citronellol Phenyl ethyl alcohol Eugenol * Linalyl acetate Nitro musks Ethyl alcohol* Diethyl phthalate Citrus oils
PRINCESS ENAMELS (Monroe Sander)	
PRINCESS EVE CHLORA STICK Deodorant (Whitehall)	Chlorophyll

Name & Use Manufacturer	Ingredients
PRINCESS PAT BATH FRAGRANCE, COLOGNE, DEODORANT CREAM, GORDON'S EX-ODOR, LIQUID ICE ASTRINGENT (Princess Pat)	
PRINCESS WHITE SHOE DRESSING (Packard Dressing)	
PRIOR-LITE ENAMEL (Payson Corp.)	
PRISMA PAINTS (New Orleans)	
PRIVATE BRANDS WARFARIN RAT & MOUSE KILLER (Private Brands)	Warfarin Corn and oat meal
PRIVATE FORMULA Analgesic (Reese Chem.)	Quinine sulfate* Camphor monobromated* Salicylamide * Caffeine
PRIVINE HYDRO-CHLORIDE JELLY 0.05% Nasal decongestant (Ciba)	Naphazoline hydrochloride 50 mg. Sodium ethyl mercurithio-salicylate 1 mg. Aromatics
PRIVINE SOLUTION Nasal decongestant (Ciba)	Naphazoline hydrochloride (0.05%) 50 mg. Phenylmercuric acetate 1-50,000
PRO-ACET DOUCHE CONCEN-TRATE (Pro-Acet)	Citric acid U.S.P. 2.5% Acetic acid U.S.P. 4.0% Lactic acid U.S.P. 2.0% Sodium lauryl sulfate U.S.P. 3.0% Dextrose U.S.P. 5.0% Lactose (beta) U.S.P. 2.5% Sodium acetate U.S.P. 2.5% Methyl paraben U.S.P. 0.5%
PROCESS 33 Paint brush cleaner (Coughlan)	
PROCTOREX Rectal lotion (Marion Pharm.)	Alcohol* 33%/v Extr. tree oil Menthol Camphor* Soft soap n-Butyl parahydroxybenzoate

*Consult Sec. II., Ingredients Index. This ingredient may be responsible for major toxic effects if poisonous amounts of this product are ingested.

- 858 -

Name & Use Manufacturer	Ingredients		Name & Use Manufacturer	Ingredients	
PROCTOREX Rectal suppositories (Marion Pharm.)	Each suppository: Extr. stramonium Ephedrine sulfate* Bismuth oxyiodide Bismuth subgallate Benzocaine n-Butyl para-hydroxybenzoate Extr. tree oil Cocoa butter	0.15 gr. 0.3 gr.	PROM HOME PERMANENT (Toni)	Ammonium thioglycolate Free ammonia Ammonium salts	
			PROMICROL Film developer (Murphy, G.)		
PRO-DERMA Skin cream (Westwood)	Silcone (polydimethyl siloxane) 52.5% Aluminum base		PRONETHSIN BURN OINTMENT (Chemical Ind.)		
PRODERMIC S.F. MFR. NO. 625 For skin (Specialists)	Acetic acid Iodine*		PRONIDE For coccidiosis (poultry) (Salsbury's)	Dinitro diphenyl sulfonyl ethylene diamine * 50% Acetyl-(paranitrophenyl) sulfanilamide 30%	
PROFESSIONAL PAINTS & VARNISHES (Pratt)			PRONTO DRAIN OPENER (Wyandotte)	Concentrated alkali*	
PROFESSOR FOSTER'S DISCOVERY Liquid detergent (Sexton)			PRONTO IGNITION SEALER (Aerosol Prod.)		
PROGESIC Analgesic (Vitec)	Sodium salicylate* 5 gr. Para-aminobenzoic acid 5 gr. Ascorbic acid 15 mg.		PRONTO INSECT KILLER (Aerosol Prod)		
PROHEXINOL Nasal decongestant (Sharp & Dohme)	Propadrine-(phenyl propanol amine hydrochloride*) 1.5% Caprokol (hexylresorcinol) 1-3000		PRONTO LIQUID ANALGESIC (Commerce)	Methyl salicylate* Menthol Isopropyl alcohol * 62%	
PRO-HYGIN Vaginal douche (Pinkham)	Benzalkonium chloride * Boric acid* Lactic acid Glucose Glycerin		PRONTO MOTH PROOFER (Aerosol Prod.)		
PROKETUSS Antiallergic antitussive (Sharp & Dohme)	Each 5 cc.: Alcohol 5% Methapyrilene hydrochloride 10 mg. Propadrine phenyl propanolamine hydrochloride 15 mg. Potassium citrate 0.15 gm. Chloroform 15 mg. Menthol 1 mg.		PRONTO-SAN PINK TABLETS Analgesic (Tosan's)	Aspirin* 3-1/2 gr. Acetophenetidin * 2-1/2 gr. Caffeine 1/2 gr.	
			PRONTO WATER PROOFER (Aerosol Prod.)		
PROKRAFT INTERIOR PAINT (Elliott)			PRO PAINTS & VARNISHES (Atlas P.&V.)		
PROLARMON JELLY (rectal) (Meco)			PROPON 4 Herbicide (Pittsburgh Coke)	Isooctyl ester of 2-(2,4,5-tri-chlorophenoxy) propionic acid* 62.9%	
PROM DYE CREAM SUEDE DRESSING (Kelly, G.J.)			PROQUANOL Douche powder (Mu-col)	Cetyl dimethyl benzyl ammonium chloride * Boric acid* Citric acid Sodium chloride Oil of eucalyptus * Methyl salicylate* Menthol * Thymol *	
PROMETIN Asthmatic antitussive (Sumlar)	Each fl. oz.: Ephedrine sulfate* 3 gr. Potassium iodide Ammonium carbonate Extr. senega and squill				

Name & Use Manufacturer	Ingredients		Name & Use Manufacturer	Ingredients	
PROQUIL Sedative (Hance)	Methapyrilene hydrochloride*	25 mg.	PROTEXALL HEP Insecticide (Pro-Tex-All)	Chlordane Oil*	2%
PRORYZA TABLETS Nasal decongestant (Clapp, Otis)	Atropine sulfate* Acetophenetidin* Acetanilid* Caffeine Sodium bicarbonate Camphor* Quinine arsenate* Arsenic	1/2000 gr. 1/4 gr. 0.175 gr. 0.025 gr. 0.05 gr. 1.4 gr. 1.100 gr. 0.0008 gr.	PRO-TEX-ALL ROACH-NOK-R Insecticide (Pro-Tex-All)	Pyrethrins Sodium fluoride* Sodium silicofluoride	0.2% 38% 0.8%
			PROTEXALL SYNTHETIC ENAMEL (Pratt Paint)		
PRO SALUS DISINFECTANT (United Chem.)			PROTEX DISINFECTANT (McVicker)		
PROSOL Ear eczema (Torch)	Mercury oleate Coal tar Salicylic acid* Phenol p-Nitrophenol Isopropyl alcohol*	0.25% 0.60% 1.50% 0.25% 0.25%	PROTEX FABRIC CEMENT (Garland)		
PROTECTIVE PASTE S.F. NO. 789 Skin protective (Specialists)	Zinc oxide Amylum Calcium lactate Sodium phosphate Petrolatum Adeps lanae		PROTEXO STUCCO CONCRETE PAINT (Sillers)		
PROTECTOLINE RUST PREVENTIVE (Magnus)			PROTEX RUST PREVENTIVE & REMOVER COMPOUND (Wayne)		
PROTEGEL For skin irritation (Wyeth Labs.)	Gel of alumina Kaolin		PROTEX (Wilke's) Protective dressing (veterinary) (Wilke)	Sulfonated linseed oil Raw linseed oil Turpentine* Resin	28.57% 25.33% 26.64% 19.46%
PRO-TEK PROTECTIVE HAND CREAM (du Pont)			PROTOSEP Food supplement (poultry) (Whitmoyer)	Cod liver oil concentrate Oil of eucalyptus * Thymol* Lactic acid Hydrochloric acid Benzoic acid Glycerin Copper gluconate* Calcium gluconate	
PRO-TEK-SHUN PAINTS, VARNISHES, ENAMELS (Steelcote)					
PROTEX Insecticide (Chem. Insect.)	Methylated naphthalene*, rotenone, and other cube extractives Acetone* Soap of petroleum sulfonates Polyethylene glycol ester of fatty acid	64.5%	PROTESEP-B For cecal coccidiosis (poultry) (Whitmoyer)	Hydrochloric acid Benzoic acid Lactic acid Thymol Oil of eucalyptus * Fortified cod liver oil Cod liver meal Dried brewers yeast Sulfur Calcium gluconate Copper gluconate	
PROTEX (Magitex) Seasonal protection (dogs) (Magitex)	Citronella oil* Lemongrass oil*		PROTO-TABS Tablets for poultry drinking water (Whitmoyer)	Copper sulfate* Calcium phenolsulfonate Sodium phenolsulfonate Zinc phenolsulfonate Boric acid*	
PROTEXAL Antibacterial (Nat'l Milling)	Sodium orthophenylphenate* Trisodium phosphate	2% 10%	PROX Rust preventative (Kano)	Resinous compounds *	

*Consult Sec. II., Ingredients Index. This ingredient may be responsible for major toxic effects if poisonous amounts of this product are ingested.

- 860 -

Name & Use Manufacturer	Ingredients
PRUBILAX Laxative (Bell Pharm.)	Each tablet: Acetophenolisatin 5 mg. Prune (powdered) 5 gr.
PRUCIDE Fungicide (medical) (Prucide)	Benzoic acid* Salicylic acid* Boric acid* Thymol * Benzyl trialkonium chloride* Isopropyl alcohol* 50%
PRUCOFF SYRUP Antispasmodic (Prucide)	Ephedrine sulfate* 1/2 gr. Potassium guaiacol sulfate 8 gr. Citric acid Sodium citrate Syrup squill Sanguinaria Alcohol 5.75%/v Menthol Glycerin
PRULEZE TABLETS, IMPROVED Cathartic (Preston Labs.)	Methyl cellulose 400 mg. Prune concentrate 100 mg. Acetophenolisatin 2 mg.
PRULOSE COMPLEX (Harrower) Laxative (Warner-Chilcott)	Each tablet: Dehydrated prune concentrate 130 mg. Methylcellulose 390 mg. Diacetylhydroxyphenylisatin 1 mg.
PRULOSE COMPLEX LIQUID (Harrower) Cathartic (Warner-Chilcott)	Each 15 cc.: Liquid prune concentrate (70% solids) 3.37 gm. Diacetyl hydroxy phenylisatin 0.002 gm. Carboxymethyl cellulose sodium 0.75 gm.
PRUNACEL Cathartic (Tutag)	Each tablet: Prune concentrate 3/4 gr. Acetophenolisatin 2 mg. Methylcellulose 1 gr.
PRUSCORBIN CAPSULES Analgesic, antipyretic (Prucide)	Phenobarbital 1/8 gr. Aspirin* 2-1/2 gr. Phenacetin* 2-1/2 gr. Caffeine 1/4 gr. Ascorbic acid 10 mg. Atropine sulfate 1/500 gr.
PRU VAGINAL JELLY (Commonwealth)	Oxyquinoline sulfate Lactic acid Alum Glycerin Boric acid Benzoic acid Gum tragacanth
PSC ALDRIN EMULSIFIABLE CONCENTRATE Insecticide (Pacific Supply)	Hexachloro hexahydro dimethano naphthalene* 23.10% Related compounds 17.40% Petroleum aromatic deriv. 52.00%
PSC ALDRIN 25% WETTABLE POWDER Insecticide (Pacific Supply)	Hexachloro hexahydro dimethano naphthalene* 23.80% Related compounds 17.90%

Name & Use Manufacturer	Ingredients
PSC AMINE WEED KILLER (Pacific Supply)	Alkanolamine salts (ethanol and isopropanol series) of 2,4-dichloro phenoxy acetic acid * 65.00%
PSC ARSENATE OF LEAD 15 & SULFUR 85 DUST Insecticide (Pacific Supply)	Lead arsenate* 15.00%
PSC BASIC COPPER SULFATE 10 DUST Fungicide (Pacific Supply)	Copper expressed as metallic* 5.25%
PSC CHLORDANE 5 DUST Insecticide (Pacific Supply)	Tech. chlordane* 5%
PSC CHLORDANE EMULSIFIABLE CONCENTRATE 72-1/2 Insecticide (Pacific Supply)	Tech. chlordane* 72.5% Aromatic petroleum deriv. solvent 15.0%
PSC CHLORDANE 5 GARDEN DUST Insecticide (Pacific Supply)	Tech. chlordane* 5.0%
PSC CHLORO IPC EMULSIVE Herbicide (Pacitic Supply)	o-Isopropyl-n-(3-chlorophenyl)-carbamate* 47.5%
PSC CO-OP ALDRIN 25% WETTABLE Insecticide (Pacific Supply)	Hexachloro hexahydro dimethano naphthalene* 23.8% Related compounds 4.00%
PSC CO-OP AMINE WEED KILLER (Pacific Supply)	Alkanolamine salts (ethanol and isopropyl series of 2,4-dichlorophenoxyacetic acid* 65.00%
PSC CO-OP CHLORO IPC EMULSIVE Herbicide (Pacific Supply)	Isopropyl-n-(3-chlorophenyl)-carbamate* 47.5%

Name & Use Manufacturer	Ingredients	Name & Use Manufacturer	Ingredients
PSC CO-OP ESTER WEED KILLER (Pacific Supply)	Isopropyl ester of 2,4-dichloro phenoxy acetic acid * (equiv. to 2,4-dichloro phenoxy acetic acid 37%) 44%	PSC CO-OP TOXAPHENE 40% WETTABLE Insecticide (Pacific Supply)	Toxaphene* 40%
PSC CO-OP GERMICIDE (Pacific Supply)	Sodium hypochlorite* 8.00%	PSC COPPER SULFATE 15 SULFUR 10 WALNUT BLIGHT DUST Fungicide (Pacific Supply)	Monohydrated copper sulfate* 15.00% Hydrated lime 30.00% Sulfur 10.00%
PSC CO-OP HEPTACHLOR 2E Insecticide (Pacific Supply)	Heptachlor* (heptachloro-tetrahydro-4,7-methanoindene) 23.22% Related compounds 9.64%	PSC CREOSOTE Wood preservative (Pacific Supply)	Neutral tar oils* 97.00%
PSC CO-OP HEPTACHLOR 2-1/2 DUST Insecticide (Pacific Supply)	Heptachlor*(heptachloro-tetrahydro-4,7-methanoindene) 2.50% Related compounds 0.97%	PSC CUPROCIDE 8 DUST Fungicide (Pacific Supply)	Cuprous oxide* 7.20%
PSC CO-OP IPC EMULSIVE Herbicide (Pacific Supply)	Isopropyl-n-phenyl-carbamate* 25.00%	PSC DDT 5 & BASIC COPPER SULFATE 10 DUST Fungicide, Insecticide (Pacific Supply)	Dichloro diphenyl trichloro-ethane* 5.00% Copper expressed as metallic* 5.25%
PSC CO-OP METHOXY-CHLOR 5 DUST Insecticide (Pacific Supply)	Methoxychlor, tech. 5.00%	PSC DDT 5 & CUPROCIDE 8 DUST Fungicide, insecticide (Pacific Supply)	Dichloro diphenyl trichloro-ethane tech.* 5.00% Yellow cuprous oxide* 7.20%
PSC CO-OP ROTENONE 5 SPRAY POWDER Insecticide (Pacific Supply)	Rotenone* 5% Other cube resins 10%	PSC DDT 5 DUST Insecticide (Pacific Supply)	Dichloro diphenyl trichloro-ethane tech.* 5.00%
PSC CO-OP SHEEP DIP Insecticide (Pacific Supply)	Phenols* 15% Sulfur dioxide extr. of petroleum 53% Soap (anhydrous) 22%	PSC DDT 10 DUST Insecticide (Pacific Supply)	Dichloro diphenyl trichloro-ethane tech.* 10.00%
PSC CO-OP SLUG PELLETS Insecticide (Pacific Supply)	Metaldehyde* 3% Calcium arsenate* 5.16%	PSC DDT 25 EMULSION Insecticide (Pacific Supply)	Dichloro diphenyl trichloro-ethane 25.00% Aromatic petroleum deriv. solvent* 65.00%
PSC CO-OP SODIUM ARSENITE 4 SOLUTION Herbicide (Pacific Supply)	Arsenic trioxide* (water-soluble form expressed as metallic 24.7%) 32.6%	PSC DDT 10 GARDEN DUST Insecticide (Pacific Supply)	DDT* 10.00%
PSC CO-OP STOCK SPRAY (Pyrenone) Insecticide (Pacific Supply)	Tech. piperonyl butoxide 0.193% Pyrethrins 0.024% Aromatic petroleum deriv. solvent* 99.783%	PSC DDT 5 SPECIAL DUST Insecticide (Pacific Supply)	Dichloro diphenyl trichloro-ethane tech.* 5.00% Petroleum oils 2.00%

*Consult Sec. II., Ingredients Index. This ingredient may be responsible for major toxic effects if poisonous amounts of this product are ingested.

Name & Use Manufacturer	Ingredients	Name & Use Manufacturer	Ingredients
PSC DDT 5 & SULFUR 50 DUST Insecticide (Pacific Supply)	Dichloro diphenyl trichloro-ethane* tech. 5.00% Sulfur* 50.00%	PSC 2,4-D & 2,4,5-T LOW VOLATILE ESTER BRUSH KILLER Herbicide (Pacific Supply)	2,4-Dichloro phenoxy acetic acid, propylene glycol butyl ether esters* 34.80% 2,4,5-Trichloro phenoxy acetic acid, propylene glycol butyl ether esters* 33.00%
PSC DDT 50% WETTABLE Insecticide (Pacific Supply)	Dichloro diphenyl trichloro-ethane* 50.00%	PSC LOW VOLATILE ESTER 70 WEED KILLER (Pacific Supply)	2,4-Dichloro phenoxy acetic acid, propylene glycol butyl ether esters* 70.50%
PSC 2,4,5-T ESTER BRAMBLE KILLER Herbicide (Pacific Supply)	2,4,5-Trichloro phenoxy acetic acid, isopropyl ester* 34.00%	PSC METHOXY-CHLOR 5 DUST Insecticide (Pacific Supply)	Methoxychlor* tech. 5.00%
PSC 2,4-D & 2,4,5-T ESTER BRUSH KILLER Herbicide (Pacific Supply)	2,4-Dichloro phenoxy acetic acid, isopropyl ester* 18.0% 2,4,5-Trichloro phenoxy acetic acid, isopropyl ester* 18.0%	PSC MONOHY-DRATED COPPER SULFATE 15 DUST Fungicide (Pacific Supply)	Monohydrated copper sulfate* 15.00%
PSC ESTER WEED KILLER (Pacific Supply)	Isopropyl ester 2,4-dichloro phenoxy acetic acid* 44.00%	PSC NICOTINE 10 DUST Insecticide (Pacific Supply)	Nicotine sulfate* 5.20%
PSC GERMICIDE (Pacific Supply)	Sodium hypochlorite* 8.00%	PSC PARATHION 25 EMULSIFIABLE Insecticide (Pacific Supply)	Parathion* 25.00% Aromatic petroleum deriv. solvent 65.00%
PSC HEPTACHLOR 2-1/2 DUST Insecticide (Pacific Supply)	Heptachlor* 2.50% Related compounds 0.97%	PSC ROTENONE 50 DUST Insecticide (Pacific Supply)	Rotenone 0.50% Other cube resins 1.25%
PSC HEPTACHLOR 2E Insecticide (Pacific Supply)	Heptachlor* 23.22% Related compounds 9.64% Aromatic petroleum deriv.* 63.66%	PSC ROTENONE 100 DUST Insecticide (Pacific Supply)	Rotenone 1.00% Other cube resins 1.75%
PSC IPC EMULSIVE Herbicide (Pacific Supply)	Isopropyl-n-phenyl-carbamate* 25.00%	PSC ROTENONE 100 GARDEN DUST Insecticide (Pacific Supply)	Rotenone 1.00% Other cube resins 2.00%
PSC LEAD ARSENATE 40 DUST Insecticide (Pacific Supply)	Lead arsenate* 40.00%	PSC ROTENONE 5 SPRAY POWDER Insecticide (Pacific Supply)	Rotenone * 5.00% Other cube resins 10.00%
PSC 2,4,5-T LOW VOLATILE ESTER 66 BRAMBLE KILLER Herbicide (Pacific Supply)	2,4,5-Trichloro phenoxy acetic acid, propylene glycol butyl ether esters* 65.30%		

*Consult Sec. II., Ingredients Index. This ingredient may be responsible for major toxic effects if poisonous amounts of this product are ingested.

Name & Use Manufacturer	Ingredients		Name & Use Manufacturer	Ingredients	
PSC SHEEP DIP Insecticide (Pacific Supply)	Total phenols* Sulfur dioxide, extr. of petroleum Anhydrous soap	15.00% 53.00% 22.00%	PULVEX ANTI-SCRATCH FLEA POWDER (Cooper)	Gamma isomer benzene hexachloride (from lindane) Hexachlorophene(2,2'-methyl- ene-bis-3,4,6-trichlorophenol) Dichlorophene(2,2'-methyl- ene-bis-4-chlorophenol)	0.5% 0.5% 0.5%
PSC SLUG PELLETS (Pacific Supply)	Metaldehyde* Calcium arsenate*	3.00% 5.16%	PULVEX ASTRINGENT TABLETS Intestinal irritation (veterinary) (Cooper)	Bismuth subcarbonate Phenyl salicylate (salol)* Zinc sulfocarbolate	3 gr. 1 gr. 1/2 gr.
PSC SODIUM ARSENITE 4 SOLUTION Herbicide (Pacific Supply)	Arsenic trioxide*	32.6%	PULVEX CAT FLEA POWDER (Cooper)	Rotenone Other cube resins	0.75% 1.0%
PSC TOXAPHENE 8 EMULSIFIABLE Insecticide (Pacific Supply)	Toxaphene* Aromatic petroleum deriv. solvent*	72.00% 20.0%	PULVEX COUGH MEDICINE FOR DOGS & CATS (Cooper)	Each fl. oz.: Fl. extr. ammonium chloride Ipecac Tinct. balsam Tolu	1 gm. 0.5 cc. 1 cc.
PSC WARFARIN CONCEN- TRATE Rodenticide (Pacific Supply)	Warfarin (3-(a-acetonylbenzyl)- 4-hydroxycoumarin)	0.5%	PULVEX DRY CLEANER FOR DOGS & CATS (Cooper)	Naphthalene* Calcium carbonate Magnesium carbonate Sulfur* Hydrous aluminum silicate	
PSC WOOD PRESERVA- TIVE (Pacific Supply)	Pentachlorophenol* Other chlorophenols Aromatic petroleum deriv. solvent *	36.08% 4.92% 40.00%	PULVEX EYE LOTION Veterinary (Cooper)	Each fl. oz.: Boric acid Zinc sulfate Phenol Camphor water	5 gr. 1 gr. 1 gr. 10 m.
P.S. LIQUID DEODORANT (Noblesse)			PULVEX FLEA SOAP (Cooper)	Soap (anhydrous) Steam-distilled pine oil Petroleum distillate Beta-thiocyanoethyl esters of mixed fatty acids (10-18 carbon atoms) B-butoxy B' thiocyano diethyl ether	80.0% 4.0% 2.0% 1.5% 0.5%
P & S UNGUENTINE (Baker, Chester)					
PTZ PASTURE MIX Food supplement (veterinary) (Hess, Dr.)	Salt Defluorinated phosphate Phenothiazine* Bone black Molasses Copper sulfate Cobalt carbonate Potassium iodide*	0.20%	PULVEX IMPROVED CONDITIONETS Food supple- ment (vet- erinary) (Cooper)	Each colored tablet: U.S.P. vitamin A 3120 units U.S.P. vitamin D 312 units Each white tablet: Tricalcium phosphate 5 gr. Manganese hypophosphite Copper sulfate	1-1/2 gr. 1/200 gr.
PTZ PELLETS WITH LEAD ARSENATE Insecticide (Hess, Dr.)	Each pellet: Phenothiazine (drench grade)* Lead arsenate (spray grade)*	7.5 gm. 0.3 gm.	PULVEX LAXATIVE TABLETS Veterinary (Cooper)	Extr. cascara Aloin	2 gr. 1/8 gr.
PULVEX AEROSOL FLEA KILLER & DEODORANT (Cooper)	Pyrethrins Piperonyl butoxide* Methoxychlor* Methylated naphthalenes* Petroleum distillate* Essential oil*	0.06% 0.48% 0.5% 4.3% 4.41% 25%	PULVEX LINIMENT Veterinary (Cooper)	Oil of turpentine Methyl salicylate* Oil of pine * Oil of sassafras * Oleoresin capsicum Alcohol*	61%
PULVEX ANALGESIC TABLETS Veterinary (Cooper)	Each tablet: Aspirin* Atropine sulfate* Caffeine	3 gr. 1/600 gr. 1/8 gr.	PULVEX PARASITIC EAR CANKER TREATMENT Veterinary (Cooper)	Phenol* Camphor*	4.5% 4.0%

*Consult Sec. II., Ingredients Index. This ingredient may be responsible for major toxic effects if poisonous amounts of this product are ingested.

Name & Use Manufacturer	Ingredients		Name & Use Manufacturer	Ingredients	
PULVEX PEPSIN & PAPAIN TABLETS Digestant (veterinary) (Cooper)	Each tablet: Pepsin Papain	2 gr. 1-1/2 gr.	PUMP LUBE (Park Chem.)	Mineral oil Soap Petroleum sulfonate	
PULVEX PINE OIL DEODORIZING DISINFEC- TANT (Cooper)	Steam-distilled pine oil* Soap	70% 20%	PUPPY LOVE COLOGNES (Manon)		
			PURASAN AD Germicide (Gallowhur)	Alkyl dimethyl benzyl ammonium chloride*	50%
PULVEX R-H-W WORM CAPSULES (Cooper)	Each capsule: n-Butyl chloride*	1.0 cc.	PURSAN DC Disinfectant (Gallowhur)	Alkyl dimethyl 3,4-dichloro- benzyl ammonium chloride *	50%
PULVEX SHAMPOO FOR DOGS Insecticide (Cooper)	Rotenone Other cube resins Methoxychlor	0.1% 0.1% 0.5%	PURASEED Disinfectant fungicide (Gallowhur)	Phenyl mercury formamide* 6.25% Anilinocadmium dilactate* 6.25%	
PULVEX TAPE WORM TABLETS (Veterinary) (Cooper)	Arecoline hydrobromide*	1/15 gr.	PURATIZED AGRICUL- TURAL SPRAY Fungicide (Gallowhur)	Phenyl mercuric triethanol ammonium lactate* (equiv. to 3% metallic mercury) 7.5%	
PULVEX TICK POWDER (Cooper)	Rotenone	3%	PURATIZED APPLE SPRAY (Puratized B) Fungicide (Gallowhur)	Phenyl mercury monoethanol ammonium acetate* 11.5%	
PULVEX TONIC TABLETS Veterinary (Cooper)	Iron sulfate U.S.P. Potassium iodide Extr. nux vomica Strychnine	2-1/2 gr. 1/2 gr. 1/60 gr. 0.000123 gr.	PURATURF Crab grass killer (Gallowhur)	Phenyl mercuri triethanol ammonium lactate* 3%	
PULVEX 6-USE DOG SOAP (Cooper)	Soap Mineral oil Oil Siberian pine needle Rotenone Other cube resins	82.7% 2.0% 1.4% 0.3% 0.6%	PURATURF 177 Fungicide (Gallowhur)	Anilinocadmium dilactate* 20%	
PULVEX WORM CAPSULES Veterinary (Cooper)	Capsule #1: Arecoline* Castor oil Capsule #2: n-Butyl chloride*	1/16 gr. 10 m. 1.0 cc.	PURE O DENT Astringent mouthwash (Purepac)	Zinc chloride * Oil of cinnamon Formaldehyde* Thymol Menthol Oil of cloves Eucalyptol *	
PULVEX WORM CAPSULES Veterinary (Cooper)	Capsule #1: Arecoline* Oil of chenopodium Castor oil Capsule #2: n-Butyl chloride *	1/32 gr. 1/2 m. 5 m. 0.5 cc.	PUREOSEPTIC 511 Mouthwash (Purepac)	Thymol Menthol Benzoic acid Methyl salicylate* Boric acid Alcohol 28%/v	
			PUREPAC ANALGESIC BALM Rubefacient, (Purepac)	Methyl salicylate* (synthetic) Camphor* Menthol* Oil of mustard (synthetic) Lanolin	
PULVIS ANTISEPTICUS FORTIOR Antiseptic douche powder (Case)	Menthol * Phenol * Oil of eucalyptus * Zinc sulfate C.P.* Boric acid* Tartaric acid Thymol * Camphor* Oil of peppermint Alkyl aryl sulfonate Salicylic acid* Alum *		PUREPAC ANTISEPTIC DOUCHE POWDER (Purepac)	Carbolic acid approx.0.01% Zinc sulfate * Eucalyptol * Boric acid* Salicylic acid* Thymol	
			PUREPAC BAY RUM (Purepac)	Alcohol 50%/v	

*Consult Sec. II., Ingredients Index. This ingredient may be responsible for major toxic effects if poisonous amounts of this product are ingested.

- 865 -

Name & Use Manufacturer	Ingredients		Name & Use Manufacturer	Ingredients	
PUREPAC BLUE OINTMENT Ectoparasiticide (Purepac)	Mercury*	10%	PUREPAC RHINITIS TABLETS (Full Strength) For colds (Hance)	Each tablet: Belladonna leaves (total alkaloids 0.000713 gr.) Quinine sulfate Camphor*	1/4 m. 1/2 gr. 1/2 gr.
PUREPAC BROWN LOZENGES PLAIN (Purepac)	Extr. licorice Tartar emetic *		PUREPAC RHINITIS (Full Strength Modified) For colds (Purepac)	Each tablet: Belladonna (1/1280 gr. alkaloids) Camphor*	1/16 gr. 1/2 gr.
PUREPAC BROWN MIXTURE N.F. Antitussive (Purepac)	Each fl. oz.: Opium* Alcohol	0.23 gr. 10%/v	PUREPAC SEIDLITZ POWDERS U.S.P. Laxative (Purepac)		
PUREPAC CARMINA- TIVE COMPOUND (Purepac)	Blackberry bark Cinnamon Cloves Ginger Glycerin Alcohol	16%/v	PUREPAC SULFUR & CREAM OF TARTAR LOZENGES (Purepac)	Sublimed sulfur Cream of tartar	
PUREPAC CASTORIA Laxative (children) (Purepac)	Fl. extr. senna Infusion of pumpkin seed Rochelle salt Sodium bicarbonate Glycerin Oil of fennel		PUREPAC SULFUR OINTMENT Fungicide (Medical) (Purepac)	Sulfur	10%
PUREPAC CCHLOROFORM LINIMENT Counter-irritant (Purepac)	Alcohol Chloroform* approx. 30%/v.	45%	PUREPAC THROAT GARGLE (Purepac)	Potassium chlorate* Ferric chloride Glycerin	
PUREPAC COLD SORE LOTION (Purepac)	Camphor benzoin* Aluminum chloride Alcohol*	60%/v	PUREPAC TINCTURE OF BENZOIN COMPOUND Inhalant (Purepac)	Alcohol* Benzoin	77%/v
PUREPAC CORN REMOVER Keratolytic (Purepac)	Alcohol Ether* Salicylic acid* Flexible collodion	12%/v 41%/v	PUREPAC TINCTURE MERTHIOLATE Antiseptic (Purepac)	Sodium ethyl mercuri thio- salicylate (Lilly) Alcohol	1-1000 50%
PUREPAC COUGH SYRUP (Purepac)	Extr. white pine bark Chloroform Spikenard root Balm Gilead buds Rectified oil of tar Extr. wild cherry Blood root		PUREPAC TOOTHACHE DROPS (Purepac)	Chlorobutanol* (chloroform derivatives) Oil of cloves * Camphor	9.5%
PUREPAC LARKSPUR LOTION WITH SABADILLA & ACETIC ACID Ectoparasiticide (Purepac)	Alkaloids of larkspur Alkaloids of sabadilla Acetic acid	0.05% 0.03% 2.40%	PUREPAC TOOTHACHE GUM (Purepac)	Benzocaine Carbolic acid*approx. 1% Oil of clove * Oil of cassia * Turpentine *	
PUREPAC RECTAL SUPPOSITORY (Purepac)	Nutgall Zinc oxide Boric acid Benzocaine Cocoa butter		PUREPAC WHITE LINIMENT (Purepac)	Turpentine* Ammonium chloride Aromatic liquid soap Ammonia Camphor*	
PUREPAC RHINITIS TABLETS 1/2 STRENGTH For colds (Hance)	Each tablet: Belladonna leaves (total alkaloids 0.000357 gr.) Quinine sulfate Camphor*	1/8 m. 1/4 gr. 1/4 gr.	PUREX BOWL CLEAN (Purex Corp.)	Acid*	
PUREPAC RHINITIS (Half Strength Modified) For colds (Purepac)	Each tablet: Belladonna (1/2560 gr. alkaloids) Camphor*	1/32 gr. 1/4 gr.	PUREX DRAIN OPENER (Purex Corp.)	Caustic*	

*Consult Sec. II., Ingredients Index. This ingredient may be responsible for major toxic effects if poisonous amounts of this product are ingested.

Name & Use Manufacturer	Ingredients	Name & Use Manufacturer	Ingredients
PUREX DRY BLEACH (Purex Corp.)	Calcium hypochlorite* 7.5%	PURITAN COCONUT SOAP (Liquid & Past) (Genesee)	Potash type soap from coconut oil
PUREX HOUSEHOLD BLEACH (Purex Corp.)	Sodium hypochlorite* approx. 5-1/4% Sodium chloride approx. 4%	PURITAN CONVEYOR LUBRICANT (Genesee)	Liquid potash soap from blend of vegetable fatty acids and potassium hydroxide*
PUREX ONE COAT WALL PAINT (Murphy Paint)		PURITAN DEODORANT (Puritan Sales)	
PURGA LAXATIVE TABLETS (K & B)	Each tablet: Aloin * 1/4 gr. Phenolphthalein 1/2 gr. Extr. belladonna leaves * 1/16 gr. Extr. cascara sagrada 1/2 gr.	PURITAN DISINFEC- TANT (Puritan Sales)	
PURI-GLOSS SELF POLISHING WAX (Puritan Chem.)		PURITAN FLUSHING FLUID FOR BRAKE SYSTEMS (Genesee)	Methanol*
PURI-KLEAN COMPOSITION FLOOR CLEANER (Puritan Chem.)		PURITAN GASKA SEAL #1 (Hardening type) (Genesee)	Alcohol*
PURINA DAIRY SPRAY (New Formula) Insecticide (Ralston)	Pyrethrins Thiocyanates* Methoxychlor * Inert ingredients*	PURITAN GASKA SEAL #2 & #3 (Non-Hardening Type) (Genesee)	
PURINA HOME SPRAY (New Formula) Insecticide (Ralston)	Pyrethrins Octyl sulfoxide of isosafrole*	PURITAN GLAD HAND SOAP (Genesee)	
PURINA INSECT KILLER (New Formula) (Ralston)	Methoxychlor Lindane* Sulfur Inert ingredients*	PURITAN HYDRAULIC BRAKE FLUIDS (Regular & Super) (Genesee)	Lubricant (synthetic or castor oil)* Glycol component Diluent (alcohol or glycol ether)*
PURI-SORB Grease absorbent compound (Puritan Chem.)		PURITAN HYDRO- LECTRIC FLUID (Hydraulic Window Fluid) (Genesee)	Synthetic type lubricant* Glycol component* Alcohol type diluent*
PURI-SYN CONCEN- TRATE SYNTHETIC FLOOR CLEANER (Puritan Chem.)		PURITAN #84 INDUSTRIAL HAND SOAP (Genesee)	
		PURITAN METAL POLISH (Genesee)	
PURITAN API THREAD COMPOUND Grease (Genesee)	Aluminum stearate base grease 20.46% Silicone compound 12.85% Silicone fluid 2.59% Graphite 18.00% Lead* 30.50% Copper 3.30% Zinc 12.30%	PURITAN OIL SOAP (Genesee)	Potash soap (40% anhydrous)
		PURITAN PENETRATING OIL (Genesee)	

*Consult Sec. II., Ingredients Index. This ingredient may be responsible for major toxic effects if poisonous amounts of this product are ingested.

Name & Use Manufacturer	Ingredients
PURITAN PLASTIC COATING (3 Types) (Genesee)	Synthetic resins Low-boiling diluents * Plasticizers Dyes * Solid dispersant (alum powder, copper)
PURITAN RUG & UPHOLSTERY CLEANER (Puritan Sales)	
PURITAN SCRUB SOAPS (Plain & Genesee)	
PURITAN SHOCK ABSORBER FLUID (Genesee)	Petroleum oil* (naphthenic base)
PURITAN SPECIAL LIQUID CONCEN-TRATE Soap (Genesee)	Anhydrous soap 36%
PURITAN SURGICAL SOAPS (Genesee)	
PURITAN VAPOR PHASE INHIBITORS (3 Types) (Genesee)	Di-isopropyl ammonium nitrite* Dicyclohexyl ammonium nitrite*
PURITAN WIRE DRAWING COMPOUND (Genesee)	
PURITOX MOTH KILLER (Chamberlain Haber)	
PURITY CROSS SHAMPOO (Fairfield)	
PURO ASPHALT PAINTS (Puroseal)	
PURO CHLOROFORM SUBSTITUTE Drycleaning spotter (Adco)	
PUROIL PAINTS, VARNISHES, ENAMELS (Murphy Paint)	

Name & Use Manufacturer	Ingredients
PURO PINE OIL DISINFEC-TANT (United Chem.)	
PURO SOLVENT & CEMENT CLEANER (Puro)	
PUROZONE DEODORANT (Brilco)	
PURPAKOTE PAINTS (Pettit)	
PURPALITE MILL WHITE Paint (Piedmont)	
PUSEY'S LOTION OR LINIMENT (Handley)	Prepared calamine Zinc oxide Glycerin Liquefied phenol 0.17%
PUSH Antacid (Gibbs)	Magnesium carbonate Calcium carbonate Sodium bicarbonate Re-distilled oil of peppermint
PUSH-BUTTON CHARCOAL LIGHTER (Bostwick)	Copper naphthenate Perfume hickory Dispersol Isopropanol * Freon
PUSH BUTTON REAL-KILL BUG KILLER (Cook Chem.)	Pyrethrins 0.046% n-Octyl sulfoxide of isosafrole 0.101% and related compounds .014% Dieldrin* 0.500% Phenyl mercuric lactate 0.016% Polymerized glycerol oleate 0.100% Petroleum distillates* 74.223%
PUTITE CAULKING COMPOUND (Ever-Plastics)	
PUTNAM BATH BLOOM (Monroe Chem.)	Sodium aryl sulfate Trisodium phosphate* Sodium tripolyphosphate* Sodium sesquicarbonate
PUTNAM DRY CLEANER (Monroe Chem.)	Soap and kerosene-like solvent*
PUTNAM FADELESS DYE (Monroe Chem.)	Aniline dyes*
PUT SPOT REMOVER (Monroe Chem.)	Naphtha*

*Consult Sec. II., Ingredients Index. This ingredient may be responsible for major toxic effects if poisonous amounts of this product are ingested.

Name & Use Manufacturer	Ingredients	Name & Use Manufacturer	Ingredients
PUZZY & SIZZY Bubble bath, shampoo (House of Puzzy)		PYRAK Burns (Germ O Form)	Thymol * Bismuth Iodine*
PYACADO FACE CREAM (Frenco)	Avacado and mineral oils Stearic acid Glycerin Triethanolamine Dow's Tego-Sept P. Paraffin Papain	PYRAMID CANVAS PRIMING (Nobema)	Hide glue Boiled linseed oil Zinc oxide Titanium oxide Calcium carbonate
PYCOPAY TOOTH POWDER (Pycope)	Sodium chloride 50% Sodium bicarbonate 35% Tricalcium phosphate 5% Calcium carbonate 7% Magnesium carbonate 2% Oil of cloves and methyl salicylate 1%	PYRAMID FINISHER Floor Varnish (O'Brien Corp.)	
PYGOLAC Dip for crucifer transplants (Hanna)	Calomel* and gypsum 1-20	PYRAMID VERMILION STUDENTS OIL COLOR (Nobema)	
PYLOX Rectal ointment (Drexel)	Oxyquinoline sulfate* Tannic acid * Menthol * Lanolin Stearic acid Ethyl aminobenzoate Camphor Glycerin	PYREFUME EMULSIFIABLE SUPER 20 Insecticide (Penick)	Pyrethrins 2.5%
PYNAMITE HOUSEHOLD CLEANER (Pine)		PYREFUME SUPER 100 Insecticide (Penick)	Pyrethrins* 11.9% Petroleum distillate* 88.1%
PYNAMITE STOVE CLEANER (Pine)	Pine oil*	PYREM DETERGENT (Bunn)	
PY-NEL PINE OIL DISINFECTANT (Winsale)		PYRENE Fire extinguisher (Pyrene)	Carbon tetrachloride*
PYNITE DISINFECTANT (Clifton)		PYRETHROL INDUSTRIAL SPRAY Insecticide (Mc Cormick)	Pyrethrins 0.29% Piperonyl butoxide tech. 2.33% Petroleum distillate* 97.38%
PYNOL PINE DISINFECTANT (Germo)		PYREXCEL LIVESTOCK CONCENTRATE 5.5 EMULSIFIABLE Insecticide (Penick)	Butoxy polypropylene glycol* 52.70% n-Octyl sulfoxide of isosafrole 4.67% Related compounds 0.63% Pyrethrins 0.53% Petroleum distillate* 27.70% Alkyl aryl polyether alcohol 7.385% Dioctyl sodium sulfosuccinate
PYRACOL Analgesic, antihistamine (Carroll Chem.)	Pyrilamine maleate* 12-1/2 mg. Acetophenetidin* 1-1/2 gr. Salicylamide* 1-1/2 gr. Caffeine 1/4 gr.		
PYRADIN Analgesic (Jenkins)	Each tablet: Acetophenetidin* 4 gr. Antipyrine* 1 gr. Caffeine 1/8 gr. Tinct. hyoscyamus 8 m. Tinct. gelsemium 4 m.	PYREXCEL EMULSIFIABLE SULFOXIDE 1-10 Insecticide (Penick)	Petroleum distillate* Polyethylene oxide sorbitan n-Octyl sulfoxide of isosafrole* (sulfoxide) Butoxy polypropylene glycol 2-Butoxy ethanol Compounds related to sulfoxide Pyrethrins*
		PYREXCEL 20 Insecticide (Penick)	Petroleum distillate* Ethanol butoxide Di-n-propyl maleate isosafrole condensate Pyrethrins
PYRA HISTAMINE Nasal spray (Mayfair)	Phenylephrine hydrochloride 0.31% Diethylene diamine hydrochloride 0.025% Methylparaben Propylparaben	PYRILAMINE MALEATE CAPSULES (West-Ward)	Pyrilamine maleate* 75 mg.

*Consult Sec. II., Ingredients Index. This ingredient may be responsible for major toxic effects if poisonous amounts of this product are ingested.

- 869 -

Name & Use Manufacturer	Ingredients		Name & Use Manufacturer	Ingredients	
PYRILATE Dietary supplement (Keenan)	Iron (ferric ammonium citrate) 25 mg. Cobalt (cobalt carbonate) 2 mg. Copper (copper citrate) 3 mg. Zinc (zinc citrate) 3 mg. Manganese (manganese citrate) 2 mg. Germanium (germanium dioxide) 1 μ gm. Molybdenum (molybdenum trioxide) 1 mg. Nickel (nickel citrate) 2 mg. Vanadium (vanadium pentoxide) 1 μ gm.		PYROCIDE BOOSTER CONCEN- TRATE D Insecticide (McLaughlin)	DDT* Pyrethrins	20.8% 1%
			PYROCIDE BOOSTER CONCEN- TRATE E Insecticide (McLaughlin)	Oil* Piperonyl butoxide Pyrethrins	91% 7.5% 1.5%
			PYROCIDE BOOSTER CONCEN- TRATE F Insecticide (McLaughlin)	Piperonyl butoxide Oil* Pyrethrins	50% 45% 5%
PYRIMALON TABLETS Analgesic (Veltex)	Each tablet: Pyranisamine maleate 25 mg. Acetylsalicylic acid* 3-1/2 gr. Acetophenetidin* 2-1/2 gr. Caffeine alkaloid 1/2 gr.		PYROCIDE BOOSTER CONCEN- TRATE G Insecticide (McLaughlin)	Piperonyl butoxide Oil* Pyrethrins	60% 37% 3%
PYRIMAL TABLETS Analgesic (Veltex)	Each brown tablet: Pyranisamine maleate* 50 mg. Each white tablet: Pyranisamine maleate* 25 mg.		PYROCIDE BOOSTER CONCEN- TRATE K Insecticide (McLaughlin)	Piperonyl butoxide Oil* Pyrethrins	50% 45% 5%
PYRINATE A-200 LIQUID Parasiticide (McKesson)	Pyrethrins 1.0% Dinitroamisole 1.0% Oleoresin parsley fruit 0.5% Sesamin 0.037% Oleic acid 3.5% Benzyl alcohol 8.0%		PYROCIDE BOOSTER CONCEN- TRATE M Insecticide (McLaughlin)	Petroleum distillate* 45% n-Octyl bicycloheptene dicarbox- imide* 50% Pyrethrins 5%	
PYRIX 10-FOG Insecticide (Chem. Insect.)	Petroleum distillate* n-Octyl bicycloheptene dicarboximide,* and pyrethrins 100%		PYROCIDE BOOSTER CONCEN- TRATE T Insecticide (McLaughlin)	Petroleum distillate 41.86% Methylated aromatic petroleum deriv.* 29.82% Beta-butoxy-beta'thiocyano- diethyl ether 10.75% Tech. methoxychlor 8.94% n-Octyl bicycloheptene dicarbox- imide 8.20% Allethrin (allyl homolog of cinerin I) 0.43%	
PYRIX 20-P.B. Insecticide (Chem. Insect.)	Petroleum distillate* Tech. piperonyl butoxide Other related compounds Pyrethrins				
PYRO CHROME PAINT (Preferred)			PYROCIDE BOOSTER CONCEN- TRATE U Insecticide (McLaughlin)	Petroleum distillate*, deodorized 76.2% n-Octyl bicycloheptene dicarbox- imide 20.0% Allethrin (allyl homolog of cinerin I) 2.2% Pyrethrins 1.6%	
PYROCIDE 20 Insecticide (McLaughlin)	Oil* Pyrethrins	97.5% 2.5%			
PYROCIDE 88 Insecticide (McLaughlin)	Oil* Pyrethrins		PYROCIDE BOOSTER CONCEN- TRATE V Insecticide (McLaughlin)	Petroleum distillate* 62.87% Methylated aromatic petroleum deriv.* 13.65% Beta-butoxy-beta'thiocyano- diethyl ether* 10.75% n-Octyl bicycloheptene dicarbox- imide* 8.20% Tech. methoxychlor 4.10% Allethrin (allyl homolog of cinerin I) 0.43%	
PYROCIDE 175 Insecticide (McLaughlin)	Oil* Pyrethrins*	80% 20%			
PYROCIDE AUTOMATIC SPRAYER CONCEN- TRATE Insecticide (McLaughlin)	Petroleum distillate* 79% n-Octyl bicycloheptene dicarbox- imide* 10% Pyrethrins 1%				
			PYROCIDE BOOSTER CONCEN- TRATE X Insecticide (McLaughlin)	Petroleum distillate, deodorized* 66.41% Methylated aromatic petroleum deriv. * 17.40% n-Octyl bicycloheptene dicarbox- imide* 10.44% Tech. methoxychlor 5.21% Allethrin 0.54%	
PYROCIDE BOOSTER CONCEN- TRATE C Insecticide (McLaughlin)	Oil* 94.37% Piperonyl butoxide 5% Pyrethrins 0.63%				

Name & Use Manufacturer	Ingredients		Name & Use Manufacturer	Ingredients	
PYROCIDE BOOSTER CONCEN-TRATE Y Insecticide (McLaughlin)	Petroleum distillate* Methylated aromatic petroleum deriv.* n-Octyl bicycloheptene dicarbox-imide* Tech. methoxychlor Allethrin Related compounds	66.44% 17.40% 10.44% 5.21% 0.27% 0.24%	PYRONYL 50-5 EMULSION CONCEN-TRATE Insecticide (Prentiss)	Pyrethrins Piperonyl butoxide	5.0% 50%
PYROCIDE BOOSTER CONCEN-TRATE Z Insecticide (McLaughlin)	Petroleum distillate*, deodorized n-Octyl bicycloheptene dicarbox-imide* Allethrin Pyrethrins	81.19% 17.00% 1.08% 0.73%	PYRONYL 50-5 OIL CONCEN-TRATE Insecticide (Prentiss)	Pyrethrins Piperonyl butoxide	5.0% 50%
PYROCIDE COMMERCIAL GROWERS SPRAY Insecticide (McLaughlin)	Pyrethrins Oil Pine oil* Dodecyl benzene sodium sulfonate	1.4% 23.6% 45% 20.0%	PYRONYL ROACH CON-CENTRATE (Prentiss)	Pyrethrins Piperonyl butoxide	1.49% 7.48%
PYROCIDE DRY Insecticide (McLaughlin)	Oil* Pyrethrins	45.8% 2.2%	PYRONYL UNIVERSAL CONCEN-TRATE Insecticide (Prentiss)	Pyrethrins Piperonyl butoxide	1.25% 5.05%
PYROCIDE DUST NO. 10 Insecticide (Sunland)	Pyrethrins	0.2%	PYRO-SANA (Mouth,throat) (Pyro-Sana)	Modified beechwood creosote *	3%
PYROCIDE-MULTICIDE DUST CONCEN-TRATE Insecticide (McLaughlin)	DDT* Pyrethrins Oil* Methylated petroleum*	10% 1.2% 22.8% 15%	PYRO-SANA OINTMENT Skin (Pyro-Sana)	Modified beechwood creosote * Petrolatum	3% 97%
PYRODERM Rubefacient (Chicago Pharm.)	Each oz.: Hyoscyamine Camphor* Oleoresin capsicum Methyl salicylate* Menthol* Oil mustard artificial	1/80 gr.	PYROTOX NO. 2 INSECTICIDE SPRAY (Mortex)	Petroleum distillates* Mineral oil Methylated aromatic petroleum deriv.* Sesame oil extractives (including 0.087% sesamin) Pyrethrins	49.144% 45.00% 5.20% 0.522% 0.134%
PYROIL Engine lubricant (Pyroil)			PYROX Insecticide (Am. Agric. Chem.)	Arsenate* Copper*	
PYRONAMEL ENAMEL (Pemco)			PYROX GARDEN SPRAY Insecticide, fungicide (Am. Agric. Chem.)	Copper expressed as metallic Calcium arsenate as tricalcium arsenate* Nicotine*	7.00% 8.75% 1.60%
PYRONOX Insecticide (Faranm)	Piperonyl butoxide tech. Pyrethrins Petroleum hydrocarbons Butoxypolypropylene glycol* Pine oil*	4.325% 0.432% 3.368% 50.320% 31.555%	PYRTOX CONTACT SPRAY Insecticide (Thompson-Hayward)	Oil* Piperonyl butoxide Pyrethrins	
PYRONYL #20 Insecticide (Prentiss)	Pyrethrins Piperonyl butoxide	0.62% 5.03%	PYRTOX NO. 20 NEW CONCEN-TRATE Insecticide (Thompson-Hayward)	Tech. piperonyl butoxide Pyrethrins Aromatic petroleum deriv. solvent* Petroleum distillate	4.73% 0.47% 25.00% 64.80%
PYRONYL DUST CONCEN-TRATE Insecticide (Prentiss)	Pyrethrins Piperonyl butoxide	0.6% 6.0%	PYRTOX WE-100 Insecticide (Thompson-Hayward)	Tech. piperonyl butoxide Pyrethrins Petroleum distillate*	10.0% 1.0% 74.0%
PYRONYL EMULSION #101 Insecticide (Prentiss)	Pyrethrins Piperonyl butoxide	1.2% 12%			

*Consult Sec. II., Ingredients Index. This ingredient may be responsible for major toxic effects if poisonous amounts of this product are ingested.

Name & Use Manufacturer	Ingredients		Name & Use Manufacturer	Ingredients	
PYSOL, PYSOLUX & PYSOLITE Paints (Pysol)			QUATROL For nose and throat (Munsch)	Menthol* Eucalyptol* Thymol iodide * Camphor* Thymol * Liquid petrolatum	
PYSOROL (Liquid) Antiseptic (Massengill)	Each fl. oz.: Gentian violet Alcohol Pine oil,*soap and rosin	0.18 gm. 1.2 cc. q.s.	QUATROSAN Vaginal douche (Veltex)	Zynamine Lactose U.S.P. Papain N.F. Cinnamic acid Menthol U.S.P. Lavender oil U.S.P. Boric acid U.S.P.* Citric acid U.S.P. Sodium lauryl sulfate U.S.P. Eucalyptol U.S.P. Magnesium carbonate	3.75% 63.35% 0.50% 0.20% 0.30% 0.80% 26.50% 0.50% 2.00% 0.10% 2.00%
PYXOLA Antiseptic (Pyxola)	Alcohol* Acetone*	60% 38%			
QB-DUST GROUND ROOT SPRAY DUST Insecticide (Bonide)	Rotenone	1%	QUEEN ANNE FURNITURE POLISH (No-Dust)		
Q.D.S. (Holcomb)	Hyamine (para di-isobutyl phenoxy ethoxy ethyl dimethyl benzyl ammonium chloride monohydrate)*		QUEEN ANNE LOTION Hand lotion (Assoc. Prod.)	Alcohol*	51%
Q.M. DISINFECTANT (Manco)			QUEEN ANNE LOTION (Peoples)	Alcohol Castile soap Diethyl phthalate Tertiary butyl alcohol Oils of bergamot, lemon and rose geranium	
QUAKER OIL SHAMPOO (Quaker)	Klearol Deo base Oil coloring Vanillin				
QUAKER POMADE (Quaker)	Petrolatum Lanolin Olive oil Oil of sage Flowers of sulfur Synth. oil of bergamot		QUEEN ANT KILLER (Drug Prod. Ga.)	Sodium arsenate*	3.29%
			QUEEN BLEACH WASHING FLUID (Wonder)		
QUAKER PRESSING OIL (Quaker)	Petrolatum Paraffin Vanillin		QUEEN CHRISTINA DEODORANT (Countess)		
QUAKERSOL (Commercial Solv.)	Ethyl alcohol*		QUEEN CHRISTINA TOILET WATER (Countess)		
QUAT-A-FOUR 4NH4 Sanitizer, disinfectant for farm and dairy (Roberts, Dr. D.)	Alkyl poly methyl trimethyl ammonium chlorides*	5%	QUEEN ESTER Hair pomade (Corpus Christi)		
QUAT-A-MONE Germicide, sanitizer, deodorant, fungicide (Russell, I.)	Methyl dodecyl benzyl trimethyl ammonium chloride*	10%	QUEEN'S PORCELAIN FINISH Paint (Howell, C.H.)		
QUATRASAL (Formerly Fungi-Treat) Fungicide (Dome)	Salicylanilide (Shirlan extra)* 5% Trimethyl octadecyl ammonium pentachloro phenate* 1% Isopropyl alcohol* 94%		QUEEN VARNISH (Federal Varnish)		
			QUEL Insecticide (Brooks Chem.)	Petroleum distillate* o-Dichlorobenzene* p-Dichlorobenzene* Piperonyl butoxide tech. Pyrethrins	
QUATRICIDE Disinfectant, fungicide, germicide (Biorganic)	Alkyl tolyl methyl trimethyl ammonium chlorides*	2-1/2%	QUELL DEODORANT (Hartlett)	Hydrous aluminum chloride	

---

*Consult Sec. II., Ingredients Index. This ingredient may be responsible for major toxic effects if poisonous amounts of this product are ingested.

Name & Use Manufacturer	Ingredients		Name & Use Manufacturer	Ingredients	
QUENATE Fungicide (Mallinckrodt)	Oxyquinoline benzoate*	10%	QUICKEE WATERLESS HAND CLEANER (Tudor)		
QUEST DEODORANT POWDER (Kimberly)	Kaolin Talc Zinc peroxide		QUICK ELASTIC Laundry starch (Hubinger)		
QUICK- ACTION GULF SPRAY Insecticide (Gulf)	Methoxychlor Pyrethrins Inert ingredients*	0.5% 0.10%	QUICK-EVAC Cathartic (Schiff)	Glycerin Sodium stearate (a fatty acid deriv.) Chlorophyll	
QUICK ACTION NON- INFLAMMABLE PAINT REMOVER (Masco)			QUICK-FLOOR Floor main- tenance and resurfacing materials (Dura Tred)		
QUICK ARROW Soap flakes (Swift)			QUICK HAIR COLOR (Goldman, M.)	Pyrogallic acid* Sodium sulfite*	
QUICK-BATH Concentrated dog cleaner (Ackerman's)	Tech. chlordane 2% Isopropyl esters of fatty acids 5% Hexachlorophene (2,2-methylene bis-3,4,6-trichlorophenol) 4%		QUICKILL INSECTICIDE, LIQUID (Warren Chem.)	DDT* Chlordane Lindane Pyrenone	6% 2% 1/2% 5%
QUICK-BRITE AUTO POLISH (Cochrane)			QUICKILL POWDER Insecticide (Warren Chem.)	DDT* Chlordane *	10% 5%
QUICK DEATH INSECTICIDE & DEODORANT (Victory Chem.)			QUICK POLISHING COMPOUND (McAleer)		
QUICK-DIP SILVER POLISH (Boyle- Midway)	Thiourea Sulfuric acid less than 2% Detergent Perfume		QUICK PRESERVA- SEAL PENETRATING FLOOR SEAL (U. S. Sanitary)		
QUICK-DRI ENAMELS (DeSoto P. & V.)			QUICK RUB For colds (Rexall)	Spirits turpentine* Camphor* Menthol Oil of eucalyptus* Oil of pine Oil of cloves	
QUICKDRY ASPHALT PAINT (Am.- Marietta)			QUICKSEAL Concrete sealer (Standard Dry)		
QUICK & EASY NON- POLISHING WAX (Internat. Chem.)			QUICK-SET For stopping leaks (Glidden Co.)		
QUICK & EASY SHAVING POWDER (Williams, J.B.)	Sodium and potassium soaps		QUICK SET COMPOUND & INKS (General Printing)		
QUICKEE Waterless Hand Cleaner (Quickee)	Oleic acid Stearic acid Amine Oil Lanolin Trisodium phosphate		QUICK-SHINE METAL POLISH (Du-Rite)		

*Consult Sec. II., Ingredients Index. This ingredient may be responsible for major toxic effects if poisonous amounts of this product are ingested.

Name & Use Manufacturer	Ingredients	
QUICKSHYNE FURNITURE POLISH (U. S. Sanitary)		
QUICKSTIKER PASTE & MUCILAGE (Ink)		
QUICK TUFEN-BRYTE FLOOR SEAL & VARNISH (U. S. Sanitary)		
QUICK WORK METAL POLISH (Nat'l. Soap)		
QUICO BRAND ENAMELS (Longman)		
QUIETABS Sedative (Commerce)	Potassium bromide* Sodium bromide* Ammonium bromide* Belladonna leaf Passiflora	
QUIETABS Sedative (Wright, M.)	Potassium bromide * 3 gr. Sodium bromide * 3 gr. Ammonium bromide * 1-1/2 gr. Powdered belladonna leaf (9/10,000 gr. alkaloids) 1/4 gr. Powdered passiflora 1 gr.	
QUIETOL Antacid, adsorbent (Commerce)	Pectin Bismuth subsalicylate Salol Kaolin Zinc sulfocarbolate Methyl salicylate	
QUIKSEEL ROOFING CEMENTS (Atlantic Paint)		
QUINAMINE CREAM For skin irritations (C & M)	Quinoform (iodochloro hydroxy quinoline)* 3% Duamine (antihistamine)* 2% Aranol penetrant Emollient cream	
QUINATROL For coccidiosis (veterinary, avian) (Whitmoyer)	Sulfaquinoxaline 25%	
QUINITABS (Harrison's)	Quinine * 1 gr./tablet Acetanilid* 1/2 gr. Cascara ext. 1/4 gr. Ext. belladonna leaves 1/16 gr. Phenolphthalein 1/4 gr. Caffeine alkaloid 1/4 gr.	
QUINK Ink (Parker Pen)		
QUINK 51 Ink (Parker Pen)		
QUINK BLUE-BLACK Ink (Parker Pen)	Dyes Iron salts* Gallic acid * Tannic acid* Mineral acids 0.1%	

Name & Use Manufacturer	Ingredients	
QUINK PERMANENT BLUE Ink (Parker Pen)	Dyes Mineral acid 0.1% Iron salts* Gallic acid *	
QUINK WASHABLE BLUE Ink (Parker Pen)	Dyes Mineral acid 0.1%	
QUINN'S HORSE LINIMENT (Davis, C.H.)		
QUINOIL HAIR TONIC FITCH'S (Fitch, F.W.)		
QUINO-JEL Antiseptic, prophylactic (Western Pharm.)	Chinosol 0.05% Boric acid 2.00% Demulcent q.s.	
QUINOLOR COMPOUND OINTMENT Antiseptic for dressings (Squibb)	White petrolatum Anhydrous lanolin Benzoyl peroxide 10% Chlor-hydroxy-quinoline 0.5%	
QUINSANA Beauty aid (Mennen)	Boric acid* Hydroxyquinoline sulfate* Magnesium stearate Talc	
QUINSEPTIKONS Antiseptic vaginal suppositories (Tablax)	Oxyquinoline sulfate Salicylic acid* Quinine hydrochloride Methyl and propyl para-hydroxybenzoates Boric acid* Cocoa butter	
QUINTALINE Nasal decongestant (Myers Labs.)	Camphor* Menthol* Boric acid*	
QUIT To discourage thumb-sucking and nail-biting (Pharmex)	Capsicum Aloes * Storax Tolu Alcohol	
QUIT ADHESIVE TAPE REMOVER (Patron)		
QUIT-IT To discourage nail-biting (Nicholson Chem.)	Sucrose Octa-acetate Acetone* Castor oil Isopropyl alcohol* 70% Capsicum 1%	
QUIX Solvent (Am. Lacquer)		
QUIX FLEA POWDER Insecticide (Bonide)	Rotenone 1.25% Other cube resins 2.50% Methyl naphthalenes * 2.04% Beta,beta dithiocyano diethyl ether 1.00%	
QUIX MIDCOAT Solvent (Am. Laquer)		
QUIXOL (Commercial Solv.)	Ethyl alcohol * Denaturant	
QUIXOL STOVE FUEL (Commercial Solv.)		

*Consult Sec. II., Ingredients Index. This ingredient may be responsible for major toxic effects if poisonous amounts of this product are ingested.

Name & Use Manufacturer	Ingredients	Name & Use Manufacturer	Ingredients
RABIN 200 LIGHTER & CLEANING FLUID (Rabin)		RADIO METAL POLISH (United Chem.)	
RAB ROWE'S ANALYZED BRAND BUILDING PAINT (Rowe)		RADNAI HAND CREAM (Gaby)	
RADGO WRITING INK REMOVER (Wilson, A. L.)		RAD PAINT & VARNISH CLEANER (Milrose)	
RAD HARDWOOD FLOOR CLEANER (Milrose)		RAD PORCELAIN, TILE & MARBLE CLEANER (Milrose)	
RADIANT FURNITURE POLISH (Boyle-Midway)	Refined petroleum oil-color water white Cedar wood oil * Turpentine* Color	RAD RUG & UPHOLSTERY CLEANER (Milrose)	
RADIANT LEMON OIL POLISH (Boyle-Midway)	Petroleum polish oil Lemon oil synthetic Citronella synthetic	RAD VENETIAN BLIND CLEANER (Milrose)	
RADIANT LIQUID WAX (Germo)		RADWAY'S READY RELIEF (Albemarle)	Camphor* 0.570 gm. Castile soap 0.428 gm. Potassium carbonate 0.280 gm. Oleoresin capsicum 0.119 gm. Dist. water 33.690 gm. Alcohol 95% Ammonia water * 4.880 gm. Caramel 0.325 gm.
RADIANT MACHINE OIL (Boyle-Midway)	Petroleum oil Vegetable oil Corrosion or rust-inhibiting agents	RAECO (Rae, J. H.)	Turpentine*
RADIANT PAINT BRUSH CLEANER (Liquid Form) (Boyle-Midway)	Naphtha* (hi flash) Turpentine*	RA-ED-O Rectal suppositories (Helm)	Aesculi semina Cinchona succirubra Phenol Benzocaine U.S.P. Oxyquinoline Benzoate
RADIANT PAINT & VARNISH REMOVER (Boyle-Midway)	Benzol* Alcohol denatured Wax	RAFEA EYE DROPS (Rafea)	Each fl. oz.: Chlorbutanol (chloroform deriv.) 1 gr. Berberine sulfate 1/8 gr. Zinc sulfate 1/4 gr. Boric acid 10 gr.
RADIANT POLISH (Boyle-Midway)	Refined petroleum oil-color water white Cedar wood oil* Turpentine*	RAFEA TABLETS Antacid, adsorbent (Rafea)	Magnesium trisilicate Aluminum hydroxide Calcium carbonate Thiamine hydrochloride Magnesium carbonate
RADIATOR STOP LEAK (Park Chem.)	Proprietary solvent	RAGGETT'S RAPID RELIEF LINIMENT (Ozark)	Spirits turpentine* Cresol* Carbolic acid* Methyl salicylate* Oil mustard (syn.) Oil eucalyptus* Camphor* Refined kerosene* Isopropanol*
RADIO-GLOSS INSIDE ENAMEL (Waterall)			
RADIOLITE BLEACH (Imperial Prod.)	Sodium hypochlorite*	RAINBOW ANILINE COLORS Dry wood stains (Murray-Williams)	
RADIOLITE WASHING FLUID (Imperial Prod.)			

*Consult Sec. II., Ingredients Index. This ingredient may be responsible for major toxic effects if poisonous amounts of this product are ingested.

Name & Use Manufacturer	Ingredients	Name & Use Manufacturer	Ingredients
RAINBOW DRY COLORS For tinting paint and cement (Murray-Williams)		RALSTON DAIRY SPRAY CONCEN-TRATE Insecticide (Ralston)	Methoxychlor* Butoxypolypropylene glycol*
RAINBOW FOAM RUG & UPHOL-STERY CLEANER (Parker, C.W.)		RALSTON DISINFECT-ANT & DIS-INFECTANT CONCEN-TRATE (Ralston)	Quaternary ammonium type*
RAINBOW READY MIXED HOUSE PAINT (Johnston)		RALSTON FLY BAIT Insecticide (Ralston)	Malathion*
RAIN DROPS WATER SOFTENER (Bu-Tay)	Sodium sesquicarbonate Sodium tripolyphosphate* Trisodium phosphate* Alkyl aryl sulfonate* Bluing (alphazurine blue* 2-G) Potassium bi-tartrate	RALSTON GRUB KILLER CONCEN-TRATE (Ralston)	Rotenone*
RAINKOTE ROOF COATING (Harrison P. & V.)		RALSTON HOME AERO SPRAY Insecticide (Ralston)	Pyrethrins Piperonyl butoxide Inert ingredients*
RAIN REM Maintenance material (Speco)	Silicone compound in aromatic solvent*	RALSTON INSECT OIL & INSECT OIL CON-CENTRATE (Ralston)	Pentachlorophenol*
RAIN-SEAL ROOF COATINGS (Pabco)		RALSTON LIN-DANE INSECTICIDE (Ralston)	Lindane*
RAINTITE ROOF COATING (Pabco)		RALSTON LIQUID BUILDING SPRAY (Ralston)	Malathion*
RAINY DAY (Protection)	Inert water-repellents Petroleum solvents *	RALSTON LIQUID PIG WORMER & POULTRY WORMER (Ralston)	Piperazine
RAKIL Rodenticide (Russell, I.)	Warfarin (3(a-acetonylbenzyl)-4-hydroxycoumarin) 0.025%		
RALEX Asthmatic antispasmodic (Partola)	Each fl. dr.: Alcohol* 47% Potassium iodide 2.453 gr. Tincture belladonna* 3.589 m. Tincture cinchona compound Aromatic spirit of ammonia	RALSTON LIQUID STOCK SPRAY Insecticide (Ralston)	Toxaphene* Lindane*
RALLAC Shellac sub-stitute (Dings)		RALSTON MANGE CONTROL Insecticide (Ralston)	Lindane*
RALSTON BLACK HEAD CONTROL Veterinary, avian (Ralston)	Nitrothiazole*	RALSTON PIGTAB GRANULES Veterinary (Ralston)	Phenothiazine Santonin*
RALSTON CAGE DROPPINGS SPRAY Insecticide (Ralston)	Malathion*	RALSTON PIG WORMER CONCEN-TRATE (Ralston)	Cadmium oxide*

*Consult Sec. II., Ingredients Index. This ingredient may be responsible for major toxic effects if poisonous amounts of this product are ingested.

Name & Use Manufacturer	Ingredients		Name & Use Manufacturer	Ingredients	
RALSTON POULTRY INSECTICIDE (Ralston)	Lindane*		RAMON'S CO-TABS For colds (Brown Mfg.)	Each tablet: Acetophenetidin* Stramonium alkaloids Sodium salicylate* Caffeine Ext. cascara Aloin Podophyllin Capsicum	1.75 gr. 1/1000 gr.
RALSTON PURINA DAIRY SPRAY (New Formula) Insecticide (Ralston)	Pyrethrins Thiocyanates* Methoxychlor		RAMON'S COVAC Antihistamine, analgesic (Brown Mfg.)	Each tablet: Pyranisamine maleate Acetophenetidin* Sodium salicylate* Caffeine	12.50 mg. 1.50 gr. 1.50 gr. 0.25 gr.
RALSTON PURINA HOME SPRAY Insecticide (Ralston)	Pyrethrins n-Octyl sulfoxide of isosafrole Inert ingredients*		RAMON'S HERBS Laxative (Brown Mfg.)	Compound of senna leaves Jalap Mandrake roots Aromatic and flavoring herbs	
RALSTON RANGE CATTLE SPRAY Insecticide (Ralston)	Toxaphene* Lindane*		RAMON'S MILD LAXATIVE WITH BILE SALTS (Brown Mfg.)	Yellow phenolphthalein not U.S.P. Cascara ext. Oleoresin capsicum Salts of bile Sodium glycocholate Sodium taurocholate	
RALSTON SCREW-WORM KILLER (Ralston)	Lindane* Chloroform* Pine tar oil		RAMON'S PINK PILLS Laxative (Brown Mfg.)	Aloin* Podophyllin Yellow phenolphthalein, not U.S.P. Ext. cascara sagrada	
RALSTON SCREW-WORM REMEDY EQ 335 (Allied Drug)	Gamma isomer of benzene hexachloride (from lindane)* Pine oil* Mineral oil	3% 35% 42%	RAMON'S RED OIL Liniment (Brown Mfg.)	Chloroform 8-3/4 m./fl. oz. Oils of origanum comm'l. tech., cedar, and camphor*sassafrass* with aromatics Petroleum base	
RALSTON SCREW-WORM SMEAR (Hess, Dr.)	Diphenylamine Benzol* Turkey red oil	35% 35% 5.5%	RAMON'S RUB For colds (Brown Mfg.)	Menthol* Camphor* Thymol* Oils of eucalyptus* Cedar leaf* Turpentine* Sassafras* Nutmeg White petrolatum base	
RALSTON SULFA-NOX (Powder, Liquid, Conc.) Veterinary (Ralston)	Sulfaquinoxaline*		RAMON'S TABS Analgesic (Brown Mfg.)	Aspirin* Caffeine	5 gr. 1/4 gr.
RALSTON WOUND PROTECTOR Veterinary (Ralston)	Lindane* Butoxypolypropylene glycol* Pine oil* Chloroform*		RAND ZONE ANTI-FREEZE (Randall)		
RALTIX For menstrual, irregularities (Tailby)	Each tablet: d-Desoxyephedrine hydro-chloride Powd. ext. viburnum opulus Salicylamide	1 mg. 30 mg. 200 mg.	RANGER ADULT CAPSULES Anthelmintic (veterinary) (Ranger)	n-Butyl chloride*capsules 16 m.	
RAMODELL'S SULFUR CREAM For dandruff (Fougera)	Precipitated sulfur*		RANGER CANKER WASH TABLETS For ear canker (veterinary) (Ranger)	Sodium borate* Boric acid*	5 gr. 5 gr.
RAMON'S BROWNIE PILLS Diuretic (Brown Mfg.)	Theobromine sodiosalicylate* Ext. uva ursi Meth. blue				

*Consult Sec. II., Ingredients Index. This ingredient may be responsible for major toxic effects if poisonous amounts of this product are ingested.

Name & Use Manufacturer	Ingredients		Name & Use Manufacturer	Ingredients	
RANGER EYE WASH TABLETS (Ranger)	Zinc sulfocarbolate Boric acid*	1/4 gr. 2 gr.	RAPIDOL CONDITION-ING SHAMPOO & HAND LOTION (Rapidol)		
RANGER FLEA POWDER (Ranger)	Rotenone Other cube resins	1% 2%	RAP-I-DOL MASTER HAIR COLORING & SHAMPOO TINT (Rapidol)		
RANGER LAXATIVE TABLETS Veterinary (Ranger)	Aloin Ext. cascara sagrada Oleoresin ginger Extract belladona leaves	1/16 gr. 1/16 gr. 1/16 gr. 1/32 gr.	RAPIDRY ENAMEL & VARNISH (Cook P. & V.)		
RANGER PUPPY CAPSULES Anthelmintic (veterinary) (Ranger)	n-Butyl chloride* capsules	8 m.	RAPONEX Rodenticide (Hydroponic)	Warfarin (3-(a-acetonylbenzyl)-4-hydroxycoumarin)	0.025%
			RAP PAINT REMOVER (Glidden Co.)		
RANGER SPECIAL EX-PECTORANT TABLETS Veterinary (Ranger)	Ipecac Terpin hydrate* Ammonium chloride Extract licorice Extract hyoscyamus*	1/10 gr. 2 gr. 1 gr. 1/2 gr. 1/8 gr.	RARE JEWEL TOILET WATER (Countess)		
RANGER TAPEWORM TABLETS Veterinary (Ranger)	Arecoline hydrobromide*	1/20 gr.	RASEMA For skin irritation (Melvin)	Resorcin Sodium salicylate* Naphthalin* Glycerin Refined distillates of coal tar * Oil of cade*	
RANOLL'S Laxative (Myers Labs.)	Aloe* Gentian mandrake Oleoresin capsicum*		RASP CHILDREN'S COUGH SYRUP (Commerce)	Alcohol Spruce Wild cherry Sanguinaria Ammonium chloride Honey Menthol	2%
RANSOM'S SYRUP COMPOUND Antitussive (Myers Labs.)	Tartar emetic* White squill Lobelia Senega root Skunk cabbage Tolu	2/5 gr.			
RAP BRUSH CLEANER (Glidden Co.)			RAT-A-KILL Rodenticide (Eradico)		
RAPID ASPHALT PAINT (Ruberoid)			RATAWAY Rodenticide (Crane)	Warfarin	0.025%
RAPID COTE VARNISH (Glidden Co.)			RAT-A-WAY Rodenticide (Miller Chem. & Fert.)	3-(a-Phenyl-b-acetyl ethyl) 4-hydroxycoumarin*	0.5%
RAPID FIXER Photographic supply (Urell)			RAT-A-WAY BAIT Rodenticide (Miller Chem. & Fert.)	3-(Alpha-acetonylbenzyl)-4-hydroxycoumarin	0.025%
RAPID FIXOL Photographic supply (FR)			RAT BALM Rodenticide (Foster's W.C.)	Acid arsenic* liquid syrup	75%
RA-PID-GRO Plant food (Ra-Pid-Gro)	Nitrogen Phosphoric acid Potash	23% 21% 17%	RAT-B-GON RAT & MICE BAIT (Calif. Spray)	Warfarin (3-(a-acetonylbenzyl)-4-hydroxycoumarin)	0.025%
RAPIDO ENAMEL (Chi-Namel)	Titanium dioxide Titanium calcium Alminum silicate Soya alkyd resin Drier Mineral spirits*	28.0 % 17.0 % 8.0 % 24.0 % 1.0 % 32.0 %	RAT-BIS-KIT PASTE Rodenticide (Rat Biscuit)	Phosphorus*	2%
			RAT CHECK Rodenticide (Chek)		
RAPIDO FLOOR VARNISH (Chi-Namel)	Chinawood oil* Modified phenolic resin Mineral spirits*	29.8% 20.7% 49.5%	RAT DEATH (Germo)		
			RAT DOOM (Crane)	Zinc phosphide*	5%

*Consult Sec. II., Ingredients Index. This ingredient may be responsible for major toxic effects if poisonous amounts of this product are ingested.

Name & Use Manufacturer	Ingredients		Name & Use Manufacturer	Ingredients	
RAT-ERASE (Burrell-Dugger)	Warfarin (3-(a-acetonylbenzyl)-4-hydroxycoumarin)	0.025%	RAVEN STOVE POLISH (Black & White Chem.)		
RATERASER Rodenticide (Crane)	Red squill*		RAWLEIGH'S INSECT DUST NO. 1 (Rawleigh)	Rotenone Sulfur	0.50% 2.92%
RAT EXIT (Wisconsin Pharm.)	Warfarin (3-(a-acetonylbenzyl)-4-hydroxycoumarin)		RAWLEIGH'S INSECT DUST NO. 2 (Rawleigh)	Rotenone Sulfur	0.75% 2.92%
RAT-KIL WITH WARFARIN (Durham's)	Warfarin (3-(a-acetonylbenzyl)-4-hydroxycoumarin)	0.025%	RAWLEIGH'S INSECT DUST NO. 3 (Rawleigh)	Rotenone Copper as metallic copper*	0.50% 7.00%
RAT KRAX Rodenticide (Koch)	Warfarin	0.025%	RAX WARFARIN Rodenticide (Prentiss)	Warfarin	0.5%
RAT LUNCHES Rodenticide (Rat)	Red squill*	10%	RAYDERM OINTMENT For dryness following irradiation (Velvet)	Euphorbia (anti-histamine) Phenyl salicylate Neatsfoot oil Cod liver oil Olive oil Lanolin Oxycholesterol Cetyl alcohol	
RAT NIP Rodenticide (Liquid)	Phosphorus	1.1%			
RAT-NOTS Rodenticide (Nott)	Red squill*	10%			
RAT-O-CIDE (Amer. Fumig.)	Red squill*				
RATOPAX Rodenticide (Biocerta)	Convallaria* Maritima scilla* Digitalis*	6.5% 3.5% 2%	RAYDEX Abrasive cleaner (Pennsylv. Salt)	Soda ash Alkaline phosphate Wetting agent	
RATRID Rodenticide (Vineland)	Warfarin (3-(a-acetonylbenzyl)-4-hydroxycoumarin)	0.5%	RAYDIZED PAINTS (Vita-Var)		
RAT RIDDER (Internat. Stock)	Warfarin* (3-(a-acetonylbenzyl)-4-hydroxycoumarin)	0.025%	RAYDUR SYNTHETIC ENAMELS & VARNISHES (Waldstein)		
RATSAULT Rodenticide (Barrett Chem.)	ANTU*	20%	RAYFLEX WEATHER WAX POLISH (Rathgeber)		
RAT SCENT Rodenticide (Woods, C. G.)	Strychnine alkaloid*	0.29%	RAY-LAX Laxative (Raymond, M.)	Aloin * Ext. belladonna leaves Strychnine* Ext. cascara sagrada	1/2 gr. 1/16 gr. 1/120 gr. 1/2 gr.
RAT SLAYER (Slayer)	Warfarin	0.025%			
RAT-STOP Rodenticide (K-R-O)	Alpha naphthyl thiourea*	15%	RAYMOND'S OINTMENT (Raymond, M.)	Petrolatum Camphor gum* Oil hemlock* Oil cajuput* Oil wormwood* Oil peppermint* Oil spearmint* Oil cade* Yellow wax	
RATTER Rodenticide (Dill)	Warfarin (3-(a-acetonylbenzyl) 4-hydroxycoumarin)	0.025%			
RAT-TOX Rodenticide (Rex Res.)	Alpha naphthyl thiourea*	20%			
RAT-TROL BAIT & CONCENTRATE (Thompson-Hayward)	Warfarin (3-(a-acetonylbenzyl)-4-hydroxycoumarin)	0.025%	RAYNO Fungicide (medical) (Purepac)	Isopropyl alcohol* Salicylic acid* Benzoic acid Methyl salicylate*	85%/v
RAT-X Rodenticide (Davis, O. D.)	Alpha naphthyl thiourea	1%	RAY-NOX Prevents sunburn (Torch)	PABA containing cream	

*Consult Sec. II., Ingredients Index. This ingredient may be responsible for major toxic effects if poisonous amounts of this product are ingested.

Name & Use Manufacturer	Ingredients	
RAYVE CREME SHAMPOO (Lever)	Duponol WA Stearic acid Lanolin Perfume	
RAZON ENAMEL (Tremco)		
R.C.B. HARDWOOD FLOOR CLEANER (Tamma)		
R & C SAL SODA WATER SOFTENER (Calif. Soda)	Tech. sal soda Sulfate Borate *	
R E A 2% CHLORDANE RESIDUAL SPRAY Insecticide (Hunter)	Tech. chlordane Petroleum hydrocarbons*	2% 98%
R E A 10% DDT DUST Insecticide (Hunter)	Pyrethrins Tech. piperonyl butoxide DDT*	0.067% 0.336% 10.000%
R E A DDT 50% WET- TABLE POWDER Insecticide (Hunter)	DDT*	50%
REAL-COAT ENAMEL (Sargent- Gerke)		
REAL-KILL BUG KILLER (Cook Chem.)	Pyrethrins n-Octyl sulfoxide of isosafrole Related compounds Dieldrin Phenyl mercuric lactate Polymerized glycerol oleate Petroleum distillates*	0.046% 0.101% 0.014% 0.500% 0.016% 0.100% 99.223%

REAL-KILL
INSECT
BOMB
(Cook Chem.)
	Pyrethrins
	Piperonyl butoxide
	Allethrin
	Beta butoxy beta thiocyano
	  diethyl ether
	n-Octyl bicycloheptene
	  dicarboximide
	Methoxychlor tech.
	Petroleum distillates*
		0.050%
		0.125%
		0.200%
		0.500%
		1.000%
		2.000%
		11.125%

REAL-KILL MOTH PROOFER (Cook Chem.)	Chlordane Petroleum distillates*	2.00% 48.00%
REALSEAL ROOF COATINGS (Detroit)		
REALTEX PLASTIC PAINT (Fox)		

Name & Use Manufacturer	Ingredients	
REALWHITE PURE WHITE PAINT (Heath & Milligan)		
R E A 7-1/2 RESIDUAL SPRAY Insecticide (Hunter)	b-Butoxy b-thiocyano diethyl ether DDT* Polymethylated naphthalenes* Petroleum distillate*	1.500% 5.000% 12.500% 81.000%
REARDON'S MOUSE SEED (Reardon, W.)	Strychnine*	0.4%
RECALSAN Analgesic (Reese Chem.)	Each tablet: Salicylamide* Sodium salicylate* Sodium para aminobenzoate Thiamine hydrochloride Ascorbic acid	3 mg. 5 mg.
R-E-C OINTMENT For hemor- rhoids (Barlow- Maney)	Carbolic acid Extract stramonium Extract arnica Hydrastis Thymol * Benzocaine Extract witch hazel Tannic acid * Menthol * Eucalyptol *	1/2% 4% 1/2%
RECREO POWDER (Plain) Dusting powder (Recreo)	Stearate of zinc compound Balsam Peru Boric acid* Talcum	
RECTAL MEDICONE Suppositories (Medicone)	Anesthesin (benzocaine) Ephedrine hydrochloride Oxyquinoline sulfate Zinc oxide Balsam Peru Cocoa butter	2 gr. 1/16 gr. 1/4 gr. 3 gr. 1 gr. q.s.
RECTALGAN For hemor- rhoids (Doho)	Benzocaine Carbolic acid Menthol Ephedrine alk.	4.5% 1.75% 0.5% 0.125%
RECTAL SUPPOSI- TORIES #35A For hemor- rhoids (Sharp & Dohme)	Each suppository: Extract stramonium Lead carbonate* Potassium alum Sol. lead subacetate * Creosote	30 mg. 60 mg. 60 mg. 0.12 cc. 30 mg.
RECTO Fungicide for aquarium water (Spratts)		
RECTOCAINE Suppositories (Kirk, C. F.)	Urea Propyl aminobenzoate Procaine Phenol	5% 5% 0.5% 1%
RECTOCAINE OINTMENT (Kirk's) For rectal irritation (Kirk, C. F.)	Propyl aminobenzoate Procaine base Phenol Benzyl alcohol Lanolin	7% 0.5% 1% 7%

*Consult Sec. II., Ingredients Index. This ingredient may be responsible for major toxic effects if poisonous amounts of this product are ingested.

- 880 -

Name & Use Manufacturer	Ingredients		Name & Use Manufacturer	Ingredients	
RECTODYNE OINTMENT For rectal irritations (Massengill)	Each oz.: Powdered opium Carbolic acid Tannic acid Ext. stramonium* Ext. hamamelis leaf Balsam Peru Tetracaine Thymol and resorcinol	2 gr. 5 gr. 20 gr. 5 gr. 20 gr. 15 gr. 2 gr. q.s.	RED CHECK BUG & ROACH POWDER (Girard, Felix)	DDT dust*	10%
			RED CHECK PREPARED BAIT FOR RATS & MICE (Girard, Felix)	Arsenic trioxide*	25%
RECTOID OINTMENT (Rectal) (Massengill)	Atropine sulfate Ephedrine sulfate Benzocaine Carbolic acid Camphor Menthol Ointment zinc oxide	0.028% 1% 3% 1.37% 0.68% 1% q.s.	RED CHECK RAT & MOUSE KILLER (Girard, Felix)	Arsenic trioxide*	99%
RED-ANKA Rubefacient (Turner's Pharm.)	Sodium salicylate* Potassium iodide* Alcohol	3%	RED CHURN LACQUER NO. 2301 (George, P.D.)		
RED ARROW D-50 WATER DISPERSIBLE POWDER Insecticide (Hy-Gro)	DDT*	50%	RED CIRCLE ANT KILLER (Red Circle)		
			RED CIRCLE GERM DESTROYER (Red Circle)		
RED ARROW DUST Insecticide (Hy-Gro)	Rotenone Other cube resins	0.75% 1.5%	RED CIRCLE INSECT KILLER (Red Circle)		
RED ARROW GARDEN SPRAY Insecticide (Hy-Gro)	Pyrethrins Piperonyl cyclonene Rotenone Other cube resins Steam distilled pine oil* Polyoxyethylene sorbitol esters of mixed fatty acids	0.50% 3.00% 1.50% 3.50% 20.0% 8.00%	RED CIRCLE ROACH DESTROYER (Powder) (Red Circle)		
			RED CLOUD BERRIES Laxative (Clarke, H.)	Colocynth N.F. (powd. ext.) Aloe U.S.P. * Aloin U.S.P.* Podophyllin U.S.P. Ipecac U.S.P. Scammony resin N.F. Cardamom U.S.P.	
RED ARROW SPECIAL GARDEN SPRAY Insecticide (Hy-Gro)	Pyrethrum Inert ingredients*	2%	RED CROSS NURSE GERMICIDE DEODORIZER (Hubbard, J.)	Alcohol * Oil lavender, oil rosemary, terpenyl acetate, oil eucalyptus,* linalyl acetate	75%/v 3%
RED ARROW TOMATO-POTATO DUST D3RC Insecticide (Hy-Gro)	Rotenone DDT* Copper*	0.75% 3% 6%	RED-DEVIL DUST Insecticide (Pearson & Co.)	Sabadilla alkaloids (derived from 20% sabadilla seed, powdered and activated)	
RED ARROW VEGETABLE GARDEN DUST Insecticide (Hy-Gro)	Rotenone Other cube resins Inert ingred.	1.00% 2.00% 97.00%	RED DEVIL FOR CLOGGED DRAINS Solvent (Babbitt)	Sodium hydroxide *	
RED ARROW WEED KILLER (Hy-Gro)	Alkanolamine salts 2, 4-Dichloro phenoxy acetic acid * Propylene glycol Butyl ether esters of 2, 4, 5-trichlorophenoxyacetic acid * 2, 4, 5-Trichlorophenoxyacetic acid*	30.00% 9.24%	RED DEVIL N 22 AUTO POLISH (Technical Color)		
RED BOAT PAINT (George, P.D.)			RED DEVIL PAINT & VARNISHES (Technical Color)		

*Consult Sec. II., Ingredients Index. This ingredient may be responsible for major toxic effects if poisonous amounts of this product are ingested.

Name & Use Manufacturer	Ingredients		Name & Use Manufacturer	Ingredients	
RED DEVIL'S LIGHTER FLUID (Devil)			RED FEATHER TICK, FLEA & LOUSE POWDER (Red Feather)	Rotenone Other cube resins Pyrethrins Sulfur*	1.0% 2.0% 0.5% 15.0%
RED DEVIL SOOT & CARBON REMOVER (Powder Form) (Marine Elect.)	Copper chloride* Lead oxide*		RED FEATHER VETERINARY V F FORMULA Insecticide (Red Feather)	Thanite* Methoxychlor Petroleum distillate*	12.0% 9.0% 69.0%
RED DEVIL SOOT REMOVER (Liquid) (Marine Elect.)	Lead naphthenate* F. O. dispersant Kerosene*		RED HEAD ANTI-POX REMEDY (Blue Ball)		
REDDI-LITE CHARCOAL LIGHTER (Reddi-Lite)			RED HEAD GERMICIDE (Blue Ball)		
RED DOT SHAVING SOAP (Mem)			RED HEADS For colds (Abbott)	Acetophenetidin * Camphor monobromated * Acetylsalicylic acid * (aspirin) Extract belladonna Total alkaloids 0.000416 gr. Strychnine sulfate	1 gr. 1 gr. 2 gr. 1/30 gr. 1/120 gr.
REDDY WATERLESS CLEANSER (Commercial Paste)			RED HEAD SOREHEAD REMEDY Veterinary (Blue Ball)		
RED FEATHER DE-WORMING POWDER Veterinary (Red Feather)	Cucurbita pepo Wormseed meal*	80% 20%	RED HEAD SULPHUR SOLUTION (Blue Ball)		
RED FEATHER DOG BATH SHAMPOO Insecticide (Red Feather)	Pure coconut oil soap base Oil of cedar leaves Phenol	 0.2%	RED HEAD WORMNOT (Blue Ball)		
RED FEATHER DOG BATH SHAMPOO WITH CHLOROPHYLL Insecticide (Red Feather)	Pure coconut oil soap base Oil of cedar leaves Phenol	 0.2%	RED HOT ALUMINUM PAINTS (Sheffield Bronze)		
RED FEATHER FORMULA 48 Antiseptic for mange (veterinary) (Red Feather)	Petroleum distillate* Pine oil* Chlordane* Dichlorophene	51% 25% 8% 8%	REDIBLEND PAINTS (Adelphi) RED-I-CAT Rodenticide (Pearson & Co.)	 Warfarin	 0.5%
RED FEATHER For heart worms (veterinary) (Red Feather)	Naphthalene* Benzoic acid * Worm oil seed * Chloroform* Iodine*		REDIMIXED ALUMINUM PAINT (Yates & Smart)		
RED FEATHER KENNEL KEEPER Insecticide (Red Feather)	Petroleum distillate* Tech. chlordane* Pyrethrum		RED JACKET NO. 465 PITLESS UNDER- GROUND DISCHARGE For sterilizing wells and pumping equipment)	Hypochlorite powder*	
RED FEATHER SPONGE BATH Insecticide (Red Feather)	Petroleum distillate* Emulsifier (polyethylene glycol oleate) Tech. chlordane* Pyrethrum		RED JASMINE PERFUME (Caswell- Massey)		

*Consult Sec. II., Ingredients Index. This ingredient may be responsible for major toxic effects if poisonous amounts of this product are ingested.

Name & Use Manufacturer	Ingredients		Name & Use Manufacturer	Ingredients	
RED KAPS Analgesic (Profant)	Calcium succinate Acid acetosalicylic* Sodium salicylate* Acetophenetidin*	3 gr. 2 gr. 2 gr. 1 gr.	RED PANTHER 1-1/2 - 0 - 0 DIELDRIN EQUIVALENT DUST Insecticide (Coahoma)	Hexachloro epoxy octahydro dimethano naphthalene* (from dieldrin) Related compounds (from dieldrin)	1.275% 0.225%
RED MARVEL METAL POLISH (Uncle Sam)	Oleic acid Oxalic acid* Alcohol Ammonia Silica		RED PANTHER 1-1/2 - 10 - 0 DIELDRIN EQUIVALENT DUST Insecticide (Coahoma)	Hexachloro epoxy octahydro dimethano naphthalene* (from dieldrin) Related compounds (from dieldrin) DDT*	1.275% 0.225% 10.000%
RED METAL ROOF PAINT (Rutland)	Pigment: Red iron oxide Aluminum silicate Vehicle: Lecithin Soya-alkyd Mineral spirits and drier*	31%/w 69%/w	RED PANTHER 10% DIELDRIN GRANULAR Insecticide (Coahoma)	Hexachloro epoxy octahydro dimethano naphthalene* Related compounds	8.50% 1.50%
RED OINTMENT S.F. MFR. NO. 730 (Specialists)	Salicylic acid* Merbromin* Boric acid*		RED PANTHER ENDRIN 1.6 LB. EMUSIFIABLE CONCEN- TRATE Insecticide (Coahoma)	Hexachloro epoxy octahydro- endo, endo-dimethano naphthalene* Petroleum hydrocarbons	19.5% 70.5%
REDOX PAINT (Continental Prod.)					
RED PANTHER ALDRIN 2 LB. EMUSIFIABLE CONCON- TRATE Insecticide (Coahoma)	Hexachloro hexahydro dimethano naphthalene* Related compounds Petroleum hydrocarbon	21.85% 16.48% 51.67%	RED PANTHER 12% GAMMA BHC WET- TABLE POWDER Insecticide (Coahoma)	Gamma isomer of benzene hexachloride* Other isomers of benzene hexachloride	12% 18%
RED PANTHER 2-1/2 - 5 - 0 ALDRIN EQUIVALENT DDT DUST (Coahoma)	Hexachloro hexahydro dimethano naphthalene* Related compounds DDT	2.375% 1.791% 5.000%	RED PANTHER 50% MALATHON EMULSIFI- ABLE CONC. Insecticide (Coahoma)	Malathion* Aromatic petroleum distillate solvent*	50% 30%
RED PANTHER CHLORO IPC EMULSIFIABLE CONCEN- TRATE Herbicide (Coahoma)	Isopropyl n-(3-chlorophenyl) carbamate*	46%	RED PANTHER 1% PARATHION DUST Insecticide (Coahoma)	Parathion*	1%
RED PANTHER 3-10-0 COTTON DUST Insecticide (Coahoma)	Gamma isomer of benzene hexachloride* Other isomers of benzene hexachloride DDT*	3% 14% 10%	RED PANTHER 1-1/2% ROTENONE CATTLE GRUB & GARDEN DUST Insecticide (Coahoma)	Rotenone Other cube resins	1.50% 1.50%
RED PANTHER 3-10-40 COTTON DUST Insecticide (Coahoma)	Gamma isomer of benzene hexachloride* Other isomers of benzene hexachloride DDT* Sulfur*	3% 14% 10% 40%	RED PANTHER 5% ROTENONE WETTABLE POWDER Insecticide (Coahoma)	Rotenone* Other cube resins	5% 10%
RED PANTHER DDT 25% EMUSIFIABLE CONCEN- TRATE Insecticide (Coahoma)	DDT Aromatic petroleum hydrocarbon*	25% 70%	RED PANTHER TOXAPHENE- LINDANE LIVESTOCK EMULSIFI- ABLE CONC. Insecticide (Coahoma)	Toxaphene* Gamma isomer of benzene hexachloride (from lindane)	60.0% 2.4%
RED PANTHER DIELDRIN 1.5 LB. EMUSIFIABLE CONCEN- TRATE Insecticide (Coahoma)	Hexachloro epoxy octahydro dimethano naphthelene* (from dieldrin) Related compounds (from dieldrin) Petroleum hydrocarbons	15.83% 2.70% 73.38%			

*Consult Sec. II., Ingredients Index. This ingredient may be responsible for major toxic effects if poisonous amounts of this product are ingested.

Name & Use Manufacturer	Ingredients	Name & Use Manufacturer	Ingredients
RED PANTHER TOXAPHENE 6 LB. EMUSIFIABLE CONCENTRATE Insecticide (Coahoma)	Toxaphene* (tech. chlorinated camphene containing 67% to 69% chlorine) 59% Petroleum distillates 31%	RED-TOP ARAMITE 25 SPRAY Insecticide (Fresno Agric.)	2-(p-tert-Butylphenoxy) isopropyl 2-chloroethyl sulfite 25% Petroleum hydrocarbons* 70%
RED PANTHER TOXAPHENE LIVESTOCK EMULSIFIABLE CONC. Insecticide (Coahoma)	Toxaphene* 61%	RED-TOP BHC 11 SPRAY Insecticide (Fresno Agric.)	Gamma isomer of benzene hexachloride* 11% Other isomers of benzene hexachloride* 30% Petroleum hydrocarbons* 54%
RED PANTHER 20-1 TOXAPHENE-PARATHION DUST Insecticide (Coahoma)	Toxaphene* 20.00% Parathion* 1.00%	RED-TOP CHLORDANE 74 SPRAY Insecticide (Fresno Agric.)	Tech. chlordane* 74%
RED POLISH (Watkins, J.)	Linseed oil Cobalt* Linoleate Mineral seal oil	RED-TOP DDT 25 SPRAY Insecticide (Fresno Agric.)	Dichloro diphenyl trichloroethane 25% Aromatic petroleum derivatives* 65%
RED RANGER FLEA, TICK & LOUSE POWDER (Coop. Seed)	Tech. piperonyl cyclonene 1.0% Pyrethrins 0.1% Rotenone 0.5% Other cube extractives 1.0%	RED-TOP DIELDRIN 15 SPRAY Insecticide (Fresno Agric.)	Hexachloro epoxy octahydro dimethano naphthalene* 15.83% Related compounds 2.79% Petroleum hydrocarbons 73.38%
RED ROBIN DUST Insecticide (Pearson & Co.)	Rotenone 1.00% Other cube resins 2.00%	RED-TOP LINDANE 20 SPRAY Insecticide (Fresno Agric.)	Lindane (gamma isomer of BHC)* 20.0% Petroleum hydrocarbons 72.0%
RED SEAL PAINTS, STAINS, VARNISHES & ENAMELS (DeSoto P. & V.)		RED-TOP MALATHION 5 SPRAY Insecticide (Fresno Agric.)	Malathion* 55%
RED SPIDER DUST Insecticide (Imperial Chem.)	Rotenone 0.80% Cube resins 1.00% Sulfur* 78.12%	RED-TOP NICOTINE 10 DUST Insecticide (Fresno Agric.)	Nicotine* expressed as alkaloid 3.6%
RED SPOT PAINTS & VARNISHES (Red Spot)		RED-TOP PARATHION 200 DDT-5 SULFUR 50 DUST Insecticide (Fresno Agric.)	Parathion* 2% DDT (setting point 89°C) 5% Sulfur 50%
RED STAR COLD CAPSULES (Commerce)	Acetophenetidin* 1 gr. Quinine Gelsemium* Podophyllin Capsicum Camphor* Aloin* Belladonna leaves 1/40 gr. Alkaloids 1/3000 gr.	RED TOP PARATHION 200 DUST Insecticide (Fresno Agric.)	Parathion (o, o-diethyl o-p-nitrophenyl thiophosphate)* 2%
RED S VARNISHES & LACQUERS (Schaefer V.)		RED-TOP PARATHION 45 SPRAY Insecticide, fungicide (Fresno Agric.)	Parathion* 45% Aromatic solvents 47%
RED-TOP ALDRIN 24 SPRAY Insecticide (Fresno Agric.)	Hexachloro hexahydro dimethano naphthalene* 22.8% Related compounds 17.2% Petroleum hydrocarbons 50.0%		

*Consult Sec. II., Ingredients Index. This ingredient may be responsible for major toxic effects if poisonous amounts of this product are ingested.

Name & Use Manufacturer	Ingredients	
RED-TOP PENTA-FOLIANT CONC. Herbicide (Fresno Agric.)	Pentachlorophenol*	32%
	Other chlorophenols	4%
RED-TOP PERTHANE 25 SPRAY Insecticide (Fresno Agric.)	Diethyl diphenyl dichloro-ethane*	25%
RED-TOP TEPP 100 DUST Insecticide (Fresno Agric.)	Tetraethyl pyrophosphate*	1.0%
	Other related organic phosphates	1.5%
RED-TOP TEPP 50 SPRAY Insecticide (Fresno Agric.)	Tetraethyl pyrophosphate*	20.0%
	Other related organic phosphates*	30.0%
RED-TOP TOXAPHENE 4-DDT 2 SPRAY Insecticide (Fresno Agric.)	Tech. toxaphene*	40%
	Dichloro diphenyl tri-chloroethane	20%
RED TOP TOXAPHENE 15-DDT 5-SULFUR 40 DUST Insecticide (Fresno Agric.)	Tech. chlorinated camphene*	15%
	Dichloro diphenyl tri-chloroethane	5%
	Sulfur	40%
RED-TOP TOXAPHENE 61 SPRAY Insecticide (Fresno Agric.)	Tech. toxaphene*	61%
	Petroleum hydrocarbons	29%
RED-TOP WOOD PRES. CONC. (Fresno Agric.)	Pentachlorophenol*	32%
	Other chlorophenols	4%
RED TOP ZEB 3-DDT 5-SULPHUR 25 DUST Insecticide, fungicide (Fresno Agric.)	Zinc ethylene-bis(dithio-carbamate)	3%
	Dichloro diphenyl tri-chloroethane*	5%
	Sulfur*	25%
REDUCER FOR FABULON For thinning and cleaning brushes (Pierce & Stevens)	Similar to FABULON solvents*	
REDUCIT ALL-PURPOSE THINNER (O'Brien Corp.)		

Name & Use Manufacturer	Ingredients	
REDUSOL THINNER (McQuade, J.)		
REDWOOD EUCALYPTOL COMPOUND Inhalant, nasal decongestant (Redwood Zone)	Gum of redwood	
	Oil of redwood*	
	Oil of eucalyptus*	
	Oil of cassai*	
	Camphor*	
	Thymol*	
	Benzoic acid	
	Boric acid*	
	Glycerin	
	Alcohol	
REDWOOD FINISH Paint (Chi-Namel)	Linseed oil	18.0%
	Alkyd resin	22.2%
	Drier	1.8%
	Petroleum spirits*	58.0%
RED-X STAINS, FILLERS, ETC. (Reliance Varnish)		
RED X 3-IN-1 RUBBER CEMENT (St. Louis Rubber)		
REEDER'S ANTI-FOULING Paint (Balto. Copper)		
REEDER'S BRAND GREEN BOOTTOP (Balto. Copper)	Chrome green containing lead chromate*	
REE-LEAF CORN REMOVER (Phenacedol)	Salicylic acid*	
	Hyoscyamus*	
	Ether*	
	Flexible collodion	
REE-LEAF TOOTHACHE DROPS (Phenacedol)	Benzyl alcohol	24%
	Oil cloves	
	Creosote*	24%
	Camphor	
	Chloroform*	
	Carbolic acid	1.2%
REESE'S BLU-TABS Nasal de-congestant (Reese Chem.)	Each tablet:	
	Ephedrine sulfate*	1/8 gr.
	Ortho iodo benzoic acid	
	Calcium lactate	
REESE'S BUNION RELIEVER (Reese Chem.)	Carbolic acid*	
	Iodine *	
	Methyl salicylate*	
	Potassium iodide	
REESE'S CALLUS REMOVER (Reese Chem.)	Salicylic acid*	
	Camphor*	
REESE'S COLD CAPSULES For colds (Reese Chem.)	Each capsule:	
	Salicylamide*	3 gr.
	Acetophenetidin*	2 gr.
	Caffeine	0.5 gr.
	Atropine sulfate	1/600 gr.
	Pyrilamine maleate	25 mg.
	Quinine sulfate	0.5 gr.

*Consult Sec. II., Ingredients Index. This ingredient may be responsible for major toxic effects if poisonous amounts of this product are ingested.

- 885 -

Name & Use Manufacturer	Ingredients		Name & Use Manufacturer	Ingredients	
REESE'S CORN REMOVER (Reese Chem.)	Salicylic acid* Camphor*		REGOE'S ANTI-SKIPPER COMPOUND Insecticide (Rigo)	Tech. piperonyl butoxide Pyrethrins	1.33% 0.10%
REESE'S SEDATIVE TABLETS (Reese Chem.)	Each tablet: Sodium bromide * Potassium bromide * Ammonium bromide* Scopolamine hydrobromide *	3 gr. 3 gr. 1-1/2 gr. 1/400 gr.	REGOE'S PINEGARD Disinfectant, deodorant (Rigo)	Pine oil* Anhydrous soap	81% 9%
REESE'S SPECIAL FORMULA Analgesic, nasal decongestant (Reese Chem.)	Acetanilid* Salicylamide* Camphor monobromated* Ephedrine sulfate*	1 gr. 1/8 gr.	REGULATORS Laxative (Wecker)	Aloin Powdered ipecac Ext. belladonna leaves Phenolphthalein	1/4 gr. 1/15 gr. 1/12 gr. 1/2 gr.
REESE'S STIMULANT DIURETIC FOR THE KIDNEYS (Reese Chem.)	Theobromine* Sodium salicylate* Potassium citrate U.S.P. Powdered ext. of buchu leaves Powdered ext. of uva ursa leaves		REGULIN Laxative (Regulin)	Jelly-forming coating of blond psyllium seed Ext. cascara Ext. licorice	
REESE'S THROAT LOZENGES (Reese Chem.)	Each lozenge: Benzocaine Tyrothricin Ammonium chloride Cetyl dimethyl benzyl ammonium chloride	5 mg. 2 mg. 1/2 gr. 1 mg.	REHISCO TABLETS For colds (Reese Chem.)	Each tablet: Aspirin* Acetophenetidin* Caffeine alkaloid Pyrilamine maleate	3-1/2 gr. 2-1/2 gr. 1/2 gr. 25 mg.
RE-FINIS-HR Cleaner for hardwood floors (Andersen)	Bleach		REID'S ANT POISON (Reid's)	Arsenic *	
REFLECT-O-LITE PASTE PAINT (Glidden Co.)			REILLY MOTH BALLS & MOTH FLAKES (Reilly)	Naphthalene*	
REFLEXIONS EAU DE TOILETTE & EXTRACT (Parfums Ciro)			REL For colds (Maryland Pharm.)	Ephedrine* Sodium benzoate Menthol Tragacanth Essence of pine needles	
REFLEX MILL WHITE PAINTS (Briggs-Maroney)			RELAXO DRAIN PIPE CLEANER (McVicker)		
REGAL OIL A (Texas Co.)	Paraffinic lubricating oil		RELIABLE AIR CLEANER Bathroom deodorant (Reliable Chem.)	Paradichlorobenzene*	
REGAL'S NO ACID SOLDERING FLUX (Regal)			RELIABLE MOTH KILLER (Reliable Chem.)	Paradichlorobenzene*	
REGAL TONE Rubber base paint (Atlantic V. & P.)			RELIABLE MOTH SQUARES (Reliable Chem.)	Refined naphthalene* Perfume oils	99-1/2% 1/2%
REGATTA PAINTS (Balto. Copper)			RELIABLE PARA-ZENE & PARA-ZENE VAPORIZER Insecticide (Reliable Chem.)	Paradichlorobenzene*	
REGLO METAL POLISH (Silver Suds)					

Name & Use Manufacturer	Ingredients	Name & Use Manufacturer	Ingredients
RELIABLE SULPHUR CANDLE FUMIGATOR (Reliable Chem.)	Sulfur*	RENOL CREAMY WHITE POLISH (Stafford)	
REL-KA-SOL Antiseptic solution (Rel-Ka-Sol)	Chlorthymol* Carbolic acid* Boric acid* Alcohol 12% Glycerin Sodium chloride Sodium saccharin Ext. calendula	RENOLWAX NO-RUB FLOOR WAX (Stafford)	
		REN-O-SAL (Salsbury's)	3-Nitro-4-hydroxyphenyl arsonic acid* 0.2 gr. Ammonium and sodium phenolsulfonates Boric acid
RELPLEXIN (For Children) Antitussive (Massengill)	Stillingia Lobelia Oil cassia (imit.) Oil cajuput	RENOVATOR Floor cleaner (Hillyard Sales)	
REM Antitussive (Maryland)		REN-O-VOTE AUTO & FURNITURE POLISH (Glidden Co.)	
REMEDOL Antacid, adsorbent (Remedol)	Each tablet: Dried aluminum hydroxide gel 5 gr. Ascorbic acid 20 mg. Pyridoxine hydrochloride 1 mg. Nicotinic acid 10 mg.	RE-NU-A-BRUSH PAINT BRUSH CLEANER (Bridges, Smith)	
REMEMBER PERFUME (Scandia)		RE-NU-ALL PAINTS, ENAMELS & STAINS (Born)	
RE-MOV-ALL OIL & GREASE REMOVER (Stull)		RENU DRAIN PIPE CLEANER (Renu)	Sodium hydroxide *
REMUVIT DRAIN PIPE CLEANER (Eastern Sanitary)		RE NU HOME TINT (Re-Nu Home)	
RENAMEL STAIN VARNISH (Becker)		RENUIT VARNISH STAINS (Jewell P. & V.)	
RE-NEER FLOOR & FURNITURE POLISH (Stafford)		RENU SPOT & STAIN REMOVER (Renu)	Carbon tetrachloride*
RENEE THORNTON SKIN LOTION (Thornton, R.)		RE-NU-WIZE POLISH (Do-Ra)	
RENEUD DEODORANT SPRAY Cosmetic (Germo)		RENUZIT ALL PURPOSE HOME DRY CLEANER & SPOT & STAIN REMOVER (Renuzit)	Petroleum distillate* Contains no carbon tetrachloride *
RENOFAB CUSTOM HOME DRY CLEANER (Renofab)	Carbon tetrachloride * Savosol #3	REN-W-WAX SELF-POLISHING WAX (Glidden Co.)	
RENO-LAC AUTO POLISH (Stafford)			

*Consult Sec. II., Ingredients Index. This ingredient may be responsible for major toxic effects if poisonous amounts of this product are ingested.

Name & Use Manufacturer	Ingredients		Name & Use Manufacturer	Ingredients	
REO LIQUID CLEANER (Internat. Chem.)			RESIDEX 2 Insecticide (Residex)	Tech. chlordane Aliphatic petroleum distillate*	2% 98%
REPABA CAPSULETS Analgesic (Reese Chem.)	Each capsule: Sodium salicylate* Para amino benzoic acid Ascorbic acid Thiamine hydrochloride	4 gr. 4 gr. 30 mg. 3 mg.	RESIDEX 70 CHLORDANE EMULSIFI- ABLE CON- CENTRATE Insecticide (Residex)	Tech. chlordane*	70%
REPELITEX KEEPS PETS OFF FURNITURE (Magitex)	Allyl isothiocyanate	0.05%	RESIDEX PIVAL Rodenticide (Residex)	2-Pivalyl-1, 3-indiandione	0.025%
REPELITEX PROTECTS PLANTS FROM DOGS & CATS (Magitex)	Allyl isothiocyanate	0.46%	RESIDEX 0.5% WARFARIN CONCEN- TRATE Rodenticide (Residex)	Warfarin	0.5%
REPELLA BUG-FIX Insecticide (Thompson Chem.)	Dimethyl phthalate 2-Ethyl hexanediol-1, 3 Butyl dimethyl dihydro gamma pyrone carboxylate Isopropanol Propellent	12.77% 3.77% 3.46% 10.00% 70.00%	RESIDEX WATER SOLUBLE WARFARIN Rodenticide (Residex)	Sodium salt of warfarin	0.54%
REPELLO INSECT REPELLENT (Binday)	Ethyl hexanediol*	100%	RESIKILL FLY SPRAY (Residex)	Petroleum distillate* n-Octyl bicycloheptene dicarboximide Tech. methoxychlor Pyrethrins Allethrin	98.31% 1.092% 0.546% 0.026% 0.026%
REPEL-O- STIK Repellent (Sintos)	Dimethyl phthalate Ethyl hexanediol Butyl dihydro gamma pyrone carboxylate	10% 4% 2%	RESIKILL FLY SPRAY CON- CENTRATE (Residex)	Petroleum distillate* n-Octyl bicycloheptene dicarboximide Tech. methoxychlor Pyrethrins Allethrin (allyl homolog of cinerin 1)	83.87% 10.44% 5.21% 0.24% 0.24%
REP-GLO SEMI-GLOSS ENAMEL (Republic)			RESIKILL LIVESTOCK SPRAY Insecticide (Residex)	Petroleum distillate* n-Octyl bicycloheptene dicarboximide Tech. methoxychlor Pyrethrins Allethrin (allyl homolog of cinerin 1)	98.31% 1.092% 0.546% 0.026% 0.026%
REP-QUIK ENAMEL (Republic)					
REQUA'S STYPTIC PENCIL (Requa)	Alum sulfate *	90%	RESIMENE (Liquid Solution) Resins for baked enamel and industrial finishes (Monsanto)	Melamine Urea	
RESCOLOR LIQUID (Thomas & Thompson)	Carbolic acid Boric acid* Fuchsin Resorcinol* Acetone*	1.9%			
RESENT CRAYON (United Crayon)	Paraffin wax Pigments		RESIMENE (Soluble Spray Dried Powder) Laminating material (Monsanto)	Melamine resin	
RESENT SEMI-MOIST WATER- COLOR PAINT SETS (United Crayon)	Earth filler Gums Pigments		RESIMUS TRACKING POWDER Insecticide (Residex)	DDT* Pyrophyllite	50.0% 50.0%
RESENT WHITE & COLORED CHALK (United Crayon)	Gypsum Pigments		RESINOL For skin irritations (Resinol)	Resorcin* Oil of cade* Prepared calamine Zinc oxide Bismuth subnitrate Boric acid*	

*Consult Sec. II., Ingredients Index. This ingredient may be responsible for major toxic effects if poisonous amounts of this product are ingested.

Name & Use Manufacturer	Ingredients	Name & Use Manufacturer	Ingredients
RESINOL OINTMENT (Resinol)	Resorcinol* Calamine Boric acid* Zinc oxide Bismuth subcarbonate Oil of cade*	RETONGA TONIC Food supplement (Package)	Iron from ferric ammonium citrate 200 mg. Vitamin B1 (thiamine chloride) 10 mg. Vitamin B2 (riboflavin) 10 mg. Niacin 15 mg. Niacinamide 30 mg. Detannated gentian extract
RESINOX Laminating material (Monsanto)	Phenolic resin Alcohol* or other organic solvent	REU-MASAN Antirheumatic (Tosan)	Each tablet: Sodium salicylate* 0.3 gm. Sodium para-aminobenzoate 0.3 gm. Ascorbic acid 20 mg.
RESIPEL LIVESTOCK PROTECTANT Insecticide (Residex)	Butoxypolypropylene glycol 50.0% Methoxychlor tech. 5.0% Methylated naphthalenes* 40.6% Mixed alkyl aryl polyether alcohol 4.4%		
RESISTO FLOOR SEALER (Upco)		REVARNCO VARNISHES (Reliance Varnish)	
RESISTOIL PAINT (Armor)		REVELRY PERFUME & EAU DE COLOGNE (Millot)	
RESP AID Veterinary (Anchor Serum)	Ammonium chloride 181.6 gm. Potassium guaiacol sulfonate 90.8 gm. Sodium iodide 4.54 gm.	REVENGE DISINFECT-ANT LIQUID DIP (Russell, I.)	Coal tar neutral oils* Soap Coal tar phenols*
RES-PER-X Antitussive (veterinary) (Wilke)	Cresote* Gum turpentine* Sulfur* Oil of tar*	REVENGE LICE DESTROYER Insecticide (Russell, I.)	Phenol and creosote from coal tar* 7% Molecular sulfur 6% Naphthalene* 3%
RESRATTUS Rodenticide (Residex)	Warfarin 0.025%	REVENGE LITTER SPRAY DIS-INFECTANT (Russell, I.)	Coal tar neutral oils* Soap Coal tar phenols*
RESTO Sedative (Harrison's)	Each dr.: Bromide* 15 gr. Antipyrine* 1/2 gr.		
RESTO FOOT CREAM (Chandler)		REVENGE ROOST PAINT Insecticide (Russel, I.)	Creosote oils Nicotine alkaloid*
RES TON For CRD, infectious sinusitis and blue comb Veterinary (avian) (Pratt Food)	Para-amino benzoic acid Procaine penicillin Dried skimmed milk and grain fermentation solubles Vitamins A and D feeding oil Niacin Choline chloride Vitamin B12 supplement	REVIVA FURNITURE POLISH & HARDWOOD FLOOR CLEANER (Jackson of London)	
RE-STO-R STOVE POLISH (Lusterine)		REVLON CAKE ROUGE (Revlon)	Talc Glycerin Tragacanth Covering agents Preservative
RESULFOLIN (Torch)	Resorcinol monoacetate* 3% Sulfur dispersion 5% Monobase	REVLON CHEEKSTICK (Revlon)	Petrolatum Lanolin Wax Covering agent Preservative
RESULTS Cathartic (Van Dyke)	Phenolphthalein (yellow)	REVLON CUTICLE OIL (Revlon)	Petrolatum
RETONE TILE REFINISHER (Lester Labs.)	Alkali*	REVLON CUTICLE REMOVER (Revlon)	Polyethoxy ether Substituted ammonium hydroxide Propylene glycol Preservative

*Consult Sec. II., Ingredients Index. This ingredient may be responsible for major toxic effects if poisonous amounts of this product are ingested.

- 889 -

Name & Use Manufacturer	Ingredients
REVLON EYEBROW PENCIL (Revlon)	Fatty acids Lanolin Waxes Vegetable oil Glycerides Resin
REVLON FACE CREAM (Revlon)	
REVLON FACE POWDER (Revlon)	
REVLON HAND COLOGNE (Revlon)	Alcohol Polyethylene glycols
REVLON HAND LOTION (Revlon)	
REVLON INDELIBLE CREAM LIPSTICK (Revlon)	Waxes Glycol Glycol ester Vegetable oils Cholesterol absorption base Covering agent Preservative
REVLON LOVE PAT Pancake make-up (Revlon)	
REVLON NAIL CREAM (Revlon)	Lanolin Petrolatum Sorbitan ester Wax Covering agent
REVLON NAIL POLISH (Revlon)	
REVLON PASTE POLISH (Revlon)	Wax Phthalate ester Lecithin Covering agents
REVLON TOUCH & GLOW FACE POWDER & MAKE-UP BASE (Revlon)	
REX AFTER SHAVE LOTION (Rex Home)	
REXALL ACID-DYSPEPSIA MIXTURE (Rexall)	Bismuth subcarbonate Magnesium carbonate Tincture capsicum Tincture cardamom compound
REXALL ANTIHISTA-MINE TABLETS (Rexall)	Pyrilamine maleate* 25 mg.

Name & Use Manufacturer	Ingredients
REXALL AQUEOUS NOSE DROPS (Rexall)	Chlorbutanol 1-3/5 gr./fl. oz. Ephedrine sulfate* Camphor* Menthol Oil of thyme Syn. oil of wintergreen* Isotonic salt solution base
REXALL BLACKBERRY & GINGER EXTRACTS Carminative (Rexall)	Alcohol 12% Flu. ext. blackberry bark Tincture of ginger Oil cinnamon Oil cloves Oil allspice Oil nutmeg
REXALL CARBOLIC SALVE Dressing for wounds (Rexall)	Carbolic acid* Petrolatum
REXALL CHERRY BARK COUGH SYRUP (Rexall)	Extractives of wild cherry bark Senega Blood root Ipecac Acetic acid
REXALL CHILDREN'S COUGH SYRUP (Rexall)	Alcohol 4% Fluid ext. of ipecac Ext. of wild cherry Tolu Camphor Benzoic acid Anethol Sugar Glycerin
REXALL COLDSORE LOTION (Rexall)	Benzoin Camphor* Menthol Carbolic acid* Alcohol* 90%/v
REXALL CORN SOLVENT Keratolytic (Rexall)	Alcohol* 22% Ether* 340 m./fl. oz. Pyroxylin Salicylic acid*
REXALL COUGH SYRUP FOR TINY TOTS (Rexall)	Ammonium bromide 1 gr./tsp. Extractives of ipecac Senega Wild cherry bark Ammonium chloride
REXALL DIURETIC COMPOUND For urinary tract irritation (Rexall)	Alcohol 10% Buchu Uva ursi Potassium nitrate* Cascara sagrada Salicylic acid* Ginger Glycerin
REXALL DIURETIC PILLS (Rexall)	Extracts of buchu Uva ursi Cascara sagrada Potassium nitrate* Podophyllin Oil juniper berries* Balsam fir*
REXALL EAR WAX DROPS (Rexall)	Carbolic acid* Urea Potassium chloride * Glycerin

*Consult Sec. II., Ingredients Index. This ingredient may be responsible for major toxic effects if poisonous amounts of this product are ingested.

Name & Use Manufacturer	Ingredients		Name & Use Manufacturer	Ingredients	
REXALL EYE DROPS (Rexall)	Camphor Boric acid Zinc sulfate		REXALL SUNBURN CREAM (Rexall)	Zinc oxide Camphor* Ethylaminobenzoate Carbolic acid* Polyvinyl alcohol Alcohol	1.7% 2.5%
REXALL FOOT BALM (Rexall)	Aqua ammonia Cottonseed oil Soap Gum arabic Beeswax Spermaceti Oil of spike lavender		REXALL THROAT GARGLE (Rexall)	Tannic acid* Potassium chlorate* Carbolic acid* Glycerin	
REXALL HYGIENIC POWDER Douche, gargle, spray (Rexall)	Borax* Boric acid* Bicarbonate of soda Thymol* Menthol Synthetic oil of wintergreen* Eucalyptol *		REXALL TRIPLE ACTION COUGH SYRUP D 417 (Rexall)	Alcohol Chloroform Salicylamide* Amm. chloride Menthol * Benzalkonium chloride * Propylene glycol Invert sugar	16% 0.9 m. fl. oz.
REXALL LIQUID CHEST RUB (Rexall)	Spirits turpentine* Camphor* Menthol Oil eucalyptus* Oil pine* Oil cloves*		REX AMERICAN BALM LOTION (Rex Home)		
REXALL MOUTH- WASH WITH CHLOROPHYLL (Rexall)	Alcohol 20% Chlorophyll Polyoxyethylene sorbitan mono-oleate Sodium citrate Menthol Oil of spearmint Oil of peppermint		REX ANT BAIT Insecticide (Rex Res.)	Thallium sulfate*	1.3%
REXALL NASAL DROPS WITH EPHEDRINE (Rexall)	Ephedrine* alkaloid Eucalyptol* Menthol * Carbolic acid* Safrol White mineral oil		REX BITTERS Cathartic (Rex Bitters)	Alcohol Cascara sagrada Senna	21%/v
REXALL PENETRAT- ING LINIMENT (Rexall)	Oleoresin of capsicum Oil of camphor* Spirits of turpentine* Refined kerosene*		REX BRILLIANTINE (Rex Home) REX DYES & SHINES SHOE POLISH (Rex Home)		
REXALL PIN-WORM RELIEF TABLETS (Rexall)	Each enteric-coated tablet: Gentian violet* 1/2 gr.		REXEL AIR CLEANERS Deodorant (Reliable Chem.)	Paradichlorobenzene*	100%
REXALL POISON IVY & OAK LOTION (Rexall)	Alcohol* 80% Grindelia resin 7-1/2%		REX FLAT ALKYD PAINT (Odorless Type) (Chi-Namel)	Titanium dioxide Calcium carbonate Aluminum silicate Soya alkyd resin Odorless mineral spirits* Drier	27.0% 33.0% 3.1% 11.3% 24.6% 1.0%
REXALL REXILLANA Antitussive (Rexall)	Alcohol 6% Fl. ext. of senega Tartar emetic* Euphorbia pilulifera Wild lettuce Menthol Cocillana		REX FLAT WALL PAINT (Chi-Namel)	Titanium calcium Calcium carbonate Aluminum silicate Heat-processed linseed oil Varnish Drier Mineral spirits*	46.3% 13.0% 2.8% 8.9% 3.3% 1.8% 23.9%
REXALL REX-RUB Counter- irritant (Rexall)	Alcohol* 25% Menthol Chlorthymol* Synthetic oil of wintergreen* Oils of chenopodium* American wormwood and tansy Acetone *		REX HEEL & SOLE ENAMEL (Rex Home)		
REXALL SKIN ANTISEPTIC (Rexall)	Thimerosal tincture* Alcohol* 47%		REX HUNTERS ANTIHISTA- MINE DOG TABLETS (Rex Hunters)	Pyrilamine maleate*	25 mg.

---

*Consult Sec. II., Ingredients Index. This ingredient may be responsible for major toxic effects if poisonous amounts of this product are ingested.

Name & Use Manufacturer	Ingredients		Name & Use Manufacturer	Ingredients	
REX HUNTERS ANTISEPTIC EYE LOTION FOR DOGS For eye, skin irritations (Rex Hunters)	Caprokol (hexylresorcinol S & D) 1-1000 solution		REXINE LIQUID HAND SOAP (Rexine)	Vegetable oil Caustic potash	
REX HUNTERS EAR MANGE LOTION FOR DOGS (Rex Hunters)	Glycerol 99% Phenol 1%		REXIT PAINT & VARNISH REMOVER (Berry Bros.)		
REX HUNTERS LAXATIVE TABLETS Veterinary (Rex Hunters)	Extract cascara sagrada		REX LIQUID CLEANER (Bonewitz)	Gluconic acid Glycolic acid Wetting agent	
			REX OIL LEATHER DYE (Rex Home)		
REX HUNTERS MANGE OINTMENT Veterinary (Rex Hunters)	Sulfur 12.28% Wool fat 8.91 % White wax 7.73 % White petrolatum 52.90% Balsam Peru 9.09 % Castor oil 9.09 %		REX OIL STAIN REMOVER (Hatch, H.)		
REX HUNTERS OINTMENT FOR DOGS For skin irritations (veterinary) (Rex Hunters)	Mercury succinimide* 0.2 gr. Wool fat White wax White petroleum Menthol* Camphor* Methyl salicylate*		REX PAINT & VARNISH REMOVER (La Place)		
			REX PASTE, SUNSEAL PASTE For wall-papering (Patent)	Processed wheat and corn materials Sodium fluosilicate trace Sodium pentachlorophenate trace	
REX HUNTERS PINE OIL DIS-INFECTANT (Rex Hunters)	Distilled pine oil* 80% Soap 10%		REX PINE CLEANER (Huntington)		
REX HUNTERS SPECIAL TAPEWORM TABLETS Veterinary (Rex Hunters)	Arecoline hydrobromide* 10%		REX ROACH POWDER (Rex Res.)	Boric acid* 27% Piperonyl cyclonene 1% Pyrethrins 0.15%	
REX HUNTERS SULFURATED FLEA POWDER (Rex Hunters)	Rotenone 1% Other derris resins 2% Pyrethrins 0.18% Sulfur 10%		REXSAN DISINFECT-ANT (Rexair Div.)	Soap Sodium 4-chloro-2-phenyl phenate* Sodium-6-chloro-2-phenyl phenate* Perfume	
REX HUNTERS WORM CAPSULES Veterinary (Rex Hunters)	C.P. tetrachloroethylene* 100%		REX SELTZER Analgesic (Rexall)	Sodium salt of aspirin* Bicarbonate of soda Citric acid	
REXIDE MOTH PROOFER Repellent (Rexair Div.)	Sodium silicofluoride 0.6%		REX SHOE DRESSING & SHOE POLISH (Rex Home)		
REXILLANA Antitussive (Rexall)	Alcohol 6% Fl. ext. of senega Tartar emetic* Euphorbia pilulifera Wild lettuce Mehtnol* Cocillana		REX SURFACE INSECTICIDE (Rex Res.)	DDT* 5%	
			REX TABLETS (White Tablets) (Rexall)	Dried oxgall	
REXIMATOR AA INSECTI-CIDE & FLY SPRAY (Rexair Div.)	Petroleum hydrocarbons Methylated aromatic petroleum deriv.* Dichloro diphenyl trichloro-ethane* Sesamin Pyrethrins		REX WALL PAPER REMOVER (Patent)	Tergitol (wetting agent) Butyl Cellosolve*	
			REX WALL SIZE (Patent)	Dextrine Animal glue Bicarbonate of soda Aluminum sulfate Bentonite	
REXINE CLEANING SOAP (Rexine)	Vegetable oil Caustic soda				

*Consult Sec. II., Ingredients Index. This ingredient may be responsible for major toxic effects if poisonous amounts of this product are ingested.

Name & Use Manufacturer	Ingredients		Name & Use Manufacturer	Ingredients	
REX WATERLESS HAND CLEANER (Bonewitz)	Potash base soap Deodorized kerosene*		RHEUMANON F-E-S CAPSULES Analgesic, antitussive (Rheumanon)	Potassium iodide Gum guaiac Aspirin*	
REZ Wood sealers, primers (Monsanto)	Synthetic resin Mineral spirits*		RHEUM REM (Steinmann's) For colds (Steinmann)	Potassium iodide Magnesium sulfate F.E. senna Colchicum Oil of peppermint	
REZIL-CLEAN, REZIL-SHINE Floor cleaner, wax (Rezilite)			RHINALGAN Nasal de- congestant (Doho)	Desoxyephedrine Antipyrine Isotonic aqueous solution with laurylamine saccharinate Methyl rosaniline chloride DOHO glycerol	0.22% 0.28% 0.02% 0.001% 2%
REZI-WAX FLOOR WAX (Standard Ind.)					
REZ WOOD SEALER & PRIMER (Aetna)			R-H 118 LIQUID Insecticide (Reasor-Hill)	Octalene* (see aldrin) DDT Oil	18.75% 22.5% 48.75%
R F CANKER DROPS (Red Feather)	Glycerin Mercresin* Acetone* Alcohol Phenol	 8% 1%	RHODE'S ANTISEPTIC SHAMPOO & HAIR TONIC (Cline)		
R-G-F INK & STAIN REMOVER (Riverside)			RHODE'S EMBROCA- TION (Cline)		
R-H 3-5-40 Insecticide (Reasor-Hill)	BHC* DDT* Sulfur*	3% 5% 40%	RHOTHANE AD-50 Insecticide (Rohm & Haas)	TDE* (dichloro diphenyl dichloroethane)	 50%
R-H-B ARSENICAL WEED KILLER Herbicide (Bogle)	Sodium arsenite*	43.17%	RHOTHANE D-3 Insecticide (Rohm & Haas)	TDE* (dichloro diphenyl dichloroethane)	 100%
R-H-B CHLORATE WEED KILLER Herbicide (Bogle)	Sodium chlorate* Calcium chloride	26.18% 14.17%	25% RHOTHANE EMULSION CONC. Insecticide (Rohm & Haas)	TDE (dichloro diphenyl dichloroethane) Aromatic petroleum deriv. solvent* and emulsifier	 25% 75%
R-H-B TCA- ARSENITE WEED KILLER Herbicide (Bogle)	Sodium arsenite* Sodium trichloroacetate	23.14% 5.88%	RHOTHANE R-30 SOLUTION Insecticide (Rohm & Haas)	TDE tech. Aromatic petroleum deriv. solvent*	2.5 lb./gal.
R-H-B TCA- CHLORATE WEED KILLER Herbicide (Bogle)	Sodium chlorate* Sodium trichloroacetate	19.99% 6.66%	RHOTHANE WP-50 (Rohm & Haas)	TDE*	50%
			R-H TOXAPHENE Insecticide (Reasor-Hill)	Toxaphene*	40%
R-H 118 DUST Insecticide (Reasor-Hill)	Octalene* (see aldrin) DDT* Gamma BHC Other isomers	2.5% 5% 0.5% 3.75%	R-H 20% TOXAPHENE DUST Insecticide (Reasor-Hill)	Toxaphene*	20%
R-H 40% EMULSIFI- ABLE CHLORDANE Insecticide (Reasor-Hill)	Chlordane*	40%	RHUBARB & PANCREATIN COMPOUND, ALKALINE (Lilly)	Each 100 cc.: Rhubarb Pancreatin Hydrastis Potassium bicarbonate Alcohol	 3.9 gm. 0.875 gm. 2 gm. 3.9 gm. 20%

---

*Consult Sec. II., Ingredients Index. This ingredient may be responsible for major toxic effects if poisonous amounts of this product are ingested.

Name & Use Manufacturer	Ingredients		Name & Use Manufacturer	Ingredients	
RHULICREAM For skin irritations (Lederle)	Zirconium oxide Benzocaine Menthol Camphor Isopropyl alcohol Methylparaben Propylparaben	1.00% 1.00% 0.70% 0.30% 8.80% 0.08% 0.02%	RICHARD ANGLIN DEODORANT POWDER, HAIR TONIC & SCALP PREPARATION (Anglin)		
RHULITOL For skin irritation due to ivy, oak, sumac poisoning (Lederle)	Tannic acid U.S.P. Chlorobutanol (chloral deriv.) Phenol Camphor Ammonium alum Isopropyl alcohol*	5% 1% 0.4% 39.5% w/v	RICHARD HUDNUT DRY-STIK, MENTHOL CREAM, SHAMPOO, HAIR & SCALP PREPARATION, PERFECTION-IST LIP BRUSH & R.S.U.P. TALCUM (Hudnut, R.)		
RHUMA-SAL Analgesic (Western Pharm.)	Sodium salicylate* Aspirin*	6 gr. 6 gr.			
RHUSTOXYLLIN For ivy poisoning, external (Kip)	Choral hydrate* Menthol Aromatics Alcohol Resinous plastic base	5% 1% q.s. 19%	RICHARD HUDNUT HAND LOTION (Hudnut, R.)		
RHU-MENTA Antacid, carminative, tonic (Whorton)	Rhubarb Cinnamon Peppermint Sodium bicarbonate Potassium bicarbonate Paw paw enzymes Calcium hydroxide to saturation Alcohol	20 gr. 20 gr. 10 gr. 12 gr. 12 gr. 1/2 gr. 12-1/2%/v	RICHARD HUDNUT LIPSTICK, FACE CREAM, BUBBLE BATHS & PERMANENT SOLUTION (Hudnut, R.)		
RHUTOCAINE (Lefcourt)	Tannic acid* Benzocaine Alcohol*		RICHARD HUDNUT PERFUMES, COLOGNES & ESSENCES (Hudnut, R.)		
RHUWIL For poison ivy, oak (Dermateen)	Metadihydroxy benzene* Grindelia Alcohol*	70%			
R-H WEED RHAP Herbicide (Reasor-Hill)	Butyl ester of 2, 4-D*	40%	RICHFIELD WEED-KILLER A, SELECTIVE WEED-KILLER NO. 1 Herbicides (Richfield)	Petroleum hydrocarbons*	
R-H 50% WETTABLE DDT Insecticide (Reasor-Hill)	DDT*	50%			
RIASOL (Shield Labs.)	Mercury* Soaps Carbolic acid Cresol	0.45% 0.5% 0.75%	RICHTER'S PAIN EXPELLER (Richter)	Alcohol* Capsicum Ammonia Camphor* Soap Essential oils*	49%
RIATABS Analgesic, antispasmodic (Halperin)	Each tablet: Salicylamides* Caffeine Ephedrine sulfate Magnesium gluconate Acetophenetidin	 1/8 gr. 1/2 gr.	RICHTER'S 3X-B Fungicide (medical) (Richter)	Alcohol* Salicylic acid* Benzoic acid*	75%
RICE R-3 READY RAT RIDDER (Rice Chem.)			RID-A-PAIN TABLETS Analgesic (Pfeiffer)	Aspirin* Phenacetin* Caffeine	3-1/2 gr. 2-1/2 gr. 1/2 gr.
RICHARD ANGLIN CORN REMEDY, WART RE-MOVER, KARAFUT POWDER & LINIMENT (Anglin)			RID DEODORANT CREAM (Lustray)		

*Consult Sec. II., Ingredients Index. This ingredient may be responsible for major toxic effects if poisonous amounts of this product are ingested.

Name & Use Manufacturer	Ingredients		Name & Use Manufacturer	Ingredients	
DR. RIDDO'S PILE OINTMENT (Improved) (Vi-Gien)	Petrolatum Lanolin Paraffin Ammonium alum Menthol Carbolic acid* U.S. certified color		RID-U Rodenticide (Smith, H. V.)	Dichloro diphenyl tri-chloroethane*	50%
RIDEX Parasiticide (Sani-Pine)	Cyanyl acetate* Methyl chavicol		RID-U BRAND INSECTICIDE CONTAINING PYRENONE INSECTICIDE (Smith, H. V.)	Petroleum distillate* Tech. piperonyl butoxide Pyrethrins	
RID-ITCH (Antiseptic) Fungicide (medical) (Thomas & Thompson)	Alcohol* Glycerin Salicylic acid* Resorcinol* Chlorothymol* Benzoic acid Biebrich scarlet red (medicinal) Boric acid*	65%	RID-U BRAND RAT KILLER (Smith, H. V.)	Warfarin (3 (a-acetonylbenzyl)-4-hydroxycoumarin)	0.025%
			RID-U BRAND RAT & MICE KILLER (Contains Pival) (Smith, H. V.)	1, 2-Pivalyl-1, 3-indandione	0.025%
RIDLEW'S F-H POWDER Feminine hygiene powder (Legendre's)	Pwd. zinc sulfate * Pwd. calamine prep. Phenol Pwd. sod. bicarb.	4% 0.4% 0.2% q.s.	RID-U WATER MISCIBLE CONCEN-TRATE Insecticide (Smith, H. V.)	Tech. piperonyl butoxide Pyrethrins Petroleum distillate*	11.8% 1.2% 72.2%
RID-O-MOTH (Moth Balls, Moth Flakes) (Standard Chlor.)	Naphthalene*	100%	RID-ZIT FOR DANDRUFF (Odell)		
RID-O-MOTH PARADI-CHLORO-BENZENE PKGS. Insecticide (Standard Chlor.)	Paradichlorobenzene*	100%	RIDZUM ROACH & ANT KILLER Insecticide (Black Panther)	Tech. chlordane Pyrethrins	2.00% 0.018%
RID-O-SOOT SOOT DESTROYER (Baker's)			RIE & NIE Rubber cement (Durkee)		
RID ROACH SPRAY Insecticide (Green Line)	Mineral oil Tech. piperonyl butoxide Pyrethrins		RIE NIE ENAMELS, PAINTS (Durkee)		
RIDSECT Insecticide (Klinzmoth)	DDT* Isobornyl thiocyanoacetate Oil*	5% 2% 93%	RIES' B.U.B. OINTMENT (Ries)	Raw linseed oil Resin Mutton tallow Natural beeswax Petrolatum Phenol	1%
RIDSECT AEROSOL Insecticide (Chipman, Ltd.)	DDT Piperonyl butoxide Pyrethrins Beta-butoxy-beta'-thiocyano diethyl ether Inert ingredients*	2.0% 0.25% 0.1% 1.0%	RIES' COLD SORE MEDI-CATION For chapped lips (Ries)	Sodium borate* Benzoic acid Salicylic acid*	
RIDSECT POWDER Insecticide (Klinzmoth)	DDT* Pyrethrins Sesame oil extractives Oil	10% 0.80% 0.30% 3%	RIES' FOOT RELIEF POWDER (Ries)	Boric acid* Zinc oxide Salicylic acid* Calcium carbonate Menthol Alum * Talc	
RIDSECT ROACH KILLER (Klinzmoth)	Petroleum distillate* Beta thiocyano ethyl esters of aliphatic acids (containing 10-18 carbon atoms) Chlordane tech.* Beta-butoxy-beta'-thiocyano diethyl ether*		RIES' OINTMENT Fungicide (medical) (Ries)	Salicylic acid* Benzoic acid* Sodium borate*	
RIDSMEL PAINT DEODORANT (Holley)			RIG Rust preventive (Rig)	Polarized emulsifying agents Hydrocarbons *	

---

*Consult Sec. II., Ingredients Index. This ingredient may be responsible for major toxic effects if poisonous amounts of this product are ingested.

Name & Use Manufacturer	Ingredients
RIGA-T Food supplement, tonic (Oliver's S-O)	Each fl. oz.: Iron (ferric) citrochloride Strychnine phosphate 1/80 gr. Vitamin B (thiamine hydrochloride) 2.9 mg. Alcohol 6%
RIGIDTEST PROTECTIVE BALM (Rigidtest)	Stearic acid Diglycol stearate Lanolin Petrolatum Ceresin Propylene glycol Carbitol Triethanolamine Methyl cellulose Zinborsal (zincborodisalicylate decahydrate with boric acid)
RIGOLADE BATH OIL (Monteil)	Perfume oils Lauric, myristic and palmitic acid alkyl esters
RIGOLADE COLOGNE (Monteil)	Perfume oil* less than 10% Specially denatured alcohol * (ethanol) Diethyl phthalate
RIGOLADE DUSTING POWDER (Monteil)	Talc Perfume oil
RIGOLADE EAU CON- CENTREE (Monteil)	Perfume oil* less than 10% Ethyl alcohol *
RIGOLADE PERFUME (Monteil)	Perfume oils* 15-30% Ethyl alcohol*
RIK RAK CLEANSER (Newport)	Silica Carbonates Sterichlor* (see hypochlorite) Perfume
RIMACO ENAMELS (Rinshed- Mason)	
RIMMEL VERBENA WATER (Rimmel)	
RING GO PORCELAIN BLEACH (United Chem.)	
RINGRINE Fungicide (medical) (Flanagan's)	Benzoic acid Salicylic acid * Oil cassia* Resorcinol monoacetate* Alcoholic-acetone* solution
RING-ROUT Fungicide (medical) (Ring-Rout)	Salicylic acid* Alcohol* 81.24% Storax Benzoin Tolu balsam Aloe * Acetone *
RINSE AWAY DANDRUFF (Skan)	Lauryl isoquinolinium bromide* Aklyl dimethyl benzyl ammonium chloride*
RINSO BLUE Detergent (Lever)	Sodium alkaryl sulfonate * Sodium polyphosphates* Fatty amide Sodium sulfate Silicate Perfume Optical dye
RIPOLIN ENAMELS (Campbell Paint)	
RIPOLIN QUICK DRY- ING PAINT & UNDERCOAT (Glidden Co.)	
RIP-ZIT LIQUID PAINT & VARNISH REMOVER (Olo)	
RISE SHAVING CREAM (Carter Prod.)	Soap Freon
RISING SUN STOVE POLISH (Prescott)	
RISPOL Respiratory decongestant (veterinary, avian) (Beebe)	Oil of eucalyptus* Guaiacol* Formalin * Menthol* Pine oil* Methyl salicylate* Oleic acid
RISTAT Stimulant, tonic (veterinary) (Salsbury's)	3-Nitro-4-hydroxyphenylarsonic acid* 400 mg./tablet
RIT Clothes dye (Rit Prods.)	
RITE-A-WAY INK (Ruxton)	
RITE-GLO DANDRUFF REMOVER (Bee Gee)	Alkyl dimethyl benzyl ammonium chloride*
RITE-GLO HENNA Hair rinse (Bee Gee)	
RITE-GLO LANOLIN AND LIQUID LANOLIN COMPOUNDS Hair, scalp preparations (Bee Gee)	Lanolin Other oils
RITEPOINT LIGHTER FLUID (Ritepointe)	

*Consult Sec. II., Ingredients Index. This ingredient may be responsible for major toxic effects if poisonous amounts of this product are ingested.

- 896 -

Name & Use Manufacturer	Ingredients		Name & Use Manufacturer	Ingredients	
RITE TONE PAINT (Pysol)			ROACHNOX Insecticide (Wisconsin Pharm.)	DDT* Pyrethrins Sesame oil extractives Petroleum hydrocarbons	10.00% 0.08% 0.30% 3.00%
RITZ DINER FOR MICE ONLY Rodenticide (Dixon-Davis)			ROACH-O BLITZ (Surface Spray) Insecticide (Blitz)	Chlordane DDT Methylated naphthalene* Petroleum distillate*	2.0% 0.5% 1.25% 36.25%
RITZ FLOOR WAX (Tumbler)			ROACHPAINT Insecticide (Bonide)	Tech. chlordane Petroleum distillate*	4% 96%
RIVAL CLEANER (Chem. Mfg. & Dist.)			ROACH POWDER WITH DDT DUST Insecticide (Allied Drug)	DDT* Pyrethrins Sesame oil extractives Petroleum hydrocarbons	10.00% 0.08% 0.30% 3.00%
R.I.W. PAINTS For damp-proofing (Toch)			ROACH SALT Insecticide (Uncle Sam)	Sodium fluoride*	90%
RIZ (Holcomb)	Santophen (sodium ortho-benzyl-parachlorophenol)*		ROACHSAULT Insecticide (Barrett Chem.)	DDT* Chlordane*	10% 5%
R-M PAINTS, ENAMELS & AUTOMOTIVE LACQUERS (Rinshed-Mason)			ROACH-X Insecticide (Davis, O. D.)	Sodium fluosilicate*	78%
R-MIR-DEK Non-slip floor coating (Miracle)			ROANT DUST Insecticide (Laconia)	Chlordane	2%
ROACH BATE Insecticide (Agkem)	Sodium borate*		ROB-A-SAN Antacid (Helm Co.)	Magnesium trisilicate Calcium carbonate Bismuth subcarbonate Saccharin	
ROACH CAFE Insecticide (Agkem)	Hydrogen borate*	50%	ROBBINS' ECONOMY SPRAY Insecticide (Robbins, G.)	DDT* Inert ingredients*	5%
ROACH CAFE Insecticide (Agkem)	Sodium borate*		ROBBINS' FLY SPRAY Insecticide (Robbins, G.)	Petroleum distillate* 2-Butoxy ethanol n-Octyl sulfoxide of isosafrole (sulfoxide) Pyrethrins Compounds related to sulfoxide	
ROACH CHEK Insecticide (Chek)					
ROACH DOOM Insecticide (Murray, E.)	Sodium fluoride*	min. 90%	ROBBINS' ROACH POWDER Insecticide (Robbins, G.)	Wheat flour Sugar Sodium chloride Sodium sulfate Other silicious matter Pyrethrum powder other than pyrethins	15.00% 5.00% 0.30% 2.00% 1.20% 14.925%
ROACHES' LAST MEAL (Maas, A.G.)	Sodium fluoride *	75%			
ROACHEX Insecticide (Florida Chem.)	Chlordane Piperonyl butoxide Allethrin Petroleum hydrocarbons*	2.5%	ROBBINS' STAIN REMOVER (Robbins, G.)		
ROACHINET ROACH POWDER (Bonrose)			ROBBINS' 2% TECHNICAL CHLORDANE Insecticide (Robbins, G.)	Tech. chlordane	2%
ROACHKILL INSECT SPRAY Insecticide (Uncle Sam)	Chlordane*		ROBBINS' VAPOR SPRAY Insecticide (Robbins, G.)	Petroleum distillate* 2-Butoxy ethanol n-Octyl sulfoxide of isosafrole (sulfoxide) Pyrethrins Compounds related to sulfoxide	

*Consult Sec. II., Ingredients Index. This ingredient may be responsible for major toxic effects if poisonous amounts of this product are ingested.

- 897 -

Name & Use Manufacturer	Ingredients		Name & Use Manufacturer	Ingredients	
ROBENE Massaging liniment (Earle)	Alcohol* Chloroform* Menthol Camphor* Witch hazel Methyl salicylate* Oil wormwood Oil sassafras *	68% 53 m./oz.	DR. DAVID ROBERTS' FOOT ROT TREATMENT Veterinary (Roberts, Dr. D.)	Crude phenols* Saponified cresylic solution* Oil of linseed	11-3/4% q.s.
DR. DAVID ROBERTS' ABSORBENT (Roberts, Dr. D.)	Alcohol Iodide of mercury* Iodide of potassium Tinct. of iodine Acetic acid	45% 5%	DR. DAVID ROBERTS' HOG MANGE OIL (veterinary) (Roberts, Dr. D.)	Gamma isomer of benzene hexachloride Other isomers of benzene hexachloride Petroleum hydrocarbons*	0.25% 0.443% 99.307%
DR. DAVID ROBERTS' CALF MEDICINE For simple scours and loose bowels (veterinary) (Roberts, Dr. D.)	Bismuth subnitrate Zinc phenolsulfonate* Tannic acid * White oak bark Chalk Anise Ginger root Tobacco dust * Ground bread crumbs		DR. DAVID ROBERTS' HOG SPRAY (Roberts, Dr. D.)	Cresol* Creosote * Eucalyptus oil* Sassafras oil* Formaldehyde* Paraffin oil	
DR. DAVID. ROBERTS' CAUSTIC DEHORNING PASTE Horn treatment (veterinary) (Dr. D. Roberts)	Potassium hydroxide* Estrol absorption base	58% 10%	DR. DAVID ROBERTS' HOOF OIL PRESCRIP- TION NO. 82 Veterinary (Roberts, Dr. D.)	Turpentine* Oil tar* Paraffin oil Color	
DR. DAVID ROBERTS' DISINFECT- ANT FOR LIVESTOCK (Roberts, Dr. D.)	Phenols*		ROBERTS' MOSQUITO REPELLENT CREAM (B & B Toil.)		
ROBERTS' ESTROGENIC HAND-ELBOW- LEG HORMONE CREME LOTION (Roberts'Labs.) Labs.)	Propylene glycol monostearate Stearic acid Oleic acid Triethanolamine Glycerin Chemosol ester of para hydroxybenzoic acid Natural estrogenic substance from gravid mares' urine		DR. DAVID ROBERTS' POULTRY SPRAY (Roberts, Dr. D.)	Cresol* Dreosote Formaldehyde* Eucalyptus oil* Sassafras oil* Paraffin oil	
ROBERTS' ESTROGENIC HORMONE CREAM (Roberts Labs.)	Yellow beeswax Spermaceti Glyceryl monostearate Anhydrous lanolin Borax Chemosol ester of para hydroxybenzoic acid Natural estrogenic substance from gravid mares' urine in sesame oil		DR. DAVID ROBERTS' SKIN OINTMENT Veterinary (Roberts, Dr. D.)	Merthiolate* Sulfur Carbolic acid Paraffin wax Petrolatum	1%
			DR. DAVID ROBERTS' SOOTHING PASTE Antitussive (veterinary) (Roberts, Dr. D.)	Cresol*comp. U.S.P. Eucalyptus oil * Glucose Sassafras oil *	70%
DR. DAVID ROBERTS' EYE LOTION Veterinary (Roberts, Dr. D.)	Zinc sulfate * Boric acid* Boiled water Pyoktannin		DR. DAVID ROBERTS' STRONG BLISTER Veterinary (Roberts, Dr. D.)	Red iodide of mercury* Petrolatum Paraffin wax	
DR. DAVID ROBERTS' FLY-OIL Insecticide (Roberts, Dr. D.)	Petroleum distillate* Pine oil* Beta-butoxy-beta' thiocyano diethyl ether* n-Octyl bicycloheptene dicarboximide Technical methoxychlor Allethrin		DR. DAVID ROBERTS' WHITE LINIMENT Veterinary (Roberts, Dr. D.)	Turpentine* Muriate of ammonia Castile soap	

---

*Consult Sec. II., Ingredients Index. This ingredient may be responsible for major toxic effects if poisonous amounts of this product are ingested.

Name & Use Manufacturer	Ingredients		Name & Use Manufacturer	Ingredients	
ROBESON FLAME-RESISTANT Flameproofing (Robeson)			ROCKLAND PENTA-PENN Wood preservative (Rockland Chem.)	Pentachlorophenol* Petroleum hydrocarbons*	5.20% 94.80%
ROBOT CLEANSER POWDER (Silver Suds)			ROCKLAND RID-O-WEED Herbicide (Rockland Chem.)	Mixed isopropyl and di-isopropanol amine salts of 2, 4-dichlorophenoxyacetic acid*	56%
ROBY'S FURNITURE POLISHES & FINISHES (Nat'l Polish)			ROCKLAND TOXAPHENE EM-6 Insecticide (Rockland Chem.)	Toxaphene* Petroleum distillate	60% 29%
ROCCAL BRAND SANITIZING AGENT (Wintrop)	Quaternary ammonium* compounds		ROCKLAND WEED KILLER (Rockland Chem.)	Sodium arsenite*	34.7%
ROCHESTER BEST BLEACH (Rochester Best)	Sodium hypochlorite*		ROCKSPAR (Glidden Co.)		
ROCHESTER LABS. SCALP LOTION FORMULA 35 (Rochester Labs.)	Alcohol Glycerin		ROCK-SPAR VARNISH (Glidden Co.)		
ROCHESTER LABS. SCALP OIL FORMULA 35 (Rochester Labs.)	Mineral oils Parawax Beeswax Petrolatum Lanolin Borax		ROCKWELL'S ROACH RID Insecticide (Private Brands)	Sodium fluoride* Sodium silicofluoride* Pyrethrin DDT*	
ROCHESTER LABS. SHAMPOO FORMULA 35 (Rochester Labs.)	Liquid soap		ROCKWELL'S SURE KILL HOUSEHOLD SPRAY Insecticide (Private Brands)	Chlordane* Lethane 384* Pyrenone 20 new Perfume Base oil	
ROCKCOTE PAINT & ENAMELS (Rockford)			ROCKY MOUNTAIN LINIMENT (Chandler)		
ROCK HARD FLOOR WAX (Golden Star)			ROCKY MOUNTAIN TEA Laxative (Myers Labs.)	Senna Sassafras Elder flowers Fennel Liver-wort Dandelion Mandrake	
ROCKLAND BRUSH KILLER (Rockland Chem.)	2, 4-Dichloro phenoxy acetic acid polyethylene glycol mono-ester 200* 36.40% 2, 4, 5-Trichloro phenoxy acetic acid polyethylene glycol mono-ester 300* 41.90% Inert ingredients: 21.70%		RO-CON Food supplement, tonic (veterinary, avian) (Whitmoyer)	Vitamin B12 Copper sulfate* Nux vomica* Gentian Anise Trace minerals Brewers' dried yeast	
ROCKLAND HOUSEHOLD AEROSOL Insecticide (Rockland Chem.)	Pyrethrins 0.45% Tech. piperonyl butoxide 1.125% Refined petroleum distillate * 13.425% Propellent 85.000%		RO-COP Insecticide (Doggett-Pfeil)	Rotenone Copper*	0.75% 5%
ROCKLAND MALATHION 50 Insecticide (Rockland Chem.)	Malathion* 57% Xylene* 33%		RO CROLITE ACID & ALKALI RESISTANT COATINGS Paint (Rowe)		

*Consult Sec. II., Ingredients Index. This ingredient may be responsible for major toxic effects if poisonous amounts of this product are ingested.

Name & Use Manufacturer	Ingredients	
RODALON 10% Fungicide (Fairfield)	Alkyl dimethyl benzyl ammonium chlorides*	10%
RODALON 50% Fungicide (Fairfield)	Alkyl dimethyl benzyl ammonium chlorides*	50%
RODALON 100% Disinfectant (Fairfield)	Alkyl dimethyl benzyl ammonium chloride*	
RODASUDS Detergent (Fairfield)		
RODENE Rodenticide (Uncle Sam)	Red squill *	90%
RODENTICIDE MICE-KILLER (Nat'l Rodent.)	Strychnine*	0.5%
RODENT KIL Rodenticide (Peters)	Warfarin (3-(a-acetonylbenzyl)- 4-hydroxycoumarin)	0.025
RODENT-RID Rodenticide (Miller Chem.)	Warfarin (3-(a-acetonylbenzyl)- 4-hydroxycoumarin)	0.025%
RODENT SLAYER Rodenticide (Slayer)	Red squill powder*	10%
RODEX Rodenticide (Am. Liquid)	Warfarin (3-(a-acetonylbenzyl)- 4-hydroxycoumarin)	0.5%
RODINE Rodenticide (Penick)	Extractives of red squill*	51%
RODITE Rodenticide (West Disinf.)	Red squill*	
RODOLON Disinfectant (Fairfield)		
RODON X AUTO POLISH & FINISH RESTORER (Wellesley)		
DR. ROGERS' AL-U-TAN Antihemor- rhagic (Texas Pheno.)	Alum*(exsiccated) Tannic acid * Iron subsulfate Iodoform Compound solution of cresol	47% 16% 35% 1% 1%
DR. ROGERS' BAG SALVE NO. 1 For udder irritation (veterinary) (Texas Pheno.)	Oil eucalyptus* Oil turpentine* Carbolic acid* Camphor Oil thuja* Methyl salicylate* Menthol Inert ingred.	2% 8% 2% 1.5% 1% 2% 0.5% 83%
DR. ROGERS' BARN M6 SPRAY Insecticide (Texas Pheno.)	Xylene* DDT* Alkyl phenoxy polyethoxy ethanol	

Name & Use Manufacturer	Ingredients	
DR. ROGERS' BONE OIL Fly repellent protectant (Texas Pheno.)	Bone oil	95.00%
DR. ROGERS' B-P-C For intestinal irritation (veterinary) (Texas Pheno.)	Kaolin Bismuth subcarbonate Pectin	3.000% 1.047% 0.523%
DR. ROGERS' BRANDING FLUID (Texas Pheno.)	Coal tar* Barium sulfide tech* Caustic soda*	50.00% 16.50% 11.50%
DR. ROGERS' CAR-BI-ZENE WOOD PRESERVER Wood pre- servative (Texas Pheno.)	Coal tar hydrocarbons*	96.00%
DR. ROGERS' C-D DUST Insecticide (Texas Pheno.)	Tribasic copper sulfate* (copper in basic copper sulfate expressed as metallic) DDT*	6% 5%
DR. ROGERS' 74% CHLORDANE EMULSIFI- ABLE CONC. Insecticide (Texas Pheno.)	Tech. chlordane* Refined petroleum oils	74.00% 15.00%
DR. ROGERS' CHLOR-DUST Insecticide (Texas Pheno.)	Tech. chlordane*	10.00%
DR. ROGERS' CHLOR 40 EMULSIFI- ABLE CONC. Insecticide (Texas Pheno.)	Tech. chlordane* Refined petroleum oil	40.00% 51.00%
DR. ROGERS' CHLOR-SPRAY Insecticide (Texas Pheno.)	Tech. chlordane Xylene* Refined petroleum oils Iso-octyl phenoxy polyethanoxy ethanol	25% 25% 20% 3%
DR. ROGERS' 5% DDT SPRAY Insecticide (Texas Pheno.)	DDT* Xylene*	5.00% 15.00%
DR. ROGERS' EZ12 LINDANE CONC. Insecticide (Texas Pheno.)	Xylene* Refined petroleum oil Gamma isomer of benzene hexachloride (from lindane)	73.00% 10.00% 10.00%
DR. ROGERS' 50WP Insecticide (Texas Pheno.)	DDT*	50%
DR. ROGERS' FORMULA NO. 1029 Insecticide (Texas Pheno.)	Pyridine* Dibutyl phthalate	10.0% 13.5%

*Consult Sec. II., Ingredients Index. This ingredient may be responsible for major toxic effects if poisonous amounts of this product are ingested.

- 900 -

Name & Use Manufacturer	Ingredients	
DR. ROGERS' GEN-SUL Antiseptic powder (veterinary) (Texas Pheno.)	Gentian violet	0.20%
	Sulfanilamide*	20.00%
	Sulfathiazole	5.00%
	Boric acid*	55.00%
ROGERS GLUE (Glidden Co.)		
DR. ROGERS' 1% LINDANE DUST Insecticide (Texas Pheno.)	Gamma isomer of benzene hexachloride (from lindane)	1.00%
DR. ROGERS' 964 DIP FOR ANGORA GOATS Insecticide (Texas Pheno.)	Pine tar	
	Xylene*	
	Iso-octyl phenoxy polyethanoxy ethanol	
	DDT*	
DR. ROGERS' OX-WARB POWDER Insecticide (Texas Pheno.)	Rotenone *	1.75%
	Other extractable cube resins	3.06%
DR. ROGERS' PHENO-THIAZINE CATTLE DRENCH Anthelmintic (veterinary)	Phenothiazine *	30.98%
DR. ROGERS' PHENO-THIAZINE DRENCH Anthelmintic (veterinary) (Texas Pheno.)	Phenothiazine *	38.21%
DR. ROGERS' PHENO-THIAZINE POWDER Anthelmintic (veterinary) (Texas Pheno.)	Phenothiazine* N.F.	98.84%
DR. ROGERS' PINK EYE POWDER (Texas Pheno.)	Sulfanilamide*	
	Azosulfamide	
	Acriflavine*	
	Boracic acid*	
DR. ROGERS' PY-RO GENERAL GARDEN & VEG. DUST Insecticide (Texas Pheno.)	Rotenone	0.25%
	Other extractable cube resins	0.44%
	Tech. piperonyl cyclonene	0.50%
	Pyrethrins	0.05%
DR. ROGERS' Q-B DIS-INFECTANT Disinfectant, deodorant (Texas Pheno.)	Para-di-isobutyl phenoxy ethoxy dimethyl benzyl ammonium chloride*	10%
DR. ROGERS' ROOST PAINT Insecticide (Texas Pheno.)	Gamma isomer of benzene hexachloride	1.35%
	Other isomers of benzene hexachloride	2.40%
	Petroleum hydrocarbons*	71.25%
	Methylated naphthalene*	25.00%

Name & Use Manufacturer	Ingredients	
DR. ROGERS' SABADILLA 20% Insecticide (Texas Pheno.)	Alkaloids of sabadilla	0.8%
DR. ROGERS' SCARLET OIL Antiseptic, protectant (Texas Pheno.)	Phenol (carbolic acid)*	3.00%
	Wood turpentine	2.00%
	Pine oil distilled	2.00%
	Oil eucalyptus	1.00%
	Gum camphor	1.00%
	Scarlet red	0.25%
	Menthol	0.25%
	Thymol	0.25%
DR. ROGERS' SCREW-WORM SMEAR EQ-335 (Texas Pheno.)	Gamma isomer of benzene hexachloride (from lindane)*	3.00%
	Pine oil*	35.00%
DR. ROGERS' SCREW-WORM SMEAR FORMULA NO. 62 (Texas Pheno.)	Diphenylamine	35.00%
	Benzol*	35.00%
	Turkey red oil	8.00%
DR. ROGERS' SCREW-WORM SMEAR 215 (Texas Pheno.)	Benzol*	34.00%
	Diphenylamine	35.00%
DR. ROGERS' SPECIAL FORMULA Anthelmintic (veterinary) (Texas Pheno.)	Phenothiazine *	37.92%
	Lead arsenate*	0.72%
DR. ROGERS' STOCK DIP & DISINFECT-ANT Disinfectant, insecticide, deodorizer (Texas Pheno.)	Coal tar acids *	11%
	Coal tar hydrocarbons *	62%
	Soap	17%
DR. ROGERS' SUL-QUO-LIQUID For coccidiosis in chickens and turkeys (Texas Pheno.)	Solution of sodium sulfaquinoxaline*	
DR. ROGERS' TICK & FLEA POWDER FOR DOGS (Texas Pheno.)	Tech. chlordane*	5.00%
	Beta, beta dithiocyano diethyl ether	1.00%
DR. ROGERS' X25 EM Insecticide (Texas Pheno.)	Xylene*	
	DDT	25%
	Alkylated aryl polyether alcohol	
	Refined petroleum oil	
ROHM & HAAS DDT Insecticide (Rohm & Haas)	DDT tech.	100%
ROHM & HAAS DITHANE D-14 Fungicide (Rohm & Haas)	Nabam* (27% as hexahydrate)	19%

Name & Use Manufacturer	Ingredients		Name & Use Manufacturer	Ingredients	
ROHM & HAAS DITHANE Z-78 Fungicide (Rohm & Haas)	Zineb	65%	RONCOVITE DROPS Dietary supplement (Lloyd)	Each 0.6 cc.: Cobalt chloride Ferrous sulfate	40 mg. 75 mg.
ROHM & HAAS D-30 SOLUTION Insecticide (Rohm & Haas)	DDT*	2.5 lb./gal.	RONDELET PERFUME (De Grasse)		
ROHM & HAAS LETHANE 60 Insecticide (Rohm & Haas)	Beta thiocyano ethyl esters of aliphatic fatty acids* containing 10-18 carbon atoms Oil*	50% 50%	RONSONOL LIGHTER FLUID (Ronson)	Hydrocarbon naphtha solvents*	
ROHM & HAAS LETHANE 384 Insecticide (Rohm & Haas)	Beta butoxy beta' thiocyano diethyl ether* Oil*	50% 50%	RONUVEX Food supplement (Kremers)	Each tablet contains: Ferrous sulfate dried Copper sulfate Thiamine hydrochloride Riboflavin Niacinamide Folic acid Vitamin B12 Liver fraction 2	100 mg. 3 mg. 2 mg. 2 mg. 10 mg. 0.25 mg. 0.50 mcg. 200 mg.
ROHM & HAAS LETHANE 384 SPECIAL Insecticide (Rohm & Haas)	Beta butoxy beta' thiocyano diethyl ether* Beta thiocyano ethyl esters of aliphatic fatty acids* containing 10-18 carbon atoms Oil*	12.5% 37.5% 50%	RONUVIN Food supplement (Kremers)	Each 3 sugar-coated tablets: Vitamin B12 with intrinsic factor concentrate 1/3 U.S.P. unit (oral) Ferrous sulfate 400 mg. Copper sulfate monohydrate 15 mg.	
ROHM & HAAS RHOTHANE (See Rhothane)				Vitamin B12 Folic acid Thiamine mononitrate Riboflavin Niacinamide Ascorbic acid Molybdenum Manganese Cobalt Zinc	2.5 mcg. 2 mg. 5 mg. 5 mg. 25 mg. 100 mg. 1.5 mg. 0.5 mg. 0.5 mg. 0.5 mg.
RO-KO LIQUID SPRAY Insecticide (Calif. Spray)	Rotenone * Other cube resins Ethylene glycol oleic esters Inert ingredients*	2.5% 2.5% 45%			
ROLAIDS Antacid (Chicle)	Dihydroxy aluminum sodium carbonate		ROOF COOLERANT Roof coating paint (Tropical)		
ROLLING TYPE SKIN LOTION (Kirby's Mineral)			ROOF DRES PAINT (Forman, Ford)		
ROMAN CLEANSER BLEACH (Roman)	Sodium hypochloride*		ROOFKOTER (Tropical)		
ROMANTIQUE EAU DE TOILETTE & PERFUMES (Parfums Corday)			ROOF LEAK Roof paint (Elliott)		
			ROOFTEX Roof coatings (Rock-Tred)		
ROMAY HOUSEHOLD CLEANER (Roman)	Trisodium phosphate* Liquid wetting agent		ROOST NO MORE Bird repellent (Nat'l Bird)		
ROMITE Window cleaner (Roman)	Butyl cellosolve* Isopropyl alcohol*		ROOST PAINT Insecticide (Watkins, J.)	Lindane* (gamma isomer of benzene hexachloride)	
RONAL Disinfectant, germicide (Argonne)	Alkyl dimethyl benzyl ammonium chloride*		ROOST SPREAD Insecticide (Salsbury's)	Gamma isomer of benzene hexachloride (from lindane) 1.3% Nicotine alkaloid* 4.0% Petroleum distillate 94.7%	
RONCOVITE Elixir (Lloyd)	Each 100 cc.: Alcohol Cobalt chloride Ferrous sulfate Propyl parahydroxy benzoate	6-1/2% 0.3 gm. 5.0 gm. 0.02%			

*Consult Sec. II., Ingredients Index. This ingredient may be responsible for major toxic effects if poisonous amounts of this product are ingested.

Name & Use Manufacturer	Ingredients	
ROOTO Sewer cleaner (Rooto)	Sodium hydroxide*	
ROOTONE (Agricultural) (Am. Chem.)		
DOCTOR ROPER FORMULA Fungicide (medical) (Sherry)	Salicylic acid* Potassium permanganate* Iso-propyl alcohol*	70%
	Oil of lavender flowers	
ROSCO FILM LACQUER & CEMENT (Rosco)		
ROSCO FILM LACQUER THINNER (Rosco)		
ROSCO LENS CLEANER (Rosco)		
ROSE BOQUET THEATRE SPRAY Deodorant (Central Chem.)	Essential oils*	
ROSE BOWL BRAND ROSE DUST Insecticide (Imperial Chem.)	Ferbam	7.00%
	Rotenone	1.00%
	Other cube resins	2.00%
	DDT	3.00%
	Dusting sulfur *	15.00%
	Beta thiocyano ethyl esters (of aliphatic fatty acids containing 10-18 carbon atoms)	0.75%
ROSE CITY ROSE PERFUME, COLOGNE & TOILET- WATER (Duvelle)	Alcohol* denatured with diethyl phthalate	
ROSE DEW Household deodorant spray (Rose Dew)	Mixed floral perfume oil compound Isopropyl alcohol* Paradichlorobenzene *	
ROSE FERBAM Fungicide (Rose Mfg.)	Ferric dimethyl dithiocarbamate	
ROSE & FLOWER GARDEN INSECT SPRAY, BOSTWICK Insecticide (Bostwick)	Pyrethrins	0.025%
	Rotenone	0.128%
	Other cube extractives	0.236%
	Tech. piperonyl cyclonene	0.256%
	Dichlone	0.120%
	Petroleum distillates	0.102%
ROSE-GLO TOILET BOWL DEODORANT (Wonder)		
ROSELL'S TOILET PREP. (Drake, J. K.)		

Name & Use Manufacturer	Ingredients	
ROSE RAT KILLER Rodenticide (Rose Ext.)	Arsenic trioxide*	99.08%
ROSE TOX Insecticide, fungicide (Bonide)	Dichloro diphenyl tri- chloroethane*	5.0%
	Gamma isomer of benzene hexachloride	1.9%
	Rotenone	0.75%
	Other cube resins	1.50%
	Sulfur* (4-5 microns)	33.40%
	Ferbam (ferric dimethyl dithiocarbamate)	5.09%
ROSE VEL SALVE (Clarke, H.)	Boric acid* Petrolatum Paraffin Wax Perfume	
ROSEWOOD Removes dandruff (Reeves, J. R.)	Potassium bicarbonate Potassium carbonate Cream tartar Alum	
	Arsenic	0.002%
	Alcohol by volume	9.0%
ROSEX (Gardner)	C. P. glycerin Boric acid* Oxyquinoline sulfate	
ROSS HOUSEHOLD & AIRPLANE CEMENT & DOPE (Ross Chem.)	Nitrocellulose solution in acetone Butyl acetate Benzol*	
ROSSIE IRON OXIDE PAINTS (Rossie)		
ROSS LIQUID GLUE (Ross Chem.)	Animal hide glue Water Thiourea Benzoic acid	
ROSS LIQUID SOLDER (Ross Chem.)	Nitrocellulose solution Acetone * Butyl acetate Benzol* Aluminum powder	
ROSS MUCILAGE (Ross Chem.)	Gum arabic Glucose Benzoic acid	
ROSS PILLS Laxative (Ross, S.)	Each pill: Powdered extract belladonna* leaves	1.32 gr.
	Total alkaloids	0.0004 gr.
	Podophyllin	1/10 gr.
	Aloin	1/4 gr.
	Oleoresin capsicum	1/32 gr.
	Powdered ipecac	1/16 gr.
ROSS RUBBER CEMENT (Ross Chem.)	Rubber dissolved in naphtha*	
ROSS WHITE PASTE (Ross Chem.)	Corn dextrine Benzoic acid	
ROTA-CAPS (Salsbury's)	Each tablet: Nicotine monoethiodide	58 mg.
	Areca nut	500 mg.
	Nicotine* (expressed as alkaloid)	22 mg.

*Consult Sec. II., Ingredients Index. This ingredient may be responsible for major toxic effects if poisonous amounts of this product are ingested.

Name & Use Manufacturer	Ingredients		Name & Use Manufacturer	Ingredients	
ROT-BAN PRESERVA-TIVE FOR WOOD Wood pre-servative (Perma Prod.)			ROTRATE 5 Insecticide (Agkem)	Pine oil* Cube resins including rotenone* Ethylene dichloride* Naphthalene* Citrus oil* Tech. piperonyl butoxide Hydrous aluminum silicate Diatomaceous earth Sodium lauryl sulfate	
ROTECIDE ROACH POWDER Insecticide (Rotenone)	Pyrethrins DDT*	0.22% 10%	ROTRATE 10 Insecticide (Agkem)	Pine oil* Cube resins including rotenone* Ethylene dichloride* Naphthalene Citrus oil* Tech. piperonyl butoxide	
ROTECIDE ROTENONE GARDEN DUST Insecticide (Rotenone)	Rotenone Other cube extractives	0.75% 1.50%	ROUGET TYPE AMERICAN MADE FUSAINS Charcoal sticks (Nobema)		
ROTECIDE ROTENONE GARDEN SPRAY Insecticide (Rotenone)	Rotenone Cube extractives Beta thiocyano ethyl esters of aliphatic acids Polymethylated naphthalenes* Non-volatile oils Camphor oil Sorbitan monooleate	1.0% 1.5% 5.0% 40.0% 32.5% 6.0% 14.0%	ROUGH ON RATS (Wells, S. C.)	Arsenic trioxide* Barium carbonate	73.9% 20.0%
			ROUGH & READY CON-CENTRATE WARFARIN Rodenticide (Eaton, J. T.)	Warfarin	0.5%
ROTENOX FARNAM GRUB SPRAY BOMB Insecticide (Farnam)	Rotenone, rotenoids and other cube resins Ethylene glycol ether of pinene Pine oil* Camphor oil* Polyisobutyl phenoxy polyethoxyethanol	0.625% 5.625% 12.250% 10.000% 5.000%	ROUGH & READY MOUSE MIX (Ritchie)		
ROTENOX TRIPLE XXX LIVESTOCK SPRAY CONC. Insecticide (Farnam)	Rotenone Technical piperonyl cyclonene Pine oil* Ethylene glycol ether of pinene Citrus oil Alkyl phenyl polyglycol Ethylene dichloride* Naphthalene* Petroleum distillate* Other cube resins	1.19% 0.20% 39.40% 3.60% 1.80% 5.00% 5.00% 2.00% 39.43% 2.38%	ROUGH & READY RAT BAIT (Eaton, J. T.)	Fortified red squill*	10%
			ROUGH & READY RAT & MOUSE BAIT (Ritchie & Janvier)		
ROTGARD WOOD PRE-SERVATIVE (Steel Treating)			ROUGH & READY RAT & MOUSE BAIT WITH WARFARIN (Eaton, J. T.)	Warfarin	0.025%
RO-TON Insecticide (Bonide)	B-butoxy B' thiocyano diethyl ether * Petroleum distillates*	3.1% 96.9%	ROUGH & READY RAT PASTE Rodenticide (Ritchie & Janvier)		
ROTOSYN INSECT DUST (Bonide)	Cube resins (including rotenone) Methyl naphthalenes	1.00% 1.30%			
ROTOX Insecticide (Doggett-Pfeil)	Rotenone Sulfur*	0.75% 25%	ROUX COLOR SHAMPOO, TINTS, DYES & TONERS (Roux)	Mildly ammoniacal, aqueous, alcoholic oil Soap emulsions Aromatic amine	
ROT-PROOF MARINE FUNGUS & MILDEW PROOFING PAINT PRODUCTS (Wilbur)			ROUX CREME HAIR-DRESSING (Roux)	Aqueous emulsion of lanolin and oil	

---

*Consult Sec. II., Ingredients Index. This ingredient may be responsible for major toxic effects if poisonous amounts of this product are ingested.

Name & Use Manufacturer	Ingredients		Name & Use Manufacturer	Ingredients	
ROUX CREME RINSE (Roux)	Aqueous dispersion of cationic and non-ionic surface-active agents		ROYAL ACTIVATED SABADILLA DUST Insecticide (Rigo)	Sabadilla alkaloids	0.40%
ROUX CREME SHAMPOO (Roux)	Aqueous dispersion of soap and synthetic detergent		ROYAL AUTO BODY POLISH & CLEANER (Richman)		
ROUX DYE SOLVENT (Roux)	Powdered mixture of citric acid and zinc reducing agent		ROYAL BAIN DE CHAMPAGNE (Caron)		
ROUX HAIR CRAYON (Roux)	Dispersion of earth pigments and emulsifying agent in blend of waxes		ROYAL BICYCLE RIM CEMENT (Richman)		
ROUX HAIR LACQUER (Roux)	Mildly alkaline solution of natural gum		ROYAL BICYCLE TIRE FLUID (Richman)		
ROUX OIL BLEACH (Roux)	Perfumed, mildly ammoniacal, aqueous, alcoholic, oil soap emulsion		ROYAL BONDING CEMENT (Richman)		
ROUX QUICK BLEACH (Roux)	Oxidizing agent* Inactive diluents		ROYAL BRAND 10% DITHANE DUST Insecticide (Southern Agric. Chem.)	Zinc ethylene-bis(dithio-carbamate)	6.50%
ROUX RINSE (Roux)	Citric acid base				
ROUX SHAMPOO TINT (Roux)	p-Phenylenediamine*		ROYAL BRAND 15% FERMATE DUST Insecticide (Southern Agric. Chem.)	Ferric dimethyl dithio-carbamate	11.40%
ROUX SIL-VER-WYTE (Roux)	Mildly acidic aqueous solution of certified colors				
ROUX STAIN REMOVER (Roux)	Hydro-alcoholic solution of solvent and detergent		ROYAL BRAND VARNISH, ENAMEL & LACQUERS (Becker)		
ROUX SUPEROXIDE (Roux)	20-Volume aqueous solution of hydrogen peroxide		ROYAL CHROMIUM POLISH (Richman)		
ROWE EYE-NOSE DROPS Nasal de-congestant (Myers Labs.)	Epinephrine hydrochloride* Boric acid* Ephedrine sulfate* Zinc sulfate*		ROYAL COPPER DUST FOR BLIGHT ON TOMATOES (Rigo)	Copper* expressed as metallic	7.00%
ROWELL'S FORMULA TEN Antacid (Rexclif)	Bismuth subnitrate Bismuth subgallate Oil peppermint Magnesium hydroxide Sodium bicarbonate				
ROWELL'S FUNGICIDAL Medical (Rexclif)	Salicylic acid* Resorcinol* Isopropyl alcohol* 50% Benzoic acid Chlorobutanol*		ROYAL CRANK CASE CLEANER & ENGINE FLUSH (Richman)		
ROWE'S ANALYZED BRAND BUILDING PAINTS (Rowe)			ROYAL CREST SHAMPOO Show animal shampoo (House of Ross)	Liquid lanolin foam shampoo	
ROXITE SYNTHETIC VARNISH & ENAMEL (Norfolk)					

*Consult Sec. II., Ingredients Index. This ingredient may be responsible for major toxic effects if poisonous amounts of this product are ingested.

Name & Use Manufacturer	Ingredients	Name & Use Manufacturer	Ingredients
ROYAL CROWN MEN'S POMADE & HAIR DRESSING (Strickland)	Petroleum jelly Olive oil	ROYAL INSTANT GLASS CLEANER (Richman)	
ROYAL CUPROCIDE DUST FOR BLIGHT ON TOMATOES (Rigo)	Yellow cuprous oxide* 5.0%	ROYAL LIQUID RADIATOR SEAL (Richman)	
ROYAL 8% DITHANE Z-78 Insecticide (Rigo)	Zinc ethylene-bis(dithio- carbamate) 5.00 %	ROYAL LIQUID WAX POLISH (Richman)	
ROYAL ENAMEL THINNER, ENGINE SEAL & ENGINE ENAMEL (Richman)		ROYAL MECHANICS' HAND SOAP (Richman)	
ROYAL FABRIC CLEANER (Richman)		ROYAL NICKEL POLISH (Richman)	
ROYAL FIRE EXTINGUISHER LIQUID (Richman)		ROYAL PALM DEODORIZER Deodorizer, germicide (Royal Palm)	Alcohol* 90%/v Oil cananga Oil bergamot Oil lavender Clary sage oil Vanillin Inone Benzoin coumarin Geraniol Amyl salicylate *
ROYAL FOAM-E-FOAM SEAT COVER & UPHOLSTERY CLEANER (Richman)		ROYAL PERMANENT TYPE HYDRAULIC BRAKE FLUID (Richman)	
ROYAL GARDEN DUST Insecticide (Rigo)	Rotenone 0.40% Other cube resins 0.80% Beta thiocyano ethyl esters of aliphatic fatty acids 0.75%	ROYAL QUICK-START GAS LINE ANTI-FREEZE (Richman)	
ROYAL GENERAL PURPOSE OIL (Richman)		ROYAL RADIATOR CLEANER (Richman)	
ROYAL GLUE (Royal Glue)		ROYAL RADIATOR SEAL COMPOUND (Richman)	
ROYAL GRAFILM OIL (Richman)		ROYAL RHOTHANE TOBACCO HORN-WORM DUST (Rigo)	DDD 10%
ROYAL GRAPHITE PENETRATING OIL (Richman)		ROYAL ROAD OIL & TAR REMOVER (Richman)	
ROYAL HEATHER AFTER SHAVE LOTION (Royal Rinse)		ROYAL RUST REMOVER & PREVENTIVE (Richman)	
ROYAL HIGH STRENGTH SODIUM FLUORIDE H Insecticide (Royal Pharm.)	Sodium fluoride* 95% Sodium silicofluoride 2-1/2%	ROYAL SABADILLA DUST Insecticide (Rigo)	Sabadilla alkaloids 0.40%

*Consult Sec. II., Ingredients Index. This ingredient may be responsible for major toxic effects if poisonous amounts of this product are ingested.

Name & Use Manufacturer	Ingredients		Name & Use Manufacturer	Ingredients	
ROYAL'S BABY COUGH SYRUP Antitussive (Royal Mfg.)	Alcohol Ext. of white pine Wild cherry Aralia Poplar buds Blood root Sassafras Menthol	6%/v	RR CRAYONS (Imperial Cray.)		
ROYAL'S LIQUID ANALGESIC (Royal Pharm.)	Alcohol* Ethyl acetate Menthol*	50%/v 12%/v	RUBALT PAINTS, LACQUERS & ENAMELS (Hague)		
ROYAL'S CARMINATIVE CORDIAL (Royal Mfg.)	Fluid ext. ginger Fluid ext. blackberry Fluid ext. rhubarb Syrup vehicle Alcohol	3%/v	RUBBER-COAT RUBBER BASE PAINTS & ENAMELS (Wilbur)		
ROYAL'S CASCARA COMPOUND TABLETS Cathartic (Royal Pharm.)	Cascara		RUBBER-CRETE CONCRETE FLOOR ENAMEL (Red Spot)		
ROYAL'S CASCARA SAGRADA EXTRACT Cathartic (Royal Pharm.)	Cascara sagrada		RUBBER FLOOR VARNISH (McMurtry)		
ROYAL'S CASTORIA Laxative (Royal Mfg.)	Senna Rochelle salt Sodium bicarbonate Anise Worm & pumpkin seed Peppermint Methyl salicylate* Sugar		RUBBERKOTE PAINTS (Pioneer)		
			RUBBER SATIN PAINTS (Mautz)		
ROYAL'S NASAL OIL (Royal Mfg.)	Ephedrine alkaloid* Menthol* Eucalyptol and camphor* in mineral oil base*		RUBBERSKIN AUTO TOP PAINT (Cochrane)		
ROYAL SOLDERING PASTE (Richman)			RUBBERTRED PORCH & FLOOR ENAMEL (Chi-Namel)	Calcium carbonate Lampblack Yellow iron oxide Red iron oxide Resin Chinawood oil* Mineral spirits* Drier	8.3% 0.1% 18.6% 1.4% 13.5% 19.1% 36.6% 2.4%
ROYAL SOSBORSZESZ Liniment (Royal Pharm.)	Alcohol* Ethyl acetate Menthol*	50%/v 12%	RUBBERTUFF FLOOR ENAMELS (Malleable)		
ROYAL'S SUN TAN OIL (Royal Mfg.)	Menthyl salicylate* Mineral oil		RUBBER-VAR Wax treatment for rubber floors (Continental Car-Na-Var)		
ROYAL WORCESTER STOVE POLISH (Royal Worcester)			RUB-BUB Caulking compound (Moore, S.)		
ROYOX HOUSEHOLD CLEANER (Royce)			RUBEROL FLOOR ENAMELS (Lehman Bros. Corp.)	All contain less than 1% lead with the exception of Tile Green	
ROZNOILE Skin antiseptic (Ni-Late)	Camphor oil* Methyl salicylate* Pine oil* Benzocaine benzoate Oxyquinoline benzoate Linseed oil Petroleum oil,* light		RUBETHERM SOLIDIFIED LINIMENT Rubefacient (Claflin)	Petrolatum Oil turpentine rectified* Oil cajuput* Camphor* Methyl salicylate* Oil cloves Oleoresin capsicum Croton oil*	

*Consult Sec. II., Ingredients Index. This ingredient may be responsible for major toxic effects if poisonous amounts of this product are ingested.

Name & Use Manufacturer	Ingredients		Name & Use Manufacturer	Ingredients	
RUBIGUENT CREAM Rubefacient (Ives-Cameron)	Methyl nicotinate Histamine dihydrochloride Glycol monosalicylate Capsicum oleoresin	1.0% 0.1% 10.0% 0.1%	THE RU-EX COMPOUND Analgesic, food supplement (Ru-Ex)	Vitamin B1 Sodium salicylate* Sodium citrate	5.87 mg.
RUBITONE For colds (Tone)	Chloroform Ascorbic acid Ammonium bromide* Ammonium salicylate* Terpin hydrate* Menthol *	1/4 m. 25 mg. 4 gr.	RUF-KOAT WRINKLE VARNISH (General Cement)		
RUB-LESS METAL POLISH (Feiner)			RUGADUB Concentrated dye solution (Chair-Loc)	Aniline dyes* Dilute acetic acid Citric acid Diethylene glycol *	
RUBMASTER RUBBING ALCOHOL COMPOUND (Drugmaster)	Ethyl alcohol Lanamine Wintergreen*	70%/v	RUG KLEEN DRY Rug and upholstery cleaner (Feemster)		
RUB-NO FLOOR WAX (Clifton)			RUG'LEAN Home carpet dry cleaner (Behlen)		
RUBOL Rubefacient (Prescript. Spec.)	Menthol * Camphor* Eucalyptol* Thymol* Mutton suet Petrolatum		RUGLYDE Rubber lubricant (Am. Grease)		
RU-BON NO. 2 For skin irritations (Ru Bon)	Salicylic acid* Resorcin* Chrysarobin Oil of myrcia in vehicle of water, glycerin and alcohol		RUGODEX Bubble type dry cleaner (Magitex)	Alkylated aryl poly-ether alcohol Sodium o-phenylphenate* Isopropyl alcohol* White vinegar	
RU-BON NO. 3 For skin irritations (Ru Bon)	Salicylic acid* Resorcin* Chrysarobin Oil of myrcia in vehicle of water, glycerin and alcohol		RUKAMOL VET. LIQUID For intestinal irritation (veterinary) (Massengill)	Each fl. oz.: Ethyl alcohol Krameria Rubus Tinct. ginger Eugenol Potassium guaiacolsulfonate	18%/v 2.6 gm. 1.6 gm. 21.5 mg. 1.04 gm.
RU-BON OINTMENT For skin and rectal irrita-tion (Ru Bon)	Chrysarobin Resorcin* Salicylic acid*		RUKO Antiseptic, rubefacient bath (Ruko)	Sulfur precipitate * Potassium iodide* Sodium sesquicarbonate Borax* Sodium sulfate	
RUBTONE VARNISH (Foy)			RUKO DOUBLE STRENGTH PINE NEEDLE BATH (Ruko)		
RUBYFLUID SOLDERING FLUX (Ruby)			RUKO LINIMENT (Ruko)	Ethyl alcohol Methyl dimethyl cyclohexanol Menthol* Camphorene Propyl. glycol Methyl salicylate* Pine needle oils*	
RUCKER'S MUTTON SUET SALVE For colds (Allied Drug)	Benzoinated suet White petrolatum Camphor* Menthol Thymol* Oil of turpentine*				
RUCKER'S TRIENA Laxative (Allied Drug)	Senna and prune extractives		RUKO-PHYLL PINE NEEDLE BATH Cosmetic (Ruko)	Pine needle oils* Chlorophyll	
RUDEK Rubefacient, (Skin-A-Fire)	Essence of comfrey root Oleoresin of capsicum* Methyl salicylate* Menthol* Oil of eucalyptus* Camphor*		RUKO SULFUR BATH For foot bath and body bath (Ruko)	Sodium sesquicarbonate Sodium hyposulfite Sulfur * Sodium sulfate Sodium borate*	

*Consult Sec. II., Ingredients Index. This ingredient may be responsible for major toxic effects if poisonous amounts of this product are ingested.

Name & Use Manufacturer	Ingredients		Name & Use Manufacturer	Ingredients	
RUKO TAR-BATH For skin irritations (Ruko)	Juniper tar* Sulfonated castor oil Water	40% q.s.100%	RUSSELL'S INCUBATOR FUMIGANT (Russell, I.)	Isopropanol* * Formaldehyde (as gas)	49.0% 18.8%
RUMADOL Analgesic (Veltex)	Salicylamide* Sodium salicylate* Manganese salicylate* Caffeine Niacin		RUSSELL'S WARFARIN CONC. Rodenticide (Russell, I.)	Warfarin (3-(a-acetonylbenzyl)- 4-hydroxycoumarin) 0.5%	
RUMAQUINE HAIR LOTION (Caswell-Massey)			RUSSELL'S WATER WORMER Veterinary (Russell, I.)	Piperazine base 97.07 gr./oz.	
RUMATAG (Tutag)	Each enteric coated tablet: Calcium glycinate Acetylsalicylic acid* Ascorbic acid Vitamin B1	 2-1/2 gr. 3 gr. 15 mg. 1 mg.	RUST-A-LOID PRIMER (General P. & C.)		
RUMEN TABLETS Intestinal stimulant (veterinary) (Globe)	Each tablet: Tartar emetic* Talc Sodium bicarbonate Citric acid Barium chloride* Starch Acacia	 44.78% 3.73% 1.5% 0.75% 44.78% 3.73% 0.74%	RUSTBAAR Rust-resisting primer (Horn)		
RUN-R-STOP (Camille)			RUSTBUSTER Rust preventative and remover (Cannon)		
DR. RUPANER'S MEDICINE (Caswell-Massey)			RUST-CHEK CORROSION RESISTANT FINISHER (Rinshed-Mason)		
RUSALCIN TABLETS Enteric, coated yellow (Haag)	Sodium salicylate* Rutin Ascorbic acid Thiamine HCl	320 mg. 5 mg. 20 mg. 3 mg.	RUSTCHROME ANTI-RUST METAL PRIMER (Claronex)		
RUSCOL KOLD KAPS For colds (Haussman)	Powd. ipecac Salol* Quinine bisulphate Phenacetin*	 2 gr.	RUST-EETER PRIMERS (Harrington)		
RUSCOL LINIMENT (Haussman)	Alcohol* Menthol* Belladonna* Capsicum Turpentine* Methyl salicylate*	55%	RUSTEND RUST PREV. COMPOUND (Rustain)		
			RUSTEX RUST RESISTING PAINT (Elliott)		
RUSCOL SPECIAL CAPSULES Antirheumatic (Haussman)	Caffeine Pepsin Aspirin* Phenacetin*	 1 gr.	RUSTEZE RUST REMOVER (Crescent Chem. Div.)		
RUSCOL WART REMOVER Keratolytic (Ruscol)	Iodine* Salicylic acid* Glacial acetic acid* Alcohol Ether	 7% 12%	RUSTFLEX BOILER COMPOUND (Flexoid)		
RUSGO VARNISH (Glidden Co.)			RUSTFLEX RUST & GREASE SOLVENT (Flexoid)		
RUSSELL'S BHC ROOST SPREAD Insecticide (Russell, I.)	Refined petroleum oil* Gamma isomer of benzene hexachloride* (from lindane) Other isomers of benzene hexachloride		RUSTGARD Liquid rust prevention (Drigard)		

*Consult Sec. II., Ingredients Index. This ingredient may be responsible for major toxic effects if poisonous amounts of this product are ingested.

Name & Use Manufacturer	Ingredients	Name & Use Manufacturer	Ingredients
RUSTICIDE Rust remover (Rusticide)	Ortho-phosphoric acid *	RUSTOPPERS RUST PREVENTIVE (Cleveland)	
RUSTIKOTE RUST PREVENTIVE COATING (Tropical)		RUST OUT LIQUID (Manatee)	
RUST-KILL Rust preventive (Liquid)		RUSTOUT RUST PRE-VENTATIVES (Flexoid)	
RUST-KURB RUST PREVENTIVE COMPOUND (Rex Oil)		RUST PREVENTIVE & REMOVER COMPOUND (Nox-Rust)	
RUST-LENE RUST PREVENTIVE (Sinclair Ref.)		RUSTREM ANTI-RUST PAINT (Speco)	Metallic pigments of chrome,* iron, aluminum, copper* titanium Lampblack Resins Plasticizers Coal tar solvents*
RUST-MASTER RUST REMOVERS (Rust Master)		RUSTREM SOLVENT & THINNER (Speco)	Coal tar aromatics*
RUST METRO PAINT (Armor)		RUSTRID Rust pre-ventive and remover compound (Val-A)	
RUSTNAUGHT ANTI-RUST PAINT (Glidden Co.)			
RUST NO RUST INHIBITOR (Morris Paint)		RUST-SELE RUST INHIBITIVE PAINT (Olo)	
RUST NOT METAL PAINT (Williamson)			
RUSTOFF FOR REMOVING RUST (Caul)		RUST-SOL Rust solvent (Rust Sol)	
		RUST-TOX RUST PREVENTIVE (Skybrite)	
RUST-OLEUM Rust preventive coating (Rust-Oleum)	Processed fish oil Essential rust-inhibiting pigments	RUSTYRASE RUST REMOVER (Hachik)	
RUST-OLEUM CLEAR-SELE Sealer (Rust-Oleum)		RU-TEL Analgesic (Ru-Tel)	Each tablet: Sodium salicylate* Thiamine Potassium citrate Ferrous sulfate Calcium levulinate
RUST-OLEUM SURFA-SELE Sealer (Rust-Oleum)			
RUST-O-LITE ALUMINUM PAINT (General P. & C.)		RUTLAND BLACK ASPHALT PAINT (Rutland)	Vehicle (varnish) 100% Gilsonite 31.2% Linseed oil 9.8% Mineral spirits* 59.0%
RUSTO LOTION (Washington Hom.)	Grindelia robusta Camphor* Isopropanol*	RUTLAND BLACK ENAMEL (Rutland)	Vehicle (varnish) 100% Gilsonite 30.9% Linseed oil 4.6% Mineral spirits* 64.5%
RUSTOP PAINTS (Coating Mat'ls.)			

*Consult Sec. II., Ingredients Index. This ingredient may be responsible for major toxic effects if poisonous amounts of this product are ingested.

Name & Use Manufacturer	Ingredients	Name & Use Manufacturer	Ingredients
RUTLAND BLACK ROOF PAINT (Rutland)	Asphalt Naphtha*	SAFE-T-GRIP PAINT (Central P. & V.)	
RUTLAND FOUNDATION COATING (Rutland)	Asphalt Asbestos Naphtha*	SAFE-T-SOL Spot remover (Patek)	Chlorinated hydrocarbons*
RUTLAND GREEN METAL ROOF PAINT (Rutland)	Pigment Chromium oxide green* Aluminum silicate Vehicle Soya alkyd resin Mineral spirits*and drier Lecithin	SAFE-T-TRED WAX (Staminite)	Ammonia*
		SAF-KIL BRAND RAT-BAIT Rodenticide (Saf-Kil)	

RYANEXCEL 96-3 Insecticide (Penick)	Ryania speciosa* 95.8%
	Di-n-propyl maleate isosafrole
	   condensate (n-propyl-isome)
	                        3.2%
		SAF-TAN CREAM Sunscreening cream (Texas Pharm.)	Digalloyl trioleate 3%
			Vanishing cream

RYANICIDE 100 Insecticide (Penick)	Ryania powder* 100%	SAF-T DRY CLEANING COMPOUND (Dural)	
RX 7-11 For dandruff (Murrell)	Sulfanilamide* Sulfathiazol* Glycerin Alcohol 35%/v	SAFTICIDE Insecticide (Residex)	Piperonyl butoxide 2.00% Pyrethrins 0.20% Petroleum distillates* 97.80%

SABIA ANTISEPTIC (Sabia)		SAFTICIDE EMULSION CONCEN- TRATE Insecticide (Residex)	Tech. piperonyl butoxide
			                        11.87%
			Pyrethrins 1.18%
			Polyoxyethylene sorbitol
			   mixed ether ester 14.94%
			Petroleum oil* 72.01%

SABIA PINE OIL Disinfectant (Sabia)	Pine oil*		
SACOTE PAINTS & SACOLUX (Saginaw)		SAF-T-ZONE Anti-freeze (McAlester)	Ethylene glycol* 93% Rust inhibitor
SAFCO SAFETY FLOOR POLISH (Legge)		SAF-T-ZONE TRAFFIC PAINT (Bownes)	
SAFE-GARD ANTISEPTIC HAND CLEANER (Safe-Gard)		SAGE AIR REFRESHER Air deodorant (Sage Labs.)	
SAFE-JEL & SAFE-CREME VAGINAL CREAM (Hychex)		SAGE SAVERS MOTH BALLS Insecticide (Sage Labs.)	

SAFE-LEX AEROSOL INSECT KILLER (Bostwick)	Methoxychlor tech. 4.000%
	Allethrin 0.10%
	n-Octyl bicycloheptene
	   dicarboximide 0.166%
	Isobornyl thiocyano
	   acetate 0.82%
	Related terpenes 0.18%
	Methylated naphthalene* 10.355%
	Petroleum distillate 4.379%
		ST. ALBAN ANTI-PAIN BALM Rubefacient (Myers Labs.)	Menthol*
			Methyl salicylate*
			Lanolin

		ST. ALBAN HERB TEA (Myers Labs.)	Senna Uva ursi Elder flowers Chamomile Fennel Centaury Sarsaparilla Triticum Sassafras Aniseed
SAFE-T-GRIP NON-SKID DECK PAINT (Marine Coatings)		ST. ANTHONY'S OIL & SALVE (Hoyt)	

*Consult Sec. II., Ingredients Index. This ingredient may be responsible for major toxic effects if poisonous amounts of this product are ingested.

Name & Use Manufacturer	Ingredients		Name & Use Manufacturer	Ingredients	
ST. JOHN'S BAY RUM (West Indies)	Alcohol Bay oil	58% 2%	SAL-C-PAR WITH COLCHICINE For gout (Vitec)	Each tablet: Salicylamide* Para-aminobenzoic acid Ascorbic acid Colchicine	5 gr. 5 gr. 30 mg. 1/250 gr.
ST. JOSEPH COUGH SYRUP FOR CHILDREN (Plough)	Sodium citrate Ipecac Menthol		SAL-C-PAR WITH MEPHENESIN Analgesic (Vitec)	Each tablet: Salicylamide* Para-aminobenzoic acid Ascorbic acid Mephenesin*	2-1/2 gr. 2-1/2 gr. 15 mg. 5 gr.
ST. JOSEPH NOSE DROPS FOR CHILDREN Nasal de-congestant (Plough)	Neosynephrine hydrochloride (brand of phenylephrine hydrochloride) Chlorobutanol* (a chloral derivative)	0.25% 0.1%	SALEM CREOL DIS-INFECTANT (Boyle-Midway)	Coal tar neutral oils* Cresylic acid* Soap	62% 11% 17%
SAK-SAK OINTMENT (Deken's)			SALETO Analgesic (Mallard)	Each tablet: Acetophenetidin* Aspirin* Salicylamide Camphor monobromated Caffeine anhydrous	2 gr. 1/4 gr.
SALAC CORN REMOVER (Salac)					
SALATONE For acid dyspepsia, hepatic torpor, etc. (Jenkins)	Each tablet: Sodium salicylate* Sodium benzoate Fluid ext. cascara sagrada	2 gr. 1/2 gr. 5 m.	SALETO INFANT Analgesic (Mallard)	Each tablet: Acetophenetidin* Aspirin* Salicylamide* Camphor monobromated Caffeine anhydrous	1/2 gr. 1/20 gr.
SALBIS ANTACID POWDER (Chase Chem.)	Bismuth subcarbonate Diastase of malt Colloidal kaolin Magnesium carbonate Calcium carbonate Sodium bicarbonate Magnesium oxide Papain Oil peppermint		SAL-FAYNE PINK CAPSULES Analegesic (Sal-Fayne)	Acetophenetidin* Aspirin* Caffeine	2-1/2 gr. 3-1/2 gr. 1/2 gr.
			SAL HEPATICA Antacid, laxative (Bristol-Myers)	Sodium chloride Citric acid Sodium sulfate Sodium bicarbonate Tartaric acid Sodium phosphate	
SAL-CAZINE Antacid (Veltex)	Sodium and potassium bicarbonates Citric acid Sodium chloride Sodium phosphate Magnesium sulfate Calcium gluconate		SALICIDIA, C.T. Analgesic (CaPhenin)	Acid acetylsalicylic* Acetophenetidin* Powd. ext. henbane Powd. ext. jamaica dogwood Powd. ext. gelsemium	2 gr. 1 gr. 1/8 gr. 1 gr. 1/21 gr.
SALCEDROX (Orange) Analgesic, antirheumatic (Massengill)	Each tablet: Sodium salicylate* Aluminum hydroxide gel dr. Calcium ascorbate Calcium carbonate	0.3 gm. 0.2 gm. 60 mg. 60 mg.	SALICYLIC ACID & GELSEMIUM COMPOUND (Lilly)	Alcohol Salicylic acid* (as sodium salicylate) Gelsemium* Cimicifuga Potassium iodide	6% 8.75 gm. 3.3 gm. 0.875 gm.
SALCIPAB (Kirkman)	Each tablet: Sodium salicylate* U.S.P. Sodium para-aminobenzoate	0.3 gm. 0.3 gm.	SALIFORM LINIMENT (Western Pharm.)	Methyl salicylate* Chloroform Diadermic menstruum	36% 8% q.s.
SALCIPAB WITH C (Kirkman)	Each tablet: Sodium salicylate* U.S.P. Sodium para-aminobenzoate Ascorbic acid U.S.P.	0.3 gm. 0.3 gm. 50.0 mg.	SALONIL Keratolytic (Torch)	Salicylic acid* Lanolin	40%
SALCOGEL-B Analgesic (Physicians Prod.)	Each tablet: Sodium salicylate* Tr. gelsemium Thiamine chloride	7-1/2 gr. 3-3/4 m. 1.5 mg.	SALPAR Analgesic (La Crosse)	Each tablet: Sodium salicylate* Para-aminobenzoic acid	4 gr. 4 gr.
SAL-C-PAR (Vitec)	Each tablet: Salicylamide* Para-aminobenzoic acid Ascorbic acid	5 gr. 5 gr. 30 mg.			

Name & Use Manufacturer	Ingredients		Name & Use Manufacturer	Ingredients	
DR. SALSBURY'S HOG-GAIN (Salsbury's)	3-Nitro-4-hydroxyphenylarsonic acid* 1.25% (corresponds to 4.7 mg. arsenic trioxide per gm.) Niacin Potassium iodide Dicalcium phosphate Copper* Iron Cobalt* Manganese* Zinc*		SALYDOL Analgesic (Eastern Pharm.)	Sodium salicylate* 40 gr. per fl. oz. Rock candy syrup Glycerin Orange flower water	
			SAMAE MIRACLE CLEANSER (Copper Clad)	Siliceous matter	
DR. SALSBURY'S IMPROVED LOUSE POWDER Insecticide (Salsbury's)	Beta,beta' dithiocyano diethyl ether * 1.35% DDT 2% Sulfur* 30%		SAMBA PERFUME & TOILET WATER (Corot)		
DR. SALSBURY'S LIQUID FUMIGANT (Salsbury's)	Formaldehyde* Orthohydroxy diphenyl* Methanol*		SAMES For coughs, hoarsness due to colds (Haussman)	Tar Menthol * Blood root Horehound Oil of eucalyptus * White pine Ammonium chloride Honey Lobelia * Chloroform 2 m./fl. oz.	
DR. SALSBURY'S 3-NITRO POWDER (Salsbury's)	3-Nitro-4-hydroxyphenyl arsonic acid* 10%		SAMPSON BARN PAINT (Peerless Paint)		
DR. SALSBURY'S PEST SPRAY Insecticide (Salsbury's)	Beta butoxy beta' thiocyanodiethyl ether 3.7% Dichloro diphenyl tri- chloroethane 25.0% Aromatic petroleum distillate * 66.3%		SAMSON DRAIN PIPE CLEANER (Internat. Plumb.)	Sodium hydroxide*	
DR. SALSBURY'S ROOST SPREAD Insecticide (Salsbury's)	Gamma isomer of benzene hexachloride (from lindane) 1.3% Nicotine alkaloid* 4.0% Petroleum distillate 94.7%		SANABALM POWDER (Sanabalm)	Boric acid* Thymol* Camphor* Formaldehyde Salicylic acid* Eucalyptol * Zinc stearate Talc	
DR. SALSBURY'S SULFA (Veterinary, avian) (Salsbury's)	4, 4'-Diaminodiphenyl sulfone* n'-Phenylsulfanilamide*		SAN-A-DOU POWDER For skin, throat mouth irritations (Euclid)	Boric acid* Alum * Menthol * Eucalyptol* Carbolic acid*	
DR. SALSBURY'S WORMAL TABLETS Anthelmintic (veterinary, avian) (Salsbury's)	Each tablet: Dibutyltin dilaurate 125 mg. Nicotine ethiodide* 55 mg. Phenothiazine 500 mg. Nicotine * 22 mg.		SANAFRIO OINTMENT For colds, muscular aches, (Crowell)	Camphor* Menthol*	
SAL SPERIN BELL Analgesic, antiheumatic (Hollings- Smith)	Calcium gluconate Acetylsalicylic acid* 3.5 gr.		SANA-GLO Cleans dishes and glassware (Sanascent)		
SAL U Laxative (San Pedro)	Sodium phosphate		SAN-A-JEL Vaginal jelly (Evons)	Lactic acid jelly	
SALVITAE Antacid, cathartic (Am. Apoth.)	Sodium sulfate Magnesium sulfate Sodium bicarbonate Potassium bicarbonate Sodium phosphate Citric acid Tartaric acid		SANALAV Douche (Kip, A.)	Benzoic, lactic, and acetic acids Phenol Thymol* Methyl salicylate* Isopropyl alcohol* 30% Menthol Eucalyptol* Aromatics Buffered propylene glycolaqueous solution	

*Consult Sec. II., Ingredients Index. This ingredient may be responsible for major toxic effects if poisonous amounts of this product are ingested.

Name & Use Manufacturer	Ingredients		Name & Use Manufacturer	Ingredients
SAN-A-LIZER Repellent, deodorizer (San-A-Lizer)	Naphthalene* 85% Methyl salicylate 5%		SAN-CURA OINTMENT For skin and scalp irrita- tions (Thompson Med.)	Chlorobutanol (chloral derivative) 1% Hexachlorophene Benzocaine Chlorothymol* Benzoic acid * Salicylic acid* Benzyl alcohol Cod liver oil Lanolin Petrolatum washable base
SANAMINE DISINFECT- ANT & GERMICIDE (Carpenter)	Methyl dodecyl benzyl trimethyl ammonium chloride* 10%			
SAN-A-MOR To sanitize poultry drink- ing water (Hilltop)	Alkyl tolylmethyl trimethyl ammonium chloride* 5.2% Propylene glycol solution 94.8%		SAN-CURA RECTAL CONES For rectal irritations (Thompson Med.)	Bismuth subcarbonate Benzocaine Bismuth subiodide Zinc oxide Boric acid
SAN-A-MOR CONCEN- TRATE To disinfect and sanitize poultry drink- ing water and combat most infectious disease germs on contact (Hilltop)	Alkyl tolyl methyl trimethyl ammonium chloride* Tetra sodium salt of ethylene diamine tetra-acetic acid Trisodium phosphate Water and sodium bicarbonate 74.4%		SANDERINE ANTISEPTIC OINTMENT For skin irritations (Sanders)	Petrolatum Oil of thyme Oxyquinoline
			SANDE'S HAND LOTION (McFarlin)	Glycerin Lin. camphor Soap U.S.P.
SANAPEL For skin irritations, ringworm, atheletes (Salinitro)	Chloral hydrate 0.2% Phenylmercuric nitrate 0.04% Benzocaine Thymol* Campho-menthol Alcohol 40%/v Benzoic acid * Salicylic acid* Resorcinol* Cresol		SANDRA CASSILL EAU DE COLOGNE (Cassill)	
			SANFORD'S BLACK INDELIBLE LAUNDRY INK, WHITE INDELIBLE INK & INDELIBLE STAMPING KIT (Sanford Ink)	Aniline oil*
SANA-SCENT Cleaner, deodorant (Sanascent)				
SANASEED Rodenticide (Bonide)	Strychnine sulfate* 0.5%		SANFORD'S DOUBLE- DUTY INK ERASER X-IT (Sanford Ink)	
SANATONE PAINTS & FINISHES (Thomson- Porcelite)			SANFORD'S GLUE & RENEW (Sanford Ink)	Polyvinyl plastic cement
SANAX Liquid wax cleaner (Finnell)			SANFORD'S GRIPPIT PAPER CEMENT (Sanford Ink)	Chlorinated hydrocarbon* Naphtha*
SANCHIA SILICONE PROTECTIVE CREAM For skin (Clapp, Otis)	Silicone (polydimethyl siloxane) 10% Lanolin 1%		SANFORD'S HOTEL & SCHOOL INK (Sanford Ink)	
SANCO PAINTS (Monroe Sander)			SANFORD'S LIQUI-STICK, LIQUI-PASTE, ROYAL CROWN MUCILAGE & TEXIT Gum arabic adhesive (Sanford Ink)	

*Consult Sec. II., Ingredients Index. This ingredient **may** be responsible for major toxic effects if poisonous amounts of this product are ingested.

Name & Use Manufacturer	Ingredients		Name & Use Manufacturer	Ingredients	
SANFORD'S MARKIT INK, BLACK STENCIL INK & DRI-LINE (Sanford Ink)	Naphtha* solvent ink		SANI-CLOR BLEACH (Lady's Choice)	Sodium hypochlorite Caustic*	5-1/4% 5-1/4%
SANFORD'S PENIT FOUNTAIN PEN INK, ALBUM & GREETING CARD INK & NUMBERING MACHINE & CHECK WRITER INK (Sanford Ink)	Phenol as a preservative less than 1%		SANIDOME DEODORANT BLOCKS (U.S. Sanitary)		
			SANIDYNE 11% DIS-INFECTANT (Schmutzler)	Para-tert-octyl-phenoxy ethoxy ethyl dimethyl benzyl ammonium chloride* 11%	
			SANI FLAT PAINT (Moore, B.)		
SANFORD'S SCHOOL & LIBRARY PASTE (Sanford Ink)	Potato dextrine adhesive		SANI-FLUSH Toilet bowl cleaner (Boyle-Midway)	Sodium bisulfate* Sodium binoxalate	82.5% 2%
SANFORD'S SOLVENE TYPE CLEANER (Sanford Ink)	Perchlorethylene* Naphtha*		SANIFUME CRYSTALS Insecticide (Royal Mfg.)	Paradichlorobenzene*	
SANFORD'S STAMP PAD INKS (Sanford Ink)	Glycerine-glycol		SANI KLEEN DISH WASHING COMPOUND Detergent (Nat'l Soap)		
SANFORD'S TEMPERA COLORS Water colors (Sanford Ink)			SANI-PHONE For the telephone (Sanford Ink)		
SANFORD'S TEXTILE PAINTS (Sanford Ink)			SANI-PHYLACTIC CREAM (Rigidtest)	Stearic acid Diglycol stearate Lanolin Petrolatum ceresin Mineral oil Propylene glycol Triethanolamine Camphor* U.S.P. Menthol* Synthetic Chlorothymol* N.F. Oil of eucalyptus* U.S.P. Zinborsal: zincborodisalicylate decahydrate with boric acid*	
SANFORD'S THINNER FOR GRIPPIT & RUBBER CEMENT (Sanford Ink)					
SANGUIDINE SYRUP Antitussive (Success)	Each fl. oz.: Codeine sulfate 2/3 gr. Squill Sanguinaria Menthol Alcohol 8.5%/v Senega Ipecac Glycerin		SANI PINE DISINFECT-ANT (Sani-Pine)	Pine oil* Soap	70% 20%
			SANI-SPRAY NON-FOG GLASS CLEANING FLUID (Allen)	Water solution of phosphates and wetting agents 4%	
SANI BOWL Cleaner (Worrell)					
SANICAP Lotion (Vogel)	Phenyl cellosolve 5% Isopropyl alcohol* 50% Aerosol OT Methyl salicylate*		SANISTAN Antiseptic (Standard Chem.)	Di-isobutyl phenoxy ethoxy ethyl dimethyl benzyl ammonium chloride* 10% Non-ionic detergent 10%	
SANI-CEN Liquid cleaner and deodorizer for toilet bowls and urinals (Central Chem.)					

*Consult Sec. II., Ingredients Index. This ingredient may be responsible for major toxic effects if poisonous amounts of this product are ingested.

Name & Use Manufacturer	Ingredients	Name & Use Manufacturer	Ingredients
SANI-STYP Antiseptic (Sanite Chem.)	Benzyl alcohol Chlorothymol* Oxyquinoline sulfate Phenylphenol Pinene* Aluminum chloride Green color in aqueous acetone solution	SANI-WAX WALL CLENE Paint cleaner (Sani-Wax)	
SANITAIRE INSTANT DEODORIZER (Campbell Chem.)	Isopropyl alcohol* Triethylene glycol Propylene glycol Para di-isobutyl phenoxy ethoxy ethyl dimethyl benzyl ammonium chloride* Freon 11 and 12	SANNETTE DOUCHE POWDER (Myers Labs.)	Boric acid* Alum* Zinc sulfate* Menthol* Methyl salicylate (synthetic oil of wintergreen)*
SANITAR DISINFECT-AND, DE-ODORANT & CLEANSER (Robbins, G.)	Neutral coal tar oils * 58% Anhydrous soap 20% Phenols* 12%	SANOCIDE WHEAT SEED PROTECTANT Insecticide, fungicide (Calif. Spray)	Hexachlorobenzene* 40% Inert ingredients*
SANITARE FOR FEMININE HYGIENE (Edru)		SAN ODORANT POWDER Embalmer's supply (Embalmers')	
SANITARY SPECIALTIES' MOTH CRYSTALS MOTH KILLER Insecticide (U.S. Sanitary)	Paradichlorobenzene*	SAN-O-FEC-D Disinfectant (Whitmoyer)	Para di-isobutyl phenoxy ethoxy ethyl dimethyl benzyl ammonium chloride* 10% Trisodium phosphate* 30% Sodium carbonate 30%
SANITARY SPECIALTIES' MOTH FLAKES Insecticide (U.S. Sanitary)	Naphthalene*	SANOHIST TABLETS (Perdue)	Pyrilamine maleate 25 mg. Aspirin* 3-1/2 gr. Acetophenetidin* 2-1/2 gr. Anhydrous caffeine 1/2 gr.
SANITEX CLEANING COMPOUND (Texo)		SAN-O-LA Disinfectant, antiseptic (Rochester Germ.)	Pine oil* Soap
SANITIZ DISINFECT-ANT & GERMICIDE (Lester Labs.)	Benzalkonium chloride* (high molecular alkyl dimethyl benzyl ammonium chlorides) 10%	SAN-O-PINE Disinfectant, deodorant (Hillyard Sales)	Pine oil* Soap
SANITONE ALKYD WALL PAINT (Am. Asbestos)		SAN-O-TABS For feminine hygiene (San-O-Tabs)	Halozone* Salt
SANI-WAX FURNITURE POLISH, HARDWOOD FLOOR, LINOLEUM, PORCELAIN, TILE, MARBLE & VENETIAN BLIND CLEANERS (Sani-Wax)		SANOVAN Powdered deodorant (Fairfield)	
		SANOZONE AIR PERFUMES (Sanozone)	
		SAN PEDRO LAXATIVE SALTS (San Pedro)	Tartaric acid Lithium carbonate Citric acid Sodium bicarbonate Table salt Ext. of lemon flavor
SANI-WAX PAINT & VARNISH CLEANER (Sani-Wax)		SAN PEDRO LAXATIVE TEA (San Pedro)	Senna Manna Peppermint Juniper berries Licorice root
SANI-WAX TILE CREME Floor wax (Sani-Wax)		SAN PEDRO TONIC Tonic (San Pedro)	Extract of beef Ammonium citrate Tinct. of gentian Aromatics Iron Tinct. of cinchone Flavored with sherry wine

*Consult Sec. II., Ingredients Index. This ingredient may be responsible for major toxic effects if poisonous amounts of this product are ingested.

Name & Use Manufacturer	Ingredients	
SAN-PHE-NOL HATCHERY SPRAY & HOUSEHOLD DISINFECT-ANT (Russell, I.)	Isopropyl alcohol*	15.33%
	Anhydrous soap	6.33%
	Terpineol	4.66%
	Chloro-2 phenylphenol*	6.00%
SAN-PHENO-X GERMICIDE (Huntington)		
SAN SEED DISINFECT-ANT Fungicide (Green Cross)	Mercury*	5%
SAN SOLVENT Cesspool cleaner (Vega)	Sodium hydroxide*	
SANTA BARBARA GOPHER POISON-ROLLED BARLEY Rodenticide (Santa Barbara)	Strychnine*	
SANTA CLARA CORROSIVE SUBLIMATE POISON Rodenticide (Santa Clara)	Corrosive sublimate*	
SANTA CLARA RAT POISON (Santa Clara)	Zinc phosphide	0.50%
SANTA CLARA SPARROW POISON (Santa Clara)	Strychnine alkaloid*	1.20%
SANTA CLARA SQUIRREL POISON (Santa Clara)	Zinc phosphide	0.50%
SANTA CLARA THALLIUM SULFATE SQUIRREL POISON (Santa Clara)	Thallium sulfate*	1.00%
SANTA CLARA WARFARIN RAT BAIT (Santa Clara)	3-(1-Phenyl-2-acetylethyl)-4-hydroxycoumarin	0.025%
SANTA CLARA ZINC CHLORIDE POISON Rodenticide (Santa Clara)	Zinc chloride*	
SANTOVAN CAPSULES (Pharmex)	Iron Vitamin B1 Liver	
SAN VEINO Embalmers' supply (Embalmers')	Chlorinated hydrocarbons*	

Name & Use Manufacturer	Ingredients	
SANYGEN GERMICIDE & DISIN-FECTANT (Miami)		
SA PAINT & VARNISH CLEANER (Simoniz)		
SAPHELLE Insecticide (Kennedy)	Tech. chlordane*	5%
	Talc	95%
SAPHEX FLY SPRAY (Kennedy)	Pyrethrins	8%
SAPHO ANTI-MOTH CRYSTALS (Kennedy)	Paradichlorobenzene*	99%
SAPHO 2% CHLORDANE LIQUID SPRAY Insecticide (Kennedy)	Chlordane tech.	2%
	Base oil*	98%
SAPHO 25% C.P.R. GARDEN DUST Insecticide (Kennedy)	Piperonyl cyclonene tech.	0.630%
	Pyrethrins	0.060%
	Rotenone	0.310%
SAPHO 5% DDT INSECT SPRAY (Kennedy)	DDT* tech.	5%
	Organic thiocyanates	2%
	Kerosene*	93%
SAPHO 10% DDT PEST DUST Insecticide (Kennedy)	DDT* tech.	10%
	Talc	
SAPHO 25% DDT WATER EMULSION SPRAY Insecticide (Kennedy)	DDT tech.	25%
	Emulsifier	7-1/2%
	Aromatic naphtha solvents*	67-1/2%
SAPHO FLOWER BOMB Insecticide (Kennedy)	Pyrethrins	0.025%
	Rotenone	0.128%
	Piperonyl cyclonene	0.256%
	Methoxychlor	3.000%
SAPHO INSECT BOMB (Kennedy)	DDT	2%
	Pyrethrins	0.1%
	Piperonyl butoxide	0.8%
	Beta butoxy beta thiocyano diethyl ether	1%
SAPHO 1% MALATHION FLY BAIT (Kennedy)	Malathion	1%
	Sugar	99%
SAPHO MOTH PROOFER BOMB (Kennedy)	Para chloraniline oleate	1.84%
	Para chloraniline salicylate	0.16%
SAPHO POWDER Insecticide (Kennedy)	Pyrethrins	9%

*Consult Sec. II., Ingredients Index. This ingredient may be responsible for major toxic effects if poisonous amounts of this product are ingested.

Name & Use Manufacturer	Ingredients		Name & Use Manufacturer	Ingredients	
SAPHO 622 REPELLENT Agric. (Kennedy)	Dimethyl phthalate Indalone Ethyl hexanediol*	60% 20% 20%	SARAN Plastic (Dow)	Polyvinylidene chloride Vinylidene chloride copolymers 1, 1-Dichloroethylene copolymers	
SAPHO REPULSEUR BOMB Insecticide (Kennedy)	Ethylhexanediol*	20%	SARA SAWYER NAIL TREAT- MENT & NAIL POLISH REMOVER (Leighton)		
SAPHO WARFARIN RAT & MOUSE KILLER Rodenticide (Kennedy)	Warfarin Corn meal	0.025% 99.075%	SARATOGA OINTMENT (Harvey, G.F.)	Boric acid* Zinc oxide Eucalyptol* Prepared suet White petrolatum	
SAPO ELIXIR CLEANING FLUID & LIGHTER FLUID (Sapo)			SARCOPTIC MANGE MEDICINE (Clayton)		
SAPOLIN ENAMELS, STAINS & PAINTS (Sapolin)			SARGENT COLORS (Am. Artists')		
SAPOLIN MEL-LUX FLAT PAINT (Sapolin)	Pigment 60%: Titanium calcium pigment Calcium carbonate Silicates Vehicle (varnish) 40%: Non-volatile (soya alkyd resin, ester gum Volatile (odorless mineral spirits)*		SARGENT NO-ROT WOOD PRE- SERVATIVE (Sargent- Gerke)	Pentachlorophenol* Mineral spirits*	5% 90%
SAPOLIN ONE COAT HOUSE PAINT (Sapolin)	Pigment 60%: Titanium magnesium Titanium dioxide Zinc oxide Basic silicate white lead 45-X Vehicle 40%: Linseed oil Drier Mineral spirits*		SARGON Cathartic (Myers)	Each pill: Powdered extract belladonna leaves* Phenolphthalein Sodium salicylate* Bile salts Aloin*	1/12 gr.
SAPOLIN TRIPLE DUTY ENAMEL (Sapolin)			SARGON Tonic (Myers Labs.)	Iron and ammonium citrate Sodium citrate Oxgall inspissated Ferrous iodide Rochelle salts Caffeine Quassia chips U.S.P. Tartaric acid Glycerin Flavor Alcohol Citric acid Cane sugar Caramel	18%/v
SAPOLIO POWDER Cleaner (Sapolio)					
SAPO ROACH SPRAY Insecticide (Sapo)			SA RUG & UPHOLSTERY CLEANER (Simoniz)		
SAPROCO CLEANSING PRODUCTS (Eastern Sanitary)			SASCO COAL TAR DIS- INFECTANT (S & S)	Coal tar neutral oils* Phenols* Soap	
SARAKA Cathartic (Union Pharm.)	Bassorin Cortex frangula		SASCO PINE OIL DIS- INFECTANT (S & S)	Pine oil* Soap Isopropyl alcohol*	
SARAKA-D Cathartic (Union Pharm.)	Bassorin Cortex frangula		SASCO RANDICIDE RESIDUAL SPRAY EMULSION TYPE Insecticide (S & S)	Tech. chlordane Inert ingredients*	2% 98%

*Consult Sec. II., Ingredients Index. This ingredient may be responsible for major toxic effects if poisonous amounts of this product are ingested.

Name & Use Manufacturer	Ingredients		Name & Use Manufacturer	Ingredients
SASCO ROACH & INSECT SPRAY (S & S)	Petroleum distillate* Tech. chlordane*		SATIN FLOW LATEX PAINT (Long Island)	
SASCO SANICIDE Insecticide (S & S)	Petroleum distillates* Tech. piperonyl butoxide Pyrethrins		SATIN FLOW PAINT (Bauer)	
SASCO-SOL LIQUID BOWL CLEANER (S & S)	Hydrogen chloride* 23% Chlorinated benzene 2.0%		SATIN GLOSS FLOOR WAX (Uncle Sam)	Waxes Resins Ammonia Triethanolamine Oleic acid
SASCO STERITONE Disinfectant (S & S)	Soap Orthobenzyl parachlorophenol* Tetrasodium ethylene diamine tetraacetate*		SATINHIDE ENAMEL (Pittsburgh Plate Glass (Paint Div.))	
SASCO WHITEEN Liquid porcelain cleaner (S & S)			SATIN-KOTE PAINT (Old Colony)	
SA SHAMPOO (Simoniz)			SATINLAC Brushing lacquer (U.S. Plywood)	Lacquer solvents*
SASHAY MOTH CRYSTALS & DEODORANT (Hy-G)	Paradichlorobenzene* 99% Perfume 1%		SATINLAC FINISH (Breinig)	
SASOCO ODORLESS DISINFECT- ANT (Sanitary Soap)			SATIN LINE FLOOR FINISHER Polish (Germo)	
SASSO CLEANER (Worrell)			SATIN LUMINALL PAINT (National Chem. & Mfg.)	
SATE ARTERIAL Embalming fluid (Embalmers')	Formaldehyde*		SATIN LUSTRE BRAND PAINT (Longman)	
SATE CAVITY Embalming fluid (Embalmers')	Formaldehyde*		SATIN LUX ENAMEL (Patterson- Sargent)	
SATINA Bluing (Baker, F.)	Paraffin wax Hydrogenated oil Dye		SATIN SCENT COLOGNE, PERFUME & SKIN BALM (Wood, A.)	
SATINALL WALL COAT- ING (Red Spot)			SATINTONE FURNITURE POLISH (Rex Home)	
SATINETTE ENAMELS (Standard- Toch)			SATSUMA ENAMEL (Heath & Milligan)	
SATINEX EGGSHELL FINISH Paint (Pierce, F.O.)			SAVABRUSH Paint brush cleaner (Glidden Co.)	
SATIN FINISH PAINTS (O'Brein, F.)				

*Consult Sec. II., Ingredients Index. This ingredient may be responsible for major toxic effects if poisonous amounts of this product are ingested.

Name & Use Manufacturer	Ingredients		Name & Use Manufacturer	Ingredients	
SAVACK SALVE (Oliver's S-O)			SAVOGRAN KUTZIT PAINT & VARNISH REMOVER, KWIKEEZE LIQUID PAINT & BRUSH CLEANER (Savogran)	Toluol* Benzol* Methanol Acetone	
SAVAGE GUN GREASE (Savage Arms)	Petroleum derivative				
SAVAGE GUN OIL Lubricating oil (Savage Arms)	Petroleum fraction		SAVOGRAN PAINT BRUSH CLEANER (Savogran)	Non-caustic alkali material	
SAVAGE GUN SOLVENT Rifle bore cleaner (Savage Arms)	Paraffin oil Solvents*		SAVOGRAN REMOVER & BLEACHER (Savogran)	Sodium perborate*	
SAV-A-LOT WALLPAPER REMOVER (LePage's)			SAVOGRAN STRYPEEZE PAINT & VARNISH REMOVER (Savogran)	Toluol* Acetone Alcohol	
SA-VA-TREE Pruning paints (South Port)					
SA-VA-TREE Wound paint (Tyson)			SAVOL Purified bleach (Savol)	Sodium hypochlorite*	3%
SAVAWALL Paint (Chi-Namel)	Titanium dioxide Aluminum silicate Hydrated chromium oxide Emulsifiable synthetic resin Drier	18.60% 27.85% 0.15% 14.00% 1.00%	SAV-ON PINE ODOR DIS- INFECTANT (Uncle Sam)	Pine oil* Soap Synthetic phenols*	
			SAV-ON PINE SCRUB SOAP (Uncle Sam)	Vegetable oil soap	
SAVE-LITE FINISHES (Sherwin- Williams)			SAVOSS Counter- irritant (veterinary) (Troy Chem.)	Isopropy alcohol* Oil wormwood* Iodine* Camphor* Tar Cedar Pine* Turpentine distillates*	15%
SAN-O-FEC- 25 Disinfectant (Whitmoyer)	Alkyl tolyl methyl trimethyl ammonium chlorides* Ethylene diamine tetra-acetic acid Tetra sodium salt Trisodium phosphate* Sodium carbonate	25.5%			
			SAVOY SATIN ENAMEL (Phelan- Faust)		
SAVE THE BABY For colds and croup (Lee, W.)	Lard Canada balsam of fir* Oil of origanum* Oil of rosemary* Camphor* Alcohol	66% 8% 13% 2% 4% 6%	SAV-YOR-WAV HAIR POMADE (Fearonce)		
			SAW PALMETTO & NUX VOMICA COMPOUND (Lilly)	Alcohol Sabal Nux vomica Sandalwood Damiana Kola Potassium acetate	26% 13.15 gm. 0.21 cc. 6.15 gm. 6.15 gm. 6.15 gm. 1.75 gm.
SAV-IT Fungicide (Cuprinol)	Ortho-hydroxybenzanilide Inert ingredients*	1% 99%			
SAVOGRAN CRACK FILLER & WOOD PUTTY (Savogran)	Calcium sulfate Silica Vegetable binder Wood flour		SAWYER'S CRYSTAL BLUE Bluing (Sawyer)	Copperas* Yellow prussiate of soda Sulfuric acid* Nitric acid*	
SAVOGRAN HEAVY DUTY CLEANER (Savogran)			SAXIN BRAND SACCHARIN TABLETS Sweetening agent (Burroughs- Wellcome)	Saccharin	1/4 gr./tablet

*Consult Sec. II., Ingredients Index. This ingredient may be responsible for major toxic effects if poisonous amounts of this product are ingested.

Name & Use Manufacturer	Ingredients	
SAXOL OINTMENT For skin irritations (Chester-Kent)	Calamine Carbolic acid* Oil wintergreen (syn.) Petrolatum Sulfur* Resorcin* Lanolin	2%
SAXON ANALGESIC BALM (Royal Mfg.)	Menthol* Methyl salicylate* Benzocaine Lanolin	
SAXON AMMONIATED MERCURY OINTMENT 5% (Royal Pharm.)	Ammoniated mercury* 24 gr./oz.	
SAXON ANTACID POWDER (Royal Pharm.)	Bismuth subcarbonate Magnesium oxide Calcium carbonate Sodium bicarbonate	
SAXON A P C TABLETS Analgesic (Royal Pharm.)	Each tablet: Aspirin* Phenacetin* Caffeine	3-1/2 gr. 2-1/2 gr. 1/2 gr.
SAXON AQUEOUS NOSE DROPS (Royal Mfg.)	Ephedrine sulfate* Chlorbutanol	1% 0.5%
SAXON ASPIRIN FOR CHILDREN (Royal Pharm.)	Aspirin*	1-1/4 gr./tablet
SAXON ASTRINGENT GARGLE (Royal Mfg.)	Alcohol Zinc chloride* Methyl salicylate* Oil of cassia* Boric acid*	10%/v
SAXON ASTRINGENT MOUTH WASH (Royal Pharm.)	Alcohol Zinc chloride* Formalin Menthol* Oil of cassia*	3%/v
SAXON BABY COUGH SYRUP (Royal Mfg.)	Alcohol Extracts of white pine Wild cherry Aralia Poplar buds Blood root Sassafras Menthol	6%/v
SAXON BAY RUM (Royal Pharm.)	Alcohol	47%/v
SAXON BEAT THE HEAT SALT TABLETS (Royal Pharm.)	Sodium chloride Corn sugar Cornstarch	70% 30% 1%
SAXON BEEF, IRON & WINE N.F. Tonic, food supplement (Royal Pharm.)	Alcohol	21%/v

Name & Use Manufacturer	Ingredients	
SAXON-BLUE OINTMENT Ectoparasiticide (Royal Pharm.)	Mercury*	10%
SAXON BRONCHIAL LOZENGES (Royal Mfg.)	Powdered extract licorice Powdered cubeb Capsicum Menthol*	
SAXON BROWN MIXTURE N.F. Antitussive (Royal Pharm.)	Opium* Alcohol	1/5 gr./fl. oz. 10%/v
SAXON CARMINATIVE CORDIAL (Royal Mfg.)	Alcohol Fl. ext. ginger Fl. ext. blackberry Fl. ext. rhubarb	3%/v
SAXON CHLOROFORM LINIMENT U.S.P. (Royal Pharm.)	Alcohol* Chloroform*	45%/v 30%/v
SAXON COLLANA SYRUP Antitussive (Royal Mfg.)	Alcohol Cocillana Euphorbia Wild lettuce Squill Senega	5%/v
SAXON CORN OUTFIT (Royal Pharm.)	Alcohol Sulfuric ether* Collodion Salicylic acid*	13%/v 284 m./fl. oz.
SAXON DOBELL'S SOLUTION N.F. Alkaline detergent, nasal douche (Royal Pharm.)	Liquified phenol	0.3%/v
SAXON DOUCHE POWDER (Royal Pharm.)	Borax* Sodium bicarbonate Thymol* Menthol* Eucalyptol*	
SAXON DRY CLEANER (Royal Pharm.)		
SAXON ELIXIR TERPIN HYDRATE & CODEINE N.F. (Royal Pharm.)	Alcohol Codeine*	40%/v 1 gr./fl. oz.
SAXON EPHEDRINE NASAL JELLY Nasal decongestant (Royal Mfg.)	Ephedrine* Menthol* Camphor* Eucalyptol* Thymol*	1%
SAXON ESSENCE OF PEPPERMINT U.S.P. Carminative, gastric stimulant (Royal Pharm.)	Alcohol*	83%/v

*Consult Sec. II., Ingredients Index. This ingredient may be responsible for major toxic effects if poisonous amounts of this product are ingested.

Name & Use Manufacturer	Ingredients	
SAXON EYE WASH (Royal Pharm.)	Boric acid Berberine hydrochloride Camphor	
SAXON F.M.C. COUGH SYRUP (Royal Mfg.)	Alcohol Chloroform Extract of ipecac Lobelia Squill Aralia Euphorbia White pine Poplar buds Wild cherry Blood root Sassafras Menthol	8%/v 3 m./fl. oz.
SAXON FOOT POWDER (Royal Pharm.)	Salicylic acid* Paraformaldehyde Boric acid* Magnesium carbonate Menthol* Zinc stearate	
SAXON GERMICIDAL SOAP 1% (Royal Pharm.)	Mercuric iodide* Anhydrous soap	1% 85%
SAXON GLYCERI-NATED ROSE WATER For chapped skin (Royal Pharm.)	Alcohol	9%/v
SAXON ICHTHAMMOL OINTMENT 10% (Royal Mfg.)	Ichthammol N.F. Petroleum base	
SAXON KREOTUS COUGH SYRUP (Royal Pharm.)	Alcohol Chloroform Beechwood creosote Extract of white pine Wild cherry Aralia Poplar buds Blood root Sassafras Tar Menthol	6%/v 3 m./fl. oz.
SAXON LARKSPUR LOTION (Royal Pharm.)	Isopropyl alcohol* Alkaloids of larkspur seed Acetic acid	20%/v 0.01% 3.00%
SAXON LAXATIVE SAX-O-COL TABLETS (Royal Mfg.)	Each tablet: Phenacetin* Ext. belladonna leaves* (1/1600 gr. or belladonna alkaloids) Ext. hyoscyamus (1/1300 gr. or hyoscyamus alkaloids) Podophyllin Quinine sulfate* Powdered capsicum Cascarin	1 gr. 1/20 gr. 1/20 gr.
SAXON LAX-O-COL CAPSULES For colds (Royal Pharm.)	Acetophenetidin* Ext. belladonna Phenolphthalein Aspirin* Quinine sulfate Oleoresin capsicum	1 gr. 1/50 gr.

Name & Use Manufacturer	Ingredients	
SAXON MOSQUITO BITE LOTION (Royal Mfg.)	Alcohol* Oil of citronella*	70%/v
SAXON MOUTH WASH & GARGLE (Royal Pharm.)	Alcohol Boric acid* Thymol* Eucalyptol* Oil of thyme* Methyl salicylate* Menthol	24%/v
SAXON NASAL OIL WITH EPHEDRINE (Royal Mfg.)	Ephedrine* alkaloid Menthol* Eucalyptol* Camphor* Mineral oil base	
SAXON OIL BERGAMOT (Imitation) (Royal Pharm.)	Volatile oil	
SAXON POISON IVY LOTION (Royal Mfg.)	Isopropyl alcohol* Glycerin Aluminum hydrate Methyl salicylate*	26%/v
SAXON RAT, MOUSE & ROACH PASTE (Royal Pharm.)	Phosphorus*	2%
SAXON RECTAL SUP-POSITORIES Astringent (Royal Pharm.)	Instrain nutgalls Zinc oxide Ethyl-amino-benzoate Cocoa butter base	
SAXON RUBBING ALCOHOL COMPD. (Royal Pharm.)	Alcohol*	70%/v
SAXON TANNIC ACID JELLY For skin burns (Royal Pharm.)	Tannic acid Carbolic acid Glycerin base	5% 0.5%
SAXON T-B-C LOZENGES WITH CHLORO-PHYLL For throat irritations (Royal Pharm.)	Each lozenge: Tyrothricin Benzocaine Sorballyn (a chlorophyllin sorbalate)	2 mg. 5 mg. 5 mg.
SAXON TERPIN HYDRATE & CODEINE LOZENGES WITH CHLORO-PHYLL Antitussive (Royal Pharm.)	Each lozenge: Terpin hydrate Codeine sulfate Sodium copper chlorophyllin (100%)	70 mg. 2.5 mg. 1 mg.
SAXON TOOTHACHE GUM (Royal Mfg.)	Oil of cloves* Phenol* Camphor* Beechwood creosote*	

*Consult Sec. II., Ingredients Index. This ingredient may be responsible for major toxic effects if poisonous amounts of this product are ingested.

Name & Use Manufacturer	Ingredients	Name & Use Manufacturer	Ingredients
SAXON TOOTHACHE OUTFIT (Royal Pharm.)	Alcohol* 67%/v Chloroform* 24 m./fl. oz. Oil of cloves* Oil cassia* Tincture of iodine*	SAYWELL'S FLEA & LICE POWDER Insecticide (Saywell)	Exhausted pyrethrum other than pyrethrins 87.25% Sodium chloride 0.05% Iron oxide 0.05%
SAXON VAPORIZING SALVE For colds (Royal Mfg.)	Camphor* Oils of turpentine* Eucalyptus* Thyme* Cedar leaf* Juniper with menthol*	SAYWELL'S INSECT SPRAY (Saywell)	Petroleum distillates Aromatic petroleum derivative solvent* DDT 5% Beta butoxy beta' thiocyano diethyl ether*
SAXON WHITFIELD'S OINTMENT Fungicide (medical) (Royal Pharm.)	Salicylic acid* Benzoic acid* Petroleum base	SAYWELL'S RAT & MICE EXTERMI- NATOR (Saywell)	Red squill compound*
SAXON W.P.T. COUGH SYRUP (Royal Pharm.)	Alcohol 6%/v Chloroform 3 m./fl. oz. Extract of white pine Aralia Poplar buds Wild cherry Blood root Sassafras Tar Menthol	SAYWELL'S ROACH FOOD (Saywell)	Sodium fluoride* 50%
		SBS-50 CLEANER- SANITIZER (Sugar Beet)	Triton X-100 Hyamine 2389 (see quaternary ammonium compounds)*
SAX-O-RUB SCENTED Rubefacient (Royal Mfg.)	Isopropyl alcohol* 90%/v	SBS-60 CREAM DEODORANT SOAP (Sugar Beet)	Cellulose and alginate gums Lanolin Fatty acid-amide condensate type Soap compatible germicide (hexachlorophene or chlorinated xylenol* type)
SAYLAB RAT & MICE KILLER Rodenticide (Saywell)	Warfarin 3-(a-acetonylbenzyl)- 4-hydroxycoumarin 0.025%		
		SBS-20 EXTRA- FINE GRANU- LATED SKIN CLEANSER (Sugar Beet)	Soda soaps Corn meal Cob Rice hulls
SAYMAN LINIMENT (Sayman)	Iso-propyl alcohol* 65% Chloroform 26 m./fl. oz. Capsicum (cayenne pepper) Camphor* Oils of cloves* Turpentine* Camphor sassafrassy Sassafras artificial Ammonia Ammonium carbonate	SBS-222 FINE GRANULATED ALL-SOLUBLE BORAX HAND SOAP (Sugar Beet)	Soda soaps Granular borax*
		SBS-15 FINE GRANULATED SKIN CLEANSER (Sugar Beet)	Soda soaps Corn meal Cob Rice hulls
SAYMAN SALVE For skin irritations (Sayman)	Camphor* Boric acid* Petrolatum Zinc oxide Lanolin Hexachlorophene	SBS-49 GENERAL PURPOSE CLEANER (Sugar Beet)	Soda ash Modified (laundry) soap Ortho- and polyphosphates Cellulose gum Synthetic detergent (fatty acid amide condensate type)
SAYWELL'S ANT FOOD Insecticide (Saywell)	Sodium fluoride* 75%	SBS-221 HEAVY DUTY ALL- SOLUBLE BORAX HAND SOAP (Sugar Beet)	Soda soap Borax*
SAYWELL'S 10% DDT POWDER Insecticide (Saywell)	DDT* 10.00% Pyrethrins 0.08% Sesame oil extract 0.30% Petroleum hydrocarbons 3.00%		

*Consult Sec. II., Ingredients Index. This ingredient may be responsible for major toxic effects if poisonous amounts of this product are ingested.

Name & Use Manufacturer	Ingredients		Name & Use Manufacturer	Ingredients
SBS-11 SKIN CLEANSER (Sugar Beet)	Soda soaps Corn meal Cob Rice hulls		SCALPOMADE Hair preparation (George, G.O.)	
SBS-30 WATERLESS HAND CLEANSER (Sugar Beet)	Paraffin type hydrocarbon Fatty acid-alkolamine soap Synthetic detergent of the fatty acid-amide condensate type Polyglycol Lanolin Cellulose gum Titanox Perfume		SCALPOULTIS SHAMPOO (George, G.O.)	
			SCANDIA EYE TONE LOTION, FRICTION LOTION, EAU DE TOILETTE (Scandia)	
SCABISOL K9 Ectoparasiticide (veterinary) (Wilke)	Calcium polysulfide* 30% Calcium thiosulphate 2%			
SCALF'S INDIAN RIVER MEDICINE Tonic (Indian River)	Alcohol 8%/v Golden seal (Hydrastis) Poplar bark Red dogwood bark Black cehosh (Cimicifuga) Yellow dock (Rumex) Tag alder (Alnus) Pipsissewa (Chimapila) Lady's slipper (Cypripedium) Blue cehosh Spignet Canada snake root False unicorn Wild cherry bark Angelica root Indian turnip Boneset Burdock Sarsaparilla Senega Senna Glycerin Sodium benzoate Caramel Pink root Queen of the meadow Propylene glycol Salicylic acid* Water		DR. SCAT CLEANSING CREAM (Scat)	
			S.C.C. LIQUID CLEANER CONCENTRATE (Solvit)	Liquid wetting agents* Complex phosphates*
			SCHALK'S DOUBLE X FLOOR CLEANER (Schalk)	Trisodium phosphate*
			SCHALK'S SAVABRUSH Brush cleaner (Schalk)	Trisodium phosphate*
			SCHALK'S WAXOFF Removes old wax (Schalk)	Trisodium phosphate*
			DR. SCHECHTER'S GRAY HAIR COLORING (Schechter)	
SCALPADE HAIR TONIC Checks dandruff (Binday)	Alcohol 60% Salicylic acid* Resorcinol* monoacetate Oleum ricini			
SCALPADE SHAMPOO Dandruff remover (Binday)	Oil of cade* Tr. green soap			
SCALP LOTION (Laird)				
SCALPO Scalp ointment (Caldo)	Ammoniated mercury* 1% Colloidal sulfur 1% Salicylic acid* 3%			

*Consult Sec. II., Ingredients Index. This ingredient may be responsible for major toxic effects if poisonous amounts of this product are ingested.

- 924 -

Name & Use Manufacturer	Ingredients
DR. SCHENCK'S MANDRAKE PILLS Cathartic (Schenck)	Aloes* (aloin) podophyllum* Colocynth* Capsicum
SCHERK FACE LOTION, PERFUMES & TOILET WATER (Scherk)	
DR. R. SCHIFFMANN'S ASTHMADOR Bronchial antispasmodic (Schiffmann)	Stramonium* Belladonna*
DR. R. SCHIFFMANN'S ASTHMADOR CIGARETTS Bronchial antispasmodic (Schiffmann)	Stramonium* Belladonna*
SCHLOTTER-BECK'S COMPOUND MIXTURE HYDRASTIS Digestant, for gastric irritation (Schlotterbeck)	Each fl. oz.: Golden seal* N.F. 30.57 gr. Rhubarb root 1.86 gr. Pepsin 2.02 gr. Potassium carbonate 1.86 gr. Traces of cinnamon, oil of peppermint; hydrochloric acid U.S.P.; glac. acetic acid, U.S.P.; tartaric acid; bicarbonate of soda Alcohol 26%
SCHLOTTER-BECK'S CORN SOLUTION Keratolytic (Schlotterbeck)	Salicylic acid* Collodion Alcohol 24% Ether* 72%
SCHLOTTER-BECK'S COMPOUND MIXTURE HELONIN Antispasmodic and uterine sedative (Schlotterbeck)	Ext. helonias (false unicorn root 4.6-1) 2.3 gr. Ext. senecio (life root 7.3-1) 3.4 gr. Ext. avena sativa (cultivated white oats, 400-1) 0.25 gr. Alcohol 34%
SCHLOTTER-BECK'S COMPOUND MIXTURE HYDRASTIS A bitter stomachic (Schlotterbeck)	Each fl. oz.: Golden seal, N.F. 30.57 gr. Rhubarb root 1.86 gr. Pepsin 2.02 gr. Potassium carbonate 1.86 gr. Alcohol 26%
SCHLOTTER-BECK'S COMPOUND SYRUP MANGANESE Tonic (Schlotterbeck)	Hypophosphites of manganese, calcium, sodium and potassium Lactate iron Quinine Alcohol 3% Strychnine 1/8 gr./oz.
SCHLOTTER-BECK'S COMP. SYR. PHOSPHO-CHLORIDE IRON Food supplement with iron (Schlotterbeck)	Tincture chloride iron Phosphoric acid* 9% Alcohol* Lime juice Sugar
SCHLOTTER-BECK'S SOL. HYPO-PHOSPHATES OF LIME & SODA Food supplement (Schlotterbeck)	Each oz.: Combined hypophosphites of lime and soda 30 gr. Alcohol 3%
SCHOENFIELD TEA Laxative, diuretic (Pfeiffer)	Senna Buckthorn Juniper berries Dog grass Uva ursi Fennel Anise Sassafras Licorice Orange peel
DR. SCHOLL'S BROMIDRO-SIS POWDER (Scholl)	Aluminum acetate Formaldehyde* Salicylic acid* Boric acid*
DR. SCHOLL'S CHLOROPHYLL FOOT LOTION (Scholl)	Isopropyl alcohol* Chlorophyll Menthol*
DR. SCHOLL'S CHLOROPHYLL FOOT POWDER (Scholl)	Aluminum chlorhydroxide Chlorophyllin Zinc stearate
DR. SCHOLL'S CORN SALVE (Scholl)	Salicylic acid* Oil of eucalyptus*
DR. SCHOLL'S FOOT BALM (Scholl)	Lanolin Methyl salicylate* Camphor* Menthol* Oil of eucalyptus* Zinc oxide
DR. SCHOLL'S FOOT LOTION (Scholl)	Alcohol* Menthol* Boric acid*
DR. SCHOLL'S FOOT POWDER Fungicide (medical) (Scholl)	Salicylic acid* Boric acid* Methyl salicylate*
DR. SCHOLL'S HALLUXOL For application to big toe joint (Scholl)	Benzoic acid* Glycerin Menthol* Camphor * Boric acid* Salicylic acid* Urea Alcohol*

*Consult Sec. II., Ingredients Index. This ingredient may be responsible for major toxic effects if poisonous amounts of this product are ingested.

Name & Use Manufacturer	Ingredients		Name & Use Manufacturer	Ingredients	
DR. SCHOLL'S LIGTONE Rubefacient (Scholl)	Alcohol* Aconite extract* Belladonna extract* Thymol* Camphor* Menthol*		SCOOT ARGENTINE ANT POISON (Lyons, I.L.)	Sodium arsenate* Tartar emetic*	3.98% 3.34%
DR. SCHOLL'S LIQUID CORN & CALLOUS REMOVER Corn & callous remedy (Scholl)			SCORPIOCIDE Insecticide (Lien)	Petroleum distillate* DDT* tech. Piperonyl butoxide tech. Methylated naphthalene* Chlordane tech.* Pyrethrins	
DR. SCHOLL'S ONIXOL Toe-nail and calloused nail groove softener (Scholl)	Sodium sulfide* Urea Triethanolamine		SCOTT'S LAWN FOOD PLUS WEED CONTROL (Scott, O.M.)	2,4-D*	
DR. SCHOLL'S PRESTO Astringent for feet (Scholl)	Alcohol* Salicylic acid* Benzoic acid* Thymol*		SCOTT'S PEST CONTROL (Scott, O.M.)	Tech. chlordane* Related compounds	9.00%
DR. SCHOLL'S SHOE DEODORIZER & FUNGICIDE (Scholl)	Isopropanol* Phenol (less than 1%) Formaldehyde*		SCOTT'S RECTAL OINTMENT (Auto-Loks)		
DR. SCHOLL'S SOLVES (Liquid) Fungicide, external (Medical) (Scholl)	Alcohol* 47% Benzoic acid* Salicylic acid* Thymol*		SCOTT'S 4-XD WEED CONTROL (Scott, O.M.)	Alkanolamine salts of 2,4-D dichlorophenoxyacetic acid 2.65%	
DR. SCHOLL'S 2-DROP CORN & CALLOUS REMOVER (Scholl)	Flexible collodion Salicylic acid* Camphor* Ether* Alcohol		SCOTT'S WEED & FEED (Scott, O.M.)	2,4-Dichloro phenoxy acetic acid 1%	
			SCRAM Insecticide (Curran)	Paradichlorobenzene* 100%	
SCHRAM'S BABY SUNTAN OIL (Schram)	Menthyl anthranilate* Oxyquinoline benzoate Mineral oil		SCRAM DOG REPELLENT (Calif. Spray)	Liquid animal bone oil 8%	
SCHUESSLER'S TRITURATED TISSUE SALTS 1 HOMEOPATHIC For nervousness (Boericke & Runyon)	Kali phosphoricum 3 x Calcarea phosphorica 3 x Magnesia phosphorica 3 x		SCRATCHEX, DR. MERRICK'S Dog powder (Westchester)	Gamma isomer of benzene hexachloride (from lindane) 1.00% Hexachlorophene 0.50% Mercaptobenzothiazole 1.50% Boric acid 3.00% Propylene glycol 3.00% Essential oil 0.20%	
SCIENCE PRODUCTS ARAMITE-15 W Insecticide Red spider (Science)	2-p-tert-Butyl phenoxy isopropyl-2-chloroethyl sulfite 15%		SC SOLVENT NO. 2 (Central Solv.)	Aromatic hydrocarbons* 75% Aliphatic hydrocarbons 25%	
			SCUFFY SHOE POLISH (Quinn)	Wax Soap Isopropanol* White pigment Starch	
SCIENOL Hemorrhoidal suppositories (G. & W.)	Istrian nutgalls Zinc oxide Ethyl aminobenzoate Cocoa butter base		SCUTL Herbicide (Scott, O.M.)	Mercury 0.25% n-1-Naphthyl phthalamic acid 0.24%	
			SEA BREEZE ANTISEPTIC AID FOR THE SKIN (Sea Breeze)	Alcohol 43%/v Gum camphor* Oil of peppermint Oil of cloves* Benzoic acid Eugenol* Oil of eucalyptus* Boric acid*	

Name & Use Manufacturer	Ingredients
SEAFORTH MEN'S TALC (McKelvy)	Cosmetic talc Inert mineral pigment Kaolin Zinc stearate Boric acid less than 2% Perfume oil Light magnesium carbonate
SEAFORTH SHAVE LOTION (McKelvy)	Alcohol 57% Menthol and benzoic acid less than 1-1/2%
SEAGULL Cesspool cleaner (Metropolitan)	Sodium hydroxide* composition
SEA LAC LACQUER THINNER (Duralac)	
SEAL COAT (Holcomb)	Mineral spirits* High flash naphtha*
SEAL COTE #279 (Durlin)	Nitrocellulose Colorless synthetic resin Dibutyl phthalate Ethyl acetate* Butyl acetate* Naphtha* fraction
SEAL-COTE NAIL & POLISH PROTECTOR (Howe & Co.)	
SEALER WOOD PRESERVATIVE (Breinig)	Linseed oil Pentachlorophenol* Mineral spirits*
SEAL REMOVER (Holcomb)	Methylene chloride*

SEAL RITE CAULKING COMPOUND (Seal Rite)	Styrenated alkyd resin and
	  chlorinated biphenyl
	           40%
	Titanium dioxide, calcium
	  carbonate and asbestos
	  fiber 40%
	Xylol* 20%

SEAL RITE EXTERIOR SUPERWHITE HOUSEPAINT (Seal Rite)	White lead* 5% Zinc oxide 15%

SEAL RITE PAINTS (Seal Rite)	Linseed, soybean, or fish
	  oil and/or alkyd resin
	           40%
	Titanium dioxide, calcium
	  carbonate and magnesium
	  silicate 40%
	Petroleum spirits* 20%
	Cobalt, manganese, lead and
	  calcium less than 1%

SEAL-TOX Wood preservative (Forman, Ford)	Pentachlorophenol* 5%

Name & Use Manufacturer	Ingredients
SEAL-TOX, INDUSTRIAL Wood preservative (Forman, Ford)	Pentachlorophenol * 3% Chlor-ortho-phenyl phenol* 2%
SEAL TREAT Wood preservative (King Chemical)	Pentachlorophenol* 5.20% Petroleum hydrocarbons* 81.80% Water repellents 13%
SEAL-TREAT PENTA Wood preservative (King Chemical)	Pentachlorophenol* 5.20% Petroleum hydrocarbons* 81.80%
SEAMSEAL #90 & #540 (Ferdinand)	Combinations of fillers ground into drying oil.
SEAPROOF ANTI-FOULING Paint (Balto. Copper)	
SEARS ROEBUCK FINE GRAIN DEVELOPER NO. 6813 Photographic supply (Tower)	
SEA & SKI TANNING CREAM (Rolley)	Glyceryl p-aminobenzoate Carbitol Triethylolamine Sesame oil Lanolin Stearic acid Glycerin U.S.P. Dye certified
SEA TRIED MARINE ENAMELS (Glidden Co.)	
SEBA-NIL for cleansing skin (Texas Pharm.)	Fat solvent Detergent Mild astringent
SEBASOL Antiseptic skin ointment (Comate)	Sulfur Sodium phenolsulfonate Resorcinol* Non-greasy base

SEBASOL GERMICIDAL SOAP (Comate)	Hexachlorophene (bis-(3,5,6-
	  trichloro-2-hydroxy phenyl)
	  methane)
	Sulfur
	Soap base

SEBORDERM For skin and scalp (Travine)	Isopropanol* 74%/v Colorless fractions of coal tar Salicylic acid 1% Resorcinol* 4% Essential oils *

*Consult Sec. II., Ingredients Index. This ingredient may be responsible for major toxic effects if poisonous amounts of this product are ingested.

Name & Use Manufacturer	Ingredients	Name & Use Manufacturer	Ingredients
SEBOROL OINTMENT & SCALP LOTION (Glenn Prod.)		SECURITY BRAND ALDRIN EQUIVALENT 25-D DUST CONCENTRATE COMP. 118 Insecticide (Woolfolk)	Hexachloro hexahydro dimethano naphthalene* 23.750% Related compounds 17.915%
SEB-O-SOL S.F. NO. 905 Face cleanser (Specialists)	Di-ethylhexyl sodium sulfosuccinate		
S.E.C. ENAMELERS (Santee)		SECURITY BRAND ANTIROT Fungicide, insecticide (Woolfolk)	Pentachlorophenol* 4.4% Other chlorophenols 0.6%
SECRET GARDEN COLOGNES, TOILET WATERS & PERFUMES (Mann, Leo)	Aromatics and essential oils* Ethyl alcohol*	SECURITY BRAND ANTIROT 10X CONCENTRATE Wood pres. (Woolfolk)	Pentachlorophenol* 37.1% Other chlorophenols 5.1%
S.E.C. ROOF PAINT (Louisville Paint)		SECURITY BRAND BENZEX Insecticide (Woolfolk)	Gamma isomer of benzene hexachloride* 6.0% Other isomers of benzene hexachloride* 30.0%
SECURITY BRAND 2-1/2-10-40 ALDRIN-DDT-SULPHUR Insecticide (Woolfolk)	Hexachloro hexahydro-endo, exo-dimethano naphthalene* 2.38% Related compounds 1.79% Dichloro diphenyl trichloroethane* 10.00% Sulfur* 40.00%	SECURITY BRAND BENZEX 10 Insecticide (Woolfolk)	Gamma isomer of benzene hexachloride* 10.0% Other isomers of benzene hexachloride* 50.0%
SECURITY BRAND 2-1/2% ALDRIN EQUIVALENT COTTON DUST Insecticide (Woolfolk)	Hexachloro hexahydro dimethano naphthalene* 2.375% Related compounds 1.791%	SECURITY BRAND BORDEAUX MIXTURE Fungicide (Woolfolk)	Copper* as metallic 12.5% Zinc as metallic 10.0%
SECURITY BRAND 2-1/2% ALDRIN EQUIV. WITH 10% COTTON DUST Insecticide (Woolfolk)	Hexachloro hexahydro dimethano naphthalene* 2.375% Related compounds 1.791% DDT (dichloro diphenyl trichloroethane)* 10.00%	SECURITY BRAND CATTLE GRUB DUST Insecticide (Woolfolk)	Rotenone 1.5% Other cube or derris resins 3.0%
		SECURITY BRAND 36% CHLORDANE Insecticide (Woolfolk)	Tech. chlordane * 36.0%
SECURITY BRAND 2-1/2% ALDRIN EQUIV. WITH 5% DDT COTTON DUST Insecticide (Woolfolk)	Hexachloro hexahydro dimethano naphthalene* 2.375% Related compounds 1.791% DDT (dichloro diphenyl trichloroethane) 5.000%	SECURITY BRAND 75% CHLORDANE Insecticide (Woolfolk)	Tech. chlordane* 75.0%
		SECURITY BRAND 5% CHLORDANE DUST Insecticide (Woolfolk)	Tech. chlordane* 5.0%
SECURITY BRAND 2-1/2% ALDRIN EQUIVALENT 5% DDT-40% SULPHUR Insecticide (Woolfolk)	Hexachloro hexahydro dimethano naphthalene* 2.375% Related compounds 1.791% DDT (dichloro diphenyl trichloroethane) 5.000% Sulfur* as elemental 40.000%	SECURITY BRAND 10% CHLORDANE DUST Insecticide (Woolfolk)	Tech. chlordane* 10.0% Sulfur* 40.00%

*Consult Sec. II., Ingredients Index. This ingredient may be responsible for major toxic effects if poisonous amounts of this product are ingested.

- 928 -

Name & Use Manufacturer	Ingredients		Name & Use Manufacturer	Ingredients	
SECURITY BRAND 10% CHLORDANE GRANULAR Insecticide (Woolfolk)	Tech. chlordane*	10.0%	SECURITY BRAND 3-5-40 COTTON DUST BHC-DDT-SULPHUR Insecticide (Woolfolk)	Gamma isomer of benzene hexachloride* 3.0% Other isomers of benzene hexachloride 15.0% DDT (dichloro diphenyl trichloro-ethane)* 5.0% Sulfur* 40.0%	
SECURITY BRAND 40% CHLORDANE WETTABLE Insecticide (Woolfolk)	Tech. chlordane*	40.0%	SECURITY BRAND 3-10-40 COTTON DUST BHC-DDT-SULPHUR Insecticide (Woolfolk)	Gamma isomer of benzene hexachloride* 3.0% Other isomers of benzene hexachloride 15.0% DDT (dichloro diphenyl trichloroethane)* 10.0% Sulfur* 40.0%	
SECURITY BRAND CHLORO 1-P-C Herbicide (Woolfolk)	Isopropyl n-3-chlorophenyl carbamate*	45.0%	SECURITY BRAND 1-1/2-5-0 COTTON DUST-DIELDRIN-DDT Insecticide (Woolfolk)	Hexachloro epoxy octahydro-endo, exo-dimethano naphtha-lene* 1.275% Related compounds 0.225% DDT (dichloro diphenyl trichloroethane)* 5.000%	
SECURITY BRAND CONDITIONED FLOUR SULPHUR Fungicide (Woolfolk)	Sulfur*	94%			
SECURITY BRAND COPPER SULPHATE SNOW CRYSTALS Fungicide (Woolfolk)	Copper sulfate*	99.0%	SECURITY BRAND 1-1/2-10-0 COTTON DUST-DIELDRIN-DDT Insecticide (Woolfolk)	Hexachloro epoxy octahydro-endo, exo-dimethano naphthalene* 1.275% Related compounds 0.225% DDT (dichloro diphenyl trichloroethane*) 10.000%	
SECURITY BRAND 20-40 COTTON DUST Insecticide (Woolfolk)	Toxaphene* 20.00% Sulfur 40.00%		SECURITY BRAND C-S-C DUST Fungicide, insecticide (Woolfolk)	Sodium aluminum fluoride* 45.0% Copper as metallic 10.0%	
SECURITY BRAND 3-5-0 COTTON DUST BHC-DDT Insecticide (Woolfolk)	Gamma isomer of benzene hexachloride* 3.0% Other isomers of benzene hexachloride 15.0% DDT (dichloro diphenyl trichloroethane)* 5.0%		SECURITY BRAND D-98 Insecticide (Woolfolk)	Petroleum oil *	98.0%
SECURITY BRAND 3-10-0 COTTON DUST BHC-DDT Insecticide (Woolfolk)	Gamma isomer of benzene hexachloride* 3.0% Other isomers of benzene hexachloride 15.0% DDT (dichloro diphenyl trichloro-ethane)* 10.0%		SECURITY BRAND 5% 3D's DUST Insecticide (Woolfolk)	DDD (dichloro diphenyl dichloro-ethane) 5.0%	
SECURITY BRAND 3-5-1 COTTON DUST BHC-DDT-PARATHION Insecticide (Woolfolk)	Parathion * 1.0% Gamma isomer of benzene hexachloride 3.0% Other isomers of benzene hexachloride 15.0% DDT (dichloro diphenyl trichloroethane) 5.0%		SECURITY BRAND 10% 3D's DUST DDD-TDE Insecticide (Woolfolk)	DDD (dichloro diphenyl dichloroethane) 10.0%	
			SECURITY BRAND 25% 3D's EMULSIFIABLE LIQUID Insecticide (Woolfolk)	DDD (dichloro diphenyl dichloroethane) 25.0% Aromatic petroleum derivative solvent* 73.0%	

*Consult Sec. II., Ingredients Index. This ingredient may be responsible for major toxic effects if poisonous amounts of this product are ingested.

Name & Use Manufacturer	Ingredients	Name & Use Manufacturer	Ingredients
SECURITY BRAND 50% 3D's WETTABLE Insecticide (Woolfolk)	DDD (dichloro diphenyl dichloroethane)* 50.0%	SECURITY BRAND 10% DIELDRIN GRANULAR Insecticide (Woolfolk)	Hexachloro epoxy octahydro dimethano naphthalene* 8.5% Related compounds 1.5%
SECURITY BRAND 25% DDT Insecticide (Woolfolk)	DDT (dichloro diphenyl trichloroethane)* 25.00%	SECURITY BRAND DIELDRIN-SOL Insecticide (Woolfolk)	Hexachloro epoxy octahydro-endo, exo-dimethano naphthalene* 15.1% Related compounds 2.4% Petroleum hydrocarbons 75.8%
SECURITY BRAND 50% DDT Insecticide (Woolfolk)	DDT (dichloro diphenyl trichloroethane*) 50.0%	SECURITY BRAND 25% DIELDRIN WETTABLE Insecticide (Woolfolk)	Hexachloro epoxy octahydro-endo, exo-dimethano naphthalene* 21.3% Related compounds 3.8%
SECURITY BRAND 5% DDT DUST Insecticide (Woolfolk)	DDT (dichloro diphenyl trichloroethane)* 5.0%	SECURITY BRAND DIMOLE SPRAY Fungicide (Woolfolk)	Ferric dimethyl dithio-carbamate* 45.0% Salicylic acid* 15.0%
SECURITY BRAND 10% DDT DUST Insecticide (Woolfolk)	DDT (dichloro-diphenyl trichloroethane)* 10.00%	SECURITY BRAND DIWEEVIL Fumigant (Woolfolk)	Ethylene dichloride 75% Carbon tetrachloride* 25%
SECURITY BRAND 25% DDT DUST Insecticide (Woolfolk)	DDT* 25.00%	SECURITY BRAND DRIN-SOL Insecticide (Woolfolk)	Hexachloro hexahydro dimethano naphthalene* 22.00% Related compounds 16.50% Xylene* 51.50%
SECURITY BRAND 5% DDT SOLUTION Insecticide (Woolfolk)	DDT (dichloro diphenyl trichloroethane*) 5.0% Petroleum hydrocarbons* 95.0%	SECURITY BRAND DRIN-SOL-DDT Insecticide (Woolfolk)	Hexachloro hexahydro dimethano naphthalene* 10.75% Related compounds 8.00% DDT (dichloro diphenyl trichloroethane) 23.00% Xylene* 48.25%
SECURITY BRAND 5% DDT-85% SULPHUR DUST Insecticide (Woolfolk)	DDT (dichloro diphenyl trichloroethane)* 5.0% Sulfur* as elemental 85.0%	SECURITY BRAND ENDRI-SOL Insecticide (Woolfolk)	Hexachloro epoxy octahydro-endo, endo-dimethano naphthalene* 19.5% Petroleum hydrocarbons 70.5%
SECURITY BRAND 10% DDT-75% SULPHUR DUST Insecticide (Woolfolk)	DDT (dichloro diphenyl trichloroethane)* 10.0% Sulfur* 75.0%	SECURITY BRAND FERBAM DUST Fungicide (Woolfolk)	Ferbam 11.4%
SECURITY BRAND DI-CHLOR-MULSION Insecticide (Woolfolk)	Ethylene dichloride* 90.0%	SECURITY BRAND 15% FERMATE DUST Fungicide (Woolfolk)	Ferbam 10.5%
SECURITY BRAND 2-1/2-10-0 DIELDRIN DUST-DDT Insecticide (Woolfolk)	Hexachloro epoxy octahydro-endo, exo-dimethano naphthalene* 2.125% Related compounds 0.375% DDT (dichloro diphenyl trichloroethane)* 10.000%	SECURITY BRAND 3% GAMMA BHC DUST Insecticide (Woolfolk)	Gamma isomer of benzene hexachloride* 3.0% Other isomers of benzene hexachloride 15.0%

Name & Use Manufacturer	Ingredients	
SECURITY BRAND 2-1/2-5-1 HEPTACHLOR Insecticide (Woolfolk)	Heptachlor Related compounds DDT (dichloro diphenyl trichloroethane) Parathion*	2.50% 0.95% 5.00% 1.00%
SECURITY BRAND 2-1/2-5-0 HEPTACHLOR COTTON DUST Insecticide (Woolfolk)	Heptachlor* Related compounds DDT (dichloro diphenyl trichloroethane)*	2.50% 0.95% 5.00%
SECURITY BRAND 2-1/2-5-40 HEPTACHLOR COTTON DUST Insecticide (Woolfolk)	Heptachlor* Related compounds DDT (dichloro diphenyl trichloroethane)* Sulfur*	2.50% 0.95% 5.00% 40.00%
SECURITY BRAND 2-1/2-10-0 HEPTACHLOR COTTON DUST Insecticide (Woolfolk)	Heptachlor* Related compounds DDT (dichloro diphenyl trichloroethane)*	2.50% 0.95% 10.00%
SECURITY BRAND 2-1/2-10-40 HEPTACHLOR COTTON DUST Insecticide (Woolfolk)	Heptachlor* Related compounds DDT (dichloro diphenyl trichloroethane)* Sulfur*	2.50% 0.95% 10.00% 40.00%
SECURITY BRAND 2-1/2 HEPTACHLOR DUST Insecticide (Woolfolk)	Heptachlor* Related compounds	2.50% 0.97%
SECURITY BRAND HEPTA-SOL Insecticide (Woolfolk)	Heptachlor* Related compounds Petroleum hydrocarbons	22.2% 8.6% 62.4%
SECURITY BRAND HEX-SOL Insecticide (Woolfolk)	Gamma isomer of benzene hexachloride* Other isomers of benzene hexachloride DDT (dichloro diphenyl trichloroethane)*	10.0% 17.8% 15.5%
SECURITY BRAND KRYAX DUST Insecticide (Woolfolk)	Sodium aluminum fluoride* Sulfur	45.00% 25.00%
SECURITY BRAND LEAD ARSENATE Insecticide (Woolfolk)	Dry lead arsenate*	98.0%

Name & Use Manufacturer	Ingredients	
SECURITY BRAND 0-10-90 LEAD ARSENATE (LIME) DUST Insecticide (Woolfolk)	Lead arsenate*	9.50%
SECURITY BRAND LIME SULPHUR SOLUTION 32° Be Insecticide (Woolfolk)	Calcium polysulfide*	30.0%
SECURITY BRAND 20% LINDANE Insecticide (Woolfolk)	Gamma isomer of benzene hexachloride* Aromatic petroleum derivative solvent*	20.0% 31.0%
SECURITY BRAND 1% LINDANE DUST Insecticide (Woolfolk)	Gamma isomer of benzene hexachloride (lindane)	1.0%
SECURITY BRAND 25% LINDANE WETTABLE Insecticide (Woolfolk)	Gamma isomer of benzene hexachloride*	25.0%
SECURITY BRAND 50% MALATHON Insecticide (Woolfolk)	Malathion*	50.0%
SECURITY BRAND 5% MALATHION DUST Insecticide (Woolfolk)	Malathion*	5.0%
SECURITY BRAND MEXIDE DUST Insecticide (Woolfolk)	Rotenone Other cube resins Sulfur*	0.75% 1.50% 25.00%
SECURITY BRAND MOP-N-MIX Insecticide (Woolfolk)	Calcium arsenate*	34.6%
SECURITY BRAND NUTONEX WETTABLE SULPHUR Fungicide, insecticide (Woolfolk)	Sulfur*	94.0%
SECURITY BRAND OIL EMULSION 66-2/3% Insecticide (Woolfolk)	Petroleum oil * Anhydrous soap	64.0% 1.0%

*Consult Sec. II., Ingredients Index. This ingredient may be responsible for major toxic effects if poisonous amounts of this product are ingested.

Name & Use Manufacturer	Ingredients	
SECURITY BRAND ORNAMENTAL SPRAY OIL Insecticide (Woolfolk)	Petroleum oil *	97.0%
SECURITY BRAND PAN APPLE SPRAY Fungicide, insecticide (Woolfolk)	Lead arsenate* Sulfur Copper Zinc	14.8% 41.0% 3.5% 5.0%
SECURITY BRAND PAN APPLE SPRAY Fungicide, Insecticide (Woolfolk)	Parathion* Dichloro diphenyl trichloro- ethane Ferbam	3.75% 12.50% 35.00%
SECURITY BRAND PAN PEACH SPRAY Fungicide, insecticide (Woolfolk)	Zinc Sulfur Lead arsenate*	9.6% 34.0% 11.5%
SECURITY BRAND PAN PLANT SPRAY Insecticide (Woolfolk)	Lead arsenate Sulfur Copper Zinc Nicotine *	9.0% 28.0% 10.0% 4.0% 2.8%
SECURITY BRAND PAN-THION Insecticide (Woolfolk)	Parathion* Zinc Sulfur	1.8% 11.2% 39.3%
SECURITY BRAND 1% PARATHION- 5% DDT DUST Insecticide (Woolfolk)	Dichloro diphenyl trichloro- ethane Parathion*	5.0% 1.0%
SECURITY BRAND 1% PARATHION- 10% DDT DUST Insecticide (Woolfolk)	Dichloro diphenyl trichloro- ethane Parathion*	10.0% 1.0%
SECURITY BRAND PARATHION 1% DUST Insecticide (Woolfolk)	Parathion*	1.0%
SECURITY BRAND 25% PARATHION EMULSIFIABLE CONCEN- TRATE Insecticide (Woolfolk)	Parathion*	25.0%
SECURITY BRAND 2-6 PARATHION- SULPHUR PEACH SPRAY Insecticide (Woolfolk)	Parathion* Sulfur	3.75% 76.25%

Name & Use Manufacturer	Ingredients	
SECURITY BRAND PARATHION 25W Insecticide (Woolfolk)	Parathion*	25.00%
SECURITY BRAND 15% PARATHION WETTABLE Insecticide (Woolfolk)	Parathion*	15.0%
SECURITY BRAND PARIS GREEN Insecticide (Woolfolk)	Copper aceto arsenite*	85.4%
SECURITY BRAND 80- 5-15 PEACH DUST Insecticide (Woolfolk)	Sulfur Lead arsenate*	75.0% 4.7%
SECURITY BRAND PEANUT DUST Insecticide (Woolfolk)	Sulfur* Copper Toxaphene*	65.00% 3.40% 10.00%
SECURITY BRAND PINK DUSTING SULPHUR Fungicide (Woolfolk)	Sulfur*	87.00%
SECURITY BRAND PIPERONYL BUTOXIDE- PYRETHRIN EMULSIFI- ABLE CONCEN- TRATE Insecticide (Woolfolk)	Tech. piperonyl butoxide Pyrethrin Emulsifying agent Petroleum oils	39.17% 3.92% 41.24% 15.67%
SECURITY BRAND POWDERED CUBE Insecticide (Woolfolk)	Rotenone* Other cube resins	5.00% 10.00%
SECURITY BRAND PYFOS TEPP Insecticide (Woolfolk)	Tetraethyl pyrophosphate* Other ethyl phosphates	40.0% 59.0%
SECURITY BRAND ROACH KILLER Insecticide (Woolfolk)	Tech. chlordane Petroleum distillate*	2.5% 97.5%
SECURITY BRAND ROSE DUST Fungicide, insecticide (Woolfolk)	Sulfur* Copper* Dichloro diphenyl trichloro- ethane* Gamma isomer of benzene hexachloride (lindane)	75.0% 5.2% 5.0% 1.0%

*Consult Sec. II., Ingredients Index. This ingredient may be responsible for major toxic effects if poisonous amounts of this product are ingested.

Name & Use Manufacturer	Ingredients	
SECURITY BRAND 1% ROTENONE DUST Insecticide (Woolfolk)	Rotenone Other cube resins	1.00% 2.00%
SECURITY BRAND 1%-25% ROTENONE-SULPHUR DUST Insecticide (Woolfolk)	Rotenone Other cube resins Sulfur*	1.00% 2.00% 25.00%
SECURITY BRAND SABANE DUST Insecticide (Woolfolk)	Sabadilla alkaloids derived from 20% sab. seed	0.8%
SECURITY BRAND SCREW-WORM REMEDY Insecticide (Woolfolk)	Gamma isomer of benzene hexachloride (lindane)* Pine oil* Mineral oil	3.00% 35.00% 42.00%
SECURITY BRAND SECURITY POISON Insecticide (Woolfolk)	Tricalcium arsenate*	56.00%
SECURITY BRAND STOCK SPRAY Insecticide (Woolfolk)	Dichloro diphenyl trichloro-ethane*	50%
SECURITY BRAND 90-10 SULPHUR-COPPER DUST Fungicide (Woolfolk)	Sulfur* Copper*	84.60% 3.40%
SECURITY BRAND 3-WAY TOBACCO DUST Insecticide (Woolfolk)	Dichloro diphenyl dichloro-ethane Parathion*	10.00% 1.00%
SECURITY BRAND TOMATO DUST Insecticide (Woolfolk)	Tri-calcium arsenate* Copper as metallic	60.0% 7.0%
SECURITY BRAND TOXAPHENE-DDT 4-2 Insecticide (Woolfolk)	Toxaphene* Dichloro diphenyl trichloro-ethane	38.5% 19.0%
SECURITY BRAND 10% TOXAPHENE DUST Insecticide (Woolfolk)	Technical chlorinated camphene*	10.0%

Name & Use Manufacturer	Ingredients	
SECURITY BRAND TOX-SOL-6 Insecticide (Woolfolk)	Toxaphene*	58.5%
SECURITY BRAND TRI-KAL DUST #20 Insecticide (Woolfolk)	Copper Tri-calcium arsenate*	7.0% 14.0%
SECURITY BRAND TRIKOP Fungicide (Woolfolk)	Copper*	25.00%
SECURITY BRAND WATERMELON DUST Fungicide, insecticide (Woolfolk)	Copper*	6%
SECURITY BRAND 40% WETTABLE TOXAPHENE Insecticide (Woolfolk)	Toxaphene*	40.0%
SECURITY BRAND ZINK-O-DUST Fungicide, insecticide (Woolfolk)	Sulfur Lead arsenate* Zinc	76.00% 4.55% 3.00%
SECURITY BRAND 80-0-20 ZINK-O-DUST Fungicide, insecticide (Woolfolk)	Zinc * Sulfur*	4.00% 79.00%
SECURITY BRAND ZINC-O-DUST 80-10-10 Fungicide, insecticide (Woolfolk)	Sulfur Lead arsenate* Zinc	77.00% 9.50% 2.00%
SECURITY BRAND Z-78 for BLUE MOLD Fungicide, insecticide (Woolfolk)	Zinc ethylene-bis(dithio-carbamate)	6.5%
SECURITY SPECIAL UDDER FORMULA Udder decongestant (veterinary) (Security)	Carbolic acid* Zinc oxide Alum* Ichthammol Lead plaster*	2%
SEDA-CITRATE (Legendre's)	Dionin Citric acid Tinct. sanguinaria Syrup of squill Glycerin Aromatics Sodium citrate Tinct. euphorbia Menthol	1/4 gr. 8 gr. 30 m. 60 m. 30 m. q.s. 60 gr. 120 m. 4/100 gr.

*Consult Sec. II., Ingredients Index. This ingredient may be responsible for major toxic effects if poisonous amounts of this product are ingested.

Name & Use Manufacturer	Ingredients
SEDAGEL Antacid, adsorbent (Pharmaceuticals)	Magnesium trisilicate Aluminum hydroxide Bismuth subsalicylate Bismuth subcarbonate Demulcent base

SEDAGEST Antacid, adsorbent (Approved)	Aluminum hydroxide gel
	  U.S.P. dried 5 gr.
	Magnesium trisilicate 4 gr.
	Magnesium phosphate tribasic
	             2 gr.
	Pectin N.F. 1/4 gr.

SEDAREX Analgesic (Sedarex)	Acetophenetidin* 2 gr./tablet Aspirin* Phenolphthalein Caffein

SEDA-STAY For motion sickness nervous tension (Stayner)	Sodium bromide* 5 gr.
	Scopolamine hydrobromide
	          1/250 gr.
	Thiamine hydrochloride
	          10 mg.

SEDATIVE LIQUID & TABLETS Veterinary (Clayton)	
SEDATOLE Sedative, antitussive (Sharp & Dohme)	Each 30 cc.: Codeine sulfate 30 mg. Wild cherry bark Sanguinaria Squill* Balm of Gilead buds Diluted phosphoric acid Menthol Alcohol 6%

SEDATUSSIN Antitussive (Lilly)	Cephalin hydrochloride
	       0.007 gm.
	Sodium benzoate 0.875 gm.
	Sanguinaria 0.83 gm.
	Squill* 10 cc.
	Tolu balsam and menthol
	       q.s.

SEEDTONE Fungicide (Am. Chem.)	n-Trichloro methylthio
	  tetrahydro phthalimide
	       50%

SEE KLEER GLASS CLEANER (Rex Home)	
SEE MORE VENETIAN BLIND, RUG & UPHOLSTERY CLEANER (Seymour)	
SELANOL Rubefacient, (Merchant Bros.)	Methyl salicylate* 11% Stearyl alcohol Cetyl alcohol Glyceryl monostearate

SELCOL Disinfectant, germicide, deodorant (Selig)	Alkyl dimethyl benzyl
	  ammonium chloride*
	      10%

SELCO WHITE STAR SPRAY Insecticide (Selig)	Petroleum distillates*
	2-Butoxyethanol di-n-propyl
	  maleate isosafrole
	  condensate*
	Pyrethrins

Name & Use Manufacturer	Ingredients

SELECTIVE WEED KILLER NO. 460 Herbicide (Pickard)	Triethanolamine salt of 2,4-
	  dichloro phenoxy acetic acid*
	    63%

SELECTIVE WEED KILLER NO. 470 Herbicide (Pickard)	Isopropyl ester of 2,4-dichloro-
	  phenoxyacetic acid
	    44%
	Aromatic petroleum naphtha*
	    51%

SELECTOL DEVELOPERS Photographic supplies (Eastman)	
SELECTOX Herbicide (Veith)	Octamethyl pyrophosphoramide*
SELIG'S ACRESEL Disinfectant for stock yards (Selig)	Cresylic acid* 23% Water 3% Glycerin
SELIG'S AKWAPINE For general disinfection (Selig)	Steam distilled pine oil* Sodium soaps
SELIG'S ALATOL DISINFECTANT (Selig)	Steam-distilled pine oil* Chloro-2,-phenylphenol* Potassium soaps Isopropyl alcohol*
SELIG'S ARSENICAL CATTLE DIP Insecticide (Selig)	Arsenic* 15.5%/w
SELIG'S FLEE FLEA Insecticide (Selig)	DDT 2% Rotenone 1% Pyrethrins 0.017%
SELIG'S FLY-GO BEADS Insecticide (Selig)	Malathion* 2%
SELIG'S GRAINFUME Fumigant (Selig)	Carbon tetrachloride* Carbon bisulfide* Sulfur dioxide
SELIG'S ORZENE Insecticide (Selig)	Orthodichlorobenzene* 100%
SELIG'S POWDERED INSECTICIDE Insecticide (Selig)	DDT* 10.00% Pyrethrins 0.08%
SELIG'S RODANTU RAT KILLER Rodenticide (Selig)	ANTU* 25%

*Consult Sec. II., Ingredients Index. This ingredient may be responsible for major toxic effects if poisonous amounts of this product are ingested.

Name & Use Manufacturer	Ingredients	Name & Use Manufacturer	Ingredients
SELIG'S SUPER SE-FLY-GO Insecticide (Selig)	Petroleum distillates* 2-Butoxyethanol Di-n-propyl maleate isosafrole condensate Pyrethrins	SEMESAN BEL SEED DISINFECTANT (du Pont)	Hydroxy mercuri nitrophenol* Hydroxy mercuri chlorophenol*
SELIG'S WEED KILLER Herbicide (Selig)	Arsenous oxide* 33.3%	SEMESAN SEED DISINFECTANT (du Pont)	Hydroxy mercuri chlorophenol*
SELIG'S WEEVI-KIL Insecticide (Selig)	Petroleum distillates* B-butoxy B'-thiocyano diethyl ether* 2-butoxyethanol Di-n-propyl maleate isosafrole condensate Pyrethrins	SEMESAN (SPECIAL) FUNGICIDE (du Pont)	Hydroxy mercuri chlorophenol* Hydroxy mercuri cresol*
SELRODO Analgesic (Stansbury)	Each tablet: Acetylsalicylic acid* 3-1/2 gr. Phenacetin* 2-1/2 gr. Caffeine alkaloid 1/2 gr. Calcium succinate 2 gr.	SEMIKON HYDRO-CHLORIDE CREAM 2% For skin irritations (Massengill)	Semikon hydrochloride* 2%
SELRODO INHALANT Antispasmodic, nasal decongestant (Stansbury)	Chlorobutanol (chloroform derivative) 0.5%	SEMINOLE WETTABLE SULFUR Insecticide (Florida Agric.)	Sulfur* 90%
SEL-TOX Herbicide (Nott)	Phenyl mercury monoethanol ammonium acetate 2.3%	SENCO ALL-PURPOSE PAINT THINNER (Senn)	Aliphatic hydrocarbon* Masking agents

SEMCOF (Syrup) Antitussive (Massengill)	Each 5 cc.:
	 Dihydrocodeinone bitartrate
	         1.8 mg.
	 Sodium citrate 0.2 gm.
	 Ammonium chloride 0.1 gm.
	 Ephedrine hydrochloride
	         5 mg.
	 Tartar emetic 1 mg.
	 Aromatics q.s.
		SENDOL Analgesic (Sendol)	Aspirin* (acetylsalicylic acid)
			 Caffeine alkaloid

SEMCOF-CP SYRUP Antitussive (Massengill)	Each 5 cc.: Codeine phosphate 10 gm. Sodium citrate 0.16 gm. Ammonium chloride 20 mg. Ephedrine hydrochloride 10 mg. Tartar emetic 0.6 mg. Aromatics q.s.	SENECA FLAKES Specialized cleaning product (Wyandotte)	Concentrated alkali*

SEMCOF EXPECTORANT SYRUP (Massengill)	Each 5 cc.:
	 Semikon hydrochloride
	    (methopyrilene hyd.)
	         15 mg.
	 Sodium citrate 0.2 gm.
	 Ammonium chloride 0.1 gm.
	 Ephedrine hydrochloride
	         10 mg.
	 Tartar emetic 1 mg.
	 Aromatics q.s.
		SENECA-X Specialized cleaning product (Wyandotte)	Concentrated alkali*

SEMCOF-M SYRUP Antitussive (Massengill)	Each 5 cc.: Morphine hydrochloride 2.5 mg. Sodium citrate 0.16 gm. Ammonium chloride 20 mg. Ephedrine hydrochloride 10 mg. Tartar emetic 0.6 mg. Aromatics q.s.	SAVOGRAN SUPERSTRIP NON-INFLAMMABLE PAINT & VARNISH REMOVER (Savogran)	Methylene chloride* Propylene dichloride* Methanol*
		SENGARIAN OINTMENT (Aschenbach)	
SEMCOQUIN (Syrup) Anti-malarial (Massengill)	Each tsp.: Quinine sulfate 0.12 gm. Chocolate syrup Aromatics	SENOKOT Cathartic (Purdue)	Cassia acutifolia pods standardized

---

*Consult Sec. II., Ingredients Index. This ingredient may be responsible for major toxic effects if poisonous amounts of this product are ingested.

Name & Use Manufacturer	Ingredients		Name & Use Manufacturer	Ingredients	
SENSATENE LINIMENT ANTISEPTIC (Dixie Labs.)	Alpha terpineol p-Cresol ethers Resorcinol ethers Anthranilic ethers Phenylethyl esters Coumarin Ionone Benzoic esters Heliotropine Guaiacol ethers Salicylic ethers Benzoic ethers Menthol esters Anisic aldehyde Cinnamic aldehyde Benzaldehyde* Benzyl alcohol Amyl cinnamic aldehyde Vanillin Acetaldehyde Denanthic ether Butyric ether Amyl butyrate Amyl acetate Essential oils*from natural sources Pine oil* Olive oil Mineral oil		SENTINEL WATER MISCIBLE LINDANE Insecticide (Sentinel Lab.)	Gamma isomer of hexachloro-cyclohexane*	20%
			SENTROCIDE Insecticide (Sentry Prod.)	Paradichlorobenzene Ethylene dichloride Carbon tetrachloride*	
			SENTRY DEODORIZING SPRAY (Sentry Prod.)	Denatured alcohol Essential oils*	
			SENTRY MOTH KILLER Insecticide (Sentry Prod.)	Paradichlorobenzene*	
			SENZODOR INCENSE (Senzodor)	Wood flours Karaya gums Vanillin U.S.P. Perfume oils	
SENTINEL ANTI FREEZE (Cliffs Dow)	Methanol* Purple dye Suitable rust inhibitors	99.85%	SEOXYL For over-indulgence and motion sickness (Robbins Corp.)	Each tablet: Cereum oxyl* Amygdalose Atropine *	1 gr. 1/50 gr. 1/300 gr.
SENTINEL EMULSIFIABLE DDT Insecticide (Sentinel Lab.)	DDT *	25%	SEPO For gargle, douche (Clapp, Otis)	Methyl salicylate Oil eucalyptus Thymol Menthol (Not U.S.P.) Boric acid * Sodium benzoate Sodium borate	9/100 m. 42/100 m. 28/100 gr. 18/100 gr. 8-1/2 gr. 1-7/10 gr. 1-7/10 gr.
SENTINEL FABRIC PEST SPRAY Insecticide (Sentinel Lab.)	Lindane DDT	1/4% 2-1/2%			
			SEPTIGYN (Septigyn)	Zinc sulfocarbolate* Copper sulfocarbolate* Sodium sulfate (dried)	
SENTINEL PHOSPHORUS PASTE Insecticide (Sentinel Lab.)	Phosphorus*	2%	SEPTISOL Liquid soap (Vestal)	Soaps and detergents derived from vegetable oils Hexachlorophene (2% of anhydrous) 0.75% Lecithin Glycerin Tetra sodium ethylene diamine tetra acetate	
SENTINEL REZ-I-DU HOUSEHOLD SPRAY Insecticide (Sentinel Lab.)	Chlordane Inert ingredients*	2%			
			SEPTO ZONE ANTISEPTIC & SALVES (Am. Pharm.)		
SENTINEL ROACH-O-EXTERMINATOR Insecticide (Pest Control Chem.)	Fluorine* Pyrethrum Pyrophyllite		SEPTRIN For skin and mucous membrane irritations (Lloyd)	Alcohol Alkyl dimethyl benzyl ammonium chloride Geranium	22% 0.1 gm. 50.0 gm.
SENTINEL WATER MISCIBLE CHLORDANE Insecticide (Sentinel Lab.)	Chlordane*	60%/w	SEQUESTRENE 330 FE IRON CHELATE To correct iron deficiency in plants growing in acid and alkaline soils (Geigy)	Tech. sodium ferric diethylene-triamine penta-acetate*	

*Consult Sec. II., Ingredients Index. This ingredient may be responsible for major toxic effects if poisonous amounts of this product are ingested.

- 936 -

Name & Use Manufacturer	Ingredients		Name & Use Manufacturer	Ingredients	
SERGEANT'S COUGH MEDICINE Veterinary (Polk Miller)	Chloroform U.S.P. Menthol Tartar emetic Ammonium chloride Potassium guaiacol sulfonate	0.47% 0.018% 0.018% 1.31% 1.31%	SERGEANT'S SKIP-FLEA SCRATCH POWDER (Polk Miller)	Chloranil Gamma isomer of benzene hexachloride Pyrethrins Tech. piperonyl butoxide	5% 1% 0.045% 0.450%
SERGEANT'S EAR CREME Veterinary (Polk Miller)	Di-isobutyl cresoxy ethyl dimethyl benzyl ammonium chloride monohydrate Carbolic acid Tyrothricin	0.1% 0.5% 0.03%	SERGEANT'S SKIP-FLEA SHAMPOO Insecticide (Polk Miller)	Tech. piperonyl butoxide Pyrethrins Ammonium lauryl sulfate Amine salt of dodecyl benzene sulfonate	0.5% 0.05% 7.5% 11.25%
SERGEANT'S EYE WASH Veterinary (Polk Miller)	Zinc sulfate Boric acid Camphor	0.15% 2.50% 0.02%	SERGEANT'S SKIP-FLEA SOAP (Polk Miller)	Anhydrous soap Beta naphthol Oil of pennyroyal	84% 3% 1%
SERGEANT'S HOUSEHOLD DISINFECTANT (Polk Miller)	Pine oil* Soap Isopropanol	77.00% 9.25% 3.75%	SERGEANT'S SKIP-TICK POWDER (Polk Miller)	Gamma isomer of benzene hexachloride Rotenone Other cube resins DDT	1% 0.80% 1.60% 2.00%
SERGEANT'S LAXATIVE TABLETS Veterinary (Polk Miller)	Calomel Ext. colocynth co.* Resin jalap	6.57% 8.82% 2.2%	SERGEANT'S SURE SHOT WORM CAPSULES Veterinary (Polk Miller)	n-Butyl chloride*	
SERGEANT'S PUPPY WORM CAPSULES (Polk Miller)	n-Butyl chloride*		SERGEANT'S TAPEWORM MEDICINE Veterinary (Polk Miller)	Arecoline hydrobromide*	
SERGEANT'S SARCOPTIC MANGE MEDICINE Ectoparasiticide, veterinary (Polk Miller)	Petroleum oils* Oil of pine tar* Tincture of cantharides Sperm oil Sulfur	72.73% 24.24% 0.01% 2.47% 0.44%	SERGEANT'S TONIC PILLS Veterinary (Polk Miller)	Arsenic trioxide* Ferrous sulfate Ext. gentian Ext. nox vomica* Strychnine*	
SERGEANT'S SKIN BALM For dogs (Polk Miller)	Parfentjevo's yeast fraction Soap Alcohol not over 3% by volume		SERTEN Antiseptic (Lloyd)	Alkyl dimethyl benzyl ammonium chlorides*	50%
SERGEANT'S SKIP-BATH DOG CLEANER Insecticide (Polk Miller)	Tech. chlordane Dipentene Para-cymene Para-menthane Terpene hydrocarbons Iso-octyl phenoxy polyethoxy ethanol	0.25% 2.30% 0.77% 0.63% 0.81% 1.00%	SERUTAN Laxative (Serutan)	Vegetable hemicellulose derived from plantago ovata Cerelose Specially refined powdered oatmeal Defatted wheat germ	

---

*Consult Sec. II., Ingredients Index. This ingredient may be responsible for major toxic effects if poisonous amounts of this product are ingested.

Name & Use Manufacturer	Ingredients	Name & Use Manufacturer	Ingredients
SERVAC Specialized cleaning product (Wyandotte)	Phosphoric acid*	SEVENTEEN HYPO- ALLERGENIC COLOGNE & ASTRINGENT (Seventeen)	
SERVACIDE Insecticide (Harvacide)	Piperonyl butoxide Pyrethrins Carbon tetrachloride*	721 SPECIAL & SUPER Specialized cleaning product (Wyandotte)	Concentrated alkali*
SERVEX NO. 2 (Servex)	Kaolin Bicarbonate of soda Nitrophenolate of mercury* 0.064 gr.	75 ROTENONE Insecticide (Chem. Form.)	Rotenone 0.75% Other cube resins 15.5% Talc 83.75%
SERVEX TRICH NO. 1 (Servex)	Boric acid* Oxyquinoline sulfate Quinine sulfate Nitrophenolate of mercury* 0.095 gr.	7-WAY COLD CAPSULES For colds (Approved)	Acetophenetidin* 1-1/4 gr. Aspirin* 1-3/4 gr. Camph. monobrom. 1/2 gr. Caffeine 1/4 gr. Phenolphthalein 1/5 gr. Atropine sulfate 1/1000 gr. Quinine sulfate 1/4 gr.
SERVEX VAGINAL JELLY (Servex)	Alcohol 5% Para-tertiary amylhydroxy benzene Sodium lauryl sulfate Boric acid	SEVERA'S ANTISEPSOL Antiseptic (Myers Labs.)	Benzoic acid* Thymol* Oil red thyme Menthol* Methyl salicylate* Eucalyptol* Boric acid* Alcohol 25%
SERVEX VAGINAL POWDER (Servex)	Quinine sulfate* Oxyquinoline sulfate* Boric acid* Nitrophenolate of mercury* 0.057 gr.	SEVERA'S BALZOL Digestant (Myers Labs.)	Gentian Calumba Alcohol 18%
SESIN 5 PELLETIZED Weed preventer (Wilson, Jack)	2,4-Dichlorophenoxy ethyl benzoate* 5%	SEVERA'S BITTERS Tonic (Myers Labs.)	Gentian Calamus Bitter orange peel Calumba
SETRETE Fungicide, insecticide (Cleary)	Phenyl mercuric ammonium acetate* 7%	SEVERA'S CATHARTIC PILLS (Myers Labs.)	Aloin* Podophyllin Resin jalap Oleoresin capsicum
SETRETE FORTIFIED Insecticide (Cleary)	Phenyl mercuric acetate* 5.0% Ethyl mercuric acetate* 1.0%	SEVERA'S COUGH BALSAM (Myers Labs.)	Tolu Wild cherry Ipecac Senega Blood root Gum arabic Alcohol 8%
SETRETE MIST Insecticide (Cleary)	Phenyl mercuric acetate* 2.25% Ethyl mercuric acetate* 1.60%	SEVERA'S GOLDEN EYE SALVE (Myers Labs.)	Yellow oxide of mercury* 2%
SET-UP SHAVE LOTION (Nestle-Le Mur)			
SEVEN-ITE CLEANER & PROTECTIVE AUTO COATING (Automotive cleaner (du Pont)			
SEVENTEEN HYPO- ALLERGENIC BRILLIAN- TINE (Seventeen)			

Name & Use Manufacturer	Ingredients	Name & Use Manufacturer	Ingredients
SEVERA'S GOTHARDOL Liniment (Myers Labs.)	Oil cajuput* Oil thyme* Capsicum mustard Soap liniment Alcohol 50% Chloroform 48 m./fl.oz.	SHACKELTON INHALER COMPOUND (Shackelton)	Gum benzoin Balsam tolu Eucalyptol* Oil of pine needles* Balsam Peru Methyl salicylate* Pine tar Terrebene Gum camphor* Vegetable coloring Alcohol ethyl* 76%/v
SEVERA'S HAIR POMADE (Myers Labs.)		SHADE TONER Preparation for dyed hair (Creative Cosm.)	
SEVERA'S HEADACHE TABLETS (Myers Labs.)	Acetopheneticin* 2-1/2 gr./tablet* Aspirin* Caffeine	SHAKTI DEODORANT LIQUID & POWDER (Coty)	
SEVERA'S OINTMENT (Myers Labs.)	Camphor* Carbolic acid* Rosin Turpentine* Linseed oil	SHAMPOOCH PET SHAMPOO Parasiticide (Kent Spec.)	Rotenone 0.04% Other ether extractives of cube 0.09%
SEVERA'S PLASTER (Myers Labs.)	Oleoresin of capsicum	SHAMPOO STRAIGHT (Altyme)	Thioglycollic acid 7-1/2% Detergent (pH 9.1) Ammonia
SEVERA'S REGALTOR Cathartic (Myers Labs.)	Black haw False unicorn Cramp bark Blue cohosh Oregon grape root Gentian Cascara Alcohol 14%	SHARLON PERFUME (House of Fragrance)	
SEVERA'S SKIN SOAP (Myers Labs.)		SHARP & DOHME ANALGESIC BALM Rubefacient (Sharp & Dohme)	Menthol* Methyl salicylate* Lanolin
SEW-A-KOTE Paints & Varnishes (Tibbets)			
S.E.X. Herbicide (Stauffer)	Sodium ethyl xanthate* and related compounds 90%	SHARP & DOHME S.T. 37 ANTISEPTIC SOLUTION For skin and mucous membranes (Sharp & Dohme)	Caprokol (hexylresorcinol) 1-1000
S.F. COSMETIC LOTION (Hulett)			
S & F LOTION For skin irritations (Humco)	Chlorothymol* Camphor* Benzoic acid* Tartaric acid Water Menthol syn. Boric acid* Salicylic acid* Citric acid	SHASTA CREME SHAMPOO (Procter & Gamble)	Ionic synthetic detergent Soap Lanolin
SG-KH Photographic supplies (Uricheck)		SHAVE WHIP BRUSHLESS LATHER Liquid soap (Campbell Prod.)	pH 10.1 Total fatty acids, free and combined as soap 4.5% Total fatty acids, as anhydrous potash soaps 5.1% Unsaponified matter 0.55%
		SHAVINE (Depilatory) (Shaving Powder)	Barium sulfide* Calcium hydroxide

*Consult Sec. II., Ingredients Index. This ingredient may be responsible for major toxic effects if poisonous amounts of this product are ingested.

Name & Use Manufacturer	Ingredients		Name & Use Manufacturer	Ingredients	
SHAVON SHAVING LOTION (George, G.O.)			SHELLACOL (Commercial Solv.)	Ethyl alcohol* (denatured)	
SHAW FINGER PAINT (Binney & Smith)			SHELL ALDREX 2 Insecticide (Shell Chem.)	Hexachloro hexahydro-endo, exo-dimethano naphthalene* 23.4% Related compounds 4.0% Petroleum hydrocarbons 65.1%	
SHEATH Rust preventative and remover (Brownell)			SHELL 25% ALDRIN WETTABLE POWDER Insecticide (Shell Chem.)	Hexachloro hexahydro-endo, exo-dimethano naphthalene* 23.8% Related compounds 4.0%	
SHED-A-LEAF Defoliant (Chipman Chem.)	Sodium chlorate* 40%		SHELL D-D Insecticide (Shell Chem.)	Chlorinated C_3 hydrocarbons* 100%	
SHED-A-LEAF L Defoliant (Chipman Chem.)	Sodium chlorate* 18.20%		SHELL DIELDREX 15 Insecticide (Shell Chem.)	Hexachloro epoxy octahydro-endo, exo-dimethano naphthalene* 15.8% Related compounds 2.8% Petroleum hydrocarbons 73.4%	
SHEERAN'S CREAM (Sheeran)	Glycerin Quince seed (Madagascar) Boric acid less than 0.05% Quince blossom perfume oil Castile soap powder Phenol 1-1/4% Denatured alcohol 10% White beeswax Spermaceti		SHELL 50% DIELDRIN WETTABLE POWDER Insecticide (Shell Chem.)	Hexachloro epoxy octahydro-endo, exo-dimethano naphthalene* 42.5% Related compounds 7.5%	
SHEERAN'S WHITE LINIMENT (Sheeran)	Ammonium carbonate Camphor gum* Oil of turpentine rectified* Pure gum spirit turpentine* Oil of thyme, red Castile soap powder		SHELL 1% ENDRIN DUST Insecticide (Shell Chem.)	Endrin (hexachloro epoxy octahydro-endo, endo-dimethano naphthalene)* 1.0%	
SHEER MAGIC LIQUID MAKE-UP (Campana)	Spermaceti wax Mineral oil Esters Triethanolamine soap		SHELL 1-1/2% ENDRIN DUST Insecticide (Shell Chem.)	Endrin (hexachloro epoxy octahydro-endo, endo-dimethano naphthalene)* 1.5%	
SHEFFIELD BRUSHLESS SHAVE CREAM (Sheffield Co.)	Fatty acids Mineral oil Lanolin Perfume		SHELL ENDRIN EMULSIBLE CONC. Insecticide (Shell Chem.)	Hexachloro epoxy octahydro-endo, endo-dimethano naphthalene* 19.5% Petroleum hydrocarbons 70.5%	
SHEFFIELD LATHER SHAVE CREAM (Sheffield Co.)	Fatty acids Vegetable oils Glycerin Caustics Inhibitor Perfume		SHELL TOX Insecticide (Shell Oil)	Beta butoxy beta' thiocyano-diethyl ether 0.5% DDT* 1% Oil* Pyrethrins	
SHEFFIELD PURE LANOLIN Skin emollient (Sheffield Co.)	Pure lanolin		SHERWIN-WILLIAMS ARSENATE OF CALCIUM Insecticide (Sherwin-Williams)	Calcium arsenate* 70%	
SHEFFIELD WATER PUTTY (Sheffield Bronze)			SHERWIN-WILLIAMS ARSENATE OF LEAD Insecticide (Sherwin-Williams)	Arsenate of lead* 98%	
SHELL A-A WEED SEED KILLER (Shell Chem.)	Allyl alcohol* 100%				

*Consult Sec. II., Ingredients Index. This ingredient may be responsible for major toxic effects if poisonous amounts of this product are ingested.

Name & Use Manufacturer	Ingredients		Name & Use Manufacturer	Ingredients	
SHERWIN-WILLIAMS BASIC COPPER ARSENATE Insecticide (Sherwin-Williams)	Basic copper arsenate*	91%	SHERWIN-WILLIAMS FLAT-RITE WHITE Enamel (Sherwin-Williams)	Pigment: Titanium calcium Titanium dioxide Calcium carbonate Silicates Vehicle: Heat bodied linseed oil Varnish Mineral spirits*	
SHERWIN-WILLIAMS BASIC COPPER SULFUR (BCS) Fungicide (Sherwin-Williams)	Copper*	50%	SHERWIN-WILLIAMS FLO-LAC Varnish stain (Sherwin-Williams)	Varnish Bitumen Inert ingredients*	
SHERWIN-WILLIAMS CHLORDANE 45% LIQUID EMULSION Insecticide (Sherwin-Williams)	Chlordane*	45%	SHERWIN-WILLIAMS FLOOR-SEAL (Sherwin-Williams)	Varnish Tung-linseed-phenolic-ester gum (non-volatile) 36% Mineral spirits* (volatile) 64%	
SHERWIN-WILLIAMS CHLORDANE 40% POWDER EMULSION Insecticide (Sherwin-Williams)	Chlordane*	40%	SHERWIN-WILLIAMS INDUSTRIAL FINISHES KEM, LUSTRAL, 42 LINE, GLOSS WHITE (Sherwin-Williams)	Pigment: Titanium dioxide Vehicle: Varnish Linseed-alkyd-soya (non-volatile) Mineral spirits* (volatile)	
SHERWIN-WILLIAMS DIELDRIN 18% EMULSIFIABLE Insecticide (Sherwin-Williams)	Dieldrin*	1.5 lb./gal.	SHERWIN-WILLIAMS INDUSTRIAL FINISHES, SAVE-LITE GLOSS WHITE (Sherwin-Williams)	Pigment: Titanium calcium Zinc oxide Titanium dioxide Vehicle: Heat-bodied linseed oil Dehydrated castor oil Driers Mineral spirits*	
SHERWIN-WILLIAMS DIELDRIN 50% WETTABLE POWDER Insecticide (Sherwin-Williams)	Dieldrin*	50%	SHERWIN-WILLIAMS INDUSTRIAL FINISHES SAVE-LITE KEM GLOSS WHITE (Sherwin-Williams)	Pigment: Titanium dioxide Zinc oxide Vehicle: Varnish Soya-alkyd resin (non-volatile) Mineral spirits* (volatile)	
SHERWIN-WILLIAMS DRY LIME-SULFUR Fungicide (Sherwin-Williams)	Calcium polysulfides* Calcium thiosulfate Sulfur	65% 5% 5%	SHERWIN-WILLIAMS KARBAM BLACK Fungicide (Sherwin-Williams)	Ferbam*	76%
SHERWIN-WILLIAMS DUSTING SULFUR Fungicide (Sherwin-Williams)	Sulfur*	93%	SHERWIN-WILLIAMS MALATHION 50% EMULSIFIABLE Insecticide (Sherwin-Williams)	Malathion*	50%
SHERWIN-WILLIAMS ENAMELOID (Sherwin-Williams)	Pigment: Titanium dioxide Titanium calcium Vehicle: Varnish Soya-alkyd (non-volatile) Mineral spirits* (volatile)		SHERWIN-WILLIAMS MALATHION 25% WETTABLE POWDER Insecticide (Sherwin-Williams)	Malathion*	25%

*Consult Sec. II., Ingredients Index. This ingredient may be responsible for major toxic effects if poisonous amounts of this product are ingested.

Name & Use Manufacturer	Ingredients		Name & Use Manufacturer	Ingredients
SHERWIN- WILLIAMS 325 MESH DUSTING SULFUR Insecticide (Sherwin- Williams)	Sulfur*	93%	SHIELD BRAND BOWL KLEAN LIQUID Cleaner for toilet bowls (Rochester Germ.)	Hydrochloric acid*
SHERWIN- WILLIAMS NON- INFLAMMABLE PAINT & VARNISH REMOVER (Sherwin- Williams)	Chlorinated hydrocarbons*		SHIELD BRAND KLIX Drain-pipe cleaner (Rochester Germ.)	Sodium hydroxide*
SHERWIN- WILLIAMS PARATHION 15% Insecticide (Sherwin- Williams)	Parathion*	15%	DR. SHIFFER'S HAIR & SCALP ANTISEPTIC (Shiffer's)	Potassium oxyquinoline sulfate*
SHERWIN- WILLIAMS PARIS GREEN Insecticide (Sherwin- Williams)	Copper aceto-arsenite*		DR. SHIFFER'S SHAMPOO (Shiffer's)	Coconut oil Olive oil Potassium hydroxide (light alkaline reaction)
SHERWIN- WILLIAMS REXPAR Spar varnish (Sherwin- Williams)	Varnish Tung-linseed-phenolic resin (non-volatile) 55% Mineral spirits* (volatile) 45%		SHILOH FOR COUGHS Antitussive (Wells, S.C.)	Chloroform 3m/fl.oz. Terpin hydrate Benzocaine Ammonium chloride Oil of peppermint Licorice Sodium citrate Sodium salicylate Oil of tar Glycerin Syrup
SHERWIN- WILLIAMS RHOTHANE 25% EMULSIFIABLE Insecticide (Sherwin- Williams)	DDD*	25%	SHILOH THROAT TABLETS For throat irritations (Wells, S.C.)	Each tablet: Tyrothricin 2 mg. Cetyl dimethyl benzyl ammonium chloride 1 mg. Ammonium chloride 1/2 gr. Benzocaine 5 mg.
SHERWIN- WILLIAMS RHOTHANE 50% WETTABLE POWDER Insecticide (Sherwin- Williams)	DDD*	50%	SHINA DISH Detergent (Tidy House)	Sodium dodecyl benzene sulfonate* 30%/w Anhydrous sodium tripolysulfate* 10% Carboxymethylcellulose 2% Sodium sulfate or Glauber's salts
SHERWIN- WILLIAMS 42-1/2% SODIUM ARSENITE SOLUTION Herbicide (Sherwin- Williams)	Arsenic trioxide*	32.5%	SHINA DISH LIQUID Dishwashing compound (Tidy House)	Sodium alkyl benzene sulfonate* 32% Xylene sulfonate* 3-4% Ethoxylated tridecyl alcohol 15% Perfume 0.1% Blue dye 5 ppm
SHERWIN- WILLIAMS TAXITE Paint and varnish remover (Sherwin- Williams)	Benzol*	more than 15%	SHINE MAGIC & SHINE MAGIC KIDDIE SHINE Leather conditioners (Shine)	
			SHINEZE LIQUID WAX (Holcomb)	Stoddard solvent*
			SHINO-CEN Cleaners (Central Chem.)	

*Consult Sec. II., Ingredients Index. This ingredient may be responsible for major toxic effects if poisonous amounts of this product are ingested.

- 942 -

Name & Use Manufacturer	Ingredients	Name & Use Manufacturer	Ingredients
SHINOLA DRESS PARADE Boot polishes (Best)		SHUPTRINE'S PILLS Cathartic (Shuptrine)	Ext. hyoscyamus (total alkaloids 0.0004 gr.) Calomel* 1 gr. Podophyllin Powd. ipecac Ext. colocynth comp.* Aloin*
SHINOLA 2-IN-1 WAX SHOE POLISH (Best)		SHUR-OFF Keratolytic (Wellman)	Alcohol 57% Ether 10% Salicylic acid* Procaine hydrochloride Phenol (carbolic acid) 1% Trichloracetic acid*
SHINO PAINTS, VARNISHES, LACQUERS, SEALERS, STAINS, FINISHES, WAXES, POLISHES (Pioneer)		SHUR SPARK (Park Chem.)	Aliphatic solvent* Oils* Resins
		SHU-SHINE WHITE CLEANER (Osmic)	
SHINO PURE OIL SOAP (Pioneer)	Vegetable oil soap	SHUTTLE Skin ointment (Grenald)	Ethyl aminobenzoate 1% Phenol 3/4% Precipitated sulfur 3% Menthol Glycerin Zinc oxide Corn starch Magma magnesia Magma of bentonite Lime water
SHINOSHEEN Cleaner (Pioneer)	Vegetable soap Gloss wax		

SHOO INSECT
REPELLENT
STICK
(Merlee)
	2-Cyclohexyl cyclohexanol*
	     3.75%
	2-Phenyl cyclohexanol*
	     8.75%		

		SIBOL (Texas Pheno.)	Diethylstilbestrol 3 mg./cc. Bland oil
DR. SHREVES A.G.S. REMEDY (Shreves)	Liquor calcis or water of lime Sassafras Quassia	SICCATIFF DE COURTRAY (Dryer) Japan quick dryer (Weber, F.)	Manganese* Lead*
DR. SHREVES S & L PILLS (Shreves)	Senna Jalap* Ginger Aloin*		
SHU-BUG Insecticide (Dolan Labs.)		S.I.C. TABLETS Enteric coated tablets for gout (Vitec)	Sodium salicylate* 10 gr. Potassium iodide 1 gr. Colchicine 1/500 gr.
SHUCO RAT POISON (Shuptrine)	Arsenic trioxide* 2.0%		

SHUFUNG
Fungicide,
spray (medical)
(Pedinol)
	Trimethyl octadecyl ammonium
	  chlorophenate* 4%
		SIDAL
		CONCEN-
		TRATE
		ANTISEPTIC
		INDUSTRIAL
		LIQUID SOAP
		(Fuld)
			Bis (3,5,6-trichloro-2-hydroxy-
			  phenyl)-methane
			Potassium soap of vegetable
			  oils

SHULTON SHAMPOO (Shulton)			

SHULTON
SOAPS
(Shulton)
		SIDAL READY
		TO USE
		ANTISEPTIC
		&
		PRESURGICAL
		LIQUID SOAP
		(Fuld)
			Bis (3,5,6-trichloro-2-hydroxy-
			  phenyl)-methane
			Potassium soap of vegetable
			  oils

SHULTS' OINTMENT For skin burns and irritations (Shults')	Zinc oxide Boric acid* Pine tar* Creolin Cresol* Vegetable oil Petrolatum		
SHU-MILK SNOW WHITE Shoe whitener (Shu-Milk)		SIDE GLANCE PERFUME & COLOGNE (Parfums Anjou)	

*Consult Sec. II., Ingredients Index. This ingredient may be responsible for major toxic effects if poisonous amounts of this product are ingested.

- 943 -

Name & Use Manufacturer	Ingredients	Name & Use Manufacturer	Ingredients
SI-DRENE Nasal decongestant (Davart)	Ephedrine sulfate* Carbolic acid Sol. hydrastine Iodo-phenol Malachite green	SILENT NIGHT PERFUME, COLOGNE STICK, DEODORANT, TOILET WATER (Countess)	
SIERRA PINE TOILET & HAND SOAP (Los Angeles Soap)	Pure soap Perfume Coal tar green dye	SILICARE Hand lotion (Revlon)	
		SILICONE AUTO WAX (Wellesley)	
SIESTA QUEEN'S Sedative (Queen)	Brominate (1-K)* 7-1/2 gr. Stearated potassium bromide	SILICONE REMOVER (Park Chem.)	Aromatic hydrocarbons* Chlorinated hydrocarbons*
SILADERM CREAM Skin protectant (Silicote)	Dimethyl polysiloxane 15% Stearic acid 8% Triethanolamine 1% Glycerol monostearate 3% Zinc stearate 2% Glycerol 5%	SILITONE CREAM Skin protectant (Silicote)	Dimethyl polysiloxane 15% Stearic acid 8% Triethanolamine 1% Glycerol monostearate 3% Zinc stearate 2% Glycerol 5%
SILADERM OINTMENT Skin protectant (Silicote)	Dimethyl polysiloxane 25% Petrolatum U.S.P. 75%	SILITONE OINTMENT Skin protectant (Silicote)	Dimethyl polysiloxane 20% Petrolatum U.S.P. 80%
SILA-FLEX COLOR PRESERVER Lacquer (Sila-Flex)		SILKY MIST CREAM LOTION (Volay)	
SILA-FLEX FERRULE CEMENT (Sila-Flex)	By-product of polystyrene	SILKY MIST HAIR TONIC (Newbro)	
SILA-FLEX ROD CEMENT (Sila-Flex)	Neoprene-based cement Methylethylketone*	SILLS CORN & CALLOUS REMOVER (Sills)	Salicylic acid* Bismuth subcarbonate Benzocaine 2.4% Castor oil Petrolatum
SILA-FLEX ROD VARNISH (Sila-Flex)	Phenolic-based varnish	SILLS POWDER TREATMENT For skin irritations (Sills)	Salicylic acid* Bismuth subcarbonate Aspirin (acetylsalicylic acid)* Ammonium alum Boric acid* Talcum
SILBE INHALEDRIN COMPOSITUM Inhalant (Radin)	Chlorbutanol* 12-1/2 gr./fl.oz. Ephedrine hydrochloride* Epinephrine Glycerin		
SILBE GLYCIRENAN Inhalant (Radin)	Chlorbutanol (chloroform deriv.) 3 gr./fl. oz. Epinephrine Glycerin	SILCO FUEL OIL SOLVENTS (Petroleum)	Aromatic solvent* comparable to xylol
SILBE GLYCIRENAN FORTE INHALANT (Radin)	Chlorbutanol 3 gr./fl.oz. Epinephrine Glycerin	SIL PI SOL OIL Antiseptic, counter-irritant (Internat. Stock)	Cresol* Thyme oil Oil of pine* Oil of turpentine* Linseed oil Gum camphor*
SILBE JODIRENAN INHALANT (Radin)	Epinephrine Iodine* Sodium iodide* Glycerin	SIL-7 Polish (Speco)	Silicone oil Gum tragacanth Diatomaceous abrasives
		SIL-9 Polish (Speco)	Silicone oil Paraffin oil
SILDEX For retarding overeating (Kal)	Dextrose Non-nutritive muciloid plantage ovata (psyllium) Collodial methycellulose	SILVA PUTZ SILVER POLISH (Am. Metal)	Infusorial earth Pure soap Mild carbonate of soda Antiseptic oil

*Consult Sec. II., Ingredients Index. This ingredient may be responsible for major toxic effects if poisonous amounts of this product are ingested.

- 944 -

Name & Use Manufacturer	Ingredients
SILVER BRITE SILVER POLISH Polish (Boyle-Midway)	Soap Abrasives Detergent Color
SILVER CLEEN Silver cleaner (Chem. Mfg. & Dist.)	
SILVER DUST BLUE DETERGENT (Lever)	Sodium alkaryl sulfonate* Sodium polyphosphates* Fatty amide Sodium sulfate Silicate Perfume Optical dye
SILVERFLEECE Silver polish (Earl Prods.)	
SILVER GATE For rectal irritation (Fletcher)	Zinc sulfate * Iodine* Lime Tannic acid* Alum Alcohol 1%
SILVER LABEL DEODORANT (Boyle-Midway)	Petroleum distillates* Freon gas
SILVER SNOW Silver polish (Welmaid)	
SILVER SUDS SILVER POLISH (Silver Suds)	
SILVO SILVER POLISH (French, R.T.)	Polishing earth Specially denatured alcohol Fatty acids Ammonia Perfume 0.06%
SIMONIZ WAXES & POLISHES (Simoniz)	

SIMON'S RHEUMATIC REMEDY (Olliffe)	Sat. sol. magnesium sulfate
	    oz. xvi
	Tincture senna oz. xx
	Syr. sarsaparilla comp.
	    oz. xxxx
	Sat. sol. potassium iodide
	    oz. x
	Fluid extract hyoscyamus
	    oz. ii & drs. iv
	Wine of colchicum oz. xxxx

SIMPLE LIFE TREATMENT LINE EYE TINT & MASCARA (Coty)	

Name & Use Manufacturer	Ingredients
SIMPLE LIFE TREATMENT LINE SPECIAL ASTRINGENT & SKIN FRESHNER (Coty)	
SINAPEX Counter-irritant (Menley & James)	Oil of mustard* Chaulmoogra oil Oil of rosemary* Oil of wintergreen (synthetic)* Menthol* Camphor*
SINEX TABLETS For sinusitis (Pharmex)	Vitamin A 100,000 units Vitamin C 500 mg. Antihistamine* 75 mg. Salicylamide* 10 gr.
SINGLE SHOT TREATMENT Laxative (Oliver's S-O)	Paregoric (opium 0.018 gr./fl. oz.) Syrup rhubarb Castor oil Alcohol 7%
SINGLETARY'S RAT & MOUSE EXTERMINATOR Rodenticide (Singletary)	Arsenic trioxide* 3.00% Arsenic as metallic 2.27%
SING SHAMPOO (Andrews, C.)	
SINO-SENE (Diefenbach)	Nebula ephedrinae* composita N.F. Oil of thyme replaced with 4-n-amyl-meta-cresol 0.1 cc./1000 cc.
SINOX SELECTIVE WEED KILLER (Standard Ag.)	Sodium dinitro ortho cresylate* 30%
SINOX GENERAL Herbicide (Standard Ag.)	Dinitro ortho secondary butyl phenol* 50% Dinitro ortho secondary amyl phenol* 10%
SINOX PE Herbicide (Standard Ag.)	Triethanolamine Isopropanolamine Salts of dinitro ortho secondary butyl phenol* 57%
SINTOS Antitussive (Sintos)	Alcohol 1% Pot. guaiacol sulfonate Wild cherry Thyme Chloroform 1/4% Ammonium chloride Pine Menthol
S-I-P PAINTS & FLOOR WASHES (Standard Ind.)	

*Consult Sec. II., Ingredients Index. This ingredient may be responsible for major toxic effects if poisonous amounts of this product are ingested.

- 945 -

Name & Use Manufacturer	Ingredients		Name & Use Manufacturer	Ingredients	
SIPPY POWDER NO. 1 Gastric antacid (Horton & Converse)	Sodium bicarbonate Calcium carbonate powder N.F.		SKAT HAND SOAP, PASTE HAND SOAP (Skat)	Mild soap base Cleaned Pennsylvania sand Marble dust Soda ash small percentage Silicate of soda Perfume	
SIPPY POWDER NO. 2 Gastric antacid (Horton & Converse)	Sodium bicarbonate Magnesium oxide powder N.F.		SKEET-CHECK Insecticide (Nott)	Indalone Dimethyl phthalate	12.5% 12.5%
SIR HAIR OIL (Allied Drug)			SKEETER DIG Insect repellent (Penslar)	Oil camphor* Oil citronella* Oil eucalyptus*	30% vol. 10% 10%
SIROIL For skin irritations (Siroil)	Mercuric oleate 4/10 of 1% Cresol* Vegetable oils Mineral oils		SKEETER SCHOO INSECT REPELLENT (Olson Co.)		
SIR SHAVING LOTION (Allied Drug)			SKEETER SKARE Insecticide (Noblesse)		
SISSON'S HOUSEHOLD OINTMENT (Sisson, P.)	Carbolic acid 7/8% Imitation oil of organum Oil of peppermint Flowers of sulfur		SKEETER SKOOT Insecticide (Rexall)	Naphthalene Camphor Menthol Oil of citronella*	0.57% 1.69% 0.27% 2.06%
6-40 DISINFECTANT Bactericide, germicide (Hilex)	Sodium hypochlorite* 6.40%			Oil of pennyroyal* Oil of lavender* Petroleum distillate* Oil of eucalyptus* Oil of sassafras* Oil of cedarleaf* B-thiocyano ethyl esters	2.12% 2.07% 81.07% 2.09% 2.45% 4.48%
SIXIDE Insecticide (Commercial Solv.)	Gamma BHC* 10% & 15%			B-butoxy B'-thiocyano diethyl ether	0.85% 0.27%
666 COLD PREPARATION (Monticello)	Antipyrine 10 gr./oz. Ammonium chloride Magnesium sulfate Citric acid		SKEETER TIS SCHOO Insecticide (Olson Co.)		
666 VAPORIZING SALVE Nasal decongestant (Monticello)	Menthol, synthetic* Camphor* Chlorthymol Safrol* Oil of turpentine* Oil of cedar leaf*		SKETTO-NOX Insect repellent (Wisconsin Pharm.)	Indalone Dimalone Dimethyl phthalate	20% 20% 60%
16-D FILM DEVELOPER & REPLENISHERS (du Pont)			SKETCHO Oil paint in stick form (Am. Crayon)		
6-12 INSECT REPELLENT (Carbide)	2-Ethyl hexanediol-1,3*		SKETOBANE Insect repellent (Commercial Chem.)		
61 VARNISH & ENAMEL (Pratt & Lambert)			SKIDOO Cleanser (Climalene)	Soap Silica flour	5% 66%
SIZIN For sizing hats (Greenville)	Sizing gum Methyl alcohol less than 2%		SKIN-A-FIRE SKIN LOTION For skin irritations (Skin-A-Fire)	Alcohol* Phenol (carbolic acid) Salicylic acid* Methyl salicylate* Glycerin	70% 2%
SIZ LAX Cathartic, carminative (Floret)	Phenolphthalein Cane sugar Milk sugar Sodium bicarbonate Tartaric acid Citric acid				

*Consult Sec. II., Ingredients Index. This ingredient may be responsible for major toxic effects if poisonous amounts of this product are ingested.

Name & Use Manufacturer	Ingredients	Name & Use Manufacturer	Ingredients
SKIN-AID For acne (Wills)	Soap Colloidal sulfur* Granulated calcium carbonate Glycerin Aerosol Stearic acid Triethanolamine Zinc oxide Sodium borate*	SKOUR-NU RUG & UPHOLSTERY CLEANER (Skour-Nu)	
		SKRAM Insect repellent (Halsey)	Dimethyl phthalate 100%
SKIN-GLO CREME Hand lotion (Bacorn)	Tragacanth	SKREEN SUN TAN LOTION (Dewey)	Salicylic acid*
SKIN-JET Fungicide (medical) (Larroque)	Alcohol* 70% Ethyl aminobenzoate Benzoic acid* Aloe * Tolu balsam Camphor* Salicylic acid* Storax Benzoin	SKRIP Ink (Sheaffer)	Synthetic dyes Humectant Iron salt Tannic acid* Phenolic compounds*
		SLA-RAT Rodenticide (Nott)	Prepared warfarin 0.025%
SKIN PAL For acne (Dermateen)	Precip. sulfur* Camphor* Special gums	SLA-RAT CONC. Rodenticide (Nott)	Concentrate warfarin 0.25%
SKIP CLEANING JELLY General purpose cleaner (Korlis)		SLEEP-EZE Sedative (Sleep-Eze)	Methapyrilene hydrochloride* 25 mg./tablet
SKIT ANT SYRUP Insecticide (Scramento)	Arsenic*	SLICK LINOLEUM COATING (Glidden Co.)	
SKIT FLY SPRAY (Sacramento)	DDT* Inert ingredients*	SLICK SET HAIR DRESS (Humbert)	
SKITO-CHASE Insect repellant (K-A-S)	Oil of sandalwood Oil of cedar Oil of citronella Terpinyl acetate Isoprop. alcohol * 93%	SLIPIT Friction eliminator (Slipit)	Paraffin Wax and oil Commercial petrolatum
SKIT REPELLENT (Sacramento)		SLOAN'S BALM (Standard Labs.) (Standard Labs.)	Oleoresin capsicum Methyl salicylate* Menthol* Oil of white camphor* Pine oil* Turpentine* Eucalyptus oil*
SKOLEX (Williams, J.B.)	Propyl p-aminobenzoate Stearic acid Triethanolamine soap Polyglycols		
SKOL SUNTAN LOTION (Williams, J.B.)	Alcohol* p-Dehydroxyethyl-amino- benzoic acid Menthol*	SLOAN'S BALM (New) Counter-irritant (Standard Labs.)	Oleoresin capsicum Methyl salicylate* Menthol* Oil of white camphor* Oil of pine* Oil of turpentine* Oil of eucalyptus *
SKOOKON Insecticide (Planetary Chem.)	Piperonyl butoxide tech. 11.89% Pyrethrins 1.19% Petroleum distillate*(deodorized) 71.99%	SLOAN'S LINIMENT (Standard Labs.)	Capsicum Methyl salicylate* Oil camphor* Turpentine* Oil pine*
SKOOT DELOUSING LEG BAND Insecticide (Lockwood)	Nicotine sulfate* 14.4% Naphthalene 21.0% Oil of tar 12.0%	SLOMONS DAB-IT Cement (Slomons)	Rubber Naphtha*
		SLOMONS FELT & FABRIC STIFFENER (Slomons)	Butyl acetate Ethyl acetate Butyl alcohol* Naphtha* Nitro cellulose cotton 1/2 second

*Consult Sec. II., Ingredients Index. This ingredient may be responsible for major toxic effects if poisonous amounts of this product are ingested.

Name & Use Manufacturer	Ingredients		Name & Use Manufacturer	Ingredients	
SLOMONS IRON BOUND CEMENT (Slomons)	Rubber Lime Rosin Naphtha*		SMARTEE NAIL POLISH REMOVER (Cameo Inc.)	Ketones* (other than acetone) Ester (acetates) Hydrocarbons (aliphatic naphtha)* Olive oil Lanolin Color Perfume	
SLOMONS PAPER CEMENT (Slomons)	Tapioca starch Phenol preservative		SMEAREX #62 Insecticide (Florida Chem.)	Diphenylamine Benzol* Turkey red oil Lampblack	35% 35% 10% 20%
SLOMONS RE CEMENT (Slomons)	Rubber Lime rosin Naphtha*		SMEAREX NO. 442 Insecticide (Florida Chem.)	Pine oil* Lindane* Mineral oil	25% 3% 50%
SLOMONS RE-KOL-IT Cement (Slomons)	Butyl acetate Ethyl acetate Butyl alcohol* Naphtha* Nitro cellulose cotton 1/2 sec.		SMEAREX NO. 505 Insecticide (Florida Chem.)	Pine oil* Lindane*	25% 3%
SLOMONS SYNTHETIC FRENCH VARNISH Fabric stiffener (Slomons)	Cotton solution Castor oil Lacquer thinner*		SMEAREX NO. 1000 Insecticide (Florida Chem.)	Diphenylamine Benzol*	30% 30%
SLOMONS THI-ON THINNER Lacquer thinner (Slomons)	Butyl acetate Ethyl acetate Denatured alcohol* Naphtha* Butyl alcohol*		SMEAREX E.Q. 3-35 Insecticide (Florida Chem.)	Lindane* Pine oil* Mineral oil Santocel C. Emulsifier	3% 35% 42% 10% 10%
SLOMONS VELVERETTE Cement (Slomons)	Polyvinyl emulsion		SMILCO RAT KISSES Rodenticide (Smico)	Red squill*	
SLUG-FEST COLLOIDAL 50 Insecticide (Crop King)	Metaldehyde* 50%		SMILING SCOT CLEANER (Ohio Labs.)	Trisodium phosphate* Sodium sesquicarbonate Sodium tripolyphosphate* Triton X100 Phenolphthalein 10 gr./1000 lb.	
SLUG-KILL Insecticide (Plant Prod.)	Metaldehyde dust* 15%		SMILING SCOT PAINT & VARNISH CLEANER (Ohio Labs.)		
SLUMBERDENT For teething babies (Durma)	Acetylsalicylic acid (aspirin)* Methyl salicylate* Eugenol*		SMILING SCOT SUDS Dishwashing compound (Ohio Labs.)	Sodium sesquicarbonate Sodium tripolyphosphate Anionic synthetic detergent* (alkyl-aryl type)	
SMAK For cold sores and fever blisters (Heritage)	Alcohol* 90%/v Chloroform 5%/v Ethyl nitrite* Glycerin		SMITH, ALSOP'S CLEAR WOOD PRESERVATIVE (Smith-Alsop)	Zinc naphthenate* 16-1/2%	
SMALL FRY BUBBLE BATH AND COLOGNE (House of Hawick)			SMITH BROTHERS COUGH SYRUP (Smith Bros.)	Benzyl alcohol 1/2 of 1% Anise Menthol Licorice	
SMARTEE NAIL POLISH (Cameo Inc.)	Pigments Cellulose nitrate Formaldehyde-amine resin Dibutyl phthalate Synthetic camphor* Esters Alcohols (ethyl, isopropyl*, butyl)* Hydrocarbons (toluene)*		SMITHER'S BALM For hemorrhoids (Smither & Hill)	Ext. witch hazel Balsam fir Acid carbolic* Sassafras Glycerin Balsam peru Camphor* Oil of eucalyptus* Wormwood Benzoin Purified animal fats Hydrocarbons*	

*Consult Sec. II., Ingredients Index. This ingredient may be responsible for major toxic effects if poisonous amounts of this product are ingested.

Name & Use Manufacturer	Ingredients	Name & Use Manufacturer	Ingredients
SMOKEY BEAR Bubble Bath (Clark, R.)	Sodium sulfate Sodium alkyl aryl sulfonate* Sodium alkyl lauryl sulfonate* Perfume	SNOWY BLEACH (Gold Seal)	
SMOOTH HAND LOTION (Caswell-Massey)		SOAKOFF WALLPAPER REMOVER (Reliable Paste)	Sulfonated oils Carbon tetrachloride
SM'S (Suppository) (S.M.)	Toluquinone 1-2500 Hydroquinone 0.01% Boric acid 0.030% Starch 0.036% Emulsifying agent 0.0025% Coconut oil stearin	SOBITAL Sedative, hypnotic (Tailby)	Sodium phenobarbital* 2 gr. Potassium bromide 30 gr. Sodium bromide 30 gr.
SM'S VAGINAL SUPPOSITORIES Spermatocide (S.M.)	Toluquinone Hydroquinone	S.O. BRONKEROL Rubefacient, counter-irritant (Olivers S-O)	Chloroform* 24 m./fl. oz. Camphor* Oil turpentine* Methyl salicylate* (syn.) Oil eucalyptus* Oil of mustard* Oil capsicum* Oil origanum Oil of peppermint
SNAROL KILLS SNAILS & SLUGS Insecticide (Boyle-Midway)	Tricalcium arsenate* 5.00% Metaldehyde 1.75%	S. O. CORN REMEDY (Oliver's S-O)	
SNO BOL Bowl cleaner (Sno-Bol)	Hydrochloric acid* 14%	SODASAN Morgan Prod.)	Magnesium carbonate Papain Malt diastase Bismuth subcarbonate Sodium bicarbonate
SNO-DRIFT PASTE (Arabol)	Corn dextrine base adhesive	SODASEPTOL Hygienic powder (Phenacedol)	Boric acid* Alum Eucalyptol* Methyl salicylate* Sodium chloride Carbolic acid* Menthol*
SNOOZE Sedative (Harwood)	Sodium bromide* 3 gr. Potassium bromide* 2 gr. Ammonium bromide* 1 gr. Powd. ext. valerian Powd. ext. passiflora		
SNOWCREME DEODORIZER (B. & P.)		SODAZYME RHUBARB COMPOUND (Pulvoid) Antacid, carminative, digestant (Drug Prod, N.Y.)	Sodium bicarbonate 0.65 gm. Rhubarb 65 mg. Papain 32 mg. Pancreatin 32 mg. Ginger 16 mg. Tartaric acid Aromatics
SNOWFLAKE CRYSTALS & SNOWFINE Water softeners (Solvay)	Crystallized sodium sesqui-carbonate		
SNO-WHITE Bleach (Selected)	Sodium hypochlorite* 5-1/4%	SO-DEF-RIN JELLY Nasal decongestant (Hance)	Ephedrine hydrochloride* Phenol sodique Menthol* Camphor Oil cassia Eucalyptol* Oil pine needles
SNOW & MASON'S SYRUP Antitussive (Claflin)	Alcohol 5%/v Squill Senega Ipecac Antimony Potassium tartrate Sanguinaria Sugar Caramel coloring	SODIBOR Dentifrice, deodorant (Sodibor)	Sodium perborate* 98% Phenol, oil of cloves, oil of peppermint small quantities Phenolphthalein Color
		SODIO-PHOS SOLUTION Cathartic (Sharp & Dohme)	Each 100 cc.: Color Exsiccated sodium phosphate N.F. 39 gm.
SNOW WHITE BLEACHING CREAM (Snow White)	Ammoniated mercury* 1.5%	SODIPHENE MOUTHWASH Antiseptic, germicide (Sodiphene)	Sodium phenolate Phenol Sodium borate Dihydroxyhexachlorodiphenyl methane, (hexachlorophene)
SNOW-WHITE SHU MILK Shoe whitener (Shu-Milk)	Neatsfoot oil	SODITE ARSENICAL POISON Insecticide (Calif. Spray)	Arsenic trioxide* 32%

*Consult Sec. II., Ingredients Index. This ingredient may be responsible for major toxic effects if poisonous amounts of this product are ingested.

- 949 -

Name & Use Manufacturer	Ingredients	Name & Use Manufacturer	Ingredients
SO-FAIR (Chap Stick)	Emollient oil Surface-active agent	SO KOOL For sunburn (K-A-S)	Tannic acid* Benzocaine Alcohol 50%
SOFENOL CREAM (C & M)	Lanolin Stearic acid Mineral oil Triethanolamine stearate Butyl and propyl para-hydroxybenzoates	SOL-AC-TAN (S.F. Mfg. No. 925) External (Specialists)	Glycerin Salicylic acid* Tannic acid* Benzoic acid* Menthol* Alcohol* 40%/v
SOF-SET HAIR SPRAY (Lee Ltd.)	Lanolin Liquid cholesterol esters	SOLARGAINE For sunburn (Lanotan)	Benzocaine Glyceryl monostearate Stearic acid Benzalkonium* Menthol camphor* Benzyl alcohol*
SOF-SET NO-LAC HAIR SPRAY (Lee Ltd.)	Lanolin Silicones Proteins		
SOFSKIN HAND CREAM & LOTION (Sofskin)		SOLAR-SCREEN Skin protective (K-R)	Alcohol* 50%/v Tannic acid* Polyethylene glycol p-Aminobenzoic acid
SOFSKIN MOISTURE MAGIC Hand cream (Vick)		SOLAXPHOS (Solution) Biliary stimulant, cathartic (Massengill)	Each 5 cc.: Sodium acid phosphate 59 gr.
SOFTO (Climalene)	Soda ash 100%	SOLDERING FLUX FORMULA NO. 415 (Kester)	Ammonium halide* solution Inert polyhydric alcohol
SOFTOL CUTICLE SET (W.B.)	Glycol 25% Potassium hydroxide* less than 2%	SOLEXTO Insecticide (Dolge)	Tech. chlordane* 48% Petroleum aliphatic hydrocarbons* 47%
SOFT SOAP U.S.P. Tincture of green soap (Massengill)	Soft soap 650 parts Oil lavender 20 parts Alcohol to make 1000 parts	SOLID SENECA & SOLID SENECA 91 Specialized cleaning product (Wyandotte)	Concentrated alkali*
SOILAX Cleaner (Economics)	Sodium phosphate* Sodium sesquicarbonate Sodium bicarbonate Synthetic wetting agent* Fluorescein color	SOLITAIR CAKE MAKE UP (Campana)	Glycerin Lanolin Petrolatum Chalk Talc Color Triethanolamine oleate Water Mineral oil Sulfonated oil Kaolin Titanium dioxide Propylene glycol Perfume
SOILCLOR Insecticide (Bonide)	Tech chlordane* 50%		
SOILENE Insecticide (Liberty Chem.)	Chlordane 2%		
SOILFUME 60-40 Fumigant (Westvaco)	Ethylene dibromide* 41.2%	SOLITAIR LIPSTICK (Campana)	Candelilla wax Beeswax Carnauba wax Deltyl (extra) Castor oil Perfume Bromo acid Ozokerite Paraffin Lanolin Mineral oil Stablizer Color
SOIL-OFF LIQUID PAINT CLEANER (Soil-Off)			
SOIL-OFF RUG & UPHOLSTERY CLEANER (Soil-Off)			
SOIREE EAU DE COLOGNE (Delex)			

Name & Use Manufacturer	Ingredients	Name & Use Manufacturer	Ingredients
SOLITAIR LOTION (Campana)	Stearic acid Tegin Lanolin Lecithin Ethyl parasept Sorbitol Alcohol Cetyl alcohol Arlacel Isopropyl myristate Butyl parasept Triethanolamine Perfume Water	SOLUMOL SCALP CREAM For seborrhea (C & M)	Oil of cade* 5% Sulfur 5% Salicylic acid* 3% Solumol (washable base)
		SOLUMOL SULFUR CREAM For dermatosis (C & M)	Sulfur 10% Resorcin* 3% Betanaphthol 1% Solumol (washable base)
SOL-LID MAN HAIR POMADE (Flora Dell)		SOLUPINE Disinfectant (Central Chem.)	Phenol co-efficient against E. typhosa 4 F.D.A. Steam-distilled pine oil* 70% Vegetable oil soap
SOL-LO CREAM For sunburn (Pfeiffer)	Benzocaine Menthol* Zinc oxide Boric acid* Propylene glycol Glycerin Chlorothymol* Camphorated phenol* Colloidal kaolin Isopropyl alcohol 0.6%	SOLUTION OF BENCHLOPHEN (Hockwald)	Phenols*
		SOLVAL GUN CLEANER (Middleton)	
		SOLV-A-TON A Ink remover (Anchor Chem.)	
SOL-LO OINTMENT For skin irritation (Pfeiffer)	Benzocaine Zinc oxide Colloidal kaolin Calamine Camphorated phenol*	SOLVAY CLEANSER NO. 600 (Solvay)	Carbonates Silicates Phosphates Wetting agents
SO-LO For repair of shoes, rubber goods (So-Lo)	Rubber Petroleum naphtha*	SOLVAY ORTHODI-CHLORO-BENZENE Insecticide (Solvay)	Orthodichlorobenzene* 85% Chlorinated benzenes (princiaplly paradichloro-benzene) 15%
SOLOMON'S LOTION (De Soto Drug)		SOLVAY PARADI-CHLORO-BENZENE Insecticide (Solvay)	Paradichlorobenzene* 99.5-100%
SOLTEX MEDICATED SHAMPOO (C & M)	Orthobenzyl parachlorophenol 0.35% Stabilized conditioner (Lecinol) Alkyl-aryl detergent	SOLVENT 7-R Insecticide (Calif. Spray)	Aromatic petroleum distillate* 95%
SOLTICE QUICK RUB For cold, muscular soreness (Chattanooga)	Menthol* Camphor* Methyl salicylate* Oil of eucalyptus*	SOLVENTOL CLEANERS (Solventol)	
SOLUCREME Ointment (Lascoff)	Cetyl alcohol Stearyl alcohol Sodium lauryl sulfate	SOLVENTOL PAINT & VARNISH CLEANER (Solventol)	
SOLULINE For coccidiocis of chickens, turkeys (Gland-O-Lac)	Sulfaquinoxaline* 25%	SOLVESOL CLEANING FLUID (Caswell-Massey)	
SOLUMOL Ointment base (C & M)	Petrolatum Spermaceti Fatty alcohols including cetyl alcohol	SOLVEX Solvent (Am. Lacquer)	
SOLUMOL CADEBERRY CREAM For dermatosis (C & M)	Oil of cadeberry 5% Sulfur 3.5% Salicylic acid 0.5% Zinc oxide 5% Solumol (washable base)	SOLVINK 1 Ink and rust stain remover (Greenville)	Oxalic acid*

*Consult Sec. II., Ingredients Index. This ingredient may be responsible for major toxic effects if poisonous amounts of this product are ingested.

Name & Use Manufacturer	Ingredients		Name & Use Manufacturer	Ingredients	
SOLVINK 2 Stain remover (Greenville)	Ammonia*		SONOMA COUNTY'S WARFARIN RAT BAIT (Sonoma)	Warfarin	0.025%
SOLVIT Cleaner (Solvit)	Phosphates Steam-distilled pine oil* Wetting agents		SONO POWDER For cecal coccidiosis in chickens, swine dysentery (Corn King)	Sodium arsanilate*	169.8 gr./oz.
SOLVURIC PILLS Diuretic (Erie)	Buchu Podophyllin Oil juniper* Asparagus seed Potassium nitrate* Apiol		SOOT CLEAN Cleaner chimney (Soot Clean)		
SOLWAY- ANNAN HYDRANGEA COMPOUND (Solway- Annan)	Each capsule: Extract hydrangea 1/2 gr. Hexamethylenamine* 1 gr. Extract broom corn seed 1 gr. Extract uva ursi 1 gr. Extract corn silk 1/2 gr. Lithium benzoate 1/4 gr. Lithium salicylate* 1/4 gr.		SOOT DESTROYER Cleaner (Toledo)		
			SOOTHENE (Our Husbands)	Pine oil* Eucalyptol* Oil of geranium Menthol* Soap made from animal fat, ashes and lye	
SOMBUTOL Sedative (Approved)	Each capsule: Sodium bromide* 3 gr. Potassium bromide* 3 gr. Ammonium bromide* 1-1/2 gr. Valerian 1/2 gr. Passion flower 1/2 gr.		SOOT-NO- MORE Soot destroyer (Camp)		
SOME ENCHANTED EVENING Cosmetics (Thornton, R.)			SOOTRID Soot destroyer (Val-A)		
SOMETHING BLUE PERFUMES & EAU DE PERFUM (House of Gourielli)			SOOVAIN Analgesic (Soovain)	Acetophenetidin* 2 gr. Aspirin* Caffeine	
SOMNI-CAPS Sedative (Randolph Labs.)	n-n-Dimethyl n' (2-thenyl)- n'(2-pyridyl) ethylene diamine hydrochloride*		SOPRONOL OINTMENT Fungicide (medical) (Wyeth Labs.)	Sodium propionate 12.3% Sodium caprylate 10% Zinc caprylate 10% Zinc caprylate 5% n-Propyl alcohol 10%	
SONATA DEODORANT (Perfumed) (Countess)			SOPRONOL POWDER Fungicide (medical) (Wyeth Labs.)	Sodium propionate 5% Sodium caprylate 10% Zinc propionate 5%	
SONATA TOILET WATER (Countess)			SOPRONOL SOLUTION Fungicide (medical) (Wyeth Labs.)	Sodium propionate 12.3% Sodium caprylate 10% Dioctyl sodium sulfosuccinate 0.1% n-Propyl alcohol 12.5%	
SONG OF INDIA PERFUME (Perkins)					
SONG OF SONGS COLOGNE & PERFUME (Wolff)			SORETONE LINIMENT Analgesic (McKesson)	Acetone* Oil of wormwood Oil of tansy Methyl salicylate* 1-Methyl-3-dimethyl- cyclohexanol-5, 4-beta- ethyl hexylphenol 0.1% Salicylic acid*	
SONOMA COUNTY'S GOPHER POISON (Sonoma)	Strychnine alkaloid* 90.5%		SORIDEX OINTMENT Fungicide, bacteriacide (medical) (Kahlenberg)	Mercury oleate* 2% Chloral hydrate* 2.2% Zinc oleate Glyceryl oleate Stearate base	

*Consult Sec. II., Ingredients Index. This ingredient may be responsible for major toxic effects if poisonous amounts of this product are ingested.

- 952 -

Name & Use Manufacturer	Ingredients	
SORTILEGE ESSENCE & PARFUM (Cigogne)		
SO-SHUR Ointment, counter-irritant (So-Shur)	Oleic acid Ammonia water Oil of turpentine* Naphtha* Alcohol Methyl salicylate*	8%
S.O. SPECIAL SKIN LOTION For skin irritations (Oliver's S-O)	Mercury bichloride Carbolic acid* Benzoic acid Salicylic acid* Alcohol	1/3 gr./fl.oz. 25%
SOS SOOT DESTROYER (SOS)		
SOURFLO & SOURFLO-TEC Laundry and textile detergents (Wyandotte)	Fluorides*	
SOUTHERN AGRIC. CHEM. 50 BRAND 5% DDT DUST Insecticide (Southern Agric.Insect.)	DDT*	5.00%
SOUTHERN AGRIC. CHEM. 50 DUST (Southern Agric. Insect.)	Rotenone Pyrethrins Sulfur*	0.50% 0.04% 18.00%
SOUTHERN AGRIC. CHEM. 100 DUST Insecticide (Southern Agric. Insect.)	Rotenone Pyrethrins Sulfur*	1.00 % 0.08 % 18.00%
SOUTHERN AGRIC. CHEM. 50 BRAND 15% FERMATE DUST Insecticide (Southern Agric. Insect.)	Ferric dimethyl dithio-carbamate	11.20%
SOUTHERN AGRIC. CHEM. 50 1% PARATHION Insecticide (Soughern Agric. Insect.)	Parathion*	1.00%

Name & Use Manufacturer	Ingredients	
SOUTHERN AGRIC. CHEM BRAND NO. 100 Insecticide (Southern Agric. Insect.)	Rotenone Sulfur*	1.00% 18.00%
SOUTHERN AGRIC CHEM. 50 BRAND 1% PARATHION Insecticide (Southern Agric. Chem.)	Parathion*	1.00%
SOUTHERN AGRIC. CHEM. 50 BRAND PRE-HEADING CABBAGE DUST Insecticide (Southern Agric. Chem.)	Parathion* Toxaphene	1.5% 10.00%
SOUTHERN AGRIC. CHEM. 1-1/2% PARATHION DUST WITH 5% DDT Insecticide (Southern Agric. Chem.)	Parathion* DDT Sulfur	1.50% 5.00% 25.00%
SOUTHERN AGRIC. CHEM. 10% RHOTHANE DUST WITH 1% PARATHION (Southern Agric. Chem.)	Parathion* DDD	1.00% 10.00%
SOUTHERN AGRIC. CHEM. 50 20% TOXAPHENE COTTON DUST Insecticide (Southern Agric. Chem.)	Toxaphene*	20.00%
SOUTHERN AGRIC. CHEM. 20% TOXAPHENE DUST Insecticide (Southern Agric. Chem.)	Toxaphene*	20.00%
SOUTHERN GIRL COLD CREAM & VANISHING CREAM (Allied Drug)		
SOUTHERN PHARMACAL pH4 VAGINAL CREME (Southern Pharm.)	Phenylmercuric acetate 0.025% Oxyquinoilne benzoate 0.025% Triethanolamine Stearic acid Boric acid Glycerin Glyceryl monostearate	

*Consult Sec. II., Ingredients Index. This ingredient may be responsible for major toxic effects if poisonous amounts of this product are ingested.

Name & Use Manufacturer	Ingredients	Name & Use Manufacturer	Ingredients
SOUTHERN PHARMACAL VAGINAL JEL (Southern Pharm.)	Phenylmercuric acetate 0.025% Oxyquinoline benzoate 0.025% Boric acid Lactic acid Glycerin in gum base (pH4)	SOUTHERN STATES 66 DUST Insecticide (Coop. Seed)	DDT 3.00% Yellow cuprous oxide* 5.64%
SOUTHERN STATES 5% ALDRIN DUST Insecticide (Coop. Seed)	Hexachloro hexahydro-endo, exo-dimethano naphthalene* 4.8% Related compounds 0.8%	SOUTHERN STATES 75 DUST (Coop. Seed)	Rotenone 0.75% Other cube resins 1.35%
SOUTHERN STATES BEAN DUST NO. 1 Insecticide (Coop. Seed)	Rotenone 0.75% Other cube resins 1.35% DDT 3.00% Sulfur* 25.00%	SOUTHERN STATES 100 DUST Insecticide (Coop. Seed)	Rotenone 1.00% Other cube resins 2.00%
SOUTHERN STATES BEAN DUST NO. 2 Insecticide (Coop. Seed)	Rotenone 0.75% Other cube resins 1.35% DDT 3.00%	SOUTHERN STATES 620 DUST Insecticide (Coop. Seed)	Yellow cuprous oxide 5.64% Calcium arsenate* 13.90%
SOUTHERN STATES BEAN DUST NO. 4 Insecticide (Coop. Seed)	Rotenone 0.75% Other cube resins 1.35% Pyrethrins 0.08%	SOUTHERN STATES 675 DUST Fungicide (Coop. Seed)	Rotenone 0.75% Other cube resins 1.35% Yellow cuprous oxide* 5.64%
SOUTHERN STATES CUPROCIDE DUST NO. 6 Fungicide (Coop. Seed)	Yellow cuprous oxide* 5.64%	SOUTHERN STATES 875 DUST Insecticide, fungicide (Coop. Seed)	Rotenone 0.75% Other cube resins 1.35% Copper expressed as metallic* 8.00%
SOUTHERN STATES D3 DUST Insecticide (Coop. Seed)	DDT 3%	SOUTHERN STATES IMPREGNATED D1 DUST Insecticide (Coop. Seed)	DDT 1.00% Aromatic petroleum deriv. solvent 0.50%
SOUTHERN STATES D3P DUST Insecticide (Coop. Seed)	DDT 3.00%	SOUTHERN STATES LIME- MONO- HYDRATED COPPER SULFATE DUST 80-20 Fungicide (Coop. Seed)	Monohydrated copper sulfate* 20.00%
SOUTHERN STATES D5 DUST Insecticide (Coop. Seed)	DDT* 5.00%		
SOUTHERN STATES D10 DUST Insecticide (Coop. Seed)	DDT* 10.00%	SOUTHERN STATES 5% MALATHION DUST Insecticide (Coop. Seed)	Malathion* 5.00%
SOUTHERN STATES 60-20-20 DUST Insecticide (Coop. Seed)	Monohydrated copper sulfate* 19.50% Calcium arsenate* 14.00%		

Name & Use Manufacturer	Ingredients
SOUTHERN STATES M5 DUST Insecticide (Coop. Seed)	Methoxychlor tech. 5.0%
SOUTHERN STATES MZ 5-39 DUST Insecticide (Coop. Seed)	Zineb (zinc ethylene-bis (dithio-carbamate)) 3.9% Methoxychlor 5.0%
SOUTHERN STATES P1 DUST Insecticide (Coop. Seed)	Parathion* 1.00%
SOUTHERN STATES PD 1-5 DUST Insecticide (Coop. Seed)	Parathion* 1.00% DDT 5.00%
SOUTHERN STATES POTATO-TOMATO DUST NO. 1-7 Insecticide (Coop. Seed)	DDT 1.00% Aromatic petroleum deriv. solvent 0.50% Copper expressed as metallic* 7.00%
SOUTHERN STATES POTATO-TOMATO DUST NO. 3-7 Insecticide (Coop. Seed)	DDT 3.00% Copper expressed as metallic* 7.00%
SOUTHERN STATES POTATO-TOMATO DUST NO. 7 Fungicide (Coop. Seed)	Copper expressed as metallic* 7.00%
SOUTHERN STATES POTATO-TOMATO DUST NO. 7.5% Fungicide (Coop. Seed)	Captan 7.5%
SOUTHERN STATES SPECIAL STRAW-BERRY DUST Insecticide (Coop. Seed)	Tech. chlordane* 5.0% DDT* 5.0%
SOUTHERN STATES TOBACCO BLUE MOLD DUST Fungicide (Coop. Seed)	Ferbam (ferric dimethyl dithio-carbamate) 11.40%
SOUTHERN STATES TOBACCO DUST NO. 10-5 Insecticide (Coop. Seed)	DDD 10.00% Tech. chlordane* 5.00%
SOUTHERN STATES TOMATO-TOBACCO DUST NO. 10 Insecticide (Coop. Seed)	DDD 10.00%
SOUTHERN STATES VEGETABLE SPRAY Insecticide (Coop. Seed)	Rotenone* 2.5% Other cube resins 4.5% Copper* 26%
SOUTHERN STATES 5% WETTABLE ROTENONE Insecticide (Coop. Seed)	Rotenone* 5% Other cube resins 9%
SOUTHERN STATES Z DUST Fungicide (Coop. Seed)	Zineb (zinc ethylene-bis (dithio-carbamate)) 3.90%
SOUTHERN STATES Z1 DUST Insecticide (Coop. Seed)	Zineb (zinc ethylene-bis (dithio-carbamate)) 3.90% DDT 1.00% Aromatic petroleum deriv. 0.50%
SOUTHERN STATES Z10 DUST Fungicide (Coop. Seed)	Zineb (zinc ethylene-bis (dithio-carbamate)) 6.50%
SOUTHLAND CHLORDANE 75% EMULSION CONC. Insecticide (Southland)	Tech. chlordane* 75.0% Aliphatic petroleum hydro-carbons 18.0%
SOUTHLAND FRUIT-ODOR QUICK KILLE HOUSEHOLD INSECTICIDE (Southland)	Tech. chlordane 2.00% Pyrethrins 0.07% Petroleum solvents* 97.43%
SOUTH PACIFIC COLOGNE (Noblesse)	
SOUTHWEST ALDRIN EMULSIFIABLE CONC. Insecticide (Southwest Sprayer)	Hexachloro-hexahydro-dimethano naphthalene* 22.5% Related compounds 17.0% Xylene* 36.5% Petroleum distillate 14.0%
SOUTHWEST ARAMITE EMULSIFIABLE Insecticide (Southwest Sprayer)	2-(p-tert-Butylphenoxy)-isopropyl 2-chloroethyl sulfite 25.8%

*Consult Sec. II., Ingredients Index. This ingredient may be responsible for major toxic effects if poisonous amounts of this product are ingested.

Name & Use Manufacturer	Ingredients	Name & Use Manufacturer	Ingredients
SOUTHWEST BHC-DDT CONC. EMULSIFIABLE Insecticide (Southwest Agric.)	Gamma isomer of benzene hexachloride* 12.25% Other related isomers of benzene hexachloride* 18.37% DDT 20.40% Xylene* 26.75%	SOUTHWEST TOXAPHENE 40% DDT 20% EMULSIFIABLE Insecticide (Southwest Sprayer)	Tech. chlorinated camphene* 40% DDT 20%
SOUTHWEST BHC EMULSIFIABLE SPRAY CONCEN-TRATE Insecticide (Southwest Agric.)	Gamma isomer of benzene hexachloride* 13.50% Other related isomers of benzene hexachloride 20.40% Xylene* 42.00%	SOUTHWEST TOXAPHENE 60% EMULSIFIABLE Insecticide (Southwest Sprayer)	Toxaphene* (tech. chlorinated camphene containing 67-69% chlorine) 60% Petroleum distillate 23%
SOUTHWEST CHLORDANE EMULSIFIABLE Insecticide (Southwest Sprayer)	Tech. chlordane* 72.00% Petroleum solvents 13.00%	SOVASOL NO. 5 Herbicide (Socony)	Petroleum naphtha* (Stoddard solvent) 100%
SOUTHWEST COTTON LEAF KILL Fungicide (Southwest Agric.)	Pentachlorophenol* 33.2% Other chlorinated phenols 4.8%	SPA INSECT KILLER (Baldwin)	Petroleum distillate* 99.70% Sesame oil extractives (including 0.04% sesamin) 0.24% Pyrethrins 0.06%
SOUTHWEST DDT 25% EMULSIFIABLE Insecticide (Southwest Sprayer)	DDT 25% Xylene* 65%	SPANDY Disinfectant, germicide (Taylor-Reed)	Dodecylamine lactate 0.40% Isopropyl alcohol 4.2% Dodecylamine salicylate 0.40%
SOUTHWEST DIELDRIN EMULSIFIABLE Insecticide (Southwest) Agric.)	Hexachloro epoxy octahydro dimethano naphthalene* 15.80% Related compounds 2.85% Petroleum hydrocarbons 73.90%	SPA STAINLESS FLYKILLER (Baldwin)	Petroleum distillate* 98.72% Pine oil 1.00% Sesame oil extractives 0.24% Pyrethrins 0.04%
SOUTHWEST FLY & ROACH SPRAY Insecticide (Southwest Sprayer)	Chlordane 2.0000% Pyrethrins 0.0025% Petroleum distillate* 97.9975%	SPARKETTE, SPARKLE Alkaline detergents (Pennyslv. Salt)	Sodium orthosilicate* Sodium hydroxide* or sodium carbonate Soap or detergents
SOUTHWEST FLY SPRAY & REPELLENT Insecticide (Southwest Sprayer)	Tech. piperonyl butoxide 10.00% Pyrethrins 1.00% Petroleum distillate* 80.00%	DR. SPATES TABLETS Cathartic (Shaffer)	Cascara sagrada Powdered extract ox bile
SOUTHWEST HEPTACHLOR EMULSIFIABLE Insecticide (Southwest Sprayer)	Heptachlor* 23.41% Related compounds 9.10% Xylene* 61.36%	SPC KITCHEN SPRAY Air purifier (Mann, Leo)	Parahydroxybenzoic acid Thymol* Beta-naphthol* Phenylethyl alcohol Formalin* Essential oils* Aromatics Isopropanol*
SOUTHWEST 25% PARATHION Insecticide (Southwest) Agric.)	Parathion* 25% Xylene 65%	SPEARHEAD'S C.C. & G. CEMENT (Spearhead)	
		SPECIAL BYCIDE OIL Insecticide (Miller Chem.)	Mineral oil Carbon bisulfide*
SOUTHWEST TEPP Insecticide (Southwest Sprayer)	Tetraethyl pyrophosphate* 40% Other related organic phosphates* 60%	SPECIAL FORMULA SKIN CREAM For dry skin (Gordon Labs.)	Cholesterol Lubricating oils Perfume

*Consult Sec. II., Ingredients Index. This ingredient may be responsible for major toxic effects if poisonous amounts of this product are ingested.

- 956 -

Name & Use Manufacturer	Ingredients
SPECIAL HANDY FLUX FOR TITANIUM (Handy)	Potassium acid fluoride* Potassium tetraborate* Boric acid*
SPECIALISTS' FORMULARY NO. 986 MEDICATED RINSE For dandruff) (Specialists)	Sodium thiosulfate Potassium sulfate Triethanolamine Benzalkonium chloride Sodium metaphosphate
SPECIALISTS UNGUENTUM MYC-O-MOL (S.F. Mfg. No. 718) Ectoparasiticide (Specialists)	Resublimed iodine* Oils Fats
SPECIAL OUTDOOR FOGGING CONC. NO. 10 Insecticide (Lorenz)	Aromatic petroleum distillate* B' butoxy b' thiocyanodiethyl ether and ethyl esters Benzene hexachloride (gamma)*
SPECIAL S-O GARGLE For throat irritations (Oliver's S-O)	Potassium chlorate* Tannic acid* Carbolic acid* Antiseptic solution N.F. Alcohol 4%
SPECIAL S-O SKIN SALVE For skin irritations (Oliver's S-O)	
SPECIAL TERMITE FLUID Insecticide (Uncle Sam)	Orthodichlorobenzene* 100%
SPECIAL THINNER 200T (Cordo)	Ketones Aromatic hydrocarbons*
SPECO SOLVENT & THINNER (Speco)	Coal tar aromatic solvent*
SPECS Paint thinner, cleaning solvent (Sunnyside)	Petroleum product classed with Stoddard solvent*
SPECTACLE PERFUME & TOILET WATER (Corot)	
SPE-DEE CLEANER (Tarbox)	
SPEDENE AUTOMOTIVE FINISHES (Glidden Co.)	

Name & Use Manufacturer	Ingredients
SPEDOLENE LUBRICATING GREASE (Tide Water)	
SPEED EASY FLAT WALL PAINT (White) (du Pont)	Resin base Resin emulsion
SPEE-DEE Paint, oil grease remover (Adco)	
SPEEDEE Wallpaper cleaner (Dover)	
SPEE-DEE CEMENTS, (China, Crockery, Glass, Furniture, Fabric, Porcelain, Model airplane, Rubber) (Owasso)	
SPEEDTONE Photographic supply (Nat'l. Chem.)	
SPEEDUP FRENCH DRY CLEANER (Globe Solvents)	Aromatics* 20% Naphthenes* 30% Paraffins 50%
SPEED-WALL GLOSS AND FLAT PAINTS (Glidden Co.)	
SPEEDWAY LINIMENT (Energy)	Gum camphor* Oil of mustard Gum benzoin Oil of spearmint Alcohol*
SPEEDY WHITE White wall tire cleaner (Modern Chem.)	
SPEEKMAN CREOSOTE Wood preser- vative (Speekman)	Coal tar neutral oils* 97%
SPEEKMAN CREOTOX Disinfectant, deodorant, cleaner (Speekman)	Petroleum aromatic oils* 53% Anhydrous soap 22% Total phenols* 15%
SPEEKMAN CREOTOX (Sheep Dip) Disinfectant (Speekman)	Petroleum aromatic oils* 53% Anhydrous soap 22% Total phenols* 15%

*Consult Sec. II., Ingredients Index. This ingredient may be responsible for major toxic effects if poisonous amounts of this product are ingested.

Name & Use Manufacturer	Ingredients		Name & Use Manufacturer	Ingredients	
SPEEKMAN DAIRY & LIVESTOCK SPRAY Insecticide (Speekman)	Mineral oil Piperonyl butoxide Tech. ether Other compounds Pyrethrins*		SPERRY'S HORN PREVENTER Veterinary (Sperry)		
SPEEKMAN GERMICIDE Disinfectant (Speekman)	Cresylic acid* Soap	51% 24%	SPERRY'S POCKET GOPHER POISON Rodenticide (Sperry)	Strychnine sulfate*	12%
SPEEKMAN INDUSTRIAL SPRAY Insecticide (Speekman)	Deodorized kerosene* Piperonyl butoxide tech. Pyrethrins*		SPERRY'S POISON WHEAT Rodenticide (Sperry)	Strychnine sulfate*	0.23%
SPEEKMAN INSECT SPRAY (Speekman)	Deodorized kerosene* Beta thiocyano ethyl esters of mixed fatty acids averaging 10-18 carbon atoms B-butoxy B' thiocyano diethyl ether*		SPERTI (Contains Bio-Dyne) Skin ointment (Whitehall)	Live yeast-cell deriv. Shark liver oil Phenylmercuric nitrate Lanolin Mineral jelly	3.0% 1-10,000
SPEEKMAN PYRECIDE Insecticide (Speekman)	Piperonyl butoxide tech. 5.92% Pyrethrins 0.59% Poloxyethylene sorbitol mixed ether ester 14.81% Petroleum oil 78.68%		SPEX-OUT (Morgan Prod.)	Carbon tetrachloride* Benzol* Toluene*	
SPEEKMAN RESIDUAL SPRAY CONTAINS 5% D.D.T. Insecticide (Speekman)	Active ingredients: 100% Deodorized kerosene* Dichloro diphenyl trichloro- ethane*		S.P.F. WOOD PRESERVER Huggins)	Free carbon Coal tar distillates*	1% 97%
			SPHINX DEODORANT (Rimmel)		
SPEEKMAN WAREHOUSE & MILL SPRAY Insecticide (Speekman)	Deodorized kerosene Carbon tetrachloride* Beta thiocyano ethyl esters of mixed fatty acids averaging 10-18 carbon atoms B-butoxy-B'-thiocyano diethyl ether*		SPHINX LIQUID GLUE (Arabol)	Animal glue Alpha naphthalene sulfonic acid	
SPERGON-DDT (Naugatuck)	Chloranil (tetrachloro-para- benzoquinone)* 93%		SPHINX METALLIC WATER COLORS (Weber, F.)	Bronze metallic powder Water-soluble gums	
SPERGON- DDT-SL (Naugatuck)	Chloranil (tetrachloro-para- benzoquinone)* 92%		SPHINX RETOUCHING VARNISH (Weber, F.)	Light varnish gums Volatile diluent*	
SPERGON-SL. (Naugatuck)	Chloranil (tetrachloro-para- benzoquinone)* 95%		SPHINX WAX CRAYONS (Weber, F.)		
SPERGON TECHNICAL Insecticide (Naugatuck)	Chloranil (tetrachloro-para- benzoquinone)* 97%		SPICE AIR Air deodorizer (Claire)	Triethylene glycol	7.5%
SPERGON WETTABLE (Naugatuck)	Chloranil (tetrachloro-para- benzoquinone)* 48%		SPICER'S COMPOUND Laxative (Spicer)	Epsom salt Cascara sagrada Senna Rhubarb Buchu Iron Jalap Juniper berries	
SPERRY'S CAUSTIC LOTION For actinomycosis (veterinary) (Sperry)	Sodium hydroxide* 65%				
SPERRY'S GOPHER GRAIN Rodenticide (Sperry)	Strychnine sulfate* 0.25%		SPICER'S PALVO POWDER Vaginal douche (Spicer)	Menthol* Glycerin Boric acid* Phenol* Thymol* Eucalyptol* Zinc sulfate*	

*Consult Sec. II., Ingredients Index. This ingredient may be responsible for major toxic effects if poisonous amounts of this product are ingested.

Name & Use Manufacturer	Ingredients	Name & Use Manufacturer	Ingredients
SPICER'S T.P.-64 Muscular analgesic, internal (Spicer)	Sodium salicylate* Cimicifuga Glycyrrhiza Potassium iodide	SPOHN'S COMPOUND Antitussive (veterinary) (Spohn)	Sulfur* Creosote* Oil of tar* Turpentine*
SPI-CO EAR TICK REMEDY Insecticide (Texas Pheno.)	Pine tar Xylene* Gamma isomer of benzene hexachloride* Other isomers of benzene hexachloride Tech. chlordane	SPOHN'S UDDER-AID Veterinary (Spohn)	Oxyquinoline benzoate Oil of camphor* Lanolin Peanut oil Petrolatum Paraffin
SPIC & SPAN CLEANER & WATER SOFTENER (Procter & Gamble)	Sodium sesquicarbonate Sodium tripolyphosphate Sodium orthophosphate Anionic synthetic detergent	SPONGE-AWAY Insecticide (Cooper)	S.D. pine oil* 43.5% Camphor oil* 6.0% Paradichlorobenzene 7.5% Rotenone 1.0% Other cube resins or extractives 2.0%
SPIC SPOT CLEANING FLUID (Norton)	Naphtha* (V.M. & P.) Stoddard solvent*	SPONGIACAINE TROCHES Antitussive (Clapp, Otis)	Extract of spongia Benzocaine 1/4 gr.
SPIGELIA & SENNA SYRUP (Hance)	Spigelia Senna Oils of caraway Oils of anise Syrup base	SPORODYNE For skin irritation (Sporodyne)	Alcohol 46% Benzoic acid* Essential oils* Menthol* Tannic acid* Benzocaine Chlorothymol Glycerin Salicylic acid*
SPIN Machine-dishwashing detergent (Climalene)		SPORTSMAN COLOGNE (Moore, J.)	Denatured alcohol* more than 70% Perfume oils Coloring matter
SPINOL Rubefacient, nasal congestion (Spinol)	Menthol* Oil amber Methyl salicylate* Cottonseed oil Oil eucalyptus* Ti tree oil Oil sassafras syn.*	SPORTSMAN D-BAR (Solidified deodorant) (Moore, J.)	Perfume oils Glycol Carbitol Hexachlorophene Denatured alcohol Soap
SPINOSE EAR TICK REMEDY Veterinary (Anchor Serum)	Gamma isomer of benzene hexachloride 0.75% Other isomers of benzene hexachloride 1.35% Pine oil* 85.0% Xylol* 12.9%	SPORTSMAN HAIR DRESSING (Moore, J.)	Denatured alcohol Benzyl benzoate Castor oil Gum benzoin
SPIRO POWDER Deodorant (Spiro)	Zinc oxide U.S.P. Magnesium carbonate U.S.P. Sierra supreme talc U.S.P.	SPORTSMAN LIQUID DEODORANT (Moore, J.)	Denatured alcohol Perfume oils Hexachlorophene
SPIX Insecticide (Dolge)	Petroleum distillates* Piperonyl butoxide Tech. essential oils* Pyrethrins*	SPORTSMAN SHAVING LOTION (Moore, J.)	Denatured alcohol approx. 70% Perfume oils Coloring matter
SPLIT-ACTION CAPSULES Anthelmintic (veterinary, avian) (Pratt Food)	Nicotine expressed as alkaloid* 2.00% Phenothiazine 10.00% Aloes 0.25%	SPORTSMAN TODDY STICK (Solidified Shave Lotion) (Moore, J.)	Perfume oils Glycol Carbitol Denatured alcohol Soap
SPLURGE WATER THINNED TEXTURE PAINT (United Gilson.)	Soya protein Water-soluble cellulose ether (sodium pentachlorophenate) 0.67%	SPOT BALM FOR DOGS For skin irritations (veterinary) (Happy Jack)	Glycerin Salycilic acid* Tannic acid* Sulfanilamide* 5% Brilliant green Isopropyl alcohol* 60%
		SPOT CHECK (Chek)	

*Consult Sec. II., Ingredients Index. This ingredient may be responsible for major toxic effects if poisonous amounts of this product are ingested.

- 959 -

Name & Use Manufacturer	Ingredients		Name & Use Manufacturer	Ingredients	
SPOT FABRIC FLUFF Rug, up-holstery, fabric cleaner (Mann, Leo)			DR. SPRAGUE'S TAKA-FLU-BRAKA CAPS Analgesic (Steinmann)	Acetophenetidin* 1 gr./tablet Aspirin* Caffeine Sod. benzoate Phenyl salicylate*	
SPOT FUMIGANT (Thompson-Hayward)	Carbon tetrachloride* 59.9% Ethylene dichloride 19.6% Ethylene dibromide* 20.5%		SPRA-KILL Insecticide (Wilkil)	Tech. chlordane 3% Inert ingredients* 97%	
SPOTLESS TOWN CLEANER (Sapolio)			SPRA-KILL Insecticide (Eagle Chem.)	Tech. chlordane 2.00% Beta-butoxy-beta-thiocyano diethylether 1.50% Inert ingredients*	
SPOTLIGHT DRY CLEANER (York Pharm.)	Naphthas* Ethylene dichloride*		SPRA-TOX Insecticide (Doggett-Pfeil)	Rotenone* Pyrethrum* Inert ingredient*	
SPOT MILL FUMIGANT (Cook Chem.)	Ethylene dichloride* 55% Carbon tetrachloride* 2.3% Ethylene dibromide* 22%		SPRATTS' BIRD LICE POWDER Insecticide (Spratts)	Pyrethrins 0.225%	
SPOT-NOT Stain preventive (Cooper)			SPRATTS' BLACKERITE (Spratts)	Lime Carbolic acid*	
SPOT OFF DRY CLEANER (Wood Labs.)			SPRATTS' CALCIUM PHOSPHATE (Tribasic) (Spratts)	Calcium min. 36.5% Phosphorus min. 17.0% pH (20% suspension) 6.5-7.2	
SPOT-REMOV-R (Goldman, R.)			SPRATTS' CAPSULES Anthelmintic for puppies and toy dogs (Spratts)	Oil chenopodium* 6.85% Santonin 0.28% Castor oil 90% Oil turpentine 1.57% Oil fennel Oil coriander U.S.P. Methyl salicylate*	
SPOTSGO Dry cleaner (Selig)					
SPOTSTIK Cosmetic (O'Leary)			SPRATTS' CAPSULES Anthelmintic for cats and kittens (Spratts)	Oil chenopodium U.S.P.* 6.24% Santonin 0.27% Castor oil 90.76% Oil turpentine 1.56%	
SPRACE OINTMENT For hemorrhoids (Shore)	Ephedrine alkaloid* 2% Benzocaine 5% Chlorothymol 1/4% Bismuth subnitrate 5% Mentholated, emollient, cholestrol base				
			SPRATTS' COUGH TABLETS Antitussive (veterinary) (Spratts)	Tinc. belladonna leaves 1/2 m. Ext glycyrrhiza Ipecac Antimony* Potassium tartrate	
SPRA-GON ANT & ROACH KILLER (Rempel)	Tech. chlordane 2.5%		SPRATTS' DIP Disinfectant (Spratts)	Coal tar hydrocarbons* Phenols* Soap	
SPRA-GON DAIRY & STOCK SPRAY Insecticide (Rempel)	Petroleum oil* Pine oil* Tech. piperonyl butoxide Pyrethrins*		SPRATTS' DIURETIC TABLETS Veterinary (Spratts)	Boric acid* Ext. uva ursi Ext. hydrangea Calcium carbonate Ext. corn silk Atropine sulfate 1/500 gr.	
SPRA-GON FLY SPRAY (Rempel)	Petroleum oil* Piperonyl butoxide Pyrethrins*				
			SPRATTS' DOG CAPSULES Anthelmintic (Veterinary) (Spratts)	Ext. areca nut 6.25% Ext. kamala Oil chenopodium* 5% Castor oil	
SPRA-GON SUPER DAIRY SPRAY Insecticide (Rempel)	Petroleum oil* 97.45% Pine oil 1.00% Tech. methoxychlor 1.00% Tech. piperonyl butoxide 0.50% Pyrethrins 0.05%				
			SPRATTS' DOG & CAT REMEDY (Spratts)		

*Consult Sec. II., Ingredients Index. This ingredient may be responsible for major toxic effects if poisonous amounts of this product are ingested.

Name & Use Manufacturer	Ingredients		Name & Use Manufacturer	Ingredients	
SPRATTS' DOG-TROT Repellent, veterinary (Spratts)	Oleum graminis citrati. br.*		SPRATTS' SARCOPTIC MANGE LIQUID Veterinary (Spratts)	Kerosene oil* Crude oil* Pine oil Nicotine* Linseed oil Oil pine tar Anhydrous soap	33% 24% 5.60% 0.0525% 24% 10% 0.66%
SPRATTS' EAR CANKER OINTMENT (Veterinary) (Spratts)	Salicylic acid* Zinc oxide Benzocaine Petrolatum Boric acid* Oil cade* Lanolin		SPRATTS' SHAMPOO (Spratts)	Cocoanut Olive oils	
SPRATTS' FLEA & INSECT POWDER (Spratts)	Pyrethrins Rotenone Other cube extractives Sulfur*	0.8% 0.25% 0.25% 25.0%	SPRATTS' SPECIAL TABLETS Diuretic (veterinary) (Spratts)	Potassium citrate Nuclein acid Powd. ext. nux vomica Strychnine Camphor	1/120 gr. 1/1600 gr.
SPRATTS' GAPINA LIQUID For bronchial parasites (veterinary, avian) (Spratts)			SPRATTS' SULFUR TABLETS Veterinary (Spratts)	Washed sulfur* Ext. ipecac Arsenic trioxide * Sodium benzoate Potassium bitartrate Ext. capsicum	1/1000 gr.
SPRATTS' LICE POWDER FOR POULTRY & GAME (Spratts)	Sulfur flour* Sodium fluoride*	44% 16%	SPRATTS' TABLETS FOR CONSTIPATION (Veterinary) (Spratts)	Cascarin bitter Aloin* Ext. belladonna* U.S.P. Total alkaloids Oleoresin ginger Podophyllin* U.S.P.	1/8 gr. 1/640 gr.
SPRATTS' LINIMENT (Spratts)	Camphor* Ammonia* Oil turpentine* Oil origanum Saponaceous base		SPRATTS' TAPEWORM TABLETS (Veterinary) (Spratts)	Arecoline hydrobromide*	4.47%
SPRATTS' MITALENE For washing cages, perches (Spratts)	Alcohol	6.80%	SPRATTS' TONIC TABLETS Veterinary (Spratts)	Po. ext. nux vomica Strychnine* Cascara sagrada Ferric hypophosphite Potassium hypophosphite	1/60 gr. 1/800 gr.
SPRATTS' OINTMENT Ectoparasiticide (veterinary) (Spratts)	Potassium bicarbonate Sulfur sublimed* Oil tar	1.6% 23% 6.2%	SPRAY-ALL DEODORANT BLOCKETTES (Elk)	Paradichlorobenzene*	
SPRATTS' OVALS WITH COD LIVER OIL Dog food (Spratts)	Wheat flour Meat meal Cod liver oil U.S.P. Iron oxide	1.5%	SPRAY-ALL DEODORANT CRYSTALS (Elk)	Paradichlorobenzene*	
SPRATTS' PENNAKURA Ectoparasiticide (veterinary, avian) (Spratts)	Quassia ext. Sodium fluoride	0.017% 0.075%	SPRAY-ALL DISINFECTANT (Elk)	Coal tar derivative*	
			SPRAY-ALL EMULSIFIABLE CONCEN-TRATE 25% Insecticide (Elk)	DDT* Aromatic hydrocarbons*	
SPRATTS' QUINELLA (Tibbs) Powder, in-testinal astringent (veterinary, avian) (Spratts)	Pulv. cranesbill Catechu Tormentil Capsicum		SPRAY-ALL GARDEN PRODUCTS (Elk)	Pyrethrum DDT*	
			SPRAY-ALL MOTH LIQUID (Elk)	Chlorinated hydrocarbons* Paradichlorobenzene	
			SPRAY-ALL PLANT LIQUID (Elk)	Pyrethrum extractives*	

*Consult Sec. II., Ingredients Index. This ingredient may be responsible for major toxic effects if poisonous amounts of this product are ingested.

Name & Use Manufacturer	Ingredients	Name & Use Manufacturer	Ingredients
SPRAY-CHEM A Wetting and spreading agent (Pacific Coast)	Alkylated aryl polyether alcohol	SPRAY-TROL BRAND SUPER-TROL Insecticide (Coyne)	Petroleum hydrocarbon* oil base Tech. piperonyl butoxide Pyrethrins*
SPRAY-DAY-LITE Paint (Glidden Co.)		SPRAYWAY Deodorizer, air sanitizer (Tru-Pine)	Triethylene glycol 7.5%
SPRAY FLO Abrasive cleaner (Pennsylv. Salt)	Alkaline silicate Phosphate Soda ash Wetting agent	SPRAYWAY Insecticide (Tru-Pine)	Pyrethrins 0.0255% Rotenone 0.128% Tech. piperonyl cyclonene 0.256% Petroleum hydrocarbon 0.102%
SPRAY GREEN Nitrogen spray for foliage feeding (Sunland)	Organic nitrogen (urea) 20%	SPRAYWAY FAST-KILL BUG KILLER Insecticide (Tru-Pine)	Tech. chlordane 2.000% Tech. piperonyl butoxide 0.115% Pyrethrins 0.046% Polymerized glycerol oleate 0.100% Petroleum distillates* 72.739% Freon 12 25.000%
SPRAYSHEEN Cleaning compound (Pioneer)			
SPRAY TAN Sunburn preventative (Spray Tan)		SPRAYWAY LIVESTOCK SPRAY Insecticide (Tru-Pine)	Pyrethrins 0.2% Tech. piperonyl butoxide 2.0% Tech. methoxychlor 3.0% Isobornyl thiocyanoacetate 1.64% Related terpenes 0.36% Methylated naphthalenes* 12.00% Petroleum distillate 10.8%
SPRAY-TROL BRAND, CONTAC-TROL Insecticide (Coyne)	Petroleum hydrocarbon oil base* Tech. piperonyl butoxide Pyrethrins		
SPRAY-TROL BRAND CONCEN-TROL Insecticide (Coyne)	Petroleum hydrocarbon* oil base Tech. piperonyl butoxide Pyrethrins	SPRAYWAY PLANT SPRAY Insecticide (Tru-Pine)	Pyrethrins 0.0255% Rotenone 0.128% Other cube extractives 0.236% Tech. piperonyl cyclonene 0.256% Petroleum hydrocarbon 0.102%
SPRAY-TROL BRAND FUMI-TROL Fumigant (Coyne)	Ethylene dichloride Carbon tetrachloride*	SPRAYWAY SPRING BLOSSOM ROOM DEODORIZER & AIR SANITIZER Household deodorant (Tru-Pine)	Triethylene glycol 7.5%
SPRAY-TROL BRAND MOTH-TROL Insecticide (Coyne)	Petroleum hydrocarbon oil base* DDT* DDD*		
SPRAY-TROL BRAND RESIDU-TROL Insecticide (Coyne)	Petroleum hydrocarbon oil base* 94.0% DDT 3.0% Tech. chlordane 3.0%	SPRAZIT AUTO & FURNITURE WAX, DEODORANTS (Plasti-Kote)	
		SPRAZIT FIRE EXTIN-GUISHER (Plasti-Kote)	
SPRAY-TROL BRAND RODEN-TROL Rodenticide (Coyne)	Warfarin (3-(a-acetonylbenzyl)-4-hydroxycoumarin) 0.5%	SPRAZIT MOTH PROOFER Repellent (Plasti-Kote)	

*Consult Sec. II., Ingredients Index. This ingredient may be responsible for major toxic effects if poisonous amounts of this product are ingested.

Name & Use Manufacturer	Ingredients
SPRAZIT PLASTIC COATING, WOOD & METAL COATING (Plasti-Kote)	
SPRED PAINT PRODUCTS (Glidden Co.)	
SPRED-RITE Sticker, spreader (agricultural) (Sherwin-Williams)	Fish oil soap
SPRING SHOWERS (Modart)	Sodium lauryl sulfate Fatty acid esters
SPRITE SPRAY DEODORANT Antiperspirant (Pharma-Craft)	Aluminum chlorhydroxide complex Aluminum chloride Urea Alcohol Perfume
SQUIBB DENTAL CREAM (Squibb)	Calcium carbonate Magnesium hydroxide Sodium alginate Sodium stearate Gelatin Glycerin Color (certified foods) Flavor (mint) Saccharin
SQUIBB LATHER SHAVE (Squibb)	
SQUIBB PHENOLOR Antiseptic, disinfectant (Squibb)	Orthophenylphenol* (hydroxy diphenyl) 13% Isopropyl alcohol 5%/v Soap 13%
SQUIRE JUNIOR'S DIAPER DEODORIZER (Curtis Squire)	Hyamine #2389
S.R.P. RUST INHIBITOR (Sonneborn)	
S.S.S. Tonic, food supplement (S.S.S.)	Queen's delight Swamp sumac Sumac Iron 33-1/3 mg./tbsp. Copper 1 mg./tbsp. Alcohol 12%
S.S.S. TONIC TABLETS Food supplement (S.S.S.)	Iron Copper Powd. root ext. rhus giabra Rhus vernix Stillingia sylvatica Betaine hydrochloride Thiamine hydrochloride
STA Paint (Testor)	Vinyl resin Dioctyl phthalate M.I.K. Toluol* Cyclohexanone

Name & Use Manufacturer	Ingredients
STA-BAC Hair dressing (Vi-Jon)	
STABCHLOR Insecticide (Chapman Chem.)	Tech. chlordane* 44.1% Petroleum distillate* 42.9%
STA-FLO LAUNDRY STARCH (Staley)	Borax Mersolite (composed largely of phenyl mercuric acetate) 0.002% Starch Color Perfume
STAG BRUSHLESS SHAVING CREAM, CREAM HAIR TONIC, MINT FREEZE DEODORANT STICK & PERFUMED HAIR OIL (Langlois)	
STAG DEODORANT CREAM (Langlois)	Aluminum chlorhydrate* Benzoic acid*
STAINFLOOR WOOD FINISH Paint product (Rogers Chem.)	
STAIN GLOSS STOVE POLISH (Satin Gloss)	
STAINTOX Wood preservative, insecticide (Abesto)	Pentachlorophenol* 5%
STA KLEAN CLEANERS (Porcelain, Tile, Marble, Linoleum, Hardwood Floor) (Staples, H.)	
STA KLEAN PAINT & VARNISH CLEANER (Staples, H.)	
STAMINE WITH A.C.A. COMPOUND (Tutag)	Each coated tablet: Pyrilamine maleate Merck* 10 mg. Acetylsalicylic acid (aspirin)* 3-1/2 gr. Acetophenetidin* 2-1/2 gr. Caffeine alkaloid 1/2 gr.

*Consult Sec. II., Ingredients Index. This ingredient may be responsible for major toxic effects if poisonous amounts of this product are ingested.

- 963 -

Name & Use Manufacturer	Ingredients
STAMINITE AMMONIATED WAX REMOVER (Staminite)	Ammonia*
STAMINITE SUPER QUALITY ENAMELS (Staminite)	Lead* Pigment* (Only Apple Green, Lettuce Green, Deep Green, and Chinese Red contain lead)
STANBACK ANALGESIC POWDERS (Stanback)	Each powder: Acetophenetidin* 5 gr. Aspirin* Caffeine
STANBACK ANALGESIC TABLETS (Stanback)	Each tablet: Acetophenetidin* 2-1/2 gr. Aspirin* Caffeine
STANDARD AEROSOL INSECT KILLER (Standard Oil)	DDT 2.00% Pyrethrins 0.10% Tech. piperonyl butoxide 0.60% B-butoxy-B'-thicyano diethyl ether 1.63% Methylated naphthalene* 5.75% Petroleum oil 4.92% Propellents 85%
STANDARD AGRIC. CHEM. SINOX-W Herbicide (Standard Ag.)	Ammonium dinitro ortho secondary butyl phenol* 13%
STANDARD AGRIC. CHEM. 90% SODIUM TCA Herbicide (Standard Ag.)	Sodium trichloracetate*
STANDARD APHID SPRAY OIL Insecticide, fungicide (Standard Oil)	Petroleum sulfonates 18.51% Soda resin soap 4.77% Highly refined coal tar creosote* 11.49% Petroleum oil* 62.50%
STANDARD BRUSH KILLER Herbicide (Standard Oil)	Isoctyl ester of 2,4-Dichloro-phenoxyacetic acid* 33.7% Isoctyl ester of 2,4,5-Trichloro-phenoxyacetic acid* 32.1%
STANDARD CRABGRASS SPRAY Herbicide (Standard Oil)	Petroleum oil* 99.99%
STANDARD 25% DDT CONCEN-TRATE (Standard Oil)	DDT 25% Petroleum xylene and deriv.* 70%

Name & Use Manufacturer	Ingredients
STANDARD DORMANT SPRAY OIL NO. 1 (Dendrol)	Petroleum oil* 90.34% Petroleum sulfonates 7.86%
STANDARD EARWORM SPRAY Insecticide (Standard Oil)	Petroleum oil* 99% DDT 1%
STANDARD ELECTRIC MOTOR OIL, FINAL HOUSE-HOLD OIL Lubricating oils (Standard Oil)	Petroleum oil* Rust and oxidation inhibitors Silicone defoamers
STANDARD ELM SPRAY Insecticide (Standard Oil)	DDT 25% Petroleum oil (paraffinic tech. white oil) 18% Petroleum xylene and related compounds* 55%
STANDARD FLOOR FINISHES, SEALER (Standard Oil)	Chinawood oil Phenolic resins Mineral spirits*
STANDARD FORMALDEHYDE Fumigant (Standard Chem.)	Formaldehyde* 37%
STANDARD FUNGICIDE (Stanofide) (Standard Oil)	Alkyl dimethyl benzyl ammonium chloride* 50%
STANDARD GARDEN DUST Insecticide, fungicide (Standard Oil)	Methoxychlor, tech. 2.500% TDE 0.500% Pyrethrins 0.020% Piperonyl cyclonene, tech. 0.125% Rotenone 0.500% Other cube extractives 1.000% Sulfur* 25.000% Ziram* 7.600%
STANDARD INSECT SPRAY WITH DDT (Standard Oil)	DDT 5.00% B-butoxy-B'-thiocyano diethyl ether 0.29% B-thiocyano ethyl esters of mixed fatty acids averaging 10-18 carbon atoms 0.89% Methylated naphthalene* 15.18% Petroleum oil* 78.64%
STANDARD LIQUID GLOSS Floor gloss (Standard Oil)	Petroleum oil Turpentine* Perfumes
STANDARD LIQUID WAX Floor polish (Standard Oil)	Solids: 12% Waxes Shellac Soap Borax Ammonia Amine soap

*Consult Sec. II., Ingredients Index. This ingredient may be responsible for major toxic effects if poisonous amounts of this product are ingested.

Name & Use Manufacturer	Ingredients	Name & Use Manufacturer	Ingredients
STANDARD LOW VOLATILE 2,4-D Herbicide (Standard Oil)	2,4-D acid, iso-octyl ester* 67.8%	STANDARD 2,4-D WEED KILLER NO. 3E (Standard Oil)	2,4-D acid, mixed butyl and isopropyl esters* 75.6%
STANDARD LOW VOLATILE 2,4,5-T Herbicide (Standard Oil)	2,4,5-T acid, iso-octyl ester* 63.2%	STANDARD 2,4-D WEED KILLER NO. 4 (Standard Oil)	Triethyl amine salt of 2,4-D acid* 16.8%
STANDARD PRESSUR-PAK PLANT SPRAY Insecticide (Standard Oil)	Rhothane (dichloro diphenyl dichloroethane) 0.20% Pyrethrins 0.05% Piperonyl butoxide 0.50% Mineral oil 24.25% Propellents 75.00%	STANDARD 2,4-D WEED KILLER NO. 5 (Standard Oil)	2,4-D acid, mixed butyl and isopropyl ester* 55.9%
STANDARD ROACH & ANT SPRAY Insecticide (Standard Oil)	Tech. chlordane 2% DDT (dichloro diphenyl trichloroethane) 2% Methylated naphthalene* 4% Petroleum distillate* 92%	STANDARD WEED KILLER Herbicide (Standard)	Petroleum* 100.0%
		STANIS Analgesic, counter-irritant (salve) (Stanis)	Oil of cajuput* Oleoresin of capsicum Menthol* Lanolin Oil of wintergreen* Oil of eucalyptus* Camphor* Petrolatum
STANDARD STOCK SPRAY WITH METHOXYCHLOR Insecticide (Standard Oil)	B-butoxy-B'-thiocyano diethyl ether 1.64% Isobornyl thiocyanoacetate 0.49% Other related terpenes 0.11% Diphenyl oxide 1.00% Methoxychlor tech. 0.50% Petroleum oil* 96.26%	STANIS COCOANUT OIL SHAMPOO (Stanis)	Cocoanut oil soap Non-toxic color
STANDARD SUMMER EMULSION CONCEN-TRATE (Verdol) Insecticide (Standard Oil)	Petroleum oil* 60% m.	STANIS COMPLEXION CREAM (Stanis)	Beeswax Spermaceti Mineral oil Lanolin White petrolatum Borax
STANDARD SUMMER SPRAY OIL NO. 1 (Superla) Insecticide (Standard Oil)	Petroleum oil* 97.3%	STANIS DERMATONE SALVE NO. 74 (Stanis)	Sulfur* Salicylic acid* Menthol* White pine tar
		STANIS FACE Powder (Stanis)	Standard talc base
STANDARD SUPER-TERMITE Insecticide (Standard Oil)	Phenols* 50% Soap 25%	STANIS IMPROVED FOOT SOAP (Stanis)	Iodine* Eucalyptus* Borax* Olive oil Bran
		STANIS SALVE #73 (Stanis)	Resorcin* Zinc oxide Camphor* Phenol* Menthol*
STANDARD TOXAPHENE CONCEN-TRATE Insecticide (Standard Oil)	Toxaphene* (tech. chlorinated camphene, chlorine content 67-69%) 60.5% Petroleum oil 36.5%	STANIS SALVE #75 For minor burns, sores, wounds (Stanis)	Boric acid* Zinc oxide Cod liver oil
		STANIS SALVE #76 Ointment (Stanis)	Comfrey root*
STANDARD 2,4-D WEED KILLER NO. 2 (Standard Oil)	Dimethylamine salt of 2,4-D acid* 49.6%	STANLEY'S ANTISEPTIC MOUTH WASH (Stanley Home)	Water Alcohol (S.D. 38B) Essential oils* Certified dye

*Consult Sec. II., Ingredients Index. This ingredient may be responsible for major toxic effects if poisonous amounts of this product are ingested.

Name & Use Manufacturer	Ingredients	Name & Use Manufacturer	Ingredients
STANLEY'S BATH SALTS (Stanley Home)		STANLEY'S METAL POLISH (Stanley Home)	Soap Plasticizer Sassafras Dowicide Silica Trisodium phosphate Bentonite Tergitol Dye
STANLEY'S BOWL CLEANER (Stanley Home)	Soda ash Sodium bicarbonate Sodium tripolyphosphate* Triton* Pine oil*		
STANLEY'S BOWL DEODORIZER (Stanley Home)	Paradichlorobenzene* Perfume	STANLEY'S NONTOX Toilet Bowl cleaner (Stanley Home)	
STANLEY'S CREME CLEANER Floor cleaner (Stanley Home)	Water Stearic acid Beeswax Estawax Cetyl alcohol Hydrocarbon solvent* Ozokerite Gersthofen wax Ammonia Monoethanolamine	STANLEY'S RUG SHAMPOO (Stanley Home)	Anionic synthetic detergent* (see quarternary ammonium compounds)
		STANLEY'S SHAMPOO (For Hard Water) (Stanley Home)	Onyxol Coconut fatty acid Monoethanolamine Versene Maprofix Red oil Triethanolamine
STANLEY'S CREME RINSE Cosmetic (Stanley Home)	Triton Maypon Aldo	STANLEY'S SHAMPOO (Regular) (Stanley Home)	Red oil Triethanolamine Tergitol Propylene glycol Coconut oil Monoethanolamine Sodium septaphosphate
STANLEY'S DENTAL PLATE CLEANER (Stanley Home)	Super floss Soap Diglycol stearate Perfume Butoben		
STANLEY'S FACE LOTION (Stanley Home)		STANLEY'S SHAVING CREAM CONCEN- TRATE (Stanley Home)	Stearic acid Myristic acid Propylene glycol Triethanolamine Monoethanolamine
STANLEY'S FLOOR CLEANER (Stanley Home)	Pine oil* Trisodium phosphate Soap Ceresine wax Ammonia* Triethanolamine	STANLEY'S SHOE POLISH (Stanley Home)	
		STANLEY'S SILENT MAID (Stanley Home)	Nonic Versene Perfume Dye
STANLEY'S FURNITURE CREAM (Stanley Home)	Polishing oil Vegetable base emulsifier Perfume		
STANLEY'S GLUE (Stanley Home)		STANLEY'S SILVER CREAM (Stanley Home)	Soap Plasticizer R-3885 Bentonite Dowicide CMC Celatom Stearic acid Titanium dioxide Tergitol Sassafras
STANLEY'S HOME PERMANENT (Stanley Home)			
STANLEY'S LIQUID DETERGENT (Stanley Home)		STANLEY'S SKIN GLO (Stanley Home)	Paraffin wax Stearic acid Triethanolamine Cetyl alcohol Butoben
STANLEY'S LIQUID METAL POLISH (Stanley Home)	Silica Pine oil* Red oil* Nonic Borax*		

*Consult Sec. II., Ingredients Index. This ingredient may be responsible for major toxic effects if poisonous amounts of this product are ingested.

Name & Use Manufacturer	Ingredients	Name & Use Manufacturer	Ingredients
STANLEY'S SPOT REMOVER Cleaner (Stanley Home)	Triton Kreelon Stearic acid Soap Borax Tetrapotassium pyrophosphate Butoben	STARDUST NAIL POLISH (Clotworthy)	
STANLEY'S STANWICK REFILL Deodorizer (Stanley Home)	Formaldehyde*	STAR 5X ALKALI Cleaning product (Wyandotte)	Conc. alkali*
STANLEY'S SURE-KYL CONCEN- TRATE Insecticide (Stanley Home)	DDT* Tech. piperonyl butoxide Pyrethrins* Methylated naphthalenes* Petroleum distillates* Freon	STARKE INHALANT (Starke)	Menthol Guaiacol Iodine* Tincture benzoin compound Alcohol* 62% Glycerin Oil of eucalyptus*
STANLEY'S TOOTH PASTE (Stanley Home)		STARK'S REDUCINE Counter- irritant (Reducine)	
STANLEY'S WINTERMINT FACIAL (Stanley Home)		STA THINNER Paint thinner (Testor)	Xylol* Toloul* Isopropyl alcohol Butyl alcohol Butyl acetate Amyl acetate M.I.K.
STANTOX 64 Herbicide (Standard Ag.)	2,4-D amine salt* (4 lbs. acid equiv./gal.)		
STANTOX 90 Herbicide (Standard Ag.)	2,4-D sodium salt (2,4-D acid* equiv. 80.5%)	STAT DOUCHE POWDER (Stat)	Vegetable oils Oil of pine* Vegetable oil soap Glycerin Camphor* Oil of eucalyptus*
STANTOX P-44 Herbicide (Standard Ag.)	2,4-D isopropyl ester* 44%	STAUFFER ALDRIN 2-E Insecticide (Stauffer)	Aldrin* 23.0% Related compounds 3.8% Xylene* range aromatic hydrocarbon 68.0%
STA-NU COPPER CLEANER (Nu Prod.)		STAUFFER ALDRIN GRANULAR Insecticide (Stauffer)	Hexachloro hexahydro-endo, exo-dimethano naphthalene* 9.5% Related compounds 7.2%
STA-OFF Repellent (Pierpont)	Isopropyl alcohol* 80% Water 14% Lemon grass oil 3% Eucalyptus oil* 3% Diethyl phthalate 1%	STAUFFER ARAMITE DUST NO. 9 Insecticide (Stauffer)	2-(p-tert-Butylphenoxy) isopropyl-2 chloroethyl sulfite 3%
STA-OFF ANTI-RABBIT EMULSION & TREE HEALANT (Niagara Hort.)	Alcohol Resin Whaleoil	STAUFFER ARAMITE 15-W WETTABLE POWDER Insecticide (Stauffer)	2-(p-tert-Butylphenoxy) isopropyl-2-chloroethyl sulfite 15%

STAPHENE Germicide (Vestal)	p-Tertiary amyl phenol soap
	Isopropanol*
	o-Benzyl-p-chlorophenol
	o-Phenylphenol*
	Tetra-sodium ethylenediamine
	  tetra-acetate
	Sodium xylensulfonate*
	    24.15%
		STAUFFER BHC-DDT EMULSIFIABLE CONCEN- TRATE Insecticide (Stauffer)	Gamma isomer of benzene
			  hexachloride 4.6%
			Other isomers of benzene
			  hexachloride 7.1%
			DDT (dichloro diphenyl
			  trichloroethane) 23.4%
			Xylene* 58.0%

STARDUST FLAME- COLORING SALTS (Standard Chem.)	Copper sulfate*
	Ammonium chloride
	Potassium chloride
	Potassium nitrate
	Vegetable fiber ash
		STAUFFER BHC-DDT EMULSIFIABLE CONCENTRATE NO. 12-20 Insecticide (Stauffer)	Gamma isomer of benzene
			  hexachloride* 12.4%
			Other isomers of benzene
			  hexachloride 19.0%
			DDT (dichloro diphenyl tri-
			  chloroethane) 20.6%
			Xylene* 41.8%

*Consult Sec. II., Ingredients Index. This ingredient may be responsible for major toxic effects if poisonous amounts of this product are ingested.

Name & Use Manufacturer	Ingredients		Name & Use Manufacturer	Ingredients	
STAUFFER BHC-DDT STOCK SPRAY Insecticide (Stauffer)	Gamma isomer of benzene hexachloride*	2.0%	STAUFFER COTTON DUST NO. 121-3 Insecticide (Stauffer)	Gamma isomer of benzene hexachloride*	3.00%
	Other isomers of benzene hexachloride	6.0%		Other isomers of benzene hexachloride	7.9%
	DDT* (dichloro diphenyl trichloroethane)	33.3%		DDT*	5.00%
	Sulfur*	15.8%			
STAUFFER BHC-DDT STOCK SPRAY NO. 12-200 EMULSIFIABLE CONCENTRATE Insecticide (Stauffer)	Gamma isomer benzene hexachloride	1.44%	STAUFFER COTTON DUST NO. 122 Insecticide (Stauffer)	Gamma isomer of benzene hexachloride*	3.00%
	Other isomers of benzene hexachloride	2.16%		Other isomers of benzene hexachloride	9%
	DDT (dichloro diphenyl trichloroethane)	24.10%		DDT*	5.00%
	Xylene*	67.00%		Sulfur*	40.00%
STAUFFER BHC 1-E EMULSIFIABLE LIQUID Insecticide (Stauffer)	Gamma isomer of benzene hexachloride*	11.8%	STAUFFER COTTON DUST NO. 301 Insecticide (Stauffer)	Hexachloro epoxy octahydro dimethano naphthalene*	1.28%
	Other isomers of benzene hexachloride	17.7%		Related compounds	0.22%
	Xylene* range aromatic hydrocarbon solvent	65.0%		Dieldrin*	1-1/2%
STAUFFER CAPTAN DUST 7.5 Fungicide, insecticide (Stauffer)	Captan (n-trichloro methyl mercapto-4-cyclohexene-1, 2-dicarboximide)	7.5%	STAUFFER COTTON DUST NO. 321 Insecticide (Stauffer)	Hexachloro epoxy octahydro dimethano naphthalene*	1.28%
				Related compounds	0.22%
				DDT*(dichloro diphenyl trichloroethane)	5.00%
				Dieldrin*	1-1/2%
STAUFFER CAPTAN 10 DUST Fungicide (Stauffer)	Captan	10.0%	STAUFFER COTTON DUST NO. 322 Insecticide (Stauffer)	Hexachloro epoxy octahydro dimethano naphthalene*	2.12%
				Related compounds	0.38%
				DDT*(dichloro diphenyl trichloroethane)	5.00%
				Sulfur*	40.00%
STAUFFER CAPTAN 50-W Fungicide (Stauffer)	n-Trichloromethylmercapto-4-cyclohexene-1,2-dicarboxmide	50%	STAUFFER COTTON DUST NO. 322-1 Insecticide (Stauffer)	Hexachloro epoxy octahydro-endo, exo-dimethano naphthalene	1.28%
				Related compounds	0.22%
				DDT* (dichloro diphenyl trichloroethane)	5.00%
STAUFFER CHLORATE BORATE LIQUID DEFOLIANT Insecticide (Stauffer)	Sodium chlorate*			Sulfur*	40.00%
				Dieldrin*	1-1/2%
			STAUFFER COTTON DUST NO. 322-2 Insecticide (Stauffer)	Hexachloro epoxy octahydro dimethano naphthalene*	1.28%
				Related compounds	0.22%
				DDT* (dichloro diphenyl trichloroethane)	10.00%
STAUFFER CHLORDANE 4-E Insecticide (Stauffer)	Tech. chlordane	43.3%		Sulfur*	40.00%
	Xylene*	51.3%	STAUFFER COTTON DUST NO. 701 Insecticide (Stauffer)	Hexachloro hexahydro-endo, exo-dimethano naphthalene*	2.4%
				Related compounds	1.8%
STAUFFER CHLORDANE 8-E Insecticide (Stauffer)	Tech. chlordane*	71.7%			
	Xylene*	21.9%	STAUFFER COTTON DUST NO. 721 Insecticide (Stauffer)	Hexachloro hexahydro dimethano naphthalene*	2.4%
				Related compounds	1.8%
STAUFFER COTTON DUST NO. 22 Insecticide (Stauffer)	DDT* (dichloro diphenyl trichloroethane)	5%		Dichloro diphenyl trichloroethane*	5.0%
	Sulfur*	82%	STAUFFER COTTON DUST NO. 821-1 Insecticide (Stauffer)	Heptachloro-4,7-methano tetrahydroindene*	2.50%
				Related compounds	0.97%
STAUFFER COTTON DUST NO. 81 Insecticide (Stauffer)	Toxaphene* (tech. chlorinated camphene, chlorine content 67-69%)	20.00%		DDT*(dichloro diphenyl trichloroethane)	10.00%

Name & Use Manufacturer	Ingredients		Name & Use Manufacturer	Ingredients	
STAUFFER COTTON DUST NO. 821-3 Insecticide (Stauffer)	Heptachloro-4,7-methano tetrahydro indene* Related compounds DDT (dichloro diphenyl tri- chloroethane)*	5.00% 1.94% 10.00%	STAUFFER 75% DDT WETTABLE CONCEN- TRATE Insecticide (Stauffer)	DDT* (dichloro diphenyl tri- chloroethane)	75%
STAUFFER COTTON DUST NO. 822 Insecticide (Stauffer)	Heptachloro-4, 7-methano tetrahydro indene* Related compounds DDT (dichloro diphenyl tri- chloroethane)* Sulfur*	2.50% 0.97% 5.00% 40.00%	STAUFFER DIELDRIN 1.5-E Insecticide (Stauffer)	Hexachloro epoxy octahydro- endo, exo-dimethano naphthalene* Related compounds Xylene*	15.9% 2.8% 75.0%
STAUFFER COTTON DUST No. 822-1 Insecticide (Stauffer)	Heptachloro-4,7-methano tetrahydro indene* Related compounds DDT (dichloro diphenyl tri- chloroethane)* Sulfur*	2.50% 0.97% 10.00% 40.00%	STAUFFER DIELDRIN EMULSIFIABLE CONCEN- TRATE NO. 151 Insecticide (Stauffer)	Hexachloro epoxy octahydro- endo, exo-dimethano naphthalene* Related compounds Xylene*	15.9% 2.8% 75.0%
STAUFFER COTTON DUST NO. 822-2 Insecticide (Stauffer)	Heptachoro-4, 7-methano tetrahydro indene* Related compounds DDT (dichloro diphenyl tri- chloroethane)* Sulfur*	5.00% 1.94% 5.00% 40.00%	STAUFFER DIELDRIN 5-W Fungicide, insecticide (Stauffer)	Hexachloro epoxy octahydro dimethano naphthalene* Related compounds	42.5% 7.5%
STAUFFER COTTON DUST NO. 822-3 Insecticide (Stauffer)	Heptachloro-4, 7-methano tetrahydro indene* Related compounds DDT (dichloro diphenyl tri- chloroethane)* Sulfur*	5.00% 1.94% 10.00% 40.00%	STAUFFER DITHANE D-14 Fungicide (Stauffer)	Nabam* (disodium ehtylene- bis (dithiocarbamate)	19%
STAUFFER DDD 2-E Insecticide (Stauffer)	DDD Xylene*	25.2% 70.0%	STAUFFER DUSTLESS 15W PARATHION Insecticide (Stauffer)	Parathion*	15%
STAUFFER DDD DUST 5 Insecticide (Stauffer)	DDD	5%	STAUFFER DUSTLESS PARATHION 25% DUST BASE Insecticide (Stauffer)	Parathion*	25%
STAUFFER DDD- SULPHUR DUST 5-50 Insecticide (Stauffer)	DDT* Sulfur*	5% 50%	STAUFFER DUSTLESS PARATHION 15-W WETTABLE POWDER Insecticide (Stauffer)	Parathion*	15%
STAUFFER DDD 5-W Insecticide (Stauffer)	DDD*	50%			
STAUFFER DDT 2-E Insecticide (Stauffer)	DDT Xylene*	25% 70%	STAUFFER DUSTLESS PARATHION 25-W WETTABLE POWDER Insecticide (Stauffer)	Parathion*	25%
STAUFFER DDT 50-W Fungicide, insecticide (Stauffer)	DDT*	50%			
STAUFFER DDT 75-W Insecticide (Stauffer)	DDT*	75%	STAUFFER ENDRIN EMULSIFIABLE CONCEN- TRATE NO. 161 Insecticide (Stauffer)	Endrin* Xylene*	19.8% 72.0%

Name & Use Manufacturer	Ingredients		Name & Use Manufacturer	Ingredients	
STAUFFER FERBAM DUST 15 Fungicide (Stauffer)	Ferbam	15.0%	STAUFFER INSECTICIDE DUST 5% DDT (Stauffer)	DDT* (dichloro diphenyl tri-chloroethane) Inert ingredients	5% 95%
STAUFFER FUNGICIDE DUST NO. 6 (Stauffer)	Zineb	3.9%	STAUFFER INSECTICIDE DUST 1% LINDANE (Stauffer)	Gamma isomer of benzene hexachloride	1%
STAUFFER FUNGICIDE DUST NO. X-170 (Stauffer)	Spergon (tetrachloro para benzoquininone)	5.0%	STAUFFER INSECTICIDE & FUNGICIDE DUST NO. 26 (Stauffer)	Zineb DDT* (dichloro diphenyl tri-chloroethane) Inert ingredients	4.0% 5.0% 91.0%
STAUFFER 80-20 GRAIN FUMIGANT (Stauffer)	Carbon tetrachloride* Carbon bisulfide*	83.5% 16.5%	STAUFFER INSECTICIDE, FUNGICIDE DUST NO. X-171 (Stauffer)	DDT (dichloro diphenyl tri-chloroethane) Tetrachloro-para-benzoquinone	3.0% 5.0%
STAUFFER HEPTACHLOR 2-E Insecticide (Stauffer)	Heptachlor* Related compounds Xylene*	23% 9% 59%	STAUFFER IRON CHELATE-6V For acid soils (Stauffer)	Chelated iron as metallic*	6-1/2%
STAUFFER INSECTICIDE BAIT NO. X-168 Insecticide (Stauffer)	Tech. chlordane Toxaphene*	2.0% 2.5%	STAUFFER IRON CHELATE-12 For acid soils (Stauffer)	Chelated iron*	12%
STAUFFER INSECTICIDE BAIT NO. X-169 Insecticide (Stauffer)	Tech. chlordane	2.0%	STAUFFER IRON CHELATE-13 For acid soils (Stauffer)	Chelated iron as metallic*	13%
STAUFFER INSECTICIDE DUST NO. 7-1 (Stauffer)	DDD (dichloro diphenyl dichloroethane) Inert ingredients	10% 90%	STAUFFER LINDANE 25-W Insecticide (Stauffer)	Gamma isomer of benzene hexachloride*	25.0%
STAUFFER INSECTICIDE DUST NO. 61-1 Insecticide (Stauffer)	Rotenone Other ethyl extractives of cube Inert ingredients	1.0% 2.0% 97.0%	STAUFFER LINDANE EMULSIFIABLE CONCEN-TRATE NO. 171 Insecticide (Stauffer)	Lindane*(gamma isomer of benzene hexachloride) Xylene*	20% 56%
STAUFFER INSECTICIDE DUST NO. 7-21-4 (Stauffer)	DDT (dichloro diphenyl tri-chloroethane) Parathion*	5.0% 2.0%	STAUFFER LINDANE STOCK SPRAY NO. 96 Insecticide (Stauffer)	Lindane (gamma isomer of benzene hexachloride)* Xylene*	12.2% 82.0%
STAUFFER INSECTICIDE DUST NO. 101 (Stauffer)	Gamma isomer of benzene hexachloride* Other isomers of benzene hexachloride Inert ingredients	5.0% 7.5% 87.5%	STAUFFER LOW VOLATILE BRUSH KILLER 1-1/3-2/3 Herbicide (Stauffer)	Isooctyl ester of 2,4-dichloro-phenoxyacetic acid* Isooctyl ester of 2,4,5-trichloro-phenoxyacetic acid*	24.5% 11.7%
STUAFFER INSECTICIDE DUST NO. 101-4 (Stauffer)	Gamma isomer of benzene hexachloride* Other isomers of benzene hexachloride Inert ingredients	4% 6% 90%	STAUFFER LOW VOLATILE BRUSH KILLER 2-2 Herbicide (Stauffer)	Isooctyl ester of 2,4-dichloro-phenoxyacetic acid* Isooctyl ester of 2,4-5-trichloro-phenoxyacetate acid*	33.7% 32.1%
STAUFFER INSECTICIDE DUST 5% CHLORDANE (Stauffer)	Tech. chlordane* Inert ingredients	5.0% 95.0%			

Name & Use Manufacturer	Ingredients	
STAUFFER MAGNETIC SULPHUR PASTE Insecticide (Stauffer)	Sulfur*	68%
STAUFFER MALATHION 5-E Insecticide (Stauffer)	o,o-Dimethyl dithiophosphate of diethyl mercaptosuccinate 56% Xylene range aromatic hydrocarbon solvent* 32%	
STAUFFER MALATHION 25-W Insecticide (Stauffer)	o,o-Dimethyl dithiophosphate of diethyl mercaptosuccinate* 25%	
STAUFFER PARATHION 2-E Insecticide (Stauffer)	Parathion* 25% Xylene 65%	
STAUFFER PARATHION NO. 401 Insecticide (Stauffer)	Parathion* 46% Xylene 41%	
STAUFFER PARATHION SULPHUR DUST 1.5-82.5 Insecticide (Stauffer)	Parathion* 1.5% Sulfur 82.5%	
STAUFFER PENTA CONCENTRATE Herbicide (Stauffer)	Pentachlorophenol* 40.0% Aromatic hydrocarbons* 40.0%	
STAUFFER S.E.X. Herbicide (Stauffer)	Sodium ethyl xanthate* and related compounds 90%	
STAUFFER TOXAPHENE DDT EMULSIFIABLE CONCENTRATE #40-20 Insecticide (Stauffer)	Toxaphene* 40% DDT (dichloro diphenyl trichloroethane) 20% Xylene* 35% Tech. chlorinated camphene	
STAUFFER 2,4-D BUTYL ESTER 265 Herbicide (Stauffer)	Butyl 2,4-dichlorophenoxy-acetate* 40.0%	
STAUFFER 2,4-D ESTER WEED KILLER 44% (Stauffer)	Isopropyl ester of 2,4-dichloro phenoxy acetic acid* 44.0%	
STAUFFER 2,4-D LIQUID SALT 400 Herbicide (Stauffer)	Dimethylamine salt of 2,4-dichloro phenoxy acetic acid* 49.4%	

Name & Use Manufacturer	Ingredients	
STAUFFER 2,4-D LOW VOLATILE ESTER 400 Herbicide (Stauffer)	Iso-octyl ester of 2,4-dichloro phenoxy acetic acid* 67.8%	
STAUFFER 2,4,5-T LOW VOLATILE ESTER 400 Herbicide (Stauffer)	Iso-octyl ester of 2,4,5-trichloro phenoxy acetic acid* 62.2%	
STA WAKE Stimulant (Approved)	Each tablet: Caffeine (anhydrous) 1.5 gr. Dextrose 5 gr.	
STA-WAKE Stimulant (Sta-Wake)	Each tablet: Caffeine alkaloid 1-3/4 gr.	
STAYBRITE For coloring concrete, cement (Horn)	Earth colors	
STAY-CUT LIQUID SANDPAPER (Reliable Paste)	Solvents* Xylol* Acetone	
STAY-DEE DUSTING POWDER Insecticide (Stayner)	DDT* 10%	
STAYNER A.P.C. TABLETS Analgesic (Stayner)	Each tablet: Aspirin* 3-1/2 gr. Acetophenetidin* 2-1/2 gr. Caffeine citrated 1/2 gr.	
STAYNER CITRATES & CARBONATES (Stayner)	Sodium bicarbonate Potassium bicarbonate Magnesium sulfate Calcium lactate Sodium phosphate Sodium chloride Citric acid Tartaric acid	
STAYNER COLD CAPSULES WITH QUININE (Stayner)	Quinine sulfate 1/2 gr. Acetophenetidin* 2 gr. Camphor* 1/4 gr. Atropine sulfate 1/2000 gr. Caffeine citrated 1/8 gr. Podophyllin 1/40 gr. Aloin 1/16 gr.	
STAYNER COLD FORMULA TABLETS (Stayner)	Acetophenetidin* 2 gr. Atropine sulfate 1/2000 gr. Camphor* 1/4 gr. Caffeine citrated 1/8 gr. Podophyllin 1/40 gr. Aloin 1/16 gr.	
STAYNER TERPIN HYDRATE & CODEINE (Stayner)	Each fl. oz.: Codeine 0.91 gr. Terpin hydrate 7.7 gr.	

*Consult Sec. II., Ingredients Index. This ingredient may be responsible for major toxic effects if poisonous amounts of this product are ingested.

- 971 -

Name & Use Manufacturer	Ingredients		Name & Use Manufacturer	Ingredients	
STAYPUT Semi-paste remover (Reliable Paste)	Benzol* Acetone Methanol		STER-BAC FORMULA S-12 Bactericide (Klenzade)	Alkyl dimethyl benzyl ammonium chloride* 	12.8%
			STERIDOL NO. 3 COOLANT GERMICIDE (Dolge)	Formaldehyde*	15%
S.T.B. FOR POULTRY (Lee, W.)	Lard approx. 66% Canada balsam of fir* approx. 8% Oil of origanum* approx. 13% Oil of rosemary* approx. 2% Camphor* approx. 4% Alcohol approx. 6%		STERIPHONE GERMICIDE (Steriphone)		
			STERLING CHALK CRAYON (Am. Crayon)		
STEARNS ELECTRIC BRAND RAT & ROACH PASTE (Stearns)	Phosphorus*		STERLING 5% CHLORDANE DUST Insecticide (Smith, C.D.)	Chlordane*	5%
STEINMAN'S CAPSULES GLYCERO- PHOSPHATES COMPOUND Tonic and appetizer (Steinmann)	Sodium Manganese Glycerosphosphates Arsenic* Calcium Iron Nux vomica* Calcium lactate		STERLING CPR DUST Insecticide (Smith, C.D.)	Piperonyl cyclonene 0.5% Pyrethrins 0.05% Rotenone 0.25% Other cube extractives 0.5% Sulfur* 25%	
STEIN'S ALPINE COLD CREAM (Stein)			STERLING DAIRY CATTLE SPRAY WETTABLE POWDER Insecticide (Smith, C.D.)	Methoxychlor*	50%
STEIN'S MAKE-UP & BEAUTY PREPARATIONS (Stein)	Beeswax Mineral oil Certified colors		STERLING DUST NO. 8 Insecticide (Smith, C.D.)	Toxaphene*	8%
STELCO ROOFING CEMENT (Stelwagon)			STERLING DUST NO. 5R ROTHANE 5% TDE Insecticide (Smith, C.D.)	TDE	5%
STELLA VITAE Laxative (Allied Drug)	Alcohol 10%/v Senecio Mitchella Black haw Helonias Caulophyllum Cramp bark Aletris Senna Gentian		STERLING LIVESTOCK SPRAY Insecticide (Smith, C.D.)	DDT* 28% Beta beta thiocyano diethyl ether 5%	
			STERLING MULTI- GARDEN DUST Insecticide (Smith, C.D.)	Nicotine alkaloid* 1.4% Rotenone 0.5% Other cube resins 1% Beta beta dithiocyano diethyl ether 0.75% Sulfur 29%	
STENCIL THINNER SOLVENT #50 (Garvery)			STERLING POISON OATS Rodenticide (Smith, C.D.)	Strychnine alkaloid* 0.37%	
STERA- KLEEN Germicide (Steriphone)			STERLING POISON WHEAT Rodenticide (Smith, C.D.)	Strychnine alkaloid* 0.18%	
STERAMINE TABLETS Germicide (Edwards- Councilor)	Para-di-isobutyl phenoxy ethoxy ethyl dimethyl benzyl ammonium chloride mono- hydrate* 50%		STERLING SABADILLA DUST NO. 80 Insecticide (Smith, C.D.)	Sabadilla*	10%

*Consult Sec. II., Ingredients Index. This ingredient may be responsible for major toxic effects if poisonous amounts of this product are ingested.

Name & Use Manufacturer	Ingredients		Name & Use Manufacturer	Ingredients
STERNO CANNED HEAT (Sterno)	Ethyl alcohol Methanol* approx. 15%		STM WOOD PRESERVA- TIVE (Speekman)	Pentachlorophenol*
STER-O-CLEAR (Continental Chemical)	Alkyl dimethyl benzyl ammonium chloride*		STOCK SPRAY & DIP Insecticide (Thompson- Hayward)	DDT* 42.20% Gamma isomer of benzene hexachloride 2.53% Other isomers of benzene hexachloride 14.20%
STEROLIN DISINFECTANT (Selig)	Coal tar neutral oils * Phenols* Sodium soaps		STOCK SPRAY CC REPELLENT Insecticide (Bonide)	Petroleum distillates* Beta-butoxy-B'-thiocyano diethyl ether*
STEROX Disinfectant, fungicide, deodorant (Pioneer)			STOCK-TOX Insecticide (Martin, C.J.)	Toxaphene* 65% Petroleum hydrocarbons 23%
STETCO DOUBLE- STRENGTH INSECT SPRAY (Stetson)	DDT* Inert ingredients		STOKE'S EXPECTORANT N.F. (Sharp & Dohme)	Each 100 cc.: Alcohol 12% Tincture opium camphorated* 17.5 cc. Fluid extract senega* 3.5 cc. Fluid extract squill* 3.5 cc. Ammonium carbonate 1.8 gm.
STETCO PYNOL DISINFECTANT (Stetson)	Steam-distilled pine oil* soap		STOMACHIC A TABLETS Antacid (Clapp, Otis)	Pectin 1 gr. Bismuth betanaphthol 1 gr. Ipecac 1/12 gr. Nux moschata 1/100 gr. Calcium carbonate 3 gr. Sodium bicarbonate 1 gr. Aromatic flavor
STETCO TRIPLE- STRENGTH INSECT SPRAY (Stetson)	DDT* Inert ingredients		STOM-AID Antacid, digestant (Steinmann)	Cascara Mixt. rhubarb Soda Bicarbonate Enzymes Lactated pepsin Aromatics
STEVENS OINTMENT Veterinary (Kopf)	Mercuric biniodide* (mercury iodide, red) Turpentine oil Cantharidin*		STOMASEPTINE Vaginal douche (StomAseptine)	Sodium perborate* Sodium bicarbonate Sodium chloride Borax* Menthol* Thymol* Eucalyptol * Methyl salicylate* Aromatics
STIK-KWIK CHINA, CROCKERY, GLASS CEMENT; RUBBER CEMENT (Rainbow)				
STILLMAN'S FRECKLE CREAM (Stillman)	Ammoniated mercury* 4% Bismuth subnitrate		STOMAX Laxative digestant (Colonial Drug)	Arom. spirits ammonia Ess. peppermint Milk magnesia
STILLMAN'S MEDICATED JELL Vaginal jelly (Stillman)	Lactic acid Boric acid* Oxyquinoline sulfate		STOP-A-LEAK STICK Waterproof glue (Ferdinand)	Asphalt Resins
STIMULATOR FOR SCALP (La Vell)			STOPETTE SPRAY DEODORANT (Montenier)	Chlorhydrol (aluminum chlor- hydroxide complex) Emulsifier fats Perfume oil
STIM-U-PLANT Plant food tablets (Stim-U-Plant)	Nitrogen 11% Phosphoric acid (available) 12% Potash 15% Vitamin B1		STOPETTE CREAM DEODORANT (Montenier)	Chlorhydrol (aluminum chlor- hydroxide complex) Urea Mineral oil Natural waxes
STIMUTOL TABLETS Food supplement (Pharmex)	Vitamin B12 25 mcg. Vitamin B1 25 mg. Ferrous gluconate 5 gr. Caffeine 1-1/2 gr.			
STIXIT PASTE (Am.Crayon)				

*Consult Sec. II., Ingredients Index. This ingredient may be responsible for major toxic effects if poisonous amounts of this product are ingested.

- 973 -

Name & Use Manufacturer	Ingredients		Name & Use Manufacturer	Ingredients
STOP-GO DRAIN CLEANER (Holcomb)	Sodium hydroxide*		STRIBLINGS' CALF PRESCRIPTION Veterinary (Stribling)	Belladonna* Stramonium* Copper phenolsulfonate Zinc phenolsulfonate
STOP GRASS GRASS GROWTH RETARDER Herbicide (Science)			STRIBLINGS' PINK EYE POWDER Veterinary (Stribling)	Acetylsalicylic acid* Calomel* Sulfonamides*
STOPIT TABLETS Analgesic (Assoc. Prod.)	Acetophenetidin* 1-3/4 gr. Aspirin* 2-3/4 gr. Caffeine 1/2 gr.		STRIBLINGS' SULFA POWDER (Stribling)	Sulfathiazole* Sulfanilamide* Sulfathiazole sodium anhydrous Sulfathiazole sodium sesqui-hydrate
STOP-MOLD B (New) Fungicide (Vis-Ko)	Sodium ortho-phenylphenate* (anhydrous) 34%		STRIDE Floor wax (Johnson, S.C.)	Natural resins Petroleum and vegetable waxes Emulsifying agents
STOP-PICK For cannibalism in poultry (Roberts, Dr.)	Belladonna* Poke root Pine tar*		STRIKE ANTISEPTIC POWDER (Coronet)	
STOP-ROT Insecticide, fungicide (Miller Chem.)	Pentachlorophenol* 5.00% Petroleum solvents* 92.79% Special solvents and impurities 2.21%		STROB-X DEVELOPER Photographic supply (Ringwood)	Metol* Hydroquinone* Sulfite Bromide* Carbonate
STOPROT Fungicide (Consumer's Chem.)	Pentachlorophenol*		STROB-X FIXER Photographic supply (Ringwood)	Ammonium thiosulfate* 60% solution Sulfite Acetic acid (small quantity)
STOP SPOT CLEANING FLUID (Wilco)	Carbon tetrachloride* Petroleum hydrocarbon fraction		STROB-X Fixer Photographic supply (Graflex)	Ammonium thiosulfate*
STOP SPOT FRENCH DRY CLEANER (Wilco)	Petroleum hydrocarbon* Surface active agents Perfume		STRONCYLATE (Upjohn)	Strontium salicylate* 5 gr. Aromatics
STORK TOILET SOAP (Armour)	Sodium salts of coco oil and palm oil		STRONG, COBB ANTISEPTIC TABLETS (Strong)	Corrosive sublimate* Ammonium chloride
STORMY WEATHER Water, mildew repellent (Protection)	2-Chlororthophenylphenol 2% Water-repellent solids Mineral spirits*		STRONG SCENT JAPANESE BEETLE LIQUID BAIT Insecticide (Goulard)	Geraniol* Eugenol* U.S.P. Clove oil* Phenyl ethyl alcohol*
STOVELINER (United Gilson.)	Fireclays Inert fillers		STRYPEEZE PAINT & VARNISH REMOVER (Savogran)	Toluol* Acetone* Alcohol
STOVOIL Rust preventive (Superior Labs.)			S.T. 37 Antiseptic (Sharp & Dohme)	Each 100 cc.: Caprokol 0.10 gm. Hexylresorcinol 1-1000 Glycerin-aqueous solution
STRAIT-LINE CARPENTER'S CHALK (Strait-Line)			S.T. 37 TOOTH PASTE (Sharp & Dohme)	Hexylresorcinol
STRE-AMBER BRILLAN-TINE (H.Q.Z.)	Tech. white mineral oil D & C yellow (oil-soluble) Oriental bouquet		STUART AFTER SHAVE STICK (Stuart)	Alcohol(S.D.A. No. 40) Sodium stearate Glycerin Menthol crystals Perfume oil

---

*Consult Sec. II., Ingredients Index. This ingredient may be responsible for major toxic effects if poisonous amounts of this product are ingested.

Name & Use Manufacturer	Ingredients	Name & Use Manufacturer	Ingredients
STUC-O-SEAL Rubber base paint (Chi-Namel)	Titanium dioxide 18.5% Zinc oxide 4.4% Mica 2.6% Magnesium silicate 26.0% Rubber and chlorinated rubber polymers 11.0% Aromatic thinner* 18.5% Aliphatic thinner* 19.0%	STULL'S MCP ESTER-LOW VOLATILE FOR WHITE BRUSH (Bee Brush) Herbicide (Stull's)	Iso-octyl ester of 2-methyl, 4-chlorophenoxyacetic acid* 23.8%
STUDIO GIRL BEAUTY MASK Face treatment (Studio)		STULL'S SPECIAL HELICOPTER SPRAY Herbicide (Stull's)	Iso-octyl ester of 2,4,5-T acid* 15.20%
STUDIO GIRL COLOGNE, PERFUME, SKIN FRESHENER, CREAM SHAMPOO (Studio)		STULL'S 2,4,5-T ESTER LOW VOLATILE Herbicide (Stull's)	Iso-octyl ester of 2,4,5-trichlorophenoxy acetic acid* 65.77%
STUDIO GIRL FACE CREAM, CLEANSING CREAM, BUBBLE BATH, ROUGE, LIPSTICK, FACE POWDER (Studio)		STUMPF'S RUST-A-WAY Combats rust (Stumpf's)	
		S-12 For vaginal irritation (Servex)	Alum* Lactose Peppermint Phenol* Boric acid* Tartaric acid Thymol* Eucalyptol* Salicylic acid* Menthol Zinc sulfate* Sodium perborate*
STUDIO GIRL FACE LOTION, SHAVING LOTION (Studio)			
STULL'S LOW VOLATILE BRUSH KILLER NO. 1 Herbicide (Stull's)	Iso-octyl ester of 2,4,5-trichlorophenoxy acetic acid* 19.50%	STYLE Liquid detergent (Iowa)	Alkyl aryl sulfonates* Non-ionic synthetic detergents
STULL'S LOW VOLATILE BRUSH KILLER NO. 2 Herbicide (Stull's)	Iso-octyl ester of 2,4-dichlorophenoxy acetic acid* 10.25% Iso-octyl ester of 2,4,5-trichlorophenoxy acetic acid* 9.77%	STYP-IT Antiseptic powder, medical (Barrett Chem.)	Oxyquinoline sulfate* Boric acid* Thymol* Bismuth subgallate Talc Thymol iodide* Zinc phenolsulfonate Bismuth oxyiodide Silene Aluminum sulfate* Potassium sulfate
STULL'S LOW VOLATILE BRUSH KILLER NO. 3 Herbicide (Stull's)	Iso-octyl ester of 2,4-dichlorophenoxy acetic acid* 19.30% Iso-octyl ester of 2,4,5-trichlorophenoxy acetic acid* 18.42%	STYPTIC Anti-hemorrhagic (Royal Mfg.)	Aluminum sulfate* Aluminum oxide
STULL'S LOW VOLATILE BRUSH KILLER NO. 4 Herbicide (Stull's)	Iso-octyl ester of 2,4-dichlorophenoxy acetic acid* 36.66% Iso-octyl ester of 2,4,5-trichlorophenoxy acetic acid* 33.78%	STYPTO-JEL Antiseptic jelly (Commerce)	Hexachlorophene* Benzocaine Aluminum sulfate*
STULL'S LOW VOLATILE WEED KILLER Herbicide (Stull's)	Iso-octyl ester of 2,4-dichlorophenoxy acetic acid* 55% Non-phytotoxic horticultural base oil 41% Emulsifier 4%	STYROLE COLD SORE LOTION (Caswell-Massey)	
		STYROWELD Plastic adhesive (Carbona)	

*Consult Sec. II., Ingredients Index. This ingredient may be responsible for major toxic effects if poisonous amounts of this product are ingested.

Name & Use Manufacturer	Ingredients	Name & Use Manufacturer	Ingredients
STYX Insecticide (Bartlett, F.A.)	Rotenone 0.53% Other cube extractives 1.06% Methylated naphthalene* 2.94% Pyrethrin 0.16% Petroleum distillate 0.65%	SULCO CAULKING COMPOUND (Sullivan)	
STYX CONCENTRATE Insecticide (Bartlett,F.A.)	Rotenone 3.19% Other cube extractives 6.37% Methylated naphthalene* 28.48% Pyrethrin 1.00% Petroleum distillate 3.97%	SULFADOL For infections (veterinary, avian) (Gland-O-Lac)	Sulfathiazole sodium U.S.P.* 100%
STYX LINE EXTRACT, TOILET WATER (Coty)		SULFADOL SOLUTION For infections (veterinary, avian) (Gland-O-Lac)	Each fl. oz.: Sulfathiazole sodium U.S.P. 58 gr.
SUAVE HAIR PREPARATIONS (Curtis, H.)	Mineral oil Esters of stearic, palmitic and lauric acid Lanolin deriv.	SULFALINE For coccidiosis, cholera (veterinary, avian) (Gland-O-Lac)	Sulfaquinoxaline* 25% Sulfur* Bentonite Dextrose
SUAVINOL OINTMENT For rectal irritation (Schoonmaker)	Steam-distilled pine oil* Eucalyptus oil*	SULFALINE SOLUTION For coccidiosis, intestinal infections (veterinary, avian) (Gland-O-Lac)	Sulfaquinoxaline sodium 3.37% Sodium hydroxide and water 96.63%
SUCRETS Antiseptic throat lozenges (Sharp & Dohme)	Each lozenge: Caprokol (hexylresorcinol) 2.4 mg.	SULFAMERAZINE POWDER VET. For intestinal infections (veterinary, avian) (Sharp & Dohme)	2-Sulfanilamide-4-methyl-pyrimidine*
SUCROCIDE Insecticide (Farmers')	Malathion (o,o-dimethyl dithio-phosphate of diethyl mercapto-succinate) 2.00%	SULFA-METHAZINE TABLETS For infections (veterinary) (Sharp & Dohme)	4,6-Dimethyl-2-sulfanilamido-pyrimidine*
SUDDEN DATE LANOLIN PLUS BEAUTIFIER & CONDITIONER (Consolid. Cosm.)	Lanolin Lanolin deriv. Silicone Perfume Freon*	SULFA-NILAMIDE TABLETS For infections (veterinary) (Fidelity Labs.)	Sulfanilamide* 60 gr. Corn starch binder
SUDDEN DEATH Insecticide (Maas, A.G.)	Cresylic acid*	SULFA-NOX (Powder, Liquid, Conc.) (Ralston)	Sulfaquinoxaline*
SUDSY SPRAY WHITE WALL TIRE CLEANER (Berry, C.H.)	Alkalis* Alcohol*	SULFA-REA For infections (veterinary) (Beebe Labs.)	Sulfanilamide* Sulfathiazole* Urea Total 80%
SUGAR & SPICE COLOGNE (Assoc. Brands)		SULF-A-SILE Grass silage additive (Hopkins Agric.)	Sodium metabisulfite*
S.U.G. #15 DROPS (S.U.G.)	Ephedrine sulfate* 1% Chloretone 1/2% C.P. dextrose 10%		
S.U.G. OINTMENT (S.U.G.)	Phenol 0.5% Pine tar ointment 9.6% Zinc oxide ointment 89.9%	SULFA-THALIDINE TABLETS For intestinal infections (veterinary) (Sharp & Dohme)	Phthalysulfathiazole* U.S.P. 4 gm.
SUICIDE WITH D.D.T. Insecticide (Koch)	Sodium fluoride* 42-1/2% DDT 5-1/2%		

*Consult Sec. II., Ingredients Index. This ingredient may be responsible for major toxic effects if poisonous amounts of this product are ingested.

- 976 -

Name & Use Manufacturer	Ingredients		Name & Use Manufacturer	Ingredients	
SULFATROL For infections (veterinary, avian) (Whitmoyer)	Sulfathiazole Urea Dried brewers yeast Natural riboflavin concentrate Animal liver meal Siliceous material	6-1/2%	SULFORCIN BASE (Half Strength) For acne (Texas Pharm.)	Sulfur Resorcinol monoacetate	4% 1-1/2%
SULFA VETERINARY For coccidosis (veterinary, avian) (Salsbury's)	4, 4'-diaminodiphenylsulfone n^1-Phenylsulfanilamide*		SULFORCIN BASE (Regular Strength) For acne (Texas Pharm.)	Sulfur Resorcinol monoacetate*	8% 3%
SULFENONE Insecticide, fungicide (Hanna)	Rotenone* Sulfur*		SULFORCIN CREAM For acne (Texas Pharm.)	Resorcinol monoacetate* Dispersible sulfur	3% 5%
SULFILL (Torch)	Sulfur* (precipitated)	40%	SULFORCIN LOTION For acne (Texas Pharm.)	Resorcinol monoacetate* Dispersible sulfur	3% 5%
SULFIX SULFUR Fungicide (Sherwin-Williams)	Sulfur*	95%	SULFORON WETTABLE SULFUR Fungicide (du Pont)	Sulfur*	
SULFOAM SHAMPOO (Lawrence Labs.)	Ethyl glycol M.S. Drew 1011 Lanolin anhydrous Duponal W.A. paste Formaldehyde Perfume Sodium bisulfite Citric acid Dispersed sulfur	trace	SULFORON X WETTABLE SULFUR Fungicide (du Pont)	Sulfur*	
SULFOCIDE Fungicide (Pratt, B.)	Sodium polysulfide* Sodium thiosulfate	40% 2%	SULFOXYDRIN (Vaso-Sulfa) Nasal Decongestant (Horton & Converse)	Sulfathiazole sodium (sesqui-hydrate) Sodium sulfite Di-desoxyephedrine HC1	2.5% 0.2% 0.125%
SULFO-CRYSTINE Cathartic (Horton & Converse)	Sodium thiosulfate Magnesium sulfate (epsom salts) Calcium sulfate Potassium sulfate	33% 27% 0.1% 0.5%	SULFUR-8 Hair and scalp preparation (Household)	Lanolin Polysulfides* Carbolic acid	
SULFODEX Insecticide, fungicide (Hanna)	DDT* Copper sulfate* dust		SULFUR-8 HAIR * SCALP CONDITIONER (Sulfur-8)		
SULFOIL For external infections (veterinary, avian) (Thoroughbred)	Each fl. oz.: Sulfathiazole Urea Chlorophyll Sulfanilamide Benzyl alcohol Propylene glycol base	3.5% 7% 3.5% 3%	SULFUR FOAM APPLICATORS Ectoparasiticide (Wyeth Labs.)	Sulfur	7%
SULFOLAN (Commerce)	Quinine Precipitated sulfur* Lanolin Castor oil Salicylic acid* Petrolatum		SUL-LATE Fungicide (Taylor)	Sulfur* Ziram* Ferbam	80% 4.5% 0.5%
SULFO-LO Antiseptic (Whorton)	Sulfur compounds of potassium and zinc* Calomine Alcohol Colloidal sulfur*	30%/v	SULMIX NO. 2 For infections (veterinary) (Wilke)	Sulfapyridine sodium Sulfathiazole sodium Sodium lactate Orthophenylphenol	6.5%/v 6.5%/v 1-6 m. 1/10,000
SULFO-MERTHIOLATE Antiseptic powder (Lilly)	Sodium p-ethyl mercuri thiophenyl sulfonate	1-1,000	SULPERCAL (Chemical Ind.)	Precipitated sulfur Peru balsam Cical base	10.00% 10.00% 80.00%

*Consult Sec. II., Ingredients Index. This ingredient may be responsible for major toxic effects if poisonous amounts of this product are ingested.

Name & Use Manufacturer	Ingredients		Name & Use Manufacturer	Ingredients	
SUL-Q-NOX SOLUTION For coccidiosis (veterinary, avian) (Greever's)	Sulfaquinoxaline sodium*		SUNLAND AGRICULTURAL POISON BAIT Insecticide (Sunland)	Calcium arsenate*	5%
SULQUIN LIQUID For coccidiosis (veterinary, avian) (Salsbury's)	Each 100 cc.: Sodium sulfaquinoxaline 3.44 gm.		SUNLAND ALDRIN SOIL TREATER 3 Soil conditioner (Sunland)	Hexachloro hexahydro dimethano naphthalene* Related compounds	2.85% 2.15%
SULQUIN SOLUBLE POWDER For coccidiosis (veterinary, avian) (Salsbury's)	Sulfaquinoxaline* 25%		SUNLAND CRYOLITE DUST NO. 50 Insecticide (Sunland)	Sodium fluoaluminate*	50%
SULTAR Laxative, tonic (Friendly Labs.)	Flowers of sulfur* Cream of tartar Sugar Flavoring		SUNLAND DDT-COPPER DUST NO. 20-25S Insecticide (Sunland)	DDT Basic copper sulfate* Sulfur	5% 20% 25%
SUMLAKIA Sedative (Sumlak)	Each tsp.: Strontium 1.80 gr. Ammonium 1.80 gr. Potassium 1.80 gr. Sodium 1.80 gr. Calcium 0.60 gr. Lithium 0.20 gr.		SUNLAND DIELDRIN DUST 1.5-50S Insecticide (Sunland)	Hexachloro epoxy octahydro-dimethano naphthalene 1.28% Related compounds 0.22% Sulfur* 50.00%	
SUMMER-AID LOTION (Corpus Christi)			SUNLAND MALATHION DUST Insecticide (Sunland)	Malathion* (o,o-dimethyl dithiophosphate of diethyl mercaptosuccinate) 4.0%	
SUMMER SPRA-OIL Insecticide (Pratt, B.)	White-oil-type spray oil 97% Emulsifier 3%		SUNLAND NICOTINE DUST NO. 10F Insecticide (Sunland)	Nicotine alkaloid*	3.6%
SUNBRITE CLEANSER (Swift)	Alkyl aryl sulfonate* Trisodium phosphate* Wedron silica		SUNLAND P.A.R. DUST 20-25S Insecticide (Sunland)	Parathion* Sulfur	2.0% 25.0%
SUNBROWN CREAM Skin protective (Carstens)	Quinine alkaloid* Crystalline sea salt Vegetable and animal fats		SUNLAND SPIDRAN DUST 5-25S Insecticide (Sunland)	p-Chlorophenyl-p-chlorobenzene sulfonate* 5.0% Sulfur* 25.0%	
SUNDAY SHOWER Dog cleaner (House of Huston)	Related compounds 0.10% Octachloro-4,7 methano-tetrahydroindane 0.15% Dichloro diphenyl dichloro-ethane 1.00% Dipentene 2.28% Para-cymene 0.77% Para-menthane 0.62% Terpene hydrocarbons 0.83%		SUNLAND SULPHUR Fungicide (Sunland)	Sulfur*	98%
			SUNLAND T.P. DUST 20 Insecticide (Sunland)	Tetraethyl pyrophosphate* 2% Other ethyl phosphates 3%	
SUN FUN SUN-TAN LOTION & INSECT REPELLENT (Dunaway)	2-Ethyl hexanediol 1-3* 22.20%		SUNLAND ZIMATE DUST 6.5 Fungicide (Sunland)	Zinc ethylene-bis (dithio-carbamate) 6.5%	
SUN-GLO PERFUME (Noblesse)			SUN'N BUG Insect repellent, sun cream (Silicote)	2-Ethylhexanediol-1,3 35% Dimethyl phthalate 12.0% Dimethyl polysiloxane 15.0% Calcium stearate 7.0% Stearic acid 10.0% Carbitol 1.0% Triethanolamine 1.0%	
SUN-GLO POLISH (Pioneer)					

*Consult Sec. II., Ingredients Index. This ingredient may be responsible for major toxic effects if poisonous amounts of this product are ingested.

Name & Use Manufacturer	Ingredients		Name & Use Manufacturer	Ingredients	
SUNNY DAY BLEACH (First National Stores)	Sodium hypochlorite* 5.25%		SUNPROTECTOL (Lamond)	Mineral oil Edible vegetable oil F.D.C. color Digaloyl-trioleate	
SUNNY DAY BLUING (First National Stores)	Oxalic acid* Prussian blue		SUN-RAY AFTER-SHAVE LOTION, BOUQUET HAIR TONIC, HAIR COLOR (Sun Ray)		
SUNNYSIDE'S GUM SPIRITS TURPENTINE (Sunnyside)	Pure gum turpentine*				
SUNNYSIDE'S LACQUER THINNER (Sunnyside)	Denatured alcohol Butyl alcohol* Butyl acetate Ethyl acetate Naphtha Toluol*		SUN-RAY COLORED CHALK, LECTURE SQUARES, POSTER CHALK (Am. Art Clay)		
SUNNYSIDE'S LINSEED OIL (Raw) Paint ingredient (Sunnyside)	Pure linseed oil		SUNSET ALL FABRIC DYE (North American)	Detergent Water softener Aniline dyes *	
SUNNYSIDE'S LINSEED OIL (Boiled) Paint ingredient (Sunnyside)	Pure linseed oil Metallic driers		SUNSET SOAP DYE (North American)	Aniline dyes* Vegetable oil Cocoanut oil soap Fabric softener Dyeing assistants	
SUNNYSIDE'S LIQUID BRUSH CLEANER Solvent (Sunnyside)	Methanol* Acetone* Benzol* Other solvents		SUNSHINE NEUTRAL CLEANER (Uncle Sam)	Vegetable oils Synthetic detergents Water softener	
SUNNYSIDE'S PAINT & VARNISH REMOVER (Sunnyside)	Methanol* Acetone* Benzol*		SUN-SOFT Water softener (Barcolene)	Distearyl dimethyl ammonium chloride* 5% Isopropyl alcohol 2%	
SUNNYSIDE'S QUAKERSOL Solvent alcohol (Sunnyside)	Denatured ethyl alcohol*		SUN SPIRITS Herbicide (Sun Oil)	Petroleum distillate* 100%	
SUNNYSIDE'S SHELLAC (Sunnyside)	Shellac Denatured ethyl alcohol*		SUPASED (Elixir) Sedative (Massengill)	Each 5 cc.: Ethyl alcohol 4%/v Potassium bromide* 0.324 gm. Sodium bromide* 0.324 gm. Ammonium bromide 0.324 gm. Zinc bromide 6.5 mg. Fluid extract belladonna (alkaloids 0.00005 gr.) 1/80 m. Fluid extract hyoscyamus (alkaloids 0.000003 gr.) 1/80 m. Fluid extract cascara sagrada 0.006 cc. Extract hops 6.5 mg.	
SUNNYSIDE'S TURPENTINE, SULFATE WOOD (Sunnyside)	Turpentine*				
SUNNY SOL (Jones, John)	Sodium hypochlorite*				
SUN-O-CAINE For skin irritations, burns (VB)	Zinc oxide Menthol* Ethyl aminobenzoate		SUPER ANAHIST ANTIBIOTIC NASAL SPRAY & NOSE DROPS (Anahist)	Thonzylamine HCl 1.0% Phenylephrine HC1 0.25% Thonzide 0.05% Gramicidin 0.005%	
SUNOCO SELF-EMULSIFYING SPRAY OIL Insecticide (Sun Oil)	Oil* 86% Naphthenic soaps 11%				

*Consult Sec. II., Ingredients Index. This ingredient may be responsible for major toxic effects if poisonous amounts of this product are ingested.

- 979 -

Name & Use Manufacturer	Ingredients	Name & Use Manufacturer	Ingredients
SUPER ANAHIST APC COMP. For colds (Anahist)	Thonzylamine hydrochloride 25 mg. Aspirin* 3.5 gr. Phenacetin* 1.5 gr. Caffeine 0.5 gr. Ascorbic acid (Vitamin C) 20 mg.	SUPER DUTY ENAMELS & STAINS (Johnston)	
SUPER ANAHIST APC. COMP. (Children's Size) For colds, hay fever (Anahist)	Thonzylamine hydrochloride 12.5 mg. Aspirin* 1.75 gr. Phenacetin* 0.75 gr. Caffeine 0.25 gr. Ascorbic acid (vitamin C) 10 mg.	SUPER-FILM INTERIOR FINISH Paint (DeSoto P. & V.)	
		SUPERFINE ENAMEL (Sargent- Gerke)	
SUPER ANAHIST COUGH SYRUP Antitussive (Anahist)	Thonzylamine HCl 6.25 mg. Ammonium chloride 50 mg. Sodium citrate 135 mg. Ascorbic acid 10 mg. Alcohol 0.5%	SUPERFINE 90% SULPHUR DUST Insecticide (Taylor)	Sulfur* 90.00
SUPER ANAHIST NOSE DROPS (Anahist)	Thonzylamine hydrochloride* Phenylephrine hydro- chloride Gramicidin Pluronic F-68	SUPERFLO PAINTS (Symolyn)	
SUPER ANAHIST RUB Rubefacient (Anahist)	Methyl nicotinate Methyl salicylate* Thonzylamine hydrochloride* Thonzide	SUPER FULDETH RA INSECTICIDE (Fuld)	DDT* Pyrethrum Oil
SUPER ANAHIST TABLETS For colds, head ache, hay fever (Anahist)	Each tablet: Thonzylamine hydrochloride 25 mg. Ascorbic acid 20 mg. Aspirin* 3-1/2 gr. Phenacetin* 1-1/2 gr. Caffeine 1/2 gr.	SUPER GLOSS NO RUB FLOOR WAX (Peerless Chem.)	
SUPER ANAHIST TABLETS (Children's Size) For colds (Anahist)	Each tablet: Thonzylamine hydrochloride 12-1/2 mg. Ascorbic acid 10 mg. Aspirin* 1-3/4 gr. Phenacetin* 3/4 gr. Caffeine 1/4 gr.	SUPER HIDING FLAT WHITE PAINT (Thompson & Co.)	
SUPERB Detergent oil (Kendall Ref.)		SUPER HIDING INTERIOR WHITE PAINTS (Barreled Sunlight) (U. S. Gutta)	
SUPERB ENAMEL (Hancock P. & V.)		SUPER HIL-BRITE Self polishing wax (Hillyard Chem.)	Soap Wax
SUPERCHLOR A PATTERSON Highly buffered salt solution (Patterson Labs.)	Sodium hypochlorite * 4%	SUPER HILCO Insecticide (Hillyard Chem.)	B-thiocyano ethyl esters of mixed fatty acids averaging 10-18 carbon atoms B-butoxy B' thiocyano diethyl ether* Essential oils* DDT*
SUPERCHROME INK (Parker Pen)	Sodium hydroxide* approx. 1%	SUPER HOUSE PAINT (Chi-Namel)	Titanium dioxide 3.3% Titanium calcium 18.2% Titanium magnesium 15.0% Zinc oxide 17.0% Basic sulfate white lead 5.7% Raw linseed oil 14.5% Heat treated linseed oil 14.5% Mineral spirits 7.8% Drier 4.0%
SUPER COPPER Fungicide (Hammond)	Copper* 15%		

*Consult Sec. II., Ingredients Index. This ingredient may be responsible for major toxic effects if poisonous amounts of this product are ingested.

Name & Use Manufacturer	Ingredients	
SUPERIOR BRAND MEDICINE Laxative (Cel-Ton-Sa)	Epsom salts (mag. sulfate) Sodium phosphate Fennel Oil cassia Cinnamic aldehyde Sodium salicylate* Iron and amm. citrate Saccharin soluble Gentian Caramel Methyl salicylate* Berberis Salicylic acid* Ammonium chloride	
SUPERIOR CHEMICAL'S 25% DDT-EMULSION CONC. Insecticide (Superior Chem.)	Oil DDT*	25%
SUPERIOR CHEMICAL'S 30% DDT OIL CONC. Insecticide (Superior Chem.)	Oil DDT*	30%
SUPERIOR FLAT WALL PAINT (Vita-Var)		
SUPERIOR INKS (Davids, C.I.)		
SUPERIOR PAINTS (Am. Paint Corp.)		
SUPERIOR PASTE (Davids, C.I.)		
SUPERIOR'S A.P.C. & GELS Analgesic (Superior Pharm.)	Each tablet: Acetophenetidin* Tinct. gelsemium N.F. Aspirin* Caffeine alkaloid	2 gr. 3 m. 3-1/2 gr. 1/4 gr.
SUPERIOR'S CALAMINE ZINC OXIDE (Plain) Skin (Superior Pharm.)	Calamine Zinc oxide* Aromatics	
SUPERIOR'S EXTRA VALUE DORMANT NUTRITIONAL SPRAY For agricultural use (Superior Fert.)	Sulfur* Zinc* Dinitro-o-cyclohexylphenol*	70% 11% 2%
SUPERIOR'S EXTRA VALUE NUTRITIONAL DUST For agricultural use (Superior Fert.)	Sulfur* Zinc* Copper*	70% 4.2% 6%
SUPERIOR'S EXTRA VALUE NUTRITIONAL SPRAY NO. 2 For agricultural use (Superior Fert.)	Sulfur* Dinitro-o-cyclohexylphenol Zinc*	63% 1.8% 7%
SUPERIOR'S EXTRA VALUE POST-BLOOM NUTRITIONAL SPRAY For agricultural use (Superior Fert.)	Sulfur* Zinc* Copper* Boron	55% 6% 8% 0.5%
SUPER KEM-TONE WHITE Latex paint (Sherwin-Williams)	Titanium dioxide Lithopone Calcium carbonate Silica and silicates Volatile thinner* water Synthetic rubber latex	19% 4% 3% 10% 44% 20%
SUPERKILL 2-1/2-0-0 ALDRIN COTTON DUST Insecticide (Taylor)	Aldrin*	2.5%
SUPERKILL 2-1/2-5-0 ALDRIN COTTON DUST Insecticide (Taylor)	Aldrin* DDT*	2.5% 5%
SUPERKILL 2-1/2-5-40 ALDRIN COTTON DUST Insecticide (Taylor)	Aldrin* DDT* Sulfur*	2.5% 5% 40%
SUPERKILL 2-1/2-10-0 ALDRIN COTTON DUST Insecticide (Taylor)	Aldrin* DDT*	2.5% 10%

*Consult Sec. II., Ingredients Index. This ingredient may be responsible for major toxic effects if poisonous amounts of this product are ingested.

Name & Use Manufacturer	Ingredients		Name & Use Manufacturer	Ingredients	
SUPERKILL 2-1/2-10-40 ALDRIN COTTON DUST Insecticide (Taylor)	Aldrin* DDT* Sulfur*	2.5% 10% 40%	SUPERKILL 5% DDT DUST Insecticide (Taylor)	DDT*	5.00%
SUPERKILL 23% ALDRIN EMULSIFIABLE CONC. Insecticide (Taylor)	Aldrin*		SUPERKILL 10% DDT DUST Insecticide (Taylor)	DDT*	10.00%
SUPERKILL 3-5 BHC-DDT EMULSIFIABLE CONC. Insecticide (Taylor)	BHC* DDT*	8.7% 14.5%	SUPERKILL 25% DDT (Miscible) Insecticide (Taylor)	DDT*	25.00%
SUPERKILL 45% CHLORDANE EMULSIFIABLE CONC. Insecticide (Taylor)	Chlordane*		SUPERKILL 35% DDT (Miscible) Insecticide (Taylor)	DDT*	35.00%
SUPERKILL CHLORO IPC Herbicide (Taylor)	Chloro IPC*	48%	SUPERKILL 25% DDT SOLUTION Insecticide (Taylor)	DDT*	25.00%
SUPERKILL 5% COPPER DUST Fungicide (Taylor)	Copper*		SUPERKILL 35% DDT SOLUTION Insecticide (Taylor)	DDT*	35.00%
SUPERKILL 7% COPPER DUST Fungicide (Taylor)	Copper*		SUPERKILL 10% DIELDRIN (Granular) Insecticide (Taylor)	Dieldrin*	10.00%
SUPERKILL 3-0-0 COTTON DUST Insecticide (Taylor)	Gamma BHC*	3%	SUPERKILL 15% DIELDRIN EMULSIFIABLE CONC. Insecticide (Taylor)	Dieldrin*	15.00%
SUPERKILL 3-5-0 COTTON DUST Insecticide (Taylor)	Gamma BHC* DDT*	3% 5%	SUPERKILL ETHYLENE DICHLORIDE EMUL. Fumigant (Taylor)	Ethylene dichloride*	90%
SUPERKILL 3-5-40 COTTON DUST Insecticide (Taylor)	Gamma isomer of BHC* DDT* Sulfur *	3.00% 5.00% 40.00 %	SUPER KILLEX Insecticide (Sherwin-Williams)	Tetraethyl pyrophosphate* 40% Other organic phosphates 60%	
SUPERKILL 3-10-0 COTTON DUST Insecticide (Taylor)	Gamma BHC* DDT*	3% 10%	SUPERKILL 11.4% FERBAM DUST Fungicide (Taylor)	Ferbam	11.4%
SUPERKILL 3-10-40 COTTON DUST Insecticide (Taylor)	Gamma BHC* DDT* Sulfur*	3% 5% 40%	SUPERKILL 2-1/2-0-0 HEPTACHLOR COTTON DUST Insecticide (Taylor)	Heptachlor*	2.5%
			SUPERKILL 2-1/2-5-0 HEPTACHLOR COTTON DUST Insecticide (Taylor)	Heptachlor* DDT*	2.5% 5%

*Consult Sec. II., Ingredients Index. This ingredient may be responsibie for major toxic effects if poisonous amounts of this product are ingested.

Name & Use Manufacturer	Ingredients	
SUPERKILL 2-1/2-5-40 HEPTACHLOR COTTON DUST Insecticide (Taylor)	Heptachlor* DDT* Sulfur*	2.5% 5% 40%
SUPERKILL 2-1/2-10-0 HEPTACHLOR COTTON DUST Insecticide (Taylor)	Heptachlor* DDT*	2.5% 10%
SUPERKILL 2-1/2-10-40 HEPTACHLOR COTTON DUST (Taylor)	Heptachlor* DDT* Sulfur*	2.5% 10% 40%
SUPERKILL 23% HEPTACHLOR EMULSIFIABLE CONC. Insecticide (Taylor)	Heptachlor*	23%
SUPERKILL LIME SULPHUR SOLUTION Insecticide (Taylor)	Calcium polysulfide* Calcium thiosulfate	29% 1%
SUPERKILL 4% MALATHION DUST Insecticide (Taylor)	Malathion*	4%
SUPERKILL 50% MALATHION EMULSIFIABLE CONC. Insecticide (Taylor)	Malathion*	50%
SUPERKILL 1% PARATHION DUST Insecticide (Taylor)	Parathion*	
SUPERKILL 23% PARATHION EMULSIFIABLE CONC. Insecticide (Taylor)	Parathion*	
SUPERKILL PEACH DUST Insecticide, fungicide (Taylor)	Parathion* Sulfur	1.5% 80%
SUPERKILL PEACH SPRAY NO. 1 Insecticide, fungicide (Taylor)	Parathion* Sulfur	2.75% 75%

Name & Use Manufacturer	Ingredients	
SUPERKILL PEACH SPRAY NO. 2 Insecticide, fungicide (Taylor)	Parathion* Sulfur	3.7% 75%
SUPERKILL PEACH SPRAY NO. 3 Insecticide, fungicide (Taylor)	Lead arsenate* Sulfur	11.5% 34%
SUPERKILL 5% PENTA-CHLORO-PHENOL Wood preservative (Taylor)	Pentachlorophenol*	5%
SUPERKILL 40% PENTA-CHLORO-PHENOL Wood preservative (Taylor)	Pentachlorophenol*	40%
SUPERKILL 0.75% ROTENONE Insecticide, fungicide (Taylor)	Rotenone Sulfur*	0.75%
SUPERKILL 1% ROTENONE Insecticide (Taylor)	Rotenone	1%
SUPERKILL 20% SABADILLA DUST Insecticide (Taylor)	Sabadilla* dust	20%
SUPERKILL 80% SULPHUR DUST Insecticide, fungicide (Taylor)	Sulfur*	80%
SUPERKILL 90% SULPHUR DUST Insecticide, fungicide (Taylor)	Sulfur*	90%
SUPERKILL 95% SULPHUR DUST Insecticide, fungicide (Taylor)	Sulfur*	95%
SUPERKILL 99% SULPHUR DUST Insecticide, fungicide (Taylor)	Sulfur*	99%

*Consult Sec. II., Ingredients Index. This ingredient may be responsible for major toxic effects if poisonous amounts of this product are ingested.

Name & Use Manufacturer	Ingredients	
SUPERKILL SUPERIOR OIL Insecticide (Taylor)	Petroleum oils*	97%
SUPERKILL 10% TDE DUST Insecticide (Taylor)	TDE	10%
SUPERKILL 24% TDE EMULSIFIABLE CONC. Insecticide (Taylor)	TDE*	24%
SUPERKILL TOBACCO DUST NO. 1 Insecticide (Taylor)	TDE Parathion*	10% 1%
SUPERKILL TOMATO DUST Insecticide (Taylor)	DDT* Copper*	5% 6%
SUPERKILL 20% TOXAPHENE COTTON DUST Insecticide (Taylor)	Toxaphene* Sulfur	20% 40%
SUPERKILL 20-40 TOXAPHENE COTTON DUST Insecticide, fungicide (Taylor)	Toxaphene* Sulfur	20% 40%
SUPERKILL 60% TOXAPHENE EMULSIFIABLE CONC. Insecticide (Taylor)	Toxaphene*	
SUPERKILL 6% WETTABLE BHC Insecticide (Taylor)	BHC*	
SUPERKILL 50% WETTABLE CHLORDANE Insecticide (Taylor)	Chlordane*	
SUPERKILL 50% WETTABLE DDT Insecticide (Taylor)	DDT*	
SUPERKILL 25% WETTABLE HEPTACHLOR Insecticide (Taylor)	Heptachlor*	

Name & Use Manufacturer	Ingredients	
SUPERKILL 25% WETTABLE MALATHION Insecticide (Taylor)	Malathion*	
SUPERKILL 15% WETTABLE PARATHION Insecticide (Taylor)	Parathion*	
SUPERKILL WETTABLE SULPHUR Insecticide, fungicide (Taylor)	Sulfur*	94%
SUPERKILL 50% WETTABLE TDE Insecticide (Taylor)	TDE*	50%
SUPERKILL ZINEB DUST Fungicide (Taylor)	Zineb	6.5%
SUPER KROME ALUM. PAINT (Sheffield Bronze)		
SUPERLASTIC HOUSE PAINT (Felton Sibley)		
SUPERLATIVE FOOT CREAM (Liquid) Fungicide (medical) (Milber)	Phenol* 5.00 cc. Zinc oxide 160.00 gm. Sodium carboxymethylcellulose 20.00 gm. Dioctyl sodium sulfosuccinate 0.65 gm. Glycerin 30.00 cc. Perfume oil	
SUPERLAX TABLETS Laxative (Univ. Nutrit.)	Carboxymethylcellulose 6 gr. Dehydrated prune concentrate 1 gr. Acetophenolisatin 1 mg.	
SUPERL POLISH (Easterday)		
SUPERPHOS ELIXIR Tonic (Success)	Sodium glycerophosphates 2 gr. Calcium glycerophosphate 2 gr. Strychnine sulfate 1/64 gr. Phosphoric acid (75%) 1.7 m. Alcohol 10%/v	
SUPER PINOL DISINFECTANT (Interstate San.)		
SUPER-PLY PAINT & ENAMEL (Glidden Co.)		

*Consult Sec. II., Ingredients Index. This ingredient may be responsible for major toxic effects if poisonous amounts of this product are ingested.

Name & Use Manufacturer	Ingredients	Name & Use Manufacturer	Ingredients
SUPER PRINT Photographic supplies (Uricheck)		SUPER- VELOXIN Embalming chemical (Eckels)	
SUPERSEAL CAULKING COMPOUND (Binzen)		SUPER WET PAINT REMOVER (Morris Paint)	
SUPER SHINE-ALL Cleaner (Hillyard Chem.)		SUPERWHITE EXTERIOR PAINT (Cook P. & V.)	
SUPERSOL Solvent (Am. Lacquer)		SUPLIGOL TABLETS (Am. Ferment)	Desiccated whole bile 4 gr. Ketocholanic acids 1 gr.
SUPER SOLAREX PAINTS (Great Lakes P. & V.)		SUPRA-GESIC Rubefacient (Superior Pharm.)	Oil of camphor* Methyl salicylate* Menthol* Oil of mustard (artifical) Turpentine*
SUPER STOCK TOX Insecticide (Martin, C.J.)	Toxaphene* 62.0% Benzene hexachloride, gamma isomer 1.89% Other isomers 3.15%	SUPREME ANTI-FREEZE (Crown Prod.)	
SUPERSTRIP NON- INFLAMM- ABLE PAINT & VARNISH REMOVER (Savogran)	Methylene chloride* Propylene dichloride* Methanol*	SUPREME LIQUID AUTO WASH (Woolsey)	
SUPER SUDS Soap powder (Colgate- Palmolive)		SUPREME PHARMA- CEUTICAL FERROUS SULFATE Food supplement with iron (Supreme Pharm.)	Each coated tablet: Ferrous sulfate U.S.P. * 5 gr.
SUPER SUDS DETERGENT (Colgate- Palmolive)			
SUPERTAH Ointment for eczema (Tailby)	Coal-tar ointment*	SUPREME SANIROID RECTAL OINTMENT (Supreme Pharm.)	Ephedrine acid oleate* Ichthynate Lanolin anhydrous S.E. Witch hazel Zinc oxide Zinc carbonate
SUPERTAH-5 OINTMENT (Tailby)	Sulfur* Salicylic acid*		
SUPER-TEX PAINT & ENAMEL (Tex Prod.)		SUPREMOLITE ACID RESISTING PAINTS & ENAMELS (Longview)	
SUPER- TOMIC DEVELOPERS Photographic supplies		SUREBRITE SUPER ALUMINUM PAINT (Panther)	
SUPER VALSPAR VARNISHES, STAINS & ENAMELS (Valentine)		SURE DEATH 23% ALDRIN EQUIVALENT EMULSIFIABLE CONC. Insecticide (Woodbury)	Hexachloro hexahydro dimethano naphthalene* 23.10% Related compounds 17.37% Petroleum hydrocarbons* 52.03%
		SURE DEATH BHC LIQUID Insecticide (Woodbury)	Gamma isomer of benzene hexachloride* 11% Other isomers of benzene hexachloride 17%

*Consult Sec. II., Ingredients Index. This ingredient may be responsible for major toxic effects if poisonous amounts of this product are ingested.

Name & Use Manufacturer	Ingredients	Name & Use Manufacturer	Ingredients
SURE DEATH CHLORDANE EMULSION CONC. Insecticide (Woodbury)	Tech. chlordane* 45% Aliphatic petroleum solvent* 45%	SURE FIRE LIGHTER FLUID (Wilco)	Petroleum hydrocarbon*
SURE DEATH DAIRY SPRAY OIL TYPE Insecticide (Woodbury)	Mineral oil 99.67% Piperonyl butoxide tech. 0.30% Pyrethrins 0.03%	SURE-GO PAINTS (Yoder)	
SURE DEATH 50% DDT Insecticide (Woodbury)	DDT* 50%	SURE-HIDE ONE COAT ENAMEL (Phelan-Faust)	
SURE DEATH DIELDRIN WE-18 Insecticide (Woodbury)	Hexachloro epoxy octahydro-endo, exo-dimethano naphthalene* 15.83% Related compounds 2.79% Petroleum hydrocarbons 73.38%	SURE-KLEAN BLEACH, GERMICIDE, CLEANER (Uddo)	
SURE DEATH EMULSIFIABLE LINDANE 12-1/2% Insecticide (Woodbury)	Gamma isomer of benzene hexachloride (from lindane) 12.50% Methylated naphthalenes 9.34% Mesityl oxide 18.41% Xylene* 48.00% Cyclohexanone 6.25%	SURE-KYL CONCENTRATE Insecticide (Stanley Home)	DDT* Tech. piperonyl butoxide Pyrethrins* Methylated naphthalenes* Petroleum distillates* Freon
		SURELIGHT CIGAR LIGHTER FLUID (Marine Labs)	
SURE DEATH INSECTICIDE 5% DDT Insecticide (Woodbury)	Petroleum hydrocarbon oils* Aromatic petroleum oil* DDT*	SURE-SHINE CLEANING COMPOUND (Safety Globe)	
SURE DEATH LINDANE SEED TREATER For agricultural use (Woodbury)	Gamma isomer of benzene hexachloride (from lindane)* 15%	SURE SHOT GUN GLUE (Casey Chem.)	Selenium* Nitric acid* Methanol*
		SURETOX FLEA POWDER (Suretox)	Rotenone 1%
SURE DEATH MALACIDE FLY KILLER Insecticide (Woodbury)	Malathion* 57% Xylene* 35%	SURETY BON HOUSE PAINT (Johnston)	
SURE DEATH MILLFUME NO. 1 Fumigant (Woodbury)	Carbon tetrachloride* Carbon bisulfide* Sulfur dioxide*	SURETY POWDERED HAND SOAP (Surety)	Soap Glycerin Coconut oil Camphor* Italian pumice
SURE DEATH MILLFUME 66 Fumigant (Woodbury)	Carbon tetrachloride* 81.3% Carbon bisulfide 12.1% Ethylene dibromide 6.6%	SURF Detergent (Lever)	Sodium alkaryl sulfonate Sodium polyphosphates Fatty amide Sodium sulfate and silicate Perfume Optical dye
SURE DEATH TDE EMULSION (Rhothane) Insecticide (Woodbury)	Dichloro diphenyl dichloro-ethane 25.0% Aromatic petroleum deriv. solvent* 71.8%	SURFACAINE (Cyclomethy-caine, Lilly) Rectal and vaginal anesthetic (Lilly)	Each suppository: 3-(2-methylpiperidino)-propyl-para-cyclohexyloxy benzoate sulfate 10 mg.
SURE DEATH TOXAPHENE EMULSION CONC. Insecticide (Woodbury)	Toxaphene* (tech. chlorinated camphene with 67-69% chlorine) 60% Aliphatic petroleum solvent 35%	SURFACAINE 0.5% (Cyclomethy-caine, Lilly) Topical anesthetic (Lilly)	3-(2-Methylpiperidino)-propyl-para-cyclohexyloxy-benzoate sulfate 0.5%

*Consult Sec. II., Ingredients Index. This ingredient may be responsible for major toxic effects if poisonous amounts of this product are ingested.

Name & Use Manufacturer	Ingredients	Name & Use Manufacturer	Ingredients
SURFACINE COMPOUND (Cyclomethy- caine Com- pound) Local anesthetic, antiseptic (Lilly)	Surfacaine (cyclomethycaine, Lilly) 0.5% Calamine 5% Zinc oxide 5% Merthiolate (Thimerosal, Lilly) 1–5,000	SURRENDER EXTRACT, EAU de TOILETTE (Parfums Ciro)	
SURFACE- KLEEN LINOLEUM & HARDWOOD FLOOR CLEANER (Staminite)		SUSPICION PERFUME, COLOGNE STICK, EAU de TOILETTE (Sardeau)	
SURFACENE (Glidden Co.)		SUSTAMIN TABLETS Analgesic, antirheumatic (Drug Research)	Sodium salicylate* Acetophenetidin* 2 gr. Anhydrous caffeine
SURFACIDE RESIDUAL INSECTICIDE (Pro–Tex–All)	Oil* DDT* Pyrethrins*	SUTTON STICK DEODORANT (Sutton)	Soap S.D.A. alcohol Hexachlorophene* Essential oils* Pure food colors
SURFLUX WALL SIZE (Vita–Var)		SUX-A-TABS Analgesic, antirheumatic (Hance)	Sodium para-aminobenzoate 1-1/2 gr. Salicylamide* 2-1/2 gr. Vitamin C 25 mg.
SURGICAL DRESSING OINTMENT (Rigidtest)	Zinborsal (zinc borodisalicylate decahydrate with boric acid) Vitamins A and D (ext. from fish liver oils) Cod liver oil Lecithin Glycerin Zinc oxide Kaolin Methyl parahydroxybenzoate Lanolin-petrolatum base	SUXION For loose dentures (Werner)	Karaya gum Mineral oils
		SUZE LIP POMADE (Sacramento)	
SURGICAL SOLUTION OF DIAPARENE CHLORIDE Antiseptic (Homemakers')	Methylbenzethonium chloride* N.N.R. Alcohol Sodium ethylene diamine tetra acetates Octyl phenoxy polyethoxy ethanol	S/V COPPER NAPHTHENATE 200-S (General Petrol.)	Copper * 2.0% Metal naphthenate W 20.0%/w Solvent* 80.0%/w
		S/V SOVACIDE F, 544-B, 544-G Insecticides (Socony)	Methylated aromatic petroleum oil*
SURGICOL For skin irritations (Claflin)	Oxyquinoline sulfate* Resorcin* Eucalyptol* Boric acid* Aluminum acetate Ointment base Lanolin	S/V SOVASPRAY NO. 1, 2, 3 Insecticides (Socony)	Paraffin base spray oil* 100%
SURIN Rubefacient (McKesson)	Methacholine chloride 0.25% Camphor* Menthol* Methyl salicylate*	S.V.W. OUTSIDE PAINTS (Standard- Toch)	
SUR-LAY HAIR TONIC (Weyer)		SWAMP ROOT Diuretic, laxative (Kilmer)	Alcohol 10-1/2% Buchu leaves Peppermint herbs Rhubarb root Mandrake root Cape aloes Scullcap leaves Colombs root Golden seal root Valerian root Sassafras* Cinnamon Oil of juniper* Oil of birch Balsam caparba Balsam tolu Syrup base
SURLIGHT PAINTS, SURNAMEL ENAMELS, SUR PACO PAINTS (St. Louis Surfacer)			

*Consult Sec. II., Ingredients Index. This ingredient may be responsible for major toxic effects if poisonous amounts of this product are ingested. ·

Name & Use Manufacturer	Ingredients		Name & Use Manufacturer	Ingredients	
SWAN BRAND FUMIGANT NO. 2 (Thompson-Hayward)	Carbon tetrachloride* Carbon bisulfide* Ethylene dibromide*		SWC NO. 2 BEN HEX DUST Insecticide (Southwest Co-op.)	Gamma isomer BHC* Other isomers	2% 13.2%
SWAN BRAND FUMIGANT NO. 3 (Thompson-Hayward)	Carbon tetrachloride* Carbon bisulfide*		SWC NO. 2-60 BEN HEX SULFUR DUST Insecticide (Southwest Co-op.)	Gamma BHC* Other isomers Sulfur*	2% 13.2% 60%
SWAN BRAND FUMIGANT NO. 6 (Thompson-Hayward)	Carbon tetrachloride* Carbon bisulfide* Methyl bromide*		SWC No. 5 CHLORDANE DUST Insecticide (Southwest Co-op.)	Chlordane	5%
SWAN BRAND FUMIGAS Fumigant (Thompson-Hayward)	Carbon tetrachloride* Carbon bisulfide* Sulfur dioxide*		SWC NO. 2-5-50 COTTON DUST Insecticide (Southwest Co-op.)	Gamma BHC* Other isomers DDT* Sulfur*	2% 14% 5% 50%
SWAN BRAND SODIUM ARSENITE SOLUTION #40 Herbicide (Thompson-Hayward)	Sodium arsenite*	40.0%	SWC NO. 5 DDT DUST Insecticide (Southwest Co-op.)	DDT*	5%
SWANEE-LAC FLOOR & LINOLEUM FINISH (Johnston)			SWC NO. 10 DDT DUST Insecticide (Southwest Co-op.)	DDT*	10%
SWAN FLOATING TOILET SOAP (Lever)			SWC NO. 5-75 DDT SULFUR DUST Insecticide (Southwest Co-op.)	DDT* Sulfur*	5% 75%
SWANSONG MOTH-PROOFING (Brilco)			SWC NO. 10-65 DDT SULFUR DUST Insecticide (Southwest Co-op.)	DDT* Sulfur*	10% 65%
SWAV LATHER SHAVING CREAM (Norwich)	Soda soap Potash soap Borax soap Saponified vegetable and animal fats		SWC NO. 5-15-40 DDT TOX-SUL DUST Insecticide (Southwest Co-op.)	DDT* Toxaphene* Sulfur*	5% 15% 40%
SWAYDEX PAINTS, VARNISH, LACQUER ENAMELS (Maas & Waldstein)			SWC NO. 10 TOXAPHENE DUST Insecticide (Southwest Co-op.)	Toxaphene*	10%
SWC NO. 2-4-0 BEN HEX D.D.T. DUST Insecticide (Southwest Co-op.)	Gamma BHC* Other isomers DDT*	2% 13.2% 5%	SWC NO. 1-1/2 VEG-HEX DUST Insecticide (Southwest Co-op.)	Gamma BHC*	1.5%
SWC NO. 1 BEN HEX DUST Insecticide (Southwest Co-op.)	Gamma BHC Other isomers	1% 6.6%			

*Consult Sec. II., Ingredients Index. This ingredient may be responsible for major toxic effects if poisonous amounts of this product are ingested.

- 988 -

Name & Use Manufacturer	Ingredients		Name & Use Manufacturer	Ingredients	
SWEENEY'S ANT-GO Insecticide (Sweeney, W.R.)	Sodium arsenate *	2.3%	SWETPAINT External analgesic (veterinary) (Thoroughbred)	Alcohol* Iodine* Potassium iodide Camphor* Methyl salicylate*	37.8%/v
SWEENEY'S MOTH BALLS (Sweeney, W.R.)	Naphthalene*	100%	SWFKILL DUST NO. 0-3-68 Insecticide (Southwest Fert.)	Gamma BHC* Other isomers Sulfur*	3% 5.25% 68%
SWEENEY'S MOTH DESTROYER (Sweeney, W.R.)	Petroleum distillates* Beta thiocyano ethyl esters of aliphatic acids (10-18 carbon atoms) B-butoxy b' thiocyano diethyl ether*		SWFKILL DUST NO. 5-0-0 Insecticide (Southwest Fert.)	DDT*	5%
SWEENEY'S NO. 1 DIP (Sweeney, W.R.)	Neutral coal tar oils* Anhydrous soap Phenols*		SWFKILL DUST NO. 5-0-41 Insecticide (Southwest Fert.)	DDT* Sulfur*	5% 41%
SWEENEY'S RAT KILLER READY MIXED (Sweeney, W.R.)	Warfarin (3-(a-acetonylbenzyl)- 4-hydroxycoumarin) 0.025%		SWFKILL DUST NO. 5-0-83 Insecticide (Southwest Fert.)	DDT* Sulfur*	5% 83%
SWEENEY'S SODIUM FLUORIDE INSECTICIDE (Sweeney, W.R.)	Sodium fluoride*	90%	SWFKILL DUST NO. 5-2-40 Insecticide (Southwest Fert.)	Gamma BHC* Other isomers DDT* Sulfur*	2% 3.5% 5% 41%
SWEEPRITE Sweeping compound (Pioneer)			SWFKILL DUST NO. 10-0-10 Insecticide (Southwest Fert.)	DDT*	10%
SWEET- AIRE HOUSEHOLD ODOR DEODORANT (Miller Protecto)			SWFKILL DUST NO. 10-0-41 Insecticide (Southwest Fert.)	DDT* Sulfur*	10% 41%
SWEET DREAMS INSECTICIDE (Altone)			SWFKILL DUST NO. 10-140 Insecticide (Southwest Fert.)	Gamma BHC Other isomers DDT* Sulfur*	1% 1.7% 10% 41%
SWEETHEART SHAMPOO (Manhattan Soap Co. (N.Y.))	Lanolin Egg		SWFKILL DUST NO. 10-2-40 Insecticide (Southwest Fert.)	Gamma BHC* Other isomers DDT* Sulfur *	2% 3.5% 10% 41%
SWEETHEART TOILET SOAP (Manhattan Soap Co.)	Sodium tallow-cocoanut oil soap Perfume 0.50-1% Titanium dioxide pigment less than 0.25%		SWFKILL DUST NO. 50-0-0 Insecticide (Southwest Fert.)	DDT*	50%
SWEET WILLIAM COLOGNES (Ayer)					

*Consult Sec. II., Ingredients Index. This ingredient may be responsible for major toxic effects if poisonous amounts of this product are ingested.

- 989 -

Name & Use Manufacturer	Ingredients		Name & Use Manufacturer	Ingredients	
SWFKILL 1% PARATHION DUST Insecticide (Pecos)	Parathion*	1%	SWIFT'S GOLD BEAR BRAND 40 (Selective weed control) Herbicide (Swift)	Triethylamine salt of 2,4-D*	
SWFKILL PURE-GAM DUST NO. 1 Insecticide (Southwest Fert.)	Gamma BHC	1%	SWIFT'S GOLD BEAR BRAND 44 (Selective weed control (Swift)	Isopropyl ester of 2,4-D*	
SWFKILL 10% TOXAPHENE DUST Insecticide (Southwest Fert.)	Toxaphene* Sulfur*	10% 46%	SWIFT'S GOLD BEAR BRAND WOODY PLANT CONTROL Herbicide (Swift)	Butoxy ethoxy propanol ester of 2,4-D* 28.00% Butoxy ethoxy propanol ester of 2,4-5-T* 13.18%	
SWFKILL 20% TOXAPHENE DUST Insecticide (Southwest Fert.)	Toxaphene* Sulfur	20% 46%	SWIFTSHEEN FLOOR WAX (Gerson-Stewart)		
SWIFT'S CLEANSER (Swift)	Alkyl aryl sulfonate Powdered trisodium phosphate Powdered tetra sodium pyrophosphate Wedron silica Magnasite Perfume Mineral oil		SWIFTSURE INSECT & MOTH SPRAY (Gerson-Stewart)		
SWIFTSEAL Wall, woodwork primer (Yarnell)			SWIFTSURE NO. 4 INSECTICIDE (Gerson-Stewart)	Beta butoxy beta' thiocyano diethyl ether* Beta thiocyano ethyl esters of fatty acids Oil Pyrethrins*	
SWIFT'S GOLD BEAR BRAND 2-2 BRUSH KILL Herbicide (Swift)	Butoxy ethoxy propanol ester of 2,4-D* 37.4% Butoxy ethoxy propanol ester of 2,4,5-T acid* 35.2%		SWIFTSURE 4 WITH DDT Insecticide (Gerson-Stewart)	Beta butoxy beta' thiocyano diethyl ether* Beta thiocyano ethyl esters of fatty acids DDT* Oil Pyrethrins*	
SWIFT'S GOLD BEAR BRAND 55 BRUSH KILL Herbicide (Swift)	Butoxy ethoxy propanol ester of 2,4,5-T acid* 69.7%		SWIRL PAINTS (Fisher, E.H.)		
SWIFT'S GOLD BEAR BRAND MALATHION FLY SPRAY Insecticide (Swift)	Malathion* 50.0% Methylated naphthalenes* 39.0%		SWIRT METAL CLEANER (Phillips Mfg.)		
			SWISH TOILET BOWL CLEANER (Paul, J.C.)	Hydrochloric acid *	
SWIFT'S GOLD BEAR BRAND 40 WEED CONTROL Herbicide (Swift)	Isopropyl and di-isopropanol amine salts of 2,4-D* 56%		SWISS ALPINE AIR DEODORANT (Hutchinson)		
SWIFT'S GOLD BEAR BRAND 44 WEED CONTROL Herbicide (Swift)	Isopropyl ester of 2,4-D* 46%		SWISS CREOSOTE Shingle stain (Phelan-Faust)		

*Consult Sec. II., Ingredients Index. This ingredient may be responsible for major toxic effects if poisonous amounts of this product are ingested.

- 990 -

Name & Use Manufacturer	Ingredients	Name & Use Manufacturer	Ingredients
SWISS KRISS Laxative (Modern Prod.)	Dried leaves of senna Licorice root Fennel Anise Caraway seed Dandelion Peppermint Papaya Strawberry and peach verbena Cyani flowers Parsley	SYNCHROME ALUMINUM PAINT (Crescent Brand)	
SWIX ROACH KILLER Insecticide (Winsale)		SYNCLOR RED LEAD PAINT (Better F. & C.)	
S.W.P. HOUSE PAINT (Sherwin-Williams)		SYN-DE CONC. SHAMPOO DETERGENT (Paglo)	Sulfated lauryl alcohol Alkylolamide
S.W.T. TABLETS Sedative (Ray Drug)	n,n-Dimethyl-n'-(a-pyridyl)-n'-(a-thenyl) ethylenediamine hydrochloride*	SYNEPHRICOL Antitussive (Winthrop)	Dihydrocodeinone bitartrate 1.33 mg. Neo-synephrine 5.0 mg. Thenfadil 4.0 mg. Potassium guaiacol sulfonate 70.0 mg. Ammonium chloride 70.0 mg. Menthol 1.0 mg. Chloroform 0.0166 cc. Alcohol 8%
SYDNEY LEE WAVE SET (Lee, S.)			
SYL-A-MANG For mange (veterinary) (Hartman)	Salicylic acid* Tannic acid* Benzyl benzoate* Oil of lavender Rubbing alcohol N.F. 66%	SYNFLEX (Alkyd Enamels) (Brown, A.)	Semi-aromatic petroleum hydrocarbons*
SYL-A-TAN For skin irritations (veterinary) (Hartman)	Rubbing alcohol compound N.F.* 66% Tannic acid* Salicylic acid* Oil of bergamot	SYN-FOR SYNTHETIC ENAMEL (O'Neil)	
SYLPHO-NATHOL (Cabot)	Caustic soda* Creosote oil* Cresylic acid* Tall oil	SYNKLOR-48-E (Naugatuck)	Tech. chlordane* 48%
		SYNKLOR-50-W (Naugatuck)	Tech. chlordane* 50%
SYLVAN WOOD VARNISH & ENAMELS (Sinclair & V.)		SYNKOTE FLOOR ENAMEL (Morris Paint)	
SYMPHONY LATEX BASE PAINT (Jacroy)		SYNLAC PAINTS (Sipe)	
SYN-A-LUX ENAMELS (Ellis Paint)		SYNODRIN NOSE DROPS (Altone)	
SYNASAL Nasal decongestant (Texas Pharm.)	1-Phenylephrine hydrochloride 1/4%	SYNOL SOAP Antiseptic, deodorant (Johnson & Johnson)	Hexachlorophene (dihydroxy-hexachlorodiphenyl methane) 1% Potassium soap base
SYN-A-TUNG PAINT (Mound City)		SYN-SUDZ Detergent (Van Vor)	

*Consult Sec. II., Ingredients Index. This ingredient may be responsible for major toxic effects if poisonous amounts of this product are ingested.

- 991 -

Name & Use Manufacturer	Ingredients
SYNTERGENT K FATTY AMINE DETERGENT (Napco)	
SYNTHALOIDS Lozenges (Buffington's)	Synthecaine (brand of ethyl aminobenzoate) 5 mg. Calpuridin (calcium iodized) 12 mg. Eucalyptol 0.35 mg. Hexamethylenamine 6.5 mg. Menthol 0.2 mg. Aromatics
SYNTHENIC AUTO ENAMEL (Morris Paint)	
SYNTROGEL Antacid (Hoffmann-La Roche)	Aluminum hydroxide 0.144 gm. Calcium carbonate, medicinal 0.071 gm. Magnesium peroxide 0.086 gm. Syntropan (Roche brand of amprotropine phosphate) 0.005 gm.
SYNVAREN PV-212 (Synvar)	Phenol-formaldehyde resin
SYNVAROL WR-513 (Synvar)	Urea Formaldehyde
SYRACOCIL SYRUP (Chase Chem.)	Alcohol 6% Tinc. cocillana Syrup of wild lettuce Syrup squill compound* Tartar emetic* Cascarin Menthol* Citric acid
SYROCOL-PM SYRUP Antitussive (Physicians Prod.)	Dihydrocodeinone bitartrate 1/6 gr. Pyrilamine maleate* 1-1/6 gr. Potassium guaiacol sulfonate 32 gr. Citric acid 4-1/2 gr.
SYROCOL SYRUP Antitussive (Physicians Prod.)	Dihydrocodeinone bitartrate 1/6 gr. Potassium guaiacol sulfonate 32 gr. Citric acid 4-1/2 gr.
SYROKOF Antitussive (Carroll Chem.)	Chloroform 4 m. White pine Wild cherry Pine tar* Ammon. chloride Honey Glycerin Ipecac* Sanguinaria Licorice Oil eucalyptus* Menthol* Simple syrup Aromatics
SYRUP CHEROUND Antitussive (Superior Pharm.)	Potassium guaiacol sulfonate 8 gr. Ammonium chloride 8 gr. Chloroform 2 m. Tartar emetic* 1/12 gr. Wild cherry Menthol Aromatics q.s.

Name & Use Manufacturer	Ingredients
SYRUP CODACOMP For bronchial irritations (Ethical)	Dihydrocodeinone bitartrate 1/6 gr. Ephedrine sulfate* 3/8 gr. Pot. guaiacol sulfonate 8 gr. Ammonium chloride 8 gr. Antimony and potassium tartrate 1/12 gr. Syrup white pine Syrup white cherry
SYRUP CODACOMP A.H. (Ethical)	Pyrilamine maleate* 90 mg. Dihydrocodeinone bitartrate 1/6 gr. Ephedrine sulfate* 3/8 gr. Potassium guaiacol sulfonate 8 gr. Ammonium chloride 8 gr. Antimony and potassium tartrate 1/12 gr. Syrup white pine Syrup wild cherry
SYRUP EUCILLANA COMPOUND Antitussive (Premo)	Ethyl morphine hydrochloride 1/4 gr. Alcohol 6% F.E. cocillana 4 m. Tr. euphorbia pilulifera 120 m. Syrup squill compound 24 m. Syrup wild lettuce 120 m. Cascarin 1 gr. Menthol 2/25 gr.
SYRUP MIGATON Antispasmodic, antitussive (San Pedro)	Methylethylamino phenylpropanol hydrochloride F.E. ipecac Ammonium chloride Menthol
SYRUP OF AMBROZOIN For throat irritations (Am. Apoth.)	Each tsp.: Alcohol 6% Terpin hydrate 1/10 gr. Potassium carbonate 1/10 gr. Sulfate 1/10 gr. Menthol Sodium benzoate Glycerin-alcohol-syrup base Oleoresins and oils Ammonium chloride 1/4 gr. Guaiacol Sanguinaria
SYRUP OF TAR COMPOUND Antitussive (Richard Drug)	Each fl. oz.: Alcohol 1% Chloroform 3 m. Pine tar * Sugar Caramel
SYRUP PEDRIN Analgesic (Broemmel)	Each 5.0 cc.: Salicylamide* 1.0 gr. Ascorbic acid 10.0 mg.
SYRUP SPONGIACAINE For throat irritations (Clapp, Otis)	Each tsp.: Alcohol 18%/v Extract of spongia Benzocaine 1/8 gr.
SYRUP SQUILLANA Antitussive (New Eng. Pharm.)	Ext. cocillana Syrup squill comp. Syrup wild lettuce Menthol
SYSTONE Tonic (Systone)	Iron and ammonium citrate Riboflavin Thiamin hydrochloride Gentian Berberis* Bitter orange Cloves Traces of copper sulfate Salicylic acid* Hydrochloric acid Flavoring oils Sarsaparilla Manganese sulfate Niacin Saccharin Caramel

*Consult Sec. II., Ingredients Index. This ingredient may be responsible for major toxic effects if poisonous amounts of this product are ingested.

Name & Use Manufacturer	Ingredients	
TABAC BLOND LOTION & EXTRACT (Caron)		
TABCIN Analgesic, antihistaminic (Miles)	Each tablet: Sodium salicylate* Acetophenetidin* Thenylpyramine hydrochloride Caffeine	200 mg. 150 mg. 25 mg. 30 mg.
TAG FUNGICIDE (Calif. Spray)	Phenyl mercuric acetate*	10%
TAHOE SUNTAN OIL (Schram)	Alcohol Tannic acid Camphor Mineral oil Menthyl anthranalate Phenol	10% 2% 1/10% 1/2 of 1%
TAILBY-NASON CALAMATUM OINTMENT Skin astringent (Tailby)	Calamine Zinc oxide Camphophenol* Calamatum with benzocaine Calamatum with antihistamine*	
TAILBY-NASON SODIUM SALICYLATE- LYMIODIN COMPOUND (Tailby)	Lymiodin (iodized lime) Sodium salicylate* Ext. calchicum root Podophyllin Capsicum Methyl salicylate*	2 gr. 3 gr. 1/4 gr. 1/150 gr. 1/64 gr.
TAJ-MAHAL ENAMELS (Davis, H.B.)	Pigment: Titanium dioxide Zinc oxide Vehicle: Soya alkyd resin solution Petroleum thinners* Driers Non volatile Volatile Toner added	34.84%
TAKA- DIASTASE (Parke, Davis)	Aspergellus oryzae enzymes	
TAKEHOLD SEALER (Johnston)		
TAKE OFF LIPSTICK STAIN REMOVER (Jeffery)	Isopropyl alcohol*	
TALBOT'S ANT POWDER (Talbot)	Pyrethrins Chlordane tech. Petroleum hydrocarbons	0.074% 3.000% 2.775%
TALBOT'S ARGENTINE ANT POISON (Talbot)	Sodium arsenite*	0.23%
TALBOT'S FLEA POWDER (Talbot)	Pyrethrins	0.7%
TALBOT'S FLY & MOTH SPRAY (Talbot)	Petroleum oil* Beta thiocyano ethyl esters of mixed fatty acids Beta butoxy beta' thiocyano diethyl ether	96.5% 2.63% 0.87%

Name & Use Manufacturer	Ingredients	
TALBOT'S FLY & MOTH SPRAY 5% DDT PLUS AA GRADE (Talbot)	Petroleum oil* DDT* Beta-butoxy-beta'-thiocyano diethyl ether	94% 5% 1%
TALI-COP COPPER PAINT (Woolsey)		
TALKIES Throat pastilles (McKesson)	Oil of eucalyptus* Methyl salicylate* Synthetic menthol* Oil of peppermint Oil of cedarleaf Oil of cloves*	
TALMIN Antacid (Jackson- Mitchell)	Dihydroxy aluminum aminoacetate Magnesium carbonate	0.324 gm. 0.124 gm.
TAMGARD MOTH & MOISTURE PREVENTIVE (Tamms)		
TAMMS SOOT DESTROYER (Tamms)		
TAMMS WALL SIZE (Tamms)		
TAM-SNO SOAP SAVER & CLEANER (Tamms)		
TAM-TABS Douche (Tech-N-Kal)	Sodium borate* Ammonium alum* Zinc sulfate* Oil eucalyptol* Menthyl salicylate Menthol* Thymol*	
TAMTEX WATER RE- PELLENT CEMENT PAINT (Tamms)		
TANAC Canker and cold sores (Nemow)	Tannic acid* Hexachlorophene* Benzocaine Propylene glycol base	
TAN-ADE To promote tan (Binday)	Salol* in a hydro- alcoholic mixture	
TANADEX Gargle (Commerce)	Benzocaine Tannic acid* Carbolic acid*	

*Consult Sec. II., Ingredients Index. This ingredient may be responsible for major toxic effects if poisonous amounts of this product are ingested.

Name & Use Manufacturer	Ingredients	Name & Use Manufacturer	Ingredients
TANCRO COUGH SYRUP (Norwich)	Chloroform 2 m./fl. oz. Wild cherry bark extractives White pine bark extractives Squill* extractives Oil pine tar* rectified Ammonium chloride Sodium citrate Menthol* Malt syrup Alcohol 6%	TANSOL SOLUTION NO. 1 Stain remover (Greenville)	Oxalic acid* Methyl alcohol*
TANCTECOL PAINT (Internat. Paint)	Denatured alcohol*	TANSOL SOLUTION NO. 2 Stain remover (Greenville)	
TANGEE FACE POWDER (Luft)		TAN-TONE EMULSION DDT 20% TOXAPHENE 40% Insecticide (Port)	Toxaphene* (tech. chlorinated Camphene, chlorine content 67-69%) 40% DDT (dichloro diphenyl trichloroethane) 20%
TANGEE LIPSTICK (Luft)	Beeswax Lanolin Castor oil Candelilla wax Certified colors Perfume oil	TANTOO REPELLENT BOMB Insecticide (Green Cross)	Ethylhexanediol* 29%
TANGEE MIRACLE MAKE-UP Make-up base (Luft)		TANTOX Skin ointment (Horton & Converse)	Tannic acid 10% Benzyl alcohol 5% p-tertiary-Amyl-phenol 0.03% Isopropy alcohol* 15%
TANGEE ROUGE (Luft)		TANTUM WAVE WITH CREAM NEU-TRALIZER (Vienna)	Neutralizer: Sodium bromate* 12% Waving solution Ammonium thioglycolate* 7-1/2%
TANG HAIR LOTION & AFTER SHAVE LOTION (House of Gourielli)		TANUROL OINTMENT Topical and rectal (Breon)	Tannic acid 3% Benzocaine 1% Carbolic acid 3/4% Lanolin and petrolatum base q.s.
TANG LEAF OIL Rubefacient (Troy Chem.)	Isopropyl alcohol* 15% Iodine* Tar distillate* Pine distillate* Oil wormwood Camphor* Cedar distillate* Turpentine distillate*	TANZALL SUN-TAN LOTION (Purepac)	Monoglyceryl p-aminobenzoate Benzocaine isopropyl alcohol* 50%/v
TAN GLO For tans (Engen)		T.A. OIL (Regular) (Tenn. Prod.)	Creosote* Guaiacol Solvent* Insecticide Hardwood creosote fraction
TANK-O-LENE (Park Chem.)	Cresylic acid* Chlorinated hydrocarbons*	TAPE-TAB POWDER Anthelmintic, veterinary, avian (Hilltop)	Nicotine alkaloid* Phenothiazine 2, 2'-Dihydroxy-5, 5'-dichloro-diphenyl methane Nux vomica 6.61% Anise
TANKOTE PAINT (Vita-Var)			
TANK SOLV (Park Chem.)	Cresylic acid* Chlorinated hydrocarbons*	TAPE-TABS Anthelmintic, veterinary, avian (Hilltop)	Nicotine alkaloid* 2.64% Phenothiazine 19.80% 2, 2'-Dihydroxy-5, 5'-dichloro diphenyl methane 14.85%
TANNER'S PAINLESS EYE WATER For eye irritations (Tanner Eye)	Berberine bisulfate Boric acid crystals Sodium biborate	TARASOL (Bailin)	
		TARGET DETERGENT (Chem. Mfg. & Dist.)	
TANOIN For burns (Lancaster, Inc.)	Tannic acid 5% Phenol 1% Camphor* Menthol* Zinc oxide	TARGO (Simoniz)	

*Consult Sec. II., Ingredients Index. This ingredient may be responsible for major toxic effects if poisonous amounts of this product are ingested.

- 994 -

Name & Use Manufacturer	Ingredients		Name & Use Manufacturer	Ingredients	
TARO Disinfectant (Central Chem.)	Minimum phenol co-efficient against E. typhosa, 7 F.D.A. Method Coal tar*		TATE-O-RUB Rubefacient ointment (Tate-Lax)	Oil eucalyptus* Methyl salicylate* Camphor* Turpentine* Carbolic acid (1 gr./oz.)	
TARR'S NEBULA RUBRA AROMATICA Spray or drops for relief of colds (Borotar)	Menthol* Camphor* Chlorobutanol*		TAT INSECT SPRAY CON- TAINING DDT Insecticide (Linck)	Petroleum distillate* DDT*	95% 5%
TARSTILL LOTION (Gorga)	Soluble coal tar distillate* 2% Isopropyl alcohol* 73%		TAT MANGE SPRAY Insecticide (Linck)	Tech. chlordane*	37%
TARSTILL OINTMENT (Gorga)	Soluble coal tar distillate* 2.5% Zinc oxide* Starch		TAT-60 ROACH KILLER Insecticide (Linck)	Tech. chlordane	2.50%
TARTAN SUNTAN LOTION (McKesson)			TAT ROACH TRAP Insecticide (Linck)	Thallium sulfate*	1%
T.A.S. SHAMPOO For dogs, Insecticide (Roben)	Rotenoids* Hydrogenated rotenone Cyclohexylamine derivatives Secondary terpene alcohol esters*		TAT SOLUTION CONC. CON- TAINING 35% DDT Insecticide (Linck)	Xylene* DDT Polyethylene glycol monoisooctyl phenyl ether	63% 35% 2%
TAT ANT BAIT Insecticide (Linck)	Thallium sulfate* 1.25%				
TAT CHLORO #8 CONC. EMULSION Insecticide (Linck)	Tech. chlordane* 72% Petroleum distillate 13%		TAUB'S QUAKER OIL LINIMENT (Auto-Loks)		
TAT CHLORO 40% W Insecticide (Linck)	Tech. chlordane* 40%		TAUB'S WILD CHERRY BALSAM (Auto-Loks)		
TAT CHLORO 5% DUST Insecticide (Linck)	Tech. chlordane* 5%		TAURCALOX Laxative (Jeffrey-Fell)	Each capsule: Sodium glycocholate Sodium taurocholate Phenolphthalein Calomel Pancreatin Powd. ext. cascara sagrada	1/8 gr. 1/50 gr. 1/8 gr. 1/20 gr. 1/2 gr. 2 gr.
TAT CHLORO REGULAR EMULSION Insecticide (Linck)	Tech. chlordane* 24%				
TATE-LAX, BITTER Tonic, laxative (Tate-Lax)	Cascara Sodium sulfate Magnesium sulfate Iron Nux vomica 0.835 gr. Strychnine alkaloid 0.009 gr./fl. oz. Sodium salicylate* Benzoic acid*		TAURO- LAXINE NO. 1 Laxative (Nelson Baker)	Each tablet: Ext. cascara sagrada Bile salts Phenolphthalein	2 gr. 1/2 gr. 1/3 gr.
			TAURO- LAXINE NO. 2 Laxative (Nelson Baker)	Each tablet: Cascarin Bile salts Phenolphthalein Pepsin Pancreatin Oil peppermint	1/2 gr. 1/2 gr. 1/3 gr. 1/2 gr. 1/2 gr. q.s. 1 gr.
TATE-LAX, SWEET Laxative (Tate-Lax)	Cascara Aromatic base Senna Stillingia Prickly ash bark Sodium salicylate Burdock root Poke root Sodium acetate		TAUROPHEN PULVOID (S.C.-Yellow) Bile stimulant, laxative (Drug Prod., N.Y.)	Purified bile salts Sodium salicylate* Sodium succinate Ext. cascara sagrada Phenolphthalein	1-1/2 gr. 1 gr. 1 gr. 1 gr. 1/2 gr.

*Consult Sec. II., Ingredients Index. This ingredient may be responsible for major toxic effects if poisonous amounts of this product are ingested.

- 995 -

Name & Use Manufacturer	Ingredients		Name & Use Manufacturer	Ingredients	
TAXITE Varnish remover (Sherwin-Williams)	Benzol*		TAYNEX SALVE For hemorrhoids (Burrough)	Each oz.: Extract stramonium Camphor* Tannic acid* Ext. witch hazel Ointment base with 2% benzocaine	30 gr.
TAXITE Paint remover (Sherwin-Williams)	Benzol*	50%	TAZ Insect repellent (H. & M.)	NMRI-448* repellent Mineral oil Alcohol	85%
TAXITE SEMI-PASTE (Sherwin-Williams)	Benzol*	30%	TEATCO PAINT (Waterall)		
TAXITE #74 (Sherwin-Williams)	Benzol* Acetone Paraffin		TEBSIN Antacid (Tebsin)	Magnesium trisilicate Aluminum hydroxide Bismuth subcarbonate Kaolin colloidal Calcium carbonate	
TAYLOR BENZENE HEXACHLORIDE COTTON DUST Insecticide (Taylor)	Gamma BHC* DDT*	3% 5%	TEBSIN TABLETS & POWDER Adsorbent, antacid (Tebsin)	Aluminum hydroxide gel powder Magnesium trisilicate Colloidal kaolin Calcium carbonate Bismuth subcarbonate	
TAYLOR BENZENE HEXACHLORIDE COTTON DUST WITH SULPHUR Insecticide (Taylor)	Gamma BHC* DDT* Sulfur*	3% 5%	TEBSON PAINTS & FINISHES (Rogers Chem.)		
			TEC-ANTI-FREEZE (Tenn. Eastman)		
TAYLOR 80-0-20 DUST MIXTURE Fungicide (Taylor)	Sulfur*	78%	TECLAC BLACK PAINT (Inter-Coastal)		
TAYLOR PARADICHLOROBENZENE Insecticide (Taylor)	Paradichlorobenzene*		TEC-LITE OIL BLEACH Hair bleach (Tecnique)	Soap base with an excess of ammonia*	
TAYLOR'S HAIR LOTION (Caswell-Massey)			TECNIQUE COLOR-TONE For hair (Tecnique)	Coloring materials Soap base Ammonia*	
			TECNIQUE HAIR COLOR (Tecnique)	Coloring materials Soap base Ammonia*	
TAYLOR TOXAPHENE COTTON DUST Insecticide (Taylor)	Toxaphene*	20%	TECNIQUE QUIK-SILVER Hair bleaching agent (LaMaur)	Sodium and potassium persulfates*	
TAYLOR TOXAPHENE COTTON DUST WITH SULPHUR Insecticide (Taylor)	Toxaphene* Sulfur	20%	TEEK Antitussive (Norwich)	Each fl. oz.: Codeine sulfate Chloroform Extracts from squill, ipecac, and sanguinaria	2/3 gr. 2 m.

Name & Use Manufacturer	Ingredients		Name & Use Manufacturer	Ingredients	
TEEL Liquid dentifrice (Procter & Gamble)	Anionic synthetic detergent Glycerin Aqueous ethyl alcohol Carboxymethylcellulose		TENDUST N DUST NO. 10 Insecticide (Calif. Spray)	Nicotine alkaloid*	3.6%
TEEN CALAMINE LOTION (Teen)			1080 POISONED BAIT Rodenticide (Santa Clara)	Sodium fluoroacetate	0.05%
TEEN HAIR COLOR, HAIR TONIC, HAIR COLOGNE, CREAM LOTION & AFTER SHAVE LOTION (Teen)			TENESTEN HORMONE CREAM FOR SCALP & HAIR (Andre)	Lanolin Cholesterol Natural estrogenic hormones 7500 I.U./oz.	
TEETHINA POWDERS Laxative (Moffett, C.J.)	Calomel* 1/18 gr. Mercury derivative* with bismuth subnitrate Sodium citrate Cassia Calcium carbonate		TENEX TAR CREAM For skin irritations (Tenex)	Benzocaine Lanolin Carbonis detergens* Menthol* Cholesterin	
TEEZ STICK COLOGNE (Stuart)	S.D.A. No. 40 alcohol* Sodium stearate Glycerin Perfume oil		TENN-CREO Wood preserver and insecticide (Tenn. Prod.)	Hardwood creosote* Oil fractions	
TEHR-FREEZE Grease (Val-A)			TENNESSEE COP-O-ZINK FUNGICIDE (Tenn. Corp.)	Copper* Zinc	48% 4%
TELES SUSPENSION For seborrheic dermatitis (Torch)	Sulfated suspension of tellurium dioxide* 2.5%		TENNESSEE COPPER CARBONATE (Basic) Fungicide (Tenn. Corp.)	Copper* as metallic	55%
TELVAR W WEED KILLER Herbicide (du Pont)	3-(p-Chlorophenyl)-1, 1-dimethylurea*		TENNESSEE COPPER SULPHATE Fungicide (Tenn. Corp.)	Copper*	
TEN-A Antiseptic ointment (B & L)	Salicylic acid* Carbolic acid* Oil of eucalyptus* Bismuth subnitrate Lanolin base		TENNESSEE DORMO-KOP Fungicide (Tenn. Corp.)	Copper in basic copper sulfate*	42%
TENA-BOV DRENCH Anthelmintic veterinary (Texas Pheno.)	Phenothiazine * 30.45% Lead arsenate* 1.14% Inert ingredients 68.41%		TENNESSEE ES-MIN-EL Soil nutrient (Tenn. Corp.)	Manganese* Copper* Zinc* Iron Boron*	
TENDERETTES Veterinary, avian (Vineland)	Diethylstilbestrol 15 mg.		TENNESSEE FERRI-FLOC Soil nutrient (Tenn. Corp.)	Metallic iron*	20%
TENDER-LEEF PLANT SPRAY Insecticide (Destruxol)	Petroleum hydrocarbons 42% Nicotine* as alkaloid 5%		TENNESSEE MONOHY-DRATED COPPER SULPHATE Fungicide (Tenn. Corp.)	Copper* as metallic	35%
TENDRA Meat tenderizer (So-Lo)	Papain Sodium benzoate Fruit acid		TENNESSEE NU-IRON For correcting nutritional deficiencies of crops (Tenn. Corp.)	Iron* as metallic	30%

*Consult Sec. II., Ingredients Index. This ingredient may be responsible for major toxic effects if poisonous amounts of this product are ingested.

Name & Use Manufacturer	Ingredients		Name & Use Manufacturer	Ingredients	
TENNESSEE NU-M For correcting nutritional deficiencies of crops (Tenn. Corp.)	Metallic manganese*	41%	TERCOL COUGH SYRUP (Commerce)	Terpin hydrate Cocillana Pot. guaiacol sulfonate Codeine Ammonium chloride	
TENNESSEE NU-Z For correcting nutritional deficiencies of crops (Tenn. Corp.)	Metallic zinc*	52-55%	TERCOL JUNIOR COUGH SYRUP FOR CHILDREN (Commerce)	Terpin hydrate Cocillana Pot. guaiacol sulfonate Codeine Ammonium chloride	
TENNESSEE TEECEE MANGANESE SULPHATE For soil treatment (Tenn. Corp.)	Manganese sulfate*	65%	TEREMOL (Whorton)	Salol* Oil of turpentine Pure pancreatin	2 gr. 2 m. 1 gr.
TENNESSEE TEECEE ZINC SULPHATE Fungicide (Tenn. Corp.)	Zinc sulfate *	89%	TERMCO WOOD GUARD (Calif. Spray)	Gamma BHC DDT Pentachlorophenol* Other chlorophenols Petroleum oils*	0.1% 2% 4.4% 0.6% 90%
			TERM-EX CLEAR WOOD PRESERVA- TIVE (Sec Mfg.)		
TENNESSEE TRI-BASIC COPPER SULPHATE Fungicide (Tenn. Corp.)	Copper* as metallic	53%	TERM-EX STAIN WOOD PRESERVA- TIVE (Sec Mfg.)		
TENNESSEE 89% ZINC SULPHATE Fungicide (Tenn. Corp.)	Zinc* as metallic	36%	TERMICIDE WOOD PRE- SERVATIVE (Atlantic Varnish)		
TEN-SOL LEG PAINT Veterinary (Thoroughbred)	Alcohol* Potassium iodide* Menthol* Oils of wormwood Peppermint Methyl salicylate* Ethyl aminobenzoate	59.17%	TERMINIX 3-4 Wood pres. (Bruce)	Mineral spirits* Butoxyethanol* Beta naphthol*	
			TERMINIX 3A3 Wood pre- servative (Bruce)	Mineral spirits* Orthodichlorobenzene* Beta naphthol* Butoxyethanol Diacetone alcohol* Pine oil*	
TEN-TOW LOTION (Perdue)	Salicylic acid* Acetone* Methyl salicylate* Benzoic acid* Tr. cudbear Isopropyl alcohol*	70%	TERMINIX D Wood pre- servative (Bruce)	Beta naphthol* Sodium orthosilicate Sodium 2-ethyl hexyl sulfate	
10-20 BRUSH KILLER Herbicide (Pittsburgh Coke)	Isooctyl ester of 2, 4- dichlorophenoxyacetic acid* Isooctyl ester of 2, 4, 5- trichlorophenoxyacetic acid*	24.2% 11.6%	TERMINIX DOVT Wood pre- servative (Bruce)	Beta naphthol* Sodium orthosilicate Sodium 2-ethyl hexyl sulfate Ethylene dibromide*	
TERBEX OINTMENT BASE (Caswell- Massey)			TERMINIX HB2 Wood pre- servative (Bruce)	Mineral spirits Aromatic hydrocarbons* Pentachlorophenol* Fuel oil Asphalt Beta naphthol*	
TERCO Lozenges (Commerce)	Terpin hydrate Codeine sulfate*		TERMITE SLAYER Wood pres. (Slayer)	Pentachlorophenol* Petroleum hydrocarbons*	5% 92%
TERCO NEW (Tailby)	Codeine phosphate* Terpin hydrate	1 gr. 8 gr.	TERMITKIL Insecticide (Faesy & Besthoff)	Orthodichlorobenzene* Paradichlorobenzene	85% 15%

Name & Use Manufacturer	Ingredients		Name & Use Manufacturer	Ingredients	
TERRATOX 218 CON- CENTRATE Wood pre- servative (Wood- Treating)	Sodium pyroarsenate* Sodium dichromate* Arsenic as metallic	71.25% 25.00% 30%	TESTOR'S DOPE THINNERS (Testor)	Xylol* Toluol* Isopropyl alcohol* Isopropyl acetate Butyl alcohol* Butyl acetate Amyl acetate M.I.K.	
TERRATOX 235 CON- CENTRATE Wood pre- servative (Wood- Treating)	Pentachlorophenol* Petroleum solvents	20.6% 70.2%	TESTOR'S HOUSEHOLD CEMENT (Testor)	Cellulose nitrate Tricresyl phosphate* Hexane* Isopropyl alcohol* Isopropyl acetate Acetone* Butyl acetate Butyl alcohol*	
TERRATOX 255 CON- CENTRATE Wood pre- servative (Wood- Treating)	Pentachlorophenol* Petroleum solvents	40% 35%	TESTOR'S MODEL AIRPLANE DOPES (Testor)	Cellulose nitrate Carbide and carbon's B-400 Xylol* Toluol* Isopropyl alcohol* Isopropyl acetate Butyl alcohol* Butyl acetate Amyl acetate M.I.K.	
TERRATOX INDUSTRIAL WEED KILLER POWDER (Assoc. Sales)	3-(p-Chlorophenyl)-1, 1- dimethylurea* Sodium chlorate* Sodium pentaborate decahydrate* Sodium tetraborate decahydrate* Sodium tetraborate pentahydrate*	8.0% 10.0% 27.0% 49.5% 2.0%			
			TESTOR'S MODEL CEMENT FORMULA A (Testor)	Cellulose acetate Tricresyl phosphate* Acetone*	
TERRAZZO- SAN TERRAZZO CLEANER (Huntington)			TESTOR'S MODEL CEMENT FORMULA B (Testor)	Cellulose nitrate Tricresyl phosphate* Hexane* Isopropyl alcohol* Isopropyl acetate Acetone* Butyl acetate Butyl alcohol* Toluol*	
TERRAZZO SEAL Polishes and waxes (Central Chem.)					
TERRO ANT KILLER Insecticide (Senoret)	Sodium arsenate*	2.27%	TESTOR'S NO. 39 HOT FUEL (Testor)	Methanol* Nitromethane* Carbide and carbon's ucon oil	
TERRO ROACH KILLER Insecticide (Senoret)	Sodium fluoride* Sodium fluosilicate	40% 10%	TESTOR'S PLA (Testor)	Short oil penta alkyd Mineral spirits* and driers Pigments the same as Testor's Colored Dopes	
			TESTOR'S STA (Testor)	Vinyl resin Dioctyl phthalate M.I.K. Toluol* Cyclohexanone	
TERSAN 75 FUNGICIDE (du Pont)	Tetramethylthiuram disulfide*				
TESTOR'S COLORED DOPES Blue Brown Cream Gold Gray Green Yellow Orange Red White (Testor)	Iron blue* and titanium dioxide Iron oxides and titanium dioxide Iron oxides and titanium dioxide Bronze powder Carbon black and titanium dioxide Iron blue and chrome yellow* Chrome yellow* Molybdate orange* Para red Titanium dioxide		TESTOR'S STA THINNER (Testor)	Xylol* Toluol* Isopropyl alcohol* Butyl alcohol* Butyl acetate Amyl acetate M.I.K.	
			TETLES Degreaser (Lester Labs.)	Chlorinated solvents* Petroleum solvents*	

*Consult Sec. II., Ingredients Index. This ingredient may be responsible for major toxic effects if poisonous amounts of this product are ingested.

Name & Use Manufacturer	Ingredients		Name & Use Manufacturer	Ingredients	
TETOR OINTMENT Antipruritic, sedative, antiseptic (Wood Chem.)	Storax Phenol* Sulfur* Pine* Camphor* Menthol* Resorcin* Tar*		TEXOLITE FLAT WALL PAINT (U.S. Gypsum)		
TETRAEROSOL Insecticide (Dao)	Tetraethyl pyrophosphate* 2.0% Other ethyl phosphates 3.0% Methyl chloride* 95.0%		TEXON LACQUERS (Texon)		
TETRAFUME, TETRAKIL GRAIN FUMIGANT, TETRA- KOTE, TETRASPOT FUMIGANT (See DOUGLAS TETRA)			TEXOPE 5 LIQUID SCRUB Soap (Texo)		

TETRA-SOL
DRY CLEAN-
ING FLUID
(Midwest)
	Amsco naphtha thinner
	Carbon tetrachloride*
			TEXRUB OIL
			Counter-
			irritant
			(Bailey)
				Menthol* crystals
				Methyl salicylate*
				Capsicum
				Oils of encalyptus*, cassia,
				   citronella, sassafras*,
				   wormwood and lavender
				   garden
				Camphor* gum
				Mustard
				Turpentine*	

TETRASPRA Insecticide (Miller Prod.)	Hexaethyl tetraphosphate*				
TETRAZETS For mouth and throat irritations (Sharp & Dohme)	Each troche: Bacitracin 50 units Tyrothricin 1 mg. Neomycin sulfate 5 mg. Benzocaine 5 mg.		TEX SEAL WAX GLAZE (Made Rite)		
			TEXSOL Dry cleaning detergent (Riverside)		
TETRO CLEANING FLUID (Wisconsin Pharm.)	Carbon tetrachloride*		TEXSPAR FLOOR CLEANER (Legge)		
TETROX Glass cleaner (Economics Lab.)			TEXTILITE CARPET CLEANER (Hockwald)		
TETSULES Insecticide (Ralston)	Tetrachloroethylene*		TEXTONE PLASTIC PAINT (U.S. Gypsum)		
TETTERINE For skin irritations (Shuptrine)	Salicylic acid* Boric acid*		T-4-L SOLUTION Skin palliative, foot deodorant	Alcohol* 90%/v Benzoic acid Salicylic acid* Camphor*	
TEX DETERGENT (Texas Acid)					
TEXINOL FLOOR CLEANER (Legge)			TG HOUSE PAINT (Lucas)		
TEXIZE WALL SIZE & SEALER (Phelan- Faust)			THA-BILO-ATE Laxative (Barlow- Maney)	Ext. nux vomica* 1/16 gr./tablet Phenolphthalein Ext. cascara sagrada Capsicum Papain Oleoresin Oxgall	
TEXO ACID RUST REMOVER (Texo)			THACHER BRAND PURE ASPIRIN (Allied Drug)	Aspirin* 5 gr./tablet	
TEXOLITE DISHWASHING COMPOUND Detergent (Texo)					

*Consult Sec. II., Ingredients Index. This ingredient may be responsible for major toxic effects if poisonous amounts of this product are ingested.

Name & Use Manufacturer	Ingredients		Name & Use Manufacturer	Ingredients	
DR. THACHER'S ANTIBIOTIC THROAT LOZENGES (Allied Drug)	Each lozenge: Tyrothricin Benzocaine	2 mg. 5 mg.	DR. THACHER'S OLD FASHIONED MUTTON SUET SALVE For colds (Allied Drug)	Suet Menthol* Thymol* Camphor Oil of cajuput* Turpentine* Petrolatum	
DR. THACHER'S ANTISEPTIC OIL For skin (Allied Drug)	Camphorated phenol* Camphor* Cottonseed Linseed oil		DR. THACHER'S PINK MIXTURE Antacid, absorbent (Allied Drug)	Bismuth subsalicylate* Salol* Zinc phenolsulfonate* Methyl salicylate* synthetic	
DR. THACHER'S ASPIRIN FOR CHILDREN (Allied Drug)	Each tablet: Pure aspirin* 1-1/4 gr. or 1/4 of a U.S.P. 5-gr. tablet		DR. THACHER'S SENNA LAXATIVE SYRUP (Allied Drug)	Alcohol Senna extractive Methyl salicylate* synthetic U.S.P. XIII	3-3/4%/v
DR. THACHER'S CHILDREN'S COUGH SYRUP (Allied Drug)	Chloroform Honey Glycerin Ammonium chloride Cherry flavor	3 m./fl. oz.	DR. THACHER'S 3-WAY FOOT POWDER Fungicide, medical (Allied Drug)	Oxyquinoline benzoate* Boric acid* Menthol* U.S.P.	
DR. THACHER'S FLEA POWDER Insecticide (Allied Drug)	Rotenone* Other cube resins	1.75% 2.00%	THALEOCO- LATES Cholagogue, laxative (Tailby)	Sodium glycocholate Sodium taurocholate Sodium succinate Phenolphthalein Cascara sagrada	
DR. THACHER'S GRUB POWDER Insecticide (Allied Drug)	Rotenone* Other cube resins	1.75% 2.0%	THALFED Asthmatic, decongestant (Massengill)	Each tablet: Phenobarbital* Theophylline,* hydrous Ephedrine hydrochloride*	8 mg. 0.12 gm. 25 mg.
DR. THACHER'S INSECT REPELLENT Repellent (Allied Drug)	Dimethyl phthalate n-Butyl mesityl oxide oxalate Cis-bicyclo (2, 2, 1)-5- heptene-2, 3-dicarboxylic acid, dimethyl ester	60% 20% 20%	THALOIN Laxative (Norwich)	Aloin* Ext. belladonna Powd. ipecac Phenolphthalein	1/4 gr. 1/24 gr. 1/15 gr. 1/2 gr.
DR. THACHER'S LINIMENT (Allied Drug)	Kerosene* Capsicum* extractive Camphor* Methyl salicylate,* syn. Allylisothiocyanate*		THANITE Insecticide (Hercules)	Isobornyl thiocyanoacetate* Other active terpenes	82% 18%
DR. THACHER'S MAGIC RUB Rubefacient (Allied Drug)	Menthol* Methyl salicylate* Camphor* Oil of eucalyptus*		THANTIS LOZENGES For throat irritations (Hynson)	Merodicein* Saligenin	1/8 gr. 1 gr.
DR. THACHER'S MEDICATED HEAT POWDER For skin irritations (Allied Drug)	Corn starch Camphor* Zinc oxide Boric acid* Oil of eucalyptus*		THANX (Calgon)	Alkaline sodium tripolyphosphate* Chlorinated trisodium phosphate*	
DR. THACHER'S MENTHO- LATED COUGH SYRUP (Allied Drug)	Chloroform Menthol* Pine tar* Honey Oil eucalyptus* Ammonium chloride Glycerin	3 m./fl. oz.	T-H CONCEN- TRATED NITROGEN, PHOSPHORUS & POTASSIUM FERTILIZER (Inorganic)		
DR. THACHER'S NOSE DROPS Antibiotic, nasal de- congestant (Allied Drug)	Tyrothricin Ephedrine hydrochloride Cetyl benzyl dimethyl ammonium chloride Methyl para-hydroxy- benzoate Propylene glycol Aquae	0.02% 0.50% 0.04% 0.20% 5.00% q.s. or 94.24%	THEOSEALS (Barnes-Hind)	Enteric coated tablet containing 3 gr. of theophyllin*	
			THEPHORIN- AC For colds (Hoffmann- LaRoche)	Each tablet: Thephorin tartrate Aspirin* Acetophenetidin* Caffeine	10 mg. 160 mg. 160 mg. 15 mg.

*Consult Sec. II., Ingredients Index. This ingredient may be responsible for major toxic effects if poisonous amounts of this product are ingested.

Name & Use Manufacturer	Ingredients		Name & Use Manufacturer	Ingredients	
THERAC For acne (C & M)	Colloidal sulfur Salicylic acid* Resorcinol*	4.0% 1.5% 1.5%	THIODOW Fungicide (Dow)	Nabam* (disodium ethylene- bis (dithiocarbamate)	
THERAPOGEN Antiseptic (Meyer, T.)	Alcohol Terpineol* Thymene Thymol* Soap Safrol Naphthalene* Bis (4 hydroxy-2, 3, 5- trichorophenyl)-methane		THIOFILM Ectoparasiti- cide (Chem. Ind.)	Sublimed sulfur*	18%
			THIOGREEN (Liquid) Fungicide (Green Cross)	Nabam*	19%
THERMOBONDS VARNISHES (Sterling Varnish)			THIONVAPOR FORMULA NO. 151 Aerosol insecticide (Edco)	Parathion* (tech. o, o-diethyl- o-p-nitrophenyl thio- phosphate)	10%
THERMODENT TOOTH PASTE (Leeming)	Calcium carbonate precipitate Sodium bicarbonate Sodium chloride Sodium sulfate Potassium sulfate Magnesium carbonate Formalin	1.4%	THIOPHOS PARATHION TECHNICAL Insecticide (Am. Cyan.)	Parathion*	98.5%
THERMOLITE 1000° ALUMINUM PAINT (Tropical)			THIOSAL Fungicide, antiseptic (Greyson)	Each 100 cc.: Sodium ethyl mercuri- thiosalicylate Salicylic acid*	0.1% 2.0%
THERMO-RUB Counter- irritant (Am. Druggists)	Eucalyptol* Spirits turpentine* Oil origanum Pine needle oil* Menthol* Oil of cloves*		DR. THOMAS' ECLECTIL OIL External and internal use (Foster- Milburn)	Spirits of turpentine* Camphor* Oil of tar Red thyme Fish oil	
THERMO RUSTCOTE RUST IN- HIBITORS (Fre-eze)			DR. THOMAS HAIR & SCALP OINTMENT (Glenn Prod.)		
THERMOTABS Salt tablets (Sharp & Dohme)	Sodium chloride Potassium chloride Calcium carbonate Dextrose	0.45 gm. 30 mg. 18 mg. 0.2 gm.	THOMAS' PREPARATION FOR COUGHS DUE TO COLDS (Thomas, W.G.)	Alcohol* Dionin Paregoric Spirits nitre* Tartar emetic* Syrup wild lettuce Menthol* Cocillana Ammonium chloride Fl. ext. licorice Euphorbia* Hive syrup Glycerin Cascarin	8% 1/8 gr./fl. oz. 28 m./fl. oz.
THERYL TABLETS Analgesic (Church)	Each tablet: Acetylsalicylic acid* (aspirin U.S.P.) Benzosulfamide (saccharin U.S.P.)	5 gr.			
THIATE WITH CODEINE Antitussive (Merrell)	Each 30 cc.: Codeine phosphate Potassium guaiacol sulfonate	60.0 mg. 2.6 gm.			
THICKOTE TOP DRESSING Automotive dressing (du Pont)			THOMAS' PREPARATION FOR DIS- COMFORTS OF COMMON COLDS (Thomas, W.G.)	Alcohol Ammonium chloride Eucalyptol* Menthol* Quinine sulfate* Spirit of peppermint Citrate of potash Fl. extract of licorice Glycerin Fl. ext. cascara aromatic	8%
THIN-X Paint thinner (Clark- Lurton)	Mineral spirits*				
THIOCAP-A Fungicide, medical (C & M)	Stabilized thioglycolic acid* Caprylic acid Salicylic acid* Propylene glycol caprylates, penetrant	30% 22.5% 5%	THOMPSON CHEMICALS ACTIVATED GRAIN WEEVIL FIX Fumigant (Thompson Chem.)	Carbon tetrachloride* Carbon disulfide* Sulfur dioxide*	

*Consult Sec. II., Ingredients Index. This ingredient may be responsible for major toxic effects if poisonous amounts of this product are ingested.

Name & Use Manufacturer	Ingredients		Name & Use Manufacturer	Ingredients	
THOMPSON CHEMICALS AFRICAN VIOLET ROOTER Insecticide (Thompson Chem.)	Alpha-naphthalene acetic acid*	140 mg.	THOMPSON-HAYWARD DAIRY CATTLE SPRAY E-10 Insecticide (Thompson-Hayward)	Butoxypolypropylene glycol* Piperonyl butoxide tech. Pyrethrins Petroleum distillate*	52.10% 5.26% 0.53% 22.11%
THOMPSON CHEMICALS DDT-32 Insecticide (Thompson Chem.)	Tech. DDT (dichloro-diphenyl-trichloroethane) Aromatic hydrocarbons*	25% 70%	THOMPSON-HAYWARD DIELDRIN (Granular) 5% Insecticide (Thompson-Hayward)	Hexachloro epoxy octahydro-endo, exo-dimethano naphthalene* Related compounds	4.3% 0.7%
THOMPSON CHEMICALS LIVESTOCK FLY BOMB Insecticide (Thompson Chem.)	Allethrin (Allyl homolog of cinerin 1) Piperonyl butoxide tech. Methoxychlor tech. Isobornyl thiocyanoacetate Other active terpenes Methylated naphthalenes* Petroleum distillate Propellent	0.2% 1.0% 3.0% 1.64% 0.36% 12.0% 11.8% 70.0%	THOMPSON-HAYWARD DIELDRIN 75W For seed treatment (Thompson-Hayward)	Hexachloro epoxy octahydro-endo, exo-dimethano naphthalene* Related compounds	63.7% 11.3%
THOMPSON CHEMICALS MH-30 PLANT GROWTH INHIBITOR Herbicide (Thompson Chem.)	Diethanolamine salt of 1, 2-dihydropyridazine-3, 6-dione*	58%	THOMPSON-HAYWARD DIELDRIN WE-15 Insecticide (Thompson-Hayward)	Hexachloro epoxy octahydro dimethano naphthalene* Related compounds Aromatic petroleum deriv. solvent*	15.83% 2.79% 73.38%
THOMPSON-HAYWARD ALDRIN SPRAY WE-40 Insecticide (Thompson-Hayward)	Hexachloro hexahydro-endo, exo-dimethano naphthalene* Related compounds Petroleum hydrocarbons	38.0% 6.4% 45.6%	THOMPSON-HAYWARD FARM BIN SPRAY INSECT KILLER (Thompson-Hayward)	Petroleum hydrocarbons* DDT* Beta butoxy beta' thiocyano diethyl ether	93.5% 5.0% 1.5%
THOMPSON-HAYWARD CATTLE GRUB DUST Insecticide (Thompson-Hayward)	Rotenone* Other cube resins	1.67% 2.50%	THOMPSON-HAYWARD FUMIGANT NO. 1 (Thompson-Hayward)	Ethylene dichloride* Carbon tetrachloride*	70.2% 29.8%
THOMPSON-HAYWARD CATTLE GRUB POWDER (Wettable) Insecticide (Thompson-Hayward)	Rotenone* Other cube resins	5.0% 7.5%	THOMPSON-HAYWARD FUMIGANT NO. 2 (Thompson-Hayward)	Carbon tetrachloride* Carbon bisulfide Ethylene dibromide	81.1% 12.0% 6.9%
THOMPSON-HAYWARD CATTLE GRUB SPRAY Insecticide (Thompson-Hayward)	Rotenone Other cube resins Pine oil Aromatic petroleum deriv. solvent*	3.6% 7.2% 30.0% 49.2%	THOMPSON-HAYWARD FUMIGANT NO. 3 (Thompson-Hayward)	Carbon tetrachloride* Carbon bisulfide	83.5% 16.5%
			THOMPSON-HAYWARD GARDEN DUST & SPRAY Insecticide (Thompson-Hayward)	Tech. methoxychlor Rotenone Other cube resins Zineb (zinc ethylene-bis (dithlocarbamate)	3.00% 0.75% 1.50% 3.90%
THOMPSON-HAYWARD DAIRY CATTLE SPRAY Insecticide (Thompson-Hayward)	Butoxypolypropylene glycol Piperonyl butoxide tech. Pyrethrins Petroleum distillate*	6.000% 0.180% 0.018% 93.802%	THOMPSON-HAYWARD HEPTACHLOR E-2 Insecticide (Thompson-Hayward)	Heptachlor* Related compounds Aromatic petroleum deriv.* solvent	22.2% 8.8% 64.0%

*Consult Sec. II., Ingredients Index. This ingredient may be responsible for major toxic effects if poisonous amounts of this product are ingested.

- 1003 -

Name & Use Manufacturer	Ingredients		Name & Use Manufacturer	Ingredients	
THOMPSON- HAYWARD MALATHION E-5 Insecticide (Thompson- Hayward)	Malathion* Aromatic petroleum deriv. solvent*	55.0% 35.0%	THOMPSON- HAYWARD TOXICHLOR DUST #10 Insecticide (Thompson- Hayward)	Tech. chlordane*	10%
THOMPSON- HAYWARD MALATHION FLY BAIT Insecticide (Thompson- Hayward)	Malathion	2.0%	THOMPSON- HAYWARD TOXICHLOR OS-20 OIL SOLUBLE CONC. Insecticide (Thompson- Hayward)	Tech. chlordane* Petroleum distillate*	20% 80%
THOMPSON- HAYWARD METHOXY- CHLOR 50-W (Thompson- Hayward)	Tech. methoxychlor*	50%	THOMPSON- HAYWARD TOXICHLOR OS-40 OIL SOLUBLE CONC. Insecticide (Thompson- Hayward)	Tech. chlordane* Petroleum distillate*	40% 60%
THOMPSON- HAYWARD METHOXY- CHLOR WE-25 Insecticide (Thompson- Hayward)	Tech. methoxychlor Aromatic petroleum deriv. solvent*	23.4% 71.6%	THOMPSON- HAYWARD TOXICHLOR WE-40 Insecticide (Thompson- Hayward)	Tech. chlordane* Petroleum distillate*	45.0% 49.0%
THOMPSON- HAYWARD SPOT FUMIGANT (Thompson- Hayward)	Carbon tetrachloride* Ethylene dichloride* Ethylene dibromide*	59.9% 19.6% 20.5%	THOMPSON- HAYWARD TOXICHLOR 40-W WETTABLE POWDER Insecticide (Thompson- Hayward)	Tech. chlordane*	40%
THOMPSON- HAYWARD STOCK SPRAY AND DIP Insecticide (Thompson- Hayward)	DDT* Gamma isomer of benzene hexachloride* Other isomers of benzene hexachloride	42.20% 2.53% 14.20%	THOMPSON MASSAGE OIL (Thompson, W. T.)	Vitamin A Unsaturated fatty acids Perfume Vitamin D Base of lanum anhydrous Vegetable lecithin Vegetable oil	
THOMPSON- HAYWARD TDE-E-2 FOR AGRICULTURE (Thompson- Hayward)	Rhothane (dichloro diphenyl dichloroethane) Aromatic petroleum deriv. solvent*	23.4% 71.6%	THOMPSON'S ANTISEPTIC LOTION For skin irritations (Thompson, W. S.)	Alcohol Mercury bichloride* Resorcin* Chloral hydrate Balsam Peru	69% 1 gr./fl. oz. 3.4 gr.
THOMPSON- HAYWARD TDE 50-W Insecticide (Thompson- Hayward)	Rhothane (dichloro diphenyl dichloroethane)*	50.0%	THOMPSON'S NASAL INHALANT Nasal de- congestant (Thompson, W. S.)	Ephedrine* Camphor* Oil of thyme Menthol* Eucalyptol* Vegetable and mineral oil base	
THOMPSON- HAYWARD TOMATO DUST SPECIAL FORMULA Insecticide (Thompson- Hayward)	Zineb Rhothane	3.9% 5.0%	THOMSON'S ALUMINUM READY- MIXED PAINT (Thomson- Porcelite)		
THOMPSON- HAYWARD TOXICHLOR DUST #5 Insecticide (Thompson- Hayward)	Tech. chlordane*	5%			

*Consult Sec. II., Ingredients Index. This ingredient may be responsible for major toxic effects if poisonous amounts of this product are ingested.

- 1004 -

Name & Use Manufacturer	Ingredients	Name & Use Manufacturer	Ingredients	
THOMSON'S BRIGHT RED OXIDE NO. 24 (Thomson-Porcelite)		THORO INSECT BOMB FOR HORSES Insecticide (Thoroughbred)	Pyrethrins Isobornyl thiocyanoacetate	0.20%
				1.64%
			Other related terpenes	0.36%
			Piperonyl butoxide tech.	
THOMSON'S HOUSE PAINT COLOR TINTS (Thomson-Porcelite)				2.00%
			Methoxychlor tech.	3.00%
			Methylated naphthalene*	
				12.00%
			Petroleum distillate	10.80%
THOMSON'S PAINTS, UNDERCOATS & ENAMELS (Thomson-Porcelite)		THOROLAC PAINTS & SEALERS (Fisher-Thorsen)		
THOMSON'S PAINT BRUSH CLEANER (Thomson-Porcelite)		THOROUGH-BRED ABSORBENT LINIMENT (Man-O-War)	Alcohol* Camphor* Iodine* Menthol* Essential oils*	85%
THORNTON'S AMALGASOL (Thornton, L. M.)	Spirit varnish Petroleum spirits Benzol* Alcohol	THOROUGHBRED ABSORBENT LINIMENT Veterinary (Man-O-War)	Alcohol Thymol* Iodine* Naphthalene* Camphor* Essential oils*	15%
THORNTON'S FRENCH LACQUER (Thornton, L. M.)	Spirit varnish Alcohol*	THOROUGH-BRED CAUSTIC BLISTER Counter-irritant, veterinary (Man-O-War)	Croton oil* Turpentine* Essential oils*	
THORNTON'S OIL CON-CENTRATE (Thornton, L. M.)	Tech. petroleum Oleic acid			
THORNTON'S VARNISH REMOVER (Thornton, L. M.)	Paraffin wax Alcohol Benzol* Acetone*	THOROUGH-BRED COUGH MEDICINE Veterinary (Man-O-War)	Potassium guaiacol sulfonate* Ammonium chloride	
THORO AMMONIA (Thoro)	Thoro ammonia*	THOROUGH-BRED DERMA STRINGE COOLING LOTION FOR HORSES LEGS (Man-O-War)	Alcohol Alum.* lead acetate* Camphor*	10%
THORO CHARCOAL STARTER (Thoro)	Cleaners naphtha*			
THORO CLEANSING AMMONIA Cleansing ammonia (Thoro)	Distilled water Aqua ammonia* Detergent	THOROUGH-BRED DIURETIC TABLETS Veterinary (Man-O-War)	Methenamine potassium nitrate*	
THOROCLEAR Invisible protection against penetration of water (Standard Dry)		THOROUGH-BRED DUAL PURPOSE LEG PAINT NO. 55 Counter-irritant, veterinary (Man-O-War)	Tincture of iodine* Oil of cedar* Potassium iodide*	
THORO DRY CLEANER (Thoro)	Ether Chloroform* Alcohol Carbon tetrachloride* Petroleum base	THOROUGH-BRED HEEL OINTMENT Veterinary (Thoroughbred)	Zinc oxide Camphor* Benzoin Lanolin Balsam Peru Menthol* Oil of eucalyptus*	

*Consult Sec. II., Ingredients Index. This ingredient may be responsible for major toxic effects if poisonous amounts of this product are ingested.

Name & Use Manufacturer	Ingredients	
THOROUGH-BRED INSECT SPRAY (Thoroughbred)	Pyrethrins	0.5%
	Sulfoxide tech.*	4.0%
	2-Butoxy ethanol	8.0%
	Pine oil steam distilled	12.5%
	Petroleum distillate*	
THOROUGH-BRED LEG PAINT NO. 36 Counter-irritant, veterinary (Man-O-War)	Iodine*	
	Mercuric iodide*	
	Alcohol	73%
THOROUGH-BRED LEG T PAINT NO. 44 Counter-irritant for horses (Man-O-War)	Alcohol	24%
	Oil of tansy*	
	Oil of wormwood*	
	Safrol*	
	Camphor*	
	Iodine*	
THOROUGH-BRED MANGE MEDICINE Sarcoptic, external, for dogs (Man-O-War)		
THOROUGH-BRED PERIOSTINE NO. 22 Counter-irritant, veterinary (Man-O-War)	Alcohol	76.5%
	Mercuric iodide*	
	Iodine*	
THOROUGH-BRED PINE DISINFECT-ANT Veterinary (Thoroughbred)	Pine oil*	
	Soap	
THOROUGH-BRED ROUND & HOOKWORM CAPSULES Veterinary (Man-O-War)	Tetrachloroethylene*	
THOROUGH-BRED SHIN & SPLINT PAINT #"11" Counter-irritant, veterinary	Mercuric iodide*	
	Iodine*	
THOROUGH-BRED SPECIAL LEG PAINT NO. 33 (Man-O-War)	Oil of cedar wood*	
	Oil of wormwood*	
	Iodine*	
	Wood alcohol*	
THOROUGH-BRED STRONGYLE-ZINE Anthelmintic, veterinary (Man-O-War)	Phenothiazine*	

Name & Use Manufacturer	Ingredients	
THOROUGH-BRED SWEAT ABSORBENT (Man-O-War)	Alcohol	67%
	Phenol*	
	Camphor*	
	Iodine*	
THOROUGH-BRED THRUSH MEDICINE External on horns, veterinary (Man-O-War)	Formaldehyde*	
THOROUGH-BRED VET-ERINARY COLIC ANODYNE (Thoroughbred)	Alcohol*	67.8%/v
	Flext. hyocyamus	
	Salicylic acid*	
	Aromatic base	
	Chloroform*	6 m./oz.
	Capsicum	
	Ammonium salicylate*	
THOROUGH-BRED VET-ERINARY DIURETIC (Thoroughbred)	Alcohol	11.10%/v
	Saw palmetto	
	Corn silk	
	Hexamethylenamine	
	Fl. ext. buchu	
	Juniper	
	Potassium acetate	
	Aromatic base	
THOROUGH-BRED VET-ERINARY LEG PAINT 22 (Thoroughbred)	Alcohol	52.4%/v
	Menthol*	
	Oil of camphor*	
	Oil cedarwood*	
	Oil peppermint	
	Iodine*	
	Potassium iodide	
	Oil turpentine*	
	Oil wormwood*	
THOROUGH-BRED VET-ERINARY LEG PAINT 36 (Thoroughbred)	Bichloride of mercury	0.156 gr./oz.
	Alcohol	36.8%/v
	Ether*	8.0%/v
	Iodine*	
	Potassium iodide*	
	Menthol*	
	Oils of camphor,* peppermint, turpentine* & cedarwood	
THOROUGH-BRED WHITE LINIMENT (Man-O-War)	Camphor*	
	Oil of wintergreen*	
	Turpentine*	
THORO WOUND LOTION Veterinary (Thoroughbred)	Methylene blue	
	Carbolic acid*	
	Thymol*	
	Menthol*	
	Boric acid*	
	Acetone*	
THORSON'S EFFER-VESCENT SOAP LAKE SALTS Antacid, carminative (Thorson)	Bicarbonate of soda	
	Tartaric acid	
	Citric acid	
	Sugar	
	Soap lake salts	
THORSON'S SOAP LAKE OINTMENT For skin irritations (Thorson)	Soap lake salts	
	Amber petrolatum	
	Powdered zinc oxide	

*Consult Sec. II., Ingredients Index. This ingredient may be responsible for major toxic effects if poisonous amounts of this product are ingested.

Name & Use Manufacturer	Ingredients		Name & Use Manufacturer	Ingredients	
THORSON'S SOAP LAKE SALTS For skin irritation, counter-irritant (Thorson)	Alumina and iron oxide Calcium carbonate Sodium sulfate Sodium carbonate Lithium sulfate Calcium sulfate Magnesium sulfate Sodium chloride Potassium carbonate		THRESHER-LAC SPRAYING LACQUERS (Thresher)		
			THRIFT UNREDUCED PAINT (Johnston)		
THOXINE CAPSULES For colds (Reese Chem.)	Each capsule: Acetanilid* Extract belladonna Camphor* Capsicum Caffeine*	1 gr. 1/3200 gr.	THROAT AID ANTIBIOTIC LOZENGES (Thompson Med.)	Tyrothricin Benzocaine Chlorophyll Cetyl dimethyl benzyl ammonium chloride	1 mg. 5 mg. 0.1 mg.
THOXINE For throat irritation (Reese Chem.)	Sodium salicylate* Ammonium chloride Fluid extract ipecac* Extract of licorice Benzocaine Menthol*		THROT-EZ LOZENGE Throat lozenge (Jeffrey-Fell)	Each lozenge: Phenyl mercuric nitrate Benzocaine Menthol Methyl salicylate Eugenol Eucalyptol* Pinene* Sucrose	1/200 gr. 1/8 gr. 1/100 gr. 1/50 gr. 1/20 gr. q.s. q.s. q.s.
THREE FLOWERS BRILLIANTINE (Solid & Liquid) (Hudnut, R.)					
THREE FLOWERS DUSTING POWDER (Hudnut, R.)			THURO-SELE Water re-pellent paint (Olo)		
			THYCO Lozenges (Manhattan Drug)	Each lozenge: Terpin hydrate Codeine sulfate Wild cherry flavor	70 mg. 2.5 mg.
THREE FLOWERS TOILET WATER (Hudnut, R.)			THYLOX SULPHUR CREAM For acne (Shulton)	Thylox sulfur Hexachlorophene Alcohol Hydrophilic absorption base	4% 0.5% 10%/w
3-IN-1 OIL (Boyle-Midway)	Petroleum lubricating oil* Corrosion or rust inhibiting agents Vegetable oil		THYLOX SULPHUR SOAP (Shulton)	Anhydrous thylox sulfur Bithionol	7-1/2% 1%
THREE LITTLE CROWNS MEN'S COLOGNE (Masie)			THYMACOL For bronchial irritations (Greyson)	Each fl. oz.: Potassium guaiacol sulfonate Ammonium chloride Saccharated extract of thyme Alcohol	8 gr. 8 gr. q.s. 9%
365 HAND CLEANER (Abradant)	Pumice, wood flour, or borax* Soap Trisodium phosphate	60% 25%	THYMERLATE, TINC. Skin antiseptic (Pharmex)	Tr. thimerosol*	
THREE STAR FLOOR CLEANERS (Sheffield Bronze)			THYMOLAC Fungicide, medical (Thymolac)	Alcohol* Thymol, U.S.P.* Salicylic acid, U.S.P.* Acetone, U.S.P.* Acid benzoic, U.S.P.*	52%
THREE STAR OIL COLORS (Sheffield Bronze)			THYOQUENT (New Formula) For sympto-matic relief of acne, pimples (Thyoquent)	Sodium polythionates Sulfur	5% 3%
THREE STAR PAINT BRUSH CLEANER (Sheffield Bronze)					
333 HOUSEHOLD SPRAY Insecticide (Campbell Chem.)	Oil* Piperonyl butoxide Pyrethrins*				

*Consult Sec. II., Ingredients Index. This ingredient may be responsible for major toxic effects if poisonous amounts of this product are ingested.

Name & Use Manufacturer	Ingredients	
THYPTOL For poison ivy, oak, sumac (Wyeth Labs.)	Kaolin in alumina gel with phenol	0.5%
TICKAWAY Ectoparasiticide (veterinary) (Goodwinol)	Rotenone Dichloro diphenyl trichloroethane Cube extractives Polyethylene glycol Methyl naphthalene*	2%/w 15% 4% 09.5% 69.5%
TICKOFF Insecticide (Red Feather)	Calcium polysulfide* Calcium thiosulfate Sulfur	
TICRO POWDER Insecticide (Wright, M.)	Gamma isomer of benzene hexachloride	0.5%
TIDE Detergent (Procter & Gamble)	Anionic synthetic detergent Sodium tripolyphosphate Sodium sulfate Sodium silicate	
TIDY General purpose cleaner (Tidy Wall)		
TIECOAT PAINTS (Vita-Var)		
TIFACIDE INDOOR FORMULA NO. 101 Insecticide (Chem. Insect.)	Halogenated hydrocarbon* Dichloro diphenyl trichlorothane* Methylated naphthalene* Chlordane tech.* Tech. piperonyl butoxide Butoxy polypropylene glycol Pyrethrins	
TIFACIDE INDOOR FORMULA NO. 102 Insecticide (Chem. Insect.)	Halogenated hydrocarbon* Methylated naphthalene* Gamma isomer of benzene hexachloride* Butoxy polypropylene glycol Perfumer	
TIFFANY FLAT PAINTS (Pierce, F.O.)		
TIGER BRAND 2-1/2% ALDRIN EQUIVALENT DDT Insecticide (Cape Fear)	Aldrin* DDT* Theoret. chlorine*	2.50% 5.00% 4.47%
TIGER BRAND 2-1/2% ALDRIN EQUIVALENT DUST Insecticide (Cape Fear)	Aldrin* Theoret. chlorine	2.50%
TIGER BRAND 3-5-40 COTTON DUST Insecticide (Cape Fear)	Gamma isomer of BHC* DDT* Sulfur*	3.00% 5.00% 40.00%

Name & Use Manufacturer	Ingredients	
TIGER BRAND 10% DDD DUST Insecticide (Cape Fear)	DDD	10.00%
TIGER BRAND 10% DDT Insecticide (Cape Fear)	DDT*	10.00%
TIGER BRAND 5% DDT DUST Insecticide (Cape Fear)	DDT*	5.00%
TIGER BRAND 10% DITHANE DUST Insecticide (Cape Fear)	Zinc ethylene-bis (dithiocarbamate)	6.50%
TIGER BRAND 15% FERMATE- 3% DDT Insecticide (Cape Fear)	Ferric dimethyl dithiocarbamate DDT	11.40% 3.00%
TIGER BRAND 15% FERMATE DUST Insecticide (Cape Fear)	Ferric dimethyl dithiocarbamate	11.40%
TIGER BRAND 1% ROTENONE WITH SULFUR Insecticide (Cape Fear)	Rotenone Sulfur*	1.00% 20.00%
TIGER BRAND 20% TOXAPHENE COTTON DUST Insecticide (Cape Fear)	Toxaphene*	20.00%
TIGER BRAND TRIPLE QUICK TOBACCO DUST Insecticide (Cape Fear)	Parathion* DDD	1.00% 5.00%
TIGER BRAND VARNISHES (Lawrence, W. W.)		
TILCO PAINT & VARNISH CLEANER (Tilton)		
TILDEN'S ANTACIDEN Antacid (Tilden)	Sodium bicarbonate Oil of peppermint Calcium carbonate Magnesium carbonate	

Name & Use Manufacturer	Ingredients		Name & Use Manufacturer	Ingredients	
TILDEN'S DANISH OINTMENT Ectoparasiticide (Tilden)	Potassium polysulfide* Sulfur* Potassium thiosulfate Lanolin Zinc hydroxide* Petrolatum Mineral oil Benzaldehyde*		TIMOFAX BRAND UNDE-CYLENATE POWDER External fungicide (medical) (Burroughs-Wellcome)	Undecylenic acid Talc Menthol* Camphor*	10%
TILETTE IRON CEMENT, WATERPROOF CEMENT FILLERS, PLASTIC CEMENT (Tilette)			TINCTURE MERCOSEPTIC Antiseptic (Horton & Converse)	Phenylmercuric nitrate* Alcohol* (isopropyl) Acetone	0.1 gm. 50% 10%
TILETTE PORCELAIN & ENAMEL RUST REMOVER (Tilette)			TINCTURE THIMEROSAL Antiseptic (Medical Chem. Corp.)	Sodium ethyl mercury thiosalicylate* (mercury 49.55%, sulfur 7.92%)	
TILETTE PORCELAIN STOVE REPAIR (Tilette)			TING Antiseptic (Pharma-Craft)	Bis (3, 5, 6-trichloro-2 hydroxyphenyl) methane	2%
TILEZE XX LIQUID FLOOR CLEANER (U.S. Sanitary)			TING Fungicide (medical) (Pharma-Craft)	Benzoic acid* Boric acid* Zinc stearate Alcohol Zinc oxide	20%
TIMBERTOX 10 CON-CENTRATE Wood preservative (Wood-Treating)	Pentachlorophenol* Other chlorophenols and related compounds Petroleum solvents Special solvents	33.20% 6.80% 35% 25%	TINNERS' RED ROOF PAINTS (Vanguard)		
TIMBERTOX 19 CON-CENTRATE Wood preservative (Wood-Treating)	Pentachlorophenol* Special solvents and plasticizers Aliphatic solvent*	17.44% 9% 49.1%	TINOSTAT For hexamitiasis in turkeys (Salsbury's)	Di-n-butyltin dilaurate* 25%	
			TINTED SATIN Latex paint (Sweeney, W. H.)		
TIMBERTOX READY-TO-USE Wood preservative (Wood-Treating)	Pentachlorophenol* Other chlorophenols and related compounds Mineral spirits* Special solvents and plasticizers	4.15% 0.85% 90% 5%	TINTEX Clothing dye (Park & Tilford)		
			TINTING COLORS Paint product (Chi-Namel)	Drop black Synthetic resin Mineral spirits* Drier	43.0% 37.0% 19.6 % 0.4
TIME SAVER LIQUID PAINT BRUSH CLEANER (Glidden Co.)			TIP TOP CEMENT For glass, crockery, china (Tip Top)	Cement Butanol* Acetone*	
TIMIT FOUR-HOUR ENAMEL (Pierce, F.O.)			TIP-TOP CRYSTAL CLEAR CEMENT (Tip Top)	Cellulose nitrate Acetone*	
TIMOFAX BRAND UNDE-CYLENATE OINTMENT External fungicide (medical) (Burroughs-Wellcome)	Undecylenic acid Vanishing cream	10%	TIP-TOP LIQUID SOLDER (Tip Top)	Aluminum powder	
			TIRE-BLANC White sidewall tire cleaner (Abradant)	Caustic potash* Denatured alcohol* Alkyl aryl sulfonate	

*Consult Sec. II., Ingredients Index. This ingredient may be responsible for major toxic effects if poisonous amounts of this product are ingested.

Name & Use Manufacturer	Ingredients		Name & Use Manufacturer	Ingredients	
TIS WITE-MILL WHITE PAINT (Otley)			T-N-T ROACH KILLER Insecticide (Vinson)	Arsenate of lead* Total arsenic (as metallic)	16.67% 3.60%
TISIT Ectoparasiticide (Pfeiffer)	Benzyl benzoate Polysorbate Benzocaine Chlorophenothane (DDT)	11.3% 80.23% 2.0% 1.0%	T-N-T WORM CAPSULES Veterinary product (T-N-T)		
TITANINE AIRPLANE DOPE & VARNISHES (Titanine)			TOBAK-O-STOP To combat tobacco habit (Ray Drug)	Tr. lobelia inflata Alcohol	11-1/2%
TITAN-O-ZINC OUTSIDE WHITE (Glidden Co.)			TOBENE UNGUENTUM For exzema (Goodwin's)	Thiourea Orthophenylphenol Benzocaine	
TITAN PASTE PAINT (Cheesman-Elliott)			TOCO PAINTS & PRIMERS, TOCONAMEL QUICK DRY-ING ENAMEL, TOCOTONE FLAT WALL-PAINT (Tropical)		
TI-TAN-Z Paste paint (Gable-Tite)					
TITESEALS Sealing compound (Radiator)	Polymerized vegetable oils Inert mineral fillers		TOE-HEEL Fungicide, external (medical) (Phenacedol)	Salicylic acid* Resorcin* Menthol* Benzoic acid Carbolic acid* Dimethyl ketone* base	1.5%
TITE-WITE PORCELAIN ENAMEL (Hommel)			TOK-TIK Insecticide (Planetary Chem.)	Toxaphene* Refined petroleum distillate	62% 26%
TIZOLEAD PREPARED HOUSE PAINT (Paragon Paint)					
TMS-10 ANTISEPTIC (Indiana)	Potassium arsenite* Dipotassium arsenate* Potassium carbonate Potassium iodide* Potassium arsenate* Alcohol	4%	TOLAZINE TABLETS (Dillard)	Mephenesin (3-ortho-toloxy-1, 2-propanediol)* Physostigmine salicylate Homatropine methylbromide*	0.5 gm. 0.5 mg. 1.2 mg.
TNEMECAULK Caulking compound (Tnemec)			TOLOXIDYNE For colds (Harvey, G. F.)	Harvamine (Phenyltoloxamine dihydrogen citrate) Acetophenetidin* Acetylsalicylic acid* Caffeine	25 mg. 0.12 gm. 0.25 gm. 30 mg.
TNEMEC COATINGS, PAINTS ETC. (Tnemec)			TOMATO FIX BOMB Aux. plant hormone (Thompson Chem.)	Parachlorophenoxyacetic acid	45 ppm.
TNEMECIDE FUNGICIDES (Tnemec)					
T-N-T ANTISEPTIC WASH Veterinary product (T-N-T)			TOMATO SAV'R Insecticide (Beebe Ness)	Basic copper arsenate* 18% Copper as metallic (from basic copper sulfate) 2% Total arsenic, expressed as metallic 4.78% Water soluble arsenic, expressed as metallic 0.05% Total copper, expressed as metallic 10%	
T-N-T FLEA POWDER Insecticide (T-N-T)					

*Consult Sec. II., Ingredients Index. This ingredient may be responsible for major toxic effects if poisonous amounts of this product are ingested.

- 1010 -

Name & Use Manufacturer	Ingredients		Name & Use Manufacturer	Ingredients	
TOMATOX Insecticide, fungicide (Bonide)	Dichloro diphenyl tri-chloroethane	3.00%	**TO-NE-KA COUGH SYRUP** (Cel-Ton-Sa)	Ammonium chloride Menthol* Chloroform	2 m.
	Copper oxychloride* (total copper content 7%)	12.00%		Beechwood creosote* White pine bark	
	Cube resins (inc. rotenone)	0.68%		Eucalyptol* Oil spruce*	
	Methyl naphthalenes	0.85%		Oil cajuput* Oil pine needles*	
TOM-SCAT To keep male cats away while females are in season (Pierpont)	Oils of all spice* Oils of eucalyptus* Mineral oil	10% 10% 80%		Glucose Saccharin Caramel Cudbear Alcohol	0.5%
				Wild cherry Spikenard Balsam poplar Bloodroot Sassafras	
TOM THUMB PAINTS, ENAMELS (Chicago Paints)			**TO-NE-KA FOOT BALM CREAM** (Cel-Ton-Sa)	Eucalyptus* Peppermint Thymol* Menthol	
TONALFA Appetite stimulant (Humphreys)	Each fl. oz.: Nux vomica* Kali arsenicosum solution*	1-1/2 m. 2 m.		Camphor* Phenol* Lanolin Glycerin Salicylic acid*	
	Cinchonidine sulfate Alfalfa Hydrastis	1/16 gr.		Benzoic acid* Special base	
	Echinacea Acidum phosphoricum Ferrum phosphoricum		**TO-NE-KA INHALANT & RUBBING OIL** (Cel-Ton-Sa)	Eucalyptus oil* Menthol* Peppermint oil* Thymol*	
	Kali phosphoricum Natrum phosphoricum Alcohol	14%		Camphor*	
TONAX Tonic (veterinary, avian) (Lee, G.)	Manganese sulfate Tobacco powder* Nux vomica* Quebracho extr. Sodium sulfate	4%	**TO-NE-KA MEDICINE** Laxative (Cel-Ton-Sa)	Sodium sulfate Aloe* Senna Buckthorn Cascara sagrada	
	Fenugreek Diammonium phosphate Cobalt sulfate Potassium iodide	0.2%		Sodium phosphate* Cinnamic aldehyde Oil cassia Methyl salicylate*	
	Malted wheat shorts Tech. copper sulfate Copperas	0.5%		Iron & ammonium citrate Salicylic acid* Benzoic acid*	
	Sulfur Natural calcium sulfate Rock phosphate Mineral oil			Saccharin sol. Berberis aquafolium Ammonium chloride Fennel Ginger	
TO-NE-KA BRAND HERBS Laxative (Cel-Ton-Sa)	Buckthorn Aloe Cascara sagrada Senna leaves			Calamus Licorice Gentian Wild cherry Caramel	
TO-NE-KA BRAND MEDICINE BALL Cathartic (Cel-Ton-Sa)	Buckthorn Senna Cascara sagrada Aloe		**TONI CREME SHAMPOO** (Toni)	Sodium lauryl sulfate Sodium stearate Lanolin Perfume	
TO-NE-KA BRAND OINTMENT For skin (Cel-Ton-Sa)	Methyl salicylate* Oil pine tar* Balsam Peru Petroleum base		**TONI HOME PERMANENT SOLUTIONS** (Toni)	Waving solution: Ammonium thioglycolate* (pH approx. 8.6) Oil creaming agent Wetting agent	
TONEKA BRAND TONIC TABLETS (Cel-Ton-Sa)	Iron (ferrous) sulfate* Gentian root			Perfume Neutralizer: Sodium perborate* Sodium hexametaphosphate	
TO-NE-KA CORN REMOVER (Cel-Ton-Sa)	Ether* Salicylic acid* Pyroaxin Acetone*	253 m.	**TONSOR** For throat irritations (Hance)	Ferric chloride Potassium chlorate* Alcohol	7%/v

*Consult Sec. II., Ingredients Index. This ingredient may be responsible for major toxic effects if poisonous amounts of this product are ingested.

Name & Use Manufacturer	Ingredients	Name & Use Manufacturer	Ingredients
TOOINWUN SEALER Undercoater (Johnston)		TOROFOR 3% CREAM (Torch)	Oleo-chlor-iodoquinoline* in monobase 5-Chloro-7-iodo-8-quinolinol Hydrophilic cream
T-O-P Insecticide (Planetary Chem.)	Dichloro diphenyl tri- chloroethane* 5% Petroleum distillate* 95%	TOROFOR OINTMENT (Torch)	Oleo-chlor-iodoquinoline* Petrolatum

TOPAMINIC For skin irritations, poison oak, ivy (Sharp & Dohme)	Each 100 gm.:
	Methapyrilene hydrochloride*
	  2.00 gm.
	Calamine, prepared 8.00 gm.
	Benzocaine 3.00 gm.
	Hexylated m-cresol 0.05 gm.
		TOSAN'S REU-MASAN Antirheumatic (Tosan)	Each tablet:
			Sodium salicylate* 0.3 gm.
			Sodium para-aminobenzoate*
			  0.3 gm.
			Ascorbic acid 20 mg.

TOPANEST Dental anesthetic (Barfred)	Hypnocaine* (brand of n-propanol
	  para amino benzyl carboxylate)
	  2%
	Benzyl alcohol N.F. 1%
	Benzalkonium chloride
	  U.S.P. 1-1000
		TOSAN SYRUP For throat irritations (Tosan)	Each fl. oz.:
			Ammonium chloride
			White pine
			Tar
			Spikenard
			Blood root
			Flaxseed
			Licorice
			Cascara
			Cocillana
			Chloroform 2-1/3 min.
			Potassium guaiacol sulfonate
			Wild cherry
			Poplar bud
			Sassafras
			Menthol
			Spruce gum
			Squill
			Wild lettuce
			Alcohol 3%
			Gomenol euphrobia

TOPATAR CREAM For skin (Sharp & Dohme)	Each 100 gm.: Coal tar solution* 5.0 cc. Colloidal sulfur 2.5 gm. Salicylic acid* 3.0 gm. Zinc oxide 5.0 gm.		
TOPEDIZER Chemical fertilizer (Assoc. Seed)			
TOP FLITE INK (Crunden)		TOSSITS Insecticide (Collins Feed)	Dichloro diphenyl tri- chloroethane* 24%
TOP FLITE MUCILAGE & PASTE (Crunden)		TOTALUME ALUMINUM PAINT (Wilbur)	
TOP HAT BLACK ENAMEL (Hilo Varnish)		TOTRUST RUST INHIBITIVE PAINT (Wilbur)	
TOPISOL Vehicle, scalp emollient (Texas Pharm.)	Alcohol 15% Propylene glycol Sorbitan monolaureate derivative	TOUCH AND GLOW Cosmetic (Revlon)	Stearic acid and its glycol ester Cholesterol bases Lecithin Triethanolamine Glycol
TOPPER FLAT WALL PAINT (Gillespie)			
TOPZOL Rodenticide (Bonide)	Red squill powder* 10%	TOUCH-OUT Ink and stain remover (Gregory)	
TOQUEN Vaginal antiseptic (Jenkins)	Each tablet: Combination of oxyquinoline benzoate* Thymol iodide Boric acid* Benzoic acid* Lactose Dextrose	TOWN & COUNTRY FLAT WHITE PAINT (du Pont)	Soya linseed alkyd resin
TOREX WATER RESISTANT ENAMELS (Inertol)		TOWN & COUNTRY OUTSIDE WHITE Paint (du Pont)	

*Consult Sec. II., Ingredients Index. This ingredient may be responsible for major toxic effects if poisonous amounts of this product are ingested.

- 1012 -

Name & Use Manufacturer	Ingredients		Name & Use Manufacturer	Ingredients	
TOWNE COLORS Latex-base tinting colors (Nat'l Gpysum)			TRACY'S TABLETS Digestant, antacid (Tracy)	Sodium bicarbonate C.P. Magnesium carbonate U.S.P. Pancreatin pure Papain Flavoring Salis effervescentis	
TOXANE Insecticide (Cotton States)	Toxaphene* Gamma isomer of benzene hexachloride	45.00% 1.00%	TRADEWINDS ANTI FOULING PAINT (Woolsey)		
TOXANOX Insecticide (Farnam)	Toxaphene* Petroleum distillate	62.00% 26.00%	TRAFCO FLOOR POLISH (Legge)		
TOXANOX PLUS LIVESTOCK SPRAY CONC. Insecticide (Farnam)	Toxaphene* Gamma isomer of benzene hexachloride (from lindane) Petroleum distillate	45.00% 1.80% 47.7%	TRAFFIC- MASTER FLOOR FINISHES (Bownes)		
TOXA-PLAN Insecticide (Planetary Chem.)	Toxaphene* (tech. chlorinated camphene containing 67-69% chlorine) Aromatic petroleum oils Emulsifying, solubilizing and stabilizing agents	60% 34.5% 5.5%	DR. TRAGER'S ANT TRAPS Insecticide (Trager)	Thallium sulfate*	1.20%
			DR. TRAGER'S 5% DDT Insecticide (Trager)	Petroleum distillate* Dichloro diphenyl tri- chloroethane* tech.	5%
TOX-ENE Insecticide (Texas Pheno.)	Toxaphene* Refined petroleum oil Xylene	51.60% 22.67% 5.73%	DR. TRAGER'S DDT 10% POWDER Insecticide (Trager)	DDT*	10%
TOXITE DISINFECT- ANT SPRAY & OINTMENT (Toxite)	Petroleum distillate* Xylenols* Cresols*	90% 8% 2%	DR. TRAGER'S DEAD SHOT Insecticide (Trager)	Petroleum distillate* n-Octyl bicycloheptene dicarboximide* Tech. methoxychlor* Pyrethrins* Allethrin* (allyl homolog of cinerin 1)	
TOX-R Insecticide (Leffingwell)	Rotenone* Other ether extractives of cube	4.0% 13.7%			
TOY HOUSEHOLD SET Shoe polish (Merry)			DR. TRAGER'S HARTSHORN AMMONIA (Trager)		
TOZE Fungicide (medical) (Allied Drug)	Chlorobutanol (chloroform derivative) Salicylic acid* Benzoic acid * Carbolic acid*	3 gr./fl. oz.	DR. TRAGER'S WARFARIN RODENTICIDE (Trager)	Warfarin (3-(a-acetonylbenzyl)- 4-hydroxycoumarin) 0.025%	
TRABUE GLUES & PASTES (Grammes)			TRAIN BRAND PAINT PRODUCTS (Trainer)		
TRACE-TONE Invigorates soil, peps up plants (Destruxol)	Copper derived from the sulfide Iron derived from the sulfide Manganese derived from the sulfide Zinc derived from the sulfide Magnesium derived from the hydroxide Organic nitrogen derived from urea Potash, water soluble	0.64% 0.56% 0.56% 0.66% 0.48% 2.25% 11.42%	TRAINER RUB Rubefacient (Lesbert)	Carbolic acid* Menthol* Thymol* Camphor* Methyl salicylate* Oil of sassafras*	
			TRAK MOTH PROOFER BOMB Insecticide (Gulf)	Dichloro diphenyl tri- chloroethane Diethyl diphenyl dichloroethane Petroleum distillates*	3.0% 3.0% 59.0%
			TRAK MOTH SPRAY Insecticide (Gulf)	DDT*	6%

*Consult Sec. II., Ingredients Index. This ingredient may be responsible for major toxic effects if poisonous amounts of this product are ingested.

Name & Use Manufacturer	Ingredients	Name & Use Manufacturer	Ingredients
TRA-LEZE WAX (Nat'l Wax)		TREDON Rubber base floor enamel (Woolsey)	
TRANSEAL FLOOR SEALER (Continental Prod.)		PLANETARY TREE MIST Insecticide (Planetary Chem.)	DDT (dichloro diphenyl trichloroethane) 32% Petroleum oil 14.5% Aromatic petroleum derivative solvent* 50.8% Emulsifying agent 2.7%
TRANSEAL INVISIBLE WATER-PROOFING For exterior masonry walls (Harrop)		TREE TANGLEFOOT Insecticide (Tanglefoot)	Castor oil Natural gum resin Vegetable wax
TRANSLUX QUICK DRYING ENAMEL (Shield Coatings)		TREET FOR ATHLETES FOOT (K-Armand)	Tr. ferric chloride* Salicylic acid*
TRANSLUX VARNISHES (Reliance Varnish)		TREE-TOX FRUIT TREE SPRAY Fungicide, insecticide (Bonide)	Sulfur* (4-5 microns) 33.4% Tech. chlordane* 6.6% Dichloro diphenyl tri-chloroethane* 6.6% Ferbam (ferric dimethyl dithiocarbamate) 5.09%
TRANS-PLANTONE Agricultural product (Am. Chemical)		TREK ANTI-FREEZE (Nat'l Carbon)	
TRANZITE SYNTHETIC ENAMEL (Hilo Varnish)		TREMCO PAINT COMPOUNDS, TREMLUX WALL PAINT, TREMCOTE HOUSE PAINT & TREMTEX CEMENT PAINT (Tremco)	
TRARISEAL Colorless waterproofing (Harrop)			
TRASK'S OINTMENT (Myers Labs.)	Lobelia Skunk cabbage Leaf tobacco Smart weed	TREND Synthetic detergent (Purex Corp.)	Sodium alkyl aryl sulfonate* Sodium tripolyphosphate* Sodium sulfate Alkanol amide
TRAVEL-AIDS (Formerly Dramacin) For motion sickness (Pharmex)		TREQUIN POWDER For pathogenic conditions of the vaginal tissues (Maurry)	Hexadecyl trimethyl ammonium bromide* Hydroxyquinoline sulfate*
TRAZ-O-TILE Cleaner terrazzo and tile (United Chem.)		TRESANOIDS' Rectal suppositories (Sharp & Dohme)	Tyrothricin 1 mg. Propadrine phenyl propanolamine hydrochloride 20 mg. Benzocaine 15 mg. Bismuth subgallate 150 mg. Zinc oxide 150 mg.
TRAX-WAX (Weatherproof)			
TREAD-SURE Anti-slip floor coating (Horn)		TREVS For motion sickness (Wright, M.)	Hyoscine hydrobromide 1/400 gr. Caffeine citrate Aspirin*
TRECO PAINTS, ENAMELS (Tredennick)		TRIANLENE HAND SOAP (Beck Eq.)	Solvents Cocoanut oil soap base
TREDENE VARNISH (Bownes)		TRIANOL PAINT STRIPPERS (Beck Eq.)	Phenol* Cresylic acid* Methylene chloride*
TREDEX VARNISH (Bownes)			

*Consult Sec. II., Ingredients Index. This ingredient may be responsible for major toxic effects if poisonous amounts of this product are ingested.

Name & Use Manufacturer	Ingredients	Name & Use Manufacturer	Ingredients
TRIANON SKIN CREME For skin irritation (Roberts Labs.)	Stearic acid Triple pressed parowax Glyceryl monostearate Glycerin Borax water Distilled stronger ammonia Menthol-Japanese* Oil eucalyptus* Hexachlorophene	TRIGON Stain remover (Patek)	Methylene chloride* Butyl acetate*
TRI-BASIC TOOTH POWDER Enzyme inhibitor (Edison)	Sodium lauroyl sarcoside Galactono-lactone-carbamide Dibasic ammonium phosphate Sodium hexametaphosphate Chlorophyll Sodium laury sulfate	TRI-KOTE SEALER (Premier)	
		TRIMAL CUTICLE REMOVERS & SHAPER Oily polish remover (Trimal)	
TRICAINAL Rectal ointment (Ciba)	Each 100 gm.: Tripelennamine hydrochloride 0.5 gm. Nupercaine base 0.125 gm. Zinc oxide Bismuth subgallate Lanolin Petrolatum Acetone sodium bisulfite 0.05%	TRIMAL LIP COVER Cosmetic (Trimal)	
		TRIMAL OILY VITA-NAIL NAIL CON-DITIONER (Trimal)	
TRICAINAL Rectal suppositories (Ciba)	Each: Tripelennamine hydrochloride U.S.P. 10 mg. Nupercaine base 2.5 mg. Zinc oxide 250 mg. Bismuth subgallate 100 mg. Acetone sodium bisulfite 1 mg. Cocoa butter	TRIM CEMENT (Park Chem.)	Aliphatic solvents* Rubber Plasticizer Filler
TRI-CHEM PACK Photographic supplies (Eastman)		TRIMSTYLE PAINTS (Egan & Hausman)	
		TRIMTONE Herbicide (Am. Chemical)	Maleic hydrazide,* sodium salt 48.3%
TRICHLORA-CAINE Ointment (Kip)	Chloral hydrate* 7% Camphor* Syn. oil of mustard Aromatics Salicylic acid* Menthol * Methyl salicylate* Petrolatum and wool fat	TRI-OGEN DIELDRIN SPRAY Insecticide (Rose Mfg.)	Hexachloro epoxy octahydro-endo, exo-dimethano naphthalene* 15.8% Related compounds 2.8% Petroleum hydrocarbons 73.4%
TRICHO-SAN VAGINAL JELLY (Milex)	Phenylmercuric acetate 0.025% Boric acid 1.00% Borax 0.700% Tragacanth 3.5%	TRI-OGEN LEAF & ROOT PLANT FOOD (Rose Mfg.)	Total nitrogen 15% Available phosphoric acid 30% Water soluble potash 15%
TRI-COP Fungicide (Chipman Ltd.)	Tribasic copper sulfate—fixed copper* 52%	TRI-OGEN ROSE & FLOWER GARDEN BOMB Insecticide, fungicide (Rose Mfg.)	Pyrethrins 0.025% Rotenone 0.128% Other cube extractives 0.236% Technical piperonyl cyclonene 0.256% Petroleum distillate 0.102% Dichlone (2, 3-dichloro-1, 4-naphthoquinone) 0.120%
TRICO WINDSHIELD WASHER SOLVENT (Trico)	Isopropyl alcohol*	TRI-OGEN ROSE DUST Insecticide (Rose Mfg.)	DDT* 5.0% Gamma isomer of benzene hexachloride (from lindane) 0.5% p-Chlorophenyl-p-chloro-benzene sulfonate 1.0% Sulfur* (200 mesh) 20.0% Ferric dimethyl dithio-carbamate (Ferbam) 3.5%
TRI-DEVELOPER PACK NO. 6817 Photographic supplies (Sears)		TRI-OGEN ROSE & FLOWER GARDEN BOMB Insecticide, fungicide (Rose Mfg.)	Pyrethrins 0.025% Rotenone 0.128% Other cube extractives 0.236% Tech. piperonyl cyclonene 0.256% Petroleum distillate 0.102% Dichlone (2, 3-dichloro-1, 4-naphthoquinone) 0.120%

*Consult Sec. II., Ingredients Index. This ingredient may be responsible for major toxic effects if poisonous amounts of this product are ingested.

Name & Use Manufacturer	Ingredients		Name & Use Manufacturer	Ingredients	
TRI-OGEN ROSE FOOD (Rose Mfg.)	Total nitrogen Available phosphoric acid Water soluble potash	5.0% 10.0% 5.0%	TRIPITE DETERGENT (McVicker)		
TRIOGEN ROSE SPRAY (Triogen No. 1) Insecticide (Rose Mfg.)	Dry lead arsenate* Pine oil Ferbam	11.70% 2.50% 3.75%	TRIPLE AAA ANALGESIC TABLETS (Triple AAA)	Acetophenetidin* Aspirin* Caffeine	2-1/2 gr.
TRIOGEN ROSE SPRAY (Triogen No. 2) (Rose Mfg.)	Rotenone Other cube resins Pyrethrins p-Chlorophenyl-p-chlorobenzene sulfonate Pine oil Triethanolamine oleate	0.50% 1.30% 0.35% 2.50% 9.00% 12.00%	TRIPLE CLEAN Cleaner for floor, walls, etc. (Feller-Jones)		
			TRIPLE D-DUST 5 Fungicide (Sunland)	DDD	5%
TRIOGEN ROSE SPRAY (Triogen No. 3) Insecticide (Rose Mfg.)	Copper (in the form of an ammoniacal copper complex) as metallic Inert ingredients*	0.80% 99.20%	TRIPLE LINK Semi-paste paint (Phelan-Faust)		
TRIO-IODINE Dressing ointment (Hand, J. A.)	Iodine* Phenol Alcohol Fat, grease and vegetable oil base	4% 1/40% 1/50%	TRIPLE PASTE (Torch)	Burow's solution Absorption base Lassar's paste	1 part 2 parts 3 parts
TRIOLITE ENAMELS (Denny)			TRIPLE SEAL PRIMER (Great Lakes P. & V.)		
TRIONA HEAVY MEDIUM SOLUBLE Fungicide (Shell Oil)	Petroleum		TRIPLE-X BRONZING LIQUID Paint (Triple-X)		
TRIOX Herbicide (Calif. Spray)	Sodium arsenite*	52.5%	TRIPLE-X CARBON TETRA-CHLORIDE CLEANER (Triple-X)	Carbon tetrachloride*	
TRIOXIN ARTERIAL CHEMICAL Embalming chemical (Eckels)			TRIPLE-X CHROME & METAL CLEANER (Triple-X)		
TRIOXIN CAVITY CHEMICAL Embalming chemical (Eckels)			TRIPLE-X CLEANERS & BLEACHERS (Triple-X)		
TRIOXIN FOR DISCOLORA-TION Embalming chemical (Eckels)			TRIPLE-X CLOSET BOWL & PORCELAIN CLEANER (Triple-X)		
TRIOXIN PRE-EMBALMING CHEMICAL (Eckels)			TRIPLE-X DANCE FLOOR WAX (Triple-X)		
			TRIPLE-X 5% DDT & 2% CHLORDANE Insecticide (Triple-X)	DDT* Chlordane	5% 2%
TRIOXITONE ARTERIAL CHEMICAL Embalming chemical (Eckels)			TRIPLE-X 5% DDT INSECTICIDE (Triple-X)	DDT*	5%

*Consult Sec. II., Ingredients Index. This ingredient may be responsible for major toxic effects if poisonous amounts of this product are ingested.

Name & Use Manufacturer	Ingredients	
TRIPLE-X 10% DDT INSECTICIDE (Triple-X)	DDT*	10%
TRIPLE-X 25% DDT INSECTICIDE (Triple-X)	DDT*	25%
TRIPLE-X 10% DDT POWDER Insecticide (Triple-X)	DDT*	10%
TRIPLE-X DRAIN-PIPE OPENER (Triple-X)		
TRIPLE-X MOTH SPRAY Insecticide (Triple-X)		
TRIPLE-X PINE OIL DISINFECT- ANT (Triple-X)		
TRIPLE-X RAT POISON (Triple-X)	Red squill*	
TRIPLE-X ROACH POWDER Insecticide (Triple-X)		
TRIPLE-X SULPHUR CANDLES Fumigant (Triple-X)	Sulfur*	
TRIPLE-X TRIPLE- ACTION DRAIN-PIPE OPENER (Triple-X)		
TRIP-LETS Antihistamine (Mayfair)	Each pink capsule: Thenylpyramine hydrochloride* 25 mg. Each white capsule: Aspirin* Caffeine Acetophenetidin* Laxarettes contain: Cascara Podophyllin* Aloin*	
TRI-6 E-12 FOR AGRI- CULTURAL USE Insecticide (Thompson- Hayward)	Gamma isomer of benzene hexachloride 13.4% Other isomers of benzene hexachloride 20.2% Aromatic petroleum deriv. solvent* 51.4%	
TRI-6 120-W Insecticide (Thompson- Hayward)	Gamma isomer of benzene hexachloride 12.0% Other isomers of benzene hexachloride* 68.0%	

Name & Use Manufacturer	Ingredients	
TRI-6 50-W Insecticide (Thompson- Hayward)	Gamma isomer of benzene hexachloride* 5.0% Other isomers of benzene hexachloride* 28.3%	
TRISOGEL (Magnesium Trisilicate & Colloidal Aluminum Hydroxide, Lilly) Antacid (Lilly)	Each fl. oz.: Magnesium trisilicate 80 gr. Aluminum hydroxide 12 gr. Chloroform 0.1%	
TRI-SPAR VARNISH (Elliott)		
TRI-SYNAR Antispasmodic (Armour Labs.)	Each tablet: Powdered extract of belladonna 4.1 mg. Phenyltoloxamine* 20.0 mg. Ethaverine hydrochloride* 20.0 mg.	
TRI-THRICIN LOZENGES (Pharmex)	Tyrothricin 2 mg. Benzocaine 5 mg. Benzalkonium chloride*	
TRITON ENAMELS (Devoe)		
TRI-TOX Fungicide, insecticide (Tritox)	Tricalcium arsenate* 7.00% Cube resins (inc. 12-1/2% rotenone) 0.45% Beta-beta' dithiocyano diethyl ether 1.35% Yellow cuprous oxide 4.50%	
TRI-TOX MOTH CRYSTALS Insecticide (Tritox)	Paradichlorobenzene* 100%	
TRITOX PARADI- CHLORO- BENZENE Insecticide (Tritox)	Paradichlorobenzene* 100%	
TRITOX ROTENONE Insecticide (Tritox)	Rotenone* 1.66% Other cube resins 3.32%	
TRITOX SPECIAL DUST MIX Insecticide (Tritox)	Rotenone 0.75% Other cube resins 1.25%	
TRIVERM CAPSULES Anthelmintic (veterinary, avian) (Gland-O-Lac)	Each capsule: Nicotine (as alkaloid)* 0.62 gr. Phenothiazine 4.61 gr. 2, 2'-Methylene bis-(5, 5'- chlorophenol) 3.46	
TRI-WEY Insecticide (Gland-O-Lac)	Nicotine (expressed as alkaloid)* 2.22% Phenothiazine 20.00% 2, 2'-Methylene bis-(5, 5'- chlorophenol) 9.18%	

*Consult Sec. II., Ingredients Index. This ingredient may be responsible for major toxic effects if poisonous amounts of this product are ingested.

Name & Use Manufacturer	Ingredients	Name & Use Manufacturer	Ingredients
TRI-X FUMIGANT Fumigant (Haertel)	Carbon tetrachloride* Ethylene dichloride Ethylene dibromide*	TRONA ESTONATE W50 Insecticide (Eston)	DDT* 50%
T.R. OINTMENT Antiseptic dressing (Gibbs)	Ammoniated mercury* 5% Zinc oxide Emollient base	TRONA ESTON CHLOROTOX Fumigant (Eston)	Ethylene dichloride 66.7% Related halogenated hydrocarbons 3.5% Carbon tetrachloride* 29.8%
TROKELLS For throat and mouth irritations (Humphreys)	Tyrothricin 2 mg. Benzocaine 5 mg.	TRONA ESTON CHLOROTOX MB Fumigant (Eston)	Ethylene dichloride 60.5% Related halogenated hydrocarbons 1.5% Carbon tetrachloride* 25.8% Methyl bromide* 12.2%
TRONA ALDRIN 2E Insecticide (Eston)	Hexachloro hexahydro-endo, exo-dimethano naphthalene* (2 lb./gal.) 23.4% Related compounds 4.0% Aromatic petroleum solvent* 65.1%	TRONA (Eston) DIELDRIN 1.5E Insecticide (Eston)	Hexachloro epoxy octahydro dimethano naphthalene* 16.0% Related compounds 2.9% Aromatic petroleum derivative solvent* 74.0%
TRONA ALKRON-25E Insecticide (Eston)	Parathion* (2 lb./gal.) 25% Aromatic petroleum solvent 70% o, o-Diethyl-o-(p-nitrophenyl) thiophosphate	TRONA ESTON ENDRIN-1.6E Insecticide (Eston)	Endrin (hexachloro epoxy octahydro-endo, endo- dimethano naphthalene)* 19.5% Aromatic petroleum solvent* 73.0%
TRONA ALKRON 25WC Insecticide (Eston)	Parathion* 25% o, o-Diethyl-o-(p-nitrophenyl) thiophosphate	TRONA ESTONMITE 50W Insecticide (Eston)	p-Chlorophenyl p-chlorobenzene sulfonate* 50%
TRONA ALKRON W25 WETTABLE PARATHION POWDER Insecticide (Eston)	Parathion* 25%	TRONA ESTONOX 60E Insecticide (Eston)	Toxaphene* 60%
TRONABOR (Borax Agricultural Pentahydrate) Herbicide (Eston)	Sodium borate pentahydrate* 92.00%	TRONA METHYL BROMIDE Fumigant (Eston)	Methyl bromide* 99.6%
TRONA BROMO- FUME-85 Fumigant (Eston)	Ethylene dibromide* (2 lb./gal.) 83%	TRONA MALAPHOS 50E Insecticide (Eston)	Malathion* (contains 5 lb./gal.) 56%
TRONA (Eston) ARATRON 25E Insecticide (Eston)	2-(p-tert-Butylphenoxy) isopropyl 2-chloroethyl sulfite* 25%	TRONA MALAPHOS- 25W Insecticide (Eston)	Malathion* 25%
TRONA (Eston) ARATRON W25 Insecticide (Eston)	2-(p-tert-Butylphenoxy) isopropyl 2-chloroethyl sulfite* 25%	TRONA MALAPHOS- 8E Insecticide (Eston)	Malathion* 80%
TRONA ESTON ARATRON W30 Insecticide (Eston)	2-(p-tert-Butylphenoxy) isopropyl 2-chloroethyl sulfite* 30%	TRONA TUMBLEAF Herbicide (Eston)	Sodium chlorate* 40%
TRONA ESTONATE 25E Insecticide (Eston)	Dichloro diphenyl tri- chloroethane 25% Aromatic petroleum solvent* 70%	TRONA TUMBLEAF ML Herbicide (Eston)	Magnesium chlorate* 17.5%

*Consult Sec. II., Ingredients Index. This ingredient may be responsible for major toxic effects if poisonous amounts of this product are ingested.

Name & Use Manufacturer	Ingredients		Name & Use Manufacturer	Ingredients	
TRONA TUMBLE-WEED 25 Herbicide (Eston)	Sodium chlorate* Sodium pentaborate decahydrate*	25% 72%	TROY DDT EMULSION SPRAY NO. 85 Insecticide (Troy Ind.)	Xylol* DDT*	
TROPICAL HEAT POWDER (Prescript. Spec.)	Calamine Talcum Corn starch Zinc oxide Rose perfume	2 parts 2 parts 4 parts	TROY DDT INSECT POWDER NO. 63 (Troy Ind.)	Sodium borate* Sodium fluoride* DDT* Pyrethrins	
TROPICAL INSECT REPELLANT Repellant (Quality Dist.)	Citronella* Oil of pine* Oil of cedar* Thanite*		TROY DDT INSECT SPRAY NO. 81 (Troy Ind.)	Petroleum distillate* DDT* Isobornyl thiocyanoacetate* Other related terpenes	
TROPICAL PAINTS, ENAMELS & VARNISHES (Tropical)			TROY DDT MOTH SPRAY NO. 84 (Troy Ind.)	Petroleum distillate* Naphthalene* DDT* Turpentine* Carbolic acid* Oil of cedar leaf*	
TROPICOP COPPER BOTTOM PAINT (Pettit)			TROY DRAIN PIPE SOLVENT NO. 127 (Troy Ind.)		
TROPILUX ODORLESS FLAT PAINT (Tropical)			TROY LIQUID STRIPPER & PAINT REMOVER NO. 92A (Troy Ind.)		
TROSAN PAINTS (Parker Paint)			TROY ODORLESS FLY SPRAY NO. 201AA (Troy Ind.)	Petroleum distillate* Isobornyl thiocyanoacetate Other related terpenes* Piperonyl butoxides Tech. pyrethrins	
TROX Insecticide (Chipman Ltd.)	Tribasic copper sulfate*-fixed copper	7.0%			
TROXIDE Insecticide, fumigant (Chipman)	Tribasic copper sulfate Calcium arsenate* Fixed copper Arsenic	7% 5%	TROY R.M.Q. MOTH SPRAY NO. 207 (Troy Ind.)	Petroleum distillate* Naphthalene* Oil of cedar leaf* Carbolic acid* Turpentine*	
TROY ANT & FLEA POWDER NO. 64 (Troy Ind.)	DDT* Pyrethrins		TROY ROACH & ANT POWDER NO. 216 (Troy Ind.)	Sodium fluoride* Sodium borate* Pyrethrins	
TROY ANTU RAT POISON COMPOUND NO. 215C (Troy Ind.)	Alpha naphthyl thiourea*		TROY SOLUBLE PINE DIS-INFECTANT NO. 194A (Troy Ind.)	Steam-distilled pine oil* Rosin soap	
TROY CARBOLE NO. 190 (Coal Tar Compound) Disinfectant (Troy Ind.)	Coal tar neutral oils* Coal tar acids* Soap		TROY SUPER DDT SPRAY NO. 80 Insecticide (Troy Ind.)	Petroleum distillate* Cresylic acid* DDT* Oil of cedar leaf*	
TROY CLOSET BOWL CLEANER NO. 126A (Troy Ind.)	Sodium bisulfate		TROY TECHNICAL LIQUOR CRESOLIS NO. 193 Disinfectant (Troy Ind.)	Cresol* Soap Alcohol*	
TROY DDD INSECTICIDE NO. 199K (Troy Ind.)	Petroleum distillate* Cresylic acid* Oil of cedar leaf*		TROY THINNERS NO. 75AC (Troy Ind.)		

*Consult Sec. II., Ingredients Index. This ingredient may be responsible for major toxic effects if poisonous amounts of this product are ingested.

Name & Use Manufacturer	Ingredients
T.R. SOLUTION Fungicide, external (medical) (Gibbs)	Each fl. oz.: Salicylic acid* Benzoic acid* Acetone* Menthol* Oil of pine* Alcohol 64.8%
TRU-AID Liquid analgesic (Tru-Aid)	Sodium salicylate* Potassium citrate Potassium iodide* Methyl salicylate* Caramel
TRUCK, TRACTOR & MACHINERY ENAMEL (Chi-Namel)	Red toner 5.8% Calcium carbonate 12.2% Chrome yellow* 0.8% Alkyd resin (100 per cent solids) 35.7% Drier 1.4% Mineral spirits* 44.1%
TRUELIGHT CEILING PAINTS (Cook P. & V.)	
TRUENESS Liquid house paint (Foy)	
DR. TRUE'S A.P.C. Analgesic (True)	Aspirin* 3-1/2 gr. Phenacetin* 2-1/2 gr. Caffeine 1/2 gr.
DR. TRUE'S ELIXIR Laxative (True)	Senna leaves Aloin*
TRUETONE LIQUID FLOOR WAX (Huntington)	
TRUE VAR Varnish (Foy)	
TRU-GLOS QUICK DRYING ENAMEL (White Co.)	Pigment: Titanium dioxide Zinc oxide Vehicle: Alkyd resin solution Hydrogenated naphtha* Dipentine Mineral spirits*
TRU-LINE INTERIOR & EXTERIOR FINISHES, PAINTS, ETC. (McGuire)	
TRUMPET VARNISH (Perfection Paint)	
TRU-PINE LIVESTOCK SPRAY Insecticide (Tru-Pine)	Pyrethrins 0.2% Tech. piperonyl butoxide 2.0% Tech. methoxychlor 3.0% Isobornyl thiocyano acetate 1.64% Related terpenes .36% Methylated naphthalenes* 12.00% Petroleum distillate 10.8% Freon 70.00%

Name & Use Manufacturer	Ingredients
TRUSCO PAINTS (Trussler)	
TRUSHAY HAND CREAM (Bristol-Myers)	Stearic acid Potassium stearate Isopropyl palmitate Glycerin Magnesium aluminum silicates Merthiolate
TRUSHAY LOTION (Bristol-Myers)	Stearic acid Triethanolamine stearate Hydrocarbons Lanolin absorption base Stearyl or cetyl alcohol Parahydroxy benzoate preservative
TRUSTY RUSTY RUST REMOVER (Comegys)	Hydrofluoric acid*
TRU-TONE CRAYONS (Bradley, M.)	
TRUTONE PAINTS & VARNISH (White Co.)	
TRU TRIM OUTSIDE COLORS Paint (Standard-Toch)	
TRY-COL Antiseptic (Gland-O-Lac)	Triethylene glycol 99.7%
TRYLON BUBBLE BATH TABLETS (Trylon)	Alkyl aryl sulfonate Sodium tripoly phosphate Sodium bicarbonate Perfume
TRYO-CREME Skin antiseptic (Pfeiffer)	Tyrothricin 0.5 mg./gm. Benzocaine 1% Zinc oxide 1% Cetyl dimethyl-benzyl-ammonium chloride 1-1000
T.S.B. SALINE Cathartic (Burns)	Soda Sulf. Magnesium carb. Magnesium sulf.
T.S.F. FOR CHICKEN LICE (Burrell-Dugger)	Sodium fluoride* 65%
T.T.D. S.F. NO. 858 Oral cleansing deodorant (Specialists)	Glycerin Sol. formaldehyde Trs. Myrrh and green soap Menthol Oils of anise and pepperment Pepsin Alcohol 8% by vol.
T.T.O. ENAMEL (O'Brien Corp.)	

*Consult Sec. II., Ingredients Index. This ingredient may be responsible for major toxic effects if poisonous amounts of this product are ingested.

Name & Use Manufacturer	Ingredients	Name & Use Manufacturer	Ingredients
TU-EX PAINTS & ENAMELS (Paintcraft)		TUMS Antacid (Lewis-Howe)	Calcium carbonate prec. Magnesium carbonate Magnesium trisilicate Oil peppermint Sugar
TUFCOTE HEAVY DUTY ENAMEL (du Pont)	Soya linseed alkyd resin	TUNG ALTUM METAL PAINT (Republic)	
TUFCOTE VARNISH STAIN (du Pont)	Phenolic resin Vegetable oil	TURBEN Paint thinner (Seidlitz)	Mineral spirits* 94% Dipentene 6%
TUF DRI ENAMEL (Central P. & V.)		TURCO BRAND PAINTS (Turco)	
TUF FLOOR VARNISH (Phelan-Faust)		TURFACIDE Herbicide (Chem. Form.)	Hexachloro epoxy octahydro dimethano naphthalene* 4.25% Related compounds from Dieldrin 0.75% Clay 95.0%
TUF-FOOT For tender feet of dogs (Bonaseptic)	Balsams Peru, tolu, styrax Aloe Benzoin	TURF CARE Insecticide (Collins Feed)	Hexachloro epoxy octahydro dimethano naphthalene* 1.70% Related compounds 0.30% Chlordane tech. 3.00%
TU-FO-LEX Food supplement (Tutag)	Each capsule: Ferrous sulfate,* dried U.S.P. 194.4 mg. Liver, desiccated, N.F. IX 200 mg. Stomach powder 100 mg. Vitamin B12 U.S.P. 10 mcg. Vitamin C (ascorbic acid U.S.P.) 50 mg. Folic acid 1 mg.	TURF-KARE Insecticide (Bonide)	Tech. chlordane 1.75%
		TURNER'S BLACK HAWK OINTMENT For skin (Eagle Chem.)	Salicylic acid* Methyl salicylate* Menthol Camphor gum*
TUF-TEX VARNISHES (Reliance Varnish)			
TUF-Y ENAMEL FINISHES (North & Judd)		TUSSAR COUGH SYRUP (Armour Labs.)	Dihydrocodeinone bitartrate* 1/6 gr. Potassium guaiacol sulfonate N.F. 8 gr. Sodium citrate U.S.P. 13.2 gr. Citric acid U.S.P. 2 gr. Prophenpyridamine maleate* 1 gr. Chloroform U.S.P. 2 m. Methyl paraben U.S.P. 0.1%
TUGASAN OINTMENT (Pyro-Sana)			
TUKOTE PAINTS (Sipe)			
TUMBL-BUG 25% DDT EMULSION CONC. Insecticide (York Pharm.)	DDT 25%/w Aromatic petroleum deriv. solvent* 70%/w	TUSS-X Antitussive (Binday)	Codeine phos. 1/2 gr./oz. Menthol Euphorbia pilulifera Wild lettuce Syr. squill comp. Cascarin Cocillana Alcohol 5%
TUMBL-BUG 5% DDT INSECTICIDE LIQUID (York Pharm.)	DDT* 5.00% Beta butoxy beta' thiocyano diethyl ether 1.06% Xylol* 7.00% Deodorized kerosene base* 86.94%	TUSSY BRILLIANTINE (Lehn & Fink)	Mineral oil Perfume
		TUSSY CREAM DEODORANT (Lehn & Fink)	Aluminum sulfate*

*Consult Sec. II., Ingredients Index. This ingredient may be responsible for major toxic effects if poisonous amounts of this product are ingested.

- 1021 -

Name & Use Manufacturer	Ingredients		Name & Use Manufacturer	Ingredients	
TUSSY FACE CREAM (Lehn & Fink)	Vegetable oils Lanolin Stearates Waxes Humectants Mineral oil Perfumes Other similar ingredients Some creams also contain estrogenic hormones		22 Fungicide (medical) (Mentho-Listine)	Rosaniline* Boric acid* Phenol* Resorcinol* Acetone*	
			TWINCOAT PAINT (Long, C.)		
TUSSY FLOZOR BLONDE Cosmetic (Lehn & Fink)	Oxygenated camomile extract Denatured alcohol* Hydrogen peroxide*		TWINKLE Copper cleaner (Drackett)		
TUSSY FLOZOR FRENCH BLUING Hair cosmetic (Lehn & Fink)	Certified dye Sulfur dioxide* Sulfurous acid*		TWIN LIGHT Insecticide (Seacoast)	Toxaphene* dust	5%
TUSSY HAND LOTIONS (Lehn & Fink)	Vegetable oils Lanolin Stearate Waxes Humectants Mineral oil Perfumes		TWIN LIGHT ARSOCOP Insecticide, fungicide (Seacoast)	Calcium arsenate* Metallic copper	20% 7%
			TWIN LIGHT ARSOCOP #30 Insecticide, fungicide (Seacoast)	Calcium arsenate* Metallic copper	30% 7%
TUSSY LIQUID DEODORANT (Lehn & Fink)	Aluminum sulfate*		TWIN LIGHT ARSORAM Insecticide, fungicide (Seacoast)	Calcium arsenate* Ziram	20% 7.6%
TUTAG ANTACID TABLETS (Tutag)	Each tablet: Aluminum hydroxide 2 gr. Magnesium phosphate tribasic 2 gr. Magnesium trisilicate 4 gr. Pectin 1/4 gr.		TWIN LIGHT ARSORAM #30 Insecticide, fungicide (Seacoast)	Calcium arsenate* Ziram	30% 7.6%
TUTAG FERROUS GLUCONATE (Tutag)			TWIN LIGHT CALOMEL ROOT DUST Insecticide (Seacoast)	Calomel*	4%
TUTAG FERROUS SULFATE (Tutag)			TWIN LIGHT CELERY DUST Fungicide (Seacoast)	Metallic copper* Sulfur*	5% 30%
TUTCH-UP FURNITURE POLISH (Dryburgh)			TWIN LIGHT CHLORDANE 45% SPRAY Insecticide (Seacoast)	Chlordane* emulsion	45%
TUTTLE'S ELIXIR Counter- irritant (veterinary) (Tuttle)	Alcohol 30% Gum camphor* P.G.S. turpentine* Oil of hemlock Ox gall Ammonia solution*		TWIN LIGHT CHLORDANE 50% W.P. Insecticide (Seacoast)	Chlordane*	50%
			TWIN LIGHT CLORO DUST Insecticide (Seacoast)	Chlordane*	5%
TWEED FACE POWDER (Lentheric)					
TWEET BIRD & AVIARY SPRAY Insecticide (House of Huston)	Piperonyl butoxide 0.6% Pyrethrins 0.06%		TWIN LIGHT CPR TRUCK CROP DUST Insecticide (Seacoast)	CPR dust base	20%
20 MULE TEAM BORAX (Pacific Coast)					

*Consult Sec. II., Ingredients Index. This ingredient may be responsible for major toxic effects if poisonous amounts of this product are ingested.

Name & Use Manufacturer	Ingredients	
TWIN LIGHT CPR TRUCK CROP DUST #30 Insecticide (Seacoast)	CPR dust base	30%
TWIN LIGHT DESPRAY Insecticide (Seacoast)	DDT*	25%
TWIN LIGHT D.R. DUST Insecticide (Seacoast)	DDT* Rotenone	5% 1/2%
TWIN LIGHT D.T. CELERY DUST Insecticide, fungicide (Seacoast)	DDT Metallic copper* Sulfur*	3% 5% 30%
TWIN LIGHT 7% DUST Fungicide (Seacoast)	Metallic copper*	7%
TWIN LIGHT 9% DUST Fungicide (Seacoast)	Metallic copper*	9%
TWIN LIGHT DUSTALL 3/4% Insecticide (Seacoast)	Rotenone Sulfur	3/4% 3%
TWIN LIGHT DUSTALL 1% Insecticide (Seacoast)	Rotenone Sulfur	1% 3%
TWIN LIGHT DUSTALL FOR ROSES Insecticide, fungicide (Seacoast)	DDT* Lindane* Ferbam Sulfur	
TWIN LIGHT DUSTALL FOR VEGETABLES Insecticide, fungicide (Seacoast)	Malathion* Methoxychlor* Captan	
TWIN LIGHT DUSTWET Insecticide (Seacoast)	Rotenone*	4%
TWIN LIGHT FERBAM DUST Fungicide (Seacoast)	Ferbam	11.4%
TWIN LIGHT GAM DUST #1 Insecticide (Seacoast)	Lindane	1%
TWIN LIGHT LINDANE 10% SPRAY Insecticide (Seacoast)	Lindane*	10%
TWIN LIGHT LINDANE 25% W.P. Insecticide (Seacoast)	Lindane*	25%
TWIN LIGHT MALATHION 50% SPRAY Insecticide (Seacoast)	Malathion*	50%
TWIN LIGHT METHOXY- ZIRAM DUST Insecticide, fungicide (Seacoast)	Methoxychlor Ziram*	3% 7.6%
TWIN LIGHT NU CU DUST Insecticide, fungicide (Seacoast)	DDT Metallic copper*	3% 7%
TWIN LIGHT NU CU DUST #5 Insecticide, fungicide (Seacoast)	DDT* Metallic copper*	5% 7%
TWIN LIGHT NU DUST #3 Insecticide (Seacoast)	DDT	3%
TWIN LIGHT NU DUST #5 Insecticide (Seacoast)	DDT*	5%
TWIN LIGHT NU DUST #10 Insecticide (Seacoast)	DDT*	10%
TWIN LIGHT NU SPRAY Insecticide (Seacoast)	DDT*	50%
TWIN LIGHT NU SPRAY S75 Insecticide (Seacoast)	DDT*	75%
TWIN LIGHT PARADUST #1 Insecticide (Seacoast)	Parathion*	1%
TWIN LIGHT RHOTHANE DUST #5 Insecticide (Seacoast)	DDD	5%
TWIN LIGHT RHOTHANE DUST #10 Insecticide (Seacoast)	DDD	10%
TWIN LIGHT ROCOP 3/4% Insecticide, fungicide (Seacoast)	Rotenone Metallic copper*	3/4% 7%

Name & Use Manufacturer	Ingredients		Name & Use Manufacturer	Ingredients	
TWIN LIGHT ROTOCU 3/4% Insecticide, fungicide (Seacoast)	Rotenone Metallic copper*	3/4% 5%	TWIN LIGHT TWO-WAY DUST #3 Insecticide (Seacoast)	Rotenone Pyrethrins	1% 0.1%
TWIN LIGHT ROTOCU 1% Insecticide (Seacoast)	Rotenone Metallic copper*	1% 5%	TWIN LIGHT ZD #783 DUST Insecticide, fungicide (Seacoast)	DDT Dithane Z-78	3% 6%
TWIN LIGHT SABADUST #40 Insecticide (Seacoast)	Sabadilla*	40%	TWIN LIGHT ZD #785 DUST Insecticide, fungicide (Seacoast)	DDT* Dithane Z-78	5% 6%
TWIN LIGHT SPRAYALL FOR FRUIT Insecticide, fungicide (Seacoast)	Lindane* DDT* Ferbam Sulfur		TWIN LIGHT ZIRAM DUST Fungicide (Seacoast)	Ziram*	7.6%
TWIN LIGHT SPRAYALL FOR TREES & SHRUBS Insecticide, fungicide (Seacoast)	Malathion* DDT* Captan Karathane		2, 4-DE-WEED Herbicide (Martin, C. J.)	Ethanol amine 2, 4-dichloro- phenoxy acetate* as triethanolamine salt 22.3%	
			2, 4-DOW Herbicide (Dow)	2, 4-Dichlorophenoxy acetic acid*	
TWIN LIGHT THANECOP Insecticide, fungicide (Seacoast)	DDD Metallic copper*	3% 7%	TWO IN ONE FLY SPRAY (Interstate Med.)	Pyrocide booster Safrol Paraffin oil* Pure creosote* Fuel oil	
TWIN LIGHT THANE DUST Fungicide (Seacoast)	Dithane Z-78	6%	217 TABLETS Relieves simple head- ache, neuralgia and pain of common colds (Frosst, C. E.)	Aspirin* Acetophenetidin* Caffeine citrate	0.23 gm. 0.15 gm. 30 mg.
TWIN LIGHT THANE DUST #10 Fungicide (Seacoast)	Dithane Z-78	10%			
TWIN LIGHT THANE-RO DUST Insecticide, fungicide (Seacoast)	DDD Dithane Z-78	3% 6%	T-X Fungicide (medical) (T-X)	Hydrophilic colloidal sulfur* Benzoic acid* Salicylic acid* Alcohol*	77%/v
			TYLAPRIN Analgesic (Tyler)	Each tsp.: Aspirin*	5 gr.
TWIN LIGHT TWO-WAY DUST #1 Insecticide (Seacoast)	Rotenone Pyrethrins	1/2% 1%	TYLON BRAND PAINTS (Balt. Paint)		
			TYON NAA-48 Holds fruit on (Crop King)	Homogenized hormone in oil Naphthalene acetic acid* 48 gm./gal.	
TWIN LIGHT TWO-WAY DUST #2 Insecticide (Seacoast)	Rotenone Pyrethrins	3/4% 0.1%	TYPEN TYPE CLEANER (Stafford)		

Name & Use Manufacturer	Ingredients		Name & Use Manufacturer	Ingredients	
TYPOLIT PRINTING INK & VARNISH, DRYERS (Maff)			U-G-L FLOOR VARNISH & SEALER (United Gilson.)	Wood oil Synthetic resin Mineral spirits*	
TYREES ANTISEPTIC POWDER (Tyree)	Zinc sulfate* Carbolic acid* Boric acid* Salicylic acid* Menthol Thymol* Eucalyptol*		U-G-L HOUSE PAINT & PRIMER (United Gilson.)	Titanium Zinc Linseed oil Mineral spirits*	
TYRO Home dairy cleanser (alkyl aryl sulfonates) (Tidy House)	Alkaline salts*		U-G-L SPAR VARNISH (United Gilson.)	Wood oil Synthetic resin Mineral spirits*	
TYROLARIS Antibiotic for mouth (Sharp & Dohme)	Tyrothricin Panthenol Alcohol	0.02% 0.02% 10%	U-IN-TAH HEAT-RESISTING PAINT (Am. Marietta)		
TYROTRON ANTI-BIOTIC LOZENGES (Tutag)	Tyrothricin Benzocaine	2 mg. 5 mg.	ULCERINE For teat ulcers (veterinary) (Roberts, Dr. D.)	Copper acetate* basic Lanolin Petrolatum Aniline*	
TYROZETS Throat antibiotic lozenges (Sharp & Dohme)	Each: Tyrothricin Benzocaine	1 mg. 5 mg.	ULMETS Antacid (Durst, S. F.)	Calcium carbonate Methyl cellulose Elm bark Saccharin	
UDDERINE Liniment (Roberts, Dr. D.)	Soap camphorated Spirits of camphor* Turpentine* Chloroform* Eucalyptus oil* Oil of cloves*	5.28%	ULTRACAIN Analgesic ointment (Herzog)	Benzocaine 0.2% Amyl para-aminobenzoate 0.7% Cod liver oil 20.0%	
UDGA TABLETS Antacid (Udga)	Bismuth subcarbonate Magnesium oxide Sodium bicarbonate		ULTRACAIN Suppositories (rectal) (Herzog)	Benzocaine 0.2% Amyl para-aminobenzoate 0.7% Cod liver oil 20.0% Phenylephrine hydrochloride U.S.P. 0.2% Cocoa-butter	
UDO ENAMELS (Utley)			ULTRA GLOSS Floor wax (Ultra Chem.)		
UDYCOTE CORROSION-RESISTANT PAINT (Udylite)			ULTRA GLOSS Pot. abrasive cleaner (Ultra Chem.)		
U-G-L ASPHALT PAINT (United Gilson.)	Asphalt Inert fillers Mineral spirits*		ULTRA KOTE SYNTHETIC ENAMEL (Haynes, C. W.)		
U-G-L CAULKING COMPOUND (United Gilson.)	Soya bean oil Fish oil Petroleum resin Inert fillers		ULTRALITE PAINT (Sipe)		
U-G-L FAST PLUG (United Gilson.)	Cement Hydrated lime*		ULTRA LUMINALL FLAT WALL PAINT (Nat'l Chem. & Mfg.)		
U-G-L FIL (United Gilson.)	Alkyd resin Aluminum stearate Inert fillers Mineral spirits*		ULTRASOL Hair preparation (Ultrasol)	Whole gland pituitary extract Cholesterin Cerebrin Natural fats Natural citric acid Lecithin Nuclein Vitellin Alkyl sulfate	

*Consult Sec. II., Ingredients Index. This ingredient may be responsible for major toxic effects if poisonous amounts of this product are ingested.

Name & Use Manufacturer	Ingredients	Name & Use Manufacturer	Ingredients
ULTRA-VAR Synthetic varnish in color (Haynes, C. W.)		UNCLE SAM SHOE POLISHES (Yankee)	Carnauba wax Paraffin Wax Beeswax Steam-distilled turpentine* Mineral oil Varsol
UMBILICARE Antiseptic for naval cord (veterinary) (Roberts, Dr. D.)	Chloride of mercury* Muriatic acid*	UNDECILLIN ATHLETE'S FOOT CREAM POWDER (Pharmex)	Zinc undecylenate* 20% Undecylenic acid 5%
UNALAC Shellac substitute (United Naval)		UNDE WASH (Stanley Home)	Water Igepal or nonic Cerfak or syntholite Versene
UNCLE HIRAM'S BUG JUICE Insecticide (New Method)	Petroleum distillate* DDT* 5% Beta thiocyano ethyl esters of alphatic acids containing 10-18 carbon atoms Beta-butoxy-beta-thiocyano diethyl ether	U-NEEK CLEANING COMPOUND (U-Neek)	
		UNGUENTINE For skin burns (Norwich)	Phenylmercuric acetate 0.01% Aluminum hydrate Zinc carbonate Zinc acetate* Carbolic acid* Zinc oxide Oil eucalyptus* Oil thyme Menthol* Eugenol* Sorbitan and polyoxyethylene sorbitan Monostearates White petrolatum
UNCLE HIRAM'S FLOOR BLEACH (New Method)			
UNCLE HIRAM'S PINE OIL DISINFECT- ANT (New Method)	Steam-distilled pine oil* 80.00% Soap 7.03% Isopropyl alcohol 3.48%		
UNCLE HIRAM'S PREMIUM WEAR GLOSS WAX (New Method)		UNGUENTINE HEMOR- RHOIDAL SUPPOSI- TORIES (Norwich)	Each cone: Anhydro para hydroxy mercuri meta cresol 0.0033 gr. Diperodon hydrochloride Aluminum hydrate Zinc carbonate Zinc acetate Zinc oxide Boric acid in mentholated cocoa butter base
UNCLE HIRAM'S TILE WHITE Cleaner for tile, marble, etc. (New Method)	Oxalic acid*		
		UNGUENTUM P. M. S. F. SPECIAL MFR. NO. 708 For skin irritations (Specialists)	Sulfathiazole* Colloidal sulfur* Crude coal tar* Zinc oxide
UNCLE SAM CREME GLOSS FURNITURE POLISH (Uncle Sam)	Sulfonated castor oil Mineral oil		
UNCLE SAM LEMON OIL POLISH (Uncle Sam)	Mineral oil Citronella*	UNGUENTUM PRIMARIUM CARBONIS COMP. S. F. MFG. NO. 712 (Specialists)	Crude coal tar*
UNCLE SAM MOTH- PROOFING (Uncle Sam)		UNI CLEANSER (Ising)	
UNCLE SAM ROACH SALT (Uncle Sam)	Sodium fluoride* 90%	UNICO ALDRIN DUST Insecticide (United Coop.)	Hexachloro hexahydro dimethano naphthalene* 19.1% Related compounds 14.4%

*Consult Sec. II., Ingredients Index. This ingredient may be responsible for major toxic effects if poisonous amounts of this product are ingested.

Name & Use Manufacturer	Ingredients		Name & Use Manufacturer	Ingredients	
UNICO ALDRIN EMULSIFIABLE CONCENTRATE Insecticide (United Coop.)	Hexachloro-hexahydro-endo, exo-dimethano-naphthalene*	22.2%	UNICO DDT WETTABLE POWDER Insecticide (United Coop.)	DDT (dichloro diphenyl trichloroethane)*	50.0%
	Related compounds	3.8%			
	Aromatic petroleum deriv. solvent *	69.5%			
UNICO ARAMITE EMULSIFIABLE CONCENTRATE Insecticide (United Coop.)	2-(p-tert-Butylphenoxy isopropyl-2-chloroethyl sulfite	24.7%	UNICO DIELDRIN EMUL. CONC. Insecticide (United Coop.)	Hexachloro epoxy octahydro-endo, exo-dimethano naphthalene*	15.3%
	Aromatic petroleum deriv. solvent*	69.8%		Related compounds	2.7%
				Aromatic petroleum deriv. solvents *	77.5%
UNICOAT GLOSS WHITE & ASBESTOS SHINGLE PAINT (Payson Corp.)			UNICO DIELDRIN WETTABLE POWDER Insecticide (United Coop.)	Hexachloro epoxy octahydro-endo, exo-dimethano naphthalene*	42.5%
				Related compounds	7.5%
UNICO AUTO-MIST SPRAY Insecticide (United Coop.)	Petroleum base oil*	94.5%	UNICO 50% DDT DUST BASE Insecticide (United Coop.)	DDT* (dichloro diphenyl trichloroethane)	50.0%
	Tech. piperonyl butoxide	5.0%			
	Pyrethrins	0.5%			
UNICO BHC EMULSIFIABLE CONCENTRATE Insecticide (United Coop.)	Gamma isomer of benzene hexachloride*	11%	UNICO FERBAM Fungicide (United Coop.)	Ferbam*	76%
	Other isomers of benzene hexachloride and related compounds	16%	UNICO FLORAL SPRAY POWDER Fungicide, insecticide (United Coop.)	DDT (dichloro diphenyl trichloroethane)*	5.00%
	Aromatic petroleum deriv. solvents*	67%		Rotenone	1.00%
UNICO BRUSH KILLER (United Coop.)	2, 4, 5-Trichloro phenoxy acetic acid, isopropyl ester*	13.6%		Other cube resins	1.86%
				Ferbam	3.80%
	2, 4-Dichloro phenoxy acetic acid, isopropyl ester*	27.9%		Ziram*	3.50%
				Dusting sulfur*	30.00%
UNICO CHLORDANE EMULSIFIABLE CONCENTRATE Insecticide (United Coop.)	Tech. chlordane*	45%	UNICO FLY FLAKES Insecticide (United Coop.)	Malathion	1.00%
	Petroleum distillate*	45%	UNICO FOUR-IN-ONE ROTENONE POWDER Insecticide (United Coop.)	Rotenone*	1.75%
UNICO 50% CHLORDANE WETTABLE POWDER Insecticide (United Coop.)	Tech. chlordane*	50%		Other cube resins*	3.25%
UNICO CHLORO IPC WEED KILLER (United Coop.)	Isopropyl-n-(3-chlorophenyl)-carbamate (Chloro-IPC)*	48%	UNICO GARDEN SPRAY POWDER Fungicide, insecticide (United Coop.)	Methoxychlor tech.	5.00%
				Rotenone	1.00%
				Other cube resins	1.86%
				Copper expressed as metallic*	7.00%
				Ferbam	5.00%
UNICO CROW DEFEAT Protects corn from crows (United Coop.)	Coal tar distillates*	98.5%	UNICO GENERAL PURPOSE FRUIT SPRAY Fungicide, insecticide (United Coop.)	DDT (dichloro diphenyl trichloroethane)	10.0%
				Lead arsenate*	25.0%
				Ferbam	11.4%
UNICO DDT EMULSIFIABLE CONCENTRATE Insecticide (United Coop.)	Dichloro diphenyl tri-chloroethane	24%	UNICO GRAIN FUMIGANT (United Coop.)	Ethylene dichloride	70.00%
	Aromatic petroleum deriv. solvent*	73%		Carbon tetrachloride*	30.00%
			UNICO HEPTACHLOR EMULSIFIABLE CONCENTRATE Insecticide (United Coop.)	Heptachlor*	22.5%
				Related compounds	8.7%
				Aromatic petroleum deriv. solvent*	66.3%

*Consult Sec. II., Ingredients Index. This ingredient may be responsible for major toxic effects if poisonous amounts of this product are ingested.

Name & Use Manufacturer	Ingredients	Name & Use Manufacturer	Ingredients
UNICO HOUSEHOLD AEROSOL Insecticide (United Coop.)	Tech. methoxychlor 3.00% Tech. piperonyl butoxide 0.60% Pyrethrins 0.24% Aromatic petroleum deriv. solvent* 16.16%	UNICO PYRENONE EMULSIFI- ABLE CON- CENTRATE Insecticide (United Coop.)	Petroleum base oil* 72.0% Polyoxy-ethylene sorbitol mixed ether ester 14.8% Technical piperonyl butoxide 12.0% Pyrethrins* 1.2%
UNICO HOUSEHOLD SPRAY Insecticide (United Coop.)	Petroleum distillate* 99.53% Dichloro diphenyl tri- chloroethane 0.25% Piperonyl butoxide 0.20% Pyrethrins 0.02%	UNICO RAT & MOUSE KILLER (United Coop.)	Sodium salt of 2-pivalyl-1, 3- indandione 0.14%
UNICO LEAD ARSENATE Insecticide (United Coop.)	Dry lead arsenate* 96%	UNICORN FLAT & GLOSS PAINTS (Eaglo)	
UNICO LINDANE EMULSIFI- ABLE CON- CENTRATE Insecticide (United Coop.)	Gamma isomer of benzene hexachloride* 20.0% Xylol* 48.0% Cyclohexanone 28.0%	UNICO ROACH & ANT KILLER (United Coop.)	Petroleum distillate* 96.78% Tech. chlordane* 2.00% Dichloro diphenyl tri- chloroethane* 1.00% Tech. piperonyl butoxide 0.20% Pyrethrins 0.02%
UNICO LINDANE WETTABLE POWDER Insecticide (United Coop.)	Gamma isomer of benzene hexachloride* 25%	UNICO RODENTICIDE CONCEN- TRATE (United Coop.)	Warfarin (3-(a-acetonylbenzyl)- 4-hydroxycoumarin) 0.5%
UNICO LO-V BRUSH KILLER (United Coop.)	Butoxy ethoxy propanol ester of 2, 4-D* 37.4% Butoxy ethoxy propanol ester of 2, 4, 5-T* 35.2%	UNICO ROOST PAINT Insecticide (United Coop.)	Gamma isomer of benzene hexachloride* 1.5%
UNICO MALATHION EMULSION CONCEN- TRATE Insecticide (United Coop.)	Malathion* 51.3% Xylol* 41.7%	UNICO SCREW- WORM REMEDY EQ-335 (United Coop.)	Gamma isomer of benzene hexachloride* 3% Pine oil* 35%
UNICO MALATHION WETTABLE POWDER Insecticide (United Coop.)	Malathion* 25%	UNICO SPRAY Insecticide (United Coop.)	DDT*
UNICO METHYL BROMIDE FUMIGANT Fumigant, insecticide (United Coop.)	Methyl bromide* 98% Chloropicrin* 2%	UNICO STOCK DIP & DIS- INFECTANT Insecticide (United Coop.)	Cresylic acids* 12% Coal tar neutral oils* 60% Soap 18%
UNICO NICOTINE SULPHATE SOLUTION Insecticide (United Coop.)	Nicotine, expressed as alkaloid* 40%	UNICO STOCK FLY SPRAY (United Coop.)	Petroleum base oil* 99.665% Piperonyl butoxide 0.300% Pyrethrins 0.035%
		UNICO SUPERIOR MISCIBLE SPRAY OIL Insecticide (United Coop.)	Petroleum distillate* 97.5%
UNICO PENTA CONCEN- TRATE Wood pre- servative (United Coop.)	Pentachlorophenol* 40% Petroleum hydrocarbons 40%	UNICO T C A-90 GRASS KILLER Insecticide (United Coop.)	Sodium trichloroacetate* 90%
UNICO PRESSURIZED CATTLE SPRAY Insecticide (United Coop.)	Methoxychlor tech. 3.0% Piperonyl butoxide tech. 2.0% Pyrethrins 0.2% Aromatic petroleum deriv. solvent* 24.8%	UNICO TDE EMULSIFI- ABLE CON- CENTRATE Insecticide (United Coop.)	Dichloro diphenyl dichloroethane tech. 25% Aromatic petroleum deriv. solvent* 69%

*Consult Sec. II., Ingredients Index. This ingredient may be responsible for major toxic effects if poisonous amounts of this product are ingested.

Name & Use Manufacturer	Ingredients		Name & Use Manufacturer	Ingredients
UNICO TOXAPHENE EMULSIFI-ABLE CON-CENTRATE Insecticide (United Coop.)	Toxaphene* 60% Aromatic petroleum derivative solvent 30%		UNIVERSAL Water pump lubricant and radiator rust inhibitor (Univ. Chem.)	
UNICO TOXAPHENE WETTABLE POWDER Insecticide (United Coop.)	Toxaphene* 40%		UNIVERSAL DRAIN PIPE CLEANER (Internat. Plumb.)	Sodium hydroxide*
UNICO 2, 4-D AMINE WEED KILLER (United Coop.)	Dimethylamine salt of 2, 4-dichlorophenoxyacetic acid* 49.5%		UNIVERSAL ENAMEL (Lawrence, W. W.)	
UNICO 2, 4-D BUTYL ESTER WEED KILLER (United Coop.)	Butyl ester of 2, 4-dichloro-phenoxyacetic acid* 57.0%		UNIVERSAL MENDING WOOD (Internat. Plumb.)	
UNICO 2, 4-D ESTER WEED KILLER (United Coop.)	Isopropyl ester of 2, 4-dichlorophenoxyacetic acid* 44%		UNIVERSAL M.Q. DE-VELOPER & STOP BATH Photographic supplies (Eastman)	
UNICO 2, 4, 5-T Lo-V ESTER Herbicide (United Coop.)	Butoxy ethoxy propanol ester of 2, 4, 5-trichloro-phenoxyacetic acid* 69.7%		UNIVERSAL MUCILAGE (Scriptex)	
UNICO 2, 4-D Lo-V ESTER WEED KILLER (United Coop.)	Butoxy ethoxy propanol ester of 2, 4-dichlorophenoxyacetic acid* 75.4%		UNIVERSAL PIPE JOINT COMPOUND (Internat. Plumb.)	
UNICO WARFARIN PELLETS Rodenticide (United Coop.)	Warfarin (3-(a-acetonylbenzyl)-4-hydroxycoumarin) 0.025%		UNIVERSAL READY MIXED PAINTS (Waterall)	
UNIGLOSS PAINT (Paragon Paint)			UNIVERSAL WATER SOFTENERS (Univ. Water)	
UNISAN WALL FINISH PAINT (Mound City)			UNI-VERSL KOTE GLOSS WHITE Paint (Central P. & V.)	
UNISYNE ENAMELS (United Finish)			UNI-WALL WASHABLE PAINT (Bauer)	
UNITED GILSONITE HT1600 ALUMINUM PAINT (United Gilson.)	Fish oil Aluminum pigment Mineral spirits* Petroleum resin		UNXLD 448 INSECT REPELLENT (Unexcelled)	
UNI-TEX ONE COAT FLAT PAINT (Elliott)			UPCO CAULK (Upco)	
UNITOL UNIVERSAL DEVELOPERS Photographic supplies (General Photo.)			UPCO SPAR EXTERIOR ENAMEL (Upco)	
UNITONE STAINS (Reliance Varnish)				

*Consult Sec. II., Ingredients Index. This ingredient may be responsible for major toxic effects if poisonous amounts of this product are ingested.

Name & Use Manufacturer	Ingredients		Name & Use Manufacturer	Ingredients	
UPJOHN'S MEDICATED FOOT POWDER For fungus infections, medical (Upjohn)	Benzoic acid Salicylic acid* Chlorothymol Boric acid* Zinc oxide Camphor Cinnamaldehyde	2.50% 2.50% 0.04% 10.00% 2.00% 0.10% 0.08%	U. S. STANDARD READY MIXED PAINTS (Eagle P. & V.)		
UPJOHN'S SPECIAL FORMULA NO. 1 (Upjohn)	Acetophenetidin* Camphor*, mono. Caffeine Atropine sulfate Acetylsalicylic acid* Phenolphthalein	1-1/4 gr. 1/2 gr. 1/4 gr. 1/1000 gr. 1-3/4 gr. 1/5 gr.	UTASED Antispasmodic, carminative, uterine sedative (Elixir)	Each 5 cc.: Viburnum opulus Wild yam Scutellaria Life root Cinnamon Clove Ginger	0.26 gm. 0.26 gm. 0.26 gm. 0.173 gm. 86.5 mg. 86.5 mg. 11 mg.
UPJOHN'S SPECIAL FORMULA NO. 2 For colds (Upjohn)	Acetophenetidin* Camphor* Aloin Quinine sulfate* Podophyllin Atropine sulfate	2 gr. 1/4 gr. 1/16 gr. 1/4 gr. 1/40 gr. 1/2000 gr.	UTERINE CAPSULES (Veterinary use) (Massengill Veterinary Division)	Each capsule: Boric acid* Ammonium alum Berberine salt Phenol* Menthol isomers* Thymol* Eucalyptol * Aromatics	
UPJOHN'S MEDICATED FOOT POWDER (Upjohn)	Benzoic acid Salicylic acid* Chlorothymol Boric acid* Zinc oxide Camphor Cinnamaldehyde	2.50% 2.50% 0.04% 10.00% 2.00% 0.10% 0.08%	UTILIVAR ENAMELS (McDougall-Butler)		
URINGO CAPSULES For uniary relief (K & B)	Formin* Powd. cubeb Acid sodium phosphate*		UTILUX HOUSE PAINTS (Jacroy)		
USANINE DISINFECT-ANT (U. S. Sanitary)			UTOL ANTIBIOTIC CREAM (McKesson)	Tyrothricin Benzocaine Hexachlorophene Zinc oxide Bismuth subsalicylate Menthol	0.05% 5% 1%
U-SEE GLASS CLEANER (United Chem.)			U-TO-NA BRAND TABLETS Laxative (Cel-Ton-Sa)	Aloin Podophyllum resin Extract cascara sagrada Extract of stramonium Total alkaloids	1/600 gr.
USI ANTIFREEZE NO. 1 (Genesee)	Ethylene glycol base*		U-TON-A IRON TONIC (Cel-Ton-Sa)	Iron and ammonium citrate Berberis Gentian Oil of sweet orange Oil of nutmegs Oil of spearmint Columbo Quassia Blue flag Yellow dock Aletris Licorice Wild cherry Benzoic acid Salicylic acid Saccharin	
USI ANTIFREEZE NO. 2 (Genesee)	Methanol base*				
U. S. METAL POLISH (Gisler)					
USP CATALYST POWDER (U.S. Plywood)	Paraformaldehyde*				
USP PHENOLIC RESIN (U.S. Plywood)	Phenol resorcinol formaldehyde resin Alcohol solution*		UXUDINE Skin ointment (Bullock-Walker)	Iodine (chemically combined with commercial oleic acid)* Methyl salicylate* Anhydrous lanolin Beeswax	5% 5%
U. S. PHOSPHORIC DUSTING SULPHUR Fungicide (U. S. Phosphoric)	Sulfur*	92%			
U. S. PHOSPHORIC WETTABLE SULPHUR Fungicide (U. S. Phosphoric)	Sulfur*	90%	V.A. DOUCHE POWDER PACKETTES (McKesson)	8-Hydroxyquinoline citrate* Boric acid* Alum * Zinc sulfate*	

*Consult Sec. II., Ingredients Index. This ingredient may be responsible for major toxic effects if poisonous amounts of this product are ingested.

Name & Use Manufacturer	Ingredients		Name & Use Manufacturer	Ingredients	
VAGAGILL Vaginal jelly (Massengill)	Phe-mer-nite (brand of phenylmercuric nitrate) (mercury prep.) Sodium lauryl sulfate Oxyquinoline sulfate Boric acid Phenol Non-greasy base	1-5000 0.3%	VALOR BRAND PRODUCTS SULPHUR CALCIUM ARSENATE DUST 50-50 Fungicide (San Joaquin)	Arsenic* Sulfur	
VAGIOBULBS Astringent vaginal suppository (Clapp, Otis)	Hydrastic canadensis Glycerin Boric acid Borax Glyco gelatin base		VAL-SALV THINNER Paint product (Valentine)		
VAK Laxative (Friendly Labs.)	Cascara sagrada aromatic fluid ext. Liquid petrolatum		VALSPAR VARNISHES, ENAMELS & LACQUERS (Valentine)		
VALDURA PAINTS, ENAMELS, COATINGS (Am. Marietta)			VAN BRITE SELF POLISHING WAX (Adco)	Carnauba wax Petroleum oxidized wax Resin Emulsifier*	
VALENTINE'S LACQUER THINNER 160075 (Valentine)	Butyl alcohol Butyl acetate Ethyl acetate Toluol* Xylol* Petroleum naphtha		VAN BRODE MOTH CHASER (Van Brode)	Naphthalene* Essential oil for perfuming	99-1/2% 1/2%
VALENTINE'S VARNISHES & ENAMELS (Valentine)			VAN BRODE MOTH CHASER (Van Brode)	Paradichlorobenzene*	100%
VALESCO Synergist (Pyro-Sana)	Each oz.: Modified creosote Sodium hypophosphite Sodium benzoate	2.7 m. 16 gr. 10 gr.	VANCIDE 51 Fungicide (Vanderbilt)	Sodium salt of dimethyl dithiocarbamic acid* Sodium salt of 2-mercaptobenzothiazole	27.6% 2.4%
VALLEY 5% DDT DUST Insecticide (Calif. Spray)	DDT*	5%	VANCO PAINTS & ENAMELS (Tredennick)		
VALLEY 10% DDT DUST Insecticide (Calif. Spray)	DDT*	10%	VAN-FLAT WALL PAINT (Vanguard)		
VALLEY 5% DDT-50% SULFUR Insecticide (Calif. Spray)	DDT* Sulfur*	5% 50%	VAN GLOSS & VAN GLOSS FINISH Paint (Vanguard)		
VALLEY 10% TOXAPHENE DUST Insecticide (Calif. Spray)	Toxaphene*	10%	VANISH TOILET BOWL CLEANER (Dunaway)	Sodium acid sulfate* Sodium carbonate Sodium chloride Talc Odorant	74.4% 10.0% 15.0% 0.3% 0.3%
VALOCITY PAINT & VARNISH REMOVER (Valentine)	Benzol*	25%	VANI-SOL BOWL CLEANSE (Nat'l Lab.)	Hydrochloric acid*	23%
VAL-OIL SEALER (Valentine)			VANO BLEACH (Chem. Inc.)		
VALON FLAT WALL PAINT (Valentine)			VANO HOUSEHOLD CLEANER (Chem. Inc.)		
			VANO LIQUID STARCH (Chem. Inc.)		

*Consult Sec. II., Ingredients Index. This ingredient may be responsible for major toxic effects if poisonous amounts of this product are ingested.

Name & Use Manufacturer	Ingredients	
VAPACON Electric vaporizer concentrate (Lamb & Berlin)	Oil of pine needles* Eucalyptus* Camphor* Menthol*	
VAPAIR Air deodorizer (Clean Home)		
VAPEX INHALANT (Fougera)	Menthol* Oils of lavender and eucalyptus* Cineol Linalyl acetate Oil of pine* Terebene Borneol	
VAPO-CEN Insecticide (Central Chem.)	Oil* Piperonyl butoxide Pyrethrins	
VAPO- CRESOLENE MEDICATED VAPOR INHALANT (Vapo- Cresolene)	Cresylic acid* fraction of coal tar	
VAPO INHALANT (Prescript. Spec.)	Alcohol* Beechwood creosote Eucalyptol Tinct. benzoin comp.	77% 0.3 cc. 0.3 cc. 30.0 cc.
VAPOL Counter- irritant, colds veterinary (Thoroughbred)	Camphor* Thymol* Oil of eucalyptus* Methyl salicylate* Menthol* Oil of turpentine* Oil of cedarwood* Petrolatum	
VAPO MIST Respiratory decongestant (veterinary, avian) (Hilltop)	Methyl phenol* Formaldehyde* Mineral oil Trichloro monofluoro methane* Dichloro difluoro methane* Oil of camphor* Methyl salicylate* Pine oil*	
VAPOMIST Use, electric vaporizors (Pharmex)	Oil solution of 5 essential oils* Menthol* Camphor*	
VAPOMITE 1-3 DUST Insecticide (Calif. Spray)	TEPP* Other ethyl phosphates Aramite	1% 1.5% 3%
VAPOMITE 1-4 DUST Insecticide (Calif. Spray)	TEPP* Other ethyl phosphates Aramite	1% 1.5% 4%
VAPO- NASALENE Nasal de- congestant (Vapo- Cresolene)	Ephedrine sulfate* Carbonyldiamide Chlorobutanol* Menthol*	1%

Name & Use Manufacturer	Ingredients	
VAPOPHOS 4 CITRUS SPRAY Insecticide (Calif. Spray)	Parathion*	46.8%
VAPOPHOS-3D 1-5 DUST Insecticide (Calif. Spray)	Parathion* DDD	1% 5%
VAPOPHOS-3D 1-10 DUST Insecticide (Calif. Spray)	Parathion* DDD	1.00% 10.00%
VAPOPHOS 1 DUST Insecticide (Calif. Spray)	Parathion*	1%
VAPOPHOS DUST NO. 1.5 Insecticide (Calif. Spray)	Parathion*	1.5%
VAPOPHOS 2 DUST Insecticide (Calif. Spray)	Parathion*	2%
VAPOPHOS 3 DUST Insecticide (Calif. Spray)	Parathion*	3%
VAPOPHOS 4 DUST Insecticide (Calif. Spray)	Parathion*	4%
VAPOPHOS-K 1-6.8 DUST Insecticide (Calif. Spray)	Parathion* Copper	1% 6.8%
VAPOPHOS-K 1-7 DUST Insecticide, fungicide (Calif. Spray)	Parathion* Copper	1% 7%
VAPOPHOS-K 1-25 DUST Insecticide, fungicide (Calif. Spray)	Parathion* Copper Zinc	1% 4.5% 4.5%
VAPOPHOS-K 2-25 DUST Insecticide (Calif. Spray)	Parathion* Zinc coposil (o, o-diethyl-o-p- nitrophenyl thiophosphate) 25% Copper expressed as metallic 4.5% Zinc expressed as metallic 4.5%	2%
VAPOPHOS LIQUID SPRAY Insecticide (Calif. Spray)	Parathion* Xylene Polyethylene glycol monoisooctylphenylether 5%	25% 68%
VAPOPHOS-S 1-50 DUST Insecticide (Calif. Spray)	Parathion* Sulfur	1% 50%

---

*Consult Sec. II., Ingredients Index. This ingredient may be responsible for major toxic effects if poisonous amounts of this product are ingested.

Name & Use Manufacturer	Ingredients		Name & Use Manufacturer	Ingredients	
VAPOPHOS-S 1-75 DUST Insecticide (Calif. Spray)	Parathion* Sulfur	1% 75%	VAPOR- BARRIER PAINTS (Walker, Norris)		
VAPOPHOS-S 2-30 DUST Insecticide, fungicide (Calif. Spray)	Parathion* Sulfur	2% 30%	VAPOR HALANT (Ontario)	Oil of wintergreen* Oil of peppermint Oil of turpentine* Oil of camphor* Oil of eucalyptus q.s.	15.3 fl. oz. 7.3 fl. oz. 32.6 fl. oz. 7.3 fl. oz. 128 fl. oz.
VAPOPHOS-S 2-50 DUST Insecticide (Calif. Spray)	Parathion* Sulfur	2% 50%	VAPORINE WONDER CLEANER (formerly called SCLEEN) (Vaporine)	Trisodium phosphate* Sesquicarbonate of soda Pine oil* Sulfonated castor oil	
VAPOPHOS-S 2-75 DUST Insecticide (Calif. Spray)	Parathion* Sulfur	2% 75%			
VAPOPHOS 2 SPRAY Insecticide (Calif. Spray)	Parathion*	25%	VAPORSPRAY Insecticide (Gerson- Stewart)	Beta-butoxy-beta'-thiocyano diethyl ether* Beta thiocyano ethyl esters of aliphatic acids Oil*	
VAPOPHOS 4 SPRAY Insecticide (Calif. Spray)	Parathion*	45.6%	VAPOR WAX (Buffalo Scient.)		
VAPOPHOS-S 3.75-70 WETTABLE Insecticide (Calif. Spray)	Parathion* Sulfur	3.75% 70%	VAPO SEAL PAINT (Walker, Norris)		
VAPOPHOS TOXAPHENE 2-10 DUST Insecticide (Calif. Spray)	Parathion* Toxaphene*	2% 10%	VAPOTONE BACCO SPRAY Insecticide (Calif. Spray)	Tetraethyl pyrophosphate* Other ethyl phosphates	40% 60%
VAPOPHOS 15 WETTABLE Insecticide (Calif. Spray)	Parathion*	15%	VAPOTONE CONC. Insecticide (Calif. Spray)	Tetraethyl pyrophosphate* Related organic phosphates*	20% 30%
VAPOPHOS 25 WETTABLE Insecticide (Calif. Spray)	Parathion*	25%	VAPOTONE- DDT 50-5 DUST Insecticide (Calif. Spray)	Tetraethyl pyrophosphate* Other ethyl phosphates DDT	0.75% 1.12% 5%
VAPOPHOS 50 WETTABLE Insecticide (Calif. Spray)	Parathion*	50%	VAPOTONE- DDT 66-3 DUST Insecticide (Calif. Spray)	TEPP* Other ethyl phosphates DDT	1% 1.5% 3%
VAPOPHOS ZINEB 1-4 DUST Insecticide, fungicide (Calif. Spray)	Parathion* Zineb	1% 4%	VAPOTONE- DDT 66-5 DUST Insecticide (Calif. Spray)	TEPP* Other ethyl phosphates DDT	1% 1.5% 5%
VAPOPHOS ZINEB 1.5-3.25 DUST Insecticide, fungicide (Calif. Spray)	Parathion* Zineb	1.5% 3.25%	VAPOTONE- DDT 66-10 DUST Insecticide (Calif. Spray)	TEPP* DDT Other ethyl phosphates	1% 10% 1.5%
VAPOPHOS ZINEB-S 1-3.25-25 DUST Insecticide, fungicide (Calif. Spray)	Parathion* Zineb Sulfur	1% 3.25% 25%	VAPOTONE- DDT 66-20 DUST Insecticide (Calif. Spray)	Tetraethyl pyrophosphate* Other ethyl phosphates DDT	1% 1.5% 20%
			VAPOTONE-3D 66-5 DUST Insecticide (Calif. Spray)	TEPP* DDD	1% 5%

*Consult Sec. II., Ingredients Index. This ingredient may be responsible for major toxic effects if poisonous amounts of this product are ingested.

- 1033 -

Name & Use Manufacturer	Ingredients	Name & Use Manufacturer	Ingredients
VAPOTONE 3D 66-10 DUST Insecticide (Calif. Spray)	Tetraethyl pyrophosphate* 1.00% Other ethyl phosphates 1.50% Dichloro diphenyl dichloro- ethane 10.00% Phosphorous expressed as elemental 0.6%	VAPOTRAN 66-5 DUST Insecticide (Calif. Spray)	Tetraethyl pyrophosphate* 1.0% Other ethyl phosphates 1.5% p-Chlorophenyl p-chloro- benzene sulfonate 5.0% Phosphorus expressed as elemental 0.6%
VAPOTONE 50 DUST Insecticide (Calif. Spray)	Tetraethyl pyrophosphate* 0.75% Other ethyl phosphates 1.12%	VAPOTRAN 66-7.5 DUST Insecticide (Calif. Spray)	Tetraethyl pyrophosphate* 1.0% Other ethyl phosphates 1.5% p-Chlorophenyl p-chloro- benzene sulfonate 7.5% Phosphorus expressed as elemental 0.6%
VAPOTONE 66 DUST Insecticide (Calif. Spray)	Tetraethyl pyrophosphate * 1.00% Other ethyl phosphates 1.50%	VAPOTRAN-S 66-5-25 DUST Insecticide (Calif. Spray)	Tetraethyl pyrophosphate* 1.0% Other ethyl phosphates 1.5% p-Chlorophenyl p-chloro- benzene sulfonate 5.0% Sulfur 25.0% Phosphorus expressed as elemental 0.6%
VAPO TONE PAINT (Walker, Norris)			
VAPOTONE- PERTHANE 66-5 DUST Insecticide (Calif. Spray)	Tetraethyl pyrophosphate* 1.00% Other ethyl phosphates 1.50% Diethyl diphenyl dichloro- ethane 4.75% Related reaction products, chiefly diethyl diphenyl trichloroethane 0.25%	VAPURE For nasal irritations (Rexall)	Menthol* Oils of spike lavender,* linaloe*, pennyroyal* and peppermint Acetone* Chlorthymol*
VAPOTONE-R 66-1 DUST Insecticide (Calif. Spray)	Tetraethyl pyrophosphate* 1.0% Other ethyl phosphates 1.5% Rotenone 1.0% Other resins from cube 1.0% Phosphorous expressed as elemental 0.6%	VAPURE DEODORIZING CAKES (Eastern Sanitary)	
VAPOTONE-S 50-30 DUST Insecticide (Calif. Spray)	Tetraethyl pyrophosphate* 0.75% Other ethyl phosphates 1.12% Sulfur 30%	VARICADE OINTMENT For skin irritations (Binday)	Ichthyol Hexachlorophene*
VAPOTONE-S 66-10 DUST Insecticide, fungicide (Calif. Spray)	TEPP* 1% Other phosphates 1.5% Sulfur 10%	VARI-TEMP REDUCER (du Pont)	
VAPOTONE-S 66-20 DUST Insecticide (Calif. Spray)	Tetraethyl pyrophosphate* 1.00% Other ethyl phosphates 1.50% Sulfur 20.00%	VAR-LAC-OID THALLIUM SULPHATE* Insecticide (Var-Lac-Oid)	Thallium sulfate*
VAPOTONE-S 66-30 DUST Insecticide, fungicide (Calif. Spray)	TEPP* 1% Other phosphates 1.5% Sulfur 30%	VARLOX TRANS- PARENT CEMENT FLOOR COATING (Tropical)	
VAPOTONE 40 SPRAY Insecticide (Calif. Spray)	Tetraethyl pyrophosphate* 40% Other ethyl phosphates 60%	VARNITON LABEL VARNISH V-21 (Varniton)	Acetone* as the main solvent n-Butyl acetate
VAPOTONE-XX SPRAY Insecticide (Calif. Spray)	Tetraethyl pyrophosphate* 20% Other ethyl phosphates 30%	VARNITON LABEL VARNISH V-21B (Varniton)	Carbon tetrachloride* Toluene*

*Consult Sec. II., Ingredients Index. This ingredient may be responsible for major toxic effects if poisonous amounts of this product are ingested.

- 1034 -

Name & Use Manufacturer	Ingredients	Name & Use Manufacturer	Ingredients
VARNITON PLASTIC PAINT (Varniton)	Coal tar hydrocarbon solvents*	VATU RUST PREVENTIVE (Am. Rust)	
VARNITON STOPCOCK LUBRICANT (Varniton)		VAZOHIST NASAL SPRAY Decongestant, antihistaminic antiseptic (Lamb & Berlin)	Phenylephrine HCl 1/2% Pyrilamine maleate 0.2% Benzalkonium chloride 1-5000 Phenyl mercuric acetate 1-50,000 Sodium bisulfite 0.2% Sodium citrate Sodium chloride
VARNO-CEMENT (Varniton)			
VARN-O-SEAL WOOD FINISH (Varn-O)		VAZOHIST TABLETS (Lamb & Berlin)	Each tablet: Pyrilamine maleate* 25 mg. Salicylamide* 1-1/2 gr. Phenacetin* 2-1/2 gr. Caffeine 1/2 gr. Ascorbic acid 20 mg.
VARN-O-SPRAY FLOOR POLISH (Varn-O)			
VARN-O-WAX FLOOR DRESSING (Varn-O)		V.B.Q. COLORS IN OIL (Thompson & Co.)	
		V-D SPOTTER Dry cleaning spotter (Adco)	
VASCO PRESERVA-TIVE Wood pre-servative (Virginia Smelt.)	Formaldehyde* Sulfur dioxide*	VEDS Cathartic (Friendly Labs.)	Each 1-1/4 gr. pill: Aloe* 3/4 gr. Podophyllin 1/16 gr. Total alkaloids 0.00078 gr. Oleoresin ginger q.s. Jalap* 1/4 gr. Ext. belladonna 1/16 gr. Croton oil* 1/32 gr.
VASEFRIN Nasal de-congestant (Hance)	Vasefrin* HCl (see ephedrine) 1% Buffered isotonic solution Sodium bisulfite 0.2% Phenyl mercuric acetate 1-50,000		
		VEEDOL LUBRICATING GREASE (Tide Water)	
VASELINE BORATED PETROLEUM JELLY (Chesebrough)	Small quantity of boric acid added to Vaseline petroleum jelly	VEG-A-PYR Insecticide (Residex)	Pyrethrins 2% Pyrethrum resins Isopropyl alcohol*
		VEG-LAX MED. PREP. (Sumlak)	
VASELINE CAMPHOR ICE (Chesebrough)	Camphor* Petrolatum Waxes and essential oils*	VEG-OIL Spreader-Sticker (G. L. F.)	Vegetable oil 90.00% B-1956 10.00%
VASELINE CARBOLATED PETROLEUM JELLY (Chesebrough)	Vaseline petroleum jelly Carbolic acid	VEG-SET (CLPA) HORMONE SPRAY Fungicide (Miller Chem. & F & Fert.)	Each 4 fl. oz.: Parachlorophenoxyacetic acid* 2 gm.
VASELINE CREAM HAIR TONIC (Chesebrough)	Lanolin Petroleum oil Waxes Emulsifier Essential oils*	VEL Detergent (Colgate-Palmolive)	
VASELINE LIP-ICE POMADE (Chesebrough)	Camphor* Petrolatum Waxes Essential oils* Homomenthyl salicylate		
VASELINE POMADE (Chesebrough)	Petrolatum Essential oils*		
VATUDRIP RUSTPROOF COMPOUNDS (Am. Rust)			

Name & Use Manufacturer	Ingredients
VELA Laxative (Battle Creek Diet.)	Rhubarb root Senna leaves Demulcents of Irish moss and okra Finely powdered concentrates of uncooked parsley, asparagus and rhubarb stalk
VELCACHOL Ointment base (Texas Pharm.)	Cholesterin Sodium lauryl sulfate Cetyl alcohol Stearyl alcohol Petrolatum U.S.P. mineral oil
VEL DURA FLAT PAINT (Stewart Paint)	
VELSICOL AR-50 Insecticide (Velsicol)	Methyl naphthalenes* Oil
VELSICOL AR-50G Insecticide (Velsicol)	Methyl naphthalene* Oil
VELSICOL AR-55 Insecticides (Velsicol)	Methyl naphthalenes* Oil
VELSICOL AR-60 Insecticide (Velsicol)	Dimethyl naphthalene* Oil
VELSICOL CHLORDANE Insecticide (Velsicol)	Chlordane*
VELSICOL HEPTACHLOR Insecticide (Velsicol)	Heptachloro-4, 7-methano tetrahydro indane*
VELSO ANTISEPTIC POWDERED HAND SOAP (Sanitary Soap)	
VELTEX CALZEMA For skin irritations (Veltex)	Benzocaine Menthol* Camphor* Carbolic acid* Zinc oxide Calamine Bentonite
VELTEX CARBOL- FUCHSIN PAINT Fungicide medical (Veltex)	Alcohol 10% Boric acid 1% Acid carbolic 4.5% Resorcinol* 10% Fuchsin 0.3% Acetone 5%
VELTEX CRC TABLETS Cathartic (Veltex)	Each tablet: Calomel (a mercury derivative)* 2 gr. Colocynth compound, pill mixture N.F. 2 gr. Rhubarb compound, pill mixture N.F. 2 gr. Oil of peppermint q.s. Oil of cloves q.s.

Name & Use Manufacturer	Ingredients
VELURE EGGSHELL FINISHES Paint (Jewell P. & V.)	
VELUX ENAMELS (Jewell P. & V.)	
VELVACAIN For skin burns (Nemow)	Tyrothricin Hexachlorophene Benzocaine Cod liver oil
VELVA GLO FLUORESCENT PAINTS (Radiant Color)	
VEL VA LITE ENAMEL (Briggs Maroney)	
VELVAPAX LIGHT DUTY Skin cleanser (Packwood)	Super-fatted powdered soap Lanolin Special skin emollients
VELVA-SHEEN Latex wall paint (Nat'l Paint)	
VELVAY DOUCHE POWDER (Commerce)	Pulvis zinci sulfatis compositus N.F. Chlorophyll
VELVENEER FLAT PAINT (Jewell P. & V.)	
VELVET ANTISEPTIC For skin (Binday)	Aqueous solution of alkyl benzyl ammonium chlorides 1-1,000
VELVET ANTISEPTIC GARGLE (Binday)	Acriflavine Benzalkonium chloride
VELVET AUTO BODY CLEANSER (Inter-Ocean)	
VELVET COLD CAPSULES (Binday)	Pyrilamine maleate* Aspirin* Caffeine Phenacetin* 2-1/2 gr./capsule
VELVETEEN ENAMEL (Monroe Co.)	
VELVETEX Synthetic rubber base paint (Mound City)	
VELVET FINISH WALL FINISHER (Morris Paint)	

*Consult Sec. II., Ingredients Index. This ingredient may be responsible for major toxic effects if poisonous amounts of this product are ingested.

Name & Use Manufacturer	Ingredients		Name & Use Manufacturer	Ingredients	
VELVET FLO FLAT PAINT (Nat'l Paint)			VERDI LOTION For skin irritations (Carmel)	Menthol* Glycerin Phenol Salicylic acid* Boric acid* Camphor* Zinc acetate Methyl salicylate* Tragacanth Ortho chloromercuriphenol Alcohol	0.0014% 0.04% 5%
VELVET GLOSS PAINT (Stewart Paint)					
VELVET LATEX-BASE WALL PAINT (Nat'l Gypsum)			VERITAS VAGINAL KREME (Veritas)	Paraformaldehyde Sodium oleate Stearic acid Glycerin Propylene glycol Triethanolamine Methyl p-hydroxybenzoate Propyl p-hydroxybenzoate	
VELVETONA PAINT (Central P. & V.)					
VEL-VE-TONE FLAT WALL PAINT (Globe Paint)			VERITHOL VAGINAL JELLY (Veritas)	Lactic acid Oxyquinoline sulfate* Boric acid* Methyl and propyl parahydroxy- benzoates Aminoacetic acid Glycerin	
VELVETONE FLAT WALL PAINT (Vane-Calvert)					
VELVE TOUCH SHAMPOO (Jewel Tea)			VERMAZINE Drinking water anthelmintic (poultry) (Whitmoyer)	Piperazine	17.0 gm./100 ml.
VELVET SHEEN Rubber base paint (Tropical)			VERMEX Pet shampoo, mange lotion (Vermex)	Soap, anhydrous Naphthalene*	6%
V-E-M NASAL OINTMENT Decongestant (Schoonmaker)	Eucalyptus oil* Menthol*		VERMICAPS Veterinary (Pharmex)	Tetrachlorethylene*	3 m.
VERACOLATE TABLETS Bile stimulant, cathartic (Standard Labs.)	Bile salts Ext. cascara sag. Phenolphthalein Oleoresin capsicum	1.07 gr. 1.00 gr. 0.50 gr. 0.05 m.	VERMIFUGE K9 Anthelmintic (veterinary) (Wilke)	Arecoline hydrobromides * Strychnine Dessicated blood meal Areca nut	1.5 gr. 1/33 gr./2 oz.
VERA-COLOR WAX BASE PAINTS (Plasti-Glaze)			VERSATILE LACQUERS FOR WOOD, GLASS & METAL (Plasti-Glaze)		
VERALON For skin and scalp irrita- tion (C & M)	Sulfur Salicylic acid Betanaphthol Resorcinol *	3% 1.6% 0.9% 3.5%	VERSATOL DEVELOPER Photographic supply (Eastman)		
VERDEFAM Fungicide (medical) (Texas Pharm.)	Sodium caprylate Sodium propionate Propionic acid Undecylenic acid Salicylic acid* Copper undecylenate Sodium dioctylsulfosuccinate Isopropyl alcohol*	2% 2% 3% 5% 5% 0.5% 0.1%	VERTEX ENAMEL, PAINTS, VARNISHES & PIPE CEMENTS (Whitlam)		

*Consult Sec. II., Ingredients Index. This ingredient may be responsible for major toxic effects if poisonous amounts of this product are ingested.

Name & Use Manufacturer	Ingredients	Name & Use Manufacturer	Ingredients
VESTAL SDC Vegetable oil soap (Vestal)	Hexachlorophene (2% of anhydrous) 0.64% Lecithin Glycerin Tetra sodium ethylene diamine tetra acetate	VICKS MEDI-TRATING COUGH SYRUP (Vick)	Sodium citrate Ammonium chloride Glycerin Cetamium (Vick brand of cetylpyridinium chloride) * Eucalyptus* Menthol* Camphor*
VETO (Cream, Spray, Stick & Aerosol) Deodorant (Colgate-Palmolive)		VICKS MEDI-TRATING THROAT LOZENGES (Vick)	Ammonium chloride Sodium citrate Benzocaine Cetamium
VETONE Tonic (veterinary) (Lloyd)	Nux vomica* (equiv. to 1.3 gr. strychnine sulfate) Strychnine sulfate* 1.26 gr. Gentian 11-1/2 gr. Lloyd's iron (iron 3/8 gr.) 24 m. Cobalt chloride 3 gr. 88 gr.	VICKS VAPORUB Rubefacient (Vick)	Camphor* Menthol* Steam-distilled wood turpentine* Oils of eucalyptus*, cedar leaf, nutmeg, thymol*
VETROLIN, THE GREEN LINIMENT (veterinary) (Thoroughbred)	Alcohol* 57%/v Camphor* Methyl salicylate* Oils of cedarwood*, sassafras* art, spike, origanum and rosemary* Castile soap	VICKS VA-TRO-NOL Nasal decon-gestant (mild) (Vick)	Menthol* Eucalyptol * Camphor* Ephedrine* Methyl salicylate*
V-14 MOTH & DEODORANT BLOCK Insecticide (Fuld)	Paradichlorobenzene*	VICKS VA-TRO-NOL (Aqeous-Isotonic) For relief of nasal con-gestion, nose and throat irritations of colds (Vick)	Ephedrine sulfate* Cetyl pyridium chloride 0.04% Chlorobutanol 0.25% Pectin
V-H POWDER Vaginal douche (Optimus)	Boric acid* Carbolic acid Ammonium alum * Menthol * Methyl salicylate* Benzoic acid * Salicylic acid* Magnesium sulfate Thymol		
		VICKS WILD CHERRY MEDICATED COUGH DROPS (Vick)	Menthol* Camphor* Tolu Thymol* Oil of eucalyptus* Benzyl alcohol* F.E. wild cherry bark
VIBRA-FLO DRAIN CLEANERS (Springfield)		VICTOR BLUING (Brate)	
VIBUR-SEAL Antispasmodic, tonic, sedative (Hurley)	Viburnum opulus 65.4 gr. Hydrastis 1/3 gr. Sodium benzyl succinate 20 gr. Aromatic vehicle q.s.1 oz. Alcohol 35%/v	VICTORIAN FLAT PAINTS (Stewart Bros.)	
		VI-DELTA EMULSION (Lederle)	Each tsp.: Vitamin A 2500 U.S.P. units Vitamin D 375 U.S.P. units Sodium benzoate 0.1% Lactic acid 1.5%
VI-CHLO-RIS Mouthwash (Vi-Jon)			
VICKS FOR COUGHS & COLDS (Vick)	Sodium citrate Ammonium chloride Glycerin Cetamium Syrup of eucalyptus Menthol* Camphor* Aromatics*	VI-DOM-A CREME For dry skin (Dome)	Synthetic vitamin A 100,000 U.S.P. units/oz. Vanishing cream
		VIENNA BETA CREAM COLD WAVES Cosmetic (Vienna)	Waving solution: Ammonium thioglycolate approx. 7-1/2% Neutralizer: Potassium bromate* 12 m.
VICKS INHALER (Vick)	Menthol * Camphor* Methyl salicylate* Bornyl acetate Oil of sassafras*	VIENNA DEEP COLD WAVE WITH CREAM NEUTRALIZER (Vienna)	Waving solution: Ammonium thioglycolate approx. 7-1/2% Neutralizer: Sodium bromate* solution approx. 12%

*Consult Sec. II., Ingredients Index. This ingredient may be responsible for major toxic effects if poisonous amounts of this product are ingested.

Name & Use Manufacturer	Ingredients	Name & Use Manufacturer	Ingredients
VIENNA 8-TEEN CREAM COLD WAVE (Vienna)	Waving solution: Ammonium thioglycolate approx. 7-1/2% Neutralizer: Potassium bromate* 12 gr.	VIKOL Bowl cleaner (Selig)	Orthodichlorobenzene 2.5% Hydrogen chloride* 23%
VIGEST (Liquid) Digestant (Massengill)	Ethyl alcohol 15%/v Papain 0.11 gm. Diastase of Malt 54 mg. Oleoresin ginger 0.004 cc. Glycerin Aromatics	VIMASCO COATINGS & PAINTS (Vimasco)	
		VINALAC LACQUER FOR VINYL PLASTIC (Schwartz)	
VI-GIEN POWDER Douche powder (Vi-Gien)	Boric acid* Menthol* Eucalyptol* Salt Glycerin Thymol* Ammonium alum Peppermint U. S. certified color Mineral oil	VINALOID PAINT (Cheesman-Elliott)	
		VINCE OXYGENAT-ING DENTI-FRICE (Standard Labs.)	Sodium borate perhydrate Calcium phosphate tribasic Magnesium trisilicate Calcium carbonate Sodium aluminum sulfate
VIGIL TYPE L To control mildew and bacteria (Patek)	Alkyl benzyl trimethyl ammonium chloride* 12.5% Sodium pentachlorophenate 3.95% Sodium salts of other chlorophenols 1.05%	VINCO SOOT DESTROYER (Vinco)	
VIGORO Plant food (Swift)	Total nitrogen 6.00% Available phosphoric acid 10.00% Water-soluble potash 4.00%	VINE FROST (Hanson)	Dinitro-sec.-butylphenol* 9.1% Mineral oil 87.9%
VIGORO CHEMICAL FERTILIZER (Swift)		VINELAND ANTI-BROOD Hormone (veterinary, avian) (Vineland)	Diethylstilbestrol 25 mg.
VI-JON Antiseptic (Vi-Jon)		VINELAND AMMONIA WATER For use by hatcheries to counteract fumes released by addition of formaldehyde to potassium permanganate (Vineland)	Ammonia water* 27%
VI-JON ASPIRIN Analgesic (Vi-Jon)	Aspirin* 5 gr.		
VI-JON HAND LOTION (Vi-Jon)			
VI-JON NAIL POLISH REMOVER PADS (Vi-Jon)		VINELAND AQUA-NOXALINE For coccidiosis of chickens and turkeys (Vineland)	Sulfaquinoxaline* 25%
VI-JON TINCTURE MERTHIOLATE (Vi-Jon)		VINELAND BLACKHEP For entero-hepalitis (veterinary, avian) (Vineland)	Amino nitrothiazole* 20%
VI-JON WAVE SET (Vi-Jon)			
VIKING DETERGENTS (Tumbler)		VINELAND BLACKHEP SOLUBLE For drinking water for enterohepatitis (veterinary, avian) (Vineland)	2-Amino-5-nitrothiazole* 45%
VIKING ENAMEL (Watervleit)			

*Consult Sec. II., Ingredients Index. This ingredient may be responsible for major toxic effects if poisonous amounts of this product are ingested.

- 1039 -

Name & Use Manufacturer	Ingredients		Name & Use Manufacturer	Ingredients
VINELAND CAPONADE Liquid hormonizer (Vineland)	Diethylstilbestrol 60 mg./cc.		VINELAND PHENO-NICOTINE WORM TABLETS Veterinary, avian (Vineland)	Arecoline hydrobromide 0.052 gr. Nicotine as alkaloid* 0.615 gr. Phenothiazine 6.67 gr.
VINELAND COAL TAR DISINFECT-ANT Phenol 5 coefficient (Vineland)	Coal tar neutral oil* 59% Soap 21% Cresylic acid* 10%		VINELAND PHENO-THIAZINE Anthelmintic (veterinary) (Vineland)	Phenothiazine* 97%
VINELAND COAL TAR DISINFECT-ANT Phenol 20 coefficient (Vineland)	Cresylic acid* 46.7% Coal tar neutral oil* 22.8% Soap 18.5%		VINELAND PINE OIL DISINFECT-ANT Phenol 6 coefficient (Vineland)	Pine oil* 80% Soap 10%
VINELAND EGG CLEANING DETERGENT (Vineland)	Wetting agents Water softeners Detergents		VINELAND PIPERAZINE WORMER Veterinary (Vineland)	Piperazine*
VINELAND FORMALDE-HYDE (Vineland)	Formaldehyde* 37%		VINELAND POTASSIUM PERMANGA-NATE Fumigant (Vineland)	Potassium permanganate 99%
VINELAND HI-LETHOL 10 Germicide, disinfectant, antiseptic, deodorant (Vineland)	Para di-isobutyl phenoxy ethoxy ethyl dimethyl benzyl ammonium chloride* monohydrate 10%		VINELAND RESPIRATORY FORMULA Respiratory decongestant (veterinary) (Vineland)	Menthol* Oil of eucalyptus* Methyl salicylate* Oil of camphor* Mineral oil
VINELAND HI-LETHOL-20 LIQUID Poultry disinfectant conc. (Vineland)	Alkyl (C_9-C_{15}) tolyl methyl trimethyl ammonium chlorides* 20% Isopropanol 10% Tetrasodium ethylenediamine tetra-acetate 3.65%		VINELAND SULFA-QUINOXALINE FEEDMIX 25% For coccidiosis in chicken flocks (Vineland)	Sulfaquinoxaline* 25%
VINELAND IMPROVED DETERGENT SANITIZER (Vineland)	Alkyl tolyl methyl trimethyl ammonium chlorides* 5% Sodium metasilicate, pentahydrate 15% Sodium carbonate 20%		VINELAND SULFA-QUINOXALINE SOLUBLE For coccidiosis of chickens and turkeys (Vineland)	Contents of package (when re-constituted with water) will make 50 gal. of solution containing 0.025% sulfaquinoxa-line in the form of sulfa-quinoxaline sodium*
VINELAND LINDANE 20% Insecticide (Vineland)	Gamma isomer of benzene hexachloride* 20.0% Xylol* 56.0% Cyclohexanone 5.5%		VINELAND WORM TABLETS Veterinary, avian (Vineland)	Arecoline hydrobromide 0.052 gr. Nicotine as alkaloid* 0.615 gr. Phenothiazine 6.67 gr.
VINELAND LIQUID SULFA-QUINOXALINE For coccidiosis in chickens and turkeys (Vineland)	2-Sulfanilamidoquinoxaline sodium* in excess sodium hydroxide		VINELAST BOTTOM PAINT (Woolsey)	
VINELAND PHENO-NICOTINE WORM POWDER Anthelmintic (veterinary, avian) (Vineland)	Each 25 pounds: Phenothiazine 5 lbs, 15.4 oz. Nicotine* as alkaloid 9.5 oz.		VIN-O-CELL RAPID DYRING FINISH (O'Neil)	

---

*Consult Sec. II., Ingredients Index. This ingredient may be responsible for major toxic effects if poisonous amounts of this product are ingested.

Name & Use Manufacturer	Ingredients	Name & Use Manufacturer	Ingredients
VINTOX Herbicide (Sherwin- Williams)	Arsenic trioxide* 32.5%	VITA-CAL SELF- SEALING FLAT WALL FINISH IN SEMI-PASTE FORM (Vita-Var)	
VINTROL Fungicide (Chipman Chem.)	Arsenic trioxide* 32.00%	VITA HAIR COLOR RESTORER (Allen, Mark)	Metallic salt, equiv. to 2.83 gr. silver nitrate* per fl. oz.
VIOFORM Dusting powder for wounds (Ciba)	Iodochlorhydroxyquin* 100%	VITALIS HAIR TONIC (Bristol- Myers)	Ethyl alcohol Castor oil or polyalkalene glycol Gum benzoin Benzyl benzoate
VIOFORM CREAM (Ciba)	Iodochlorhydroxyquin cream* 3%	VITALIZED CLEANER (Holcomb)	Caustic potash*
VIOFORM OINTMENT For skin irritations (Ciba)	Iodochlorohydroxyquin ointment* 3%	VITA-LUX ENAMELS, PAINTS & VARNISHES (Vita-Var)	
VIOLET & LILAC TOILET WATER (Cassebeer)		VITA-PINE CLEANER (Holcomb)	Caustic potash*
VIOLET SEC DUSTING POWDER (Hudnut, R.)		VITAPLASTIC Wall primer (Patterson- Sargent)	
VIOLET SEC TALCUM (Hudnut, R.)		VITATONE MEDICINES (Senoret)	
VIOLET SEC TOILET WATER (Hudnut, R.)		VITA-VAR OIL COLORS (Vita-Var)	
VIOL-OGEN Insecticide (Rose Mfg.)	Rotenone 0.90% Other cube resins 1.90% Mannitan monolaurate 30.00% Pine oil 5.00%	VITA-VAR PAINTS & VARNISHES (Vita-Var)	
VIOL-OGEN PLANT FOOD (Rose Mfg.)	Nitrogen 13% Phosphorus 26% Potash 13%	VITA-VAR WOOD SEALER (Vita-Var)	
VIPOL-AQUA- NOXALINE For coccidiosis of chickens and turkeys (Vineland)	Sulfaquinoxaline* 25%	VITOLIN Tonic (Humphreys)	Nux vomica 5 m. Kali arsenicosum solution 1 m. Hydrastis Acidum phosphoricum Galangal Echinacea Ferrum phosphoricum Kali phosphoricum Natrum phosphoricum Alcohol 14%
VIRGINIA ZINC SULFATE Fungicide (Virginia Smelt.)	Zinc sulfate* as anhydrous 89%		
VIRGIN WHITE ENAMEL (Thompson & Co.)		VI-TOSIS Fungicide, external (medical) (Vi-Tosis)	Boric acid* Eucalyptol* Menthol* Salicylic acid* Ammonium alum Carbolic acid* Magnesium carbonate Tricalcium phosphate
VITABRONZE FOR CLEANING BRONZE (Caul)			

*Consult Sec. II., Ingredients Index. This ingredient may be responsible for major toxic effects if poisonous amounts of this product are ingested.

Name & Use Manufacturer	Ingredients	
VITRA-CARLITE ENAMEL QUICK BAKING SYN. (Hilo Varnish)		
VITRALEX AUTOMOTIVE FINISHES (Pratt & Lambert)		
VITRALITE Enamel undercoating (Pratt & Lambert)		
VITRALOID AUTO LACQUER ENAMEL (Pratt & Lambert)		
VITRIC ENAMELS (Bishop-Conklin)		
VI-VA ALUM. PAINT & VARNISH (Johnston)		
VIVINGER Uterine sedative (Clapp, Otis)	Alcohol Sodium salicylate* Viburnum opulus (cramp bark) Oleoresin of ginger Aromatics*	25% by volume 1 gr.
VIXOL Fumigant, bowl cleaner (Selig)	Orthodichlorobenzene Hydrogen chloride*	2.5% 23%
VOCALINE For throat irritations (Assoc. Prod.)	Guaiacum Ammonium carbonate Cinchona Glycerin Honey Acacia Serpentaria	
VOL-A-TENE PAINT THINNER (Pioneer)		
VOLCK CONC. FLOWABLE Insecticide (Calif. Spray)	Petroleum oils*	80%
VOLCK CONCEN-TRATE PASTE EMULSION Insecticide (Calif. Spray)	Petroleum oils*	80%
VOLCK 90 FLOWABLE OIL EMULSION Insecticide (Calif. Spray)	Petroleum oils*	90%

Name & Use Manufacturer	Ingredients	
VOLCK GREENHOUSE SPRAY Insecticide (Calif. Spray)	Petroleum oils*	96%
VOLCK OIL SPRAY Insecticide (Calif. Spray)	Petroleum oils*	97%
VOLTAFLAT PAINTS (Voltax)		
VOLTALAC INSULATING VARNISH (Standard-Toch)		
VOLTALITE ENAMEL (Voltax)		
VOLTAX PAINTS, ENAMELS, VARNISHES (Voltax)		
VOLUME OINTMENT-CRAFT For poison ivy and oak (Bullock-Walker)	Carbolic acid Zinc oxide Lead subacetate* solution Ammonium alum Ichthammol Oil of tar Camphor*	4/5% 10-1/2% 3% 4/5% 2-1/2% 6% 2-1/2%
VONEDRINE INHALER (Merrell)	Phenylpropylmethyl amine Aromatics	0.250 gm.
VON'S PINK TABLETS Antacid (New York Von)	Bismuth subnitrate Magnesium hydroride Sodium bicarbonate	
VOO DOO 42 KILLS RATS & MICE Rodenticide (Xterminator)	Warfarin (3-(a-acetonylbenzyl)-4-hydroxycoumarin)	0.025%
VOO DOO MOUSE-KIL TRACKING POWDER (Xterminator)	Micronized DDT*	50%
VOO DOO WHITE MAGIC INSECTICIDE Insecticide (Xterminator)	Tech. chlordane	2%
VORCO BRANDS PAINTS (Vortex)		
VORCOLITE FLAT WALL PAINT (Vortex)		

*Consult Sec. II., Ingredients Index. This ingredient may be responsible for major toxic effects if poisonous amounts of this product are ingested.

Name & Use Manufacturer	Ingredients	Name & Use Manufacturer	Ingredients
VORLAC FLOOR PAINT (Vorac)		WALLBOARD ADHESIVE (Miracle)	Resinous materials Pigments Aliphatic petroleum hydrocarbon *
VOR-NAMEL ENAMEL (Vorac)		WALL BOND SEMI-GLOSS INTERIOR (Warren Paint)	
VOTOL Insecticide (Waltham)	Tech. chlordane 2% Aliphatic petroleum solvent* 98%	WALL CHARM SELF-SEALING FLAT PAINT (Harrison P. & V.)	
V & P SOLVENT PAINT & VARNISH REMOVERS (Vane-Calvert)		WALLGARD-ONE COAT PAINT (Vita-Var)	
VULCALOCK Adhesive (Goodrich, B. F.)	Benzol*	WALLHIDE INTERIOR PAINTS, FLAT, SEMI-GLOSS, GLOSS WALL, RUB-BERIZED SATIN FINISH (Pittsburgh Plate Glass)	
VULCANOL STOVE POLISH (Prescott)			
VULCANX PAINT & VARNISH (Atlas P.&V.)		WALLTONE WASHABLE FLAT WALL PAINT (Dunn)	
VULKAN Washing compound (Central Chem.)		WALLUSTRE INTERIOR MILL FINISH (Devoe)	
WAIKIKI TAN LAHONI Cosmetic (Morgan, H.)	Camphor* Phenol* Tannin* Gums Preservative	WALTHAM BLACKBOARD CHALK CRAYON (Am. Crayon)	
WALDEX Paint cleaner (Lester)	Detergents Phosphates*	WAMPOLE'S CREO-TERPIN COMPOUND Antitussive (Wampole)	Each fl. oz.: Chloroform 1 m. Creosote 2 m. Terpin hydrate 2 gr. Calcium glycerophosphate 4 gr. Sodium glycerophosphate 4 gr.
WALDSTERN HEADACHE TABLETS (Craighill)			
MADAM C. J. WALKER HAIR & SCALP PREPARATION (Walker, Mme.)	Copper sulfate* Precipitated sulfur*		
MADAM C. J. WALKER SKIN BRIGHTENER (Walker, Mme.)	Ammoniated mercury* 5% Bismuth subnitrate	WAMPOLE'S PREPARATION Stimulant tonic (Wampole)	Alcohol 12% Strychnine sulfate* 1/80 gr./tbsp.
MADAM C. J. WALKER TEMPLE SALVE (Walker, Mme.)	Precipitated sulfur* Petrolatum	WAMPOLE'S VAGINAL CONES (Wampole)	Each cone: Ichthammol (ammonium ichthosulfonate) 10 gr. Zinc sulfate 7/16 gr. Boric acid 1-1/2 gr. Sodium benzoate Thymol Eucalyptol in a base of glycerinated gelatin
WALKO TABLETS Drinking water antiseptic for poultry (Walker Rem.)	Potassium permanganate* 40%		
		WARBICIDE 5 Insecticide (Chipman, Ltd.)	Rotenone* 5%

*Consult Sec. II., Ingredients Index. This ingredient may be responsible for major toxic effects if poisonous amounts of this product are ingested.

Name & Use Manufacturer	Ingredients	Name & Use Manufacturer	Ingredients
WARCIN Rodenticide (Warcin)	Warfarin (3-(a-acetonylbenzyl)-4-hydroxycoumarin) 0.025%	WASHINGTON SHOE POLISH (Manhattan Kreole)	
WARD'S OIL Furniture polish (Montgomery Ward)		WATCH DOG LYE (Babbit)	Sodium hydroxide* 94% Sodium carbonate 2%
WARD'S PASTE WAX Furniture wax (Montgomery Ward)		WATCO READY MIXED PAINTS & VARNISHES (Waterall)	
WARFARAT Rodenticide (Hess, Dr.)	Warfarin 0.025%	WATE-ON (Wate-On)	Each 100 cc.: Vegetable oil 40% Dextrose 10% Vitamin D 1665 I.U. Vitamin B12 U.S.P. 5.55 mg. Sodium benzoate 0.1%
WARFAR-MOR (Hilltop)	Warfarin (3-(a-acetonylbenzyl)-4-hydroxycoumarin) 0.025%		
WARFET WITH WARFARIN AND T.M.F. Rodenticide (Vineland)	Warfarin (3-(a-acetonylbenzyl)-4-hydroxycoumarin) 0.025%	WATERALL PAINTS (Waterall)	
WARFORIN FOR RATS & MICE (York Chem.)		WATERBURY'S COMPOUND Antitussive (Standard Labs.)	Alcohol 10% Potassium guaiacol sulfonate Potassium creosote sulfonate Balsam tolu Malt syrup Corn syrup Glycerin
WARNER'S COMPOUND TABLETS Diuretic (Meyers Labs.)	Salol (phenyl salicylate)* Po. ext. buchu Po. ext. gentian Theobromine* Po. ext. uva ursi	WATERBURY'S NUTRITIVE (formerly known as Waterbury's Compound Plain) (Standard Labs.)	Alcohol 10% Thiamine hydrochloride Niacinamide Iron ammonium citrate Calcium hypophosphite Calcium lactate Magnesium chloride Malt syrup Corn syrup Glycerin Lactic acid Soluble saccharin Imitation sherry wine flavor Caramel
WAR-RAT Rodenticide (Davis, O. D.)	Pivalyl-1, 3 indandione 0.025%		
WARREN'S RODENT KILLER (Warren Chem.)	Warfarin 0.025%		
WARREN-TEED For skin irritation, poison ivy, insects (Warren-Teed)	Thenylpyramine hydrochloride* 2% Hexachlorophene (2, 2-dihydroxy-3, 5, 6-hexa-chlorodiphenyl methane) 3% Benzocaine 3% Calamine Vanishing base	WATERLOX ENAMEL, PAINTS, SEALERS, STAINS (Empire Varnish)	
WARTINE POISON FOR WARTS Veterinary (Roberts, Dr. D.)	Formaldehyde* Bichromate of potash* Coloring	WATERPROOF FLOOR WAX (Uncle Sam)	Resins Ammonia Morpholine Oleic
WASH-ER CLEAN (Wilson-Imperial)	Carbon tetrachloride* 80%	WATERSPAR FURNITURE POLISH, FLOOR & POLISHING WAX (Pittsburgh Plate Glass)	
WASH-FREE KUT-KOTE STRIPPER (Day)	Toluol* Methyl acetone Diacetone		

*Consult Sec. II., Ingredients Index. This ingredient may be responsible for major toxic effects if poisonous amounts of this product are ingested.

Name & Use Manufacturer	Ingredients	Name & Use Manufacturer	Ingredients
WATERSPAR QUICK- DRYING ENAMELS, CLEAR AND COLORED VARNISHES, LACQUERS (Pittsburgh Plate Glass)		WATKINS LINDANE CONEN- TRATE Insecticide (Watkins, J.)	Lindane* 10% Emulsifiable base oil
WATER-WASH Paint and varnish remover (Savogran)	Methylene chloride* Synthetic detergents	WATKINS LIQUID CLEANER (Watkins, J.)	Soap Ammonia* Ethylene glycol* Isopropyl alcohol*
WATER WOR-MOR Drinking water anthelmintic (veterinary) (Hilltop)	Piperazine citrate base* 32.3% Magnesium sulfate 5%	WATKINS LIQUID WAX (Watkins, J.)	Oleic acid Wax Triethanolamine Borax* Ammonia* Shellac*
WATKINS 25% DDT CONCEN- TRATE Insecticide (Watkins, J.)	DDT* 25% Emulsifiable base oil	WATKINS LIVESTOCK SPRAY CON- CENTRATE Insecticide (Watkins, J.)	Methoxychlor* Butoxypolypropylene glycol* Emulsifiable base oil
WATKINS DDT PYRETHRUM FLY & MOTH SPRAY (Watkins, J.)	Petroleum hydrocarbons* DDT* Sesame Pyrethrum	WATKINS 50% MALATHION CONCEN- TRATE Insecticide (Watkins, J.)	Malathion* Emulsifiable base oil
WATKINS FLY BAIT (Watkins, J.)	Malathion* 2%	WATKINS MOSQUITO- CHIGGER REPELLENT (Watkins, J.)	
WATKINS FLY & MOTH SPRAY (Watkins, J.)	Pyrethrum extract Piperonyl butoxide Inert ingredient*	WATKINS MOTH CRYSTALS (Watkins, J.)	Paradichlorobenzene*
WATKINS FLY SPRAY (Watkins, J.)	Methoxychlor* Lethane* Thanite* Petroleum distillate*	WATKINS ROACH & ANT SPRAY (Watkins, J.)	Chlordane 3% Deodorized base oil*
WATKINS GARDEN DUST Insecticide (Watkins, J.)	Copper* Rotenone* Pyrethrins Piperonyl butoxide	WATKINS ROACH, FLEA & LOUSE POWDER (Watkins, J.)	DDT* 10%
WATKINS GARDEN DUST (Triple Duty) (Watkins, J.)	Rotenone* Sabadilla* Copper*	WATKINS SARCOPTIC MANGE OIL (Watkins, J.)	Orthophenylphenol* Petroleum hydrocarbons*
WATKINS INSECT DUST (Watkins, J.)	Rotenone*	WATKINS SPOT REMOVER (Watkins, J.)	Carbon tetrachloride* Naphtha
WATKINS INSECTICIDE AEROSOL (Watkins, J.)	DDT* Allethrin Lethane 384* Freon propellant	WATKINS UNGUENT For skin (Watkins, J.)	2, 2'-Dihydroxy-5, 5'-dichloro diphenyl methane Petrolatum Lanolin Cetyl alcohol Isopropyl esters of fatty acids
WATKINS INSECT SPRAY (Watkins, J.)	DDT* 5% Deodorized base oil*	WATSON STANDARD 44 VARNISHES & ENAMELS (Watson- Standard)	

---

*Consult Sec. II., Ingredients Index. This ingredient may be responsible for major toxic effects if poisonous amounts of this product are ingested.

Name & Use Manufacturer	Ingredients	Name & Use Manufacturer	Ingredients
WAX-SEAL PASTE WAX (Upco)		WEBER CREMNITZ WHITE Artists' color (Weber, F.)	Basic lead carbonate*
WAXTANE STAIN & WAX (Warren Paint)		WEBER DAMAR VARNISH Artists' material (Weber, F.)	Singapore white Damar Gum Turpentine*
W & B CUTTING OIL 1749 (White & Bagley)	Petroleum oils* Especially processed (sulfurized) fatty oils		
W & E ALL ROUND PRESCRIP- TION Cathartic (Etheridge)	Phenacetin* 10 gr. Tinct. belladonna* 40 m. Acetylsalicylic acid* Cascara sagrada aromatic Alkaloidal Caffeine Syrups Aromatics	WEBER DARK DRYING OIL Artists' supply (Weber, F.)	Linseed oil Siccatiff
		WEBER DECORA- COLOR SOLVENT Artists' material (Weber, F.)	
WEARMASTER PAINTS (Standard Ind.)			

WEATHERBEST
HOUSE PAINT
(Staminite)
	Lead* (in all colors except the
	  red and brown, which are
	  iron oxides)
		WEBER
		DECORA
		FABRIC
		PAINTING
		COLORS
		(Weber, F.)
			Dye in lacquer

WEBER AUREOLIN Artists' color (Weber, F.)	Double nitrite of cobalt* and potassium*		
WEBER CHINESE WHITE Artists' color (Weber, F.)	Zinc oxide	WEBER EGG EMULSION, FOR TEMPERA PAINTING Artists' material (Weber, F.)	Linseed oil Damar varnish Poppy oil Egg
WEBER CHROME YELLOWS Artists' color (Weber, F.)	Lead chromate* Lead sulfate*	WEBER EMERALD GREEN Organic lake pigment (Weber, F.)	
WEBER CLE-PO-SIL POLISH (Weber Dental)	Carnauba wax Oleic acid Silicone oil	WEBER EMERAUDE GREEN Artists' color (Weber, F.)	Oxide of chromium*
WEBER CLE-PO-WAX CREAM POLISH (Weber Dental)	Sulfonated castor oil White mineral oil Mineral oil Essential oil*	WEBER ETCHERS' PRINTING INK (Weber, F.)	Frankfort, vine and lamp blacks
WEBER COBALT BLUE Artists' color (Weber, F.)	Oxide of cobalt* and aluminum	WEBER FLAKE WHITE Artists' color (Weber, F.)	White lead*
WEBER COBALT GREENS Artists' color (Weber, F.)	Oxide of cobalt* Zinc oxide	WEBER GLAZING MEDIUM Artists' material (Weber, F.)	Damar varnish Linseed oil
WEBER COPAL VARNISH, PICTURE STRENGTH Artists' material (Weber, F.)	Synthetic gums Drying oil Turpentine*	WEBER INDIAN YELLOW Organic pigment of yellow dye (Weber, F.)	

---

*Consult Sec. II., Ingredients Index. This ingredient may be responsible for major toxic effects if poisonous amounts of this product are ingested.

Name & Use Manufacturer	Ingredients	Name & Use Manufacturer	Ingredients
WEBER INTENSE BLUE, INTENSE CERULEAN BLUE, INTENSE GREEN Artists' color (Weber, F.)	Copper phthalocyanine*	WEBER OXIDE OF CHROMIUM TRANS- PARENT Artists' color (Weber, F.)	Hydrated sesquioxide of chromium*
WEBER LEMON YELLOW Artists' color (Weber, F.)	Strontium chromate*	WEBER PAINTING OIL NO. 1 Artists' material (Weber, F.)	Gum damar Refined oil Turpentine*
WEBER LEMON YELLOW (Barytes) Artists' color (Weber, F.)	Barium chromate*	WEBER PERMANENT VIOLETS Artists' color (Weber, F.)	Double salt of phosphoric acid Manganese* Ammonium
WEBER LIGHT DRYING OIL Artists' supply (Weber, F.)	Linseed oil Turpentine* Drying oil	WEBER PRUSSIAN BLUE Artists' color (Weber, F.)	Ferric ferrocyanide*
WEBER MALACHITE GREEN Artists' color (Weber, F.)	Native basic copper carbonate*	WEBER PRUSSIAN GREEN Artists' color (Weber, F.)	Gamboge* Prussian blue
WEBER MARS COLORS Artists' color (Weber, F.)	Hydrate and oxide of iron*	WEBER PURE SCARLET Artists' color (Weber, F.)	Mercuric iodide*
WEBER MASTIC VARNISH, FULL STRENGTH Artists' material (Weber, F.)	Gum mastic Turpentine*	WEBER RAW UMBER Artists' color (Weber, F.)	Iron oxide* Manganese oxide*
WEBER MEGILP Artists' color (Weber, F.)	Gum mastic Turpentine* Drying oil	WEBER RED LEAD Artists' color (Weber, F.)	Oxide of lead*
WEBER NAPLES YELLOWS Artists' color (Weber, F.)	Compounds of lead* antimoniate	WEBER RESIN-OIL PAINTING MEDIUM Artists' material (Weber, F.)	Damar varnish Stand oil Venice turpentine*
WEBER NUT OIL Artists' material (Weber, F.)	Pale oil expressed from walnuts	WEBER RES-N-GEL Mixing medium in oil painting (Weber, F.)	Colloidal synthetic resin gel
WEBER OXIDE OF CHROMIUM OPAQUE Artists' color (Weber, F.)	Sesquioxide of chromium*	WEBER SILVER WHITE Artists' color (Weber, F.)	Barium sulfate Zinc sulfide*

*Consult Sec. II., Ingredients Index. This ingredient may be responsible for major toxic effects if poisonous amounts of this product are ingested.

Name & Use Manufacturer	Ingredients	Name & Use Manufacturer	Ingredients
WEBER STAND OIL, DUTCH TYPE Artists' material (Weber, F.)	Polymerized linseed oil	WEBER WHITE LEAD FOR MOUNTING Artists' material (Weber, F.)	White lead* Bodied linseed oil
WEBER SUGAR OF LEAD Dryer for oil paints (Weber, F.)	Acetate of lead*	WEBER ZINC WHITE Artists' color (Weber, F.)	Oxide of zinc*
WEBER TRANS- PARENT MEDIUM Extends lake colors in oil (Weber, F.)	Alumina hydrate ground Poppy oil	WEBER ZINC YELLOW Artists' color (Weber, F.)	Zinc chromate*
WEBER VERDIGRIS Artists' color (Weber, F.)	Basic copper acetate*	W-E-B FLY KILLER (Southland)	Malathion* (o, o-dimethyl dithiophosphate of diethyl mercaptosuccinate) 2.00%
WEBER VERMILIONS Artists' color (Weber, F.)	Varieties of sulfide of mercury*	W-E-B INSECT REPELLENT (Liquid) (Southland)	Dimethyl phthalate Alpha, alpha-dimethyl alpha-carbobutoxy dihydro-gamma pyrone* 2-Ethylhexanediol-1, 3* Bicyclo-(2, 2, 1)-5-heptene-2, 3-dicarboxylic acid, dimethyl ester
WEBER VIRIDIAN Artists' color (Weber, F.)	Oxide of chromium*	W-E-B INSECT SPRAY (Southland)	Petroleum distillate* 94.6% Diethyl diphenyl di- chloroethane 2.85% Related compounds 0.15% Tech. chlordane 2.00% Tech. piperonyl butoxide 0.33% Pyrethrins 0.07%
WEBER WATER- PROOF DRAWING INK BLACK Artists' material (Weber, F.)	Carbon ink		
WEBER WHITE LEAD Artists' color (Weber, F.)	Basic lead carbonate*		

*Consult Sec. II., Ingredients Index. This ingredient may be responsible for major toxic effects if poisonous amounts of this product are ingested.

- 1048 -

Name & Use Manufacturer	Ingredients	Name & Use Manufacturer	Ingredients
WEBTEX BLACK ASPHALTUM Proofer (Webster, W.F.)	Petroleum naphtha* 35% Gilsonite and petroleum asphalt 65%	WEEDICIDE 32 Herbicide (Thompson Chem.)	Diethanolamine salt of 2,4-D*
WEED A BOMB Herbicide (Thompson Chem.)	Isooctyl ester of 2,4-dichloro phenoxy acetic acid 4.50% Isooctyl ester of 2,4,5-tri-chloro phenoxy acetic acid 0.75% Propellent gas 50.00%	WEEDICIDE 64 Herbicide (Thompson Chem.)	Diethanolamine salt of 2,4-D*
WEEDAR 64 Herbicide (Am. Chemical)	2,4-D alkanolamine salt* (41% 2,4-D acid, 4 lb. 2,4-D acid/gal.) 68%	WEEDICIDE 50% BUTYL ESTER Herbicide (Thompson Chem.)	Butyl ester of 2,4-D*
WEEDAR MCP Herbicide (Am. Chemical)	2-Methyl 4-chloro phenoxy acetic acid* 2 lb./gal.	WEEDICIDE I AMINE CONC. Herbicide (Thompson Chem.)	Isopropylamine salt of 2,4-D*
WEEDAR MCP CONCENTRATE Herbicide (Am. Chemical)	Diethanolamine salt of 2-methyl 4-chlorophenoxyacetic acid* 60.8%	WEEDICIDE LV I.0-80 2,4-D ESTER Herbicide (Thompson Chem.)	Iso-octyl 2,4-dichloro phenoxy acetates* 67.8%
WEEDAWAY, BRUSH KILLER, CHLORO IPC #4, LIQUID (See Miller Weedaway)		WEEDICIDE 2,4-D Herbicide (Thompson Chem.)	2,4-Dichloro phenoxy acetic acid* 60%
WEED-B-GON IMPROVED Herbicide (Calif. Spray)	Tetrahydro furfuryl ester of 2,4,5-trichloro phenoxy acetic acid* 6.6% Tetrahydro furfuryl ester of 2,4-dichlorophenoxy acetic acid* 13.8%	WEED N FEED Fertilizer (French Ren.)	
WEED-B-GON 64-X WEED KILLER Herbicide (Calif. Spray)	Dimethylamine salt of 2,4-dichlorophenoxy acetic acid* 49.4%	WEED-NO-MORE Herbicide (Acme Q.P.)	Iso-octyl ester of 2,4-D* 12% Oils Emulsifiers
WEED-B-GON 88-X WEED KILLER Herbicide (Calif. Spray)	Dimethylamine salt of 2,4-dichlorophenoxy acetic acid* 64%	WEED-NO-MORE Herbicide (Green Cross)	2,4-Dichloro phenoxy acetic acid* equiv. 16 oz./gal.
WEEDETH Herbicide (Miller Chem. Co.)	Dimethylamine salt of 2,4-dichloro phenoxy acetic acid* 49.4%	WEED-NOTS Herbicide (Nott)	Sodium salt monohydrate of 2,4-D* 35%
WEEDEATH 40 Herbicide (Hanson, H.)	Ethylamine salt of 2,4-D* 57%	WEEDONE AERO-CONCENTRATE 96 Herbicide (Am. Chemical)	Ethyl ester 2,4-D*
WEEDEATH 44 Herbicide (Hanson, H.)	Isopropyl ester of 2,4-D* 44%	WEEDONE BRUSH KILLER 32 Herbicide (Am. Chemical)	2,4,5-T butoxy ethanol ester* 11%
WEEDESTER Herbicide (Miller Chem. Co.)	Butyl ester of 2,4-dichloro phenoxy acetic acid* 40%	WEEDONE BRUSH KILLER 64 Herbicide (Am. Chemical)	Butoxy ethanol ester 2,4,5-T* acid equiv. 1.33 lb./gal. Botoxy ethanol ester 2,4-D* acid equiv. 2.67 lb./gal.
WEEDETTE Herbicide (Linck)	Triethanolamine salt of 2,4-dichloro phenoxy acetic acid* 67%	WEEDONE BRUSH KILLER 977 (Am. Chemical)	Butoxy ethanol ester of 2,4-dichloro phenoxy acetic acid* 21.5% Butoxy ethanol ester of 2,4,5-trichloro phenoxy acetic acid* 10.4%
WEEDICIDE Herbicide (Thompson Chem.)	Isopropyl 2,4-dichloro phenoxy acetate* 45%		

*Consult Sec. II., Ingredients Index. This ingredient may be responsible for major toxic effects if poisonous amounts of this product are ingested.

Name & Use Manufacturer	Ingredients	Name & Use Manufacturer	Ingredients
WEEDONE CHICKWEED KILLER (Am. Chemical)	Potassium cyanate* 52.0%	WEEDUST 2,4 Herbicide (Am. Chemical)	2,4-Dichloro phenoxy acetic acid ethyl ester 2.0%
WEEDONE CONC. 48 Herbicide (Am. Chemical)	2,4-D ethyl ester* 39%	WEEVIL GO MILL SPRAY Insecticide (Adco)	Petroleum distillate* Tech. piperonyl butoxide Pyrethrins*
WEEDONE CRAB GRASS KILLER (Conc.) (Am. Chemical)	Potassium cyanate* 86%	WEEVIL KILL Insecticide (Thompson-Hayward)	Carbon tetrachloride* 68.1% Ethylene dichloride 24.7% Ethylene dibromide 7.2%
WEEDONE CRAB GRASS KILLER CONTAINING SODAR (Am. Chemical)	Sodar (disodium methylarsonate)* 31.65%	WEKILL Herbicide (Planetary Chem.)	Amyl ester of 2,4,5-trichloro phenoxy acetic acid* 55.9%
WEEDONE CRAB GRASS KILLER IMPROVED (Am. Chemical)	Potassium cyanate* 53.8% MCP 11.1%	WELCH'S AEGOPODIUM Anti-rheumatic (Welch)	Each fl. oz.: Wine of colchicum seed* 0.2 fl. oz. Potassium iodide* 0.08 oz.
WEEDONE IMPROVED (Am. Chemical)	Butoxy ethanol esters 2,4-D* and 2,4,5-T	WELDONA TABLETS Analgesic (Weldona)	Sodium salicylate* 2-1/2 gr. Powdered extract of cimicifuga 1/8 gr. Powdered extract of pokeroot (phytolacca) 1/8 gr.
WEEDONE INDUSTRIAL BRUSH KILLER (Am. Chemical)	Butoxy ethanol esters 2,4-D* and 2,4,5-T* 2 lbs. ea./gal.	WELDWOOD CONTACT CEMENT (U. S. Plywood)	Neoprene rubber Phenolic resins Plasticizers Volatile Organic solvents*
WEEDONE IPC Herbicide (Am. Chemical)	IPC* 3 lb./gal.	WELDWOOD GLUE (U. S. Plywood)	Urea formaldehyde resins Inert cellulosic fillers
WEEDONE LV4 Herbicide (Am. Chemical)	Butoxy ethanol ester 2,4-D* 4 lb. acid/gal.	WELDWOOD PLASTIC RESIN GLUE (U. S. Plywood)	Urea formaldehyde resin Cellulose flour
WEEDONE 2,4,5-T Herbicide (Am. Chemical)	Butoxy ethanol ester 2,4,5-T* 4 lbs. acid equiv. per gal.	WELDWOOD PRESTO-SET GLUE (U. S. Plywood)	Polyvinyl acetate resin
WEEDOUT Herbicide (Doggett-Pfeil)	2,4-D amine salt*	WELLCOME BRAND BENZYL BENZOATE EMULSION Ectoparasiticide (Burroughs-Wellcome)	Benzyl benzoate* 50% Emulsifying agents (oleic acid and triethanolamine)
WEEDOUT TURF FOOD Herbicide (Doggett-Pfeil)	2,4-D amine salt*	WELLCOME BRAND TOILET LANOLINE OINTMENT (Burroughs-Wellcome)	Lanolin Solid and liquid petrolatum
WEEDUST 2% Herbicide (Am. Chemical)	Ethyl ester 2,4-D*	WELMAID Silver polish (Welmaid)	

*Consult Sec. II., Ingredients Index. This ingredient may be responsible for major toxic effects if poisonous amounts of this product are ingested.

- 1050 -

Name & Use Manufacturer	Ingredients	Name & Use Manufacturer	Ingredients
WENZELMANN RUG & UPHOLSTERY CLEANER (Wenzelmann)		WESTVACO NO. 8 GRAIN & MILL FUMIGANT (Westvaco)	Carbon tetrachloride* 65% Ethylene dichloride 30% Ethylene dibromide 5%
WERNET DENTU CREME Cosmetic (Wernet)	Sodium soaps of coconut oil fatty acids Lactose Sodium benzoate Glycerin Saccharin Stearic acid	WESTVACO NO. 9 GRAIN & MILL FUMIGANT (Westvaco)	Carbon tetrachloride* 80% Carbon bisulfide* 15% Ethylene dibromide 5%
WERNET DENTURE CREAM (Wernet)	Inert polishing agent Coconut oil Stearic acid soaps Gum tragacanth Glycerin Saccharin Flavor	WEST-WARD CARBOXY METHYL CELLULOSE Laxitave (West-Ward)	Sodium carboxy methyl cellulose 0.5 gm./tablet
WESTAN CREAM Anti-sunburn cream (Western Pharm.)	Monoglyceryl para-amino-benzoate 2% Lanolin	WET-O-DRY PAINT & GREASE REMOVER (Midland Color)	
WESTAN LOTION Anti-sunburn lotion (Western Pharm.)	Monoglyceryl para-amino-benzoate 2%	WETSPOT Drycleaning spotter (Adco)	
WESTERN GENTLEMAN (for Men) (Studio)		WHD SPECIAL MEDICINE Laxative (Myers Labs.)	Sodium bicarbonate Calcium carbonate Magnesium oxide heavy
WESTERN SOLVENTS STA Anti-Freeze (Western Solvents)	Methanol* Borax*	DR. WHETZEL'S CIGARETTES Asthmatic antispasmodic (Myers Labs.)	Stramonium and lobelia herb Total alkaloids 0.175%
WESTERN WAX WORKS LINOLEUM CLEANER (Western Wax)		DR. WHETZEL'S LIQUID PRESCRIPTION Antitussive (Myers Labs.)	Potassium iodide Tinc. cardamom comp. Salicylic acid* Tinc. gentian comp. Sodium salicylate*
WESTPHAL'S HAIR COLOR RENEWER AID (Westphal)	Metallic salts*	DR. WHETZEL'S POWDER Asthmatic antispasmodic (Myers Labs.)	Each avoir. oz.: Powd. stramonium leaves (containing 0.55 gr. stramonium alkaloids) 42.02% Powd. lobelia herb
WESTPINE Disinfectant (West Disinf.)	Pine oil* Soap Alcohol	WHITE ACE White Shoe Polish (Old Dutch)	
WESTVACO 3-5-40 COTTON DUST Insecticide (Westvaco)	DDT* BHC* Sulfur*	WHITE ACE FLAT PAINTS (Paramount)	
WESTVACO NO. 3 GRAIN & MILL FUMIGANT (Westvaco)	Carbon tetrachloride* 80% Carbon bisulfide* 20%	WHITE CLOVERINE SALVE For skin irritations (Wilson Chem.)	Rectified oil of turpentine * White petrolatum White refined wax
WESTVACO NO. 6 SPOT FUMIGANT (Westvaco)	Carbon tetrachloride* 60% Ethylene dichloride 25% Ethylene dibromide 15%	WHITE KIND COLD CREAM TOILET SOAP (Los Angeles Soap)	Pure soap Perfume Cold cream

*Consult Sec. II., Ingredients Index. This ingredient may be responsible for major toxic effects if poisonous amounts of this product are ingested.

Name & Use Manufacturer	Ingredients	Name & Use Manufacturer	Ingredients
WHITE DIAMOND WAX (Butcher)	Waxes Solvent* (Socony-Vacuum Sovasol #5) Gum turpentine*	WHITE'S HYDROLITE CASEIN WALL PAINT (White Co.)	Pigment: Titanium dioxide Diatomaceous silica Aluminum silicate Vehicle 64.78% Casein-resin emulsion solution
WHITE KIND D DETERGENT (Los Angeles Soap)	Alkyl aryl sulfonate* (from petroleum source) Polyphosphates* Sodium sulfate	DR. WHITE'S HYGIENIC POWDER (First National Labs.)	Menthol* Thymol Phenol* Sodium bicarbonate Eucalyptus Methyl salicylate* Borax* Sodium chloride
WHITE KING CLEANSER (Los Angeles Soap)	Silica Alkyl aryl type detergent* Sodium phosphate*		
WHITE KING WATER SOFTENER (Los Angeles Soap)	Sodium polyphosphate* Sodium sesqui carbonate	WHITE'S LONG LEADER COUGH SYRUP (First National Labs.)	Alcohol 6% Wild cherry bark White pine bark Oil pine tar Sodium citrate Menthol Malt syrup Chloroform 2 m./fl. oz. Squill Ammonium chloride Potassium guaiacol sulfonate
WHITE LADY BLEACH Bleach, cleaning compound (Howerton)	Sodium hypochlorite* 5.25%		
WHITE LINIMENT Veterinary (Roberts, Dr. D.)	Turpentine* Muriate of ammonia Castile soap Soft water	WHITE'S METHENE COUGH SYRUP (First National Labs.)	Each fl. oz.: Alcohol 1-1/2% Horehound Squill Thyme Benzocaine Glycerin Chloroform 2 m. Tolu Senega Capsicum Menthol Syrup base
WHITE MAGIC BLEACH (Home Needs)	Sodium hypochlorite*		
WHITE'S APPLIDERM-2 For skin disorders (White Labs.)	Menthol 0.2% Hexachlorophene 0.25% Hydrophilic emulsion base		
WHITE'S BABY COUGH SYRUP (First National Labs.)	Chloroform 2 m./fl. oz. Squill Ipecac Wild cherry bark Squill Sanguinaria	DR. WHITE'S MOTH KILLER (White, R.C.)	Cedar oil* Petroleum oil* Organic thiocyanates*
		DR. WHITE'S OIL-O-YUTH LINIMENT (First National Labs.)	Alcohol* 70% Chloroform* 4% Ether 2% Oils of cloves, origanum, sassafras* and wintergreen* Gum camphor* Phenol* Menthol* Capsicum Ammonia water
WHITE'S BLACK CROW COLD PILLS (First National Labs.)	Acetophenetidin* 2 gr. Aloin* Podophyllin quinine sulfate 2/5 gr. Camphor* Oleoresin capsicum		
DR. WHITE'S HEM-O-RO PILE OINTMENT (First National Labs.)	Aluminum acetate* Benzocaine Extract belladonna Phenol* Petrolatum base Zinc oxide Bismuth subgallate Menthol* Lanolin	WHITE'S PINK LAXATIVE PILLS (First National Labs.)	Each pill: Ext. belladonna leaf 1/12 gr. Phenolphthalein Aloin* Podophyllin Ipecec
		DR. WHITE'S PREPARATION FOR MINOR IRRITATIONS OF THE THROAT (First National Labs.)	Potassium chlorate* Boric acid* Balsam tolu Iron chloride* Glycerin

*Consult Sec. II., Ingredients Index. This ingredient may be responsible for major toxic effects if poisonous amounts of this product are ingested.

- 1052 -

Name & Use Manufacturer	Ingredients
WHITE'S PREPARED PAINT (White Co.)	Pigment: 37.00% Leaded zinc oxide * Barium sulfate Magnesium silicate Vehicle: Raw linseed oil Heat-treated linseed oil Mineral spirits *
WHITE'S VAGINAL SUPPOSITORIES (First National Labs.)	Boric acid* Benzoic acid * Oxyquinoline* Alkaloid Cocoa butter base
WHITE'S VARNISHES (White Co.)	Synthetic resins Vegetable oils Mineral spirits* and driers

WHITE'S
VARNISHES,
BAKELITE
FLOOR SEAL
(White Co.)
	Non-volatile (penarithyrol
	  resin, linseed and chinawood
	  oil) 38.00%
	Volatile(mineral spirits)*
	        62.00%

WHITE TAR DEODORANT PARADI- CHLORO- BENZENE VAPORIZER CAKES Insecticide (Reliable Chem.)	Paradichlorobenzene*
WHITE TAR MOTH BALLS (Koppers)	Refined naphthalene* 100%
WHITE TAR MOTH CAKE (Reliable Chem.)	Refined naphthalene*
WHITE TAR PARA NAP MOTH FLAKES (Reliable Chem.)	Refined naphthalene* Paradichlorobenzene
WHITE TAR TOILET BOWL BLOCK Deodorizer (Reliable Chem.)	Perfume naphthalene*
WHITE TAR TOILET BOWL ODORIZER (Reliable Chem.)	Perfume paradichlorobenzene*
WHITFIELD'S OINTMENT Fungicide (Boyle & Co.)	Benzoic acid 12% Salicylic acid* 6%
WHITFIELD'S OINTMENT (Purepac)	Benzoic acid 12% Salicylic acid* 6%
WHITMAN K-95 DISINFECTANT ANTISEPTIC DEODORANT CLEANSER (Whitman)	Pine oil* Soap

Name & Use Manufacturer	Ingredients

WHITMIRE'S
FLEAS-OFF
Repellent
(Whitmire)
	Pyrethrins I and II 0.136%
	Rotenone 0.084%
	Rotenoids & other cube resins
	        0.166%
	Tech. piperonyl butoxide 0.375%
	Ethylene glycol ether of pinene
	        4.750%
	Pine oil 2.000%
	Butoxy polypropylene glycol*
	        17.589%
	Para di-isobutyl phenoxy ethoxy
	  ethyl dimethyl benzyl ammonium
	  chloride 0.200%
	Isopropanol 13.200%
	Petroleum distillate 1.500%
	Propellent gas 60%

WHITMIRE'S
TICKS-OFF
INSECT
REPELLENT
BOMB
(Mine)
	Hydrogenated rotenone and other
	  cube resins 0.108%
	Rotenone and other cube resins
	  (Rotenone 0.098%; other
	  cube resins 0.229%) 0.327%
	Butoxy polypropylene glycol*
	        28.014%
	Ethylene glycol ether of pinene
	        0.981%
	Mineral oil refined 10.355%
	Isopropanol 14.715%
	Propellent gas 45.500%

WHITMOYER
BHC ROOST
PAINT
(Whitmoyer)
	Petroleum oils* 98.42%
	Gamma isomer of benzene
	  hexachloride* 1.50%
	Other isomers of benzene
	  hexachloride 0.08%

WHITMOYER B-T POWDER Anthelmintic (veterinary, avian) (Whitmoyer)	Nicotine (expressed as alkaloid)* 3.3% Phenothiazine 30.0% Strychnine* 0.16 gr./oz.
WHITMOYER CROW REPELLENT (Whitmoyer)	Tar oils* 96%
WHITMOYER INCUBATOR FUMIGANT (Whitmoyer)	Furfuraldehyde* Formaldehyde*

WHITMOYER
S Q S
For poultry
drinking water
(Whitmoyer)
	Solution of sulfaquinoxaline
	  sodium* (2-sulfanilamido-
	  quinoxaline sodium) in excess
	  sodium hydroxide 3.44 gm./100

WHITMOYER SULFA-T For poultry drinking water (Whitmoyer)	Sulfathiazole-sodium* 12.7% (w/v)
WHITMOYER TEKERESOL Disinfectant antiseptic cleanser (Whitmoyer)	Cresylic acid* Soap emulsifier
WHITMOYER VERMEX TABLETS Anthelmintic (Veterinary, avian) (Whitmoyer)	Nicotine alkaloid* 2.64% Phenothiazine 19.80% 2,2' Dihydroxy-5,5" dichloro diphenyl methane 14.85%

*Consult Sec. II., Ingredients Index. This ingredient may be responsible for major toxic effects if poisonous amounts of this product are ingested.

Name & Use Manufacturer	Ingredients	Name & Use Manufacturer	Ingredients
WHITMOYER WHIT-NIK Anthelmintic (veterinary, avian) (Whitmoyer)	Nicotine* (expressed as alkaloid) 5.0%	WHITTEMORE SCUFF (Shoe Polish (Liquid)) (Whittemore)	
WHITMOYER WHITOLINEUM Wood preservative (Whitmoyer)	Coal tar distillates* 97%	WHITTEMORE WAX SHOE POLISH (Whittemore)	
		WHIZ Fire extinguisher (Hollingshead)	Carbon tetrachloride*
WHITMOYER WHIT-PELS Chemical caponizing pellets for chickens, turkeys (Whitmoyer)	Diethylstilbestrol 15 mg./pellet	WHYTECOTE LIQUID PORCELAIN Paint (White Co.)	Pigment: Titanium dioxide Zinc oxide Vehicle: Alkyd resin solution Hydrogenated naphtha Mineral spirits and driers
WHITMOYER WHITPINE Disinfectant (Whitmoyer)	Steam distilled pine oil* Soap emulsifier	WHYTECOTE SEMI-GLOSS FOR INTERIOR WALL Paint (White Co.)	Pigment: Titanium calcium pigment Titanium dioxide Calcium carbonate Diatomaceous silica Zinc stearate Vehicle: Alkyd resin solution Varnish* Mineral spirits and driers*
WHITMOYER WHIT-SAN Detergent, sanitizer for washing eggs (Whitmoyer)	Alkyl (C_9-C_{15}) tolyl methyl trimethyl ammonium chlorides* 5% Sodium metasilicate, penta- hydrate 15% Sodium carbonate 20%		
WHITMOYER WHITSPRAY Insecticide (Whitmoyer)	Petroleum distillate* Tech. piperonyl butoxide Steam-distilled pine oil* Oil of eucalyptus* Pyrethrins*	WIGGS WATERLESS CLEANSER Cleanser, disinfectant (Wiggs)	Sodium palmitate Sodium stearate Trisodium phosphate Silicate of soda Sassafras perfume
WHITSPHILL Fungicide (medical) (Torch)	Salicylic acid* 6% Benzoic acid 12% Monobase	WILBERT'S DOT Abrasive cleaner (Wilbert)	
WHITSPHILL HALF STRENGTH Fungicide (medical) (Torch)	Salicylic acid* 3% Benzoic acid 6% Monobase	WILBERT'S FRESH-PINE DISINFECTANT CLEANER & DEODORANT (Wilbert)	Steam-distilled pine oil * Liquid soap
WHITSYN-5 For coccidiosis (veterinary, avian) (Whitmoyer)	2,4-Diamino-5-(p-chlorophenyl)- 6-ethylpyrimidine* Sulfaquinoxaline* Hydrated aluminum silicates	WILBERT'S NO-RUB FLOOR WAX (Wilbert)	Carnauba wax Synthetic resins Morpholine Oleic acid (red oil) Ammonia
WHITSYN-10 For coccidiosis (veterinary, avian) (Whitmoyer)	2,4-Diamino-5-(p-chlorophenyl)- 6-ethylpyrimidine* Sulfaquinoxaline*	WILBERT'S NO-RUB FURNITURE CREAM (Wilbert)	Sulfonated castor oil Mineral oil
WHITSYN-10 (With arsanilic acid) For coccidiosis (veterinary, avian) (Whitmoyer)	2,4-Diamino-5-(p-chlorophenyl)- 6-ethylpyrimidine Sulfaquinoxaline Arsanilic acid*	WILBERT'S SHOE POLISH (Paste) (Wilbert)	
WHITSYN-S For coccidiosis (veterinary, avian) (Whitmoyer)	2,4-Diamino-5-(p-chlorophenyl)- 6-ethylpyrimidine* Sulfaquinoxaline* Monoethanolamine Polyoxyethylene alkyl aryl ether Isopropyl alcohol* Propylene glycol	WILBERT'S SHOE WHITE (Wilbert)	Titanium dioxide Zinc oxide Talc Carboxymethylcellulose Gum acacia Sodium benzoate
		WILBUR'S ATHLETES FOOT LOTION Fungicide (medical) (Halsey)	Benzoic acid Salicylic acid* Boric acid* Glycerin Acetone* Non-greasy solvent

*Consult Sec. II., Ingredients Index. This ingredient may be responsible for major toxic effects if poisonous amounts of this product are ingested.

Name & Use Manufacturer	Ingredients	Name & Use Manufacturer	Ingredients
WILCO 55 FAST DRYING FLOOR FINISH (Wilson- Imperial		WILHOLD FLASH GLUE (Acorn Adh.)	Vinyl acetate Phenolic component
WILCO SEAL PENETRATING FLOOR FINISH (Wilson- Imperial)		WILHOLD GLUE WITH ORTHONOL (Acorn Adh.)	Polyvinyl acetate polymer Plasticizers 2% Hydrocarbons 1%
WILCOXSON'S PERFECTION LINIMENT Rubefacient (veterinary) (Wilcoxson)	Oil turpentine* Potassium iodide* Camphor* Alcohol	WILHOLD REE-STIK CEMENT (Acorn Adh.)	Latex rubber cement Hydrocarbon solution*
		WILHOLD WATERPROOF GLUE (Acorn Adh.)	Phenol-formaldehyde resin Compound of paraformaldehyde Walnut-shell flour

WILDFLOWER
COLOGNE
(Assoc.
Brands)
		WILKE'S
		CANINE FLEA
		POWDER
		(Wilke)
			Rotenone* 1.48%
			Other cube resins 2.94%
			Gamma isomer of benzene
			  hexachloride (from lindane)
			    1.00%
			DDT* 5.00%

WILDFLOWER PERFUME (Assoc. Brands)		WILKE'S 50% DDT WETTABLE POWDER Insecticide (Wilke)	DDT* 50%

WILDROOT
CREAM-OIL
Hair tonic
(Wildroot)
	Refined lanolin
	Liq. petrolatum
	Oxycholesterol
		WILKE'S
		HOUSEHOLD
		FLY SPRAY
		(Wilke)
			Beta thiocyano ethyl esters of
			  aliphatic acids containing
			  10-18 carbon atoms 0.625%
			Beta butoxy beta' thiocyano
			  diethyl ether 1.875%
			DDT* 5.000%
			Petroleum distillates*
			    92.500%

WILDROOT HAIR TONIC (Wildroot)			
WILDROOT SHAMPOO (Wildroot)		WILKE'S KAP-ETTES Tenderizer for poultry (Wilke)	Diethylstilbestrol 15 mg./pellet
WILHELM INSTANT Paint & Varnish Remover (Wilhelm)	Benzol volatile solvent* Higher aromatic solvents* Petroleum wax	WILKE'S PINK EYE POWDER For infections (veterinary) (Wilke)	Sulfanilamide* Neoprontosil* Sulfadiazine Sulfathiazole* Calomel*, mercury prep. 0.5%

WILHELM
WIL-STRIP
NON-
FLAMMABLE
PAINT,
VARNISH &
LACQUER
REMOVER
(Wilhelm)
	Methylene chloride*
	Thickeners, wetting agents
		WILKE'S
		POULTRY
		ROOST PAINT
		& SPRAY
		Insecticide
		(Wilke)
			Gamma isomer of benzene
			  hexachloride* (from lindane)
			    1.5%
			Inert ingredients*

WILHOLD BUILDERS ADHESIVE (Acorn Adh.)	Vinyl acetate Alkyd resins Plasticizers Portland cement Asbestos Other fibers	WILKE'S SHAMPOO Ectoparasiticide (veterinary) (Wilke)	Soap, anhydrous 25.00% Acetone* 12.50%
WILHOLD CEMENT RESIN (Acorn Adh.)	Polyvinyl acetate polymer solution Acetic acid	WILKE'S SULFA BALM For skin irritations, infections (veterinary) (Wilke)	Sulfanilamide 5% Sulfathiazole 5% Lanolin (wool fat) 15% Petrolatum 75%
WILHOLD CONTAX CEMENT (Acorn Adh.)	Neoprene rubber-based cement Toluol* Methyl ethyl ketone*		

---

*Consult Sec. II., Ingredients Index. This ingredient may be responsible for major toxic effects if poisonous amounts of this product are ingested.

Name & Use Manufacturer	Ingredients	Name & Use Manufacturer	Ingredients
WILLAT ALL-PURPOSE COLD PERMANENT WAVE LOTION (Heatless)	Ammonium thioglycolate* (pH 8.94)	WILLIAMSBURG DEEP TONES INTERIOR FINISH PAINTS (Atlantic V. & P.)	
WILLAT CIRCLETTE COLD WAVE LOTIONS Clear, opal golden (Heatless)	Ammonium thioglycolate*	WILLIAMS SHAVING CREAM (Williams, J.B.)	Potassium and sodium soaps Glycerin Boric acid*
		WILLIAMS SKAT (Williams, J.B.)	Ethyl hexanediol* Perfume Alcohol*
WILLAT DYNA CURL COLD WAVE LOTIONS (Heatless)	Three strength, X, XX and XXX, mono-thioglycerol* (pH 9.35)	WILL-KILL Insecticide (Miller Chem.)	Petroleum distillates*97.839% Tech. chlordane 2.000% Tech. piperonyl butoxide 0.115% Pyrethrins 0.046%
WILLAT GLIST'N AIRE Hair oil in aerosol can (Heatless)	Fine mineral oil	WILLOW PAINTS (Hoboken)	
WILLAT JUNIOR MISS COLD WAVE LOTION (Heatless)	Ammonium thioglycolate* (pH 9.3)	WILSO General purpose cleaner (Williams Co. (Mich.))	
WILLAT MAGIC RAIN COLD WAVE LOTION (Heatless)	Thioglycerol*	WILSON'S O.K. PLANT SPRAY Insecticide (Wilson, Andrew)	Potassium oleate 7.00% Emulsified oils of citronella and turpentine 2.00% Nicotine alkaloid* 1.60%
WILLAT MAGNAWAVE COLD WAVE LOTIONS (Heatless)	Mono-thioglycolate*	WINCHESTER SHOT GUN & RIFLE GREASE (Olin)	
WILLAT NEUTRALIZER Cosmetic (Heatless)	2 packages: 1 citric acid, mild 1 sod. perborate,* mild	WINDEX Window cleaner (Drackett)	
WILLAT PLYON COLD WAVE LOTIONS (Heatless)	Sodium thioglycolate* (pH 9.25)	WINDO-CEN Window cleaner (Central Chem.)	
WILLAT SKIN-KOTE Hand protective creme (Heatless)	Aluminum stearate	WINDO-CLEAN Cleaner (Hillyard)	Organic solvents*
WILLAT TONE-UP HAIRDRESSING (Heatless)	Triethanolamine stearate	WINDOW CLEAN (Stanley Home)	Snow floss Ammonia* Hydrated lime Carnauba wax Tergitol Dowicide Hydrocarbon solvent * Bentonite Wintergreen * Japan wax Vegetable emulsifier Dye
WILLAT WANDA COLD WAVE LOTIONS (Heatless)	Ammonium thioglycolate* (pH 9.03)		

---

*Consult Sec. II., Ingredients Index. This ingredient may be responsible for major toxic effects if poisonous amounts of this product are ingested.

Name & Use Manufacturer	Ingredients		Name & Use Manufacturer	Ingredients	
WINDOW CLEANER CONCENTRATE (Holcomb)	Dioxan*		WINRU C.P.R. VEGETABLE SPRAY CONC. Insecticide (Winru)	Piperonyl cyclonene tech.	2.12%
				Pyrethrins	0.21%
				Rotenone	1.06%
				Other cube resins	2.12%
				Pine oil, steam distilled*	30.68%
WINDOW WAX (Uncle Sam)	Oleic acid			Polymethyl naphthalenes*	12.77%
	Silica			Isothymoxy chloroethyl ether	1.70%
	Ammonia *			Mono- and di-isopropyl cresols	0.64%
	Naphtha *			Polyoxyethylene sorbitol mixed fatty acid ester	15.96%
WIND-O-WIPE Cleaner (Graham)				Soya bean oil refined	15.96%
				Petroleum oil	16.78%
WIND-O-WIPE WINDOW CLEANER (Henry Eng.)			WINRU DDT CHLORDANE CONCENTRATE Insecticide (Winru)	DDT	25%
				Tech. chlordane	10%
				Methylated naphthalenes*	42.5%
WINDSHIELD WASHER SOLVENT SUPER DRI (Park Chem.)	Ethyl or isopropyl alcohol*			Petroleum distillate	22.5%
			WINRU DDT CHLORDANE SPRAY Insecticide (Winru)	DDT*	5%
				Tech. chlordane	2%
WINDSOR PAINT & VARNISH CLEANER, RUG & UPHOLSTERY CLEANERS, VENETIAN BLIND CLEANER (Windsor Wax)				Methylated naphthalenes*	8.5%
				Petroleum distillates*	84.5%
			WINRU DDT-LINDANE CONC. Insecticide (Winru)	DDT	25%
				Gamma isomer of benzene hexachloride (from lindane)	2.5%
				Aromatic petroleum deriv. solvent*	67.5%
WINDY DAY LOTIONS Skin preparations (Assoc. Brands)			WINRU DDT-LINDANE SPRAY Insecticide (Winru)	DDT	2.50%
				Gamma isomer of benzene hexachloride (from lindane)	0.25%
				Aromatic petroleum deriv. solvent*	6.75%
WINERY SPECIAL Specialized cleaning product (Wyandotte)	Concentrated alkali*			Petroleum distillate*	90.50%
			WINRU 25% DDT OIL CONCENTRATE Insecticide (Winru)	DDT	25%
				Aromatic petroleum solvents*	75%
WING INSECTICIDE (Clean Home)	DDT*	5%	WINRU 5% DDT SPRAY Insecticide (Winru)	DDT*	5%
	Pyrethrum	5%		Methylated naphthalenes*	8.5%
WINNEBAGO BRAND PAINT (Parker, I.)				Petroleum distillates*	86.5%
			WINRU 90% EMULSIFIABLE CHLORDANE Insecticide (Winru)	Tech. chlordane*	90%
WINRU 20% CHLORDANE CONC. Insecticide (Winru)	Tech. chlordane*	20%	WINRU 45% EMULSIFIABLE CHLORDANE CONC. Insecticide (Winru)	Tech. chlordane*	45%
	Petroleum distillate*	80%		Polyoxyethylene sorbitol esters of mixed fatty acids	10%
				Petroleum distillate*	45%

*Consult Sec. II., Ingredients Index. This ingredient may be responsible for major toxic effects if poisonous amounts of this product are ingested.

Name & Use Manufacturer	Ingredients	Name & Use Manufacturer	Ingredients
WINRU 25% EMULSIFIABLE DDT Insecticide (Winru)	DDT 25% Aromatic petroleum solvent* 70%	WINRU PYRENONE FLY SPRAY (Winru)	Tech. piperonyl butoxide 0.25% Pyrethrins 0.03% Petroleum distillate* 99.72%
WINRU LINDANE 5 Insecticide (Winru)	Gamma isomer of benzene hexachloride (from lindane) 0.5% Aromatic petroleum deriv. solvent 1.9% Petroleum distillate* 97.6%	WINRU PYRENONE FOGGING SPRAY Insecticide (Winru)	Tech. piperonyl butoxide 1.26% Pyrethrins 0.16% Petroleum distillate* 98.58%
WINRU 20% LINDANE Insecticide (Winru)	Gamma isomer of benzene hexachloride (from lindane)* 20% Aromatic petroleum deriv. solvent* 75%	WINRU PYRENONE INDUSTRIAL SPRAY Insecticide (Winru)	Tech. piperonyl butoxide 3.00% Pyrethrins 0.30% Petroleum distillate* 96.70%
WINRU METHOXANE CONC. Insecticide (Winru)	Methoxychlor 24% Gamma isomer BHC (from lindane) 4% Aromatic petroleum deriv. solvent* 67%	WINRU PYRENONE LIVESTOCK SPRAY Insecticide (Winru)	Tech. piperonyl butoxide 11.55% Pyrethrins 1.16% Polyoxyethylene sorbitol ester of mixed fatty acids 8.78% Petroleum oil* 78.51%
WINRU METHOXANE SPRAY Insecticide (Winru)	Gamma isomer of benzene hexachloride (from lindane) 0.5% Methoxychlor 3.0% Aromatic petroleum deriv. solvents* 8.4% Petroleum distillate* 88.1%	WINRU PYRENONE MILL SPRAY Insecticide (Winru)	Tech. piperonyl butoxide 1.0% Pyrethrins 0.1% Petroleum distillate* 98.9%
WINRU METHOXY- CHLOR CONC. Insecticide (Winru)	Tech. methoxychlor 24% Aromatic petroleum deriv. solvent* 71%	WINRU PYRENONE OIL SPRAY CONC. Insecticide (Winru)	Tech. piperonyl butoxide 6.32% Pyrethrins 0.32% Petroleum distillate* 93.36%
WINRU PYRENONE CONC. 101 Insecticide (Winru)	Tech. piperonyl butoxide 12.15% Pyrethrins 1.22% Petroleum distillate* 86.63%	WINRU PYRENONE OIL SPRAY SPECIAL Insecticide (Winru)	Tech. piperonyl butoxide 3.16% Pyrethrins 0.16% Petroleum distillate* 96.68%
WINRU PYRENONE CONTACT SPRAY (Winru)	Tech. piperonyl butoxide 0.50% Pyrethrins 0.06% Petroleum distillate* 99.44%	WINRU PYRENONE ROACH SPRAY (Winru)	Petroleum distillate* Tech. piperonyl butoxide Pyrethrins*
WINRU PYRENONE DAIRY SPRAY Insecticide (Winru)	Tech. piperonyl butoxide 0.24% Pyrethrins 0.03% Mineral oil 99.73%	WINRU PYRENONE T-143 Insecticide (Winru)	Tech. piperonyl butoxide 10.0% Pyrethrins 1.0% Polyoxyethylene pentalaurate 4.5% Petroleum distillate* 84.5%
WINRU PYRENONE EMULSIFIABLE CONC. QUICK BREAKING Insecticide (Winru)	Tech. piperonyl butoxide 11.8% Pyrethrins 1.18% Polyoxyethylene sorbitol esters of mixed fatty acids 0.60% Petroleum distillate* 86.42%	WINRU PYRENONE VAPORIZER CONC. NO. 1 Insecticide (Winru)	Tech. piperonyl butoxide 2.5% Pyrethrins 0.31% Petroleum distillate* 97.19%
WINRU PYRENONE EMULSIFIABLE CONC. STABLE Insecticide (Winru)	Tech. piperonyl butoxide 11.8% Pyrethrins 1.18% Polyoxyethylene sorbitol esters of mixed fatty acids 14.75% Petroleum distillate* 72.27%	WINRU PYRENONE VAPORIZER CONC. NO. 2 Insecticide (Winru)	Tech. piperonyl butoxide 3.74% Pyrethrins 0.75% Petroleum distillate* 95.51%

*Consult Sec. II., Ingredients Index. This ingredient may be responsible for major toxic effects if poisonous amounts of this product are ingested.

- 1058 -

Name & Use Manufacturer	Ingredients	Name & Use Manufacturer	Ingredients
WINRU PYRENONE WATER EMULSION Insecticide (Winru)	Tech. piperonyl butoxide 1.47% Pyrethrins 0.15% Petroleum distillate 9.15% Polyoxyethylene sorbitol esters of mixed fatty acids 1.84%	WISK CREAM HAIR REMOVER (Sales)	
WINRU SPECIAL BIN SPRAY Insecticide (Winru)	DDT* 5% Tech. chlordane 2% Methylated naphthalenes* 8.5% Chloropicrin 0.05% Petroleum distillate* 84.45%	WISP-STICK HAIR DRESSING (Good Grooming)	
		WISTARIA SCENTED LOTION (Abbott)	Tragacanth Glycerin Boric acid Alcohol 7.2% Acetone 0.8%
WINRU SPECIAL RESIDUAL SPRAY Insecticide (Winru)	Petroleum distillate* Tech. chlordane* Tech. piperonyl butoxide Pyrethrins*	WITCH'S BREW For skin irritation (veterinary) (Kent Spec.)	Pure lard Kerosene* Petrolatum Coal tar oil* Castor oil Coal tar phenols Cresylic acid 0.40% Coal tar hydrocarbons 0.50% Sulfur* 35.00%
WINRU SPECIAL ROACH SPRAY (Winru)	Petroleum distillate* Tech. chlordane* Tech. piperonyl butoxide Pyrethrins*		
WINRU TWO-IN-ONE GRAIN FUMIGANT (Winru)	Carbon tetrachloride* 81.3% Carbon bisulfide* 12.1% Ethylene dibromide 6.6%	WIZARD GLASS & METAL POLISH (Boyle-Midway)	Silicone oil Petroleum naphtha Emulsifiers Siliceous abrasives
WINTER BALM Cosmetic (Smither & Hill)	Alcohol 30%	WIZARD GREASE REMOVER (Hatters)	
WINTERGREEN GERMICIDE (Uncle Sam)	Methyl salicylate* Emulsifiers Synthetic phenols*	WIZARD HAIR SPRAY (Boyle-Midway)	
WINTER-PHENE Bactericide (Varley)	Isopropyl alcohol* Vegetable oil soaps o-Benzyl p-chlorophenol Methyl salicylate* Essential oils*	WIZARD INK ERADICATOR (Ward's)	
WINTER VAPOROL SPRAY Insecticide (Calif. Spray)	Petroleum oils* 97%	WIZARD SPRAY DEODORIZER (Boyle-Midway)	Deodorant oil (essential oil type)* Emulsifiers
WIPE-ON (New improved super) Polish (Embree)	Plastic resin varnish*	WIZARD WICK DEODORIZER (Boyle-Midway)	Emulsifiers of the alkyl poly-oxyethylene glycol ester or hydroxypolyethoxy propyl stearate type Deodorant oils* Alcohol Formaldehyde Anti-oxidant
WISCONSIN PENTA PRESERVATIVE Controls chicken mites (Wisconsin Solv.)	Pentachlorophenol* 4.2% Other chlorophenols 0.6% Petroleum hydrocarbons* 95.0%		
		W. & L. FORMULA NO. 9 For scalp (Peau Seche)	Cholesterol Oil lavender Eugenol Oil thyme Oil nutmeg Balsam Peru Oil bay Oil neroli Oil bergamot Oil cassia Chloroform Denatured ethyl alcohol #40
WISCONSIN VETERINARY SALVE (Wisconsin Pharm.)	Zinc oxide Carbolic acid Hydroxyquinoline sulfate Lanolin Petrolatum		
WISK Liquid detergent (Lever)		W.O. INSULATING VARNISH (Standard-Toch)	

*Consult Sec. II., Ingredients Index. This ingredient may be responsible for major toxic effects if poisonous amounts of this product are ingested.

Name & Use Manufacturer	Ingredients	Name & Use Manufacturer	Ingredients
WOLTRA CAUSTIC PENCIL (Woltra)	Silver nitrate*	WONDER KOTE SEMI GLOSS WALL FINISH (Standard-Toch)	
WOLVERINE ANTI-FREEZE COMPOUND (Wolverine)		WONDER-LAC LACQUERS (Pennsylv. Lacquer)	
WOLVERINE PENTA-CHLOR Wood preservative (Wolverine)	Pentachlorophenol*	WONDER LIQUID SOAP (Uncle Sam)	Cochin cocoanut oil
WONDER-ALL FINISHES Paint (Egan & Hausman)		WONDER METAL POLISH (Uncle Sam)	Oxalic acid* Alcohol* Ammonia* Silica in water (contains no free acid)
WONDER BAR OIL POLISH (Uncle Sam)	Mineral oil Wax	WONDER ODORLESS DISINFECTANT (Uncle Sam)	Quaternary ammonium salts*
WONDERCOTE SEMI-INTERIOR PAINT (Sonneborn)		WONDER ODORLESS DISINFECTANT & SANITIZER (Uncle Sam)	Quaternary ammonium salts* Non-ionic detergent
WONDER CREME FURNITURE & AUTO POLISH (Wonder)		WONDER PINEAIR DISINFECTANT (Uncle Sam)	Steam-distilled pine oil* 15% Soap Synthetic phenols*
WONDER FLOOR OIL (Uncle Sam)	Paraffin base oil	WONDER PINE AROMA DISINFECTANT (Uncle Sam)	Steam-distilled pine oil* 40% Soap Isopropanol*
WONDERFUL DREAM BRAND SALVE (Wonderful)	Phenyl mercury benzoate 1-5000 Oil of tar Turpentine Olive oil Linseed oil Rosin Burgundy pitch Gum thus Camphor Beeswax Mutton tallow	WONDER PINE ODOR DEODORANT (Uncle Sam)	Pine oil* Soap
		WONDER PREPARED LIQUID WAX (Uncle Sam)	Carnauba Beeswax Ozokerite
WONDER GLO CLEANER & WATER SOFTENER (Wonder)		WONDER PREPARED PASTE WAX (Uncle Sam)	Carnauba Ozokerite wax
WONDER-GLOSS FURNITURE POLISH (Uncle Sam)	Mineral oil Wax Borax	WONDER RUG & UPHOLSTERY CLEANER (Uncle Sam)	Vegetable oils Potassium hydroxide* Synthetic detergent Naphtha*
WONDERGRO Chemical fertilizer (Flower City Plant)		WONDER SALVE For skin irritations (Drexel)	Oxyquinoline sulfate* Benzocaine Urea Menthol Camphor* Eucalyptol* Lanolin
		WONDER SCRUB SOAP (Uncle Sam)	Neutral vegetable oil base

*Consult Sec. II., Ingredients Index. This ingredient may be responsible for major toxic effects if poisonous amounts of this product are ingested.

Name & Use Manufacturer	Ingredients		Name & Use Manufacturer	Ingredients	
WONT-BURN FIRE RETARDENT PAINT (Resistall)			WOOD'S C-GO For colds (Wood Chem.)	Alcohol 5% Sodium salicylate* F.E. cascara aromatic Elix lactated pepsin Syrup of tolu F.E. belladonna 2 m./oz. Menthol * Essence peppermint	
WOODBRITE Furniture polish (Boyle-Midway)			WOOD'S DIXIRUB LINIMENT (Wood Chem.)	Menthol* Camphor gum* Eucalyptol* Pine oil*	
WOODBURY SHAMPOO (Liquid) (Woodbury, John H.)			WOOD'S HED'S TABLETS Analgesic (Wood Chem.)	Aspirin * gr. iiiss Phenacetin* gr. iiss Caffeine citrate gr. ss	
WOODBURY TOILET SOAP (Jergens)			WOOD'S HISTO For colds (Wood Chem.)	Alcohol 5% Sodium salicylate* F.E. cascara aromatic Elix. lactated pepsin Syrup of tolu Thonzylamine-HCl* 15 mg./tsp. Menthol* Essence peppermint	
WOOD FIX Wood preservative (Thompson Chem.)	Pentachlorophenol* 40% Petroleum solvents 35%				
WOODLAND'S RAT & MOUSE REPELLENT POWDER (Woodland)	Sodium fluosilicate*		WOOD'S PEP-LAX Laxative (Wood Chem.)	F.E. cascara aromatic F.E. podophyllin Essence peppermint Elixir lactated pepsin	
WOODLEY'S EYE DROPS For ophthalmic irritation (Carolina)	Berberine sulfate Boric acid Zinc sulfate		WOODTREAT NO. 112 READY-TO-USE Wood preservative (Wood-Treating)	Zinc naphthenate* 10% Tetrachlorophenol 0.2% Coconutamine 0.18% Oil* 77%	
WOODLIFE Wood preservative (Protection)	Pentachlorophenol* 3.0% Tetrachlorophenol 1.5% 2-Chlororthophenylphenol 0.5% Petroleum solvent* 85.0%		WOODTREAT 113 READY-TO-USE Wood preservative (Wood-Treating)	Zinc naphthenate* 12.5% Water repellents 4% Mineral spirits* 83.5%	
WOOD-REM Wood preservative (Speco)	Hydrocarbon vehicle* Resins Plasticizers Coal tar solvents* Creosote*		WOODTOX NO. 116 CONC. Wood preservative (Wood-Treating)	Pentachlorophenol* 11% Pine oil* 11% Oil 42%	
WOOD'S ALA For malaria (Wood Chem.)	Quinine sulfate solution of iron chloride Magnesium sulfate Citric acid				
WOOD'S A.T.O. OINTMENT Fungicide (medical) (Wood Chem.)	Carbolic acid* 5 m./oz. Menthol * Iodoform calamine Salicylic acid* Sulfur prec.* Zinc oxide		WOODTOX NO. 116 READY TO USE Wood preservative (Wood-Treating)	Pentachlorophenol* 5% Pine oil* 11% Oil 42%	
WOOD'S BABALAX (For colds) mild laxative (Wood Chem.)	Sodii salicylate* 20 gr./oz. F.E. cascara aromatic F.E. senna Syrup tolu		WOODTOX 120 CONCEN-TRATE Wood preservative (Wood-Treating)	Pentachlorophenol* 17.68% Other chlorophenols and related compounds 3.12% Pine oil 4.20% Mineral spirits* 41.30% Water repellents 33.70%	
WOOD'S BISMOMIX Antacid, digestant (Wood Chem.)	Milk of bismuth Tr. opii camphorated Lactated pepsin Tr. gambir				

*Consult Sec. II., Ingredients Index. This ingredient may be responsible for major toxic effects if poisonous amounts of this product are ingested.

Name & Use Manufacturer	Ingredients	Name & Use Manufacturer	Ingredients
WOODTOX 120 READY-TO-USE Wood preservative (Wood-Treating)	Pentachlorophenol 4.15% Other chlorophenols and related compounds 0.85% Mineral spirits* 86.0% Inactive ingred: Water repellents and special solvents 9.00%	WRIGHT'S SILVER CREAM (Wright, J.)	Diatomaceous earth Soap Soda ash
WOODWARD-WANGER'S Drain clean (Woodward-Wanger)	Sodium hydroxide*	WRISLEY WATER SOFTENER (Wrisley)	Baking soda Washing soda Sodium borate* Phosphates*
		WUNDER-SKIN For acne (Purepac)	2,2'-Methylene bis (3,4,6-trichlorophenol)* Sulfur* Resorcinol* Alcohol* 10%
WOOLSEY ANTI-FOULING HARD RACING FINISH (Woolsey)	Toluidine red 9% Acetomercuri benzene* 7% Soya alkyd resin 42% Mineral spirits* 42%	WUN FLAT PAINT (Parker Paint)	
WOOSTER PAINT BRUSH CLEANER (Wooster)		WYAMINE INHALER (Wyeth Labs.)	Each inhaler: Mephentermine* (N-methyl-phenyl-tert-butylamine) 250 mg. Menthol 10 mg. Aromatics
WORKMASTER WALLPAPER CLEANER (Cincy)	Wheat flour Refined kerosene oil Vegetable dye Salt Preservatives	WYAMINE SULFATE, NASAL SOLUTION Nasal decongestant (Wyeth Labs.)	Wyamine sulfate* 0.5% Chlorobutanol 0.5%
WORMAL GRANULES (Salsbury's)	Dibutyltin dilaurate (butynorate) 7% Nicotine* 3% Phenothiazine 29%		
WORMIX Anthelmintic (veterinary, avian) (Salsubry's)	Phenothiazine 55.0% Nicotine* (expressed as alkaloid) 5.5%	WYAMINE-TYROTHRICIN NASAL SOLUTION Nasal decongestant (Wyeth Labs.)	n-Methyl-tert-butylamine sulfate 0.5% Tyrothricin 0.02% Chlorobutanol 0.5%
WOR-MOR POWDER Anthelmintic (veterinary, avian) (Hilltop)	Phenothiazine Copper sulfate 26% Nicotine sulfate* Nux vomica 9% Capsicum Oil of anise U.S.P. Kamala Iron sulfate Areca nut 4-1/2%	WYANDOTTE BAKERY PAN CLEANER (Wyandotte)	Sodium chromate*
WORM-X-BALL Anthelmintic (veterinary) (Thoroughbred)	Phenothiazene*	WYANDOTTE CALCIUM CHLORIDE* Used for laying dust, melting ice, dehumidifying basements, etc. (Wyandottee)	Calcium chloxide*
W.P.T. COUGH SYRUP Antitussive (Royal Pharm.)	Alcohol 6%/v Chloroform 3m/fl. oz. Extract of white pine Aralia Poplar buds Wild cherry Blood root Sassafras Tar with menthol	WYANDOTTE NO. 91 FLAKE ALKALI Cleaning product (Wyandotte)	Conc. alkali*
WRIGHT FURNITURE CREAM (Shield-All)	Sulfonated castor oil Mineral oil Artifical oil of citronella	WYANDOTTE K-5 Laundry and textile detergent (Wyandotte)	Conc. alkali*
WRIGHT'S PAINT & VARNISH CLEANER (Wright, J.)			

*Consult Sec. II., Ingredients Index. This ingredient may be responsible for major toxic effects if poisonous amounts of this product are ingested.

- 1062 -

Name & Use Manufacturer	Ingredients		Name & Use Manufacturer	Ingredients	
WYANDOTTE 770 Laundry and textile detergent (Wyandotte)	Conc. alkali*		X BOILER LIQUID Plumbing and heating product ("X")	Tannins* Asbestos Isopropyl alcohol*	37-38%
WYANOID OINTMENT For relief of hemorrhoids (Wyeth Labs.)	Zinc oxide Ephedrine sulfate Balsam Peru Boric acid Benzocaine Emollient base		X BOILER RUSTOFF Plumbing and heating prod. ("X")	Sodium carbonate monohydrate 50% Potassium bichromate* 50% Orange dye	
WYANOIDS Suppositories for hemorrhoids (Wyeth Labs.)	Ext. belladonna 0.5% Zinc oxide Bismuth oxyiodide Balsam Peru Ephedrine sulfate 0.1% Boric acid Bismuth subcarbonate Cocoa butter		X-CELL-ALL LIQUID BRUSH CLEANER (Nat'l Chem. & Mfg.)	Alcohol Benzol* Methanol	
WYETH CASCARA PETROGALAR Cathartic (Wyeth Labs.)	Aqueous extract cascara sagrada (not U.S.P.) 13.2% Mineral oil 65%		X-CELL-ALL LIQUID PAINT & VARNISH REMOVER (Nat'l Chem. & Mfg.)	Alcohol Benzol* Methanol Wax	
WYETH COLLYRIUM Eye lotion (Wyeth Labs.)	Antipyrine 0.4% Boric acid Borax Sodium ethyl-mercuri-thio- salicylate 0.002%		X-CELL-ALL NO-WASH, NON- FLAMMABLE PAINT & VARNISH REMOVER (Nat'l Chem. & Mfg.)	Methylene chloride* Methanol*	
WHETH COLLYRIUM WITH EPHEDRINE Eye drops (Wyeth Labs.)	Boric acid Borax Antipyrine 0.4% Ephedrine 0.1% Sodium ethyl-mercuri-thio- salicylate 0.002%		X-CELL-ALL SEMI-PASTE PAINT & VARNISH REMOVER (Nat'l Chem. & Mfg.)	Alcohol Benzol* Methanol Wax	
WYETH FIRST AID POWDER Veterinary antiseptic dry dressing (Wyeth Labs.)	Bismuth oxyiodide Zinc phenolsulfonate Phenol* Menthol* Alum Bismuth subgallate Allantoin Thymol* Eucalyptol * Boric acid* Ortho-benzyl-para-chlorophenol Zinc oxide Bismuth subcarbonate Magnesium carbonate		X-ECUTE INSECTICIDE BOMB (Beebe Ness)	Allethrin (allyl homolog of cinerin 1) 0.15% DDT (dichloro diphenyl tri- chloroethane) 1.00% Methoxychlor tech. 1.00% Beta butoxy beta thiocyano diethyl ether 1.00% n-Octyl bicycloheptene dicarboximide 1.00% Methylated aromatic petroleum deriv.* 5.00% Petroleum distillates 5.85%	
WYETH POISON IVY-OAK- SUMAC COMBINED EXTRACT (Wyeth Labs.)	Almond oil Resins of poison ivy, oak and sumac Chlorobutanol 0.5%		X FABRIC COAT Automotive product ("X")	Titanium dioxide 13% Aluminum stearate 1% Calcium carbonate 13% Mineral spirits * 33% Cobalt (6%) 0.5% Lead (24%) 0.5%	
X BLOCK LIQUID Automotive product ("X")	Tannins* 37-38% Asbestos Isopropyl alcohol*		X-L AIR CLEANERS Bathroom deodorant (Reliable Chem.)	Paradichlorobenzene* 100%	
X BOILER FLUSH Plumbing and heating product ("X")	Asbestine 50% Sodium carbonate monohydrate 25% Trisodium phosphate 15% Tannins 5% Sodium bichromate* appx. 5%		X LIQUID KARWASH Cleaner ("X")	Salt of dodecylbenzene sulfonate Sodium sulfate Lauryl diethanolamide Diethanolamine	

*Consult Sec. II., Ingredients Index. This ingredient may be responsible for major toxic effects if poisonous amounts of this product
are ingested.

Name & Use Manufacturer	Ingredients	Name & Use Manufacturer	Ingredients
X LIQUID SEALER (Blonde) Automotive product ("X")	Starch Asbestos Isopropyl alcohol* Cellulose gum (high viscosity form of sodium carboxy-methylcellulose) Soda ash	X-38 SCREW-WORM CONTROL (veterinary) (Lee, G.)	Dichloro diphenyl trichloro-ethane tech. 25.0% Gamma isomer of benzene hexachloride (from lindane) 4.5% Xylene tech.* 57.0%
X LIQUID SEALER (Regular & Dark) Automotive product ("X")	Tannins * 35% Asbestos Isopropyl alcohol* Cresylic acid 0.5%	X WATER PUMP LUBRICANT & RUSTOFF Lubricant and rust and scale inhibitor ("X")	Water-soluble emulsifying oil 20%/v
X-L-O DDT MOTH SPRAY NO: 83 (Troy Ind.)	Orthodichlorobenzol* Petroleum distillate Ethylene dichloride DDT*	XX MOTH KILL CYRSTALS & LIQUID (United Chem.)	
X-PANDOTITE FURNITURE CEMENT & FILLER (X-Pando)	Oxychloride type	XX ROACH POWDER (United Chem.)	
X-PANDOTITE PATCHING CEMENT (X-Pando)	Oxychloride type	XXX PLASTIC WALL FINISH Paints (Muralo)	
X PIPECUT OIL Plumbing and heating product ("X")	Esso Pennex #40 cutting oil	XXX (Triple) AGRIFUME INSECT SPRAY 50 (Leffingwell)	Tetraethyl pyrophosphate* 20% Other related organic phosphates 30%
X PIPEJOIN Plumbing and heating product ("X")	Mineral oil 42%/w Bentonite 15%/w Vermiculite 29%/w Lithopone* 14%/w Turpentine 1%/w	XXX (Triple) ALCUFE Fungicide (Leffingwell)	Copper (expressed as metallic)* 6.0%
X POWDER KARWASH Cleaner ("X")	Sodium salt of docylbenzene sulfonate 40% Sodium sulfate 60%	XXX (Triple) ARAMITE-DDT DUST 3-5 Insecticide (Leffingwell)	2-(p-tert-Butylphenoxy) isopropyl-2-chloroethyl sulfite 3.0% DDT* 5.0%
X RADIATOR FLUSH Scale and sludge remover ("X")	Soda ash Sodium bichromate 1%/w Caustic soda 1/3 of 1% Kerosene 9%/w Steam-distilled pine oil 3%/w Red oil (oleic acid) 3% Isopropyl alcohol 2%/w Caustic potash 0.3%/w	XXX (Triple) COPPER BORDEAUX 12-1/2 Fungicide (Leffingwell)	Copper (expressed as metallic)* 12.5%
X SUPER FLUSH Scale and sludge remover ("X")	Top compartment: Oxalic acid* (flake form) Boric acid, granular* DuPont's Milori blue dye Bottom compartment: Sodium carbonate monohydrate 85% Potassium bichromate* 15% Orange pigment	XXX (Triple) COPPER BORDEAUX 22 Fungicide (Leffingwell)	Copper (expressed as metallic)* 22.0%
		XXX (Triple) DDT SPRAY 45 Insecticide (Leffingwell)	DDT* 4.5%
X-TERMIN-8 Wood preservative (Planetary Chem.)	Tech. pentachlorophenol* 5% Petroleum solvent* 90%	XXX (Triple) DDT-SULPHUR DUST 5-50 Insecticide (Leffingwell)	DDT* 5.0% Sulfur* 50.0%

---

*Consult Sec. II., Ingredients Index. This ingredient may be responsible for major toxic effects if poisonous amounts of this product are ingested.

Name & Use Manufacturer	Ingredients		Name & Use Manufacturer	Ingredients	
XXX (Triple) FLOWABLE HEAVY MEDIUM Insecticide (Leffingwell)	Petroleum oil*	82%/w	XXX (Triple) NUTRA-SPRAY 20-4 Fungicide (Leffingwell)	Zinc (expressed as metallic)* 20.0% Copper (expressed as metallic)* 4.0%	
XXX (Triple) KLOROMITE 50 WETTABLE Insecticide (Leffingwell)	p-Chlorophenyl p-chlorobenzene sulfonate*	50%	XXX (Triple) PARATHION 50W Insecticide (Leffingwell)	Parathion (o,o-diethyl-o-(p-nitrophenyl) thiophosphate)* 50%	
XXX (Triple) KLOROMUL Insecticide (Leffingwell)	p-Chlorophenyl p-chlorobenzene sulfonate*	20.0%/w	XXX (Triple) ROTO-FLO 50R Insecticide (Leffingwell)	Petroleum oil* 82.00%/w Rotenone 0.20% Other extractive of cube and/or derris 0.40%	
XXX (Triple) LINDANE DUST 1 Insecticide (Leffingwell)	Gamma isomer of benzene hexachloride (from lindane)	1.00%	XXX (Triple) TOXAPHENE PARATHION 10-2 DUST Insecticide (Leffingwell)	Toxaphene 10.0% Parathion* 2.0%	
XXX (Triple) LIQUID 2,4-D (64) Herbicide (Leffingwell)	Alkanolamine salts of 2,4-dichloro phenoxy acetic acid*	66.8%	XXX (Triple) UNICIDE 60 Insecticide (Leffingwell)	Petroleum oil* 99.0%/w	
XXX (Triple) LIQUID THRIP-TOX Insecticide (Leffingwell)	Sabadilla alkaloid complexes	0.50%	XXX (Triple) ZINC MANGANESE NUTRA-SPRAY 18-7 Agricultural use (Leffingwell)	Zinc (expressed as metallic)* 18.5% Manganese (expressed as metallic)* 7.0%	
XXX (Triple) MALATHION 25-W Insecticide (Leffingwell)	Malathion*	25.0%	XXX (Triple) ZINC NUTRA-SPRAY 20 Agricultural use (Leffingwell)	Zinc (expressed as metallic)* 20.5%	
XXX(Triple) NUTRA-PHOS 5 Agricultural use (Leffingwell)	Zinc (expressed as metallic)* 16.5% Manganese (expressed as metallic)* 7.0% Phosphoric acid 5.0%		XZIT SOOT DESTROYER (Xzit)		
XXX (Triple) NUTRA-PHOS 10 Agricultural use (Leffingwell)	Zinc (expressed as metallic)* 14.0% Manganese (expressed as metallic)* 7.0% Phosphoric acid * 10.0%		YAGER'S LINIMENT For skin irritations, rubefacient (Yager)	Ammonia Camphor* Oil of camphor* Sassafras Turpentine*	
XXX (Triple) NUTRA-SPRAY 14-14 Agricultural use (Leffingwell)	Zinc* 14.0% Manganese* 14.0%		YANKY CLOVER COLOGNE & TOILET WATER (Hudnut, R.)		
XXX (Triple) NUTRA-SPRAY 17-4-4 Agricultural use (Leffingwell)	Zinc* 17.5% Manganese* 4.0% Copper* 4.0%		YARDLEY BOND STREET ENGLISH COMPLEXION POWDER (Yardley)		
			YARDLEY HAND CREAM (Yardley		

*Consult Sec. II., Ingredients Index. This ingredient may be responsible for major toxic effects if poisonous amounts of this product are ingested.

- 1065 -

Name & Use Manufacturer	Ingredients
YARDLEY OLD ENGLISH LAVENDER TOILET SOAP (Yardley)	
YARDLEY SHAVING CREAM (Yardley)	Stearic acid soft soap Lavender essential oils
YARDLEY SHAVING LOTION (Yardley)	Menthol Alcohol Lavender essential oils
YDROZINCOL Ointment for external use (San Pedro)	Ammoniated mercury* 1-1/3% Ichthammol Zinc oxide Camphor*
YERBA SANTA TROCHES Antitussive (Boericke & Runyon)	Eriodictyon Extract of glycyrrhiza
YODORA DEODORANT CREAM (McKesson)	
YOST'S ORIGINAL SCALP FORMULA (House of Yost)	Lecithin combined with neutral and essential oils * Oxyquinoline benzoate* Isopropyl alcohol * Fluid extract capsicum Hexachlorophene*
YOUELL'S LIQUID RAT & MOUSE EXTERMINATOR (Allen)	Arsenic trioxide* 3.20%
YOUNG FOLKS COLOGNE, BUBBLE BATH, EASY CLEAN & SHAMPOO (Hudnut, R.)	
YOUNG SKIN LINE DEODORANT (Laird)	
ZALKON WET DRESSING (Gordon Labs.)	Benzalkonium chloride 1-2000 Sodium borate* Sodium bicarbonate Sodium chloride Menthol * Thymol * Oil of eucalyptus *
ZAN-Z-LAC Q.D. ENAMEL Paint (Davis, H.B.)	Titanium dioxide Zinc oxide Soya alkyd resin solution Petroleum thinners* Non volatile driers Volatile (petroleum thinners)

Name & Use Manufacturer	Ingredients
ZAT 448 Insect repellent (H. & M.)	NMRI-448 repellent* 80% Ethyl alcohol
Z.B.T. BABY POWDER WITH OLIVE OIL (Centaur- Caldwell)	Talc Olive oil
ZEAL For burns (Carolina)	Boric acid * Tannic acid * Glycerin Carbolic acid 1% Menthol Isopropyl alcohol 1.5%
ZEEMADE For skin irritations (veterinary) (Binday)	Salicylic acid* Coal tar* Sulfur* Alcohol 4%
ZEEN RUG & UPHOLSTERY CLEANER (Zeen)	
ZEETONE PAINT REMOVER & STAIN (Riverside)	
ZEF-IR DEODORIZER (Huntington)	
ZEHRUNG ESTER BRUSH KILLER (Zehrung)	Isopropyl ester of 2,4-D* Isopropyl ester of 2,4,5-T*
ZEHRUNG 2,4-D ESTER WEED KILLER (Zehrung)	Isopropyl ester of 2,4-D*
ZEHRUNG 2,4-D SELECTIVE AMINE WEED KILLER (Zehrung)	Dimethylamine salt of 2,4-D*
ZEHRUNG 2,4,5-T BLACKBERRY VINE KILLER (Zehrung)	Isopropyl ester of 2,4,5,-T*
ZEHRUNG WEED BLITZ Herbicide (Zehrung)	Dimethylamine salt of 2,4-D* Dimethylamine salt of 2,4,5-T*
ZEMACOL For chapped skin (Norwich)	Zyloxin (ortho-chloro-mercuri- phenol) 0.04% Zinc acetate Salicylic acid* Carbolic acid* Alcohol 2%

*Consult Sec. II., Ingredients Index. This ingredient may be responsible for major toxic effects if poisonous amounts of this product are ingested.

Name & Use Manufacturer	Ingredients		Name & Use Manufacturer	Ingredients	
ZEMO Antiseptic (Rose, E.W.)	Alcohol Carbolic acid* Sodium salicylate* Methyl salicylate* Borax* Menthol* Boric acid* Benzoic acid * Thymol * Eucalyptol* Essential oils *	35%	ZERONE ANTI-RUST ANTI-FREEZE (du Pont)	Methanol base*	
ZEMO OINTMENT (Rose, E.W.)	Bismuth subnitrate G-11 (hexachlorophene)* Zinc oxide Menthol* Iodobenzoic acid Methyl salicylate* Boracic acid*		ZERO-10 For colds (Dacus)	Alcohol Fl. ext. cascara sagrada aromatic Sodium salicylate* Menthol* Elixir lactated pepsin Chloroform Syrup ipecac Balsam Peru	2-6/10%
ZENE-A-TROL Anthelmantic (Pratt Food)	Phenothiazine N.F.* Lorol alcohol Polyvinyl alcohol Algin Coumarin N.F.	98.8% 0.5% 0.4% 1.2%	Z-G-G PASTE Ointment (CaPhenin)	Zinc oxide Gelatin Glycerin	
ZEN-O-PHEN Anthelmintic (veterinary, avian) (Corn King)	Phenothiazine*	100%	ZILATONE TABLETS Cathartic, choleretic (Drew Pharm.)	Extract nux vomica (strychnine 1/217 gr.) 1/16 gr. Phenolphthalein 1/2 gr. Bile salts compound 1-1/8 gr. Ext. cascara sagrada 3/4 gr. Pancreatin 7/8 gr. Pepsin (triple strength) 3/20 gr. Capsicum 1/10 gr.	
ZEN-O-PHEN POWDER Anthelmintic (veterinary) (Corn King)	Phenothiazine*	100%	ZIMATE DUST 5-50S Fungicide (Sunland)	Zinc ethylene-bis(dithiocar- bamate) 5% Sulfur* 50%	
ZEN VITREOUS CLEANER (Holcomb)	Hydrochloric acid*		ZIN-AL-COL LIQUID For skin irritations and sun burn (Drug Prod., N.Y.)	Carbolic acid 1% Colloidal zinc hydroxide Solution aluminum acetate * Menthol * Glycerin Lime water Rose water	
ZEO-DUR (Permutit)	Complex alumino-silicate compound Ion exchanges used in water softeners		ZINC CHLORIDE POISON Rodenticide (Santa Clara)	Zinc chloride*	
ZEO-KARB (Permutit)	Sulfonated bituminous coal				
ZEPHIRAN CHLORIDE Antiseptic, germicide (Winthrop)	High molecular, alkyl dimethyl- benzyl ammonium chlorides*		ZINC COPOSIL FUNGICIDE (Calif. Spray)	Copper (expressed as metallic)* 19%	
ZEREX ANTI-RUST ANTI- FREEZE (du Pont)	Ethylene glycol base*		ZINCFRIN For eye irritations (Alcon)	Zinc sulfate 0.25% Benzalkonium chloride* Phenylephrine hydrochloride U.S.P. 0.12%	
ZERLATE ZIRAM FUNGICIDE (du Pont)	Zinc dimethyl dithiocarbamate*		ZINC FUNGICIDE DUST 5 (Sunland)	Complex ferric-zinc ethylene- bis(dithiocarbamate) 5.0%	
ZERO CAULKING COMPOUND (Monroe Co.)			ZINCOFAX For skin irritations (Burroughs- Wellcome)	Zinc oxide 15% Lanolin	
ZERO (Liquid Cleaning Composition (Hood)	Synthetic organic detergent materials* Phosphates*		ZIN-EMUL #1 For skin irritations (Texas Pharm.)	Zinc oxide Corn starch Glycerin	
			ZIN-EMUL #2 For skin irritations (Texas Pharm.)	Zinc oxide Zinc carbonate Corn starch Cholesterin U.S.P. mineral oil	

*Consult Sec. II., Ingredients Index. This ingredient may be responsible for major toxic effects if poisonous amounts of this product are ingested.

Name & Use Manufacturer	Ingredients	Name & Use Manufacturer	Ingredients
ZING Insecticide (Planetary Chem.)	Refined chlordane 2% DDT* (dichloro diphenyl tri-chloroethane) 3% Petroleum distillate (deodorized)* 95%	ZONITE Antiseptic, deodorant (Zonite)	Sodium hypochlorite* Sodium hydroxide* Sodium chloride
ZINK-O-DUST Insecticide (Woolfolk)	Sulfur 74% Lead arsenate* 4.55% Zinc 2% DDT 5%	ZONITORS Vaginal suppositories (Zonite)	Chloramine *
ZIP KILL INSECT KILLER (Allied Home)	DDT 3.000% Methoxychlor tech. 1.00% Allethrin 0.100% n-Octyl bicyloheptene dicarboximide 0.166% Isobornyl thiocyanoacetate 0.820% Other related terpenes 0.180% Aromatic petroleum deriv.* 12.000% Petroleum distillate 2.734%	ZORATOR TOILET BOWL DEODORANT (Curran)	Naphthalene* 100%
		ZOTOX CRAB GRASS KILLER (Garden Prod.)	Arsenic acid * 37.5%
		ZOTOX WITH ZIRCONIUM For poison ivy, oak, sumac (Zotox)	Hydrous zirconia
		ZUDS AUTO WASH (Wellesley)	
ZIP-OFF Paint remover (Andersen)	Methylene chloride* (paint-remover grade) Methanol*	ZUD SPECIALTY CLEANER & RUST REMOVER (Rustain)	
ZIPOLA Zipper lubricant (High Chem.)	Petroleum waxes Perchlorethylene base	ZURD Rodenticide (Murd)	Warfarin 0.025%
ZIPPY LIQUID LAUNDRY STARCH (Zippy)	Corn starch Salt Pine oil * Sodium fluoride *	ZX-7 For acne and skin irritations (Nemow)	Pyrilamine maleate* Tyrothricin Hexachlorophene Benzocaine Zinc oxide Bismuth subsalicylate Menthol *
ZIRADRYL CREAM For poison ivy or oak (Parke Davis)	Benadryl hydrochloride* (diphenhydramine hydrochloride) 2% Zirconium oxide (as the carbonate) in cream base 4%	ZYLAX TABLETS Laxative (Glidden, O.)	Acetophenolisatin 5 mg. Debittered brewers dried yeast 160 mg. Sodium carboxymethylcellulose 0.3 gm.
ZIRCOCARB LOTION For poison ivy, sumac and oak (Vogel)	Carbonated hydrous zirconia 4.5% Zirconium acetate 1.0% Glycerin	ZYLON CLOSET BOWL CLEANER ZYLON DRAIN CLEANER, ZYLON PIPE & TRAP CLEANER (Zylon)	
ZIRNOX For skin irritations; poison ivy,oak (Bristol Labs.)	Bristamin (brand of phenyl-toloxamine) dihydrogen citrate 1% Zirconium oxide 4%	ZYMELOSE GRANULES Laxative (Glidden, O.)	Each 1/2 tsp: Debittered brewers dried yeast 0.64 gm. Sodium carboxymethylcellulose 2.0 gm.
ZIZ-O Drain pipe and sewer cleaner (Hillyard)	Potassium hydroxide*	ZYMELOSE TABLETS Laxative (Glidden, O.)	Each tablet: Debittered brewers dried yeast 160 mg. Sodium carboxymethylcellulose 0.5 gm.
Z-M-O For muscular aches, neuralgia, sprains, bruises, insect bites, etc. (Mace)	Camphor* Safrol * Oil of eucalyptus * Menthol* Methyl salicylate* Turpentine* Cotton seed oil Mineral oil	ZYMENOL Laxative (Glidden, O.)	Brewers yeast culture 12% Mineral oil 50%
ZOKON PAINT REMOVER (Lester)	Mild alkali* Methylene chloride*	ZYMOLE TROKEYS (Consolid. Royal)	Menthol * Oil of eucalyptus * Oil of red thyme Oil of peppermint Gum acacia

*Consult Sec. II., Ingredients Index. This ingredient may be responsible for major toxic effects if poisonous amounts of this product are ingested.

General Formulations

Introduction

In this section are given in alphabetical order several hundred formulas for products and preparations commonly found in households and on farms. These formulas are offered when ingredients and composition of a product are not listed in the *Trade Mark Index*, Section V. A precise statement is not important; formulas are needed only to orient the physician. His questions are:

What kinds of materials are usually employed?

Are there any highly toxic components?

About what percentage of the product is the toxic component?

What can be said about its nature?

Directions for use

I. Use this Section VI *if ingredients are unknown*
   a. Specifically, if the trade name is known and the category of use (furniture polish, laundry bleach) is known but ingredients are not listed in the Trade Mark Index; or,
   b. If the category of use is known but trade name is unknown.

II. *See Index (i.e., Table of Contents) on p. 1073*
   Alphabetical listing of categories of use.

III. *Consult appropriate formula*
   a. Note toxicity rating.
   b. Note ingredients starred (asterisks). (The starred ingredient may be responsible for major toxic effects.)

IV. *Consult Ingredients Index, Section II*

The Index

The key to the General Formulations Section lies on p. 1073. This thoroughly cross-indexed list should be examined for the common name, category of use, or type of product responsible for the poisoning. The index category refers by page number to a statement of composition. Here is given a formula and a list of constituents.

The Formula

The formula is a "typical" or basic" or "representative" one. In many formulas, the percentages of each constituent are indicated; these are at best only approximations. The formulas obviously cannot literally describe all products, but they can illustrate for each category something

of the proportions that are frequently employed. The formulas do give considerable guidance when ingredients are not known and cannot easily be found, for example, specific ingredients are not listed for many products in the Trade Mark Index, Section V. A number of reasons may be cited for these omissions. Sometimes the coverage is incomplete and the product is not listed. In some cases the composition is a trade secret and information is deliberately withheld; in others the composition varies with the availability or with the market price of raw materials, and the manufacturer cannot vouch for the formula a month or a year hence and therefore says nothing.

As presented here the "formulations" are heterogeneous; some merely list "standard" or well-known ingredients (for example, linoleum cements: phenolic resin and denatured ethyl alcohol); others give a prototype formula[1] (for example, baby oil: peanut oil—98.9, maleic anhydride—0.1, hexachlorophene—1.0). There is no guarantee that any of these formulas is actually used or is available on the market. Many were adapted from encyclopedias, reference books, or text books, some from correspondence with manufacturers. Some are composites made from scanning the formulas in the Trade Mark Index. Ideally these formulations should have been prepared by well qualified technologists who could authoritatively cite ranges of composition based on types of materials and select the formulas characteristic of products in each category. Ideally the toxicity ratings should then be made by an equally expert industrial toxicologist who could draw on special privileged information. The first edition of this compilation has had too many such problems for solution; this one has not been solved. An attempt to obtain this invaluable assistance is planned; offers of help are urgently solicited. A specific instance of the power of experience may be mentioned; a major manufacturer of soaps and cleaning products gave the opinion that from animal tests many such products probably would be rated as "2," i.e., lethal dose range of a pint to a quart, whereas in humans, the effective rating based on clinical experience probably should be "1," i.e., lethal dose greater than a quart.

The "May Contain" List

In addition to the formula or list under each category title, there is a second list headed "may contain." These substances have been compiled from many sources: a) product labels, b) letters from manufacturers, c) reference books, d) personal communications. No consistent screening has been applied to remove obsolescent, rare, or experimental materials. There is no guarantee on the other hand that the lists are exhaustively complete. Imperfect as they are, no better source of readily available information is known to us. On occasion data may be found here to explain a puzzling reaction, for instance, these lists should be of help to allergists.

---

[1] In most cases the formulas are given in percentages, the cosmetics section is an exception; for cosmetic formulas, the numbers are grams of solids and cubic centimeters of liquids.

Toxicity Rating

Each general formulations category has been given a toxicity rating to assist the physician in making a prognosis when his patient has ingested some product for which the composition is unobtainable. If the toxicity rating is low (1 or 2), the hazard is low. For certain formulations, one or more ingredients are starred (asterisk). Starred ingredients are in our opinion probably responsible for the toxic effects. These ingredients may be found in the *Ingredients Index*, Section II. References are provided in the *Ingredients Index* to the *Therapeutic Index* for a description of toxic symptoms and of recommended treatment.

In assigning a toxicity rating, the point of view has been conservative. By this is meant that the toxicity rating describes the most toxic of several alternative formulations. As an example, the toxicity rating of denture adhesives may be considered. These mixtures, containing casein glue, karaya gum, mineral oil and a flavor, would be rated "1" or "2," except that some brands contain sodium borate or sodium fluoride, each of which as a substance has a toxicity rating of "4." Depending on the percentage composition, the toxicity rating of a particular adhesive might be "2" or even "3." Therefore this rating (2 or 3) is given to the category. The toxicity rating may thus be interpreted as "probably not more toxic than" the estimate given. A corollary is that certain products may have toxicities less than that listed for the category. Although this may appear to be a discrimination against the safer formulas, the part of caution demands such an advice. Since our intent is solely to assist the doctor in planning emergency treatment, a conservative position is the only defensible one. It is obviously difficult to guess the toxicity of a mixture where the percentage composition is not given; the difficulty is heightened for mixtures in which the percentage of one component may vary over wide ranges (for example, alcohol content in cleaning fluids). In fact the uncertainties are so great that we have been repeatedly tempted to omit the toxicity ratings in this section. The decision to offer them is based on day-to-day experience. When calls come from the emergency department, the toxicologist is always asked to evaluate the toxicity of ingested material regardless of acknowledged imperfections in his knowledge.

Toxicity ratings are not always given for agricultural products because the active components are always known (from the label) and because the active components are listed in the *Ingredients Index*, Section II.

Acknowledgment is gladly made of the essential help given by Kenneth E. Lauterbach who compiled most of the formulas, by Clifton J. Latiolais who selected the formulas for cosmetic preparations, by John D. Gabourel who prepared the material on paints and pigments, by Mrs. Mary June Soffer who listed the "may contain" constituents and by Dr. Edward LeB. Gray who assessed the toxicity ratings. Mrs. Veronica Conley, Assistant Secretary, Committee on Cosmetics, American Medical Association, prepared for us extensive lists of basic categories and constituents of cosmetics. The first efforts to bring together the material of this section by Dr. Robert

O. Jensen deserves mention. The help of Mrs. Marie Spiegl is also acknowledged. Many companies have given time and advice to assist in preparing
this section, only a few can be mentioned: Procter and Gamble Company
(Dr. R. E. Hauber), Niagara Chemical Company (Dr. S. K. Reed),
Genesee Research Corporation (Dr. Chester M. White), and Shell Chemical Company (Dr. Norman G. White).

TABLE OF CONTENTS

ABRASIVES

WHITE ROUGES . . . . Toxicity rating 1
  Silica . . . . 96 to 97%
  Alumina 1.3%
  Iron oxide 0.2%
  Magnesia 0.1%
  Potassium hydroxide . . . . 0.0 to 0.3%
  Sodium carbonate 0.1%
  Calcium oxide 0.01%
  Barium stearate 0.7%
  Other rouges (toxicity rating 1) consist mainly of
    aluminum oxide abrasive with a binder of greases,
    waxes, and some fatty acids such as stearic acid.

ADHESIVES

BUILDERS' ADHESIVES . . . . Toxicity rating 2
  Binder
    Vinyl acetate
    Alkyd resins
    Plasticizers
  Hardner
    Portland cement
    Asbestos

CANVAS CEMENTS . . . . Toxicity rating 4
  Pentachlorophenol*
  May contain:
    Petroleum solvents*
    Resins

CASEIN GLUES . . . . Toxicity rating 2
  Casein glue
  Borax
  Oleic acid
  Ammonium hydroxide
  May also contain:
    Latex
    Soybean oil

CHINA CEMENTS . . . . Toxicity rating 2
  Polyvinyl acetate
  Plasticizer 2%

DENTURE ADHESIVES . . . . Toxicity rating 2 or 3
  Casein glue
  Karaya gum
  Mineral oil
  Oil of peppermint
  Sodium borate*
  Sodium fluoride*
  Sodium oxalate*
  Sodium sulfite
  Trisodium phosphate

FABRIC CEMENTS . . . . Toxicity rating 2 or 3
  Latex emulsion 98.0%
  Sulfur 0.5%
  Zinc 0.5%
  May also contain:
    Benzene*

FISHING ROD CEMENTS . . . . Toxicity rating 3
  Neoprene
  Methyl ethyl ketone*

FURNACE CEMENTS . . . . Toxicity rating 1
  Sodium silicate 40%
  Asbestos . . . . ⎫
  Carbon black . . . . ⎪
  Clay . . . . ⎬ 60%
  Silicon dioxide . . . . ⎪
  Water . . . . ⎭

ADHESIVES (Cont.)

GASKET CEMENTS . . . . Toxicity rating 2
  May contain:
    Alcohol
    Asbestos
    Blown vegetable oil
    Mica
    Plasticizer
    Resins
    Talc

GLUES, GENERAL PURPOSE . . . . Toxicity rating 2 or 3
  Glue 40%
  Urea . . . . ⎫
  Sodium β-naphthalenesulfonate . . . . . . ⎪
  Calcium chloride or nitrate . . . . ⎬ 10 to 20%
  Magnesium chloride or nitrate . . . . . . ⎪
  Zinc chloride or nitrate* . . . . ⎭
  Water . . . . 40 to 50%
  Phenol . . . . trace
  May also contain:
    Ammonium thiocyanate*
    Borax*
    Latex
    Magnesium oxide
    Oleic acid
    Sodium hydroxide
    Sodium molybdate
    Zinc oxide

LINOLEUM CEMENTS . . . . Toxicity rating 3
  Phenolic resin
  Denatured ethyl alcohol*

LIQUID SOLDERS . . . . Toxicity rating 3
  Cellulose nitrate
  Aluminum powder
  Acetone*

MODEL AIRPLANE CEMENTS . . . . . . Toxicity rating 3
  Cellulose nitrate 15%
  Acetone* 49%
  Amyl acetate* 22%
  Butyl acetate 7%
  Ethyl acetate 7%
  May also contain:
    Benzene*
    Butyl alcohol*
    Cyclohexanone*
    Dibutyl phthalate
    Hexane*
    Isopropyl acetate
    Isopropyl alcohol*
    Toluene*
    Tricresyl phosphate*
    Urea
    Xylene*

MUCILAGE . . . . Toxicity rating 1 or 2
  Gum arabic 6%
  Rice starch 6%
  Sugar 25%
  Water 63%
  Salicylic acid . . . . very small amount
  May contain:
    Tapioca gum

PASTES . . . . Toxicity rating 1 or 2
  Corn and wheat dextrin
  Sodium fluosilicate . . . . trace
  Sodium pentachlorophenate . . . . trace
  Phenol . . . . trace
  Water

PATCHING CEMENTS . . . . Toxicity rating 1
  Cement
  Sand

Starred ingredients (*) may be responsible for major toxic effects; consult Sec. II.

ADHESIVES (Cont.)

PIPE JOINT CEMENTS . . . . . . Toxicity rating 1 or 2
  Black strap molasses 50%
  Amorphous graphite 50%
  Other formulations contain various combinations of:
    Calcium carbonate
    Calcium hydroxide
    Casein
    Petroleum wax
    Sodium carbonate
    Sodium pentachlorophenate . . . . . . trace
    Soya protein
    Titanium dioxide
    Vegetable drying oils

PLASTIC CEMENTS . . . . Toxicity rating 3 or 4
  Nitrocellulose
  Acetone*
  Ethylene dichloride*
  Toluene*
  May also contain:
    Carbon tetrachloride*
    Chloroform*
    Dibutyl phthalate
    Polyvinyl acetate
    Urea-formaldehyde resin
    Wood flour

RESINOUS ADHESIVES . . . . Toxicity rating 3 or 4
  May contain:
    Alcohol
    Benzene*
    Butyl alcohol*
    Cellulose
    Chalk
    Glycerin
    Ketones*
    Manila gum
    Phenolic, melamine and resorcinol resins
    Phenols*
    Polystyrene
    Polyvinyl acetate
    Rosin
    Urea-formaldehyde resins
    Wood flour

ROOFING CEMENTS . . . . Toxicity rating 3
  Asphalt
  Asbestos
  Mineral spirits*

RUBBER CEMENTS . . . . Toxicity rating 3
  Rubber latex
  Acetone*
  Amyl acetate*
  Carbon disulfide*
  Methyl ethyl ketone*
  Petroleum ether*
  Toluene*

SHOE CEMENTS
                          Toxicity rating 3

  1. Rubber
      Petroleum ether*
                       Toxicity rating 3 or 4
  2. Cellulose nitrate
      Acetone*
      Aromatic solvents*

THERMOPLASTIC ADHESIVES . . . . . Toxicity rating 2
  May contain:
    Aluminum stearate
    Asphaltum rubber
    Binders
    Glues
    Lamp black
    Paraffin oil
    Powdered silica
    Sugar
    Sulfur
    Wood flour

ADHESIVES (Cont.)

TILE CEMENTS . . . . Toxicity rating 3 or 4
  May contain:
    Calcium carbonate
    China clay
    Dryer (containing lead)*
    Magnesium oxide
    Magnesium silicate
    Mercuric oxide (red or yellow)*
    Mineral thinner*
    Phenyl mercurial oleate*
    Titanium calcium pigment
    Vegetable oil

WALL SIZES . . . . Toxicity rating 2 or 3
  Dextrin
  Animal glue
  Sodium bicarbonate
  Aluminum sulfate*
  Bentonite
  May also contain:
    Methyl alcohol*
    Vinyl acetate

WATERPROOF ADHESIVES (a two component adhesive)
  Powder . . . . Toxicity rating 3
    Paraformaldehyde*
    Walnut shell flour
  Liquid . . . . Toxicity rating 3
    Alcohol
    Phenol-formaldehyde resin
    Water
    May contain:
      Asphalt
      Lime hydrate
      Lime rosin
      Petroleum solvents*
      Resorcinol*
      Sodium fluoride*
      Trisodium phosphate

AGRICULTURAL PRODUCTS

ANIMAL BAITS AND REPELLENTS
  Rabbit, Deer, Wolf, Coyote
    Zinc dithiocarbamate-amine complex*
    Sulfur*

BIRD BAITS AND REPELLENTS
  Strychnine*
  Petroleum hydrocarbons*
  Sometimes Fish oil, Linseed oil, Soap, Sulfur*,
    Turpentine*

BLOSSOM THINNERS
  Dinitro o-secondary butyl phenol*

BRANDING FLUIDS
  Barium sulfide*
  Sodium hydroxide*

DEBARKING COMPOUNDS
  Arsenic*

DEFOLIANTS
  Sodium chlorate*
  Magnesium chlorate*
  Sometimes Ammonium borate*, Aromatic hydrocarbons*,
    Pentachlorophenol*, Sodium metaborate*

DEHORNING PASTES
  Sodium hydroxide*
  Calcium hydroxide
  Glycerin
  Lime

Starred ingredients (*) may be responsible for major toxic effects; consult Sec. II.

AGRICULTURAL PRODUCTS (Cont.)

DISINFECTANTS, SEED AND PLANT
Mercury*
Thiram*
Dieldrin*
Benzene hexachloride*
Sometimes Aliphatic petroleum hydrocarbons*,
   Ammonium sulfate, Helione orange,
   8-Hydroxyquinoline sulfate*, Magnesium sulfate,
   Malachite green*, Manganese sulfate*, Piperonyl
   butoxide, Pyrethrins*

DISINFECTANTS, STOCK AND POULTRY
Organic ammonium chlorides* (Quaternary ammonium
   compounds)
Petroleum hydrocarbons*
Sodium hypochlorite*

EGG DETERGENTS
Alkyl ammonium chlorides* (Quaternary ammonium
   compounds)
Sodium carbonate
Sodium silicate

FERTILIZERS
Nitrogen (fixed)
Phosphoric acid
Potassium salts
Petroleum hydrocarbons
Zinc salts*
Copper salts*
Manganese salts*
Chlorophenoxy acetic acid
Iron salts*
Sulfur
Boric acid*
Sometimes Aluminum silicate, Ammonium phosphate,
   Bacteria (non-pathogenic), Benzene hexachloride*,
   Calcium polyphosphate, Chlorinated petroleum
   hydrocarbon*, Cobalt*, Lime, Mercury, Potassium
   iodide*, Sodium carbonate, Sodium molybdate,
   Turpentine

FRUIT DROP INHIBITORS
α-Naphthaleneacetic acid*
α-2,4,5-Trichlorophenoxypropionic acid,*
   triethanolamine salt
p-Chlorophenoxy acetic acid

LIVESTOCK FEEDS
Calcium phosphate
Cobalt salts*
Copper salts*
Iron salts*
Magnesium salts
Manganese salts*
Sometimes Calcium carbonate, Oil of anise,
   Potassium iodide*, Shell flour, Zinc salts*

NEST LITTER
Magnesium aluminum sulfate*

PLANT-TREE FOODS
Available nitrogen (as urea, ammonium nitrate)
Available phosphoric acid (as monoammonium
   phosphate, as monopotassium polyphosphate,
   as monosodium polyphosphate)
Available potash (as potassium nitrate* or chloride,
   monopotassium phosphate)
Cornstarch
α-Naphthalene acetic acid*

POULTRY TENDERIZERS
Diethylstilbestrol (stilbesterol)

ROOST PAINTS
Petroleum hydrocarbons* (petroleum oils, benzene
   hexachloride*, anthracene oil)*

AGRICULTURAL PRODUCTS (Cont.)

SOIL CONDITIONERS
Iron salts*
Manganese salts*
Zinc salts*
Copper salts*
Phosphate
Aluminum sulfate*
Boron salts*
Ethylene tetrachloride*
Hexachloro, hexahydro, dimethano naphthalene*
Magnesium sulfate
Mercuric chloride
Nitrogen (fixed)
Piperonyl butoxide
Potassium salts*
Pyrethrins*
Sodium benzoate
Sulfer
Sodium ferric ethylenediamine tetraacetate*
Urea

SPREADERS, STICKERS
Sulfonated oil
Vegetable oil

SPROUT INHIBITORS
Methyl ester of naphthalene acetic acid*

WOOD PRESERVATIVES
Chlorophenols*
Chlorobenzene*
Chlorinated coal tar oil*
Petroleum hydrocarbons (aliphatic and aromatic)*
Zinc or copper naphthenate*
Turpentine*
Titanium salts
Benzene hexachloride*
Chlordane*
Water repellents
Sometimes Boric acid*, Calcium carbonate, Coconut
   amine, Copper salts*, Piperonyl butoxide, Pyrethrins*,
   Resin, Resin acids, Aluminum salts, Arsenic*, DDT*,
   Rosin, Silica, Sulfur dioxide*, Zinc salts*

ANTIFREEZES

PERMANENT . . . . Toxicity rating 3
   Ethylene glycol* . . . .   90 to 100%
   Dye
   Rust inhibitor* (see below)

METHANOL . . . . Toxicity rating 3
   Methyl alcohol* 99.9%
   Dye
   Rust inhibitor
Some of the compounds used as rust inhibitors are:
   Inorganic
      Borates*
      Chromates* (not used with alcohol or glycol)
      Molybdates*
      Nitrites*
      Phosphates
      Tungstates
      Zinc chloride*
   Organic
      Amines
      Animal fats
      Mineral oils
      Soap
      Sulfonated oils
      Vegetable oils
   Calcium chloride and sodium chloride are used for
      refrigeration brines. Calcium chloride solutions
      are also used in tractor tires for added weight.
   Glycerol and ethyl alcohol are used as antifreezes
      for cosmetics.
   Lubricating oils have been used as cooling agents
      in specially prepared engines.

ANTIFREEZES (Cont.)

Foam suppressors used are:
Alkyl lactates
Amyl alcohol*
Calcium acetate
Calcium ricinoleate
Castor oil soap
Dibutyl phthalate
Ethyl oleate
Phenyl stearate
Vegetable oils

BLEACHES, LAUNDRY

LIQUID .... Toxicity rating 3
Sodium hypochlorite* .... 3 to 6%
Sodium chloride .... 4 to 5%
Sodium hydroxide and/or sodium
carbonate .... 0.2 to 0.5%
Water .... 89 to 93%

POWDER

Toxicity rating 3
1. Calcium hypochlorite* .... 8 to 9%
   Alkaline cleaning powders 90%
2. Sodium perborate tetrahydrate* .. 20 to 30%
   Sodium sesquicarbonate .... 70 to 80%
   Fluorescent dye .... 0.2 to 0.4%

TABLETS .... Toxicity rating 5
Calcium hypochlorite*........... 68%
Inert ingredients 32%
For calcium and sodium hypochlorite see Hypochlorite,
Section III
Laundry bleaches may contain:
Oxalic acid*
Sodium hyposulfite*
Sodium perborate*
Sodium peroxide*
Sodium or potassium bichromate*
Trisodium phosphate*

BLUINGS

GUN BLUINGS .... Toxicity rating 4
Potassium nitrate 3.5%
Mercuric chloride* 2.4%
Potassium chlorate* 3.0%
Ferric chloride 0.9%
Sodium nitrate 0.9%
Cupric chloride 0.5%
Spirit of ethyl nitrite 6.5%
Water 82.3%
Sometimes contain:
Nitric acid
Selenium*

LAUNDRY BLUINGS .... Toxicity rating 2
Soap 92%
Borax ....⎫
Sodium tripolyphosphate ....⎬ 6 to 8%
Trisodium phosphate............⎭
Denatured alcohol .... minute quantities
Prussian blue .... minute quantities
May contain:
Alkyl aryl sulfonates
Paraffin wax
Sodium sulfate
Minute amounts of:
Acetic acid
Aniline blue*
Nitric acid
Oxalic acid*
Sodium ferrocyanide
Sulfuric acid
Ultra marine blue

BRAKE FLUIDS

BRAKE FLUIDS .... Toxicity rating 3
Lubricant .... 15 to 20%
Castor oil
Castor oil soap
Butyl or glyceryl ether of polyoxyethylene
propylene glycol
Polypropylene glycol
Solvent .... 80 to 85%
Methyl, ethyl and butyl ethers of ethylene
glycol* and related glycols
Brake fluids may contain:
Ethyl alcohol*
Isopropyl alcohol*
Propyl alcohol*
n-Butyl alcohol*
Isobutyl alcohol*
Mixed amyl alcohols*
Hexylene glycol*
Diethylene glycol*
Ethylene glycol*
Butylene glycol*
Inhibitors:
Amine soaps
Potash soaps
Antioxidants:
Hydroquinone
Bisphenol A
Dyes*

BRAKE SYSTEM FLUSHING FLUIDS... Toxicity rating 3
Methyl, ethyl or isopropyl alcohol*

CANDLES

HOUSEHOLD .... Toxicity rating 1
Stearic acid
Paraffin
Dye (minute amount)

CHURCH .... Toxicity rating 1
Beeswax
Paraffin
The candle wick is treated with:
Ammonium chloride
Ammonium phosphate
Ammonium sulfate
Borax
Boric acid
Potassium nitrate

CAULKING COMPOUNDS

CAULKING COMPOUNDS
Toxicity rating 3
1. Styrenated alkyd resin ....⎫
   Chlorinated biphenyl* ....⎬ 40%
   Titanium dioxide ....⎭
   Calcium carbonate ....⎫ 40%
   Asbestos fibre ....⎭
   Xylene* 20%
Toxicity rating 1
2. Polyvinyl acetate
   Titanium dioxide
   Calcium carbonate

Toxicity rating 3
3. Vegetable oils (edible)
   Mineral thinner*
   Drier (containing 5% lead)*
   Titanium dioxide
   Calcium carbonate
   Asbestos fibre
   May contain:
   Aluminum or calcium stearate
   Asphalt
   Chromium*
   Cork
   Iron oxide
   Petroleum sulfonate
   Polybutane
   Wax
   Zinc oxide

Starred ingredients (*) may be responsible for major toxic effects; consult Sec. II.

CAULKING COMPOUNDS (Cont.)

CHALKS . . . . Toxicity rating 1 or 2
  Calcium carbonate
  Calcium sulfate
  Pigments

CLEANERS

ABRASIVE CLEANERS . . . . Toxicity rating 3
  Silica abrasive . . . . }
  Soap . . . . } 94%
  Moisture . . . . }
  Trisodium phosphate 3%
  Dodecyl benzene sodium sulfonate . .   2%
  Nonyl benzene sodium sulfonate 0.9%
  Sodium perborate* 5%
  May contain:
    Aluminum oxide
    Colloidal clay
    Fatty acids
    Kerosene*
    Long chain hydrocarbons
    Pumice
    Rouge
    Sodium hydroxide*

ALUMINUM CLEANERS . . . . Toxicity rating 3
  Sometimes contain:
    Ammonium chloride
    Calcium carbonate
    Magnesium oxide
    Petroleum naphtha*
    Powdered pumice
    Red iron oxide
    Soda soap
    Sodium sesquicarbonate
    Sodium silicate
    Tartaric acid*
    Trisodium phosphate*
    Whitening

ASPHALT TILE CLEANERS . . . . Toxicity rating 2
  Sodium carboxymethylcellulose
  Santomerse S
  Perfume
  Dye
  Water

AUTOMOBILE CLEANERS . . . . Toxicity rating 3
  Alkyd aryl sodium sulfonate* 40%
  Sodium sulfate 60%
  Sometimes contain:
    Diethanolamine
    Lauryl diethanolamide

BOILER CLEANERS . . . . Toxicity rating 3
  Trisodium phosphate* 66.5%
  Sodium sulfate, anhydrous 33.0%
  Sodium dichromate 0.5%
  Other formulations may contain sodium carbonate
  or sodium hydroxide.*

CARBURETOR CLEANERS . . . . Toxicity rating 4
  Sometimes contain:
    Chlorinated hydrocarbons* (toxic if inhaled in a
      confined area)
    Coal tar distillates*
    Corrosion inhibitors (usually borax or chromates)*
    Detergents*

DAIRY CLEANERS . . . . Toxicity rating 3 or 4
  China clay
  Chlorine compounds* (see Hypochlorite, Section III)
  Hydrocarbon sulfonate
  Phosphoric acid*
  Quaternary ammonium compounds*
  Sodium aluminate
  Sodium carbonate
  Sodium hydroxide*
  Sodium metaphosphate*
  Sodium metasilicate

CLEANERS (Cont.)

  Sodium sulfite*
  Trisodium phosphate*
The toxicity rating of chlorine compounds and the
quaternary ammonium compounds is 4; that of
phosphates is 3.

DETERGENTS—(Synthetic)
  The term "detergent" meaning originally cleaner, is
    now widely used to specify the synthetic detergents
    (non-soap cleaning products) which have such popular
    household use today.
  All purpose household powder. . . . Toxicity rating 2 or 3
    Synthetic anionic detergent*
    Sodium silicate
    Sodium sulfate
    Sodium polyphosphate*
    Trisodium phosphate*
    Perfume
  Dishwashing, germicidal (commercial)
                                     Toxicity rating 3 or 4
    1. Quaternary, ammonium compound* greater than 10%
                                     Toxicity rating 3 or 4
    2. Hypochlorite*
  Dishwashing (mechanical) . . . . Toxicity rating 3
    Synthetic anionic detergent (small amount)
    Sodium polyphosphate*
    Sodium silicate
    Sodium carbonate
    Sodium sesquicarbonate
    Trisodium phosphate*
    May contain:
      Sodium hydroxide* (over 10%)
  Liquid (all purpose) . . . . Toxicity rating 2 or 3
    Synthetic anionic detergent* (or nonionic detergent)
    Denatured ethyl alcohol
    Fatty acid amides (small amount)
    Water
    May contain:
      Ethylene glycol* and perfume
  Scouring powders or cleansers . . . . . . Toxicity rating 2
    Abrasive material 80%
      (such as Feldspar, Pumice or Quartz)
    Sodium carbonate
    Sodium tripolyphosphate
    Tetrasodium pyrophosphate
    Synthetic anionic detergent

DRAIN AND PIPE CLEANERS . . . . Toxicity rating 4 or 5
  1. Sodium or potassium hydroxide*   94 to 100%
     (see Alkali, Section III)
     Sodium carbonate . . . .   0.8 to 2.0%
  2. Sodium bisulfate 80%
     Sodium chloride 15%
     Steatite (talc) 5%
  Sometimes contain:
    Aluminum particles (metallic)
    Hydrochloric acid* (see Acid, Section III)
    Sodium sulfate
    Sulfuric acid* (see Acid, Section III)

DRY CLEANERS . . . . Toxicity rating 4
  1. Carbon tetrachloride* 100%
  2. Carbon tetrachloride* . . . . . .   20 to 80%
     With any of the following:
       Alcohol
       Benzene*
       Chloroform*
       Ether*
       Naphtha*
       Stoddard solvent*
       Toluene*
       Xylene*
  3. Various combinations of the following solvents are
     also in use:
       Alcohol
       Benzene*
       Chloroform*
       Kerosene*
       Methylene chloride*
       Perchloroethylene*

Starred ingredients (*) may be responsible for major toxic effects; consult Sec. II.

CLEANERS (Cont.)

        Petroleum hydrocarbons*
        Stoddard solvent*
        Toluene*
        Trichloroethylene*
        Xylene*
All of the above aromatic hydrocarbons and chlorinated
    hydrocarbons, with the execption of methylene chloride,
    have a toxicity rating of 4. All the above aliphatic
    hydrocarbons, ethers and alcohols have a toxicity rat-
    ing of 3.

ENGINE AND MOTOR CLEANERS Toxicity rating 3 or 4
Caustic potash* (see Alkali, Section III)
Chlorinated hydrocarbons*
Coal tar distillates*
Corrosion inhibitor
Detergent
Petroleum solvent*
The coal tar distillates have a toxicity rating of 4, the
    chlorinated hydrocarbons of 3 or 4 and the petroleum
    solvent of 3.

FUR CLEANERS . . . . Toxicity rating 4
Alcohol
Benzene*
Carbon tetrachloride*
Petroleum ether*

FURNACE CLEANERS (Soot Destroyers)
                                  Toxicity rating 2
Charcoal
Potassium nitrate

FURNITURE CLEANERS . . . . Toxicity rating 3
Alkyl aryl sodium sulfonate*
Ammonium hydroxide*
Isopropyl alcohol*
Methyl alcohol*
Sodium hydroxide*

GENERAL PURPOSE CLEANERS . . . Toxicity rating 3
Trisodium phosphate* . . . .   50 to 60%
Sodium sesquicarbonate . . . .   25 to 35%
Sodium pyrophosphate . . . .   5 to 10%
Sodium alkyl aryl sulfonate . . . .   0.5 to 1.5%
Sometimes contain:
    Kerosene*
    Pine oil*
    Silicates
    Sodium bicarbonate

GLASS AND WINDOW CLEANERS . Toxicity rating 2 or 3
Isopropyl alcohol 12%
Detergent . . . .   1 to 2%
Phosphate salt . . . .   1 to 2%
Water . . . .   84 to 86%
Ammonia, dye, perfume . . . .   trace
Sometimes contain:
    Borax
    Carbon tetrachloride*
    Glycerin
    Kerosene*
    Lemongrass oil
    Sodium bicarbonate
    Sodium oleate
    Tannic acid

JEWELRY CLEANERS . . . . Toxicity rating 3
Ammoniated soap
Isopropyl alcohol*
Perfume
Dye

LEATHER CLEANERS . . . . Toxicity rating 2
Borax
Carnauba wax
Denatured alcohol
Japan wax
Oil of citronella
Palm oil
Rosin

CLEANERS (Cont.)

Sodium carbonate
Sodium hydroxide
Tallow

LENS CLEANERS . . . . Toxicity rating 2
1. Detergent . . . . } 4%
   Phosphate salt . . . . }
   Water 96%
2. Isopropyl alcohol 12%
   Wetting agent . . . .   2 to 4%
   Water . . . .   84 to 86%

METAL CLEANERS (Rust Removers)
                    Toxicity rating 4 (with cyanide 5)
1. Ammonium fluoride*
   Hydrofluoric acid*
                    Toxicity rating 4 (with cyanide 5)
2. Sodium fluosilicate*
   Sodium bifluoride*
                    Toxicity rating 3 or 4 (with cyanide 5)
3. Phosphoric acid
   Detergents*
   May contain:
      Ammonium hydroxide*
      Ammonium oxalate*
      Aniline dye*
      Borax*
      Calcium carbonate
      Cresylic acid*
      Cyanide*
      Emery
      Ethylene dichloride*
      Ferric oxide
      Glycerin
      Isopropyl alcohol*
      Kerosene*
      Naphthalene*
      Nitric acid*
      Oleic acid
      Petroleum hydrocarbons*
      Pine oil*
      Potassium soap
      Pumice
      Rouge
      Silica
      Silver nitrate*
      Soda ash
      Sodium bicarbonate
      Sodium chromates*
      Sodium dichromate*
      Stearic acid
      Sulfuric acid*
      Tetrachloroethylene*
      Thiourea
      Turpentine*

OVEN CLEANERS . . . . Toxicity rating 3 or 4
Sodium hydroxide base*

PAINT BRUSH CLEANERS . . . . . . Toxicity rating 3 or 4
Kerosene* 57%
Oleic acid 29%
Ammonium hydroxide, conc. 7%
Denatured ethyl alcohol 7%
May also contain:
    Acetone*
    Benzene*
    Borax*
    Butyl alcohol*
    Diglycol oleate
    Isopropyl alcohol*
    Methyl alcohol*
    Methylene chloride*
    Naphtha*
    Naphthalene*
    Sodium chromate*
    Stoddard solvent*
    Toluene*
    Trisodium phosphate
    Xylene*

Starred ingredients (*) may be responsible for major toxic effects; consult Sec. II.

CLEANERS (Cont.)

PAINT CLEANERS . . . . Toxicity rating 3 or 4
  Emulsifying and suspending agents
  Isopropyl alcohol*
  Kerosene*
  Methylene chloride*
  Petroleum ether*
  Xylene*

PORCELAIN, MARBLE, TILE AND ENAMEL
CLEANERS . . . . Toxicity rating 2
  Abrasive 88%
  Sodium tripolyphosphate 5%
  Alkyl aryl sufonate 5%
  Trisodium phosphate 2%

RADIATOR CLEANERS

                            Toxicity rating 4
1. Oxalic acid* or sodium bisulfate
                            Toxicity rating 4
2. Hydrochloric acid*
                            Toxicity rating 3 or 4
3. Chlorinated hydrocarbons
    Detergent
    May contain:
      Sodium bisulfite*

RUG CLEANERS . . . . Toxicity rating 4
  Sawdust
  Trichloroethylene*

SEWER, CESSPOOL AND SEPTIC TANK
CLEANERS . . . . Toxicity rating 5
  Sodium hydroxide* or potassium
    hydroxide* (see Alkali, Section III) .   100%

SHOE CLEANERS . . . . Toxicity rating 2 or 3
  Titanium dioxide
  Trisodium phosphate*

SOAPS
  Bar soaps . . . . Toxicity rating 2
    Anhydrous soap 86.5%
    2,2-Thiobis (4,6-dichlorophenol) . . .   1.6%
    Glycerin 0.7%
    Sodium chloride 0.5%
    Water 10.0%
    May also contain:
      Borax*
      Bran
      Eucalyptus oil*
      Hexachlorophene
      Iodine
      Mercuric iodide*
      Olive oil
      Sulfur
  Industrial hand cleaners (used with water)
                        Toxicity rating 2
    Pumice, wood flour or borax . . . . .   60 to 75%
    Powdered soap 25%
    Trisodium phosphate
    May contain:
      Alcohol
      Coconut oil
      Colloidal clay
      Dioxane for stain removal
      Glycerin
      Hexachlorophene
      Lanolin
      Mineral spirits
      Perfume
      Sodium bicarbonate
      Synthetic detergent
  Industrial hand cleaners (used without water)
                        Toxicity rating 2 or 3
    Agar-agar alkalized
    Alcohol
    Ammonium hydroxide* (3%)
    Casein
    Cellulose derivatives
    Cottonseed fatty acid
    Diethylene glycol*
    Dioxane for stain removal

CLEANERS (Cont.)

  Egg albumin
  Essential oil*
  Glycerol monstearate
  Kerosene-like hydrocarbons*
  Lanolin
  Lime
  Mineral oil
  Paraffin wax
  Potassium hydroxide
  Sodium alkyl aryl sulfonate
  Sodium carbonate
  Sodium hexametaphosphate
  Sodium hydroxide
  Spermaceti
  Stearic acid
  Tallow soap
  Water
  White soap chips
  Liquid soaps . . . . Toxicity rating 2 or 3
    Anhydrous soap . . . .   15 to 40%
    Glycerin 3%
    Hexachlorophene 1%
    Lecithin 1%
    Water . . . .   55 to 80%
    May also contain:
      Ammonium hydroxide*
      Isopropyl alcohol*
      Lanolin
      Methyl salicylate*
      Pine oil*
      Potassium hydroxide
      Potassium oleate
      Sodium lauryl sulfate
      Sodium polyphosphate
      Sulfur
      Tetrasodium ethylenediaminetetraacetate
      2,2-Thiobis (4,6-dichlorophenol)
  Soap powders . . . . Toxicity rating 2
    Anhydrous soap . . . .   33 to 85%
    Lanolin
    Oil of sassafras
    Pine oil
    Sodium pyrophosphate
    Sodium sulfate
    Sodium tripolyphosphate
    Tall oil-ethylene oxide condensate
    May also contain:
      Glycerin
      Sodium alkyl aryl sulfonate
      Sodium carbonate
      Sodium silicate

STAIN REMOVERS
  Coffee stain removers . . . . Toxicity rating 3
    Sodium hypochlorite* 8%
    Water 92%
  General use . . . . Toxicity rating 3
    1. Ammonium hydroxide*
    2. Hydrocarbon solvents*
      Soap
      May contain:
        Alcohol*
        Ammonium chloride
        Ammonium persulfate
        Amyl and ethyl acetate*
        Benzene*
        Butyl acetate*
        Carbon tetrachloride*
        Chloroform*
        Glacial acetic acid*
        Glycerin
        Lactic acid
        Methylene chloride*
        Naphtha*
        Oxalic acid*
        Perchloroethylene*
        Tetrahydrofurfural
        Toluene*
        Trichloroethylene*
  Iodine stain removers . . . . Toxicity rating 2
    Sodium thiosulfate 10%
    Water 90%

Starred ingredients (*) may be responsible for major toxic effects; consult Sec. II.

CLEANERS (Cont.)

Lipstick removers

                                    Toxicity rating 3

  1. Isopropyl alcohol*

                                      Toxicity rating 3

  2. Isoamyl acetate*
     Petroleum hydrocarbons*

                                      Toxicity rating 4

  3. Carbon tetrachloride*
     Butyl cellosolve*
     Chloroform*
     Alcohol

Rust and ink removers . . . . Toxicity rating 3
  Oxalic acid*
  Methyl alcohol*
  Water

TAR REMOVERS . . . . Toxicity rating 4
Xylene*
Chlorinated hydrocarbons*

TIRE CLEANERS . . . . Toxicity rating 3
Potassium hydroxide* (see Alkali,
  Section III) . . . . }
Denatured alcohol . . . . } about 20%
Alkyl aryl sulfonate . . . . }
Water 80%

TOILET BOWL CLEANERS

                                    Toxicity rating 5

  1. Sodium hydroxide* 100%
     (see Alkali, Section III)

                                    Toxicity rating 3

  2. Hydrochloric acid* . . . . 14 to 23%
     (see Acid, Section III)
     Dichlorobenzene 2.5%

                                    Toxicity rating 3

  3. 1,3-Dichloro-3,5-dimethylhydantoin* 95%

                                    Toxicity rating 2

  4. Sodium bisulfate. . . . . 75 to 100%
     Sodium chloride. 15%
     Sodium carbonate. 10%
     Talc, odorant 0.5%

WALL CLEANERS . . . . Toxicity rating 3
Ammonium hydroxide*
Borax*
Colloidal clay
Diglycol stearate
Kerosene*
Powdered dry soap
Silica
Soda ash
Sodium lauryl sulfate
Sulfated fatty alcohol
Trisodium phosphate*

WALLPAPER CLEANERS . . . . . . Toxicity rating 1 to 3
Wheat flour . . . . }
Water . . . . } 80.00%
Salt 17.00%
Mineral spirits 1.00%
Ammonium aluminum sulfate 0.06%
Methyl salicylate 0.02%
Dye 0.005%
May contain:
  Alkali metal salts for preservative (slight amount)
  Ammonium hydroxide*
  Borax*
  Coconut oil soap
  Ethyl ether*
  Ethylene dichloride*
  Ethylene glycol monobutyl ether
  Glycerin
  Kerosene oil (slight amount)
  Naphthalene*
  Oleic acid
  Potash
  Sawdust
  Soda ash
  Triethanolamine
  Trisodium phosphate*

CLEANERS (Cont.)

WINDSHIELD CLEANERS . . . . Toxicity rating 3
Ethyl alcohol or isopropyl alcohol*

COSMETICS

BABY PREPARATIONS
Baby creams . . . . Toxicity rating 1
  Lanolin, anhydrous 6.0
  Paraffin 10.0
  Mineral oil 70.0
  Zinc stearate 6.0
  Cetyl alcohol. 4.0
  Beeswax 4.0
                                      100.0
Baby lotions . . . . Toxicity rating 1
  Sodium alginate 0.35
  Butyl p-aminobenzoate 0.01
  Methyl p-aminobenzoate 0.09
  Triethanolamine 0.5
  Stearic acid 0.9
  Stearyl alcohol 0.9
  Cetyl alcohol. 0.5
  Lanolin, anhydrous 1.0
  Liquid petrolatum, light 30.0
  Water, q.s. 100.0
May contain:
  Glycerin
  Glyceryl monostearate
  Perfume
Baby oils

                                    Toxicity rating 1

  1. Mineral oil 94.0
     Oxyquinoline benzoate or sulfate . . 1.0
     Lanolin, anhydrous 5.0
                                  100.0
                         Toxicity rating 1 or 2
  2. Peanut oil. 98.9
     Maleic anhydride 0.1
     Hexachlorophene 1.0
                                  100.0

    May contain:
      Olive and vegetable oils
      Perfume
      Cetyl alcohol
      Sorbitol
      Triethanolamine stearate
Baby powders

                                    Toxicity rating 2

  1. Talc 70.0
     Kaolin 20.0
     Hydroxyquinoline sulfate 1.0
     Magnesium carbonate or stearate . 7.0
     Hexachlorophene 1.0
     Chalk. 1.0
                                    100.0
                                Toxicity rating 3
  2. Talc 49.0
     Magnesium carbonate or stearate . 1.0
     Zinc stearate 20.0
     Boric acid* 30.0
                                  100.0

    May contain:
      Perfume
      Titanium dioxide
Baby soaps   Toxicity rating 1
  Sodium soaps of coconut and palm oil

BATH PREPARATIONS
Bath oils

                                    Toxicity rating 2

  1. Perfume. . . . . 0.1 to 0.2
     Sulfonated oil, q.s. 100.1
                                  Toxicity rating 3
  2. Pine oil 20.0
     Sulfonated castor oil 40.0
     Water, q.s. 100.0
     Bath oils may contain:
      Attar of flowers
      Cetyl alcohol
      Essential oils*
      Lanolin

Starred ingredients (*) may be responsible for major toxic effects; consult Sec. II.

COSMETICS (Cont.)

Oil of bergamot
Petrolatum
Stearate
Tar

Bath salts

Toxicity rating 2

1. Sodium sesquicarbonate 60.0
   Magnesium sulfate 2.0
   Sodium metaphosphate 3.0
   Trisodium phosphate 1.0
   Sodium bicarbonate 24.0
   Citric or tartaric acids....... 10.0
   ___
   100.0

   Toxicity rating 3

2. Sodium borate* (borax) 20.0
   Sodium hexametaphosphate 1.0
   Sodium bicarbonate 35.0
   Corn starch 44.0
   ___
   100.0

Bubble bath

Powder .... Toxicity rating 3
Sodium alkyl aryl sulfonate* 50.0
Sodium sulfate............. 25.0
Sodium carbonate........... 24.0
Perfume oil 1.0
___
100.0

Liquid .... Toxicity rating 3
Triethanolamine lauryl sulfate* .. 40.0
Propylene glycol 8.0
Perfume oil 2.0
Sodium alginate solution (2%) 50.0
___
100.0

Bubble baths may contain:
Alcohol
Methyl p-hydroxy benzoate
Phosphates

CREAMS

Astringent creams

Toxicity rating 2

1. Witch hazel extract 50.0
   Stearic acid 16.0
   Sodium carbonate........... 1.0
   Glycerin 6.0
   Water, q.s. 100.0

   Toxicity rating 2

2. Aluminum potassium sulfate ... 4.0
   Zinc sulfocarbolate (or sulfate) . 2.0
   Stearic acid 16.0
   Sodium carbonate........... 1.0
   Glycerin 6.0
   Water, q.s. 100.0

   Toxicity rating 2

3. Tannic acid............... 2.0
   Stearic acid 16.0
   Sodium carbonate........... 1.0
   Glycerin 6.0
   Water, q.s. 100.0

Barrier creams (protective)

Toxicity rating 1

1. Stearic acid 10.0
   Beeswax................. 1.5
   Glycerin................. 5.0
   Casein.................. 0.3
   Ammonium hydroxide 0.5
   Water, q.s............... 100.0

   Toxicity rating 2

2. Zinc oxide 10.0
   Zinc stearate 5.0
   Titanium dioxide 10.0
   Butyl stearate 5.0
   Liquid petrolatum 10.0
   White petrolatum 60.0
   ___
   100.0

   Toxicity rating 2

3. Silicone, high viscosity 25.0
   White petrolatum 75.0

   Toxicity rating 2

4. Polyethylene glycol 1540
   monostearate 5.0
   Butyl stearate 5.0
   Petrolatum 3.0

COSMETICS (Cont.)

Diglycol stearate (neutral) 4.0
Paraffin 3.0
Potassium hydroxide 7.0
Magnesium stearate 15.0
Water 58.0
___
100.0

Barrier creams may contain:
Aluminum compounds*
Benzoic acid
Borates
Ceresin
Lanolin
Salicylates*
Sodium silicate
Talc
Triethanolamine

Bleach and freckle creams

Bleach creams .... Toxicity rating 3
Hydrogen peroxide* (5%) 8.0
Lanolin, anhydrous............ 10.0
Spermaceti 10.0
Petrolatum, q.s. 100.0

Freckle ointments .... Toxicity rating 4
Bismuth subnitrate 6.0
Ammoniated mercury* 6.0
Precipitated chalk 6.0
Zinc oxide 6.0
Camphor, powder* 6.0
Cold cream, q.s. 100.0

Skin bleaches .... Toxicity rating 3
Zinc peroxide or Sodium perborate* 8.0
Magnesium carbonate 50.0
Titanium dioxide 2.0
Zinc oxide 40.0
___
100.0

Bleach and freckle creams may contain:
Oxalic acid*

Cleansing creams (all-purpose, 4 type creams)

Toxicity rating 2

1. Liquid petrolatum 3.0
   Spermaceti 2.0
   Glycerin................. 6.0
   Sodium borate 1.0
   Diglycol stearate 14.0
   Ceresin 2.0
   Stearic acid 10.0
   Sodium lauryl sulfate 1.0
   Water, q.s................ 100.0

   Toxicity rating 2

2. Beeswax................. 5.0
   Triethanolamine stearate 12.0
   Lanolin 2.0
   Triethylene glycol 8.0
   Petrolatum 5.0
   Water, q.s................ 100.0

Cleansing creams may contain:
Boric acid
Cetyl alcohol
Gum karaya
Gum tragacanth
Magnesium sulfate
Soap
Sodium carbonate

Cold creams (all-purpose creams, 4 purpose creams)

Toxicity rating 1

1. Ceresin (or ozokerite) 3.5
   Spermaceti 10.0
   Beeswax 10.0
   Mineral oil (or olive, persic,
   almond) 45.0
   Sodium borate (borax) 0.5
   Sodium benzoate 1.0
   Perfume.................. 0.1
   Water 30.0
   ___
   100.0

   Toxicity rating 2

2. Stearic acid 15.0
   Liquid petrolatum 16.0
   Cholesterin................ 2.0
   Triethanolamine 2.0
   Carbitol.................. 8.0
   Methyl parahydroxybenzoate 0.1

Starred ingredients (*) may be responsible for major toxic effects; consult Sec. II.

COSMETICS (Cont.)

```
        Perfume................      0.1
        Water, q.s.              100.0
        Cold creams may contain:
          Cetyl alcohol
          Glycerin
          Menthol
Cucumber creams ............    Toxicity rating 2
  Fresh cucumber juice..........    24.0
  Sodium benzoate .............     4.0
  Lanolin, anhydrous............    48.0
  Cold cream base, q.s. ........   100.0
Emollient creams (lubricating)
                                Toxicity rating 1
  1. Lecithin ................      6.0
     Lanolin .................     10.0
     Cocoa butter ...........       4.0
     Cholesterin.............        2.0
     Cold cream base ..........     78.0
                                   100.0
                                Toxicity rating 1
  2. Lecithin ................      3.0
     Lanolin ................       5.0
     Sorbitol or mannitol, fatty acid
       esters ...............       5.0
     Spermaceti .............       5.0
     Glyceryl monostearate .......  12.0
     Methyl p-hydroxybenzoate .....  0.1
     Water, q.s...............     100.0
     Emollient creams may contain:
       Animal oils
       Boric acid
       Camphor
       Castor oil
       Cetyl alcohol
       Soybean oil
       Sperm oil
       Triethanolamine
       Turpentine
       Undecylenic acid
       Vegetable oils
       Zinc oxide
Hand creams.................    Toxicity rating 1
  Glyceryl monostearate .........  12.0
  Liquid petrolatum .............   6.0
  Lanolin ..................       4.0
  Cocoa butter ..............       2.0
  Methyl p-hydroxybenzoate .......  0.1
  Water, q.s..................     100.0
  May contain:
    Aluminum silicate
    Ammonium hydroxide
    Benzyl alcohol
    Boric acid
    Castor oil
    Cetyl alcohol
    Hexachlorophene
    Magnesium silicate
    Sodium alginate
    Sodium benzoate
    Sodium bicarbonate
    Sodium carbonate
    Sodium metabisulfate
    Witch hazel
    Zinc oxide
Hormone creams
  Creams with combinations of cholesterin and
  lecithin have been erroneously known as hormone
  creams. The more popular terms for these
  preparations are tissue or nourishing creams.
                                Toxicity rating 1
  1. Cholesterin .............      2.0
     Lecithin ................      1.0
     Beeswax.................       4.0
     Stearic acid .............     4.0
     Lanolin .................     10.0
     Cocoa butter .............     4.0
     Olive oil ...............     40.0
     Sodium borate ...........      1.0
     Sodium benzoate ...........    0.6
     Water, q.s...............     100.0
```

COSMETICS (Cont.)

```
                                Toxicity rating 1
  2. Estrogenic substances .......  25,000 units
     Stearyl alcohol ...........    1.0
     Beeswax.................      15.0
     Sodium borate ............     0.7
     Vegetable oil ............    20.0
     Wool wax ................     10.0
     Water, q.s................    100.0
Lanolin creams (cold cream with high lanolin content)
                                Toxicity rating 3
  Lanolin ..................      12.0
  White wax.................       7.5
  Spermaceti ...............       5.0
  Oil of peach kernel* .........   31.0
  Sodium borate ............       0.5
  Perfume .................        0.1
  Water ...................       43.9
                                  100.0
Liquifying creams .............   Toxicity rating 1
  Paraffin ..................      6.0
  White wax.................      12.0
  Liquid petrolatum ..........    54.0
  Stearic acid ..............      1.0
  Sodium borate .............      1.0
  Water ...................       26.0
                                  100.0
Massage creams ..............   Toxicity rating 2
  1. Beeswax.................     12.0
     Spermaceti .............     12.0
     Lanolin ................      8.0
     Peanut oil..............     32.0
     Sodium borate ...........     1.0
     Camphor ...............       1.0
     Water, q.s..............     100.0
  2. Stearic acid ............     9.0
     Cocoa butter ...........      1.0
     Wheat or corn starch .....   14.0
     Sodium borate ...........     2.5
     Glycerin...............       3.0
     Ammonium hydroxide (6%) .....  1.0
     Water .................      66.5
Shave creams (brushless)
                                Toxicity rating 1
  1. Stearic acid ............    23.0
     Anhydrous lanolin .........   4.0
     Triethanolamine ..........    0.8
     Sodium borate ...........     0.8
     Carbitol ...............      1.5
     Water, q.s...............    100.0
                                Toxicity rating 2
  2. Stearic acid ............    16.0
     Cetyl alcohol............     2.0
     Sulfonated castor oil..........  2.0
     Sodium hydroxide ..........    0.4
     Ammonium hydroxide ........    6.0
     Glycerin...............       4.0
     Diethylene glycol ..........   6.0
     Water, q.s................    100.0
     Brushless shave creams may contain:
       Alcohol
       Lard
       Linseed oil
       Menthol
       Phenol
       Soap
       Sodium alginate
       Sodium salicylate
       Tallow
       Zinc compounds
Shave creams (lathering) .........  Toxicity rating 1
  Stearic acid ...............     24.0
  Peanut oil ................       6.0
  Coconut oil ..............        6.0
  Sodium hydroxide............     10.0
  Propylene glycol ............    12.0
  Sodium lauryl sulfate ..........  0.5
  Water, q.s. ...............     100.0
  May contain:
    Alcohol
    Lard
```

Starred ingredients (*) may be responsible for major toxic effects; consult Sec. II.

COSMETICS (Cont.)

Linseed oil
Menthol
Phenol
Soap
Sodium alginate
Sodium salicylate
Tallow
Zinc compounds
Vanishing creams

	Toxicity rating 2
1. Stearic acid	15.2
Potassium hydroxide	0.8
Cetyl alcohol	2.0
Glycerin	10.0
Perfume	0.1
Water, q.s.	100.0
2. Stearic acid	12.0
Sodium borate	1.0
Spermaceti	2.0
Glyceryl monostearate	5.0
Diethylene glycol	5.0
Water, q.s.	100.0

Vanishing creams may contain:
Ammonium stearate
Mineral oil
Potassium carbonate
Soap
Sodium carbonate

Vitamin creams	Toxicity rating 1
Cod liver oil	20.0
Lanolin, anhydrous	30.0
Petrolatum	50.0
	100.0

"Waterless" hand cleaners	Toxicity rating 1
Polyoxyethylene sorbitan monooleate	6.2
Sorbitan sedquioleate	1.2
Methyl p-hydroxybenzoate	0.1
Sodium carboxymethylcellulose	2.5
Perfume	q.s.
Water, q.s.	100.0

DENTAL PREPARATIONS

Denture adhesives	Toxicity rating 2
Tragacanth powder	75.0
Karaya gum powder	24.0
Sassafras oil	1.0
	100.0

Denture cleaners	Toxicity rating 3
Sodium perborate*	32.4
Sodium chloride	60.0
Magnesium sulfate	2.5
Calcium chloride	2.5
Sodium carbonate	2.5
Methyl salicylate	0.01
Menthol	0.02
Peppermint oil	0.1
	100.0

Liquid dentrifices	Toxicity rating 2
Sodium alginate	0.8
Saccharin sodium	0.1
Flavor	1.5
Alcohol	20.0
Glycerin	8.0
Sodium lauryl sulfate	4.0
Amaranth solution (5%)	0.2
Water, q.s.	100.0

Toothpastes

Ammoniated	Toxicity rating 2
Ammonium phosphate, dibasic	3.0
Urea	13.0
Tricalcium phosphate	38.7
Sorbitol solution (70%)	14.5
Glycerin	10.0
Sodium lauryl sulfoacetate	2.0
Aminoacetic acid	0.3
Carboxymethylcellulose	0.3
Flavor oil	1.1
Saccharin	0.2
Dichlorophene	0.2
Water, q.s.	100.0

COSMETICS (Cont.)

Chlorophyll	Toxicity rating 1
Chlorophyllin (potassium copper derivative)	0.2
Calcium carbonate	20.0
Soap, neutral	5.0
Tragacanth powder	6.0
Polyoxyethylene sorbitan monostearate	4.0
Glycerin	20.0
Saccharin sodium	0.1
Water, q.s.	100.0

Fluoride	Toxicity rating 2
Stannous fluoride to give fluoride	0.1
Regular toothpaste, q.s.	100.0

Regular	Toxicity rating 2
Calcium carbonate	20.0
Magnesium carbonate	6.0
Magnesia magma	12.0
Sodium chloride	40.0
Saccharin	0.2
Soap powder	1.0
Tragacanth	1.0
Glycerin	12.0
Water, q.s.	100.0

Toothpastes may contain:
Alkyl aryl sulfonate
Alkyl sarcosinate
Alumina hydrate
Formalin
Galacto-lactone-carbamide
Hydroxybenzoates
Irish moss extractives
Menthol
Methyl salicylate
Mineral oil
Oil of cloves
Papain
Potassium sulfate
Sodium alginate
Sodium benzoate
Sodium bicarbonate
Sodium hexametaphosphate
Sodium lauryl sulfate
Sodium oxalate
Sodium perborate
Sodium phosphate
Sodium stearate
Sodium sulfate
Tetrasodium pyrophosphate
Titanium dioxide

Toothpowders

Ammoniated	Toxicity rating 2
Ammonium phosphate, dibasic	5.0
Urea	22.5
Bentonite	5.0
Calcium carbonate	63.2
Sodium lauryl sulfoacetate	3.0
Saccharin	0.3
Peppermint oil	1.0
	100.0

Chlorophyll	Toxicity rating 2
Chlorophyllin (potassium copper derivative)	2.0
Calcium phosphate, tribasic	44.0
Magnesium carbonate	11.0
Calcium carbonate	40.0
Soap, neutral	0.5
Saccharin sodium	0.2
Calcium stearate	2.0
Flavor oils	0.3
	100.0

Regular	Toxicity rating 3
Calcium carbonate	50.0
Sodium perborate*	16.0
Zinc peroxide	24.0
Soap powder, q.s.	100.0

Starred ingredients (*) may be responsible for major toxic effects; consult Sec. II.

COSMETICS (Cont.)

DEODORANTS

Antiperspirants

Cream . . . . Toxicity rating 2
Aluminum chlorhydroxide complex	15.0
Glycol distearate	14.0
Liquid petrolatum	5.0
Beeswax	2.0
Sodium lauryl sulfate	1.0
Pectin	0.5
Citric acid	2.0
Propylene glycol	6.0
Water, q.s.	100.0

Liquid . . . . Toxicity rating 2 or 3
Aluminum chloride*	20.0
Alcohol	10.0
Propylene glycol	10.0
D & C color	0.01
Water, q.s.	100.0

Powder . . . . Toxicity rating 2 or 3
Aluminum potassium sulfate*	35.0
Zinc stearate	8.0
Titanium dioxide	2.0
Talc	55.0
	100.0

Stick . . . . Toxicity rating 2
Aluminum chloride	10.0
Beeswax	10.0
Paraffin	32.0
Petrolatum	24.0
Cocoa butter, q.s.	100.0

Simple

Creams (paste) . . . . Toxicity rating 2
Oxyquinoline sulfate	4.0
Formaldehyde	1.0
Zinc sulfocarbolate	2.0
Propylene glycol	4.0
Glyceryl monostearate	20.0
Liquid petrolatum	8.0
Water, q.s.	100.0

Liquid . . . . Toxicity rating 2
Oxyquinoline sulfate	4.0
Formaldehyde	1.0
Alcohol	10.0
Water, q.s.	100.0

Powder . . . . Toxicity rating 3
Boric acid*	32.0
Zinc peroxide	20.0
Zinc stearate	10.0
Talc or starch	38.0
	100.0

Stick
		Toxicity rating 2
1. Oxyquinoline sulfate	2.0	
Zinc sulfocarbolate	2.0	
Talc	20.0	
Beeswax	10.0	
Paraffin	32.0	
Petrolatum	24.0	
Cocoa butter, q.s.	100.0	
		Toxicity rating 3
2. Hystrene T-70 fatty acid	5.0	
Sorbitol	2.0	
Alcohol*	85.4	
Sodium hydroxide	0.6	
Hexachlorophene	2.0	
Water	5.0	
	100.0	

Deodorants and antiperspirants may contain:
Bentonite
Benzoic acid*
Calcium borate*
Candelilla wax
Chloral hydrate
Glycerin
Lanolin
Magnesium salts
Zinc oxide

Depilatories

Cream . . . . Toxicity rating 4
Barium sulfide*	15.0
Lanette wax S X	20.0
Spermaceti	3.0

COSMETICS (Cont.)

Stearic acid	2.0
Triethanolamine	0.2
Cetyl alcohol	20.0
Sesame oil	20.0
Perfume	q.s.
Water	19.0
	100.0

Liquid . . . . Toxicity rating 3
Sodium sulfide*	8.0
Starch, soluble	4.0
Sugar	4.0
Glycerin	5.0
Sodium borate	1.0
Sodium lauryl sulfate	1.0
Water, q.s.	100.0

Powder
		Toxicity rating 4
1. Strontium sulfide*	32.0	
Calcium sulfide*	24.0	
Precipitated chalk	32.0	
Menthol	1.0	
Talc, q.s.	100.0	
		Toxicity rating 4
2. Barium sulfide*	24.0	
Zinc oxide	32.0	
Soap powder	6.0	
Talc, q.s.	100.0	

Wax . . . . Toxicity rating 2
Rosin	50.0
Beeswax	24.0
Paraffin	20.0
Benzocaine	2.0
White petrolatum, q.s.	100.0

EYE PREPARATIONS

Eye creams (eye tissue creams, eye wrinkle creams)
Toxicity rating 1
Lecithin	6.0
Cholesterin	2.0
Beeswax	24.0
Lanolin	6.0
Sodium benzoate	1.0
Almond oil, q.s.	100.0

Eye shadows . . . . Toxicity rating 2
Beeswax	10.0
Spermaceti	8.0
Cetyl alcohol	4.0
Lanolin	8.0
Petrolatum, q.s.	100.0
Color (iron oxide pigments)	q.s.

Eyebrow pencils . . . . Toxicity rating 1
Lampblack	10.0 to 20.0
Petrolatum	40.0
Paraffin, q.s.	100.0

Eyebrow plucking creams . . . . . Toxicity rating 2
Benzocaine	2.0
Cold cream	98.0
	100.0

Eyelash and eyebrow dyes . . . . Toxicity rating 2
Brown, black and blue certified oil soluble dyes
Eyelash creams . . . . Toxicity rating 3
Lanolin	5.0
Cocoa butter	4.0
Paraffin	10.0
Cetyl alcohol	2.0
Peach kernel oil,* q.s.	100.0

Eyelash oils . . . . Toxicity rating 1
Lanolin	8.0
Cocoa butter	4.0
Cetyl alcohol	8.0
Alcohol	2.0
Water	10.0
Olive oil, q.s.	100.0

Mascaras
Cake . . . . Toxicity rating 2
Lampblack	40.0
Diethylene glycol stearate	25.0
Kaolin	20.0
Sulfonated castor oil	15.0
	100.0

Starred ingredients (*) may be responsible for major toxic effects; consult Sec. II.

COSMETICS (Cont.)

Cream	Toxicity rating 1
Stearic acid	10.0
Petrolatum	6.0
Liquid petrolatum	10.0
Triethanolamine	3.0
Lampblack	10.0
Water	61.0
	100.0

FACE MASKS

Beauty clays	Toxicity rating 1
Purified siliceous earth	10.0
Kaolin	40.0
Glycerin	6.0
Water, q.s.	100.0
Face packs	Toxicity rating 2
Zinc stearate	4.0
Zinc oxide	4.0
Glycerin	8.0
Tragacanth	4.0
Alcohol	10.0
Limewater, q.s.	100.0

May contain:
Acacia
Balsam of Peru
Glyceryl monostearate
Magnesium carbonate
Mercurized wax
Salicylic acid
Spermaceti
Sulfonated castor oil
Talc
Titanium oxide
Zinc sulfocarbolate

HAIR PREPARATIONS

Hair brillinatines

Cream hair dressing	Toxicity rating 2
Polyethylene glycol 400 monostearate	3.0
Liquid petrolatum	20.0
Alcohol	10.0
Water, q.s.	100.0
Perfume	q.s.
Liquid	Toxicity rating 2
Lanolin	2.0
Liquid petrolatum	50.0
Castor oil	16.0
Alcohol, q.s.	100.0
Perfume	q.s.

May contain:
Amine soap
Apricot kernel oil
Beeswax
Benzyl benzoate
Brucine sulfate
Ceresin
Cetyl alcohol
Copper chloride
Fatty esters
Ferric chloride
Glycerin
Gum benzoin
Gum tragacanth
Kerosene
Menthol
Olive oil
Paraffin
Polyglycols
Pyrogallic acid
Stearates
Thymol

Solid	Toxicity rating 1 or 2
Lanolin	5.0
Petrolatum	50.0
Ceresin (ozokerite)	8.0
Liquid petrolatum, q.s.	100.0

May contain:
Borax
Boric acid
Camphor
Ceresin
Cholesterin
Esters

COSMETICS (Cont.)

Essential oils
Extract of mullein
Glycerin
Glyco B
Glycols
Hexachlorophene
Lead acetate
Menthol
Methyl parasept
Oil of bergamot
Oil of sage
Paraffin
Pilocarpine
Quinine
Resin
Spermaceti
Sulfur
Tar
Triethanolamine
Waxes

Hair dyes

Metallic salt type

Black (iron dye)	Toxicity rating 3
Pyrogallol*	6.0
Alcohol*	32.0
Acetic acid (99%)	0.4
Ferric chloride	1.0
Sugar	1.0
Water	16.0
Ether,* q.s.	100.0

Blond (nickel dye)

Solution No. 1	Toxicity rating 3
Pyrogallol*	6.0
Alcohol	20.0
Water, q.s.	100.0
Solution No. 2	Toxicity rating 3
Nickel ammonium sulfate*	6.0
Sugar	1.0
Ammonium hydroxide (10%)*	20.0
Water, q.s.	100.0
Brown (manganese dye)	Toxicity rating 3
Manganese acetate	10.0
Pyrogallol*	10.0
Acetic acid (99%)	0.2
Water, q.s.	100.0

Silver

Solution No. 1	Toxicity rating 3
Silver nitrate*	10.0
Ammonium hydroxide (10%)*	32.0
Water, q.s.	100.0
Solution No. 2	Toxicity rating 3
Pyrogallol*	6.0
Alcohol	24.0
Water, q.s.	100.0

Oxidizing type

Black	Toxicity rating 3
p-Phenylenediamine HCl*	2.0
Water, q.s.	100.0
Blond	Toxicity rating 1
p-Phenylenediamine HCl	0.1
Diamidophenol	0.1
Water, q.s.	100.0
Brown	Toxicity rating 2
p-Phenylenediamine HCl	0.5
Diamidophenol	0.5
Water, q.s.	100.0

Vegetable type

Black (hair color)	Toxicity rating ?
Indigo	83.0
Henna	17.0
	100.0
Dark Brown (hair color)	Toxicity rating ?
Indigo	75.0
Henna	25.0
	100.0
Light Brown (hair color)	Toxicity rating ?
Indigo	70.0
Henna	30.0
	100.0

Starred ingredients (*) may be responsible for major toxic effects; consult Sec. II.

COSMETICS (Cont.)

Hair dyes (metallic salt and vegetable types)
may contain:
  Aminohydroxybenzene*
  Bismuth salts
  Borax*
  Cadmium salts*
  Cobalt*
  Copper chloride*
  Glycerin
  Hydrogen peroxide*
  Lead acetate*
  Metal (p-methyl aminophenol sulfate)
  Potassium dichromate*
  Sodium hydroxide*
  Sodium persulfate*
  Sodium thiosulfate
  Tin salts

Hair lacquers	Toxicity rating 2
Polyvinyl pyrolidone	2.0
Shellac	0.2
Absolute alcohol	17.5
Perfume	0.3
Freon gas propellants	83.0
	100.0

May contain:
  Boric esters
  Casein
  Cholesterol esters
  Gum acacia
  Gum benzoin
  Karaya gum
  Lanolin
  Silicones
  Sodium alginate
  Sodium bromate*

Hair straighteners	Toxicity rating 2
Polyethylene glycol 6000	2.1
Cetyl alcohol	13.0
Stearyl alcohol	8.6
Triethanolamine lauryl sulfate	1.1
Propylene glycol	16.0
Ammonium thioglycolate (53%)	10.5
Ammonium hydroxide (28%)	3.3
Perfume	2.0
Water	43.4
	100.0

May contain:
  Beeswax
  Castor oil
  Formaldehyde
  Glycerin
  Paraffin
  Permanganate*
  Potassium bromate*
  Rosin
  Soap
  Sodium hydroxide
  Starch
  Tallow gums
  Tragacanth

Hair tints or color rinses	Toxicity rating 2
Propylene glycol monostearate, S.E.	10.0
Sodium lauryl sulfate	1.0
Rhodamine	4.0
Cholesterol	8.0
Lecithin	12.0
Ammonium hydroxide (20%)	5.0
Perfume	0.5
Water, q.s.	100.0

Black hair rinse	Toxicity rating 2 or 3
D & C Black No. 1	16.0
D & C Red No. 13	2.4
D & C Brown No. 1	1.6
Tartaric acid, USP (use 30 grains to 1 gallon of water)	80.0
	100.0

Hair tints or rinses may contain:
  Chloramine T
  Citrate
  Oxalic acid
  Triton-400

COSMETICS (Cont.)

Hair tonics	Toxicity rating 3
1. Euresol	2.0
Castor oil	4.0
Tincture of cantharides*	12.0
Spirits of lavender, q.s.	100.0
2. Resorcinol	1.0
Beta naphthol	1.0
Chloral hydrate*	4.0
Tincture of capsicum	1.2
Tincture of cantharides*	1.2
Castor oil	1.0
Alcohol*	80.0
Water, q.s.	100.0

Hair tonics may contain:
  Acetyl methyl pyrandione
  Arsenic*
  Balsam of Peru
  Benzalkonium chloride*
  Benzyl benzoate
  Calveynth
  Camphor*
  Capsicum
  Cholesterol
  Citrus oils
  Copper sulfate*
  Dihydroxy hexachlorodiphenyl methane
  Essential oils*
  Extracts of figwort
  Glycerin
  Gum benzoin
  Hexachlorophene
  Lanolin
  Lecithin
  Mercuric chloride*
  Mineral oil
  Mullein
  Mutton tallow
  Nutgalls
  Nux vomica*
  Olive oil
  Organic ammonium chloride*
  Paraffin
  Potassium oxyquinoline sulfate
  Quinine sulfate
  Resorcinol monoacetate
  Salicylic acid
  Silicone
  Soapbark
  Sodium caprylate
  Sodium undecylenate
  Stone root
  Strychnine*
  Tannic acid
  Turpentine
  Waxes
  Witch hazel

Permanent waves

Waving solution	Toxicity rating 2
Thioglycollic acid (75%)	6.0
Ammonium hydroxide (28%)	6.0
Sulfatate B	0.1
Water, q.s.	100.0

Neutralizing solution	Toxicity rating 3 or 4
Hydrogen peroxide (6%)*	50.0
Tartaric acid	3.0
Water, q.s.	100.0

Some neutralizers included in wave sets are in
solid form. The most widely used solid
neutralizer is potassium bromate.* These
neutralizers have a toxicity rating of 5.

Permanent wave solutions may contain:
  Ammonium carbonate
  Ammonium phosphate
  Ammonium sulfate
  Borax
  Citric acid
  Duponol M.E. or C
  Ethanolamine
  Lanolin
  Mineral oil
  Monothioglycerol

Starred ingredients (*) may be responsible for major toxic effects; consult Sec. II.

COSMETICS (Cont.)

NOPCO 1408
Sodium bromate*
Sodium hexametaphosphate
Sodium perborate*
Sodium phosphate
Urea

LIPSTICKS

Liquid lipsticks	. . . .	Toxicity rating 2 or 3
Ethyl cellulose	. . . .	3.0
Rosin	. . . .	2.5
Shellac	. . . .	1.0
Castor oil	. . . .	4.5
Petroleum ether*	. . . .	15.0
Alcohol	. . . .	72.0
Rhodamine B	. . . .	1.0
Saframine	. . . .	0.5
Saccharin	. . . .	0.05
Perfume flavor	. . . .	0.5
		100.0

Tube lipsticks	. . . .	Toxicity rating 2
Beeswax	. . . .	40.0
Tetrahydrofurfuryl acetate	. . . . . .	30.0
Cocoa butter	. . . .	20.0
Lanolin	. . . .	5.0
Bromo acid	. . . .	2.0
p-Hydroxybenzoic acid	. . . .	0.1
Red cosmetic lakes	. . . .	q.s.
Perfume	. . . .	q.s.
		100.0

Lipsticks may contain:
Beeswax
Candelilla wax
Carnauba wax
Ceresin
Cetyl alcohol
Cholesterol
Ozokerite
Eosin dyes
Glycol esters
Glycols
Lard
Lecithin
Mineral oil
Paraffin
Sodium dioctyl sulfocyanate
Sodium lauryl sulfate
Spermaceti
Stearates
Vegetable oil

LIQUID MAKE-UPS

Liquid cosmetic stockings	. . . .	Toxicity rating 2
Propylene glycol monostearate	. . . .	4.0
Oleic acid	. . . .	2.0
Liquid petrolatum	. . . .	1.0
Bentonite suspension (5%)	. . . .	20.0
Color pigments	. . . .	14.0
Triethanolamine	. . . .	1.5
Propylene glycol	. . . .	6.0
Methyl p-hydroxybenzoate	. . . .	0.2
Water, q.s.	. . . .	100.0

Liquid powders

1. Titanium dioxide	. . . .	Toxicity rating 1
		2.0
Talc	. . . .	1.0
Stearic acid	. . . .	10.0
Liquid petrolatum	. . . .	12.0
Triethanolamine	. . . .	3.0
Water, q.s.	. . . .	100.0
Perfume	. . . .	q.s.

2. Cetyl alcohol	. . . .	Toxicity rating 2
		0.2
Lanolin, anhydrous	. . . .	0.2
Glyceryl stearate	. . . .	0.8
Sodium hydroxide	. . . .	0.2
Stearic acid	. . . .	7.5
Propylene glycol	. . . .	15.0
Titanium dioxide	. . . .	5.0
Color pigments	. . . .	5.0 to 12.0
Water, q.s.	. . . .	100.0

COSMETICS (Cont.)

Liquid powders may contain:
Alcohol
Boric acid
Calcium carbonate
Candelilla wax
Carnauba wax
Clay
Essential oils
Esters
Ethyl parasept
Glycerin
Glycols
Iron oxide
Lecithin
Magnesium carbonate
Magnesium oleate
Oils
Sorbitol
Spermaceti
Waxes
Zinc oxide
Zinc stearate

LOTIONS

Astringent lotions	. . . .	Toxicity rating 2 or 3
1. Alum	. . . .	1.0
Lactic acid	. . . .	1.0
Propylene glycol	. . . .	6.0
Alcohol	. . . .	16.0
Water, q.s.	. . . .	100.0
Perfume	. . . .	q.s.
2. Menthol	. . . .	0.2
Benzoin tincture	. . . .	4.0
Tragacanth	. . . .	1.0
Glycerin	. . . .	4.0
Oil of cinnamon	. . . .	0.6
Water, q.s.	. . . .	100.0

Astringent lotions may contain:
Aluminum chloride*
Boric acid*
Camphor*
Chromium salts*
Ferric salts
Glycol
Lead acetate*
Tannic acid
Zinc oxide
Zinc sulfate*
Zinc sulfocarbolate

Bleach lotions	. . . .	Toxicity rating 3
Hydrogen peroxide (5%)*	. . . .	64.0
Tincture of benzoin	. . . .	4.0
Water, q.s.	. . . .	100.0

Freckle lotions

		Toxicity rating 3
1. Potassium chlorate*	. . . .	2.0
Potassium carbonate	. . . .	6.0
Sodium borate	. . . .	1.0
Sugar	. . . .	6.0
Glycerin	. . . .	16.0
Rose water, q.s.	. . . .	100.0

		Toxicity rating 2
2. Acetic acid (dilute)	. . . .	4.0
Alcohol	. . . .	4.0
Citric acid	. . . .	6.0
Glycerin	. . . .	6.0
Water, q.s.	. . . .	100.0

Hand lotions

		Toxicity rating 1
1. Propylene glycol monostearate	. . .	6.0
Oleic acid	. . . .	2.0
Mineral oil	. . . .	1.0
Cetyl alcohol	. . . .	1.0
Lanolin	. . . .	1.0
Triethanolamine	. . . .	1.0
Glycerin	. . . .	5.0
Methyl p-hydroxybenzoate	. . . . .	0.1
Water, q.s.	. . . .	100.0

		Toxicity rating 1
2. Stearic acid	. . . .	6.4
Propyl p-hydroxbenzoate	. . . .	0.1

Starred ingredients (*) may be responsible for major toxic effects; consult Sec. II.

COSMETICS (Cont.)

Isopropyl myristate	1.5
Polyethylene glycol 600 monostearate	0.3
Potassium hydroxide	0.2
Carboxymethylcellulose solution (0.8%)	41.2
Water	50.3
	100.0

Toxicity rating 1

3. Stearic acid	7.0
Lanolin	0.5
Sorbitan monooleate	0.5
Polyoxyethylene sorbitan monostearate	2.5
Sorbitol	5.0
Methyl p-hydroxybenzoate	0.1
Perfume	0.1
Water, q.s.	100.0

Hand lotions may contain:
- Acetone
- Alcohol
- Alginates
- Almond oil
- Aluminum chloride
- Ammonium hydroxide
- Bay rum
- Beeswax
- Benzoic acid
- Boric acid
- Calcium thioglycollate
- Camphor
- Carbamide
- Carbowax
- Cholesterol
- Citric acid
- Clay
- Cocoa butter
- Diethyl phthalate
- Essential oils
- Ethers
- Formaldehyde
- Gum acacia
- Gum karaya
- Gum tragacanth
- Iron oxide
- Lecithin
- Neatsfoot oil
- Olive oil
- Oxyquinolin sulfate
- Phenol
- Potassium cetyl palmitate
- Potassium sulfate
- Quince seed
- Resorcinol monoacetate
- Sesame oil
- Soap
- Sodium benzoate
- Sodium lauryl sulfate
- Sodium stearate
- Spermaceti
- Sulfur
- Thymol
- Titanium dioxide
- Turpentine
- Urea
- Vegetable oil
- Waxes
- Witch hazel

Mouth washes

Toxicity rating 2

1. Zinc chloride	0.8
Oil of eucalyptus	0.2
Methyl salicylate	0.2
Eucalyptol	0.06
Menthol	0.1
Thymol	0.1
Fluid extract of hydrastis	0.2
Glycerin	4.0
Alcohol	32.0
Orange water, q.s.	100.0

COSMETICS (Cont.)

Toxicity rating 3

2. Phenol*	2.0
Sodium sulfocarbolate	2.5
Sodium bicarbonate	3.5
Glycerin	21.0
Carmine to color	q.s.
Orange water, q.s.	100.0

Toxicity rating 2

3. Benzalkonium chloride solution (10%)	0.6
Saccharin sodium	0.05
Amaranth solution (5%)	0.1
Cinnamon oil	0.2
Polyoxyethylene sorbitan monolaurate	1.2
Water, q.s.	100.0

Mouth washes may contain:
- Benzoic acid
- Boric acid
- Formaldehyde
- Indigo root
- Oil of ceryeph
- Tannic acid
- Turpentine
- Zinc chloride*

Shaving lotions **Toxicity rating 2**

1. Menthol	0.1
Alum	1.0
Camphor	0.2
Boric acid	2.0
Propylene glycol	6.0
Alcohol	12.0
Water, q.s.	100.0
Perfume	q.s.
2. Benzoin tincture	2.0
Boric acid	2.0
Witch hazel extract	32.0
Glycerin	6.0
Alcohol	4.0
Water, q.s.	100.0
Perfume	q.s.

Shaving lotions may contain:
- Bay rum
- Benzocaine
- Benzoic acid
- Cantharides
- Capsicum
- Citric acid
- Essential oils
- Formaldehyde
- Gum tragacanth
- Lactic acid
- Lavender
- Lilac
- Rose Water
- Titanium dioxide
- Zinc carbonate
- Zinc oxide
- Zinc stearate

Skin fresheners **Toxicity rating 2**

Hamamelis water	60.0
Camphorated alcohol (10%)	15.0
Citric acid	1.0
Alcohol	24.0
	100.0

May contain:
- Arnica
- Bay rum
- Boric acid
- Brucine sulfate
- Chamomile
- Esters
- Floral waters
- Glycerin
- Hexachlorophene
- Lactic acid
- Magnesia
- Menthol
- Oil of lavender
- Phosphoric acid
- Talc
- Tincture of benzoin

Starred ingredients (*) may be responsible for major toxic effects; consult Sec. II.

COSMETICS (Cont.)

NAIL PREPARATIONS

Cuticle creams (softener)

Liquid .... Toxicity rating 3	
Potassium hydroxide*	4.0
Glycerin.	24.0
Water, q.s.	100.0
Cream .... Toxicity rating 3	
Salicylic acid*	6.0
Lactic acid	6.0
Beeswax.	20.0
Lanolin	20.0
Petrolatum	16.0
Liquid petrolatum	20.0
Water, q.s.	100.0

Cuticle creams may contain:

Boric acid*
Cetyl alcohol
Cocoa butter
Glycol ether
Glycols
Olive oil
Paraffin
Perfume oil soap
Polyethoxy ether
Potassium tetrapyrophosphate*
Sorbitan ester
Stearic acid
Triethanolamine
Trisodium phosphate*
Wax
Wetting agent

Nail bleaches .... Toxicity rating 2	
Citric acid	4.0
Potassium binoxalate	1.0
Water, q.s.	100.0
Nail enamel .... Toxicity rating 3	
Nitrocellulose	11.4
Tricresyl phosphate*	8.3
Dibutyl phthalate	13.5
Ethyl acetate*	31.5
Butyl acetate*	30.0
Ethyl alcohol.	4.9
D & C Red No. 19	0.1
D & C Red No. 31	0.2
Oil pink	0.1
	100.0
Nail finishes .... Toxicity rating 3	
Celluloid	6.0
Amyl acetate*	75.0
Acetone*, q.s.	100.0
Nail polishes .... Toxicity rating 3	
Nitrocellulose	10.0
Resorcinol diacetate*	10.0
Ethyl lactate	20.0
Alcoholic carmine solution (1%) ...	0.2
Methyl acetate*, q.s.	100.0

May contain:

Acetone*
Amyl acetate*
Benzoin
Benzyl abietate
Butyl acetyl ricinoleate
Camphor*
Carnauba wax
Castor oil
Cellulose acetate
Cellulose acetobutyrate
Cellulose acetopropionate
Dibutyl phthalate
Ethyl cellulose
Ethyl formate*
Ester gum
Formaldehyde - amine resin
Hydrocarbons*
Gum dammar
Lake colors
Lecithin
Lithopone
Mastic sandarac
Pontianas
Shellac
Titanium dioxide

Toluene*
Wax
Xylene*

Nail polish removers

	Toxicity rating 4
1. Acetone*	32.0
Alcohol	20.0
Benzene*	40.0
Ethyl acetate, q.s.	100.0
	Toxicity rating 3
2. Amyl acetate*	100.0
Perfume.	q.s.
Cream type .... Toxicity rating 3	
Stearic acid	9.0
Castor oil.	2.0
Triethanolamine	3.5
Butyl acetate*	70.0
Water	15.5

Nail polish removers may contain:

Almond oil
Beeswax
Butyl acetyl ricinoleate
Butyl stearate
Cetyl alcohol
Cottonseed oil
Cyclohexanol (or methyl derivative)
Ethyl oleate
Glyceryl ricinoleates
Glycol
Glycol stearate
Isopropyl alcohol*
Ketones*
Lanolin
Magnesium oleate
Mineral oil
Oleyl alcohol
Olive oil
Paraffin
Spermaceti
Stearyl alcohol
Triethanolamine stearate

Nail whites

Cream .... Toxicity rating 1	
Titanium dioxide	2.0
Beeswax.	12.0
Cetyl alcohol.	4.0
Oxycholesterin	16.0
Petrolatum	24.0
Cocoa butter	4.0
Sodium borate	0.6
Tincture of benzoin	6.0
Water, q.s.	100.0
Liquid .... Toxicity rating 1	
Titanium dioxide	1.0
Glyceryl monostearate	4.0
Beeswax.	1.0
Almond oil	10.0
Petrolatum	6.0
Water, q.s.	100.0

PERFUMES

Cologne waters .... Toxicity rating 3	
Oil of lavender flowers	0.2
Oil of lemon	0 8
Oil of neroli	0.1
Alcohol,* q.s.	100.0
Concentrated perfume extracts ..... Toxicity rating 3	
Floral odor*	3.0 to 5.0
Alcohol, q.s.	100.0

Bouquets and blends of floral odors are offered
as perfume extracts under such names as
Chypre, L'Origan, Muse, and Narcisse Noir.

Floral odors

French rose ₊ .... Toxicity rating 4	
Rose, absolute	20.0
Citronellol*	15.0
Isoeugenol	5.0
Phenylethyl alcohol	10.0
Phenylpropyl alcohol	10.0
Aldehyde (C_8) 10%	1.0

₊See Essential Oils*

COSMETICS (Cont.)

Rhodinol.................	14.0
Geraniol,* q.s.	100.0
Heliotrope †.......... Toxicity rating 4	
Heliotropine	20.0
Coumarin	10.0
Ylang-Ylang (Bourbon)	5.0
Tuberose, absolute liquid	5.0
Terpineol*.................	20.0
Vanillin	10.0
Benzyl acetate..............	10.0
Rose, absolute..............	5.0
Jasmine (synthetic), q.s.	100.0
Jasmine†.......... Toxicity rating 4	
Jasmine, absolute	5.0
Aldehyde, C10	2.0
Phenylethyl alcohol	10.0
Rhodinol.................	10.0
Heliotropine	10.0
Ylang-Ylang (Bourbon)	5.0
Hydroxycitronellal	10.0
Linalool	10.0
Linalyl acetate	5.0
Benzyl acetate..............	30.0
Benzyl alcohol, q.s.	100.0
Lilac †................ Toxicity rating 4	
Anisic aldehyde	5.0
Cinnamic alcohol	10.0
Heliotropine	10.0
Phenylethyl alcohol*	20.0
Phenyl acetaldehyde* (50%)	10.0
Phenylpropyl aldehyde	2.0
Linalool	10.0
Hydroxycitronellal	10.0
Benzyl acetate..............	10.0
Jasmine, absolute	5.0
Rhodinol.................	5.0
Terpineol, q.s.	100.0
Muguet (lily of the valley)† ...... Toxicity rating 4	
Benzyl acetate*.............	15.0
Linalool	10.0
Cinnamic acetate	5.0
Phenylethyl alcohol	10.0
Hydroxycitronellal*	15.0
Ionone	10.0
Jasmine, absolute	5.0
Rose, absolute..............	5.0
Rhodinol	10.0
Terpineol,* q.s.............	100.0

†See Essential Oils*

Florida waters................ Toxicity rating 3	
Oil of neroli	0.5
Oil of lavender flowers	0.5
Oil of bergamot	3.0
Oil of clove	0.2
Oil of cinnamon	0.3
Oil of rose	0.5
Orange flower water	10.0
Alcohol,* q.s.	100.0
Sachets	
Potpourri .... Toxicity rating 2	
Lavender flowers	65.0
Rose petals...............	29.4
Vanilla..................	1.2
Clove buds, powdered	1.2
Storax resin, powdered	1.2
Benzoin (Siam) powdered......	1.2
Ambergris, powdered	0.4
Oil of rose	0.4
	100.0
Ylang-ylang sachet .... Toxicity rating 2	
Orange peel, granular	50.00
Rose petals	46.62
Coumarin	0.01
Vanillin	0.02
Tincture of civet	0.10
Tincture of musk	0.05
Oil of ylang-ylang	0.30
Oil of rose	0.01
Oil of bergamot	0.05
Oil of rose geranium	2.84
	100.0

COSMETICS (Cont.)

Solid eau de cologne .... Toxicity rating 2 or 3	
Sodium stearate.............	8.0
Isopropyl myristate	10.0
Glycerin	3.0
Cologne perfume oil	3.0
Ethyl alcohol,* q.s.	100.0
Stick colognes .... Toxicity rating 3	
Hystrene T-70 fatty acid	5.0
Sorbitol	2.0
Alcohol*.................	87.4
Sodium hydroxide...........	0.6
Water	5.0
Perfume..................	q.s.
	100.0
Toilet waters .... Toxicity rating 3	
Floral odor*..............	1.0
Alcohol (65 to 75%), q.s.	100.0

POWDERS

After shave powders .... Toxicity rating 3	
Menthol	0.6
Boric acid*.................	20.0
Talc, q.s.................	100.0
Perfume	q.s.
Compact (cake make-up) powders	
	Toxicity rating 2
1. Talc	54.0
Kaolin	26.0
Zinc oxide	10.0
Titanium dioxide	3.0
Tragacanth mucilage	6.0
Mineral oil	2.0
Perfume and color	q.s.
	100.0
	Toxicity rating 2
2. Diethylene glycol stearate	25.0
Titanium dioxide	20.0
Kaolin	10.0
Talc	25.0
Sulfonated castor oil	15.0
Color pigment	5.0
	100.0
	Toxicity rating 2
3. Titanium dioxide and color pigments	30.0
Talc	10.0
Carnauba wax	8.0
Isopropyl myristate	52.0
	100.0
Face powders .... Toxicity rating 2	
Titanium dioxide	3.0
Zinc oxide	12.0
Calcium carbonate	4.0
Zinc stearate	2.0
Talc, q.s.................	100.0
Iron dioxide pigments, q.s. to color (up to 5%)	
Rice powders .... Toxicity rating 2	
Rice starch	16.0
Magnesium carbonate	1.0
Magnesium stearate	.12.0
Kaolin	8.0
Titanium dioxide	4.0
Talc, q.s.................	100.0
May contain:	
Aluminum stearates	
Barium sulfate	
Bismuth subcarbonate	
Calcium sulfate	
Cetyl alcohol	
Color	
Lithopone	
Magnesium oxide	
Metallic soaps	
Mineral oil	
Perfume	
Starch	
Sulfur	
Zinc sulfide	
Talcum powders .... Toxicity rating 2	
Boric acid	2.0
Magnesium carbonate	4.0
Talc, q.s.................	100.0
Perfume..................	q.s.

Starred ingredients (*) may be responsible for major toxic effects; consult Sec. II.

COSMETICS (Cont.)

May contain:
  Ammonium alum
  Ammonium chloride
  Barium sulfide
  Benzoic acid
  Calcium carbonate
  Calendula extract
  Camphor
  Hydroxyquinoline sulfate
  Iron oxide
  Kaolin
  Magnesium stearate
  o-Benzyl phenol
  Potassium soap
  Sodium perborate
  Sodium soap
  Sulfur
  Titanium dioxide
  Turpentine
  Zinc oxide
  Zinc stearate

ROUGES

Cake (compact) . . . . Toxicity rating 2
  Talc 40.0
  Kaolin 20.0
  Brilliant red lake (certified) 10.0
  Zinc oxide 20.0
  Zinc stearate 4.0
  Liquid petrolatum 3.0
  Tragacanth mucilage 3.0
  Perfume. . . . . q.s.
                                          100.0
Cream

                                Toxicity rating 2
1. Erythrosin to color 4.0
  Stearic acid 24.0
  Cetyl alcohol. 6.0
  Potassium hydroxide 1.0
  Glycerin 6.0
  Water, q.s. 100.0
                              Toxicity rating 2 or 3
2. Sorbitan sesquioleate 2.0
  Lanolin 2.0
  Mineral oil 16.0
  Petrolatum 30.0
  Color pigment* 10.0
  Sorbitol 6.0
  Perfume. . . . . q.s.
  Water 34.0
                                          100.0
Liquid . . . . Toxicity rating 2
  Carmine 4.0
  Ammonium hydroxide (28%) 6.0
  Glycerin. 12.0
  Water, q.s. 100.0
Liquid lip rouges . . . . Toxicity rating 2
  Ethyl alcohol. 88.0
  Ethyl cellulose 3.5
  Oleic acid monoglyceride 3.5
  Red color pigment 5.0
                                          100.0
Paste. . . . . Toxicity rating 2
  Carmine 4.0
  Ammonium hydroxide 4.0
  Beeswax. 6.0
  Cetyl alcohol. 4.0
  Stearic acid 8.0
  Cocoa butter 4.0
  Petrolatum, q.s. 100.0

SHAMPOOS

Cream. . . . . Toxicity rating 3
  Sodium alkyl sulfate paste* 54.0
  Stearic acid 10.0
  Triethanolamine stearate 12.0
  Glyceryl monostearate 3.0
  Diglycol laurate. 2.0
  Sodium borate* 7.0
  Perfume oil 1.0
  Water, q.s. 100.0

COSMETICS (Cont.)

Foaming . . . . Toxicity rating 3
  Sulfonated castor oil* 90.0
  Sodium lauryl sulfate 5.0
  Liquid petrolatum 5.0
                                          100.0
Jelly or paste . . . . Toxicity rating 2
  Castille soap shavings 40.0
  Olive oil 4.0
  Soft soap 4.0
  Potassium carbonate solution (5%) . . 4.0
  Triethanolamine 1.0
  Alcohol (50%), q.s. 100.0
Soap. . . . . Toxicity rating 2 or 3
  Coconut oil 15.0
  Palm oil 5.0
  Potassium hydroxide* (90%) 3.0
  Sodium hydroxide (90%) 1.0
  Alcohol 7.0
  Ethylenediaminetetraacetic acid
    (sodium salt). 0.5
  Water, q.s. 100.0
Soapless . . . . Toxicity rating 3
  Sulfonated castor oil* 63.0
  Sulfonated olive oil* 30.0
  Liquid petrolatum 5.0
  Ethylene glycol 2.0
  Perfume . . . . q.s.
Shampoos may contain:
  Alkylamine lauryl sulfate*
  Ammonium hydroxide
  Ammonium thioglycollate*
  Benzoic acid
  Castor oil
  Cholesterol
  Coal tar
  Cottonseed oil
  Diethylaminoethyloleylamide as phosphate,
    benzoate, acetate, borate, citrate
  Extract of mullein
  Formaldehyde
  Glycerin
  Glycol monostearate
  Hexachlorophene
  Karaya gum
  Lanolin
  Lecithin
  Magnesium silicate
  Methyl cellulose
  Mineral oil
  Myristic acid
  Oil of cade*
  Oxycholesterol
  p-Hydroxybenzoate
  Potassium pyrophosphate
  Propylene glycol
  Sodium alginate
  Sodium alkyl aryl polyether sulfonates*
  Sodium citrate
  Sodium dihexylsulfosuccinate
  Sodium-N-methyl-N-oleoyl taurate
  Sodium salt of isothionic acid reaction
    product with oleic acid
  Sodium stearate
  Soybean oil
  Sulfonated naphthalenes*
  Sulfonated condensation product of mono-
    ethanolamine and coconut fatty acids
  Thioglycollic acid*
  Triethanolamine myristate
  Triethanolamine oleate
  Trisodium phosphate*
  Tween - 20
  Vegetable oils

SUNTAN PREPARATIONS, FILM FORMING AGENTS

Alcoholic solutions . . . . Toxicity rating 2
  Isobutyl p-aminobenzoate 5.0
  Glycerin. 10.0
  Water 25.0
  Alcohol 60.0
                                          100.0

Starred ingredients (*) may be responsible for major toxic effects; consult Sec. II.

COSMETICS (Cont.)

Aqueous solutions . . . . Toxicity rating 3
Sodium p-aminobenzoate	5.0
Polyoxyethylene sorbitan mono-	
oleate	2.0
Water	50.0
Alcohol,* q.s.	100.0

Creams . . . . Toxicity rating 2
Methyl p-aminobenzoate	5.0
Glyceryl monostearate, S.E.	14.0
Isopropyl myristate	25.0
Lanolin	5.0
Propylene glycol	5.0
Titanium dioxide	3.0
Iron oxide pigment	2.2
Methyl p-hydroxybenzoate	0.2
Water, q.s.	100.0

Oily solutions . . . . Toxicity rating 3
Iron oxide pigments	2.0
Homomenthyl salicylate*	20.0
Ethyl p-aminobenzoate	2.0
Alcohol	20.0
Olive oil.	30.0
Peanut oil, q.s.	100.0

Suntan preparations may contain:
Animal fat
Beeswax
Borates
Camphor*
Castor oil
Chondrus
Cocoa butter
Coconut oil
Cottonseed oil
Cydonium
Formaldehyde*
Glycols
Heliophan
Hydroquinone*
Methyl salicylate*
Mineral oil
Neatsfoot oil
Oil of lavender*
Perfume
Petrolatum
Phenol*
Poppyseed oil
Quince seed
Quinine alkaloid*
Sesame oil
Stearic acid
Sulfonated ils*
Tannic acid*
Triethanolamine
Turpentine*
Vegetable oil
White oil

CRAYONS

CRAYONS. . . . . Toxicity rating 2
Paraffin wax
Stearic acid
Pigments
Children's Crayons are made from products known to be "non-toxic," although the term has no strict meaning. Children, babies in particular, seem to react differently from adults at times. For example, para red seems harmless to adults and animals, but sometimes poisons small children who eat products which contain it.
Industrial Crayons: Most crayons for industrial use are of two types, water insoluble and water soluble (indelible). The insoluble pencil leads and lumber crayons, in general, have non-toxic pigments. The exceptions might be the yellows and greens which may contain lead chromate.
The dyes used in leads for water soluble pencils are of various types. Harmless dyes are most commonly used, although there is a possibility that some manufacturers use para red. Indelible or copying leads contain methyl violet (gentian violet). The amount likely to be taken orally is

CRAYONS (Cont.)

small, but the appearance of the child's mouth may frighten the parents. The only ill effects that are attributable to methyl violet are nausea and headache for a few hours, although vomiting, diarrhea, liver and kidney injuries may occur rarely.

DECORATIONS

DECORATIONS (Christmas spray for trees, etc.)
Toxicity rating 3
Freon
Lucite
Methylene chloride*
Perfume

DECORATIONS . . . . Toxicity rating 3 or 4
Christmas tree ornaments of the "bubble light" variety frequently have such substances as carbon tetrachloride*, ethyl alcohol*, methyl chloride*, methylene chloride*, or ethyl ether*.

DEGREASERS

POWDER . . . . Toxicity rating 4
Kaolin
Naphtha
Carbon tetrachloride*

LIQUID . . . . Toxicity rating 3 or 4
Petroleum solvent*
Emulsifier
Pine oil*
Chlorinated hydrocarbons*

DEODORIZERS

CLEANSER TYPE . . . . Toxicity rating 3
Pine oil*	70 to 80%
Soap	10%
Water and coloring.	10 to 20%

DEODORANT BLOCKS
	Toxicity rating 3
1. p-Dichlorobenzene	100%
	Toxicity rating 4
2. Naphthalene	100%

REFRIGERATOR DEODORIZER. . . . . . Toxicity rating 1
Activated charcoal 100%

SPRAY TYPE
Toxicity rating 3
1. Isopropyl alcohol*	
Triethylene glycol	
Propylene glycol	42.5%
p-Diisobutyl phenoxy ethoxy ethyldimethyl benzyl ammonium chloride*	
Inert ingredients, water	57.5%
	Toxicity rating 2
2. Triethylene glycol.	7 to 90%
May have freon propellant	

WICK TYPE . . . . Toxicity rating 2 or 3
Formaldehyde*	0.0 to 5.0%
Water	90 to 92%
Emulsifier	
Deodorant oils* (see essential oils)	
Alcohol	
Antioxidant	

DISINFECTANTS

ACIDS . . . . Toxicity rating 4
Alkyl (C_8 to C_{18}) dimethylbenzyl-
ammonium chloride* . . . . 30 to 50%
Ammonium chloride
Sodium bicarbonate
Sometimes contain:
Acetic acid
Benzoic acid*
Boric acid*
Butyric acid

Starred ingredients (*) may be responsible for major toxic effects; consult Sec. II.

DISINFECTANTS (Cont.)

Carbonic acid
Chloroacetic acid*
Citric acid
Formic and related acids*
Lactic acid
Propionic acid
Pyroligneous acid
Salicylic acid*
Sulfurous acid*
see also Acid, Section III

ALKALIES

		Toxicity rating 3 or 4
1. Ammonium hydroxide*		3 to 29%
Water		71 to 97%
		Toxicity rating 5
2. Sodium hydroxide*		94%
Sodium carbonate		2%

Sometimes contain:
Calcium hydroxide*
Sodium silicates
Trisodium phosphate*
see also Alkali, Section III

HALOGENS

		Toxicity rating 4
1. Calcium hypochlorite*		50%
Inert ingredients		50%
		Toxicity rating 3
2. Sodium hypochlorite*		3 to 5%
Sodium chloride		less than 5%
Sodium phosphate*		92%

Sometimes contain:
Chloramines
Iodine*
see also Hypochlorite, Section III

PHENOLS .... Toxicity rating 4

1. Cresol*	50%
Soap	23 to 31%
Glycerin	3%
2. Coal tar phenols*	8 to 30%
Coal tar hydrocarbons*	44 to 58%
Soap	15 to 25%
Water	10%

Sometimes contain:
Alcohol
Ammonium hydroxide*
Borax*
Formaldehyde*
Orthophenylphenol*
Sodium bicarbonate

MISCELLANEOUS

	Toxicity rating 3 or 4
1. Alkyl dimethylbenzylammonium chloride*	2 to 20%
Trisodium phosphate*	30%
Sodium carbonate	30%
Isopropyl alcohol*	20%
Pine oil	9%
	Toxicity rating 3
2. Pine oil*	70 to 85%
Anhydrous soap	7 to 20%
Water	8 to 18%
Isopropyl alcohol	3 to 6%
3. Garbage can sprays	Toxicity rating 4
o-Dichlorobenzene*	60%
Petroleum distillate	10%
Pine oil	5%
4. Seed disinfectants	Toxicity rating 4
Phenylmercuric acetate*	3 to 7%
Inert ingredients	95%
5. Vegetable germicides	Toxicity rating 3
Alcohol*	85%
Thymol, oil origanum, oil cajeput*, oil lavender*, oil rosemary*, oil pine	10%
Inert ingredients	5%
	Toxicity rating 3 or 4
6. Formaldehyde*	15 to 37%
Inert ingredients	63 to 85%

DISINFECTANTS (Cont.)

7. Dyes	Toxicity rating
Acridine dyes	?
Brilliant green	4
Crystal violet	4
Methylene blue	3
Pyridine compounds	?
Sulfonamides	3
8. The Metals and their salts	
Arsenic and arsenical compounds	5
Copper and copper salts	4
Mercury and mercurials	5
Silver and silver compounds	4
Metallic silver	
Simple silver salts	
Colloidal silver compounds	
Zinc	4
Sulfur	3
Oxidizing agents	
Ozone	?
Hydrogen peroxide	3 or 4
Sodium perborate	4
Benzoyl peroxide	3?
Dichromate	4
Sodium azide	5
Potassium permanganate	corrosive 4?

The following list of chemically named compounds are used specifically as disinfectants: many use the compounds already named under the general categories.

	Toxicity rating
Alkylated tolylmethyltrimethylammonium chloride	4
Sodium p-toluenesulfonechloramide	?
Monohydroxymercuridiiodoresorcin- sulfonphthalein	?
Octadecenyl dimethylethylammonium bromide (see alkyl dimethylethyl- ammonium bromide)	4
m-Cresyl acetate (see cresol)	4
N-dichlorosulfamylbenzoic acid	3
Phenylmercuric borate	5
Sodium pentachlorophenate	4
Tridecyl benzylhydroxyethylimida- zolinium chloride (see alkyl hydroxyethylimidazolinium chloride)	4
Polyalkylnaphthalene methyl pyridinium chloride (see quaternary ammonium chloride)	4
Mercury salicylophenylformic acid	5
Anhydride of 4-nitro-3-hydroxymercuri- o-cresol (nitromersol)	?
Secondary amyltricresol (see cresol)	4
Nitrofurazone (5-nitro-2-furaldehyde semicarbazone)	4
Quaternary ammonium salt	4
Alkyl dimethylbenzylammonium chloride	4
2,8 diaminoacridine	?
Cetylpyridinium chloride	4
Sodium metasilicate pentahydrate	3
2,8-diamino-10-methylacridium chloride	?

DRIERS

AIR DEHUMIDIFIERS

	Toxicity rating 2
1. Calcium chloride	100%
	Toxicity rating 2 or 3
2. Aluminum chloride	
Calcium chloride	
Potassium chloride*	100%
Sodium tripolyphosphate*	

FUEL TANK DRIERS (to absorb water in gasoline)

	Toxicity rating 3
Methyl alcohol*	100%

DYES

EASTER EGG DYES .... Toxicity rating 1 or 2	
Lactose and dextrose	97%
U.S. certified coal tar colors	3%

Starred ingredients (*) may be responsible for major toxic effects; consult Sec. II.

DYES (Cont.)

May contain:
  Alum
  Aluminum sulfate
  Dextrin
  Sodium sulfate

LEATHER DYES . . . . Toxicity rating 4
Methyl, ethyl or isopropyl alcohol* . .   30%
Xylene*
Aniline dye*
May contain:
  Nitrobenzene*
  Tannic acid*

RUG DYES . . . . Toxicity rating 2 or 3
Aniline dye*
Acetic acid
Citric acid
Diethylene glycol*
Sodium chloride

SHOE DYES . . . . Toxicity rating 3 or 4
Isopropyl alcohol*
o-Dichlorobenzene*
Diethylene glycol monoethyl ether
Nigrosine* (aniline black)

EMBALMING FLUIDS

EMBALMING FLUIDS . . . . Toxicity rating 3
1. Methyl formate* 30.0%
   Formamide 1.0%
   Sodium borate 2.5%
   Sodium nitrate 0.5%
   Glycerin 10.0%
   Water 56.0%
2. Glyoxal (40%)* 20.0%
   Formaldehyde solution*† 20.0%
   Sodium borate 2.0%
   Sodium nitrate 5.0%
   Glycerin 6.0%
   Methyl alcohol* 20.0%
   Water 27.0%
†Commercial grade (formalin) containing 40% by volume
of formaldehyde gas.
3. Highly concentrated forms of embalming fluid are
   also available and used for injection into internal
   cavities.

FILLERS

1. Magnesium carbonate . . . . Toxicity rating 3
2. Magnesium oxide . . . . Toxicity rating 3
3. Mercuric oxide (red and yellow) . . Toxicity rating 5

FIRE EXTINGUISHERS

CARBON DIOXIDE FIRE EXTINGUISHERS
Compressed carbon dioxide gas 100%

DRY CHEMICAL FIRE EXTINGUISHERS
                               Toxicity rating 2
Sodium bicarbonate 99%
Magnesium stearate . . . . trace
Tricalcium phosphate . . . . trace

FOAM FIRE EXTINGUISHERS . . . Toxicity rating 2 or 3
Charge A Aluminum sulfate*
Charge B Sodium bicarbonate
         Licorice
         Potassium phosphate

LIQUID FIRE EXTINGUISHERS . . . . . . Toxicity rating 1
1. Calcium chloride solution
                           Toxicity rating 4
2. Carbon tetrachloride* 100%
                           Toxicity rating 4
3. Carbon tetrachloride* . . . . }
   Trichloroethylene* . . . . } 100%
                           Toxicity rating 3
4. Chlorobromomethane 100%
   (see dichloromethane*)

FIRE PROOFING COMPOUNDS

FIRE PROOFING COMPOUNDS . . . . . Toxicity rating 2
Ammonium sulfate
Magnesium carbonate
Magnesium oxide

FIRE WORKS

OXIDIZING AGENTS . . . . Toxicity rating 4
Potassium nitrate*
Potassium chlorate*
Barium nitrate*
Potassium perchlorate*

FUEL AND BINDERS
Charcoal
Fossil gums
Gelatin
Glue
Iron powder
Lampblack
Lead nitrate*
Magnesium
Milk sugar
Petroleum
Resins
Shellac
Starch
Stearin
Sugar
Suflur
Zinc powder

COLORS . . . . Toxicity rating 4 or 5
Phosphorus*, mercury*, sulfocyanate, antimony*,
copper* salts, e.g., arsenate*, carbonate, oxalate*,
oxide, sulfate, sulfide*, and chloride.

FIREPLACE COLORS

FIREPLACE COLORS

		Toxicity rating 3
1. Copper chloride*		10.0%
Coke dust, sawdust		90.0%
2. Flame colorations may contain	Toxicity rating	
Violet		
Potassium compounds	3	
Rubidium compounds	3?	
Cesium compounds	3?	
Blue		
Copper chloride or bromide . . .	4	
Lead compounds	5	
Arsenic compounds	5	
Selenium compounds	6	
Green		
Copper compounds	4	
Thallium compounds	5	
Tellurium compounds	5?	
Barium compounds	4 or 5	
Molybdenum coumpounds	5?	
Antimony compounds	5	
Ammonium compounds	?	
Zinc compounds	4	
Borates	4	
Phosphates	3	
Red		
Lithium compounds	3	
Strontium compounds	2	
Calcium compounds	2	
Yellow		
Sodium compounds	?	

FUELS

FIRE KINDLERS

	Toxicity rating 3
1. Naphtha*	100%
	Toxicity rating 3
2. Copper naphthenate	
Perfume hickory	
Isopropyl alcohol*	
Freon	

Starred ingredients (*) may be responsible for major toxic effects; consult Sec. II.

FUELS (Cont.)

Flares used for lighting fires, so called "kindle flares" are made from bagasse of sugar cane, petrolatums, and candle wax.

LIGHTER FLUIDS . . . . Toxicity rating 3
Naphtha* 100%
Perfume . . . . trace

MODEL AIRPLANE FUELS . . . . Toxicity rating 3
Methyl alcohol*
Nitromethane*
Oil

MOTOR FUELS . . . . Toxicity rating 3
Gasoline*
Kerosene*
Alcohols*
Ethers*
Petroleum ether*
May contain:
Gum inhibitor 0.003%
  2,6-Ditertiary butyl-4-methyl phenol
  N,N'-disecondary butyl paraphenylenediamine
  2,4-Dimethyl-6-tertiarybutylphenol
Dye 0.0003%
  Blue   1,4-Di(isopropylamino) anthraquinone
  Yellow p-Dimethylaminoazobenzene
  Red   Methyl derivatives of azobenzene-4-
          azo-2-naphthol
Tetraethyl lead 0.0002%
Metal deactivator
  N,N'-disalicylidene-1,2-propanediamine
                                          0.0004%

FUMIGANTS

GENERAL USE
Following are the ingredients which appear most frequently in the products listed in Section V. They are arranged according to the frequency of their appearance in that list. This does not indicate the frequency of their use. A popular product may be purchased and used many times more frequently than a less popular or more selective material. For toxicity ratings, see the Ingredients Index, Section II.
                                          Toxicity rating
Carbon tetrachloride*)
Ethylene dichloride*   } used frequently }
Ethylene dibromide*   ) in combination) . .   4
Methyl bromide   4
Sulfur   3
Carbon bisulfide   4
Calcium cyanide   6
Formaldehyde and furfuraldehyde   4
Chloropicrin . . . .   5?
Nicotine   6
Acrylonitrile, Monochloroacetonitrile,
  Trichloroacetonitrile . . . .   4 or 5
Ethylene oxide . . . .   ?
Benzene   4
Azobenzene   4
Hydrocyanic acid   6
Other chlorinated compounds . . . .   4 or 5
May contain:
  Chloro-3-bromopropene-1*
  Dichloroethyl ether*
  Dichloro-1-nitroethane*
  Naphthalene*
  Orthodichlorobenzene*
  Pentachlorobenzene*
  Pentachlorophenol*
  Propylene dichloride* (dichloroporpene and
    propane)
  Tetrachloroethylene*

FUNGICIDES AND INSECTICIDES

For toxicity ratings, see Ingredients Index, Section II

FUNGICIDES AND INSECTICIDES (Cont.)

GENERAL USE
DDT*, and other chlorinated compounds such as aldrin
  and dieldrin*
Copper compounds*
Sulfur*
Zinc compounds*
Rotenone*
Ferric dimethyldithiocarbamate*
BHC, Lindane (hexachlorocylohexane)*
Organic phosphorous compounds (parathion*,
  malathion*, TEPP*, HETP*, OMPA*, systox)*
Arsenicals*
Pyrethrins*
Methoxychlor (paramethoxyphenol)*
Petroleum distillates*
Sodium aluminum fluoride (cryolite)*
Dinitro-ortho-cresol*
Phygon (2,3-dichloro-1,4-naphthoquinone)*
Bordeaux mixture*
Mercurous and mercuric chloride*
Organic mercury compounds*

HERBICIDES

For toxicity ratings, see Ingredients Index, Section II.

GENERAL USE
2,4-D (2,4-dichlorophenoxyacetic acid)* (weed killer)
2,4,5-T (2,4,5-trichlorophenoxyacetic acid)* (brush
  and poisonous plant and vine killer)
These two herbicides, with their esters and salts,
  are usually used in combination.
Sodium chlorate* (soil sterilant, weed killer)
Dinitrophenol* and derivatives (selective weed killers)
Petroleum distillates* (aquatic and general weed
  killers)
Borates* (weed and grass killers)
Potassium cyanate* (crab grass, chick weed and
  general weed killers)
Isopropyl chlorophenyl carbamate* (grass killer)
Pentachlorophenol* (weed killer and fungicide)
Sodium arsenate* (weed killer and insecticide)
Phenyl mercuric acetate* (crab grass and weed killer)
Trichloroacetic acid* (grass killer)
Arsenic trioxide* (defoliant and insecticide)
Disodium 3,6-endoxohexahydrophthalic acid* (endothal)
  (defoliant)
Maleic hydrazide* (1,2-dihydropyridazine-3,6-dione in
  water soluble diethanolamine salt) (plant inhibitor)
Nitro-phenols
Sometimes: Calcium or sodium cyanamide*,
  Dichloralurea, Ethyl xanthogen disulfide*,
  Potassium thiocyanate*, Sodium arsenate* and
  Sodium arsenite*, Sodium isopropyl xanthate*,
  Tetrachloroethane*

INCENSE (Punk)

INCENSE . . . . Toxicity rating 2
Wood flour
Karaya gum
Vanillin
Perfume oils

INKS

HECTOGRAPH INKS. . . . . Toxicity rating 2 or 3
Mineral acid* . . . . less than 10%
Dyes* . . . . less than 10%
Water . . . . less than 50%

INK ERADICATORS
                                          Toxicity rating 3
1. Sodium hypochlorite* . . . .   3 to 6%
   Sodium chloride . . . .   4 to 5%
   Sodium hydroxide and/or sodium
     carbonate . . . .   0.2 to 0.5%
   Water . . . .   89 to 93%

Starred ingredients (*) may be responsible for major toxic effects; consult Sec. II.

INKS (Cont.)

                                                    Toxicity rating 2
2. Tartatic acid*
   Water
                                                    Toxicity rating 4
3. Alcohol
   Potassium oleate
   Oil of mirbane*

LAUNDRY INDELIBLE INKS ...... Toxicity rating 4
Xylene* .... over 50%
Dye .... less than 10%

MUSIC INKS .... Toxicity rating 3
Chromic acid*................ less than 10%
Pigment* .... less than 10%
Phenol .... trace

OPAQUE INKS .... Toxicity rating 3
Glycols and alcohols* .... 1 to 50%
Synthetic resins .... less than 10%
Dyes* .... less than 10%

REDUCERS AND THINNERS .... Toxicity rating 2
May contain:
   Lanolin
   Driers containing very small amounts of lead,
      manganese, or cobalt
   Petrolatum
   Petroleum oils
   Waxes

STAMPING INKS .... Toxicity rating 3
Propylene glycol .... less than 50%
Glycerin .... less than 50%
Phenol .... trace
Dyes* .... less than 10%
Water
May contain:
   Butyl carbitol* .... less than 50%

WRITING INKS
Federal specifications for blue-black ink:
                                    Toxicity rating 2 or 3
Tannic acid................. 1.2%
Gallic acid 0.4%
Ferrous sulfate 1.5%
Hydrochloric acid (dilute) 1.2%
Phenol 0.1%
Blue dye.................. 0.3%
Water 95.3%
May contain:
   Dyes .... 0.5 to 2.0%
   Mineral acid .... about 0.1%
   Methyl alcohol .... less than 2.0%
   Sodium hydroxide........... about 1.0%
   Bis(2-hydroxyethyl) sulfonamide of copper
      phthalocyanine
   Carbon black
   Diethylcyclohexylamine lauryl sulfate*
   Ethylene glycol
   Glycerin
   N,N-Disalicylethylenediamine*
   Oxalic acid*
   Prussian blue
   Silver nitrate*
   Tartaric acid
   Thymol*

INSECTICIDES

For toxicity ratings, see Ingredients Index, Section II.

ALFALFA AND GRAIN PEST
Sometimes Chlordane, DDT*, Aromatic hydrocarbons*

ANT
Arsenic*
Chlordane*
Thallium sulfate*
Petroleum distillates* (aliphatic)

INSECTICIDES (Cont.)

Fluorides*
Pyrethrins*
Gamma isomer of benzene hexachloride*
Rotenone*
Sometimes Chloroethane*, Cyanides*, DDT*, Aldrin*,
   Aliphatic thiocyanates, Boric acid*, Carbon
   tetrachloride*, Aromatic hydrocarbons*, and Sesame
   oil

APHID
Organic phosphorus insecticides*
Gamma isomer of benzene hexachloride*
DDD*
Nicotine*
Phosphates*
Sometimes Aromatic hydrocarbons*, DDT*, Soap,
   Pine oil*

AVIARY AND BIRD SPRAYS
Sometimes Piperonyl butoxide, Pyrethrins

BARN, MILL, BIN SPRAYS
Pyrethrins*
Petroleum distillates (aliphatic)*
Piperonyl butoxide
Aromatic hydrocarbons*
DDT*
Aliphatic thiocyanates*
Gamma isomer of benzene hexachloride*
Methoxychlor*
Sometimes Chlordane,*N-octyl bicycloheptene
   dicarboximide,*Sesame oil extractives, Sulfur,*
   Toxaphene*

BEDBUG
Sometimes DDT*, Aliphatic thiocyanates*, Aromatic
   hydrocarbons*

BEETLE
Rotenone* and other cube resins and extractives
DDT*
Sulfur*
Aromatic hydrocarbons*
Petroleum distillates* (aliphatic)
Chlordane*
Sometimes Chlorobenzene*, Methoxychlor*, Organic
   phosphorous insecticides*

BOOSTER CONCENTRATES
Petroleum distillates* (aliphatic)
N-octyl bicycloheptene dicarboximide *
Allethrin*
Aromatic hydrocarbons*
Methoxychlor*
Pyrethrins*
Aliphatic thiocyanates*
Sometimes Piperonyl butoxide

BORER
Sometimes Aromatic hydrocarbons*, DDT*, Petroleum
   distillates* (aliphatic), Soap

CATERPILLAR
Sometimes DDD*

CHINCH BUG
Chlordane*
DDT*
Sometimes Nicotine *

CITRUS PEST
Aramite
Zinc*
Sometimes Copper*, Sulfur*, Organic phosphorous
   insecticides*, Chlorophenyl-chlorobenzene sulfonate*

CORN EAR WORM
Sometimes Petroleum distillates* (aliphatic),
   Pyrethrum

Starred ingredients (*) may be responsible for major toxic effects; consult Sec. II.

INSECTICIDES (Cont.)

COTTON PEST
DDT*
Gamma isomer of benzene hexachloride*
Sulfur*
Heptachlor*
Aldrin*
Toxaphene*
Aromatic hydrocarbons*
Organic phosphorous insecticides*
Dieldrin*
Sometimes Arsenic*, Chlordane*, Rotenone*

CRANBERRY PEST
Sometimes Organic phosphorous insecticides,*
    Aromatic hydrocarbons*

CUCUMBER PEST
Copper*
Gamma isomer of benzene hexachloride*
Methoxychlor*
Sometimes Nicotine*

CUTWORM
Arsenic*
Sometimes Chlordane*, Toxaphene*, Petroleum distillate*
    (aliphatic)

DAIRY STOCK SPRAYS
Petroleum distillates* (aliphatic)
Pyrethrins*
Methoxychlor*
Piperonyl butoxide
Gamma isomer of benzene hexachloride*
N-octyl bicycloheptene dicarboximide*
Sometimes Pine oil, Allethrin, Aromatic hydrocarbons*

DIPS AND DISINFECTANTS
Aromatic hydrocarbons*
Soap
Arsenic*
Gamma isomer of benzene hexachloride*
DDT*
Petroleum distillates* (aliphatic)
Sometimes Chlordane*, Sulfur*, Turpentine*, Aliphatic
    thiocyanates*, Chlorophenol*, Mercury*, Methoxychlor*,
    Nicotine*, Quarternary ammonium compounds*,
    Rotenone*, Toxaphene*

DOG AND CAT FLEAS AND LICE
Rotenone*
Petroleum distillates* (aliphatic)
Pyrethrins*
Gamma isomer of benzene hexachloride*
Aromatic hydrocarbons*
Chlordane*
Piperonyl butoxide
Pine oil*
DDT*
Soap
Sometimes Anise oil, Camphor,*Tetrachlorquinone,
    Chloromethane,*Piperonyl cyclonene, Dichlorophene,
    Aliphatic thiocyanates,*Amino salt of dodecyl
    benzene sulfonate, Boric acid, Chlorobenzene,*
    Hexachlorophene, Ipepac, Jalap powder, N-octyl
    bicycloheptene dicarboximide,*Oil of pennyroyal,
    Quaternary ammonium compounds,*Sulfonated
    castor oil

DRENCHES
Aluminum silicate
Phenothiazine*
Sometimes Chloroethane*, Copper*, Nicotine*, Zinc*

EARWIG
Sometimes Gamma isomer of benzene hexachloride,*
    Chlordane, Fluorides*

EARWORM
DDT*
Petroleum distillates*(aliphatic)
Sometimes Chloroethyl ether,*Aromatic hydrocarbons*

INSECTICIDES (Cont.)

FLEA
Rotenone* and other cube resins, extractives
Pyrethrins*
Aliphatic thiocyanates*
DDT*
Aromatic hydrocarbons*
Petroleum distillates* (aliphatic)
Gamma isomer of benzene hexachloride*
Chlordane*
Fluorides*
Sulfur*
Chlorophenols*
Toxaphene*
Sometimes Allethrin, Chlorophene*, Iron, Nicotine*,
    Piperonyl cyclonene, Quaternary ammonium
    compounds*, Pini oil*, Sesame oil extractive

FLORAL GARDEN PEST
Rotenone* and other cube resins, extractives
DDT*
Sulfur*
Gamma isomer of benzene hexachloride*
Ferbam*
Pyrethrins*
Copper*
Petroleum distillates* (aliphatic)
Piperonyl cyclonene*
Arsenic*
Aliphatic thiocyanates*
Captan
p-Chlorobenzene sulfonate*
Nicotine*
Organic phosphorous insecticides*
Pine oil*
Sometimes Aramite, Chloranil, Chlorobenzoquinone,
    Dichlone*, Magnesiu, Zinc*

FLORAL PEST (House)
Rotenone* and other cube resins, extractives
Sometimes Aliphatic thiocyanates*, Pyrethrins*, Zinc*

FLY
Petroleum distillates* (aliphatic)
Pyrethrins*
Aliphatic thiocyanates*
Piperonyl butoxide
Organic phosphorous insecticides*
DDT*
Aromatic hydrocarbons*
Pine oil*
Methoxychlor*
Gamma isomer of benzene hexachloride*
Rotenone* and other cube resins, extractives
Sometimes Chlordane*, Citrus oils, Sesame oil
    extractives, Pyrocide booster, Thanite*, Bone oil,
    Nicotine*, Resin

FRUIT PEST
DDT*
Sulfur*
Organic phosphorous insecticides*
Arsenic*
Aromatic hydrocarbons*
Gamma isomer of benzene hexachloride*
Ferbam*
Petroleum distillates* (aliphatic)
Zinc*
Methoxychlor*
Thiophosphates*
Chlordane*
Rotenone* and other cube resins, extractives
Captan
Sometimes Copper*, Aliphatic thiocyanates*, Chloro-
    ethyl sulfite*, Dinitrophenol*, Nicotine*, Pyrethrins*

GARDEN PEST
Rotenone* and other cube resins, extractives
Copper*
DDT*
Pyrethrins*
Petroleum distillates* (aliphatic)

INSECTICIDES (Cont.)

Aromatic hydrocarbons*
Sulfur*
Methoxychlor
Aliphatic thiocyanates*
Gamma isomer of benzene hexachloride*
Chlordane*
Organic phosphorous insecticides*
Piperonyl cyclonene*
Zineb
Zinc*
Ziram*
Sometimes Pine oil*, Arsenic*, Nicotine*, Carbon
tetrachloride*, Citrus oil, Dieldrin*, Phenothiazine*,
Resin, Sabadilla*, Toxaphene*

GENERAL USE
The following ingredients are compiled according to
the frequency of their appearance in insecticides for
general use.
DDT* and other chlorinated hydrocarbons, such as:
Aldrin*
Dieldrin*
TDE*
Petroleum distillates*
BHC*
Sulfur*
Organic phosphorous compounds:
Parathion*
TEPP*
HETP*
OMPA*
Systox*
Malathion*
Rotenone*
Pyrethrin*
Copper compounds*
Chlordane*
Zinc compounds*
Arsenates*
Aliphatic thiocyanates*
Piperonyl butoxide
Nicotine*
Sodium aluminum fluoride* (cryolite)
Formaldehyde*
Azobenzene*

GRASSHOPPER
Chlordane*
Petroleum distillates* (aliphatic)
Sometimes Aromatic hydrocarbons*, Chloronaphthalene*,
DDT*

GREENHOUSE PEST
Organic phosphorous insecticides*
DDT*
Sometimes Aramite, Aromatic hydrocarbons*,
Ferbam*, Methoxychlor*, Nicotine*, Petroleum
distillates* (aliphatic), Sulfur*

GRUB
Rotenone* and other cube resins, extractives
Sulfur
Pine oil*
Sometimes Aromatic hydrocarbons*, DDT*, Petroleum
distillates* (aliphatic), Camphor*, Piperonly
cyclonene*, Terpenes*

HORNFLY
Sometimes Aromatic hydrocarbons*, DDT*, Petroleum
distillates* (aliphatic)

HORSEFLY
Sometimes Gamma isomer of benzene hexachloride*

HOUSEHOLD SPRAYS
Petroleum distillates* (aliphatic)
Pyrethrins*
DDT*
Aliphatic thiocyanates*
Aromatic hydrocarbons*
Chlordane*
Piperonyl butoxide

INSECTICIDES (Cont.)

Gamma isomer of benzene hexachloride*
Sulfoxide*
Dieldrin*
Sometimes Cyanides*, Organic phosphorous compounds*,
Sesame oil extractives

HOUSE PLANT INSECT SPRAYS
Sometimes Rotenone* and other cube resins and
extractives, Methoxychlor*, Piperonyl cyclonene*,
Pyrethrins*

INDUSTRIAL SPRAYS
Petroleum distillates* (aliphatic)
Pyrethrins*
Piperonyl butoxide
DDT*
Rotenone* and other cube resins and extractives
Aliphatic thiocyanates*
Sometimes Allethrin, Aromatic hydrocarbons*, Gamma
isomer of benzene hexachloride*, Sulfoxide*

INSECTICIDAL PAINTS
Aromatic petroleum distillates*
DDT*
Sometimes Gamma isomer of benzene hexachloride*,
Methoxychlor*, Organic phosphorous insecticides*,
TDE*

LARVICIDES
DDT*
Aluminum silicofluoride*
Sometimes Chlorobenzene*, Chloropicrin*, Fluorides*

LAWN PEST
Chlordane*
DDT*
Dieldrin*
Gamma isomer of benzene hexachloride*
Petroleum distillates* (aliphatic)
Sometimes Aromatic hydrocarbons*, Sulfur*

LICE
Sulfur*
Aromatic hydrocarbons*
Rotenone* and other cube resins, extractives
Gamma isomer of benzene hexachloride*
Fluorides*
Pyrethrin*
DDT*
Nicotine*
Methoxychlor*
Petroleum distillates* (aliphatic)
Aliphatic thiocyanates*
Sabadilla*
Sometimes Cyanides*, Di-octyl sodium sulfosuccinate*,
Heptachlor*, Organic phosphorous insecticides*

LIVESTOCK AND POULTRY SPRAYS
Petroleum distillates* (aliphatic)
Pyrethrins*
Piperonyl butoxide
Aromatic hydrocarbons*
Aliphatic thiocyanates*
Gamma isomer of benzene hexachloride*
Pine oil*
Rotenone* and other cube resins, extractives
DDT*
Methoxychlor*
Toxaphene*
Sulfur*
Chlordane*
Ethylene dichloride*
Sometimes Benzene hexachloride*, Citrus oil,
Chlordane*, Chlorobenzene*, Sassafras oil*

MAGGOT
Sometimes Mercury* and Aldrin*

MANGE TREATMENT
Sometimes Petroleum distillates* (aliphatic), Aromatic
hydrocarbons*, Gamma isomer of benzene hexachloride*, Chlordane*, Sulfur*, Turpentine*, Wool fat

---

Starred ingredients (*) may be responsible for major toxic effects; consult Sec. II.

INSECTICIDES (Cont.)

MEALY BUG
Sometimes Aliphatic thiocyanates*

MITE
Aramite
Aromatic hydrocarbons*
Organic phosphorous insecticides*
DDT*
Sulfur*
Chlorobenzene*
Petroleum distillates* (aliphatic)
Gamma isomer of benzene hexachloride*
Chlordane*
DDD*
Piperonyl butoxide
Pyrethrins*
Sometimes Captan, Chlorophenol*, Dieldrin*,
    Dinitrophenol*, Fluorides*, Pine oil*, Rotenone*

MOSQUITO
DDT*
Pyrethrins*
Aromatic hydrocarbons*
Petroleum distillates* (aliphatic)
Aliphatic thiocyanates*
Methoxychlor*
Sesame oil extractive
Sometimes Chlordane*, Organic phosphorous
    insecticides*, Piperonyl butoxide, Rotenone*, TDE*

MOTH
Chlorobenzene*
Aromatic hydrocarbons*
Petroleum distillates* (aliphatic)
DDT*
Aliphatic thiocyanates*
Pyrethrins*
Pine oil*
Methoxychlor*
Chloroaniline esters*
Silicofluorides*
Chlordane*
Carbon tetrachloride*
Ethylene dichloride*
Piperonyl butoxide
DDD*
Fluorides*
Sometimes Benzene hexachloride*, Red cedar chips,
    Sesame oil extractives

MUSHROOM PEST
Sometimes Pyrethrin*

OIL
Petroleum distillates* (aliphatic)
Aromatic hydrocarbons*
Rotenone*
Chlordane*
DDT*
Dinitro-o-cresol*
Resins
Sometimes Allethrin, Piperonyl butoxide,
    Pyrethrins*, Soap, Sulfonated oils*, Sulfur*

ORCHARD SPRAYS
DDT*
Ferbam
Sometimes Aramite, Gamma isomer of benzene
    hexachloride*, Chlordane*, Sulfur*

ORCHID PEST
Sometimes DDT*, Nicotine*, Petroleum distillates*
    (aliphatic)

PEANUT PEST
Sulfur*
DDT*
Copper*
Isodrin*

PLANT SPRAYS
Rotenone* and other cube resins, extractives

INSECTICIDES (Cont.)

Petroleum distillates* (aliphatic)
Pyrethrins*
Piperonyl cyclonene*
Nicotine*
Arsenic*
Sometimes Copper*, Lead, Piperonyl butoxide,
    Rhothane*, Soap, Sulfur*, Zinc*

POTATO PEST
Copper*
DDT*
Arsenic*
Aromatic hydrocarbons*
Cuprous oxide*
Chloroethane*
Zinc*
Zineb
Sometimes Copper-zinc-chromate complex*, Rotenone*

REPELLENTS
Aromatic hydrocarbons*
Petroleum distillates* (aliphatic)
Pine oil*
Citronella oil*
Bone oil
Pyrethrins*
Chlorobenzene*
Piperonyl butoxide
Sulfonated castor oil*
Sometimes Chloromethane*, Methoxychlor*, Oil of
    lavender*, Rotenone*, Thanite*

RESIDUAL SPRAYS
Petroleum distillates* (aliphatic)
DDT*
Chlordane*
Aromatic hydrocarbons*
Pyrethrins*
Aliphatic thiocyanates*
Piperonyl butoxide
Sometimes Terpenes*

ROACH
Chlordane*
Pyrethrins*
Petroleum distillates* (aliphatic)
Sodium fluoride*
DDT*
Aliphatic thiocyanates*
Boric acid*
Piperonyl butoxide
Fluosilicates*
Aromatic hydrocarbons*
Piperonyl cyclonene*
Gamma isomer of benzene hexachloride*
Sesame oil extractives
Sometimes Arsenic*, Carbon tetrachloride*,
    Chlorobenzene*, Dichlorodifluoromethane*, Terpenes*

ROOST PAINT AND SPRAYS
Gamma isomer of benzene hexachloride*
Aromatic hydrocarbons*
Petroleum distillates* (aliphatic)
Nicotine*
Rotenone* and other cube resins, extractives
Pine oil
Sometimes DDT*, Sassafras oil*, Sulfur*

ROOT TREATMENTS
Sometimes Rotenone*, Chlordane*, Mercury*,
    Petroleum distillates* (aliphatic), Sulfur*

ROUND WORM
Sometimes Nicotine*

SCALE OIL
Sometimes Petroleum distillates* (aliphatic), Aromatic
    hydrocarbons*, Vegetable oils, Spray oil

SCREW WORM
Aromatic hydrocarbons*
Gamma isomer of benzene hexachloride*
Pine tar oil*

Starred ingredients (*) may be responsible for major toxic effects; consult Sec. II.

INSECTICIDES (Cont.)

Chloroform*
DDT*
Sulfonated castor oil*
Sulfur*
Rotenone*
Sometimes Carbon tetrachloride*, Resin

SEED, BULB, GRAIN TREATMENTS
Gamma isomer of benzene hexachloride*
Mercury*
Captan
Chlorobenzene*
Chlorobenzoquinone*
Sometimes Aromatic hydrocarbons*, Dieldrin*,
  Piperonyl butoxide, Pyrethrins*

SILVERFISH
DDT*
Fluorides*
Pyrethrins*

SKIPPER
Sometimes Capsicum, Nitrates, Piperonyl butoxide,
  Pyrethrins*

SLUG
Petroleum distillates* (aliphatic)
Arsenic*
Sometimes Copper*, Rotenone*, Sulfur*

SMEAR
Aromatic hydrocarbons*
Benzene hexachloride*
Pine oil*
Petroleum distillates* (aliphatic)
Sometimes Santocel C, Sulfonated castor oil*

SOIL TREATMENTS
Isodrin*
Petroleum distillates* (aliphatic)
DDT*
Benzene hexachloride*
Chlordane*
Chloronaphthalenes*
Nicotine*
Aldrin*
Sometimes Aromatic hydrocarbons*, Copper*, Ferbam*,
  Gypsum, Sulfur*

SPIDER
Rotenone* and other cube resins, extractives
Sulfur*
Aramite
Sometimes Chlordane*, Chlorophenyl chlorobenzene
  sulfonate*, Chlorophenyl methyl carbinol*, Pyrethrins*

SQUASHBUG, HARLEQUINBUG
Sometimes Sabadilla*

SWEET POTATO PEST
Sometimes Aldrin*, Xylene*

TERMITE
Petroleum distillates* (aliphatic)
Chlordane*
Chlorobenzene*
Chlorophenol*
Aromatic hydrocarbons*
Gamma isomer of benzene hexachloride*
Alkyl aryl sulfonate*
DDT*
Sometimes Arsenic*, Copper*, Copper naphthenate*,
  Sulfur

THRIP
Sometimes Alkali*, Fish oil, Nicotine*, Resin, Sabadilla*,
  Pine oil*

TICK
Gamma isomer of benzene hexachloride*
Chlordane*
Rotenone* and other cube resins, extractives

INSECTICIDES (Cont.)

Pine oil*
Aromatic hydrocarbons*
DDT*
Pyrethrins*
Sulfur*
Vegetable waxes
Sometimes Aliphatic thiocyanates*, Ammonia*,
  Methoxychlor*, Piperonyl cyclonene*, Thanite*,
  Toxaphene*, Vegetable Oil

TOBACCO PEST
DDT
Organic phosphorous insecticides*
DDD*
Zineb
Aromatic hydrocarbons*
Arsenic*
Gamma isomer of benzene hexachloride*
TDE*
Nicotine*
Rotenone* and other cube resins, extractives
Fluoaluminates*
Sometimes Chlordane*, Copper*, Lead*, Petroleum
  distillates* (aliphatic), Sulfur*, Toxaphene*

TOMATO PEST
Copper*
Arsenic*
DDT*
Rotenone*
Zineb
Aromatic hydrocarbons*
Chloroethane*
Methoxychlor*
Sometimes Aliphatic thiocyanates*, p-Chlorophenoxy
  acetic acid*, Sulfur*, Ziram*

TREE-CLIMBING PEST
Sometimes Gamma isomer of benzene hexachloride*,
  DDT*, Petroleum distillates* (aliphatic), Rezo wax

TREE SPRAYS
Petroleum distillates* (aliphatic)
DDT*
Aromatic hydrocarbons*
Pine oil*
Rotenone*
Gamma isomer of benzene hexachloride*
Ferbam
Nicotine*
Pyrethrins*
Sulfur*
Sodium di-nitro-o-cresylate*
Sometimes Aramite, Captan, Piperonyl cyclonene*,
  Turpentine*

VEGETABLE PEST
Rotenone* and other cube resins, extractives
DDT*
Organic phosphorous insecticides*
Copper*
Sulfur*
Aromatic hydrocarbons*
Gamma isomer of benzene hexachloride*
Chlordane*
Pyrethrum
Petroleum distillates* (aliphatic)
Methoxychlor*
Piperonyl cyclonene*
DDD*
Sometimes Captan, Dieldrin*, Heptachlor*, Zineb,
  Arsenic*, p-Chlorophenyl p-chlorobenzene sulfonate*,
  Clay, Mercury*, Toxaphene*, Turpentine*, Vegetable
  oil, Zinc*

VINEYARD PEST
Sometimes Copper*, DDT*

WALNUT PEST
Sometimes Arsenic*, DDT*

Starred ingredients (*) may be responsible for major toxic effects; consult Sec. II.

INSECTICIDES (Cont.)

WATERBUG
Sometimes Boric acid*, Pyrethrins*, Fluorides*,
Thallium sulfate*

WEEVIL
Petroleum distillates* (aliphatic)
Aromatic hydrocarbons*
Pyrethrins*
Fluorides*
Aliphatic thiocyanates*
Dieldrin*
Heptachlor*
Sometimes Carbon tetrachloride*, Chlordane*,
Ethylene dibromide*, Ethylene dichloride*, Toxaphene*

LAUNDRY STARCHES

LIQUID
1.   Toxicity rating 1
   Sodium carboxymethylcellulose ..   3.0%
   Formaldehyde 0.2%
   Water
                     Toxicity rating 2
2. Starches
   Sodium chloride
   Terpineol . . . . less than 1.0%
   Perfume oils . . . . less than 1.0%
   o-Phenylphenol . . . . less than 1.0%
                     Toxicity rating 3
3. Polyvinyl acetate
   Tricresyl phosphate*
   Water

POWDER . . . . Toxicity rating 2
Starch 93.0%
Calcium chloride 0.1%
Boric acid 5.0%
Deactivated enzyme 0.5%
Laundry starches may contain:
Phenyl mercuric acetate . . . . trace
Soap powder 0.5%
Soda ash 0.5%
Sodium fluoride . . . . trace

LUBRICANTS

CUTTING OILS . . . . Toxicity rating 2
Sulfur . . . . less than 10%
Lard oil . . . . ⎫
Mineral oil . . . . ⎬ 90%

GENERAL PURPOSE OILS . . . . . Toxicity rating 2 or 3
Petroleum lubricating oil
Corrosion inhibitor
May contain:
Borax*
Silicone

GRAPHITE LUBRICANTS . . . . . . Toxicity rating 1 or 2
Carbon . . . . 70 to 98%
Inert ingredients . . . . 5 to 30%
Silica . . . . 0 to 0.5%
Alumina . . . . trace
May contain:
Iron oxide

GREASES . . . . Toxicity rating 2 or 3
Petroleum grease
Soap
Graphite
May contain:
Borax*
Chromate*
Zinc salt*

LUBRICATING PENCILS . . . . Toxicity rating 2
Paraffin wax and oil
Petrolatum . . . . small amount
Coloring . . . . trace

PENETRATING OILS . . . . Toxicity rating 3 or 4
Low viscosity petroleum oil*
Oleic acid

LUBRICANTS (Cont.)
Carbon tetrachloride*
Butyl alcohol*
Higher fatty alcohols

PUMP LUBRICANTS . . . . Toxicity rating 2
Mineral oil
Soap
Petroleum sulfonate
Water

RUBBER LUBRICANTS . . . . Toxicity rating 2 or 3
Isopropyl alcohol*
Grease
Oils

THREAD LUBRICANTS (A.P.I. Grease)
                  Toxicity rating 3 or 4
Aluminum stearate grease 20.5%
Silicone compound 12.8%
Silicone fluid 2.6%
Graphite 18.0%
Lead* 30.5%
Copper 3.3%
Zinc* 12.3%

VASELINES . . . . Toxicity rating 2
Borated petroleum jelly
Boric acid . . . . small amount
Carbolic acid . . . . small amount
Camphor
Waxes
Oils

WIRE DRAWING COMPOUNDS . . . Toxicity rating 2 or 3
Paste soap
Trisodium phosphate*

MATCHES

MATCHES . . . . Toxicity rating 3
Potassium chlorate*
Glue (animal)
Red phosphorus*
Phosphorous sesquisulfide*
Ground glass
Corn starch
Sulfur*
Wood rosin
Coloring dyes
Paraffin wax
May contain:
Clay
Diatomite
Formaldehyde
Glycol
Iron peroxide
Manganese dioxide
Plaster of Paris
Potassium chlorate*
Potassium dichromate*
Zinc oxide
The striking surface of the strike-on-the-box match
consists of: . . . . Toxicity rating 3
A binder, e.g., gum arabic
Amorphous phosphorus *
An abrasive, e.g., quartz or ground glass
May contain:
Antimony sulfide*
Iron sulfide*
Tin trisulfide*

MODELING CLAYS

MODELING CLAYS . . . . Toxicity rating 1
Kaolin
Gypsum
Petrolatum
Wax
Castor oil
Vegetable dye

Starred ingredients (*) may be responsible for major toxic effects; consult Sec. II.

PAINTS

ANTI-ALGAE PAINTS . . . . Toxicity rating 4
  Cuprous oxide*. . . . . copper as metal 7%
  Copper soap
  Arsenic oxide* . . . . arsenic as metal 7%
  Copper sulfate pentahydrate *
  Mercury soap . . . . mercury as metal 0.3%
  2,2,-dihydroxy-5,5-dichloro-
    diphydroxy-5,5-dichloro-
    diphenylmethane* or 2,2-
    methylenebis(4-chlorophenol)*

ANTI-CORROSION PAINTS
  Pigment   Toxicity rating
    Zinc chromate* 4
    Lead chromate* 4
    Red lead oxide* 3
    Basic lead carbonate* . . . : 4
    Zinc oxide . . . . 2 or 3
    Lead monoxide* 3
  Vehicle
    Rosin 2
    Pine oil*. 3
    Coal tar* 4
    Petroleum ether* 3
  Anti-corrosion paints may contain:
    Ammonium hydroxide* 3
    Arsenic* 5
    Cuprous oxide* 4
    Ethyl alcohol 3
    Kerosene*. 3
    Mercuric oxides* 5
    Metallic soap . . . . ?
    Methylene chloride* 3
    Paraffin
    Plastic thickener
    Rust retardant

ASPHALT PAINTS . . . . Toxicity rating 3
  Varnish
  Linseed oil
  Mineral spirits*
  Asphalt
  Petroleum ether*

CARBOFUCHSIN PAINTS . . . . Toxicity rating 3
  Phenol* 4.5%
  Boric acid 1.0%
  Resorcinol* 10.0%
  Fuchsin 0.3%
  Acetone 5.0%
  Alcohol 10.0%
  Water 8.5%

DISINFECTING WHITE PAINTS . . . . . Toxicity rating 2
  Gamma isomers of benzene hexa-
    chloride (lindane) . . . . less than 0.3%
  Phenols . . . . less than 2.0%
  Neutral oils . . . . less than 2.0%

DRIERS   Toxicity rating
  Vanadium compounds*. . . . . 3 or 4
  Manganese compounds* . . . . : . . . 3
  Zinc compounds* 4
  Iron compounds* 3
  Cobalt compounds* 4
  Potassium hydroxide* 4
  Lead naphthenate* . . . . 3?
  Lead octoate*. . . . . 3?
  Lead tallate* . . . . 3?
  Other lead compounds* 4

ENAMEL . . . . Toxicity rating 3 or 4
  Titanium oxide
  Melamine resin
  Glyceryl phthalate resin
  Maleated resin
  Petroleum aromatics*

FINGERPAINTS . . . . Toxicity rating 2 or 3
  Corn starch base
  Vegetable pigments for color
  Wetting agents

PAINTS (Cont.)

  Chalk
  Methyl cellulose
  Methyl salicylate*

GRAPHITE PAINT PIGMENT . . . . Toxicity rating 2
  Carbon
  Silica
  Alumina
  Iron oxide

LACQUER THINNERS . . . . Toxicity rating 4
  Ethyl alcohol . . . . 0 to 5%
  Ethyl acetate* . . . . 20 to 21%
  Butyl alcohol* . . . . 10 to 11%
  Butyl acetate* . . . . 20 to 23%
  Toluene* . . . . 25 to 28%
  Aliphatic hydrocarbons* . . . . 16 to 20%
  May contain:
    Amyl acetate*
    Isopropyl acetate*
    Isopropyl alcohol*
    Pigment
    Xylene*

LACQUERS . . . . Toxicity rating 2 or 3
  Nitrocellulose
  Ester gum (glyceryl, methyl and ethyl esters of
    rosin acids)
  Cottonseed oil
  Synthetic resins made from cotton and oil
  Synthetics made from soya beans
  Pigments
  Nitric acid
  Lead acetate*
  Magnesium oxide

OILS . . . . Toxicity rating 2
  Linseed oil
  Soybean oil
  Fish oil
  Castor oil
  Synthetic oil
  Tung oil
  Perilla oil
  Oiticica oil

PAINT REMOVERS
                               Toxicity rating 4
  1. Benzene* . . . . 15 to 70%
     Ethyl alcohol . . . . 30 to 85%
     Acetone* . . . . 30 to 85%
     Paraffin wax . . . . 30 to 85%
                               Toxicity rating 3
  2. Petroleum naphtha* 44%
     Methyl ethyl ketone* 14%
     Ethyl acetate* 14%
     Ethyl alcohol. 14%
     Paraffin wax 14%
     Paint removers may also contain:
       Carbon tetrachloride*
       Ethylene dichloride*
       Methyl alcohol*
       Methylene chloride*
       Propylene dichloride*

PLASTICIZERS . . . . Toxicity rating 3
  Tricresyl phosphate*
  Diethyl phthalate
  Diamyl phthalate
  Dibutyl phthalate
  Linseed oil
  Soy oil
  Camphor*
  Castor oil

RESINS . . . . Toxicity rating 2
  Synthetic
    Hydrocarbons
    Alkyd
    Maleic
    Urea

Starred ingredients (*) may be responsible for major toxic effects; consult Sec. II.

PAINTS (Cont.)

Phenolic
Vinyl
Melamine
Coumarone
Indene
Ester gum
Natural
Asphaltum
Shellac
Rosin
Dammar
Singapore
Kaurie
Pontianak
Manila
Congo
East India

SOLVENTS AND THINNERS

		Toxicity rating 4
1. Paraffin hydrocarbons*		56.8%
Naphthalenes*		30.6%
Aromatics		12.6%
		Toxicity rating 3
2. Petroleum ether*		90 to 100%
Acetone, benzene* or toluene*		0 to 10%

Solvents and thinners may contain:
Pine oil*
Terpene derivatives*

STAINS . . . . Toxicity rating 3

Oleo resinous varnishes
Mineral spirits*

TIRE PAINTS . . . . Toxicity rating 3

Aliphatic solvents*
Rubber
Plasticizer
Pigments

VARNISHES AND SHELLACS . . . . Toxicity rating 3 or 4

Resins
Methyl alcohol*
Ethyl alcohol*
Gasoline*
Benzene*
Sodium hydroxide
Turpentine*
Lead*

WHITE WASH PAINTS . . . . Toxicity rating 2

Dimethoxydiphenyltrichloroethane	2.0 to 3.0%
Sodium pentachlorophenate	1.0 to 2.0%
Sodium salts of other chlorophenates	less than 0.5%
Calcium hydroxide	

PENCILS

INDELIBLE PENCIL LEAD . . . . Toxicity rating 3

Methyl violet*

LEAD PENCILS . . . . Toxicity rating 1

"Lead"	
Wax	
Clay	
Graphite	
Finish	
Lacquer	
Eraser	
Natural rubber	
Sulfur	
Color	
Titanium	small amount

PET CARE

DRY CLEANERS, DOG AND CAT . Toxicity rating 3 or 4

Naphthalene*
Calcium carbonate
Magnesium carbonate
Sulfur*
Aluminum silicate

PET CARE (Cont.)

May contain:
Borax*
Degreased starch
Glycerin
Phenol*
Pine oil*
Sodium carbonate
Zinc oxide

SOAPS, DOG AND CAT . . . . Toxicity rating 2

Vegetable oil soap	30%
Camphor oil	1.8%
Rotenone	0.1%
Cube resins	0.2%
Pyrethrins	0.1%

SPRAYS, DOG . . . . Toxicity rating 2

Pyrethrins	0.03%
Cube resins	0.2%
Petroleum distillate	0.1%
Rotenone	0.1%
Ethyl alcohol	24.0%
Butoxypolypropylene glycol	15.0%
Propellant	60.0%

PHOTOGRAPHIC PRODUCTS

DESENSITIZERS . . . . Toxicity rating ?

Pinacryptol green
Pinacryptol yellow

DEVELOPERS . . . . Toxicity rating 2 or 3

Elon or metol	0.1 to 1.0%
Sodium sulfite	2.0 to 9.0%
Hydroquinone or catechol	0.6 to 1.1%
Sodium carbonate	1.3 to 12.0%
Potassium bromide	0.1 to 0.5%
Water	77.0 to 97.0%

May contain:
Sodium hydroxide	1.6%
Balanced alkali	1.9%
Sodium thiocyanate	0.7%
Sodium bisulfite	1.4%
Borax	0.2%
Sodium hexametaphosphate*	0.3%
Parahydroxyphenyl glycine	2.0%
Paraphenylenediamine	1.0%
Orthophenylenediamine	1.0%
Trisodium phosphate	11.0%
1,4-Dihydroxy-2-chlorobenzene	4.7%
2,4-Diaminophenol dihydrochloride	0.6%

May also contain:
Benzotriazol*
Boric acid*
Citric acid
Ethyl alcohol*
Methyl alcohol*
Paraformaldehyde*
Potassium metabisulfite
Sodium sulfate
Sulfuric acid

FILM CLEANERS . . . . Toxicity rating 3 or 4

May contain:
Ammonium hydroxide*
Chlorinated solvents*
Denaturant
Ethyl alcohol
Methyl alcohol*
Petroleum ether*
Trichloroethane*
Wax
Carbon tetrachloride*

FIXING BATHS . . . . Toxicity rating 3

Sodium thiosulfate*	4.0 to 37.0%
Sodium sulfite	0.7 to 7.0%
Acetic acid (28%)	2.0 to 21.0%
Boric acid	0.6 to 3.0%
Potassium aluminum sulfate	1.0 to 9.0%
Water	57.0 to 96.0%

Starred ingredients (*) may be responsible for major toxic effeces; consult Sec. II.

PHOTOGRAPHIC PRODUCTS (Cont.)

May contain:
Ammonium chloride	4.0%
Sodium bisulfite	2.0%
Borax	4.0%
Potassium chromium sulfate	1.0%
Sulfuric acid (conc.)	0.3%
Potassium metabisulfite	5.0%
Potassium thiocyanate	9.0%
Citric acid	0.4%

HARDENING BATHS

Formalin-carbonate hardening bath . . Toxicity rating 2
Formaldehyde (37% solution)	0.9 to 1.0%
Sodium carbonate	0.5 to 0.6%
Water	98.0%

May contain:
Aluminum chloride*

Chrome alum bisulfite hardening bath
Toxicity rating 3
Potassium chromium sulfate*	2.0 to 3.0%
Sodium sulfate or bisulfite	2.0 to 6.0%
Water	91.0 to 96.0%

May contain:
Acetic acid (28%)	5.0%

Boric acid*
Sodium sulfite*
Potassium alum*

HYPO ELIMINATORS
Toxicity rating 2
Hydrogen peroxide (3% solution)	13.3%
Ammonium hydroxide (28%)	1.1%
Water	85.6%

INTENSIFIERS
Chromium intensifiers
Bleach . . . . Toxicity rating 3
Potassium dichromate*	0.9 to 9.0%
Hydrochloric acid* (conc.)	0.7 to 7.0%
Water	84.0 to 98.0%

Redeveloper . . . . Toxicity rating 2 or 3
Standard developer* (see developer)
Mercury intensifiers
Bleach . . . . Toxicity rating 3 or 4
Potassium bromide	1.0 to 2.0%
Mercuric chloride*	1.0 to 2.0%
Water	96.0 to 98.0%

Redeveloper†
Solution A . . . . Toxicity rating 5
Sodium cyanide*	3.0%
Water	97.0%

Solution B . . . . Toxicity rating 3
Silver nitrate*	4.0%
Water	96.0%

†May be any standard developer
Quinone-thiosulfate intensifiers
Solution A . . . . Toxicity rating 2 or 3
Potassium dichromate*	2.0%
Sulfuric acid (conc.)	5.0%
Water	92.0%

Solution B . . . . Toxicity rating 2
Sodium bisulfite	0.4%
Hydroquinone	1.0%
Wetting agent	0.4%
Water	98.0%

Solution C . . . . Toxicity rating 2
Sodium thiosulfate	2.0%
Water	98.0%

The intensifier is prepared by mixing solutions A, B,
and C in equal proportions.
Silver intensifiers
Stock solution A . . . . Toxicity rating 3
Silver nitrate*	6.0%
Water	94.0%

Stock solution B . . . . Toxicity rating 2
Sodium sulfite	6.0%
Water	94.0%

Stock solution C . . . . Toxicity rating 2
Sodium thiosulfate	10.0%
Water	90.0%

PHOTOGRAPHIC PRODUCTS (Cont.)

Stock solution D . . . . Toxicity rating 2
Sodium sulfite	0.5%
Elon	0.8%
Water	98.7%

The intensifier is prepared by mixing solutions A, B,
C and D in proportions of 1:1:1:3 respectively.
Intensifiers may contain:
Lead nitrate*
Potassium permanganate*

REDUCERS
Farmer's reducer
Solution A . . . . Toxicity rating 2
Potassium ferricyanide	0.7 to 7.0%
Water	93.0 to 99.3%

Solution B   Toxicity rating 2 or 3
Sodium thiosulfate*	3.0 to 21.0%
Water	79.0 to 97.0%

Flattening reducers
Bleach . . . . Toxicity rating 2
Potassium ferricyanide	1.3 to 3.0%
Potassium bromide	1.0 to 3.0%
Ammonium hydroxide	0.1%
Water	96.0%

Redeveloper
Solution A . . . . Toxicity rating 3
p-Aminophenol hydrochloride*	10.0%
Water	90.0%

Solution B . . . . Toxicity rating 2
Potassium bromide	10.0%
Water	90.0%

Persulfate reducers . . . . Toxicity rating 2 or 3
Ammonium persulfate	3.0 to 6.0%
Sulfuric acid (conc.)	0.5 to 0.6%
Water	93.4 to 96.5%

Other reducers may contain:
Potassium permanganate*	0.02 to 5.0%
Potassium citrate	6.0%
Ferric ammonium sulfate	4.0%
Sodium sulfite	3.0%
Citric acid	2.0%

May contain:
Ferric chloride*

STAIN REMOVERS
Solution A . . . . Toxicity rating 1
Potassium permanganate	0.5%
Water	99.5%

Solution B . . . . Toxicity rating 2 or 3
Sulfuric acid*	3.0%
Sodium chloride	7.0%
Water	90.0%

May contain:
Sodium sulfite	3.0%
Sodium bisulfite	3.0%

STOP BATHS . . . . Toxicity rating 2 or 3
Acetic acid (28%)	3.0 to 12.5%
Sodium sulfate	4.0%
Water	87.5 to 95.0%

May contain:
Potassium chromium sulfate*

TESTS FOR HYPO
Permanganate test . . . . Toxicity rating 1
Potassium permanganate	0.05%
Sodium hydroxide	0.1%
Water	99.8%

Mercuric chloride test . . . . Toxicity rating 4
Mercuric chloride*	2.0%
Potassium bromide	2.0%
Water	95.0%

Lead azide test . . . . Toxicity rating 4
Solution A
Iodine*	9.0%
Potassium iodide	9.0%
Water	82.0%

Solution B
Sodium azide*	10.0%
Water	90.0%

Starred ingredients (*) may be responsible for major toxic effects; consult Sec. II.

PHOTOGRAPHIC PRODUCTS (Cont.)

Silver nitrate test. . . . . Toxicity rating 2
  Silver nitrate 1.0%
  Water 99.0%
  Other tests for hypo may contain:
  Formaldehyde*
  Starch
  Hydrochloric acid*

TONERS

Blue toners . . . . Toxicity rating 2
  Sodium thiosulfate . . . . 10.0 to 12.0%
  Potassium aluminum sulfate 3.0%
  Silver nitrate . . . . 0.03 to 0.1%
  Sodium chloride. . . . . 0.03 to 0.1%
  Potassium bromide 0.03%
  Potassium iodide 0.03%
  Water . . . . 85.0 to 87.0%
Dye bath. . . . . Toxicity rating 3 or 4
  Safranine A* (red)
  Chrysoidine* (orange)
  Auramine* (yellow)
  Victoria green* (green)
  Methylene blue* B.B. (blue)
  Methyl violet* (violet)
  Acetic acid*
Single solution dye toner . . . . Toxicity rating 3
  Methyl alcohol* (wood alcohol)
  Acetone*
  Acetic acid*
  Dye* (one of above mentioned - see Dye Bath)
Varigam toners . . . . Toxicity rating 2 or 3
  Potassium ferricyanide*
  Potassium bromide*
  Potassium iodide*
  Sodium chloride
  Nitric acid*
  Thiocarbamide (thiorea)
  Sodium hydroxide
  Sodium carbonate
  Potassium carbonate
  Gold chloride*
  Potassium thiocyanate*
Gold toners . . . . Toxicity rating 2
  Solution A
    Sodium thiosulfate 19.0%
    Potassium persulfate 2.0%
    Silver nitrate 0.1%
    Sodium chloride. 0.1%
    Water 78.0%
  Solution B
    Gold chloride 0.4%
    Water 99.5%
Iron toners . . . . Toxicity rating 2
  Ferric ammonium citrate 0.4%
  Oxalic acid 0.4%
  Potassium ferricyanide. 0.4%
  Water 98.0%
  May contain:
  Acetic acid
Polysulfide toners . . . . Toxicity rating 2
  Potash sulfurated. 0.7%
  Sodium carbonate 0.2%
  Water 99.0%
Selenium toners . . . . Toxicity rating 2 or 3
  Sodium sulfide 1.0%
  Selenium metal 0.1%
  Sodium thiosulfate 15.0%
  Sodium bisulfite. 5.0%
  Water 78.9%
Sulfide sepia toners . . . . Toxicity rating 3
  Bleaching solution
    Potassium ferricyanide. . . . . 1.0 to 2.0%
    Potassium bromide . . . . 2.0 to 3.0%
    Potassium oxalate* 5.0%
    Acetic acid (28%) 1.0%
    Ammonium hydroxide (28%) 1.0%
    Water . . . . 91.0 to 96.0%
  Toning sulition
    Sodium sulfide . . . . 0.7 to 1.0%
    Water 99.0%

PHOTOGRAPHIC PRODUCTS (Cont.)

Uranium toners . . . . Toxicity rating 2
  Uranium nitrate . . . . 0.2 to 0.8%
  Potassium oxalate or oxalic acid . . . 0.2 to 0.4%
  Potassium ferricyanide. . . . . 0.1 to 0.4%
  Ammonium aluminum sulfate 0.6%
  Hydrochloric acid 0.05%
  Water . . . . 98.0 to 99.0%
  Other toners may contain:
    Nitric acid (conc.) 1.5%
    Thiorea 0.5%
    Potassium thiocyanate 10.0%
    Borax 3.0%
    Sodium phosphate
    Sodium hydroxide

TRAY CLEANERS . . . . Toxicity rating 4
  Potassium dichromate* 8.0%
  Sulfuric acid* 16.0%
  Water 76.0%

PIGMENTS

BLACK	Toxicity rating
Carbon black.	1
Bone black (animal charcoal)	1
Lampblack	1
Iron blue (Ferric ferrocyanide)*	3
Asphalt	2

BLUE	
Iron blue (Ferric ferrocyanide)*	3
Titanium dioxide	1
Calcium carbonate	1
Silica	1
Calcium sulfate	2

BROWN	
Burnt umber (iron and manganese oxides, and clay)	2
Burnt sienna (iron oxide and clay) . . .	2
Ferric oxide*	3 ?
Chrome orange*	4
Yellow iron oxide*	3 ?
Titanium calcium pigment	1
Silica and silicates	1
Calcium carbonate	1
Titanium magnesium pigment	2
Zinc oxide*	3
Basic sulfate of white lead*	4
Lampblack (trace)	1

BUFF	
Titanium dioxide	1
Yellow iron oxide*	3 ?

GOLD	
Bronze powder	3 ?

GRAY	
Carbon black.	1
Titanium dioxide	1
Calcium carbonate	1
Zinc oxide	3 ?
Barium sulfate	1

GREEN	
Iron blue (Ferric ferrocyanide)*	3
Lead chromate*	4
Chromium oxide	2
Magnesium silicate	2
Titanium calcium pigment	1
Calcium carbonate	1
Silica	1
Yellow iron oxide*	3 ?
Titanium dioxide	1
Zinc chromate*	4

MAPLE	
Yellow iron oxide*	3 ?
Ferric oxide*	3 ?

Starred ingredients (*) may be responsible for major toxic effects; consult Sec. II.

PIGMENTS (Cont.)

	Toxicity rating
Titanium dioxide	1
Silica and silicates	1

OAK
Titanium dioxide	1
Ferric oxide*	3?
Yellow iron oxide*	3?
Calcium carbonate	1

RED
Toluidine red*	4
Chrome orange (basic lead chromate)*	4
Calcium carbonate	1
Para red*	4
Ferric oxide*	3?
Titanium calcium pigment	1
Molybdate orange (lead chromate, sulfate, and molybdate)*	4
Toluidine toner	?
Silica	1

PIGMENTS (Cont.)

	Toxicity rating
TANGERINE (Orange)	
Chrome orange (lead chromate)	4
Titanium dioxide	1
Lead chromate	4

WHITE
Titanium dioxide	1
Calcium carbonate	1
Lithopone (zinc sulfide* and barium sulfate)	3
Titanium caclium pigment	1
Titanium magnesium pigment	2
Basic sulfate of lead*	4
Zinc oxide*	3
Silicates	1
Mica	1

YELLOW
Lead chromate*	4
Titanium dioxide	1
Calcium carbonate	1
Silica	1

COMMON PIGMENTS AND DYES[††]
(as found in paints, inks, etc.)

Common Name	Chemical Ingredients	In Section II See Under:
A. VIOLET:		
Benzyl violet	A basic triphenylmethane dye	Gentian violet
Cobalt violet	Cobalt phosphate and cobalt arsenite	Cobalt and arsenic
Crystal violet	A basic triphenylmethane dye	Gentian violet
Manganese violet	Manganese ammonium phosphate	Manganese salts
Methyl violet	A basic triphenylmethane dye	Gentian violet
Nürnberg	Manganese ammonium phosphate	Manganese salts
Permanent violet	Manganese ammonium phosphate	Manganese salts
Ultramarine violet		
B. BLUE:		
Alizarine blue	Anthraquinone	Alizarine
Alkali blue	An acid triphenylmethane dye	(not in ing. index)
Azurite	Basic copper carbonate	Copper salts (cupric)
Blue basic lead sulfate	Basic lead sulfate, lead sulfite, lead sulfide and carbon	Lead salts
Blue bice	Basic copper carbonate	Copper salts (cupric)
Blue frit	Copper calcium silicate	Copper salts (cupric)
Blue lead	Basic lead sulfate, lead sulfite, lead sulfide and carbon	Lead salts
Blue verditer	Basic copper carbonate	Copper salts (cupric)
Bronz blue	Ferric ferrocyanide	Ferric salts
Celestial blue	Ferric ferrocyanide	Ferric salts
Cerulean blue	Cobaltous stannate	Cobalt salts, stannic salts
Chinese blue	Ferric ferrocyanide	Ferric salts
Cobalt blue	Cobalt aluminate	Cobalt salts
Cobalt ultramarine	Cobalt aluminate	Cobalt salts
Copper blue	Cupric sulfide	Copper salts (cupric) and sulfides
Copper phthalocyanine blue	Phthalocyanine	Copper salts
Copper phthalocyanine lakes	Phthalocyanine	Copper salts
Covellite	Cupric sulfide	Copper salts (cupric) and sulfides
Egyptian blue	Copper calcium silicate	Copper salts (cupric)
Erioglaucine blue	An acid triphenylmethane dye	(not in ing. index)
Glacier blue	A basic triphenylmethane dye	Gentian violet
Green shade blacktone iron blue	Ferric ferrocyanide	Ferric salts
Green shade iron blue	Ferric ferrocyanide	Ferric salts
Indanthrene blue	Insoluble anthroquinone	(not in ing. index)
Indigo blue	Anthraquinone	(not in ing. index)
Indulines		
Iron blue	Ferric ferrocyanide	Ferric salts
King's blue	Cobalt aluminate	Cobalt salts
Laquer blue	Ferric ferrocyanide	Ferric salts
Manganese blue	Sodium sulfate, potassium permanganate and barium nitrate	Barium and manganese
Miloir blue	Ferric ferrocyanide	Ferric salts
Mineral blue	Basic copper carbonate	Copper salts (cupric)

[††]Modified from the analysis of J. J. Mattiello, Protective and Decorative Coatings, Vol. II, pp. 50-57, John Wiley and Sons, New York, 1942, with written permission of the publisher.

Starred ingredients (*) may be responsible for major toxic effects; consult Sec. II.

PIGMENTS AND DYES (Cont.)

Mineral gray	Hydrated aluminum silicate and silica	Aluminum oxide
Non-bronz blue	Ferric ferrocyanide	Ferric salts
Patent blue		(not in ing. index)
Peacock blue	Barium or aluminum lake of an acid triphenylmethane dye	(not in ing. index)
Phthalocyanine blue	Phthalocyanine	(not in ing. index)
Pompeian blue	Copper calcium silicate	Copper salts (cupric)
Prussian blue	Ferric ferrocyanide	Ferric salts
Red shade blacktone iron blue	Ferric ferrocyanide	Ferric salts
Red shade iron blue	Ferric ferrocyanide	Ferric salts
Smalt	Potassium silicate and cobalt oxide	Cobalt salts
Setoglaucine blue	A basic triphenylmethane dye	Gentian violet
Setopaline blue	A basic triphenylmethane dye	Gentian violet
Steel blue	Ferric ferrocyanide	Ferric salts
Sublimed blue lead	Lead sulfate, lead sulfite, lead sulfide and carbon	Lead salts
Sulfonated indulines		
Thenards blue	Cobalt aluminate	Cobalt salts
Toning blue	Ferric ferrocyanide	Ferric salts
Ultramarine blue	(Mostly silicate)	Silica
Victoria blue	A basic triphenylmethane dye	Gentian violet

C. GREEN:

Acetate chrome green	Lead chromate and ferrocyanide	Lead chromate
Acid green	A barium lake of an acid triphenylmethane dye	Gentian violet and barium
Brilliant green	A basic triphenylmethane dye	Gentian violet
Cadmium green	Chromium oxide and basic copper carbonate	Copper salts and chrome green
Chlorinated copper phthalocyanine	Phthalocyanine	(not in ing. index)
Chlorophyll	Vegetable chlorophyll	Chlorophyll
Chrome green	Lead chromates and ferrocyanide	Lead chromate
Chromium oxide	Chromic oxide and sodium bichromate fused with boric acid, hydrolyzed in water	Chromate salts and boric acid
Cobalt green	Calcined product containing cobalt, zinc, and aluminum oxide	Zinc oxide and cobalt salts
Copper phthalocyanine green	Phthalocyanine	
Copper resinate	Copper acetate and turpentine or balsam	Copper salts and turpentine
Emerald green	Copper acetoarsenite	Paris green
Green earth	Hydrous iron, magnesium, aluminum potassium silicate	Ferric salts
Guignets green	Sodium bichromate fused with boric acid, hydrolyzed with water	Chromate salts and boric acid
Hookers green	Ferrocyanide and a natural green resin called gamboge	Gamboge
Hydrated chromium oxide	Sodium bichromate fused with boric acid and hydrolyzed in water	Chromate salts and boric acid
Imperial green	Copper acetoarsenite	Paris green
Indanthrene green	An anthraquinine dye	Alizarin
Malachite green	A basic triphenylmethane dye	Gentian violet
Metal-free phthalocyanine	Phthalocyanine	
Naphthol green B (D and C)		(not in ing. index)
Nitrate chrome green	Lead chromate and ferrocyanide	Lead chromate
Olive green	Basic lead chromate ferrocyanide	Lead chromate
Paris green	Copper acetoarsenite	Paris green
Permanent green	Chromium oxide and cadmium sulfide or cadmium sulfoselenide or zinc chromate	Chrome green, cadmium salts, chromate salts, selenium, sulfide
Phthalocyanine green	Phthalocyanine	
Rinmann's green	Calcined cobalt, zinc and aluminum oxide	Zinc oxide, cobalt salts
Scheele's green	Acid copper arsenite	Paris green
Schweinfurt green	Copper acetoarsenite	Paris green
Ultramarine green	China clay (aluminum silicate), sulfur, soda ash, charcoal - all heated together at 1500°F.	
Verdigris	Copper dibasic acetate	Copper salts
Victoria green	A basic triphenylmethane dye	Gentian violet
Zinc green	Zinc chromate + ferrocyanide	Zinc chromate

D. YELLOW AND BROWN:

Annatto	Vegetable dye	(not in ing. index)
Antimony yellow	Lead antimoniate	Lead salts, antimony
Auramine yellow	A basic triphenylmethane dye	Gentian violet
Aureolin	Potassium cobaltinitrite	Cobalt and nitrites
Barium yellow	Barium chromate	Barium salts and chromate salts
Benzidine yellow	Insoluble azo dye	(not in ing. index)
Brown hydrated iron oxide	Iron oxide	Ferric salts
Burnt umber	Calcined - ferric oxide (45-55%), silica (13%), manganese dioxide (8-16%), plus smaller % of aluminum, calcium and magnesium oxides	Manganese and ferric salts
Cadmium yellow	Cadmium sulfide, cadmium sulfoselenide, barium sulfate	Cadmium salts, selenium, and sulfide
Cadmium yellow lithopone	Cadmium sulfide, cadmium sulfoselenide, barium sulfate	Cadmium salts, selenium, and sulfide

PIGMENTS AND DYES (Cont.)

Cassel yellow	Lead oxychloride (PbCl$_2$· 7 PbO)	Lead salts
Catechu	Vegetable	(not in ing. index)
Chrome yellow	Lead chromates, zinc chromates, lead molybdate, lead sulfate	Lead chromate, lead salts, zinc chromate
Cobalt yellow	Potassium cobaltinitrite	Cobalt and nitrites
Cutch	Vegetable	(not in ing. index)
Domestic ocher	Ferric oxide, silica, aluminum oxide	Ferric salts
Domestic raw sienna	Ferric oxide, silica, aluminum oxide	Ferric salts
Fluorescein yellow (D and C)	Fluoresceins	(not in ing. index)
French ocher	Ferric oxide, silica, aluminum oxide	Ferric salts
Fustic	Vegetable	(not in ing. index)
Hansa yellow	Insoluble azo dye	
Helio yellow	An anthraquinone dye	Alizarin
Hypernic	Vegetable	(not in ing. index)
Indanthrene yellow	An anthraquinone dye	Alizarin
Italian raw sienna	Ferric oxide, silica, aluminum oxide	Ferric salts
Kings yellow	Arsenic sulfide (As$_2$S$_3$)	Arsenic trisulfide
Lead chromate	Lead chromate	Lead chromate
Logwood extract	Vegetable	(not in ing. index)
Manganese brown	Manganic hydroxide, manganous oxide, manganese dioxide	Manganese
Manganite	Manganic hydroxide, manganous oxide, manganese dioxide	Manganese
Mercuric oxide	Mercuric oxide	Mercury compounds
Metallic brown	Ferric oxide (80%), silica and aluminum oxide	Ferric salts
Mineral brown	Ferric oxide (80%), silica and aluminum oxide	Ferric salts
Mosaic gold	Stannic sulfide	Stannic salts

D. YELLOW AND BROWN (Cont.):

Naphthol yellow	(structure)	(not in ing. index)

$$\left[2OH \underset{NO_2}{\overset{O^-}{\bigcirc}} SO_3^- \right] Ba^{++}$$

Naples yellow	Lead antimoniate	Lead salts, antimony
Natural yellow oxide	Ferric oxide, silica, and aluminum hydroxide	Ferric salts
Nitroso dyes (yellow)		(not in ing. index)
Ocher	Ferric oxide, silica and aluminum oxide	Ferric salts
Orpiment	Arsenic sulfide (As$_2$S$_3$)	Arsenic
Pure cadmium yellow	Cadmium sulfide, cadmium sulfoselenide	Cadmium salts and selenium
Quercitron lakes	Vegetable	(not in ing. index)
Raw sienna	Ferric oxide, silica, aluminum oxide	Ferric salts
Raw umber	Ferric oxide (50%), silica (13%), manganese dioxide (15%)	Manganese
Sepia	Sepia occurs in ink bag of cuttlefish--dry ink is extracted with a boiling soda ash solution and ppt. with acid	(not in ing. index)
Strontium yellow	Strontium chromate	Chromate salts
Tartrazine yellow (F, D and C)	Soluble azo dye	(not in ing. index)
Thioflavine yellow	(structure)	(not in ing. index)

$$\underset{CH_3}{\overset{S}{\bigcirc}}C-\bigcirc-N-(CH_3)_2 \quad [Cl]$$
(a thiazole)

Toluidine yellow	Insoluble azo dyes	(not in ing. index)
Turkey umber	Ferric oxide (50%), silica (13%), manganese dioxide (15%), plus aluminum, calcium and magnesium oxides	Ferric salts and manganese
Vandyke brown	Vegetable	(not in ing. index)
Yellow hydrated iron oxide	Ferric oxide (hydrated)	Ferric salts
Zinc yellow	Zinc chromate	Zinc chromate

E. ORANGE:

Algol orange	An anthraquinone dye	Alizarin
Antimony sulfide	Antimony sulfide	Antimony compounds
Antimony vermilion	Antimony sulfide	Antimony compounds
Cadmium orange	Cadmium sulfide, cadmium sulfoselenide, barium sulfate	Cadmium salts, selenium, and sulfide
Chrome orange	Basic lead chromate	Lead chromate
Hansa orange	An insoluble azo dye	(not in ing. index)
Molybdate chrome orange	Lead chromate, lead sulfate, and lead molybdate	Lead chromate, lead molybdate and lead salts
Orange mineral	Lead tetraoxide	Lead salts
Orthonitraniline orange	An insoluble azo dye	(not in ing. index)

$$\underset{}{\overset{NO_2}{\bigcirc}}-N=N-\overset{OH}{\bigcirc}$$

Permanent orange (D and C)	An insoluble azo dye	(not in ing. index)
Persian orange	Soluble azo dye	(not in ing. index)
Realgar	Arsenic sulfide (As$_2$S$_2$)	Arsenic trisulfide
Sodium lithol	A soluble azo dye	(not in ing. index)

PIGMENTS AND DYES (Cont.)

F. RED

Acid scarlet	A soluble azo dye	(not in ing. index)
Algol red	An anthraquinone dye	Alizarin
Alizarine	An anthraquinone dye	Alizarin
Alizarine red	An anthraquinone dye	Alizarin
Bromo acids	Bromo fluoresceins (eosine)	(not in ing. index)
Bromo fluoresceins	Bromo fluoresceins (eosine)	(not in ing. index)
Burnt sienna	Iron oxide, silica, aluminum oxide	Ferric oxide
Cadmium red	Cadmium sulfide, cadmium sulfoselenide	Cadmium salts, selenium and sulfide
Cadmium red lithopone	Cadmium sulfide, cadmium sulfoselenide, barium sulfate	Cadmium salts, selenium and sulfide
Carmine	An anthraquinone dye	Alizarin
Chinese vermilion	Mercuric sulfide	Mercury compounds
Chlorinated paranitraniline	An insoluble azo dye	(not in ing. index)
Cinnabar	Mercuric sulfide	Mercury compounds
Cochineal	An anthraquinone dye	Alizarin
Cuprous oxide	Cuprous oxide	Cuprous oxide
Domestic hematite	Iron oxide (60%), silica (20%), and alumina, lime and magnesia	Ferric oxide
Dutch pink	Vegetable dye	(not in ing. index)
English vermilion	Mercuric sulfide	Mercury compounds
Eosines (Y and YSK, D and C)	Bromo fluorescein	(not in ing. index)
Erythrosine (F, D and C)	Iodo fluorescein	(not in ing. index)
Fuchsine red	A basic triphenylmethane dye	Gentian violet
Helindones	An anthraquinone dye	Alizarin
Indian red	Calcined ferrous sulfate (i.e., ferric oxide)	Ferric salts
Lithol	A soluble azo dye	(not in ing. index)
Lithol rubines (D and C)	A soluble azo dye	(not in ing. index)
Madder lake	An anthraquinone dye	Alizarin
Magenta	A basic triphenylmethane dye	Gentian violet
Paras (red)	An insoluble azo dye	
Persian berries	Vegetable dye	(not in ing. index)
Persian gulf oxide	Ferric oxide (60%), silica (20%), plus alumina, lime and magnesia	Ferric salts
Phloxine toner	Lead ppt. of bromofluoresceins (eosines)	Lead salts bromo-fluoresceins (not in ing. index)
Pigment scarlets (D and C)	A soluble azo dye	(not in ing. index)
Pure cadmium red	Cadmium sulfide and cadmium sulfoselenide	Cadmium salts, selenium, and sulfide
Red chalk	Aluminum silicate colored by ferric oxide	Aluminum silicate
Red iron oxide	Ferric oxide	Ferric salts
Red lake C lakes	Soluble azo dye	(not in ing. index)
Red lake D lakes (D and C)	Soluble azo dye	(not in ing. index)
Red lake P lakes	Soluble azo dye	(not in ing. index)
Red lake R lakes	Soluble azo dye	(not in ing. index)
Red lead	Lead tetraoxide (Pb_3O_4) and lead oxide (PbO)	Lead salts

Rhodamines (BaD and C)

$(C_2H_5)_2-N-\ \cdots\ -N(C_2H_5)_2$ ... COOH ... [Cl] ... O

(not in ing. index)

Safranine red

$H_3C\ \cdots\ N\ \cdots\ CH_3$
$H_2N\ \cdots\ \cdots\ NH_2$
N [Cl]

(not in ing. index)

Spanish oxide	Ferric oxide (60%), silica (20%), plus alumina, lime and magnesia	Ferric salts
Thioindigos	An anthraquinone dye	(not in ing. index)

$S\ \cdots\ C=C\ \cdots\ S$ ... O ... O

Toluidines (Red 1 D and C)	An insoluble azo dye	Toluidine
Turmeric	Vegetable dye	(not in ing. index)
Venetian red	Ferric oxide (40%), calcium sulfate (60%)	Ferric salts, calcium salts

G. MAROON

Amaranth maroon	A soluble azo dye	(not in ing. index)
Azo bordeaux	A soluble azo dye	(not in ing. index)
Cadmium maroon	Cadmium sulfide and cadmium sulfoselenide	Cadmium salts, selenium, and sulfide
Helio bordeaux	A soluble azo dye	(not in ing. index)
β-Hydroxynaphthoic maroons	A soluble azo dye	(not in ing. index)
α-Naphthylamine maroon	An insoluble azo dye	(not in ing. index)
Pyrites cinder	Iron oxide (from calcined iron sulfide)	Ferric salts
Toluidine maroons	Insoluble dyes	Toluidine

PIGMENTS AND DYES (Cont.)

H. WHITE:

Alumina hydrate	Aluminum hydroxide	Aluminum oxide
Aluminum hydroxide	Aluminum hydroxide	Aluminum oxide
American process zinc oxide	Zinc oxide	Zinc oxide
Anhydrite	Anhydrous calcium sulfate	Calcium salts
Antimony oxide	Antimony oxide	Antimony compounds
Abestine	Magnesium silicate	Talc
Barite	Barium sulfate	Barium salts, insoluble
Barium carbonate	Barium carbonate	Barium salts, water or acid soluble
Barytes	Barium sulfate	Barium salts, insoluble
Basic carbonate white lead	Basic lead carbonate	Lead salts
Basic magnesium carbonate	Basic magnesium carbonate	Magnesium salts
Basic sulfate white lead	Basic lead sulfate	Lead salts
Bentonite	A colloid clay	
Blanc fixe	Barium sulfate	Barium salts, insoluble
Calcium magnesium carbonate silicate	Complex calcium magnesium carbonate silicate	Magnesium salts
Chalk	Calcium carbonate	Calcium salts
China clay	Aluminum silicate	
Diatomaceous earth	Silica	Silica
French process zinc oxide	Zinc oxide	Zinc oxide
Gloss white	Aluminum hydroxide (25%) barium sulfate (75%)	Aluminum oxide
Ground limestone	Calcium carbonate	Calcium salts
Gypsum	Calcium sulfate	Calcium salts
High strength lithopone	Zinc sulfide (50%), barium sulfate (50%)	Zinc salts and sulfides
Infusorial earth	Silica	Silica
Kaolin	Aluminum silicate	
Lead titanate	Lead titanate (93%), lead sulfate (7%)	Lead salts
Leaded zinc oxide	Zinc oxide and lead sulfate	Lead salts and zinc oxide
Lead-free zinc oxide	Zinc oxide	Zinc oxide
Light carbonate of magnesia	Basic magnesium carbonate	Magnesium salts
Lithopone	Zinc sulfide (29%), barium sulfate (71%)	Zinc salts, sulfides
Magnesite	Magnesium carbonate	Magnesium salts
Magnesium oxide	Magnesium oxide	Magnesium salts
Magnesium silicate	Magnesium silicate	Talc
Mica	Potassium aluminum silicate	
Natural anhydrite	Anhydrous calcium sulfate	Calcium salts
Permanent white	Barium sulfate	Barium salts, insoluble
Precipitated barium carbonate	Barium carbonate	Barium salts, soluble
Precipitated calcium carbonate	Calcium carbonate	Calcium salts
Precipitated gypsum	Calcium sulfate	Calcium salts
Precipitated magnesium carbonate	Magnesium carbonate	Magnesium salts
Pumice	Aluminum, potassium and sodium silicates	
Pure titanium dioxide	Titanium dioxide	Titanium dioxide
Quartz	Silica	Silica
Satin white	Aluminum hydroxide and calcium sulfate	Calcium salts
Silica	Silica	Silica
Silk white	Calcium chloride and sodium silicate	Calcium salts and sodium silicate
Talc	Magnesium silicate	Talc
Titanated lithopone	Zinc sulfide, barium sulfate, titanium dioxide	Barium and zinc salts and sulfides
Titanated barium	Titanium dioxide (30%), barium sulfate (70%)	Barium salts, insoluble and titanium dioxide
Titanated calcium	Titanium dioxide (30%), calcium sulfate (70%)	Calcium salts
Titanium dioxide	Titanium dioxide	Titanium dioxide
Titanated magnesium	Titanium dioxide (30%) magnesium silicate (70%)	Titanium dioxide and talc
Tripoli	Silica	Silica
Tripolite	Silica	Silica
White basic lead sulfate	Basic lead sulfate	Lead salts
Whiting	Calcium carbonate	Calcium salts
Witherite	Barium carbonate	Barium salts
Zinc oxide	Zinc oxide	Zinc oxide
Zinc sulfide	Zinc sulfide	Zinc sulfide
Zinc sulfide barium	Zinc sulfide (50%) barium sulfate (50%)	Zinc sulfide, barium salts
Zinc sulfide magnesium	Zinc sulfide (50%) magnesium silicate (50%)	Zinc sulfide

I. BLACK:

Animal black	Carbon (10-20%) and calcium phosphate (80-90%)	Calcium salts
Asphalt	Asphalt	
Birch black	Carbon (50-90%) and mineral	
Black iron oxide	Black iron oxide (Fe_3O_4)	Ferric salts
Black lead	Graphite	
Blue black	Carbon (50-90%) and mineral	
Bone black	Carbon (10-20%) and calcium phosphate (80-90%)	
Carbon black	Carbon	
Channel black	Carbon	
Colloidal carbon	Carbon	
Graphite	Carbon	

PIGMENTS AND DYES (Cont.)

Iron oxide black	Black iron oxide (Fe_3O_4)	Ferric salts
Ivory black	Carbon (10-20%) and calcium phosphate (80-90%)	
Lampblack	Carbon	
Low oil absorption lampblack	Carbon	
Magnetic oxide	Black iron oxide (Fe_3O_4)	Ferric salts
Manganese black	Manganese dioxide	Manganese
Mineral black	Carbon (15-85%) and silicates or iron oxide	Ferric salts
Natural black iron oxide	Black iron oxide (Fe_3O_4)	Ferric salts
Nigrosines		
Plumbago	Carbon (graphite)	
Precipitated black iron oxide	Black iron oxide (Fe_3O_4)	Ferric salts
Soft black	Carbon (50-90%) and mineral	
Stove black	Carbon (graphite)	
Sulfonated nigrosines		
Sulfur colors		
Swedish black	Carbon (50-90%) and mineral	
Thermal black	Carbon	
Vegetable black	Carbon (50-90%) and mineral	
Vine black	Carbon (50-90%) and mineral	
Willow black	Carbon (50-90%) and mineral	
Wood pulp black	Carbon (50-90%) and mineral	

J. METALLIC:

Aluminum powder	Aluminum	Aluminum
Copper alloy	Copper, zinc, aluminum, tin	Copper, zinc, aluminum, tin
Copper bronze powder	Copper (97-98%), zinc (1%) and iron	Copper
Dendritic copper powders	Copper (98%), zinc (1%) and traces of other metals	Copper
Green gold bronze	Copper (68%), zinc (31%) and aluminum (0.25%)	Copper
Lining bronzes	Finest grade bronze	Copper
Metallic aluminum powder	Aluminum	Aluminum
Metallic copper powder	Copper	Copper
Metallic gold	Gold	Gold
Metallic lead	Lead	Lead
Metallic nickel	Nickel	Nickel
Metallic silver	Silver	Silver
Metallic tin	Tin	Tin
Metallic zinc	Zinc and 1-2% zinc oxide	Zinc
Molding bronze	Medium grade	Copper
Pale gold bronze	Copper (92%), zinc (6%), aluminum (2%)	Copper
Rich gold bronze	Copper (77%), zinc (22%), aluminum (10%)	Copper
Rich pale gold bronze	Copper (90%), zinc (9%), aluminum (1%)	Copper
Standard bronze		Copper
Zinc dust	Zinc plus 1 to 4% zinc oxide	Zinc

PLATING COMPOUNDS

CHROME FINISH . . . . Toxicity rating 5 or 6
Silver nitrate*
Sodium cyanide*

POLISHES

ALUMINUM POLISHES . . . . Toxicity rating 3
Potassium hydroxide*
Benzene*
Equal parts of rum and olive oil
Pumice stone
Emery paste mixed with tallow
Rouge powder with oil of turpentine*

AUTOMOBILE POLISHES . . . . Toxicity rating 3
Ammonium hydroxide
Boiled linseed oil
Cedar oil*
Citronella oil*
Oil of caraway seeds
Petroleum solvent (usually kerosene)*
Phenol (1%)
Turpentine*
Vegetable wax

CHROME CLEANERS

Toxicity rating 3 or 4
1. Abrasive
   Ammonium hydroxide*
   Ammonium oxalate*

Toxicity rating 3
2. Abrasive
   Alcohol*
   Naphtha*
   Petroleum oil
   Water

FLOOR POLISHES (Shellac Type) . . . Toxicity rating 3
Methyl and ethyl alcohol
Gums
Mineral spirits*

FURNITURE POLISHES . . . . Toxicity rating 2 or 3
Mineral oil 55%
Emulsifying oil 3%
Isopropyl alcohol 4%
Water 38%
May contain:
   Ammonium hydroxide
   Diglycol laurate
   Kerosene*
   Methyl cellulose
   Perfume
   Petroleum ether*
   Sassafras oil*
   Silicone oils
   Sodium alkyl sulfate
   Stearic acid
   Sulfonated castor oil*
   Triethanolamine
   Wax

LEATHER POLISHES . . . . Toxicity rating 2
Carnauba wax
Animal and vegetable oils
Triethanolamine

METAL POLISHES . . . . Toxicity rating 2 or 3
Water 54.5%
Silica 34.0%
Soap 5.5%
Ammonium oxalate* 3.0%
Isopropyl alcohol 1.0%
Glycerin 2.0%
May contain:
   Alcohol
   Ammonium hydroxide*
   Charcoal
   Emery flour levigated
   Lye*
   Mutton suet
   Oleic acid

POLISHES (Cont.)

Oxalic acid*
Petroleum ether*
Pine oil*
Red lead oxide*
Sawdust
Sodium carbonate
Sulfric acid*
Turpentine*
Vaseline

PLASTIC POLISHES . . . . Toxicity rating 4
Paraformaldehyde* 100%

PORCELAIN AND METAL POLISHES . . Toxicity rating 2
Silica abrasive
Soda soap
Pine oil . . . .   less than 1%
Ammonium hydroxide . . . .   less than 1%
Oxalates . . . .   less than 1%

SCRATCH REMOVER POLISHES . . . . . Toxicity rating 3
Petroleum spirits*
Wood stains

SHOE POLISHES
Colored . . . . Toxicity rating 3 or 4
   Methyl, ethyl, isopropyl alcohol*
   Aniline*
   Nitrobenzene*
   Turpentine
   Wax (vegetable, animal, bee)
   Tar and tar color*
   Oleate soap
   Detergent
   Lanolin
White . . . . Toxicity rating 2
   Titanium dioxide
   Zinc oxide
   Talc
   Carboxymethylcellulose
   Gum acacia
   Sodium benzoate
   Water

SILVER POLISHES
Burnishing type . . . . Toxicity rating 2
   Water
   Diatomaceous earth
   Soap
   Sodium carbonate
   Ammonium hydroxide*
   Perfume
Dip type . . . . Toxicity rating 3
   Thiourea
   Sulfuric acid*
   Wetting agent
   Dye
   Silver polishes may contain:
      Petroleum ether*
      Pine oil*

STOVE POLISHES . . . . Toxicity rating 3
Carbon black
Graphite
Naphtha*

SUEDE DRESSINGS . . . . Toxicity rating 3
Aniline dye*
Isopropyl alcohol*

WOOD POLISHES
Cream polish . . . . Toxicity rating 2
   Mineral oil 55%
   Emulsifying oil 3%
   Isopropyl alcohol 4%
   Water 38%
Oil polish . . . . Toxicity rating 3
   Petroleum oil* . . . .   90 to 100%
   Cedar wood oil . . . .   small amount
   Oil of turpentine . . . .   small amount
   Color . . . .   trace

Starred ingredients (*) may be responsible for major toxic effects; consult Sec. II.

PORCELAIN GLAZING COMPOUNDS

PORCELAIN GLAZING COMPOUNDS. . Toxicity rating 1
  Fish oil
  Lard oil
  Inert fillers

PRESERVATIVES

Brush (paint) . . . . Toxicity rating 3
  Turpentine*
  Kerosene*
  Linseed oil
  Gelatin
  Glycerin
  Ammonium alum*
  Potash alum*
  Citric acid
Canvas. . . . . Toxicity rating 3
  Pentachlorophenol* (less than 5%)
  Tetrachlorophenol* (less than 5%)
  2-Chlorophenylphenol* (less than 5%)
  Petroleum solvents*
  Ortho dichlorobenzene 1%
  Synthetic resins
  Diacetone alcohol*
Concrete . . . . Toxicity rating 4
  Calcium (calcined solution)
  Colloidal resins
  Coal tar solvents*
Floor (wood) . . . . Toxicity rating 4
  Magnesium fluorosilicate*
  Sodium zinc silicate
  Sulfates
Foundation . . . . Toxicity rating 3
  Asphalt
  Asbestos
  Petroleum ether*
Polish . . . . Toxicity rating 2 or 3
  Gum tragacanth
  Bentonite
  Alcohol*
  Mineral oil
  Sulfonated castor oil*
  Glycerin
  Wintergreen*
  Oil (hydrocarbon)*
Roof . . . . Toxicity rating 3
  Asphalt (cut back with solvents)
  Asbestos
  Slate filler
  Petroleum ether*
Rust (protection against) . . . . Toxicity rating 3
  Phosphoric acid*
  Aniline dye*
Wood . . . . Toxicity rating 3
  Gum resin
  Zein (corn protein)
  Denatured alcohol*
  Ethyl triethanol amine
  Glycol humectant
  Naphthenic acid*
  Copper hydrate*
  Mineral spirits*
  Copper naphthenate*
  Zinc naphthenate
  Copper linoleate*
  Copper oleate*

PUTTIES

SYNTHETIC WOOD PUTTIES . . . . . . Toxicity rating 2
  1. Calcium sulfate
    Silica
    Vegetable binder
    Wood flour
  2. Gypsum
    Dextrin
    Inert fillers
  Synthetic wood putties may contain:
    Asbestos
    Metallic soaps
    Mineral oil
    Nitrocellulose lacquer

PUTTIES (Cont.)

  Organic solvents
  Pigments

WHITE LEAD PUTTIES . . . . Toxicity rating 3 or 4
  Note: 5, 10, 20, and 30% putties are sold. The per-
  centages refer to the weight percentage of basic lead
  carbonate* in the pigment.
  Ground limestone. . . . . }
  Asbestos fibre. . . . . }
  Talc . . . . } 90%
  Titanium dioxide . . . . }
  Linseed oil . . . . }
  Soybean oil . . . . } 8%
  Mineral oil 2%

REPELLENTS

BIRD REPELLENTS . . . . Toxicity rating 3 ?
  Water gas tar 88.6%
  Turpentine 7.4%
  Inert ingredients 4.0%

DOG AND CAT REPELLENTS
               Toxicity rating 3 (with nicotine 5)
  Isopropyl alcohol 80%
  Water 14%
  Lemon grass oil 3%
  Eucalyptus oil 3%
  Diethyl phthalate* 1%
  Dog and cat repellents may contain:
    Allyl isothiocyanate*
    Animal bone oil
    Citral and associated terpenes
    Mineral oil
    Nicotine sulfate*
    Oil of allspice
    Oil of mustard
    Soap

INSECT REPELLENT STICKS . . . . Toxicity rating 3
  2-Phenylcyclohexanol*
  2-Cyclohexylcyclohexanol*
  Sodium stearate
  Denatured alcohol
  Perfume
  Water

INSECT REPELLENTS	Toxicity rating
Dimethyl phthalate	2
Citronella oil*	3
Benzocaine	2
Cisbicyclo-heptene dicarboxylic acid, dimethyl ester.	?
Butyl dimethyl dihydrogamma pyrone carboxylate.	2
Butoxy polypropylene glycol*	3
2-ethylhexanediol-1,3*	3
Pyrethrin*	3
Piperonyl butoxide	2
Petroleum distillates*	3
Lavender*	?
Camphor	4
Phenol*	4
Cresylic acid*	4
Pine tar*	3
Indalone	2
Oil of eucalyptus*	4
Paradichlorobenzene* (moth balls and flakes)	3
Naphthalene*.	4

RODENTICIDES

BAT REPELLENTS . . . . Toxicity rating 3
  Paradichlorobenzene*

GENERAL USE
  Warfarin
  Strychnine*
  Antu*
  Extractives of red squill*
  Phosphorous

Starred ingredients (*) may be responsible for major toxic effects; consult Sec. II.

RODENTICIDES (Cont.)

Arsenic*
Pival (2-pivalyl-1,3-inandione) and other inandiones
Zinc phosphide*
DDT*
Thallium
May contain:
  Barium carbonate*
  Chlordane*
  Paradichlorobenzene*
  Sodium fluoride*
  Sodium fluosilicate*
  Sulfur*

GOPHER POISONS

1. Strychnine or strychnine sulfate
                  0.2 to 90.5% (usually 0.5%)
   Inert ingredients . . . . balance

	Toxicity rating
Strychnine* content 20-90.5%	6
Strychnine* content 2-19%	5
Strychnine* content 0.2-1.9%	4

2. Arsenic trioxide*
   Inert ingredients

Content 10-90%	5
Content 1-9%	4
Content less than 1%	3 or 2

3. Phosphorus*
   Inert ingredients

Content 34-100%	6
Content 3.4-33%	5
Content 0.34-3.3%	4

MOLE POISONS . . . . Toxicity rating 4

1. Strychnine* or strychnine sulfate . 0.5 to 0.8%
   Inert ingredients . . . . 99.2 to 99.5%
2. Ricin* 0.3%
   Inert ingredients 99.7%

MOUSE BAITS AND POISONS

Pellets . . . . Toxicity rating 5
  Strychnine* 2.1%
  Inert ingredients 97.9%
Powders
  The following ingredients are arranged according to
  their frequency of use by rodenticide manufacturers.
                  Toxicity rating 4

1. Strychnine and strychnine
   sulfate* . . . . 0.2 to 0.8%
   Inert ingredients . . . . 99.2 to 99.8%
                  Toxicity rating 4
2. DDT* 50.0%
   Inert ingredients 50.0%
                  Toxicity rating 2
3. Warfarin 0.025%
   Inert ingredients 99.975%
                  Toxicity rating 3
4. Thallium sulfate* 1.0%
   Inert ingredients 99.0%
                  Toxicity rating 2
5. Pival (2-pivalyl-1,3-inandione). . 0.025%
   Inert ingredients 99.975%
                  Toxicity rating 4
6. Sodium fluoride* 70.0%
   Powdered silica 30.0%
The inert ingredients may be corn meal, ground grain,
bird seed, silica or talc.

RAT AND MOUSE POISONS

The following ingredients are arranged according to
their frequency of use by rodenticide manufacturers.
                  Toxicity rating 2
1. Warfarin 0.025%
   Inert ingredients 99.975%
   Concentrate:
    Warfarin 0.5%
    Inert ingredients 99.5%
                  Toxicity rating 2
2. Pival (2-pivalyl-1,3-inandione). . 0.025%
   Inert ingredients 99.975%
   Concentrate:
    Pival 0.5%
    Inert ingredients 99.5%

RODENTICIDES (Cont.)

                  Toxicity rating 4
3. Arsenic trioxide* . . . . 2.0 to 3.2%
   Arsenic, metallic . . . . 0.0 to 2.5%
   Inert ingredients . . . . 95.3 to 98.0%
                  Toxicity rating 5
4. Arsenic trioxide* . . . . 25.0 to 99.0%
   Inert ingredients . . . . 1.0 to 75.0%
                  Toxicity rating 4
5. Sodium arsenite* 2.3%
   Inert ingredients 97.7%
                  Toxicity rating 4
6. Thallium sulfate* 2.9%
   Inert ingredients 97.1%
                  Toxicity rating 4
7. Sodium fluoride* 70.0%
   Silica, powdered 30.0%
8. Sodium fluosilicate
The inert ingredients may be corn meal, ground grain,
bird seed, silica or talc.

RAT AND ROACH PASTE . . . . Toxicity rating 4
Phosphorus* 2.5%
Inert ingredients 97.5%

RAT BAITS AND POISONS

Liquids . . . . Toxicity rating 5
  Acidic arsenic solution* 75.0%
  Extract of red squill
Pastes
                  Toxicity rating 4
1. Phosphorus* . . . . 2.0 to 2.5%
   Inert ingredients . . . . 97.5 to 98.0%
                  Toxicity rating 3
2. Zinc phosphide* 5.0%
   Inert ingredients 95.0%
                  Toxicity rating 3
3. Extractives of red squill* 2.0%
   Inert ingredients 98.0%
Powders
The following ingredients are arranged according to
their frequency of use by rodenticide manufacturers.
                  Toxicity rating 2
1. Warfarin 0.025%
   Inert ingredients 99.975%
   Concentrate:
    Warfarin 0.5%
    Inert ingredients 99.5%
2. Antu* . . . . 1.0 to 99.0% (usually 20%)
   Inert ingredients . . . . balance
   Antu* content 100% . . . . Toxicity rating 3
   Antu* content 20% . . . . Toxicity rating 3
                  Toxicity rating 3
3. Extractives of red squill . . . . 5.0 to 10.0%
   Inert ingredients . . . . 90.0 to 95.0%
                  Toxicity rating 4
4. Phosphorus . . . . 1.0 to 2.0%
   Inert ingredients . . . . 98.0 to 99.0%
5. Phosphorus
   Phosphorus* content 100% . . . . . . Toxicity rating 6
   Phosphorus* content 10% . . . . Toxicity rating 5
   Phosphorus* content 1% . . . . Toxicity rating 4
   Warfarin
6. Arsenic trioxide . . . . 2.0 to 99.0%
   Arsenic, metallic . . . . 0 to 0.7%
   Arsenic* oxide content 100% . . . . Toxicity rating 5
   Arsenic* oxide content 10% . . . . . Toxicity rating 4
   Arsenic* oxide content 1% . . . . . . Toxicity rating 3
                  Toxicity rating 5
7. Arsenic trioxide* 73.9%
   Barium carbonate* 20.0%
   Inert ingredients 6.1%
                  Toxicity rating 4
8. Strychnine* 0.3%
   Inert ingredients 99.7%
9. Zinc phosphide . . . . 0.5 to 94.0%
   Inert ingredients . . . . balance
   Zinc phosphide* content 100% . . . . Toxicity rating 4
   Zinc phosphide* content 10% . . . . Toxicity rating 3
   Zinc phosphide* content 1% . . . . . Toxicity rating 2
                  Toxicity rating 2
10. Pival 0.025%
    Inert ingredients 99.975%

Starred ingredients (*) may be responsible for major toxic effects; consult Sec. II.

RODENTICIDES (Cont.)

11. Sodium fluosilicate*
    Content 100% . . . . Toxicity rating 4
    Content 10% . . . . Toxicity rating 3
    Content 1% . . . . Toxicity rating 2

RAT BISCUITS . . . . Toxicity rating 4
Arsenious oxide* 10.5%
Rat baits and poisons may contain:
    Convallarin 7.0%
    Digitalis* 2.0%

SQUIRREL POISONS

                                        Toxicity rating 3
1. Thallium sulfate* 1.0%
   Inert ingredients 99.0%
                                        Toxicity rating 2
2. Zinc phosphide 0.5%
   Inert ingredients 99.5%
                                        Toxicity rating 2
3. Sodium fluoroacetate 0.05%
   Inert ingredients 99.5%

SEALING COMPOUNDS

SEALING COMPOUNDS   Toxicity rating
Polyvinyl acetate   1
Limestone   1
Titanium dioxide   1
Polymerized vegetable oil   2
Volatile diluents* . . . . 3 or 4
Synthetic rubber   1
Lacquer adhesive
Preservatives
    Oil of sassafras*
    p-Chlorometacresol
    Sodium pentachlorophenate
Hexamethylenetetramine   3

SHOCK ABSORBER FLUIDS

DELCO TYPE . . . . Toxicity rating 2
Naphthenic or paraffinic petroleum oil

HOUDAILLE TYPE . . . . Toxicity rating 2 or 3
Glycerin
Alcohol
Glucose
Water

SOLDERING FLUXES

LEAD SOLDERING
Liquid . . . . Toxicity rating 2 or 3
Zinc chloride* . . . . }
Ammonium chloride . . . . } 17 to 30%
Water . . . . 70 to 83%
May contain:
    Hydrochloric acid*
    Rosin
    Acetone*
Paste . . . . Toxicity rating 2 or 3
Zinc* and ammonium chloride
Petrolatum
Water

SILVER SOLDERING . . . . Toxicity rating 4
Potassium acid fluoride*
Potassium tetraborate*
Boric acid*

TITANIUM SOLDERING . . . . Toxicity rating 4
Potassium acid fluoride*
Potassium tetraborate*
Boric acid*

SOLVENTS

Organic solvents fall into the following distinct chemical
groups:
    Alcohols . . . . Toxicity rating
    Glycols* . . . .   2 or 3

SOLVENTS (Cont.)

                                        Toxicity rating
Alcohol amines
    Monoethanolamine   2
    Diethanolamine   2
Chlorinated solvents
    Carbon tetrachloride*   4
    Methylene chloride*   3
    Ethylene dichloride*   3
    Propylene dichloride*   4
    Trichloroethylene*   4
    Perchloroethylene*   3
    Monochlorobenzene*   3
    Orthodichlorobenzene*   4
    Trichlorobenzene*   4
    Methyl chloroform (1,1,1-trichloro-
        ethane)* . . . .   3 or 4
Esters
    Ethyl acetate*   3
    Isopropyl acetate*   3
    Secondary butyl acetate*   3
    Amyl acetate*   3
Hydrocarbons
    Aliphatics*   3
    Aromatics*   4
    Terpenes and cyclics of terpene
        structure*   3
Ketones
    Methyl ethyl ketone*   3
    Methyl isobutyl ketone*   3
    Diacetone*   3
    Glycol ethers* . . . .   2 or 3
Other common solvents are:
    Turpentine*   3
    Kerosene*, gasoline*, and other
        petroleum solvents*   3
    Cresylic acid*   4
    Mineral spirits* (Stoddard solvents)   3

SHELLAC THINNERS, OR METAL CLEANERS

                                        Toxicity rating 3
Ethyl alcohol* 92%
Methyl alcohol 5%
Methyl isobutyl ketone 1%
Ethyl acetate 1%
Naphtha 1%

WALL PAPER REMOVERS . . . . Toxicity rating 4
1. Butyl cellosolve*
   Sodium tetradecyl sulfate
   Water
2. Sulfonated oils*
   Carbon tetrachloride*

VANILLA, IMITATION

VANILLA, IMITATION . . . . Toxicity rating 3
Vanillin*
Ethyl vanillin
Glycerin
Carmel

VAPOR PHASE CORROSION INHIBITOR

VAPOR PHASE CORROSION INHIBITOR
                                        Toxicity rating 4?
Diisopropylammonium nitrite*
Dicyclohexylammonium nitrite*

WATER SOFTENERS

INSOLUBLE RESIN . . . . Toxicity rating 2
Polymeric resin . . . . }
Sulfonated polystyrene . . . . } 100%
May contain:
    Sulfonated bituminous coal

SOLUBLE TYPE . . . . Toxicity rating 3
1. Trisodium phosphate* 100%
2. Sodium carbonate* 100%
   May contain:
       Alkyl aryl sulfonate*
       Aniline dye*

Starred ingredients (*) may be responsible for major toxic effects; consult Sec. II.

WATER SOFTENERS (Cont.)

    Phosphorus pentoxide*
    Sodium bicarbonate
    Sodium hexametaphosphate
    Sodium metasilicate*
    Sodium monoxide*
    Sodium sesquicarbonate
    Sodium sesquisilicate*
    Sodium tripolyphosphate*

ZEOLITE . . . . Toxicity rating 2?
    Complex sodium aluminum silicate   100%

WATERPROOFING COMPOUNDS

WATERPROFFING COMPOUNDS . . . . Toxicity rating 4
    Wax . . . . }
    Carbon tetrachloride* . . . . } 100%

WAXES

FLOOR, SELF-POLISHING WAXES . . . Toxicity rating 2
    Carnauba wax . . . . }
    Synthetic resins . . . . }. 10 to 15%
    Morpholine 1.0%
    Oleic and stearic acids 1.0%
    Borax 0.2%
    Water . . . .   83 to 88%
    May contain:
      Isopropyl alcohol*

GENERAL PURPOSE . . . . Toxicity rating 2 or 3
    Turpentine*
    Mineral spirits*
    Waxes
    May contain:
      Coloring

WAXES (Cont.)

    Detergent
    Emulsifier
    Mineral waxes (may be chlorinated)
    Perfume
    Vegetable waxes (e.g., carnauba, curicury)
    Wood preservative
    Zinc stearate

PASTE WAXES . . . . Toxicity rating 2
 1. Carnauba wax . . . . }
    Paraffin . . . . } 39%
    Stearic acid soap . . . .
    Borax . . . .   less than 1%
    Ammonium hydroxide . . . .   less than 1%
    Water 60%
                                              Toxicity rating 3
 2. Natural and petroleum waxes . . . . . }
    Naphtha* . . . . } 100%
    May contain:
      Coloring
      Perfume
      Sugar cane resin
      Turpentine*

WINDOW WAXES . . . . Toxicity rating 2 or 3
    Silica abrasive
    Amine soaps
    Waxes
    Petroleum solvent*
    Ammonium hydroxide . . . .   trace

WELDING FLUXES

WELDING FLUXES . . . . Toxicity rating 4
    Alkaline fluorides*
    Alkaline earth metals

Starred ingredients (*) may be responsible for major toxic effects; consult Sec. II.

A

ABBOTT LABS., 14th & Sheridan Rd., N. Chicago, Ill.

ABELMAN, M., CO., 84 Stonely Rd., Boston, Mass.

ABESTO MFG. CORP., 131 Wabash St., Michigan City, Ind.

ABLON FINISHES, INC., 80 Waydele St., Newark, N.J.

ABRADANT PRODUCTS CO., INC., 1048 Niagara St., Buffalo, N.Y.

ACE PHOTO LABS., 316 W. Washington St., Chicago 6, Ill.

ACETO CHEMICAL CO., INC., 40-40 Lawrence St., Flushing 54, L.I., N.Y.

ACKERMAN'S DAR LAB., 279 Hempstead Ave., Malverne, L.I., N.Y.

ACME FERTILIZER CO., Wilmington, N.C.

ACME QUALITY PAINTS, INC., 8250 St. Aubin Ave., Detroit 11, Mich.

ACME WHITE LEAD & COLOR WORKS, 8250 St. Aubin Ave., Detroit 11, Mich.

ACORN ADHESIVES CO., INC., 678 Clover St., Los Angeles 31, Calif.

ACORN REFINING CO., 8001 Franklin Blvd., Cleveland 2, Ohio.

ADAMS CO., 100 S. Broad St., Philadelphia 10, Pa.

ADCO, INC., Sedalia, Mo.

ADELL CHEMICAL CO., Holyoke, Mass.

ADELPHI PAINT & COLOR WORKS, INC., 86-00 Dumont Ave., Ozone Park 17, L.I., N.Y.

ADMIRALTY MFG. CO., Box 49, Fruitvale Station, Oakland, Calif.

ADVANCE CHEM. CO., 6210 W. State St., Milwaukee, Wis.

ADVANCE MERCHANDISING CO., Toledo, Ohio.

ADVANCE PAINT CO., 601 Kentucky Ave., Indianapolis, Ind.

ADVANCE RESEARCH CORP., 20 S. Peoria St., Chicago 7, Ill.

AERO-SANITATION CO., 325 W. Pacific Ave., St Louis 19, Mo.

AEROSOL PRODUCTS CORP., 371 E. 116th St., Chicago 28, Ill.

AETNA PLYWOOD & VENEER CO., 1733 N. Elston Ave., Chicago, Ill.

AFRICANO LABS., INC., 156 Chambers St., New York 7, N.Y.

AGAVA PRODUCTS INC., 32-36 Exchange Pl., Jersey City 2, N.J.

A-GENE LAB., 616 Blow St., St. Louis 11, Mo.

AGICIDE, INC., Racine, Wis.

AGKEM, INC., 506 Maine St., Quincy, Ill.

AGOL CHEM. CO., INC., 826 17th St., N.W., Washington 5, D.C.

AGRICULTURAL LABS., INC., 1147 Chesapeake Ave., Columbus 16, Ohio.

AGRICULTURAL PROCESSING INDUSTRIES, INC., P.O. Box 2251, Denver, Colo.

AGSCO INC., 700 N. 3rd St., Grand Forks, N.Dak.

AHLGRENS, F., Tekn. Fabrik A.B., Gavle, Sweden

AIRCRAFT-MARINE PRODUCTS, Inc., 2100 Paxton St., Harrisburg, Pa.

AIREM CO., 408 Main St., Winchester, Mass.

AIRKEM, INC., 241 E. 44th St., New York 17, N.Y.

AIRLINE CHEMICALS, INC., Main at Azorb, Ann Arbor, Mich.

AIROSOL CO., INC., 823 Main St., Neodeska, Kans.

AIX OLEIN CO., 1247 61st St., Brooklyn, N.Y.

AKERITE CO., 3161 Clybourn Ave., Chicago 18, Ill.

AKRON PAINT & VARNISH CO., Firestone Pkwy. & Beck Ave., Akron, Ohio.

ALABAMA PAINT CO., 3601 10th Ave. N., Birmingham, Ala.

ALABASTINE PAINT PRODUCTS, Chicago Bronze & Color Works, 2601 W. Grand Ave., Chicago 12, Ill.

ALADDIN LABORATORIES, INC., 620 S. 8th St., Minneapolis 4, Minn.

ALADDIN PAINT CO., INC., 2473 Enterprise, Los Angeles, Calif.

ALASKA FERTILIZER CO., 84 Seneca St., Seattle, Wash.

ALBERMARLE PHARMACEUTICAL CO., 130 East 38th St., New York 16, N.Y.

ALBERTO-CULVER CO. OF HOLLYWOOD, 4201 W. Grand Ave., Chicago 51, Ill.

ALBI CHEMICAL CORP., 9 Park Pl., New York 7, N.Y.

ALBURGER RESEARCH PRODUCTS CO., 7354 Santa Monica Blvd., Los Angeles 46, Calif.

ALCATRAZ CO., INC., 1902 Ellen Rd., Richmond, Va.

ALCON LABS., INC., P.O. Box 1959, Fort Worth, Tex.

ALGAEDERM, INC., 1635 Hinman Ave., Evanston, Ill.

ALKAID CORP., 70 E. 45th St., New York 17, N.Y.

ALKALITHIA CO., 312 W. Lombard St., Baltimore 1, Md.

ALKALOL CO., Taunton, Mass.

ALKA-VITA CO., 1752 Westwood Blvd., Los Angeles 24, Calif.

ALKEM PRODUCTS CO., Box 95, Bogota, N.J.

ALLAN & CO., 4454 Easton, St. Louis, Mo.

ALLCOCK MFG. CO., N. Water St., Ossining, N.Y.

ALLEN CO., Pittstown, N.J.

ALLEN, L. B., CO., 6722 Bryn Mawr Ave., Chicago, Ill.

ALLEN, MARK, CO., 2109 2nd Ave., Detroit 1, Mich.

ALLEN OPTICAL CO., 85 Allen, Buffalo, N.Y.

ALLENTOWN PAINT MFG. CO., Allentown, Pa.

ALLIED COMPOSITIONS CO., INC., 11-15 44th Rd., Long Island City 1, L. I., N.Y.

ALLIED DISTRIBUTORS, 907 Penn Ave., Pittsburgh 22, Pa.

ALLIED DRUG PRODUCTS CO., 16th & Pierse Sts., Chattanooga, Tenn.

ALLIED HOME PRODUCTS, C-Z Chemical Co. Division, Beloit, Wis.

ALLIED PAINT MFG. CO., 2300 N. Lewis, Tulsa 1, Okla.

ALLIED PRODUCTS CO., 4265 Duncan Ave., St. Louis 10, Mo.

ALLIED PRODUCTS CO., 1133 W. Newport Ave., Chicago, Ill.

ALL-WINTER ANTI-FREEZE CO., 333 E. Dong St., Columbus, Ohio

ALLYN & CO., INC., 271 Vance St., Memphis 5, Tenn.

ALMA LABS., INC., 421 Audubon Bldg., New Orleans 16, La.

ALMAR CHEMICAL CO., 2050 8th Ave., New York 26, N.Y.

ALMAY, INC., Division Schieffelin & Co., 22 Cooper Sq., New York 3, N.Y.

ALMKLOV'S PHARMACY, Cooperstown, N.Dak.

ALMOLINE CO., 107 Grant St., Pawnee City, Nebr.

ALOISE PHARMACEUTICALS, 1682 2nd Ave., New York 28, N.Y.

ALOX CORP., Buffalo Ave. & Iroquois St., Niagara Falls, N.Y.

ALPHA ASSOCIATES, 60 E. 42nd St., New York 17, N.Y.

ALPHA CHEMICAL CO., 143 S. Kings Rd., Los Angeles 48, Calif.

ALTONE CHEMICAL CO., 3941 Tehoupitoulas St., New Orleans 15, La.

ALTON PRODUCTS, INC., Yonkers, N.Y.

ALTYME PRODS., INC., 105 E. 29th St., New York 16, N.Y.

ALUMATONE CORP., Grande Vista Ave. & E. Pico, Los Angeles, Calif.

ALUMINUM CO. OF AMERICA, E. St. Louis, Ill.

ALUMINUM INDUSTRIES, INC., 2438 Beekman St., Cincinnati 25, Ohio

ALVEO CORP., Box 922, St. Petersburg, Fla.

AMALGAMATED CHEM. CORP., Rorer & Ontario Sts., Philadelphia 34, Pa.

AMALGAMATED PAINT CO., 90 West St., New York, N.Y.

AMAZOL CO., 1025 W. Washington Blvd., Los Angeles 15, Calif.

AMBASSADOR PAINT SPECIALTIES CO., 6440 DeBuel Ave., Detroit 11, Mich.

AMBER LION CO., P.O. Box 267, Torrence, Calif.

AMBROID CO., 305 Franklin St., Boston 10, Mass.

AMEND DRUG & CHEMICAL CO., 117 E. 24th St., New York, N.Y.

AMERICAINE INC., 1316 Sherman Ave., Evanston, Ill.

AMERICAN ABRASIVE METALS CO., Sayre & Coit, Irvington, N.J.

AMERICAN AEROSOL CORP., 406 W. 16th St., Holland, Mich.

AMERICAN AGRICULTURAL CHEMICAL CO., 50 Church St., New York 7, N.Y.

AMERICAN APOTHECARIES CO., 29-28 41st Ave., Long Island City 1, L. I., N.Y.

AMERICAN ART CLAY CO., 4717 W. 16th St., Indianapolis 24, Ind.

AMERICAN ARTISTS' COLOR WORKS, INC., 5610 1st Ave., Brooklyn, N.Y.

AMERICAN ASBESTOS PRODUCTS CO., 8000 Franklin Blvd., Cleveland, Ohio

AMERICAN BRANDS CO., 1812 Ellen Rd., Richmond 20, Va.

AMERICAN CELCURE WOOD PRESERVING CORP., 1074 E. 8th St., Jacksonville 6, Fla.

AMERICAN CHEMICAL PAINT CO., Ambler, Pa.

AMERICAN CHICLE CO., 405 Lexington Ave., New York, N.Y.

AMERICAN CRAYON CO., 1706 Hayes Ave., Sandusky, Ohio.

AMERICAN CYANAMID CO., 1937 W. Main St., Stamford, Conn.

AMERICAN DISINFECTANT CO., 928 Eye Street, N.W., Washington 1, D.C.

AMERICAN DRUGGISTS SYNDICATE, INC., 503 E. 72nd St., New York 21, N.Y.

AMERICAN FELSOL CO., Lorain, Ohio.

AMERICAN FERMENT CO., 1450 Broadway, New York 36, N.Y.

AMERICAN FLOOR SURFACING MACHINE CO., 539 S. St. Clair, Toledo, Ohio.

AMERICAN FLUID CO., 4002 Woodland, Kansas City, Mo.

AMERICAN FLURESIT CO., INC., 4011 Red Bank Rd., Cincinnati 27, Ohio.

AMERICAN FUMIGATING CO., INC., 4553 Delmar Ave., St. Louis 8, Mo.

AMERICAN GREASE STICK CO., Muskegon, Mich.

AMERICAN INDUSTRIES, INC., 10 P.O. Sq., Boston 9, Mass.

AMERICAN LACQUER SOLVENTS CO., P.O. Box 271, Phoenixville, Pa.

AMERICAN-LA FRANCE-FOAMITE CORP., 101 East La France St., Elmira, N.Y.

AMERICAN LIQUID FERTILIZER CO., Marietta, Ohio.

AMERICAN LITHOGRAPH VARNISH CO., Kearny, N.J.

AMERICAN MARIETTA CO., 101 E. Ontario, Chicago, Ill.

AMERICAN MARINE PAINT CO., 311 California, San Francisco, Calif.

AMERICAN METAL POLISH CORP., 13-15 Custom House St., Boston 10, Mass.

AMERICAN OIL CO., American Bldg., Baltimore 2, Md.

AMERICAN PAINT CO., 902 N. Larrabee St., Chicago, Ill.

AMERICAN PAINT CORP., Duluth, Minn.

AMERICAN PHARMACAL CO., 101 W. Mitchell St., Milwaukee 4, Wis.

AMERICAN PHENOLIC CORP., 1830 S. 54th Ave., Chicago 50, Ill.

AMERICAN RUST PROOF CO., INC., 302 Butler St., Brooklyn, N.Y.

AMERICAN SCIENTIFIC LAB., INC., P.O. Box 232, Madison 1, Wis.

AMERICAN SERUM CO., 2117 Leech St., Sioux City 1, Iowa.

AMERICAN SHELLAC CO., 4-62 47th Rd., Long Island City, L. I., N.Y.

AMERICAN SOLVENTS CO., Perkiomen & Grice, Pheonixville,Pa.

AMERICAN VARNISH CO., 1138 N. Branch St., Chicago, Ill.

AMERICAN VETERINARY LAB., 1336 Truman Rd., Kansas City, Kans.

AMERICAN WRITING INK CO., 15 Hathaway St., Boston, Mass.

AMES CO., INC., Elkhart, Ind.

AMES DRUG CO., 630 Divisadero St., San Francisco 17, Calif.

AMES LABS., INC., South Norwalk, Conn.

AMFRE DRUG CO., INC., 121 E. 24th St., New York 10, N.Y.

AMLEX CO., 1016 Central Ave., Cincinnati, Ohio.

AMM-I-DENT, INC., 390 Wayne St., Jersey City 2, N.J.

AMPION CORPORATION, 4-88 47th Ave., Long Island City, L. I., N.Y.

A-M-R CHEMICAL CO., 985 E. 35th St., Brooklyn 10, N.Y.

AMSCO SOLVENTS & CHEMICALS CO., 4619 Reading Rd., Cincinnati, Ohio.

ANAHIST CO., INC., 21 Gray Oaks Ave., Yonkers 2, N.Y.

ANBESOL CO., 807 Mt. Prospect Ave., Newark 4, N.J.

ANCHOR CHEMICAL CO., INC., 827 Bergen St., Brooklyn, N.Y.

ANCHOR SERUM CO., Livestock Exchange Bldg., S. St. Joseph, Mo.

ANDERSEN SPECIALTY MFG. CORP., 5618 S. Harper Ave., Chicago 37, Ill.

ANDERSON-CAMPBELL CORP., Stoneleigh Rd., Carmel, N.Y.

ANDERSON-PRICHARD OIL CORP., 1000 Liberty Bank Bldg., Oklahoma City 2, Okla.

ANDICAL SCALP LOTION MFG. CO., 918 New Lots Ave., Brooklyn 8, N.Y.

ANDRÉ COSMETICS, INC., 18 E. 49th St., New York 1, N.Y.

ANDREW, WILSON, INC., Springfield, N.J.

ANDREWS, A. H., CO., 37 S. Wabash, Chicago, Ill.

ANDREWS, CYNTHIA, INC., Lexington Ave., Bethpage, L. I., N.Y.

ANGLIN, RICHARD, SR., P.O. Box 568, Bridgeport 5, Conn.

ANSCO, 175 Clinton St., Binghamton, N.Y.

ANSUL CHEMICAL CO., 3300 Hegely, Marinette, Wis.

ANTARA CHEMICALS, Sales Div. of General Aniline & Film Corp., 435 Hudson St., New York 14, N.Y.

ANTE-FERMEN CO., INC., 305 Maple St., Clinton, S.C.

ANTELL, CHARLES, INC., Mount & Cole Sts., Baltimore, Md.

ANTHRON PRODUCTS, 313 S. Orange St., Newark 3, N.J.

ANTI-BORAX COMPOUND CO., Fort Wayne, Ind.

ANTI-HYDRO WATERPROOFING CO., 265-277 Badger Ave., Newark 8, N.J.

ANTISEPTAL CO., 5524 N. Northwest Hgwy., Chicago, Ill.

ANT-ROACH POWDER CO., 262 W. 26th St., New York 1, N.Y.

ANZIO CHEMICAL CO., 600 Michigan Bldg., Detroit 26, Mich.

A & P, see Great Atlantic & Pacific.

APCO LABS., 940 W. Peachtree St., Atlanta, Ga.

A-PENN OIL CO., Butler, Pa.

APEX ALKALI PRODUCTS CO., Main & Rector Sts., Philadelphia 27, Pa.

APEX CHEMICAL MFG. CORP., 1745 W. Grand Blvd., Detroit 8, Mich.

APHINE MFG. CO., Madison, N.J.

APOTHECARIES HALL CO., 28 Benedict St., Waterbury 88, Conn.

APPLETON PRODUCTS CO., 10215 Jos. Campau Ave., Detroit 12, Mich.

APPROVED PHARM. CORP., 407-09 Hickory St., Syracuse 3, N.Y.

ARABOL MFG. CO., 1829 S. 54th Ave., New York, N.Y.

ARCHER-DANIELS-MIDLAND, 29th Ave., S.E., & Great Western Tracks, Minneapolis 2, Minn.

ARCO CO., 7301 Bessemer St., Cleveland 27, Ohio.

ARDEN, ELIZABETH, 581 5th Ave., New York, N.Y.

AREM, INC., 5259 W. Fullerton Ave., Chicago 39, Ill.

AREND DRUG CO., 677 N. Michigan Ave., Chicago 11, Ill.

AR-EX PRODUCTS CO., 1036 W. Van Buren St., Chicago 7, Ill.

ARGO & CO., INC., 2714 Southern Ave., Memphis 11, Tenn.

ARGONNE PRODUCTS, P.O. Box 461, Sacramento, Calif.

ARIZONA FERTILIZERS, INC., 734 E. S.P. Dr., Phoenix, Ariz.

AR-JAY LABS., INC., 304 E. 6th St., Ontario, Calif.

ARKANSAS CO., INC., P.O. Box 210, Newark 1, N.J.

ARLENGE LABS., 156 Chambers St., New York 7, N.Y.

ARLINGTON-FUNK LABS., Division of U. S. Vitamin Corp., 250 E. 43rd St., New York 17, N.Y.

ARLO CO., Cedar Rapids, Iowa.

ARMAND CO., 124 Des Moines St., Des Moines 6, Iowa.

ARMOUR & CO., 1355 W. 31st St., Chicago 9, Ill.

ARMOUR FERTILIZER WORKS, 350 Hunt Bldg., Chicago, Ill.

ARMOUR LABS., Box 511, Kankakee, Ill.

ARMSTRONG CHEMICAL CO., INC., Canandaigua, N.Y.

ARMSTRONG CO., 1001 E. 103rd St., Chicago 28, Ill.

ARMSTRONG CORK CO., Lancaster, Pa.

ARMSTRONG PAINT & VARNISH CO., 1318-1500 S. Kilbourn Ave., Chicago 23, Ill.

ARNAR-STONE LABS., INC., 225 E. Prospect Ave., Mount Prospect, Ill.

ARNESTO PAINT CO., 550 W. 46th St., New York, N.Y.

ARNOLD'S DRUG PRODUCTS, INC., 3722 Poplar Ave., Brooklyn 24, N.Y.

ARRESTINE SALES AGENCY, P.O. Box 3315, S. Highland St., Birmingham, Ala.

ART CHEMICAL PRODUCTS INC., Huntington, Ind.

ARTCO PRODUCTS CO., 1350 Watson Ave., Wilmington, Calif.

ARTLOOM CARPET CO., INC., Philadelphia, Pa.

ARTO MFG. CO., 410 Callowhill, Philadelphia, Pa.

ARTRA COSMETICS, INC., see Union Pharm.

ARZEN-ARDENT CO., 120 W. Platt St., Maquoketa, Iowa.

ASCATCO LABS., 5760 Melrose Ave., Hollywood 28, Calif.

ASCHENBACH & MILLER, INC., 346 N. Orianna St., Philadelphia 6, Pa.

ASEPTICO LABS., INC., 58 N. Fitzhugh St., Rochester 14, N.Y.

ASEPTINOL MFG. CO., 8 S. Dearborn St., Chicago 3, Ill.

ASHWORTH CHEMICAL CO., 590 S. Main St., Memphis 3, Tenn.

ASSOCIATED BRANDS, INC., 35 Clover Pl., Brooklyn 16, N.Y.

ASSOCIATED JUST DISTRIBUTORS, Baltimore 31, Md.; Los Angeles 13, Calif.

ASSOCIATED PRODUCTS CO., 77 P St., N.E., Washington 2, D.C.

ASSOCIATED SALES & SUPPLY CO., 5137 Southwest Ave., St. Louis, Mo.

ASSOCIATED SEED GROWERS, INC., New Haven 2, Conn.

ASTHMA NEFRIN CO., INC., 6049 N. Interstate Ave., Portland 11, Oreg.

ASTOR EXTERMINATING CO., 808 Memorial Dr., Cambridge 39, Mass.

ASTRA LABS., INC., 44 Mohawk Ave., Scotia, N.Y.

ATHEA LABS., INC., 223 E. Detroit St., Milwaukee 2, Wis.

ATHELSTAN PRODUCTS CO., 4700 Aldrich Ave., Minneapolis 9, Minn.

ATHLOID LABS., 735 Park Ave., Rochester 7, N.Y.

ATLANTIC PAINT CO., 185 Madison Ave., New York, N.Y.

ATLANTIC VARNISH CO., 100 E. Santa Anita Ave., Burbank, Calif.

ATLANTIC VARNISH & PAINT CO., INC., 3000 North Blvd., Richmond, Va.

ATLAS DRUG CO., 8416 Hudson Blvd., North Bergen, N.J.

ATLAS LABS., 1603 Delia Ave., Akron, Ohio.

ATLAS PAINT & VARNISH CO., INC., 32 Buffington Ave., Irvington, N.J.

ATLAS POWDER CO., Wilmington 99, Del.

ATLAS PUTTY PRODUCTS CO., 1515 W. Carroll Ave., Chicago 7, Ill.

ATOMIX, INC., Wilmington, Del.

AUBRY SISTERS, 104 5th Ave., New York 11, N.Y.

AULT & WILBORG CORP., Dana & Thomas Aves., Cincinnati, Ohio.

AUNT LOU MEDICINE CO., Main St., Oak Grove, La.

AURINE CO., INC., 6224 N. Broadway, Chicago, Ill.

AUSTIN LABS., INC., 15 Woodbine St., Providence 6, R. I.

AUTHORIZED BRANDS, 70 Central Ave., S.W., Atlanta 2, Ga.

AUTO-LOKS MFG. CO., INC., 175 Park Row, New York 7, N.Y.

AUTOMOTIVE FINISHES, INC., 8747 Brandt, Dearborn, Mich.

AVON-ALLIED PRODUCTS, INC., 30 Rockefeller Plaza, New York, N.Y.

AVON PRODUCTS CO., Suffern, N.Y.

AYARS, HELEN, CO., 3719 N. 14th St., St. Louis 7, Mo.

AYER, HARRIET HUBBARD, INC., 505 Park Ave., New York 22, N.Y.

AYERST LABORATORIES, 22 E. 40th St., New York 16, N.Y.

A-ZEE-O PRODUCTS, INC., 1500 Elmwood Ave., Folcroft, Pa.

B

BAALMANN, J., 129 Tehama St., San Francisco 3, Calif.

BABBITT, B. T., INC., 386 4th Ave., New York 16, N.Y.

BABE-EEZ CO., 11 Beacon St., Boston, Mass.

BACORN CO., P.O. Box 3, Elmira, N.Y.

BAER BROTHERS BRONZE POWDER CO., Stamford, Conn.

BAER BROS. PAINT & VARNISH, Div. of Adelphi Pt. & Color Works, 86-00 Dumont Ave., Ozone Pk. 17, L.I., N.Y.

BAER DRUGS, INC., 2206 South St., Philadelphia 46, Pa.

BAILEY, TEX, CO., Troy, N.Y.

BAILIN CHEMICAL CO., 143 Dahill Rd., Brooklyn 18, N.Y.

BAIRD & McGUIRE, INC., Holbrook, Mass.

BAKER, CHESTER LABS., INC., 295 Huntington Ave., Boston 15, Mass.

BAKER, C. P., & CO., 503 N. 11th St., Philadelphia 23, Pa.

BAKER, FRANKLIN, Division of General Foods Corp., 15th & Bloomfield Sts., Hoboken, N.J.

BAKER, John C., Co., 1017 N. 4th St., Philadelphia 23, Pa.

BAKER PAINT & VARNISH CO., 224 Suydam Ave., Jersey City, N.J.

BAKER, W. A., LABS., 660 Arlington St., San Francisco 12, Calif.

BAKER'S SERVICE CO., 191 E. Main St., Malone, N.Y.

BALDWIN CHEMICAL LABS., Broad St., Saegerstown, Pa.

BALDWIN LABS., 1 N. Grand Ave., Baldwin, L. I., N.Y.

BALL LABS., 1709 N. Kenmore, Los Angeles 27, Calif.

BALM BARR, INC., 727 W. Lake St., Chicago 6, Ill.

BALTIMORE COPPER PAINT CO., Key Hgwy., Baltimore 30, Md.

BALTIMORE PAINT & COLOR WORKS, 2325 Annapolis Ave., Baltimore 30, Md.

BALTZ, ROBERT N., & CO., 1009 Harvard Terr., Evanston, Ill.

BANAY, INC., 205 W. Highland Ave., Milwaukee 3, Wis.

BANDINI FERTILIZER CO., 4139 Bandini Blvd., Los Angeles 23, Calif.

BANFI PRODUCTS CORP., 503 W. Broadway, New York 12, N.Y.

BANNER MFG. CO., 3551 Blake St., Denver, Colo.

BARBASOL CO., 846 N. Senate Ave., Indianapolis 7, Ind.

BARBER, W. H., CO., Minneapolis 14, Minn.

BARBO MFG. CO., 220 W. 19th St., New York 11, N.Y.

BARCO CHEMICAL PRODUCTS, 701 S. La Salle St., Chicato 5, Illinois.

BARCO CHEMICALS INC., 61 Butner St., Des Moines 15, Iowa.

BARCOLENE CO., 200 Camden St., Boston, Mass.

BARDEX MED. CO., 237 E. Spring St., Columbus 15, Ohio.

BAR F PRODUCTS, 6028 Troost Ave., Kansas City 4, Mo.

BARFRED RESEARCH LABS., P.O. Box 428, Coconut Grove Sta., Miami 33, Fla.

BARIBEAU & SON, Levis, Que., Canada.

BARKER, MOORE & MEIN CO., 541 N. Orianna St., Philadelphia 23, Pa.

BARKER, WM. JAY, 160 E. 127th St., New York 35, N.Y.

BARLOW-MANEY LABS., Cedar Rapids, Iowa.

BARNES, A.C., see Zonite Prod.

BARNES-HIND LABS. INC., 895 Kifer Rd., Sunnyoak, Calif.

BARNSDALL PRODUCTS CORP., Tulsa, Okla.

BARR, G., & CO., 1134 W. 37th St., Chicago, Ill.

BARRELED-SUNLIGHT PAINT CO., 41 Dudley, Providence, R. I.

BARRETT CHEMICAL CO., 1331 N. Robinson St., Philadelphia 31, Pa.

BARRETT DIVISION, Allied Chemical & Dye Corp., 40 Rector St., New York 6, N.Y.

BARRETT VARNISH CO., 1532 S. 50th Ct., Cicero 50, Ill.

BARTELDES SEED CO., 3770 E. 40th Ave., Denver 16, Colo.

BARTLETT, F. A., TREE EXPERT CO., Stamford, Conn.

BARTLETT, N. M., MFG. CO., LTD. Beamsville, Ont., Canada.

BARTLEY, JOHN T., & CO., Beaver Falls, Pa.

BARTON CHEM. CO., 3907 S. Langley Ave., Chicago 15, Ill.

BARTON MFG. CO., 4157 N. Kingshighway, St. Louis 15, Mo.

BARTZ DRUG CO., 87-89 Monroe Ave., Grand Rapids 2, Mich.

BASCH, GEORGE, CO., Longfellow & Randall Aves., New York 59, N.Y.

BATTLE CREEK DIETETIC CO., Battle Creek, Mich.

BATTLE CREEK FOOD CO., Battle Creek, Mich.

BAUER & BLACK, Division of Kendall Co., 2500 S. Dearborn St., Chicago 16, Ill.

BAUER, J. E., CO., 1021 N. Mission Rd., Los Angeles, Calif.

BAUGH SONS CO., 20 S. Delaware Ave., Philadelphia 6, Pa.

BAXTER, DON, INC., 1015 Grandview Ave., Glendale 1, Calif.

BAXTER MFG. CO., Dubuque, Iowa.

BAYBANK DRUG CO., 84-40 101st St., Richmond Hill 18, L. I., N.Y.

BAYER CO., Division of Sterling Drug, Inc., 1450 Broadway, New York 18, N.Y.

BAY STATE DRUG CO., INC., 419 Main St., Palmer, Mass.

B & B DRUG CO., 116 Clinton Pl., Newark 8, N.J.

B & B TOILETRIES, 2750 N. California Ave., Chicago 47, Ill.

B. C. REMEDY CO., 423 Morris St., Durham, N.C.

BEACON CO., 33 Richdale Ave., Cambridge 40, Mass.

BEAR MFG. CO., INC., Winfield, Kans.

BEAU PEEP PRODUCTS, 5642 Lake Park Ave., Chicago 37, Ill.

BEAUMONT CO., St. Louis, Mo.

BEAUTÉ-VUES CORP., 3333 N. San Fernado Blvd., Burbank, Calif.

BEAUTY AFFILIATES, 117-18 240th St., Elmont, L. I., N.Y.

BEAUTY COUNSELORS, INC., Grosse Pointe, Mich.

BEAUTY PRODUCTS, LTD., 450 Lincoln St., Denver 9, Colo.

BECK EQUIPMENT CO., 3360 W. 137th St., Cleveland 11, Ohio.

BECK, I. & SONS, INC., 256 Mott St., New York 12, N.Y.

BECK PRODUCTS CO., P.O. Box 8579, Pittsburgh 20, Pa.

BECKER, R. A., CO., 2217 Langdon Farm Rd., Cincinnati, Ohio.

BECTON, DICKINSON & CO., Rutherford, N.J.

BEEBE LABS., INC., P.O. Box 2106, St. Paul 9, Minn.

BEEBE NESS CO., Division of Geo. H. Lee Co., Omaha, Nebr.

BEECHEM, EMMA LAB., Oscawana on Hudson, N.Y.

BEECHAM LABS., 1102 W. State St., St Johns, Mich.

BEE DEE PRODUCTS, Chattanooga 9, Tenn.

BEE GEE LABS., 1613 W. 54th St., Los Angeles 37, Calif.

BEEMAN'S LAB., INC., 758 Ponce de Leon Pl., N.E., Atlanta 6, Ga.

BEHLEN, H., & BRO., Christopher & Gay Sts., New York, N.Y.

BELLAIRE PRODUCTS, INC., Houston, Tex.

BELL CHEMICAL CO., INC., 730 15th St., N.W., Washington, D.C.

BELL CHEMICAL CO., 435 W. 59th St.; Chicago 21, Ill.

BELL & CO., INC., Orangeburg, N.Y.

BELLE MOSS CO., 9509 Gratiot Ave., Detroit 13, Mich.

BELLEVUE PHARMACAL CO., 407 1st Ave., New York 10, N.Y.

BELL, H. O., Tyngsboro, Mass.

BELL LABS., Tracy, Calif.

BELL-O-SAL MFG. CO., 1340 N. 12th St., Philadelphia 22, Pa.

BELL PHARMACAL CO., 1007 Avenue G., Lubbock, Tex.

BELL TRAP MFG. CO., 1932 N. 11th St., Fort Smith, Ark.

BELMONT LABS, INC., 4730 Market St , Philadelphia 39, Pa.

BELVA MFG. CO., 4038 Easton Ave., St. Louis 13, Mo.

BELVIDERE LABS., 700 W. Locust St., Belvidere, Ill.

BENDEL, HENRI, INC., 10 W. 57th St., New York 19, N.Y.

BENDIX PRODUCTS, Division of Bendix Aviation Corp., South Bend 20, Ind.

BENE VIM CORP., 145 Nassau St., New York 38, N.Y.

BENGAL CO., 570 W. 131st St., New York 27, N.Y.

BENGUE, INC., 2023 Kerrigan Ave., Union City, N.J.

BENNETT, E.W., & CO., 16th & Utah Sts., San Francisco 3, Calif.

BENNETTS-BARNETT LAB., 517 Harrison Ave., Fresno 3, Calif.

BEN-THOL CO., 201 E. 2nd St., Hastings, Minn.

BERJON CO., 2074 Union Ave., Memphis 4, Tenn.

BERLOU MANUFACTURING CO., Marion, Ohio.

BERMAN CHEMICAL CO., 698 Superior, Toledo, Ohio.

BEROSOL CO., 116 John St., New York 38, N.Y.

BERRY BROTHERS, INC., 211 Leib St., Detroit 7, Mich.

BERRY, C. H., MFG. CO., 2507-2509 S. 3rd St., St. Louis 4, Mo.

BEST FOODS, INC., 1 E. 43rd St., New York 17, N.Y.

BESTOSEAL CO., 16 Bridge St., New York, N.Y.

BETA CIBUS CO., 1751 Lawrence, Detroit 6, Mich.

BETALAX CO., INC., 508 Franklin Ave., Mt. Vernon, N.Y.

BETHESDA PHARMICAL CO., 6402 Georgia Ave., N.W., Washington 11, D.C.

BETTER FINISHES & COATINGS INC., 268 Doremus Ave., Newark, N.J.

BETTER WAY BRANDS, INC., 220 Miracle Mile, Coral Gables, Fla.

BICKMORE CO., 119 S. Main St., Old Town, Maine.

BICKUM, DOROTHY, 295 5th Ave., New York 16, N.Y.

BIDETAL PHARM. CO., 427 Fort Washington Ave., New York 33, N.Y.

BIG DRIP, St. Charles, Ill.

BIHN & WOLFF CO., Ash & Almond Sts., Philadelphia, Pa.

BI-LETS PRODUCTS, INC., 1123 Church St., Nashville, Tenn.

BINDAY LABS., INC., 723 Fulton Ave., Hempstead, L. I., N.Y.

BINNEY & SMITH INC., 41 E. 42nd St., New York 17, N.Y.

BINZ, EDW. G., CO., 1554 Thompson Ave., Glendale, Calif.

BINZEN HARDWARE MFG. CO., 211 E. 141st St., New York 51, N.Y.

BIOCERTA CORP., 303 5th Ave., New York 16, N.Y.

BIORGANIC LABS., INC., 75 Chamberlain Ave., East Patterson, N.J.

BIRD & SON, INC., East Walpole, Mass.

BIRMINGHAM APOTHECARY, INC., 1021 S. 20th St., Birmingham 5, Ala.

BISHOP-CONKLIN CO., 3949 Medford, Los Angeles, Calif.

BISHOP, HAZEL, INC., Paramus, N.J.

BISHOP LAB., INC., 374 50th St., Brooklyn 20, N.Y.

BISONITE CO., 126 Lakeview Ave., Buffalo, N.Y.

BLACK CAT, INC., 512 E. James St., Tampa 3, Fla.

BLACKMAN, HARRY I., Ph. G., 1918 Vera Ave., Redwood City, Calif.

BLACKMAN STOCK MEDICINE CO., 717 E. Main St., Chattanooga 8, Tenn.

BLACKO MEDICINE CO., Box 991, Charleston 24, W. Va.

BLACK PANTHER CO., INC., P.O. Box 132, Sanford, N.C.

BLACK'S MEDICINE CO., Box 991, Charleston 24, W. Va.

BLACK SWAN MFG. CO., 2235 W. Grand Ave., Chicago, Ill.

BLACK WHIRLING ENAMELS, Division of Glidden Co., 10999 Madison Ave., Cleveland, Ohio.

BLACK & WHITE CHEMICAL CO., 130 Walnut Ave., New York, N.Y.

BLACK & WHITE CO., Division of Plough Inc., Memphis, Tenn.

BLAIR, R. H., PHARMACIST, 16411 E. Warren Ave., Detroit 24, Mich.

BLAISDELL PENCIL CO., Bethayres, Pa.

BLANCHARD, INC., 50 W. 17th St., New York 11, N.Y.

BLANCHARD, JOSEPH, Pawhuska, Okla.

BLAND, E. R., CO., 666 9th Ave., San Diego 1, Calif.

B & L DISTRIBUTING CO., INC., 718 Ritchie Ave., Silver Spring, Md.

BLEECKER CO., Ghent, N.Y.

BLEMO CO., 212 3rd St., N.W., Canton 2, Ohio.

BLIND-X-CO., 2833 Hennepin Ave., Minneapolis 8, Minn.

BLISS, ALONZO O., MEDICAL CO., 1811 Columbia Rd., N.W., Washington 9, D.C.

BLISTEX CO., 3132 S. Canal St., Chicago 16, Ill.

BLITZ PRODUCTS, INC., 945 George St., Chicago 14, Ill.

BLIZ PRODUCTS CO., Fairfield, Conn.

BLOCK DRUG CO., 257 Cornelison Ave., Jersey City 2, N.J.

BLOSSER CO., Distributor, Atlanta, Ga.

BLOTEX CO., 124 S. Broadmoor Blvd., Springfield, Ohio.

BLUE BALL CHEMICAL CO., 2504 S. Kuhl Ave., Orlando, Fla.

BLUE CROSS PRODUCTS, 1827 Pacific St., Brooklyn 33, N.Y.

BLUE DEVIL LAB., 1915 Morris Ave., Bronx 53, N.Y.

BLUE-JAY PRODUCTS, Division of Kendall Co., 131 S. Franklin St., Chicago 6, Ill.

BLUE RIDGE FRUIT EXCHANGE, Waynesboro, Pa.

BLUE SEAL CHEMICAL CO., Roselle Park, N.J.

BLUE SUDS CO., 1520 Spruce St., Philadelphia 2, Pa.

BLUM, D. & CO., INC., 36-59 36th St., Long Island City 6, L. I., N.Y.

BOATWRIGHT PAINT & VARNISH WKS., 1103 Marietta, N.W., Atlanta, Ga.

BOBBI COSMETICS, Division of Gillette Co., Merchandise Mart, Chicago 54, Ill.

BOCHNER, A. M., MED. CO., P.O. Box 483, Vincennes, Ind.

BODEKER DRUG CO., 1416 E. Main St., Richmond 73, Va.

BODKIN CO., 7546 196th St., Flushing, L. I., N.Y.

BOEHMER, A. L., PAINT CO., Covington, Ky.

BOERICKE & RUNYON, Division of Humphreys Medicine Co., Inc., 273 Lafayette St., New York 12, N.Y.

BOGLE, R. H., CO., INC., Alexandria, Va.

BOHMAN BROTHERS, INC., 98 Monroe Ave., Rochester, N.Y.

BOLDT LABS., 107 Pine St., Sheboygan Falls, Wis.

BOMBI PERFUMER, INC., 135 E. 50th St., New York 22, N.Y.

BON AMI CO., 17 Battery Pl., New York 4, N.Y.

BONASEPTIC CO., Box 144, Station C, Atlanta, Ga.

BONDRITE MFG. CO., 4022 Neosho St., St. Louis, Mo.

BONEWITZ CHEMICALS, INC., Burlington, Iowa

BONIDE CHEMICAL CO., Utica 4, N.Y.

BONNEAU DYE CO., 2004 St. Clair Ave., Cleveland 14, Ohio.

BONROSE DRUG CO., 301 3rd Ave., New York 10, N.Y.

BORAX CONSOLIDATED LTD., 102 Park Ave., New York, N.Y.

BORDEN CO., Chemical Division, 350 Madison Ave., New York 17, N.Y.

BORDMAN CO., THE, Umbria & Lemonte Sts., Manayunk, Philadelphia 27, Pa.

BORN, L., Hampton, Va.

BORNE-SCRYMSER CO., 632 S. Front St., Elizabeth, N.J.

BOROCYL CO., 1241 N. Ashland Ave., Chicago 22, Ill.

BOROPHENIQUE CO., 506 Chateau Ave., Baltimore 12, Md.

BOROTAR CHEM. CO., 11315 Durant Ave., Cleveland 8, Ohio.

BOSTON PUTTY WORKS, INC., 11 Roland, Charlestown, Mass.

BOSTWICK LABS., INC., 706 Bostwick Ave., Bridgeport 5, Conn.

BOTANY, Passaic, N.J.

BOTTS MFG. CO., 79 Crosby St., New York, N.Y.

BOURJOIS INC., 33 Capron St., Rochester 2, N.Y.

BOURLAND, JIM, 910 Elysian St., Houston 10, Tex.

BOVAC CO., 1045 1st Ave., New York 22, N.Y.

BOWEN MFG. CO., Prairie City, Iowa.

BOWES SEAL FAST CORP., Indianapolis 7, Ind.

BOWNES, FRANK, CO., Chelsea, Mass.

BOYD MFG. CO., INC., 2608 2nd Ave., N., Birmingham 3, Ala.

BOYER CHEMICAL LABS., Drug Trade Division, 2700 S. Wabash Ave., Chicago 16, Ill.

BOYER PRODUCTS CO., 1440 Madison St., Kansas City 6, Mo.

BOYLE & CO., 356 S. Mission Rd., Los Angeles 33, Calif.

BOYLE-MIDWAY INC., South Ave. & Hale St., Cranford, N.J.

BOZEMAN DRUG CO., Montgomery, La.

B. & P. CO., P.O. Box 2632, Lakewood 7, Ohio.

BRADFIELD CO., see S.S.S. Co.

BRADFORD OIL CO., Palmer, Mass.

BRADLEY, C.E., LABS., INC., 45 Elm, Brattleboro, Vt.

BRADLEY, MILTON, CO., 74 Park St., Springfield 2, Mass.

BRADSHAW, PRAEGER & CO., 3250 D. 47th Pl., Chicago, Ill.

BRANDENFELS, CARL, St. Helens, Oreg.

BRANOWER CHEM. CO., 210 E. 68th St., New York 21, N.Y.

BRANT, J. W., CO., Albion, Mich.

BRATE, W. C., Co., 121-131 Tivoli St., Albany 4, N.Y.

BRATER, JOHN K., & CO., INC., 150 Havon Ave., Port Washington, N.Y.

BRAUN CORP., 1363 S. Bonnie Beach Pl., Los Angeles, Calif.

BRAUN KNECHT-HEIMAN CO., 1400 16th St., San Francisco 19, Calif.

BRAY PHARMACEUTICAL CORP., 133 E. 58th St., New York 22, N.Y.

BRAYTON CHEMICALS, INC., Burlington, Iowa.

BREAKSTONE & CO., 2155 W. Harrison St., Chicago 12, Ill.

BRECK, JOHN H., INC., 115 Dwight St., Springfield 3, Mass.

BRECK, JOS., & SONS CORP., 401 Summer St., Boston 10, Mass.

BREDENBECK PRODUCTS, 1900 Euclid Ave., Cleveland 15, Ohio.

BREINIG BROS., INC., Hoboken, N.J.

BREITENBACH, M.J., CO., DISTRIBUTOR, New York, N.Y.

BRENNAN PHARMACAL CO., 103 Columbia St., Albany 10, N.Y.

BREON, GEORGE A., & CO., 1450 Broadway, New York 18, N.Y.

BRETOCOL LABS., 500 Grand St., Brooklyn 11, N.Y.

BRIDGEPORT BRASS CO., Insecticide Division, 30 Grand St., Bridgeport 2, Conn.

BRIGGS LABORATORY., 420 Congress Ave., New Haven, Conn.

BRIGGS MARONEY CO., Everett, Mass.

BRIGHTO CHEMICAL CO., 385 Arnett Blvd., Rochester 11, N.Y.

BRILCO LABS., 1555 63rd St., Brooklyn, N.Y.

BRISTOL LABS., INC., 401 W. Taylor St., Syracuse 1, N.Y.

BRISTOL-MYERS CO., 630 5th Ave., New York 20, N.Y.

BRITTON HERB CO., 333 Genesee St., Cincinnati 2, Ohio.

BROADY OINTMENT CO., 1333 Nicholson Ave., Lakewood 7, Ohio.

BROEMMEL PHARM., 1235 Sutter St., San Francisco 9, Calif.

BRONCHI-LYPTUS CORP., 732 Ceres Ave., Los Angeles 21, Calif.

BRONDOW, INC., 26 E. 1st St., Mt. Vernon, N.Y.

BROOKFIELD LABS., Brookfield, Ill.

BROOKLINE CHEMICAL CO., 79 Sudbury St., Boston, Mass.

BROOKLINE PHARMACY, 652 Fremont St., Boston 18, Mass.

BROOKLYN PAINT & VARNISH CO., INC., 50 Jay St., Brooklyn 1, N.Y.

BROOKS CHEMICALS, INC., 3304 E. 87th St., Cleveland 27, Ohio.

BROOKS MEDICINE CO., 328 Sumner Ave., Brooklyn 21, N.Y.

BROSIS, 17 N. Wabash Ave., Chicago 2, Ill.

BROWN, ANDREW, CO., 5431 S. District Blvd., Los Angeles 22, Calif.

BROWN, EDWARD A., CO., 749 Boylston St., Newton Highlands 61, Mass.

BROWN MFG. CO., Le Roy, N.Y.

BROWN MEDICINE CO., P.O. Box 416, Morristown, Tenn.

BROWN-VAUGHN PHARM. CO., 1045 Oak St., San Francisco 17, Calif.

BROWNELL INDUSTRIES, see Casey Chem. Products.

BRUCE, E. L., CO., 1700 Thomas St., Memphis 1, Tenn.

BRUNSWICK CHEMICAL CO., P.O. Box 437, Brunswick, Ga.

BRUSH-NU CO., 618 Hanover St., Baltimore, Md.

BRYAN LABS., 805 E. Mulberry St., Bryan, Ohio.

B & S SALES CO., 7202 W. Vienna Ave., Milwaukee 16, Wis.

BUCKEYE CHEMICAL & SPECIALTY CO., 29 E. 21st St., New York 10, N.Y.

BUCKEYE PAINT & VARNISH CO., 716-22 15th St., Toledo, Ohio.

BUCKINGHAM WAX CO., Van Dam St. & Borden Ave., Long Island City, L. I., N.Y.

BUCKLEY PHARMACAL CO., Burbank, Calif.

BUCKMAN LABS., INC., 1256 N. McLean Blvd., Memphis 8, Tenn.

BUFF MFG. CO., 87 Union Ave., Pittsburgh 5, Pa.

BUFFALO FIRE APPLIANCE CORP., 200 Crane St., Dayton, Ohio.

BUFFALO SCIENTIFIC CO., Norris-Hertel St., Buffalo, N.Y.

BUFFINGTON'S, INC., Worcester 8, Mass.

BUG-A-BOO PRODUCTS, INC., Dover, N.H.

BUILDING CHEMICALS CORP., 51 E. 42nd St., New York, N.Y.

BULL, DR. JOHN, MEDICINE CO., 423-25 Greenup St., Covington, Ky.

BULLARD, E. D., CO., 275 8th St., San Francisco 3, Cal.

BULLOCK-WALKER MFG. CO., 910 Cherry St., S.E., Grand Rapids 6, Mich.

BUNN, JOHN, CORP., 167 Ashland Ave., Buffalo, N.Y.

BURMA-VITA CO., 2318 Chesnut Ave., W., Minneapolis 5, Minn.

BURNHAM LABS., INC., 431 S. Dearborn St., Chicago 5, Ill.

BURNHAM SOLUBLE IODINE CO., 160 E. 127th St., New York, N.Y.

BURNS, T. S., & BOYS CO., 447 Main St., Buffalo, N.Y.

BURR CHEMICAL CO., 3329 Auburn St., Rockford, Ill.

BURRELL-DUGGER CO., 229 E. South St., Indianapolis 25, Ind.

BURROUGH BROS. MFG. CO., 123
Market Pl., Baltimore 2, Md.
BURROUGHS WELLCOME & CO.
(U.S.A.), INC., Tuckahoe, N.Y.
BURTON, PARSONS & CO., 1515 U St.,
N.W., Washington 9, D.C.
BURTON PRODUCTS CO., 8441 S.
Chicago Ave., Chicago 17, Ill.
BUSCHMAN, A.C., & CO., 410
Frelinghuysen Ave., Newark 5, N.J.
BU-TAY PRODUCTS LTD., 5832
Garfield Ave., Los Angeles 22, Calif.
BUTCHER POLISH CO., 183
Commercial St., Malden 48, Mass.
BUZZE'S PHARM. CO., 32 E. St., N.W.
Washington 1, D.C.
BYON PHARMACAL CORP., Brooklyn,
N.Y.

C

CABELL CHEMICAL CO., Huntington
3, W. Va.
CABOT, SAMUEL, INC., 1371 Oliver
Bldg., Boston, Mass.
CACTUS REMEDY CO., P.O. Box 1251,
San Francisco 1, Calif.
CALBAR PAINT & VARNISH CO.,
2612-26 N. Martha, Philadelphia, Pa.
CALDO CO., 110 Riverside Ave.,
Buffalo 7, N.Y.
CALGON, INC., Hagan Bldg., 323 4th
Ave., Pittsburgh 22, Pa.
CALIFORNIA CHEMICAL CO., 217-
235 Birch Ave., Sacramento 15, Calif.
CALIFORNIA FARM SUPPLY CO.,
2223 Fulton St., Berkeley 4, Calif.
CALIFORNIA SODA CO., 355 Cypress
St., Oakland 20, Calif.
CALIFORNIA SPRAY CHEMICAL
CORP., Lucas & Ortho Way, Rich-
mond, Calif.
CALLAHAN, GEO., & CO., INC.,
Herbert Ave., Claster, N.J.
CALOTABS CO., INC., 54 11th St.,
N. E., Atlanta, Ga.
C. A. L. PRODUCTS CO., 610 S.
Broadway, Los Angeles 14, Calif.
CALSO WATER CO., 333 12th St., San
Francisco 3, Calif.
CALUMET DIVISION, Calumet &
Hecla Inc., Calumet, Mich.
CALUMET REFINING CO., 13921
Mackinaw Ave., Chicago, Ill.
CALVIN CHEMICAL CORP., 2891 N.W.
75th St., Miami 47, Fla.
CALVITAL PHARMACEUTICAL &
COSMETIC CORP., 117 N. 2nd Ave.,
Mount Vernon, N.Y.
CAMDEN COKE PLANT, Public Service
Electric & Gas Co., Front & Chestnut
Sts., Camden, N.J.
CAMEO CORP., N. Ravenwood Ave.,
Chicago 77, Ill.
CAMEO, INC., 3116 Bellevue Rd.,
Toledo 6, Ohio.
CAMILLE SPECIALTIES CO., 22 W.
21st St., New York 11, N.Y.
CAMP CHEMICAL CO., INC., 1560
62nd St., Brooklyn 19, N.Y.
CAMPANA SALES CO., Campana Bldg.,
Batavia, Ill.
CAMPAU, MARIE, 532 Cottage Grove,
S.E., Grand Rapids 2, Mich.
CAMPBELL CHEMICALS, INC., 3807
S. Kingshighway Blvd., St. Louis 9, Mo.

CAMPBELL COOK MEDICINE
CO., 1501 Augusta Rd., Green-
ville, S.C.
CAMPBELL, M. L., CO.,
2909 Chrysler Rd.,
Kansas City 15,
Kans.
CAMPBELL PAINT & VARNISH CO.,
Division of Glidden Co., Main &
Gratiot Sts., St. Louis, Mo.
CAMPBELL PHARMACAL CO.,
P.O. Box 2324, Dearborn, Mich.
CAMPBELL PRODUCTS CO., 505
W. Main St., Bensenville, Ill.
CANDO CO., INC., 13-15 Custom
House St., Boston 10, Mass.
CANDY & CO., INC., 35th & S.
Maplewood Ave., Chicago Ill.
CANISOL LABS., 1368 St. Nicholas
Ave., New York 33, N.Y.
CANNON CHEMICAL CO., INC., 181
Portland Ave., Cambridge 41,
Mass.
CAPATONE PRODUCTS CO., INC.,
543 10th Ave., New York 18, N.Y.
CAPE FEAR CHEMICAL, INC.,
P.O. Box 543, Elizabethtown, N.C.
CaPHENIN CHEMICAL CO.,
Waverly, Iowa.
CAPITOL CEMENT CO., Ossining,
N.Y.
CAPITOL CHEMICAL CO., 3255
Prospect Ave., Washington, D.C.
CAPUDINE CHEM. CO., P.O. Box
526, Raleigh, N.C.
CARAGOL LABORATORIES, INC.,
26011 Kinsman Rd., Cleveland 22,
Ohio.
CARAJON CHEMICAL CO., 27 W.
Main St., Fremont, Mich.
CARA NOME, see Langlois.
CARBIDE & CARBON CHEMICALS
CO., Division of Union Carbide &
Carbon Corp., 30 E. 42nd St., New
York 17, N.Y.
CARBISULPHOIL CO., 2917 Swiss
Ave., Dallas, Tex.
CARBOLA CHEMICAL CO., INC.,
Natural Bridge, N.Y.
CARBOLINEUM WOOD PRESERVING
CO., 528 W. Highland Ave.,
Milwaukee 3, Wis.
CARBONA PRODUCTS CO., 30-50
Greenpoint Ave., Long Island City
1, L. I., N.Y.
CARBO-SEPTIC CORP., 48-20 43rd
Ave., Long Island City 4, L. I., N.Y.
CARBOZINE LAB., 315 S. Broadway,
St. Louis 2, Mo.
CARDINELL CORP., 13 Label St.,
Montclair, N.J.
CAREY, PHILIP, MFG. CO.,
Cincinnati, Ohio.
CARLAY DIVISION, Campana Corp.,
Batavia, Ill.
CARMA LABS., Route No. 5,
Waukesha, Wis.
CARMEL & CO., 606 Dartmouth Dr.,
N.E., Albuquerque, N. Mex.
CAROLINA MEDICINE CO., 806
Dixon Ave., Asheboro, N.C.
CARON CORP., 730 5th Ave., New
York 19, N.Y.
CAROSANTI, INC., 2158 Church St.,
Philadelphia, Pa.

CARPENTER-MORTON CO., 376 3rd
St., Everett 49, Mass.
CARPENTER, W. D., CO., INC., 111
Irving Ave., Syracuse 3, N.Y.
CARROLL CHEMICAL CO., 2301
Hollins St., Baltimore 23, Md.
CARROLL SHELLAC & VARNISH CO.,
2656 Salmon, Philadelphia 25, Pa.
CARR'S DRUG CO., 21 Main St.,
Centerville, Miss.
CARSTENS, H. GOSLAR, 30 E. 20th St.,
New York 3, N.Y.
CARTER CO., 1729 13th St., N.W.,
Washington 9, D.C.
CARTER-LUFF CHEM. CO., 738
Warren St., Hudson, N.Y.
CARTER PAINT CO., Liberty, Ind.
CARTER PRODUCTS, INC., New
Brunswick, N.J.
CARTER'S INK CO., Cambridge 42,
Mass.
CARVER, BROOKS, 702 W. Main St.,
New Albany, Ind.
CASE, G. M., LABS., San Diego, Calif.
CASEY CHEMICAL PRODUCTS, 4400
Glen Pl., Minneapolis 10, Minn.
CASEY, D., P.O. Box 731, Portland,
Oreg.
CASITE CORP., Hastings, Mich.
CASMITH REMEDY CORP., 730 15th
St., N.W., Washington 5, D.C.
CASSEBEER, H. A., 953 Madison Ave.,
New York 21, N.Y.
CASSILL DISTRIBUTING CO., 7955
Melrose Ave., Los Angeles 46, Calif.
CASTILLA PRODUCTS, INC., 230
Grand St., New York 13, N.Y.
CASTLE, JAMES M., INC., South &
Water Sts., Philadelphia, Pa.
CASWELL-MASSEY CO., LTD., 106 E.
19th St., New York 3, N.Y.
CAUL, PHILIP M., CO., 460 Woodland,
Cleveland, Ohio.
CAVALIER CO., Jackson & West St.,
Key Hgwy., Baltimore 30, Md.
CAWTHON-COLEMAN DRUG CO., 23
Broad St., Selma, Ala.
C. C. G. PRODUCTS CO., Carla Ct.,
Powell Rd., Essexville, Mich.
C & D PRESCRIPTION PHARMACY,
P.O. Box 711, Texas City, Tex.
CEDACOTE CORP., 261 Gayoso,
Memphis, Tenn.
CEDAR HILL FORMULAE CO., New
Britain, Conn.
CEDAR-LUX PRODUCTS CO., INC.,
703 Main St., Kansas City 6, Mo.
CEL-TON-SA MEDICINE CO., 1016
Central Ave., Cincinnati 2, Ohio.
CENTAUR-CALDWELL CO., Division
of Sterling Drug, Inc., 1450 Broadway,
New York 18, N.Y.
CENTRAL CHEMICAL CO., INC., 510
W. 5th St., Kansas City 5, Mo.
CENTRAL CITY CHEM. CO., 2501 W.
Washington Blvd., Chicago 12, Ill.
CENTRAL PAINT & VARNISH WORKS,
INC., 63 Prospect St., Brooklyn 1,
N.Y.
CENTRAL SOAP CO., Hampden &
Wabash Aves., St. Paul, Minn.
CENTRAL SOLVENTS & CHEMICALS
CO., 2540 W. Flournoy St., Chicago
12, Ill.
CENTRAL SUPPLY CO., 322 Grove St.,
Brooklyn 27, N.Y.

CENTURY NATIONAL CHEM. CO., 45 Ward St., Paterson 1, N.J.

CEREAL SOAPS CO., INC., 334 E. 27th St., New York 16, N.Y.

CERIBELLI & CO., Fair Lawn, N.J.

CERTA-VIN MEDICINE CO., Court & Walnut Sts., Cincinnati 2, Ohio.

CERTOX CHEMICAL CO., Brooklyn 2, N.Y.

CHAIR-LOC CO., Old Lakewood Rd., Lakehurst, N.J.

CHAMBERLAIN, F. B., CO., 41 Branch St., St. Louis 7, Mo.

CHAMBERLAIN HABER CHEMICAL CO., 1105 W. 11th St., Cleveland 13, Ohio.

CHAMBERLAIN SALES CO., 702 6th Ave., Des Moines, Iowa.

CHAMPION BRONZE POWDER & PAINT CO., 2526 W. Van Buren, Chicago, Ill.

CHAMPION CHALK MANUFACTURING CO., Topsfield, Mass.

CHAMPO PRODUCTS CO., 163 N. High St., Columbus 15, Ohio.

CHANDLER DISTRIBUTORS, 9 S. Broadway, St. Louis 2, Mo.

CHAPIN MEDICAL SUPPLY CO., INC., 72 Needham St., Newton Highlands 61, Mass.

CHAPMAN CHEMICAL CO., Memphis, Tenn.

CHAPMAN'S PHARMACY, Fairlee, Vt.

CHAP STICK CO., 2101 Hudson St., Lynchburg, Va.

CHARLES OF THE RITZ, 11 E. 58th St., New York, N.Y.

CHASE, DR. A. W., CO., INC., 43-44 21st St., Long Island City, L. I., N.Y.

CHAS, CHEMICAL CO., 280 Chestnut St., Newark 5, N.J.

CHASE PRODUCTS CO., 1816 St. Charles Rd., Maywood, Ill.

CHASE VARNISH CO., INC., 248 Green St., Brooklyn, N.Y.

CHATHAM PHARMACEUTICALS, INC., 901 Broad St., Newark 2, N.J.

CHATTANOOGA MEDICINE CO., 1715 W. 38th St., Chattanooga 9, Tenn.

CHEESEMAN MEDICINE CO., 11 E. 12th St., New York 3, N.Y.

CHEESMAN-ELLIOTT CO., 645 Kent Ave., Brooklyn, N.Y.

CHEK PRODUCTS CO., INC., 31 Nassau Pl., East Orange, N.J.

CHEMAGRO CORP., 101 Park Ave., New York 17, N.Y.

CHEMCO CO., 2932 Cleveland Blvd., Louisville, Ky.

CHEM-CRAFT, INC., 450 Market St., Perth Amboy, N.J.

CHEMDRUG CORP., 730 5th Ave., New York 19, N.Y.

CHEMICAL CORP. OF COLORADO, W. 12th at Quivas, Denver, Colo.

CHEMICAL & EXTERMINATING CO., 3410 Broadway, New York 31, N.Y.

CHEMICAL FORMULATORS, INC., P.O. Box 10035, Station C, Charleston, W. Va.

CHEMICAL INDUSTRIES OF CALIFORNIA, Santa Barbara, Calif.

CHEMICAL INSECTICIDE CORP., 129 Montague St., Brooklyn 1, N.Y.

CHEMICAL MFG. & DISTRIB. CO., 6th & Bushkill Dr., Easton, Pa.

CHEMICAL PRODUCTS CO., Ellsworth, Minn.

CHEMICAL PRODUCTS CO., INC., Aberdeen, Md.

CHEMICAL SPECIALTIES, INC., 54 Waltham Ave., Springfield 9, Mass.

CHEMICALS, INC., 2601 Wood St., Oakland, Calif.

CHEMIPURE LABS., 170-06 Hillside Ave., Jamaica 3, L. I., N.Y.

CHEMURGIC CORP., P.O. Box 630, Turlock, Calif.

CHENEY MEDICINE CO., 2227 Barrington Dr., Toledo 6, Ohio.

CHERAMY, 539 W. 45th St., New York 36, N.Y.

CHERING, S., Bloomfield, N.J.

CHERRY'S FAMOUS SALVE CO., 136 Greenland Ave., Trenton 8, N.J.

CHESEBROUGH-POND'S, INC., 17 State St., New York 4, N.Y.

CHESTER-KENT, INC., 96-102 S. Wabash St., St. Paul 1, Minn.

CHEWALLA CO., 7816 S. Claiborne Ave., New Orleans 18, La.

CHICAGO PAINTS, INC., 4500 W. 14th St., Chicago, Ill.

CHICAGO PHARMACAL CO., 5547 N. Ravenswood Ave., Chicago, Ill.

CHICAGO SHOW PRINTING CO., Mystik Adhesives Prod. Division, 2635 N. Kildare Ave., Chicago 39, Ill.

CHICHESTER CHEM. CO., 2317 Madison Sq., Philadelphia 46, Pa.

CHIEF TWO MOON HERB CO., 33 Wales St., Waterbury 42, Conn.

CHILTON LABS., INC., 68 Forest St., Montclair, N.J.

CHILTON PAINT CO., College Point, N.Y.

CHI-NAMEL PAINT & VARNISH CO. 1101 3rd St., S. Minneapolis 15, Minn.

CHIPMAN CHEM. CO., INC., Bound Brook, N.J.

CHIPMAN, LTD., Montreal, Canada.

CHLORO CHEMICALS, I. Beck & Sons, Inc., New York 3, N.Y.

CHLOROLIN SALES CO., 733 Broadway, New York 3, N.Y.

CHURCH CHEM. CO., 1814 E. 40th St., Cleveland 3, Ohio.

CIBA PHARMACEUTICAL PRODUCTS, INC., Summit, N.J.

CIGOGNE, INC., 60 E. 56th St., New York 22, N.Y.

CINCY PRODUCTS, CO., 2817 Highland Ave., Cincinnati 12, Ohio.

CITADEL PRODUCTS, 1601 Sheepshead Bay Rd., Brooklyn 35, N.Y.

CITIES SERVICE OIL CO., 70 Pine St., New York 5, N.Y.

CITROX LABS., INC., P.O. Box 22, Chesterland, Ohio.

CITY FUMIGATING & EXTERMINATING CO., 213 Monroe Ave., Rochester, N.Y.

CLAFLIN CO., 40 Mathewson St., Providence 3, R. I.

CLAIRE MFG. CO., 7642 Vincennes Ave., Chicago 20, Ill.

CLANTZ, N., & SONS, 289 Broadway, New York, N.Y.

CLAPP, OTIS, & SON, INC., 439 Boylston St., Boston 16, Mass.

CLARK-CLEVELAND, INC., Binghamton, N.Y.

CLARK-LURTON CORP., 40 Water St., E. Cambridge 41, Mass.

CLARK-MILLNER SALES CO., 549 W. Washington St., Chicago 6, Ill.

CLARK, ROBERT H., CO., 9330 Santa Monica Blvd., Beverly Hills, Calif.

CLARKE, H., & SONS, 6400 Rhode Island Ave., Riverdale, Md.

CLARKE SANDING MACHINE CO., 30 E. Clay Ave., Muskegon, Mich.

CLARONEX PRODUCTS, INC., 239 Java, Brooklyn, N.Y.

CLAYTON, GEO. W., CO., 1810 S. Wabash Ave., Chicago 16, Ill.

CLEAN HOME PRODUCTS, INC., 507 N. Cardinal Ave., St. Louis 3, Mo.

CLEAN PRODUCTS CO., 815 E. Mound St., Columbus 5, Ohio.

CLEAN SURFACE PRODUCTS CO., 311 N. Desplaines St., Chicago 6, Ill.

CLEARY, W. A., CORP., New Brunswick, N.J.

CLEVELAND CLEANER & PASTE CO., 7275 Neville Ave., S.W., Cleveland, Ohio.

CLEVELAND HEATER CO., 2312 Superior Ave., N.E., Cleveland, Ohio.

CLIFFS DOW CHEMICAL CO., Marquette, Mich.

CLIFTON CHEMICAL CORP., 62 William St., New York, N.Y.

CLIMALENE CO., Canton 1, Ohio.

CLINE, E. E., 114 Higgins Rd., Park Ridge, Ill.

CLINIC HYGIENIC CO., Lancaster, Pa.

CLINTON METALLIC PAINT CO., Clinton, N.Y.

CLO-FILL PRODUCTS, INC., 20 Greene St., New York 13, N.Y.

CLOROX CHEMICAL CO., 850 42nd Ave., Oakland 1, Calif.

CLOTWORTHY, H. A., P.O. Box 3334, Miami 21, Fla.

CLOVER LEAF PAINT & VARNISH CORP., 43rd & Vernon Blvd., Long Island City, L. I., N.Y.

C & M PHARMACAL, INC., 927 Porter St., Detroit 26, Mich.

COAHOMA CHEMICAL CO., P.O. Box 728, Clarksdale, Miss.

COAST LABS., 2 N. Vermont Ave., Atlantic City, N.J.

COATING MATERIALS LAB., INC., Belleville, N.J.

COCHRANE CHEMICAL CO., 153 Main St., Matawan, N.J.

COFFELT CHEMICAL CO., INC., 700 Elton Ave., New York 55, N.Y.

COFFEY, W. M., MFG. CO., P.O. Box 564, Texarkana, Ark.-Tex.

COLBTRANS CO., INC., 652 E. 54th St., Brooklyn 3, N.Y.

COLE CHEMICAL CO., 3715-31 Laclede Ave., St. Louis 8, Mo.

COLE, J. W., CO., 6918 Oleander Ave., Chicago 31, Ill.

COLGATE-PALMOLIVE CO., 105 Hudson St., Jersey City 2, N.J.

COLIT LABS., 2231 Broadway, New York 24, N.Y.

COLLINS-BENTON CO., INC., 200 Washington St., Hoboken, N.J.

COLLINS FEED & SUPPLY CO., N.E. 94th St. & F. E. C. R.R., Miami 38, Fla.

COLLINS, MIRIAM, PALM BEACH LABS. CO., 2508 Nicollet Ave., Minneapolis 4, Minn.

COLLOIDAL PRODUCTS CORP., 2598 Taylor St., San Francisco, Calif.

COLONIAL ALLOY CO., Ridge & W. Cranford Sts., Philadelphia, Pa.

COLONIAL DAMES CO., LTD., 1060 S. Vail Ave., Montebello, Calif.

COLONIAL DRUG CO., 15th & Race Sts., Philadelphia 2, Pa.

COLONIAL WORKS, Norman & Russell Aves., Brooklyn, N.Y.

COLORADO PAINT CO., 3551 Blake St., Denver, Colo.

COLOTONE CO., 724 W. Park Ave., Waterloo, Iowa.

COLUMBIA CHEM. CO., INC., 154 Erie St., Chicago 11, Ill.

COLUMBIAN HOG & CATTLE POWDER CO., 1457 Genesee St., Kansas City 2, Mo.

COMATE LABS., INC., 20 W. 45th St., New York 36, N.Y.

COMEGYS CHEMICAL CO., Philadelphia, Pa.

COMET MODEL HOBBYCRAFT, INC., 129 W. 29th St., Chicago 16, Ill.

COMFORT MFG. CO., 500 S. Throop St., Chicago 7, Ill.

COMMERCE DRUG CO., INC., 505 Court St., Brooklyn 31, N.Y.

COMMERCIAL CHEMICALS, LTD., Division of Standard Chemical, Ltd., Pier H, Ft. Carrall St., Vancouver 4, B. C.

COMMERCIAL PASTE CO., Columbus, Ohio.

COMMERCIAL SOLVENTS CORP., 17 E. 42nd St., New York 17, N.Y.

COMMON SENSE MFG. CO., 1392 Niagara St., Buffalo 13, N.Y.

COMMONWEALTH RESEARCH LABS., 811 Peoples National Bank Bldg., Grand Rapids 2, Mich.

COMSTOCK CO., LTD., Comstock Bldg., Brockville, Ont., Canada.

CONCIALDI, JOSEPH G., JR., 412 Dover Rd., Rockaway, N.J.

CON-FERRO PAINT & VARNISH CO., 3228 N. Broadway, St. Louis, Mo.

CONGOLEUM-NAIRN, INC., Kearny, N.J.

CONNORS, HARRY J., 233 E. 75th St., Chicago 19, Ill.

CONQUERINE CO., Lynchburg, Va.

CONSOLIDATED CHEM. CO., 835 Cherry St., S.E., Grand Rapids 6, Mich.

CONSOLIDATED COSMETICS, 30 W. Hubbard St., Chicago 10, Ill.

CONSOLIDATED ROYAL CHEMICAL CORP., 657 W. Chicago Ave., Chicago 10, Ill.

CONSUMER'S CHEMICAL PRODUCTS, P.O. Box 411, Summit, N.J.

CONSUMERS GLUE CO., 1515 N. Hadley St., St. Louis 6, Mo.

CONTINENTAL CAR-NA-VAR CORP., 1676 E. National Ave., Brazil, Ind.

CONTINENTAL CHEMICAL CO., 417-1/2 U St., Sacramento, Calif.

CONTINENTAL CHEMIST CORP., 2068 W. Ogden Ave., Chicago 12, Ill.

CONTINENTAL DRUG CO., 1005 Patapsco Ave., Baltimore 25, Md.

CONTINENTAL LABS., INC., 100 Beekman St., New York 38, N.Y.

CONTINENTAL PRODUCTS CO., St. Clair & Bliss Aves., Cleveland, Ohio.

CONTRA CO., Division of Severna Labs., Inc., 13 W. 46th St., New York 36, N.Y.

COOK CHEMICAL CO., P.O. Box 78, Kansas City 41, Mo.

COOK & DUNN PAINT CORP., 109 St. Francis St., Newark, N.J.

COOK PAINT & VARNISH CO., 1412 Knox, N. Kansas City, Mo.

COOK, THOMAS E., CHEMICAL CO., 305 N. Main St., Springfield, Tenn.

COOPERATIVE ASSOCIATION, INC., Columbus, Ohio.

COOPERATIVE SEED & FARM SUPPLY SERVICE, INC., Richmond 13, Va.

COOPER, WM., & NEPHEWS, 1909 Clifton Ave., Chicago 14, Ill.

COPLEY OF BOSTON, INC., Bolton 14, Mass.

COPPCO CO., INC. (see King Chemical Co.), Memphis, Tenn.

COPPER BRITE, INC., 1109 N. Poinsettia Pl., Los Angeles, Calif.

COPPER CLAD PRODUCTS, INC., 276 Passaic St., Newark 4, N.J.

COP-R-NU, INC., 117 W. Grand Ave., Chicago 10, Ill.

CORDO CHEM. CORP., 230 Park Ave., New York 17, N.Y.

CORNELL CHEMICAL & EQUIPMENT CO., 224 N. Franklin Rd., Baltimore 23, Md.

CORNELL MEDICINE CO., Edgewood, Ohio.

CORNER, JAMES, & SONS, 438 N. Front St., Baltimore, Md.

CORN KING CO., INC., Cedar Rapids, Iowa.

CORN OFF CO., 3240 Ellenda Ave., Los Angeles 34, Calif.

CORN PRODUCTS REFINING CO., 17 Battery Pl., New York, N.Y.

CORONA CHEMICAL DIVISION, Pittsburgh Plate Glass Co., Moorestown, N.J.

CORONA FOOTHILL LEMON CO., P.O. Box B, Corona, Calif.

CORONA MFG. CO., 215 S. Detroit St., Kenton, Ohio.

CORONET CHEMICAL CO., Ramshorn Dr., Allenwood, N.J.

COROT, LES PARFUMS, 36 W. 33rd St., New York 1, N.Y.

CORPUS CHRISTI MEDICINE CO., P.O. Box 1712, Corpus Christi, Tex.

CORTISOL CO., 327 Washington St., Buffalo 3, N.Y.

CORT-LIVINGSTON, INC., 68 Joy St., Brooklyn 1, N.Y.

COSMATA CO., 301 Wallabout St., Brooklyn 6, N.Y.

COSMETIC DISTRIBUTORS, INC., 109 Academy St., Jersey City, N.J.

COTTON PRODUCERS' ASSN., P.O. Box 2210, Atlanta 1, Ga.

COTTON STATES CHEMICAL CO., INC., P.O. Box 3186, West Monroe, La.

COTY INC., 730 5th Ave., New York 19, N.Y.

COUGHLAN, G. N., CO., West Orange, N.J.

COUGLELARE, G.N., CO., 29 Spring St., West Orange, N.J.

COULTER, L. B., CO., 201 S. Main St., Salisbury, N.C.

COUNTESS MARITZA COSMETIC CO., INC., 250 W. 55th St., New York 19, N.Y.

COURTLEY, LTD., 113 W. 18th St., New York 11, N.Y.

COVAGRAY LABS., 69 W. 46th St., New York 36, N.Y.

COWEN, R. S., CO., 9 East 38th St., New York 16, N.Y.

COWLES CHEMICAL CO., 7016 Euclid Ave., Cleveland, Ohio.

COWLEY PHARMACEUTICAL, INC., 65 Southbridge St., Auburn, Mass.

COWLEY, S. L., & SONS, P.O. Box 454, Hugo, Okla.

COWMAN-CAMPBELL PAINT CO., 5232 Shilsole Ave., Seattle, Wash.

COYNE CHEMICAL CO., Los Angeles, Calif.

CRAFTINT MANUFACTURING CO., 1615 Collamer Ave., Cleveland 10, Ohio.

CRAIGHILL & JONES, Lynchburg, Va.

CRANE CHEM. CO., 24 8th St., San Francisco 3, Calif.

CRANOLENE CO., Girard, Kans.

CRAYOFF CORP., 34 Roberts St., Pasadena 3, Calif.

CRAZY WATER CO., Mineral Wells, Tex.

CREATIVE CHEMICAL CO., 4618-22 Friendship Ave., Pittsburgh 24, Pa.

CREATIVE COSMETIC CO. OF HOLLYWOOD, 7029 Willoughby, Los Angeles 38, Calif.

CREOMULSION CO., P.O. Box 1214, Atlanta 1, Ga.

CRESCENT BRAND BRONZE POWDER CO., 116-122 W. Illinois St., Chicago, Ill.

CRESCENT CHEMICAL CORP., 450 Market St., Perth Amboy, N.J.

CRESCENT CHEMICAL DIVISION, 233 Oliver Ave., Pittsburgh, Pa.

CRESCENT OIL CO., INC., 514 W. Wyoming St., Indianapolis 2, Ind.

CRESCENT PHARM. CORP., 21-12 Newtown Ave., Long Island City 2, L. I., N.Y.

CRESCENT PRODUCTS CO., 315 N. 14th St., Terre Haute, Ind.

CREST MFG. CO., 4-65 48th Ave., Long Island City, L. I., N.Y.

CRETE-TREAT CO., R.D. 1, Peninsula, Ohio.

CREVISTON & CO., INC., 5161 N. Ashland Ave., Chicago 40, Ill.

CRISP, S. A., CANINE CO., Shelby St., Blacksburg, S.C.

CRISTY CHEMICAL CORP., Worcester, Mass.

CROCKENBERG, F. X., 519 Main St., Honesdale, Pa.

CROOKES LABS., INC., Union & Liberty Sts., Mineola, L. I., N.Y.

CROP KING CO., Yakima, Wash.

CROSBY LABS., 3010 W. Burbank Blvd., Burbank, Calif.

CROWELL DISTRIBUTING CORP., 833 E. 6th St., Los Angeles 21, Calif.

CROWN PRODUCTS CO., P.O. Box 427, Douglas, Ga.

CRUNDEN MARTIN MFG. CO., 2nd & Gratiot, St. Louis, Mo.

CRYSTAL SOAP & CHEMICAL CO., INC., 6300 State Rd., Philadelphia 35, Pa.

CUDAHY PACKING CO., Anchor Glue Division, Dept. 1, 221 LaSalle St., Chicago, Ill.

CULLIGAN, INC., Northbrook, Ill.

CUMMER CO., 22 High St., Brattleboro, Vt.

CUPRINOL DIVISION, Darworth, Inc., Simsbury, Conn.

CURLCARE CO., 303 5th Ave., New York 16, N.Y.

CURLEY CO., INC., 1432 N. Randolph St., Philadelphia 22, Pa.

CURRAN, FRANK J., CO., 8100 S. Main St., Downes Grove, Ill.

CURRIER'S TABLETS, INC., 200 S. Los Angeles St., Los Angeles, Calif.

CURTIS, HELENE, INDUSTRIES, INC., 4401 W. North Ave., Chicago 39, Ill.

CURTIS LABS., INC., 2718 Griffith Park Blvd., Los Angeles 27, Calif.

CURTIS MFG. & ASBESTOS CO., 29-30 Lewis Wharf, Boston, Mass.

CURTIS-PARKER CO., P.O. Box 187, San Jose, Calif.

CURTIS SQUIRE, INC., 415 1st Ave., N., Minneapolis 1, Minn.

CUSHING MFG. CO., 65 W. Main St., Sandy, Utah.

CUSHMAN & DENISON MFG. CO., INC., 153 W. 23rd St., New York 11, N.Y.

CUSTOMS COLORS CORP., 9229 E. Prairie Rd., Evanston, Ill.

CUTISENE CO., 1207 Water St., Santa Cruz, Calif.

CUZILINA DRUG CO., 201 E. Grand Ave., Ponca City, Okla.

CYCLEWELD CEMENT PRODUCTS PLANT, Division of Chrysler Corp., P.O. Box 775, Trenton, Mich.

C-Z CHEMICAL CO., see Allied Home Products

D

DACAR CHEMICAL PRODUCTS CO., McCartney & Datesh Sts., Pittsburgh, Pa.

DACUS DRUG CO., INC., 108 Le Sieur Ave., Portageville, Mo.

DAGGETT & RAMSDELL, INC., 420 Frelinghuysen Ave., Newark 5, N.J.

DAINTY-MAID, INC., Powder Hill, Middlefield, Conn.

DAIRY ASSOCIATION CO., INC., Depot St., Lyndonville, Vt.

DAIRY REMEDIES, 120 High St., Montclair, N.J.

DALY-HERRING CO., Adkin & University Sts., Kinston, N.C.

DAME NATURE CO., INC., 420 Madison Ave., New York 17, N.Y.

DAMPNEY CO., Hyde Park, Boston 36, Mass.

DAMSCHINSKY, CARL, INC., 253-22 85th Rd., Bellrose 26, N.Y.

DANA, C. H., CO., INC., Hyde Park, Vt.

DANDOK PRODUCTS CO., 746 Exchange St., Vermillion, Ohio.

DANDRICIDE GO., Division of King Research, Inc., 114 12th St., Brooklyn 15, N.Y.

DAND-RID'R CO., 261 5th Ave., New York 16, N.Y.

DANIEL, JNO. B., INC., 76 Central Ave., S.W., Atlanta 1, Ga.

DANIELS, DR. A. C., INC., 172 Milk St., Boston 9, Mass.

DANIELS, ROBERT & CO., INC., 1205 Harrod Ave., New York 72, N.Y.

DANIELS, ROSS, INC., 713-15 Mulberry St., Des Moines 9, Iowa.

DANMAR, INC., 4438 N. 20th St., St. Louis 7, Mo.

DANTOL CO., 286 S. 2nd St., Memphis, Tenn.

DAO CORP., Terre Haute, Ind.

DARA PRODUCTS, 1005 Plum St., Cincinnati 2, Ohio.

D'ARCY OILS, 446 W. 125th St., New York, N.Y.

DARK-EYES CO., 3319 W. Carrol Ave., Chicago 24, Ill.

DARLING, RUTH, INC., 11 E. 44th St., New York 17, N.Y.

DARWORTH, INC., (see Cuprinol Division), Simsbury, Conn.

DATTILO COSMETICS, INC., 82-96 61st Rd., Elmhurst, L. I., N.Y.

DAUGHTER, DR. J. W., CO., 6 Morley Rd., Wollaston 70, Mass.

DAVART PRODUCTS, Ashland, Ky.

DAVEY TREE EXPERT CO., Kent, Ohio.

DAVI, H. R., CO., 1111 W. Grand Ave., Oakland, Calif.

DAVIDS, C. I., & SONS, INC., 325 W. 66th St., New York, N.Y.

DAVIDS, THADDEUS, INKS CO., 325 W. 66th St., New York, N.Y.

DAVIES-YOUNG SOAP CO., 705 Albany St., Dayton, Ohio.

DAVIN LABS., P.O. Box 513, New Milford, N.J.

DAVIS, C. H., CO., Rome, N.Y.

DAVIS, C. T., 1530 E. Blount St., Pensacola, Fla.

DAVIS, H. B., CO., Bayard & Severn Sts., Baltimore 30, Md.

DAVIS LABS., P.O. Box 1919, Oakland 4, Calif.

DAVIS & LAWRENCE CO., 75 Main St., Dobbs Ferry, N.Y.

DAVIS-LLOYD DRUG CO., 191 Main St., Ridgefield Park, N.J.

DAVIS, O. D., CHEM. CO., Kuntz Rd., Erie, Pa.

DAVISON CHEMICAL CO., Division of W. R. Grace & Co., Baltimore 3, Md.

DAVIS PAINT CO., S.E. 14th & Iron Sts., Kansas City, Mo.

DAVIS PHARMACAL CO., 105 Market St., Marianna, Fla.

DAVIS WHOLESALE DRUG CO., 206 S. 14th St., Baton Rouge 1, La.

DAY, JAMES B., & CO., 1872 Clybourn Ave., Chicago 14, Ill.

DAY-KINGSLEY DRYER CO., Cleveland, Ohio.

DAYTON LABS. CORP., 684 Broadway, New York 12, N.Y.

DAYTON PHARMACAL CO., Chicago, Ill.

D. C. LABS., INC., P.O. Box 836, Newark, N.J.

d-CON CO., INC., 112 E. Walton St., Chicago 11, Ill.

DEAM CORP., 41 Beale Ave., Memphis 3, Tenn.

DEAN'S KING CACTUS OIL CO., 723 Randolph St., Waterloo, Iowa.

DEARBORN CHEMICAL CO., Chicago, Ill.

DEARBORN SUPPLY CO., 2350 Clybourn Ave., Chicago 14, Ill.

DEB CO., 110 Gillett St., Hartford, Conn. (No longer in existence.)

DEBEVOISE CO., Department S, 74-84 20th St., Brooklyn, N.Y.

DECO DEVELOPMENT ENGINEERING CO., 724 S. Wise St., Decatur, Ill.

DEE, GEORGE H., & CO., Omaha, Neb.

DEER-O PAINTS & CHEMICALS, LTD., 2431 E. Van Buren, Phoenix, Ariz.

DE GRASSE GRANDEE CORP., 39 W. 60th St., New York 23, N.Y.

DEKEN'S PRODUCTS, P.O. Box 666, Newark 1, N.J.

DELAGAR PRODUCTS, INC., 270 Park Ave., New York 17, N.Y.

DELANCEY CHEMICAL CO., 359 Bedford Ave., Brooklyn 11, N.Y.

DELCO PAINT & VARNISH WORKS, 2469 Enterprise, Los Angeles, Calif.

DELEX PRODUCTS, 30 W. 15th St., New York 11, N.Y.

DELK PEST CONTROL, P.O. Box 1093, Fresno 14, Calif.

DE LOSTE, JOS. S., CO., Madison, Ind.

DELTEX INDUSTRIES, New York, N.Y.

DENNIS CHEMICAL CO., 2701 Papin St., St. Louis 3, Mo.

DENNY, HILBORN & ROSENBACH, INC., 12th & Vine Sts., Philadelphia, Pa.

DENT & CO., C. S., Division of Grandpa Soap Co., 912 Sycamore St., Cincinnati 2, Ohio.

DENTA-FLUR CO., Bellflower, Calif.

DENTAL PRODUCTS CORP., Penn & Stiegel Sts., Manheim, Pa.

DENTA PRODUCTS, Division of Vick Chem. Co., 122 E. 42nd St., New York 17, N.Y.

DENTON MEDICINE CO., 1523 McGavock St., Nashville 3, Tenn.

DENVER CHEM. MFG. CO., 163 Varick St., New York 13, N.Y.

DENVER RADIUM SERVICE, 1671 Logan St., Denver 5, Colo.

DE-PASS CHEMICAL CO., 412 E. 47th St., Chicago 15, Ill.

DE PREE CO., Holland, Mich.

DERMAL PRODUCTS CO., 523 Mills Bldg., Topeka, Kans.

DERMATEEN CO., 104 Carbonton Rd., Sanford, N.C.

DERMA VIVA CO., 1873 Burton Lane, Park Ridge, Ill.

DERMEX LABS., 1619 Euclid Ave., Cleveland, Ohio.

DESITIN CHEM. CO., 70 Ship St., Providence 2, R. I.

DE SOTO CHEMICAL CO., Arcadia, Fla.

DE SOTO DRUG & CHEMICAL CO., 172 Vance Ave., Memphis 3, Tenn.

DE SOTO PAINT & VARNISH CO., Southern R.R. & Somerville, Memphis, Tenn.

DESTRUXOL CORP., LTD., 497 S. Arroyo Pkwy., Pasadena 1, Calif.

DETHOL MFG., CO., 3800 37th Pl., Brentwood, Md.

DETREX CORP., P.O. Box 501, Detroit 32, Mich.

DETROIT GRAPHITE CO., 550 12th St., Detroit, Mich.

DEVIL LABS CO., 557 E. 8th St., Cincinnati 2, Ohio.

DEVOE & RAYNOLDS CO., INC., P.O. Box 328, Louisville 1, Ky.

DE WANS, INC., P.O. Box 506, Minneapolis 1, Minn.

DE WEESE CHEMICAL CO., 513 Liberty St., Findlay, Ohio.

DEWEY PRODUCTS CO., 532-558 Cottage Grove, S.E., Grand Rapids 2, Mich.

DE WITT, E. C., & CO., INC., 2835 Sheffield Ave., Chicago 14, Ill.

DEWITT PRODUCTS CORP., 5860 Plummer Ave., Detroit 9, Mich.

DE WOLF, C. H., CO., 35 Dodge Ave., East Haven 12, Conn.

DEXTER BROS. CO., 86 Broad St., Boston, Mass.

DIAMOND ALKALI CO., Union Commerce Bldg., Cleveland 14, Ohio.

DIAMOND BLACK LEAF CO., Union Commerce Bldg., Cleveland 14, Ohio.

DIAMOND CHEMICAL PRODUCTS, 17 E. 48th St., New York 17, N.Y.

DIANOL, INC., 4760 Freemont Terr., S., St. Petersburg, Fla.

DIAPERWITE, INC., 99 Hudson St., New York 13, N.Y.

DIAPHRAGM & CHEMICAL CO., 235 E. Ontario St., Chicago, Ill.

DICKEY DRUG CO., 8-1/2 Front St., Bristol, Va.

DICKEY EYE WATER CO., P.O. Box 771, Montgomery 2, Ala.

DICKINSON, E. E., CO., Essex, Conn.

DICKS-PONTIUS CO., 5300 Old Springfield Pike, Dayton, Ohio.

DIE-DEAD PRODUCTS CO., P.O. Box 164, Winter Haven, Fla.

DIEFENBACH LABS., INC., 80 Hamilton St., Rochester 7, N.Y.

DIENER, GEO. W., MFG. CO., 427 N. Monticello Ave., Chicago, Ill.

DIEZ, H., CO., 5006 Pitt St., New Orleans 15, La.

DIF CORP., Garwood, N.J.

DILL CO., Norristown, Pa.

DILLARD, R. YATES, & CO., Memphis 3, Tenn.

DINET & DELFOSS, INC., 30 N. Michigan Blvd., Chicago, Ill.

DINGS & SCHUSTER, 17 John St., New York, N.Y.

DIOPTRON CO., P.O. Box 1313, Milwaukee 1, Wis.

DITZLER COLOR DIVISION, Pittsburgh Plate Glass Co., 8000 W. Chicago Ave., Detroit 4, Mich.

DIVERSEY CORP., 1820 Roscoe St., Chicago 13, Ill.

DIXIE LABS., INC., P.O. Box 129, Martinsville, Va.

DIXIE-RUB CO., INC., 8 S. Union, Concord, N.C.

DIXON-DAVIS CO., 2702 Monroe St., Madison 5, Wis.

D-K SALES CO., 113 S. Baker St., Granbury, Tex.

D-MOTH CO., 2214 Summer St., Dallas 2, Tex.

DOAK PHARMACAL CO., INC., 295 Madison Ave., New York 17, N.Y.

DOBBS CO., Legonier, Pa.

DODDS MED. CO., INC., OF U. S., 52 Highland Ave., Hamburg, N.Y.

DODGE CHEMICAL CO., 656 Beacon St., Boston, Mass.

DOGGETT-PFEIL CO., 642 Morris Turnpike, Springfield, N.J.

DOGTOWN PRODUCTS CO., 3711 Bienville Ave., New Orleans 19, La.

DOHO CHEMICAL CO., 100 Varick St., New York 13, N.Y.

DOLAN LABS., 7370 Dale Ave., St. Louis 17, Mo.

DOLAN, V. J., & CO., 1828 N. Laramie Ave., Chicago, Ill.

DOLCIN CORP., New York, N.Y.

DOLGE, C. B., CO., Ferry Lane, Westport, Conn.

DOLLE, FRED, INC., 2712 S. Kedzie Ave., Chicago 23, Ill.

DOME CHEMICALS, INC., 109 W. 64th St., New York 23, N.Y.

DOMESTIC CHEMICAL CO., 3350 San Fernando Rd., Los Angeles 41, Calif.

DOMINANT PRODUCTS CO., INC., 359 Pearl St., New York 7, N.Y.

DONAHUE, F. J., VARNISH CO., Knodell Ave. & G.T. R.R., Detroit, Mich.

DONFIELD CO., 1154 N. Glencove Rd., Syracuse 6, N.Y.

DON JUAN CO., INC., 67 Vestry St., New York 13, N.Y.

DONTÉ CHEM. CO., 80 Allenwood Rd., Great Neck, L. I., N.Y.

DOOR-O-WESTERN PAINTS, INC., Amarillo, Tex.

DO-RA MFG. CO., INC., Minneapolis, Minn.

DORITE MFG. CO., Charleston, Ill.

DORMIN, INC., New York, N.Y.

DORVAL CHEMICAL CO., 429 Hicks St., Brooklyn 2, N.Y.

DOSALAC CHEMICAL CO., 830 Magnolia Ave., Elizabeth, N.J.

DOUBLE B. PRODUCTS CO., INC., 29 Bartholomew Ave., Hartford 6, Conn.

DOUGLAS CHEM. CO., 620 E. 16th Ave., North Kansas City, Mo.

DOUGLAS LABS., CORP., 2360 N.W. 23rd St., Miami 42, Fla.

DOUGLAS MILLER CO., Philadelphia, Pa.

DOUGLAS PHARM. CO., 40 S. Las Robles Ave., Pasadena 1, Calif.

DOUGLAS PHARMACAL CO., 5 Douglas St., Hartford, Conn.

DOUGLAS PRODUCTS CO., 7208 Sepulveda Blvd., Van Nuys, Calif.

DOVER PRODUCTS CO., 815 Warthington, Chicago, Ill.

DOW CHEMICAL CO., Midland, Mich.

DOX CO., 1953 University Ave., St. Paul, Minn.

DRACKETT PRODS. CO., 5020 Spring Grove Ave., Cincinnati 32, Ohio.

DRAKE, J. K., EST. OF, Troy, N.Y.

DRAKE LABS., 1377 Broadway, Detroit 26, Mich.

DREW, E. F., & CO., INC., 15 E. 26th St., New York 10, N.Y.

DREW PHARM. CO., 1450 Broadway, New York 18, N.Y.

DREXEL LABS., 4007 Garrett Rd., Drexel Hill, Pa.

DREYFUSS CO., 307 Delaware Ave., Buffalo 2, N.Y.

DRI-FOOT LABS., 209 N. Main St., West Bend, Wis.

DRIGARD PRODUCTS CORP., 112 E. 19th St., New York 3, N.Y.

DRISCOLL, A. D., Park St., Whitney Point, N.Y.

DRI-SEAL PRODUCTS, INC., 2326 N. 3rd St., Milwaukee, Wis.

DRISKELL DRUG CO., 416 Main St., Carrollton, Ky.

DRITZ, JOHN, & SONS, 1115 Broadway, New York 10, N.Y.

D & R LABS., INC., 39 W. Adams St., Chicago 3, Ill.

DROBINSKI, F., PHARMACIST, 700 5th Ave., Brooklyn 15, N.Y.

DRUGMASTER, INC., St. Louis, Mo.

DRUG PRODUCTS CO., 1419 Talbotton Rd., Columbus, Ga.

DRUG PRODUCTS CO., INC., 1663 Weirfield St., Brooklyn 27, N.Y.

DRUG RESEARCH CORP., 369 Lexington Ave., New York, N.Y.

DRYBURGH & SONS, INC., 106 E. Mason St., Milwaukee 2, Wis.

DRYCO CO., P.O. Box 7092, Dallas, Tex.

DRY-PITS LOTION CO., 3522 Hawthorne Blvd., St. Louis 4, Mo.

DUFFY MEDICINE CO., 423-1/2 Wood St., New Bern, N.C.

DUKE PRODUCTS CO., 1628 W. Venice Blvd., Los Angeles 6, Calif.

DUMAS-WILSON & CO., 4821 Fairview Ave., St. Louis 16, Mo.

DUNAWAY, JUDSON, CO., Dover, N.H.

DUNCAN CO., 2328 N.W. 21st St., Oklahoma City 7, Okla.

DUNMIRE, J. H., CO., 304 Maple St., Kennett, Mo.

DUNN EDWARDS CORP., 1838 S. Flower St., Los Angeles, Calif.

DUNNE, FRANK W., CO., 41st & Linden, Oakland, Calif.

DUNTON, M. W., CO., Eddy & Halligan Sts., Providence 3, R.I.

DUNWODY, R. G., & Sons, 235 Forsyth St., S.W., Atlanta 3, Ga.

du PONT, E. I., de NEMOURS & CO., INC., 1007 Market St., Wilmington 98, Del.

DUPREE MEDICINE CO., 20 E. 17th St., New York 3, N.Y.

DURA TRED CO., 359 No. Central Park Blvd., Chicago, Ill.

DURAKO PAINT & COLOR CORP.,
6315 E. 7 Mile at Nedding, Detroit,
Mich.

DURAL COMPANY, INC., 115 E.
Seeboth, Milwaukee 4, Wis.

DURALAC CHEMICAL CORP., 86
Lister St., Newark 5, N.J.

DUREX PRODUCTS, INC., 684
Broadway, New York, N.Y.

DURFEE CO., 43 National Dr., N.W.,
Grand Rapids, Mich.

DURHAM CHEMICAL CO., 4124 E.
Pacific Way, Los Angeles 23, Calif.

DURHAM'S DRUG PRODS., CO.,
Comanche, Tex.

DU-RITE CHEMICAL CO., Brentwood,
Md.

DURKEE-ATWOOD CO., 217 N.E. 7th
St., Minneapolis, Minn.

DURLIN CO., 744 Broad St., Newark
2, N.J.

DURMA PRODS. CO., INC., 267
Irving Ave., N. Minneapolis 8, Minn.

DURST MANUFACTURING CO., INC.,
409 Lafayette St., New York, N.Y.

DURST, S. F. & CO., 5317 N. 3rd St.,
Philadelphia 20, Pa.

DUSHARME PRODUCTS, INC., Sexton
Bldg., Minneapolis 15, Minn.

DUVEEN SOAP CORP., Long Island
City 6, L. I., N.Y.

DUVELLE, Box 7525, Portland 20,
Oreg.

DYRUD LABORATORIES, Prairie Du
Chien, Wis.

DYSPEPTOL CO., 44 Main St., Hunter,
N.Y.

E

EAGLE CHEMICAL CO., Cameron,
Tex.

EAGLE OIL AND SUPPLY CO., 77 W.
2nd, Boston, Mass.

EAGLE PAINT & VARNISH WORKS OF
PITTSBURGH, 225 Galveston Ave.,
Pittsburgh, Pa.

EAGLE PHARMACAL CO., Mayville,
Mich.

EAGLE PHOTO SUPPLY CO., 57 E.
9th St., New York 3, N.Y.

EAGLO PAINT & VARNISH CORP.,
49-20 5th St., Long Island City, L. I.,
N.Y.

EARLE CHEMICAL CO., 1125 Market
St., Wheeling, W. Va.

EARL PRODUCTS CO., Chappaqua,
N.Y.

EASE, INC., Burbank, Calif.

EASTCO, INC., 110 Mamaroneck Ave.,
White Plains, N.Y.

EASTERDAY SUPPLY CO., 1150 W.
4th St., Los Angeles, Calif.

EASTER MORN COSMETICS, 9145 S.
Leavitt St., Chicago 20, Ill.

EASTERN PHARMACAL CO., INC.,
P.O. Box 104, Mt. Vernon, N.Y.

EASTERN SANITARY PRODUCTS &
PAPER CORP., 68 33rd St., Brooklyn,
N.Y.

EASTERN STATES FARMERS'
EXCHANGE INC., West Springfield,
Mass.

EASTERN STATES PAINT & VARNISH
CO., Swanson & Mefflin Sts.,
Philadelphia, Pa.

EASTMAN KODAK CO., 343 State
St., Rochester 4, N.Y.

EASYDO, INC., 30 W. Washington
Ave., Chicago 2, Ill.

EATON CHEMICAL & DYESTUFF
CO., 1490 Franklin St., Detroit 7,
Mich.

EATON, J. T., & CO., INC., 1106
Lakeview Rd., Cleveland 8, Ohio.

EATON LABORATORIES, Norwich,
N.Y.

EBREY CHEM. WORKS, P.O. Box
6, Miami 1, Fla.

EBY REMEDY CO., Marengo, Iowa.

E-C CO., 2475 Broadway, San Diego
2, Calif.

ECKELS, H. S., & CO., 231 N. 16th
St., Philadelphia 2, Pa.

ECKMAN LAB., INC., Wyndmoor,
Pa.

ECONOMICS LABORATORY, INC.,
Guardian Bldg., St. Paul 1, Minn.

ECONOMY PLUMBER CO., 39
Lispenary, New York, N.Y.

EDCO CORPORATION, Childs Rd.,
Elkton, Md.

EDCO INTERNATIONAL CORP.,
9993 Broadstreet Ave., Detroit 4,
Mich.

EDELMAN, S. CO., P.O. Box 68,
Mt. Vernon, N.Y.

EDGERLY, J. W., & CO., Ottumwa,
Iowa.

EDISON CHEMICAL CO., 2710 S.
Parkway, Chicago 16, Ill.

EDKINS LABS., 708 S. Manhattan
Pl., Los Angeles 5, Calif.

EDLICH LABS, 896 1st Ave., New
York 22, N.Y.

EDROLAX, INC., New York, N.Y.

EDRU PRODUCTS CO., 219 W.
Broad St., Quakertown, Pa.

EDWAL SCIENTIFIC PRODUCTS
CORP., 420 W. 111th St., Chicago
28, Ill.

EDWARDS, GEORGE, Livingston,
Mont.

EDWARDS-COUNCILOR CO.,
Norfolk, Va.

EGAN & HAUSMAN CO., INC., 9-02
43rd Rd., Long Island City, L. I.,
N.Y.

EGYPTIAN LACQUER MFG. CO.,
P.O. Box 444, Newark 1, N.J.

8 IN 1 PET PRODUCTS, INC., 107
Bleecker St., New York 12, N.Y.

ELAINE LABS., 1629 E. 12th St.,
Brooklyn 29, N.Y.

ELARS PRODUCTS, INC., 1601 E.
Grace St., Richmond 19, Va.

ELECTRIC REDUCTION COMPANY
OF CANADA, LTD., 137 Wellington
St., W., Toronto 1, Ontario, Canada.

ELECTRONS, INC., Platteville, Wis.

ELENE OF VIENNA, INC., 110 E.
42nd St., New York 17, N.Y.

ELGIN SOFTENER CORP., 142 N.
Grove Ave., Elgin, Ill.

ELK, B. R., & CO., INC., 179
Palisade Ave., Garfield, N.J.

ELLENI COSMETIC LABS., 133 E.
Carrillo St., Santa Barbara, Calif.

ELLIOTT PAINT & VARNISH CO.,
4525 W. 5th Ave., Chicago, Ill.

ELLIS CHEMICAL CO., W. Concord,
Mass.

ELLIS, H. G., CO., 58 Main St.,
Camden, N.Y.

ELLIS PAINT CO., 718 W. Anaheim,
Long Beach, Calif.

ELL-VEE PRODUCTS, Bethel, Tenn.

ELM, J. GEO., 132 Ohio River Blvd.,
Pittsburgh 2, Pa.

ELMO, INC., Tulip & Rhaun Sts.,
Philadelphia, Pa.

EL-MONTE MANUFACTURING CO.,
322 N. Foothill Blvd., Pasadena 8,
Calif.

ELMS, J. C., EUROPEAN HAIR CO.,
INC., 5612 S. Kingshighway, St.
Louis 9, Mo.

ELROY NAVAL STORE CO., INC.,
Vidalia, Ga.

ELY, CHAS. S., Millville, Pa.

EMBALMERS' SUPPLY CO., Westport,
Conn.

EMBREE MFG. CO., 10 W. Mravlag
Pl., Elizabeth 4, N.J.

EMERGENCY LABS., Jersey City, N.J.

EMEROL MFG. CO., INC., 242 W.
69th St., New York, N.Y.

EMERSON DRUG CO., Bromo-Seltzer
Tower Bldg., Baltimore 1, Md.

EMPIRE CHEMICAL PRODUCTS CO.,
8 Longworth, Newark, N.J.

EMPIRE STATE VARNISH CO., 40
Varick St., Brooklyn, N.Y.

EMPIRE VARNISH CO., 2640 E. 76th
St., Cleveland, Ohio.

EMULSO CORP., Ellicott & Mohawk
Sts., Buffalo, N.Y.

EMULSOL CHEMICAL CORP., 59 E.
Madison St., Chicago 3, Ill.

END-O-CORN, End-O-Corn Bldg.,
Rutland, Vt.

ENERGY DRUG CO., 1762 E. 12th St.,
Cleveland 14, Ohio.

ENGEN. ALF., 309 E. 2nd South St.,
Salt Lake City 2, Utah.

ENGINE LIFE PRODUCTS CORP., S.
Granada & W. Valley, El Morete,
Calif.

ENJAY CO., INC., 15 W. 51st St., New
York 19, N.Y.

ENO-SCOTT & BOWNE, Bloomfield,
N.J.

ENTERPRISE CHEMICAL CO., P.O.
Box 147, Troy, Mo.

ENTERPRISE PAINT MFG. CO., 2841
S. Ashland Ave., Chicago, Ill.

EPIDERMICIDE CO., P.O. Box 432,
Minot, N. Dak.

EPTOL CO., 650 N. Rush St., Chicago
11, Ill.

ERADICO CO., 690 E. Congress St.,
Detroit 26, Mich.

ERIE DRUG CO., 417 State St., Erie,
Pa.

ERNECKE & SALMSTEIN CO., 1611 N.
Sheffield Ave., Chicago, Ill.

ERWIN VETERINARY PRODS., 803
Deerfield Rd., P.O. Box No. 1,
Deerfield, Ill.

ESAMAR PRODS. CO., 6118 Gambleton
Place, St. Louis 14, Mo.

ESSENIC MFG. CO., 902 North Ave.,
Plainfield, N.J.

ESSEX CHEMICAL CO., McCarter
Hgwy., Newark, N.J.

ESSO STANDARD OIL CO., 15 W. 51st
St., New York 19, N.Y.

ESS-TEE-DEE HAIR DRESSING CO., 2120 W. Van Buren St., Chicago 12, Ill.

ESTES CO., L. W. 3713 New Hampshire Ave., N.W., Washington 10, D.C.

ESTON CHEMICALS DIVISION, American Potash & Chemical Corp., 3030 W. 6th St., Los Angeles 54, Calif.

ETHERIDGE, S. B., DRUG STORE, 169 W. Main St., Washington, N.C.

ETHICAL SPECIALTIES, INC., 2603-A Midlothian Pike, Richmond, Va.

ETHIX CORP., P.O. Box 115, Inwood 96, L. I., N.Y.

ETIWAN FERTILIZER CO., Charleston, S.C.

EUCLID MEDICINE CO., 408 W. St. Clair Ave., Cleveland, Ohio.

EUPRAXINE CO., 5877 Janet St., W. Dearborr, Mich.

EVANS DEPILATORY CO., Mitten Bldg., Philadelphia 2, Pa.

EVANS, GEORGE B. LABS., Philadelphia, Pa.

EVERCRETE, INC., 424 W. 42nd St., New York, N.Y.

EVER-DRY CORP., 2568 San Fernando Rd., Los Angeles 65, Calif.

EVERETT & BARRON CO., 359 Eddy St., Providence 3, R.I.

EVER-PLASTICS CORP., 420 Lexington Ave., New York, N.Y.

EVERSEAL MFG. CO., INC., 258 W. 57th St., New York, N.Y.

EVERT'S DRUG STORE, 2 N. Main St., Knox, Ind.

EVER YOUTH, INC., 1737 E. 172nd St., New York 72, N.Y.

EVONS, LOUIS E. CO., 4007 Garrett Rd., Drexel Hill, Pa.

EWING, FOX M., CO., 240 E. 136th St., New York, N.Y.

EXCELLO DRUG PRODUCTS, 2002 Morris Ave., Union, N.J.

EXCELSIOR LABORATORY, Atlantic City, N.J.

EXELENTO MEDICINE CO., 391 Pryor St., S.W., Atlanta 1, Ga.

EX-LAX, INC., 423 Atlantic Ave., Brooklyn 17, N.Y.

EXOLON CO., 950 E. Niagara St., Tonawanda, N.Y.

EXPORT CHEM. CORP. OF COLORADO, W. 12th Ave. at Quivas, Denver 4, Colo.

EXSORA CO., 117 Five Oaks Ave., Dayton 5, Ohio.

EYLAX LABS., 1003 E. Arcadia Ave., Peoria 4, Ill.

E. Z. CHEMICAL CO., Rm. 505, American Security and Trust Bldg., 730 15th St., N.W., Washington, D.C.

EZALL PRODUCTS CO., 1447 Boston Rd., New York 60, N.Y.

F

FABERGÉ, INC., 395 S. Broad Ave., Ridgefield, N.J.

FABTECO PRODUCTS, Div. of Bartlett Tree Research Labs., Stamford, Conn.

FACIALS' LIMITED, 1680 N. Vine St., Los Angeles 28, Calif.

FACTOR, MAX, & CO., 1666 N. Highland Ave., Los Angeles 28, Calif.

FAESY & BESTHOFF, INC., 325 Spring St., New York 13, N.Y.

FAHRNEY, DR. PETER & SONS CO., Chicago, Ill.

FAIRFIELD LABS., INC., 417 Cleveland Ave., Plainfield, N.J.

FALCON CHEM. CO., 1312 Benton Ave., Pittsburgh 12, Pa.

FALK CO., Wayzata, Minn.

FALLS CHEM CO., P.O. Box 962, Memphis 12, Tenn.

FAN TAN CO., INC., 118 S. Clinton St., Chicago 7, Ill.

FANT, INC., 2259 N. Foster Ave., Chicago, Ill.

FARBOIL CO., Key Hgwy. & Montgomery Sts., Baltimore 30, Md.

FARENGA CO., INC., 105-04 Jamaica Ave., Richmond Hill 18, L. I., N.Y.

FARM BUREAU COOP. ASSOC., INC., Columbus 16, Ohio.

FARMCRAFT, INC., P.O. Box 309, Portland 7, Oreg.

FARMERS COOPERATIVE EXCHANGE, INC., Statesville, N.C.

FARNAM CO., P.O. Box 2151, Phoenix, Ariz.

FATHER JOHN'S MED. CO., INC., 73 Market St., Lowell, Mass.

FATSCO, 251 N. Fair Ave., Benton Harbor, Mich.

FAULTLESS STARCH CO., 1025 W. 8th St., Kansas City 7, Mo.

FEARONCE BEAUTY PRODUCTS, 1835 W. Colombia Ave., Philadelphia 21, Pa.

FEDERAL CHEMICAL CO., 2701-5 Winthrop Ave., Indianapolis 5, Ind.

FEDERAL PAINT CO., INC., 263 42nd St., Brooklyn 32, N.Y.

FEDERAL VARNISH CO., 2841 S. Ashland Ave., Chicago, Ill.

FEEMSTER, W. R., CO., Brooklyn, Mich.

FEINER CHEMICAL MFG. CO., 239 Mill St., Springfield, Mass.

FELLER-JONES CORP., 270 Park Ave., New York 17, N.Y.

FELLOWS MED. MFG. CO., INC., 26 Christopher St., New York 14, N.Y.

FELS & CO., 73rd St., & Woodland Ave., Philadelphia 42, Pa.

FELTON SIBLEY CO., INC., 136 N. 4th St., Philadelphia 6, Pa.

FERDINAND, L. W., & CO. (FERDICO) Mica Lane, Newton Lower Falls 62, Mass.

FERGUSON FUMIGANTS, INC., 810 S. Florissant Rd., Ferguson 21, Mo.

FERRUBRON PAINT CO., 548 W. Highland Ave., Milwaukee, Wis.

F. & F. LABS., INC., 3501 W. 48th Pl., Chicago 32, Ill.

FIDELITY CHEMICAL PRODUCTS CORP., 473 Frelinghuysen Ave., Newark, N.J.

FIDELITY LABS., INC., 4303 S. Halsted St., Chicago 9, Ill.

FIEBING CHEM. CO., 516 S. 2nd St., Milwaukee 4, Wis.

FINNELL SYSTEM, INC., 515 East St., Elkhart, Ind.

FIRESTONE TIRE & RUBBER CO., 1200 Firestone Pkwy., Akron 17, Ohio.

FIRST NATIONAL LABS., INC., 123 Iron St., Lehighton, Pa.

FIRST NATIONAL STORES, 5 Middlesex Ave., Somerville 45, Mass.

FISHER, E. H., INC., 826 S. 18th St., St. Louis, Mo.

FISHER EQUIPMENT CO., 2014 Livernois Ave., Detroit, Mich.

FISHER SCIENTIFIC CO., Eimer & Amend Div., Greenwich & Morton Sts., New York 14, N.Y.

FISHER-THORSEN CO., 2100 N.W. 22nd Ave., Portland, Oreg.

FISKE BROS. REFINING CO., 129 Dockwood, Newark 5, N.J.

FITCH, A. PERLEY, CO., 24 Depot St., Manchester, N.H.

FITCH, F. W., DIV. GROVE LABORATORIES, 2650 Pine St., St Louis 3, Mo.

FITZPATRICK BROS., INC., 1300 W. 32nd Pl., Chicago 8, Ill.

FIX-ALL PRODUCTS, INC., 325 W. 16th St., New York, N.Y.

FLACH LAB., 1800 Washington Ave., New Orleans 13, La.

FLAG-SULPHUR & CHEMICAL CO., 1007 Wallace S. Bldg., Tampa 2, Fla.

FLANAGAN'S, 57 S. Washington St., Wilkes-Barre, Pa.

FLASH CHEMICAL CO., 160 2nd St., Cambridge 42, Mass.

FLEAFOAM CO., 215 Harding St., Syracuse 8, N.Y.

FLEET, C.B., CO., INC., Lynchburg, Va.

FLEMMINGS, A. C., MFG. CO., 503 25th Ave., Meridan, Miss.

FLETCHER, LYLE M., CO., Rt. 1, P.O. Box 1121, Elk Grove, Calif.

FLEXOID PRODUCTS, INC., 170 Summer St., Boston, Mass.

FLOMAR PRODUCTS CO., 259 E. Erie St., Milwaukee 2, Wis.

FLOQUIL PRODUCTS, INC., 1993 Broadway, New York 23, N.Y.

FLORA DELL LABS., 392 Tarrytown Rd., White Plains, N.Y.

FLORATOSE LABORATORIES, Salisbury, Conn.

FLORES, I. D., DRUG CO., Floresville, Tex.

FLORET PRODS. CO., INC., 45 Lispenard St., New York 13, N.Y.

FLORIDA AGRICULTURE SUPPLY CO. (FASCO), 1611 Talleyrand, Jacksonville, Fla.

FLORIDA CHEM. INDUSTRIES, INC., P.O. Box 1630, W. Palm Beach, Fla.

FLOROZONE CO., 62-28 Forest Ave., Brooklyn 27, N.Y.

FLOWER CITY LABORATORIES, 511 Dewey Ave., Rochester, N.Y.

FLOWER CITY PLANT FOOD CO., INC., Pittsford, N.Y.

FLURENE CHEM. LTD., 100 W. Main St., Washington, N.C.

FOARD, F. C., & CO., INC., 26 Wells St., Bridgeport, Conn.

F. O. B. INC., 1010 George St., Chicago 13, Ill.

FOLEY & CO., Chicago, Ill.

FOMOS LABS., INC., 100 Beekman St., New York 38, N.Y.

FOOT-RITE PRODS. CORP., 3560 Broadway, New York 31, N.Y.

FORMAN, FORD & CO., 111 S. 2nd St., Minneapolis, Minn.

FORT DODGE CHEMICAL CO., 111 S. 14th St., Fort Dodge, Iowa.

FORT DODGE LABS., INC., Fort Dodge, Iowa.

FORT ORANGE CHEMICAL CO., 264 Bradford St., Albany, N.Y.

"42" PRODUCTS, LTD., 11500 Tennessee Ave., Los Angeles 25, Calif.

FOSTER, BENJAMIN CO., 4635 W. Girard Ave., Philadelphia 31, Pa.

FOSTER-DACK CO., 8704 S. Winchester Ave., Chicago 20, Ill.

FOSTER-MILBURN CO., Buffalo, N.Y.

FOSTER'S, W. C., LINIMENT CO., 1034 Green St. Circle, Gainesville, Ga.

FOUGERA, E., & CO., INC., 75 Varick St., New York 13, N.Y.

FOUNDRY RUBBER, INC., Bethesda, Md.

FOUNTAIN SQUARE PHARMACY, INC., 610 Georgia Ave., Chattanooga, Tenn.

FOUR PENNY PRODUCTS CO., INC., 1218-20 N. Bosworth Ave., Chicago 22, Ill.

FOX MFG. CO., Fort Smith, Ark.

FOY PAINT CO., INC., 1775 Mentor Ave., Cincinnati, Ohio.

FR CORP., 951 Brook Ave., New York 56, N.Y.

FRAGRANTAIRE CO., 118 E. 28th St., New York 17, N.Y.

FRANCO AMERICAN HYGIENIC CO., 1576 Maple Ave., Evanston, Ill.

FRANKAY LABORATORIES, INC., Nutley 10, N.J.

FRANKLIN, BENJAMIN, PAINT & VARNISH CO., 4820 Langdon, Philadelphia, Pa.

FRANKLIN GLUE CO., Chestnut & Water Sts., Columbus, Ohio.

FRANKLIN LABORATORIES, INC., Englewood, N.J.

FRANKLIN MINERAL PRODUCTS CO., Franklin, N.C.

FRANKLIN, O. M., SERUM CO., 409 Live Stock Exch. Bldg., Denver 16, Colo.

FRATELLI BRANCA & CO., INC., 12 Desbrosses St., New York 13, N.Y.

FRAZER PAINT CO., 2475 Hubbard St., Detroit, Mich.

FREDENBURGH-HECHT CO., 7 Hawthorne Rd., Concord, Mass.

FREEDOL REMEDY CO., 60 K St., Boston 27, Mass.

FRE-EZE CHEMICAL CORP., 1019A Virginia Ave., Atlanta, Ga.

FRENCH-BELL CO., 2429 Grand River Ave., Detroit 1, Mich.

FRENCH LABS., 529 S. 7th St., Minneapolis 15, Minn.

FRENCH RENOVATING CO., 1260 W. 4th, Cleveland, Ohio.

FRENCH, R. T., CO., 1 Mustard St., Rochester 9, N.Y.

FRENCO LABS., Nogales, Ariz.

FRESHENOL CO., 87 Beekman Rd., Summit, N.J.

FRESNO AGRICULTURAL CHEMICAL CO., Fresno, Calif.

FRESNOL MANUFACTURING CO., 2201 Yates Ave., Los Angeles 22, Calif.

FREY YENKIN PAINT CO., 251 N. Sandusky, Columbus, Ohio.

FRIENDLY LABS., 200 E. Main St., Shawnee 3, Okla.

FROMEYER & CO., 606 Reading Rd., Cincinnati, Ohio.

FROSST, CHAS. E. & CO., U. S. A., INC., 3571 St. Antoine St., Montreal, Que., Canada.

FROST LABORATORIES, INC., 430 Lexington St., Auburndale, Boston 66, Mass.

FROST PAINT & OIL CO., 1209 N.E. Tyler St., Minneapolis 13, Minn.

FRYE MFG. CO., 26th & Dean Ave., Des Moines, Iowa.

FULD BROS., INC., 702-710 S. Wolfe St., Baltimore 31, Md.

FULLER BRUSH CO., Hartford 2, Conn.

FULLER, C.F., CO., 71 Atwood Ave., Sausalito, Calif.

FULLER, H. B., CO., 181 W. Kellogg Blvd., St. Paul 2, Minn.

FULLER SYSTEM, INC., Woburn, Mass.

FULLER, W. P., & CO., Mission & Beale Sts., San Francisco, Calif.

FULTON SPECIALTY CO., 200 5th Ave., New York, N.Y.

G

GABLE-TITE PRODUCTS CO., P.O. Box 96, Miami, Fla.

GABY CO., 1825 N. 6th St., Philadelphia 22, Pa.

GADDY, R. L., PHARMACIST, P.O. Box 742, Jacksonville, Fla.

GAGNON-HASKELL, INC., Auburn, Maine.

GAIL, JEAN, PARFUMS, 106 E. 19th St., New York 3, N.Y.

GALEN LABS., 907 Penn Ave., Pittsburgh 22, Pa.

GALENOL CO., INC., 77 Auburn Ave., N.E., Atlanta 1, Ga.

GALLOWHUR CHEMICAL CORP., N. Water St., Ossining, N.Y.

GANE BROS. & LANE, INC., 1341 W. Lake St., Chicago, Ill.

GARD INDUSTRIES, INC., 733 Green Bay Rd., Wilmette, Ill.

GARDEN HOSE SPRAY CO., 7 Upland Rd., Cambridge 4, Mass.

GARDEN PRODUCTS CO., 3247 S. Grand Blvd., St. Louis, Mo.

GARDINER MFG. CO., 160 Van Renesselaer, Buffalo, N.Y

GARDNER CO., P.O. Box 5425, Cleveland 1, Ohio.

GARDNER LABS., 917 Airport Rd., Ferguson 21, Mo.

GARFIELD TEA CO., INC., Hewlett, N.Y.

GARLAND CO., 3748 E. 91st St., Cleveland, Ohio.

GART PHARM. CO., 61-18 Laurel Hill Blvd., Woodside 77, L. I., N.Y.

GARVERY FOUNTAIN BRUSH & INK CO., Newstead & Clayton Aves., St. Louis, Mo.

GASFLUX CO., 198 Wayne St., Mansfield, Ohio.

GASTOM CHEMICAL CO., Newark, N.J.

GATES PAINT MFG. CO., Charleston, W. Va.

GATES RUBBER CO., 1001 S. Broadway, Denver, Colo.

GATEWAY CHEMICAL CO., 1412 Walnut, Kansas City, Mo.

GEBAUER CHEMICAL CO., 9408 St. Catherine Ave., Cleveland 4, Ohio.

GEIGY AGRICULTURAL CHEMICALS, Div. Geigy Chemical Corp., 89 Barclay St., New York 8, N.Y.

GEM PRODUCTS CO., 323 Market St., Camden, N.J.

GENA LABS., INC., 1343 Plowman St., Dallas 8, Tex.

GENERAL ANILINE & FILM (see Antara Chemicals)

GENERAL CEMENT MFG. CO., 921 Taylor Ave., Rockford, Ill.

GENERAL CHEMICAL DIVISION, Allied Chemical & Dye Corp., 40 Rector St., New York, N.Y.

GENERAL ELECTRIC CO., Chemical Div., One River Rd., Schenectady 5, N.Y.

GENERAL FINISHES INC., Div. of Forman, Ford & Co., 111 S. 2nd St., Minneapolis 1, Minn.

GENERAL FOODS CORP., Hoboken, N.J.

GENERAL PAINT AND CHEMICAL CO., New Albany, Ind.

GENERAL PAINT CORP., Tulsa, Okla.

GENERAL PAINT CORP., Army at Potrero, San Francisco, Calif.

GENERAL PAINT & VARNISH CO., 2001 N. Mendell St., Chicago, Ill.

GENERAL PETROLEUM CORP., 612 S. Flower St., Los Angeles 54, Calif.

GENERAL PHOTOGRAPHIC SUPPLY CO., 138 Charles St., Boston 14, Mass.

GENERAL PLATING 6547 St. Paul St., Detroit, Mich.

GENERAL PRINTING INK CO., 44th Ave. & 10th St., Long Island City, L. I., N.Y.

GENERAL PRODUCTS CO., 1243 S. Wabash Ave., Chicago 5, Ill.

GENERAL SOLVENTS CO., 926 Exchange St., Rochester, N.Y.

GENERAL VITAMIN & MINERAL CO., 131 Shonnard St., Syracuse, N.Y.

GENESEE RESEARCH CORP., 961 Lyell Ave., Rochester 6, N.Y.

GEORGE, P. D., CO., 5100 N. 2nd St., St. Louis, Mo.

GEORGES SUPPLY CO., 614 12th St., N.W., Washington 5, D.C.

GEORGIA O. GEORGE, c/o Hawkins Distributing Co., 1483 N. Vine St., Los Angeles 28, Calif.

GERMADOL PRODUCTS CORP., 698 Broadway, New York 3, N.Y.

GERMOFORM CHEM. CO., 2859 S. Pulaski Rd., Chicago 23, Ill.

GERMO MFG. CO., 1470 S. Vandeventer, St. Louis, Mo.

GERSON-STEWART CORP., Ft. of Lisbon Rd., Cleveland, Ohio.

GESELL, R., INC., 200 W. Houston St., New York 14, N.Y.

"GETS-IT", INC., Subsidiary of Plough, Inc., Memphis, Tenn.

GETZUM PRODUCTS, 1310 Lehnder St., Summer, Wash.

G. G., INC., 1726 S. Del Mar Ave., San Gabriel, Calif.

GIBBS, T. R., MED. CO., 3056 Q St., S.E., Washington 20, D.C.

GIBSON-HOMANS CO., 2366 Woodhill Rd., Cleveland, Ohio.

G. I. DRUG CO., 79 E. 95th St., Brooklyn 12, N.Y.

GIES, WALTER G., CO., Crownsville, Md.

GILBERT, B. S., PHARM. CO., 304 W. Market St., York, Pa.

GILBERT LABS., INC., Morristown, N.J.

GILL, THOMAS, SOAP CO., Brooklyn, N.Y.

GILLESPIE VARNISH CO., 126 Dey St., Jersey City, N.J.

GILLETTE SAFETY RAZOR CO., 15 W. 1st St., Boston, Mass.

GINGISOL LABS., 557 Leader Bldg., Cleveland 14, Ohio.

GINO PILL CO., INC., 1415 Hertel Ave., Buffalo 16, N.Y.

GIRARD, FELIX, CO., INC., 2108 4th Ave., S., Minneapolis 4, Minn.

GISLER POLISH, INC., 557 E. Washington St., Indianapolis 4, Ind.

GLAMORENE CORP., 10 E. 44th St., New York 17, N.Y.

GLAMUR PRODUCTS, INC., Syracuse, N.Y.

GLAND-O-LAC CO., 1818 Leavenworth, Omaha 1, Nebr.

GLAZO, INC., P.O. Box 285, Port Chester, N.Y.

GLENDON PYROPHYLLITE CO., P.O. Box 2414, Greensboro, N.C.

GLENMORE CO., 1036 Broadway, Brooklyn 21, N.Y.

GLENN COUNTRY AGR. COMM., Memorial Bldg., Willows, Calif.

GLENN PRODUCTS CO., 110 Observer Hgwy. Hoboken, N.J.

GLEN-STAR MFG. CO., 440 Windsor Ave., Wilson 5, Conn.

GLENWAY CO., 4429 San Fernando Rd., Glendale 4, Calif.

GLESSNER CO., 230 E. Sandusky St., Findlay, Ohio.

G.L.F. SOIL BUILDING SERVICE, Terrace Hill, Ithaca, N.Y.

GLIDDEN CO., 1396 Union Commerce Bldg., Cleveland 14, Ohio.

GLIDDEN, OTIS E., & CO., INC., Waukesha, Wis.

GLISS'N PRODUCTS CO., INC., 11131 Michigan Ave., Chicago 28, Ill.

GLISTEN CO., Hillsdale, Mich.

GLOBAL MFG. SALES AGENCY, INC., Detroit, Mich.

GLOBE LABS., 116 Commerce St., Fort Worth 2, Tex.

GLOBE PAINT WORKS, INC., 212 Market St., Williamsport, Pa.

GLOBE SANITARY SUPPLY CO., 2249 E. 38th St., Los Angeles, Calif.

GLOBE SOLVENTS CO., INC., 7th & Fishers Ave., Philadelphia, Pa.

GLOBE VARNISH CO., Kelly & La Schall Sta., Pittsburgh, Pa.

GLORIA-FAY CO., 18820 Eureka St., Detroit, Mich.

GLOVER, H. CLAY, CO., INC., Meadowbrook National Bank Bldg., West Hempstead, N.Y.

GOBBERDIEL, J. P., 306 S. Wabash St., Chicago 4, Ill.

GODEFROY MFG. CO., 3510 Olive St., St. Louis 3, Mo.

GOLD BOND STERLIZING POWDER CO., INC., 47 Main St., Fairhaven, Mass.

GOLD MEDAL HAARLEM OIL CO., Jersey City, N.J.

GOLD SEAL CO., Bismark, N. Dak.

GOLDEN CHURN LABS., 2307 N. 11th St., St. Louis 6, Mo.

GOLDEN GLINT CO., INC., P.O. Box 3366, Seattle 14, Wash.

GOLDEN PEACOCK, INC., P.O. Box 31, Paris, Tenn.

GOLDEN STAR POLISH MFG. CO., 2901 E. 13th St., Kansas City, Mo.

GOLDEN WEST CO., Box 22, Knoxville, Tenn.

GOLDEN-YOUTH MFG. CO., 923 N. Rockwell, Chicago 22, Ill.

GOLDMAN, MARY T., Box 40, Quincy, Ill.

GOLDMAN, RALPH H., ENTERPRISES, 11 W. 42nd St., New York 36, N.Y.

GOLD SEAL CO., Bismark, N. Dak.

GOMPES, HENRI S., INC., 381 4th Ave., New York 16, N.Y.

GONZALEZ, ESPIRIDION, P.O. Box 4271, Sta. A., San Antonio 7, Tex.

GOODE-CAGE DRUG CO., INC., 401 Spring St., Shreveport 90, La.

GOOD GROOMING PRODUCTS, Detroit, Mich.

GOOD JAMES, CO., 2120 E. Susquehanna Ave., Philadelphia, Pa.

GOODMAN CHEM., NEW YORK CORP., 232 6th St., Brooklyn 15, N.Y.

GOODRICH, B. F., CHEMICAL CO., Div. of B. F. Goodrich Co., Rose Bldg., 2060 E. 9th St., Cleveland 15, Ohio.

GOODRICH DRUG CO., 500 Robert St., St. Paul 1, Minn.

GOODRICH-GAMBLE CO., 56 Emerald St., Minneapolis 14, Minn.

GOODWINOL PRODS. CORP., Wappingers Falls, N.Y.

GOODWIN'S N. C., LAB., INC., New York, N.Y.

GORDON LABORATORIES, 475 Commonwealth Ave., Boston 15, Mass.

GORDON THOMAS SALES CORP., 345 Kings Hgwy., Brooklyn 23, N.Y.

GORGA DRUG CO., 115 E. 61st St., New York 21, N.Y.

GORHAM CO., 333 Adelaide Ave., Providence 7, R.I.

GOTHAM PHARMACEUTICAL CO., INC., 1207 Kings Hgwy., Brooklyn 29, N.Y.

GOTTLIEB CHEMICAL CO., 142 Central Ave., Ridgefield Park, N.J.

GOULARD & OLENA, INC., Skillman, N.J.

GOULD, BARBARA, SALES CORP., 35 W. 34th St., New York 1, N.Y.

GOWAN CHEM. CO., 116 S. Calvert St., Baltimore 2, Md.

GRAFF MOTOR CO., Rapid City, S. Dak.

GRAFLEX, INC., 320 W. Ohio St., Chicago 10, Ill.

GRAHAM MFG. CO., Holyoke, Mass.

GRAMMES, L. F., & SONS, INC., 380 Union St., Allentown, Pa.

GRANDPA SOAP CO., Cincinnati 2, Ohio.

GRANT MFG. CO., 2 S. Pennsylvania, Oklahoma City 8, Okla.

GRAPHIC ECONOMY DEVELOPER CO., 1624 S. Trumbull Ave., Chicago 23, Ill.

GRATNY DRUG CO., INC., 1324 Southwest Blvd., Kansas City 3, Kans.

GRAVES PAINT & VARNISH CO., Chester, Pa.

GRAY, DOROTHY, LTD., 192 Bloomfield Ave., Bloomfield, N.J.

GRAY FOX, INC., 406 Westport Rd., Kansas City 6, Mo.

GRAYLENE CO., 529 S. Franklin St., Chicago 7, Ill.

GRAY'S LABORATORIES, 1690 Broadway, New York 19, N.Y.

GREAN-RUB CO., 3731 Laclede Ave., St. Louis 8, Mo.

GREAT ATLANTIC & PACIFIC TEA CO., 420 Lexington Ave., New York 17, N.Y.

GREAT LAKES LABS., see Great Lakes Pharm. Corp.

GREAT LAKES PAINT & VARNISH CO., 2215 N. Pulaski Rd., Chicago, Ill.

GREAT LAKES PHARMACAL CORP., 5026 Woodland Ave., Cleveland 4, Ohio.

GREAT NORTHERN CHEMICAL CO., 222 Clara St., San Francisco 7, Calif.

GREAT STUFF PRODUCTS CO., 530 57th St., West New York, N.J.

GREAT WESTERN INSECTICIDE CO., 24 Horatio St., New York 14, N.Y.

GREDAG, INC., 3949 Streeter Bldg., Niagara Falls, N.Y.

GREEN CROSS PRODUCTS DIV., Sherwin Williams Co., of Canada Ltd., P.O. Box 489, Montreal 22, Que., Canada.

GREENE SALES CO., INC., Arley, Ala.

GREEN LINE CHEM. CORP., 2329 Olive St., St. Louis 3, Mo.

GREEN OIL SOAP CO., 5524 N. Northwest Hgwy., Chicago, Ill.

GREENVILLE CHEMICAL CO., Greenville, S.C.

GREENWOOD, T. H., CO., North Hills, Pa.

GREEVER'S INC., Chilhowie, Va.

GREGORY FOUNT-O-INK CO., 3501 Eagle Rock Rd., Los Angeles 65, Calif.

GREIL DRUG & CHEMICAL CO., Pittsburgh, Pa.

GREINER, EMIL, CO., 20-26 N. Moore St., New York 13, N.Y.

GRELLVA, INC., 22 W. 48th St., New York 19, N.Y.

GRENALD LABS., Louisville, Ky.

GREYSON LABS., Lynn, Mass.

GRIFFIN MFG. CO., INC., 410 Willoughby Ave., Brooklyn 5, N.Y.

GRIFFITH LABS. INC., 1415 W. 37th, Chicago, Ill.

GRISSMER, EARL, CO., Indianapolis, Ind.

GRISWOLD MEDICINE CO., INC., 2811 School St., Des Moines 11, Iowa.

GRISWOLD SALVE CO., 729 Main St., Hartford 2, Conn.

GROSS, WM. H., CHEM. CO., 1915 S. Hackberry St., San Antonio 10, Tex.

GROVE LABS., INC., 8877 Ladue Rd., St. Louis 24, Mo.

GRUMBACHER, M., INC., 466 W. 34th St., New York, N.Y.

GUARANTEE PRODS. CO., 301 Chestnut St., Grand Fork, N.Dak.

GUILD, J. H., CO., INC., Rupert, Vt.

GUILMARD CO., INC., 2101 Ponce de Leon Blvd., Coral Gables 32, Fla.

GUITARE LABS., 652 N. Robertson Blvd., Los Angeles 46, Calif.

GULF OIL CO., 264 Gulf Bldg., Pittsburgh 30, Pa.

GULF STATES SALES CORP., 101 S. 21st St., Birmingham, Ala.

GUSTAFSON, E. B., 547 S. Marengo Ave., Pasadena 5, Calif.

G. W. DISTRIBUTING CORP., 41 N. 2nd Ave., Mt. Vernon, N.Y.

G. & W. LABS., 372 Ocean Ave., Jersey City 5, N.J.

GYNECOLOGICAL SPECIALTIES, INC., 413 E. Broadway, Altona, Ill.

GYPSY FIRE FOLKE COMPANY, INC., Delmar, N.Y.

H

HAACK LABS., INC., 1415 S.W. Harbor Dr., Portland 1, Oreg.

HAAG, INC., 1509 E. Main St., Richmond 19, Va.

HAAS PHARMACY, 376 Park Ave., New York 22, N.Y.

HABER, HARRY D., 211 E. Broadway, New York 2, N.Y.

HACHIK BLEACH CO., 50th above Wynnfield Ave., Philadelphia, Pa.

HACK PAINT & CHEMICAL WORKS, Phoenixville, Pa.

HAERTEL, WALTER PROD. CO., 2840 4th Ave., S., Minn. 8, Minn.

HAEUSER SHELLAC CO., INC., 55 St., Brooklyn, N.Y.

HAGUE, ALFRED, & CO., 226 34th St., Brooklyn, N.Y.

HAINES PRODUCTS CO., Carey, Ohio.

H. A. INK ERADICATOR CO., 1707 Zerega Ave., New York, N.Y.

HAIR, DR. B. W., MEDICINE CO., 314 N. 12th St., Richmond, Ind.

HAIR SPECIALTY CO., 112 E. 23rd St., New York 10, N.Y.

HAIRTEX CO., 721 Larkin St., San Francisco 9, Calif.

HAKES, CYRUS D. 7557 Marion Ave., New York 58, N.Y.

HALABY CO., SAMUEL, 482 Clinton Ave., S., Rochester 7, N.Y.

HALE PRODUCTS, P.O. Box 1052, Glendale 5, Calif.

HALGAR, INC., 251 E. Grand Ave., Chicago 11, Ill.

HALITOSINE CO., INC., 5156 Delmar Blvd., St. Louis 8, Mo.

HALOID CO., Rochester 3, N.Y.

HALPERIN, A. E., CO., INC., 75 Northampton St., Boston 18, Mass.

HALSEY DRUG CO., INC., 1827 Pacific St., Brooklyn 33, N.Y.

HALWELL CO., 69 N. Central Ave., Valley Stream, N.Y.

HAMMOND PAINT & CHEM. CO., Beacon, N.Y.

HAMPDEN COLOR & CHEMICAL CO., Springfield, Mass.

HAMPSHIRE SOLVENTS CO., Concord, N.H.

HAMPTON-CROSS CO., 120 S. 10th St., Louisville, Ky.

HANCE BROS., AND WHITE CO., 12th and Hamilton St., Philadelphia, Pa.

HANCOCK, JOHN F. & SON, INC., 521 W. Lombard St., Baltimore 1, Md.

HANCOCK PAINT & VARNISH CO., North Quincy, Mass.

HAND, J. A., & SON CO., 614 3rd St., Moosic, Pa.

HANDLEY LABS., 37 Golden Ave., Arlington, Mass.

HAND MEDICINE CO., 1530 Spring-Garden St., Philadelphia, Pa.

HANDY AND HARMON, 82 Fulton St., New York 38, N.Y.

HANLON DRUG PRODUCTS, Poughkeepsie, N.Y.

HANNA, LESTER W. Route 1, Box 210, Forest Grove, Oreg.

HANSON, HOWARD, & CO., 715 3rd St., S.E., Roanoke 3, Va.

HANSON, W. T., CO., 4 E. 39th St., New York 16, N.Y.

HAPPY JACK, INC., Snow Hill, N.C.

HARALSON, W. L., & SONS, Fort Payne, Ala.

HARDIG PAINT CO., 1111 Harrison Ave., Cincinnati, Ohio.

HARDY SALVE CO., P.O. Box 155, Claremont, N.H.

HAROLD SUPPLY CO., see 8 in 1 Pet Products, Inc.

HARRINGTON PAINT CO., 1628 Collander Ave., Cleveland, Ohio.

HARRIS, B., CO., 7472 Melrose Ave., Los Angeles 46, Calif.

HARRIS HAIR TONIC CO., 3883 S. Orange Dr., Los Angeles 56, Calif.

HARRIS, P. F., MFG. CO., 624 E. Washington Ave., North Little Rock, Ark.

HARRIS PRODS. CO., INC., P.O. Box 4, Miami Beach 39, Fla.

HARRIS STANDARD PAINT CO., 1026 N. 19th St., Tampa, Fla.

HARRISON, A. S., CO., P.O. Box 568, South Norwalk, Conn.

HARRISON PAINT & VARNISH CO., Harrison Ave., S.W., & Walters, Canton, Ohio.

HARRISON PRODUCTS, INC., 610 Folsom St., San Francisco 7, Calif.

HARRISON'S DRUG STORE, 4700 Williamsburg Ave., Richmond 23, Va.

HARROP CHEMICAL CO., 125 Hoboken Ave., Jersey City, N.J.

HARROWER LAB., INC., see Warner-Chilcott.

HARSHAW CHEMICAL CO., 1945 E. 97th St., Cleveland 6, Ohio.

HART, A. THOMAS, CO., INC., Buffalo, N.Y.

HARTLETT, M., CO., 2604 Oriole Tr., Long Beach, Michigan City, Ind.

HARTMAN PRODUCTS, 1901 Sylvania Ave., Toledo 13, Ohio.

HARTZ, J. F., 780 W. Eight Mile Rd., Ferndale 20, Mich.

HARTZ MOUNTAIN PRODUCTS, 36 Cooper Sq., New York, N.Y.

HARVEY, G. F., CO., Saratoga Springs, N.Y.

HARVEY LABS., INC., 5109 Germantown Ave., Philadelphia 44, Pa.

HARVEY PAPER PRODUCTS CO., Sturgis, Mich.

HARVEY PHOTOCHEMICALS, INC., Newton, N.J.

HARWOOD PHARMACAL CO., INC., 507 Central Ave., Newark 7, N.J.

HALSAM, FENTON, J., CO., 21 Prospect St., Cambridge 39, Mass.

HASTINGS MANUFACTURING CO., Casite Div., Hastings, Mich.

HATCH, HENRY C., CO., Brockton, Mass.

HATCH, ORA, Bloomington, Wis.

HATTERS SUPPLY CO., 404 S. Wells, Chicago, Ill.

HAUG DRUG CO., Milwaukee 3, Wis.

HAUSMAN DRUG CO., 122 W. 1st St., Trinidad, Colo.

HAUSSMAN PHARMACY, 3196 3rd Ave., New York 56, N.Y.

HAVILAND, ANN, 1 W. 52nd St., New York 19, N.Y.

HAVILAND PRODUCTS CO., 421 Ann St., N.W., Grand Rapids 2, Mich.

HAWLEY, C. D., Berlin, Wis.

HAYES-SAMMONS CO., 718 Holland Ave., Mission, Tex.

HAYNER, NORMAN C., CO., 194 Edinburgh St., Rochester, N.Y.

HAYNES, C. W., LABS., INC., Springfield, Mass.

HAYNES, PIERRE E., 5946 Norwaldo Ave., Indianapolis 20, Ind.

HAYR CHEMICAL CO., INC., Newark, N.J.

HAYSMA CO., 333 N. Michigan Ave., Chicago 1, Ill.

HAYS-TAYLOR INC., 3343 Flanagan Ave., Tonawanda, N.Y.

HEALTH PRODS. CO., 807 W. Wisconsin Ave., Milwaukee 3, Wis.

HEARN SALVE CO., P.O. Box 23, Carrollton, Ga.

HEATH & MILLIGAN MFG. CO., 1833 S. Normal, Chicago, Ill.

HEATLESS PERMANENT WAVE CO., 512 2nd St., San Francisco 7, Calif.

HEIDT INSECTICIDE CO., E. 9th Ave., Cordele, Ga.

HEIFLER & HEIFLER, 3069 Brighton First St., Brooklyn 35, N.Y.

HEIL PROCESS EQUIPMENT CORP., 12900 Elmwood Ave., Cleveland, Ohio.

HEINL'S GREENHOUSES, Toledo, Ohio.

HELDER CHEMICAL CO., Columbus, Ohio.

HELD & GUSTAFSON, 547 Marengo Ave., Pasadena 5, Calif.

HELLER LABS., INC., Div. B. Heller & Co., Calumet Ave. & 40th St., Chicago 15, Ill.

HELLWIG, A. T., & CO., 98 Park Place, New York 7, N.Y.

HELM CO., 1340 Rocky Gap Rd., Benton Harbor, Mich.

HELM GOAT MILK PRODUCTS, 148 Vista Dr., Jackson, Mich.

HEMMERDINGER, L., & CO., 438 E. 123rd St., New York, N.Y.

HEMORR-AID CORP., P.O. Box 243, Oshkosh, Wis.

HENLAN CO., P.O. Box 34, Hackensack, N.J.

HENNEN PRODUCTS, 1325 Chapline St., Wheeling, W. Va.

HENNESSY ASSOCS., 201 Verona Ave., Newark, N.J.

HENRY ENGRAVING CO., 5346 River Dr., Moline, Ill.

HENRY LABS., INC., 2906 West End Ave., Nashville 5, Tenn.

HEPA, INC., 2483 Lee Blvd., Cleveland Heights 18, Ohio.

HERB FARM SHOP, LTD., 347 5th Ave., New York 16, N.Y.

HERBOLD LAB., INC., 8008 W. 3rd St., Los Angeles 48, Calif.

HERCULES POWDER CO., Wilmington, Del.

HERITAGE PHARMACALS, 360 N. Michigan Ave., Chicago 1, Ill.

HERMANN CHEMICAL CO., St. Paul, Minn.

HEROCK MFG. CO., Phoenixville, Pa.

HERP PHARMACAL CO., 723 Dearborn Ave., Louisville 11, Ky.

HERPICIDE CO., 805 E. 140th St., New York 54, N.Y.

HERRIOTT POLISH CO., St. Louis, Mo.

HERSHEY ESTATES, Soap and Extraction Div., Hershey, Pa.

HERSHKOWITZ, J. INC., 247 Centre St., New York 13, N.Y.

HERZOG LABS., INC., Buffalo 4, N.Y.

HESS, DR., & CLARK, INC., Orange & 7th Sts., Ashland, Ohio.

HESS, E. E., CO., Brook, Ind.

HESS HAIR MILK LABS., Rice St. & County Rd., A2, St. Paul 2, Minn.

HEUN, E. W., CO., St. Louis 16, Mo.

HEWITT SOAP CO., INC., Dayton, Ohio.

HEXOL, INC., 1500 17th St., San Francisco 7, Calif.

HEYWOOD LABS., 126 E. Teany, Louisville 9, Ky.

H.G.O. MEDICINE CO., 2345 Dresden Rd., Zanesville, Ohio.

H. & H. CLEANER CO., 134 E. Locust St., Des Moines 9, Iowa.

HIGGINS INK CO., 271 9th St., Brooklyn 15, N.Y.

HIGH CHEMICAL CO., 1760 N. Howard St., Philadelphia 22, Pa.

HIGH POINT PAINT & FINISHES CORP., High Point, N.C.

HIKE CHEMICAL CO., 7634 Gannon Ave., St. Louis 5, Mo.

HILD FLOOR MACHINERY CO., Washington & Halstead Sts., Chicago, Ill.

HILEX CO., 319 E. Kellogg Blvd., Saint Paul 1, Minn.

HILGERS, J., & CO., see Rex Hunters Prods. Co.

HILL LABS., Jacksonville 7, Fla.

HILL LABS., INC., 3008 Caroline St., Houston 4, Tex.

HILL MFG. CO., 1500 Jonesboro Rd., S.E., Atlanta, Ga.

HILLMAN PHARM. CO., 185 N. Wabash Ave., Chicago 1, Ill

HILLSHIRE FARMS, INC., R.F.D., Killingly, Conn.

HILLTOP LABS., 718 Washington Ave., N., Minneapolis 1, Minn.

HILLYARD CHEMICAL CO., St. Joseph 1, Mo.

HILLYARD SALES CO., St. Joseph, Mo.

HILO CO., P.O. Box 246, Norwalk, Conn.

HILO VARNISH CORP., 376 3rd St., Everett, Mass.

HIMROD MFG. CO., 35 York St., Brooklyn 1, N.Y.

HINKLE DRUG CO., 3rd & Locust Sts., Columbia, Pa.

HINZE AMEROSIA, INC., 30 Rockefeller Plaza, New York 20, N.Y.

HIRESTRA LABS, INC., Lexington Ave., Bethpage, L. I., N.Y.

HISCOX CHEMICAL WORKS, INC., P.O. Drawer 1220, Bradenton, Fla.

H. & M. PRODS. CO., 1618 Elm St., Cincinnati 10, Ohio.

HOAG-FARMER MFG. CO., 1021 W. Lake, Chicago, Ill.

HOBART LABORATORIES, 900 N. Franklin St., Chicago 10, Ill.

HOBO MED. CO., 950 Grand Ave., Beaumont, Tex.

HOBOKEN WHITE LEAD & COLOR WORKS, Hoboken, N.J.

HOBS LABS., Passaic, N.J.

HOCKWALD CHEMICAL CO., Mississippi & Mariposa Sts., San Francisco, Calif.

HOFER CHEM. CO., Main St., Freeman, S. Dak.

HOFFMANN-LaROCHE, INC., Nutley, N.J.

HOLCOMB, J. I., MFG. CO., 4401 Cold Spring Rd., Indianapolis 8, Ind.

HOLDFAST RUBBER CO., 1486 Lakewood Ave., S.E., Atlanta, Ga.

HOLLAND-RANTOS CO., 145 Hudson St., New York 13, N.Y.

HOLLEY CHEMICAL CO., 126 E. 25th St., New York, N.Y.

HOLLINGSHEAD, R. M., CORP., Camden 2, N.J.

HOLLINGS-SMITH CO., Orangeburg, N.Y.

HOLLISTER'S, Warren, Pa.

HOLMES, E. S., CO., 1747 Victory Blvd., Glendale 1, Calif.

HOLMES, E. T., & CO., Cleveland, Ohio.

HOLT PRODUCTS CO., 820 E. Locust St., Milwaukee 12, Wis.

HOMEMAKERS' PRODS., 380 2nd Ave., New York 10, N.Y.

HOMMEL, O., CO., 211 4th St., Pittsburgh, Pa.

HOME NEEDS CO., 5950 Walker Ave., Los Angeles 22, Calif.

HOOD CHEMICAL CO., INC., 80 Rittenhouse Place, Ardmore, Pa.

HOOKER ELECTROCHEMICAL CO., Niagara, N.Y.

HOOKER ELECTROCHEMICAL CO., CORP., 1650 Luett Ave., Indianapolis 22, Ind.

HOOVER LINIMENT CO., Carlisle, Ind.

HOPKINS AGRICULTURAL CHEM. CO. 740 Williamson St., Madison 3, Wis.

HOPKINS PRODUCTS, INC., 1300 Race St., Baltimore, Md.

HORN, A. C., INC., 10th St. & 44th Ave., Long Island City 1, L. I., N.Y.

HOROWITZ, A. G., Standard Cut Rate Drugs, 507 Central Ave., Newark, N.J.

HORTON & CONVERSE, 621 W. Pico Blvd., Los Angeles 15, Calif.

HOSID PRODUCTS INC., Hosid Bldg., Syracuse, N.Y.

HOTOPF VARNISH CO., 265 Gates Ave., Jersey City, N.J.

HOUCK & CO., Cleveland, Ohio.

HOUSE FOR MEN, INC., 609 N. La Salle St., Chicago 10, Ill.

HOUSE OF BRISTOL, INC., 2610 N. 83rd St., Milwaukee, Wis.

HOUSE OF FRAGRANCE, 3757 N. 73rd Ave., Chicago 34, Ill.

HOUSE OF GABLER, 128-130 E. King St., Chambersburg, Pa.

HOUSE OF GOURIELLI, 655 5th Ave., New York 22, N.Y.

HOUSE OF HAWICK, 68 Jay St., Brooklyn 1, N.Y.

HOUSE OF HUSTON, INC., 351 San Lorenza Ave., Coral Gables, Fla.

HOUSE OF LOWELL, 421 S. College St., Piqua, Ohio.

HOUSE OF MARSHALL, P.O. Box 188, Mt. Vernon, N.Y.

HOUSE OF PUZZY, 40 Hopkins Place, Baltimore 1, Md.

HOUSE OF ROSE, P.O. Box 603, Des Moines, Iowa.

HOUSE OF YOST, Lake Tomahawk, Wis.

HOUSEHOLD PRODUCTS, Stamford, Conn.

HOUSTON DRUG CO., 404 Caroline St., Houston, Tex.

HOWARD BROS. CHEM. CO., 70 Niagara St., Buffalo 2, N.Y.

HOWARD LABS., INC., 28 E. 1st St., Mt. Vernon, N.Y.

HOWE AND CO., 911 Western Ave., Seattle, Wash.

HOWE AND FRENCH, INC., Weymouth 88, Mass.

HOWE CO., Stony Creek, Conn.

HOWELL BROTHERS CHEM. LAB.,
5414 Girard Ave., Philadelphia 31,
Pa.

HOWELL, C. H., & CO., 212 Race St.,
Philadelphia, Pa.

HOWELL CO., INC., 1104 Magazine
St., New Orleans 9, La.

HOWERTON GOWEN COMPANY,
Roanoke Rapids, N.C.

HOWES MFG. CO., 111 Hudson,
Jersey City, N.J.

HOYT APOTHECARIES CO., 89
Ashbury Terr., San Francisco 17,
Calif.

H. Q. Z. DIST., INC., 1750 S. Smith
Ave., San Jose, Calif.

H. S. SPECIALITY, 1206 S. 11th St.,
Tacoma, Wash.

HUBBARD, CHAS., & SON CO., 211 W.
Water, Syracuse, N.Y.

HUBBARD CO., 2819 Southwest Blvd.,
Kansas City 8, Mo.

HUBBARD, J., & CO., 94 Ash St.,
Nashua, N.H.

HUBERE COSMETICS, 9 W. Illinois
St., Chicago 10, Ill.

HUBINGER CO., Keokuk, Iowa.

HUDNUT, ALEX., PHARMACEUTICAL
OF NEW YORK, 1020 3rd Ave., New
York 21, N.Y.

HUDNUT, RICHARD, 113 W. 18th St.,
New York, N.Y.

HUDSON & CO., Peninsula Blvd.,
Pokomoke City, Md.

HUDSON CORP., Chicago, Ill.

HUENELATOR CORP., 9256 Beverly
Blvd., Beverly Hills, Calif.

HUGGINS, JAMES, & SON, INC.,
239 Medford St., Malden 48, Mass.

HUGHEL, C., CO., INC., Academy St.,
Madison, N.C.

HUGHES GLUE CO., 3500 St. Aubin
St., Detroit 7, Mich.

HULET, ARTHUR G., 133 N. Wilton
Pl., Los Angeles 4, Calif.

HUMBERT PETROLEUM PRODUCTS,
223 Glen St., Glen Cove, L. I., N.Y.

HUMCO LAB., 1220 Main St.,
Texarkana, Tex.

HUMPHREYS MEDICINE CO., INC.,
273 Lafayette St., New York 12, N.Y.

HUNCKE, MAX, CHEM. CO., 626 4th
Ave., Brooklyn, N.Y.

HUNTER, WILFRED A., INC., 7315
Goff Ave., Richmond Hts. 17, Mo.

HUNTERS, REX, PRODUCTS CO.,
Rockport, Mass.

HUNTINGTON LABS. INC., 900 E.
Tipton, Huntington, Ind.

HURLEY, H. O., CO., INC., 2560
Tophill Rd., Louisville 6, Ky.

HUSH CO., 148 N. 2nd St.,
Philadelphia 6, Pa.

HUTCHINSON, W. & E., INC., 1233
S. San Pedro St., Los Angeles 15,
Calif.

HUTTIG SASH & DOOR CO., 1206 S.
Vandeventer Ave., St. Louis, Mo.

HUXLEY PHARMACEUTICALS, 121
No. Hanley Rd., Clayton, St. Louis
5, Mo.

HY-BEAUTE CHEM. CO., 268 Auburn
Ave., N.E., Atlanta, Ga.

HYCHEX PROD., 3935 W. Irving Rd.,
Chicago 18, Ill.

HYDROPONIC CHEMICAL CO.,
INC., Copley, Ohio.

HYDROSAL CO., 717 Sycamore St.,
Cincinnati, Ohio.

HYDROTEX INDUSTRIES, 4333 N.
Central Expressway, P.O. Box
2400, Dallas 21, Tex.

HY-G CORP., 222 Clara St., San
Francisco 7, Calif.

HYG-A-TABS LABS., 351 Eastern
Pkwy., Brooklyn 16, N.Y.

HYGENA CO., 77 Auburn Ave.,
Atlanta 1, Ga.

HYGIENE RESEARCH, INC., 684
Broadway, New York 12, N.Y.

HY-GRO CORP., 1101 Maryland
Ave., Baltimore 1, Md.

HYGIENIC PRODS. CO., see Boyle-
Midway.

HY-LIFE MINERAL CO., 2145
Blake St., Denver 2, Colo.

HYNSON, WESTCOTT & DUNNING,
INC., 1030 N. Charles St.,
Baltimore 2, Md.

HY-PHEN CORP., Box 272,
Matoaka, W. Va.

HY-TROUS CORP., 50 Cross St.,
Boston, Mass.

I

IDEAL PASTE & CHEMICAL CO.,
3559 W. 140th St., Cleveland, Ohio.

IDEAL STENCIL MACHINE CO.,
Bellville, Ill.

ILLINOIS BRONZE POWDER CO.,
2023 S. Clark St., Chicago, Ill.

ILLINOIS CLAY PRODUCTS CO.,
116 Chicago St., Joliet, Ill.

IMPERIAL CHEM. CO., W. 6th &
Grass Sts., Shenandoah, Iowa.

IMPERIAL CRAYON CO., 649
Lexington Ave., Brooklyn, N.Y.

IMPERIAL FLOORING & WATER-
PROOFING CO., Melrose Park,
Ill.

IMPERIAL PAPER & COLOR CORP.,
Glens Falls, N.Y.

IMPERIAL PHARM. CO., 130-02
101st Ave., Richmond Hill 19, L. I.,
N.Y.

IMPERIAL PRODUCTS CO., 1600
Fountain St., Philadelphia, Pa.

IMPERVIOUS VARNISH CO., P.O.
Box 340, Rochester, Pa.

INDIANA LABORATORIES INC.,
1505 S. D St., Richmond, Ind.

INDIANAPOLIS PAINT AND COLOR
CO., P.O. Box 1259, Indianapolis,
Ind.

INDIAN REFINING CO.,
Lawrenceville, Ill.

INDIAN RIVER MEDICINE CO., 143
N. Tennessee Ave., Lafollette,
Tenn.

INDIA PAINT AND LACQUER CO.,
728 E. 59th St., Los Angeles 1,
Calif.

INDUSTRIAL MARINE PRODUCTS
INC., 1018 E. 46th St., Brooklyn,
N.Y.

INDUSTRIAL MATERIALS CO., 1017
McCall St., Houston, Tex.

INERTOL CO., 490 Frelinghuysen
Ave., Newark, N.J.

INK RIBBON MFG. CORP., 884
Valencia, San Francisco, Calif.

INMAN DRUG CO., 2217 Bull St.,
Savannah, Ga.

INNER-AID MEDICINE CO., 129 W.
3rd St., Covington, Ky.

INNERCLEAN CO., 833 E. 6th St.,
Los Angeles, Calif.

INNER-TONE MEDICINE CO.,
Covington, Ky.

INNIS, SPEIDEN & CO., see Larvacide
Prods.

INORGANIC BIOELEMENTS, INC.,
15037 Shore Acres Dr., Cleveland 10,
Ohio.

INSECT CONTROL & RESEARCH INC.,
Johnnycake Rd., Baltimore 7, Md.

INSL-X CO., 100 Water St., Ossining,
N.Y.

INSTANT PRODS. CO., INC., 702
Swan St., Buffalo 10, N.Y.

INTER-COASTAL PAINT CORP.,
East St., E. St. Louis, Ill.

INTERNATIONAL BIOTICAL CORP.,
95 5th Ave., New York, N.Y.

INTERNATIONAL CELLUCOTTON
PRODUCTS CO., see Kimberly-
Clark Corp.

INTERNATIONAL CHEMICAL CO.,
3140 S. Canal St., Chicago, Ill.

INTERNATIONAL LABS., INC., 80
Main St., W., Rochester 14, N.Y.

INTERNATIONAL METAL POLISH
CO., 1910 Quill St., Indianapolis 7,
Ind.

INTERNATIONAL MUTOSCOPE CORP.,
44 11th St., Long Island City 1, L. I.
N.Y.

INTERNATIONAL NICKEL CO., INC.,
67 Wall St., New York 5, N.Y.

INTERNATIONAL PAINT CO., 21 West
St., New York, N.Y.

INTERNATIONAL PLUMBING MFG.
CO., INC., 45 Murray St., New York
7, N.Y.

INTERNATIONAL RESEARCH CORP.,
Danbury, Conn.

INTERNATIONAL RUSTPROOF CORP.,
12509 Broadway & Destrehan, St.
Louis, Mo.

INTERNATIONAL SILVER CO.,
Meriden, Conn.

INTERNATIONAL SISAL CO., 722 N.
1st St., Minneapolis, Minn.

INTERNATIONAL STOCK FOOD CO.,
1316 S. 6th St., Minneapolis 4, Minn.

INTER-OCEAN OIL CO., 50 S. James
St., Kansas City, Mo.

INTERSTATE MED. CO., Kingsley,
Iowa.

INTERSTATE SANITATION CO., 433
Elm St., Cincinnati, Ohio.

IODENT CHEMICAL CO., 2233 Park
Ave., Detroit 1, Mich.

IODOBOR CO., 230 E. 61st St., New
York 21, N.Y.

IODISE CO., 1 Martin Ave., Clifton,
N.J.

I-ODORAL, INC., Pittsburgh 20, Pa.

IOSALINE CO., P.O. Box 1749,
Washington 13, D.C.

IOWA SOAP CO., Burlington, Iowa.

I. P. A. MFG. CO., 810 Parker St.,
McKinney, Tex.

IRWIN PAINT CO., 4th & Addison Sts., Berkeley, Calif.

ISANA PRODUCTS, INC., 1512 N. Fremont St., Chicago, Ill.

ISING, C. E., CORP., Flushing, L. I., N.Y.

I-SIS CHEM. CO., Springdale, Conn.

IT SHOE POLISH PRODUCTS, INC., 111 N. Greene St., Baltimore, Md.

IVES-CAMERON CO., Philadelphia, Pa.

IVY CORP., The Crescent, Montclair, N.J.

IVY-OFF CORP., P.O. Box 365, Framingham, Mass.

J

JACKS MFG. CO., 2029 St. Anthony Ave., St. Paul, Minn.

JACKSON, E. B., & CO., 4116 Ruckle St., Indianapolis 5, Ind.

JACKSON-MITCHELL PHARM-ACEUTICALS CO., Culver City, Calif.

JACKSON OF LONDON PRODUCTS, 68 W. 58th St., New York, N.Y.

JACKSON, S., & SON, INC., P.O. Box 137, New Orleans 3, La.

JACROY CO., Bedford, Ohio.

J. A. K. CO., INC., P.O. Box 3232, Sta. F., Atlanta, Ga.

JAMAICA LABORATORIES CO., 182 Peace St., Jamaica, L. I., N.Y.

JAMES, LEONARD, CO., San Saba, Tex.

JAMOL CO., 101 Maiden Lane, New York 7, N.Y.

JANNEY, SEMPLE, HILL & CO., Minneapolis, Minn.

JAYBRA PRODUCTS INC., 84 Pitts St., New York 2, N.Y.

JAYE MFG. CO., 6200 Grand Ave., Cleveland, Ohio.

JAY'S LABORATORIES, Orange, N.J.

JEFFERSON PHARMACAL CO., 8847 Gratiot Ave., Detroit 13, Mich.

JEFFERY LABS., 13310 Oxnard St., Van Nuys, Calif.

JEFFREY-FELL CO., 1700 Main St., Buffalo 9, N.Y.

JENKINS LABS., INC., 17 Wall St., Auburn, N.Y.

JERGENS, ANDREW, CO., Cincinnati, Ohio.

JERIS SALES CO., 100 Jersey Ave., New Brunswick, N.J.

JEWELL PAINT & VARNISH CO., 349 N. Western Ave., Chicago, Ill.

JEWELL PHARMACEUTICALS, INC., 508 Franklin Ave., Mt. Vernon, N.Y.

JEWEL TEA CO., Barrington, Ill.

JIFFY REMEDIES CO., see J. R. Co.

JIFFY-WAY, INC., Owatonna, Minn.

J & J REMEDY CO., 1752 Westwood Blvd., Los Angeles 24, Calif.

JOHNSON, C. E., & CO., see Welmaid Mfg.

JOHNSON & JOHNSON, New Brunswick, N.J.

JOHNSON, J. W., CO., 3100 W. Randolph St., Bellwood, Ill.

JOHNSON, MATT J., CO., Lakota, N. Dak.

JOHNSON OIL REFINING CO., 20 N. Wacker Dr., Chicago, Ill.

JOHNSON, OLIVER, & CO., Providence, R.I.

JOHNSON PRODUCTS CO., 5350 Broadway, Chicago 40, Ill.

JOHNSON, S. C., & SON, INC., Racine, Wis.

JOHNSON'S CLEANER CO., 16 W. Utica St., Buffalo, N.Y.

JOHNSTON, GASTON, CORP., 24-64 45th St., Long Island City, L. I., N.Y.

JOHNSTON, R. F., PAINT CO., 3925 Huston Ave., Cincinnati, Ohio.

JOLY LOTION, 1452 N.W. 24th St., Miami 42, Fla.

JONCAIRE TOILETRIES, 30 W. 24th St., New York 11, N.Y.

JONES, JOHN WILEY, CO., Caledonia, N.Y.

JONES PRODUCTS, INC., 167 2nd St., Cambridge, Mass.

JONJEEMS LABS., New Bern, N.C.

JORDEAU, JEAN, INC., 7 3rd St., South Orange, N.J.

JOY CHEMICAL, INC., 133 Webster St., Pawtucket, R.I.

JOYCE, JO ANN, 4317 Bell St., Kansas City 2, Mo.

J. N. T. MFG. CO., INC., New York, N.Y.

J. P. PRODUCTS CO., INC., 30 Douglas St., Hammond, Ind.

J. R. CO., Downers Grove, Ill.

J. R. PHARM CO., 2011 Edgmont Ave., Chester, Pa.

JULIENNE COSMETICS, 16 Main St., Tewksbury, Mass.

K

KADOL PHARM CO., 3312 DuBois Pl., S.E., Washington 19, D.C.

KAHLENBERG LABS., INC., Maine, Higel & Lodge, Sarasota, Fla.

K & B DRUG CO., 4246 Maxwell St., Detroit 14, Mich.

K AND W PRODUCTS, INC., 8319 Allport Ave., Whittier, Calif.

KANO LABORATORIES, 1000 S. Thompson Lane, Nashville 11, Tenn.

KANSAS CITY HOMEOPATHIC PHARMACY, 1408 Grand Ave., Kansas City 6, Mo.

KAOLOID CO., 154 E. Erie St., Chicago 11, Ill.

KARITH CHEMICAL CO., 815 W. Arthington St., Chicago 7, Ill.

K-ARMAND CO., P.O. Box 363, Lake Charles, La.

KARNAK CHEMICAL CO., Virginia Ave. & New St., West Chester, Pa.

KARRER CO., 810 N. Plankinton Ave., Milwaukee, Wis.

KARSEAL CORP., Hollywood, Calif.

K-A-S LABORATORY, 381 Flatbush Ave., Brooklyn 17, N.Y.

KAS-MO REMEDY CO., 949 7th St., Port Arthur, Tex.

KATCO PHARMACAL CO., P.O. Box 298, Montclair, N.J.

KAY PREPARATIONS CO., INC., 522 5th Ave., New York 36, N.Y.

KAZ MFG. CO., INC., 540 12th Ave., New York 36, N.Y.

KEEBER, DR., LABS, INC., 110 S. Bishop St., Dallas, Tex.

KEENAN LABORATORIES, INC., Frostproof, Fla.

KELLER CO., 28 S. Main St., Mechanicsburg, Ohio.

KELLEY, WALTER T., CO., Clarkson, Ky.

KELLOGG'S INSECTICIDE CO., P.O. Box 3145, Terminal Annex, Los Angeles 54, Calif.

KELLY AGRICULTURAL PRODUCTS CO., McKeesport, Pa.

KELLY, GEORGE J., INC., Lynn, Mass.

KEMP & LANE, INC., LeRoy, N.Y.

KENDALL, DR. B. J. CO., 532 Main St., Enosburg Falls, Vt.

KENDALL, C. B., CO., INC., 2039 Madison Ave., Indianapolis 6, Ind.

KENDALL REFINING CO., 1177 Kendall Ave., Bradford, Pa.

KENITE LABORATORY, 23 Samson Ave., Madison, N.J.

KENMORE PHARMACY INC., 500 Commonwealth Ave., Boston 15, Mass.

KENNEDY, W. ALAN, LTD., 112 McGill St., Montreal 1, Canada.

KENT CHEMICAL CO., INC., P.O. Box 154, Reading, Pa.

KENT CO., INC., 1324 Southwest Blvd., Kansas City 3, Kans.

KENTON PHARM. CO., INC., 423 Greenup St., Covington, Ky.

KENT SPECIALTIES CO., P.O. Box 408, Los Angeles, Calif.

KENYON PRODS., 420 Lexington Ave., New York 17, N.Y.

KEPEC CHEM. CORP., 4th & Cherry Sts., Milwaukee, Wis.

KEROS LABS., INC., 100 Beekman St., New York 38, N.Y.

KESSLER REMEDY CO., 417 State St., Erie, Pa.

KESTER SOLDER CO., 4201 Wrightwood Ave., Chicago 39, Ill.

KEY CO., P.O. Box 494, East St. Louis, Ill.

KEYSTONE CHEM. CO., INC., 2019 Center St., N.W., Cleveland 13, Ohio.

KEYSTONE LABS., INC., 491 S. 3rd St., Memphis 2, Tenn.

KEYSTONE PAINT & VARNISH CORP., 71 Otsego St., Brooklyn 31, N.Y.

KEYSTONE PLASTICS CO., 701 Painter St., Media, Pa.

KEYSTONE REFINING CO., 4821 Garden St., Philadelphia, Pa.

KIL BALM CO., 5578 N. 3rd St., Milwaukee 9, Wis.

KILGORE SEED CO., 1039 W. Cypress St., Gainesville, Fla.

KILMER & CO., INC., 375 Fairfield Ave., Stamford, Conn.

KIMBALL, C. M., CO., Board of Trade Bldg., 131 State St., Boston 9, Mass.

KIMBERLY-CLARK CORP., Neenah, Wis.

KINDL PRODUCTS, Ridgewood, N.J.

KINDLE-LITE CORP., 159 West St., Brooklyn 22, N.Y.

KING CALCIUM PRODUCTS, Campbellville, Ontario, Canada.

KING CHEMICAL CO., 2342 S. Lauderdale, Memphis 6, Tenn.

KING, E. & F., CO., INC., 640 Pleasant St., Norwood, Mass.

KING MANUFACTURING CO., 2601 Davison Rd., Flint 6, Mich.

KING RESEARCH, INC., 144 12th St., Brooklyn 15, N.Y.

KING, W. H. DRUG CO., 117 S. Wilmington St., Raleigh, N.C.

KING'S MEN, LTD., 11500 Tennessee Ave., Los Angeles 25, Calif.

KINRECO PRODUCTS, 720 W. 4th St., Topeka, Kans.

KIP, ALDRICH & CO., INC., 132 E. 2nd St., Mineola, L. I., N.Y.

KIP, INC., 778 E. Pico Blvd., Los Angeles 21, Calif.

KIRBY, GEO., JR., PAINT CO., 14 Wall St., New Bedford, Mass.

KIRBY'S MINERAL PRODUCTS, 15 Fike Ave., Union, S.C.

KIRCHNER LABS., INC., 11231 Superior Ave., Cleveland 6, Ohio.

KIRK, C. F., CO., 521 W. 23rd St., New York 11, N.Y.

KIRKMAN PHARM. CO., 1436 Elliott Ave., W., Seattle, Wash.

KIWI POLISH CO., PTY. LTD., 99 High St., Pottstown, Pa.

KLAUSS-WHITE CO., 1441 W. Poplar, San Antonio 7, Tex.

KLEAN-STRIP CO., INC., 2336 S. Lauderdale St., Memphis 6, Tenn.

KLEEN-A-SKIN LAB., 381 Flatbush Ave., Brooklyn 17, N.Y.

KLEER CO., P.O. Box 68, Bradford, Pa.

KLEEREX, INC., 2459 University Ave., St. Paul 4, Minn.

KLENZADE PRODUCTS, INC., Beloit, Wis.

KLINK CHEM. CORP., 463 Keap St., Brooklyn 11, N.Y.

KLINZMOTH CHEM. CORP., 519 E. 72nd St., New York 21, N.Y.

KLUTCH CO., Elmira, N.Y.

KNAPP MONARCH CO., Bent & Potomac Sts., St. Louis 16, Mo.

KNIGHT, MAURICE A., 171 Kelly Ave., Akron, Ohio.

KNOCK-EM STIFF PRODUCTS CO., 588 Crescent St., Brockton 44, Mass.

KNOMARK MANUFACTURING CO., INC., 330 Wythe Ave., Brooklyn 11, N.Y.

KNOX CO., 1651 N. Argyle, Los Angeles 28, Calif.

KOCH SUPPLIES, INC., 2520 Holmes St., Kansas City 8, Mo.

KOEHLER & KOEHLER LABS., 815 W. St. Paul Ave., Milwaukee, Wis.

KOEHLER'S LAB., 4133 La. Crosse Ave., Cincinnati 27, Ohio.

KOENIG LABS., 116 N. Paulina St., Chicago 12, Ill.

KOHLER MFG. CO., INC., 220 W. 19th St., New York 11, N.Y.

KOHLER-McLISTER PAINT CO., 1275 Osage, Denver, Colo.

KOHNSTAMM, H. & CO., INC., 83 Park Place, New York 7, N.Y.

KOJENE PRODS. CORP., 80 Main St., W., Rochester 11, N.Y.

KOKEN CO., Broadway & Tyler Sts., St Louis 6, Mo.

KOMPOLITE CO., INC., 11 44th Rd., Long Island City 1, L. I., N.Y.

KONDON MFG. CO., 2608 Nicollet Ave., Minneapolis 8, Minn.

KONGO CHEM. CO., INC., 204 W. 124th St., New York 27, N.Y.

KOPERTOX LABS., Simsbury, Conn.

KOPF MFG. CO., INC., 49 Warren St., New York 7, N.Y.

KOPP, RUTH N. 334 E. Poplar St., York 1, Pa.

KOPPERS CO., INC., Pittsburgh 19, Pa.

KOREX CO., 523 W. Nine Mile Rd., Ferndale 20, Mich.

KORLIS, LTD., 285 Broadway, New York, N.Y.

KORY PRODUCTS, INC., 236 W. 15th St., New York, N.Y.

KOSS, PAUL, SUPPLY CO., 900 Folsom St., San Francisco 7, Calif.

KOTALKO SALES CO., 111 Academy St., Jersey City, N.J.

K PRODUCTS CO., 910 Boston Bldg., Salt Lake City 1, Utah.

K-R LABORATORIES, 511 Olive St., Seattle 1, Wash.

KRAUPNER & KRAUPNER, INC., 1375 Myrtle Ave., Brooklyn 37, N.Y.

KRAUPNER PHARMACEUTICAL CO., Brooklyn, N.Y.

KREMBS & CO., 669 W. Ohio St., Chicago 10, Ill.

KREMERS-URBAN CO., Milwaukee 1, Wis.

KRESO-TOL CORP., Jamestown, N.Y.

KRESS AND OWEN CO., P.O. Box 167, Middletown, N.J.

KRIEGER CO., P.O. Box 13, St. Joseph, Mich.

KRISTEE PRODUCTS CO., 44 N. Summit, Akron 8, Ohio.

K-R-O CO., 19 N. Limestone St., Springfield 99, Ohio.

KROMALL CHEMICAL & DISPERSIONS CORP., 10-20 46th Ave., Long Island City, L. I., N.Y.

KROY PRODUCTS, INC., 153 W. 27th St., New York 1, N.Y.

KRYLON, INC., Ford & Washington Sts., Norristown, Pa.

KUDYMERN SALES ORG., (Cuzalina Drug Co.), 201 E. Grand Ave., Ponca City, Okla.

KUHN MEDICINE CO., 935 Hollywood Way, Burbank, Calif.

KUHN PAINT CO., Houston, Tex.

KUMFORT DRUG PRODUCTS CO., 1362 W. 6th St., Cleveland 13, Ohio.

KURFEES, J. F. PAINT CO., 201 E. Market, Louisville, Ky.

KURLASH CO., INC., 128 South Ave., Rochester 4, N.Y.

KWIK-FYRE KINDLER CO., 204 W. 4th St., Royal Oak, Mich.

L

LABCO PET PRODUCTS CO., 285 Franklin St., Boston 10, Mass.

LACONIA LABORATORIES, Laconia, N.H.

LACO PRODUCTS, INC., 4201 Pulaski Hgwy., Baltimore, Md.

LA CROSSE PHARM. CO., 101 State St., LaCrosse, Wis.

LA DANA LABS., INC., 705 S. 16th St., Omaha 2, Neb.

LADY AMERICA, INC., 326 W. Kalamazoo Ave., Kalamazoo, Mich.

LADY ANDRES PERFUMERS, INC., 1344 U St., N.W., Washington, D.C.

LADY ESTHER, 7171 W. 65th St., Chicago, Ill.

LADY LENNOX CO., 544 S. Main St., Memphis 2, Tenn.

LADY'S CHOICE FOODS, 1237 Minnesota St., San Francisco 7, Calif.

LAFAYETTE PHARM., INC., 526 N. Earl Ave., Lafayette, Ind.

LA FORD CHEM. CO., INC., 105 N. Bradley Ave., Indianapolis 1, Ind.

LA FRE LABS., INC., 308 York Ave., Philadelphia 6, Pa.

LAIRD, R. H., CO., 785 5th Ave., New York 22, N.Y.

LAKE CHEMICAL CO., 3070 W. Carroll Ave., Chicago, Ill.

LAKE COUNTRY AGR. COMM., P.O. Box 2, Kelseyville, Calif.

LAKE LABORATORIES, Box 3925, Strathmoor Station, Detroit, Mich.

LAMAC PROCESS CO., 1253 W. 12th St., Erie 6, Pa.

LA MAUR, INC., Minneapolis 2, Minn.

LAMB & BERLIN PHARMACEUTICALS, 901 Pershing Dr., Silver Spring, Md.

LAMBERT PHARM. CO., Div. of Warner-Lambert Pharm., St. Louis 6, Mo.

LA-MO LABS, INC., 2015 E. 65th St., Cleveland 3, Ohio.

LAMOND PRODS., INC., 954 Rogers Ave., Brooklyn 26, N.Y.

LANCASTER, INC., 6700 11th Ave., Los Angeles 43, Calif.

LANCASTER PAINT AND GLASS CO., Lancaster, Pa.

LANDEN PUTTY WORKS, INC., 45 Irving St., Malden, Mass.

LANDON LABORATORIES, 117 W. 67th St. Terr., Kansas City, Mo.

LANGLOIS, Boston, Mass.

LANIKOL CO., 217 N. Water St., Milwaukee, Wis.

LANMAN & KEMP-BARCLAY & CO., INC., 135 Water St., New York 5, N.Y.

LANOLAVE LABS., Box 89, Waco, Tex.

LAN-O-SHEEN INC., 804 Finch Bldg., St. Paul 1, Minn.

LANOTAN, INC., (formerly Peau D'Or Sales Corp.), 601 N.E. 13th St., Miami 32, Fla.

LA PLACE, L. J. & M., 10 Lediart Lane, Paterson, N.J.

LA PLAYA PRODUCTS, INC., 122 W. 26th St., New York 1, N.Y.

LARKIN PRODUCTS, INC., 191 Van Rensselaer St., Buffalo 10, N.Y.

LARROQUE DRUG CO., 1317 Main St., Jeanerette, La.

LARSON LABS., INC., P.O. Box 484, Erie, Pa.

LA RUE-AXTELL PUMICE CO., Eustis, Nebr.

LARVACIDE PRODUCTS, INC., 117 Liberty St., New York 6, N.Y.

LA SALLE LABS., INC., 3021 Wabash Ave., Detroit 16, Mich.

LASCOFF, J. LEON, & SON, INC., 1209 Lexington Ave., New York 28, N.Y.

LASCOFF LABORATORIES, INC., 150 E. 82nd St., New York 28, N.Y.

LASER LABS., Foshay Tower, Minneapolis 2, Minn.

LASTIK PRODUCTS CO., INC., Forbes & Meyrau Ave., Pittsburgh 13, Pa.

LASTING PRODUCTS CO., Franklintown Rd., Baltimore, Md.

LA VAL LABS., 411 N. Charles St., Baltimore 1, Md.

LA VELL LABS., 6 River St., Dundee, Ill.

LAVO COMPANY OF AMERICA, 300 N. 7th St., Milwaukee, Wis.

LAVOPTIK CO., 661 Western Ave. N., St. Paul 3, Minn.

LAVORIS CO., 918 3rd St., N., Minneapolis 1, Minn.

LAWRENCE LABORATORIES, INC., 55 W. 42nd St., New York 36, N.Y.

LAWRENCE, W. W. & CO., 1124 W. Carson St., Pittsburgh, Pa.

LAWRENCE-WILLIAMS CO., Cleveland, Ohio.

LAWTER CHEMICALS, INC., 3550 Touby Ave., Chicago 45, Ill.

LAXA-PIRIN CO., INC., 366 S. Meridian St., Indianapolis, Ind.

LAZARIN CO., 99 Tracy Pl., Hewlett, L. I., N.Y.

LEA MANUFACTURING CO., 16 Cherry Ave., Waterbury 20, Conn.

LEAF OIL LABORATORIES, LTD., Sutton, Nebr.

LEAVENS PRODS. CO., 1324 South West Blvd., Kansas City 3, Kans.

LEBANON CHEMICAL CORP. (See Central Chemical), Lebanon, Pa.

LE BLANC CORP., Lafayette, La.

LECKENBY, HARRY N., CO., Duvall, Seattle, Wash.

LEDERLE LABS.DIV., American Cyanamid Co., 30 Rockefeller Pl., New York, N.Y.

LEE, GEO. H., CO., 1115 Harney St., Omaha 8, Nebr.

LEE LIMITED, 25 W. 45th St., New York 36, N.Y.

LEE RUBBER & TIRE CORP., Conshohocken, Pa.

LEE, SYDNEY, BEAUTY REQUISITES, 15 Intervale Rd., Wellesley Hills 82, Mass.

LEE, WM. W., & CO., INC., Watervliet, N.Y.

LEECH PRODUCTS CO., 4th & Hendricks St., Hutchinson, Kans.

LEEMING, THOMAS, & CO., INC., 155 E. 44th St., New York 17, N.Y.

LEFCOURT PHARMACEUTICAL, 400 Forest Ave., W. New Brighton, L. I., N.Y.

LE FEVRE CHEMICAL CO., 1639 W. Main St., Oklahoma City, Okla.

LE FEVRE, JOSEPHINE CO., 6734 Woolston St., Philadelphia 38, Pa.

LEFFINGWELL CHEMICAL CO., Whittier, Calif.

LE GEAR, DR. L. D., MED. CO., 4161 Beck Ave., St. Louis 16, Mo.

LEGENDRE'S, INC., 124 Baronne St., New Orleans 12, La.

LEGGE, WALTER A., CO., INC., 101-A Park Ave., New York, N.Y.

LEGULO, 5618 W. Eddy St., Chicago 34, Ill.

LEHMAN BROS., 1830 St. Clair Ave., Cleveland 14, Ohio.

LEHMAN BROS. CORP., 22 Halladay St., Jersey City, N. J.

LEHN & FINK PRODUCTS CORP., 445 Park Ave., New York 22, N.Y.

LEHON CO., 4411 S. Oakley Ave., Chicago, Ill.

LEIGHTON, SARA S., LABS., 1220 W. 104th St., Cleveland 2, Ohio.

LEKTROLITE CORP., 545 5th Ave., New York 17, N.Y.

LENASON CO., 1260 W. 4th St., Cleveland 13, Ohio.

LENEVA LABS., 1266 S. 13th St., Omaha, Neb.

LENK MANUFACTURING CO., 30 Cummington St., Boston 15, Mass.

LENTHÉRIC, INC., 745 5th Ave., New York, N.Y.

LEONARD CO., 506 3rd St., Des Moines, Iowa.

LEONARDI, S. B. & CO., INC., 27 Railroad Ave., New Rochelle, N.Y.

LEONHARDT, DR., CO., 327 Washington St., Buffalo 3, N.Y.

LEONID DE LESCINSKIS, 49 W. 46th St., New York 36, N.Y.

LE PAGE'S, INC., Essex Ave., Gloucester, Mass.

LE PRINCE, INC., 799 Broadway, New York 3, N.Y.

LESBERT DRUG CO., 1598 Laclede Rd., Cleveland 21, Ohio.

LESLIE & CO., 20 E. 53rd St., New York 22, N.Y.

LESLIE PHARMACAL CO., 9 E. Blackwell St., Dover, N.J.

LESTER DRUG CO., INC., 241 Main St., Buffalo 3, N.Y.

LESTER LABS., LTD., P.O. Box 4897, Atlanta 2, Ga.

LETHELIN PRODUCTS CO., INC., 15 MacQuesten Parkway, S., Mt. Vernon, N.Y.

LETO REMEDY CO., 503 Taft Blvd., San Antonio 11, Tex.

LEVER BROTHERS CO., 390 Park Ave., New York 22, N.Y.

LEVIS, JOHN A., & SONS, INC., 330 Lyell Ave., Rochester 6, N.Y.

LEWAL INDUSTRIES, INC., 150 E. 35th St., New York 16, N.Y.

LEWAL PHARMACEUTICAL CO., 2735 N. Ashland Ave., Chicago 14, Ill.

LEWIS-HOWE CO., 319 S. 4th St., St. Louis 2, Mo.

LEWY CHEMICAL CO., 707 Broadway, New York 3, N.Y.

LIBBY OIL & CHEMICAL CO., Rockford, Ill.

LIBBY, Research Division, 66 Phoenix Row, Haverhill, Mass.

LIBERTY CHEMICAL LAB., Division of Liberty Insecticides, Inc., P.O. Box 156, Franklin Park, Ill.

LICK, INC., 3929 Kipling Ave., Minneapolis, Minn.

LIEBERT, HELEN, 767 5th Ave., New York 22, N.Y.

LIEBICH, G. I., CO., 931 N. Ogden Ave., Chicago, Ill.

LIEN CHEM. CO., 9229 W. Grand Ave., Franklin Park, Ill.

LILLY, ELI & CO., Indianapolis 6, Ind.

LINCK, O. E. CO., INC., Clifton, N.J.

LINCO PRODUCTS CORP., 2155 W. 80th St., Chicago, Ill.

LINK CHEMICAL CO., 206 W. 82nd St., Kansas City 5, Mo.

LINO-PASTE CO., 1948 Carroll Ave., Chicago, Ill.

LINTON, McINTOSH, Hadley, N.Y.

LINTON PENCIL CO., Lewisburg, Tenn.

LIQUID VENEER CORP., 144-172 Urban St., Buffalo 11, N.Y.

LITLE, T. J., INC., 118 Meadow Lane, Grosse Pointe 30, Mich.

LITTLE BEAR SPECIALTIES CO., INC., 3840 Bennington Ave., Kansas City 3, Mo.

LITTLE WONDER CO., 613 Bonham St., Grand Prairie, Tex.

LIX CO., Distributors, 3112 Guardian Bldg., Detroit 26, Mich.

L. & K. LABORATORIES & CO., 500 N. Robert St., St. Paul 5, Minn.

LLOYD BROTHERS, Cincinnati 3, Ohio.

LOCKHART, P. O., Perry, Fla.

LOCKWOOD, LAWRENCE A., CO., 232 E. Erie St., Chicago 11, Ill.

LONDON'S, DR., PRODUCTS, INC., College Grove, Tenn.

LONG, CHARLES R., JR., Louisville, Ky.

LONG ISLAND PAINT & CHEMICAL CO., Glen Cove, L. I., N.Y.

LONG MFG. CO., 991 Williams St., San Leandro, Calif.

LONGMAN & MARTINEZ, INC., N. 9th & Roebling Sts., Brooklyn, N.Y.

LONGO, INC., 37 E. 19th St., New York 3, N.Y.

LONGVIEW PAINT & VARNISH CO., Longview, Wash.

LORD, F. T., POLISH CO., 14 Alden St., Boston, Mass.

LORENZ CHEMICAL CO., 17th & Nicholas Sts., Omaha 2, Nebr.

LORR LABS., 200 Godwin Ave., Paterson 1, N.J.

LOS ANGELES CHEMICAL CO., 1960 Santa Fe Ave., Los Angeles 21, Calif.

LOS ANGELES SOAP CO., WHITE KING SOAP CO., 617 E. 1st St., Los Angeles 54, Calif.

LOTSHAW, ANDY, CO., 126 N. Clinton St., Chicago 6, Ill.

LOUISIANA DRUG CO., INC., Lombard & Cherry Sts., Opelousas, La.

LOUISVILLE PAINT MFG. CO., 1110 W. Main St., Louisville, Ky.

LOUISVILLE VARNISH MFG. CO., 1400 Maple St., Louisville 10, Ky.

L & R MFG. CO., 577 Elm St., Arlington, N.J.

L. & S. LABS., INC., 236 N. Broad St., Fremont, Nebr.

LUCA PRODUCTS CO., W. 4th & Hendricks Sts., Hutchinson, Kans.

LUCAS, JOHN & CO., INC., 1617 Pennsylvania Blvd., Philadelphia 3, Pa.

LUCERNE CORP., Pulaski, Va.

LUCKY STAR MFG. CO., 441 W. 6th St., Cincinnati 3, Ohio.

LUCKY TIGER MFG. CO., 544 W. 6th St., Cincinnati 3, Ohio.

LUEBERT, A. G., 126 S. 5th Ave., Coatesville, Pa.

LUFT, CO., GEORGE W., 34-12 36th Ave., Long Island City 1, L. I., N.Y.

LURA-GLO LABS., 1504 32nd St., Oakland 8, Calif.

LUSTERINE MFG. CO., INC., 36 River St., Bridgeport, Conn.

LUSTRAY LABS., 127 Green St., Brooklyn 22, N.Y.

LUSTRO-LEAF, INC., 538 Madison Ave., New York, N.Y.

LUXURY IMPORTS, INC., 385 5th Ave., New York 16, N.Y.

LUZIER'S, INC., 3210 Gillham Plaza, Kansas City, Mo.

LYK-NU CO., INC., 279 E. 139th St., New York 54, N.Y.

LYNWOOD CO., INC., 7716 W. North Ave., Chicago 35, Ill.

LYON, J. C., 10 Pine St., South Norwalk, Conn.

LYONS, I. L. & CO., LTD., 800 Tehoupitoulas St., New Orleans 11, La.

LYONS, J., & CO., LTD., INC., 812 Jersey Ave., Jersey City 2, N.J.

M

MAAS, ALBERT G., CO., 155 E. Maryland St., Indianapolis 4, Ind.

MAAS & WALDSTEIN CO., 2121 Mc Carter Hgwy., Newark, N.J.

MAC DERMID, W. D., CHEMICAL CO., Bristol, Conn.

MAC DONALD'S REMEDIES, 53 Washington St., Binghamton, N.Y.

MACE LABS., INC., 319 Main St., Neenak, Wis.

MAC ESLIN & CO., 214 W. Market St., York, Pa.

MAC GREGOR, INC., 1513 N. Larrabee St., Chicago 10, Ill.

MACKLANBURG-DUNCAN CO., P.O. Box 1197, Oklahoma City, Okla.

MACK'S MEDICAL CO., INC., Waltham, Mass.

MACLEAN, NEIL A., CO., INC., 470 8th St., San Francisco 3, Calif.

MACNEAL, JAMES B., & CO., Warner & Worcester Sts., Baltimore, Md.

MACY'S, New York, N.Y.

MADE RITE PRODUCTS CO., 2408 7th St., St. Louis, Mo.

MADEMOISELLE TOILETRIES, INC., 6237 S. Prairie Ave., Chicago 37, Ill.

MAFF, JOHN, INC., 80 E. Peddle St., Newark, N.J.

MAGAY CORP., P.O. Box 74, Bayside 60, N.Y.

MAGIC-FOAM SALES CORP., 15 W. Pearl St., Cincinnati 2, Ohio.

MAGIC FUT-EZ CO., INC., West Bend, Wis.

MAGIC IRON CEMENT CO., 1366 E. 34th St., Cleveland 14, Ohio.

MAGICLEANER CO., 55 Jones St., Newark 3, N.J.

MAGIC POLISH CO., INC., New York, N.Y.

MAGIC SEAL INDUSTRIES, P.O. Box 1032, Oakland 4, Calif.

MAGITEX CO., INC., 144 Main St., Saco, Me.

MAGNUS CHEMICAL CO., 3 Kreie St., Garwood, N.J.

MAHDEEN CO., 260 North St., Nacogdoches, Tex.

MAID-EASY CLEANSING PRODUCTS, CORP., 25 Elm Ave., Mount Vernon, N.Y.

MAINES, E. L., CO., Rutland, Mass.

MAJESTIC DRUG CO., 2061 Bronx St., Bronx 60, N.Y.

MAKERS OF KAL, INC., 256 N. New Hampshire Ave., Los Angeles 4, Calif.

MAKO PHARM. CO., 132 S. Highland Ave., Pittsburgh 6, Pa.

MALEX CHEMICAL CORP., 1109 E. 8th St., Los Angeles 21, Calif.

MALLARD, INC., 3021 Wabash Ave., Detroit 16, Mich.

MALLEABLE, INC., 546 W. Washington St., Chicago, Ill.

MALLINCKRODT CHEMICAL WORKS, 72 Gold St., New York 8, N.Y.

MALLON DIV., Doho Chemical Corp., 100 Varick St., New York 13, N.Y.

MALTBIE LABS., 240 High St., Newark 1, N.J.

MANATEE CHEMICALS, INC., 2000 27th St., E., Bradenton, Fla.

MANCO CHEMICAL CO., 500 Santa Fe Dr., Denver 4, Colo.

MANHATTAN DRUG CO., 156 Tillary St., Brooklyn 1, N.Y.

MANHATTAN KREOLE PRODUCTS, INC., N. 10th St. & Bedford Ave., Brooklyn, N.Y.

MANHATTAN SOAP CO., INC., Bristol, Pa.

MANHATTAN SOAP CO., 441 Lexington Ave., New York, N.Y.

MANN CHEMICAL CO., 2972 Rochester St., Detroit 6, Mich.

MANN, LEO, & CO., 160 N. Washington St., Boston 14, Mass.

MANNING POWDER CO., P.O. Box 1201, Fort Worth 1, Tex.

MANON FRERES, INC., 440 Pearl St., New York 7, N.Y.

MAN-O-WAR REMEDY CO., P.O. Box 22, Lima, Pa.

MANSON DISTRIBUTORS, 220 Fox St., Aurora, Ill.

MARCELLE COSMETICS, INC., 1741 N. Western Ave., Chicago 47, Ill.

MARCHAND, CHARLES, CO., 521 W. 23rd St., New York 11, N.Y.

MARCUS-LESOINE, Whitehouse Station, N.J.

MARIETA MFG. CO., 4000 E. 16th St., Indianapolis, Ind.

MARIN COUNTY AGR. COM., 519 4th St., San Rafael, Calif.

MARINE COATINGS, INC., 63 Prospect St., Brooklyn, N.Y.

MARINE ELECTROLYSIS ELIMINATOR CO., 617 Dearborn St., Seattle 4, Wash.

MARINE LABS. OF AMERICA, INC., 109 3rd St., Brooklyn, N.Y.

MARION LABS., INC., Grand Ave. at 29th St., Kansas City, Mo.

MARION PHARMACAL LABS., P.O. Box 3, Sunnyside Sta., Long Island City, L. I., N.Y.

MARK LABS., INC., 120 S. Homewood Ave., Pittsburgh 8, Pa.

MARKWELL MFG. CO., 200 Hudson St., New York, N.Y.

MARLENE'S, INC., 349 W. Ontario, Chicago, Ill.

MARLO PRODUCTS CO., 1430 W. 9th St., Cleveland 13, Ohio.

MAR-O-MIST, INC., 3033 N. Clark St., Chicago 14, Ill.

MAR-O-VEL CO., 207 S. Broadway, Oklahoma City 2, Okla.

MAR-PRODS. CO., P.O. Box 2548, Jacksonville, Fla.

MARRIOTT LAB., S. Grand & McArthur Blvd., Springfield, Ill.

MARROW'S, INC., 657 W. Chicago, Chicago, Ill.

MARTIN, C. J., & SONS, INC., P.O. Box 1133, Austin, Tex.

MARTIN DENNIS CO., Newark, N.J.

MARTIN HERB CO., P.O. Box 65, Parnassus Sta., New Kensington, Pa.

MARTIN, L., CO., INC., 380 Madison Ave., New York 17, N.Y.

MARTIN-PARRY CORP., P.O. Box 954, Toledo 1, Ohio.

MARTIN-SENOUR PAINTS, 2520 Quarry St., Chicago 8, Ill.

MARTIN VARNISH CO., 900 W. 49th St., Chicago, Ill.

MARTINDALE ELECTRIC CO., 1365 Hird Rd., Cleveland, Ohio.

MARTO PRODUCTS CO., Cleveland, Ohio.

MARVAN PRODUCTS, 1834 E. 2nd St., Brooklyn 23, N.Y.

MARVEL INDUSTRIES, INC., 134 Crosby St., San Antonio 8, Tex.

MARVELL PHARMACAL CO., 55 W. 16th St., New York 11, N.Y.

MARYLAND PHARM. CO., 2419 Greenmount Ave., Baltimore 18, Md.

MASCO CHEMICAL CO., Kearny, N.J.

MASIE, H. H., TOILETRIES, 24 E. 21st St., New York 10, N.Y.

MASON HAIR DYE CO., 1403 Hawthorne Pl., St. Louis 17, Mo.

MASSENGILL, S. E., CO., 527 5th St., Bristol, Tenn.

MASTER BRONZE POWDER CO., 5009 Calumet Ave., Hammond, Ind.

MASTER LABS., 2523 Leavenworth, Omaha 1, Nebr.

MASURY, JOHN W., & SON, INC., 1700 Bayard St., Baltimore, Md.

MATERIALS & TREATMENT CO., INC., North Ave. & 3rd St., Milwaukee, Wis.

MATTHEW PRODUCTS, INC., 117 E. 24th St., New York 10, N.Y.

MAURRY, H. E., BIOLOGICAL CO., 6109 S. Western Ave., Los Angeles 47, Calif.

MAUTZ PAINT & VARNISH CO., Madison, Wis.

MAXWELL INSECTICIDE CO., P.O. Box 5627, Raleigh, N.C.

MAY, D. R., SEED CO., Knoxville 7, Tenn.

MAYBELLINE CO., 5900 N. Ridge Ave., Chicago, Ill.

MAYER, F. G., DRUG, Division of Zotox Pharmacal Co., Inc., Stamford, Conn.

MAYFAIR LABS., 900 Hansen Pl., Park Ridge, Ill.

MAYNARD, INC., 2341 Milwaukee Ave., Chicago 47, Ill.

MAYO, D. R., SEED CO., 4718 Kingston Pike, Knoxville 7, Tenn.

MAYOR CO., Lake Quivira, Kansas City, Mo.

MAYOR PHARMACAL CO., Rochester, Minn.

MAYPINKS CO., 300 Main St., Avon-By-The-Sea, N.J.

M. B. C. CHEMICAL SERVICE CO., 341 Wall St., Tracy, Calif.

MC ADAMS & MORFOD, INC., 200 W. Main St., Lexington 6, Ky.

MC ALEER MFG. DIV., McAleer Sq., Rochester, Mich.

MC ALESTER FUEL CO., P.O. Box 783, McAlester, Okla.

MC CAMBRIDGE & MC CAMBRIDGE CO., 6400 Rhode Island Ave., Riverdale, Md.

MC CLELLAN, C. U., LABS., CORP., 321 W. Redondo Beach Blvd., Gardena, Calif.

MC CONNON & CO., Division of the Mackwin Co., Winona, Minn.

MC CORMICK & CO., INC., Baltimore 2, Md.

MC DONALD O'BRIAN CO., 581 Boylston St., Boston, Mass.

MC DOUGALL-BUTLER CO., INC., 2825 Main St., Buffalo, N.Y.

MC FARLIN, FAYE, 326 Alderson Ave., Billings, Mont.

MC GUIRE-WOODLOCK PAINT CO., 1620 W. Monroe St., Chicago, Ill.

MC ILLWAIN DRUG CO., 111 W. Main St., Parsons, Tenn.

MC KELVY, ALFRED D., CO., 60 West St., Bloomfield, N.J.

MC KESSON & ROBBINS, INC., Bridgeport 9, Conn.; 155 E. 44th St., New York 17, N.Y.

MC KESSON & ROBBINS, INC., Van Vleet-Ellis Division, 109 S. 2nd St., Memphis 11, Tenn.

MC KEWEN, G. E., & CO., 1-3 N. Carey St., Baltimore 23, Md.

MC LAUGHLIN GORMLY KING CO., 1715 S. E. 5th St., Minneapolis 14, Minn.

MC MURRAY DRUG CO., Abbeville, S.C.

MC MURTRY MFG. CO., 1533 Arapahoe, Denver, Colo.

MC NEIL DRUG CO., INC., 849 Florida Ave., Jacksonville 3, Fla.

MC PHAIL PRODUCTS CO., 2021 Kuhl Ave., Orlando 10, Fla.

MC QUADE DRUG STORE, 22 Clifton Ave., Ansonia, Conn.

MC QUADE, JOHN, & CO., 229 E. 42nd St., New York, N.Y.

MC VICKER, W. B., CO., 295 Douglas St., Brooklyn, N.Y.

MECHANICAL PROCESS CO., 388 Valley St., S. Orange, N.J.

MECO PRODUCTS CO., Chicago, Ill.

MEDICAL ARTS LABORATORIES, INC., P.O. Box 432, Tuscaloosa, Ala.

MEDICAL CHEMICALS CORP., 4122 W. Grand Ave., Chicago 51, Ill.

MEDICAL CHEMICALS, INC., 406 E. Water St., Baltimore 2, Md.

MEDICO CHEM. CORP. OF AMERICA, 15 E. 40th St., New York, 16, N.Y.

MEDICONE CO., 225 Varick St., New York 14, N.Y.

MEDI-PED LABS., INC., P.O. Box 145, Westwood, N.J.

MEDIPHAR LABS., INC., 308 W. Lombard St., Baltimore 1, Md.

MEHRON, INC., 150 W. 46th St., New York 19, N.Y.

MEL-O-WAX PRODUCTS, INC., 331 E. Lancaster Ave., Wynnewood, Pa.

MELVIN CO., 1608 Mission St., South Pasadena, Calif.

MEM CO., 67 Irving Pl., New York 3, N.Y.

MENLEY & JAMES, LTD., 91-27 138th Pl., Jamaica 35, L. I., N.Y.

MENNEN CO., 345 Central Ave., Newark 4, N.J.

MENTHOLATUM CO., 1360 Niagara St., Buffalo 13, N.Y.

MENTHO-LISTINE CHEM. CO., 1211 Willard St., Houston 6, Tex.

MENTOS PRODUCTS CO., INC., 6010 Haverford Ave., Philadelphia 31, Pa.

MEN-ZO-LIN PRODUCTS CO., INC., P.O. Box 153, Fredonia, N.Y.

M. E. PHARMACAL CO., 4420 Old York Rd., Philadelphia 40, Pa.

MERCHANT BROS., 14 East St., Danvers, Mass.; 30 E. Main St., Gloucester, Mass.

MERCHANTS & MFRS. PAINT CO., 108 S. 2nd St., Louisville, Ky.

MERCIREX CO., Milford, Del.

MERCK & CO., INC., Rahway, N.J.

MERIX CHEMICAL CO., 1021 E. 55th St., Chicago 15, Ill.

MERKIN, M. J., PAINT CO., 1441 Broadway, New York, N.Y.

MERLEE, INC., 300 Roanoke Bldg., Minneapolis 2, Minn.

MERRELL, WM. S., CO., Lockland Station, Cincinnati 15, Ohio.

MERRICK MEDICINE CO., 501 S. 8th St., Waco, Tex.

MERRY MFG. CO., 952 Gest St., Cincinnati 3, Ohio.

MERSON PRODUCTS CO., 67 Essex St., Jersey City, N.J.

MERTENS & SON, 2000 Terrace Pl., Nashville 3, Tenn.

METAL TRIMS, INC., 2857 Wilson Ave., Youngstown, Ohio.

METROPOLITAN REFINING CO., INC., 50 23rd St., Long Island City 1, L. I., N.Y.

MEYER & CO., 16361 Mack Ave., Detroit 24, Mich.

MEYER BROS. DRUG CO., 217 S 4th St., St. Louis 2, Mo.

MEYER, CHAS., 11 E. 12th St., New York 3, N.Y.

MEYER, THEODORE, EST., 213 S. 10th St., Philadelphia 7, Pa.

MEZZACON PRODUCTS CO., 17510 St. Clair Ave., Cleveland 10, Ohio.

M & H LABS., 2705 Archer Ave., Chicago, Ill.

MIAHATI, INC., 381 4th Ave., New York 16, N.Y.

MIAMI PRODUCTS & CHEMICAL CO., 530 Lonoke St., Dayton, Ohio.

MICHIGAN CHEMICAL CORP., St. Louis, Mich.

MIDCONTINENT PAINT & LACQUER CO., 1921 Central St., Kansas City, Mo.

MIDDLETON, BASIL, Culver, Ind.

MIDLAND COLOR & CHEMICAL CO., 15 Greene St., Jersey City, N.J.

MIDLAND LABS., Dubuque, Iowa.

MIDWEST MFG. CO., 17126 Schaeffer Hgwy., Detroit 35, Mich.

MIGHTY MENDER CO., 103 S. Jefferson St., Kittanning, Pa.

MILBER DRUG PRODUCTS, 2669 N. 76th St., Milwaukee 10, Wis.

MILBURN CO., 3246 E. Woodbridge Ave., Detroit 7, Mich.

MILES LABS., INC., Elkhart, Ind.

MILEX PRODUCTS, 3935 Irving Park Rd., Chicago 18, Ill.

MILLER CHEMICAL & FERTILIZER CORP., 2226 N. Howard St., Baltimore 18, Md.

MILLER CHEMICAL CO., 525 N. 15th St., Omaha 2, Nebr.

MILLER PAINT & WALL PAPER CO., 317 S.E. Grand St., Portland, Ore.

MILLER PRODUCTS CO., Ft. of S.W. Caruthers, Portland, Oreg.

MILLER PROTECTO PRODUCTS CO., 1317 S. Westnedge Ave., Kalamazoo 41, Mich.

MILLIGAN BROS. SYSTEM, 117 S. Wilson Ave., Jefferson, Iowa.

MILLOT, F., 683 5th Ave., New York 22, N.Y.

MILNER PRODUCTS CO., P.O. Box 4465, Fondren Sta., Jackson, Miss.

MILROSE PRODUCTS CO., 306 W. 117th St., New York 26, N.Y.

MINE SAFETY APPLIANCES CO., 201 N. Braddock Ave., Pittsburgh, Pa.

MINER-HILLARD MILLING CO., 1426 W. 3rd St., Wilkes-Barre, Pa.

MINER'S, INC., 36 E. 12th St., New York 3, N.Y.

MINNESOTA CHEMICAL CO., 2885 Hampden Ave., St. Paul, Minn.

MIRACLE ADHESIVES CORP., 214 E. 53rd St., New York 22, N.Y.

MIRRORLIKE MFG. CO., Queens Blvd., Long Island City, L. I., N.Y.

MISCIBLE PRODUCTS, INC., Belmar, N.J.

MISSION PHARMACAL CO., P.O. Box 1676, San Antonio 6, Tex.

MISSOURI PAINT & VARNISH CO., 5125 N. 2nd St., St. Louis, Mo.

MITCHELL SEED & GRAIN CO., 601 N. Virginia, Roswell, N. Mex.

MODART, INC., 520 Plymouth Bldg., Minneapolis 2, Minn.

MODERN CHEMICAL SPECIALITIES
CORP., 86 Industrial St., Rochester,
N.Y.

MODERN METAL PRODUCTS CO.,
18 Ames, Cambridge 42, Mass.

MODERN PRODUCTS INC., 1428 N.
24th St., Milwaukee 5, Wis.

MODERN SUPPLY CO., 837 W. North
Ave., Pittsburgh 33, Pa.

MOFFETT, C. J., MEDICINE CO.,
Columbus, Ga.

MONROE CHEMICAL CO., 301 Oak
St., Quincy, Ill.

MONROE CO., INC., 10700 Quebec
Ave., Cleveland, Ohio.

MONROE SANDER CORP., 10-20 46th
Ave., Long Island City, L. I., N.Y.

MONSANTO CHEMICAL CO., 445
Park Ave., New York 22, N.Y.

MONTE CHRISTO COSMETIC CO.,
12 E. 22nd St., New York 10, N.Y.

MONTEIL MFG. CORP., 38-14 30th
St., Long Island City 1, L. I., N.Y.

MONTENIER, JULES, INC., 440 W.
Superior St., Chicago 10, Ill.

MONTGOMERY WARD, New York,
N.Y.

MONTICELLO DRUG CO., 45 Broad
St., Viaduct, Jacksonville 4, Fla.

MOORE, BENJAMIN & CO., 511
Canal St., New York, N.Y.

MOORE, JOHN HUDSON, CO.,
Division of Lambert Co., 681 5th
Ave., New York 22, N.Y.

MOORE-LELAND PAINT & OIL CO.,
Charleston, S.C.

MOORE MFG. CO., 128 Mt. Vernon
St., Springfield, Vt.

MOORE, SAMUEL, CHEMICAL CO.,
INC., Mantua, Ohio.

MORETEX CHEMICAL PRODUCTS,
314 W. Henry St., Spartanburg, S.C.

MORGAN, HARRY D., LABS., 707 N.
Vine St., Los Angeles 38, Calif.

MORGAN PRODUCTS CORP., 160 E.
127th St., New York 35, N.Y.

MORRIS DRUG CO., 7 E. Market St.,
York, Pa.

MORRIS PAINT & VARNISH CO.,
E. St. Louis, Ill.

MORTELL, J. W., CO., Kankakee, Ill.;
Lyndhurst, N.J.; Detroit, Mich.

MORTON PAINT MFG. CORP.,
Zanesville, Ohio.

MORTON PHARMACEUTICALS, 1625
N. Highland St., Memphis 8, Tenn.

MOSS CO., 183 St. Paul St.,
Rochester 4, N.Y.

MOSSO, C. A., CO., 215 S. Leavitt
St., Chicago 12, Ill.

MOTH KING CORP., Detroit, Mich.

MOTHER'S REMEDIES CORP., 30 S.
Washington St., Chicago, Ill.

MOTOMCO, INC., 10 Murray St.,
New York 7, N.Y.

MOUND CITY PAINT & COLOR CO.,
202 S. 9th St., St.Louis, Mo.

MOYER, J. BIRD, CO., INC., 117 N.
5th St., Philadelphia 6, Pa.

MU-COL CO., INC., 156 E. Tupper St.,
Buffalo 3, N.Y.

MUNSCH & CO., 2815 Decatur Ave.,
New York 58, N.Y.

MURALO CO., INC., Haskell, N.J.

MURD CO., 37 N. Mascher St.,
Philadelphia 6, Pa.

MURINE CO., INC., 660 N. Wabash
Ave., Chicago 11, Ill.

MURPHY, GEORGE, INC., 57 E. 9th
St., New York 3, N.Y.

MURPHY LABS., INC., 6908 Market
St., Upper Darby, Pa.

MURPHY PAINT DIVISION,
Interchemical Corp., Wooster,
Ohio.

MURPHY-PHOENIX CO., 9505
Cassius Ave., Cleveland 5, Ohio.

MURRAY, EDGAR A., CO., Division
of Fairfax Bio. Labs., Willow
Brook Rd., Clinton Corners, N.Y.

MURRAY-WILLIAMS COLOR &
CHEMICAL CO., 353 Boyden Ave.,
Maplewood, N.J.

MURRELL LABS., INC., P.O. Box
28, Norman, Okla.

MUSKEGON PAINT & VARNISH CO.,
Muskegon, Mich.

MUSTEROLE CO., 1748 E. 27th St.,
Cleveland 14, Ohio.

MY-ALGINE LABS., 897-899
Tonawanda St., Buffalo 7, N.Y.

MYERS LABORATORIES, INC.,
Warren, Pa.

MYERS, LOUIS H. 802 Martin Ave.,
Bryn Mawr, Pa.

MY-KO CHEMICAL CORP., 312 N.
Water St., Milwaukee 2, Wis.

MYSTIC FOAM CORP., 2003 St.
Clair Ave., Cleveland 14, Ohio.

N

"NA-CHURS" PLANT FOOD CO.,
421 Monroe St., Marion, Ohio.

NACOR MED. CO., 15 E. Washington
St., Indianapolis 4, Ind.

NACTO CLEANER CORP., 1200 E.
156th St., New York 59, N.Y.

NAPCO CHEMICAL CO., INC.,
Lewis & Carter Sts., Harrison, N.J.

NASH, C. A., & SON, INC., Norfolk,
Va.

NASH KELVINATOR CORP., Detroit,
Mich.

NASON CO., Kendall Sq. Station,
Boston, Mass.

NATIONAL BEAUTY SUPPLY CO.,
52 W. 125th St., New York 27, N.Y.

NATIONAL BIRD CONTROL LABS.,
5315 W. Touhy Ave., Skokie, Ill.

NATIONAL BROOM MFG. CO.,
Pueblo, Colo.

NATIONAL CANINE PRODUCTS,
INC., 1133 McDonald Ave.,
Brooklyn 30, N.Y.

NATIONAL CARBON CO., See
Carbide & Carbon.

NATIONAL CHEMICAL CO., 1516
Industrial St., Los Angeles 21,
Calif.

NATIONAL CHEMICAL LABS.,
INC., West Palm Beach, Fla.

NATIONAL CHEMICAL &
MANUFACTURING CO., 3617 S.
May St., Chicago 9, Ill.

NATIONAL CRAYON CO., Easton,
Pa.

NATIONAL DENTAL CO.,
Convent, N.J.

NATIONAL DRUG CO., Philadelphia,
Pa.

NATIONAL GYPSUM CO., INC., 192
Delaware Ave., Buffalo, N.Y.

NATIONAL JAYGOL DISTRIBUTORS,
INC., 293 24th St., Brooklyn 32, N.Y.

NATIONAL LAB., INC., 4934 Lewis
Ave., Toledo 12, Ohio.

NATIONAL MFG. CORP., 3343
Flanagan St., Tonawanda, N.Y.

NATIONAL MILLING & CHEMICAL
CO., 4601 Nixon St., Philadelphia 27,
Pa.

NATIONAL PACKAGE DRUGS, INC.,
St. Louis, Mo.

NATIONAL PAINT PRODUCTS, INC.,
498 Chancellor Ave., Irvington, N.J.

NATIONAL POLISH CO., Van Wert,
Ohio.

NATIONAL PRODUCTS CO., 409 Main
St., Eau Claire, Wis.

NATIONAL REMEDY CO., 82 Lake
Ave., Tuckahoe, N.Y.

NATIONAL RODENTICIDE CO., 285
Van Brunt St., Brooklyn 31, N.Y.

NATIONAL SANITARY PRODUCTS,
INC., 3411 Locust St., St. Louis, Mo.

NATIONAL SOAP CO., 9029 Norcross
Ave., Detroit, Mich.

NATIONAL TOILET CO., Paris, Tenn.

NATIONAL VULCANIZED FIBRE CO.,
Wilmington 99, Del.

NATIONAL WAX CO., 1300 W.
Division St., Chicago, Ill.

NATRIPHENE CO., 424 Book Bldg.,
Detroit 26, Mich.

NAUGATUCK CHEMICAL, Division of
U. S. Rubber Co., Naugatuck, Conn.

NAVAL STORES RESEARCH SECTION,
U. S. Dept. of Agriculture, Naval
Stores Station, Olustee, Fla.

NAYLOR, H. W., CO., Morris, N.Y.

NELSON BAKER & CO., 503 E. 72nd
St., New York 21, N.Y.

NELSON, DETROIT, INC., see Nelson,
Baker.

NEMOW CO., 505 Court St., Brooklyn
31, N.Y.

NEOCO CO., 1001 N. McCadden Pl.,
Los Angeles, Calif.

NEPHRON CO., 1005 South K St.,
Tacoma 3, Wash.

NESTLE CO., INC., 2 William St.,
White Plains, N.Y.

NESTLE-LE MUR CO., 902 Broadway,
New York 10, N.Y.

NEUHAUS PRODS. CO., 824 S. Kingsley
Dr., Los Angeles 5, Calif.

NEUSHAFER, HELEN, INC., 14th Ave.
& 111th St., College Point, L. I., N.Y.

NEVASCO LAB., 2671 Flower St.,
Huntington Park, Calif.

NEVIN, T. H., CORP., Island-Preble at
Morehouse, Pittsburgh, Pa.

NEWBRO MFG. CO., 199 Walker St.,
S.W., Atlanta 55, Ga.

NEWCOMB LABS., 385 Harrison Ave.,
Boston 18, Mass.

NEW ENGLAND LACQUER CO., 10
King Philip Rd., East Providence, R.I.

NEW ENGLAND PHARMACEUTICAL
CO., 130 Ward St., New Haven, Conn.

NEW IDEA CHEMICAL CO., 24 Frost
Ave., Boston 22, Mass.

NEW JERSEY ZINC CO., 160 Front St.,
New York 38, N.Y.; San Francisco,
Calif.

NEW METHOD VARNISH CO., Elmira,
N.Y.
NEW ORLEANS PAINT & COLOR CO.,
700 Barrone, New Orleans, La.
NEWPORT SOAP CO., 1100 78th Ave.,
Oakland 21, Calif.
NEWSKIN CO., 882 3rd Ave., Brooklyn
32, N.Y.
NEWTON CHEMICAL & SUPPLY CO.,
Bridgeville, Del.
NEWTON HORSE MED. CO., 13976 St.
Marys Ave., Detroit 4, Mich.
NEWTON, PAUL D. & CO., INC.,
Newark, N.J.
NEW YORK PHARMACEUTICAL CO.,
Bedford Springs, Bedford, Mass.
NEW YORK VON CO., 82 Lake Ave.,
Tuckahoe, N.Y.
NIAGARA CHEM. DIV., Food
Machinery Corp., Middleport, N.Y.
NIAGARA HORTICULTURAL
PRODUCTS, St. Catharines, Ontario,
Canada.
NICHOLSON CHEMICAL CO., INC.,
2024 W. 6th St., Los Angeles 5, Calif.
NICHOLSON DRUG CO., 849 W.
Roosevelt Rd., Chicago 8, Ill.
NICO-STOP LABS., Modesto, Calif.
NI-LATE MFG. CO., 342 Marietta
St., N.W., Atlanta, Ga.
NISSY PARFUMS, INC., 56 16th St.,
New York 3, N.Y.
NIX CO., 46 N. 3rd St., Memphis 1,
Tenn.
NIXON, STUART & BARKER, INC.,
329 Fulton St., Peoria, Ill.
NOBEMA PRODUCTS CORP., 141
Greene St., New York 12, N.Y.
NOBLE PINE PRODUCTS CO., 12
Chapel St., Newark 5, N.J.
NOBLESSE COSMETICS, 35 S.
Dearborn St., Chicago 5, Ill.
NO-DUST MFG. CO., Marietta, Ohio.
NOGRAY HAIR REMEDY CO., 516
5th Ave., New York 18, N.Y.
NOONAN, T., SONS CO., 38 Portland
St., Boston 14, Mass.
NOPCO CHEMICAL CO., Harrison,
N.J.
NORAMEX CO., INC., 125 E. 46th St.,
New York 17, N.Y.
NORCRAFT-WESTWARE, INC., 4411
Appleton St., Cincinnati 9, Ohio.
NORDICSON ENTERPRISES, LTD.,
Toronto, Canada.
NOREEN, INC., 450 Lincoln St.,
Denver 9, Colo.
NOREX LABS., INC., 350 5th Ave.,
New York 1, N.Y.
NORFOLK PAINT & VARNISH CO.,
Quincy, Mass.
NO-RINSE LABS., 455 Livingston Ave.,
Dayton 10, Ohio.
NORITO CO., 225 N. Michigan Ave.,
Chicago 1, Ill.
NORTH AMERICAN DYE CORP., 22
North St., Danbury, Conn.
NORTH & JUDD MFG. CO., 498 E.
Main St., New Britain, Conn.
NORTHAM WARREN CORP.,
Stamford, Conn.
NORTHRUP, KING & CO., 1500
Jackson St., N.E., Minneapolis,
Minn.
NORTON PRODUCTS CO., 2333
Enterprise St., Los Angeles 21, Calif.

NORWICH PHARM. CO., 17 Eaton
Ave., Norwich, N.Y.
NOTT MFG. CO., 14 N. 2nd Ave.,
Mt. Vernon, N.Y.
NOURISHINE SALES CO., 4863 W.
Adams Blvd., Los Angeles 16,
Calif.
NOURSE OIL CO., Kansas City 8,
Mo.
NOVA LABS., 511 W. Houston St.,
San Antonio 7, Tex.
NOXACORN CO., INC., 75 Varick,
New York 13, N.Y.
NOXEM PRODUCTS CO., 101 W.
Mitchell St., Milwaukee 4, Wis.
NOXON INC., 812 Jersey Ave.,
Jersey City 2, N.J.
NOX-RUST CORP., 2425 S.
Halstead St., Chicago 8, Ill.
NOXZEMA CHEMICAL CO.,
Baltimore 11, Md.
NU-AGE PRODUCTS, INC.,
Brooklyn, Mich.
NUMOTIZINE, INC., 900 N.
Franklin St., Chicago, Ill.
NU PRODUCTS CO., 700 S. Flower,
Burbank, Calif.
NURLBURT, W. B., 3434 Wabash
Ave., Cincinnati 7, Ohio.
NU STEEL CO., 1714 S. Ashland
Ave., Chicago 8, Ill.
NU-TONE PRODUCTS CORP., 26 E.
22nd St., New York 10, N.Y.
NYCOL PRODUCTS, INC., 721 W.
Washington St., Ionia, Mich.

O

OAKES SEED & FEED STORE, Rio
Hondo, Tex.
OAKITE PRODUCTS, INC., 22
Thames St., New York 6, N.Y.
OAKLEY PAINT MFG. CO., 727
Antonio Ave., Los Angeles, Calif.
O'BRIEN CORP., 101 N. Johnson
St., South Bend 21, Ind.
O'BRIEN, FREDERICK, CO.,
Huntington Park, Calif.
OCCASION COSMETIC CO., 1100
Isabel St., Burbank, Calif.
O-CEDAR CORP., 2246 W. 49th St.,
Chicago 9, Ill.
OCTOGEN PHARMACAL CO., 1928
Storrs Ave., Utica, N.Y.
OCULINE CO., 9538 Brighton Way,
Beverly Hills, Calif.
ODELL CO., INC., 230 Wright St.,
Newark 5, N.J.
ODOL CHEMICAL CORP., 90 W.
Broadway, New York 17, N.Y.
ODOR-NEVER CO., 94 Ash St.,
Nashua, N.H.
OELWEIN CHEMICAL CO., INC.,
Oelwein, Iowa.
OGILVIE SISTERS, 227 E. 45th St.,
New York 17, N.Y.
OHIO LABS., INC., 1266 Goodale
Blvd., Columbus 8, Ohio.
OHIO PHARMACAL CO., 1291 W. 6th
St., Cleveland, Ohio.
OHIO SOLVENTS & CHEMICALS
CO., 3470 W. 140th St., Cleveland
11, Ohio.
OHIO VALLEY DRUG CO., 1305
Main St., Wheeling, W. Va.

OIL-DRI CORP. OF AMERICA, 520 N.
Michigan Ave., Chicago, Ill.
OIL OF INDIA CO., 116 W. Illinois St.,
Chicago, Ill.
OLD COLONY PAINT & CHEMICAL
CO., 620 Lamar, Los Angeles, Calif.
OLD DUTCH INDUSTRIAL PRODUCTS
CO., INC., Harrison, N.J.
OLD HICKORY MED. CO., 406 Guild
Dr., Chattanooga 4, Tenn.
OLD 97 CO., 2306 35th St., Tampa 5,
Fla.
O'LEARY, LYDIA, INC., 41 E. 57th
St., New York 22, N.Y.
OLEIDE PRODUCTS CO., 147-20 75th
Ave., Flushing 67, L. I., N.Y.
OLEUM PRODUCTS CO., 1129
Capouse Ave., Scranton 9, Pa.
OLIN INDUSTRIES, INC., New Haven
4, Conn.
OLIN MATHIESON CHEMICAL CORP.,
Mathieson Bldg., Baltimore 3, Md.
OLIVE TABLET CO., 29 E. 5th Ave.,
Columbus, Ohio.
OLIVER CHEMICAL CO., 1918
Freeman Ave., Cincinnati, Ohio.
OLIVER'S S-O DRUG CO., 219 S. 1st,
Union City 1, Tenn.
OLIVO CO., Philadelphia 34, Pa.
OLLIFFE, W. M., 6 Bowery, New York
13, N.Y.
OLO PAINT CORP., 9810 Meech Ave.,
Cleveland, Ohio.
OLSON CO., Box 2430, Sarasota, Fla.
OLSON PRODUCTS CORP., 620 S.
Broadway, Albert Lea, Minn.
OMAR PRODUCTS CO., 1770 Genesse,
Columbus, Ohio.
OMEGA CHEMICAL CO., 76 Mill Rd.,
Jersey City , N.J.
OMNI PRODUCTS, INC., Queens
Village, L. I., N.Y.
ONALIM CO., INC., 2295 2nd Ave.,
New York 35, N.Y.
O'NEIL DURO CO., Becher & 4th Sts.,
Milwaukee, Wis.
ONE-SPOT CO., Jessup, Md.
ONOX, INC., 121 2nd St., San Francisco
5, Calif.
ONTARIO CHEMICAL CO., 4119 N.
Tryon, Charlotte, N.C.
ONTHANK, G. W., CO., 11 Cherry,
Des Moines, Iowa.
ONYX OIL & CHEMICAL CO.,
Industrial Division, Warren & Morris
Sts., Jersey City 2, N.J.
OPITZ, JOHN, INC., 50 39th St., Long
Island City 4, L. I., N.Y.
OPTIMUS PHARM. CO., INC., P.O.
Box 444, Taylors, S.C.
ORBIS PRODUCTS CORP., 215 Pearl
St., New York, N.Y.
OR-BLOS-CO., INC., 1763 Geraldine
Dr., Jacksonville 5, Fla.
ORBOLENE CO., 325 Olive St., St.
Louis 2, Mo.
ORJENE CO., INC., 395 Broadway,
New York 13, N.Y.
ORTHO PHARMACEUTICAL CORP.,
Raritan, N.J.
OSGOOD PRODUCTS CO., 42 Eden
Ave., West Newton 65, Mass.
OSMIC CHEMICAL CO., 18 Court St.,
Brockton 17, Mass.
OSSAR & SHAPIRO, 402 Long Lane,
Stonehurst Hills, Upper Darby, Pa.

OSTREX CO., New York, N.Y.

OTALGAN CORP., Somerset, Mass.

OTHINE CORP., 775 Main St., Buffalo 3, N.Y.

OTLEY PAINT MFG. CO., 1742 N. Winchester Ave., Chicago, Ill.

OUR HUSBANDS CO., 825 Exchange Ave., Lyndon, Vt.

OUTERS LABS., Onalaska, Wis.

OVERTON HYGIENIC MFG. CO., 3653 S. State St., Chicago 9, Ill.

OWASSO PRODUCTS, Owasso, Mich.

OWEN DRUG CO., 1015 S. Fulton St., Salisbury, N.C.

OWENS, MINOR & BODEKER, INC., 1000 East Cary St., Richmond, Va.

OWL DRUG CO., 1101 Sherman St., Decatur, Ala.

OXFORD LABORATORIES, INC., Dayton, Va.

OXIDERMO PRODUCTS, INC., Springport, Mich.

OZANE CO., 555 W. 22nd St., New York 11, N.Y.

OZARK CO., 940 Fatherland St., Nashville 6, Tenn.

P

PABCO PRODUCTS, INC., 4th & Brannan Sts., San Francisco, Calif.

PACIFIC CHEMICAL CO., 114 W. College St., Los Angeles, Calif.

PACIFIC COAST BORAX CO., 100 Park Ave., New York 17, N.Y.

PACIFIC GRAPHITE COMPANY, INC., 40th & Linden St., Oakland 8, Calif.

PACIFIC GUANO CO., 2nd St. & Hearst Ave., Berkeley 2, Calif.

PACIFIC PAINT & VARNISH CO., 4th & Cedar St., Berkeley, Calif.

PACIFIC SUPPLY COOPERATIVE, Chemicals Division, P.O. Box 3819, Portland 8, Oreg.

PACKAGE PRODUCTS, INC., Atlanta, Ga.

PACKARD DRESSING CO., Stoughton, Mass.

PACKARD PAINT & VARNISH CO., 99 Potter St., Boston, Mass.

PACKERS TAR SOAP, INC., Mystic, Conn.

PACKWOOD, G. H., MFG. CO., 1545 Tower Grove Ave., St. Louis 10, Mo.

PACQUIN, INC., 155 E. 44th St., New York 17, N.Y.

PAGE BARKER DIST. OF AMERICA, 911 Western Ave., Seattle 4, Wash.

PAGE, E. R., CO., INC., 117 S. Jefferson St., Marshall, Mich.

PAGLO LABS., 78 5th Ave., New York 11, N.Y.

PAINTCRAFT CO., Galesburg, Ill.

PAISLEY PRODUCTS, INC., 1770 Canalport Ave., Chicago 16, Ill.

PALMER PAINT SALES, 21600 Wyoming Ave., Oak Park 37, Mich.

PALMER SHOW CARD PAINT CO., INC., 21650 Wyoming Ave., Detroit 20, Mich.

PALMER, SOLON, 39 Division St., Newark 2, N.J.

PAN DERMA LABS., 272 Saratoga Ave., Brooklyn 33, N.Y.

PANOGEN, INC. (Research Dept.), Woodstock, Ill.

Panther Oil & Grease Mfg. Co., 840 N. Main, Fort Worth, Tex.

PAPER PRODUCTS, INC., 4423 Fruitland Ave., Los Angeles 58, Calif.

PAPSOMAX CO., 27 Railroad Ave., New Rochelle, N.Y.

PARADERM LABS., INC., 79 Sudbury St., Boston 14, Mass.

PARADISE CHEMICAL CO., 43 W. Barkley St., Hicksville, N.Y.

PARADISE PRODUCTS CORP., 378 Bergen Blvd., Fairview, N.J.

PARAEUSAL CO., 4498 Lahm, Akron 19, Ohio.

PARAFFINE COMPANIES INC., 4th & Brannan Sts., San Francisco, Calif.

PARAGON DISTRIBUTING CORP., 1841 Park Ave., New York 35, N.Y.

PARAGON PAINT & VARNISH CORP., 5-59 46th Ave., Long Island City, L. I., N.Y.

PARAMOUNT PAINT & VARNISH CO., 141 League St., Philadelphia, Pa.

PARFUM L'ORLE, INC., 6 E. 39th St., New York 16, N.Y.

PARFUMS ANJOU, Batavia, Ill.

PARFUMS CHARBERT, INC., 630 5th Ave., New York 20, N.Y.

PARFUMS CIRO, INC., 693 5th Ave., New York 22, N.Y.

PARFUMS CORDAY, INC., 730 5th Ave., New York 19, N.Y.

PARFUMS DE RENEL, INC., 224 Central Pkwy., Mt. Vernon, N.Y.

PARFUMS PECHEUR, 208 W. 23rd St., New York 11, N.Y.

PARIS COSMETICS, INC., Roosevelt Ave. & 99th St., Corona 68, L. I., N.Y.

PARK-ADAMS, INC., 40 Somerset St., Plainfield, N.J.

PARK CHEMICAL CO., 8074 Military Ave., Detroit 4, Mich.

PARKE, DAVIS & CO., Jos. Campau Ave. at the River, Detroit 23, Mich.

PARKER BROS, INC., Salem, Mass.

PARKER, C. W., CO., INC., 1415 2nd St., Des Moines, Iowa

PARKER HERBEX CORP., 167 Brown Ave., Stamford, Conn.

PARKER, IRA & SONS CO., Oshkosh, Wis.

PARKER PAINT & VARNISH MFG. CORP., Crowley Ave., Valparaiso, Ind.

PARKER PEN CO., Court & Division Sts., Janesville, Wis.

PARKER, W. J., CO., 2329 Harford Rd., Baltimore 18, Md.

PARK PHARMACY, 533 Rutledge Ave., Charleston 20, S.C.

PARKS-BARNES, INC., 530 6th St., Hermosa Beach, Calif.

PARK & TILFORD, 485 5th Ave., New York 17, N.Y.

PARR PAINT & COLOR CO., Syracuse & Brussells Rd., Cleveland, Ohio.

PARROT CHEMICAL CO., Stamford, Conn.

PARSONS AMMONIA CO., 19 Rector St., New York 6, N.Y.

PARSONS CHEMICAL WORKS, 226 N. Bridge St., Grand Ledge, Mich.

PARTOLA PRODUCTS CO., 2020 Montrose Ave., Chicago 18, Ill.

PASSAIC ANALYTICAL LABS., INC., Passaic Ave., Caldwell, N.J.

PASSONNO-HUTCHEON CO., 9808 Meech Ave., Cleveland, Ohio.

PASTOL LAB., 1044 Gerard Ave., New York, N.Y.

PATAKY, MADAME OLGA, P.O. Box 7406, Philadelphia 4, Pa.

PATCH, E. L., CO., Stoneham 80, Mass.

PATEK & CO., 1900 16th St., San Francisco, Calif.

PATENT CEREALS CO., Geneva, N.Y.

PATRICK'S INDUSTRIES, 1507 Saratoga Ave., W., Ferndale 20, Mich.

PATRON CHEM. CORP., 1145 Clover Ave., Los Angeles 34, Calif.

PATTERSON LABS., INC., 11930 Pleasant Ave., Detroit 17, Mich.

PATTERSON-SARGENT CO., St. Clair, Kopp & 38th, Cleveland, Ohio.

PATTY REMOVER & CHEMICAL CORP., 19 Gay St., New York, N.Y.

PAUL, J. C., & CO., 8140 N. Ridgeway Ave., Skokie, Ill.

PAUL LABS., 2018 E. 177th St., New York 61, N.Y.

PAULEN CHEMICAL CO., 54th Ave. & Berwyn Rd., Berwyn, Md.

PAWNEE CO., P.O. Box 228, Austin, Tex.

PAXTON, F. H., & SONS, INC. 469 E. Ohio St., Chicago, Ill.

PAYSON CORP., 418 Lexington Ave., New York, N.Y.

PAYSON'S INDELIBLE INK CO., Northampton, Mass.

PEARL POLISHES, INC., 85 Leroy Ave., Buffalo, N.Y.

PEARL PRODUCTS CO., Buffalo, N Y.

PEARSON & CO., 103 N. Water St., Mobile 3, Ala.

PEARSON PHARMACAL CO., INC., 33-00 Northern Blvd., Long Island City 1, L. I., N.Y.

PEAU D'OR SALES CORP., (see Lanotan Inc.)

PEAU SECHE, INC., 24 N. Wabash Ave., Chicago 2, Ill.

PECK & STERBA, INC., 80 Main St., W., Rochester 14, N.Y.

PECK'S PRODUCTS CO., St. Louis, Mo.

PECORA PAINT CO., 3501 N. 4th St., Philadelphia 40, Pa.

PECOS VALLEY FERTILIZER & CHEMICAL CO., Division of Southwest Fertilizer & Chemical Co., Clint, Tex.

PED-EX CO., Covington, Ky.

PEDINOL LABS., 152 W. 42nd St., New York 36, N.Y.

PED-I-RUB CO., 1700 Exchange St., Oklahoma City 8, Okla.

PEDRICK, V. O. PHM., P.O. Box 4139, Miami 25, Fla.

PEELE, W. R., CO., INC., Clayton, N.C.

PEERLESS BARBER & BEAUTY SUPPLY CO., 432 S. State St., Salt Lake City 1, Utah.

PEERLESS CHEMICAL CO., 3856-60 Oakman Blvd., Detroit, Mich.

PEERLESS CO., P.O. Box 216, Jourdanton, Tex.

PEERLESS PAINT MFG. CO., Appleton, Wis.

PEKTAMOL LABS., 505 Court St., Brooklyn 31, N.Y.

PEMCO CORP., Eastern & Pemco Aves., Baltimore, Md.

PENICK, S. B., & CO., 50 Church St., New York 8, N.Y.

PENN-CHAMP OIL CORP., 808 Butler Savings & Trust Bldg., Butler, Pa.

PENN CO., Boston, Mass.

PENN CRETE PRODUCTS CO., 20th & Lippincott Sts., Philadelphia, Pa.

PENNEX PRODUCTS CO., INC., 3941 Sennott St., Pittsburgh 13, Pa.

PENNSYLVANIA ENGINEERING CO., 1119 N. Howard St., Philadelphia 23, Pa.

PENNSYLVANIA LACQUER WORKS, 145 N. 4th St., Philadelphia, Pa.

PENNSYLVANIA REFINING CO., 104 S. Main St., Butler Pa.

PENNSYLVANIA SALT MFG. CO., 3 Penn Center Plaza, Philadelphia 2, Pa.

PENOLA OIL CO., 15 W. 51st St., New York 19, N.Y.

PENSLAR CO., INC., 503 E. 72nd St., New York 21, N.Y.

PEOPLES DRUG STORES, INC., 61 P St., N. E., Washington 2, D.C.

PEPSINIC SELTZER CORP., 58 Front St., Worcester 8, Mass.

PEPSODENT DIVISION, Lever Bros. Co., 390 Park Ave., New York 22, N.Y.

PERDUE, P. K., PHARMACAL CO., 2356 Minto St., Augusta, Ga.

PERES, FREDERICK, & CO., INC., 431 S. Dearborn St., Chicago 5, Ill.

PERFECTION MODEL PRODUCTS, 4145 W. Kinzie, Chicago 24, Ill.

PERFECTION PAINT & COLOR CO., 715 E. Maryland, Indianapolis, Ind.

PERKINS, DOROTHY, CO., 5114 Southwest Ave., St. Louis 10, Mo.

PERMA-NAIL CO., 1100 Isabel St., Burbank, Calif.

PERMANENT WAVE PROCESS CO., 22 Kenwood St., Brookline 46, Mass.

PERMA PRODUCTS CO., 699 Morgan Ave., Cleveland, Ohio.

PERMA-STRATE, 271 Vance Ave., Memphis 2, Tenn.

PERMATEX COMPANY, INC., 1702 Ave. Y, Brooklyn 35, N.Y.

PER-MO PRODUCTS CO., 3604 Woodland Ave., Kansas City 3, Mo.

PERMUTIT CO., 330 W. 42nd St., New York 36, N.Y.

PEROLIN CO., INC., 10 E. 40th St., New York 16, N.Y.

PERRIGO, L., CO., Allegan, Mich.

PERRY & DERRICK CO., 109 Corwine, Cincinnati, Ohio.

PESSL, HELENE, INC., 785 5th Ave., New York 22, N.Y.

PEST CONTROL EQUIPMENT CO., 24 N. Bond St., Mount Vernon, N.Y.

PEST CONTROL PRODUCTS CO., 6144 Santa Monica Blvd., Los Angeles 38, Calif.

PETERS CO., 101 Francis St., Steven Point, Wis.

PETERSON OINTMENT CO., INC., 257 Franklin St., Buffalo 2, N.Y.

PETROLEUM SOLVENTS CORP., 331 Madison Ave., New York 17, N.Y.

PETROZOIN PRODUCTS CO., P.O. Box 2051 D, Pasadena, Calif.

PETTEL, R. S., & CO., 601 N. 63rd St., Philadelphia, Pa.

PETTIT PAINT CO., 507-519 Main St., Belleville, N.J.

PFANTSTIEHL DETERGENT CHEMICALS, INC., 2843 W. 19th St., Chicago 23, Ill.

PFEIFFER, S., MFG. 3965 Laclede Ave., St. Louis 8, Mo.

PFIZER, CHARLES, & CO., Terre Haute, Ind.

PFIZER LABS., Brooklyn 6, N.Y.

PHARMACEUTICALS, INC., 278 Jeliff Ave., Newark 1, N.J.

PHARMACIA LABS., INC., 270 Park Ave., New York 17, N.Y.

PHARMACO, INC., Galloping Hill Rd., Kenilworth, N.J.

PHARMA-CRAFT CORP., INC., 405 Lexington Ave., New York 17, N.Y.

PHARMART DRUG PRODUCTS, 121 Liberty Ave., Richmond Hill, L. I., N.Y.

PHARMASEAL LABS., 1015 Grandview Ave., Glendale, Calif.

PHARMEX, INC., DISTRIBUTORS, 296 Andrews St., Rochester 5, N.Y.

PHELAN-FAUST PAINT MFG. CO., 932 Loughborough Ave., St. Louis, Mo.

PHELPS DODGE REFINING CORP., 40 Wall St., New York 5, N.Y.

PHENACEDOL CO., 2536 S. Galvez St., New Orleans 25, La.

PHENOPLAST CORP., 115 E. 23rd St., New York 17, N.Y.

PHILADELPHIA WHOLESALE DRUG CO., 10th & Spring Garden St., Philadelphia, Pa.

PHILLIPS, CHARLES H., CO., Division of Sterling Drug Co., Inc., 1450 Broadway, New York, N.Y.

PHILLIPS MFG. CO., 3406 W. Touhy Ave., Chicago, Ill.

PHOENIX CHEMICAL CO., P.O. Box 1232, Phoenix, Ariz.

PHYSICIANS & HOSPITAL SUPPLY CO., INC., 1400 Harmon Pl., Minneapolis, Minn.

PHYSICIANS PHARMACY, 30 Douglas St., Hammond, Ind.

PHYSICIANS PRODUCTS CO., INC., Petersburg, Va.

PICKARD, A. E., Mt. Vernon, Ill.

PIEDMONT PAINT MFG. CO., Greenville, S.C.

PIED PIPER PRODUCTS, LTD., 3129 Kingsway, Vancouver, B. C., Canada.

PIERCE & STEVENS, INC., 710 Ohio St., Buffalo 3, N.Y.

PIERCE, F. O., CO., 2-33 50th Ave., Long Island City, L. I., N.Y.

PIERCE, S. S., CO., 133 Brookline Ave., Boston 17, Mass.

PIERCE'S PROPRIETARIES, INC., Buffalo, N.Y.; Toronto, Ont., Canada.

PIERPONT PRODUCTS CO., 312 Stuart St., Boston 16, Mass.

PIERRE, DR., CHEMICAL CO., 2020 Montrose Ave., Chicago 18, Ill.

PIKE, J. J., & CO., R.D. No. 1, P.O. Box 74, Glen Rd., Sparta, N.J.

PINAUD, ED., INC., 902 Broadway, New York, N.Y.

PINE, MORTON S., CO., 406 Caxton Bldg., Cleveland 15, Ohio.

PINE-OX-GEN MFG. CO., 31 Lynn St., Malden 48, Mass.

PINETRINE CO., INC., 180 Lafayette St., New York 13, N.Y.

PINEX CO., 123 W. Columbia St., Ft. Wayne, Ind.

PINGO CO., 79 Sudbury St., Boston 14, Mass.

PINKHAM, LYDIA E., MED. CO., 271 Western Ave., Lynn, Mass.

PINKY PRODUCTS, INC., 285 Madison Ave., New York 17, N.Y.

PINO PRODS. CO., Deland, Fla.

PINOL MFG. CO., INC., Hancock & Berks, Philadelphia, Pa.

PINOLATOR, INC., 1809 Minnehaha Ave., Minneapolis 4, Minn.

PIONEER MANUFACTURING CO., 3053 E. 87th St., Cleveland, Ohio.

PISO CO., 211 Market St., Warren, Pa.

PITMAN-MOORE CO., Division of Allied Labs., Inc., 1220 Madison Ave., Indianapolis 6, Ind.

PITTSBURGH COKE & CHEMICAL CO., Agricultural Chemicals Division, Neville Island, Pa.

PITTSBURGH PLATE GLASS CO., Paint Division, 420 DuQuesne Bldg., Pittsburgh, Pa.

PLANETARY CHEMICAL CO., Ballas Rd., Creve Coeur, Mo.

PLANTABBS CORP., 1101 Maryland Ave., Baltimore 1, Md.

PLANTERS CHEMICAL CORP., 3111 Broad Creek Rd., Norfolk 12, Va.

PLANT PRODUCTS CORP., Kennedy Ave., Blue Point, L. I., N.Y.

PLANT SHINE CO., St. Louis, Mo.

PLASTEX CO., 446 Arsenal, Watertown 72, Mass.

PLASTICLEAR CO., 814 Elm St., Manchester, N.H.

PLASTI-GLAZE CO., IND., Ventura, Calif.

PLASTI-KOTE, INC., 400 Lakeside Ave., N.W., Cleveland 13, Ohio.

PLOUGH, INC., 3022 Jackson Ave., Memphis 1, Tenn.

PLUNKETT CHEMICAL CO., 3500 S. Morgan St., Chicago 9, Ill.

PLUTO CORP., French Lick, Ind.

PLYMOUTH MFG. CO., Plymouth, Mass.

POLANA SOAP WKS., Anniston, Ala.

POLINEL CO., P.O. Box 848, Hollywood, Fla.

POLK, CHAS. F., CO., P.O. Box 212, Troy, N.Y.

POLK MILLER PRODUCTS CORP., 2007 N. Hamilton St., Richmond 20, Va.

POLORIS CO., INC., 12 High St., Jersey City, N.J.

POND PHARMACAL CO., INC., DISTRIBUTORS, 50-19 47th Ave., Woodside, L. I., N.Y.

POND'S EXTRACT CO., 380 Madison Ave., New York 17, N.Y.

POPE LABS., Hallowell, Maine.

PORT FERTILIZER & CHEM. CO., Los Fresnos, Tex.

PORTER CHEMICAL CO., Hagerstown, Md.

PORTER MFG. & SUPPLY CO., 2836 Sunset Blvd., Los Angeles 26, Calif.

PORTER PAINT CO., 419 S. 14th St., Louisville, Ky.

POSNER, I., INC., 111 W. 128th St., New York 7, N.Y.

POTTER DRUG & CHEMICAL CORP., 123 Medford St., Malden 48, Mass.

POWERS, E. C., CO., P.O. Box E., Dorchester Center Sta., Boston 24, Mass.

PRATT, B. G., CO., 204 21st Ave., Paterson 3, N.J.

PRATT FOOD CO., Hammond, Ind.

PRATT & LAMBERT, INC., 92 Tonawanda, Buffalo, N.Y.

PRATT PAINT & VARNISH CO., P.O. Box 1134, Dallas, Tex.

PREACHERS, INC., Parsons, Tenn.

PRECISION-COSMET CO., INC., 529 S. 7th St., Minneapolis, Minn.

PREFERRED UTILITIES MFG. CORP., 1862 Broadway, New York, N.Y.

PREMIER LABS., Birmingham, Ala.

PREMO PHARMACEUTICAL LABS., INC., 3 Leuning St., S. Hackensack, N.J.

PRENTIL CORP., 20 Bonnie Brae, Utica 3, N.Y.

PRENTISS DRUG & CHEMICAL CO., INC., 110 William St., New York 38, N.Y.

PRESCOTT, J. L., CO., 27 8th St., Passaic, N.J.

PRESCRIPTION LAB., 1629 College Ave., Lubbock, Tex.

PRESCRIPTION PHARMACY, 723 Fulton Ave., Hempstead, L. I., N.Y.

PRESCRIPTION SPECIALTIES CO., 317 Main Ave., N. San Antonio 5, Tex.

PRESERVATIVE PAINT CO., 5410 Airport Way, Seattle, Wash.

PRESTO MANGE REMEDY CO., P.O. Box 604, Oklahoma City, Okla.

PRESTON DRUG CO., Superior, Nebr.

PRESTON LABS., INC., 814 W. North Ave., Chicago 22, Ill.

PRETONE CO., Camden, N.J.

PRICELESS PRODUCTS CO., 3115 S. Dixie Hgwy., W. Palm Beach, Fla.

PRINCE MATCHABELLI, 60 West St., Bloomfield, N.J.

PRINCESS PAT, LTD., 2709 S. Wells St., Chicago 16 Ill.

PRIVATE BRANDS, INC., 300 S. 3rd St., Kansas City 18, Kans.

PRO-ACET INC., 290 41st St., Oakland 11, Calif.

PROCTER & GAMBLE CO., Gwynne Bldg., Cincinnati, Ohio.

PRODUCTS, INC., 7 W. 22nd St., New York, N.Y.

PRODUCTS SALES, INC., 6400 Herman Ave., Cleveland, Ohio.

PROFANT, O. F., 746 Lyman Ave., Oak Park, Ill.

PROFESSIONAL PRODUCTS, P.O. Box 409, Shawnee, Okla.

PROM COSMETICS, Division of Gillette Co., Chicago 54, Ill.

PROOF PRODUCTS CORP., 118 Meadow Land, Grosse Pointe 30, Mich.

PROTECTION PRODUCTS MANUFACTURING CO., Kalamazoo 99, Mich.

PROTECTIVE COATINGS, INC., P.O. Box 3985, Detroit 27, Mich.

PROT-EGG PRODS., 136-30 41st Ave., L. I., N.Y.

PRO-TEX-ALL CO., INC., 205 Court, Evansville, Ind.

PRUCIDE LABORATORIES, INC., 5824 Myrtle Ave., Brooklyn 27, N.Y.

PUHL, JOHN, PRODUCTS CO., 5900 W. 51st St., Chicago, Ill.

PURDUE FREDERICK CO., 135 Christopher St., New York 14, N.Y.

PURDUM CO., Danville, Va.

PURE DRUG & CHEMICAL CORP., Ft. of Lamokin St., Chester, Pa.

PUREPAC CORP., 511 E. 72nd St., New York 21, N.Y.

PUREX CORPORATION, LTD., 9300 Rayo Ave., South Gate, Calif.

PUREX PRODUCTS, INC., Ridgely, Carey, & Scott Sts., Baltimore, Md.

PURITAN CHEMICAL CO., 926 Ashby St., N.W., Atlanta, Ga.

PURITAN SALES CO., 209 Peters St., Atlanta, Ga.

PURITY CHEMICAL PRODUCTS CO., 1005 Cleveland Ave., Santa Rosa, Calif.

PURO CHEM., INC., 2600 W. Madison, Cleveland, Ohio.

PUROSEAL PRODUCTS CO., New Market, N.J.

PYCOPE, INC., 392 Wayne St., Jersey City 2, N.J.

PYRENE MFG. CO., 540 Belmont Ave., Newark, N.J.

PYRO-SANA LAB., 1503 Chestnut St., St. Louis 3, Mo.

PYROIL COMPANY, INC., LaCrosse, Wis.

PYSOL PAINT MFG. CORP., East Paterson, N.J.

PYXOLA LABS., Main St., Yazoo City, Miss.

Q

QUAKER HAIR GOODS CO., 1920 South St., Philadelphia 46, Pa.

QUALITY CHEMISTS, INC., 2646 Arthur Ave., St. Louis 17, Mo.

QUALITY COSMETICS CORP., 316 Dean St., Brooklyn 17, N.Y.

QUALITY DISTRIBUTING CO., Orange City, Fla.

QUEEN LABS., P.O. Box 1294, South Side Sta., Springfield, Mo.

QUEL PRODUCTS, INC., 3304 E. 87th St., Cleveland 4, Ohio.

QUICKEE PRODUCTS, INC., 141 Woodworth Ave., Yonkers, N.Y.

QUINN, K. J. & CO., INC., 209 Canal St., Malden 48, Mass.

QURET MFG. CO., 908 Sanford St., Muskegon Heights, Mich.

R

RABIN CO., 4800 DeKalb Ave., Los Angeles, Calif.

RADIANT COLOR CO., Oakland, Calif.

RADIANT FINISH CO., 612 N. Michigan Ave., Chicago, Ill.

RADIATOR SPECIALTY CO., 1700 Dowd Rd., Charlotte 1, N.C.

RADIN, THEODORE INC., 299 Madison Ave., New York 17, N.Y.

RAE CHEMICAL CO., P.O. Box 137, Cincinnati 33, Ohio.

RAE, J. H. OIL CO., 10 Ambrose St., Rochester, N.Y.

RAFEA PHARMACAL CO., 141 E. 44th St., New York 17, N.Y.

RAINBOW RUBBER CO., Butler, Pa.

RALSTON PURINA CO., 835 8th St., St. Louis 2, Mo.

RAMEAU, PAUL & GREGORY, 475 5th Ave., New York 16, N.Y.

RANDALL PRODUCTS MFG. CO., 2095 Broadway, New York, N.Y.

RANDALL-THOMSON CORP., Royal Center, Ind.

RANDOLPH LABS., P.O. Box 63, Wellesley Branch, Boston 81, Mass.

RANDOLPH-TENNY, INC., 27 E. Monroe St., Chicago 3, Ill.

RANGER PRODUCTS CO., INC., 735 Dixwell Ave., New Haven 11, Conn.

RANSOM, D., SON & CO., Buffalo, N.Y.

RA-PID-GRO CORP., Dansville, N.Y.

RAPIDOL DISTRIBUTING CORP., 1750 Plaza Ave., New Hyde Park, N.Y.

RAT BISCUIT CO., Division of KRO Co., 19 N. Limestone St., Springfield, Ohio.

RATHGEBER LABS., New Haven, Conn.

RAT LUNCHES CO., 1497 Ogden St., Denver, Colo.

RAWLEIGH, W. T., CO., S. Liberty Ave., Freeport, Ill.

RAY-CLAW LABS., INC., Orlando, Fla.

RAY DRUG CO., P.O. Box 855, Oakland 18, Calif.

RAYMOND, CHAS., & CO., INC., 381 4th Ave., New York 16, N.Y.

RAYMOND, M. E., INC., 56 E. High St., Ballston Spa, N.Y.

R-B LABS., 1911 Waverly St., Palo Alto, Calif.

REARDEN CO., 473 Broadway, Bayonne, N.J.

REARDON CO., 7501 Page St., St. Louis, Mo.

REARDON, W. G., LABS., INC., 330 Main St., Port Chester, N.Y.

REASOR-HILL CORP., Jacksonvile, Ark.

RECREO MFG. CO., INC., 804 Chestnut St., Utica 4, N.Y.

RECSEI LABS., 47 Tabor Lane, Santa Barbara, Calif.

RED CIRCLE PRODUCTS CO., 1309 St. Emanuel St., Houston 3, Tex.

REDDI-LITE CO., Elmira, N.Y.

RED FEATHER PRODUCTS, P.O. Box 52, Melrose, Fla.

RED HAND COMPOSITION CO., 1 Broadway, New York, N.Y.

RED JACKET MFG. CO., 1051 S. Rolff St., Davenport, Iowa.

REDOLENT PRODUCTS CO., 3115 S. Dixie Hgwy., West Palm Beach, Fla.

RED SPOT PAINT & VARNISH CO., 110 Main St., Evansville, Ind.

REDUCINE CO., INC., Otsego 1, Mich.

REDWOOD ZONE INHALANT CO., 317 Neondocino Ave., Santa Rosa, Calif.

REEDER, OLIVER & SONS., INC., 501 Key Hgwy., Baltimore, Md.

REED LABS., 2163 Palm Ave., San Mateo, Calif.

REED, L. L., 31 Chenango St., Cazenovia, N.Y.

REEFER-GALLER, INC., 225 5th Ave., New York 10, N.Y.

REESE CHEMICAL CO., 10617 Frank Ave., Cleveland 6, Ohio.

REEVES, J. R., CO., INC., 126 W. Court St., Anderson, Ind.

REGAL METAL CO., 83 Woodbine St., Hartford, Conn.

REGULIN DIVISION, S. F. Durst & Co., Inc., 5317 N. 3rd St., Philadelphia 20, Pa.

REID'S LAB., 419 Laurel St., Modesto, Calif.

REILLY TAR & CHEMICAL CORP., 1615 Merchants Bank Bldg., 11 South Meridian St., Indianapolis 4, Ind.

RELIABLE CHEMICAL CO., 10 N. Ball Terr., Passaic, N.J.

RELIABLE PASTE & CHEMICAL CO., 3560 Shields Ave., Chicago 9, Ill.

RELIANCE PENCIL CORP., 6th Ave. & Vine St., Mt. Vernon, N.Y.

RELIANCE VARNISH CO., 4730 Crittenden Dr., Louisville, Ky.

RELIANCE WHITING CO., Alton, Ill.

REL-KA-SOL CHEM. CO., 303 Runnymede Ave., Jenkintown, Pa.

REMEDOL CO., 4108 Moss Rose Dr., Nashville 2, Tenn.

REMPEL CHEMICAL PRODUCTS, INC., P.O. Box 1185, Fresno, Calif.

RENOFAB PRODS. CO., 755 E. 134th St., New York 54, N.Y.

RE-NU HOME TINT PRODUCTS, 729 W. Wisconsin Ave., Milwaukee 3, Wis.

RENU PRODUCTS INC., 1846 Park Ave., New York 35, N.Y.

RENUZIT HOME PRODS. CO., 1724 Chestnut St., Philadelphia 3, Pa.

REPUBLIC PAINT & VARNISH CO., 1330 S. Kilbourn Ave., Chicago, Ill.

REQUA MFG. CO., INC., 1193 Atlantic Ave., Brooklyn 16, N.Y.

RESEARCH DES-TEX, INC., 2884 Bird Ave., Miami 33, Fla.

RESEARCH PRODUCTS CORP., 1015 E. Washington Ave., Madison 10, Wis.

RESEARCH SPECIALTIES CO., P.O. Box 1129, Santa Monica, Calif.

RESIDEX CORP., 1500 W. Elizabeth Ave., Linden, N.J.

RESINOL CHEM CO., 517 W. Lombard St., Baltimore 1, Md.

RESISTALL PAINT MFG. CO., 34 Park Row, New York, N.Y.

RETORT PHARMACEUTICAL CO., INC., 42-25 9th St., Long Island City 1, L. I., N.Y.

REVLON PRODUCTS CORP., 745 5th Ave., New York 22, N.Y.

REXAIR DIVISION, Martin-Parry Corp., 1455 W. Alexis Road, Toledo 1, Ohio.

REXALL DRUG CO., Rexall Sq., Beverly at La Cienga, Los Angeles 48, Calif.

REX BITTERS CO., 3321 W. Armitage Ave., Chicago 47, Ill.

REX-CLEANWALL CORP., Brazil, Ind.

REXCLIF PRODUCTS CO., 1718 S.E. 47th Ave., Portland 15, Oreg.

REX HOME SUPPLY CO., 181 Ferndale Rd., Scarsdale, N.Y.

REX HUNTERS PRODS., Rockport, Mass.

REXINE CO., P.O. Box 186, Sheboygan, Wis.

REX OIL & CHEMICAL CO., 9100 Loren Ave., Cleveland, Ohio.

REX RESEARCH CORP., 600 Montrose Ave., Toledo 7, Ohio.

REZILITE MFG. CO., 2436 Greenleaf Ave., Chicago, Ill.

RHEUMANON CO., 8847 Gratiot Ave., Detroit 13, Mich.

RHODES, A., CO., INC., 95 Bridge St., Lowell, Mass.

RHODES PHARM. CO., INC., 1814 E. 40th St., Cleveland 3, Ohio.

RHODES, PRESTON T., 520 N. 61st St., Philadelphia, Pa.

RICE CHEMICAL CO., 125 W. Main St., Ardmore, Okla.

RICHARD DRUG LAB., P.O. Box 203, Burlington, Vt.

RICHARDS BROS., 104 Front St., Marietta, Ohio.

RICHARDS, CARYL, INC., 10 Box St., Brooklyn 22, N.Y.

RICHARDS PHARMACEUTICAL CO., Santa Monica, Calif.

RICHELIEU, MARIE, 45 W. 45th St., New York 36, N.Y.

RICHFIELD OIL CORP., 555 S. Flower St., Los Angeles, Calif.

RICHMAN CHEMICAL PRODUCTS CO., 2632 W. 19th St., Chicago 8, Ill.

RICHTER, F. AD., & CO., INC., P.O. Box 351, Staten Island 7, N.Y.

RID CO., Corpus Christi, Tex.

RIDD LAB., P.O. Box 266, Edmonds, Wash.

RIEGER, PAUL, & CO., 220 Commercial St., San Francisco, Calif.

RIES HAMLY, INC., 14579 Longacre Rd., Detroit 27, Mich.

RIGIDTEST PRODUCTS, INC., 4455 N. Malden Ave., Chicago, Ill.

RIGO MFG. CO., P.O. Box 1188, Nashville 2, Tenn.

RIG PRODUCTS CO., Oregon, Ill.

RIKER, CLARK, CO., 144 E. Kelso Rd., Columbus 2, Ohio.

RIMMEL, INC., 565 5th Ave., New York 17, N.Y.

RING PRODUCTS CO., 536 Clifford Ave., Rochester 21, N.Y.

RING-ROUT, INC., P.O. Box 208, New Orleans 3, La.

RINGWOOD CHEMICAL CORP., 120 S. La Salle St., Chicago, Ill.

RINSHED-MASON CO., Milford & Epworth Sts., Detroit, Mich.

RITCHIE, HAROLD F., INC., Clifton, N.Y.

RITCHIE & JANVIER, INC., 60 Orange St., Bloomfield, N.J.

RITEPOINTE CO., 4350 S. Kingshighway Blvd., St. Louis 9, Mo.

RITE-WAY PRODUCTS CO., 1241 Belmont Ave., Chicago 13, Ill.

RITORNELLE, INC., 366 Madison Ave., New York 17, N.Y.

RIT PRODS. CORP., 1437 W. Morris St., Indianapolis, Ind.

RIVERSIDE MFG. CO., 4919 Connecticut Ave., St. Louis, Mo.

ROACH TRAP CO., 1932 N. 11th St., Fort Smith, Ark.

ROBBINS, ANATOLE, INC., 5533 Sunset Blvd., Los Angeles 28, Calif.

ROBBINS CORP., 505 Savings & Loan Bldg., Middletown, Ohio.

ROBBINS ETHOL CORP., 19 W. S. Temple, Salt Lake City, Utah.

ROBBINS, GEO. B., DISINFECTANT CO., 42 Carleton St., Cambridge 42, Mass.

ROBEN PRODUCTS, INC., 1011 6th Ave., Des Moines 14, Iowa.

ROBERTS CO., 1049 Broadway, Burlingame, Calif.

ROBERTS, DR. DAVID, VET. CO., 728 N. Grand Ave., Waukesha, Wis.

ROBERTS LABS., 1427 16th St., Denver 2, Colo.

ROBERTSON, THEO. B., PRODUCTS CO., INC., 700 W. Division St., Chicago 10, Ill.

ROBERTS PAINT CORP., 515 Bryant Ave., New York, N.Y.

ROBESON PRESERVO CO., Port Huron, Mich.

ROBINSON BROS. CHEMICALS, INC., 255 Randolph St., Brooklyn 37, N.Y.

ROCHAS, MARCEL, PARFUMS, INC., 1 E. 57th St., New York 22, N.Y.

ROCHESTER BEST WASHING FLUID CO., 133 Hartford St., Rochester 5, N.Y.

ROCHESTER GERMICIDE CO., 333 Hollenbeck St., Rochester 21, N.Y.

ROCHESTER LABS., 16 6th St., S.W., Rochester, Minn.

ROCKFORD PAINT MFG. CO., 200 Sayre St., Rockford, Ill.

ROCKLAND CHEMICAL CO., 839 N. 6th St., Newark 7, N.J.

ROCK-TRED CORP., 7444 N. St. Louis Ave., Stokie, Ill.

ROCKWELL LABS., INC., 300 S. 3rd St., Kansas City 18, Kans.

ROEMER DRUG CO., 606 N. Broadway, Milwaukee 2, Wis.

ROGERS CHEMICAL CORP., 9727 Conan Blvd., Detroit, Mich.

ROGERS & HUBBARD CO., Portland, Conn.

ROGERS PAINT, INC., 8250 Aubin Ave., Detroit, Mich.

ROGERS PARK DRUG CO., 4504 Garrison Blvd., Baltimore 15, Md.

ROHM & HAAS CO., Washington Sq., Philadelphia 5, Pa.

ROLLEY, INC., 182 Geary St., San Francisco, Calif.

ROLLINS, F. E., CO., 41 Hanover St., Boston 13, Mass.

ROMAN CLEANSER CO., 2700 E. McNichols Rd., Detroit 12, Mich.

ROMERO DRUG CO., 912 W. Russell Pl., San Antonio 1, Tex.

RONSON CORP., 31 Fulton St., Newark 2, N.J.

ROOTO CORP., 17319 Wyoming Ave., Detroit 21, Mich.

RORER, WILLIAM H., INC., Pharmaceutical Chemicals, 5th & Chestnut Sts., Philadelphia 6, Pa.

ROSCO LABS., 367 Hudson Ave., Brooklyn 1, N.Y.

ROSE DEW PRODUCTS, 2416 S. Garvey Blvd., Alhambra, Calif.

ROSE, E. W., CO., 1750 E. 27th St., Cleveland 14, Ohio.

ROSE EXTERMINATOR CO., 1809 W. North Ave., Chicago 22, Ill.

ROSE MFG. CO., 6 Main St., Beacon, N.Y.

ROSENFELD, HENRY, COSMETICS CO., INC., 498 7th Ave., New York 18, N.Y.

ROSEWELL, ELIZABETH, COSMETICS, 545 5th Ave., New York 17, N.Y.

ROSS CHEMICAL & MFG. CO., 8459 Melville St., Detroit 17, Mich.

ROSS, SYDNEY, CO., 1450 Broadway, New York 18, N.Y.

ROSSIE IRON ORE PAINT CO., Ogdensburg, N.Y.

ROSSMAR LABS., 1806-8 E. Venango St., Philadelphia 34, Pa.

ROTENONE PRODS., CO., INC., 110 Eaton Pl., East Orange, N.J.

ROTHENBERGER, C. B., PHARMACIST, West Leesport, Pa.

ROUX DISTRIBUTING CO., INC., 1841 Park Ave., New York 35, N.Y.

ROWE PAINT & VARNISH CO., INC., College & Crowell Sts., Niagara Falls, N.Y.

ROWLAND, WEIL & CO., P.O. Box 398, Madison, N.J.

ROYAL GLUE CO., 709 S. Caton Ave., Baltimore, Md.

ROYAL MFG. CO., (see Royal Pharm. Corp.)

ROYAL PALM PRODUCTS, INC., 9 Eliot St., Somerville 43, Mass.

ROYAL PHARM. CORP., 12 N. 1st St., Duquesne, Pa.

ROYAL RINSE CO., P.O. Box 4515, West Park Sta., Philadelphia 31, Pa.

ROYAL WORCESTER CO., 12 Alden St., Boston 14, Mass.

ROYCE CHEMICAL CO., Herrick & Carlton Aves., Carlton Hill, N.J.

RUBBERCRAFT CORP. OF CALIF., LTD., 1800 W. 220th St., Torrance, Calif.

RUBEROID CO., 502 5th Ave., New York, N.Y.

RUBINSTEIN, HELENA, INC., 655 5th Ave., New York 22, N.Y.

RU BON CHEMICAL CO., INC., 3610 Woodland Ave., Kansas City 3, Mo.

RUBY CHEMICAL CO., Glenn & McDowell St., Columbus, Ohio.

RUDD PAINT & VARNISH CO., 1608 15th, W., Seattle, Wash.

RU-EX CO., 2459 University Ave., St. Paul 4, Minn.

RUKO CHEMICAL CO., 84 Talbot St., Kew Gardens 15, L. I., N.Y.

RUMFORD CHEMICAL WORKS, 12 Newman Ave., Rumford, R.I.

RUNDLE, GEORGE H., CO., 419 Caldwell St., Piqua, Ohio.

RUSCOL MFG. CO., 3196 3rd Ave., New York 56, N.Y.

RUSSELL, A. F., & CO., 2 Depot Plaza, Tuckahoe 7, N.Y.

RUSSELL, I. D., CO., LABS., 2463 Harrison St., Kansas City, 10, Mo.

RUSTAIN PRODUCTS, 240 E. 152nd St., New York 51, N.Y.

RUSTICIDE PRODUCTS CO., 3125 Perkins Ave., Cleveland 14, Ohio.

RUST MASTER CHEMICAL CO., 56 Creighton St., Boston, Mass.

RUST-OLEUM CORP., Evanston, Ill.

RUST SOL, P.O. Box 671, Hagerstown, Md.

RUTLAND FIRE CLAY CO., Rutland, Vt.

RU-TEL CO., 2459 University Ave., St. Paul 4, Minn.

RUXTON PRODUCTS, INC., 6315 Warrick St., Cincinnati, Ohio.

RYSTAN CO., INC., 7 N. MacQuesten Pkwy.; Mount Vernon, N.Y.

S

SABIA PRODUCTS CO., 2202 N. 29th St., Philadelphia 32, Pa.

SACHS MFG. CO., 1639 Forbes St., Pittsburgh 19, Pa.

SACHS, W. D., 878 Nostrand Ave., Brooklyn 25, N.Y.

SACRAMENTO PHARMACAL CO., 3900 Broadway, Sacramento, Calif.

SAFE-GARD MFG. CO., 1285 W. 6th St., Cleveland, Ohio.

SAFETY GLOBE & MFG. CO., Columbus, Ohio.

SAFETY REMEDY CO., 1215 22nd St., N.W., Canton 9, Ohio.

SAFEWAY CHEMICAL CO., 5709 Walworth Ave., Cleveland 2, Ohio.

SAF-KIL CO., 347 Pipestone St., Benton Harbor, Mich.

SAGE LABS., INC., 53 W. 36th St., New York 18, N.Y.

SAGE, PEGGY, 50 E. 57th St., New York 22, N.Y.

SAGER BROS., 42 W. 15th St., New York 11, N.Y.

SAGINAW PAINT MFG. CO., Saginaw, Mich.

ST. LAWRENCE CHEMICAL CO., Harmon, N.Y.

ST. LOUIS RUBBER CEMENT CO., St. Louis, Mo.

ST. LOUIS SURFACER & PAINT CO., 4210 Arlington Ave., St. Louis, Mo.

SALAC FOOT COMFORT CO., 532 Cottage Grove, S.E., Grand Rapids 2, Mich.

SALES AFFILIATES, INC., 801 2nd Ave., New York 17, N.Y.

SAL-FAYNE CORP., 801 S. Patterson Blvd., Dayton 2, Ohio.

SALINITRO LABS., 237 E. 116th St., New York 29, N.Y

SALSBURY'S, DR., LABS., Charles City, Iowa.

SAN-A-LIZER CORP., 3051 Rosslyn St., Los Angeles 41, Calif.

SANABALM CO., 3257 Friendship St., Philadelphia 49, Pa.

SANASCENT CO., 15 Courtney Ave., Newburgh, N.Y.

SANDERS LABS., INC., 402 W. Highland St., Tecumseh, Okla.

SAN-EQUIP. INC., see Vega Ind.

SANFORD & SON, 6332 Warner Dr., Los Angeles 48, Calif.

SANFORD INK CO., 2740 Washington Blvd., Bellwood, Ill.

SANI-PINE CORP., 1285 McDonald Ave., Brooklyn 30, N.Y.

SANIS CHEMICAL CO., 325 Broadway, Chico, Calif.

SANITARY SOAP CO., Paterson, N.J.

SANITE CHEMICAL CO., 813 Roseneath Rd., Richmond 21, Va.

SANI-WAX CO., Dallas, Tex.

SAN JOAQUIN SULPHUR CO., P.O. Box 127, Lodi, Calif.

SAN-O-TABS CO., 8516 Walnut Dr., Los Angeles 46, Calif.

SANOZONE CO., 1127 Roy St., Philadelphia, Pa.

SAN PEDRO LABS., 110 Produce Row, San Antonio 7, Tex.

SANTA BARBARA COUNTY AGRICULTURAL COMMISSIONER, Court House, Santa Barbara, Calif.

SANTA CLARA COUNTY AGRIC. COMMISSIONER, Hall of Justice, San Jose, Calif.

SANTEE ENAMELING CO., Santee & E. 14th Sts., Los Angeles, Calif.

SANTISEPTIC CO., 2829 N.E. Glisan Ave., Portland 12, Oreg.

SAPO ELIXIR CHEMICAL CO., 800 E. Big Bend Rd., Kirkwood 22, Mo.

SAPOLIN PAINTS, INC., 229 E. 42nd St., New York, N.Y.

SAPOLIO PRODUCTS CO., 439 West St., New York 14, N.Y.

SARAVIL DRUGS, 132 2nd Ave., New York 3, N.Y.

SARDEAU, INC., 522 5th Ave., New York 36, N.Y.

SARGEANT ACNOID PHARM. CO., INC., Highland Mills, N.Y.

SARGENT-GERKE CO., 323 W. 15th St., Indianapolis, Ind.

SARTORIUS, A., & CO., 80 5th Ave., College Point, L. I., N.Y.

SATIN GLOSS POLISH CO., 10 Alden St., Boston 14, Mass.

SAVAGE ARMS CORP., Chicopee Falls, Mass.

SAVOGRAN CO., 25 Huntington Ave., Boston 16, Mass.

SAVOL BLEACH CO., East Hartford, Conn.

SAWYER CRYSTAL BLUE CO., 13 Custom House St., Boston, Mass.

SAYMAN PRODUCTS CO., 2101 Locust St., St. Louis 3, Mo.

SAYWELL LABS., 2004 St. Clair Ave., Cleveland 14, Ohio.

SCANDIA COSMETIC CORP., 44 E. 52nd St., New York 22, N.Y.

SCAT, DR., CHEMICAL CO., Chicago, Ill.

SCHAEFER VARNISH CO., 15th & Magnolia Sts., Louisville, Ky.

SCHAEFFER MFG. CO., Baston & Kosciusko Sts., St. Louis, Mo.

SCHAFFER LABS., 3512 Ocean View Blvd., Glendale 8, Calif.

SCHAFFNER, GUS J., CO., Herron Ave., Pittsburgh, Pa.

SCHALK CHEMICAL CO., 351 E. 2nd St., Los Angeles 12, Calif.

SCHECHTER & CO., 3213 Snyder Ave., Brooklyn 26, N.Y.

SCHENCK, J. H., & SON, Memphis, Tenn.

SCHERING CORP., 2 Broad St., Bloomfield, N.J.

SCHERK CORP., 157 Atlantic Ave., Brooklyn 2, N.Y.

SCHIEFFELIN & CO., 16 Cooper Sq., New York 3, N.Y.

SCHIFF BIO-FOOD PRODUCTS, INC., 80 Montgomery St., Jersey City 3, N.J.

SCHIFFMANN, R. CO., 1734 N. Main, Los Angeles 31, Calif.

SCHLOTTERBECK & FOSS CO., 117 Preble St., Portland 3, Maine.

SCHMIDT, A. O., CO., 2100 Bryant St., San Francisco 10, Calif.

SCHMUTZLER MFG. CO., 1123 S. 16th St., Quincy, Ill.

SCHOLL MFG. CO., INC., 213 W. Schiller St., Chicago 10, Ill.

SCHOONMAKER LABS., 132 Central Ave., Caldwell, N.J.

SCHRAM PRODUCT CO., 1522 2nd Ave., San Mateo, Calif.

SCHUEMANN-JONES CO., 2134 E. 9th St., Cleveland 15, Ohio.

SCHWARTZ CHEMICAL CO., INC., 326 W. 70th St., New York, N.Y.

SCIENCE PRODUCTS CO., 1230 E. 63rd St., Chicago, Ill.

SCIENTIFIC INDUSTRIES INC., 132 Front St., New York 5, N.Y.

SCOTT JAY CO., 2750 N. Wolcott Ave., Chicago 14, Ill.

SCOTT, L. E., CO., 277 Water St., Warren, R.I.

SCOTT, O. M. & SONS CO., Marysville, Ohio.

SCRIPTEX PRODUCTS CO., 523 S. 2nd St., Philadelphia, Pa.

SCRIPTO, INC., P.O. Box 4847, Atlanta 2, Ga.

SEABOARD SUPPLY CO., 830 Clinton Ave., Newark, N.J.

SEA BREEZE LABS., INC., 122 Meyran Ave., Pittsburgh 13, Pa.

SEACOAST LABORATORIES, INC., 156 Perry St., New York 14, N.Y.

SEAGER, HELAINE, INC., 355 S. Robertson Blvd., Beverly Hills, Calif.

SEAL RITE CAULKING CO., INC., 17300 Wyoming Ave., Detroit 21, Mich.

SEARS, ROEBUCK & CO., Chicago 7, Ill.

SEC MFG. CO., 59 N.E. 26th St., Miami, Fla.

SECURITY SEAL CO., 144 W. 27th St., New York 1, N.Y.

SEDAREX CO., INC., 1010 St. Paul St., Baltimore 2, Md.

SEECK & KADE, INC., 440 Washington St., New York 13, N.Y.

SEED-TREET LABS., see Pearson & Co.

SEELY MFG. CO., 1900 E. Jefferson Ave., Detroit 7, Mich.

SEEMAN BROS., see Airkem, Inc.

SEIBERLING LATEX CO., 1945 Barberton St., Akron, Ohio.

SEIBERT CORP., 10 Market St., Camden 2, N.J.

SEIDLITZ PAINT & VARNISH CO., 18th & Garfield Ave., Kansas City, Mo.

SELECTED PRODUCTS, INC., 308 W. Washington St., Chicago, Ill.

SELIG CO., 336 Marietta St., N.W. Atlanta 1, Ga.

SEMLER, R. B., INC., New Canaan, Conn.

SENDOL CO., 115 Grand Ave., Kansas City 6, Mo.

SENN, GEORGE, INC., 2200 E. Westmoreland St., Philadelphia 34, Pa.

SENORET CHEMICAL CO., 610 Gratiot St., St. Louis 2, Mo.

SENTINEL CHEMICAL CO., P.O. Box 853, Oakland 4, Calif.

SENTINEL LAB., 213 E. Jefferson St., Springfield, Ill.

SENTRY PRODUCTS CO., 70 Locust St., Boston 25, Mass.

SENZODOR, INC., 2180 Monroe Ave., Rochester 18, N.Y.

SEPTIGYN CO., 2821 Bryan St., Dallas, Tex.

SERIVER & QUINN, 1336 Willow St., Los Angeles, Calif.

SERUTAN CO., 290 Jelliff Ave., Newark 8, N.J.

SERVEX, INC., 5107 N. Figueroa St., Los Angeles 42, Calif.

SERVICE DRUG INC., 101 Summit St., Toledo, Ohio.

SEVENTEEN COSMETICS, Milton Rd., Rye, N.Y.

SEVRAN RESEARCH, INC., 605 Lincoln Rd., Miami Beach, Fla.

SEWALL PAINT & VARNISH CO., 1009 W. 8th St., Kansas City, Mo.

SEWERAGE COMMISSION, P.O. Box 2097, Milwaukee, Wis.

SEXAUER, J. A. MFG. CO., 2503 3rd Ave., New York 51, N.Y.

SEXTON, JOHN, & CO., Chicago, Ill.

SEYMOUR PRODUCTS CO., INC., 2416 W. Roosevelt Rd., Chicago, Ill.

SHACKELTON INHALER CO., INC., 44 Ionia, S.W., Grand Rapids 2, Mich.

SHAFFER LABS., INC., 10259 Helendale Ave., Tulunga, Calif.

SHANNON LUMINOUS MATERIALS CO., 7356 Santa Monica Blvd., Los Angeles 46, Calif.

SHAPIRO, IRA J., CO., INC., 45 E. 11th St., New York 3, N.Y.

SHARP & DOHME, INC., 640 N. Broad St., Philadelphia 1, Pa.

SHARP, J. C., PRODUCTS, Chattanooga, Tenn.

SHAVING POWDER CO., P.O. Box 1164, Savannah, Ga.

SHAW, JOHN, DRUG CO., Blooming Prairie, Minn.

SHEAFFER, W. A., PEN CO., Fort Madison, Iowa.

SHEERAN DRUG CO., 106 N. Main St., New Lexington, Ohio.

SHEFFIELD BRONZE PAINT CORP., 17814 Waterloo Rd., Cleveland, Ohio.

SHEFFIELD CO., 3850 Congress Expressway, Broadview, Ill.; 500 5th Ave., New York, N.Y.; New London, Conn.

SHELL CHEMICAL CORP., 50 W. 50th St.; New York 20, N.Y.

SHELL CHEMICAL CORP., Agricultural Division, 460 Park Ave., New York, N.Y.

SHELL OIL CO., 50 W. 50th St., New York, N.Y.

SHERRY, INC., 11671 N.W. 7th Ave., Miami 38, Fla.

SHERWIN-WILLIAMS CO., 101 Prospect Ave., N.W., Cleveland 1, Ohio.

SHIELD-ALL CO., Middle Country Rd., Coram, L. I., N.Y.

SHIELD COATINGS CORP., Verona, N.J.

SHIELD LABS., 12850 Manafield Ave., Detroit, Mich.

SHIFFER'S, DR., LABS., 203 Colonial Arcade, Cleveland 15, Ohio.

SHINE MAGIC CO., St. Louis, Mo.

SHORE CHEMICAL CO., INC., Boston Post Rd., Madison, Conn.

SHREVES, DR., MEDICINE CO., P.O. Box 382, Newton, Iowa.

SHULTON, INC., Route U. S. 46, Clifton, N.J.

SHULTS' OINTMENT CO., Box 243, Newtown Square, Pa.

SHUPTRINE CO., P.O. Box 644, Savannah, Ga.

SHY PRODUCTS CO., 180 N. Wacker Dr., Chicago 6, Ill.

SIGMA CHEMICAL CO., 4648 Easton Ave., St. Louis, Mo.

SILA-FLEX, 1919 Placentia, Costa Mesa, Calif.

SILICOTE CORP., P.O. Box 359, Oshkosh, Wis.

SILLERS PAINT & VARNISH CO., INC., 3325 S. Garfield Ave., Los Angeles, Calif.

SILLS CO., 223 E. Illinois St., Vinita, Okla.

SILVER SUDS CO., 829 N. 19th St., Philadelphia 30, Pa.

SIMONIZ CO., 2100 Indiana Ave., Chicago 16, Ill.

SINCLAIR PHARMACAL CO., INC., Fishers Island, N.Y.

SINCLAIR REFINING CO., 600 5th Ave., New York, N.Y.

SINCLAIR & VALENTINE CO., 611 W. 129th St., New York, N.Y.

SINGLETARY, F. B., JR., & CO., 208 S. Washington St., Rocky Mount, N.C.

SINTOS CO., 220 E. 21st St., New York 10, N.Y.

SIPE, JAMES B., & CO., 115 Vanadium Rd., Pittsburgh, Pa.

SIROIL LABS., INC., Santa Monica, Calif.

SISSON DRUG CO., 729 Main St., Hartford 2, Conn.

SISSON, P. H. MFG. CO., 294 N. Main St., Canandaigua, N.Y.

SISSON'S DRUG STORE, 73 Oak St., Decker, Ind.

SKAN LABORATORIES, INC., 1312 N. Fair Oaks, Pasadena 3, Calif.

SKAT CO., Hartford 6, Conn.

SKIN-A-FIRE CORP., 5259 W. Fullerton Ave., Chicago 39, Ill.

SKOUR-NU, INC., 42 W. 15th St., New York, N.Y.

SKYBRITE CO., 3215 Perkins Ave., Cleveland, Ohio.

SLAYER PRODUCTS CO., 3410 Broadway, New York 31, N.Y.

SLEEP-EZE CO., INC., 1067 E. Anaheim St., Long Beach 13, Calif.

SLICK SHINE CO., 207 Astor St., Newark 5, N.J.

SLIPIT PRODUCTS, INC., 169 Water St., New York, N.Y.

SLOMONS LABS., INC., 31-27 Thomson Ave., Long Island City 1, L. I., N.Y.

S. M. LABS. CO., 2013 4th Ave., Seattle 1, Wash.

SMICO PRODUCTS, 1123 Draper St., Cincinnati, Ohio.

SMITH-ALSOP PAINT & VARNISH CO., INC., Terre Haute, Ind.

SMITH BROTHERS, INC., Poughkeepsie, N.Y.

SMITH, CARROLL DUNHAM, PHARMACAL CO., New Brunswick, N.J.

SMITH, C. D., CHEMICAL DIV., Grand Junction, Colo.

SMITH-CORWIN, INC., Irvington, N.J.

SMITH, H. V., & CO., 1910 University Ave., St. Paul 4, Minn.

SMITH, KLINE & FRENCH LABS., 1530 Spring Garden St., Philadelphia 1, Pa.

SMITH LAB., INC., 718 Baltimore St., Kansas City 6, Mo.

SMITH, UPSHER, CO., 529 S. 7th St., Minneapolis 15, Minn.

SMITHER AND HILL DRUG CO., 2339 Main St., Buffalo 14, N.Y.

SNO-BOL CO., Pontiac, Mich.

SNOW WHITE PRODUCTS CO., 2101 Hudson, Lynchburg, Va.

SNOWWHITE CHEMICAL CO., Toledo, Ohio.

SNYDER, M. L., & SON, INC., Boston Ave. & Jaspar St., Philadelphia, Pa.

SOCONY MOBIL OIL COMPANY, INC., 26 Broadway, New York 4, N.Y.

SODIBOR LABS., 173 Mamaroneck Ave., White Plains, N.Y.

SODIPHENE CO., 2555 Southwest Blvd., Kansas City 8, Mo.

SOFSKIN, Division of Vick Chemical Co., 60 West St., Bloomfield, N.J.

SOIL BLDG. SERVICE, Ithaca, N.Y.

SOIL-OFF MFG. CO., 628 Vine St., Glendale 4, Calif.

SOLAR PRODUCTS CO., 2258 S. Drake Ave., Chicago 23, Ill.

SOLARINE CO., 625-49 S. Smallwood St., Baltimore, Md.

SO-LO MARX RUBBER CO., Cincy Ave., Loveland, Ohio.

SOLVAY PROCESS DIVISION, Allied Chemical & Dye Corp., P.O. Box 271, Syracuse 1, N.Y.

SOLVENT MFG. CO., 388 Race St., Holyoke, Mass.

SOLVENTOL CHEMICAL PRODUCTS, INC., 15841 2nd Blvd., Detroit, Mich.

SOLVIT CHEMICAL CO., INC., 3734 Speedway Rd., Madison 5, Wis.

SOLWAY-ANNAN CO., 6400 Rhode Island Ave., Riverdale, Md.

SOMNYL PHARMACAL CORP. OF AMERICA, 475 5th Ave., New York 17, N.Y.

SONNEBORN, L., Bldg. Products Division, 80 8th Ave., New York, N.Y.

SONOMA COUNTRY AGR. COMM., Santa Rosa, Calif.

SOOT CLEAN CO., Sanford, N.C.

SOOVAIN CO., 522 Market, San Diego, Calif.

SORBOL CO., 28 S. Main St., Mechanicsburg, Ohio.

SO-SHUR OINTMENT CO., 733 W. Commerce St., Oklahoma City 9, Okla.

SOS PRODUCTS, 282 Nassau Ave., Brooklyn, N.Y.

SOUTH BEND BAIT CO., South Bend 23, Ind.

SOUTH PORT PAINT CO., 555 Lathrop Ave., Savannah, Ga.

SOUTHERN AGRICULTURAL CHEMICALS, INC., Box 191, Kingtree, S.C.

SOUTHERN AGRICULTURAL INSECTICIDES, INC., Box 1130, Hendersonville, N.C.

SOUTHERN CHEMICAL SALES & SERVICE CO., see Diamond Black Leaf Co.

SOUTHERN COATINGS & CHEMICAL CO., Sumter, S.C.

SOUTHERN LABS., INC., P.O. Box 1204, Macon, Ga.

SOUTHERN LACQUER CO., 1426 Philpot, Baltimore, Md.

SOUTHERN PHARM. CO., INC., 8901 W. Lawn Ave., Brentwood 17, Mo.

SOUTHERN PINE CHEMICAL, Division of Glidden Co., P.O. Box 389, Jacksonville 1, Fla.

SOUTHERN PINE EXTRACT CO., Tallahasse, Fla.

SOUTHERN RESEARCH LABS., Starkville, Miss.

SOUTHLAND PRODUCTS CO., P.O. Box 455, Lake Worth, Fla.

SOUTHWEST AGRICULTURAL CHEMICAL CO., Waco, Tex.

SOUTHWEST CO-OPERATIVE WHOLESALE, 1821 E. Jackson St., Phoenix, Ariz.

SOUTHWEST DISTRIBUTING CO., See Lien Chem.

SOUTHWEST FERTILIZER & CHEMICAL CO., Clint, Tex.

SOUTHWEST SPRAYER & CHEMICAL CO., P.O. Box 487, Waco, Tex.

SPEARHEAD BOILER PLUG & SPECIALTY CO., 704 Woodland Ave., Cleveland 15, Ohio.

SPECIAL FORMULA CORP., 445 Park Ave., New York 22, N.Y.

SPECIALISTS FORMULARY, 907 Penn Ave., Pittsburgh 22, Pa.

SPECIALTY PRODUCTS CO., 433 Bourbon St., New Orleans 16, La.

SPECO, INC., 7308 Associate Ave., Cleveland 9, Ohio.

SPEEKMAN, F. M., CO., 241 Quint St., San Francisco 24, Calif.

SPENCE-MC CORD DRUG CO., LaCrosse, Wis.

SPERRY, J., CO., 210 E. 10th St., Sioux Falls, S. Dak.

S.P.F. WOOD PRESERVING CO., Division of James Huggins & Son, Inc., Malden 48, Mass.

SPICER, CHAS. R., CO., INC., 357 N. Main St., Memphis 3, Tenn.

SPINOL CO., 213 Mahantongo St., Pottsville, Pa.

SPIRO POWDER CO., 290 Larkin St., Buffalo, N.Y.

SPOHN MEDICAL CO., 202 N. Main St., Goshen, Ind.

SPORODYNE CO., 201 Cincinnati St., Dayton 8, Ohio.

SPRATTS AMERICA, LTD., 18 Congress St., Newark 5, N.J.

SPRAY TAN, INC., 2 Sherwood Ave., Baltimore 8, Md.

SPRINGFIELD PRODUCTS CO., Springfield, Ohio.

SQUIBB, E. R., & SONS, Div. of Olin Mathiesin Chem. Corp., 745 5th Ave., New York 22, N.Y.

S & S CO., INC., Albany, Ga.

S.S.S. CO., P.O. Box 4447, Atlanta 2, Ga.

STACOAT PAINT & VARNISH CO., 1821 Daly St., Los Angeles, Calif.

STADLER FERTILIZER CO., 1010 Denison Ave., Cleveland 9, Ohio.

STAFFORD, S. S., INC., 609 Washington St., New York, N.Y.

STALEY, A. E., MFG. CO., Decatur, Ill.

STAMINITE CORP., 109 Water St., New Haven 11, Conn.

STANBACK CO., LTD., Salisbury, N.C.

STANDARD AG. CHEMICALS, INC., 429 Forum Bldg., Sacramento 14, Calif.; Hoboken, N.J.

STANDARD CHEMICAL CO., 236 2nd St., Oakland 7, Calif.

STANDARD CHLORINE CHEMICAL COMPANY, INC., Jacobus Ave., South Kearny, N.J.

STANDARD DRUG CO., 408 W. St. Clair Ave., Cleveland 13, Ohio.

STANDARD DRY WALL PRODUCTS INC., New Eagle, Penn.

STANDARD INDUSTRIAL PRODUCTS, INC., 1500 Park, Evansville, Ind.

STANDARD LABORATORIES, INC., 113 W. 18th St., New York 11, N.Y.

STANDARD MEDICAL SUPPLY CO., 735 N. High St., Columbus 8, Ohio.

STANDARD MEDICINES CO., see Standard Medical.

STANDARD OIL CO., (Indiana), 910 S. Michigan Ave., Chicago 80, Ill.

STANDARD PASTE & GLUE CO., 3622 W. 38th St., Chicago, Ill.

STANDARD-TOCH CHEMICAL INC., Port Richmond, S. I., N.Y.

STANDARD WOOD PRESERVER CO., 4624 D'Hemecourt St., New Orleans 19, La.

STANHOPE MFG. CO., 1628 W. Venice Blvd., Los Angeles 6, Calif.

STANIS, Z. G., CO., 2822 Archer Ave., Chicago 8, Ill.

STANLEY HOME PRODUCTS, INC., Easthampton, Mass.

STANLEY INDUSTRIES, 13415 24th Ave., S., Seattle 88, Wash.

STANLEY, JOHN T., CO., 642 W. 30th St., New York, N.Y.

STANSBURY CHEMICAL CO., 1929 Aurora Ave., Seattle 9, Wash.

STAPLES, H. F., & CO., INC., 33 Ship Ave., Medford, Mass.

STARKE, LEWIS E., PHARMACAL CO., 4910 Delor St., St. Louis 9, Mo.

STAR SHEEN COSMETIC CO., 4602 Hollywood Blvd., Los Angeles 27, Calif.

STAT LABS., 123 McTyere St., Jackson, Miss.

STATLER PHARMACY, Statler Hotel, Buffalo 2, N.Y.

STAUFFER CHEMICAL CO., Chauncey, N.Y.

STA-WAKE CORP. OF AMERICA, 127 S. San Vicente St., Los Angeles 48, Calif.

STAYNER CORP., 2100 Ward St., Berkeley 5, Calif.

STAZE, INC., 375 Fairfield Ave., Stamford, Conn.

STEARNS ELECTRIC PASTE CO., 111 W. Washington St., Chicago 2, Ill.

STEELCOTE MFG. CO., Theresa Ave. & Gratiot St., St. Louis, Mo.

STEEL TREATING EQUIPMENT CO., Dearborn Mich.

STEIN, M., COSMETIC CO., 430 Broome St., New York, N.Y.

STEINMANN PHARMACAL LAB., 14 Rossmore Ave., Bronxville, N.Y.

STELWAGON MFG. CO., 19th St. & Washington Ave., Philadelphia, Pa.

STEMPEL FIRE EXTINGUISHER MFG. CO., Boston Ave. & Jasper St., Philadelphia, Pa.

STENTON LABS., INC., P.O. Box 575, Wilkes-Barre, Pa.

STERIPHONE CO., INC., 103 Park Ave., New York 17, N.Y.

STERLING PAINT & VARNISH CO., Malden, Mass.

STERLING PRODUCTS DIVISION, Sterling Drug, Inc., Monticello, Ill.

STERLING PRODUCTS, INC., Distributors, Wheeling, W. Va.

STERLING PRODUCTS INTER-NATIONAL, INC., 1450 Broadway, New York 18, N.Y.

STERLING VARNISH CO., 1953 Zenderoll Ave., Sewickley, Pa.

STERNO, INC., 9 E. 37th St., New York 16, N.Y.

STETSON, M. D., CO., c/o Boston Chemical Industries, Inc., 64 E. Brookline St., Boston, Mass.

STEVENS CHEMICAL CO., 2240 W. Baltimore St., Baltimore 23, Md.

STEVENS INDUSTRIES, INC., N. Main St., Dawson, Ga.

STEVENS, WM. H. & SONS, 2621 Arnold Rd., Des Moines 10, Iowa.

STEWART BROTHERS PAINT CO., Alliance, Ohio.

STEWART-LUNHAL CO., 7349 Coldwater Canyon Ave., Los Angeles, Calif.

STEWART PAINT MFG. CO., 1730 Washington Ave., Minneapolis, Minn.

STEWART-SIMMONS, INC., P.O. Box 459, Mason City, Iowa.

STEWART-WARNER CORP., 1826 Diversey Pkwy., Chicago, Ill.

STIEH, WILLIAM M., & CO., INC., 20 Vesey St., New York 7, N.Y.

STILLE-YOUNG CORP., 3950 N. Lincoln Ave., Chicago, Ill.

STILLMAN CO., 323 Main St., Aurora, Ill.

STIM-U-PLANT LABS., INC., 2077 Parkwood, Columbus 16, Ohio.

STODDARD, G. S., & CO., INC., 121 E. 24th St., New York 10, N.Y.

STOKER, H. L., CO., P.O. Box 112, Claremont, Calif.

STOM ASEPTINE CORP., 150 W. 28th St., New York 1, N.Y.

STONHARD CO., 501 Stonhard Bldg., 1306 Spring Garden St., Philadelphia, Pa.

STRAIT-LINE PRODUCTS, Santa Ana, Calif.

STRAND PRODUCTS CO., 118 S. Clinton St., Chicago 6, Ill.

STRASENBURGH, R. J., 195 Exchange St., Rochester, N.Y.

STRATFORD-COOKSON CO., 4058 Haverford Ave., Philadelphia 4, Pa.

STRIBLING, JOHN B., & SON, LTD., 1507 S. Oakes St., San Angelo, Tex.

STRICKLAND, J.R., CO., 1400 Ragan St., Memphis, Tenn.

STRONG, COBB & CO., INC., 2654 Lisbon Rd., Cleveland 4, Ohio.

STUART, INC., Rossmor Bldg., St. Paul 1, Minn.

STUCCO PRODUCT CO. OF FLORIDA, INC., 2592 Priscilla, Jacksonville, Fla.

STUDEBAKER CHEMICAL CO., Elyria, Ohio.

STUDIO GIRL - HOLLYWOOD, INC., Glendale, Calif.

STULL, A. J., & CO., 5821 Tacony St., Philadelphia, Pa.

STULL'S CHEMICALS, INC., 109 S. Flores St., San Antonio 5, Tex.

STUMPF'S, JOHN, SONS, 614 1st St., Gretna 1, La.

STURTEVANT, F. C., CO.,21-23 Mechanic St., Hartford 5, Conn.

SUBOX, INC., 5 Fairmount Park, Hackensack, N.J.

SUCCESS CHEMICAL CO., 2145 Pitkin Ave., Brooklyn 7, N.Y.

SUDBURY LAB., Dutton Rd., South Sudbury, Mass.

S. U. G. CHEMICAL CO., 121 W. Packer Ave., Sayre, Pa.

SUGAR BEET PRODUCTS CO., Saginaw, W.S., Mich.

SULFUR-8 CHEMICAL CO., 41 Albany Ave., Brooklyn 13, N.Y.

SULLIVAN & CO., 212 E. Trigg Ave., Memphis 2, Tenn.

SULPHO-NAPTHOL CO., 131 Milk St., Boston 9, Mass.

SUMLAK CO., 3562 Vine St., Cincinnati 20, Ohio.

SUMLAR CO., 3120 Tilden Ave., Brooklyn 26, N.Y.

SUMMERS FERTILIZER CO., INC., & KELLY AGRIC. PRODS. CO., Mc Keesport, Pa.

SUNDURE PAINT CORP., Sundure Bldg., Syracuse, N.Y.

SUNLAND INDUSTRIES, INC., P.O. Box 1669, Fresno, Calif.

SUN OIL CO., 1608 Walnut St., Philadelphia 3, Pa.

SUN RAY HAIR PREPARATION CO., 2404 Fuller St., New York 61, N.Y.

SUNNYSIDE OIL CO., 5530 N. Wolcott Ave., Chicago 40, Ill.

SUNSET SALES CORP., 1660 N. Hobart Blvd., Los Angeles 27, Calif.

SUNSHINE, JOHN, CHEMICAL CO., INC., 600 W. Lake St., Chicago 6, Ill.

SUPER-TOMIC PRODUCTS CO., 6411 Hollywood Blvd., Los Angeles 28, Calif.

SUPERIOR CHEMICAL PRODUCTS, INC., 47 N. 2nd St., Philadelphia 6, Pa.

SUPERIOR FERTILIZER CO., P.O. Box 1021, Tampa, Fla.

SUPERIOR LABS., Grand Rapids, Mich.

SUPERIOR PAINT & LACQUER WORKS, 6231 Maywood Ave., Huntington Park, Calif.

SUPERIOR PHARMACAL CO., 823 E. 5th St., Dayton 2, Ohio.

SUPREME PHARMACEUTICAL CO., 354 Mercer St., Jersey City 2, N.J.

SURBIN LABS., 1350 New York Ave., Brooklyn 3, N.Y.

SURETOX CO., P.O. Box 704, New Brunswick, N.J.

SURETY MFG. CO., 215 W. Illinois St., Chicago 10, Ill.

SURF LAB., 2 N. Vermont Ave., Atlantic City, N.J.

SUTLIFF & CASE CO., INC., Peoria, Ill.

SUTTON COSMETICS, INC., 385 5th Ave., New York 16, N.Y.

SUTTON LABORATORIES, Chapel Hill, N.C.

SUWANEE DRUG CO., Newberry, Fla.

SWAMP & DIXIE LABS., INC., 1622 N. Lewis St., Tulsa, Okla.

SWANSON CO., 68 E. Locust St., Newark, Ohio.

SWEDISH SHAMPOO LABS., 880 Broadway, New York 3, N.Y.

SWEENEY, W. H., & CO., 43 E. Water St., St. Paul, Minn.

SWEENEY, W. R., Salisbury, Mo.

SWIFT & CO., Plant Food Division, Chicago, Ill.

SYMOLYN PAINT MAKERS, INC., 6316 Northwest Hgwy., Chicago, Ill.

SYNVAR CORP., Wilmington, Del.

SYSTEM PRODUCTS CO., 6407 S. Park Ave., Chicago, Ill.

SYSTONE MEDICINE CO., 39 E. Court St., Cincinnati 2, Ohio.

T

TABLAX CO., Union Sq., New York, N.Y.

TAFT INDUSTRIAL CHEMICAL CO., INC., 203 E. 18th St., New York 3, N.Y.

TAILBY-NASON CO., 49 Amherst St., Boston 42, Mass.

TALBOT MFG. CO., 465 E. 31st St., Los Angeles 11, Calif.

TAMMS INDUSTRIES, INC., Builders Bldg., Dept. T, 228 N. LaSalle St., Chicago, Ill.

TAMPA DRUG CO., Florida Ave. & Washington St., Tampa 2, Fla.

TANGLEFOOT CO., 314 Straight Ave., S.W., Grand Rapids 4, Mich.

TANNER EYE WATER CO., Douglas, Ga.

TARBOX, L. B., CO., Batavia, N.Y.

TARKAN PHARMACAL CO., Steubenville, Ohio.

TATE-LAX MEDICINE CO., Rt. 9, Box 440, Waco, Tex.

TATTOO, INC., 16 W. 60th St., New York 23, N.Y.

TAYLOR CHEMICAL CO., P.O. Box 337, Aberdeen, N.C.

TAYLOR-REED CORP., Glenbrook, Conn.

TEBSIN, INC., 1636-38 Silverlake Blvd., Los Angeles 26, Calif.

TECHNICAL COLOR & CHEM. WKS., INC., 439 3rd Ave., Brooklyn, N.Y.

TECHNICAL PRODUCTS CO., 1395 Main St., Walnut Creek 13, Calif.

TECHNICAL SUPPLY CO., 1911 University Ave., Palo Alto, Calif.

TECH-N-KAL, 12925 Auburn Ave., Detroit 23, Mich.

TECHNO-CHEMICAL LAB., 95 Manhattan St., Rochester, N.Y.

TECNIQUE, INC., 520 Plymouth Bldg., Minneapolis 2, Minn.

TEEN LABS., P.O. Box 28, Arlington, Tex.

TENEX LABS., INC., Cedar Rapids, Iowa.

TENNESSEE CORPORATION, 617 Grant Building, Atlanta 1, Ga.

TENNESSEE EASTMAN CHEMICAL PRODUCTS, INC., Kingsport, Tenn.

TENNESSEE PRODUCTS & CHEMICAL CORP., 512 First American National Bank Bldg., Nashville 3, Tenn.

TESTOR CHEMICAL CO., 615 Buckbee St., Rockford, Ill.

TETRA "D" SALES CO., 715 Lincoln Pl., Brooklyn 16, N.Y.

TEWI PERFUME CO., 100-30 67th Dr., Forest Hills, L. I., N.Y.

TEXAS ACID & CHEMICAL CO., Beaumont, Tex.

TEXAS CO., 135 E. 42nd St., New York 17, N.Y.

TEXAS PHARM. CO., P.O. Box 1659, San Antonio 6, Tex.

TEXAS PHENOTHIAZINE CO., 2021 N. Grove, Fort Worth 6, Tex.

TEXO CORP., 3710 Floral Ave., Cincinnati, Ohio.

TEXON INDUSTRIAL CORP., 5-50 49th Ave., Long Island City, L. I., N.Y.

TEX PRODUCTS, INC., Newark, N.J.

THAYER, HENRY, CO., 100 Inman St., Cambridge 39, Mass.

THEOBALD INDUSTRIES, Kearny, N.J.

THIBAULT & WALKER CO., 5-48 46th St., Long Island City, L. I., N.Y.

THOMAS CHEMICAL CO., INC., Lynchburg, Va.

THOMAS CO., 1645 Hennepin Ave., Minneapolis 3, Minn.

THOMAS, I. P., DIVISION, Pennsylvania Salt Mfg. Co., Paulsboro, N.J.

THOMAS PRODUCTS, INC., 45 N. Division St., Buffalo 3, N.Y.

THOMAS & THOMPSON CO., E. Baltimore St., Baltimore 2, Md.

THOMAS, W. G., PHM., Varina, N.C.

THOMPSON CHEMICALS CORP., 3600 Monon St., Los Angeles 27, Calif.

THOMPSON & CO., 1085 Edwards Blvd., Oakmont, Pa.

THOMPSON-HAYWARD CHEMICAL CO., Thompson Bldg., Kansas City, Mo.

THOMPSON LABORATORIES, INC., Richmond, Indiana.

THOMPSON MEDICAL CO., INC., 224 W. 28th St., New York 1, N.Y.

THOMPSON, W. S., PRODUCTS CO., 77 P St., N.E., Washington, D.C.

THOMPSON, WM. T., CO., 2727 Hyperion Ave., Los Angeles 27, Calif.

THOMSON-PORCELITE PAINT CO., 330 Race St., Philadelphia 6, Pa.

THORNTON, L. M., MFG., INC., 2821 E. 18th St., Kansas City, Mo.

THORNTON, RENEE, COSMETICS, INC., 2 W. 47th St., New York 36, N.Y.

THORO PRODUCTS CO., 3240 Larimer St., Denver 5, Colo.

THOROUGHBRED REMEDY CO., Elmont, L. I., N.Y.

THORSON SOAP LAKE PRODUCTS CO., P.O. Box 98, Soap Lake, Wash.

THREE P PRODUCTS, P.O. Box 3291, Hill Sta., Augusta, Ga.

THRESHER PAINT & VARNISH DIVISION, 1100 E. Monument St., Dayton, Ohio.

THYMOLAC CO., 54 Gill Pl., Buffalo, N.Y.

THYOQUENT LABS., Division of Clark-Cleveland Inc., Binghamton, N.Y.

TIBBETS CORP., 1624 E. 14th St., Los Angeles, Calif.

TIDE WATER ASSOC. OIL CO., 79 New Montgomery St., San Francisco 20, Calif.

TIDY HOUSE PRODUCTS CO., 1400 Evans St., Omaha, Nebr.

TIDY WALL CO., Royal Oak, Mich.

TILDEN CO., New Lebanon, N.Y.

TILETTE CEMENT CO., INC., 401 Lafayette St., New York 3, N.Y.

TILTON PRODUCTS, 1100 Illinois Ave., Pittsburgh 16, Pa.

TIP TOP PRODUCTS CO., 1515 Cuming St., Omaha 2, Nebr.

TITANIME, INC., Elmwood & Morris Aves., Union, N.J.

T-LAX PRODUCTS CO., Birmingham, Ala.

TNEMEC CO., 121 W. 23rd St., Kansas City, Mo.

T-N-T DOGGIE REMEDIES, 18820 Eureka St., Detroit 12, Mich.

TOCH BROS. CO., Elm Park, S.I., N.Y.

TOGSTAD, C. D., CO., Kokomo, Ind.

TOLEDO PT. & CHEMICAL CO., 23 Blucher St., Toledo, Ohio.

TONE PROFESSIONAL PRODUCTS, 677 Amsterdam Ave., New York 25, N.Y.

TONGUE, R. E., & BROS. CO., INC., Allegheny Ave. & Ambler St., Philadelphia, Pa.

TONI CO., Research Lab., 222 W. N. Bank Dr., Chicago 54, Ill.

TORCH LABS., INC., 110 Chestnut St., Philadelphia 6, Pa.

TOSAN DRUG CO., 3419 Broadway, New York 31, N.Y.

TOWER, Distributors for Sears Roebuck & Co., Photographic Materials Division, 925 S. Homan Ave., Chicago, Ill.

TOXITE LABORATORIES, INC., Cumberland, Ind.

TRACY CO., INC., New London, Conn.

TRAGER MFG. CO., 1015-1059 Price St., Scranton 4, Pa.

TRAINER, WALTER L., CO., Germantown & Rising Sun Aves., Philadelphia, Pa.

TRANSOGRAM CO., INC., Coudersport, Pa.

TRAVINE LAB., 395 W. Passaic Ave., Bloomfield, N.J.

TREDENNICK PAINT MFG. CO., 450 Pratt, Meriden, Conn.

TREMCO MFG. CO., 8701 Kinsman Rd., Cleveland, Ohio.

TRIANGLE CHEMICAL CO., 1115 Charlotte Ave., Nashville 4, Tenn.

TRICKER, WILLIAM, INC., Independence, Ohio.

TRICO PRODUCTS CORP., 817 Washington St., Buffalo 3, N.Y.

TRIMAL LABS., 7029 Willoughby Ave., Los Angeles 38, Calif.

TRIPLE AAA TABLETS, INC., 370 Genesee St., Buffalo 24, N.Y.

TRIPLE-X CHEMICAL LABS., INC., 2803 S. Calumet Ave., Chicago 16, Ill.

TRITOX CHEM. CO., Washington, Ind.

TROPICAL PAINT & OIL CO., 1210-52 W. 70th St., Cleveland, Ohio.

TROUT, FREDERICK, CO., 974 W. Peachtree St., N.W., Atlanta, Ga.

TROY CHEMICAL CO., INC., 110 E. 42nd St., New York 17, N.Y.

TROY INDUSTRIAL PRODUCTS, Division of Globe Sanitary Supply Co., 2249 E. 38th St., Los Angeles 58, Calif.

TRU-AID MEDICINE CO., 212 E. 13th St., Cincinnati 10, Ohio.

TRU-LEX MEDICINE CO., P.O. Box 632, Covington, Ky.

TRU-PINE CO., 7638 Vincennes Ave., Chicago 20, Ill.

TRUE, DR. J. F., & CO., INC., Lynn, Mass.

TRUSCON LABS., Carriff St., Detroit, Mich.

TRYLON PRODUCT CORP., 2750 N. Wolcott Ave., Chicago 14, Ill.

TUBED CHEMICALS CORP., 2 Pine St., Easthampton, Mass.

TUDOR CHEMICAL SPECIALTIES, INC., 141 Woodworth Ave., Yonkers 2, N.Y.

TUMBLER, J. A., LAB., INC., 423 S. Hanover St., Baltimore, Md.

TURCO PAINT & VARNISH CO., 315 Market St., Philadelphia, Pa.

TURNER HALL CORP., 142 5th Ave., New York 11, N.Y.

TURNER'S PHARM., 2100 E. Main St., Richmond 23, Va.

TUTAG, S. J., & CO., 19180 Mt. Elliott Ave., Detroit 34, Mich.

TUTTLE ELIXER CO., 188 Hanover St., Boston 13, Mass.

TWIN CITY SHELLAC CO., INC., 334 Flushing Ave., Brooklyn 5, N.Y.

TWITTY BROS., 779 Broadway, New York, N.Y.

T-X PHARMACAL CO., Akron, Ohio.

TYLER, A. G., INC., New York, N.Y.

TYREE, J. S., CHEMISTS, INC., 743 15th St., N.E., Washington, D.C.

TYSON ORCHARD SERVICE, Flora Dale, Pa.

U

UDDO, F., & SONS, 200 Bienville, New Orleans, La.

UDGA, INC., 2459 University Ave., St. Paul, Minn.

UDYLITE CORP., 1653 Grand Blvd., Detroit, Mich.

ULMER PHARMACAL CO., 1400 Harmon Pl., Minneapolis 3, Minn.

ULTRA CHEMICAL WORKS, INC., 2 Wood St., Paterson 4, N.J.

ULTRASOL SALES CORP., 140 Overlook Pl., Newburgh, N.Y.

ULTRA-VIOLET PRODUCT, INC., 5114 Walnut Grove Ave., San Gabriel, Calif.

UNCLE SAM CHEMICAL CO., INC., 575 W. 131st St., New York 27, N.Y.

UNDERTAKERS SUPPLY CO., 337 S. Peoria St., Chicago, Ill.

U-NEEK MANUFACTURING CO., Newton, Iowa.

UNEXCELLED CHEMICAL CORP., 350 5th Ave., New York, N.Y.

UNION CARBIDE & CARBON CO., see Carbide & Carbon.

UNION OIL CO. OF CALIF., Los Angeles, Calif.

UNION PAINT & VARNISH CO., 1206 Shore Ave., Pittsburgh, Pa.

UNION PHARMACEUTICAL CO., INC., Bloomfield, N.J.

UNION RUBBER & ASBESTOS CO., Trenton 6, N.J.

UNITED CHEMICAL CO., 401 Delaware St., Kansas City, Mo.

UNITED COOPERATIVES, INC., 450 W. Ely St., Alliance, Ohio.

UNITED CRAYON, 115 4th Ave., Brooklyn 17, N.Y.

UNITED FINISH CO., Peabody, Mass.

UNITED GILSONITE LABS., Scranton 1, Pa.

UNITED NATIONAL CO., 549 W. Randolph St., Chicago 6, Ill.

UNITED NAVAL STORES CO., 82 Blauer St., New York, N.Y.

UNITED SALES & MFG. CO., Division of Foster-Milburn Co., Buffalo, N.Y.

U. S. CHEMICAL PRODUCTS CO., P.O. Box 212, Columbus, Ohio.

U. S. GUTTA PERCHA PAINT CO., 41 Dudley St., Providence, R.I.

U. S. GYPSUM CO., 300 W. Adams St., Chicago, Ill.

U. S. PACKAGING CORP., Bridgeport, Conn.

U. S. PLYWOOD CORP., 55 W. 44th St., New York 36, N.Y.

U. S. PHOSPHORIC PRODS. DIV., Tennesee Corp., Tampa, Fla.

U. S. REFINING CO., 2695 E. 55th St., Cleveland, Ohio.

U. S. RODENT DESTROYER CO., Los Gatos, Calif.

U. S. RUBBER CO., Naugatuck Chemical Division, Naugatuck, Conn.

U. S. SANITARY SPECIALTIES CORP., 1001 S. California Ave., Chicago, Ill.

U. S. SPECIALTY MFG. CO., West Somerville, Mass.

UNIVERSAL MEDICAL CO., 1400 S. Pulaski Rd., Chicago 23, Ill.

UNIVERSAL NUTRITIONS, INC., 16 Hudson St., New York 13, N.Y.

UNIVERSAL PAINT & VARNISH CORP., Bedford, Ohio.

UNIVERSAL REFINING PRODUCTS CO., INC., 1133 Broadway, New York, N.Y.

UNIVERSAL WATER SOFTENER CO., 1005-1007 S. 5th Ave., Maywood, Ill.

UPCO CO., 4800 Lexington Ave., Cleveland, Ohio.

UPJOHN CO., Kalamazoo 99, Mich.

URELL, INC., 2630 Humboldt St., Los Angeles 31, Calif.

URICHECK PHOTO CO., 951 Burton St., Freeland, Pa.

UTILITY CO., INC., 636 W. 44th St., New York 36, N.Y.

UTLEY PAINT CO., INC., Hardwick, Vt.

V

VAL-A CO., 700 W. Root St., Chicago 9, Ill.

VALBAR CHEMICAL CORP., 247 Greenwich Ave., Greenwich, Conn.

VALENTINE & CO., Jacobus Ave., South Kearny, N.J.

VALMAS DRUG CO., Lima, N.Y.

VAN BRODE MILLING CO., INC., Clinton, Mass.

VAN CLEEF BROS., INC., 7800 Woodlawn Ave., Chicago 19, Ill.

VANDERBILT, R. T., CO., 230 Park Ave., New York 17, N.Y.

VAN DYKE SALES CO., Atlantic City, N.J.

VANE-CALVERT PAINT CO., 1601 N. Broadway, St. Louis, Mo.

VANGUARD PAINTS & FINISHES, INC., Marietta, Ohio.

VAN PATTON PHARMACEUTICAL CO., 1104 W. Belmont, Chicago, Ill.

VAN SICKLE GLASS & PAINT CO., 143 S. 10th St., Lincoln, Nebr.

VAN-S LABS., 1681 8th St., Oakland, Calif.

VAN STAN, V. F., CO., 3844 Germantown Ave., Philadelphia, Pa.

VANTINES, INC., 34 W. 15th St., New York 11, N.Y.

VAN VOR CHEMICAL CO., Box 671, Hagerstown, Md.

VAPO-CRESOLINE CO., Division of Grandpa Brands Co., 912 Sycamore St., Cincinnati 2, Ohio.

VAPORINE CO., 83 S. Water Market, Chicago 8, Ill.

VARCROFT WORKS, INC., Pottstown, Pa.

VAR-LAC-OID CHEMICAL CO., 116 Broad St., New York 4, N.Y.

VARLEY, JAMES, & SONS, INC., 1200 Switzer Ave., St. Louis 15, Mo.

VARNITON CO., 416 N. Varney St., Burbank, Calif.

VARN-O WAX CO., Newburgh, N.Y.

VB LABS., 269 Monticello Ave., Jersey City 6, N.J.

VEGA INDUSTRIES, INC., San-Equip Div., Syracuse 5, N.Y.

VEGETRATES CO., 4361 Melrose Ave., Los Angeles 29, Calif.

VEITH CHEMICAL CO., INC., 2050 McKinley Ave., Fresno 3, Calif.

VELAND PRODS., INC., Cleveland, Ohio.

VELODENT PRODUCTS MFG. CO., INC., 1 Union Sq., W., New York 3, N.Y.

VELSICOL CORP., 330 E. Grand Ave., Chicago 11, Ill.

VELTEX CO., 1811 1st Ave., N., Birmingham 3, Ala.

VELVET PHARM. PRODUCTS CO., INC., 11 Park Pl., New York 7, N.Y.

VERITAS PRODUCTS CO., INC., 41 Union Sq., New York, N.Y.

VERMEX CO. OF AMERICA, 163a S. Glenwood Pl., Burbank, Calif.

VERNON DRUG CO., 129 Wickham Ave., Middletown, N.Y.

VESTAL INC., 4963 Manchester Ave., St. Louis 10, Mo.

VICK CHEMICAL CO., 60 West St., Bloomfield, N.J.

VICTORIA CHEMICAL CO., Newark, N.J.

VICTOR SALES CO., P.O. Box 1021, Petersburg, Va.

VICTORY CHEMICAL CO., 148 Fairmount Ave., Philadelphia 23, Pa.

VICTORY SPRAY EMULSION CO., 18 Channing Rd., Burlingame, Calif.

VIENNA BEAUTY PRODUCTS, INC., 216 N. Clinton St., Chicago 6, Ill.

VI-GIEN LABS., 149 Collingwood Ave., Detroit 2, Mich.

VI-JON LABS., INC., St. Louis, Mo.

VIMASCO CORP., Charleston, W. Va.

VINCO CO., INC., 305 E. 45th St., New York, N.Y.

VINELAND POULTRY LABS., E. Landis Ave., Vineland, N.J.

VINSON CHEM. PRODUCTS CO., INC., 4435 N.W. 2nd Ave., Miami 37, Fla.

VIRGINIA SMELTING CO., West Norfolk, Va.

VIS-KO INC., Sumner, Wash.

VITAL DRUG PRODUCTS, 27 Tuckahoe Rd., Yonkers 2, N.Y.

VITA-VAR CORP., 48 Albert Ave., Newark, N.J.

VITEC CORP., 412 E. 10th St., Kansas City 6, Mo.

VI-TOSIS LABS., 149 Collingwood Ave., Detroit 2, Mich.

VIVAUDOU, JEAN, CO., INC., 10 W. 33rd St., New York 1, N.Y.

VOGARELL PRODUCTS CO., 1212 W. Washington Blvd., Los Angeles 7, Calif.

VOGEL LABS., Mohegan Lake, N.Y.

VOLAY OF PARIS CO., P.O. Box 1097, Greenwich, Conn.

VOLTAX CO., 3 Reservoir Ave., Bridgeport, Conn.

VON SCHRADER MFG. CO., 16th St. & Junction Ave., Racine, Wis.

VORAC CO., Rutherford, N.J.

VORTEX MFG. CO., 1960 W. 77th St., Cleveland, Ohio.

VULCAN VARNISH CO., 1112 W. Main St., Louisville, Ky.

W

WADE, JIM, & CO., 1507 Marshall St., Shreveport 50, La.

WADSWORTH-HOWLAND & CO., 141 Federal St., Boston, Mass.

WAGNER ELECTRIC CORP., St. Louis 4, Mo.

WAILES-DOVE-HERMISTON CORP., 1941 Linden St., Westfield, N.J.

WALBUCK CRAYON CO., Andover, Mass.

WALDSTEIN CO., 2121 McCarter Hgwy., Newark, N.J.

WALKER, MADAM C. J., MFG. CO., 617 Indiana Ave., Indianapolis 2, Ind.

WALKER, CORP. & CO., INC., 406 Ash St., Syracuse 8, N.Y.

WALKER, NORRIS, PAINT MFG. CO., Salem, Oreg.

WALKER PHARMACAL CO., 4200 Laclede Ave., St. Louis 8, Mo.

WALKER REMEDY CO., 224 Commercial St., Waterloo, Iowa.

WALLACE LABS., INC., Division of Carter Products, Inc., New Brunswick, N.J.

WALTHAM CHEMICAL CO., 817 Moody St., Waltham 54, Mass.

WAMBAUGH CHEMICAL CO., Goshen, Ind.

WAMPOLE, HENRY K., & CO., INC., 440 Fairmount Ave., Philadelphia, Pa.

WANDER CO., 105 W. Adams St., Chicago 3, Ill.

WARCIN CO., 121 W. Wacker Dr., Chicago 1, Ill.

WARD'S, 52 Franklin St., Boston, Mass.

WARNER-CHILCOTT LABS., Division of Warner Hudnut, Inc., Morris Plains, N.J.

WARNER'S REMEDY CO., see Meyers Labs.

WARREN CHEMICAL PRODUCTS CO., 576 E. Market St., Warren, Ohio.

WARREN PAINT & COLOR CO., Nashville, Tenn.

WARREN REFINING & CHEMICAL CO., 5151 Denison Ave., Cleveland 2, Ohio.

WARREN-TEED PRODUCTS CO., Columbus 8, Ohio.

WASHBURN, W. O., & SONS, INC., 500 Robert St., St. Paul 1, Minn.

WASHINGTON BARBER & BEAUTY SUPPLY CO., Washington, Pa.

WASHINGTON HOMOEPATHIC PHARMACY, 724 11th St., N.W., Washington 1, D.C.

WASHINGTON LABS., North End Pier 66, Bell St. Terminal, Seattle 1, Wash.

WATE-ON CO., 230 N. Michigan, Chicago, Ill.

WATERALL, WM., & CO., 118 N. Front St., Philadelphia, Pa.

WATERPROOF PAINT & VARNISH CO., Watertown, Mass.

WATERVLEIT PAPER CO., Watervleit, Mich.

WATKINS, J. R., CO., Winona, Minn.

WATKINS, R. L., CO., Division of Sterling Drug Co., Inc., New York 18, N.Y.

WATSON-STANDARD CO., Galveston & Steppler Sts., Pittsburgh, Pa.

WATTERS CO., 1106 S. Flower St., Burbank, Calif.

WAVAL-THERMAL 3333 N. San Fernando Blvd., Burbank, Calif.

WAYNE CHEMICAL PRODUCTS CO., Copeland & M.C.R.R., Detroit, Mich.

W. B. ASSOCIATES, 22 E. 49th St., New York, N.Y.

W.-B. CHEM. CO., INC., 15 MacQuesten Pkwy., S., Mt. Vernon, N.Y.

WEARTEST CHEMICAL CO., New York, N.Y.

WEATHERPROOF CO., Cleveland, Ohio.

WEAVER-WALL CO., 3700 Brookpark Rd., Cleveland, Ohio.

WEBB PRODUCTS CO., 214 G. St., San Bernardino, Calif.

WEBER COSTELLO CO., Chicago Heights, Ill.

WEBER DENTAL MANUFACTURING CO., 2206 13th St., N.E., Canton 5, Ohio.

WEBER, F., CO., 1220 Buttonwood St., Philadelphia 23, Pa.

WEBSTER, W. F., CEMENT CO., 224 Thorndike St., Cambridge 41, Mass.

WECKER PHARM., 3859 Broadway, New York 32, N.Y.

WELCH, W. C., M.D., & CO., 80 Maple Ave., White Plains, N.Y.

WELDONA, INC., Broadwalk Arcade, Atlantic City, N.J.

WELIN-SATER CO., 64 S. Lake Ave., Pasadena, Calif.

WELLESLEY SOAP & CHEMICAL CO., Wellesley, Mass.

WELLMAN CO., 127 Arch St., Sunbury 1, Pa.

WELLS, E. B., 340 W. Chicago St., Coldwater, Mich.

WELLS S. C. & CO. (Brown Manufacturing Co.), 1-3 Church St., Le Roy, N.Y.

WELMAID MFG. CORP., 41 Pineapple Ave., Sarasota, Fla.

WENZELMANN CHEMICAL WORKS, Galesburg, Ill.

WERNER DR., LABS., c/o Rainbow, Inc., 1354 Boston Rd., New York 56, N.Y.

WERNET DENTAL MFG. CO., INC., 105 Academy St., Jersey City 2, N.J.

WESTCHESTER VETERINARY PRODUCTS, 110 Mamaroneck Ave., White Plains, N.Y.

WEST COAST SOAP CO., 2505 Poplar St., Oakland, Calif.

WEST DISINFECTING CO., 42-16 West St., Long Island City 1, L. I., N.Y.

WESTERN CHEMICAL & MFG. CO., 3270 E. Washington St., Los Angeles, Calif.

WEST INDIES BAY CO., 600 Oak Grove St., Minneapolis 3, Minn.

WESTERN PHARMACAL CO., 121 W. Commonwealth Ave., Salt Lake City 15, Utah.

WESTERN ROSIN & TURPENTINE CO., 6472 Selkirk St., Detroit, Mich.

WESTERN SOLVENT & CHEMICALS CO., 6472 Selkirk Ave., Detroit 11, Mich.

WESTERN STATES LACQUER CO., 4450 E. Washington St., Los Angeles, Calif.

WESTERN WAX WORKS, 118 4th St., Oakland, Calif.

WESTPHAL, PAUL, INC., 653 11th Ave., New York, N.Y.

WESTVACO CHLOR-ALKALI DIVISION, Food Machinery & Chemical Corp., 161 E. 42nd St., New York 17, N.Y.

WEST-WARD INC., New York, N.Y.

WESTWARE, INC., Cincinnati 9, Ohio.

WESTWOOD PHARMACEUTICALS, 468 Dewitt St., Buffalo 13, N.Y.

WETHERILL, GEORGE D., & CO., Arch & Waterloo Sts., Philadelphia, Pa.

WEYER, GEO. H., INC., 1219 Main St., Kansas City 6, Mo.

WHAYNE MFG. CO., 120 Main St., Leparto, Ark.

WHEELER, REYNOLDS & STAUFFER, Division of Stauffer Chemical Co., 636 California St., San Francisco 8, Calif.

WHITE, A. J., LTD., 91-27 138th Pl., Jamaica 35, L. I., N.Y.

WHITE & BAGLEY CO., 100 Foster St., Worcester 8, Mass.

WHITE CO., 3200 E. Biddle St., Baltimore 13, Md.

WHITEHALL PHARMACAL CO., 22 E. 40th St., New York 16, N.Y.

WHITE, H. KIRK, CO., Oconomowoc, Wis.

FIRST AID & GENERAL EMERGENCY TREATMENT

INGREDIENTS INDEX • THERAPEUTIC INDEX

SUPPORTIVE TREATMENT • TRADEMARK INDEX

GENERAL FORMULATIONS • MANUFACTURERS INDEX

FIRST AID & GENERAL EMERGENCY TREATMENT

INGREDIENTS INDEX • THERAPEUTIC INDEX

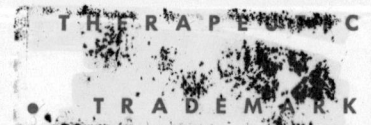

TOXICITY RATING CHART

Date Due

Toxicity Rating or Class	mg./kg.	nan (150 lbs.)
6 super toxic	less than 5	a taste (less than 7 drops)
5 extremely toxic	5–50	between 7 drops and 1 teaspoonful
4 very toxic	50–500	between 1 teaspoonful and one ounce
3 moderately toxic	500–5 gm./kg.	between 1 ounce and 1 pint (or 1 lb.)
2 slightly toxic	5–15 gm./kg.	between 1 pint and 1 quart
1 practically non-toxic	above 15 gm./kg.	more than 1 quart

FIRST AID & GENERAL EMERGENCY TREATMENT

INGREDIENTS INDEX • THERAPEUTIC INDEX

SUPPORTIVE TREATMENT • TRADEMARK INDEX

GENERAL FORMULATIONS • MANUFACTURERS INDEX

FIRST AID & GENERAL EMERGENCY TREATMENT

INGREDIENTS INDEX • THERAPEUTIC INDEX

SUPPORTIVE TREATMENT • TRADEMARK INDEX